MÜLLER'S IMAGING OF THE CHEST

2nd
EDITION

MÜLLER'S IMAGING OF THE CHEST

EDITORS

CHRISTOPHER M. WALKER, MD
Associate Professor of Radiology
University of Kansas Medical Center
Kansas City, Kansas

JONATHAN H. CHUNG, MD
Associate Professor
Section Chief of Thoracic Radiology
Interim Vice Chair for Quality
Department of Radiology
The University of Chicago Medicine
Chicago, Illinois

ASSOCIATE EDITORS

STEPHEN B. HOBBS, MD
Assistant Professor
Department of Radiology and Medicine
University of Kentucky
Lexington, Kentucky

BRENT P. LITTLE, MD
Division of Thoracic Imaging
Department of Radiology
Massachusetts General Hospital
Boston, Massachusetts

CAROL C. WU, MD
Associate Professor
Department of Diagnostic Radiology
The University of Texas MD Anderson Cancer Center
Houston, Texas

ELSEVIER

ELSEVIER

1600 John F. Kennedy Blvd.
Ste 1600
Philadelphia, PA 19103-2899

MÜLLER'S IMAGING OF THE CHEST, SECOND EDITION ISBN: 978-0-323-46225-9

Previous editions copyrighted 2008 by Saunders, an imprint of Elsevier Inc.

Library of Congress Control Number: 2018953443

Publisher: Russell Gabbedy
Senior Content Development Specialist: Ann Ruzycka Anderson
Publishing Services Manager: Catherine Albright Jackson
Senior Project Manager: Claire Kramer
Design Direction: Ryan Cook

Printed in China

Last digit is the print number: 9 8 7 6 5 4 3 2 1

To Eunhee, thank you for your constant support and pushing me to take on this project.
You truly make me a better man.
To Elsie, thank you for always loving me and making me aware of the things
that matter most in life.
To Lillian, thank you for always making me laugh and giving the biggest
hugs a dad could ever ask for.

CMW

To my parents, Kyu Youl and Bok Hee: Thank you for endlessly encouraging my curiosity.
To my daughter, Alexandra: Thank you for always being so excited to see me
when I come home; it is the only time I have felt like a rock star.
And to my loving wife, Aimee-Sue: Thank you for being the backbone of our family.
Your unending support and love always inspire me.

JHC

CONTRIBUTORS

Kiran Batra, MD
Assistant Professor
Department of Radiology
UT Southwestern Medical Center
Dallas, Texas

Matthew Bentz, MD
Assistant Professor
Department of Diagnostic Radiology
Oregon Health and Science University
Portland, Oregon

Marcelo F. Benveniste, MD
Associate Professor
Department of Diagnostic Radiology
Thoracic Section
The University of Texas MD Anderson Cancer Center
Houston, Texas

Anupama Brixey, MD
Department of Diagnostic Radiology
Oregon Health and Science University
Portland, Oregon

Juliana Bueno, MD
Assistant Professor of Radiology
Department of Radiology and Medical Imaging
University of Virginia
Charlottesville, Virginia

Suzanne C. Byrne, MD, FRCPC
Clinical Assistant Professor of Radiology
Department of Radiology
Memorial University
St. John's, Newfoundland, Canada

Brett W. Carter, MD
Associate Professor
Department of Diagnostic Radiology
The University of Texas MD Anderson Cancer Center
Houston, Texas

Jonathan H. Chung, MD
Associate Professor
Section Chief of Thoracic Radiology
Interim Vice Chair for Quality
Department of Radiology
The University of Chicago Medicine
Chicago, Illinois

Patricia M. de Groot, MD
Associate Professor
Department of Diagnostic Radiology
The University of Texas MD Anderson Cancer Center
Houston, Texas

Stephane L. Desouches, DO
Assistant Professor of Radiology
Medical College of Wisconsin
Milwaukee, Wisconsin

Robert M. DeWitt, MD, Major, USAF MC
Assistant Professor of Radiology
Uniformed Services University of the Health Sciences
Bethesda, Maryland
Landstuhl Regional Medical Center
Landstuhl, Germany

Jeremy J. Erasmus, MD
Professor
Department of Diagnostic Radiology
The University of Texas MD Anderson Cancer Center
Houston, Texas

Stephen K. Frankel, MD
Chief Medical Officer
Professor of Medicine
Division of Pulmonary, Critical Care, and Sleep Medicine
Department of Medicine
National Jewish Health
Denver, Colorado

Tomás Franquet, MD
Chief, Section of Thoracic Imaging
Department of Radiology
Hospital de Sant Pau
Barcelona, Spain

Cristina S. Fuss, MD
Associate Professor
Department of Diagnostic Radiology
Oregon Health and Science University
Portland, Oregon

Sherief Garrana, MD
Resident Physician
Department of Thoracic Radiology
University of Missouri–Kansas City/Saint Luke's Hospital of Kansas City
Kansas City, Missouri

Matthew D. Gilman, MD
Division of Thoracic Imaging and Intervention
Massachusetts General Hospital
Boston, Massachusetts

J. David Godwin, MD
Professor of Radiology
Department of Radiology
University of Washington
Seattle, Washington

Daniel R. Gomez, MD
Associate Professor
Department of Radiation Oncology
The University of Texas MD Anderson Cancer Center
Houston, Texas

Ashish Gupta, MD
Assistant Professor
Department of Medical Imaging
University of Ottawa
Ottawa, Ontario, Canada

Vedant Gupta, MD
Assistant Professor of Medicine
University of Kentucky College of Medicine
Lexington, Kentucky

Thomas E. Hartman, MD
Professor
Department of Radiology
Mayo Clinic
Rochester, Minnesota

Stephen B. Hobbs, MD
Assistant Professor
Department of Radiology and Medicine
University of Kentucky
Lexington, Kentucky

Yeon Joo Jeong, MD
Department of Radiology
Pusan National University Hospital
Pusan National University School of Medicine
Busan, South Korea

Michael A. Kadoch, MD
Assistant Professor of Clinical Radiology
Department of Radiology
University of California–Davis
Sacramento, California

Jeffrey S. Klein, MD
A. Bradley Soule and John P. Tampas Green and Gold Professor of Radiology
Department of Radiology
University of Vermont College of Medicine
Burlington, Vermont

Sarah T. Kurian, MD
Department of Radiology
University of Missouri–Kansas City
Kansas City, Missouri

Kyung Soo Lee, MD
Department of Radiology
Samsung Medical Center
Sungkyunkwan University School of Medicine
Seoul, South Korea

John P. Lichtenberger, MD
Associate Professor of Radiology
Uniformed Services University of the Health Sciences
Bethesda, Maryland

Rebecca M. Lindell, MD
Assistant Professor
Department of Radiology
Mayo Clinic
Rochester, Minnesota

Brent P. Little, MD
Division of Thoracic Imaging
Department of Radiology
Massachusetts General Hospital
Boston, Massachusetts

Jaume Llauger, MD
Chief, Section of Musculoskeletal Imaging
Department of Radiology
Hospital de la Santa Creu i Sant Pau
Universitat Autònoma de Barcelona
Barcelona, Spain

Andrea L. Magee, MD
Resident Radiologist
Department of Radiology
The University of Chicago
Chicago, Illinois

Victorine V. Muse, MD
Assistant Professor of Radiology
Harvard Medical School
Massachusetts General Hospital
Boston, Massachusetts

Justin M. Oldham, MD, MS
Assistant Professor
Department of Internal Medicine
Division of Pulmonary, Critical Care, and Sleep Medicine
University of California–Davis
Sacramento, California

Melissa Price, MD
Instructor in Radiology
Division of Thoracic Imaging and Intervention
Massachusetts General Hospital
Boston, Massachusetts

Steven L. Primack, MD
Professor and Vice Chair
Department of Diagnostic Radiology
Oregon Health and Science University
Portland, Oregon

Bradley S. Sabloff, MD
Professor
Department of Diagnostic Radiology
The University of Texas MD Anderson Cancer Center
Houston, Texas

Jean M. Seely, MDCM, FCRPC
Associate Professor
University of Ottawa
Head of Breast Imaging Section
Department of Medical Imaging
The Ottawa Hospital
Clinician Investigator
Ottawa Hospital Research Institute
Ottawa, Ontario, Canada

Phillip A. Setran, MD
Radiology Resident
Department of Diagnostic Radiology
Oregon Health and Science University
Portland, Oregon

Girish S. Shroff, MD
Associate Professor
Department of Diagnostic Radiology
The University of Texas MD Anderson Cancer Center
Houston, Texas

Justin T. Stowell, MD
Resident
Department of Radiology
University of Missouri–Kansas City
Kansas City, Missouri

Nicola Sverzellati, MD, PhD
Professor of Radiology
Department of Medicine and Surgery
University of Parma
Parma, Italy

Mylene T. Truong, MD
Professor
Department of Diagnostic Radiology
The University of Texas MD Anderson Cancer Center
Houston, Texas

Emily B. Tsai, MD
Department of Radiology
Stanford University
Stanford, California

Chitra Viswanathan, MD
Professor
Department of Diagnostic Radiology
Division of Diagnostic Imaging
The University of Texas MD Anderson Cancer Center
Houston, Texas

Christopher M. Walker, MD
Associate Professor of Radiology
University of Kansas Medical Center
Kansas City, Kansas

Charles S. White, MD
Professor
Department of Diagnostic Radiology
University of Maryland
Baltimore, Maryland

Carol C. Wu, MD
Associate Professor
Department of Diagnostic Radiology
The University of Texas MD Anderson Cancer Center
Houston, Texas

FOREWORD

The aim of this second edition of *Imaging of the Chest* is to provide a succinct, state-of-the art overview of imaging of the thorax. We congratulate Drs. Christopher Walker and Jonathan Chung in achieving this goal by combining their outstanding talents as editors and their ability to obtain the collaboration of an exceptional team of internationally renowned chest radiologists to write chapters in their fields of expertise. The new edition includes a truly up-to-date review of the clinical, radiologic, and pathologic manifestations of lung diseases and several hundred new images that provide excellent illustrations of the latest technologic advances.

The emphasis of this book, similar to daily practice, is on chest radiography and computed tomography (CT). However, as is also required in clinical practice, it includes the indications and characteristic findings on magnetic resonance imaging and, when applicable, scintigraphy, positron emission tomography (PET), integrated PET-CT imaging, and ultrasound. The book also provides a summary of the clinical manifestations and pathologic findings. The clinical history is always helpful and often essential for an accurate diagnosis or appropriate differential diagnosis, while knowledge of the pathologic findings allows a better understanding of the patterns of abnormalities seen on the radiologic images.

As the editors, we were delighted with the quality of the first edition and very thankful to the numerous authors who were responsible for its success. There have been, however, many major changes and new developments since the publication of that edition in 2008, which led to the need for a major revision and update. We chose to pass on the new edition to a young team of editors with the talent, energy, and dedication required in planning, organizing, and completing this monumental endeavor. We are very pleased to see that they managed to improve the quality of the book and believe that it will be extremely useful to radiology residents, chest radiology fellows, pulmonary physicians, thoracic surgeons, and general radiologists with an interest in chest imaging.

Nestor L. Müller
C. Isabela Silva Müller

PREFACE

We are honored and humbled to be the editors of the second edition of *Müller's Imaging of the Chest.* We are indebted to the previous editors, Drs. Nestor Müller and Isabela Silva, as well as their Associate and Assistant Editors, Drs. David Hansell, Kyung Soo Lee, and Martin Rémy-Jardin, for their extraordinary work in directing and creating the first edition of this textbook and organizing a team of some of the most esteemed chest radiologists. The authoritative and comprehensive content in the first edition of *Imaging of the Chest* made it the clear gold standard reference in thoracic imaging. When we were first offered the opportunity to edit this textbook, we were reluctant because the first edition was a hard act to follow. However, the opportunity to have a hand in the second iteration of the textbook, which we used as our personal go-to reference, was too hard to turn down. Thankfully, our wives urged us to take on this project lest we kick ourselves in the future. Given the daunting task of updating and editing the authoritative content assembled by the previous world-class team of chest radiologists, we knew we would need help. Our associate editors, Drs. Stephen Hobbs, Brent Little, and Carol Wu, were all obvious choices to help us direct this endeavor given their superior clinical training, unique clinical backgrounds, and complementary clinical and academic interests.

Chest radiography continues to be the most commonly obtained imaging study throughout the world. In many patients, a high-quality chest radiograph, combined with appropriate clinical information, allows for accurate diagnosis. However, in many cases, it is helpful to obtain chest computed tomography (CT) imaging given its higher contrast resolution. In recent years, the line between high-resolution CT of the chest and standard CT has blurred as volumetric helical CT acquisition becomes the norm, allowing for reconstruction of images in any plane and in virtually any slice thickness. Contrast-enhanced chest CT and chest CT angiography are highly valuable tools in the assessment of suspected malignancy, vascular abnormalities, and thromboembolic disease. Magnetic resonance imaging (MRI) and positron emission tomography (PET) imaging are useful adjuncts in thoracic imaging, specifically in the setting of known or suspected malignancy. Although specialized centers have used MRI and PET imaging for evaluation of nonmalignant pulmonary abnormalities, these are still mostly avenues for research rather than accepted clinical standards.

In the second edition of this textbook, we aim to provide a comprehensive review of thoracic imaging while simultaneously compressing the size of the textbook from a two-volume set to a single-volume reference. Needless to say, this was challenging, but we are quite proud of the end product and hope you will agree that essential content has not been excluded. The first part of this book deals with normal imaging appearance of the thorax on chest radiography and CT with detailed discussions of thoracic anatomy. Truly, one does not know what abnormal is until one knows what normal is. The second part of this book approaches thoracic imaging from the "findings" aspect rather than from the diagnosis side. This is likely most relevant to readers of this textbook, given that this is how patients present: with an unknown diagnosis but with abnormalities on chest imaging. Finally, the third part is arranged in a diagnosis or diagnostic category approach, as is typical of most textbooks.

Specific highlights include updates on lung cancer screening and an updated review of pulmonary fibrosis and interstitial lung disease management and diagnosis. In addition, four new chapters were created to more fully include topics pertinent to chest imagers: Leukemia, Idiopathic Pleuroparenchymal Fibroelastosis, Interstitial Pneumonia with Autoimmune Features, and Noninfectious Lung and Stem Cell Transplantation Complications.

This book would not have been possible without the support of our colleagues and mentors. We thank, first, all our mentors at the University of Washington and the Massachusetts General Hospital for cultivating our passion for cardiopulmonary imaging and guiding us in the gauntlet of academic radiology; second, specific leaders in the field, including Drs. David A. Lynch and J. David Godwin, whom we had the pleasure of working with and who continually provided their support and advice on all matters; and third, our trainees, who have always kept us honest in regard to what we knew (or thought we knew). We hope you enjoy reading this textbook (although based on your track record, we assume you will get around to it next rotation). Finally, we thank the wonderful staff at Elsevier who have made this endeavor possible, including but not limited to Robin Carter, Ann Anderson, Claire Kramer, and Margaret Nelson.

This book is aimed at clinical radiologists, pulmonologists, trainees, and any other health care professionals interested in thoracic imaging. It provides a concise but comprehensive overview of imaging findings of thoracic diseases. We hope that the second edition of *Müller's Imaging of the Chest* will be a valuable resource for the thoracic health care community and will ultimately improve patient care.

Jonathan H. Chung, MD
Christopher M. Walker, MD

CONTENTS

MÜLLER'S IMAGING OF THE CHEST

1 Normal Chest Radiography and Computed Tomography*

JULIANA BUENO | CHRISTOPHER M. WALKER | JONATHAN H. CHUNG

Radiography

Technique

PROJECTIONS

The standard radiographic views for evaluation of the chest are the posteroanterior (PA) and lateral projections with the patient standing; such projections provide the essential requirement for proper three-dimensional (3D) assessment (Fig. 1.1). In patients who are unable to stand, anteroposterior (AP) upright or supine projections offer alternative but considerably less satisfactory views. The AP projection is of inferior quality because of the shorter focal-detector distance, the greater magnification of the heart, and the restricted ability of many such patients to suspend respiration or achieve full inspiration.

BASIC RADIOGRAPHIC TECHNIQUES

Diagnostic accuracy in thoracic pathology is related partly to the quality of the radiographic images themselves, and multiple variables require attention.

Patient Positioning and Respiration

Images are ideally acquired at full inspiration to avoid magnification of the cardiomediastinal silhouette and vascular crowding, which decrease diagnostic capability.

A well-centered x-ray beam, lack of rotation, and exclusion of the scapulae from the field of view are essential for adequate positioning. The distance between the medial ends of the clavicles (anterior structures) and the spinous processes of the thoracic vertebrae (posterior structures) are reliable landmarks to assess position. In a properly centered radiograph the medial ends of the right and left clavicles are equidistant from the spinous processes (Fig. 1.2). The American College of Radiology standards for performance of standard chest radiography in adults specify the use of at least a 72-inch (1.8-m) tube-detector distance for PA radiographs and a minimum of 40 inches in portable radiographs.[1,2]

Exposure

Exposure factors should be such that there is faint visualization of the thoracic spine and the intervertebral disks on the PA radiograph so that lung markings behind the heart are clearly visible.[1]

Kilovoltage

A high-kilovoltage technique (115–150 kVp) should be used for PA and lateral chest radiographs.[1] The high kVp allows better penetration of the mediastinum and shorter exposure times, thus minimizing cardiac motion artifacts and providing sharper outline of the pulmonary and mediastinal structures.[1]

IMAGE ACQUISITION

Conventional screen-film radiography has a number of limitations and therefore has been replaced by computed radiography (CR) and digital radiography (DR).

The process of acquisition, transmission, display, and storage of digital images has many advantages over conventional screen-film systems,[3,4] and it is widely used as the primary technology in conventional radiographic studies. A potential disadvantage of CR and DR is that patients may receive unnecessarily high radiation doses, which may not be detected because they do not result in perceivable alterations in image quality. The wider latitude of digital systems allows them to be used under a much broader range of exposure conditions and makes them an ideal choice for applications in which exposure is highly variable or difficult to control, such as bedside radiography. This results in a reproducible quality and considerable decrease in the repeat rate for bedside chest radiographs when using CR, compared with screen-film radiography.[5]

Two main types of digital systems are available commercially: systems based on photostimulable storage phosphor image receptors, known as CR, and systems based on flat-panel x-ray detectors or array of detectors that directly capture the radiographic image, known as DR.

Computed Radiography

CR (storage phosphor radiography) involves the use of a reusable photostimulable phosphor plate rather than film to record the image. Plates coated with the phosphor are loaded into special cassettes that are outwardly similar to screen-film cassettes. During exposure the receptor stores the x-ray energy and is then scanned by a laser beam, which results in the creation of visible or infrared

*The editors and the publisher would like to thank Drs. Nestor L. Müller and C. Isabela Silva Müller for contributing material on this topic to the prior edition of this work. It has served as the foundation for the current chapter.

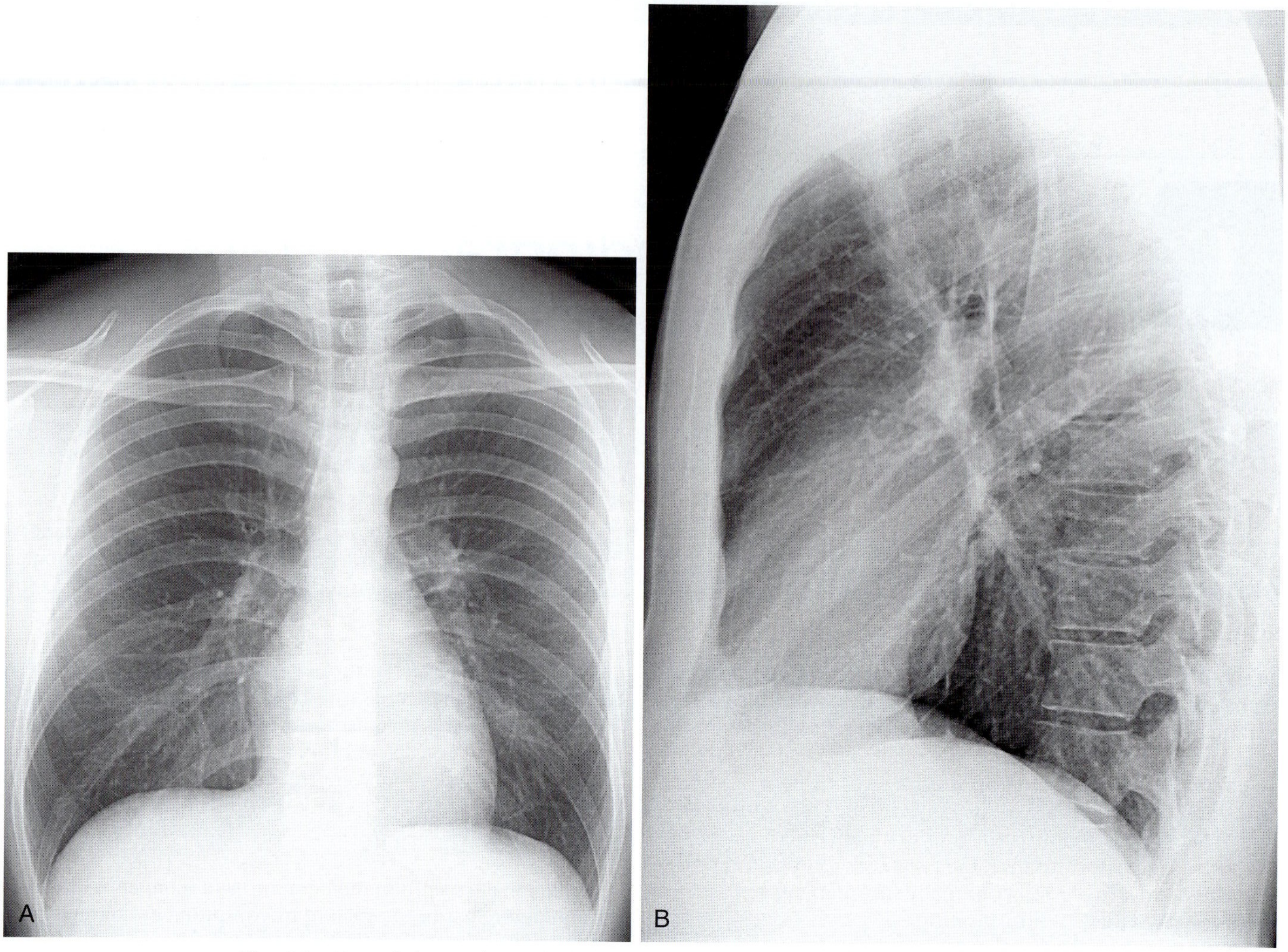

Fig. 1.1 Normal chest radiograph. (A) Posteroanterior projection. (B) Lateral projection.

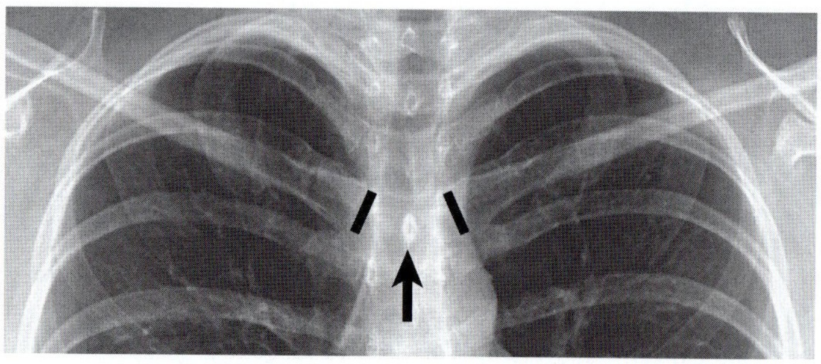

Fig. 1.2 Properly centered chest radiograph. A view from a frontal radiograph shows that the medial ends of the right and left clavicles (highlighted in black) are equidistant to the spinous process *(arrow)* of the vertebra at the same level, thus indicating that the radiograph is properly centered.

radiation, the intensity of which corresponds to the absorbed x-ray energy. The resultant luminescence is measured and recorded digitally.[6]

Digital Radiography

DR uses a flat-panel x-ray detector or an array of detectors to directly capture the radiographic image numerically, thus eliminating the step of reading out the detector. The detectors in DR are selenium based and provide the additional advantage of having considerably greater quantum efficiency than conventional screen-film systems and photostimulable phosphor detectors do,[7,8] which results in an image quality superior to that of screen-film systems and existing storage phosphor detectors at a comparable or lower radiation dose.[9]

Normal Anatomy of the Chest

AIRWAYS

Trachea and Bronchi

The trachea is a midline structure, and the tracheal walls are parallel except on the left side just above the bifurcation, where the aorta commonly causes a smooth indentation (Fig. 1.3). The trachea measures 10 to 12 cm in length and has 16 to 20 C-shaped cartilage rings on its lateral and anterior aspects and a fibromuscular posterior margin. Calcification of the cartilage rings is a common normal finding in patients older than 40 years, particularly women, but it is seldom evident on radiographs (Fig. 1.4). The upper limits of normal for coronal and sagittal

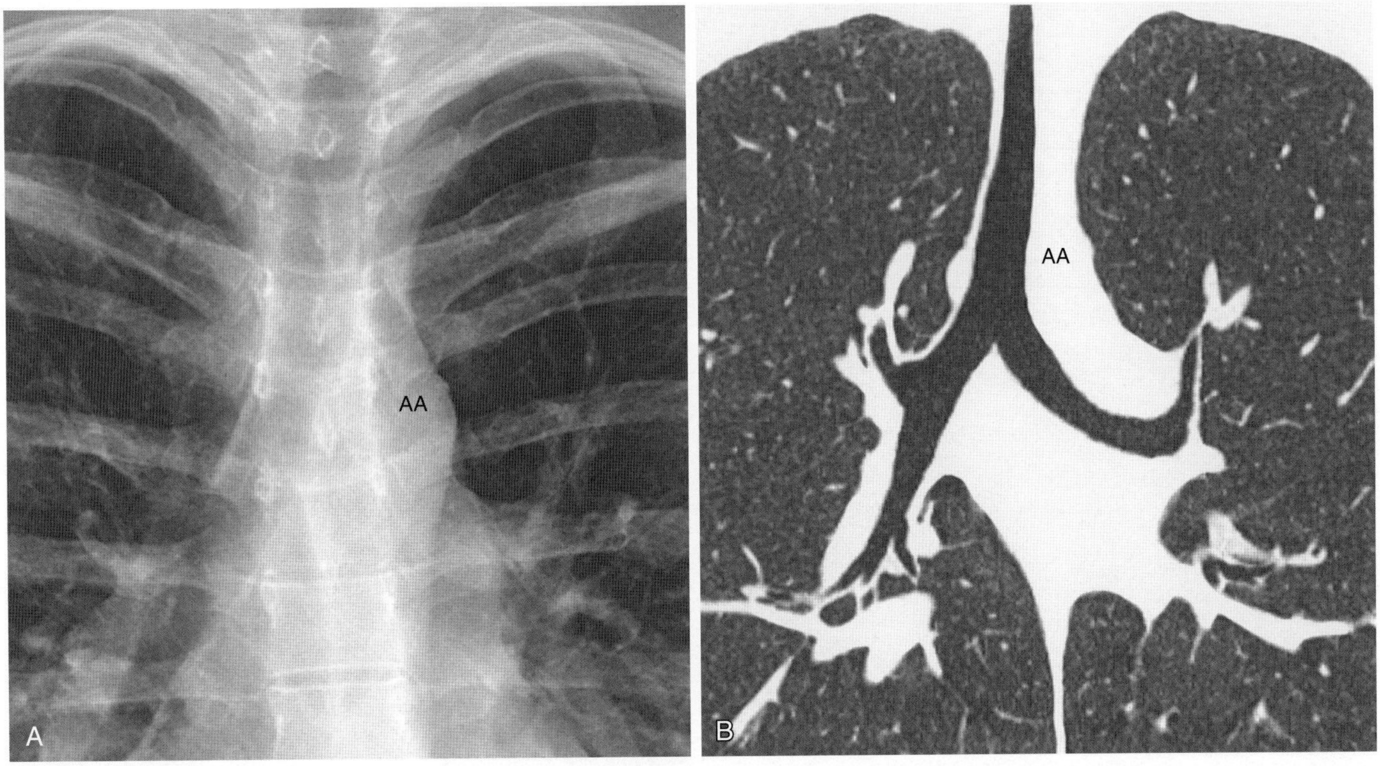

Fig. 1.3 Normal trachea and main bronchi. (A) Frontal radiograph shows that the tracheal air column is fairly straight and located in the midline except at the level of the aortic arch *(AA)*, where the trachea is indented and may be slightly deviated to the right. The trachea divides into a short right main bronchus and a longer and more horizontal left main bronchus. (B) Coronal reformatted image from a CT scan demonstrating the normal anatomy of the trachea, the slight indentation at the level of the aortic arch *(AA)*, and the main bronchi. Approximately 2 cm after its origin, the right main bronchus branches into the right upper lobe bronchus and the bronchus intermedius.

diameters of the trachea in men are 25 and 27 mm, respectively; in women, they are 21 and 23 mm, respectively.[10] The lower limit of normal for both dimensions is 13 mm in men and 10 mm in women.[10]

The trachea divides into the left and right main bronchi at the carina, at approximately the level of the fifth thoracic vertebra. The subcarinal angle ranges widely from 35 to 90 degrees (mean, 61 degrees)[11]; thus routine measurement of this angle has no diagnostic value.

The right main bronchus measures approximately 2 cm in length and has a more vertical course than the left main bronchus does (see Fig. 1.3). It divides into the right upper lobe bronchus and the bronchus intermedius. The bronchus intermedius continues distally for 3 to 4 cm from the takeoff of the right upper lobe bronchus and then bifurcates into bronchi to the middle and lower lobes. The left main bronchus is approximately 5 cm in length and divides into the left upper and lower lobe bronchi.

The lobar bronchi branch into segmental bronchi. Segmental bronchi are visible on chest radiographs only when they are seen end-on as ring shadows or when they are abnormally thickened. The most commonly seen segmental bronchi on a chest radiograph are the anterior segmental bronchi of the upper lobes; seen as ring shadows adjacent to the accompanying segmental pulmonary artery (Fig. 1.5).

KEY POINTS: TRACHEA

- Normal diameter in men is 13–27 mm.
- Normal diameter in women is 10–23 mm.
- The tracheal cartilages are C shaped and spare the posterior tracheal wall, which is membranous.

PULMONARY ARTERIAL AND VENOUS CIRCULATION

Pulmonary Arteries

The pulmonary trunk or main pulmonary artery originates in the mediastinum at the pulmonary valve and extends cranially and slightly to the left for 4 to 5 cm before bifurcating within the pericardium into the shorter left and longer right pulmonary arteries (Fig. 1.6). The left pulmonary artery continues until it reaches the hilum, where it arches over the left main bronchus and gives off the left upper lobe and interlobar arteries, from which segmental and subsegmental branches arise. The left interlobar artery lies posterolateral to the upper lobe bronchus.

The right pulmonary artery courses behind the ascending aorta before dividing in front of the right main bronchus into ascending (truncus anterior) and descending (interlobar) branches.

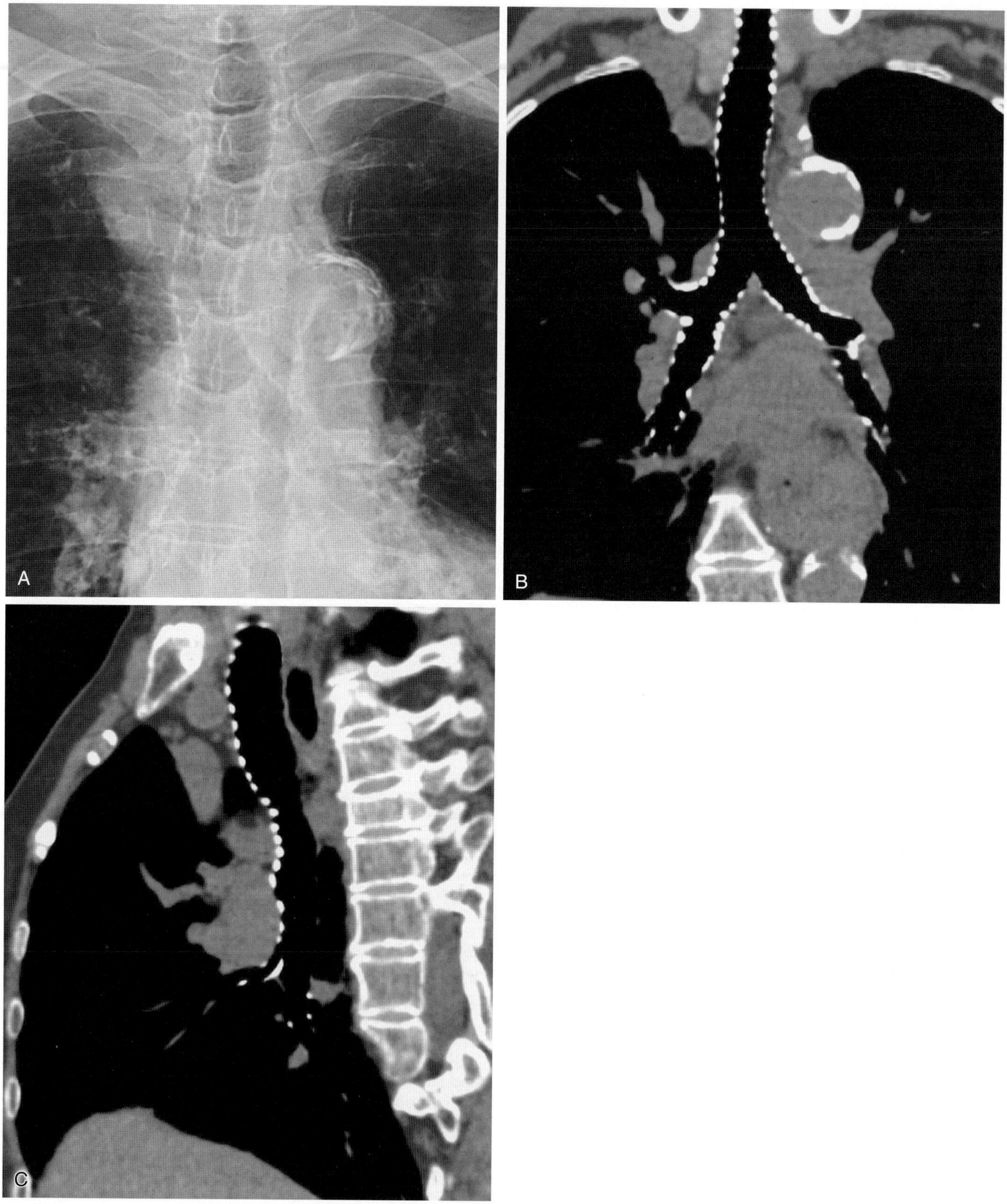

Fig. 1.4 Tracheal and bronchial wall calcification. A magnified view from a posteroanterior chest radiograph (A) in an elderly patient shows calcification of the tracheal and bronchial walls. Coronal (B) and sagittal (C) reformatted images from a CT scan show the extent of tracheal and bronchial calcification. Airway wall calcification is a normal finding in elderly patients.

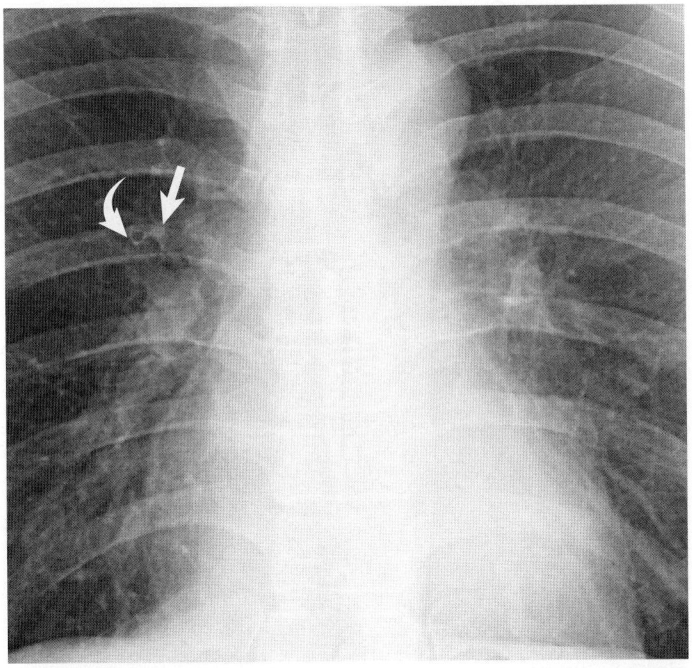

Fig. 1.5 Anterior segmental bronchus of the right upper lobe seen end-on. A view from a frontal radiograph shows a ring shadow *(curved arrow)* corresponding to the anterior segmental bronchus of the right upper lobe seen end-on and the adjacent anterior segmental pulmonary artery *(straight arrow)*. The outer diameter of the bronchus on the upright chest radiograph is slightly larger than that of the adjacent artery.

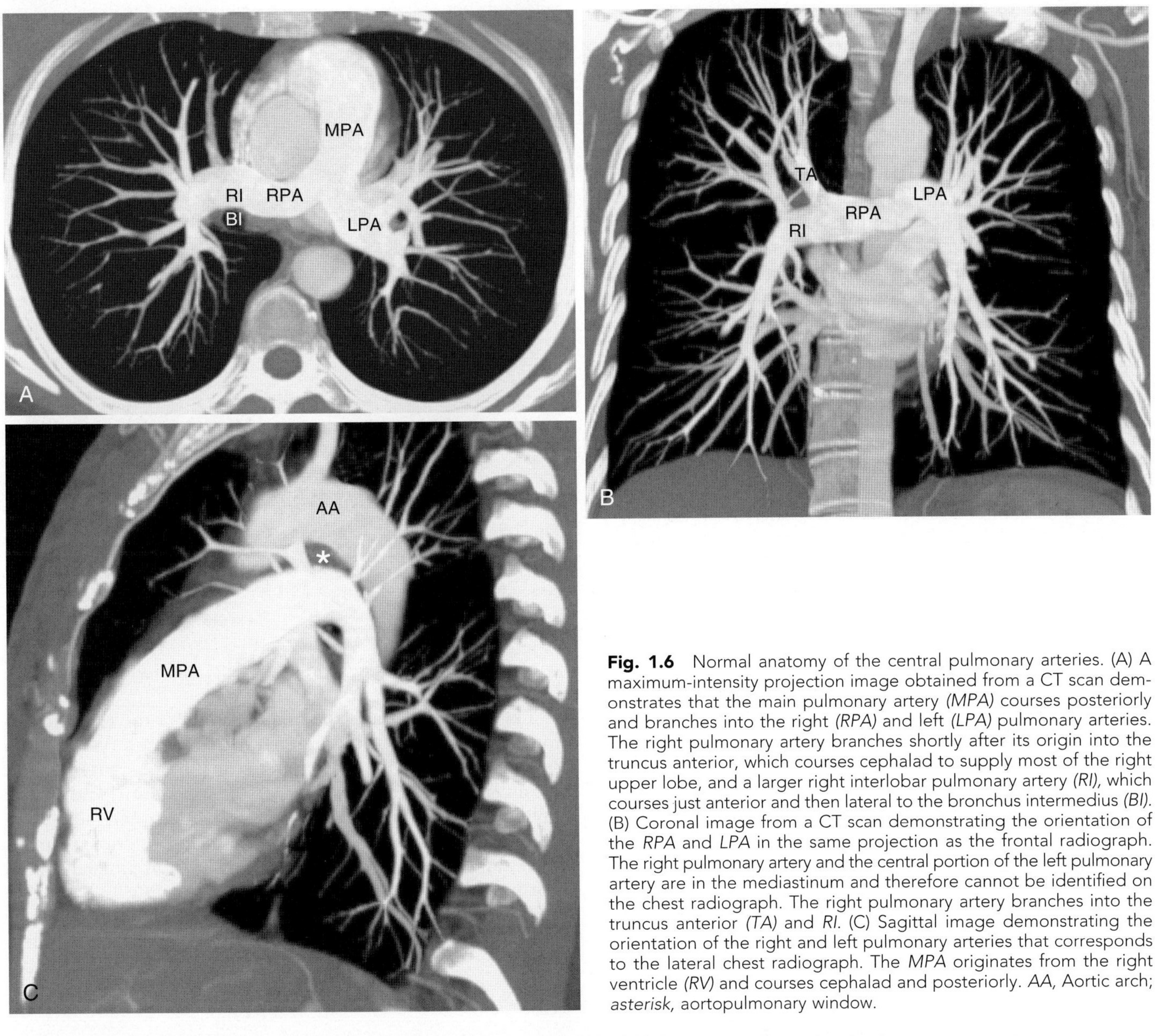

Fig. 1.6 Normal anatomy of the central pulmonary arteries. (A) A maximum-intensity projection image obtained from a CT scan demonstrates that the main pulmonary artery *(MPA)* courses posteriorly and branches into the right *(RPA)* and left *(LPA)* pulmonary arteries. The right pulmonary artery branches shortly after its origin into the truncus anterior, which courses cephalad to supply most of the right upper lobe, and a larger right interlobar pulmonary artery *(RI)*, which courses just anterior and then lateral to the bronchus intermedius *(BI)*. (B) Coronal image from a CT scan demonstrating the orientation of the *RPA* and *LPA* in the same projection as the frontal radiograph. The right pulmonary artery and the central portion of the left pulmonary artery are in the mediastinum and therefore cannot be identified on the chest radiograph. The right pulmonary artery branches into the truncus anterior *(TA)* and *RI*. (C) Sagittal image demonstrating the orientation of the right and left pulmonary arteries that corresponds to the lateral chest radiograph. The *MPA* originates from the right ventricle *(RV)* and courses cephalad and posteriorly. *AA*, Aortic arch; *asterisk*, aortopulmonary window.

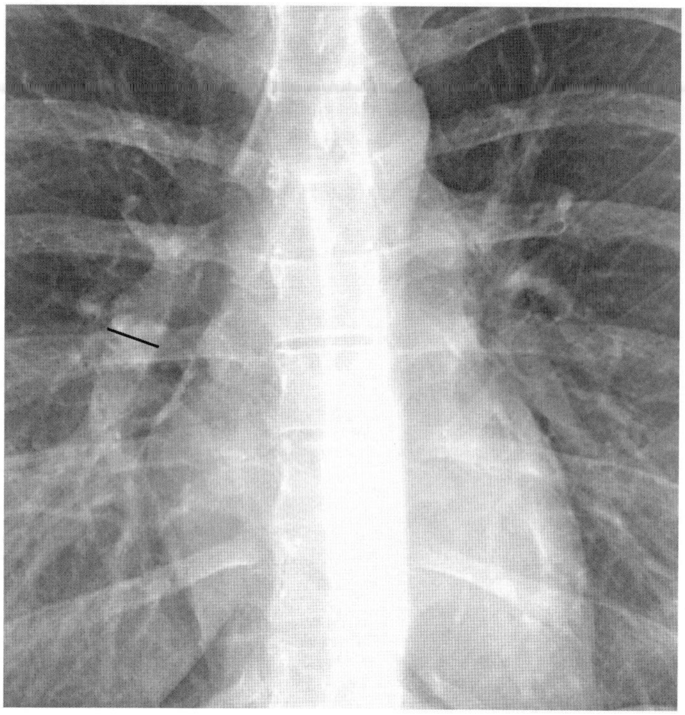

Fig. 1.7 Normal right interlobar artery visualized on a frontal chest radiograph. The upper limit of normal of the transverse diameter of the interlobar artery measured from its lateral aspect to the air column of the bronchus intermedius *(black bar)* is 16 mm in men and 15 mm in women.

Measurements of pulmonary arterial diameter can be helpful in the assessment of pulmonary vascular disease, although in conventional radiography, it is limited to the measurement of the right interlobar artery. The upper limit of normal of the transverse diameter of the right interlobar artery (measured from its lateral aspect to the air column of the bronchus intermedius) is 16 mm in men and 15 mm in women (Fig. 1.7).[12] Dilation of the interlobar pulmonary artery may result from increased pressure (e.g., pulmonary arterial hypertension), increased flow (e.g., left-to-right shunts), or aneurysm formation (e.g., Behçet disease) (Fig. 1.8).

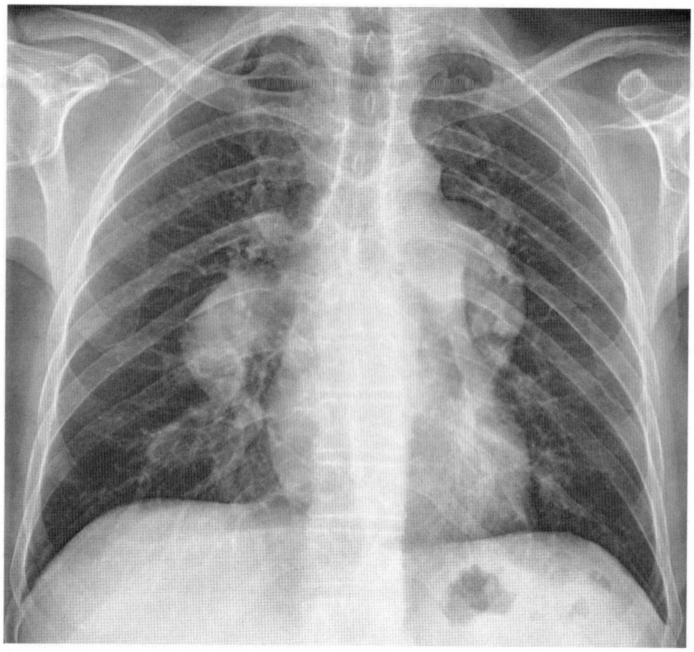

Fig. 1.8 Enlarged central pulmonary arteries from severe pulmonary arterial hypertension. A frontal radiograph shows markedly enlarged central pulmonary arteries.

KEY POINTS: PULMONARY ARTERIES

- The pulmonary trunk or main pulmonary artery is not normally visualized on radiography in adults.
- Normal diameter of the right interlobar pulmonary artery is <16 mm.

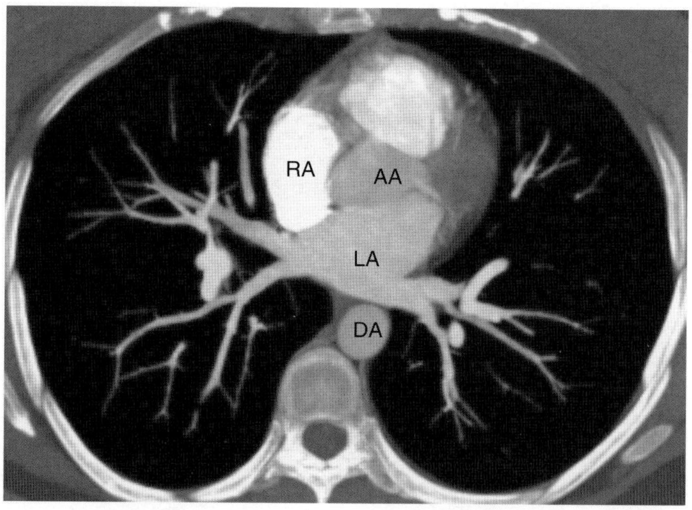

Fig. 1.9 Inferior pulmonary veins. A maximum-intensity projection image obtained from a CT scan shows two main right and left inferior pulmonary veins as they drain into the left atrium *(LA)*. *AA*, Ascending aorta; *DA*, descending aorta; *RA*, right atrium.

Pulmonary Veins

The pulmonary veins arise from venules that drain the alveolar capillaries and the capillary network of the pleura. In contrast to the pulmonary arteries, they are not associated with the airways. Although their final course is variable, there are usually two main superior and two main inferior vessels, the former draining the middle and upper lobes on the right and the upper lobe on the left and the latter draining the lower lobes (Fig. 1.9).

PULMONARY HILA

The anatomic structures rendering the hila visible on radiographs are primarily the pulmonary arteries and veins, with lesser contributions from the bronchial walls, surrounding connective tissue, and lymph nodes (Fig. 1.10).

On a PA radiograph the main shadow of the right hilum is formed by the vertically oriented interlobar artery. Right hilar structures immediately cephalad to the interlobar artery include the ascending pulmonary artery (truncus anterior) and superior pulmonary vein (Fig. 1.11). The end-on opacity and radiolucency of the contiguous anterior (and occasionally posterior) segmental artery and bronchus can be identified in approximately 80% of normal individuals (see Fig. 1.5).[13]

On the left the upper hilar opacity is formed by the distal left pulmonary artery, the proximal portion of the left interlobar

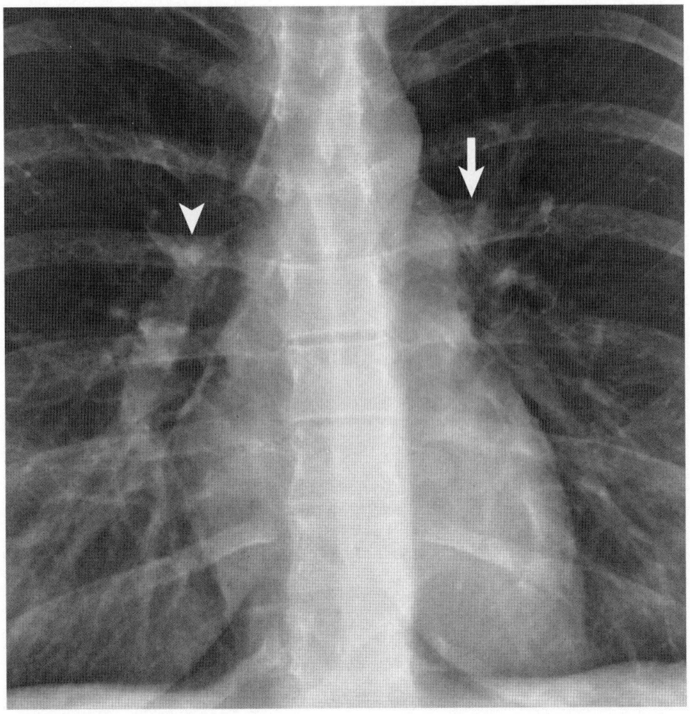

Fig. 1.10 Normal hila. A view from a frontal radiograph shows that the main shadow of the right hilum is formed by the vertically oriented interlobar artery *(arrowhead)* and that of the left hilum by the distal left pulmonary artery *(right arrow)* and descending left pulmonary artery. Because the left pulmonary artery arches above the left main and left upper lobe bronchi, the left hilum is normally 1–2 cm higher than the right hilum.

artery and its segmental arterial branches, and the left superior pulmonary vein and its major tributaries. Because the left pulmonary artery arches over the left main and left upper lobe bronchi, the left hilum is typically 1 to 2 cm higher than the highest point of the right hilum (right interlobar artery) (see Fig. 1.10).

Surrounding the hilar vessels and bronchi are small amounts of fat and small lymph nodes, which cannot normally be distinguished from other structures on the radiograph. Enlargement of the hilar lymph nodes leads to increased size and opacity of the hilum, a lobulated contour, and obscuration of the interlobar artery. Hilar fullness from lymphadenopathy can be differentiated from hilar fullness from pulmonary arterial enlargement by carefully examining the adjacent hilar vessels. In lymphadenopathy the vessels will be visible through the region of hilar fullness (Fig. 1.12), whereas the vessels will converge on the margins of the hilar fullness in the setting of pulmonary arterial enlargement (see Fig. 1.8). This finding is known as the *hilar convergence sign* (see Fig. 1.12).

The radiographic anatomy of the hila on a *lateral projection* is complex because the right and left hilar components are to a large degree superimposed (Fig. 1.13).[14,15] The trachea is usually well seen down to the level of the carina, where the air column can be seen to taper. At the level of the carina the left pulmonary artery can be seen as a curved structure as it courses above the left main bronchus and continues as the descending left pulmonary artery; consequently, the left upper lobe bronchus is seen in about 75%[15] because it is completely surrounded by vessels (the left pulmonary artery above, the descending artery behind, and the mediastinal component of the left superior pulmonary

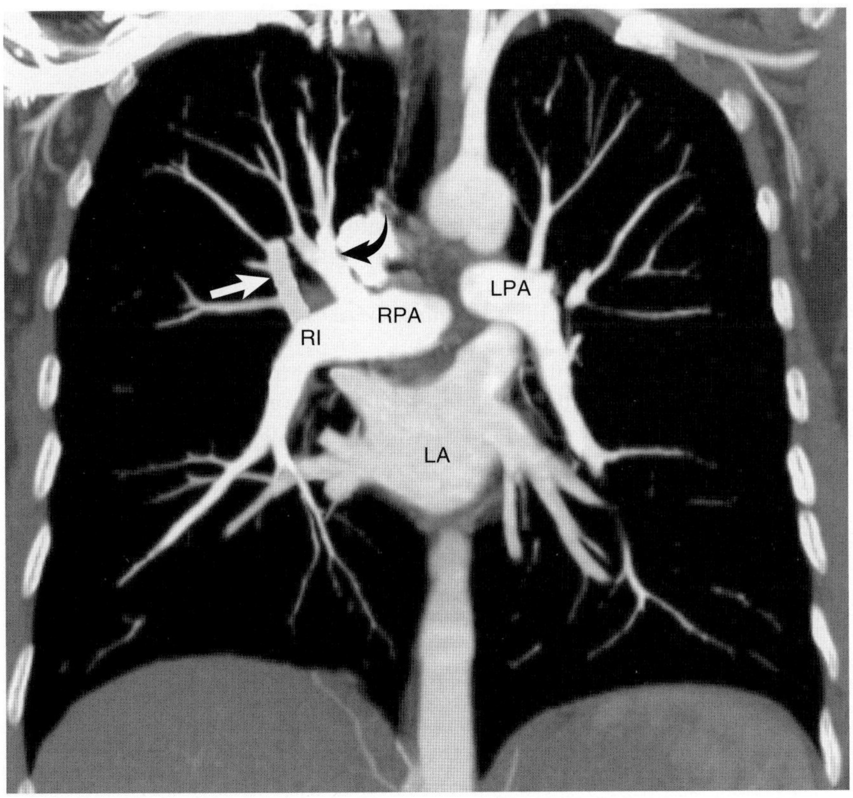

Fig. 1.11 Normal hilar anatomy. A coronal image from a CT scan demonstrates the hilar anatomy as seen on a radiograph. The right pulmonary artery *(RPA)* is in the mediastinum and therefore not visible on the frontal radiograph. On a frontal radiograph the main shadow of the right hilum is formed by the vertically oriented interlobar artery *(RI)*. Right hilar structures immediately cephalad to the interlobar artery include the ascending pulmonary artery (truncus anterior) *(curved arrow)* and the right superior pulmonary vein *(straight arrow)*. Most of the left hilum is formed by the distal left pulmonary artery *(LPA)* and left descending pulmonary artery. *LA,* Left atrium.

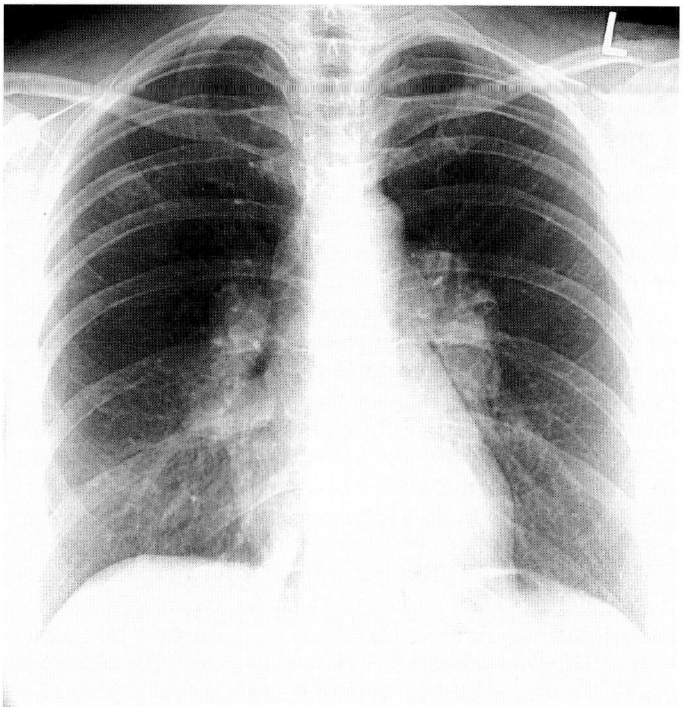

Fig. 1.12 Enlarged bilateral hilar lymph nodes from sarcoidosis. A frontal chest radiograph shows a lobulated contour of the hila and increased size and opacity, findings characteristic of hilar lymph node enlargement. Note that the hilar vessels course through the convex hilar opacities (absence of the hilar convergence sign), indicative of the nonpulmonary artery origin of the hilar opacities.

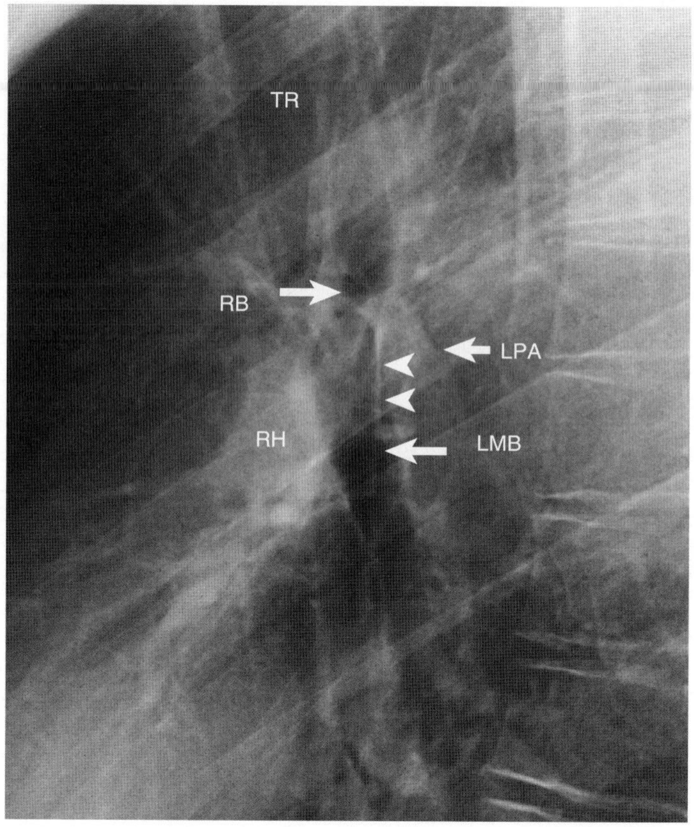

Fig. 1.13 Normal hilar anatomy on a lateral chest radiograph. A magnified view of the hila from a lateral radiograph shows the trachea *(TR)* tapering off at the level of the carina immediately above the level of the left pulmonary artery *(LPA)*, which is seen as a curved structure as it courses above the left main bronchus *(LMB)* and continues as the descending left pulmonary artery. The air column of the right upper lobe bronchus *(RB)* is seen at the level of the carina. The posterior wall of the trachea is continuous with the posterior wall of the right main and bronchus intermedius, which form the intermediate stem line *(arrowheads)*. The right hilum *(RH)* is located anterior to the right bronchus intermedius.

vein in front). The air column of the normally more cephalic right upper lobe bronchus can be identified end-on as a rounded radiolucency in 50% of subjects because it is devoid of vascular envelopment on its posterior aspect such that aerated upper or lower lobe parenchyma normally abuts its wall. Consequently, clear identification of the right upper lobe bronchial lumen en face constitutes highly suggestive evidence that the airway is completely surrounded by soft tissue, most likely enlarged lymph nodes.

Below the level of the carina, a line continuous with the posterior tracheal wall represents the posterior wall of the right main and intermediate bronchi and is known as the *intermediate stem line* (see Fig. 1.13). The posterior wall of the right upper lobe and bronchus intermedius is rendered visible by air in their lumina in front and by aerated lung parenchyma in the azygoesophageal recess behind. On a well-centered lateral projection the intermediate stem line transects the middle or posterior third of the circular, radiolucent left upper lobe bronchus. The intermediate stem line is visible in 95% of individuals and normally measures 1 to 3 mm in thickness.[15,16] The intermediate stem line can become abnormally thickened in patients with interstitial edema or in the presence of right hilar disease, most commonly right hilar lymphadenopathy.[17]

On a lateral view the right hilar opacity is composed of the superior pulmonary vein anteriorly, the ascending and descending right pulmonary arteries posteriorly, and surrounding connective tissue and lymph nodes. The right pulmonary artery is a mediastinal vessel enveloped by other vessels or soft tissue elements and is therefore not seen on the lateral radiograph. The major portion of the left hilar vasculature is visible behind the intermediate stem line. The top of the left pulmonary artery is seen in 95% of subjects, usually as a sharply marginated opacity above and behind the radiolucency of the left upper lobe bronchus (see Fig. 1.13).

The right and left inferior pulmonary veins are commonly imaged end-on as a result of their horizontal orientation, with a nodular opacity created below and behind the lower portion of the hila. Fortunately, vessels can generally be identified as they converge toward the opacity, thereby permitting their distinction from a true parenchymal mass.

The shadows of the right hilum in front of the main bronchi and left pulmonary artery, as it courses over the left main and upper lobe bronchi, result in an inverted U appearance that delineates the radiolucent "inferior hilar window" (see Fig. 1.13). Normally, there are no large vessels coursing immediately below the middle and lower lobe bronchi on the right and the upper and lower lobe bronchi on the left. Therefore any rounded opacity greater than 1 cm in the inferior hilar window on a lateral view is likely to be an enlarged node or a mass (Fig. 1.14).

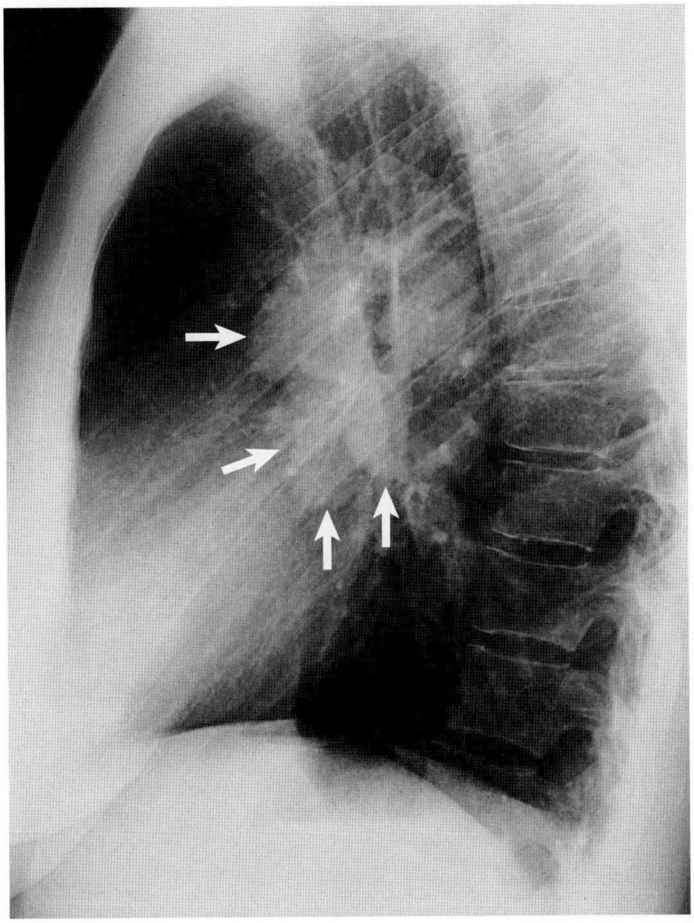

Fig. 1.14 Enlarged hilar lymph nodes on a lateral projection. A magnified view of a lateral chest radiograph in a patient with sarcoidosis shows a lobulated contour and increased opacity in the hila *(arrows)*, characteristic of hilar lymph node enlargement.

LUNG PARENCHYMA

Secondary Lobule

The secondary lobule is the smallest discrete portion of the lung that is surrounded by connective tissue septa.[18] The normal secondary lobule cannot be identified on a chest radiograph. Only when the interlobular septa are rendered visible as septal lines as a result of thickening by fluid or tissue, such as edema or carcinoma, can the lung between two lines be recognized as a secondary lobule.[19] Septal lines (Kerley lines) are identified most commonly in the anterior and lateral aspects of the lungs, where they are best developed (Fig. 1.15).

SEGMENTS AND LOBES

The normal anatomy of the pulmonary segments is variable, complex, and difficult to appreciate on radiographs (Fig. 1.16); it can, however, be readily assessed on computed tomography (CT). An approximate location of an abnormality within a given segment can often be determined by careful analysis of its location on frontal and lateral radiographs.

RADIOGRAPHIC DENSITY

The radiopacity of the lungs is a result of the absorptive power of each of its components: gas, blood, and tissue. Nonaerated lung in vivo consists of approximately half blood and half tissue,[20–23]

On a properly positioned radiograph the radiographic density of the right and left lungs is symmetric. If the patient is rotated, the lung closer to the detector is more uniformly radiopaque (whiter) than the other lung; conversely, the lung that is farthest away from the detector is uniformly less radiopaque (more black).[19] Provided that the patient is not rotated and the x-ray beam is centered properly, any discrepancy in the density of the two lungs must be interpreted as being abnormal. The cause varies from such benign conditions as scoliosis and congenital absence of the pectoral muscles to more significant disorders such as Swyer-James-McLeod syndrome.

PULMONARY MARKINGS

Correct interpretation of the chest radiograph requires a thorough knowledge of the pattern of linear markings throughout the normal lung. These markings are created by the pulmonary arteries, bronchi, veins, and accompanying interstitial tissue. The pulmonary arteries fan outward from both hila and gradually taper as they proceed distally, up to about 1 to 2 cm from the visceral pleural surface.

The PA chest radiograph of a normal erect individual invariably shows some discrepancy in the size of the pulmonary vessels in the upper lung zones compared with the lower zones as a result of the apicobasal pressure gradient.[19] In a recumbent individual a decrease in the influence of gravity renders this discrepancy in vascular size minimal.

PLEURA

The pleural space is enclosed by the visceral pleura, which is tightly attached to the lungs, and by the parietal pleura, which lines the chest wall, diaphragm, and mediastinum. The two join at the hila. The visceral pleura consists of mesothelial cells overlying two layers of elastic tissue that separate a small amount of connective tissue and lymphatic vessels. Because the combined thickness of the normal parietal and visceral pleural layers is approximately 0.2 mm, the pleura over the convexity of the lungs and over the diaphragmatic and mediastinal surfaces is not normally visible on CR or CT. Each pleural space normally contains 8.4 ± 4.3 mL of fluid.[24] Control of the volume and composition of pleural liquid is affected by a number of mechanisms, including Starling forces (providing filtration through the parietal and absorption through the visceral mesothelium), lymphatic drainage, and the activity of mesothelial cells.[25] Fluid is usually produced in the parietal pleura and drained at the visceral pleura, and it tends to be drawn into the space because recoil of the lung and chest wall acts as an opposing force over most of the range of respiratory volumes.

Interlobar Fissures

Fissures are invaginations of the pleura that extend from the outer surface of the lung into its substance. They are traditionally considered in two groups: those that separate the lungs into the three right-sided and two left-sided lobes (*normal* fissures) and those that occur within one of the lobes themselves (*accessory* fissures). The normal fissures are the *minor fissure* (located between the right middle and upper lobes), the *right major fissure* (between the combined right upper and middle lobes and the right lower lobe), and the *left major fissure* (between the left

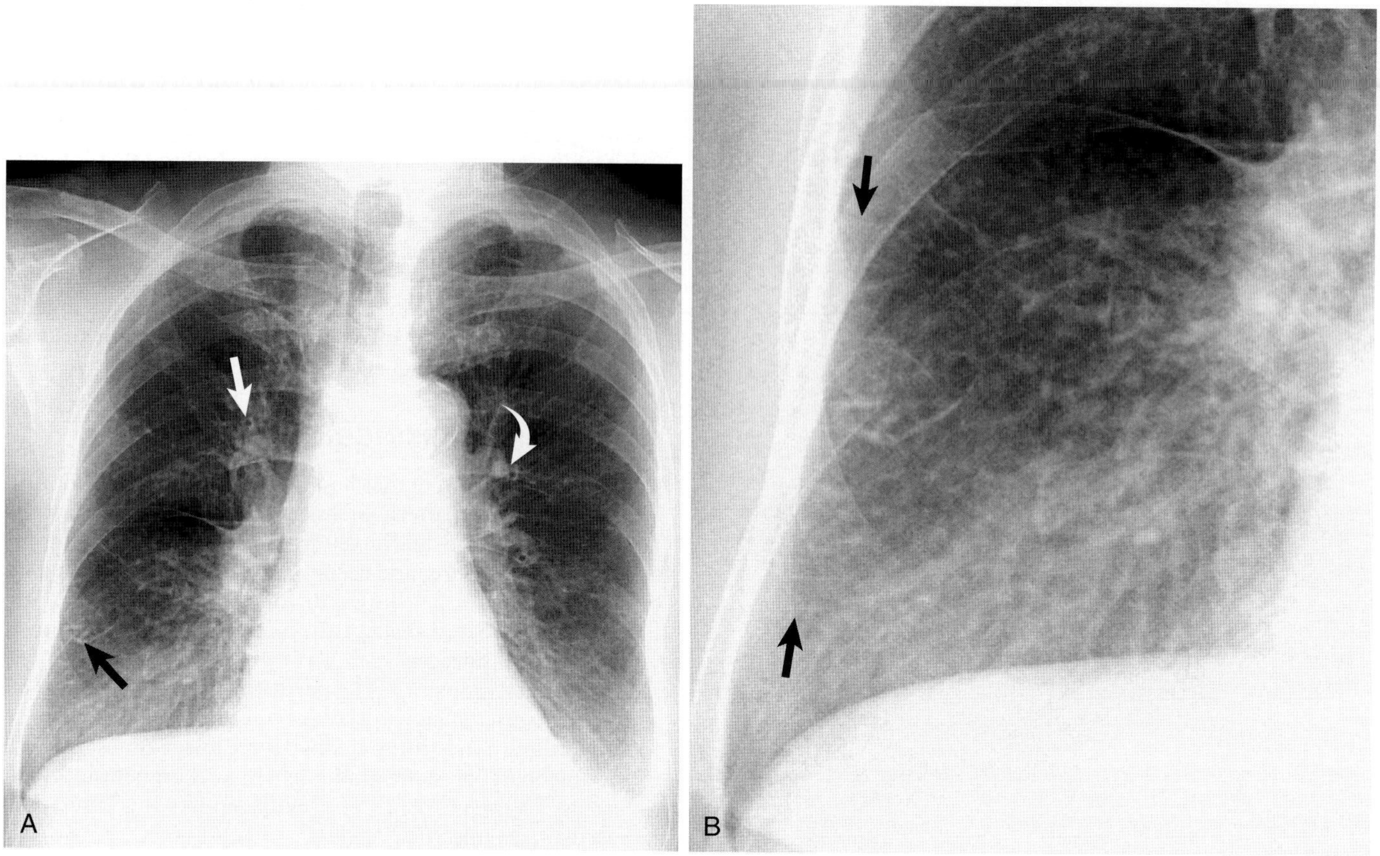

Fig. 1.15 Thickening of the interlobular septa in interstitial pulmonary edema. (A) A frontal chest radiograph in a patient with left heart failure and interstitial pulmonary edema shows septal (Kerley B) lines *(black arrow)*. Also noted is bronchial cuffing as a result of edema *(straight arrow)* and increased size of the anterior segmental left upper lobe pulmonary artery *(curved arrow)*, which has a greater diameter than the adjacent bronchus does. Also noted are small bilateral pleural effusions. (B) A magnified view of the right lower lung region better demonstrates the septal lines *(arrows)*.

upper and lower lobes) (Fig. 1.17). On a lateral chest radiograph the major fissures can be seen as lines that extend obliquely downward and forward from the level of the fifth thoracic vertebra and end at the diaphragm a few centimeters behind the anterior pleural gutter (Fig. 1.18). In the majority of cases the interlobar fissures are incomplete, and the incidence of accessory fissures is variable.

Accessory Fissures

Azygos Fissure. The azygos fissure is one of the most recognized accessory fissures, created by downward invagination of the azygos vein through the apical portion of the right upper lobe.[26] It is manifested radiographically as a curvilinear shadow that extends obliquely across the upper portion of the right lung and terminates at a variable distance above the right hilum in a *teardrop* shadow caused by the azygos vein itself (Fig. 1.19). Because the vein runs outside the parietal pleura, four pleural layers (two parietal and two visceral) form the fissure.

Inferior Accessory Fissure. This fissure separates the medial basal segment from the remainder of the lower lobe. It is seen on 5% to 13% of chest radiographs, most commonly on the right, as a thin line extending from the medial aspect of the hemidiaphragm (most commonly right) obliquely cephalad and medially toward the right hilum (Fig. 1.20).[27,28]

Superior Accessory Fissure. The superior accessory fissure separates the superior segment from the basal segments of the lower lobes, more commonly on the right. The fissure can be identified on approximately 3% of lateral chest radiographs.[27]

Left Minor Fissure. The left minor fissure is present in 8% to 18% of individuals but is seen on radiographs in only 1.6% of cases. The left minor fissure tends to be in a slightly more cephalad location than the right minor fissure and, like the right minor fissure, tends to be dome shaped (convex superiorly).[29,30]

Pulmonary Ligament

The pulmonary ligament consists of a double layer of pleura that tethers the medial aspect of the lower lobe to the adjacent mediastinum and diaphragm.[31] It is formed by the mediastinal parietal pleura as it reflects over the main bronchi and pulmonary arteries and veins onto the surface of the lung as the visceral pleura. Although the pulmonary ligament is anatomically extraparenchymal, it is contiguous laterally with a cleavage plane in the parenchyma of the lower lobe known as the *intersegmental (intersublobar) septum,* which separates the medial from the posterior basal segments. The pulmonary ligament is not seen on PA or lateral chest radiographs, although it determines the shape of the collapsed lower lobe in patients with atelectasis and the shape of the collapsed lung in patients with pneumothorax.

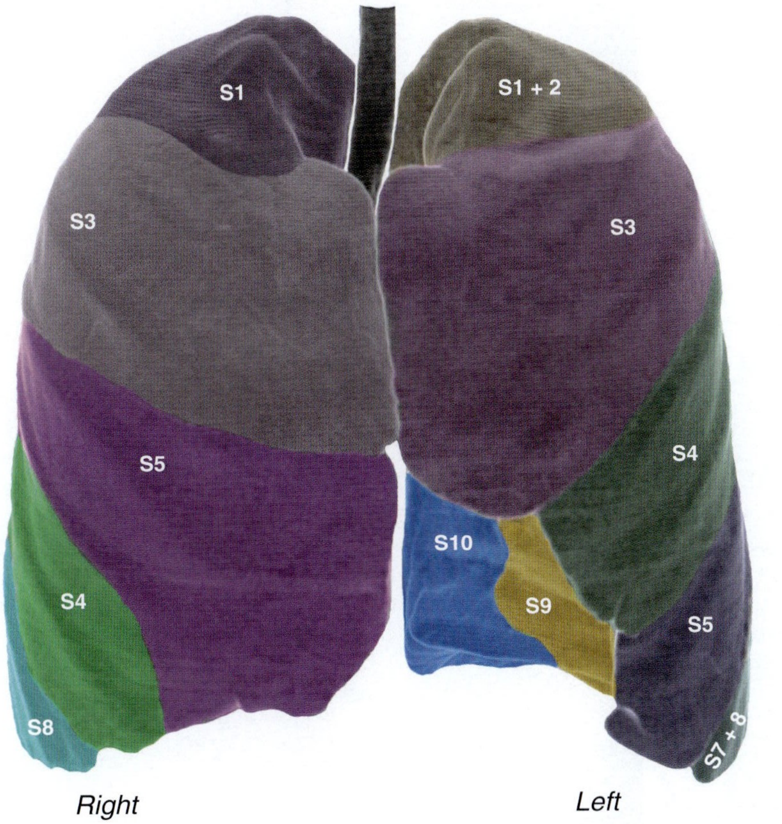

A

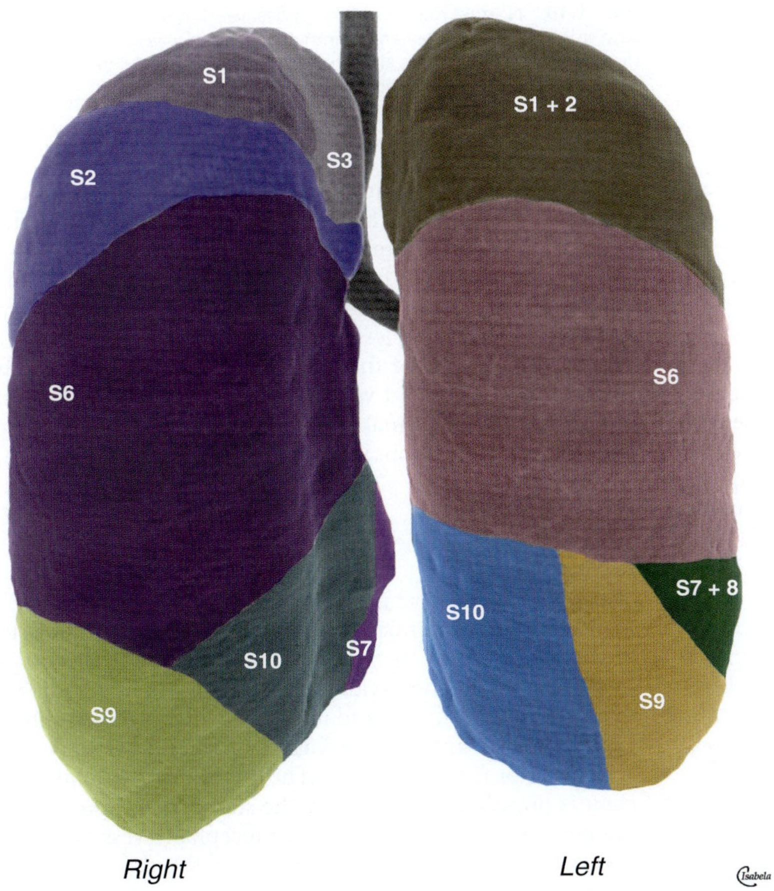

B

Fig. 1.16 (A) Pulmonary lobes and segments: anterior view. A schematic drawing superimposed on a three-dimensional surface reformatted image obtained with a multidetector CT scanner shows the location of the pulmonary segments and lobes on the anterior surface of the right and left lungs. The segments that form the anterior surface of the right lung include the apical *(S1)* and anterior *(S3)* segments of the right upper lobe, the lateral *(S4)* and medial *(S5)* segments of the right middle lobe, and the anterior basal (S8) segment of the right lower lobe. The anterior view of the left lung shows the location of the apicoposterior segment *(S1 + 2)*, anterior *(S3)* segment, and superior *(S4)* and inferior *(S5)* lingular segments of the left upper lobe, as well as the anteromedial basal *(S7 + S8)* segment. Because the heart was removed from the original image, the lateral basal *(S9)* and posterior basal *(S10)* segments of the left lower lobe are also demonstrated on this image. (B) Pulmonary lobes and segments: posterior view. The segments that form the posterior surface of the right lung include the apical *(S1)*, posterior *(S2)*, and anterior *(S3)* segments of the right upper lobe and the superior *(S6)*, lateral basal *(S9)*, posterior basal *(S10)*, and (adjacent to the heart, which is not shown) medial *(S7)* basal segments of the right lower lobe. The segments that form the posterior surface of the left lung include the apicoposterior *(S1 + S2)* segments of the left upper lobe and the superior *(S6)*, anteromedial basal *(S7 + S8)*, lateral basal *(S9)*, and posterior basal *(S10)* segments of the left lower lobe.

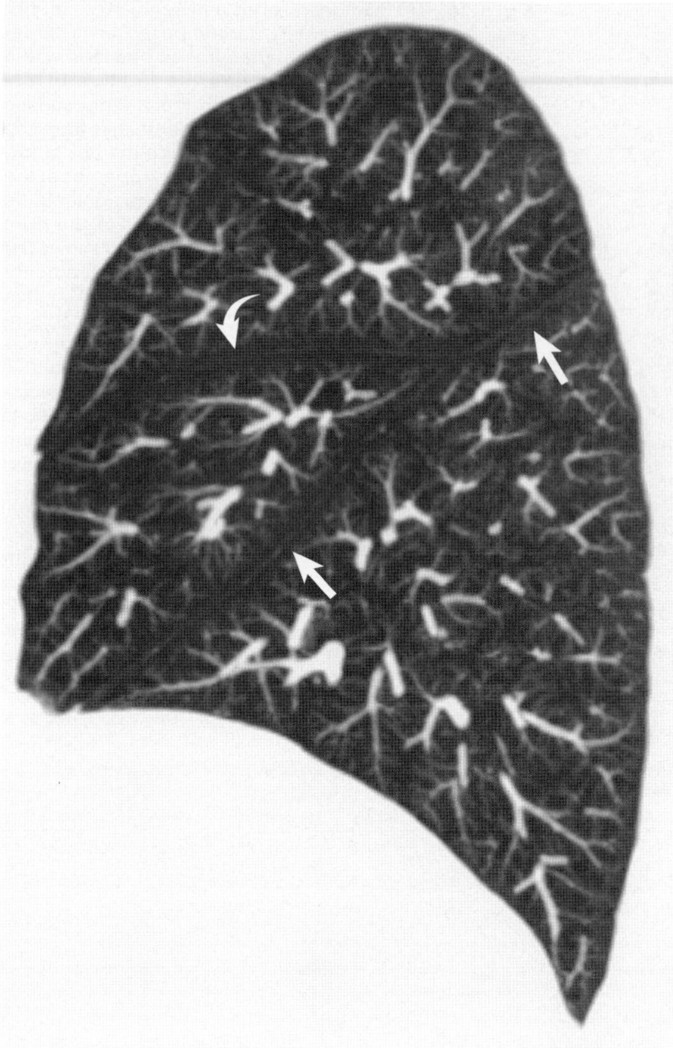

Fig. 1.17 Normal right interlobar fissures. A sagittal maximum-intensity projection image obtained from a CT scan shows normal position of the right major *(straight arrows)* and minor *(curved arrow)* interlobar fissures.

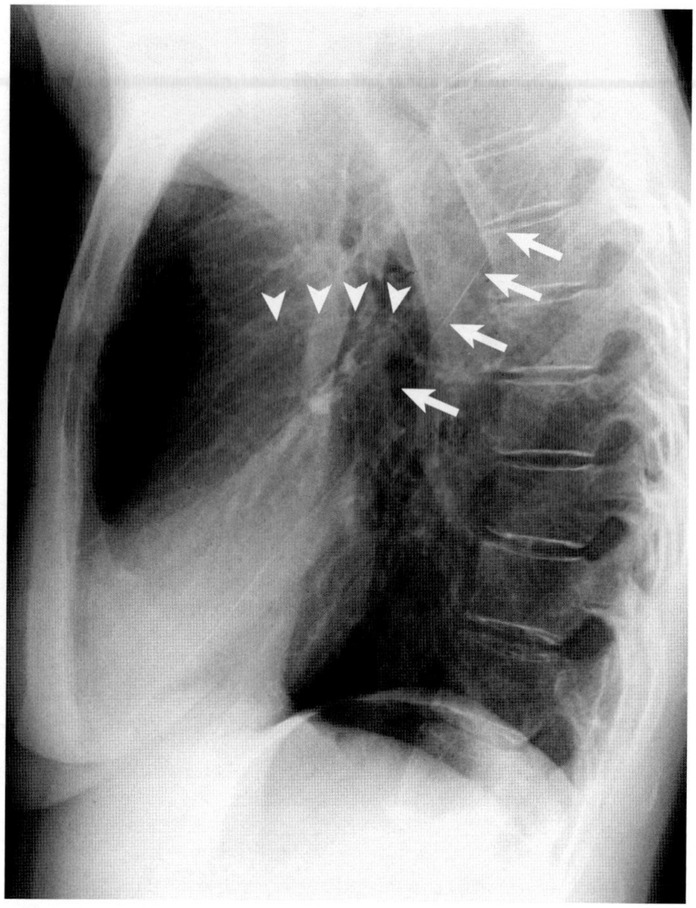

Fig. 1.18 Normal major and minor fissures. Lateral radiograph showing the right major *(arrows)* and minor *(arrowheads)* fissures. The left major fissure normally projects slightly posterior to the right major fissure and is not well seen on this radiograph.

THORACIC INLET

The thoracic inlet represents the junction between structures at the base of the neck and those of the thorax. It parallels the first rib and is higher posteriorly than anteriorly (Fig. 1.21). Therefore, on a frontal chest radiograph, an opacity that is effaced on its superior aspect and that projects at or below the level of the clavicles must be situated anteriorly, whereas one that projects above the clavicles is retrotracheal and posteriorly situated. These characteristic findings together have been termed the *cervicothoracic sign* by some authors.

From front to back, structures occupying the thoracic inlet include the right and left brachiocephalic veins (which join behind the right side of the manubrium to form the superior vena cava [SVC]), the supraaortic branches, the trachea, the esophagus, and the recurrent laryngeal nerves on either side of the esophagus (Figs. 1.22).

The overall shadow of the great systemic veins and arteries as seen on a frontal chest radiograph extending from below the level of the thoracic inlet to the heart is known as the vascular pedicle. The width of the vascular pedicle is measured from the lateral edge of the SVC as it crosses the right main bronchus to a vertical line drawn inferiorly from the point where the left subclavian artery arises from the aortic arch (Fig. 1.23).[32] Although variable, the vascular pedicle in a normal upright PA chest radiograph measures less than 6 cm. Widening (>7 cm) may result from dilation of the great vessels (supine position, pregnancy, increased blood volume, left heart failure), mediastinal abnormality (mediastinal lipomatosis, lymph node enlargement, masses, fluid collections), or pleural disease.[33]

MEDIASTINUM

Anatomy

The mediastinum separates the thorax vertically into two compartments and can be defined anatomically as the partition between the lungs. Although there is variability in the description of the mediastinum, the most widely used classification on radiography divides it anatomically (and for diagnostic purposes) into three compartments: anterior (prevascular), middle (cardiovascular), and posterior (postvascular).[34] The *anterior mediastinal compartment* is bounded anteriorly by the sternum and posteriorly by the pericardium, aorta, and brachiocephalic vessels. It merges superiorly with the anterior aspect of the thoracic inlet and extends down to the level of the diaphragm. The compartment

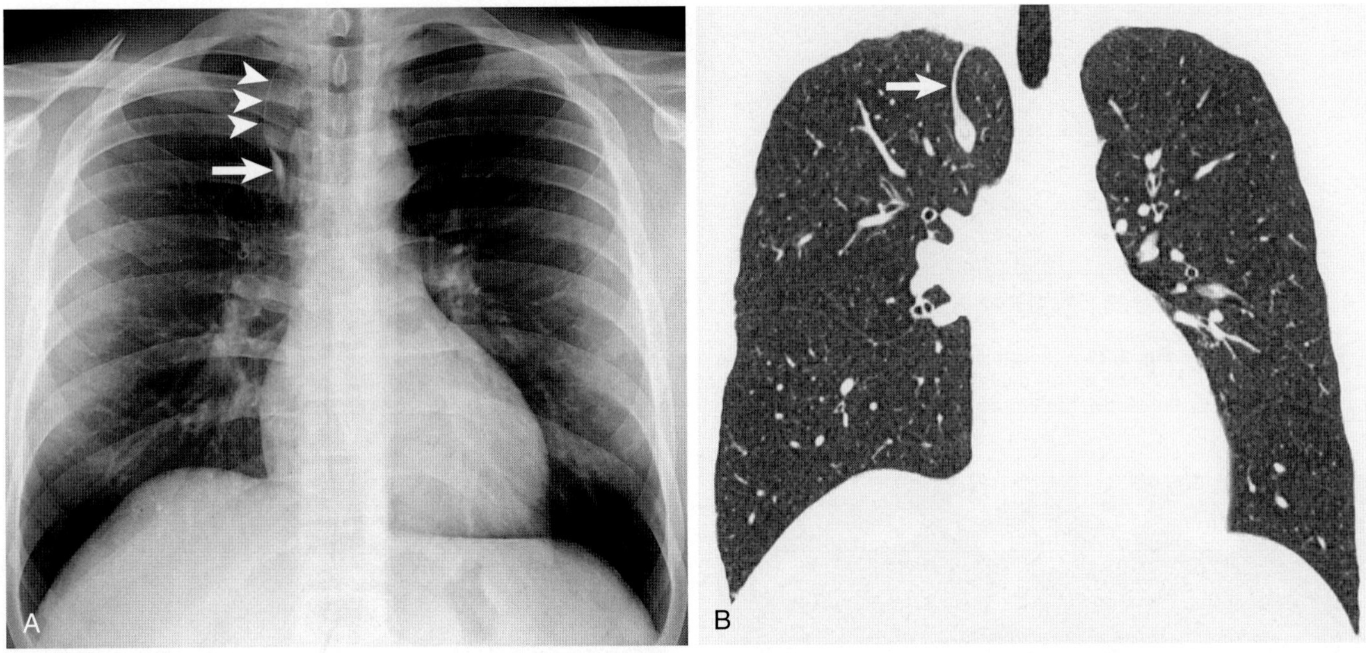

Fig. 1.19 Azygos fissure. (A) Posteroanterior chest radiograph showing the azygos fissure as a curvilinear line *(arrowheads)* extending obliquely across the upper portion of the right lung. Note the azygos vein *(arrow)* coursing within the fissure. (B) Coronal reformatted image from a CT scan showing the azygos fissure *(arrow)*.

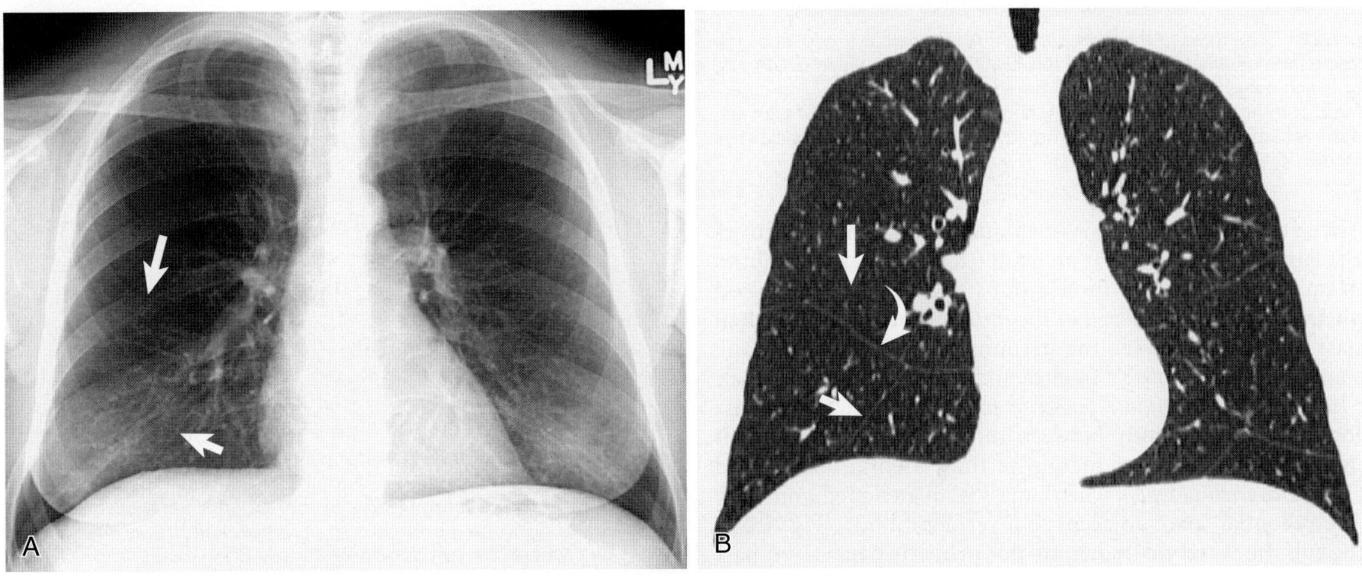

Fig. 1.20 Accessory fissures. (A) Posteroanterior chest radiograph showing the right minor fissure *(long arrow)* and right inferior accessory fissure *(short arrow)*. (B) Coronal reformatted CT image showing the right minor fissure *(long straight arrow)*, right inferior accessory fissure *(short straight arrow)*, and right superior accessory fissure *(curved arrow)*. Also noted are several accessory fissures in the left lung.

contains the thymus gland, branches of the internal mammary artery and vein, lymph nodes, the inferior sternopericardial ligament, and variable amounts of fat. On a chest radiograph the thymus is visible only in infants and young children, in whom it fills much of the anterior mediastinal space.

The *middle mediastinal compartment* contains the pericardium and its contents, the ascending and transverse portions of the aorta, the superior and inferior venae cavae, the brachiocephalic (innominate) arteries and veins, the phrenic nerves and the cephalad portion of the vagus nerves, the trachea and main bronchi and their contiguous lymph nodes, and the main pulmonary arteries and veins. The *posterior mediastinal compartment* is bounded anteriorly by the pericardium and the vertical part of the diaphragm, laterally by the mediastinal pleura, and posteriorly by the bodies of the thoracic vertebrae. It contains the descending thoracic aorta, esophagus, thoracic duct, azygos and hemiazygos veins, autonomic nerves, fat, and lymph nodes.

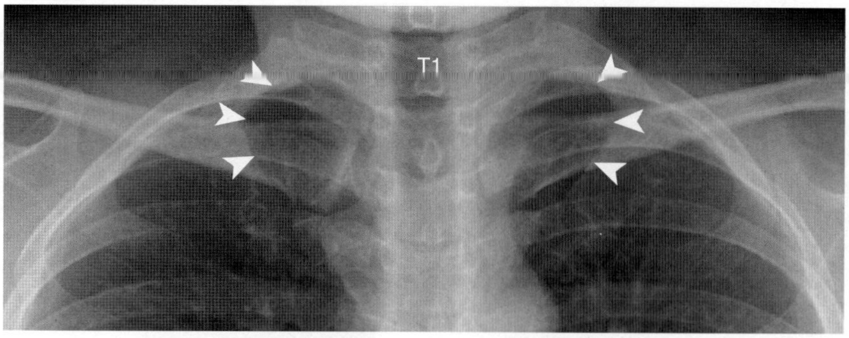

Fig. 1.21 Thoracic inlet. A detailed view from a posteroanterior chest radiograph shows the right and left first ribs as they originate posteriorly from the first thoracic vertebra *(T1)* and course anteriorly and inferiorly. The thoracic inlet parallels the first ribs *(arrowheads)* and is therefore higher posteriorly.

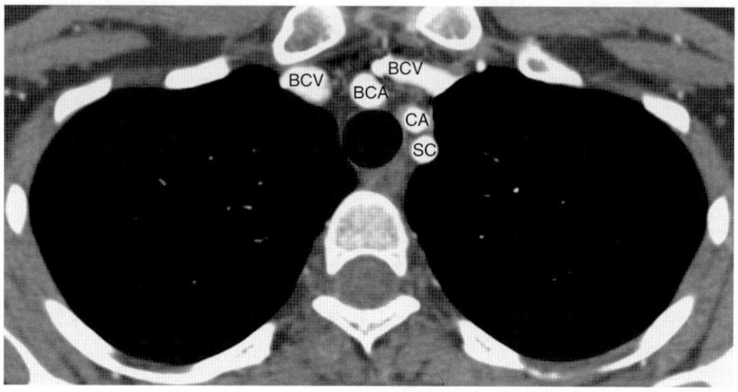

Fig. 1.22 Structures in the thoracic inlet. A CT scan at the level of the thoracic inlet shows the right and left brachiocephalic veins *(BCV)*, the right brachiocephalic artery *(BCA)* immediately anterior to the trachea, the left common carotid artery *(CA)* slightly to the left of the trachea, and the left subclavian artery *(SC)* more posteriorly. The esophagus lies posterior to the trachea.

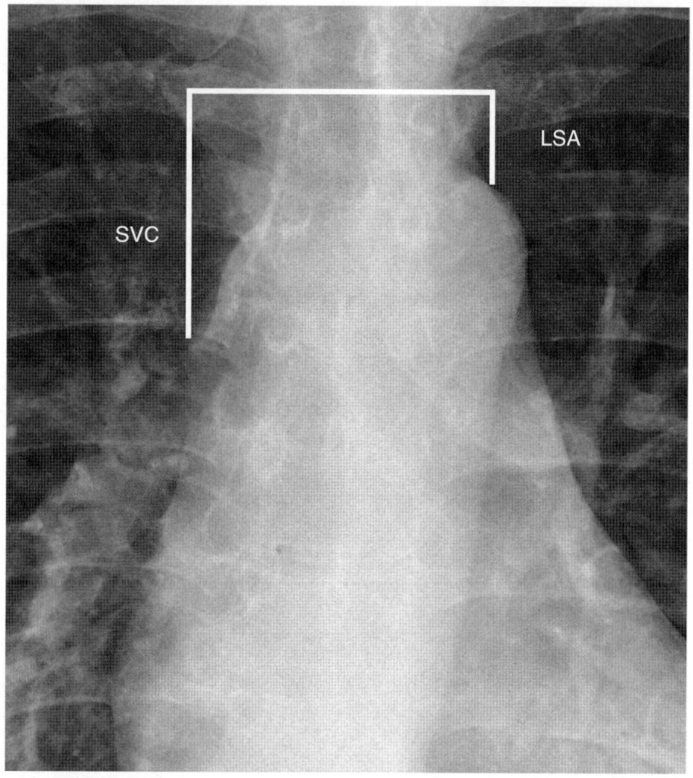

Fig. 1.23 Vascular pedicle. A detailed view from a posteroanterior (PA) chest radiograph shows the width of the vascular pedicle, which is measured from the lateral edge of the superior vena cava *(SVC)* as it crosses the right main bronchus to a vertical line drawn inferiorly from the point where the left subclavian artery *(LSA)* arises from the aortic arch. The normal width of the vascular pedicle on an upright PA chest radiograph is less than 6 cm.

Given the variability in the visualization of anatomic structures in the lateral radiograph, it is preferable to classify abnormalities seen on radiographs into three groups based on the likelihood of their anatomic location: (1) the *anterior mediastinum* when a mass is situated between the sternum and a line drawn along the anterior border of the trachea and the posterior border of the heart,[35] (2) the *middle-posterior mediastinum* when a mass is located predominantly between this line and a line drawn 1 cm behind the anterior margin of the vertebral bodies, and (3) the *paravertebral region* when a mass is situated predominantly in the potential space adjacent to a vertebral body (Fig. 1.24). Although the vertebral bodies are not properly considered part of the posterior mediastinum, lesions in the paravertebral region are not infrequent causes of opacities projecting over the posterior mediastinal compartment on the lateral chest radiograph and thus should be considered within the differential diagnosis. Accurate assessment of the anatomic location of these abnormalities can readily be accomplished with CT or magnetic resonance imaging (MRI).

Frontal Chest Radiograph

On a frontal chest radiograph the mediastinal shadow to the right of the trachea is formed by the right brachiocephalic vein and the SVC, and the contour of the lower mediastinal shadow is formed by the right atrium (Fig. 1.25). The interface between the right brachiocephalic vein and the SVC is seen in almost all patients from the level of the medial end of the right clavicle to the level of the right bronchus (see Fig. 1.25). The density of the SVC is generally less than that of the aortic arch, and its interface with the lung is normally slightly concave laterally.[36] Increased opacity in the region of the SVC and the lateral convexity of its interface with the lung may result from increased size of the SVC (supine position, pregnancy, and right heart failure), paratracheal lymph node enlargement, a mediastinal mass, mediastinal hemorrhage, or a pleural abnormality.[36]

The trachea is normally bordered on its right lateral aspect by pleura covering the right upper lobe. Contact of the right lung in the supraazygos area with the right lateral wall of the trachea

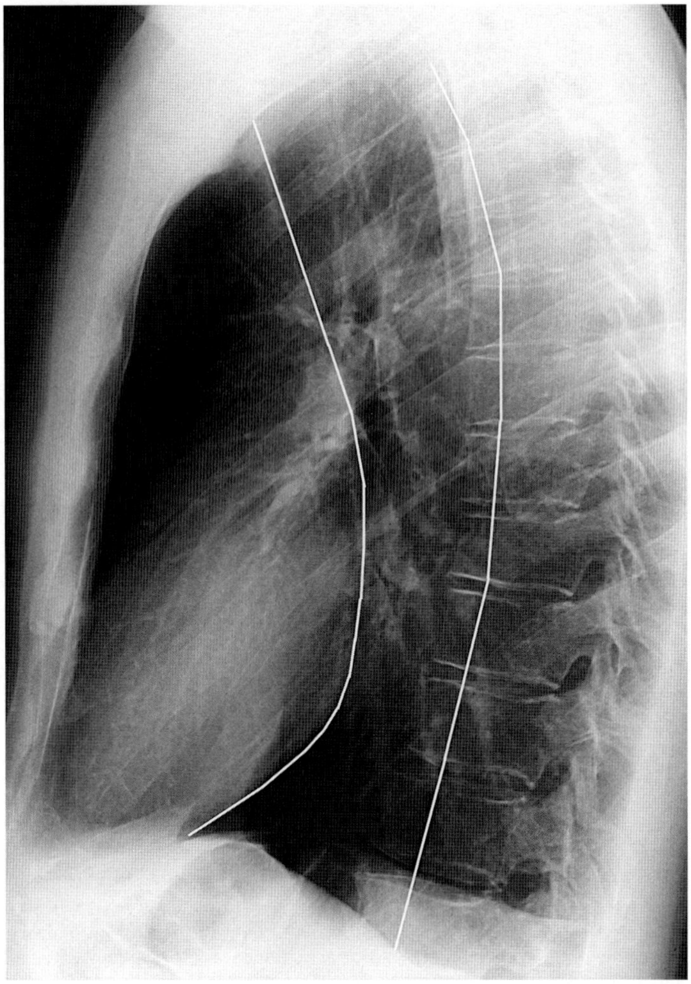

Fig. 1.24 Mediastinal compartments on a lateral chest radiograph. A mass can be considered to probably lie in the anterior mediastinum if it is situated predominantly in the region in front of a line drawn along the anterior border of the trachea and the posterior border of the heart. A mass probably lies in the middle or posterior mediastinum if it is situated between this line and a line drawn 1 cm posterior to the anterior aspect of the vertebral bodies. Extrapulmonary masses posterior to this line are typically paravertebral in location.

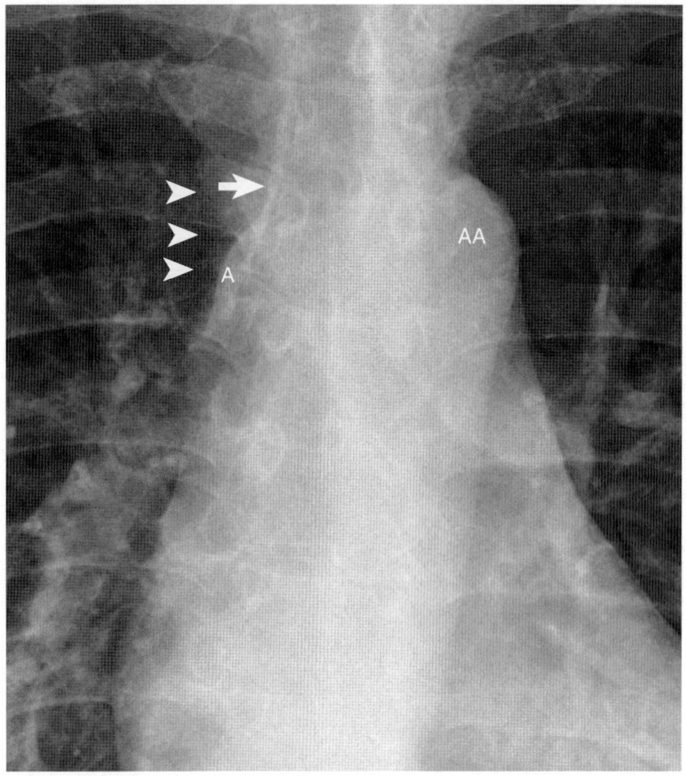

Fig. 1.25 Normal right paratracheal region. A detail view from a frontal chest radiograph shows a normal mediastinum at the level of the aortic arch *(AA)*. The right lateral border is delimited by the faint opacity of the superior vena cava (SVC) *(arrowheads)*. The SVC normally has a straight outer contour and lower opacity than the aortic arch does. Note the right paratracheal stripe *(arrow)* and the azygos vein *(A)* at the level of the right tracheobronchial angle.

creates a thin stripe of soft tissue density that is usually visible on frontal chest radiographs and is known as the *right paratracheal stripe* (see Fig. 1.25).[37] This stripe is formed by the right wall of the trachea, contiguous parietal and visceral pleura, and a variable quantity of mediastinal fat. The thickness of this stripe above the level of the azygos vein generally ranges from 1 to 4 mm. Widening of the paratracheal stripe (>5 mm) may be due to thickening of the tracheal wall by inflammation or space-occupying lesions, paratracheal lymph node enlargement, mediastinal hemorrhage, or pleural disease.[36,37] Widening of the paratracheal stripe is not a particularly sensitive sign for lymphadenopathy in that it is present in only approximately 30% of patients who demonstrate paratracheal lymph node enlargement on CT.[36]

A slightly flattened elliptical opacity can frequently be seen in the region of the right tracheobronchial angle corresponding to the azygos vein being viewed tangentially as it enters the SVC (see Fig. 1.25).

The *azygos vein* originates in the upper lumbar region at the level of the renal veins as a continuation of the right ascending lumbar vein. Along its course the vein receives tributaries from the 5th to 11th intercostal veins on the right, the right subcostal vein, the right superior intercostal vein, the right bronchial veins, and the superior and inferior hemiazygos veins.[38] It drains into the SVC.

Contact of the right lower lobe with the esophagus and the ascending portion of the azygos vein results in the *azygoesophageal recess.*[38,39] This recess is frequently identified on a well-penetrated PA radiograph as an interface that extends from the diaphragm to the level of the azygos arch (Fig. 1.26). A focal right-sided convexity of the azygoesophageal recess interface should raise suspicion of an underlying pathologic process, such as a hiatal hernia, esophageal tumor or duplication cyst, azygos vein dilation, or subcarinal lymph node enlargement.

The left lateral wall of the trachea is rarely visible on a PA chest radiograph because of contiguity of the left subclavian artery and mediastinal fat. On a frontal chest radiograph the mediastinal shadow to the left of the trachea above the level of the aortic arch is typically a low-density arcuate opacity (concave laterally) extending from the aortic arch to a point at or just above the medial end of the clavicle (Fig. 1.27). The lateral margin of this density corresponds to the course of the left subclavian artery and may be formed by the artery or, more commonly, by adjacent fat. The first convexity of the left aspect of the mediastinum is formed by the posterior portion of the aortic arch. Contact of the lateral aspect of the descending aorta and the left lung results in the left paraaortic interface. A lateral

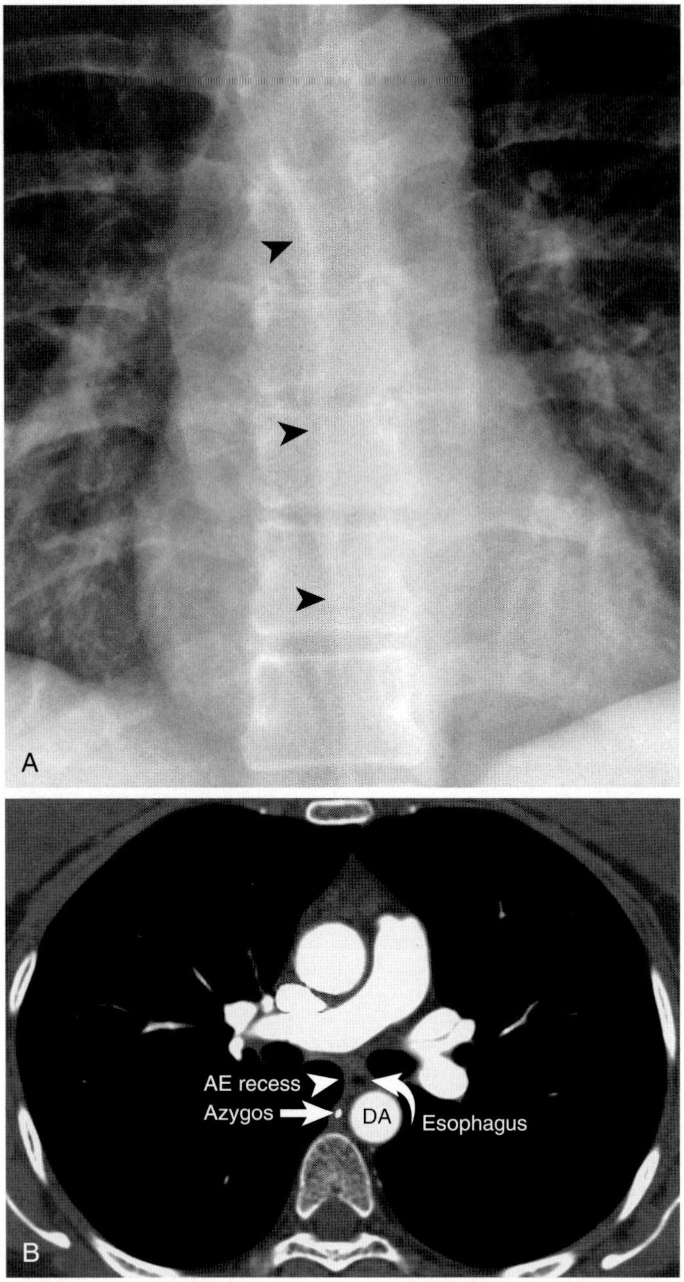

Fig. 1.26 Azygoesophageal recess. (A) Detail view from a frontal chest radiograph showing the azygoesophageal recess as a smooth continuous arc *(arrowheads)* as it extends from the diaphragm to the level of the azygos arch. (B) Contrast-enhanced CT scan showing the azygos vein and the esophagus forming the medial border of the azygoesophageal *(AE)* recess. *DA,* Descending thoracic aorta.

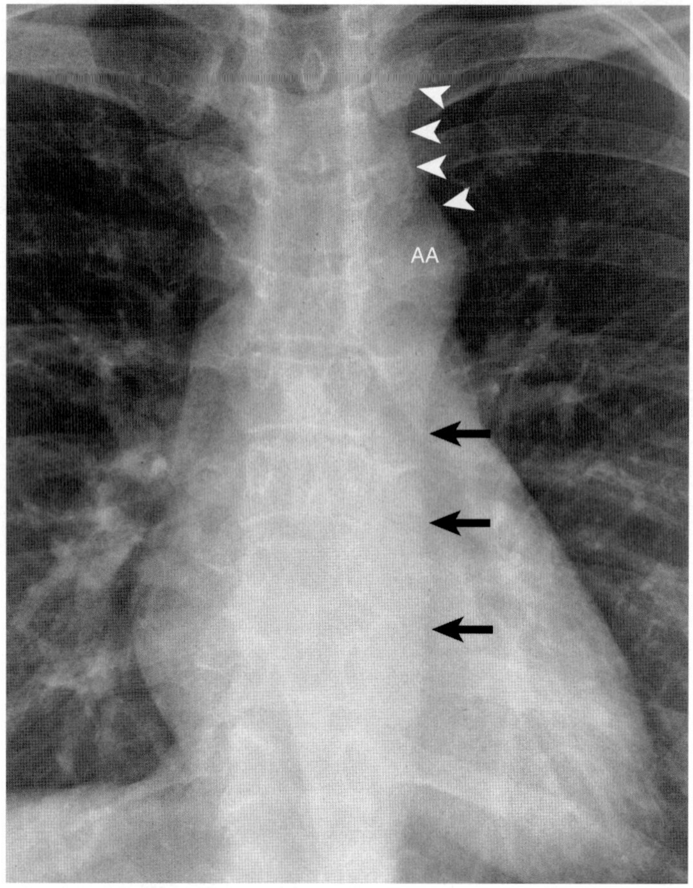

Fig. 1.27 Normal left mediastinal shadow. A detail view from a frontal chest radiograph shows the outer margin of the left mediastinum above the aortic arch *(AA)* as an arcuate opacity concave laterally *(arrowheads)* and extending from the aortic arch to a point just above the medial end of the clavicle. The lateral margin of this opacity corresponds to the course of the left subclavian artery and may be formed by the artery or, more commonly, by adjacent fat. The first convexity of the left aspect of the mediastinum is formed by the posterior portion of the aortic arch. Extending from the aortic arch, the left border of the descending aorta *(arrows)* can be seen coursing medially down to the level of the diaphragm.

convexity of the left paraaortic interface may result from tortuosity of the aorta (normally seen in the elderly), an aortic aneurysm, a paraaortic mediastinal mass, hemorrhage, or enlarged lymph nodes.

A small triangular or round opacity is seen immediately lateral to the aortic arch on approximately 1% of chest radiographs.[27] This opacity, known as the "aortic nipple," is caused by the left superior intercostal vein as it courses cephalad and forward to enter the left brachiocephalic vein (Fig. 1.28).

The opacity seen immediately below the level of the aortic arch and above the left main bronchus is the main pulmonary artery. The space between the arch of the aorta and the left pulmonary artery is known as the aortopulmonary window, which is usually concave or straight (Fig. 1.29). It is occupied largely by mediastinal fat; its medial boundary is the ductus ligament, and its lateral boundary is the mediastinal and visceral pleura over the left lung, which creates the aortopulmonary window interface. Convexity of the aortopulmonary window interface may result from lymph node enlargement, a mediastinal tumor, or an aortic aneurysm. Because the left recurrent laryngeal nerve courses in the aortopulmonary window, pathologic processes in this region may be associated with left vocal cord palsy and hoarseness.

The interfaces between the anterior and posterior mediastinal contents and the lungs just inferior to the thoracic inlet result in linear shadows known as the anterior and posterior junction lines, respectively.

The anterior junction line is formed by contact of the right and left lungs with the adjacent prevascular mediastinum in the retrosternal space. On a PA chest radiograph this line is typically oriented obliquely from upper right to lower left behind the sternum (Fig. 1.30), seen in approximately 20% of cases.

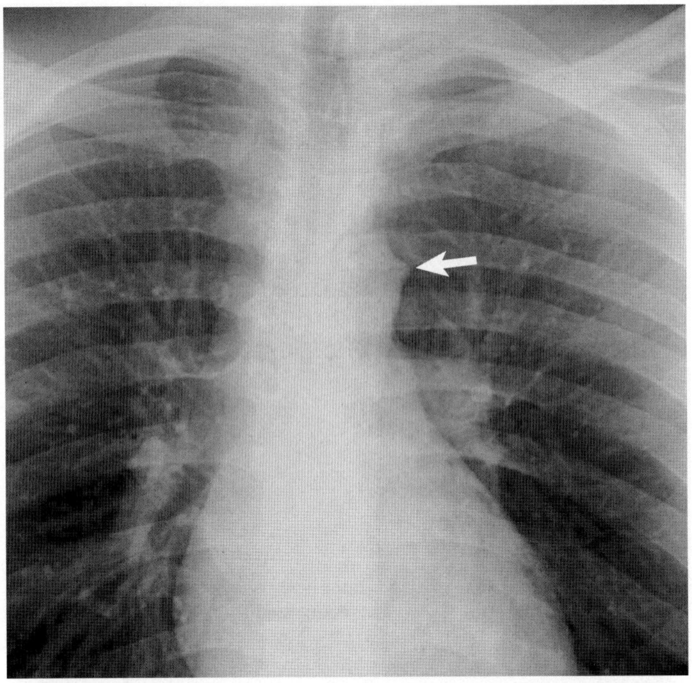

Fig. 1.28 Aortic nipple. Detail view from a frontal radiograph showing a small triangular opacity *(arrow)* immediately lateral to the aortic arch. This opacity, known as the aortic nipple, is caused by the left superior intercostal vein as it courses cephalad and forward to enter the left brachiocephalic vein.

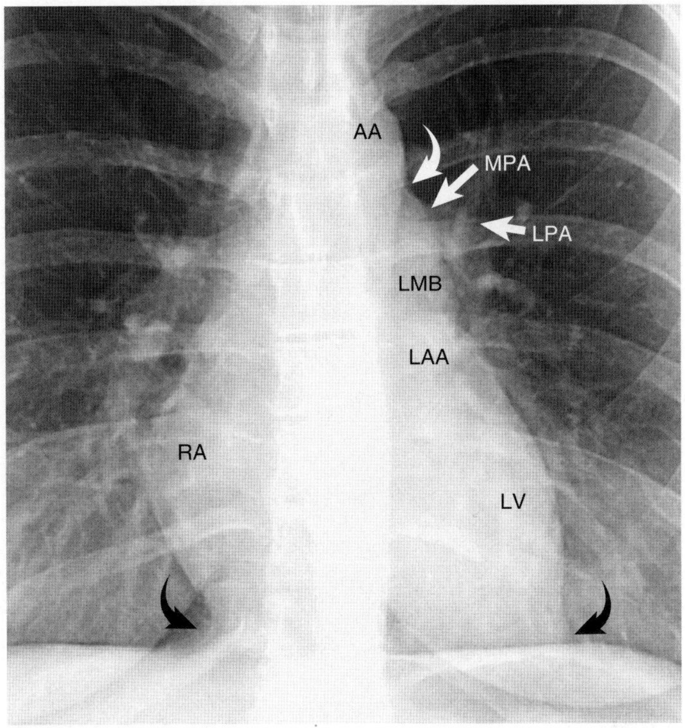

Fig. 1.29 Normal mediastinum and heart. A detail view from a frontal radiograph shows the aortic arch *(AA)*. The opacity seen immediately below the level of the aortic arch and above the left main bronchus is the main pulmonary artery *(MPA)*. At this level the main pulmonary artery appears as an oval or elliptical opacity medial to the left pulmonary artery *(LPA)*. From the level of the aortic arch to the level of the pulmonary artery, the lateral border of the mediastinum is normally concave laterally or straight *(white curved arrow)*. The space between the arch of the aorta and the pulmonary artery is known as the aortopulmonary window. The main and left pulmonary arteries are located immediately above the level of the left main *(LMB)* and left upper lobe bronchi. The lateral border immediately below the left main bronchus is formed by the left atrial appendage *(LAA)* and is usually slightly concave or straight. The remaining left border of the heart is formed by the left ventricle *(LV)*. The right border of the heart is formed by the right atrium *(RA)*. The cardiophrenic angles or sulci *(black curved arrows)* are located at the junction of the cardiopericardial silhouette and the diaphragm. Variable amounts of mediastinal fat are normally present in this region.

The pleural apposition between the upper lobes and along with any intervening mediastinal tissue creates the *posterior junction line* (see Fig. 1.30). On a PA radiograph the posterior junction line usually projects through the air column of the trachea; it may be straight or slightly convex to the left.

Lateral Chest Radiograph

The trachea can be readily seen on a lateral radiograph as it descends in a straight course obliquely caudally and posteriorly (Fig. 1.31). The anterior wall of the trachea is seldom visible because it is obscured by the mediastinum, but the posterior wall can usually be seen because it abuts the lung. The posterior wall together with adjacent fat forms the posterior tracheal stripe or band, which generally measures less than 4 mm in diameter. Measurement of this stripe, however, is seldom helpful because the esophagus may be interposed between the posterior trachea and lung and result in a stripe thickness of 1 cm or greater.

The region posterior to the tracheal stripe and anterior to the spine above the level of the aortic arch is known as the retrotracheal triangle (Fig. 1.31), which is a characteristically lucent space, and it contains the esophagus, lymph nodes, and posterior segments of the upper lobes. Increased opacity in the retrotracheal triangle in the lateral radiograph is abnormal, and although commonly resulting from an aberrant subclavian artery, other entities, such as an esophageal tumor, a thyroid mass, lymph node enlargement, or a foregut duplication cyst, may cause an abnormal density.

KEY POINTS: HILA AND MEDIASTINUM

- Left hilum normally 1–2 cm higher than the right
- Normal diameter of the vascular pedicle: <7 cm
- Normal right paratracheal stripe: 1–4 mm

HEART

In normal individuals the transverse diameter of the heart measured on standard PA radiographs is generally in the range of 11.5 to 15.5 cm.[19] A commonly used measurement to assess overall heart size is the ratio of the widest cardiac diameter to the widest inside thoracic diameter, known as the cardiothoracic ratio. A cardiothoracic ratio greater than 50% on a PA radiograph with the patient upright has a specificity of approximately 80% for the detection of left ventricular dilation but a sensitivity of only 50%.[19] The cardiothoracic ratio is not helpful in detecting left atrial or right ventricular enlargement because neither of these chambers is reflected in the transverse dimension.

Cardiac size and contour of the heart are influenced by five main factors:

1. *Cardiac cycle:* The diameter is largest at end diastole and smallest at peak systole. The change in heart width between systole and diastole is usually less than 1 cm.
2. *Height of the diaphragm,* which in turn is influenced by lung volumes. The lower the position of the diaphragm, the longer and narrower the cardiovascular silhouette.

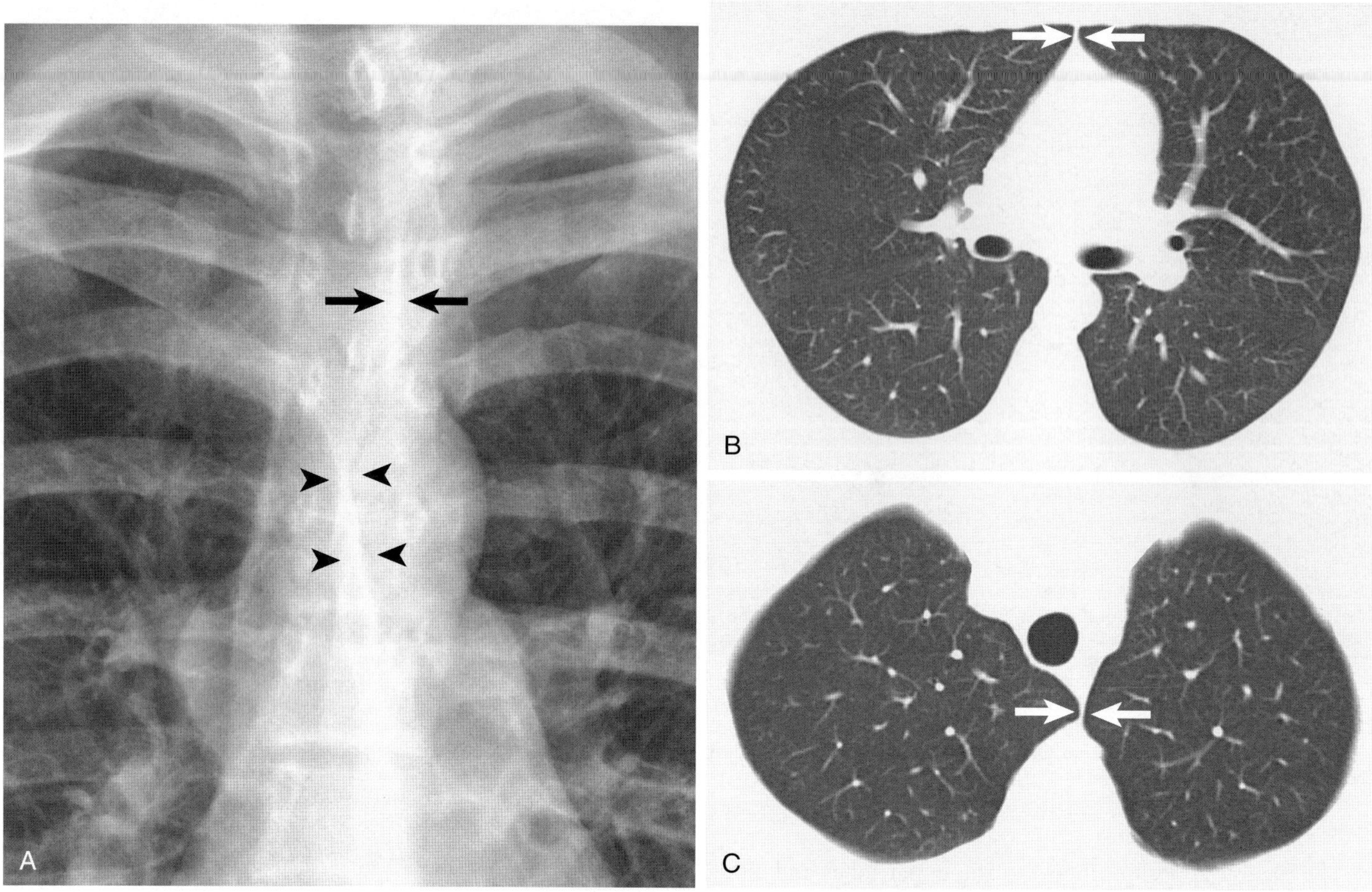

Fig. 1.30 Anterior and posterior junction lines. (A) Detail view of a chest radiograph showing the anterior junction line *(arrowheads)* extending from the level of the aortic arch inferiorly and obliquely to the left and posterior junction line *(arrows)* above the level of the aortic arch. (B) CT scan at the level of the bronchus intermedius showing contact of the right and left lungs *(arrows)* in the retrosternal space. This contact results in the anterior junction line seen on the radiograph. (C) CT scan in the region of the thoracic inlet showing contact of the right and left lungs *(arrows)* posterior to the esophagus, which results in the posterior junction line.

3. *Intrathoracic pressure,* which influences not only cardiac size but also the appearance of the pulmonary vascular pattern.
4. *Body position:* Assuming equality of all other factors, the heart is broader when a subject is recumbent than when erect.
5. *PA versus AP radiograph:* The heart is magnified and appears larger on radiographs performed with AP projection of the x-ray beam.

The right border of the heart on a frontal radiograph is formed by the right atrium as it abuts the right middle lobe. Adjacent to the diaphragm, the inferior vena cava (IVC) may be seen as it enters the right atrium. The right ventricle is not visible on a frontal radiograph.

The heart border immediately below the level of the left bronchus is typically concave or straight (see Fig. 1.29). A focal convexity at this level is most suggestive of enlargement of the left atrial appendage, a finding seen most commonly in mitral heart disease. Enlargement of the left atrium may elevate the left main bronchus and cause splaying of the tracheal carina.

The junction of the right and left heart borders with the anterior hemidiaphragms results in the right and left cardiophrenic angles or recesses (see Fig. 1.29). These recesses contain fat (mediastinal fat pad) and lymph nodes and are usually concave laterally. A focal convexity of the cardiophrenic angle may result from the accumulation of fat (prominent mediastinal fat pad), a pericardial cyst, enlarged anterior diaphragmatic lymph nodes, or a Morgagni hernia (Fig. 1.32).

On a lateral view the anterior border of the heart is formed by the right ventricle. Normally, the right ventricle contacts only the lower half of the sternum (Fig. 1.33). The earliest sign of right ventricular enlargement on the radiograph is loss of the retrosternal clear space superiorly. The posterior heart border is formed in its upper third by the left atrium and in its lower two-thirds by the left ventricle. In some patients the IVC may be seen entering the posterior border of the right atrium.

DIAPHRAGM

On a chest radiograph the upper surface of the dome-shaped diaphragm is normally visualized as it forms an interface with the lung; the soft tissues of the abdomen obscure its inferior surface. In approximately 95% of normal adults the level of the cupola of the right hemidiaphragm is projected in a

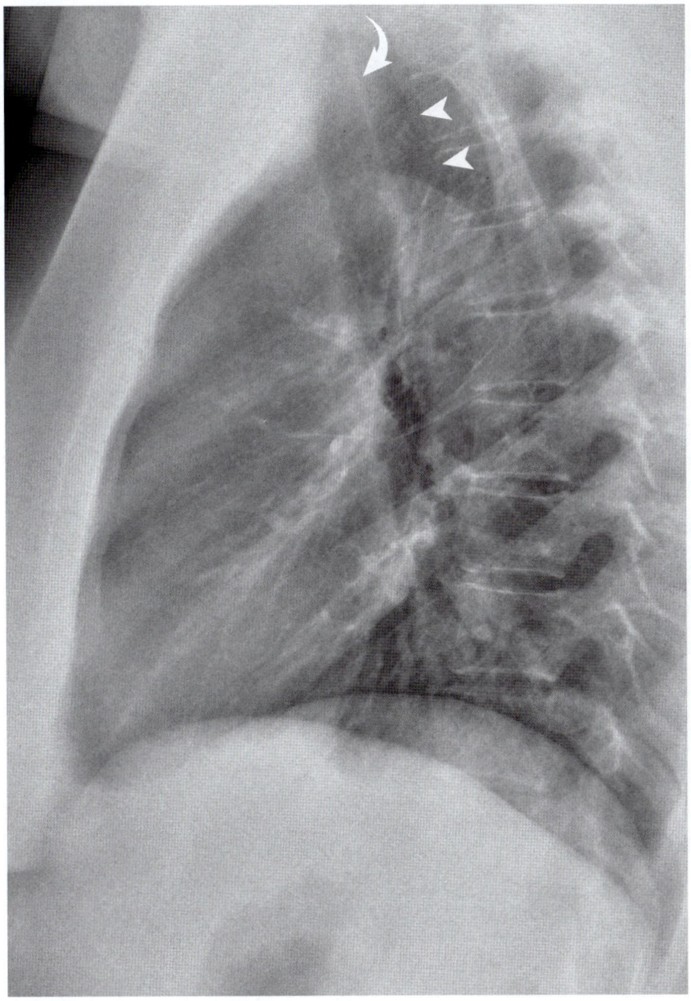

Fig. 1.31 Trachea and retrotracheal triangle. A lateral radiograph shows the trachea as it descends in a straight course obliquely caudally and slightly posteriorly. The posterior wall together with adjacent fat forms the posterior tracheal stripe *(arrow)*. The region posterior to the tracheal stripe and anterior to the spine above the level of the aortic arch is known as the retrotracheal triangle *(arrowheads)*.

plane ranging from the anterior end of the fifth rib to the sixth anterior interspace.[40] On a left lateral view of the chest the right hemidiaphragm is seen along its entire length, whereas the anterior portion of the left hemidiaphragm is obscured by the heart (Fig. 1.34).

CHEST WALL

On a frontal radiograph of the thorax the soft tissues, including the skin, subcutaneous fat, and muscles, are usually distinguishable over the shoulders and along the thoracic wall. In the absence of pulmonary or pleural disease, deformity of the spine, or congenital anomalies of the ribs themselves, the rib cage should be symmetric.

The intercostal arteries, veins, and nerves are situated in the inferior inner surface of the ribs. By convention, a lateral chest radiograph is taken with the left side against the radiographic detector to avoid cardiac magnification. Therefore the right ribs, being further away, are magnified and appear bigger than the left ribs (the *big rib* sign).[41]

In approximately 0.5% of the population unilateral or bilateral cervical ribs can be seen arising from the seventh cervical vertebra (Fig. 1.35).[42] These are generally incidental findings, although they may result in thoracic outlet syndrome—pain and weakness in the C8 nerve root distribution, variation in pulse intensity in the two arms when the affected extremity is in certain positions. Other supernumerary ribs are rare.

The sternum forms the anterior midline portion of the thoracic cage. It is made up of the manubrium, which articulates with the clavicles; the body; and the xiphoid process. The most common congenital abnormality of the sternum is a depression of the sternum known as pectus excavatum, or "funnel chest," which may cause leftward displacement and axial rotation of the heart when severe.[43] In these cases obscuration of the right heart border on frontal radiographs may mimic right middle lobe airspace disease (Fig. 1.36).

A less common congenital abnormality is abnormal protrusion of the sternum known as pectus carinatum, or "pigeon breast" (Fig. 1.37), which is seen with increased frequency in patients with cyanotic congenital heart disease.[43]

The sternum is difficult to assess on a frontal view and best seen on lateral or oblique views. Retrosternal lung allows identification of a stripe between the posterior cortex of the sternal body and the lung. This retrosternal stripe is composed primarily of fat and ranges from 1 to 3 mm in thickness. Indentation of the lung by parasternal structures, particularly costal cartilage, may result in a lobulated contour posterior to the parasternal stripe. A focal convexity or lobulation that is not at the level of a costal cartilage is suggestive of an abnormality, most commonly enlarged internal mammary lymph nodes.

On an optimal chest radiograph exposure factors should be such that the thoracic spine and intervertebral disks are faintly visible, with the spinous processes being in the midline. Contact between the lower lobes and the paravertebral soft tissues results in paravertebral interfaces or stripes that are commonly visible on a frontal radiograph, particularly in the lower part of the chest, usually thin and parallel to the spine. Displacement of the paravertebral stripe may occur with a vertebral abnormality (osteophyte, fracture, infection, neoplasm), paravertebral masses (hematoma, neurogenic tumor, paravertebral abscess), or lymph node enlargement.

Computed Tomography

Technical Aspects

The CT image is a two-dimensional representation of a 3D cross-sectional slice, the third dimension being the section or slice thickness. The slice thickness also is known as the collimation width and was traditionally defined by collimators between the x-ray tube and the patient. Current technology allows acquisition of submillimetric slice thickness, which results in an isometric voxel and thus allows reconstruction of CT data in any imaging plane (sagittal, coronal, oblique, curved). The CT image is composed of multiple picture elements (typically 512 × 512) known as pixels. A pixel is a unit area (i.e., each square on the image matrix); it reflects the attenuation of a unit volume of tissue, or voxel, which corresponds to the area of the pixel multiplied by the section thickness. The x-ray attenuations of the structures within a given voxel are averaged to produce the image. The CT image reflects the absorption of x-rays by tissues

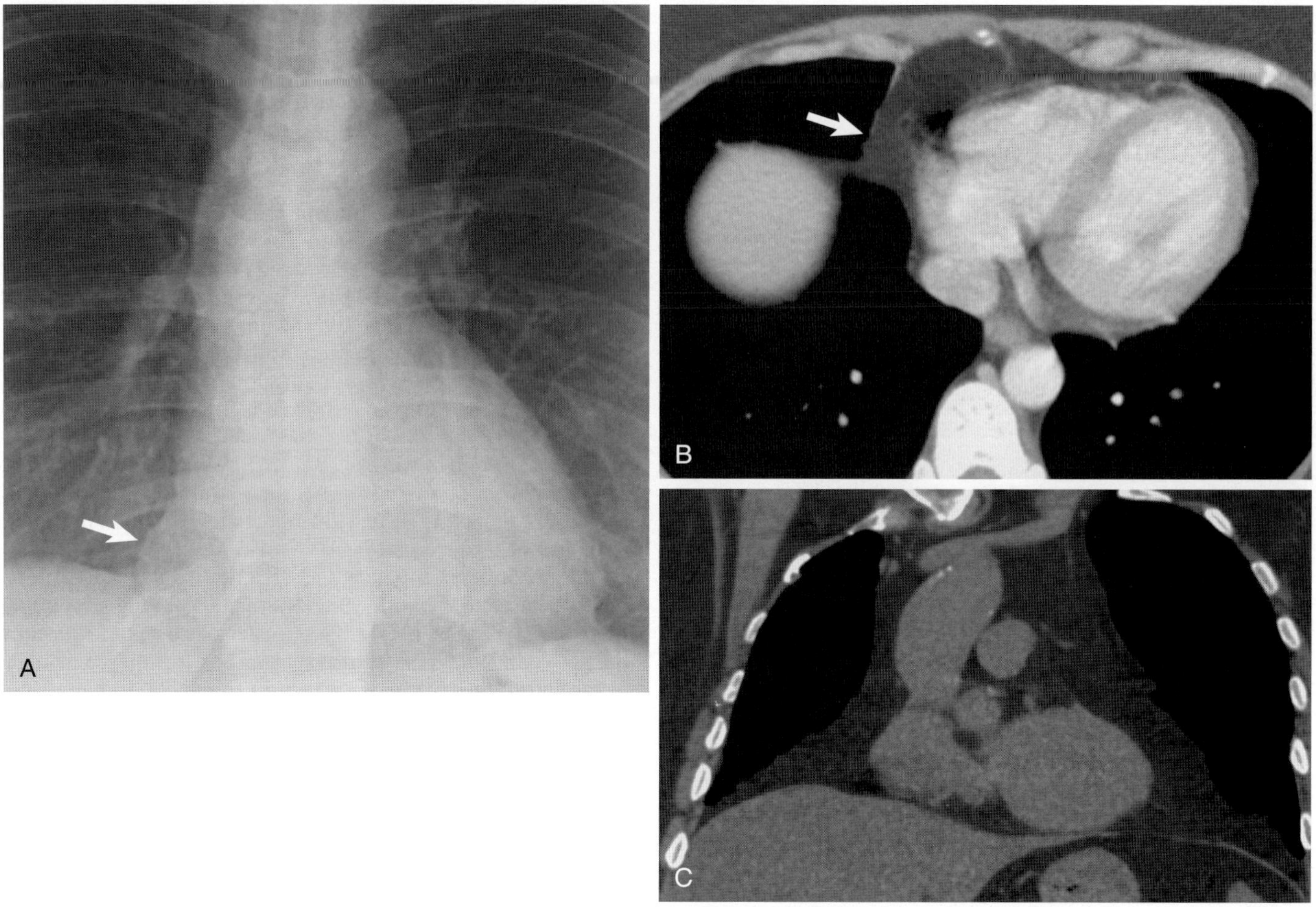

Fig. 1.32 Mediastinal fat pads and mediastinal lipomatosis. (A) A posteroanterior chest radiograph shows the right mediastinal fat pad *(arrow)*. (B) A CT image demonstrates the right mediastinal fat pad *(arrow)*. (C) A coronal reformatted CT image demonstrates extensive mediastinal lipomatosis and increased size of the mediastinal fat pads. The heart size is within normal limits.

of differing atomic number (radiographic density) within the CT section. The x-ray tube and the detectors are placed on opposite sides of the patient in a ring-like structure known as the CT gantry, which surrounds the patient, who is positioned on the CT table located in the center of the gantry. The gantry rotates around the patient, producing a series of projections that are mathematically reconstructed by a computer to form the CT image.

INCREMENTAL AND CONTINUOUS VOLUME (SPIRAL) COMPUTED TOMOGRAPHY

Spiral (helical) volumetric CT was an important technical advance introduced in the early 1990s that allows continuous scanning while the patient is moved continuously through the CT gantry.[44] Current spiral CT scans of the chest are typically completed during a single breath-hold. The continuous nature of the data acquisition allows true volumetric scanning, increased spatial resolution in the longitudinal axis, and the production of high-quality multiplanar and 3D reformations without additional radiation exposure. Because spiral CT allows the entire chest to be scanned during a single breath-hold, it virtually eliminates artifacts caused by respiratory motion that otherwise degrade image quality.

Major developments were the introduction of faster rotational times (subsecond CT scans) and multiple detector arrays (multidetector CT).[45,46] Faster rotational times make it possible to increase the anatomic coverage for any given section thickness and result in a marked reduction in cardiac motion artifacts and improvement in the evaluation of the pulmonary and systemic vessels. The advantages of multidetector CT scanners include improved temporal resolution, improved spatial resolution in the z-axis, increased efficiency in x-ray tube use, and decreased image noise.

Multidetector CT scanners generate isotropic data sets (i.e., 3D voxels with nearly identical measurements along their individual x-, y-, and z-axes). The increased spatial resolution in the z-axis (cephalocaudad plane) results in considerable improvement in the multiplanar and 3D reconstructions.

Multiplanar image displays allow better appreciation of the spatial relationships of various structures than a series of individual cross-sectional images. Use of graphics-based software systems and volume-rendering techniques allows depictions of the luminal surface of the airways that resemble the images

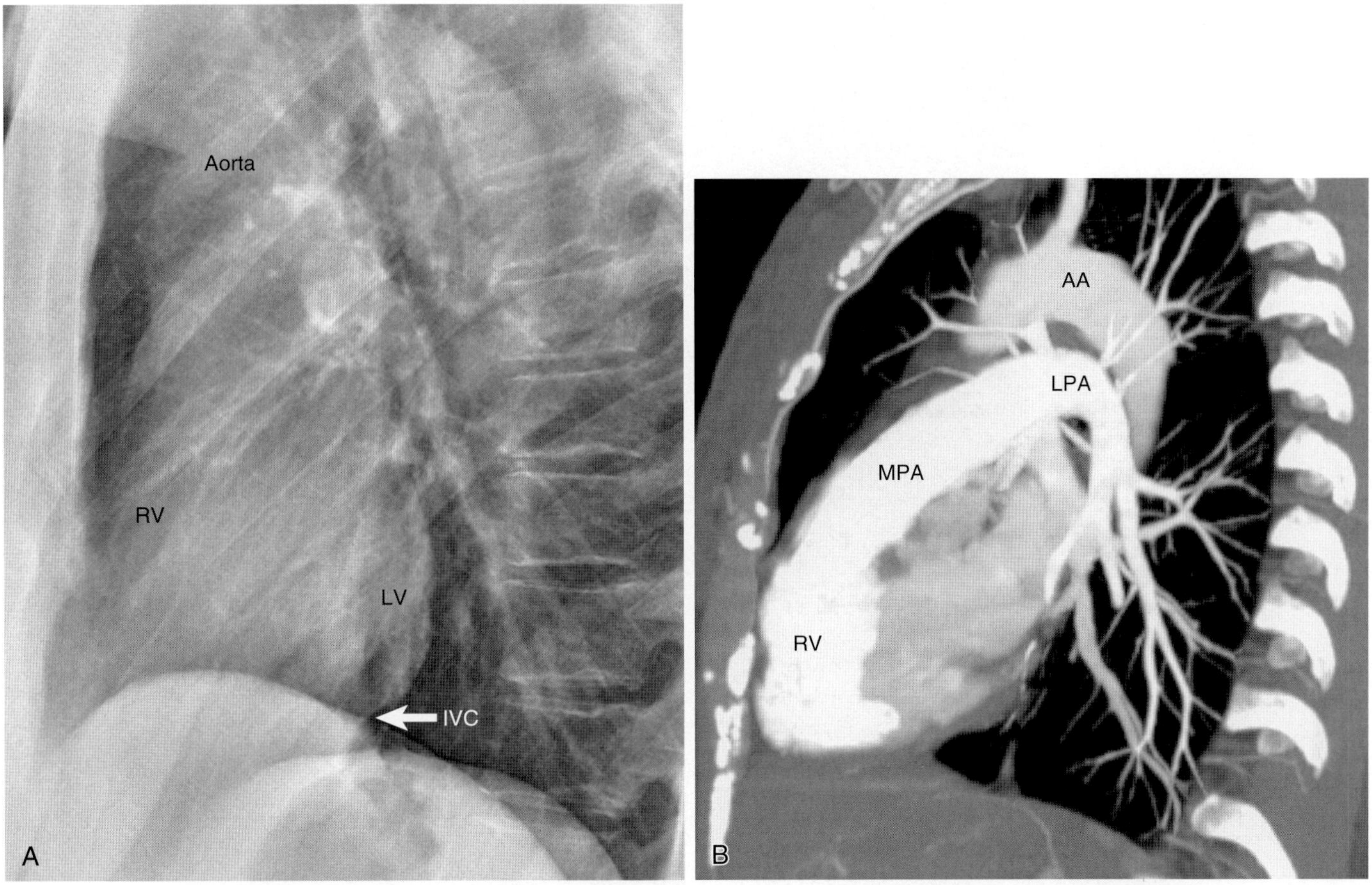

Fig. 1.33 (A) Normal cardiac anatomy on a lateral radiograph. A lateral radiograph shows the anterior border of the heart formed by the right ventricle *(RV)*, which contacts less than the lower half of the sternum. The lower two-thirds of the posterior heart border are formed by the left ventricle *(LV)* and the upper third by the left atrium. The faint opacity *(arrow)* seen in the posterior cardiophrenic angle represents the inferior vena cava *(IVC)* as it drains into the right atrium. The ascending aorta, aortic arch, and proximal descending aorta are well seen in this elderly patient. The aorta is not as well seen in normal young adults. (B) Sagittal reformatted CT image shows the *RV*, pulmonary outflow tract, and main pulmonary artery *(MPA)* forming the anterior contour of the heart. *AA*, Aortic arch; *LPA*, left pulmonary artery.

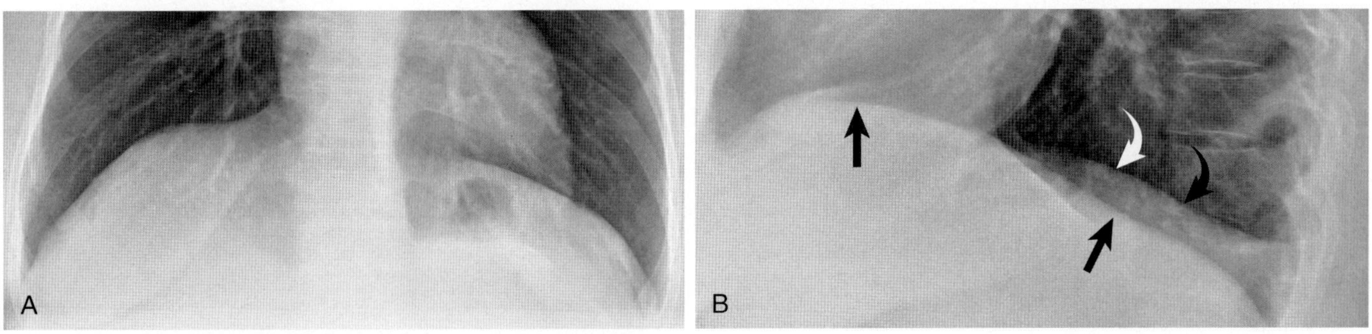

Fig. 1.34 Normal diaphragm. (A) Detail view from a frontal radiograph showing the upper surface of the dome-shaped right and left hemidiaphragms. The right hemidiaphragm is normally 1–3 cm above the level of the left hemidiaphragm. (B) Detail view from a lateral radiograph showing the entire length of the right hemidiaphragm *(straight arrows)*. The anterior portion of the left hemidiaphragm *(curved arrows)* is obscured by the heart.

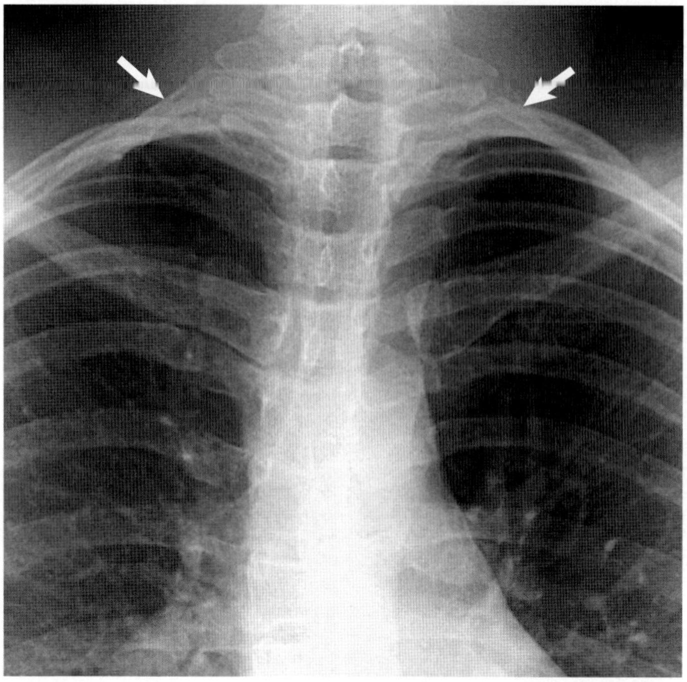

Fig. 1.35 Bilateral cervical ribs in a woman with thoracic outlet syndrome. A detail view from a frontal chest radiograph shows bilateral cervical ribs *(arrows)* arising from the seventh cervical vertebral body.

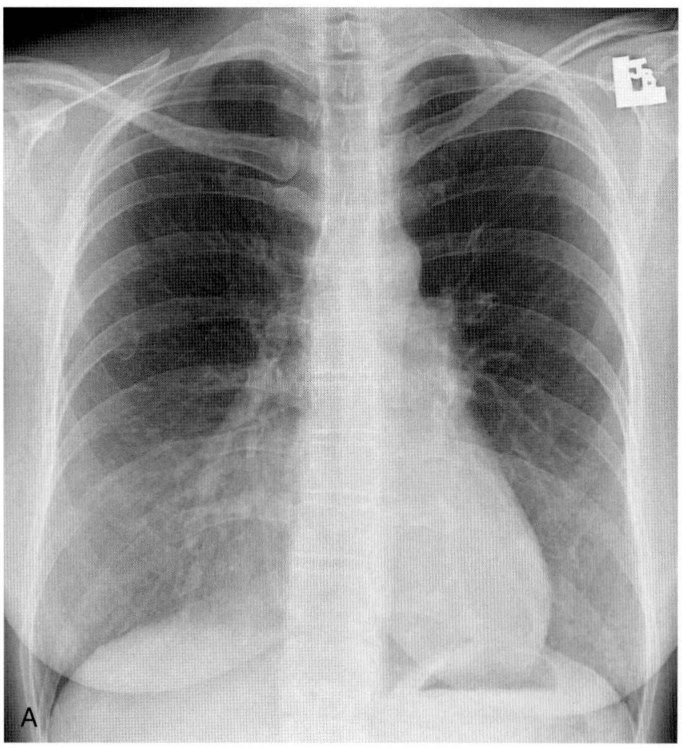

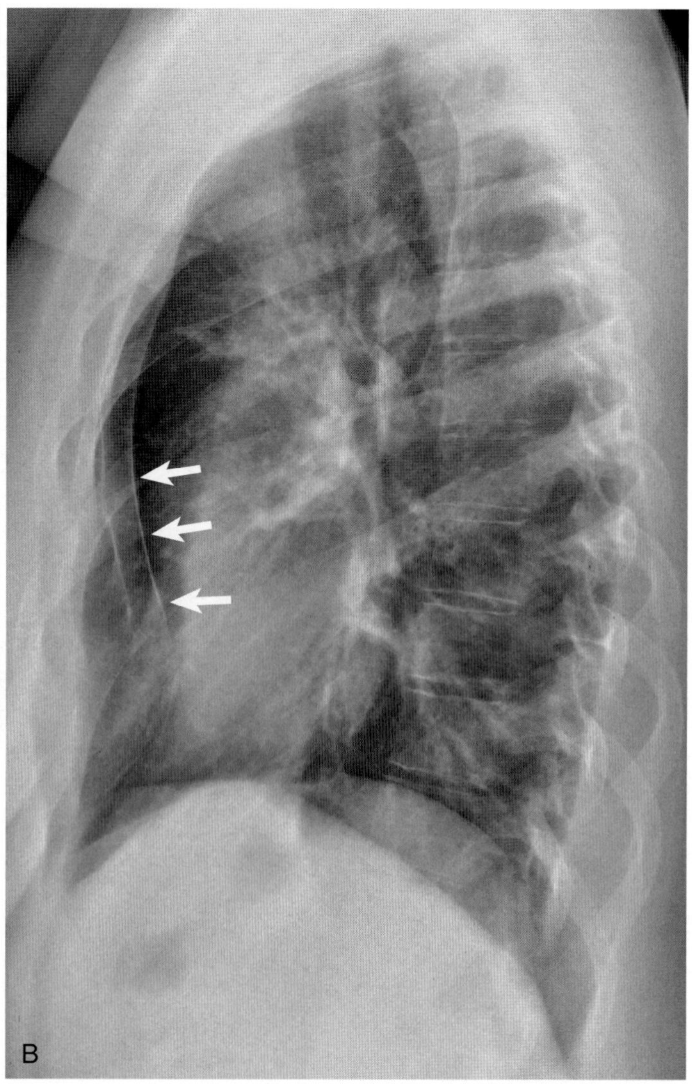

Fig. 1.36 Pectus excavatum. (A) Posteroanterior chest radiograph demonstrating displacement of the heart to the left and obscuration of the right heart border. (B) Lateral chest radiograph showing abnormal depression of the sternum *(arrows)* known as pectus excavatum, or "funnel chest."

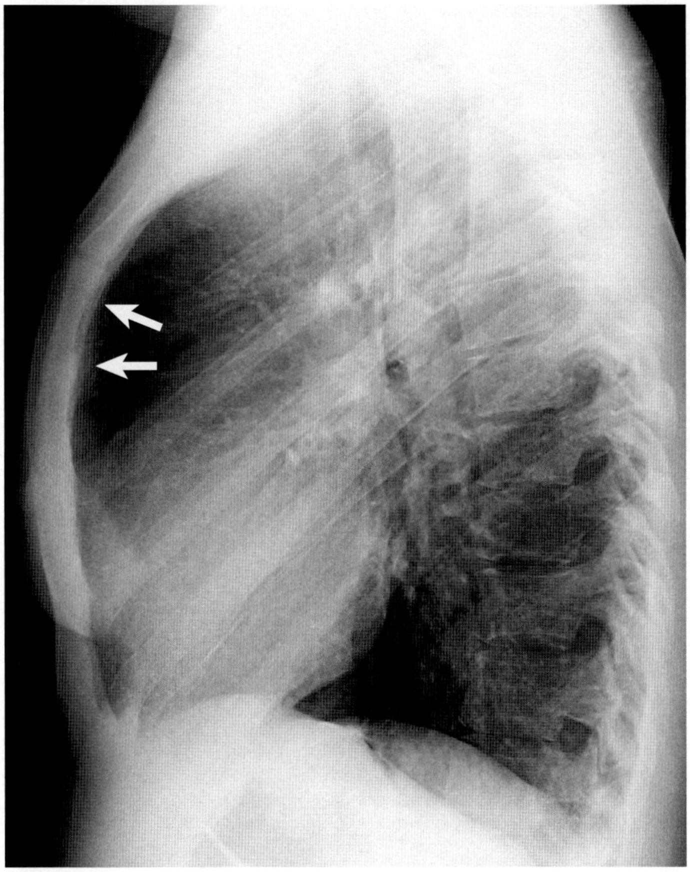

Fig. 1.37 Pectus carinatum. A lateral chest radiograph shows abnormal protrusion of the sternum *(arrows)* known as pectus carinatum, or "pigeon breast."

seen by bronchography or during bronchoscopy (Figs. 1.38 and 1.39).

Several techniques have been used to depict the entire volume of data. A technique that is particularly helpful in CT angiography and in the detection of lung nodules is maximum-intensity projection (MIP) (Fig. 1.40).[47] MIP images display the structures of interest that are brighter than the adjacent structures in any given stack (slab) of preselected axial images. The resolution inherent to the axial images from which it is created is maintained. The major pitfall with MIP slabs is that only the highest density object contributes to the final image.[47] Hypodense structures are hidden inside hyperdense structures, therefore limiting the efficacy of MIP images in diagnosing pulmonary embolism. Thicker slabs (3–10 mm) are most helpful in the assessment of pulmonary nodules (Fig. 1.41). A related technique is minimum-intensity projection, which highlights the structures with minimal density within a given slab of axial images. Sliding minimum-intensity projection with 5 to 10 mm thick slab images improves conspicuity of small areas of hypoattenuation and is particularly helpful in detecting mild emphysema (Fig. 1.42).[48]

Volume rendering uses all of the data from the multidetector CT acquisition in the final image (Fig. 1.43). It is a truly 3D reconstruction that conveys depth perception. All voxels contained within the reconstructed volume are included in the display, and voxels outside the boundaries of the reconstruction are invisible on the final image. Current workstations allow volume rendering to be performed routinely in real time and in concert with multiplanar reformatting images and MIP slabs. Volume rendering is most helpful in assessing changes in vascular morphology (e.g., strictures) and in clarifying complex 3D anatomic relationships.[49]

IMAGING PARAMETERS

Several operator-dependent parameters influence the information provided by chest CT. The main ones are slice thickness, field of view, reconstruction algorithm, and image display settings (window width and level). In selected cases intravenous (IV) contrast medium may be used to distinguish vessels from soft tissue lesions or to detect intravascular abnormalities, such as pulmonary emboli.

The attenuation value of each picture element (pixel) of the CT image represents the average of all the attenuation values within the unit volume of tissue, or voxel, which corresponds to the area of the pixel multiplied by the section thickness. The section thickness determines the number of structures or tissues that are averaged to produce each pixel. Decrease in section thickness leads to decrease in volume averaging and increase in spatial resolution.

The optimal slice thickness is determined by the size of the structure being assessed and by the number of scans required to evaluate the patient. It has been well established that thin sections (≤2 mm) are required for adequate assessment of the pulmonary parenchyma and peripheral bronchi (Fig. 1.44).[50,51] Although thicker sections (e.g., 3–5 mm) provide adequate assessment of most mediastinal abnormalities, thin sections allow more detailed evaluation of the lung parenchyma and are now used almost routinely in chest imaging.

CT scans are routinely performed during suspended full inspiration, which provides optimal contrast between normal aerated lung parenchyma and abnormal soft tissue and minimizes transient atelectasis, a finding that may mimic or obscure parenchymal disease. In patients with obstructive lung disease additional scans may be obtained during or after forced expiration to detect airway abnormalities, such as tracheobronchomalacia, and to delineate areas of air-trapping (Fig. 1.45).

In most cases the scans are done with the patient supine. Scans with the patient prone occasionally are required to detect subtle parenchymal abnormalities in the dorsal lung regions that may be otherwise obscured by normal dependent density or atelectasis. Prone scans are most helpful in patients with suspected parenchymal disease and normal chest radiographs,[52] in patients with suspected asbestosis, and in patients with clinically suspected interstitial lung disease in whom the CT scan in the supine position shows only questionable abnormalities limited to the dependent lung regions (Fig. 1.46).

CT numbers in the thorax range from approximately −1000 Hounsfield units (HUs) for air in the trachea to approximately 700 HUs for dense bones. The display of the CT image on the monitor is determined by the window level and width and is limited to 256 shades of gray. No single window setting can display adequately all of the information available on a chest CT scan. To display the large number of attenuation values (HUs) within a limited number of shades of gray, a CT number is selected that corresponds to approximately the mean attenuation value of the tissue being examined. This center CT attenuation value is called the window level. The computer is instructed to assign one shade of gray to a certain number of CT attenuation values above and below the window level. The range of CT

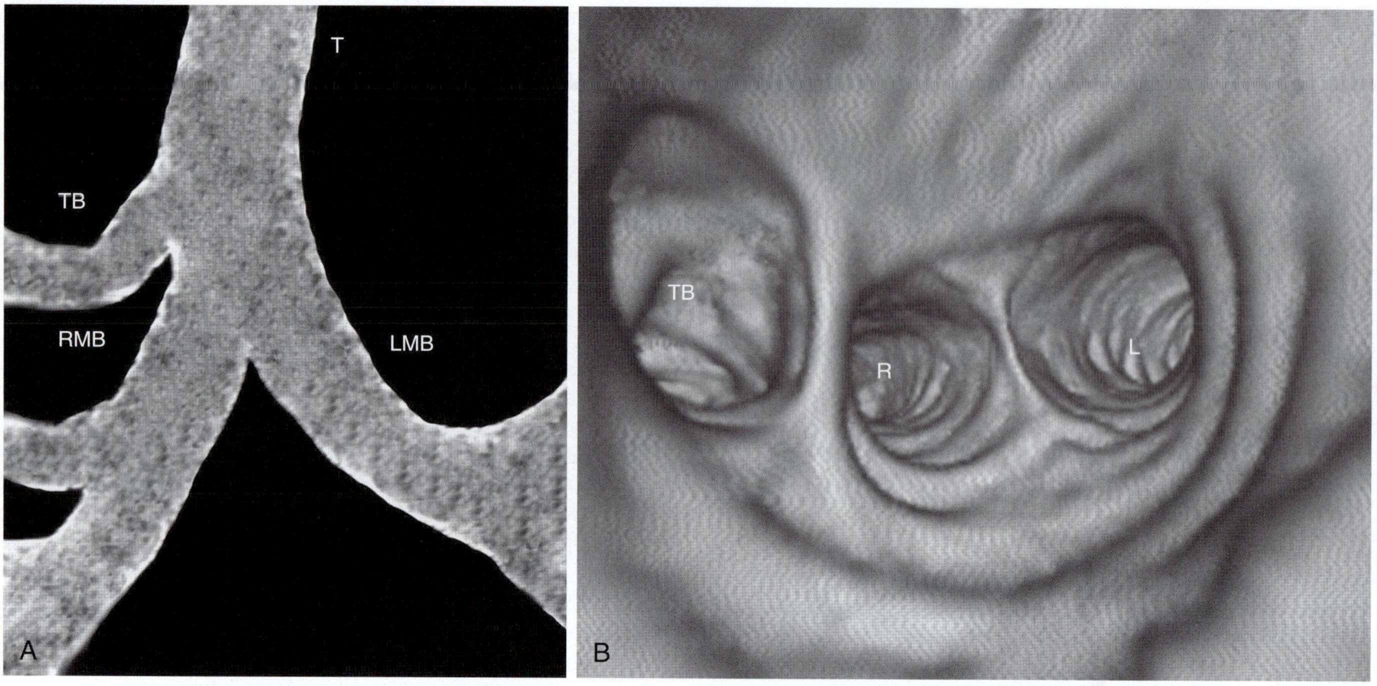

Fig. 1.38 Volume-rendering techniques (CT bronchography and CT bronchoscopy): tracheal bronchus. (A) Three-dimensional external volume-rendering reformation of airways viewed from an anterior perspective shows tracheal bronchus *(TB)* originating from the lower trachea *(T)*. Also noted are the right main bronchus *(RMB)* and left main bronchus *(LMB)*. The reformation resembles a bronchogram (CT bronchography). (B) CT reformation using volume-rendering technique shows view of the tracheal and bronchial lumina that resembles the view seen at bronchoscopy (CT bronchoscopy or virtual bronchoscopy). The image shows *TB*, right main *(R)* bronchus, and left main *(L)* bronchus as "seen" from the level of the lower trachea.

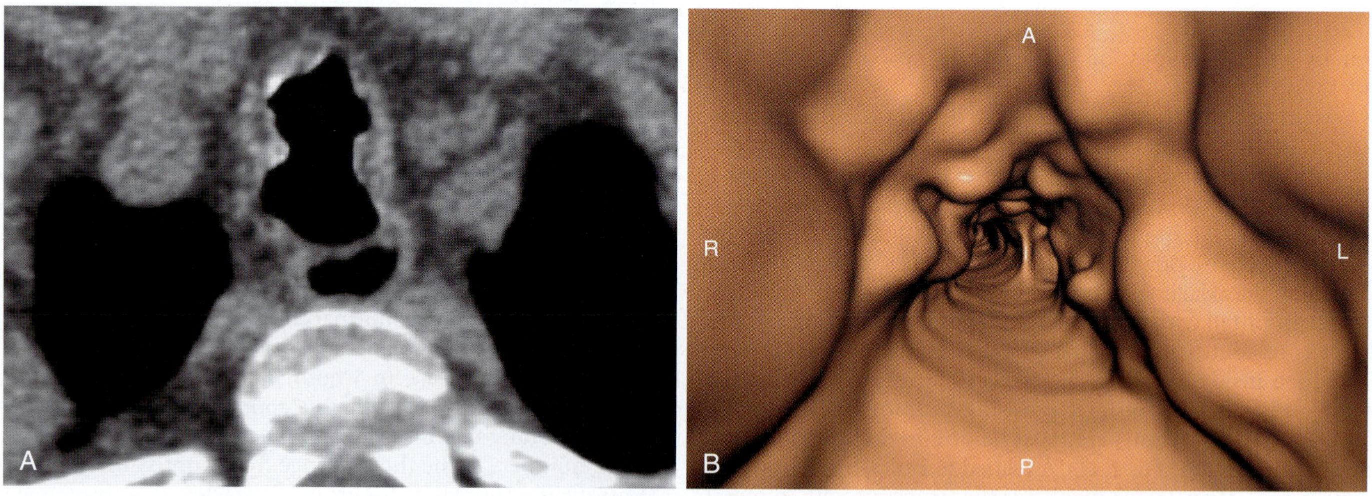

Fig. 1.39 Volume-rendering techniques (CT bronchoscopy): tracheobronchopathia osteochondroplastica. (A) Transverse magnified view of the upper trachea from a CT scan shows nodular protrusions arising from the anterior and lateral walls of the trachea and projecting into the tracheal lumen. (B) CT bronchoscopy better shows the diffuse nodularity that results in diffuse luminal narrowing. Note sparing of the posterior *(P)* tracheal wall. The findings are characteristic of tracheobronchopathia osteochondroplastica. *A*, Anterior; *L*, left; *R*, right.

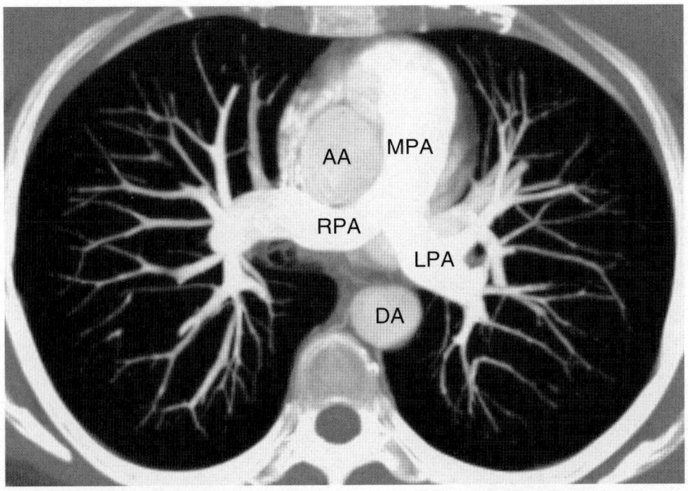

Fig. 1.40 Maximum-intensity projection (MIP) reconstruction. Axial MIP image better shows the branching pattern of the central pulmonary arteries and their relationship to the adjacent structures. *AA*, Ascending aorta; *DA*, descending aorta; *LPA*, left pulmonary artery; *MPA*, main pulmonary artery; *RPA*, right pulmonary artery.

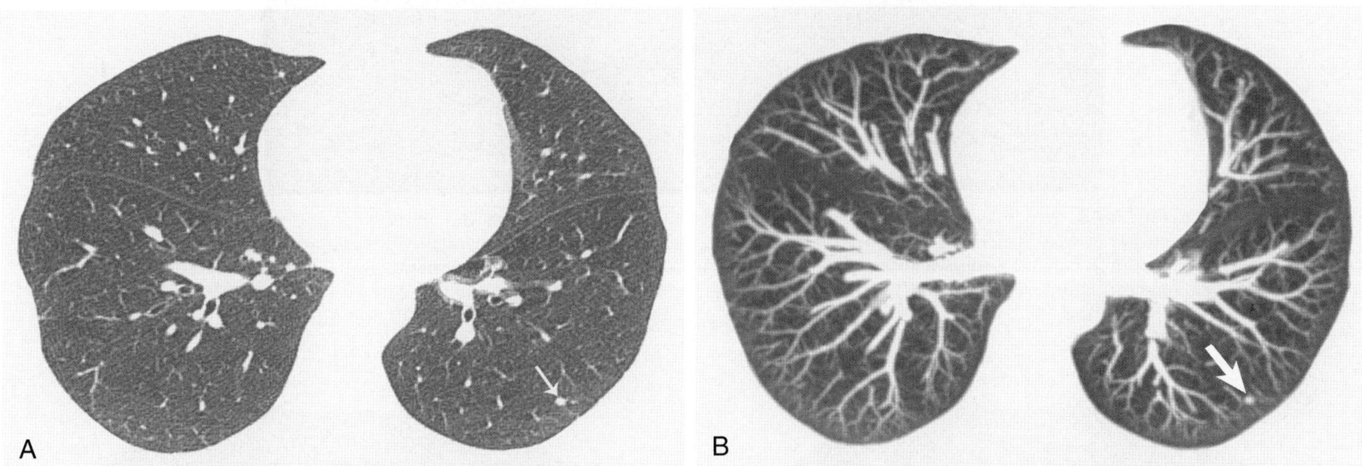

Fig. 1.41 Value of maximum-intensity projection (MIP) reconstruction in the detection of small lung nodule. (A) CT scan shows small subpleural nodule in the left lower lobe *(arrow)*. (B) MIP reconstruction of a 5-mm thick slab of lung at similar level allows easier distinction of the nodule *(arrow)* from the pulmonary vessels.

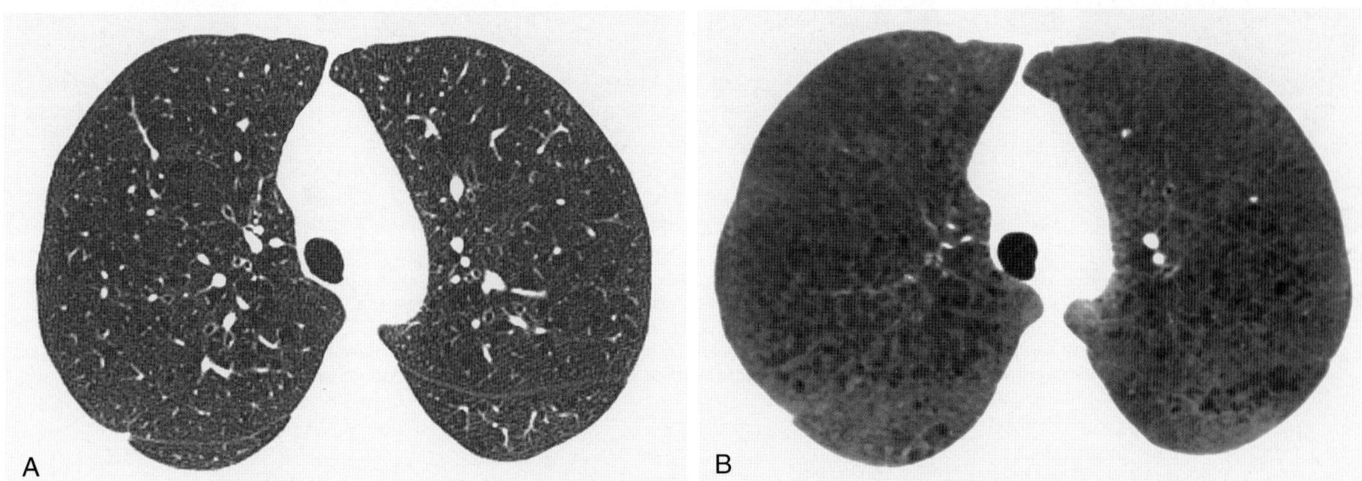

Fig. 1.42 Minimum-intensity projection reconstruction (MIP). (A) High-resolution CT (HRCT) at the level of the aortic arch shows mild emphysema in the upper lobes. The areas of emphysema are difficult to distinguish from normal lung. (B) MIP reconstruction of a 5-mm thick slab of lung shows numerous areas of abnormally low attenuation characteristic of emphysema. Even in retrospect, the extent of emphysema is underestimated on the HRCT image.

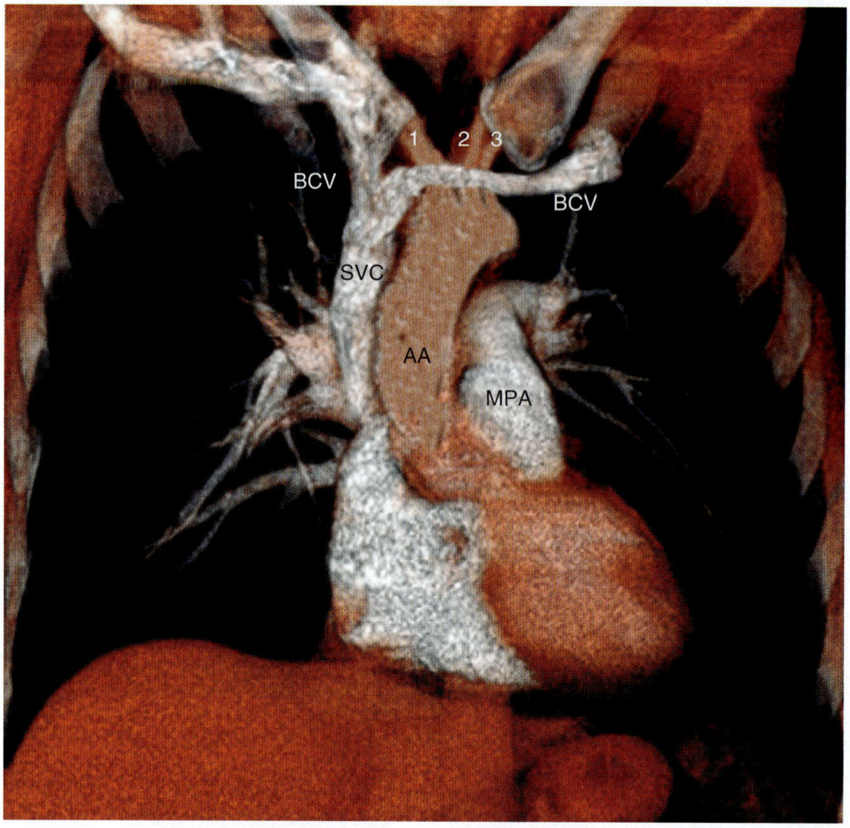

Fig. 1.43 Volume-rendering three-dimensional (3D) imaging. Coronal 3D volume-rendering image shows normal structures of the mediastinum and thoracic inlet. *1,* Right brachiocephalic artery; *2,* left common carotid artery; *3,* left subclavian artery; *AA,* ascending aorta; *BCV,* brachiocephalic vein; *MPA,* main pulmonary artery; *SVC,* superior vena cava.

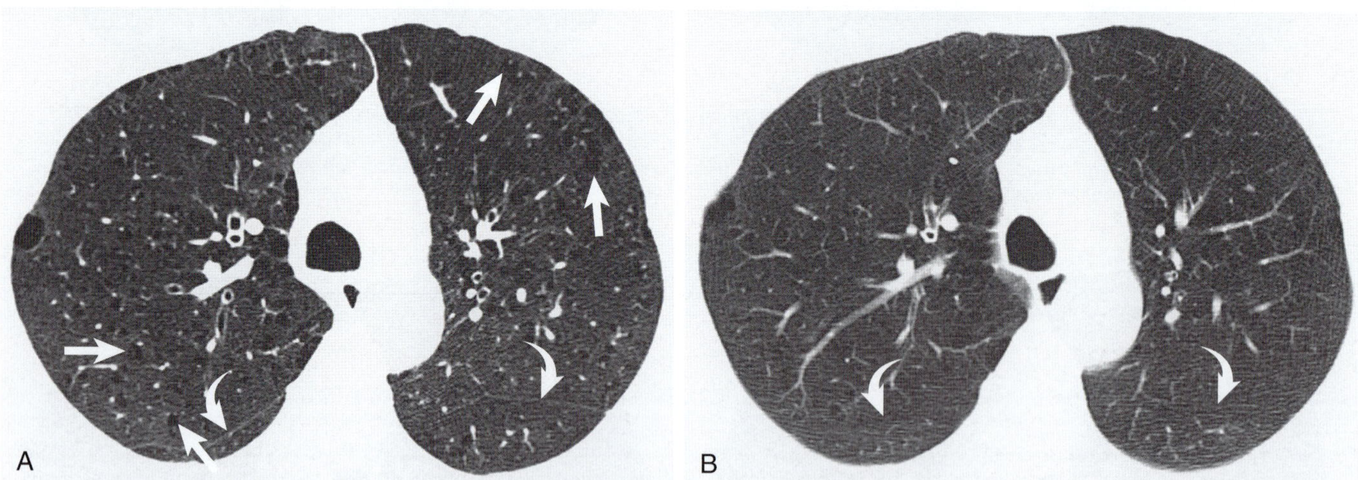

Fig. 1.44 Thin-section versus thick-section CT. (A) Thin-section (1 mm) CT scan shows numerous focal areas of decreased attenuation *(straight arrows)* characteristic of emphysema. The interlobar fissures are seen as sharply defined lines *(curved arrows).* (B) Thick-section (5 mm) CT scan does not allow adequate assessment of the small focal areas of emphysema. The interlobar fissures at this level are poorly seen as broad bands of slightly increased or decreased attenuation *(curved arrows).*

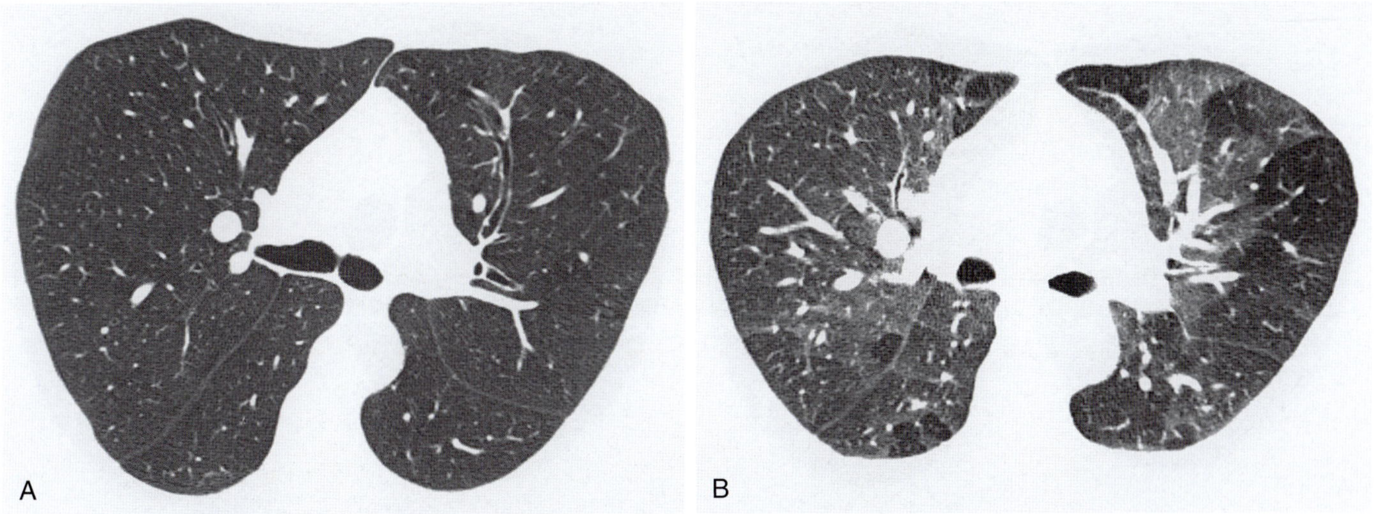

Fig. 1.45 Inspiratory and expiratory CT. (A) Low-dose high-resolution CT scan performed at full inspiration shows subtle areas of decreased attenuation and vascularity. (B) Low-dose CT scan performed after maximal expiration shows extensive bilateral air-trapping.

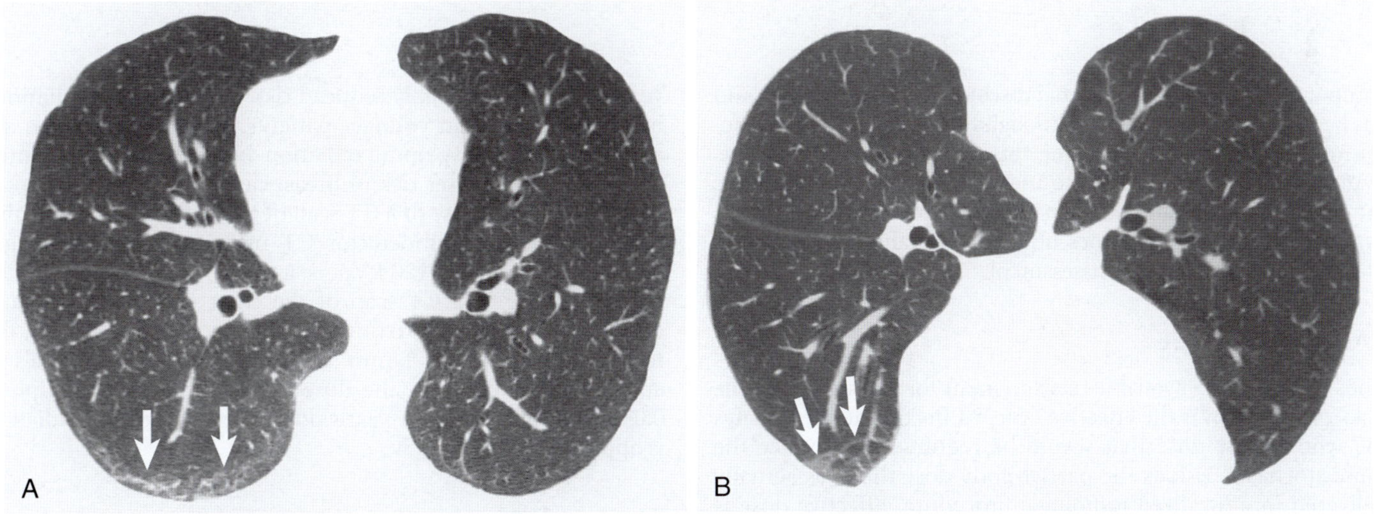

Fig. 1.46 Value of prone CT in patients with dependent opacity in the supine position. (A) High-resolution CT (HRCT) with the patient supine shows focal linear and ground-glass opacities *(arrows)* in the dorsal regions of the right lower lobe. (B) HRCT at the same level with the patient prone shows resolution of the opacity in the dorsal regions of the lower lobe and development of focal opacities *(arrows)* in dependent regions of the right middle lobe. The distribution of the findings and their resolution with change in position are characteristic of dependent atelectasis.

numbers above and below the window level is called the window width. To depict the lungs adequately, a window level of −600 to −700 HUs and a window width of 1000 to 1500 HUs are recommended. Window levels of 30 to 50 HUs and window widths of 350 to 500 HUs usually provide the best assessment of the mediastinum, hila, and pleura, as a general although not absolute guideline of values.

HIGH-RESOLUTION COMPUTED TOMOGRAPHY

The distinction between a "normal CT' scan and high-resolution CT (HRCT) scan continues to blur as CT technology advances and lung imaging protocols have evolved to maximize the available technology. CT scan data are routinely reconstructed using a standard or soft tissue algorithm, which smoothens the image and reduces visible image noise; such an algorithm is preferred in the assessment of abnormalities of the mediastinum and chest wall. Use of a high spatial–frequency reconstruction algorithm is required for optimal assessment of the lung parenchyma.[53,54] This algorithm reduces image smoothing and increases spatial resolution, allowing better depiction of normal and abnormal parenchymal interfaces and better visualization of small vessels, airways, and subtle interstitial abnormalities (Fig. 1.47). The combination of thin-section CT scan (0.5–1 mm collimation) and a high spatial–frequency reconstruction algorithm provides the optimal assessment of interstitial and airspace lung disease,

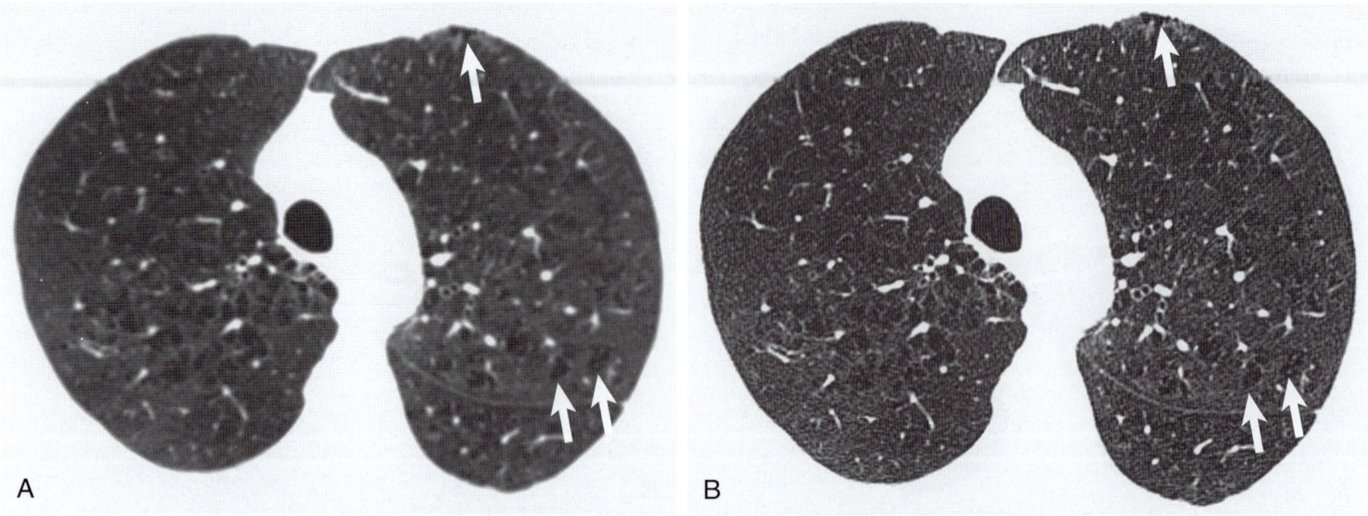

Fig. 1.47 Standard and high-resolution reconstruction algorithms. (A) CT image reconstructed using a standard or soft tissue algorithm shows poor definition of the pulmonary vessels and of the interface between focal areas of emphysema *(arrows)* and normal lung parenchyma. (B) CT image from the same data set but reconstructed using a high-resolution, edge-enhancing algorithm shows sharp definition of the pulmonary vessels and sharp demarcation between areas of emphysema *(arrows)* and normal lung.

comparable to that of gross (macroscopic) lung pathology, and has been referred to as HRCT, although now standard reconstruction of any chest CT scan using this methodology is possible. Typically, HRCT protocols also include images obtained while the patient is prone and also during end expiration. IV contrast is not administered as it does not add any value in the setting of interstitial lung disease assessment.

RADIATION DOSE

The best currently available measurement for assessment of the risks of radiation is the effective dose.[55] Effective dose estimates the whole-body dose that would be required to produce the same stochastic risk as the partial-body dose that was actually delivered in a localized radiologic procedure. Effective dose is useful because it allows comparison with other types of radiation exposure, such as whole-body radiation exposure secondary to natural background radiation. Effective dose is calculated by summing the absorbed doses to individual organs weighted for their radiation sensitivity. The measurement unit is the sievert (Sv). When the effective dose has been calculated, risk estimates for stochastic effects can be produced by using a linear extrapolation of radiation exposure data from Japanese atomic bomb survivors.

The main risk of radiation used in diagnostic x-rays, including CT, is the development of fatal cancers. The International Commission on Radiological Protection has recommended the use of a conservative risk of 50 additional fatal cancers induced per 1 million people of the general population exposed to 1 millisievert (mSv) of medical radiation.[55] Although this is the average risk, there is a pronounced age effect on the risk of cancer from ionizing radiation. Children may be an order of magnitude more sensitive than adults to the risk of cancer induction from the same effective dose of ionizing radiation as they have more time to express the cancer, and they have more rapidly dividing cells than adults have.[56,57] For the same reason, adults older than 50 years have a considerably reduced risk of developing radiation-induced cancer than younger patients. At all ages, women are at higher risk of developing radiation-induced cancer than men because of the greater risk of breast cancer.[58]

The radiation dose of a CT scan of the chest performed volumetrically using multidetector CT using 300 milliamperage-seconds (mAs) and 120 kVp is approximately 7 mSv.[58] The radiation dose of a CT scan of the chest performed for lung cancer screening is approximately 1.5 mSv. By comparison, the radiation dose using 1-mm sections at 10-mm intervals is approximately 0.7 mSv, the dose of a PA chest radiograph is 0.05 mSv, and the average yearly dose from background radiation is approximately 2.5 mSv.[58]

Normal Anatomy

AIRWAYS

Trachea and Main Bronchi

The tracheal wall is typically seen as a 1- to 2-mm soft tissue stripe on CT (Fig. 1.48). Cartilage calcification is commonly seen in older subjects, particularly women. Cartilage calcification may also occur prematurely in patients undergoing prophylactic warfarin therapy for anticoagulation. The cross-sectional appearance of the trachea varies but is most commonly rounded or oval. The posterior tracheal wall is typically flat or convex posteriorly on CT scans performed at maximal inspiration and convex anteriorly on expiratory CT (Fig. 1.49). The upper limits of normal for the transverse (coronal) and AP (sagittal) diameters of the trachea in men are 25 and 27 mm, respectively, and in women are 21 and 23 mm, respectively.[59] The lower limit of normal for both dimensions is 13 mm in men and 10 mm in women. Because of the increase in the intrathoracic pressure, the diameter of the intrathoracic trachea decreases during expiration. The decrease in the AP diameter is mainly due to invagination of the posterior tracheal membrane, a finding that is useful in confirming that an adequate expiration has occurred on expiratory CT.

The trachea divides into the left and right main bronchi at the carina (Fig. 1.50). For a short distance, the main bronchi contain horseshoe-shaped cartilage rings, similar to the trachea. More distally, the cartilage plates become less regularly shaped.

Lobar Bronchi and Bronchopulmonary Segments

The lobar bronchi give origin to segmental bronchi. Although the segmental bronchial anatomy varies, in most patients the right lung contains 10 segmental bronchi, and the left contains 8 (Fig. 1.51). There are two widely accepted nomenclatures for bronchopulmonary anatomy: the Jackson-Huber and Boyden classifications. The Jackson-Huber nomenclature is the most widely adopted terminology in North America and the one used throughout this book.[60,61] The Boyden classification uses a numerical system for identifying the bronchial segments. The segmental bronchi are designated by B, followed by a number (e.g., B1), and subsegmental bronchi are indicated by the segmental number, followed by a lowercase letter (e.g., B1a). The numbering of the segmental bronchi corresponds to their order of origin from the airway. The segments of lung that the bronchi supply are identified by the letter "S," followed by the corresponding number.

The right upper lobe usually has three segments: apical (S1 in the Boyden classification), anterior (S3), and posterior (S2). The middle lobe has two segments: lateral (S4) and medial (S5). The right lower lobe has five segments: superior (S6), medial basal (S7), anterior basal (S8), lateral basal (S9), and posterior basal (S10) (see Fig. 1.16).

The left upper lobe usually has two segments: apicoposterior (S1 and S2) and anterior (S3). The lingula has two segments—superior (S4) and inferior (S5), and the left lower lobe has four—superior (S6), anteromedial basal (S7 and S8), lateral basal (S9), and posterior basal (S10).

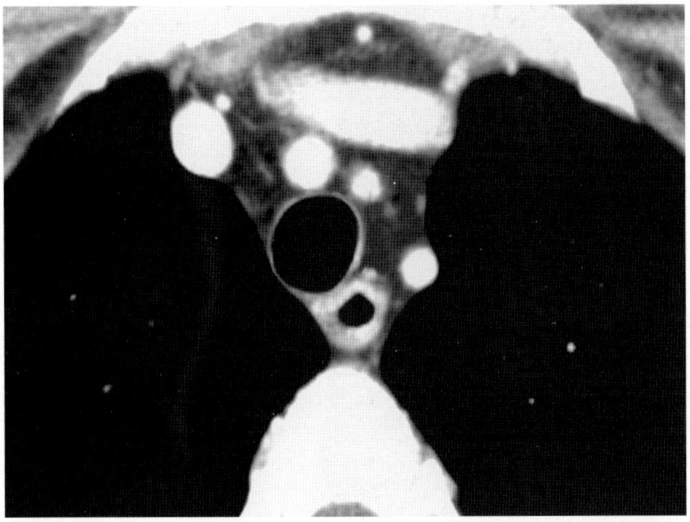

Fig. 1.48 Normal trachea. CT scan shows normal trachea. The tracheal wall is seen as a soft tissue stripe measuring 1–2 mm in thickness. The anterior and lateral walls are formed by horseshoe-shaped cartilaginous rings, which frequently calcify with age. The posterior wall consists of a fibromuscular noncartilagenous membrane.

NORMAL BRONCHI ON COMPUTED TOMOGRAPHY

The outer diameter of the bronchus is normally approximately equal to that of the adjacent pulmonary artery (Fig. 1.52). Bronchi may appear larger than the adjacent pulmonary artery if the artery bifurcates before the corresponding bronchus or if it is narrowed because of vasoconstriction. The measurement also is influenced by altitude, presumably as a result of a combination of hypoxic vasoconstriction and bronchodilation.[62]

The airways divide by asymmetric dichotomous branching, with approximately 23 generations of branches from the trachea to the alveoli. As they branch, the bronchi become smaller and have thinner walls. The wall thickness of the bronchi is approximately 10% to 15% of its diameter. Because their walls become progressively thinner, smaller bronchi are difficult to see. The smallest bronchi that can be seen on HRCT (≈1-mm slice thickness) are typically 1.5 to 2 mm in diameter (Fig. 1.53). In normal individuals no airways can be visualized within 1 cm of the costal or paravertebral pleura.

Text continued on p. 37

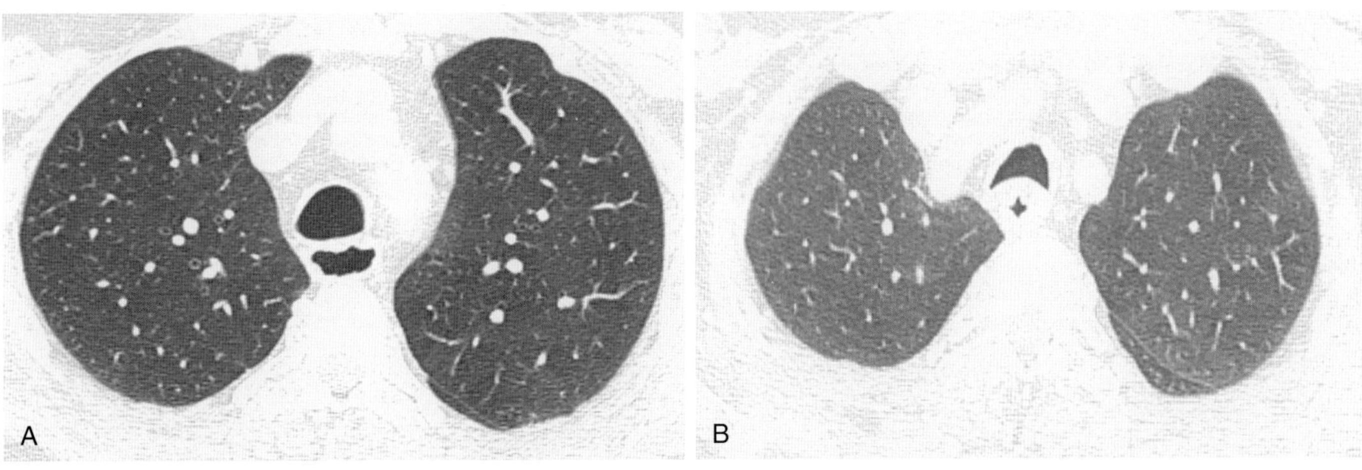

Fig. 1.49 Normal trachea on inspiration and expiration. (A) Inspiratory CT scan shows slight posterior convexity of the posterior tracheal wall. (B) Expiratory CT scan shows decreased diameter of the trachea and anterior convexity of the posterior tracheal wall. Also note normal increase in lung attenuation.

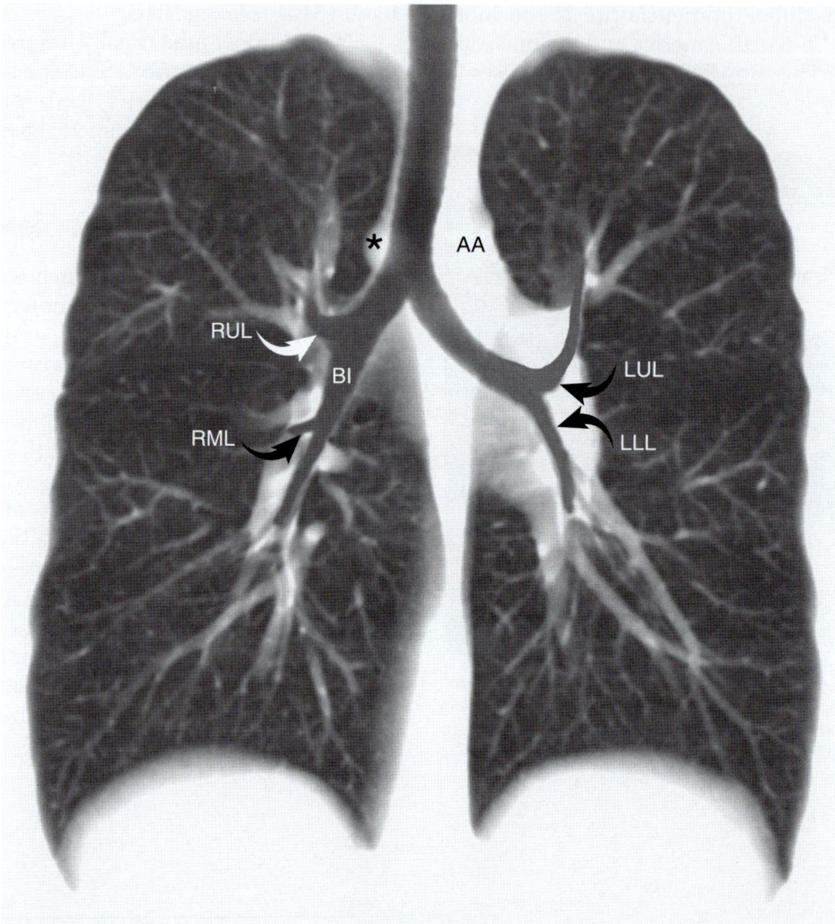

Fig. 1.50 Normal trachea, main and lobar bronchi. Coronal reformation from a CT scan shows trachea dividing into right and left main bronchi. Approximately 2 cm after its origin, the right main bronchus divides into right upper lobe *(RUL)* bronchus and bronchus intermedius *(BI)*. The left main bronchus measures approximately 5 cm in length and gives origin to the left upper *(LUL)* and lower lobe *(LLL)* bronchi. *Asterisk* indicates azygos vein. *AA,* Aortic arch; *RML,* right middle lobe bronchus.

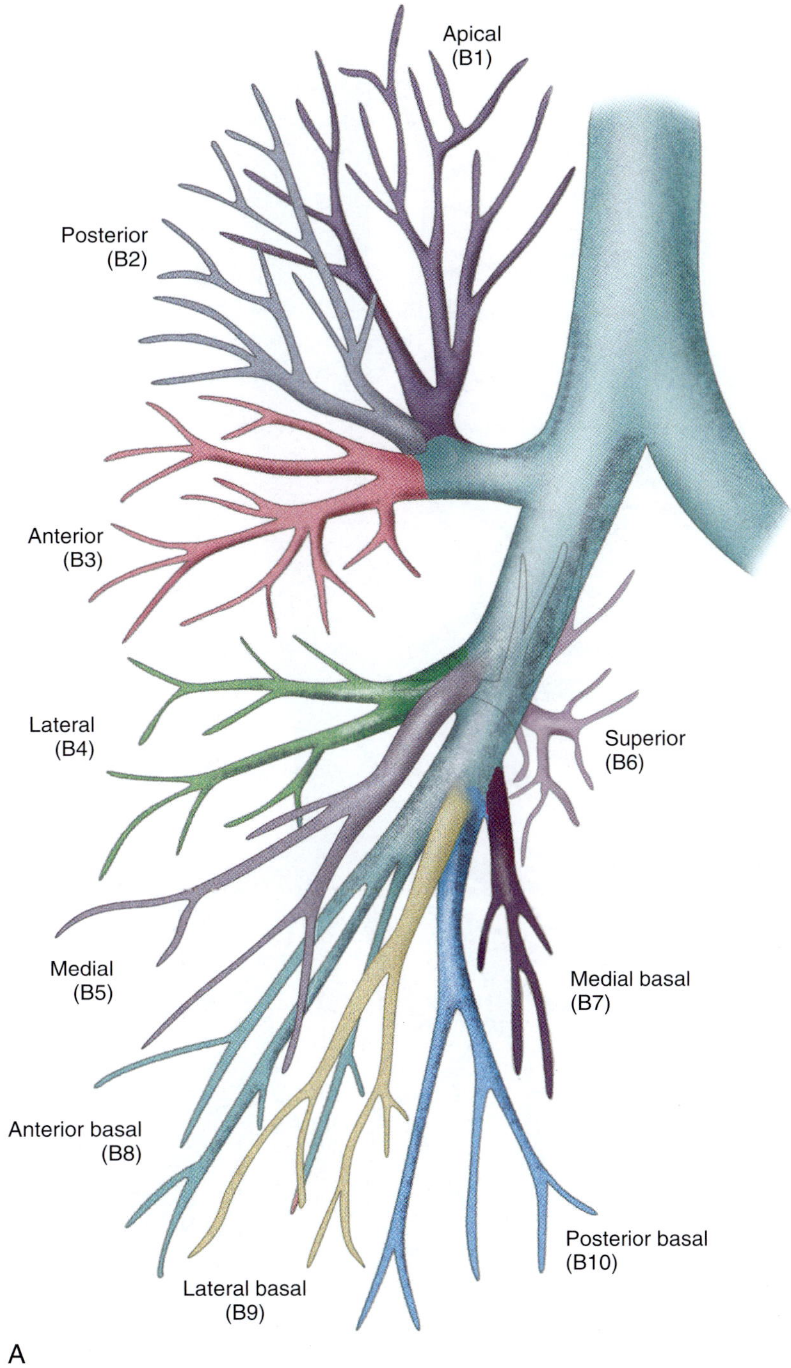

Fig. 1.51 Schematic drawings of the bronchial tree and pulmonary segments. (A) Right bronchial tree (frontal projection). Schematic drawing shows the normal location of the segments *(B1–B10)* of the right bronchial tree in frontal projection.

Continued

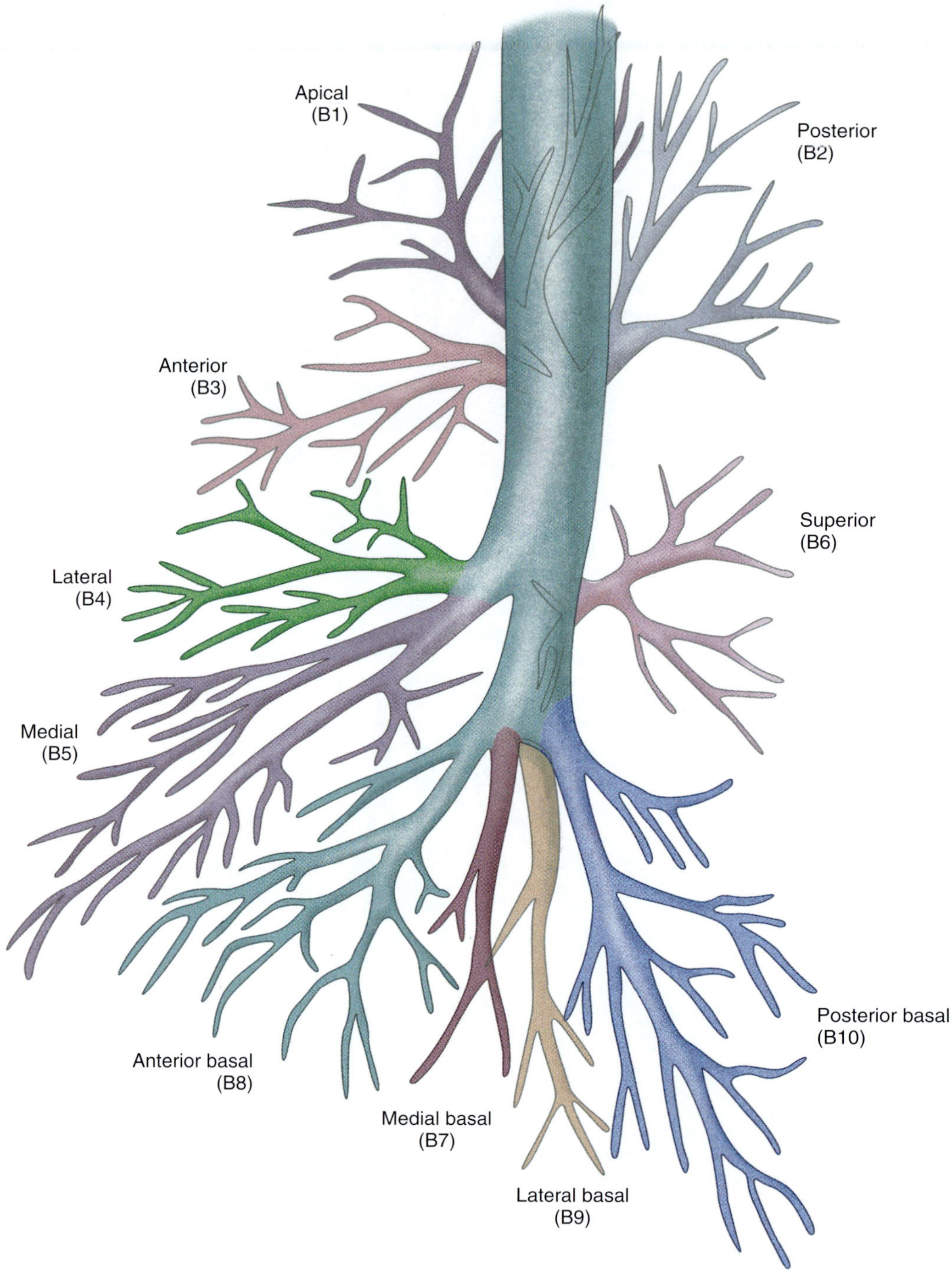

B

Fig. 1.51, cont'd (B) Right bronchial tree (lateral projection). Schematic drawing shows the normal location of the segments *(B1–B10)* of the right bronchial tree in lateral projection.

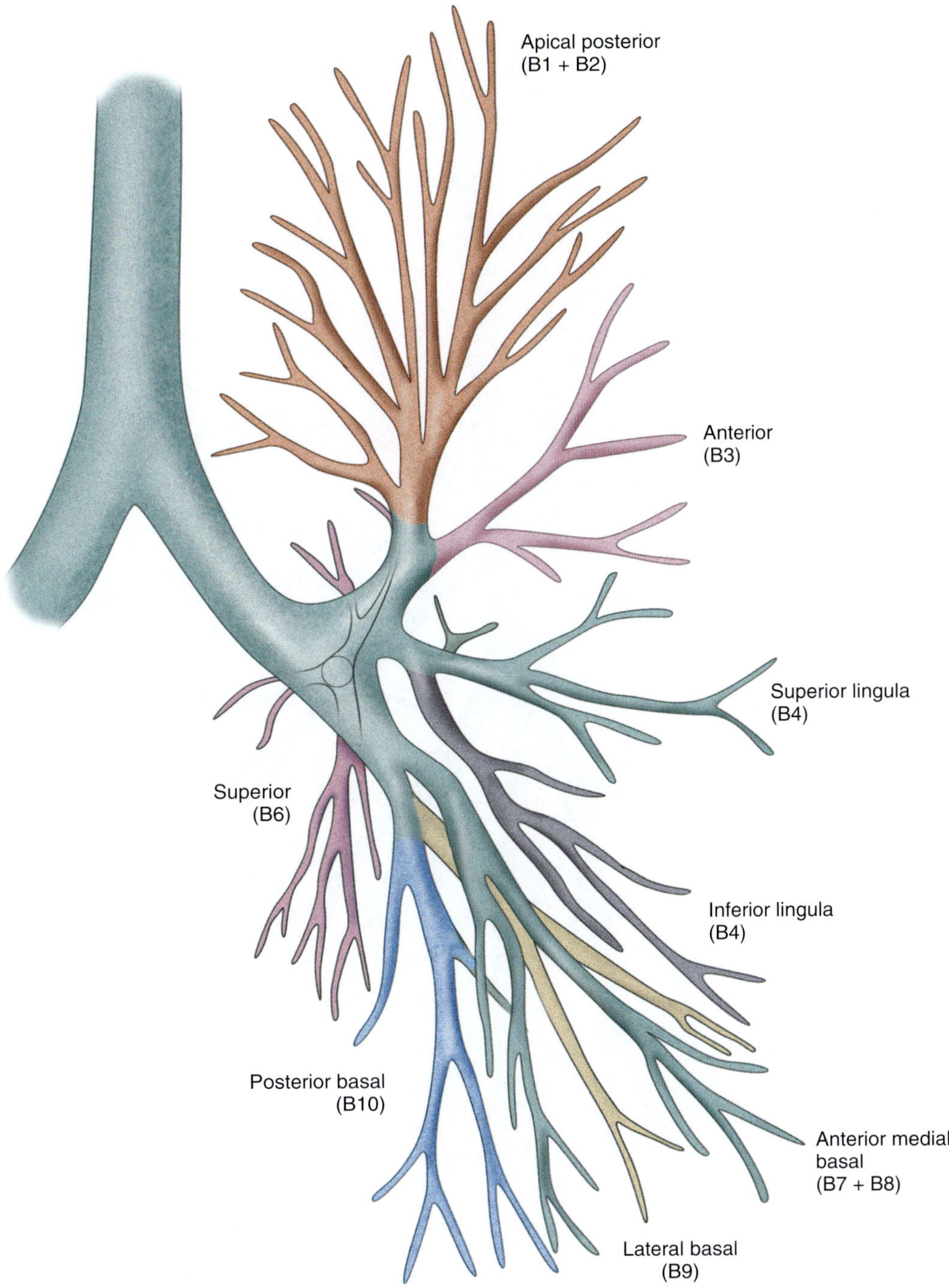

Fig. 1.51, cont'd (C) Left bronchial tree (frontal projection). Schematic drawing shows the normal location of the segments *(B1–B10)* of the left bronchial tree in frontal projection.

Continued

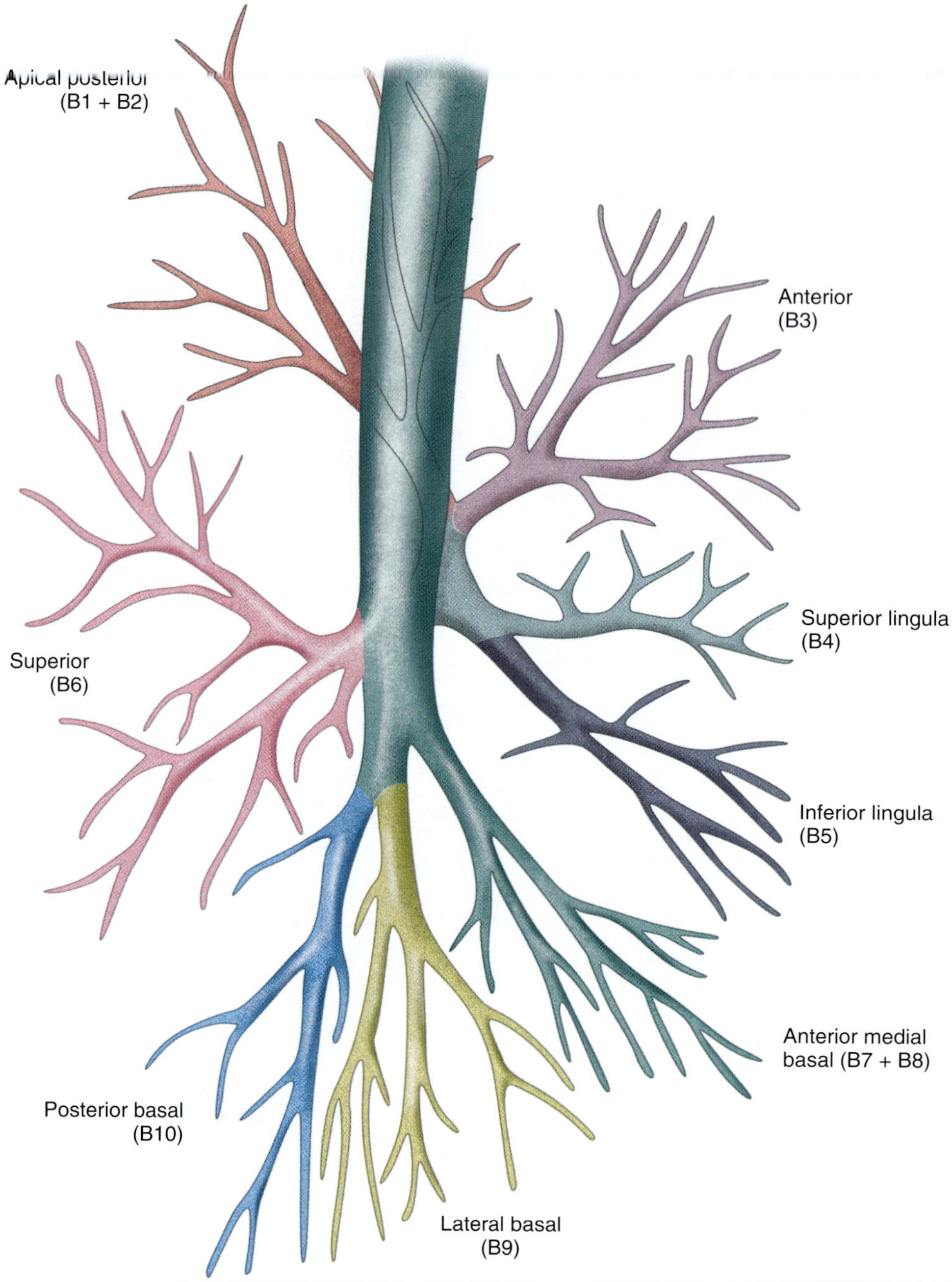

D

Fig. 1.51, cont'd (D) Left bronchial tree (lateral projection). Schematic drawing shows the normal location of the segments *(B1–B10)* of the left bronchial tree in lateral projection.

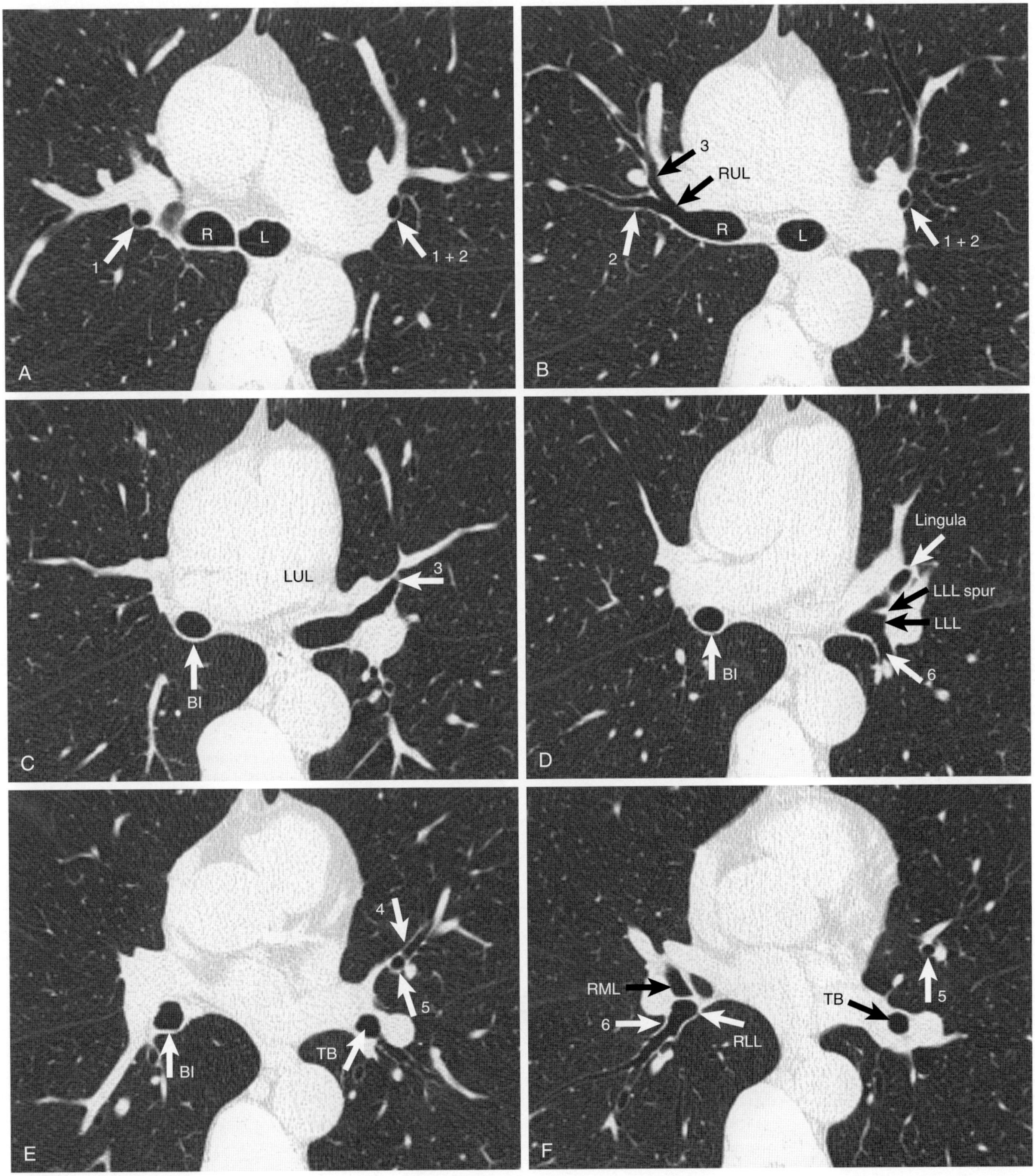

Fig. 1.52 Normal segmental anatomy on CT. (A) CT scan at the level of the proximal right *(R)* and left *(L)* main bronchi shows apical segmental bronchus (1) of right upper lobe and apicoposterior segmental bronchus *(1 + 2)* of left upper lobe. (B) CT scan at level of the right upper lobe bronchus *(RUL)* shows posterior *(2)* and anterior *(3)* segmental bronchi of right upper lobe and an apicoposterior segmental bronchus *(1 + 2)* of left upper lobe. (C) CT scan at level of the left upper lobe bronchus *(LUL)* shows anterior *(3)* segmental bronchus of left upper lobe and bronchus intermedius *(BI)*. (D) CT scan slightly caudal to (C) shows lingular bronchus (lingula), left lower lobe bronchus *(LLL)*, superior segmental bronchus *(6)* of left lower lobe, and bronchus intermedius *(BI)*. (E) CT scan slightly caudal to (D) shows bifurcation of lingular bronchus into the more horizontal superior lingular segmental bronchus *(4)* (seen along its long axis) and the more vertical oriented inferior lingular segmental bronchus *(5)* (seen in cross-section). The superior lingular segmental bronchus can be seen to be bifurcating into subsegmental bronchi shortly after its origin. Also visualized at this level are the left truncus basalis (left lower lobe bronchus distal to the takeoff of the superior segmental bronchus) *(TB)* and the bronchus intermedius *(BI)*. (F) CT scan slightly caudal to (E) shows right middle lobe *(RML)* and right lower lobe *(RLL)* bronchi, superior segmental bronchus *(6)* of right lower lobe, truncus basalis of left lower lobe *(TB)*, and inferior lingular segmental bronchus *(5)*.

Continued

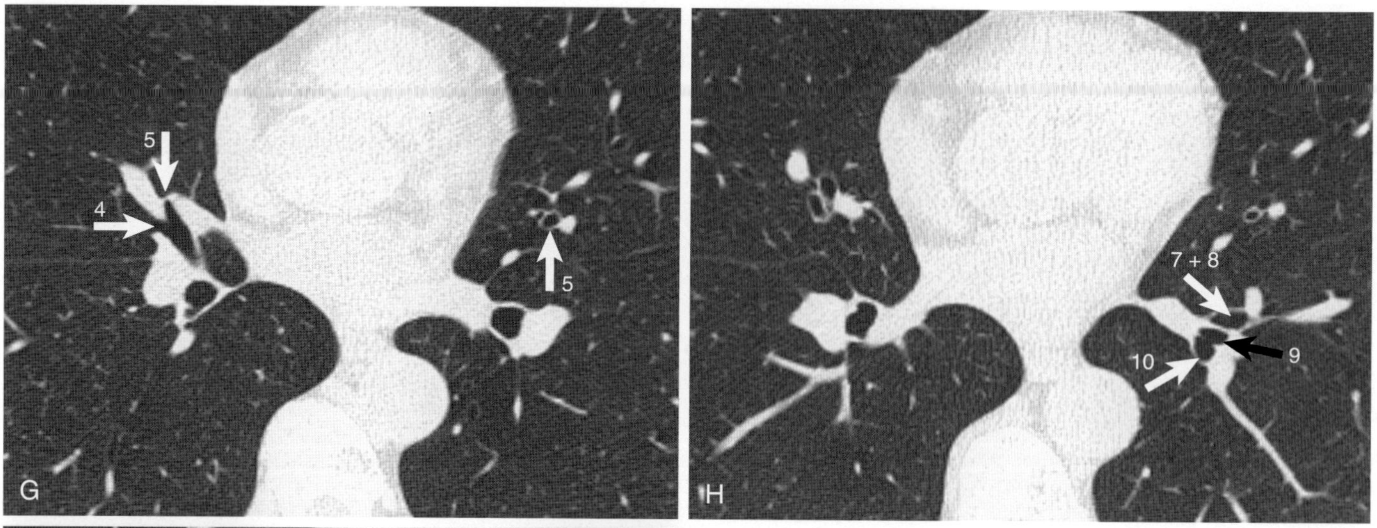

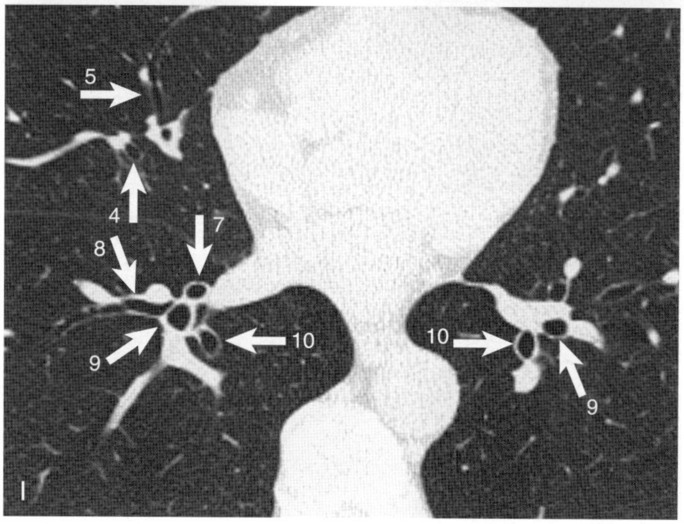

Fig. 1.52, cont'd (G) CT scan at bifurcation of right middle lobe bronchus shows lateral *(4)* and medial *(5)* segmental bronchi of right middle lobe, inferior lingular segmental bronchus *(arrow; 5)*, and truncus basalis of right and left lower lobe. (H) CT scan at the level of the inferior pulmonary veins shows anteromedial *(7 + 8)*, lateral *(9)*, and posterior *(10)* basal segmental bronchi of left lower lobe. (I) CT scan slightly caudal to (H) shows medial *(7)*, anterior *(8)*, lateral *(9)*, and posterior *(10)* basal segmental bronchi of right lower lobe; lateral *(4)* and medial *(5)* segmental bronchi of right middle lobe; and lateral *(9)* and posterior *(10)* segmental bronchi of left lower lobe.

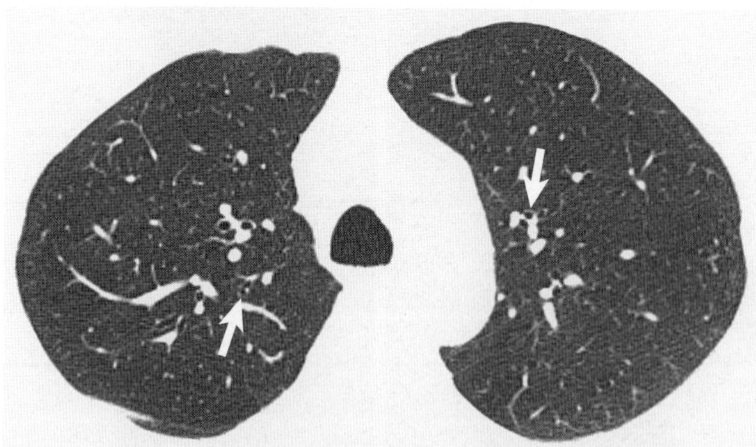

Fig. 1.53 Normal bronchi on high-resolution CT (HRCT). HRCT scan at the level of the upper lobes shows several small bronchi *(arrows)*. The smallest bronchi that can be identified measure 1.5–2 mm in diameter. No bronchi are normally seen within 1 cm of the costal pleura or abutting the mediastinum.

BRONCHIOLES

Bronchioles are airways whose walls lack cartilage. They are classified into membranous bronchioles, which do not contain alveoli, and respiratory bronchioles, which are lined partly by alveoli. The membranous bronchiole immediately proximal to a respiratory bronchiole is called the terminal bronchiole. Approximately two to three additional generations of respiratory bronchioles are present after the most proximal branch. Terminal bronchioles measure about 0.6 mm in diameter, and distal respiratory bronchioles measure about 0.4 mm.[63] Because their walls are less than 0.1 mm thick, normal bronchioles cannot be visualized on CT.

PULMONARY ARTERIAL AND VENOUS CIRCULATION

Pulmonary Arteries

The pulmonary trunk or main pulmonary artery originates in the mediastinum at the pulmonary valve and extends cranially before bifurcating within the pericardium (Fig. 1.54). The normal diameter of the main pulmonary artery varies depending on the

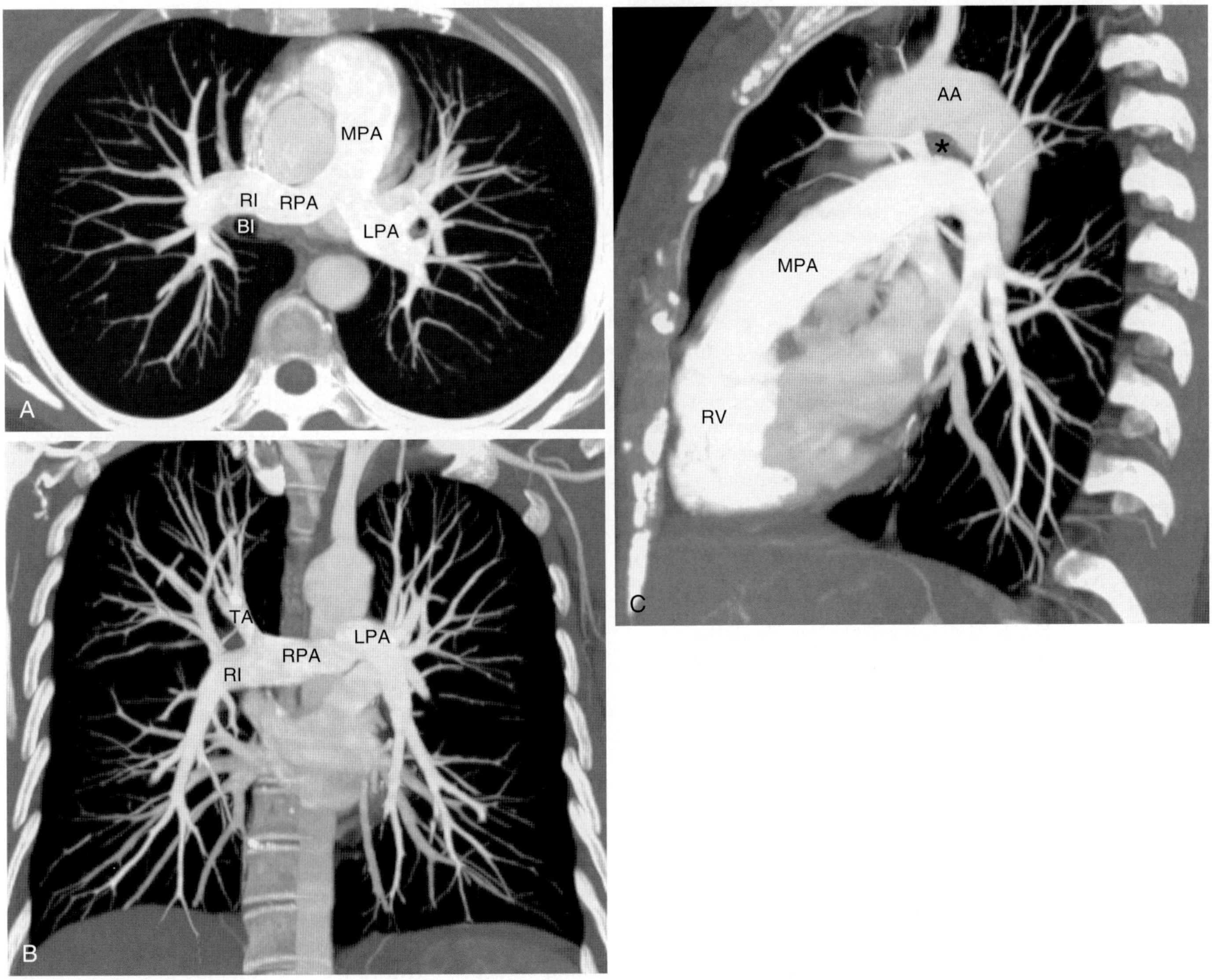

Fig. 1.54 Normal anatomy of the central pulmonary arteries. (A) Maximum-intensity projection (MIP) reconstruction CT image shows that the main pulmonary artery *(MPA)* courses posteriorly and branches into the right *(RPA)* and left *(LPA)* pulmonary arteries. The right pulmonary artery branches shortly after its origin into the truncus anterior, which courses cephalad to supply most of the right upper lobe, and a larger right interlobar pulmonary artery *(RI)* that courses just anterior and then lateral to the bronchus intermedius *(BI)*. (B) MIP image in the coronal plane shows the orientation of the *RPA* and *LPA* in the same projection as the frontal radiograph. The right pulmonary artery and the central portion of the left pulmonary artery are in the mediastinum and cannot be identified on the chest radiograph. The right pulmonary artery branches into the truncus anterior *(TA)* and *RI*. (C) MIP image in the sagittal plane shows the orientation of the right and left pulmonary arteries that correspond to the lateral chest radiograph. The *MPA* originates from the right ventricle *(RV)* and courses cephalad and posteriorly. *Asterisk* indicates aorticopulmonary window. *AA,* Aortic arch.

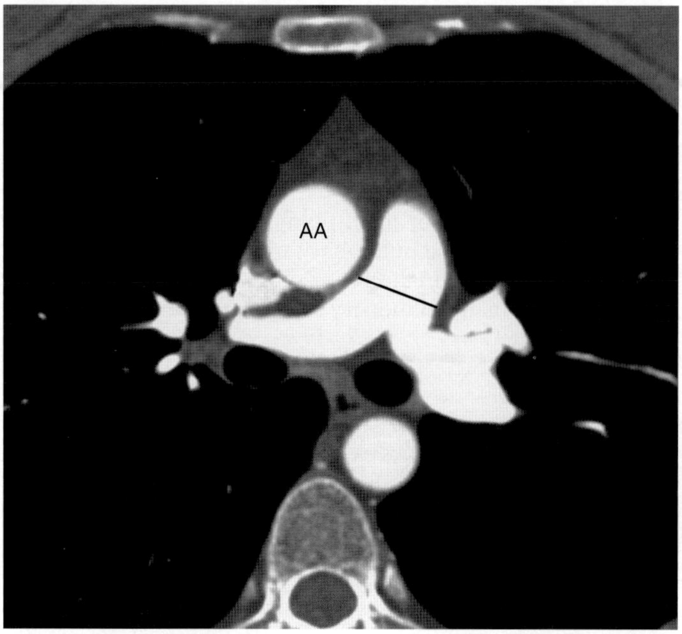

Fig. 1.55 Normal diameter of main pulmonary artery. The normal diameter of the main pulmonary artery, measured at the level of its bifurcation *(black line)*, is less than 32.5 mm and smaller than the ascending aorta *(AA)* at the same level.

study cited but is usually less than or equal to 32.5 mm and slightly smaller than the ascending aorta at the same level.[64–67] The measurement of the main pulmonary artery is best made at a right angle to the long axis of the main pulmonary artery at the level of its bifurcation (Fig. 1.55). There is no significant difference between measurements in men and women.

The left pulmonary artery continues in more or less the same line as the pulmonary trunk until it reaches the hilum, where it arches over the left main bronchus. Subsequently, the artery sometimes gives off a short ascending branch that divides into segmental branches to the upper lobe; more commonly, it continues directly into the vertically oriented left interlobar artery, from which the segmental arteries to the upper and lower lobes arise directly. The left interlobar artery lies posterolateral to the upper lobe bronchus.

The right pulmonary artery divides into the ascending (truncus anterior) and descending (interlobar) branches (see Fig. 1.54). Although variable, the common pattern is for the ascending artery to subdivide into the segmental branches that supply the right upper lobe and for the descending branch to contribute the segmental arteries to the middle and right lower lobes.

Although the course of the most proximal pulmonary arteries is fairly constant, the origin and branching pattern of lobar and segmental arteries show considerable variation. Despite this variation, the pulmonary arterial system invariably is related intimately to the airways and divides with them, a branch always accompanying the adjacent airway down to the level of the distal respiratory bronchioles. In addition to these conventional vessels, many supernumerary (accessory) branches of the pulmonary artery arise at points other than corresponding airway divisions and penetrate the lung parenchyma directly.

Pulmonary Veins

There are usually two main superior and two main inferior vessels, the former draining the middle and upper lobes on the right side and the upper lobe on the left and the latter draining the lower lobes. In a significant percentage of patients, the right middle lobe vein drains directly into the left atrium or into the confluence of right inferior pulmonary veins as they enter the left atrium (Fig. 1.56). The right-sided superior and inferior pulmonary veins course beneath the main pulmonary artery posterior to the SVC and enter the left atrium separately. The left-sided veins pass anterior to the descending aorta and enter the atrium separately as on the right or join within the pericardial cavity to enter the atrium as a common channel. As in the pulmonary arterial system, numerous supernumerary vessels join the veins as they course through the lung.

BRONCHIAL CIRCULATION

There is considerable variation in the number and origin of human bronchial arteries, with a relatively common pattern being one on the right (originating as a common intercostal–bronchial artery trunk, which is the first right intercostal artery that arises directly from the aorta) and two on the left, arising directly from the descending aorta.[19,68] The right and left bronchial arteries arise at the level of or slightly lower than the tracheal carina[69] and measure about 1 to 1.5 mm in diameter. The intrapulmonary bronchial arteries are situated within the peribronchial connective tissue and branch with the airways to the terminal bronchioles.

The bronchial circulation is unique in that it has dual venous drainage. One portion, related predominantly to the trachea and large bronchi, drains through the bronchial veins to the right side of the heart via the azygos and hemiazygos systems. A second portion, related to the major portion of the intrapulmonary bronchial flow, is derived from extensive anastomoses with the pulmonary circulation at precapillary, capillary, and postcapillary sites and drains into the left atrium via the pulmonary veins (bronchopulmonary anastomotic flow).

Bronchial arteries become enlarged in patients with bronchiectasis (Fig. 1.57) and patients with decreased pulmonary artery blood flow (e.g., patients with severe chronic pulmonary thromboembolism) (Fig. 1.58).

LUNG PARENCHYMA

Secondary Pulmonary Lobule

The secondary pulmonary lobule is the smallest discrete portion of the lung that is surrounded by connective tissue septa (Fig. 1.59).[70] Normal interlobular septa are identified easily on HRCT scan as straight lines 1 to 2.5 cm in length and slightly more than 0.1 mm in thickness that often extend to the pleural surface. They are identified most commonly in the anterior and lateral aspects of the lungs, where they are best developed. Although less well visualized in the more central regions of the lungs, they can be identified when they are thickened by edema or inflammatory or neoplastic tissue (Fig. 1.60). The pulmonary parenchyma between the interlobular septa and the centrilobular pulmonary arteries (lobular core) contains small vessels and airways and their accompanying interstitium that are below the resolution of CT. This area is seen as a region of homogeneous attenuation slightly greater than air.

There are two major reasons for considering the secondary lobule the fundamental unit of lung structure from a radiologic point of view: (1) It is the smallest anatomic unit that can be identified clearly on HRCT, and (2) assessment of the distribution

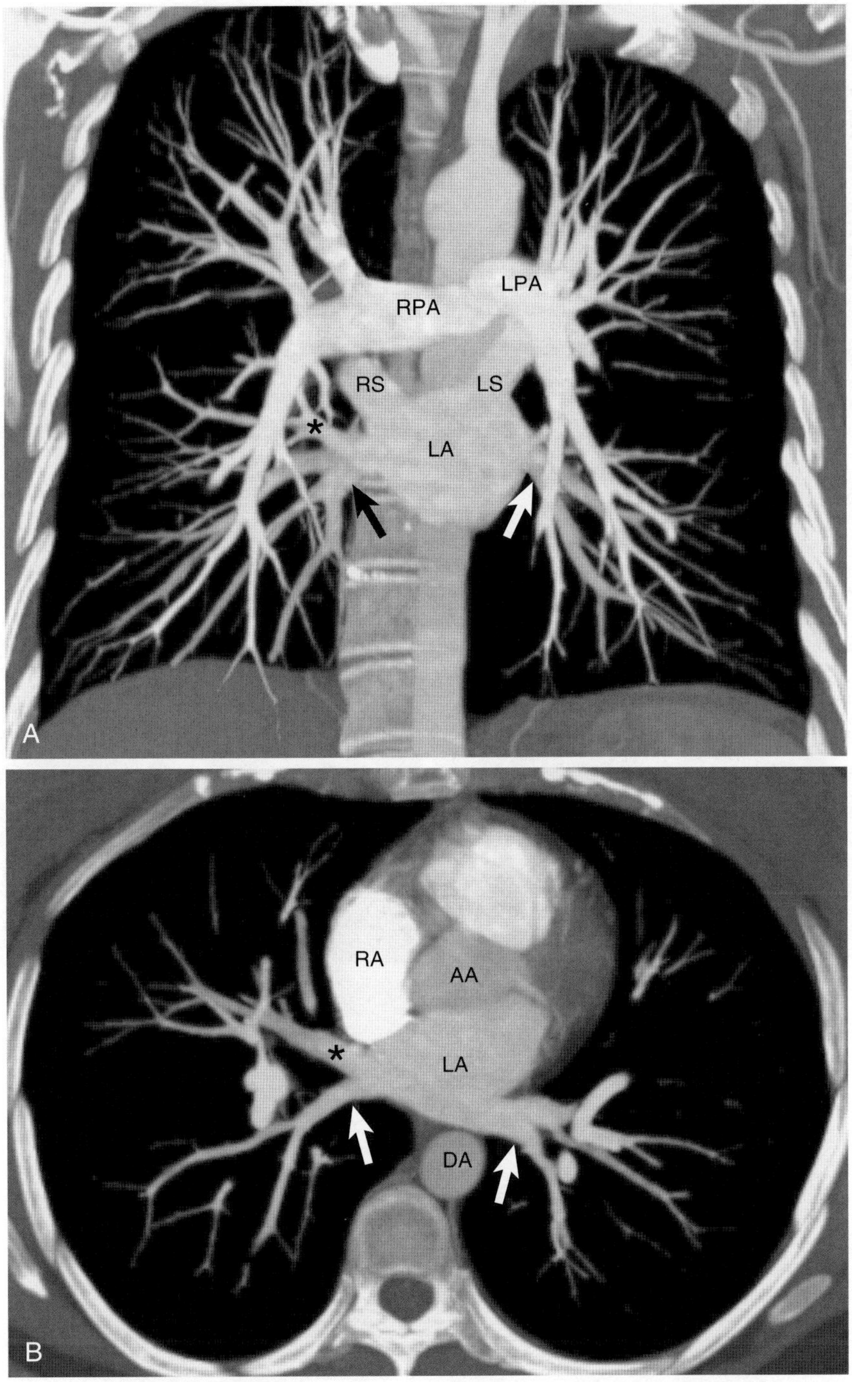

Fig. 1.56 Pulmonary veins and left atrium. (A) Maximum-intensity projection (MIP) coronal reformation CT scan shows the right *(RS)* and left *(LS)* superior pulmonary veins, right middle lobe pulmonary vein *(asterisk)*, and inferior pulmonary veins *(arrows)* as they join the left atrium *(LA)*. *LPA*, Left pulmonary artery; *RPA*, right pulmonary artery. (B) MIP axial reformation shows the confluence of the inferior pulmonary veins *(arrows)* and right middle lobe vein *(asterisk)* as they drain into the left atrium *(LA)*. *AA*, Ascending aorta; *DA*, descending aorta; *RA*, right atrium.

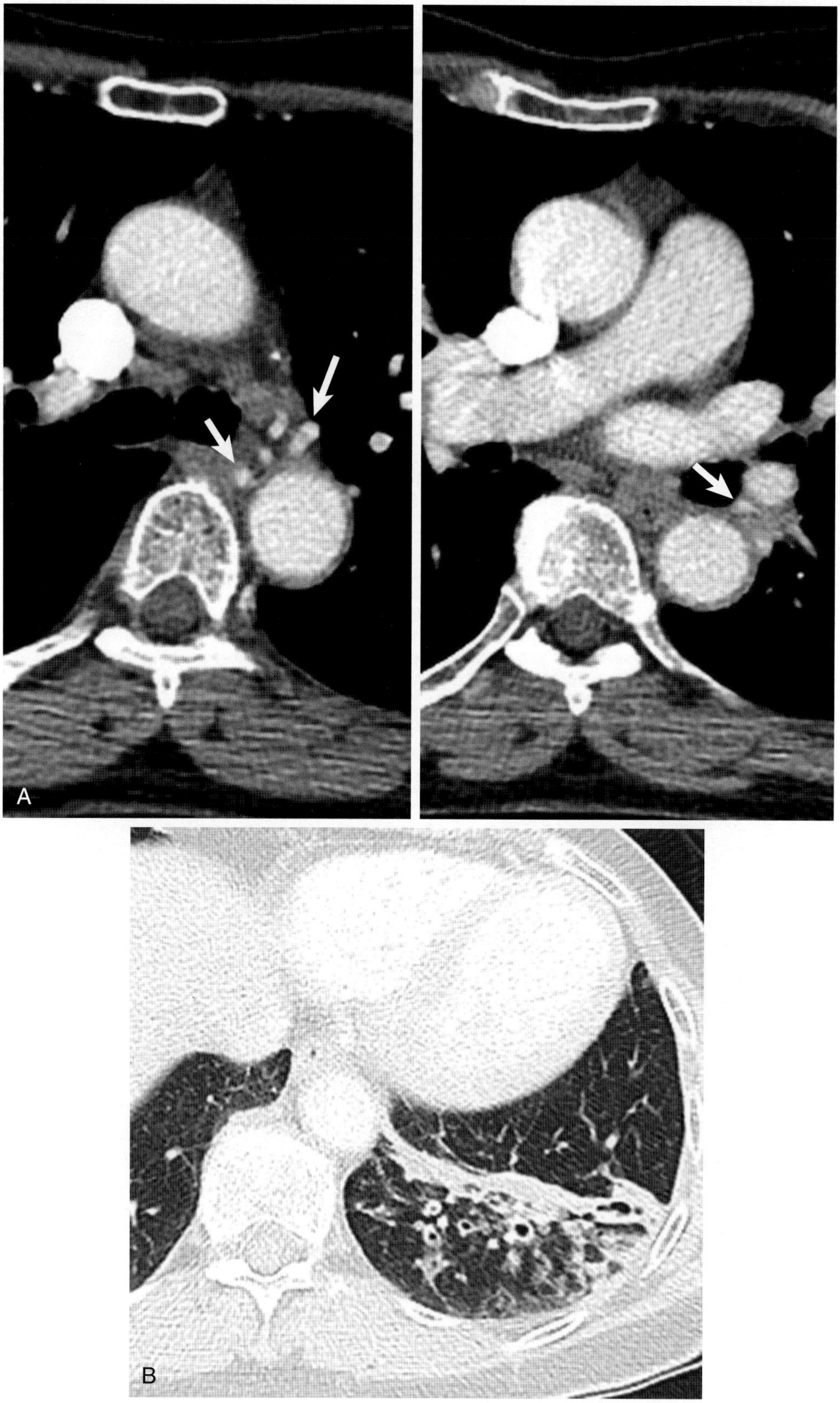

Fig. 1.57 Enlarged bronchial arteries in bronchiectasis. (A) Axial CT angiograms show marked dilation of the left bronchial arteries *(arrows)*, which enter the hilum of the left lung to supply the bronchiectatic lower lobe airways seen on the axial CT scan in (B). *(From Walker CM, Rosado-de-Christenson ML, Martínez-Jiménez S, et al. Bronchial arteries: anatomy, function, hypertrophy, and anomalies.* Radiographics. *2015;35:32–49.)*

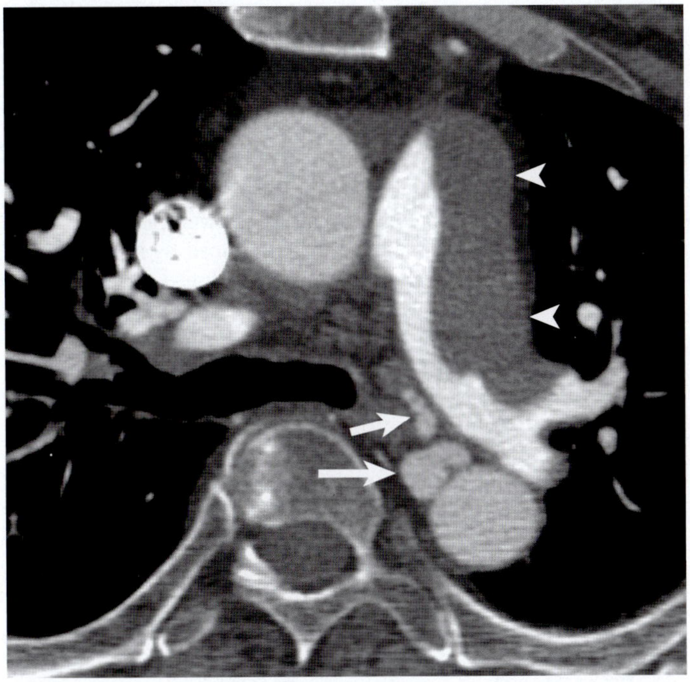

Fig. 1.58 Enlarged bronchial arteries in chronic pulmonary thromboembolic disease. Axial CT angiogram shows a large eccentric filling defect *(arrowheads)* in the main pulmonary artery and left pulmonary artery, with dilated tortuous left bronchial arteries *(arrows)*. *(From Walker CM, Rosado-de-Christenson ML, Martínez-Jiménez S, et al. Bronchial arteries: anatomy, function, hypertrophy, and anomalies.* Radiographics. *2015;35:32–49.)*

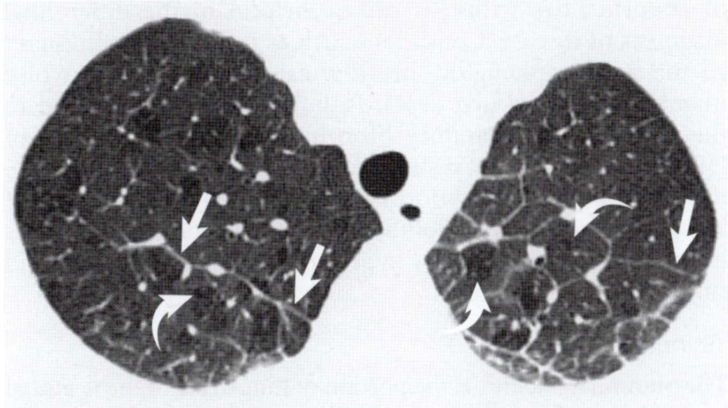

Fig. 1.60 Interstitial pulmonary edema and centrilobular emphysema. High-resolution CT scan shows extensive thickening of the interlobular septa *(straight arrows)*. Also noted are focal areas of increased lucency *(curved arrows)* near the center of the secondary lobules characteristic of centrilobular emphysema. Although the emphysema is initially limited to the central regions of the lobule, it eventually involves the entire lobule.

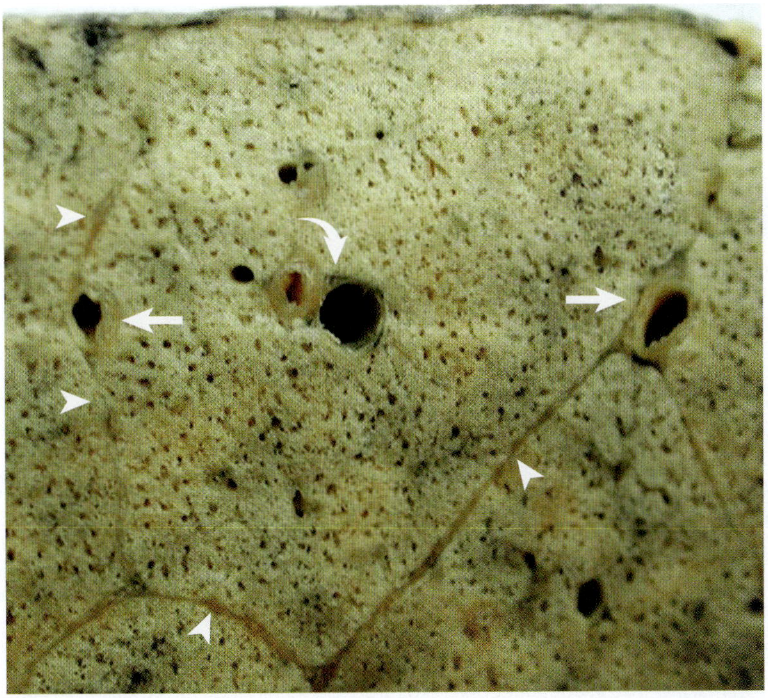

Fig. 1.59 Normal pulmonary lobule. Lung specimen shows secondary lobule surrounded by connective tissue septa *(arrowheads)*. The lobular bronchiole and pulmonary artery *(curved arrow)* are located in the center of the lobule, and the draining pulmonary veins *(straight arrows)* are located in the interlobular septa. *(Courtesy Dr. Reynaldo T. Rodrigues, Federal University of São Paulo, São Paulo, Brazil.)*

of abnormalities within it can be helpful in the differential diagnosis of disease. Conditions such as interstitial pulmonary edema and lymphangitic spread of carcinoma tend to involve mainly the interlobular septa. Pathologic processes related to the terminal or respiratory bronchioles are characterized on HRCT by predominant distribution near the center of the lobule. Examples of specific abnormalities include localized areas of low attenuation in centrilobular emphysema and micronodules in infectious bronchiolitis, hypersensitivity pneumonitis, and silicosis.

Acinus

The pulmonary acinus is the portion of lung distal to the terminal bronchiole and is composed of respiratory bronchioles, alveolar ducts, alveolar sacs, alveoli and their accompanying vessels, and connective tissue. Reported measurements of acinar diameter vary from 6 to 10 mm, depending to some extent on the technique by and pressure at which the lung is inflated.[71,72] Depending on its size, a secondary pulmonary lobule may contain 3 to 24 acini.[73]

LUNG DENSITY ON COMPUTED TOMOGRAPHY

The measurement of lung density with CT is based on the existence of an approximately linear relationship between the attenuation of the x-ray beam and the density of materials of low atomic number (ranging from nitrogen to water). Attenuation on a CT scan is expressed in terms of the Hounsfield unit scale, in which water is 0 HUs and air is −1000 HUs. Measurements of lung attenuation on CT scans performed at end inspiration in normal individuals typically range from −700 to −900 HUs.[74–76] The attenuation in the upper lung zones tends to be slightly more negative than of the lower lung zones, the upper zones having a mean attenuation of −859 HUs compared with −847 HUs for the lower lung zones in a study of healthy subjects who underwent spirometrically gated CT at 90% of vital capacity.[75]

An AP gradient is normally present, the attenuation in dependent lung regions being typically 50 to 100 HUs greater than that in nondependent regions.[76,77] This gradient is attributable primarily to the influence of gravity on blood flow and lung inflation. Although the normal AP lung attenuation gradients are nearly linear, with attenuation increasing gradually from anterior to posterior lung, the lingula and superior segments of the lower lobes tend to be relatively lucent in many normal subjects.[78] It has been suggested that these segments may be less well ventilated than adjacent lung and less well perfused.[78]

The CT attenuation is markedly influenced by lung volume, progressively increasing as lung volume is reduced during expiration. The mean attenuation change between full inspiration and expiration ranges from approximately 100 to 300 HUs.[79,80] Although measurements of lung attenuation and gradients on inspiration and expiration are seldom used in clinical practice, it is important to be aware that any decrease in lung volume results in increased attenuation. CT scans obtained after an incomplete inspiratory effort or during expiration may result in apparent ground-glass opacities that can mimic lung disease (Fig. 1.61).

Dependent lung regions usually show a greater increase in lung attenuation during expiration than do nondependent lung regions.[78,79] As a result, the AP attenuation gradients normally seen on inspiration are greater on expiratory scans (see Fig. 1.61). The increase in attenuation on expiratory CT scans is usually inhomogeneous because some areas of lung do not increase in attenuation as much as others and appear relatively lucent. These areas of normal air-trapping usually involve a small proportion of lung and are most typically seen in the superior segments of the lower lobes, the anterior middle lobe or lingula, or involving individual pulmonary lobules, particularly in the dependent regions of the lower lobes (Fig. 1.62).[78,81,82]

PLEURA

Anatomy

Most of the normal pleura is not visible on CT. A 1- to 2-mm thick line of soft tissue attenuation normally is seen, however,

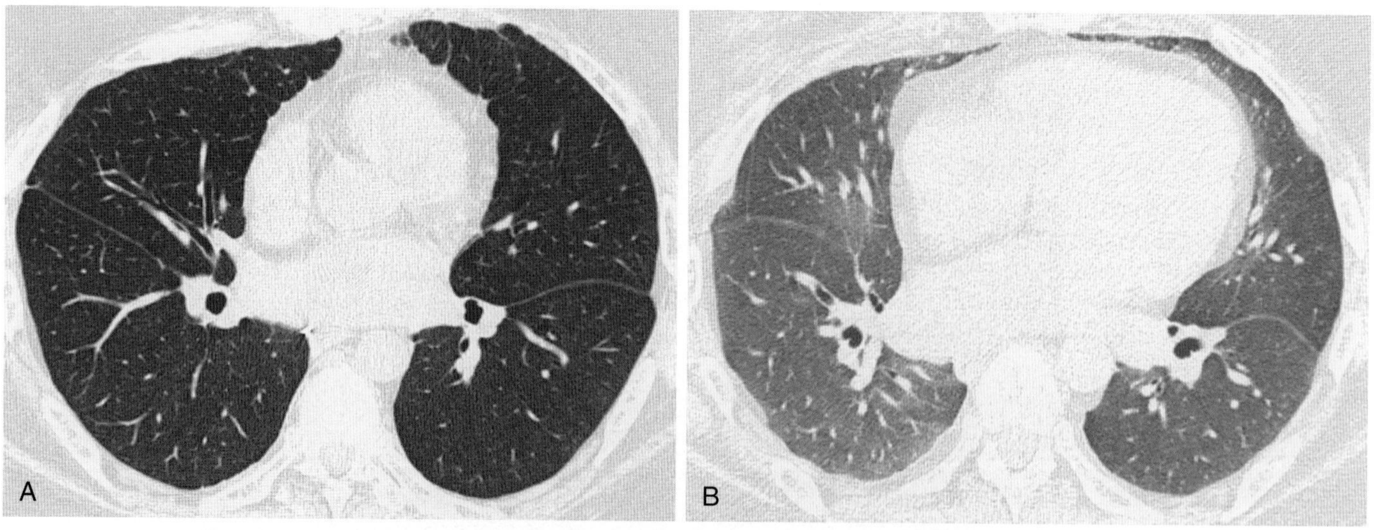

Fig. 1.61 Normal increase in attenuation on expiratory CT mimicking lung disease. (A) High-resolution CT (HRCT) performed at end inspiration shows minimal anteroposterior gradient in lung attenuation. (B) HRCT performed at end expiration shows marked increase in attenuation, particularly in the right middle and lower lobes, resulting in ground-glass opacification. Such a normal increase in attenuation at low lung volumes may mimic parenchymal disease.

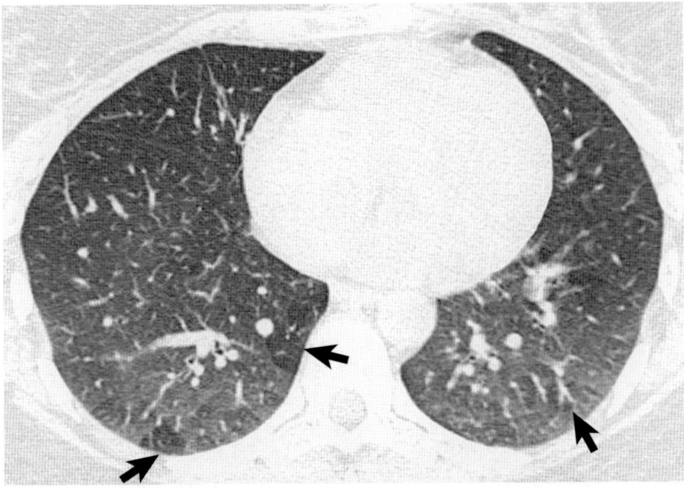

Fig. 1.62 Normal lobular air-trapping. High-resolution CT performed at end expiration shows normal increase in attenuation, particularly in the lower lobes, and a few lobular areas of air-trapping *(arrows)*. Such small focal areas of air-trapping in the dependent lung regions are commonly present in normal individuals and do not represent airway disease.

between the lung and chest wall between the inner edges of the ribs in the intercostal spaces. This line represents the combined thickness of the visceral pleura, normal pleural fluid, parietal pleura, endothoracic fascia, and innermost intercostal muscle (Fig. 1.63), and it is known as the *intercostal stripe*.[83]

Interlobar Fissures

Fissures are invaginations of the pleura that extend from the outer surface of the lung into its substance. The anatomy of the interlobar and accessory fissures has been described in the radiography section of this chapter.

Interlobar fissures are manifested in three ways on CT scan: lucent bands, dense bands, and lines. This variable appearance is related to the section thickness and the plane of the fissure on the cross-sectional CT image. On CT scans performed using 5-mm thick sections, a perpendicular fissure (e.g., in the upper thorax) is likely to produce a linear configuration, whereas a more oblique orientation causes a well-defined, dense (ground-glass) band. Because the minor fissure and the plane of the CT scan are more or less tangential to one another, the fissure typically is manifested as a lucent area relatively devoid of vessels compared with the same region in the left lung. On thinner sections (1–2 mm thick) the major fissures are visualized as continuous smooth lines measuring less than 1 mm in thickness. The minor fissure usually is visualized as a curvilinear line or band of increased attenuation that forms a quarter circle or semicircle in its highest aspect (located slightly cephalad to the level of the origin of the middle lobe bronchus) (Fig. 1.64).

Accessory Fissures

Any portion of lung may be separated partly or completely from adjacent pulmonary tissue by an accessory fissure. Accessory fissures are seen anatomically in about 50% of lungs.[83] They vary in their degree of development from superficial slits not more than 1 cm deep to complete fissures. The most common are the azygos, inferior, and superior.

Azygos Fissure. The azygos fissure is created by downward invagination of the azygos vein through the apical portion of the right upper lobe.[84] The fissure is seen on CT in approximately 1% of individuals[85] as a thin, curved line or band extending from the right lung apex to the level of the T4 or T5 vertebral body (Fig. 1.65).

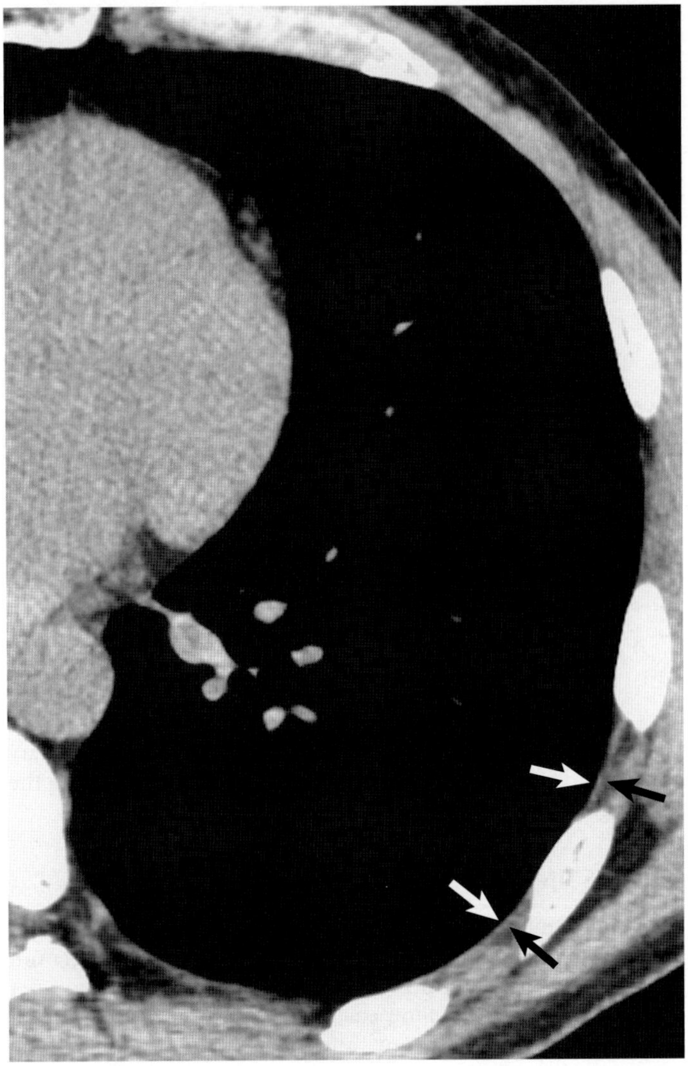

Fig. 1.63 Normal pleura and intercostal stripe. High-resolution CT scan shows normal intercostal stripe as a thin white line *(arrows)* that represents the combined thickness of the visceral and parietal pleura, normal fluid within pleural space, endothoracic fascia, and innermost intercostal muscle. The normal pleura adjacent to the ribs is too thin to be seen.

Inferior Accessory Fissure. The inferior accessory fissure separates the medial basal segment from the remainder of the lower lobe (Fig. 1.66). The inferior accessory fissure is seen on CT in approximately 10% of patients, usually in the right lower lobe.[85,86]

Superior Accessory Fissure. The superior accessory fissure separates the superior segment from the basal segments of the lower lobes, more commonly on the right; as they are oriented in the horizontal plane, it is often easiest to identify them on coronal or sagittal reformatted CT images. They are seen on CT in approximately 5% of patients.

Pulmonary Ligament

The appearance of the pulmonary ligament on CT varies but usually consists of a small peak or pyramid on the mediastinal

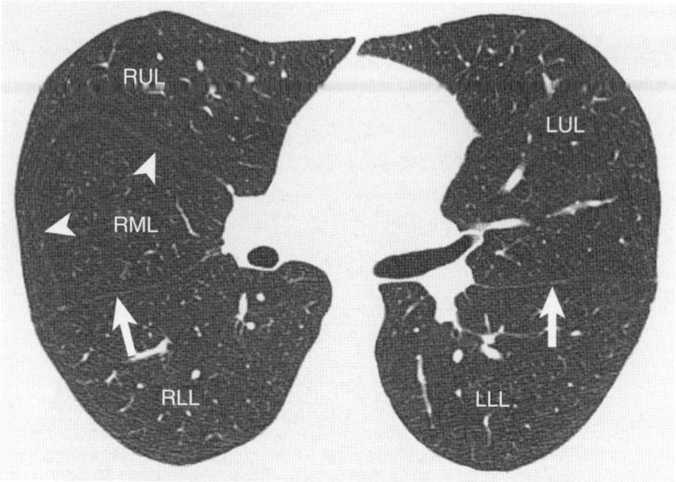

Fig. 1.64 Normal interlobar fissures on high-resolution CT. High-resolution CT scan shows right and left major *(straight arrows)* and right minor *(arrowheads)* fissures. The lung parenchyma surrounded by the minor fissure corresponds to the right middle lobe *(RML)*, whereas the parenchyma lateral and anterior to the minor fissure represents the right upper lobe *(RUL)*. *LLL*, Left lower lobe; *LUL*, left upper lobe; *RLL*, right lower lobe.

surface that represents the ligament and a thin linear opacity that extends from the apex of the peak to the lung, marking the intersegmental septum (Fig. 1.67).

MEDIASTINUM

The mediastinum is the compartment or partition that separates the right and left pleural sacs. It is situated between the sternum and the vertebral column and extends from the thoracic inlet to the diaphragm. CT allows accurate depiction of the normal and abnormal mediastinum and precise localization of the mediastinal masses as to site of origin, extent, and relationship to specific mediastinal structures. The mediastinum is divided anatomically into three compartments on lateral radiography. The International Thymic Malignancy Interest Group (ITMIG) has developed a new classification model of the mediastinal compartments based on cross-sectional imaging that has been accepted as a new standard and is discussed in detail in Chapter 77. On CT it is often easier to base the differential diagnosis of a mediastinal mass on a direct observation of the tissue or structure from which the mass is arising (e.g., lymph nodes, aorta, thymus, trachea, esophagus).

Although adequate images often can be obtained without the use of IV contrast media, IV contrast medium is required for optimal depiction of vascular structures and distinction between vascular and nonvascular structures. The systemic and pulmonary vessels as they course in the mediastinum together with the trachea and main bronchi are helpful landmarks to localize other mediastinal structures.

For purposes of review of normal mediastinal anatomy as seen on CT, the mediastinum can be divided into three regions: (1) supraaortic region, (2) aortic arch down to tracheal carina, and (3) subcarinal region.

Supraaortic Region

The thoracic inlet represents the junction between structures at the base of the neck and structures of the thorax. The most cephalad portion of the mediastinum, adjacent to the thoracic inlet, has a narrow AP diameter. The mediastinal structures in this region, from front to back, include the right and left brachiocephalic (innominate) veins, the common carotid arteries (lying immediately anterior to the subclavian arteries), the trachea (situated immediately behind the supraaortic vessels), the esophagus (located behind the trachea and in front of the spine), and the recurrent laryngeal nerves on either side of the esophagus (Fig. 1.68). The esophagus is usually collapsed but may contain small amounts of air.

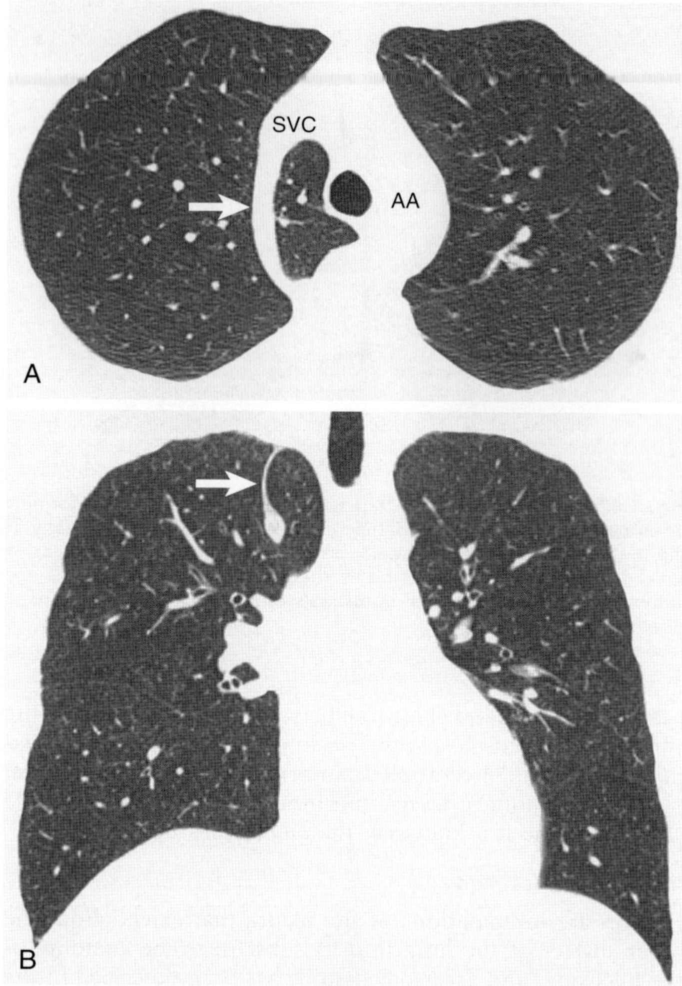

Fig. 1.65 Azygos fissure. (A) Cross-sectional CT scan shows the azygos arch *(arrow)* as it extends anteriorly from the paravertebral region to drain into the superior vena cava *(SVC)*. *AA*, Aortic arch. (B) Coronal reformation shows the azygos fissure *(arrow)*.

The right brachiocephalic vein has a nearly vertical course throughout its length. Below the thoracic inlet, the left brachiocephalic vein crosses from left to right to join the right brachiocephalic vein to form the SVC (Fig. 1.69).

Other normal structures that may be seen in the supraaortic mediastinum include small lymph nodes and small vascular branches, particularly the internal mammary veins. In some patients the thyroid gland may extend into the supraaortic mediastinum above the level of the left brachiocephalic vein. Because of its iodine content, the thyroid has greater attenuation than soft tissue, allowing easy recognition on CT (Fig. 1.70).

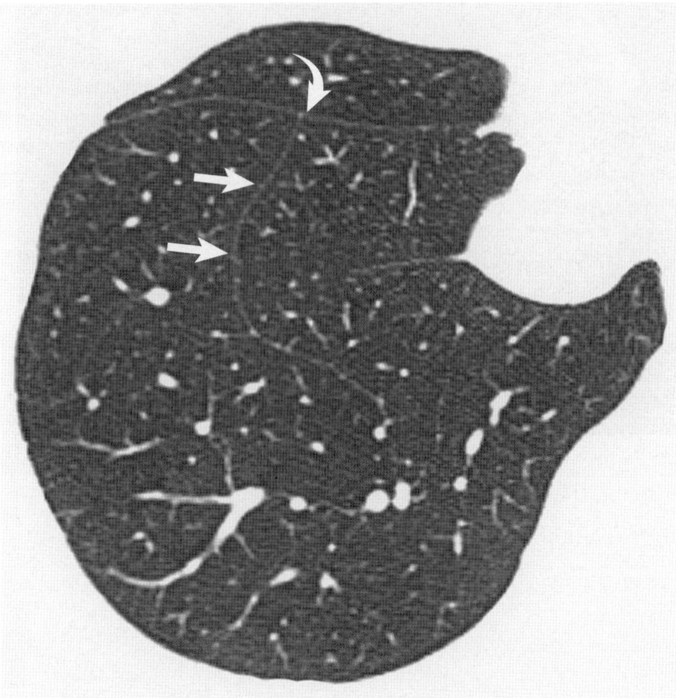

Fig. 1.66 Inferior accessory fissure. View of the right lung from a high-resolution CT scan shows inferior accessory fissure *(straight arrows)* separating the medial from the anterior basal segments of the right lower lobe and attaching to the major fissure *(curved arrow)*.

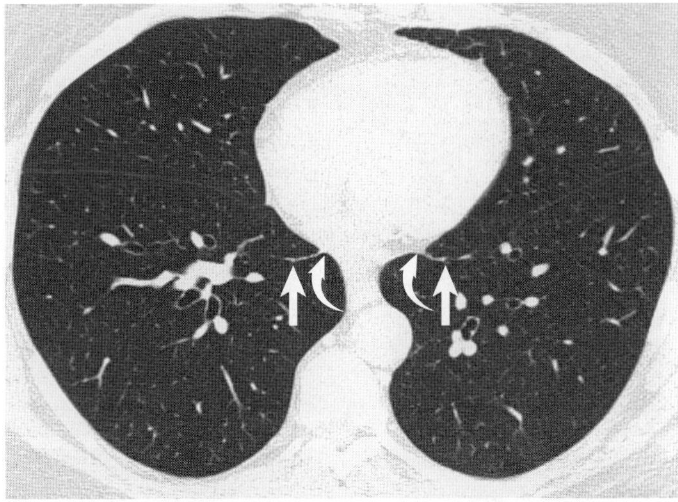

Fig. 1.67 Inferior pulmonary ligament. High-resolution CT scan 2 cm below the level of the inferior pulmonary veins shows a small peak on the mediastinal surface *(curved arrows)* that represents the right and left inferior pulmonary ligaments. The thin linear opacity that extends from the apex of the pulmonary ligament represents the intersegmental septum *(straight arrows)*, which separates the medial basal from the posterior basal segments of the lower lobes.

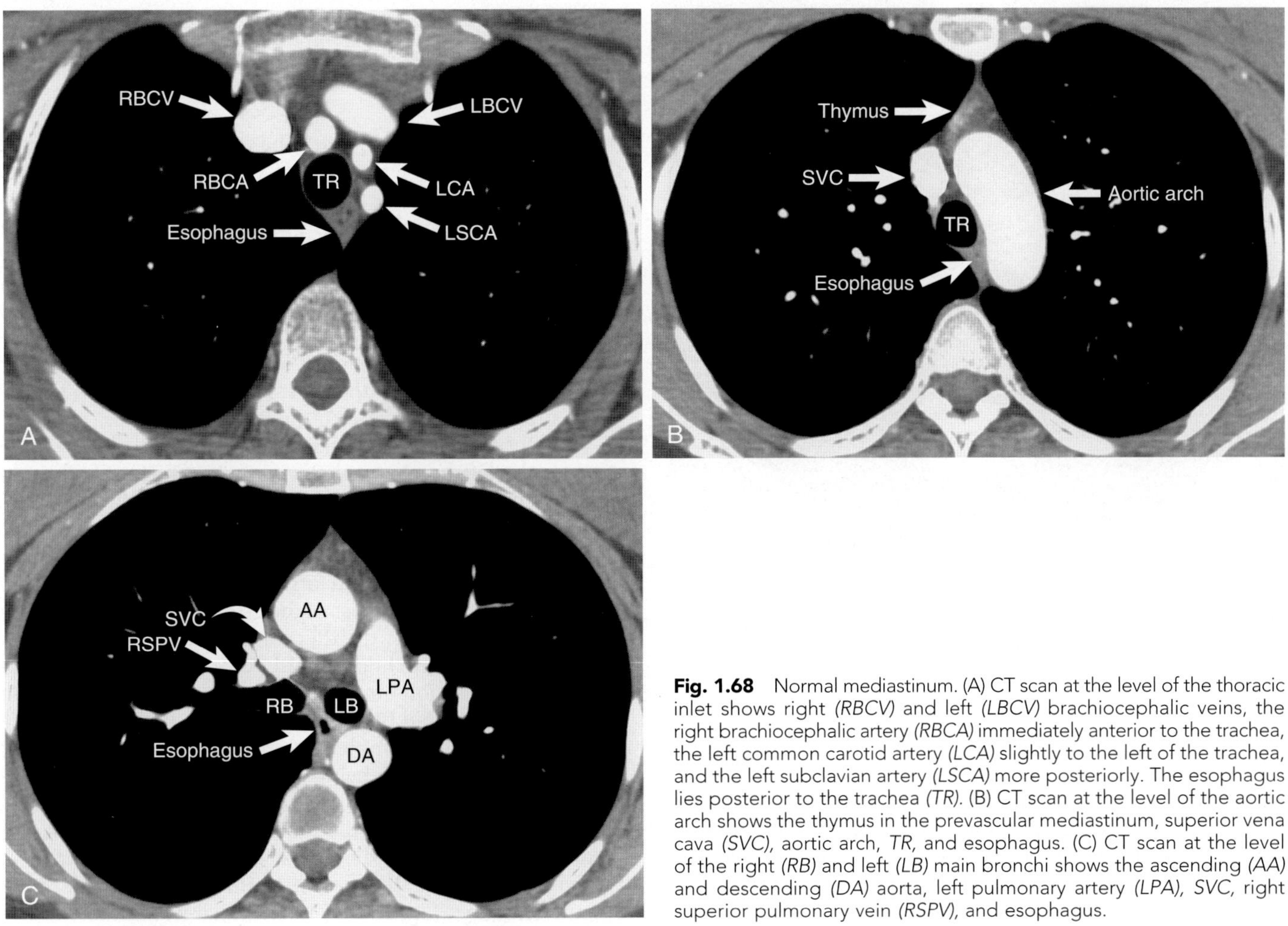

Fig. 1.68 Normal mediastinum. (A) CT scan at the level of the thoracic inlet shows right *(RBCV)* and left *(LBCV)* brachiocephalic veins, the right brachiocephalic artery *(RBCA)* immediately anterior to the trachea, the left common carotid artery *(LCA)* slightly to the left of the trachea, and the left subclavian artery *(LSCA)* more posteriorly. The esophagus lies posterior to the trachea *(TR)*. (B) CT scan at the level of the aortic arch shows the thymus in the prevascular mediastinum, superior vena cava *(SVC)*, aortic arch, *TR*, and esophagus. (C) CT scan at the level of the right *(RB)* and left *(LB)* main bronchi shows the ascending *(AA)* and descending *(DA)* aorta, left pulmonary artery *(LPA)*, *SVC*, right superior pulmonary vein *(RSPV)*, and esophagus.

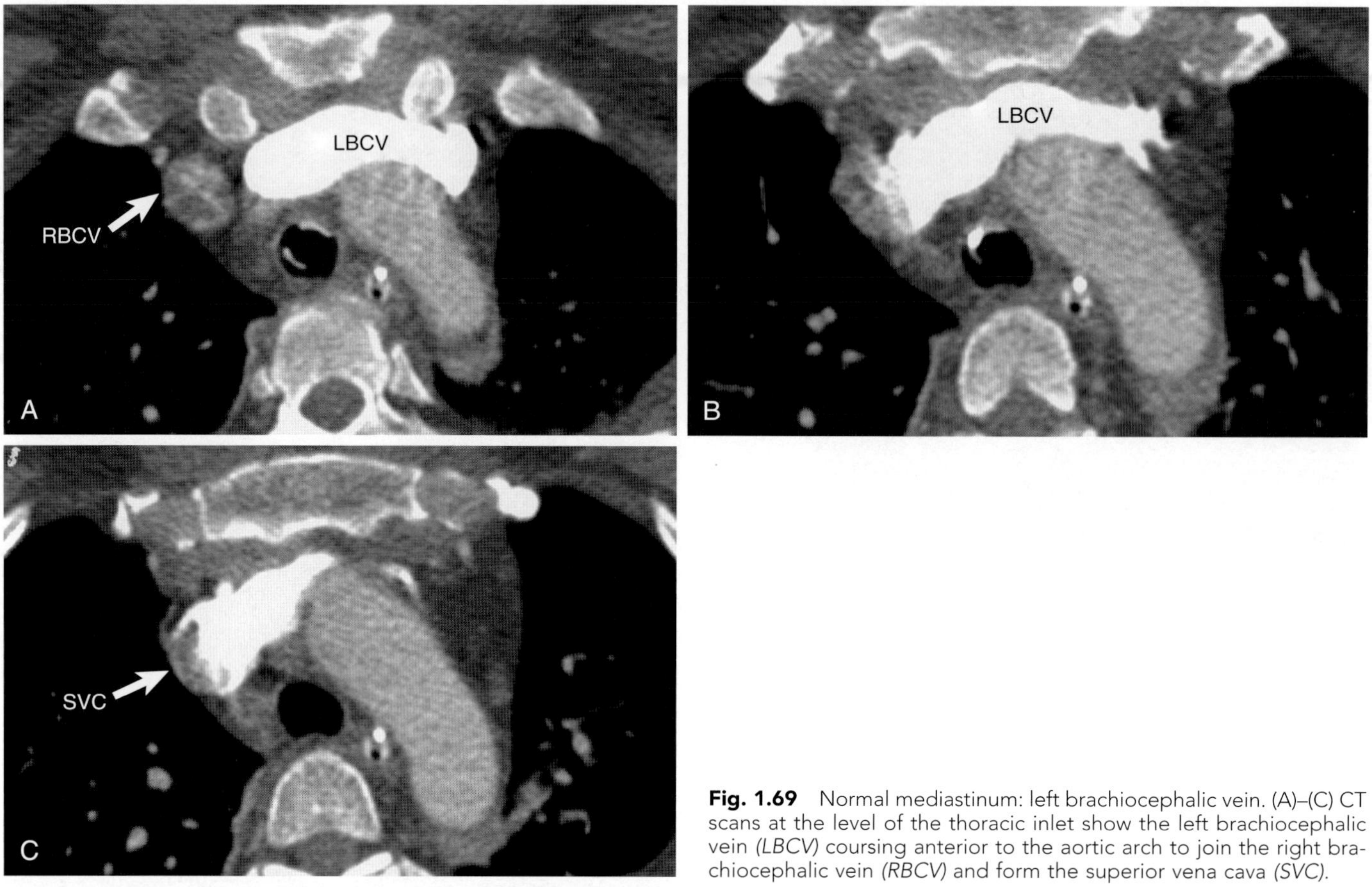

Fig. 1.69 Normal mediastinum: left brachiocephalic vein. (A)–(C) CT scans at the level of the thoracic inlet show the left brachiocephalic vein *(LBCV)* coursing anterior to the aortic arch to join the right brachiocephalic vein *(RBCV)* and form the superior vena cava *(SVC)*.

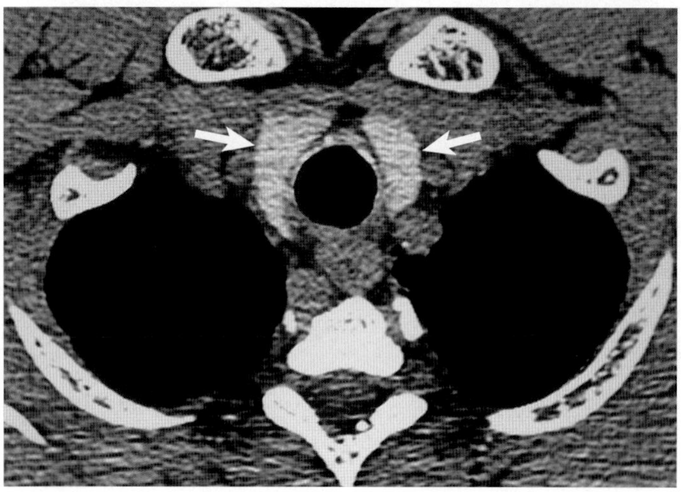

Fig. 1.70 Normal thyroid gland. Nonenhanced CT scan shows normal thyroid gland *(arrows)* with attenuation greater than the soft tissue as a result of its iodine content.

Aortic Arch to Tracheal Carina

The region of the mediastinum spanning the aortic arch to the tracheal carina contains the aorta, SVC, pulmonary arteries, thymus, left recurrent laryngeal nerve, esophagus, and several important lymph node groups (see Fig. 1.68B and C). The aortic arch begins at the brachiocephalic artery and consists of a proximal and a distal segment. The proximal arch gives rise to the brachiocephalic, left common carotid, and left subclavian arteries; variations in the branching pattern of these vessels and their divisions are common. The distal part of the arch, between the origin of the left subclavian artery and the ligamentum arteriosum, is known as the aortic isthmus. Distal to the ligamentum arteriosum is the descending thoracic aorta.

The anterior aspect of the aortic arch (proximal portion) is located anterior and to the right of the trachea. It courses to the left and posteriorly, with the most posterior portion of the arch being situated anterior and to the left of the spine.

The left superior intercostal vein courses cephalad and forward to enter the left brachiocephalic vein (Fig. 1.71). The location of the vein adjacent to the lateral convexity of the aortic arch results in a focal opacity that is well seen on CT.

Anterior to the aorta and SVC is a triangular space that contains lymph nodes, the thymus, and fat. The thymus is usually smoothly molded to the anterior aspect of the great vessels and may extend cephalad to the level of the thyroid gland and inferiorly to the base of the heart. In children and adolescents the thymus has soft tissue attenuation on CT. The thymus increases in size until puberty, after which it begins to involute. In patients older than 30 years it is almost completely replaced by fat, with only thin strands of thymic tissue being seen within the prevascular fat. On CT the thymus often appears bilobed or arrowhead shaped, with each of the two thymic lobes contacting the mediastinal pleura (see Fig. 1.68B). The most useful measurement of the thymus on CT is the thickness (measured perpendicular to the length) of a lobe (Fig. 1.72). The maximal normal thickness of

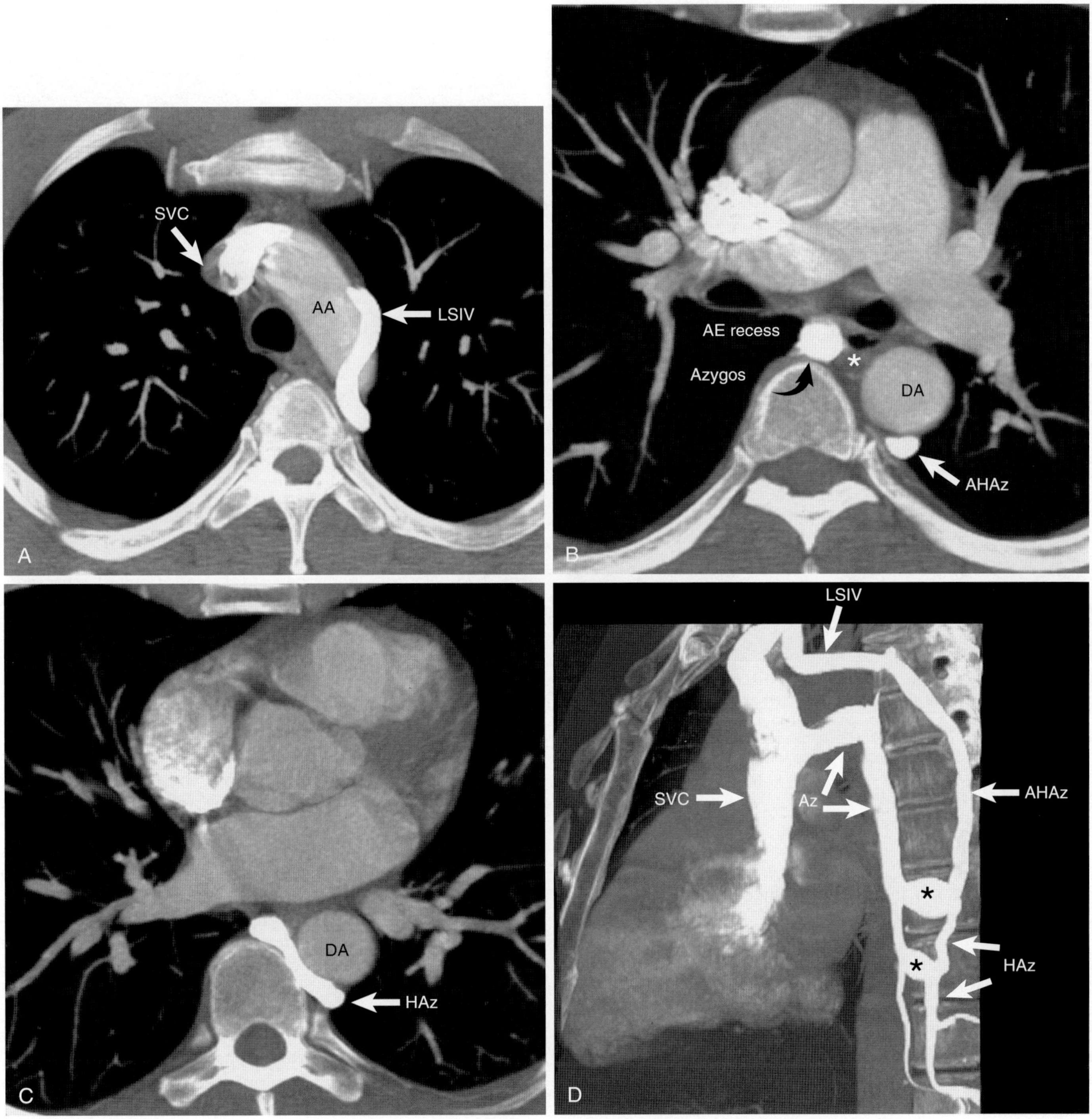

Fig. 1.71 Left superior intercostal vein and the azygos and hemiazygos systems on CT. (A) Contrast-enhanced maximum-intensity projection (MIP) CT image at the level of aortic arch *(AA)* shows prominent left superior intercostal vein *(LSIV)*. *SVC*, Superior vena cava. (B) CT scan at the level of the main pulmonary artery shows the azygos vein *(curved arrow)* and the esophagus *(asterisk)* forming the medial border of the azygoesophageal *(AE)* recess. The accessory hemiazygos vein *(AHAz)* lies posterior to the descending aorta *(DA)* and within the paravertebral space. (C) CT scan at the level of the inferior pulmonary veins shows a communicating vein between the hemiazygos vein *(HAz)* and the azygos vein. (D) Oblique sagittal MIP image shows the normal course of the superior vena cava *(SVC)*; left superior intercostal vein *(LSIV)*; and azygos *(Az)*, accessory hemiazygos *(AHAz)*, and hemiazygos *(HAz)* veins. Note the communicating veins *(asterisks)* between the hemiazygos and azygos veins.

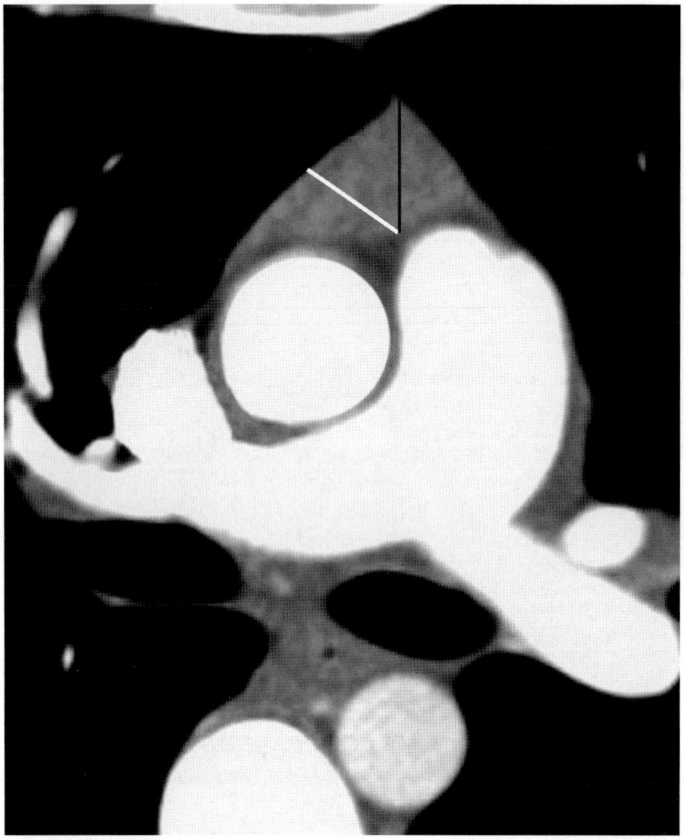

Fig. 1.72 Measurement of thymic size. The thymus typically has a triangular or arrowhead shape. For measurement purposes, the thymus is divided in half by a line through the anterior apex of the gland and perpendicular to it *(black line)*. The thickness of each thymic lobe corresponds to the short-axis diameter of the lobe *(white line)*. The maximal normal thickness of the thymus is 1.8 cm in patients younger than 20 years and 1.3 cm in older patients.

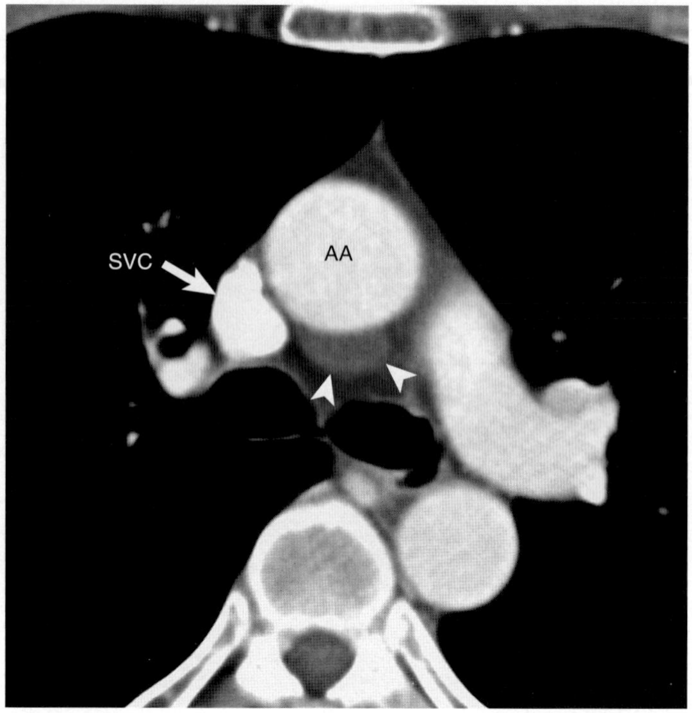

Fig. 1.73 Normal superior pericardial recess. Contrast-enhanced CT scan shows normal amount of pericardial fluid *(arrowheads)* contiguous with the posterior wall of the ascending aorta *(AA)*. The location and low attenuation are characteristic for the superior pericardial recess, allowing it to be distinguished from paratracheal lymph node enlargement. *SVC*, Superior vena cava.

the thymus is 1.8 cm in patients younger than 20 years and 1.3 cm in older patients.[87,88]

Anterior to the trachea and posterior to the SVC and the aortic arch is a space known as the pretracheal or anterior paratracheal space. This space normally contains variable amounts of fat and small lymph nodes (paratracheal lymph nodes). On the left side the mediastinal region immediately caudal to the aortic arch and cephalad to the main pulmonary artery is termed the aorticopulmonary window. The aorticopulmonary window is marginated medially by the ductus ligament (ligamentum arteriosum) and laterally by the mediastinal and visceral pleura over the left lung. The aorticopulmonary window (see Fig. 1.54C) contains fat, the aorticopulmonary lymph nodes, and the left recurrent laryngeal nerve.

Below the level of the aortic arch, the ascending aorta and descending aorta are visible as separate structures. The ascending aorta is slightly larger (mean diameter, ≈3.5 cm; range 2.5–4.5 cm) than the descending aorta (mean diameter, ≈2.5 cm; range, 1.5–3.5 cm).[89] At the level of the proximal ascending aorta, a small amount of pericardial fluid often can be seen immediately posterior to the aorta and projecting into the pretracheal space, known as the superior pericardial recess (Fig. 1.73).

The trachea bifurcates into the right and left main bronchi. At the level of the tracheal carina, the azygos vein can be seen forming an arch as it courses forward and passes over the right main bronchus to enter the posterior wall of the SVC.

Subcarinal Region

Immediately below the tracheal carina are the subcarinal lymph nodes and a variable amount of fat. At the level of the tracheal carina or slightly more caudally, the azygos vein parallels the esophagus along the right side of the mediastinum. This portion of the mediastinum contacts the medial pleural reflections of the right lower lobe and is known as the azygoesophageal recess. On the left side the hemiazygos vein lies parallel and posterior to the descending aorta and within the paravertebral space (see Fig. 1.71B). The left paravertebral space contains the hemiazygos vein, paravertebral nodes (seldom seen in normal individuals), and fat.

LYMPHATIC SYSTEM OF THE LUNGS, PLEURA, AND MEDIASTINUM

Parietal pleural lymphatics are distributed extensively over the costal and diaphragmatic surfaces. Visceral pleural lymphatics course within the connective tissue layer, where they form a plexus of channels whose major tributaries roughly follow the pleural lobular boundaries. The anterior pleura is drained by the internal mammary and the anterior and middle peridiaphragmatic lymph nodes, the posterior pleura is drained by extrapleural lymph nodes adjacent to vertebral bodies, the anterior and lateral diaphragm is drained by the internal mammary and anterior peridiaphragmatic nodes, and the posterior diaphragm is drained

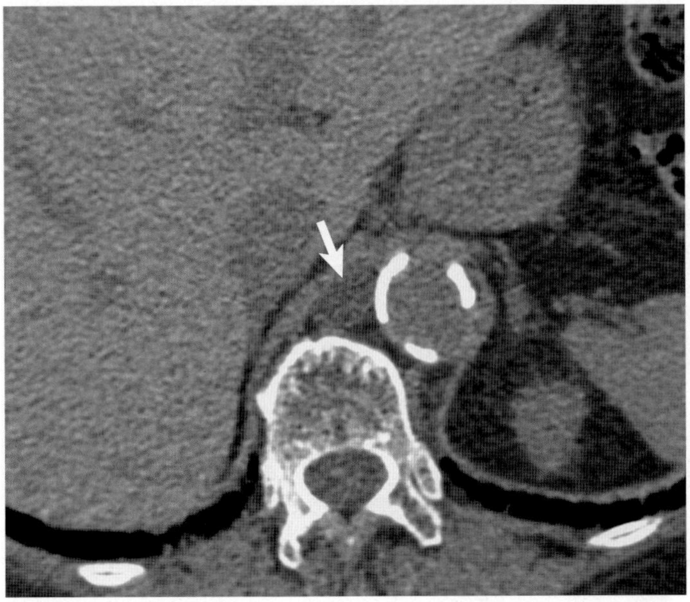

Fig. 1.74 Cisterna chyli. CT scan shows low-attenuation retrocrural opacity *(arrow)* immediately to the right of the aorta; this is the characteristic location of the cisterna chyli.

by the paraaortic and posterior mediastinal (e.g., retrocrural) nodes. The anterior and lateral chest wall lymphatics drain to the anterior or pectoral nodes, and the posterior chest wall lymphatics drain to the axillary nodes.

Within the lung, lymph flows along two major pathways, one in the peribronchovascular connective tissue and the other in the interlobular septal connective tissue. In the former it flows centripetally toward the hilum, eventually reaching the peribronchial and hilar lymph nodes; in the interlobular septa it often drains into the pleural lymphatics. Anastomotic channels connect the interlobular lymphatics with the lymphatics in the bronchoarterial sheath.

Thoracic Duct and Right Lymphatic Duct

The thoracic duct is a continuation of the cisterna chyli, which is formed by the junction of the two lumbar lymphatic trunks on the anterior aspect of the vertebral column at the level of T12 to L2 (Fig. 1.74).[90] The duct enters the thorax through the aortic hiatus of the diaphragm, and, in most individuals, it lies to the right of the aorta and follows its course cephalad; in the lower portion of the thorax, it lies roughly in the midline or slightly to one side of the vertebral column. At about the level of the carina, the duct crosses the left main bronchus and runs cephalad in a plane parallel to the left lateral wall of the trachea and slightly posterior to it. The duct leaves the thorax between the esophagus and left subclavian artery and runs posterior to the left brachiocephalic vein. It joins the venous system most commonly at the internal jugular vein but sometimes drains into the subclavian, brachiocephalic, or external jugular veins. The radiologic anatomy of the right lymphatic duct has been documented poorly because it cannot be opacified easily, and it is an inconstant channel.

Lymph Nodes. Although pleuropulmonary lymphatics are not normally visible radiologically, their intrathoracic repository, the hilar and mediastinal lymph nodes, frequently is discernible. Lymph nodes are identified on CT scans as round or oval structures of soft tissue attenuation, with or without central or eccentric radiolucent fat, in a location that does not correspond to normal vascular or neural structures.

Parietal and Visceral Groups of Thoracic Lymph Nodes. Intrathoracic lymph nodes can be classified into parietal and visceral groups; the former reside outside the parietal pleura in extramediastinal tissue, where they drain the thoracic wall and other extrathoracic structures, whereas the latter are located within the mediastinum between the pleural membranes and drain primarily the intrathoracic tissues.[90] The Mountain-Dresler regional lymph node classification for lung cancer staging (Mountain-Dresler/American Thoracic Society maps) has long been used in North America in the staging of lung cancer (Fig. 1.75). However, this has now been replaced with a revised mediastinal lymph node map created by the International Association for the Study of Lung Cancer (IASLC)[90a] to resolve discrepancies between the Mountain-Dresler system and other similar schema. This new model was adopted during the 7th revision of the tumor-node-metastasis (TNM) Classification of Malignant Tumors in the same year (Figs. 1.76 to 1.80; Table 1.1).[90b]

The most important modification of the IASLC lymph node map is the definition of the left lateral wall of the trachea as the new anatomic boundary between right- and left-sided lymph nodes (Fig. 1.81) and regrouping of mediastinal lymph nodes into seven specific zones: supraclavicular, upper, aorticopulmonary, lower, subcarinal, interlobar, and peripheral.[91] Each of these zones is further assigned to a nodal station numbered from 1 to 14 and described as right (R) or left (L).

The relevance of this classification and its inclusion in the TNM system is the prognostic implication that these lymph nodes have in the case of metastatic involvement, specifically in the staging of lung cancer. Patients without regional metastatic lymphadenopathy are designated as N0. Patients with metastatic lymph node involvement of ipsilateral peripheral or hilar zones (stations 10–14) are designated as N1. The presence of ipsilateral mediastinal (upper, aortopulmonary, and lower) or subcarinal metastatic lymph nodes (stations 2–9) is considered N2 disease, and the metastatic involvement of any nodes in the contralateral mediastinal, hilar-interlobar, and peripheral zones, as well as any ipsilateral or contralateral supraclavicular zone lymph nodes (station 1), is considered N3 disease.

Although no longer included in the lymph node map or considered in the staging system, parietal lymph nodes, such as the internal mammary and peridiaphragmatic lymph nodes, are important nodal stations commonly involved in other neoplasms, such as lymphoma, malignant pleural mesothelioma, esophageal cancer, and breast cancer.

The internal mammary lymph nodes are located in the upper portion of the thorax behind the anterior intercostal spaces bilaterally, medial or lateral to the internal mammary vessels. They drain the anterior chest wall, breasts, anterior pleura, and anterior diaphragm and communicate with prevascular lymph nodes and peridiaphragmatic lymph nodes.

The peridiaphragmatic lymph nodes include the anterior (pericardiophrenic), middle (lymph nodes adjacent to the IVC), and the posterior (retrocrural) lymph nodes.

Lymph Node Size. Lymph nodes are usually ovoid in shape. Assessment of their size usually is based on the measurement of the smallest nodal diameter (short axis) as seen on the transverse CT image because it shows much less variability than

Text continued on p. 54

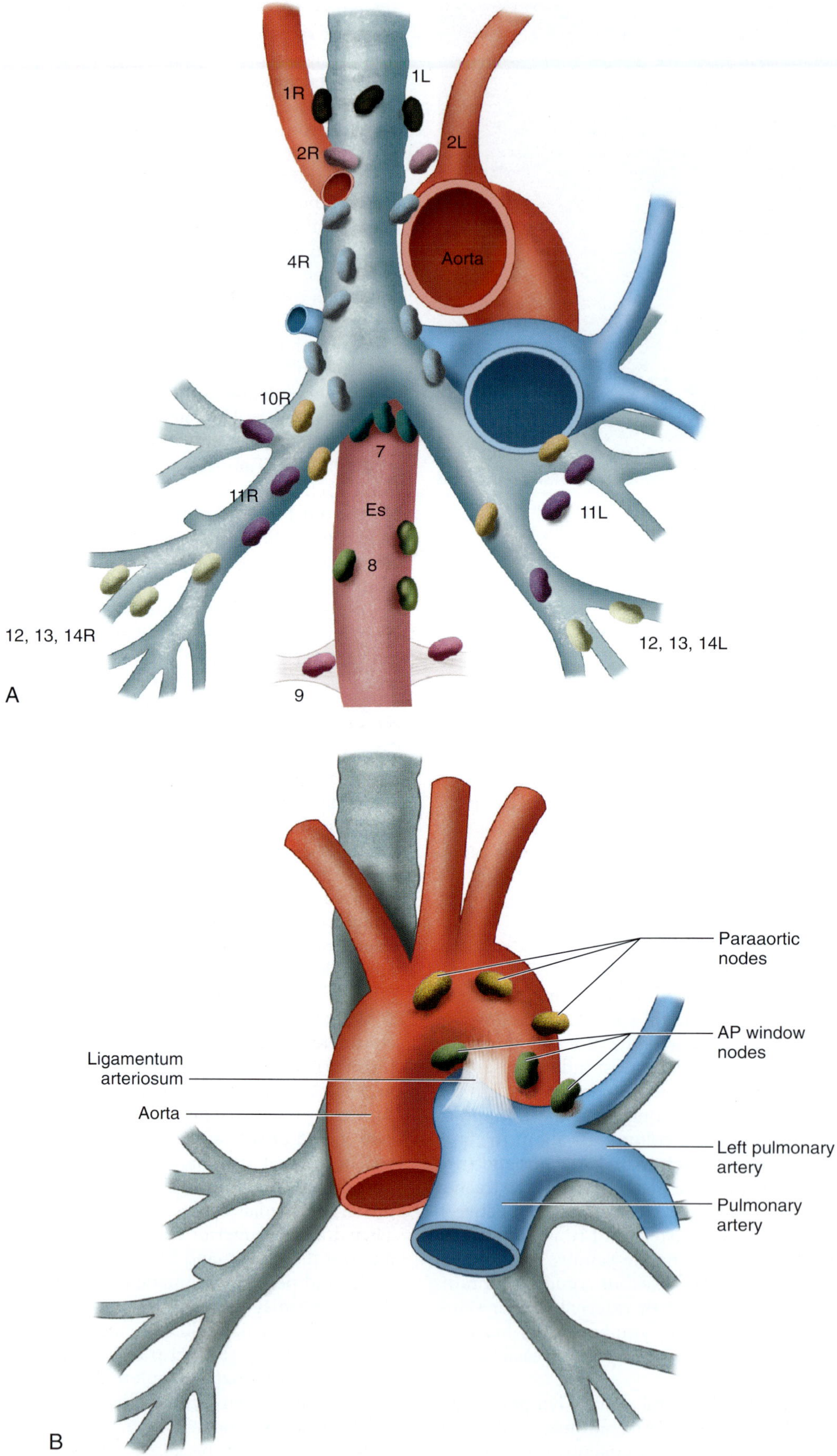

Fig. 1.75 Mediastinal and hilar lymph node map. (A) and (B) Schematic drawings show the mediastinal and hilar lymph node stations. *AP*, Aortopulmonary; *Es*, Esophagus. *(Modified from Mountain CF, Dresler CM: Regional lymph node classification for lung cancer staging.* Chest. *111:1719, 1997.)*

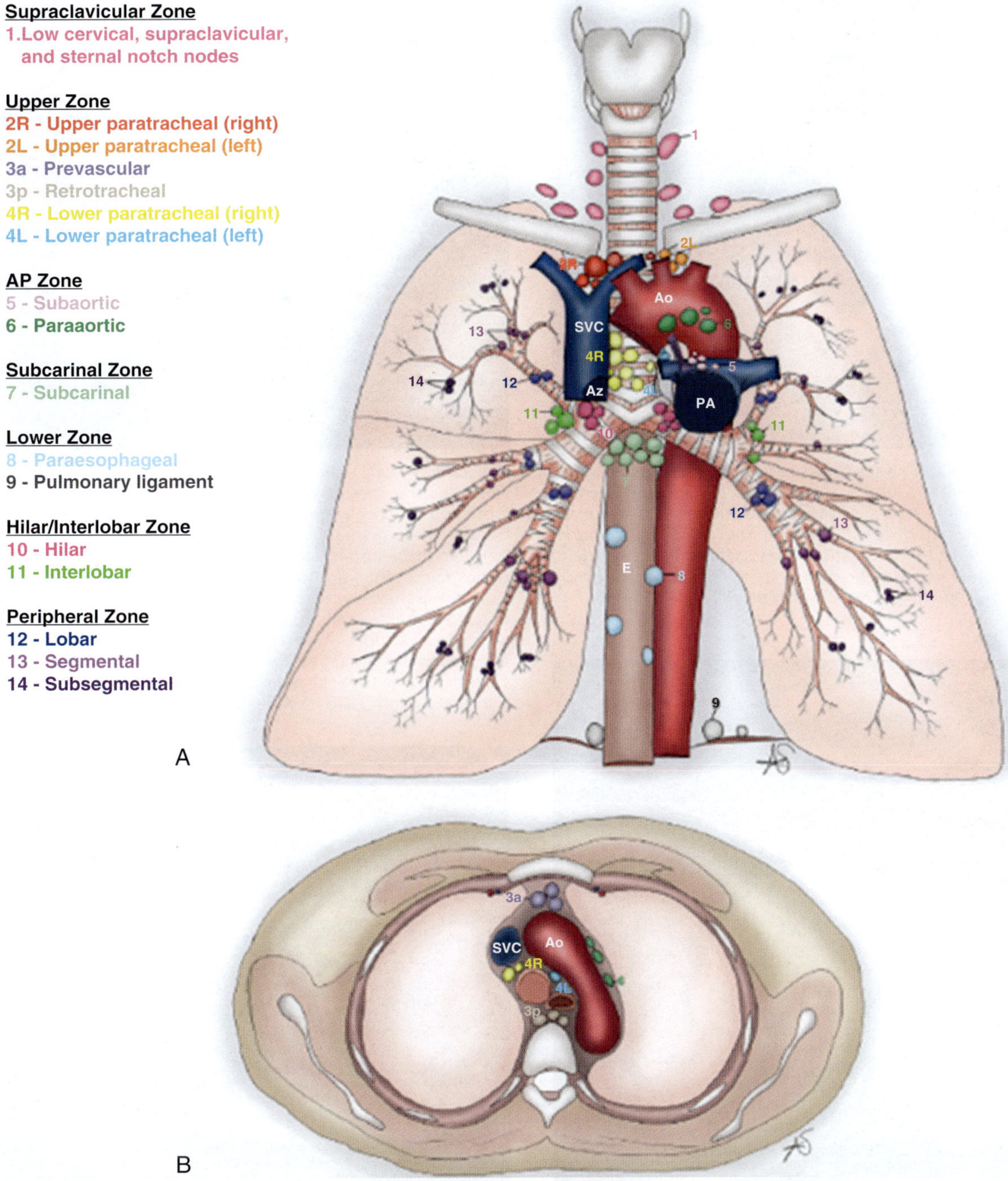

Fig. 1.76 Diagram of the International Association for the Study of Lung Cancer Lymph Node Map. Coronal illustration (A) demonstrates the distribution and location of the lymphatic groups as defined by the new classification system. Image (B) illustrates an axial image of the chest at the level of the aortic arch and the position of the nodal groups in relationship to the mediastinal organs at this level. Refer to Table 1.1 for anatomic details of nodal stations. *Ao,* Aorta; *AP,* aortopulmonary; *Az,* azygos vein; *PA,* pulmonary artery; *SVC,* superior vena cava. *(From Jawad H, Sirajuddin A, Chung JH. Review of the International Association for the Study of Lung Cancer Lymph Node Classification System: localization of lymph node stations on CT imaging.* Clin Chest Med. *2013;34:353–363; Fig. 2.)*

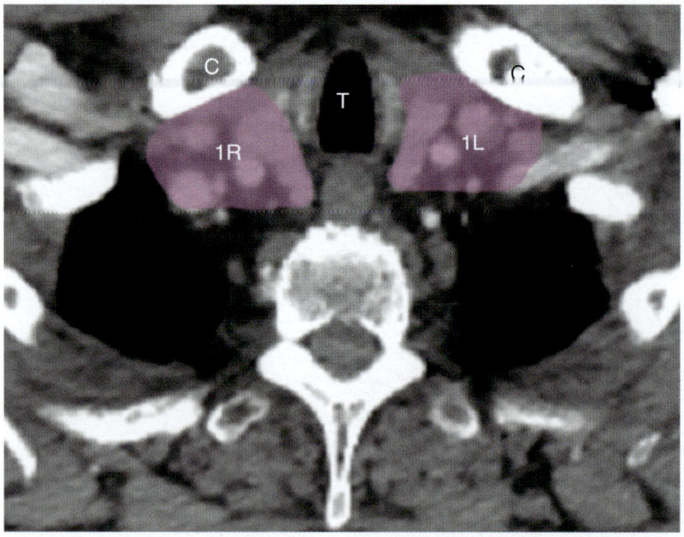

Fig. 1.77 Station 1 lymph nodes (supraclavicular zone) are illustrated in this axial CT image at the level of the thoracic inlet. Station 1 lymph nodes are localized behind the clavicles *(C)* and superior to the sternal notch *(pink areas highlighted)*. *L*, left; *R*, right. *(From Jawad H, Sirajuddin A, Chung JH. Review of the International Association for the Study of Lung Cancer Lymph Node Classification System: localization of lymph node stations on CT imaging.* Clin Chest Med. *2013;34:353–363; Fig. 3A.)*

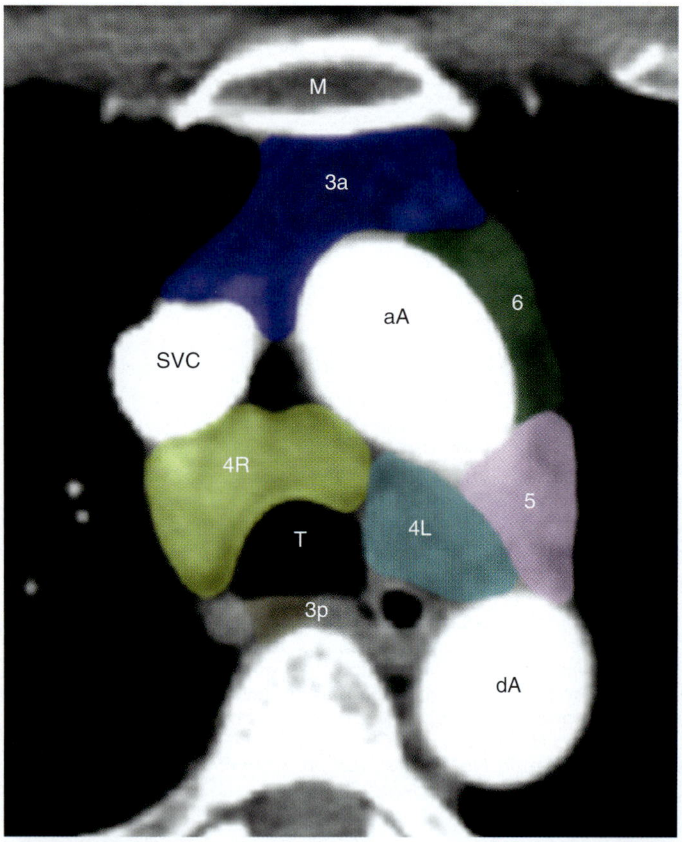

Fig. 1.79 Location of nodal stations *3a, 3p, 4R, 4L, 5,* and *6.* Axial CT of the chest at the level of aorticopulmonary window highlights the location of stations *3a (blue-violet), 3p (brown), 4R (yellow), 4L (teal), 5 (pale pink),* and *6 (green). aA,* Ascending aorta; *dA,* descending aorta; *M,* manubrium; *SVC,* superior vena cava; *T,* trachea. *(From Jawad H, Sirajuddin A, Chung JH. Review of the International Association for the Study of Lung Cancer Lymph Node Classification System: localization of lymph node stations on CT imaging.* Clin Chest Med. *2013;34:353–363; Fig. 7a.)*

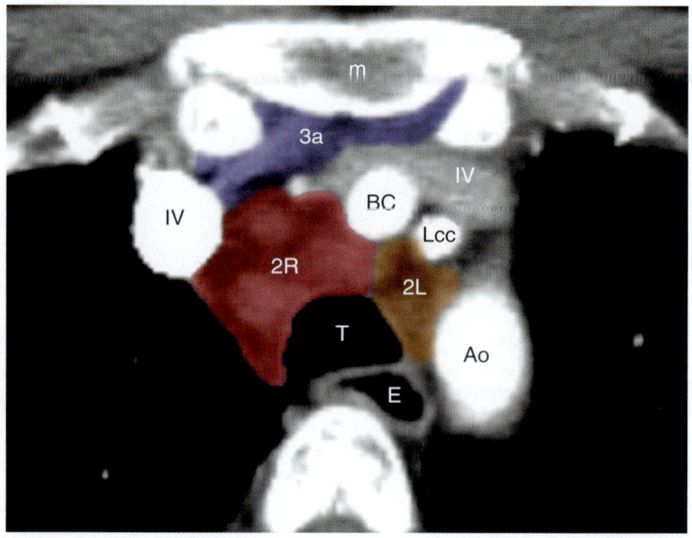

Fig. 1.78 Axial CT image of the chest coned in the superior mediastinum illustrates the location of nodal stations *2* and *3.* Stations *2R* and *2L* (upper paratracheal, right *[red]* and left *[orange]*) lie inferior to the superior border of the manubrium *(m),* which serves as the anatomic landmark between these nodes and station *1* lymph nodes. The prevascular lymph nodes *(3a, purple)* are localized posterior to the sternum and anterior to the superior vena cava and innominate vein *(IV). Ao,* Aorta; *BC,* brachiocephalic artery; *E,* esophagus; *Lcc,* left common carotid artery; *T,* trachea. *(From Jawad H, Sirajuddin A, Chung JH. Review of the International Association for the Study of Lung Cancer Lymph Node Classification System: localization of lymph node stations on CT imaging.* Clin Chest Med. *2013;34:353–363; Fig. 4.)*

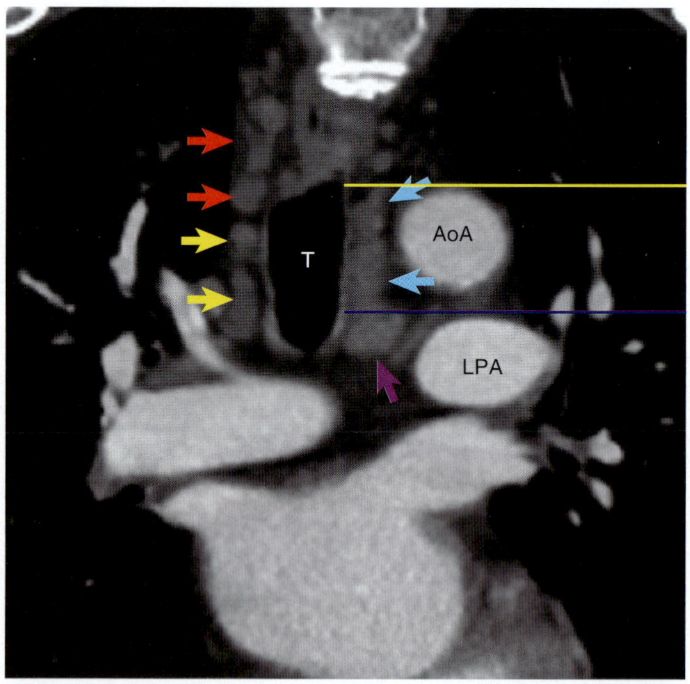

Fig. 1.80 Coronal chest CT scan shows the anatomic landmarks used to define stations 2R *(red arrows),* 4R *(yellow arrows),* and 4L *(blue arrows).* Superior border of the aortic arch *(yellow line)* forms the superior margin of station 4L; superior rim of left main pulmonary artery *(blue line)* forms the inferior border of station 4L. Below the superior rim of the *LPA,* surgical treatment of the nodes anterior to the tracheal bifurcation is similar to mediastinal lymph nodes and are therefore often grouped into the lower paratracheal stations despite the ambiguity of the International Association for the Study of Lung Cancer Classification (station *4, magenta arrow*). *AoA,* Aortic arch; *LPA,* left main pulmonary artery; *T,* trachea. *(Modified from Jawad H, Sirajuddin A, Chung JH. Review of the International Association for the Study of Lung Cancer Lymph Node Classification System: localization of lymph node stations on CT imaging.* Clin Chest Med. *2013;34:353–363; Fig. 9.)*

TABLE 1.1 IASCL LYMPH NODE CLASSIFICATION

			ANATOMIC BOUNDARIES		
Nodal Zone	**Lymph Node Group**	**IASCL Station**	**Superior Border**	**Inferior Border**	**Other Important Anatomic Descriptors**
Supraclavicular	Lower cervical; supraclavicular; sternal notch nodes	1R and 1L	Lower margin of cricoid cartilage	Laterally: both clavicles Medially: upper border of the manubrium	Border between 1R and 1L nodes: midline of trachea
Upper	Upper paratracheal	2R	Medially: superior border of manubrium Laterally: apex of right lung and pleural space	Intersection of caudal margin of left brachiocephalic (innominate) vein with trachea	Border between 2R and 2L: left lateral border of trachea
		2L	Medially: superior border of manubrium Laterally: apex of right lung and pleural space	Superior border of the aortic arch	
	Prevascular (3a) and	3a	Apex of the chest	Carina	Anterior border: sternum Posterior border: SVC (on the right) and left carotid artery (on the left)
	retrotracheal (3p)	3p	Apex of the chest	Carina	
	Lower paratracheal	4R	Intersection of caudal margin of left brachiocephalic vein with trachea	Lower border azygos vein	Anterior boundary: posterior aspect of trachea Demarcation between 4R and
		4L	Superior border of the aortic arch	Superior rim of the main pulmonary artery	4L: left lateral border of trachea Left-lateral limit of 4L: ligamentum arteriosum
Aorticopulmonary	Subaortic	5	Lower border of aortic arch	Upper rim of left main pulmonary artery	Lateral to ligamentum arteriosum
	Para-aortic	6	Horizontal line drawn tangentially to the upper border of aortic arch	Lower border of aortic arch	Located anterior and lateral to ascending aorta and aortic arch
Subcarinal	Subcarinal	7	Carina of the trachea	Left: upper border of the left lower lobe bronchus Right: lower border of the bronchus intermedius	
Lower	Paraesophageal	8	Left: upper border of left lower lobe bronchus Right: lower border of bronchus intermedius	Diaphragm	Adjacent to esophageal wall; can be either side of midline
	Pulmonary ligament	9	Inferior pulmonary vein	Diaphragm	Lie within the pulmonary ligament (which is formed by inferior extension of mediastinal pleural reflections)
Hilar–Interlobar	Hilar	10	Left: superior rim of main pulmonary artery Right: caudal border of azygos vein	Interlobar regions	Includes lymph nodes adjacent to mainstem bronchi and hilar vessels
	Interlobar	11			Located distal to the bifurcation regions of mainstem bronchi
Peripheral	Lobar	12			Adjacent to lobar bronchi
	Segmental	13			Adjacent to segmental bronchi
	Subsegmental	14			Adjacent to subsegmental bronchi

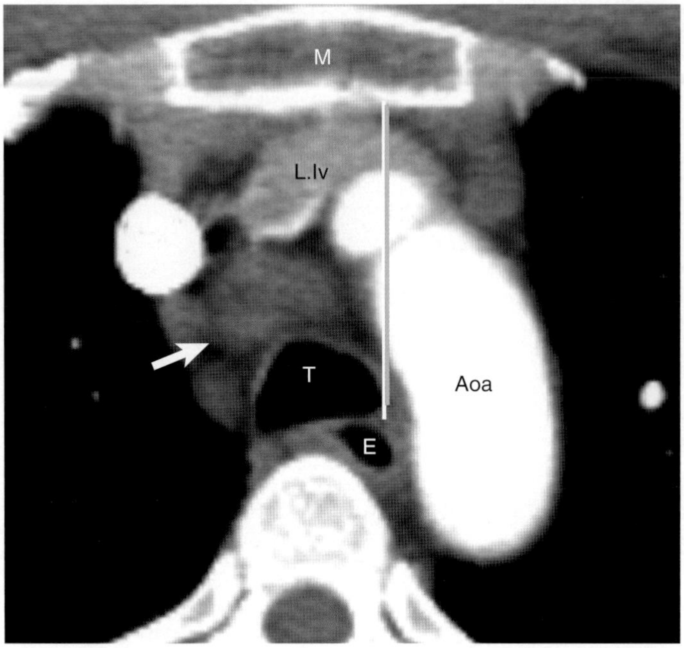

Fig. 1.81 Axial CT image at the level of the aortic arch demonstrates the left lateral wall of the trachea *(green line)* as the anatomic landmark that defines right and left according to the new classification scheme. The *white arrow* points to an enlarged 2R lymph node. *Aoa,* Aortic arch; *E,* esophagus; *L.Iv,* left innominate vein; *T,* trachea. *(Modified from Jawad H, Sirajuddin A, Chung JH. Review of the International Association for the Study of Lung Cancer Lymph Node Classification System: localization of lymph node stations on CT imaging.* Clin Chest Med. *2013;34:353–363; Fig. 5.)*

the long axis. The short-axis diameter above which a node should be considered enlarged depends on its location.[92] Upper paratracheal and left paraesophageal nodes should be considered enlarged when the short-axis diameter is greater than 7 mm. The threshold value for anterior mediastinal nodes is 8 mm; for lower paratracheal and right paraesophageal nodes, 10 mm; and for subcarinal nodes, 11 mm. A more pragmatic and commonly used approach, although less accurate, is to consider all mediastinal lymph nodes as being normal in size unless they exceed 10 mm in short-axis diameter.

Diaphragm. The diaphragm is a musculotendinous structure that separates the thoracic and abdominal cavities. Its costal muscle fibers arise anteriorly from the xiphoid process and around the convexity of the thorax from ribs 7 to 12; posteriorly, the crural fibers arise from the lateral margins of the first, second, and third lumbar vertebrae on the right side and from the first and second lumbar vertebrae on the left. These fibers converge toward the central tendon and are inserted into it nearly perpendicular to its margin.

On CT the diaphragm can be seen only where the upper surface interfaces with the lung and the inferior surface interfaces with intraperitoneal or retroperitoneal fat. Although it is not seen where it abuts structures of similar soft tissue attenuation, such as the liver and spleen, the position of the diaphragm can be readily inferred because at all levels the lungs and pleura lie adjacent and peripheral to it, whereas the abdominal viscera lie central to it (Fig. 1.82).

The posterior or lumbar portion of the diaphragm is well visualized where the fibers arising from the crura and arcuate ligament arch forward to insert into the central tendon

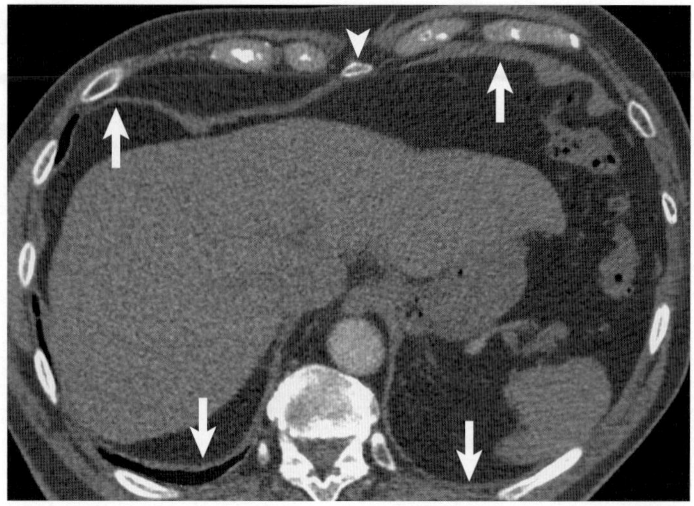

Fig. 1.82 Normal diaphragm. CT scan at the level of the xiphoid *(arrowhead)* shows normal cross-sectional anatomy of the diaphragm *(arrows),* which is outlined by the lung and abdominal fat.

(Fig. 1.83). The right crus is longer than the left and arises from the anterolateral surface of the first, second, and third lumbar vertebrae; the left crus arises from the first and second lumbar vertebrae.[93] Although the most anterior aspect of the crura can be identified in the preaortic position, laterally the crural fibers usually merge smoothly and indistinguishably with the fibers arising from the medial arcuate ligaments. The median arcuate ligament connecting the two crura forms the anterior margin of the aortic hiatus, and the crura form the lateral border. The aorta, azygos, and hemiazygos veins and the thoracic duct course across the diaphragm through this hiatus. The esophageal hiatus lies anterior to the aortic hiatus and contains the esophagus and vagus nerve. The third diaphragmatic hiatus is the hiatus for the IVC. This is the most anterior hiatus, being situated within the central tendon immediately inferior to the right atrium.[94]

The mean thickness of the diaphragm is slightly greater in men than in women and slightly greater on the right than on the left (≈5 mm on the right and 4 mm on the left).[95] Although there is no significant relationship between thickness and age, a generalized increase in diaphragmatic nodularity and irregularity is seen in older individuals. This presumably results from increased laxity of the connective tissues that bind the diaphragm with age.[95] Focal diaphragmatic defects occur mainly in older individuals (70–79 years of age) and are mainly seen in the posterior portion of the diaphragm.[95] Herniation of omental fat through the diaphragmatic defect, often seen in otherwise normal elderly individuals (Fig. 1.84), may cause diagnostic difficulties by mimicking a lung tumor on the radiograph or a traumatic diaphragmatic hernia on CT.[96]

Chest Wall. Because of the characteristic oblique orientation of the ribs, only a small portion of any given rib is seen on a single cross-sectional CT section. The ribs can be well seen, however, on multiplanar and volumetric reconstructions.

Because of the fat planes separating the various muscle groups, CT images allow identification of most individual chest wall muscles. The outer anterior chest wall musculature is composed mainly of the pectoralis major (larger and more superficial) and the pectoralis minor (Fig. 1.85). The serratus anterior is located immediately superficial to the ribs on the lateral aspect of the thorax. The posterior chest wall musculature is more complex

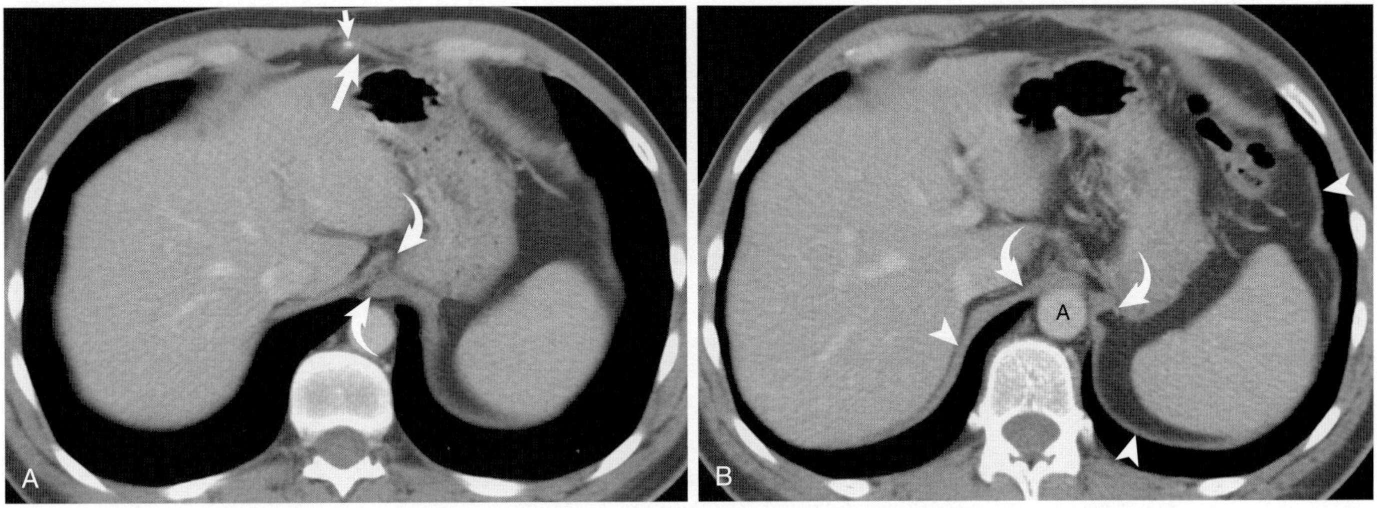

Fig. 1.83 Normal diaphragm. (A) CT scan at the level of the xiphoid *(small straight arrow)* shows the anterior muscle fibers of the left hemidiaphragm *(large straight arrow)* as they insert into the xiphoid. Although there is apparent discontinuity of the anterior fibers of the right hemidiaphragm at this level, there was normal continuity and insertion into the sternum at a slightly more cephalad level. Posteriorly, the diaphragmatic crura *(curved arrows)* can be seen at the level of the esophageal hiatus. (B) CT scan slightly caudal to A shows right and left crura *(curved arrows)* converging immediately anterior to the aorta *(A)*. The right crus is smooth, whereas the left crus has a nodular appearance. This is a normal variant that may be unilateral or bilateral and should not be confused with lymph node enlargement. The diaphragm can be seen only where its upper surface interfaces with the lung and the inferior surface interfaces with intraperitoneal or retroperitoneal fat *(arrowheads)*. Although it is not seen where it abuts structures of similar soft tissue attenuation, such as the liver and spleen, its position can be readily inferred because at all levels the lungs and pleura lie adjacent and peripheral to it, whereas the abdominal viscera lie central to it.

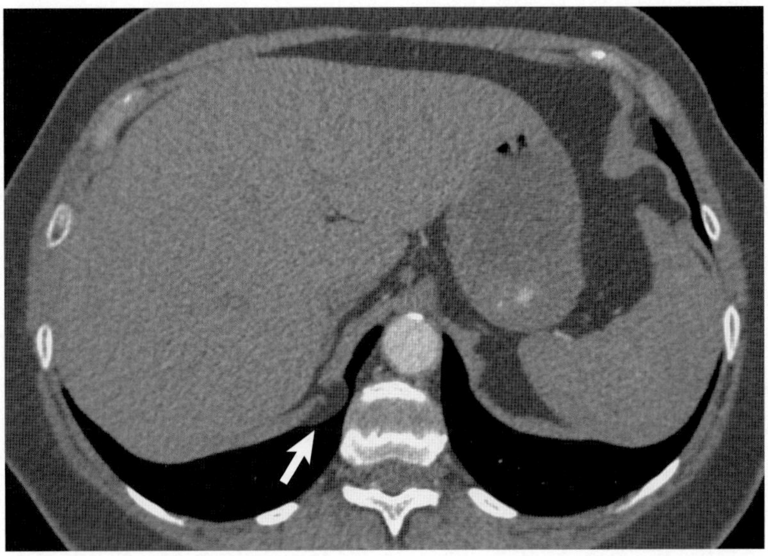

Fig. 1.84 Normal diaphragmatic defect with age. CT scan shows incidental herniation of omental fat *(arrow)* through a small right hemidiaphragmatic defect.

and includes superficial, intermediate, and deep muscles.[97] The first of these muscle groups controls arm motion and includes the trapezius, latissimus dorsi, levator scapulae, and rhomboid muscles. The intermediate muscles are inspiratory and include the superior and inferior serratus posterior muscles. The deep muscles lie adjacent to the vertebral column and regulate its motion.

The external and internal intercostal muscles lie between the ribs and usually cannot be distinguished from each other on CT. The innermost intercostal muscles, together with the parietal pleura and endothoracic fascia, are seen as a 1- to 2-mm thick line or stripe in the interspaces along the anterior and posterior costal pleural surfaces known as the endothoracic fascia, which was described previously.[83]

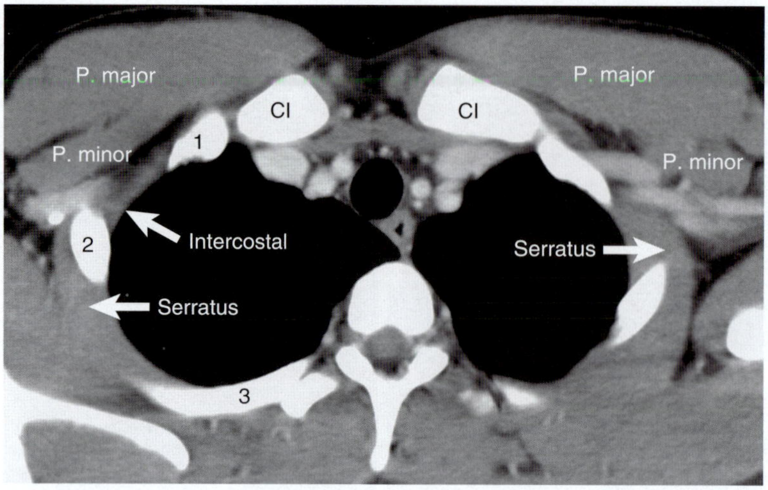

Fig. 1.85 Normal cross-sectional CT anatomy of the chest wall. CT scan at the level of the medial end of the right and left clavicles *(Cl)* shows first *(1)*, second *(2)*, and third *(3)* right ribs and the first and second left ribs. The outer anterior chest wall musculature is composed of the pectoralis major *(P. major)* and the pectoralis minor *(P. minor)* muscles. The internal and external intercostal muscles *(Intercostal)* lie between the ribs, and the serratus anterior *(Serratus)* is located immediately superficial to the ribs on the lateral aspect of the thorax.

SUGGESTED READINGS

Cole TJ, Henry DA, Jolles H, Proto AV. Normal and abnormal vascular structures that simulate neoplasms on chest radiographs: clues to the diagnosis. *Radiographics*. 1995;15:867–891.

Gibbs JM, Chandrasekhar CA, Ferguson EC, Oldham SA. Lines and stripes: where did they go? From conventional radiography to CT. *Radiographics*. 2007;27(1):33–48.

MacMahon H. Digital chest radiography: practical issues. *J Thorac Imaging*. 2003;18:138–147.

Mayo JR, Aldrich J, Müller NL. Radiation exposure at chest CT: a statement of the Fleischner Society. *Radiology*. 2003;228:15–21.

Nason LK, Walker CM, McNeeley MF, Burivong W, Fligner CL, Godwin JD. Imaging of the diaphragm: anatomy and function. *Radiographics*. 2012;32(2):E51–E70.

Schaefer-Prokop C, Uffmann M, Eisenhuber E, Prokop M. Digital radiography of the chest: detector techniques and performance parameters. *J Thorac Imaging*. 2003;18:124–137.

Sussmann AR, Ko JP. Understanding chest radiographic anatomy with MDCT reformations. *Clin Radiol*. 2010;65(2):155–166.

The full reference list for this chapter is available at ExpertConsult.com.

2 Consolidation*

JONATHAN H. CHUNG | CHRISTOPHER M. WALKER

Airspace consolidation is defined as replacement of gas within the airspaces by fluid, protein, cells, or other material. Consolidation is characterized on radiographs and computed tomography (CT) by the presence of one or more fairly homogeneous opacities associated with obscuration of the pulmonary vessels and little or no loss of volume. Homogeneous opacities that do not obscure the underlying pulmonary vessels are referred to as ground-glass opacities. Although ground-glass opacities may result from partial filling of the airspaces, they frequently reflect the presence of predominantly interstitial abnormalities and are therefore discussed in Chapter 5.

The differential diagnosis of airspace consolidation must take into consideration the pattern and distribution of the consolidation, the presence of associated findings such as lymph node enlargement, patient age, recent travel history, and symptoms such as fever or hemoptysis. The differential diagnosis should consider the various substances that may fill the airspaces, namely, water (e.g., edema), blood (e.g., pulmonary hemorrhage), pus (e.g., pneumonia), cells (e.g., adenocarcinoma, lymphoma, organizing pneumonia), fat (e.g., lipoid pneumonia), or protein (e.g., alveolar proteinosis). Although in the vast majority of cases consolidation seen radiologically reflects airspace filling, consolidation may occasionally result from encroachment of the airspaces by extensive interstitial disease, as may be seen, for example, in some patients with sarcoidosis. Furthermore, several conditions classified as interstitial lung diseases, such as acute interstitial pneumonia and organizing pneumonia, have a major airspace component histologically and radiologically. Although it has been suggested that the terms *airspace filling* or *airspace shadowing* are preferable to consolidation,[1] these terms are seldom used in clinical practice.

In most cases the differential diagnosis of parenchymal consolidation is based on a combination of clinical, laboratory, and chest radiographic findings. CT is performed mainly in patients with suspected underlying disease (e.g., endobronchial tumor, bronchiectasis, pulmonary thromboembolism) or complications (e.g., abscess formation, empyema) and in patients with progressive consolidation who are not responding to therapy. In this chapter we consider the radiographic and CT findings and differential diagnosis of consolidation.

Chest Radiograph

Consolidation is characterized on radiographs by the presence of one or more fairly homogeneous opacities associated with obscuration of the pulmonary vessels and little or no loss of volume (Fig. 2.1). The margins of the consolidation are usually poorly defined except where the consolidation abuts the pleura, such as a fissure. The poor definition of the margins results from partial filling of the airspaces as the consolidation spreads to involve adjacent normal lung. Air-containing bronchi (air bronchograms) are frequently visible within the consolidation. Air bronchograms may not be seen if there is complete bronchial obstruction (e.g., distal to a tumor) or filling of the bronchi with blood (e.g., pulmonary infarction) or inflammatory secretions and pus (e.g., bronchopneumonia).

SILHOUETTE SIGN

The mediastinal and diaphragmatic contours are normally seen on the chest radiograph where they abut contiguous air-containing lung. When the consolidation is situated in any portion of lung adjacent to a mediastinal or diaphragmatic border, that border can no longer be seen radiographically. Obscuration of the silhouette of the heart, aorta, or diaphragm by an adjacent opacity is known as the silhouette sign (see Fig. 2.1).[2] The corollary is that an opacity within the lungs that does not obliterate the mediastinal or diaphragmatic contour cannot be situated within lung contiguous to these structures. Although the silhouette sign is most useful in the differentiation of middle lobe and lingular disease (which obscures the silhouette of the adjacent heart) from lower lobe disease (which obscures the silhouette of the adjacent diaphragm), it may also provide precise anatomic information in other sites. Such information includes obliteration of the diaphragm by consolidation in the adjacent lower lobe (Fig. 2.2), obliteration of the aortic arch on the left side by airlessness of the apicoposterior segment of the left upper lobe, obliteration of the ascending arch of the aorta and the superior vena cava by consolidation of the anterior segment of the right upper lobe, and obliteration of the posterior paraspinal line by contiguous airless lung in the left posterior gutter.[2] Assessment of the silhouette sign is reliable only on radiographs performed with proper technique. Underpenetration may result in loss of visibility of a normal border. Another potential pitfall is the presence of pectus excavatum, which may result in obscuration of the right heart border because of replacement of aerated lung along the right cardiac border by the depressed thoracic wall (Fig. 2.3).

FOCAL AND MULTIFOCAL CONSOLIDATION

Consolidation may be focal, patchy, or distributed widely throughout both lungs. Focal consolidation may be segmental or nonsegmental in distribution; occasionally, it involves an entire

*The editors and the publisher would like to thank Drs. Nestor L. Müller and C. Isabela Silva Müller for contributing material on this topic to the prior edition of this work. It has served as the foundation for the current chapter.

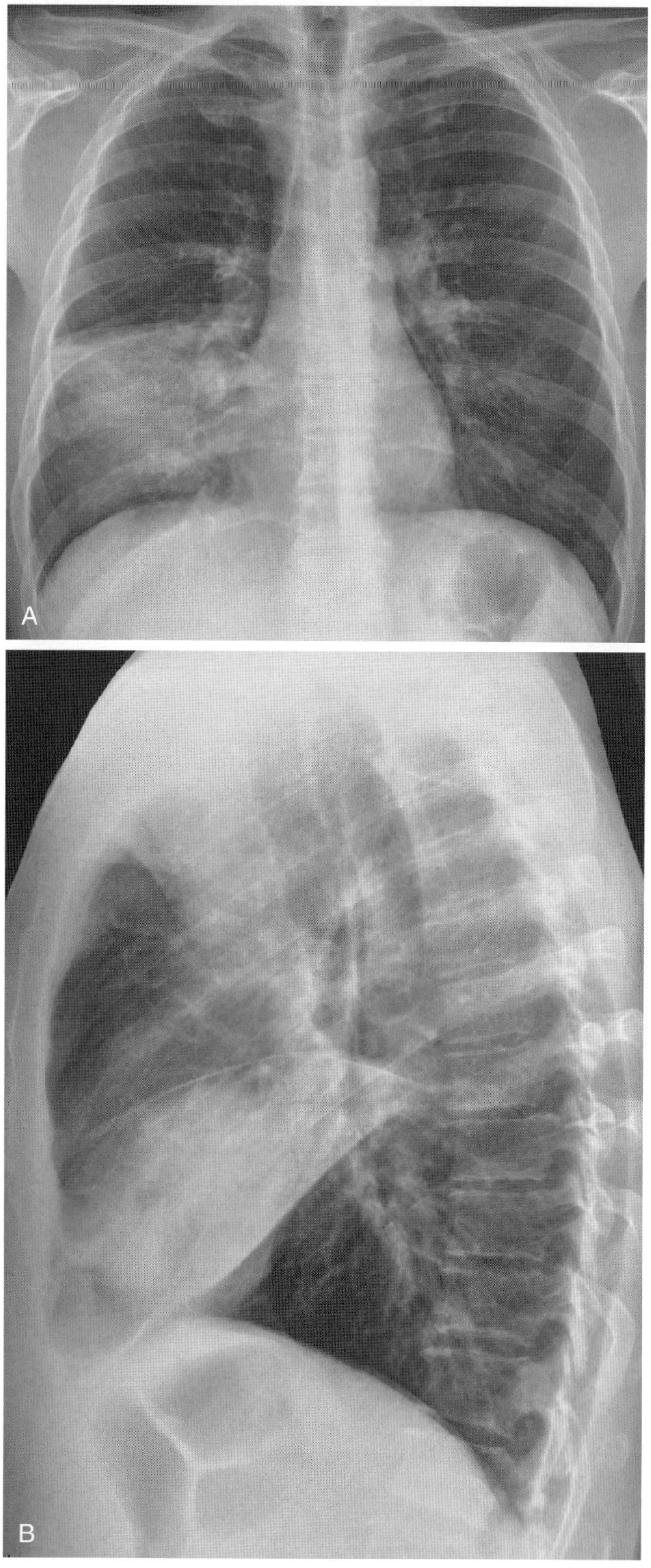

Fig. 2.1 Parenchymal consolidation and silhouette sign from middle lobe pneumonia. (A) Posteroanterior chest radiograph showing consolidation in the right lower lung zone. Note obscuration of the right heart border (silhouette sign), consistent with consolidation in the right middle lobe. The dome of the right hemidiaphragm is clearly seen, consistent with sparing of the basal segments of the lower lobes. (B) Lateral chest radiograph showing dense consolidation in the right middle lobe.

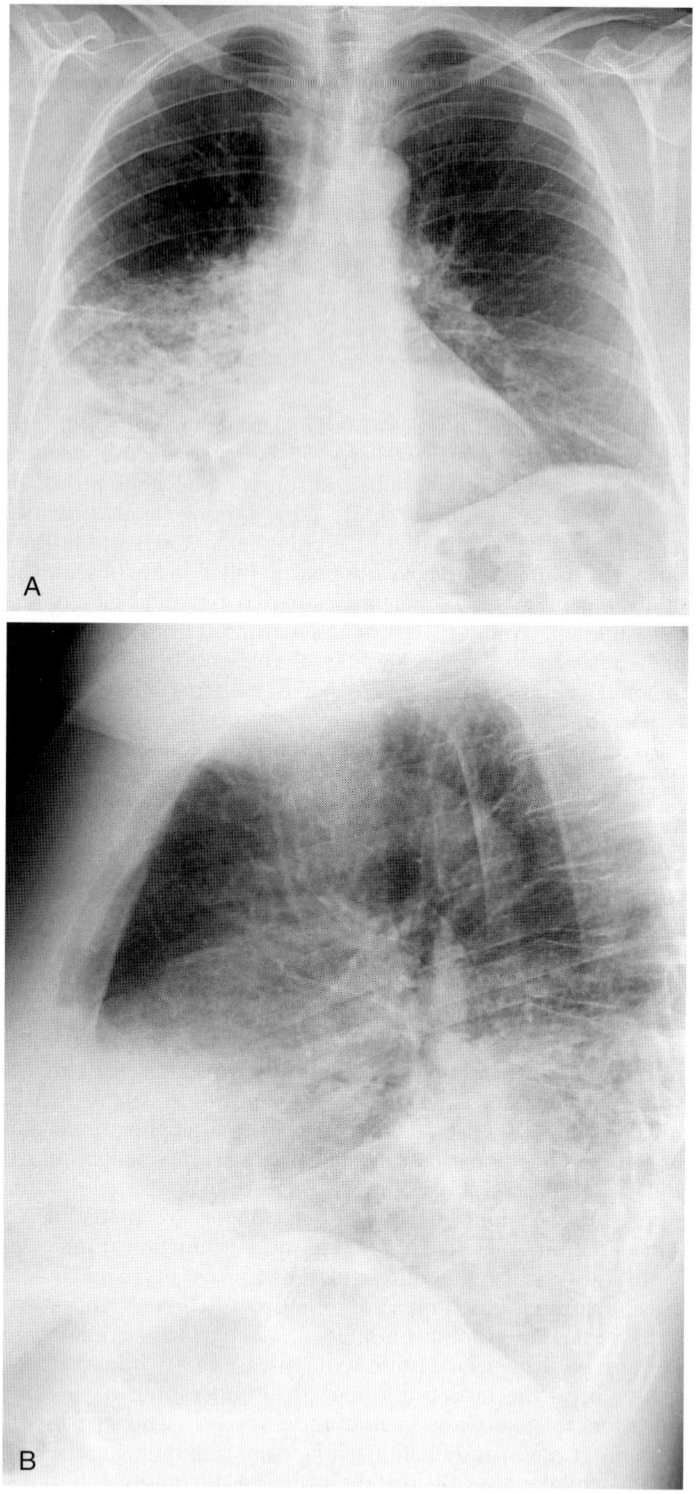

Fig. 2.2 Parenchymal consolidation and the silhouette sign in right middle and lower lobe pneumonia. (A) Posteroanterior chest radiograph showing parenchymal consolidation in the right lower lung zone with obscuration of the silhouettes of the right heart border and the right hemidiaphragm. (B) Lateral chest radiograph confirming the presence of consolidation in the right middle lobe, which accounts for obscuration of the right heart border on the frontal view, and consolidation in the lower lobe, which obscures the silhouette of the right hemidiaphragm. The left hemidiaphragm is clearly seen as outlined by lung on both the frontal and lateral views.

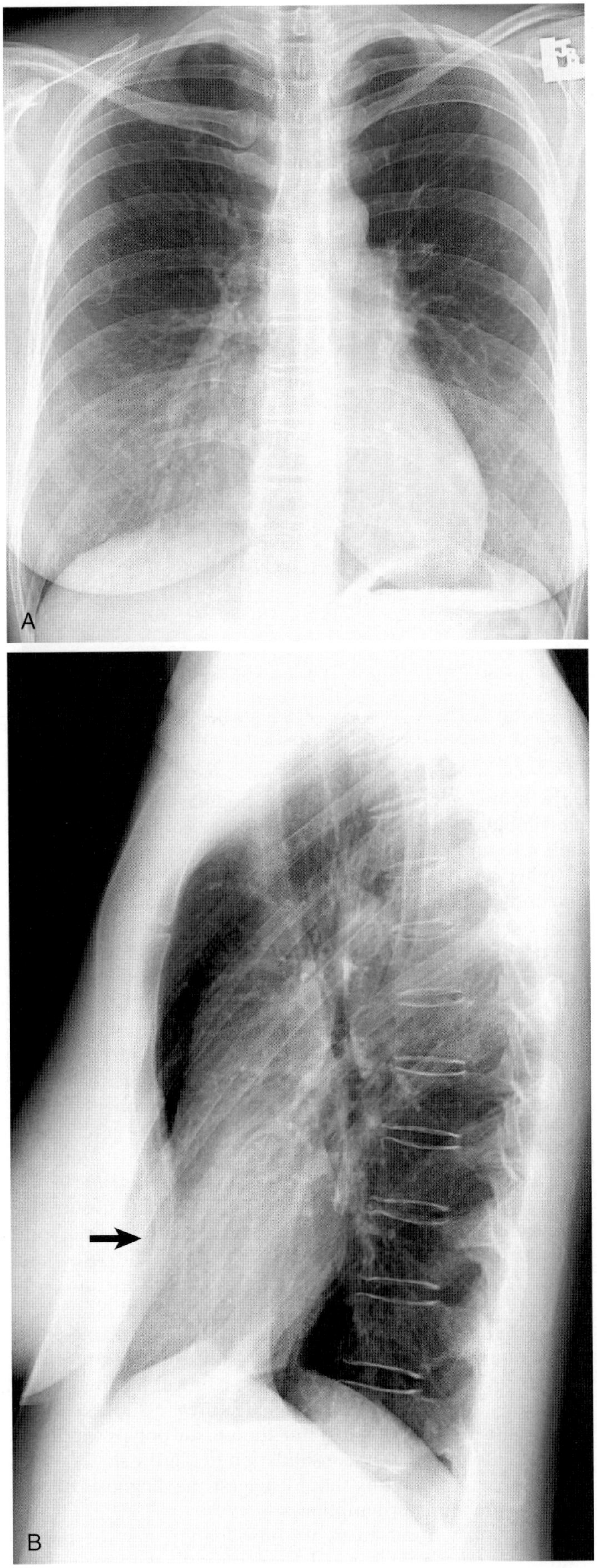

Fig. 2.3 Silhouette sign in pectus excavatum. (A) Posteroanterior chest radiograph showing increased opacity in the right lower lung zone with obscuration of the right heart border. (B) Lateral chest radiograph showing a pectus excavatum deformity *(arrow)*. Ancillary findings of pectus excavatum on the frontal radiograph include increased opacity, shift of the heart to the left, and vertical course of the anterior ribs.

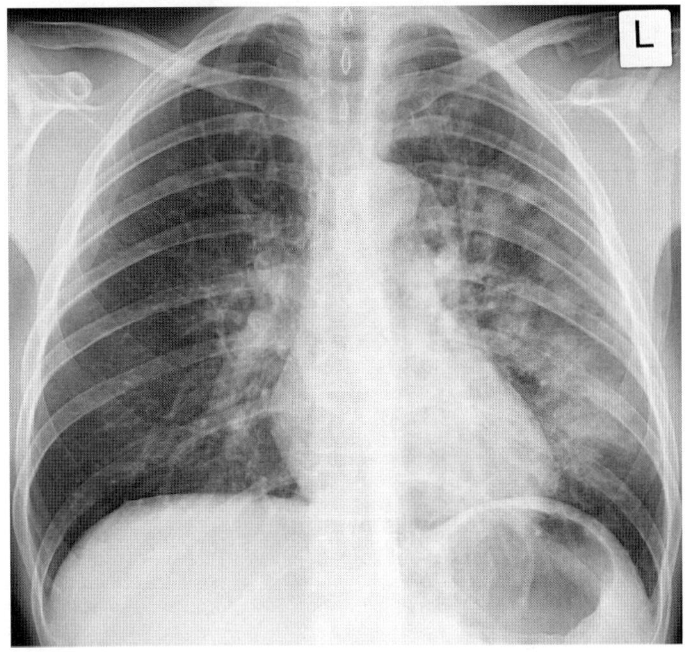

Fig. 2.4 Multifocal consolidation in bronchopneumonia. Posteroanterior chest radiograph showing patchy consolidation in the left upper and lower lobes. Note the inhomogeneous increased opacity of the left heart compared with the region of the right atrium, consistent with consolidation in the retrocardiac region of the left lower lobe.

lobe or lung. Segmental consolidation with or without associated volume loss typically results from endobronchial obstruction (e.g., pulmonary carcinoma) or from pulmonary infarction (e.g., thromboembolism or angioinvasive aspergillosis). A segmental distribution can also be seen after aspiration and with pneumonia caused by *Staphylococcus aureus, Streptococcus pyogenes,* or a variety of gram-negative bacteria. These organisms more commonly cause multifocal or patchy bilateral consolidation (bronchopneumonia), however (Fig. 2.4). A similar distribution may be seen in severe fungal pneumonia, particularly in immunocompromised patients. Lobar (nonsegmental) consolidation is most commonly due to pneumonia, typically secondary to *Streptococcus pneumoniae* or *Klebsiella pneumoniae,* in which case it is associated with air bronchograms and normal (see Fig. 2.1) or, occasionally, increased lung volume (lobar expansion). Lobar expansion results in convexity of the interlobar fissure (bulging fissure sign) (Fig. 2.5). Less commonly, lobar or segmental consolidation is secondary to bronchial obstruction (e.g., pulmonary carcinoma), in which case it is typically associated with atelectasis and a lack of air bronchograms.

Parenchymal consolidation may also result in poorly defined 5- to 10-mm nodular opacities known as airspace nodules (Fig. 2.6). They have been shown to represent involvement of respiratory bronchioles and surrounding alveoli and are particularly common in patients with infectious bronchiolitis and

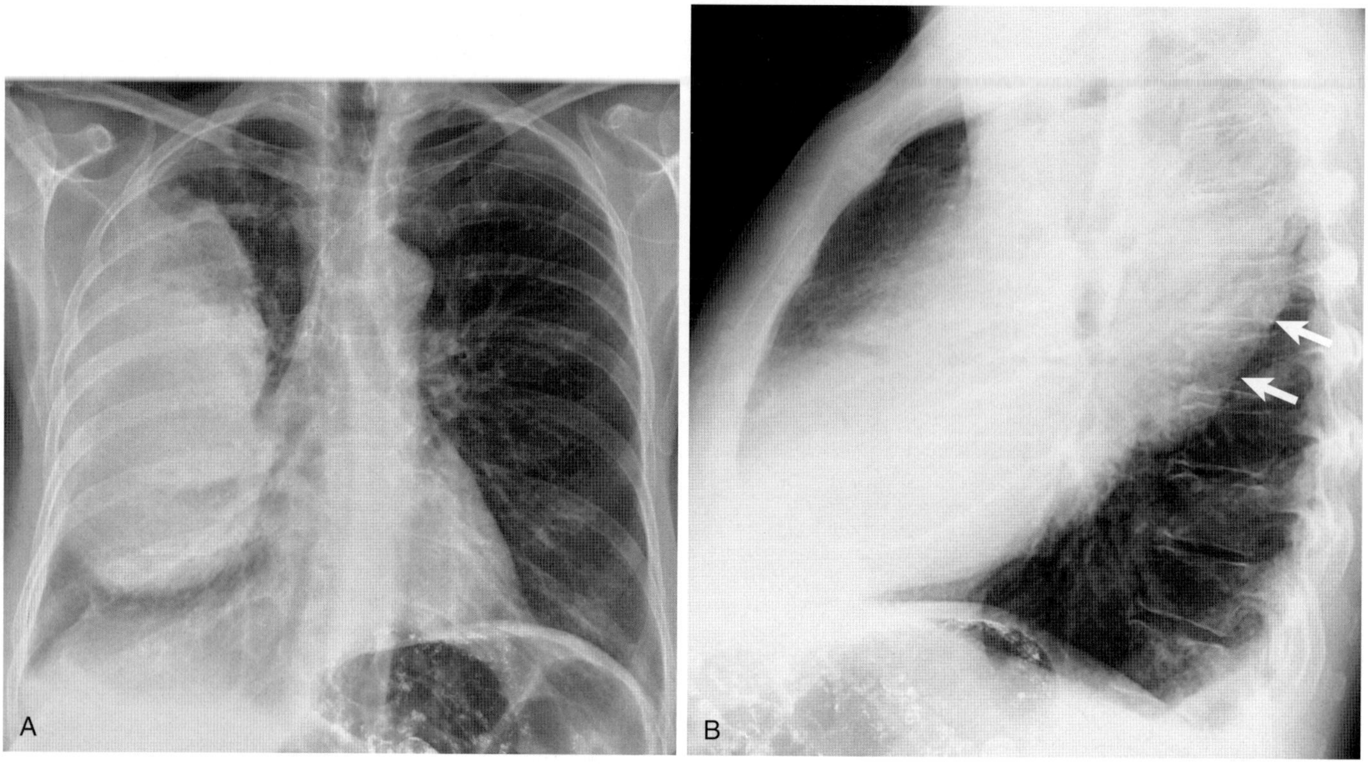

Fig. 2.5 Severe pneumonia with lobar expansion and the "bulging fissure sign." (A) Posteroanterior chest radiograph showing dense consolidation in the right upper and middle lobes. (B) Lateral chest radiograph demonstrating posterior convexity of the major fissure *(arrows)* (bulging fissure sign), characteristic of lobar expansion. Also noted are a small right pleural effusion and residual barium in the splenic flexure.

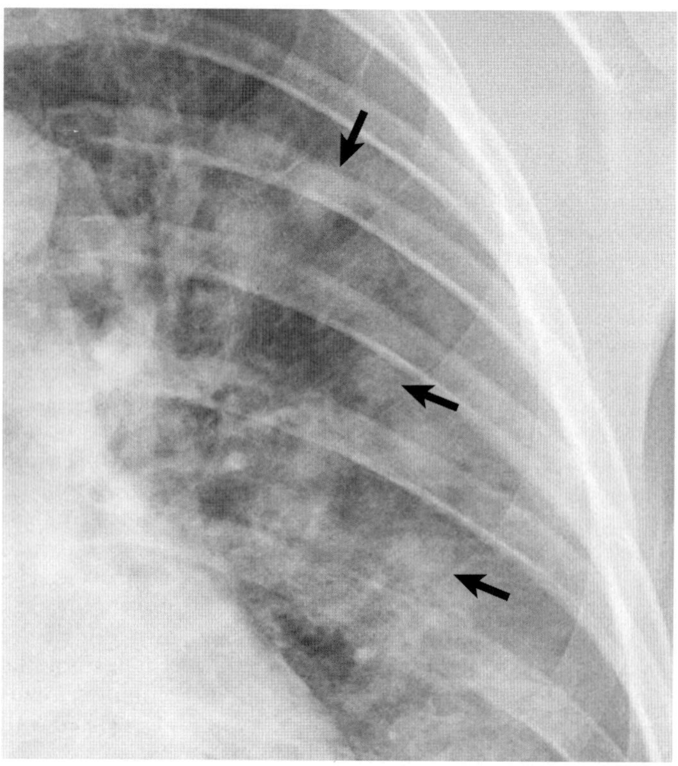

Fig. 2.6 Airspace nodules. A magnified view of the left upper lobe in a patient with bronchopneumonia (same patient as in Fig. 2.4) shows several round opacities with poorly defined margins *(arrows)*. These opacities represent airspace nodules and have been shown to histologically reflect the presence of peribronchiolar (centrilobular) consolidation.

early bronchopneumonia.[3] These nodular opacities have a centrilobular distribution and are more commonly seen on high-resolution CT than on radiographs.

Spherical (round) areas of consolidation may occur in pneumonia ("round pneumonia") (Fig. 2.7), septic embolism, focal organizing pneumonia, atelectasis ("round atelectasis"), and neoplasms (particularly adenocarcinoma and lymphoma), as well as occasionally in the early phases of acute respiratory distress syndrome (ARDS). Round pneumonia occurs much more frequently in children than in adults. Although round pneumonia in adults may result from bacterial infection (particularly *S. pneumoniae* and *Haemophilus influenzae*), most commonly no organism is identified.[4] Occasionally, round pneumonia may result from viral infection (e.g., severe acute respiratory syndrome [SARS] caused by coronavirus) or from Q fever, a zoonosis caused by *Coxiella (Rickettsia) burnetii.*[4,5] Patients with round pneumonia usually have acute to subacute symptoms of community-acquired pneumonia. However, some patients may be asymptomatic or exhibit nonspecific symptoms.[4] Because most cases of round pneumonia are easily treated with antibiotics, this diagnosis should be considered in all patients with a rounded area of consolidation.[6] Focal organizing pneumonia is a distinct entity that may result from incomplete or delayed resolution of bacterial, viral, or fungal pneumonia, or it may be idiopathic. The histologic features include a chronic inflammatory infiltrate and granulation tissue polyps within the airspaces. Round areas of consolidation that grow slowly over a period of several months should suggest the diagnosis of pulmonary carcinoma or lymphoma.

Occasionally, focal areas of consolidation may be due to pulmonary edema. This is seen most typically with myocardial infarction, resulting in papillary muscle dysfunction or rupture.[7] Affected patients have acute mitral regurgitation toward the orifice of the right superior pulmonary vein, causing preferential distribution of edema to the right upper lobe. The consolidation in these patients is typically nonsegmental and may range from mild, predominantly perihilar upper lobe consolidation to dense consolidation involving the entire right upper lobe. Less common causes of focal or multifocal consolidation include pulmonary vein occlusion, edema in patients with extensive pulmonary vascular obstruction (e.g., severe acute pulmonary embolism resulting in edema in regions of lung with less extensive disease), and reexpansion pulmonary edema. Reexpansion pulmonary edema is an iatrogenic complication that occurs after rapid reexpansion of a collapsed lung following drainage of pneumothorax or hydrothorax (Fig. 2.8). It typically appears suddenly within 1 hour after lung reexpansion. The process usually involves the entire reexpanded lung, although on rare occasions only a single lobe or segment may be involved. In most cases reexpansion pulmonary edema increases in severity for 24 to 48 hours and then slowly resolves over the next 5 to 7 days.[8]

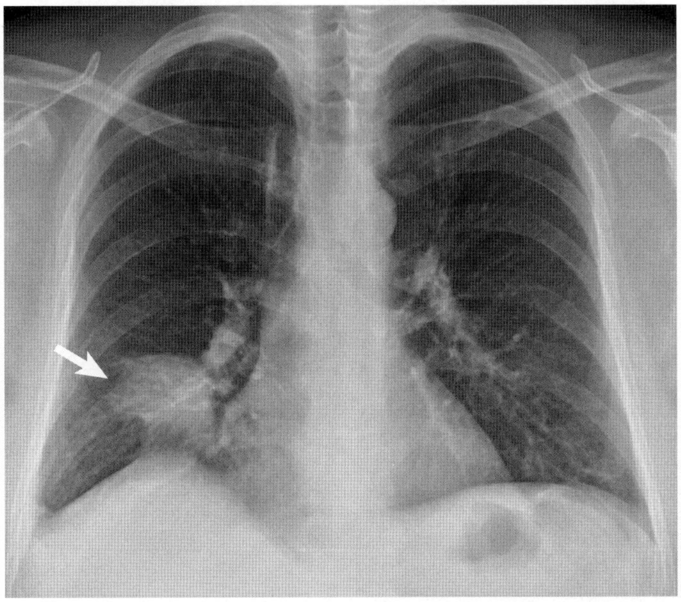

Fig. 2.7 Round pneumonia. Posteroanterior chest radiograph showing a round mass-like area of consolidation *(arrow)* in the right middle lobe.

Hemorrhage should be considered, particularly in patients with hemoptysis and in those with blunt chest trauma. Causes of focal pulmonary hemorrhage and hemoptysis include pulmonary carcinoma, bronchiectasis, pulmonary embolism, and infarction. Causes of multifocal or diffuse areas of hemorrhage include granulomatosis with polyangiitis (formerly Wegener granulomatosis), Goodpasture syndrome, microscopic polyangiitis, and systemic lupus erythematosus (Fig. 2.9).

Multifocal consolidation is most commonly due to viral, bacterial, or fungal bronchopneumonia (see Fig. 2.4). The consolidation may be unilateral or bilateral.

Chronic conditions typically associated with multifocal consolidation include simple pulmonary eosinophilia (Loeffler syndrome), chronic eosinophilic pneumonia, and organizing pneumonia. Simple pulmonary eosinophilia is characterized by blood eosinophilia and transient and migratory areas of consolidation that typically clear spontaneously within 1 month.[9] Organizing pneumonia is most frequently manifested as patchy nonsegmental unilateral or bilateral areas of consolidation (Fig. 2.10).[10,11] The consolidation may involve any lung zone but

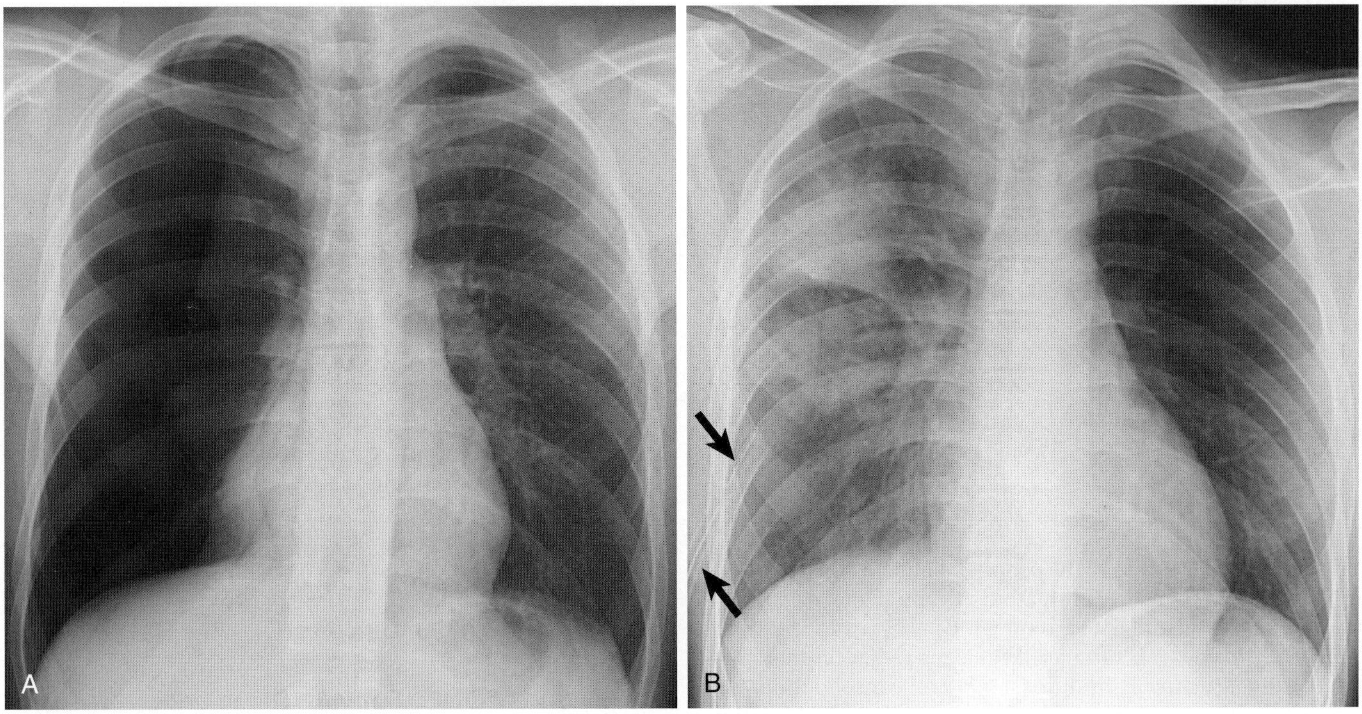

Fig. 2.8 Reexpansion pulmonary edema. (A) Posteroanterior chest radiograph showing a large right pneumothorax. (B) A chest radiograph 36 hours after insertion of a right chest tube *(arrows)* shows areas of consolidation and extensive hazy areas of increased opacity (ground-glass opacities) in the right lung consistent with reexpansion pulmonary edema.

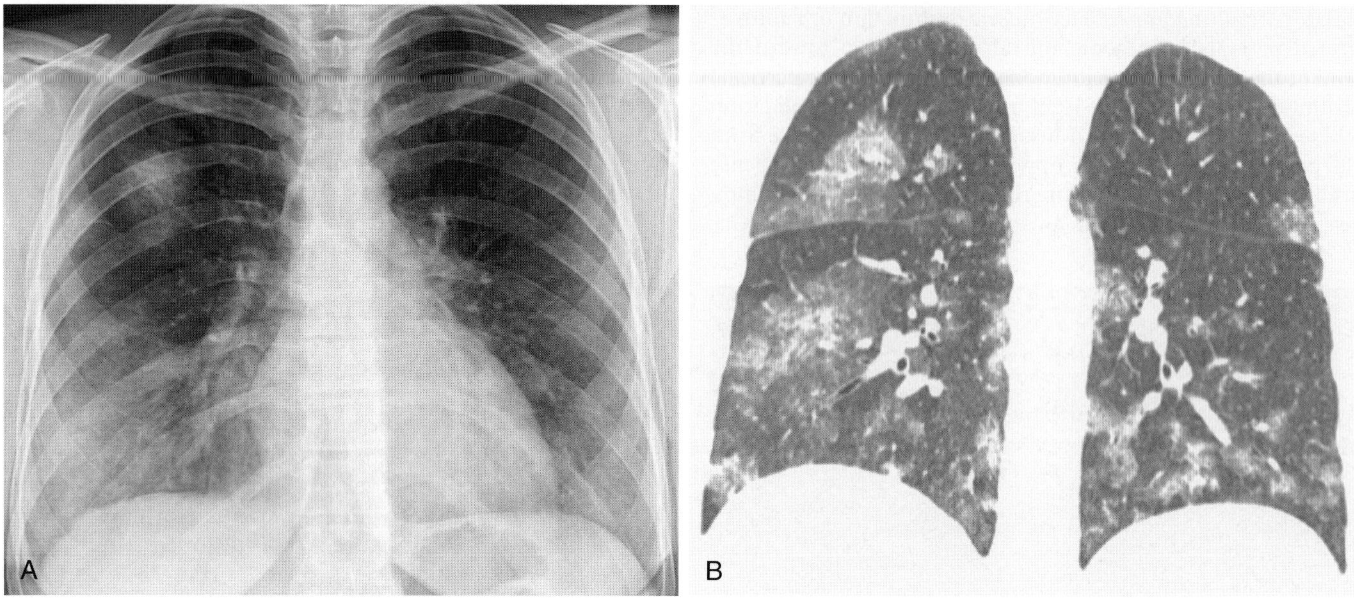

Fig. 2.9 Multifocal consolidation in diffuse pulmonary hemorrhage in granulomatosis with polyangiitis. (A) Posteroanterior chest radiograph showing dense consolidation in the right upper lobe and poorly defined areas of consolidation and ground-glass opacities in the lower lung zones. (B) Coronal reformatted CT image demonstrating multifocal areas of consolidation and ground-glass opacities.

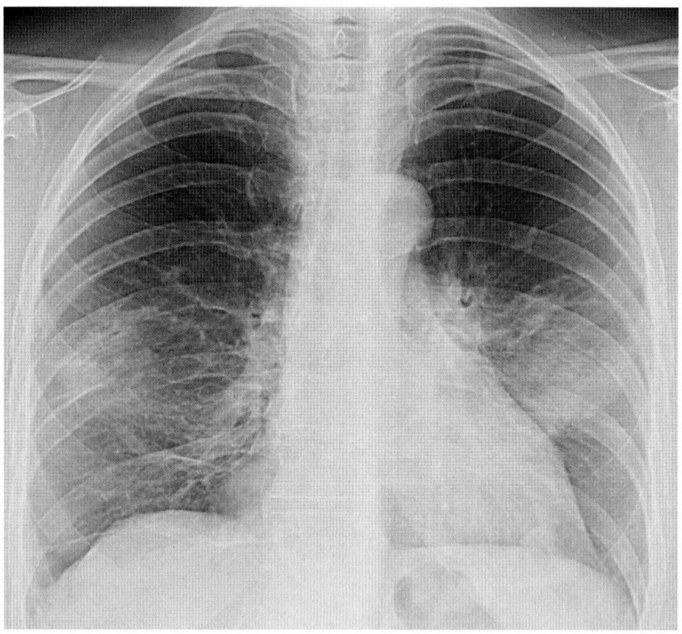

Fig. 2.10 Cryptogenic organizing pneumonia. A posteroanterior chest radiograph shows patchy bilateral areas of consolidation and ground-glass opacities.

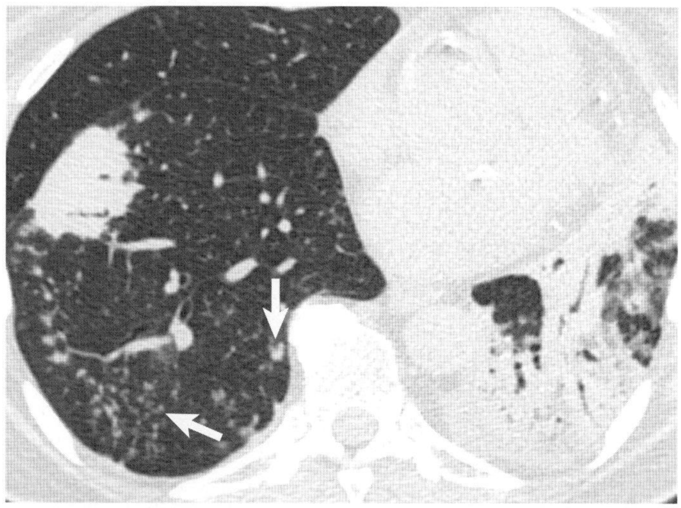

Fig. 2.11 Adenocarcinoma. Axial image from noncontrast chest CT shows left greater than right multifocal lung consolidation with air bronchograms. Mild centrilobular and tree-in-bud nodularity *(arrows)* in the right lower lobe is consistent with aerogenous spread of cancer.

tends to be most extensive in the peripheral lung regions. Organizing pneumonia may be idiopathic (cryptogenic organizing pneumonia) or secondary to a known cause such as infection, drug reaction, collagen vascular disease, or radiation therapy.

Occasionally, chronic multifocal bilateral consolidation may be due to adenocarcinoma or lymphoma.[12] The consolidation in adenocarcinoma may be focal or multifocal and confluent and is usually associated with air bronchograms (Fig. 2.11). The consolidation results from tumor growth along the alveolar walls combined with secretion of mucin. Occasionally, production of copious amounts of mucin may result in expansion of the lobe and bulging of the interlobar fissures (bulging fissure sign).[12] Pulmonary lymphoma may result in single or multiple mass-like areas of consolidation or, less commonly, extensive confluent areas of consolidation (Fig. 2.12).[13,14] The areas of consolidation usually contain air bronchograms.

EXTENSIVE CONFLUENT AND DIFFUSE CONSOLIDATION

A number of conditions may result in extensive or diffuse bilateral consolidation. Because the radiologic appearance is often similar

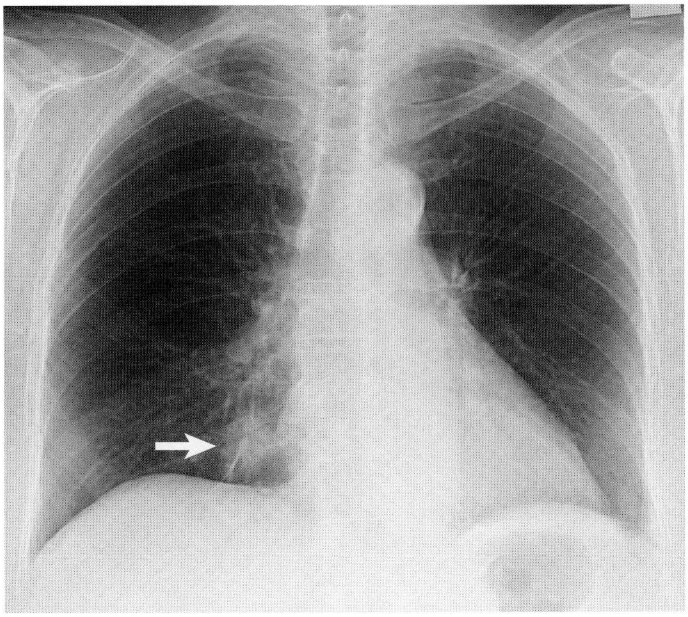

Fig. 2.12 Primary pulmonary lymphocytic MALT lymphoma of the lung. Posteroanterior chest radiograph showing focal consolidation in the right lower lung zone *(arrow)*. Note the focal obliteration of the right heart border (silhouette sign) at the level of the consolidation indicating origin in the middle lobe.

KEY POINTS: CAUSES OF FOCAL OR MULTIFOCAL AIRSPACE CONSOLIDATION

ACUTE

- Pneumonia
  - Bacteria, mycobacteria, fungi, viruses
  - Aspiration
- Hemorrhage
  - Secondary to focal disease such as bronchiectasis or carcinoma
  - Contusion (trauma)
  - Vasculitis
  - Infarct (pulmonary thromboembolism)
- Pulmonary edema
  - Reexpansion edema
  - Papillary muscle dysfunction (right upper lobe edema)
  - Blood flow redistribution in severe pulmonary thromboembolism
  - Pulmonary vein occlusion

CHRONIC

- Pneumonia
- Eosinophilic pneumonia
- Organizing pneumonia
- Lipoid pneumonia
- Neoplasm
  - Postobstructive pneumonitis distal to endobronchial carcinoma
  - Adenocarcinoma, lymphoma

regardless of cause, it is essential to know the clinical history (e.g., trauma, known systemic disease), presence or absence of fever, and immune status of the patient.

Extensive or diffuse bilateral consolidation is seen most commonly in patients with hydrostatic pulmonary edema, permeability edema such as ARDS, diffuse pulmonary hemorrhage, and *Pneumocystis* pneumonia. In hydrostatic pulmonary edema the consolidation tends to involve mainly the perihilar regions (known as a *butterfly* or *batwing* distribution) and is commonly associated with thickening of the interlobular septa (septal lines) and cardiomegaly (Fig. 2.13). Other conditions that may result in a predominantly perihilar distribution include diffuse pulmonary hemorrhage, inhalational lung injury, alveolar proteinosis, and *Pneumocystis jirovecii* pneumonia (Fig. 2.14). *P. jirovecii* pneumonia, seen most commonly in patients with AIDS, typically progresses radiographically from a subtle perihilar haze to diffuse bilateral consolidation. Pleural effusions are typically absent.[15,16]

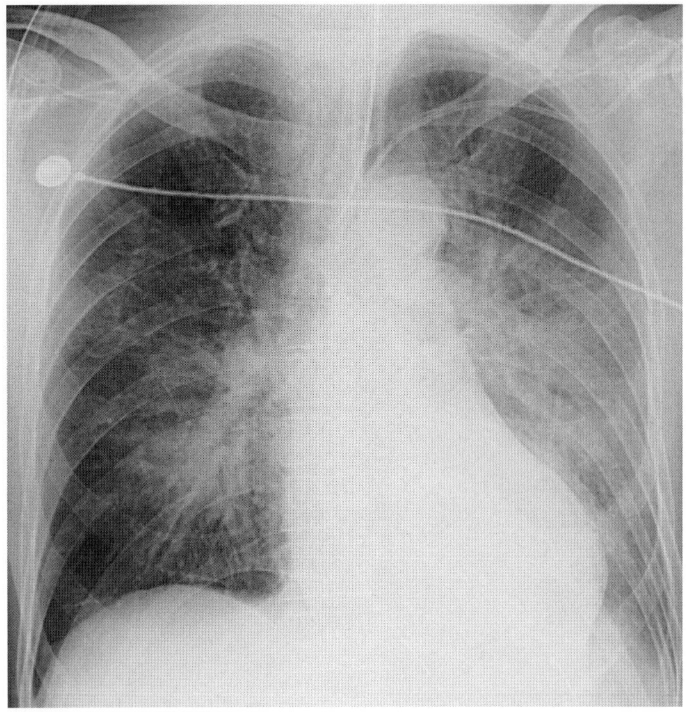

Fig. 2.13 Hydrostatic pulmonary edema from left heart failure. A posteroanterior chest radiograph shows extensive consolidation with relative sparing of the subpleural regions. A central venous catheter and an endotracheal tube are in place.

The consolidation in ARDS may initially be patchy but tends to become rapidly confluent and diffuse (Fig. 2.15).[8] Air bronchograms are commonly seen. Septal lines are seldom evident on the radiograph unless the patient has superimposed hydrostatic pulmonary edema. Common causes of ARDS include shock, trauma, sepsis, pancreatitis, pneumonia, and drug reactions. A similar pattern may be seen in acute interstitial pneumonia, which is essentially an idiopathic form of ARDS.

Diffuse pulmonary hemorrhage is most commonly seen in patients with systemic vasculitis, including Goodpasture syndrome, granulomatosis with polyangiitis, and microscopic polyangiitis. Diffuse hemorrhage can also be seen in some collagen vascular diseases, particularly systemic lupus erythematosus. Diffuse pulmonary hemorrhage may result in patchy or confluent bilateral areas of consolidation that tends to involve mainly the middle and lower lung zones (Fig. 2.16; see also Fig. 2.9).[17] The consolidation may have a predominantly perihilar distribution and typically spares the lung apices and the region of the costophrenic angles.[17]

The characteristic radiologic pattern of chronic eosinophilic pneumonia consists of bilateral areas of consolidation predominantly involving the outer thirds of the lungs ("reverse

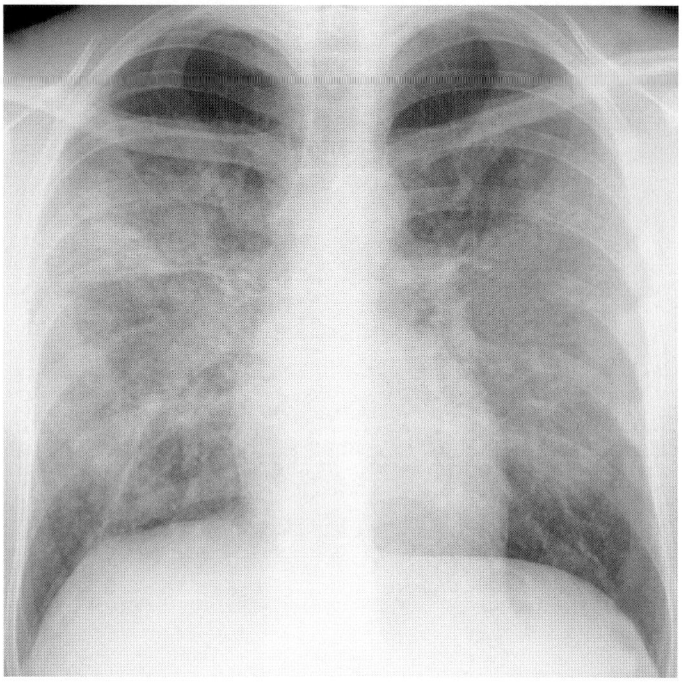

Fig. 2.14 *Pneumocystis jirovecii* pneumonia in the setting of AIDS. A posteroanterior chest radiograph shows bilateral areas of consolidation and ground-glass opacities in a predominantly perihilar distribution.

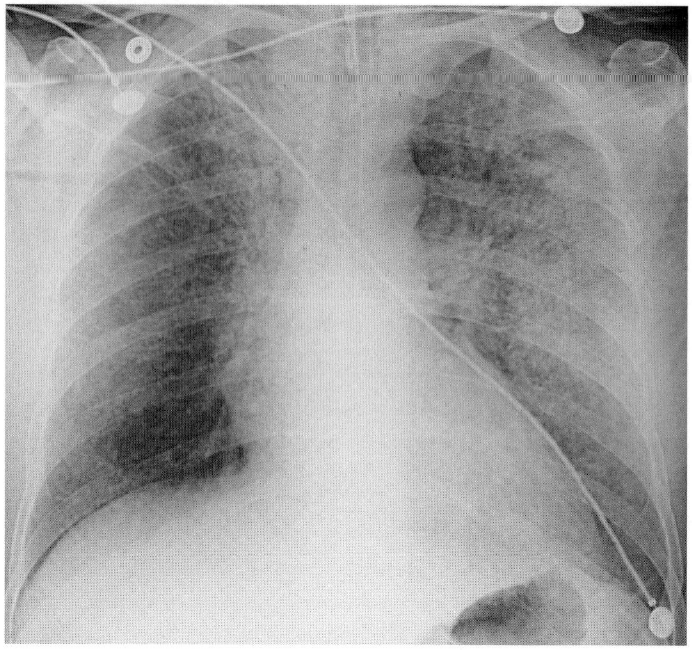

Fig. 2.16 Diffuse pulmonary hemorrhage in granulomatosis with polyangiitis. An anteroposterior chest radiograph shows extensive bilateral areas of consolidation and ground-glass opacities. Endotracheal and nasogastric tubes are in place.

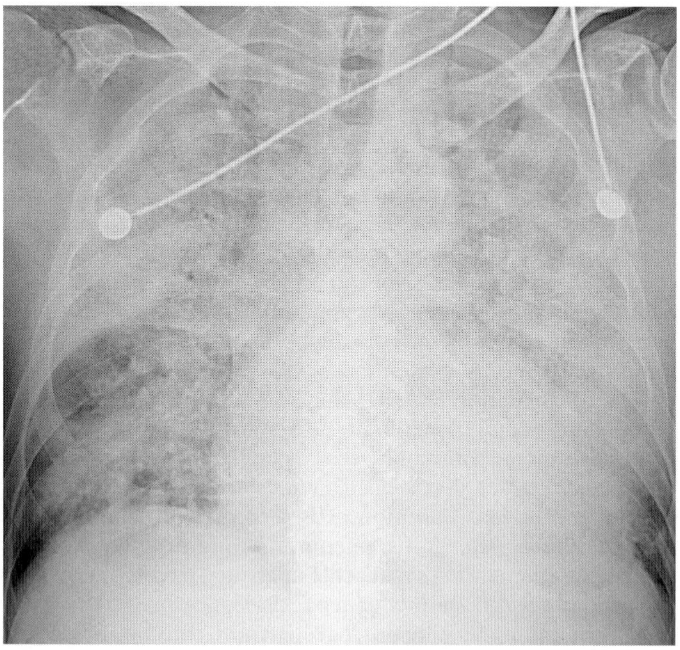

Fig. 2.15 Acute respiratory distress syndrome. An anteroposterior chest radiograph shows extensive bilateral areas of consolidation.

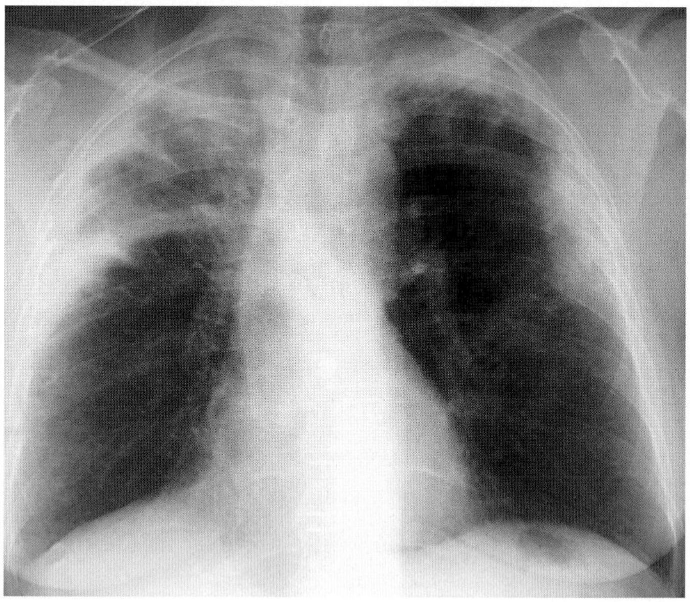

Fig. 2.17 Chronic eosinophilic pneumonia. A posteroanterior chest radiograph shows bilateral areas of consolidation involving the peripheral regions of the upper and middle lung zones.

pulmonary edema pattern") and typically involving mainly the upper lobes (Fig. 2.17).[18] Approximately 50% of patients have a history of atopy, most often asthma, and most have peripheral eosinophilia.[18] Organizing pneumonia is usually multifocal (Fig. 2.18; see also Fig. 2.10), but occasionally it may be diffuse. In approximately 60% of patients, organizing pneumonia has a predominantly peripheral distribution similar to chronic eosinophilic pneumonia or a peribronchial distribution (or both). This distribution is more readily seen on CT than on radiographs.[19]

Diffuse bilateral consolidation on the chest radiograph may also result from alveolar proteinosis (Fig. 2.19). The consolidation often has a slightly granular appearance. High-resolution CT typically shows bilateral ground-glass opacities with superimposed interlobular septal thickening and intralobular lines, a pattern known as "crazy-paving" (see Chapter 5).

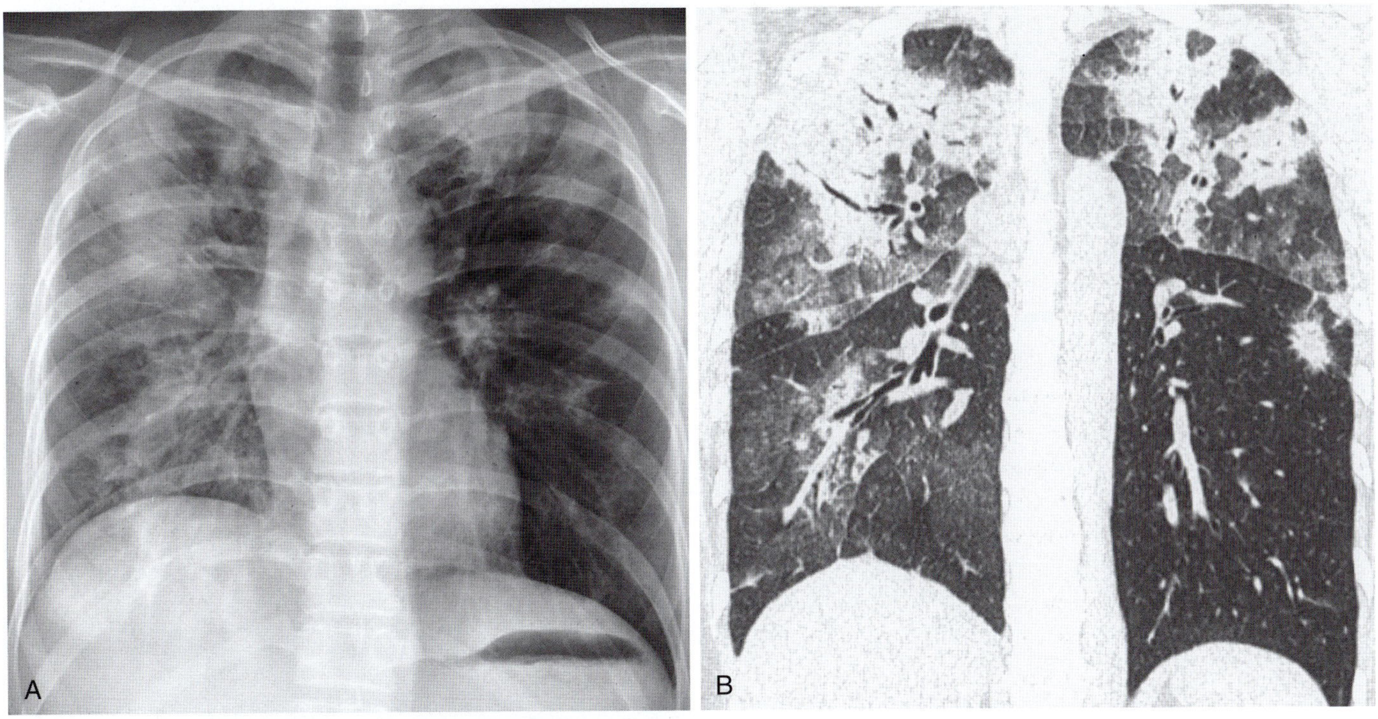

Fig. 2.18 Cryptogenic organizing pneumonia. (A) Posteroanterior chest radiograph showing bilateral multifocal and confluent consolidation involving mainly the upper lobes. (B) A coronal reformatted CT image shows a predominant peribronchial and peripheral distribution of the consolidation.

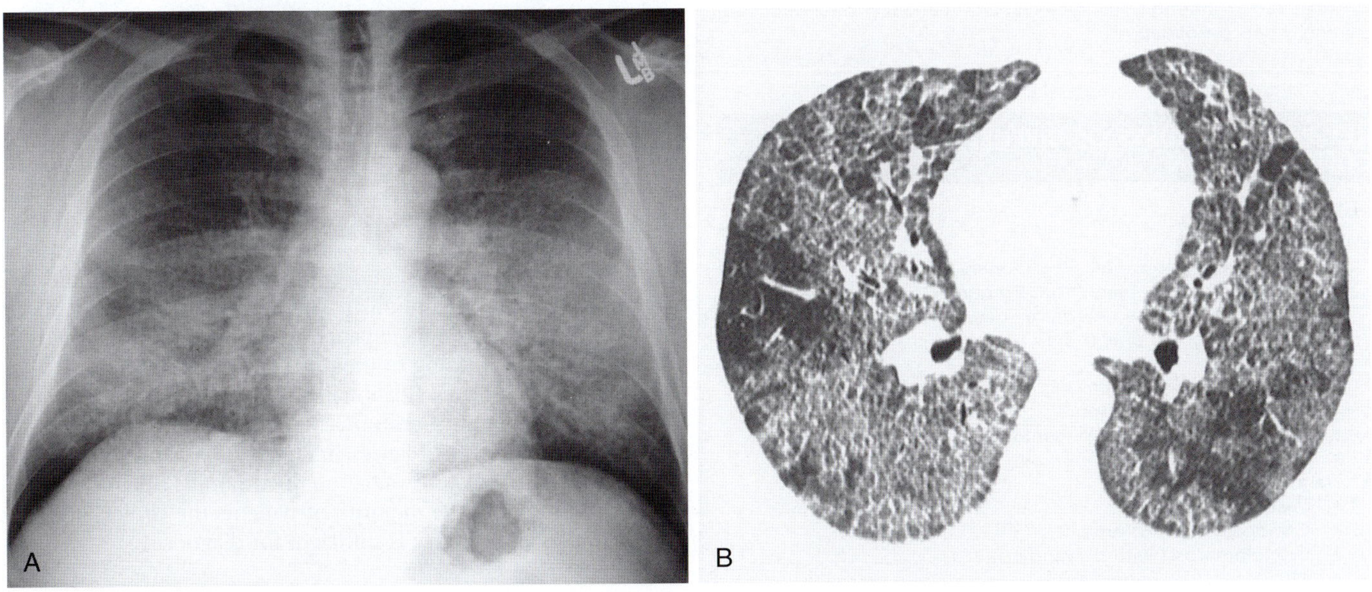

Fig. 2.19 Alveolar proteinosis. (A) Posteroanterior chest radiograph showing extensive bilateral areas of consolidation and ground-glass opacities with relative sparing of the lung apices and bases. (B) High-resolution CT scan demonstrating bilateral ground-glass opacities with superimposed smooth septal lines and intralobular lines resulting in a pattern known as "crazy-paving."

Computed Tomography

Consolidation on CT is defined as a homogeneous increase in pulmonary parenchymal attenuation that obscures the margins of vessels and airway walls.[1] An air bronchogram is frequently present. A homogeneous increase in opacity without obscuration of vessels and airway walls is referred to as ground-glass opacity.

In most patients with consolidation, the findings are readily apparent on radiographs, and CT adds little additional information. However, CT may be helpful in the differential diagnosis, in the detection of underlying disease, and in the evaluation of complications. For example, CT frequently demonstrates localized collections of fat in patients with patchy or diffuse consolidation caused by lipoid pneumonia (Fig. 2.20).[21] It may also be helpful in patients with suspected amiodarone lung by demonstrating the characteristic increased attenuation caused by accumulation of this iodinated agent within the lung parenchyma.[22] The characteristic peripheral distribution of chronic eosinophilic pneumonia is evident on

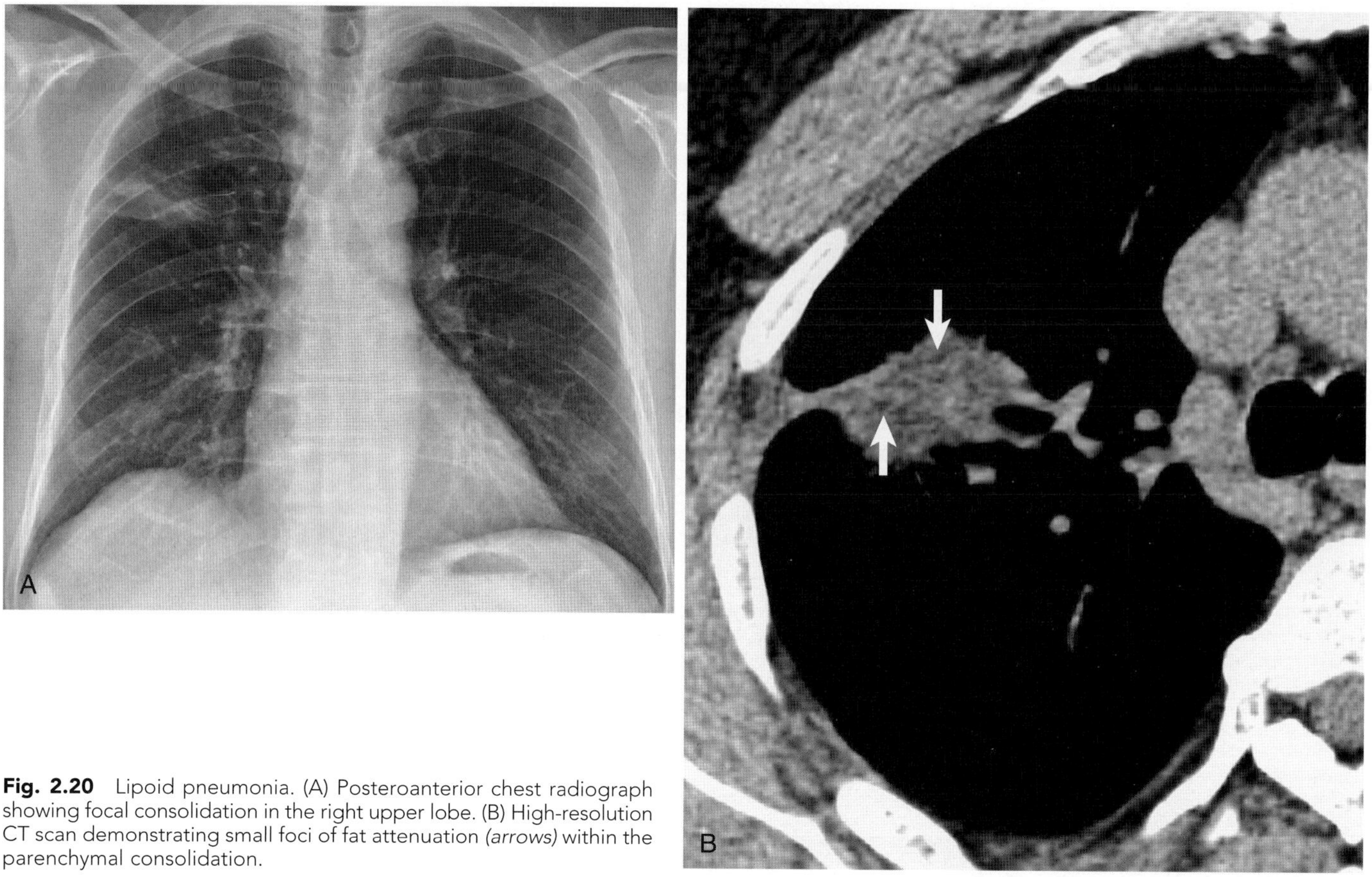

Fig. 2.20 Lipoid pneumonia. (A) Posteroanterior chest radiograph showing focal consolidation in the right upper lobe. (B) High-resolution CT scan demonstrating small foci of fat attenuation *(arrows)* within the parenchymal consolidation.

KEY POINTS: CAUSES OF DIFFUSE PARENCHYMAL CONSOLIDATION

ACUTE

- Edema
  - Hydrostatic (cardiogenic) pulmonary edema
  - Increased-permeability (noncardiogenic) pulmonary edema
  - Any cause of acute respiratory distress syndrome
  - Acute interstitial pneumonia
- Pneumonia
  - Severe bacterial pneumonia
  - Influenza virus pneumonia
  - *Pneumocystis jirovecii* pneumonia
  - Cytomegalovirus pneumonia
- Hemorrhage
  - Vasculitis
  - Goodpasture syndrome
  - Granulomatosis with polyangiitis
  - Microscopic polyangiitis
  - Systemic lupus erythematosus
  - Bleeding diathesis
  - Chemotherapy
  - Anticoagulation

CHRONIC

- Pneumonia
  - Chronic eosinophilic pneumonia
  - Organizing pneumonia
  - Lipoid pneumonia
- Neoplasm
  - Primary or metastatic adenocarcinoma, lymphoma
- Metabolic disease
  - Pulmonary alveolar proteinosis

radiographs in only about 50% of cases but is seen on CT in virtually all cases.[23,24] High-resolution CT may also demonstrate parenchymal abnormalities, including small foci of consolidation in patients with apparently normal radiographs.[25,26] In addition, CT may be helpful in the assessment of patients with suspected underlying disease (e.g., endobronchial tumor, bronchiectasis, pulmonary thromboembolism) or complications (e.g., abscess formation, empyema) and in patients with progressive consolidation who are not responding to therapy.

Acute causes of consolidation include bacterial, tuberculous, viral, and fungal pneumonia; pulmonary edema; ARDS; and pulmonary hemorrhage. Chronic causes include organizing pneumonia, eosinophilic lung disease, radiation pneumonitis, adenocarcinoma, and lymphoma. In the majority of patients the clinical and chest radiographic appearance is sufficient for diagnosis.

ACUTE CAUSES OF PARENCHYMAL CONSOLIDATION

Pneumonia

Pneumonia may result in two main patterns: lobar (nonsegmental) consolidation and segmental consolidation (bronchopneumonia). Lobar pneumonia is characterized by the presence of homogeneous airspace consolidation involving adjacent segments of a lobe (Fig. 2.21). The consolidation tends to occur initially in the periphery of the lung beneath the visceral pleura and to spread across segmental boundaries; it may eventually involve the entire lobe. The bronchi usually remain patent, which results in air bronchograms within the areas of consolidation. On high-resolution CT, areas of ground-glass opacity denoting incomplete

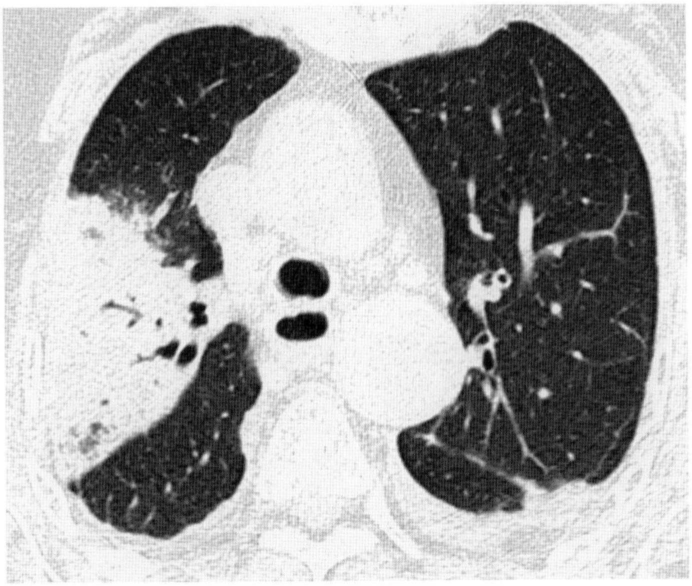

Fig. 2.21 Lobar pneumonia. Axial CT scan showing consolidation in the right upper lobe, which contains several air bronchograms. Incidental note is made of esophageal dilation, aortic dilation, and a small left pleural effusion.

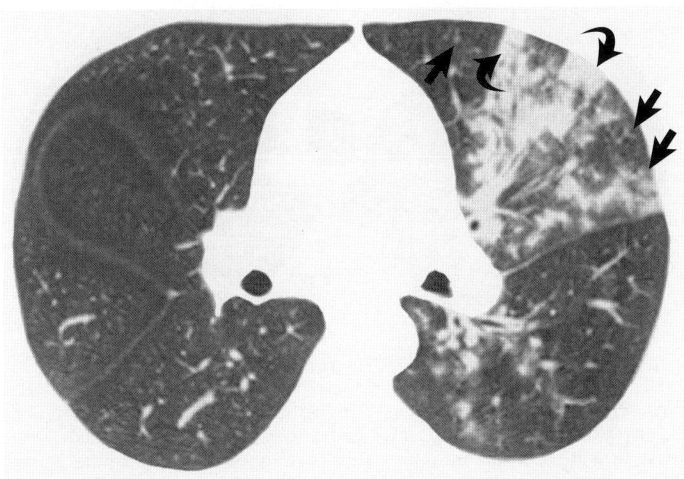

Fig. 2.22 Bronchopneumonia from *Mycoplasma pneumoniae*. A high-resolution CT scan shows centrilobular nodular and branching opacities *(straight arrows)* and lobular areas of consolidation *(curved arrows)* in the lingula and left lower lobe. *(Courtesy Dr. Atsushi Nambu, Department of Radiology, University of Yamanashi, Japan.)*

filling of alveoli can often be seen adjacent to the airspace consolidation.[27,28] The vast majority of cases of lobar pneumonia are caused by bacteria, most commonly *S. pneumoniae* and less commonly *K. pneumoniae, Legionella pneumophila, H. influenzae,* and *Mycobacterium tuberculosis.*[29]

The characteristic CT manifestations of bronchopneumonia consist of multifocal lobular areas of consolidation, centrilobular nodules and branching linear opacities, and airspace nodules (Fig. 2.22).[27,28] The areas of consolidation tend to involve entire pulmonary lobules and to spare adjacent lobules (lobular distribution). As the consolidation progresses, it becomes confluent and may involve entire segments or lobes. The centrilobular nodular and branching linear opacities result in an appearance resembling a tree in bud ("tree-in-bud" pattern) and reflect the presence of

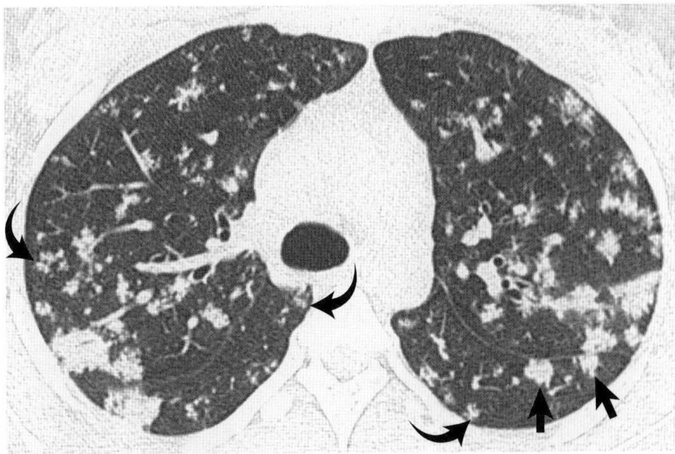

Fig. 2.23 Tree-in-bud pattern and airspace nodules in tuberculosis. A high-resolution CT image shows branching centrilobular nodular opacities ("tree-in-bud" pattern) *(curved arrows)*, airspace nodules 4–10 mm in diameter *(straight arrows)*, and focal areas of consolidation.

inflammatory exudate in the lumen and walls of membranous and respiratory bronchioles and the lung parenchyma immediately adjacent to them (Fig. 2.23).[29] The airspace nodules typically measure 4 to 10 mm in diameter and have poorly defined margins. A large number of organisms may result in bronchopneumonia, including various bacteria (most commonly *S. aureus, H. influenzae,* and *Pseudomonas aeruginosa*), fungi, viruses, and *Mycoplasma pneumoniae.*[29,30]

CT is particularly helpful in the detection, differential diagnosis, and management of immunocompromised patients with pulmonary complications.[25,31,32] Focal areas of consolidation secondary to infection in immunocompromised AIDS and non-AIDS patients are most commonly due to bacterial pneumonia.[33] Fungal infection needs to be considered, particularly in neutropenic patients with hematologic malignancies.[32]

Pulmonary Edema and Acute Respiratory Distress Syndrome

The most common manifestations of hydrostatic pulmonary edema on CT are septal thickening and ground-glass opacities.[34] The edema tends to have a perihilar and gravitational distribution (Fig. 2.24). Areas of consolidation involving mainly the dependent lung regions may be present in patients with severe edema. Commonly associated findings include small pleural effusions and cardiomegaly.

ARDS is manifested on CT by the presence of bilateral consolidation or ground-glass opacities (or both) that may be patchy or diffuse and tend to involve mainly the dependent lung regions (Fig. 2.25).[35,36] Septal thickening may be superimposed on the ground-glass opacities and result in the "crazy-paving" pattern.[37]

Acute interstitial pneumonia is a fulminant disease of unknown cause that usually occurs in a previously healthy person and produces histologic findings of diffuse alveolar damage.[38] The clinical, radiologic, and histologic findings are identical to those of ARDS.[39]

Diffuse Pulmonary Hemorrhage

The high-resolution CT findings of diffuse pulmonary hemorrhage consist of bilateral patchy or confluent areas of consolidation or ground-glass opacities, or both.[17,40] Interlobular septal thickening and poorly defined centrilobular nodular opacities are

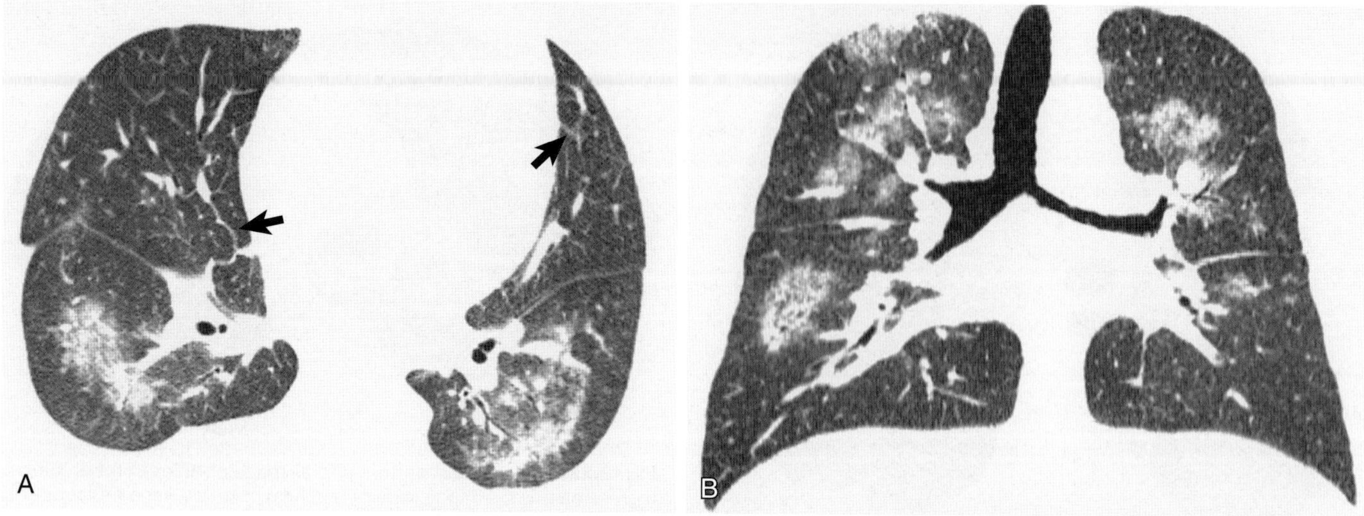

Fig. 2.24 Perihilar distribution of hydrostatic pulmonary edema from left heart failure. (A) High-resolution CT image showing consolidation and ground-glass opacities in the lower lobes. Note mild interlobular septal thickening *(arrows)* and small pleural effusions. (B) Coronal reformatted image demonstrating a predominantly perihilar (batwing) distribution of the consolidation and ground-glass opacities.

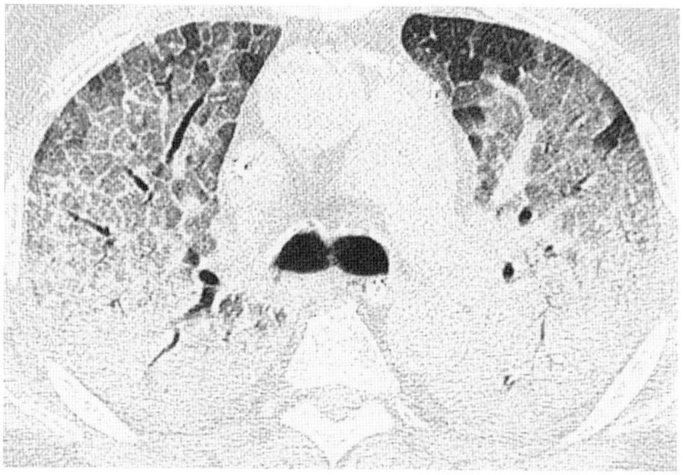

Fig. 2.25 Acute respiratory distress syndrome. A high-resolution CT image shows bilateral consolidation with air bronchograms in the dependent regions of the lungs. Also noted are extensive ground-glass opacities with superimposed smooth septal thickening ("crazy-paving" pattern).

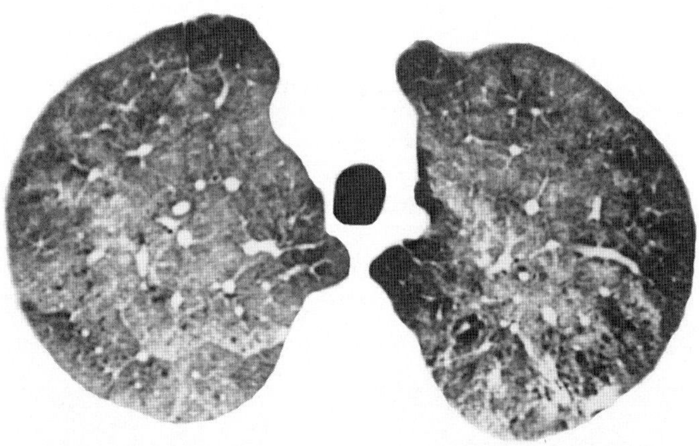

Fig. 2.26 Diffuse pulmonary hemorrhage in granulomatosis with polyangiitis. A high-resolution CT scan shows extensive bilateral ground-glass opacities, small areas of consolidation, and poorly defined small nodular opacities.

frequently seen over the following few days as the hemorrhage resolves (Fig. 2.26). These abnormalities presumably result from resorption of the hemorrhage via the lymphatics.

CHRONIC CAUSES OF PARENCHYMAL CONSOLIDATION

Organizing Pneumonia

Organizing pneumonia is a condition characterized pathologically by the presence of buds of loose granulation tissue within the alveolar ducts and airspaces. Bronchiolar involvement may or may not be present.[41] Although many cases are idiopathic (cryptogenic organizing pneumonia), half or more of cases of organizing pneumonia occur in the setting of pulmonary infection, drug reaction, radiation therapy, collagen vascular disease, or inhalation of toxic fumes.[41,42]

The CT manifestations of organizing pneumonia usually consist of patchy bilateral consolidation, which in approximately 60% to 80% of cases are peribronchial or subpleural in distribution (Figs. 2.27 and 2.28).[43–45] In about 60% of patients with organizing pneumonia, some of the areas of consolidation involve mainly the perilobular regions and may surround areas with ground-glass opacity, thereby resulting in a "reversed halo sign."[45,46]

Eosinophilic Lung Disease

The term *eosinophilic lung disease* is used to describe a group of entities characterized by abundant accumulation of eosinophils in the pulmonary interstitium and airspaces.[47] Peripheral blood eosinophilia is commonly present. The two most common conditions are simple pulmonary eosinophilia, also known as *Loeffler syndrome,* and chronic eosinophilic pneumonia. Simple pulmonary eosinophilia is characterized by the presence of

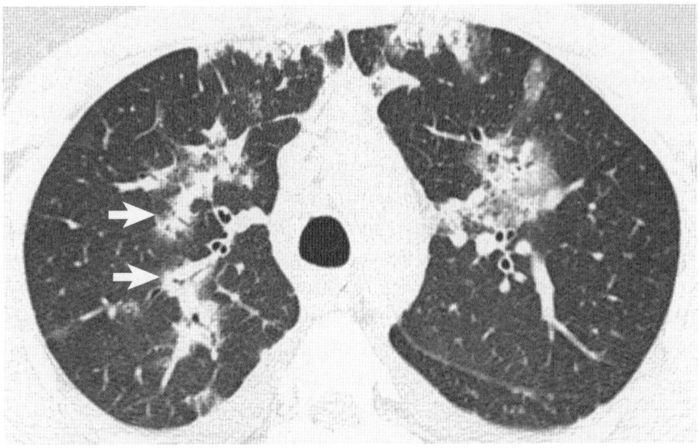

Fig. 2.27 Cryptogenic organizing pneumonia. A high-resolution CT scan shows bilateral areas of consolidation in a peribronchial *(arrows)* and subpleural distribution.

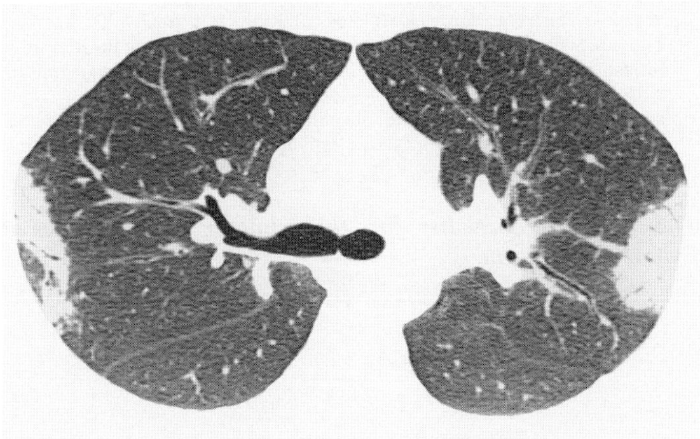

Fig. 2.28 Organizing pneumonia secondary to a drug reaction (5-aminosalicylic acid derivate (mesalamine) for the treatment of ulcerative colitis). A high-resolution CT scan shows patchy bilateral airspace consolidation in a peripheral distribution with associated air bronchograms. *(From Silva CI, Müller NL. Drug-induced lung diseases: most common reaction patterns and corresponding high-resolution CT manifestations.* Semin Ultrasound CT MR. *2006;27:111-116; with permission).*

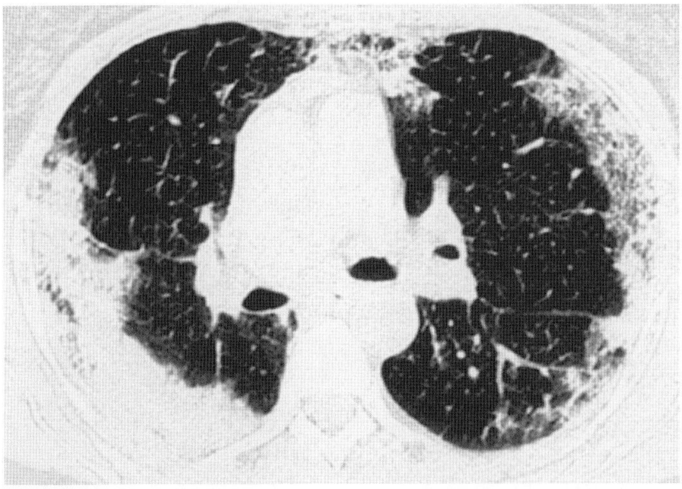

Fig. 2.29 Chronic eosinophilic pneumonia. A high-resolution CT scan shows bilateral peripheral areas of consolidation.

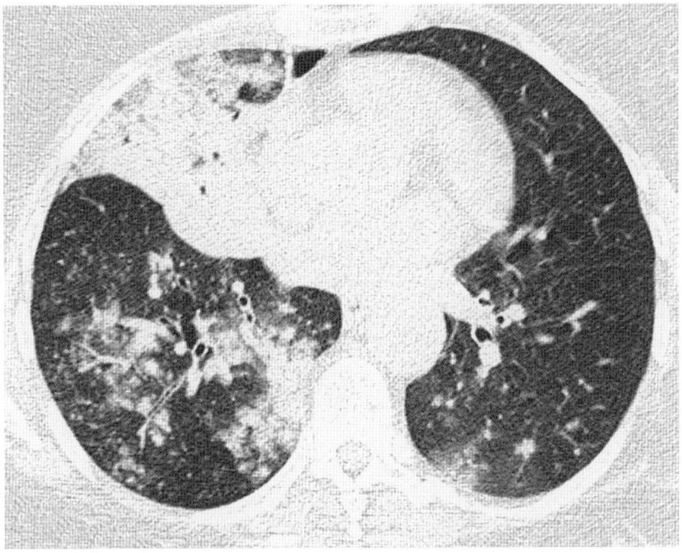

Fig. 2.30 Adenocarcinoma. A high-resolution CT image shows extensive consolidation and mild volume loss in the right middle lobe and patchy consolidation, ground-glass opacities, and small nodular opacities in the lower lobes.

transient and migratory bilateral areas of consolidation. On CT the areas of consolidation often have a predominantly peripheral distribution[47]; areas of ground-glass opacity are also frequently seen.[48] Chronic eosinophilic pneumonia is characterized by the presence of homogeneous consolidation involving mainly the peripheral lung regions ("the photographic negative of pulmonary edema") of the middle and upper lung zones. This characteristic finding is seen on chest radiographs in only approximately 50% of cases[9,18] but is evident on CT in virtually all cases (Fig. 2.29).[23,24] The majority of patients have ground-glass opacities adjacent to the areas of consolidation. Chronic eosinophilic pneumonia may be a manifestation of eosinophilic granulomatosis with polyangiitis (formerly Churg-Strauss syndrome), an eosinophilic vasculitis seen almost exclusively in patients with asthma.[49] Consolidation in a peripheral distribution identical to that of chronic eosinophilic pneumonia may be seen in patients with organizing pneumonia and, occasionally, in those with sarcoidosis and adenocarcinoma.

Lipoid Pneumonia

Exogenous lipoid pneumonia results from the aspiration of mineral, vegetable, or animal oil. Radiographic and CT findings include single or multiple nodules or masses and localized or confluent areas of consolidation.[21,50] In approximately 80% of patients, focal areas of fat attenuation can be seen on CT (see Fig. 2.20).[21,50] A less common manifestation consists of ground-glass opacities with superimposed interlobular septal thickening and intralobular lines ("crazy-paving" pattern).[51]

Adenocarcinoma

Primary lung or metastatic adenocarcinoma can be manifested as a solitary nodule or mass, as patchy or confluent areas of ground-glass opacity or consolidation, or, less commonly, as numerous ground-glass and soft tissue nodules (Fig. 2.30).[12,52] Diffuse lung involvement may result from a multifocal origin,

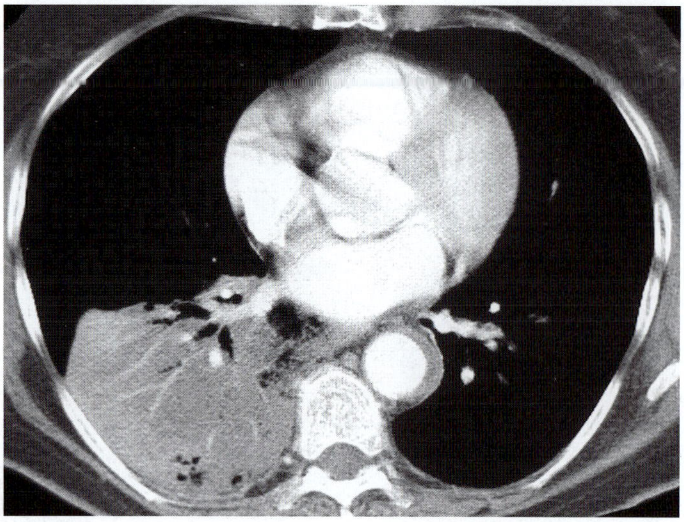

Fig. 2.31 Adenocarcinoma and the CT angiogram sign. Contrast-enhanced CT image demonstrates low attenuation consolidation with well-visualized opacified vessels within the consolidation (CT angiogram sign).

endobronchial spread of tumor from a primary focus, or hematogenous metastases.

Ground-glass opacity results from the tendency of the tumor to spread locally along the alveolar walls (a pattern known as lepidic growth) and from consolidation secondary to mucin and fluid produced by the tumor.[53] Air bronchograms are commonly visible. Centrilobular nodules are commonly associated, presumably reflecting the presence of bronchogenic spread of tumor. Because the fluid and mucus produced by the tumor are of low attenuation, if CT is performed with infusion of contrast medium, the enhanced pulmonary vessels can be seen within the consolidation. This has been referred to as the CT angiogram sign (Fig. 2.31).[54] This sign, however, is not specific because it is also seen in other causes of consolidation, including bacterial pneumonia, lipoid pneumonia, pulmonary lymphoma, pulmonary infarction, and pulmonary edema.[55] The CT angiogram sign is therefore of limited value in the differential diagnosis. It can be considered suggestive of adenocarcinoma in patients without infectious symptoms only if the mean attenuation of the consolidated lung is less than that of the chest wall musculature.[56]

Adenocarcinoma should be suspected in patients with ground-glass opacities or consolidation that progresses over a period of several months. Features that favor the diagnosis of adenocarcinoma rather than infection on CT include the presence of coexisting nodules, a peripheral distribution of the consolidation, and the presence of small focal ("bubble-like") areas of lucency.[57,58]

SUGGESTED READINGS

Sverzellati N, Lynch DA, Hansell DM, Johkoh T, King TE Jr, Travis WD. American Thoracic Society-European Respiratory Society Classification of the Idiopathic Interstitial Pneumonias: Advances in Knowledge since 2002. *Radiographics*. 2015;35(7):1849–1871.

Walker CM, Abbott GF, Greene RE, Shepard JA, Vummidi D, Digumarthy SR. Imaging pulmonary infection: classic signs and patterns. *AJR Am J Roentgenol*. 2014;202(3):479–492.

The full reference list for this chapter is available at ExpertConsult.com.

3 Atelectasis*

BRENT P. LITTLE

Atelectasis is defined as less than normal inflation of all or part of the lung with a corresponding diminution in lung volume.[1] Although the term *collapse* is often used synonymously with atelectasis, it should be reserved for complete atelectasis.

Mechanisms of Atelectasis

Mechanisms of atelectasis can be classified into five types: obstructive (resorptive), passive, compressive, adhesive, and cicatrization (scar).

OBSTRUCTIVE ATELECTASIS

Obstructive or resorptive atelectasis occurs when airflow to a region of lung is interrupted as a result of airway obstruction (Fig. 3.1). As oxygen is resorbed, alveoli decrease in volume, with their pressure remaining atmospheric. Consequently, the partial pressure of carbon dioxide and nitrogen in the alveoli rises relative to capillary blood, and both gases diffuse into blood to maintain equilibrium. Thus alveolar volume is further reduced, with a consequent rise in the alveolar-capillary blood PO_2 gradient; oxygen diffuses into capillary blood, and the cycle is repeated until all alveolar gas is absorbed. In healthy lungs breathing atmospheric air, complete air absorption occurs within 24 hours. In intubated patients breathing a high concentration of inspired oxygen, complete air absorption often occurs within an hour. The end result of such airway obstruction is complete collapse of the involved lobe or lung unless, as is often the case, pneumonitis develops distal to the obstruction. *Obstructive pneumonitis* (e.g., distal to pulmonary carcinoma) frequently leads to consolidation severe enough to limit loss of volume; this condition is often referred to as "drowned lung." The characteristic radiographic picture of obstructive pneumonitis (i.e., homogeneous opacification of a segment, lobe, or lung without air bronchograms) is highly suggestive of an obstructing endobronchial lesion.

Computed tomography (CT) often provides valuable additional information in patients with obstructive atelectasis, particularly with regard to the precise location and extent of the obstructing process (see Fig. 3.1). CT performed after the administration of intravenous contrast material may distinguish a proximal obstructing tumor from collapsed lung or adjacent mediastinal structures.[2,3] In some patients, magnetic resonance imaging (MRI) or positron emission tomography (PET) can provide comparable or complementary information by depicting the mass and adjacent collapsed lung.[3,4]

*The editors and the publisher would like to thank Drs. Nestor L. Müller and C. Isabela Silva Müller for contributing material on this topic to the prior edition of this work. It has served as the foundation for the current chapter.

PASSIVE ATELECTASIS

Passive atelectasis denotes loss of volume as the lung retracts in the presence of pneumothorax (Fig. 3.2). The lung has a natural tendency to collapse and does so when removed from the chest. While the lungs are in the thoracic cavity, this tendency is opposed by the chest wall. At the resting respiratory position (functional residual capacity), the tendency for the lung to collapse and the chest wall to expand is equal and opposite. In the presence of pneumothorax the lung retracts and its volume decreases. Provided that the pleural space is free (i.e., without adhesions), atelectasis of any portion of lung is proportional to the amount of air in the adjacent pleural space. As the lung shrinks adjacent to a pneumothorax, its density does not increase appreciably until it is almost completely collapsed. This presumably occurs because the reduction in lung volume is approximately balanced by a reduction in blood content and accounts for the difficulty commonly experienced in identifying the lung edge in cases of small or moderate spontaneous pneumothorax.

COMPRESSIVE ATELECTASIS

Compressive atelectasis (also called relaxation atelectasis by some radiologists) results from compression of the lung by an adjacent space-occupying process. Any intrathoracic space-occupying process, such as a bronchogenic cyst, bulla, neoplasm, pleural effusion, or large osteophyte, induces airlessness of a thin layer of contiguous lung parenchyma (Fig. 3.3).

On CT atelectasis is seen commonly in the dependent lung regions as an ill-defined area of increased attenuation or subpleural curvilinear opacities (Fig. 3.4). The former measures from a few millimeters to 1 cm or more in thickness and has been called *dependent opacity* or *dependent density.* Subpleural curvilinear opacities, also known as *subpleural lines,* are linear areas of increased attenuation measuring several centimeters in length and located within 1 cm of the pleura and parallel to it. Both manifestations of dependent atelectasis characteristically disappear when the patient changes position; differentiation of dependent atelectasis from true interstitial or airspace disease can be established easily by scanning the patient in the supine and prone positions (see Fig. 3.4).

ROUND ATELECTASIS

Round atelectasis (also called rounded atelectasis) is a distinct form of atelectasis characteristically associated with focal pleural thickening.[5] The majority of cases of round atelectasis are seen in patients exposed to asbestos.[6] Other causes include pleural effusion or thickening from tuberculosis, infections other than tuberculosis, pulmonary infarction, left heart failure, hemothorax, surgery (mainly cardiac surgery), and malignant tumor.[5,6] On

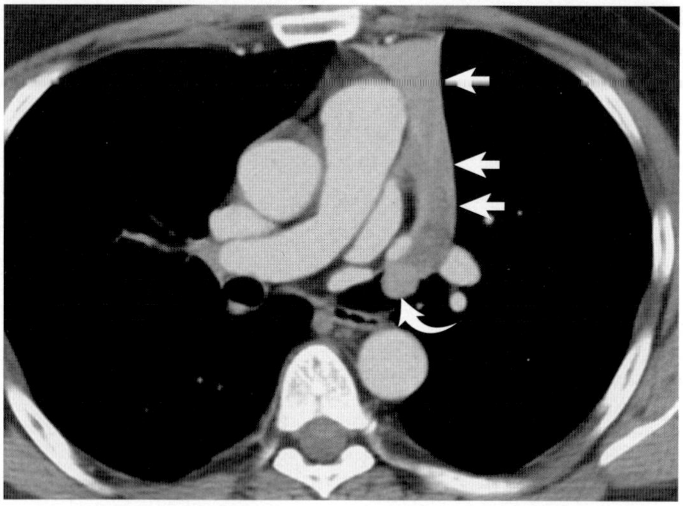

Fig. 3.1 Obstructive (resorptive) atelectasis of the left upper lobe from endobronchial carcinoid. A contrast-enhanced CT scan shows tumor *(curved arrow)* obstructing the left upper lobe bronchus with associated complete left upper lobe atelectasis *(straight arrows)*. Note the anterior and medial shift of the left major fissure *(straight arrows)*.

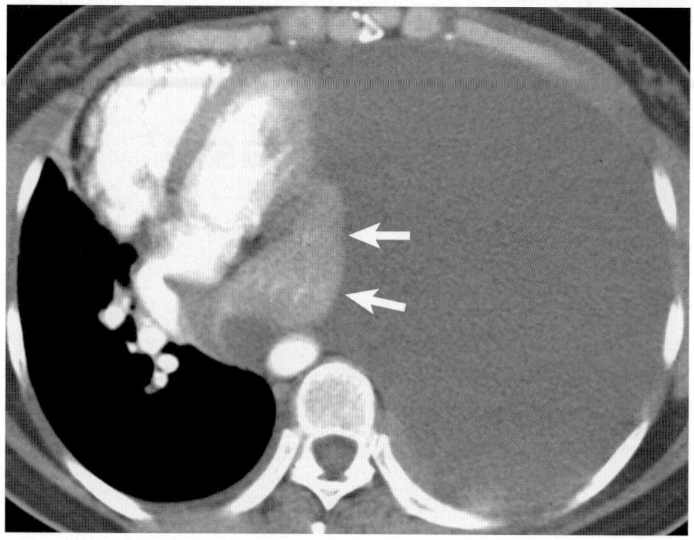

Fig. 3.3 Compressive or relaxation atelectasis in malignant pleural effusion secondary to metastatic adenocarcinoma. A contrast-enhanced CT scan shows a large left pleural effusion with rightward shift of the mediastinum and complete compressive atelectasis of the left lower lobe *(arrows)*.

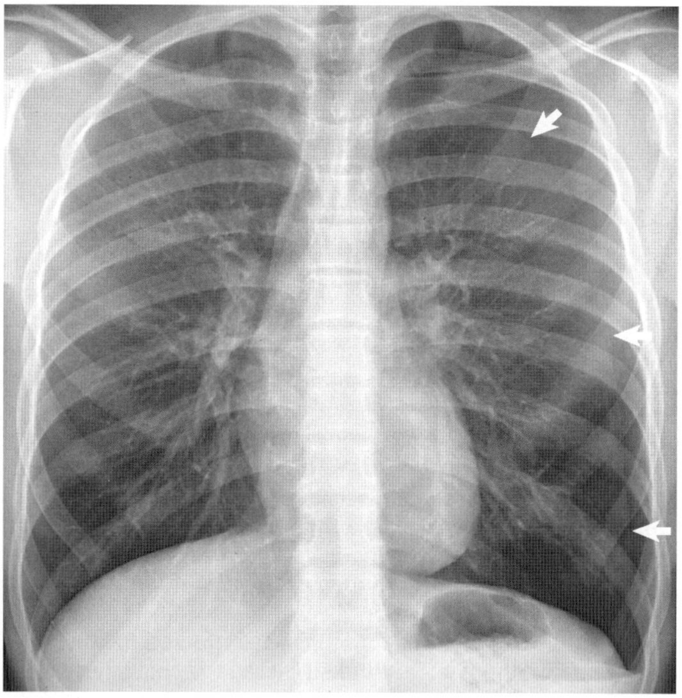

Fig. 3.2 Passive atelectasis in pneumothorax. A posteroanterior chest radiograph shows a moderate left-sided pneumothorax and a small amount of left pleural fluid resulting in a fluid level in the left costophrenic sulcus. The pneumothorax can be recognized by noting the margin of the visceral pleura *(arrows)*. Although left lung volume has decreased, there is no apparent increase in left lung opacity.

conventional radiographs round atelectasis is seen as a fairly homogeneous round, oval, wedge-shaped, or irregularly shaped mass in the peripheral lung adjacent to thickened pleura (Fig. 3.5).[5] It usually measures 3 to 6 cm in greatest diameter, although it may involve an entire lobe, and is associated with loss of volume of the affected lobe. The bronchi and vessels in the vicinity of the mass are gathered together in a curvilinear fashion as they pass toward the mass, similar to the tail of a comet (comet tail sign), a feature best appreciated on CT. The abnormality occurs most commonly in the lower lobes.[6]

The characteristic CT features consist of bronchi and vessels curving and converging toward a round or oval mass that abuts an area of pleural thickening and is associated with evidence of volume loss in the affected lobe; vessels and bronchi curve into the periphery of the mass, which forms the basis for the comet tail sign (Fig. 3.6).[5,7] The hilar (central) aspect of the mass usually has indistinct margins as a result of blurring by the entering vessels. Air bronchograms are identified within the mass in approximately 60% of cases. Hypertrophy of extrapleural fat may be identified adjacent to the mass, a feature that reflects chronicity and is therefore not seen in all cases.

In most patients the CT findings are sufficiently characteristic that neither biopsy nor further investigative procedures are necessary to exclude more ominous disease.[5,7] ^{18}F-fluorodeoxyglucose (FDG) PET usually shows little or no uptake (i.e., uptake equal to or less than mediastinal blood pool) and may be helpful in distinguishing round atelectasis from carcinoma in confusing cases.[8] Follow-up of patients who have round atelectasis has shown that the majority of lesions are stable for many years. Occasionally, a lesion decreases in size, resolves within a few weeks to several years, or enlarges.[6,9] Needle biopsy may rarely be required to rule out carcinoma.[10]

ADHESIVE ATELECTASIS

The term *adhesive atelectasis* is used to describe atelectasis caused, at least in part, by deficiency of surfactant.[11] Surfactant reduces the surface tension of the alveoli as their surface area or volume decreases; thus the critical closing pressure of alveoli occurs at a lower volume and distending pressure, thereby effectively protecting against collapse. Causes of adhesive atelectasis in adults include radiation pneumonitis, smoke inhalation injury, acute respiratory distress syndrome, and pulmonary thromboembolism.[11] Atelectasis in radiation pneumonitis is usually limited to the irradiated portions of the lungs; occasionally, it is seen outside the regions of the radiation ports, particularly on CT.[12] The radiographic

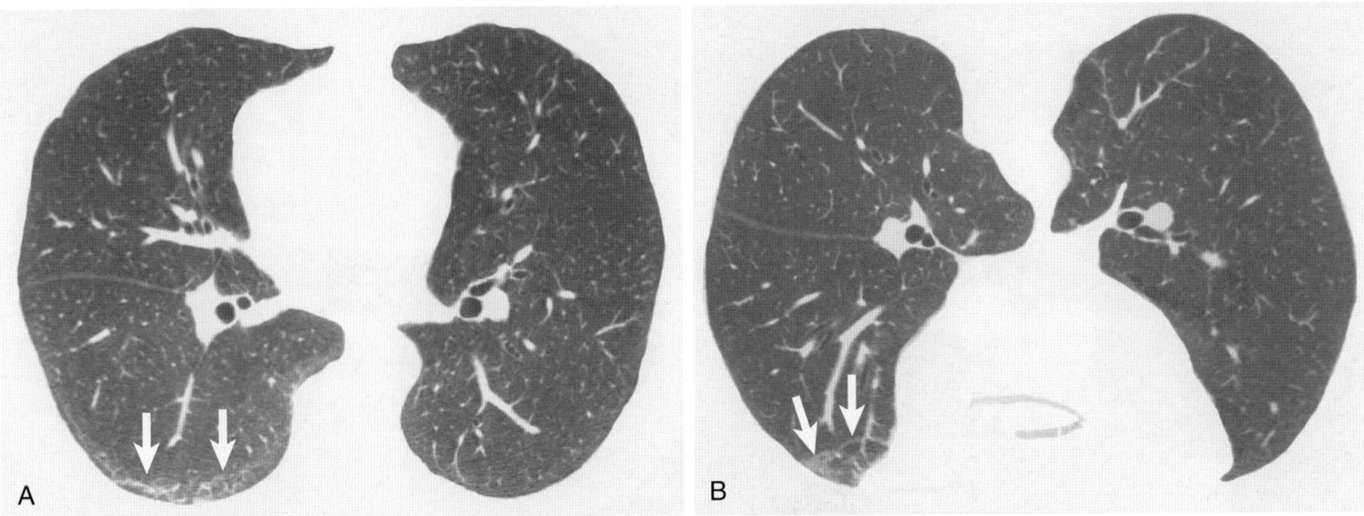

Fig. 3.4 Dependent atelectasis. A high-resolution CT scan (A) with the patient supine shows focal linear and ground-glass opacities *(arrows)* in the dorsal regions of the right lower lobe. A high-resolution CT scan (B) at the same level with the patient prone shows resolution of the opacity in the dorsal regions of the lower lobe and the development of focal opacities *(arrows)* in dependent regions of the right middle lobe. The distribution of the findings and resolution with change in position are characteristic of dependent atelectasis.

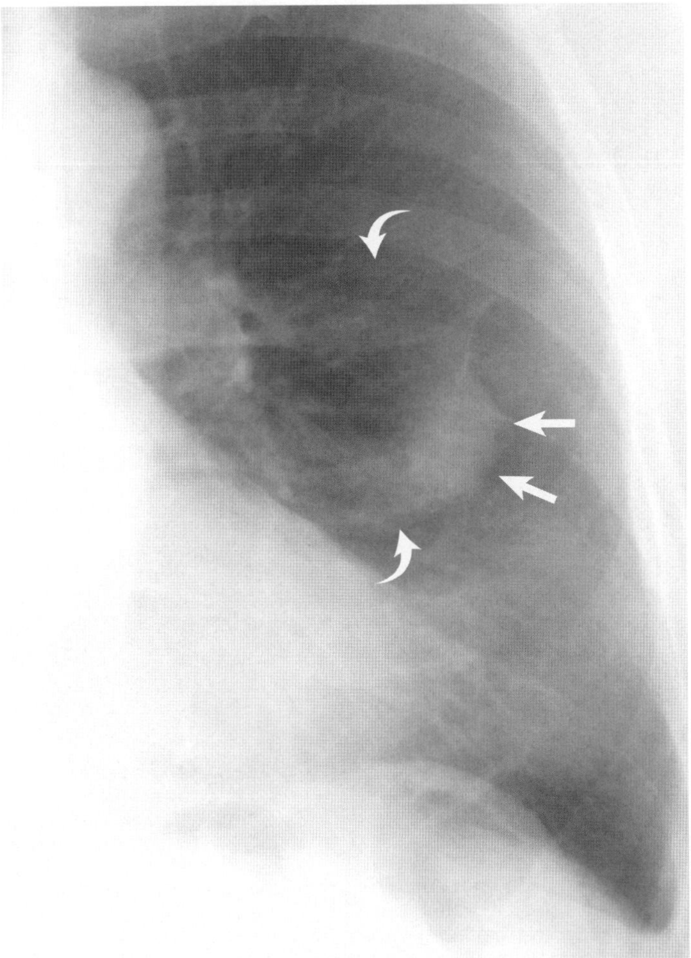

Fig. 3.5 Round atelectasis in a man with asbestos-related pleural disease. A magnified view of the left lung from a posteroanterior chest radiograph shows an oval opacity. The lateral margins *(straight arrows)* are well defined (where the opacity abuts the lung), and the medial margins are poorly defined (where the opacity abuts the pleura). Pulmonary vessels *(curved arrows)* can be seen to curve toward the opacity (comet tail sign).

and CT findings consist of areas of ground-glass opacification or consolidation with associated loss of volume (Fig. 3.7). The radiologic manifestations of radiation pneumonitis usually occur approximately 1 to 6 months after the completion of radiation therapy.[12] Focal ischemia distal to pulmonary thromboembolism may lead to a local reduction in surfactant that results in subsegmental, segmental, or, less commonly, lobar atelectasis.[11]

Atelectasis, particularly of the left lower lobe, is seen in the majority of patients after cardiac surgery. It is likely that adhesive atelectasis also plays a part in loss of volume postoperatively and accounts for the marked arteriovenous shunting that may occur even when the chest radiograph is relatively normal.[13]

CICATRIZATION ATELECTASIS

Although for the sake of completeness we have included loss of volume associated with pulmonary fibrosis in the section on atelectasis, the term *atelectasis* is seldom used in this context. The fundamental pathologic process is one of fibrosis, the fibrous tissue undergoing retraction as it matures and resulting in loss of volume of the affected portion of lung. The fibrosis may be localized, best exemplified by long-standing tuberculosis and radiation fibrosis (see Fig. 3.7), or diffuse, as seen in idiopathic pulmonary fibrosis.

The bronchi and bronchioles within the affected lung are dilated because of the increased elastic recoil from the surrounding pulmonary fibrosis, a phenomenon known as *traction bronchiectasis and bronchiolectasis* (see Fig. 3.7).[14] The radiologic signs are as might be expected: a segment or lobe occupying a volume smaller than normal with a density rendered inhomogeneous by dilated, air-containing bronchi and with irregular thickened strands extending from the atelectatic segment to the hilum. Compensatory signs of chronic loss of volume are usually evident and include local mediastinal shift (frequently manifested by a marked deviation of the trachea when segments of the upper lobe are involved), displacement of the hilum (which may be severe in upper lobe disease), and compensatory overinflation of the remainder of the affected lung.

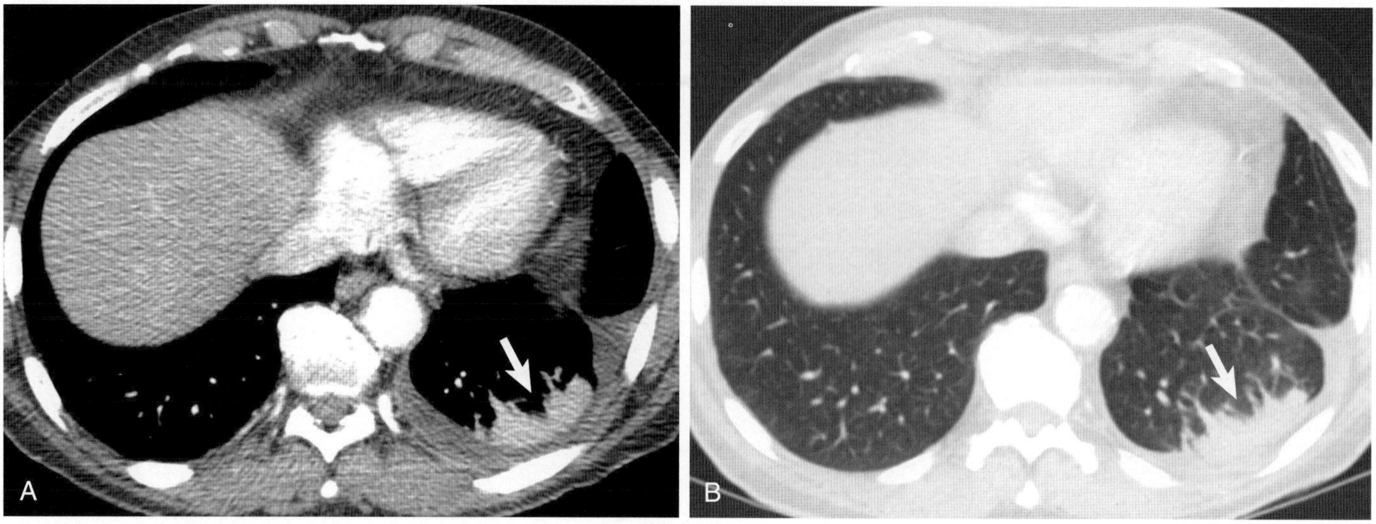

Fig. 3.6 Round atelectasis, stable for several years. (A) A high-resolution CT scan at soft tissue windows shows a uniformly enhancing irregular mass *(arrow)* in the left lower lobe adjacent to a small chronic left pleural effusion, with mild pleural thickening. (B) At lung windows the mass has a "comet tail" appearance at the medial border *(arrow)* with retraction of adjacent vessels toward the mass.

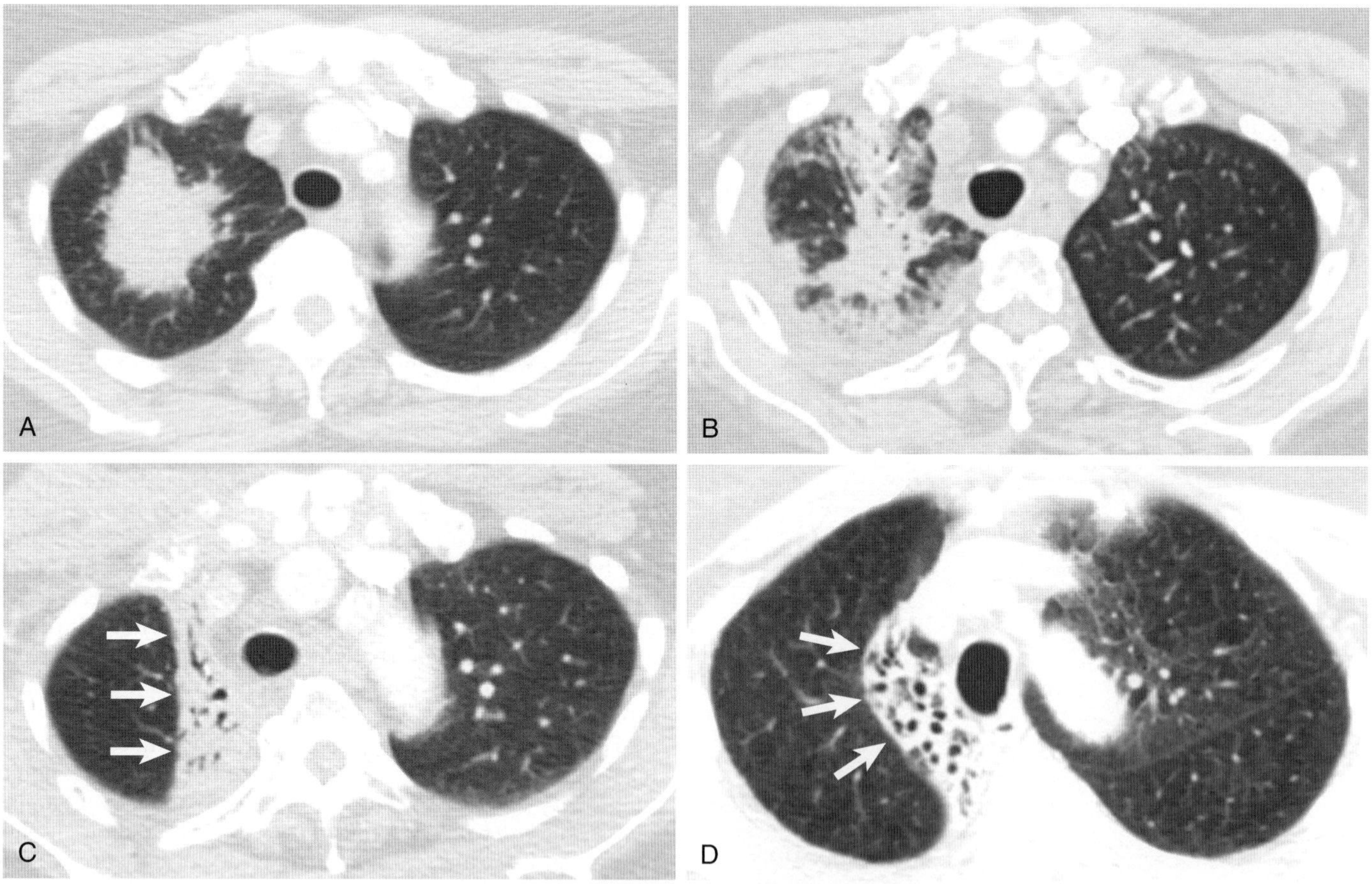

Fig. 3.7 Adhesive and cicatrization atelectasis after radiotherapy. A CT scan (A) shows a right upper lobe mass, proven on lung biopsy to be pulmonary carcinoma. The size of the upper lobes is fairly symmetric. A CT scan (B) 6 months after radiotherapy shows extensive ground-glass opacities in the right upper lobe in the radiation portal, characteristic of radiation pneumonitis. A CT scan (C) 2 years later shows a typical appearance of radiation fibrosis (cicatrization atelectasis) with straight outer borders *(arrows)*. Note the presence of dilated and distorted bronchi within the areas of fibrosis (traction bronchiectasis) and compensatory overinflation of the adjacent lung. (D) Another patient 2 years after radiotherapy for right upper lobe lung cancer shows severe right upper lobe cicatricial atelectasis; there is posteromedial and superior displacement of the right major fissure *(arrows)*.

KEY POINTS: MECHANISMS OF ATELECTASIS

- **Obstructive atelectasis**
  - Distal to obstruction of a bronchus
- **Passive atelectasis**
  - Retraction of lung in the presence of pneumothorax
- **Compressive atelectasis**
  - Compression by a space-occupying process, such as a pleural effusion, pulmonary mass, or bulla
- **Adhesive atelectasis**
  - Caused by deficiency of surfactant (e.g., radiation pneumonitis)
- **Cicatrization atelectasis**
  - Caused by contraction of fibrous tissue as it matures; can be focal (e.g., tuberculosis) or diffuse (e.g., idiopathic pulmonary fibrosis)

Radiologic Signs of Atelectasis

The radiologic manifestations of atelectasis may be classified into direct and indirect signs.[15,16] Direct signs include displacement of the interlobar fissures and crowding of bronchi and vessels within the area of atelectasis; indirect signs include pulmonary opacification and signs related to shift of other structures to compensate for the loss of volume (Fig. 3.8).

DIRECT SIGNS

Displacement of Interlobar Fissures

Displacement of the fissures that form the boundary of an atelectatic lobe is one of the most dependable and easily recognized signs of atelectasis (see Fig. 3.8). For each lobe the position and configuration of the displaced fissures are predictable for a given loss of volume; these factors are considered later in relation to specific patterns of lobar and segmental atelectasis.

Crowding of Vessels and Bronchi

As the lung loses volume the vessels and bronchi in the atelectatic area become crowded together. This finding is one of the earliest signs of atelectasis and can be recognized most readily when comparison is made with previous radiographs. Increased opacification of the atelectatic lobe may result in obscuration of the vessels; however, except in patients who have obstructive atelectasis, crowded air bronchograms are visible within the area of atelectasis on radiographs or CT.

INDIRECT SIGNS

Apart from the presence of increased opacity, the main indirect radiologic signs of atelectasis include mechanisms that compensate for the reduction in pleural pressure, such as diaphragmatic elevation, mediastinal shift, hilar displacement, and overinflation of the remainder of the lung (see Fig. 3.8). The more acute the atelectasis, the greater the predominance of diaphragmatic and mediastinal displacement; the more chronic the atelectasis, the more that compensatory overinflation of nonatelectatic lung predominates.

The local increase in opacity results from a combination of resorption of air and accumulation of fluid. The volume of an airless lobe or segment depends not only on which order of bronchus is obstructed but also on the amount of sequestered fluid within the obstructed parenchyma. Because the lung contains a large amount of air and normal lung density is only 0.12 g/mL, the lung must become almost completely collapsed before increased opacification from loss of volume is apparent on the chest radiograph.

KEY POINTS: RADIOLOGIC SIGNS OF ATELECTASIS

- **Direct**
  - Displacement of interlobar fissures
  - Crowding of vessels and bronchi
- **Indirect**
  - Local increase in opacity
  - Elevation of the hemidiaphragm
  - Shift of the mediastinum
  - Compensatory overinflation of remaining lung
  - Displacement of the hila

Elevation of the hemidiaphragm is more marked in lower than in upper lobe atelectasis. In the lower lung zones, elevation tends to occur in the area contiguous to the lobe involved—posterior elevation in lower lobe atelectasis and anterior elevation in middle lobe or lingular atelectasis, although, in the latter two situations the diaphragmatic displacement is seldom severe.

When assessing diaphragmatic elevation, it is important to be aware of possible variations in the relationship of the two hemidiaphragms. Although the right dome is normally 1 to 2 cm higher than the left, in approximately 10% of normal subjects the two hemidiaphragms are at the same level, and in 2% the right hemidiaphragm is more than 3 cm higher than the left.[17]

The anterior and middle mediastinal compartments are more mobile than the posterior compartment and therefore shift to a greater extent in patients with atelectasis.

Overinflation of the remainder of the ipsilateral lung is one of the most important and reliable indirect signs of atelectasis. It seldom occurs rapidly and, in the early stages of lobar atelectasis, is usually of less diagnostic help than the other compensatory phenomena, such as diaphragmatic elevation and mediastinal displacement. As the period of atelectasis lengthens, however, overinflation becomes more severe and the diaphragmatic and mediastinal changes regress.

When an entire lung becomes atelectatic after obstruction of a main bronchus, the resultant loss of volume of the hemithorax must be compensated for largely by overinflation of the contralateral lung (Fig. 3.9). In this situation the mediastinal shift may be large; because the mediastinum is less stable anteriorly than elsewhere, the anterior septum is rotated laterally and posteriorly, the normal lung overinflating to such an extent that it occupies the whole anterior portion of the thorax. Thus the heart and the collapsed lung are displaced into the posterior portion of the ipsilateral hemithorax.

Hilar displacement occurs more commonly in atelectasis of the upper than the lower lobes and is usually more marked the more chronic the atelectasis; for example, scarring of the upper lobes as a result of tuberculosis commonly causes severe upward displacement of the ipsilateral hilum. Downward displacement of the right hilum in cases of lower lobe atelectasis is seldom as clearly appreciated. Downward displacement of only the left hilum, however, is more readily apparent, particularly if it brings the left hilum level with the right—an appearance seen in only 3% of normal individuals.[17]

A cardinal sign of lower lobe atelectasis is loss of visibility of the interlobar artery; because the lung parenchyma adjacent to the artery is airless, the air-tissue interface is lost and the vessel

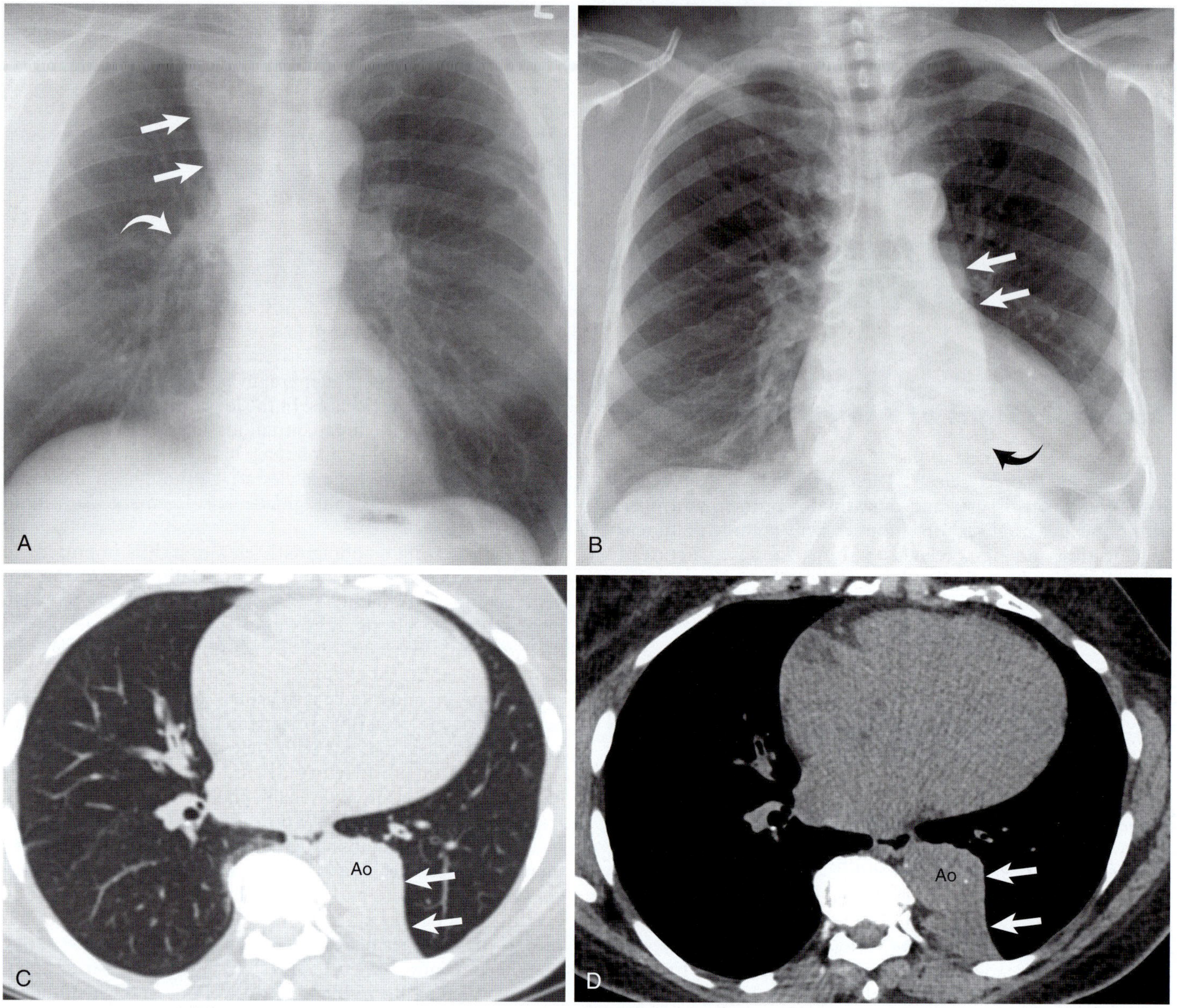

Fig. 3.8 Direct and indirect signs of atelectasis in obstructing lung cancer. A view from a chest radiograph (A) shows cephalad and medial displacement of the minor fissure *(straight arrows)*, a direct sign of right upper lobe atelectasis. Also note several indirect signs, including increased opacity of the atelectatic lobe, superior displacement of the right hilum, lateral displacement of the right interlobar pulmonary artery *(curved arrow)*, and elevation of the right hemidiaphragm. (B) Radiograph of a different patient with asthma and a mucus plug shows several indirect signs of left lower lobe atelectasis. Although the descending aortic contour is distinct superiorly *(straight arrows)*, the distal descending aortic silhouette is obscured *(curved arrow)* because of the adjacent collapsed left lower lobe. Increased opacity at the left cardiophrenic angle corresponds to the collapsed lobe, and subtle increased lucency of the remaining left lung represents compensatory left upper lobe overinflation. CT of the same patient shown in lung (C) and soft tissue (D) windows illustrates posterior and medial shift of the left major fissure *(arrows)*, with the collapsed left lower lobe draped over the aorta *(Ao)*.

becomes invisible. A helpful sign in detecting lower lobe atelectasis is medial displacement of the interlobar and lower lobe pulmonary arteries. This sign is particularly valuable on the left side, where pleural effusion sometimes creates a triangular shadow in the posterior paravertebral zone that simulates total left lower lobe atelectasis. Preservation of the shadow of the interlobar artery establishes the pleural origin of the opacity, whereas its obliteration indicates lobar atelectasis.

Patterns of Atelectasis

Because the degree of atelectasis of a lobe is governed to a large extent by the amount of fluid and cells that it contains, the radiographic image varies from a consolidated lobe with only minimal loss of volume to a state of total collapse; therefore the anatomic-spatial relationships in each lobe range from normal volume to total atelectasis.

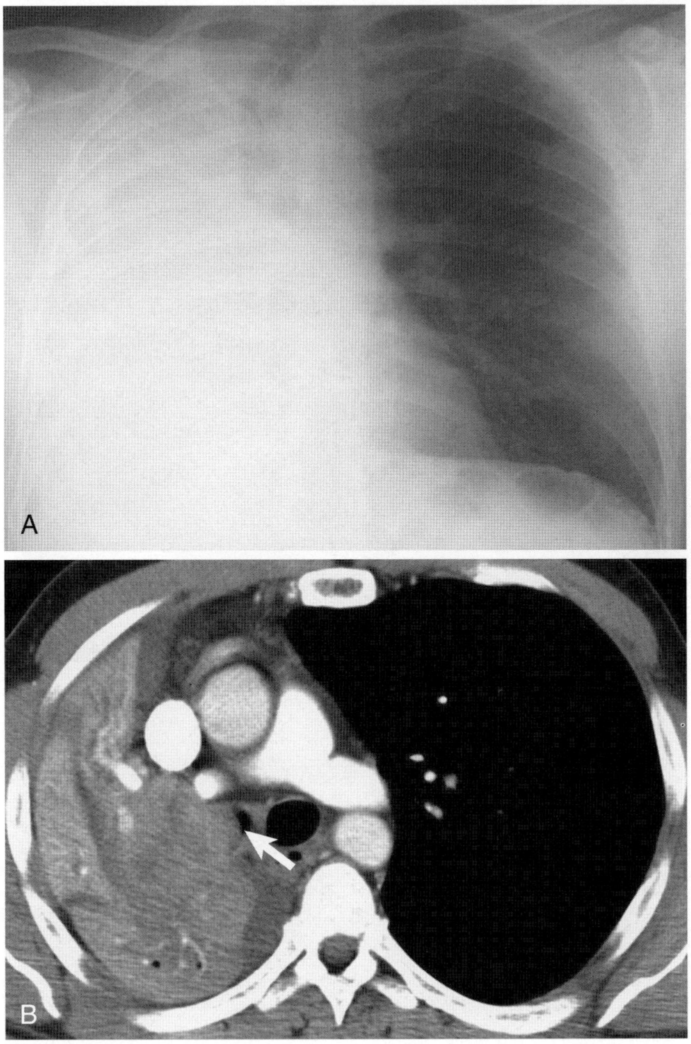

Fig. 3.9 Obstructive atelectasis of the right lung from squamous cell carcinoma. A chest radiograph (A) shows opacification and decreased volume of the right hemithorax. The trachea and mediastinum are shifted to the right, and the left lung shows compensatory overinflation. The lack of air bronchograms within the opacified atelectatic right lung is consistent with obstructive atelectasis. A contrast-enhanced CT scan (B) demonstrates complete obstruction of the right main bronchus by tumor *(arrow)*, as well as distal atelectasis and obstructive pneumonitis. Note that the descending aorta is essentially in its normal position, whereas the anterior and middle mediastinal compartments are markedly displaced to the right.

Provided that there is no pneumothorax or pleural effusion, in the majority of cases the visceral pleura covering an atelectatic lobe continues to relate intimately to the parietal pleura, regardless of the severity of atelectasis; the visceral pleural surface usually maintains contact with the parietal pleura over either the convex or the mediastinal surface of the hemithorax. Because the medial aspect of the lobe is relatively fixed, the forms that the atelectatic lobe can adopt are limited. The resultant shape is partly affected by the relatively rigid components of the lung (bronchi, arteries, and veins), which can be crowded together in very close apposition in one plane but have limited capacity to foreshorten. Thus any pulmonary lobe in its fully inflated state may be likened to a pyramid with its apex at the hilum and its base contiguous to the parietal pleura; as the lobe loses volume, two surfaces of the pyramid approximate, the end result of total atelectasis being a flattened triangle or triangular "pancake" whose apex and base tend to maintain contiguity with the hilum and parietal pleura, respectively.

On CT atelectatic lobes become wedge shaped rather than hemispheric in cross section, with the apex situated at the origin of the affected bronchus.[18,19] The atelectatic lobe tapers smoothly toward the hilum except when the atelectasis is due to a large central tumor, in which case there is a focal lateral convexity (S sign of Golden; see later). Other signs suggestive of an obstructive tumor on CT include the presence of an endobronchial or peribronchial soft tissue mass and absence of air bronchograms within the atelectatic lobe.

TOTAL PULMONARY ATELECTASIS

When an entire lung becomes atelectatic because of obstruction of a main bronchus, the compensatory phenomena are identical in character to those that develop with less severe pulmonary atelectasis (see Fig. 3.9). Elevation of the ipsilateral hemidiaphragm is recognizable only on the left side, the stomach bubble indicating its position. The hemithorax generally shows evidence of retraction. As the normal contralateral lung overinflates, the whole mediastinum moves to the affected side, with the greatest shift occurring anteriorly, where the mediastinum is most mobile.

Atelectasis of an entire lung is generally secondary to complete obstruction of a main bronchus and is associated with increased opacity of the affected lung. However, in patients with partial obstruction, previous tuberculosis, or pneumothorax, loss of volume may occur with normal or even decreased opacity of the atelectatic lung.

LOBAR ATELECTASIS

The patterns created by atelectasis of the right and left upper lobes differ and are therefore described separately; the lower lobes have almost identical patterns and are considered together.

Right Upper Lobe

The minor fissure and the upper half of the major fissure approximate by shifting upward and forward, respectively (see Fig. 3.8A). On a lateral projection both fissures appear gently curved, the minor fissure assuming a concave configuration inferiorly, whereas the major fissure may be convex, concave, or flat; the minor fissure shows roughly the same curvature in a posteroanterior projection. As volume diminishes further the visceral pleural surface sweeps upward over the apex of the hemithorax so that the lobe comes to occupy a flattened position contiguous to the superior mediastinum. When completely atelectatic, its volume is so small that in a posteroanterior projection its shadow creates no more than a slight widening of the superior mediastinum. In a lateral projection the collapsed lobe may appear as an indistinctly defined triangular shadow with its apex at the hilum and its base contiguous to the parietal pleura just posterior to the apex of the hemithorax.

Another sign commonly associated with right or left upper lobe atelectasis or lobectomy (less commonly with middle lobe atelectasis) is the *juxtaphrenic peak* (Fig. 3.10),[20] which consists of a small, sharply defined triangular opacity that projects upward from the medial half of the hemidiaphragm at or near the highest point of the dome. In the vast majority of cases the juxtaphrenic peak is related to an inferior accessory fissure.[21] The juxtaphrenic

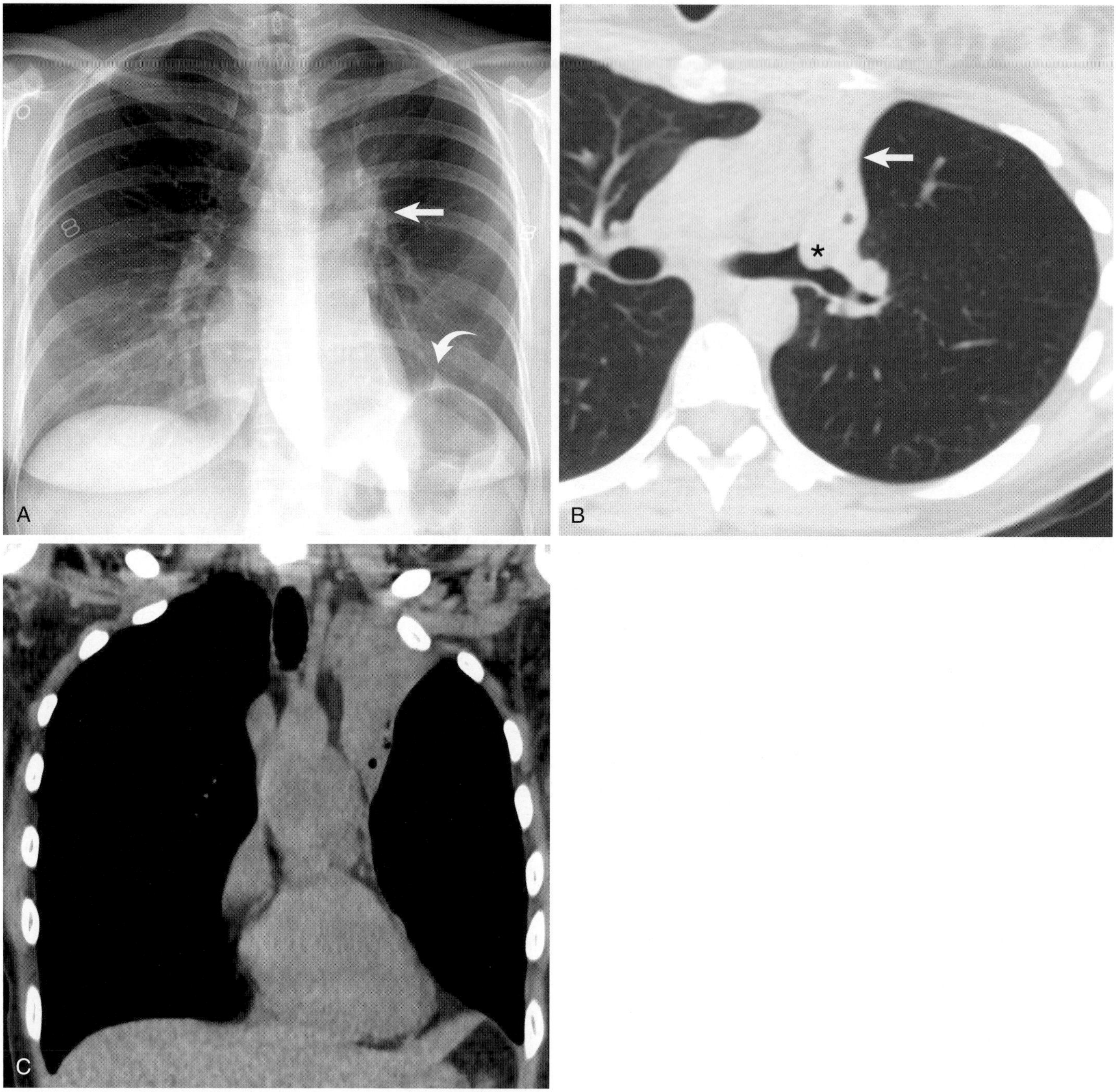

Fig. 3.10 Juxtaphrenic peak caused by left upper lobe collapse in the setting of endobronchial carcinoid tumor. A chest radiograph (A) shows a decrease in size of the left hemithorax, elevation of the left hilum *(straight arrow)*, elevation of the left hemidiaphragm, and a juxtaphrenic peak representing traction upon the inferior pulmonary ligament *(curved arrow)*. Axial image from CT scan in lung windows (B) shows the endobronchial tumor *(asterisk)* with left upper lobe collapse causing medial and superior shift of the left major fissure *(arrow)*. Coronal CT image in soft tissue windows (C) shows the collapsed left upper lobe with superior and medial shift of the major fissure.

peak presumably results from upward retraction of the portion of the visceral pleura (and associated extrapleural fat) that protrudes into a recess on the basal surface of the lung. The tethering effect is presumably greater at this pleural extension into the inferior accessory fissure because the pleural extension is less distensible than the adjacent lung parenchyma.[21]

Right upper lobe atelectasis caused by large hilar tumors may be associated with a characteristic downward bulge in the medial portion of the minor fissure. This feature, combined with the concave appearance of the lateral aspect of the minor fissure, results in a reverse S configuration of the minor fissure and is known as the *S sign of Golden,* also called the *reverse S sign of*

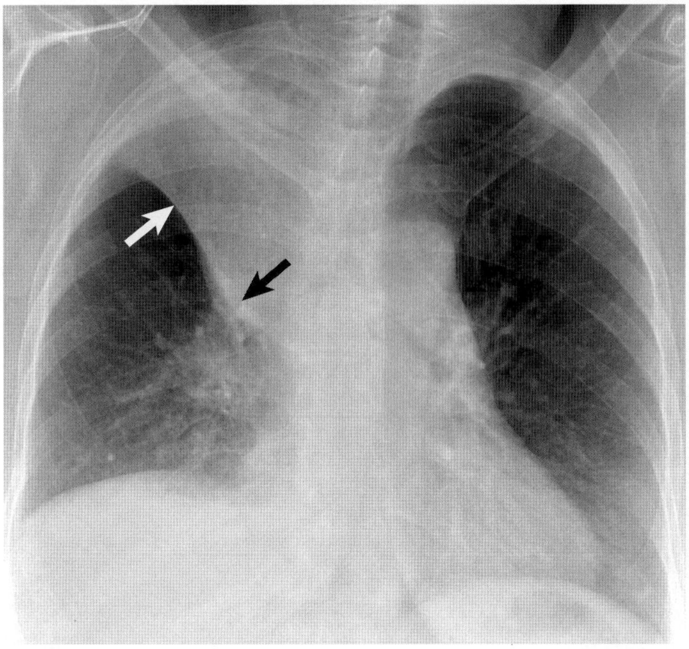

Fig. 3.11 Right upper lobe atelectasis and the *S sign of Golden* caused by an obstructing right hilar mass. A chest radiograph demonstrates right upper lobe atelectasis. Note the focal downward bulge *(black arrow)* in the medial portion of the displaced minor fissure, corresponding to the lower margin of the hilar mass, and a concave appearance of the lateral aspect of the minor fissure *(white arrow)*, resulting in a reverse S configuration known as the S sign of Golden. Also note the mild elevation of the right hemidiaphragm.

Golden (Fig. 3.11).[16,22] This sign is highly suggestive of pulmonary carcinoma as the cause of atelectasis. Although initially described for right upper lobe atelectasis, the Golden S sign is in fact applicable to atelectasis of any lobe.[16]

On CT the medial margin of the atelectatic right upper lobe abuts the mediastinum and is associated with superior and medial displacement of the minor fissure (Fig. 3.12). With elevation of the minor fissure the overinflated middle lobe shifts upward laterally alongside the atelectatic upper lobe. Compensatory overinflation of the right lower lobe results in superior, anterior, and medial displacement of the major fissure.

Left Upper Lobe

The major difference between atelectasis of the left and right upper lobes is related to the absence of a minor fissure on the left; all lung tissue anterior to the major fissure is involved (Fig. 3.13). This fissure, which is slightly more vertical than the major fissure on the right, is displaced forward in a plane roughly parallel to the anterior chest wall, a relationship depicted particularly well on a lateral radiograph. As volume loss increases the fissure moves further anteriorly and medially, until on lateral projection the shadow of the lobe is no more than a broad linear opacity contiguous and parallel to the anterior chest wall. The contiguity of the atelectatic lobe to the mediastinum obliterates the left cardiac border in frontal projection (the "silhouette sign").

As the apical segment moves downward and forward, the space that it vacates is occupied by the overinflated superior segment of the lower lobe; the apex of the hemithorax thus contains aerated lung. Sometimes, this lower lobe segment inserts itself medially between the apex of the atelectatic upper lobe and the mediastinum, thereby creating a sharp interface with the medial edge of the atelectatic lobe and allowing visualization of the aortic arch. The overinflated superior segment is then seen on a frontal radiograph as a crescent of hyperlucency, hence the term *Luftsichel* ("air crescent") in the German literature.[16] This feature is more often seen on the left than on the right (see Fig. 3.13).[23]

On CT the atelectatic left upper lobe can be seen to abut the anterior chest wall and mediastinum. The major fissure is shifted cephalad and anteriorly. The posterior margin of the atelectatic left upper lobe has a V-shaped contour or a small peak from the apex of the lung to the hilum as a result of tethering of the major fissure by the hilum (Fig. 3.14).

Atelectasis of the upper division of the left upper lobe with sparing of the lingula results in findings similar to those of right upper lobe atelectasis. The interface between the atelectatic upper division and the overinflated lingula is usually arcuate and bowed in an upward direction, even in the absence of a left minor fissure. Lingular atelectasis resembles right middle lobe atelectasis and is associated with obscuration of the left heart border on posteroanterior radiographs and a triangular opacity with the apex at the hilum on lateral views. The inferior margin of the atelectatic segment is well defined, being bordered by the major fissure; however, because a left minor fissure is uncommon, the superior margin is usually irregular or poorly defined.[16]

Right Middle Lobe

The diagnosis of right middle lobe atelectasis is one of the most difficult to make on a frontal radiograph and one of the easiest on a lateral radiograph. With progressive loss of volume the minor fissure and the lower half of the major fissure approximate and are almost in contact when collapse is complete (Fig. 3.15). The resultant triangular "pancake" of tissue has its apex at the hilum and its base apparently contiguous to the parietal pleura over the anterolateral convexity of the thorax and is well seen on a lateral radiograph.

In a posteroanterior projection, there may be no discernible increase in opacity, the only evidence of disease being obliteration of part of the right cardiac border as a result of contiguity of the right atrium with the medial segment of the atelectatic lobe (the silhouette sign). The difficulty in detecting atelectasis in this projection is related to the obliquity of the atelectatic lobe in a superoinferior plane and the thickness of the collapsed lobe itself.

The CT appearance of right middle lobe atelectasis consists of a broad triangular or trapezoidal opacity with the apex directed toward the hilum (Fig. 3.16).[18] As the lobe loses volume the minor and major fissures move toward each other, the former downward and the latter upward and forward. The posterior border of the atelectatic middle lobe is usually defined because the major fissure is almost perpendicular to the plane of section.

Lower Lobes

The findings of right and left lower lobe atelectasis are similar. The lower lobes are bounded anteriorly by the major fissures and are attached to the lower mediastinum and medial aspect of the hemidiaphragm by the inferior pulmonary ligament.[16] They therefore collapse medially, toward the mediastinum, and contact with the hemidiaphragms is generally maintained. The upper half of the major fissure swings downward and the lower half backward. This displacement is best appreciated on a lateral

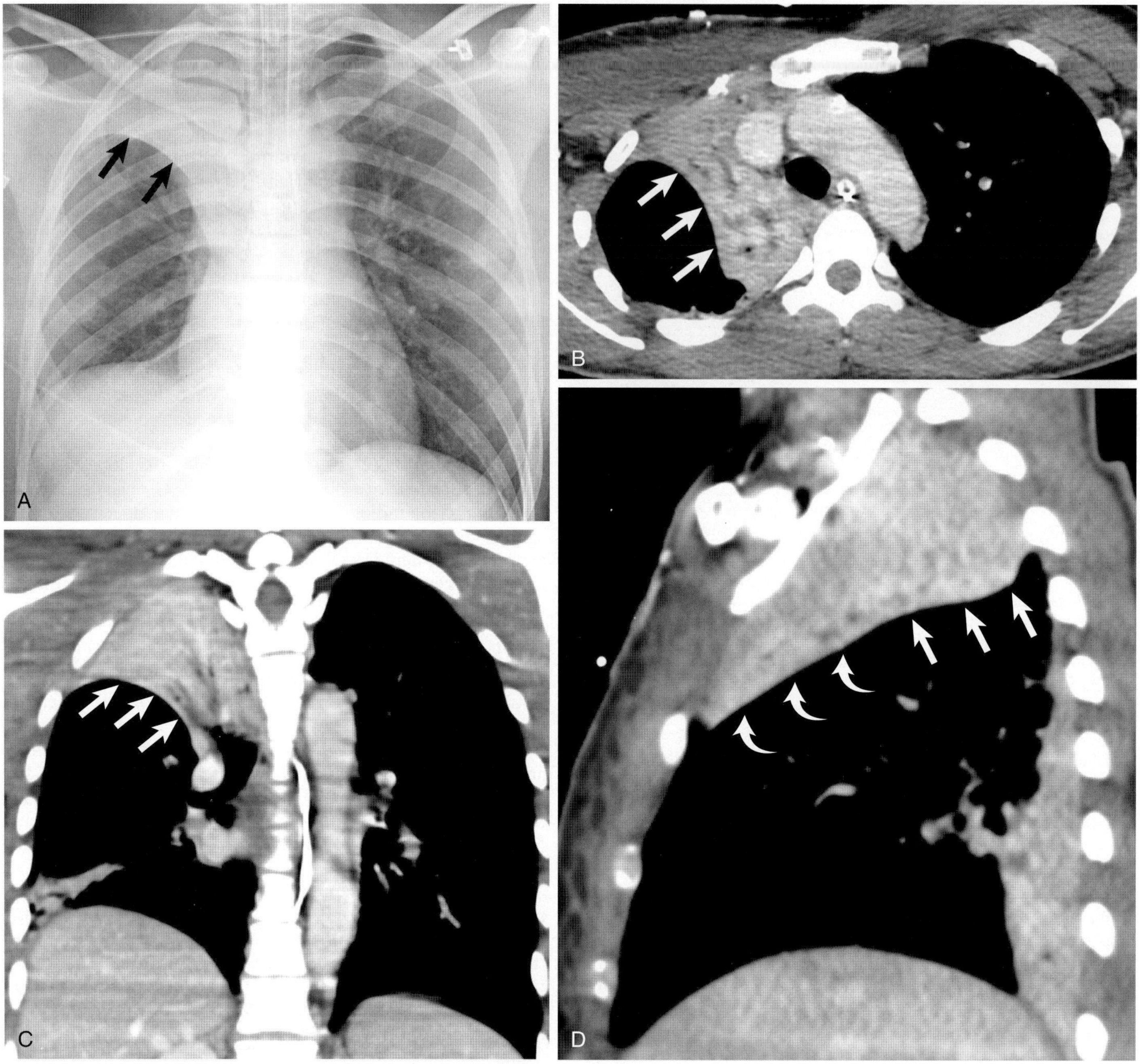

Fig. 3.12 Right upper lobe atelectasis resulting from aspiration and mucus plugging. Chest radiograph (A) shows right upper lobe atelectasis, with superior displacement of the minor fissure *(arrows)*. Axial CT image (B) demonstrates an atelectatic right upper lobe as enhancing soft tissue density lying against the mediastinum and outlined laterally by the minor fissure *(arrows)* that is displaced superiorly and medially. Note the fluid within the right upper lobe bronchi resulting from aspiration and proximal bronchial obstruction. Coronal CT image (C) in soft tissue windows shows right upper lobe atelectasis with superior and medial retraction of the minor fissure *(arrows)*. Sagittal CT image (D) shows a combination of superior displacement of the right minor fissure *(curved arrows)* and anterior and superior displacement of the right major fissure *(straight arrows)*.

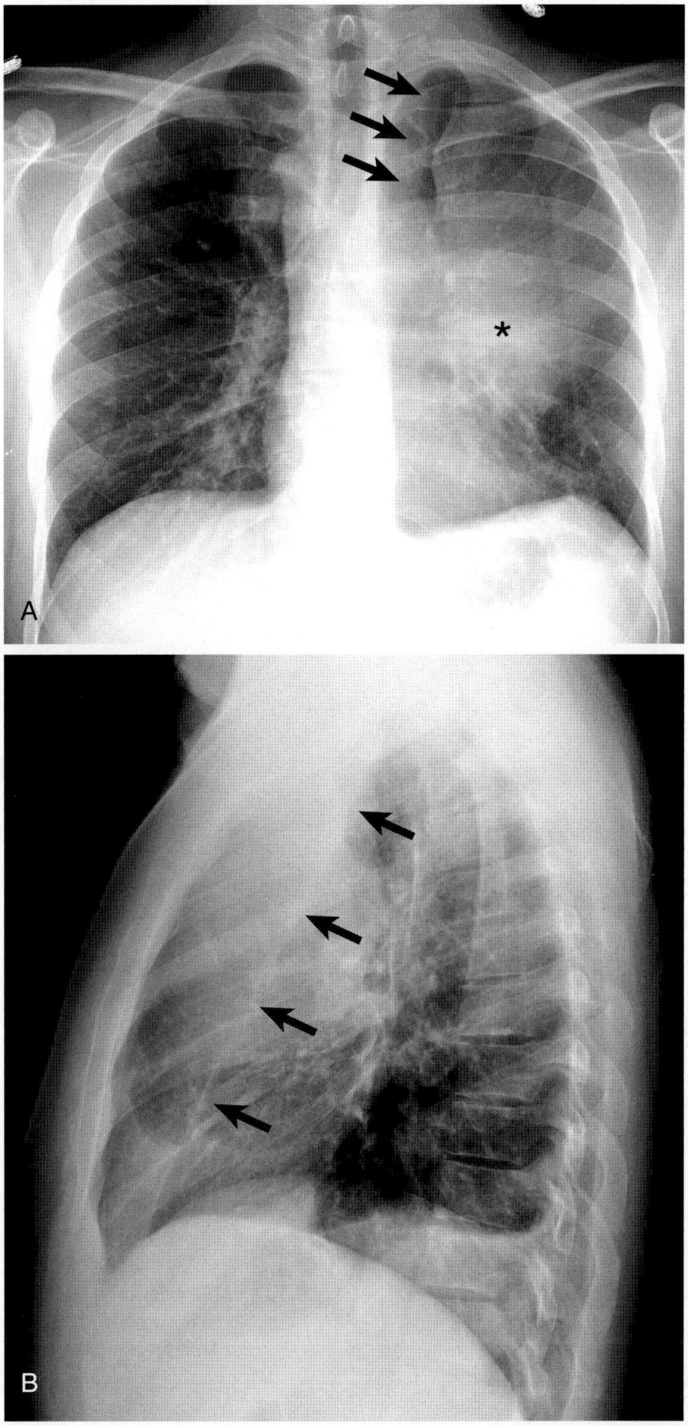

Fig. 3.13 Left upper lobe atelectasis and the *Luftsichel* sign. A posteroanterior chest radiograph (A) shows a left hilar mass *(asterisk)*. Poorly defined increased opacity of the left upper hemithorax is associated with obliteration of the left heart border ("silhouette sign"), loss of volume in the left hemithorax, elevation of the left hemidiaphragm, and superior displacement of the left hilum, characteristic of left upper lobe atelectasis. Note the crescent-shaped radiolucency between the apex of the atelectatic left upper lobe and the aortic arch, the Luftsichel sign *(arrows)*. A lateral radiograph (B) shows anterior displacement of the left major fissure *(arrows)*. Compensatory overinflation of the left lower lobe causes the superior segment to outline the region of the aortic arch, thus accounting for the crescent-shaped lucency on the frontal radiograph.

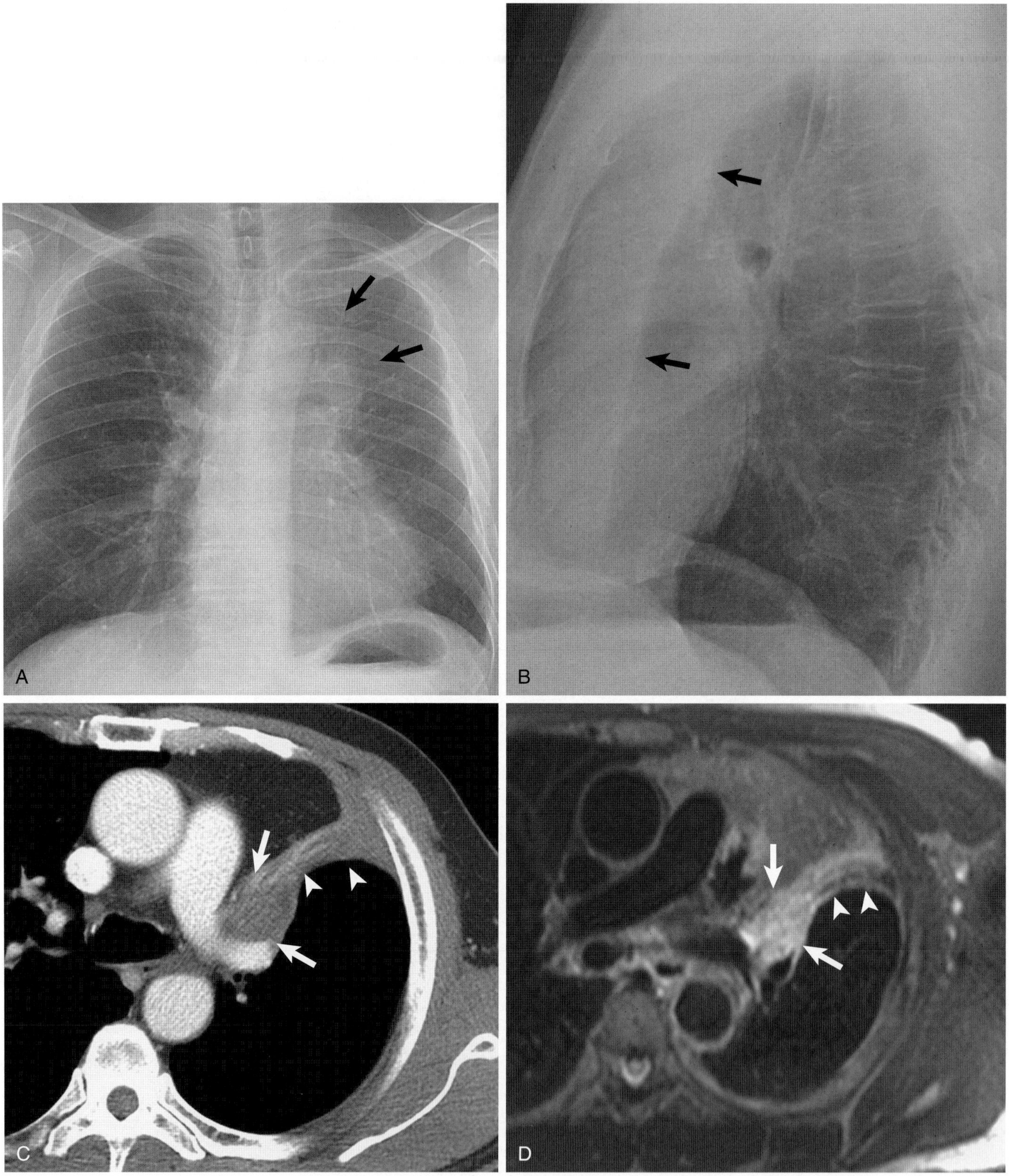

Fig. 3.14 Left upper lobe atelectasis from endobronchial squamous cell carcinoma. A posteroanterior chest radiograph (A) shows subtle increased opacity of the left hemithorax and a poorly defined opacity in the left suprahilar region *(arrows)*. A lateral view (B) shows anterior displacement of the left major fissure *(arrows)*. A contrast-enhanced CT scan (C) demonstrates an obstructing mass *(arrows)* and distal atelectasis with associated superior and medial displacement of the left major fissure *(arrowheads)*. A T2-weighted MR image (D) shows a high–signal intensity tumor *(arrows)* and a lower-intensity atelectatic left upper lobe *(arrowheads)*. *(Courtesy Dr. Kyung Soo Lee, Samsung Medical Center, Seoul, South Korea.)*

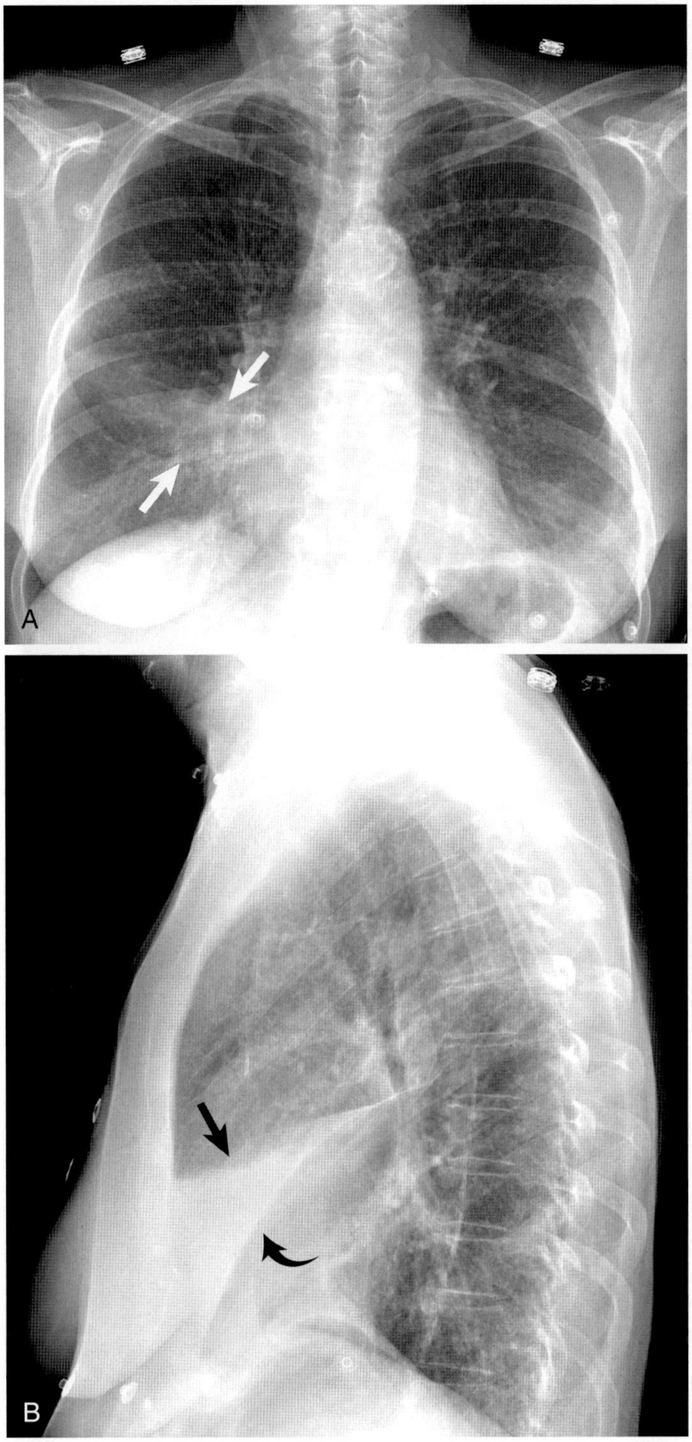

Fig. 3.15 Right middle lobe atelectasis. A posteroanterior radiograph (A) shows a poorly defined area of increased attenuation associated with obscuration of the right heart border (silhouette sign, *arrows*). A lateral (B) view shows downward shift of the minor fissure *(straight arrow)* and forward shift of the right major fissure *(curved arrow)*, leading to a triangular area of increased opacity characteristic of right middle lobe atelectasis.

projection. On a posteroanterior view the hilum and main bronchus are displaced inferiorly and medially; the interlobar artery is displaced medially and is often not visible because it is obscured by the surrounding airless lung. The atelectatic lobe also obscures the hemidiaphragm.

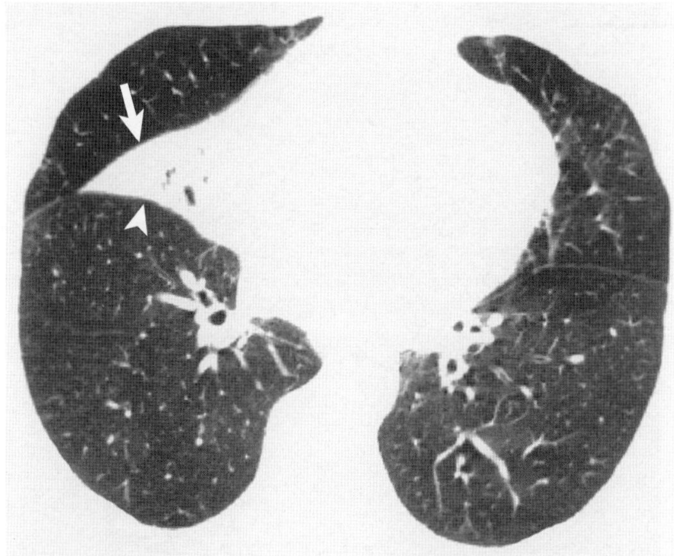

Fig. 3.16 Right middle lobe atelectasis on CT from chronic bronchiectasis. A high-resolution CT scan shows a characteristic broad triangular configuration of the atelectatic right middle lobe. The anterior border of the atelectatic lobe is outlined by the minor fissure *(arrow)*, which is displaced downward, and the posterior border is outlined by the major fissure *(arrowhead)*, which is displaced upward and forward.

During its downward displacement, the upper half of the fissure usually becomes clearly evident on a posteroanterior projection as a well-defined interface extending obliquely downward and laterally from the region of the hilum (Fig. 3.17). The minor fissure may remain in a normal position or be displaced inferiorly. As the atelectasis progresses the lobe moves posteromedially to occupy a position in the posterior costophrenic gutter and medial costovertebral angle. Because the flat surface of the triangular "pancake" lies against the mediastinum, the thickness of tissue traversed by the x-ray beam in a lateral projection may be insufficient to cast a shadow; indeed, when the atelectasis is severe, the only abnormal feature may be a subtle increase in opacity of the lower thoracic vertebrae (see Fig. 3.17) (normally, the vertebrae become relatively more radiolucent from above downward). Provided that exposure factors ensure adequate penetration of the heart, the atelectatic lobe should be plainly visible on a frontal projection as a diminutive triangular opacity in the costovertebral angle.

On CT atelectatic lower lobes can be seen to lose volume in a posteromedial direction and to subsequently pull the major fissure downward (Fig. 3.18).[18] The lateral portion of the major fissure demonstrates a greater degree of mobility because the medial aspect is fixed to the mediastinum by the hilar structures and the pulmonary ligament.

Combined Lobar Atelectasis

Because involvement of the two lobes of the left lung results in total pulmonary collapse, atelectasis of two lobes simultaneously produces a distinctive radiologic pattern only in the right lung.[24]

Combined Right Middle and Lower Lobe Atelectasis. Combined atelectasis of the right middle and lower lobes results from obstruction of the bronchus intermedius. On a posteroanterior radiograph, an atelectatic right lower lobe obscures the right hemidiaphragm, whereas an atelectatic right middle lobe obscures the right heart border (Fig. 3.19). The major and minor fissures

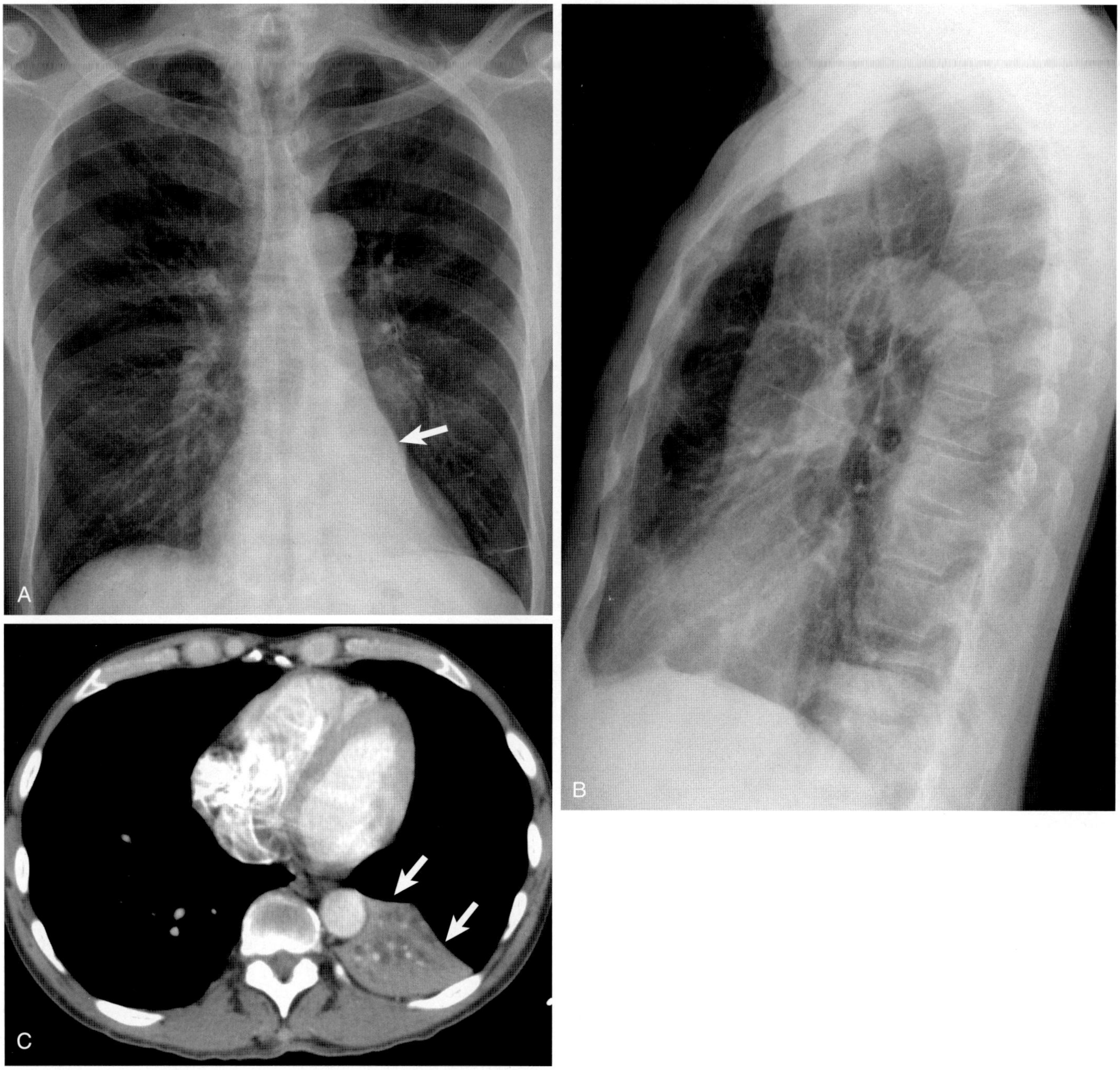

Fig. 3.17 Left lower lobe atelectasis secondary to mucus plugging related to asthma. A chest radiograph (A) shows inferior and medial displacement of the left major fissure that results in a well-defined interface extending obliquely downward and laterally from the region of the hilum *(arrow)*, a finding characteristic of left lower lobe atelectasis. The atelectatic left lower lobe obscures the silhouette of the left descending pulmonary artery and the medial left hemidiaphragm. A lateral view (B) demonstrates a subtle increase in opacity of the lower thoracic vertebrae caused by the atelectatic lower lobe as it moved posteromedially to occupy a position in the posterior costophrenic gutter. Normally, the lower vertebrae are more radiolucent than the higher ones because of superimposition of the shoulder musculature over the upper thoracic vertebrae. (C) Axial CT image shows the atelectatic left lower lobe with posterior and medial displacement of the left major fissure *(arrows)*. Note endobronchial fluid and close spacing of the vessels and bronchi.

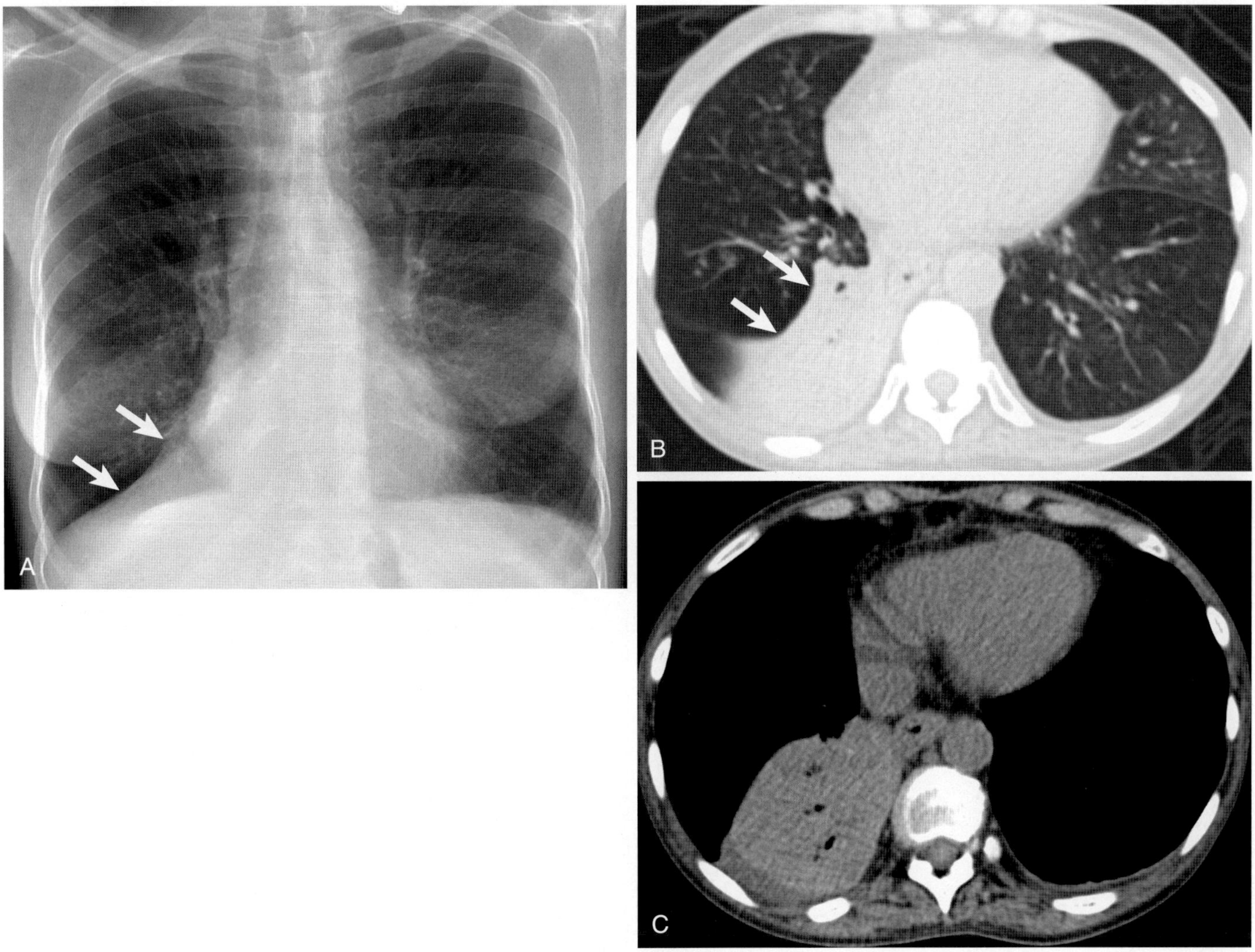

Fig. 3.18 Right lower lobe atelectasis resulting from aspiration and mucus plugging. A posteroanterior chest radiograph (A) shows medial and inferior displacement of the right major fissure *(arrows)*, with obscuration of the lateral portion of the right hemidiaphragm. Note that the right heart border, which would be obscured in right middle lobe atelectasis, is still visible. Axial CT images in lung (B) and soft tissue (C) windows show right lower lobe atelectasis with posterior and medial displacement of the right major fissure *(arrows)*; the right middle lobe remains aerated.

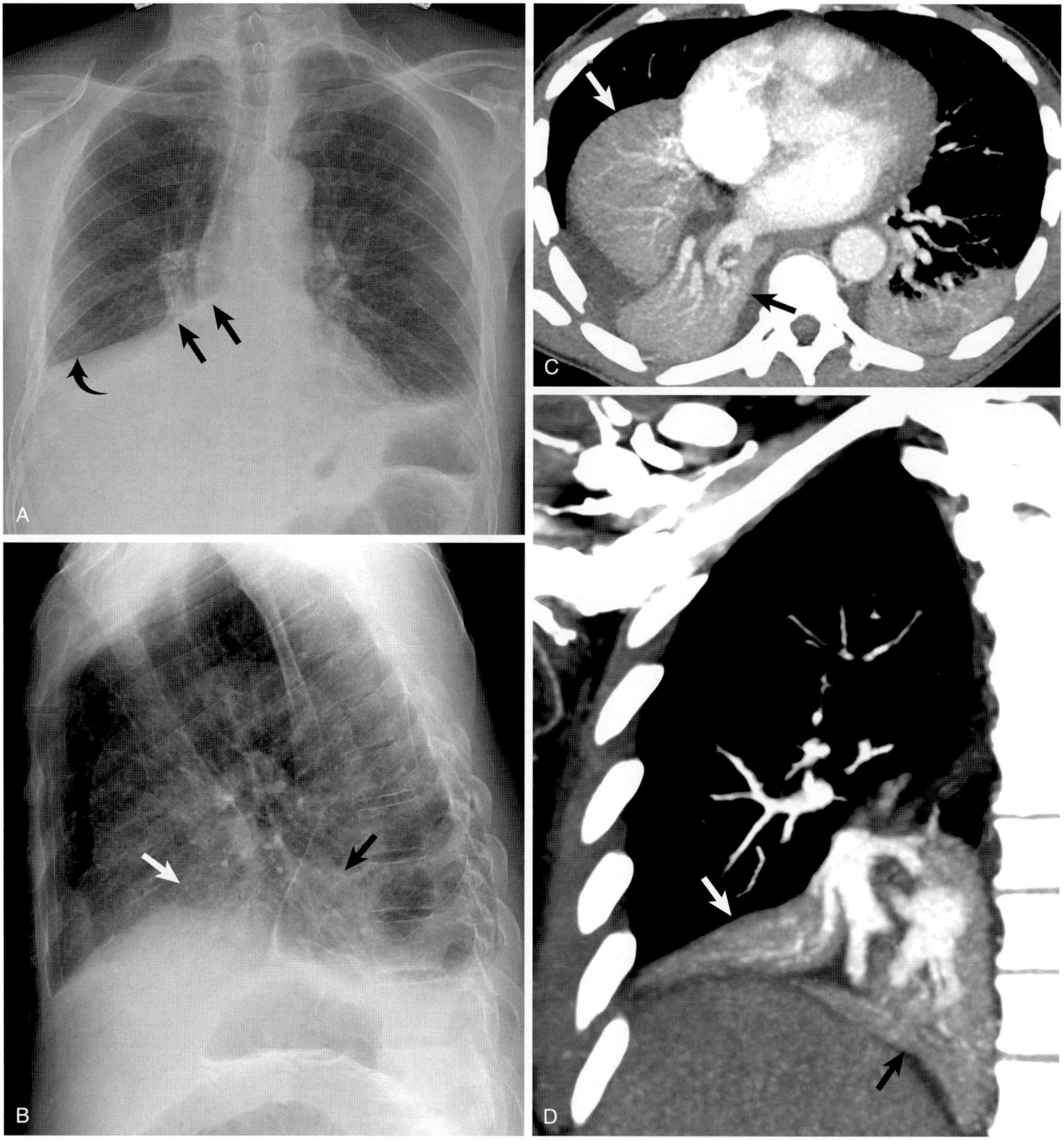

Fig. 3.19 Combined right middle lobe and lower lobe atelectasis from carcinoid tumor in the bronchus intermedius. A posteroanterior chest radiograph (A) shows inferior displacement of the right major *(straight arrows)* and minor *(curved arrow)* fissures. Inferior displacement of the right hilum and overinflation of the right upper lobe are also evident. The silhouettes of the right atrium and right hemidiaphragm are obscured by the atelectatic middle and lower lobes. A lateral view (B) reveals increased opacity throughout the right lower lung zone with obscuration of the right hemidiaphragm. Increased opacity anteriorly corresponds to the atelectatic right middle lobe *(white arrow)*, whereas posterior opacity corresponds to the atelectatic right lower lobe *(black arrow)*. Axial CT image (C) demonstrates the collapsed right middle lobe anteriorly *(white arrow)*, and right lower lobe posteriorly *(black arrow)*; a right pleural effusion extends along the interlobar fissures, separating the two lobes. Sagittal reformatted CT image (D) shows the collapsed right middle lobe anteriorly *(white arrow)* and the right lower lobe posteriorly *(black arrow)*.

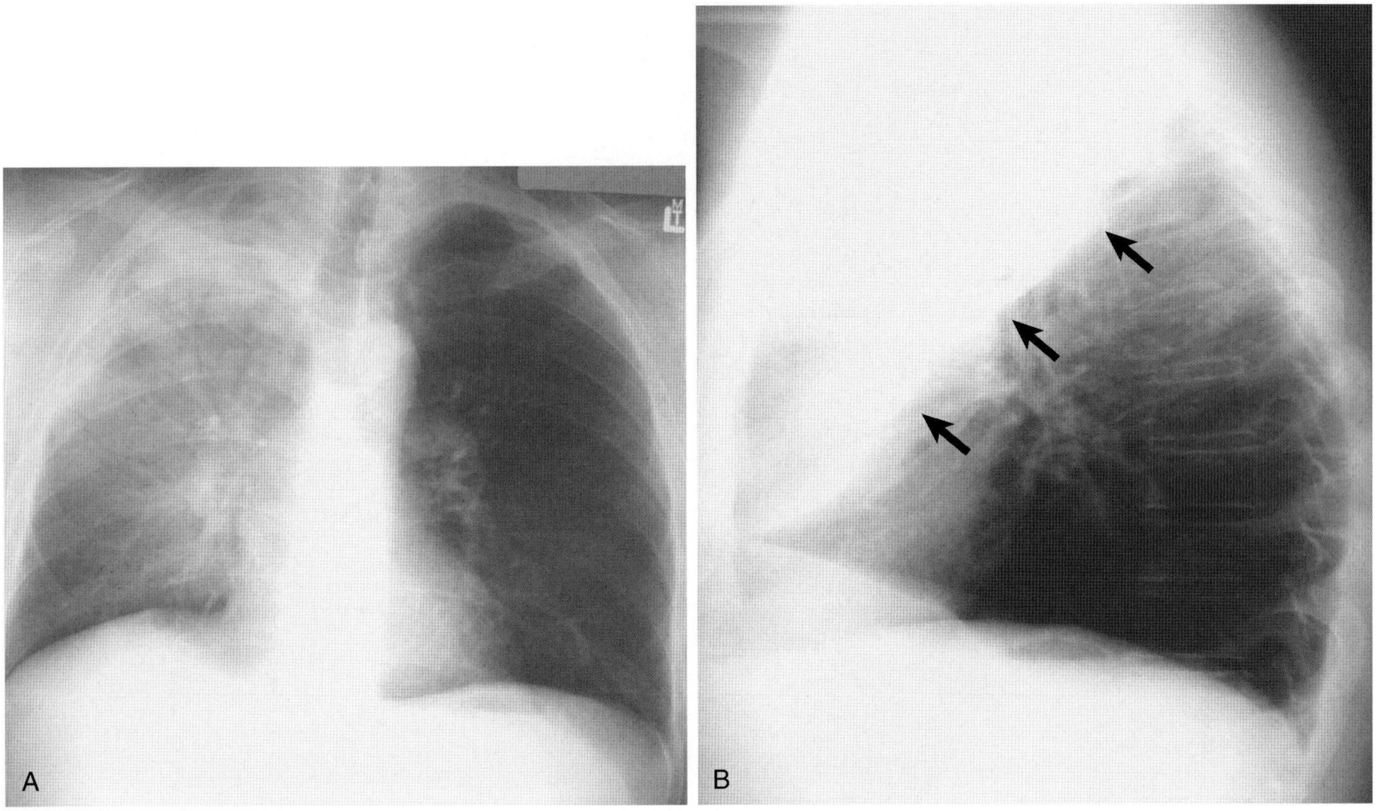

Fig. 3.20 Combined right upper and middle lobe atelectasis from obstructing small cell carcinoma. A posteroanterior chest radiograph (A) shows opacification of the right upper half of the chest with superior displacement of the right hilum and obscuration of the right heart border. A lateral view (B) shows marked anterior and superior displacement of the major fissure *(arrows)*.

are displaced downward and backward so that the opacity occupies the posteroinferior portion of the hemithorax. The opacity may possess an upper surface that is concave or convex upward.[24]

On CT the atelectatic right middle and lower lobes occupy the lower hemithorax and abut the right cardiac border medially and the right hemidiaphragm inferiorly.[24] The right major fissure borders the lateral margin of the atelectatic lobes, and the minor fissure borders the anteromedial margin.

Combined Right Upper and Middle Lobe Atelectasis. Because of the independent and sometimes remote origin of the lobar bronchi of these lobes, such an occurrence is uncommon. Separate causes or a single cause operating at two anatomic locations must be invoked to explain coincidental involvement; it has been described most commonly with mucus plugs and pulmonary carcinoma and, less commonly, with carcinoid tumors, metastatic tumors, and inflammatory processes.[24]

The radiographic findings of combined atelectasis of the right upper and middle lobes are similar to those of left upper lobe atelectasis (Fig. 3.20). On a posteroanterior radiograph it appears as an opacity that obscures the outline of the mediastinum and fades laterally. Cephalad and lateral displacement, as well as rotation of the hilar vessels, may be apparent and is usually associated with obscuration of the silhouettes of the ascending aorta and right atrium. On a lateral radiograph the major fissure can be seen to be displaced anteriorly (see Fig. 3.20). The major fissure may be straight, convex anteriorly, or convex posteriorly.[24]

CT shows anterior displacement of the major fissure, with the hyperinflated lower lobe filling most of the right hemithorax. The atelectatic lobes cause a wedge-shaped area of soft tissue attenuation that abuts the chest wall anteriorly and the ascending aorta and right heart border medially.[24]

Combined Right Upper and Lower Lobe Atelectasis. Combined atelectasis of the right upper and lower lobes is rare. It may result from mucus plugs occurring simultaneously in the bronchi of the right upper and lower lobes. There is also an example in a patient with mucinous adenocarcinoma without any CT or bronchoscopic evidence of bronchial obstruction.[24] The radiologic and CT findings of combined atelectasis of the right upper and lower lobes are similar to those of isolated atelectasis of either lobe.

Migrating Lobar Atelectasis

Uncommonly, heavy atelectatic lobes filled with fluid, pneumonic consolidation, or tumor may migrate within the hemithorax with changes in body position. In one series of six cases, migrating atelectasis involved the right upper lobe in three cases and the right upper and middle lobes in three cases.[25] On supine anteroposterior radiographs the atelectatic lobe or lobes occupied the right upper lung zone, with a wedge shape abutting the right mediastinal border. On erect posteroanterior radiographs the heavy atelectatic lobe or lobes migrated downward and formed a perihilar or infrahilar area of increased opacity that obscured the right cardiac margin (Fig. 3.21). Erect lateral radiographs showed inferior shift of the anterosuperiorly located

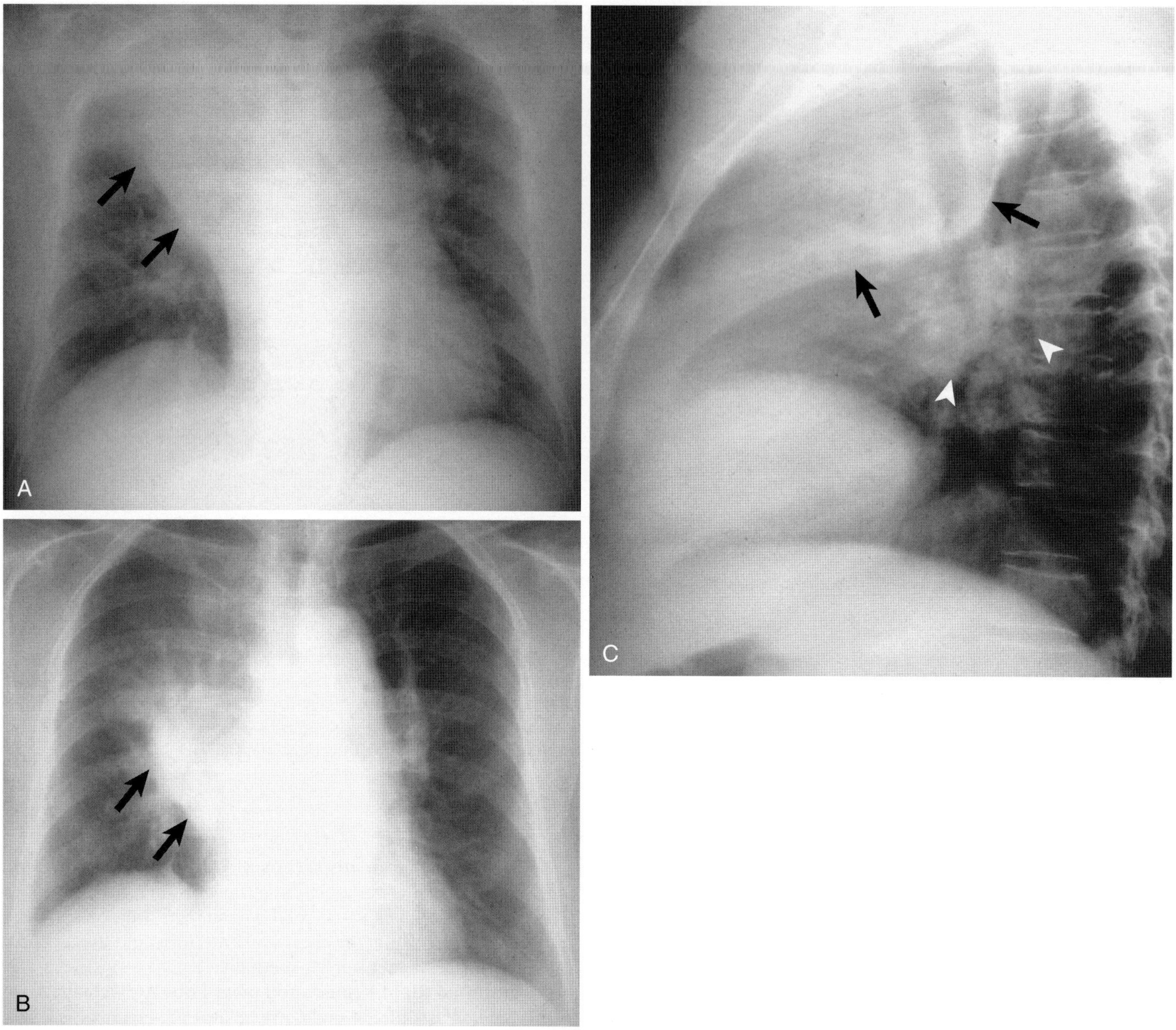

Fig. 3.21 Migrating atelectasis. A chest radiograph with the patient supine (A) shows a parenchymal opacity *(arrows)* in the right upper and middle lung zones and elevation of the right hemidiaphragm. A chest radiograph with the patient upright (B) shows downward migration of the increased opacity *(arrows)*. A lateral view (C) demonstrates anterior displacement of right major fissure *(arrows)*, characteristic of combined right upper and middle lobe atelectasis. Also noted is hilar lymphadenopathy *(arrowheads)*. *(Courtesy Dr. Kyung Soo Lee, Samsung Medical Center, Seoul, South Korea.)*

atelectatic lobe or lobes to the anteroinferior portion of the hemithorax. Migrating lobar atelectasis per se has little clinical and radiologic significance. However, when a lobe or lobes are migrating and occupying a dependent position on erect posteroanterior and lateral radiographs, they may mimic a hilar or mediastinal mass.

SEGMENTAL ATELECTASIS

Segmental atelectasis usually results from bronchial obstruction and is associated with obstructive pneumonitis. Thus a homogeneous opacity that conforms to the anatomic distribution of a bronchopulmonary segment and in which no air bronchogram is identifiable should immediately alert the physician to the presence of an obstructing endobronchial lesion associated with obstructive pneumonitis and atelectasis. Occasionally, bronchiectasis develops distal to an obstruction lesion (Fig. 3.22). As might be anticipated, the opacity resulting from segmental obstructive pneumonitis depends not only on the original volume of lung parenchyma affected but also on the volume of inflammatory tissue that has replaced it. Thus the shadow can vary from a large conical opacity in which there is very little loss of volume to little more than a broad linear opacity in which atelectasis has predominated.

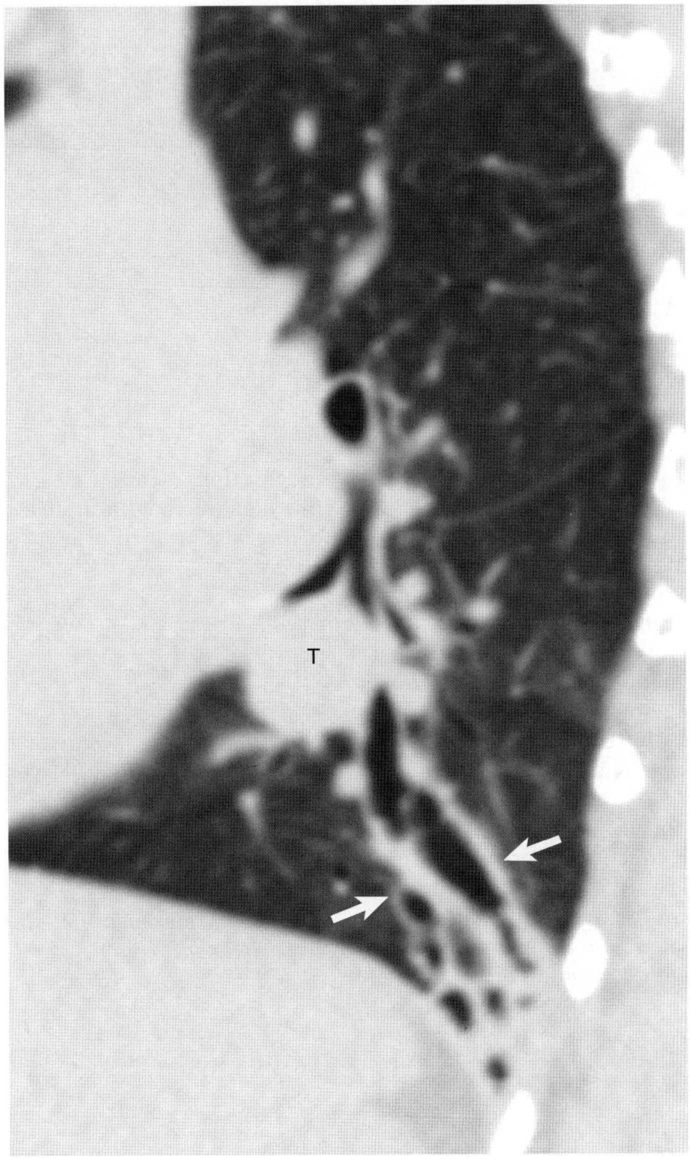

Fig. 3.22 Segmental atelectasis and bronchiectasis within the right lower lobe due to a carcinoid tumor. The tumor *(T)* obstructs segmental bronchi within the right lower lobe, causing distal segmental atelectasis and bronchiectasis *(arrows)*. The remainder of the right lower lobe remains aerated, but the overall volume of the lobe is decreased. The slow growth typical of carcinoid tumors often allows distal bronchiectasis to develop over time through a ball-valve mechanism.

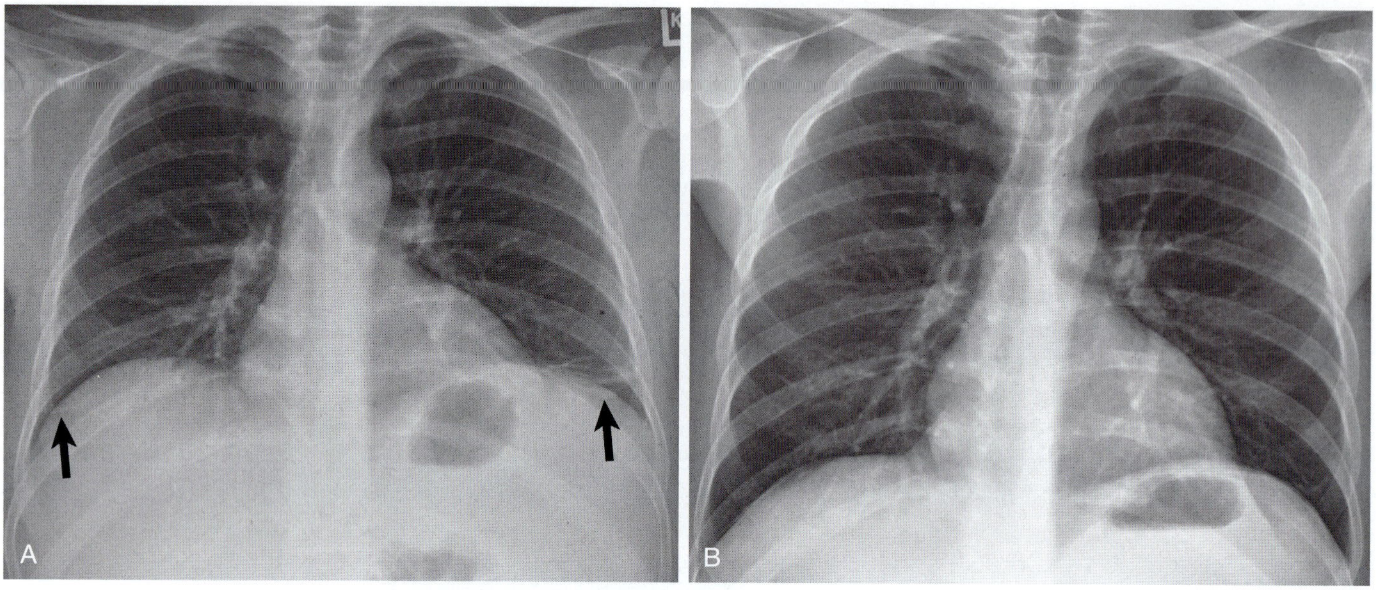

Fig. 3.23 Linear atelectasis. A chest radiograph performed at low lung volumes (A) shows linear opacities in both lower lobes *(arrows)*, characteristic of linear atelectasis. A chest radiograph performed at full inspiration (B) is normal.

LINEAR (PLATE-LIKE) ATELECTASIS

Linear atelectasis (discoid atelectasis, plate-like atelectasis) is typically manifested as linear soft tissue opacities ranging from 1 to 3 mm in thickness and 4 to 10 cm in length; they are situated in the middle and lower lung zones, most commonly the latter (Fig. 3.23). Although usually oriented in a roughly horizontal plane, they may be obliquely oriented, depending on the zone of lung affected. They may be single or multiple, unilateral or bilateral. Linear atelectasis is typically seen in conditions that diminish diaphragmatic excursion, such as intraabdominal surgery or inflammatory disease.

In 10 patients in whom a linear opacity was present on their last antemortem radiograph and subsequently underwent autopsy, linear areas of atelectasis extended to the pleural surface and were associated with invagination of the overlying pleura, with foci of subpleural atelectasis associated with invagination of the adjacent pleura.[26] An association with congenital pleural clefts, indentations, scars, and incomplete fissures suggested to the investigators that linear atelectasis develops preferentially at sites of preexisting pleural invagination; bronchial obstruction was absent.

SUGGESTED READINGS

Lee KS, Logan PM, Primack SL, Müller NL. Combined lobar atelectasis of the right lung: imaging findings. *AJR Am J Roentgenol*. 1994;163:43–47.

Molina PL, Hiken JN, Glazer HS. Imaging evaluation of obstructive atelectasis. *J Thorac Imaging*. 1996;11:176–186.

Proto AV. Lobar collapse: basic concepts. *Eur J Radiol*. 1996;23:9–22.

Woodring JH, Reed JC. Types and mechanisms of pulmonary atelectasis. *J Thorac Imaging*. 1996;11:92–108.

Woodring JH, Reed JC. Radiographic manifestations of lobar atelectasis. *J Thorac Imaging*. 1996;11:109–144.

The full reference list for this chapter is available at ExpertConsult.com.

4 Nodules and Masses*

SARAH T. KURIAN | CHRISTOPHER M. WALKER | JONATHAN H. CHUNG

Solitary Lung Nodule or Mass

A pulmonary nodule is defined as any pulmonary lesion that is well-defined, discrete, approximately circular, and 3 cm or less in diameter.[1,2] The term *mass* is used for lesions greater than 3 cm in diameter. The differential diagnosis of a nodule or mass detected on a radiograph or CT is very broad (Table 4.1). However, more than 95% fall into one of three groups: malignant neoplasms (primary or metastatic), infectious granulomas (tuberculosis or endemic fungi), or less commonly, benign tumors (neoplastic or nonneoplastic). Approximately 40% of solitary lung nodules detected on a chest radiograph represent primary lung cancer.[3,4]

Most of the nodules detected radiographically measure more than 1 cm in diameter. Noncalcified nodules less than 7 mm in diameter are seldom visible on radiographs. In contrast, nodules as small as 1 to 2 mm in diameter are readily seen on CT. More than 50% of smokers who undergo thin-section CT have small lung nodules, almost all of which measure less than 7 mm in diameter.[5] The vast majority of these small nodules are benign.[6,7]

The first step in assessing a lesion detected on a chest radiograph is to determine that it is indeed a lung nodule rather than a pleural or chest wall abnormality, such as a healing rib fracture, pleural neoplasm, or skin lesion projecting over the lung (Fig. 4.1). The next step is to evaluate the imaging characteristics of the nodule to determine whether there are findings that favor a benign or a malignant lesion. After this, one must integrate the imaging characteristics with clinical findings such as patient age, risk factors such as cigarette smoking or a known primary extrathoracic neoplasm, recent travel history, and symptoms such as fever or hemoptysis. For example, a nodule in an adolescent patient is likely to be benign, regardless of its margin characteristics. A growing noncalcified nodule in an older smoking patient is likely to be malignant even though it has smooth borders. In the vast majority of cases, pulmonary metastases are multiple. However, single lung metastases may also occur, particularly with sarcomas and testicular tumors.

Advances in multidetector CT have improved nodule detection and characterization with thin-section imaging, acquisition within a single breath-hold, high-quality volumetric image data, as well as multiplanar and maximum intensity projection (MIP) reconstructions (Fig. 4.2).[8,9] Of note, multiplanar CT images should be fully used in assessing a nodule's shape and appearance because linear opacities, as seen with atelectasis or scar, may appear nodular in a single plane. In the vast majority of cases, no intravenous contrast material is necessary for nodule characterization.

In evaluating lung nodules, it is useful to divide them into two categories: (1) those that are clearly benign, as determined by rigidly defined radiologic signs,[10] and (2) those of indeterminate nature, which represent all other lesions. This allows one to distinguish benign from malignant nodules with a reasonable degree of confidence.

LOCATION OF THE LESION

An intrapulmonary nodule tends to form an acute angle with the contiguous pleura and to have well-defined margins when seen en face (see Fig. 4.1A and B). A nodule originating within the pleural space, rib, or chest wall displaces the pleura and underlying lung inward (see Fig. 4.1C and D). It therefore tends to have tapered margins and form an obtuse angle with the chest wall and to have one side demonstrating a well-defined margin and the opposite side a poorly defined margin when seen en face (incomplete border sign). Similar to all other radiologic signs, this sign is fallible. Occasionally, an extrapulmonary nodule relates to the lung at an acute angle and an intrapulmonary mass at an obtuse angle.

Imaging Characteristics of Lung Nodules

Distinction between benign and malignant lesions can often be established with a reasonable degree of confidence from the clinical and radiographic findings, although findings are seldom pathognomonic. The main diagnostic radiologic criteria are nodule size, change in size over time, attenuation (including presence of calcification or fat), margin characteristics, and ^{18}F-fluorodeoxyglucose (FDG) avidity.

Size

The prevalence of malignancy typically varies by size with less than 1% for nodules less than 5 mm, 0.5% to 28% for nodules 5 to 10 mm, and 64% to 82% for nodules greater than 20 mm.[11,12] When interpreting these figures it is important to remember that the likelihood of carcinoma is influenced strongly by other factors such as age and smoking history.

Change in Size

Because uncontrolled growth is a characteristic feature of cancer, in the absence of an infectious or inflammatory process, an enlarging pulmonary nodule should be considered malignant until proven otherwise by tissue sampling. However, because some benign lesions such as hamartoma and histoplasmoma can enlarge and some adenocarcinomas can grow slowly, an increase in the size of a nodule, by itself, should not be the sole consideration governing the therapeutic approach. Traditionally, 2-year stability in size has been considered a reasonably reliable criterion of benignity; however, the validity of this statement has been questioned, particularly with respect to ground-glass or part-solid nodules, in which a slight change in size may be difficult to appreciate. Patients with ground-glass and part-solid

*The editors and the publisher would like to thank Drs. Nestor L. Müller and C. Isabela Silva Müller for contributing material on this topic to the prior edition of this work. It has served as the foundation for the current chapter.

TABLE 4.1 SOLITARY PULMONARY NODULE OR MASS: DIFFERENTIAL DIAGNOSIS

Etiology	Features
CONGENITAL	
Bronchogenic cyst	Water density on CT (50%). Almost all have high signal intensity on T2-weighted MRI
Pulmonary arteriovenous malformation	Round, oval, or slightly lobulated. CT shows a feeding artery and draining vein
INFECTIOUS/INFLAMMATORY	
Tuberculosis	Common. Mainly upper lobes. Frequently calcifies
Histoplasmosis	Common in endemic areas. Frequently calcifies
Coccidioidomycosis	Common in endemic areas. Frequently cavitates. Rarely calcifies
Echinococcus	Water density on CT
Lung abscess	Cavitation or low-attenuation center on CT
Focal (round) pneumonia	Less common in adults than in children. Tends to have ill-defined margins
Granulomatosis with polyangiitis	A solitary nodule is uncommon
Rheumatoid nodules	Necrobiotic rheumatoid nodules most commonly multiple
Organizing pneumonia	Tends to have ill-defined margins
Lipoid pneumonia	Irregular margins. Foci of fat density on CT (80%)
Conglomerate fibrosis in sarcoidosis	Uncommon. Typically bilateral, perihilar, and upper lobes. Air bronchograms
Conglomerate fibrosis in talcosis	Intravenous drug user. Typically upper lobes. Characteristic high attenuation because of talc deposition
PNEUMOCONIOSIS	
Progressive massive fibrosis in silicosis	Typically perihilar, bilateral, and upper lobes. Other findings of silicosis
NEOPLASTIC	
Pulmonary carcinoma	Smooth, lobulated, or most commonly, spiculated margins
Carcinoid tumor	Relatively uncommon. Usually smooth margins
Hamartoma	Uncommon. Tends to have lobulated margins. Sixty percent have areas of fat density on CT. Popcorn calcification characteristic but uncommon
Metastasis	Solitary metastasis uncommon except for sarcoma. Tends to have smooth margins
TRAUMATIC	
Hematoma	Uncommon. Smooth margins. Usually in a peripheral location. Slow but progressive decrease in size

TABLE 4.2 FLESICHNER CRITERIA FOR SOLID NODULES

SOLID NODULE					
	<6 mm	<6 mm	6–8 mm	6–8 mm	>8 mm
	Low Risk	**High Risk**	**Low Risk**	**High Risk**	**Any Risk**
Solitary	No follow-up	12-mo CT if suspicious[a]	6- to 12-mo CT, consider 18- to 24-mo CT if suspicious[a]	Both 6- to 12-mo CT and 18- to 24-mo CT	Consider CT, PET/CT, or tissue sampling at 3 mo
Multiple	No follow-up	12-mo CT if suspicious[b]	3- to 6-mo CT, consider 18- to 24-mo CT if suspicious[b]	Both 3- to 6-mo CT and 18- to 24-mo CT	3- to 6-mo CT; additional 18- to 24-mo CT if high risk or suspicious[b]

[a]Suspicious by morphology or with upper lobe location.
[b]Based on most suspicious nodule.
Modified from MacMahon H, Naiditch NP, Goo JM, et al. Guidelines for management of incidental pulmonary nodules detected on CT images: from the Fleischner Society 2017. *Radiology*. 2017;284:228-243.

nodules require longer monitoring as outlined by the Fleischner criteria (Tables 4.2 and 4.3).[11,13]

Use of the doubling time provides a more accurate assessment of the nature of a pulmonary nodule than a simple increase in size does. Doubling refers to volume, not diameter. Assuming a nodule to be spherical, its diameter must be multiplied by 1.25 to obtain the diameter of a sphere whose volume is double (e.g., the volume of a nodule 2 cm in diameter is doubled by the time that its diameter reaches 2.5 cm). A doubling of diameter represents an eightfold increase in volume. Measurement of doubling time requires at least two serial chest radiographs or CT scans showing a roughly spherical lesion whose diameter can be averaged from measurements in at least two planes. In a study of 218 pulmonary nodules (177 malignant and 41 benign), virtually all nodules whose doubling time was 7 days or less or 465 days or longer were benign.[14] A pulmonary nodule whose rate of growth falls between these limits is often malignant. A pitfall to be aware of is indolent lung cancer (particularly adenocarcinoma), which may manifest as a ground-glass nodule gradually enlarging over 5 years or longer. For this reason, ground-glass nodules merit longer follow-up, per the Fleischner criteria (see Table 4.3). Perhaps the most useful application of the growth rate

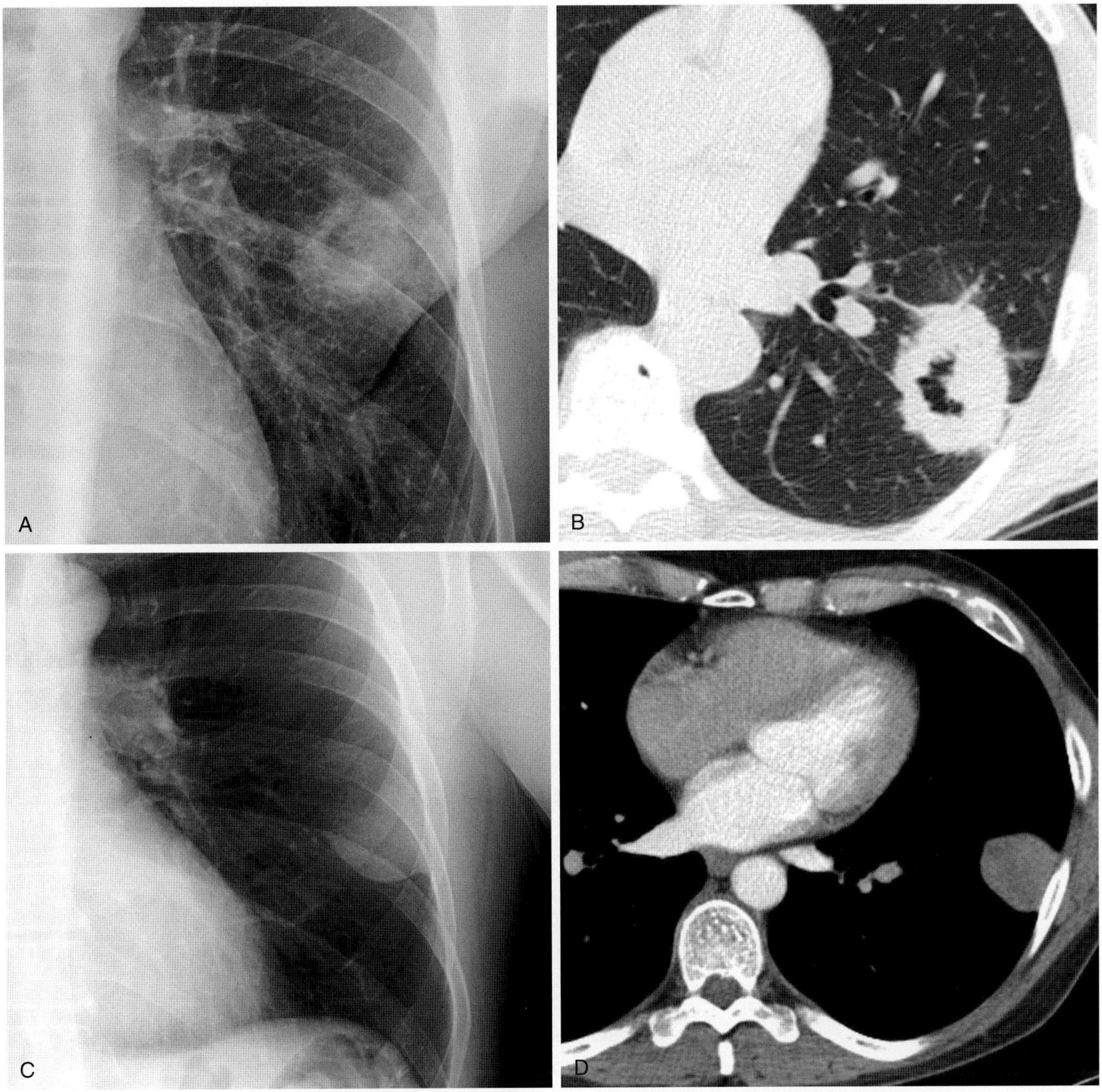

Fig. 4.1 Lung nodule or mass versus a pleural or chest wall nodule or mass. (A) Frontal chest radiograph shows a cavitary left lower lobe nodule. All the margins of the nodule are well seen, suggesting a lung origin. (B) Axial CT scan confirms the intraparenchymal location of the cavitary left lower lobe nodule in a man with lung cancer. (C) Frontal chest radiograph from a different patient with localized fibrous tumor of the pleura shows a nodular opacity with tapered margins that forms an obtuse angle with the chest wall. Note that the inferior margins of the nodule are well defined, indicative of contact with lung, whereas the upper and outer margins are poorly defined, indicative of contact with the pleura and chest wall. This is called the "incomplete border sign" and helps suggest a pleural or chest wall location of a lesion. (D) Axial CT image from the same patient as (C) confirms the pleural origin of the abnormality. *(Fig. 4.1C reproduced with permission from Walker CM, Takasugi JE, Chung JH, et al. Tumorlike conditions of the pleura.* Radiographics. *2012;32:971-985.)*

TABLE 4.3 FLEISCHNER CRITERIA FOR SUBSOLID (GROUND-GLASS AND PART-SOLID) NODULES

SOLITARY SUBSOLID NODULE			
	<6 mm	**≥6 mm**	
		Initial follow-up:	*Additional follow-up if stable:*
Ground-glass	No follow-up	6- to 12-mo CT	Biannual CT until 5 years
Part-solid	No follow-up	3- to 6-mo CT	Annual CT at least 5 years (Note: Solid component must remain <6 mm; persistent part-solid nodules with solid component measuring ≥6 mm should be considered highly suspicious for adenocarcinoma.)
MULTIPLE SUBSOLID NODULES			
	<6 mm	**≥6 mm**	
Initial follow-up	3- to 6-mo CT	3- to 6-mo CT	
Additional follow-up (if stable)	Consider 24- and 48-mo CT	Per most suspicious nodule	

Modified from MacMahon H, Naiditch NP, Goo JM, et al. Guidelines for management of incidental pulmonary nodules detected on CT images: from the Fleischner Society 2017. *Radiology*. 2017;284:228–243.

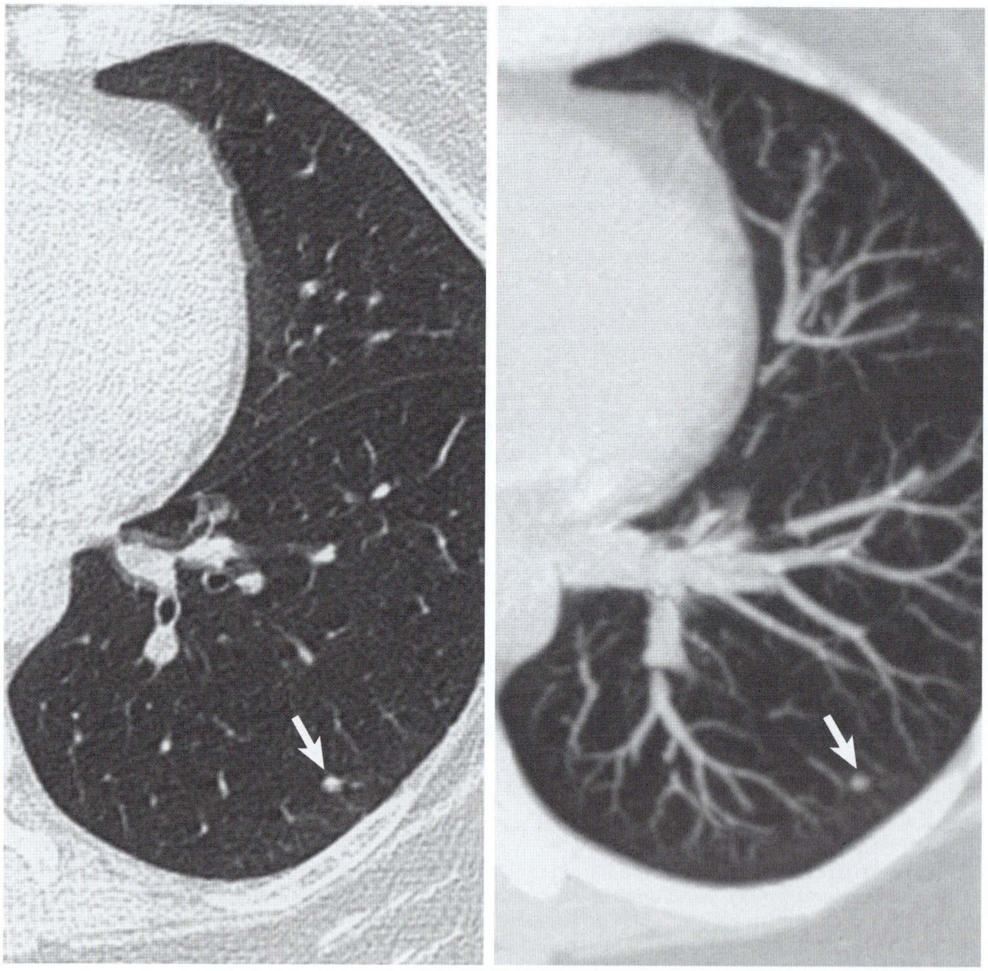

Fig. 4.2 Value of a maximum intensity projection (MIP) reconstruction in the detection of a small lung nodule. Composite image with axial CT image *(left image)* and MIP reconstruction *(right image)* shows a small left lower lobe nodule *(arrows)*, better visualized on the MIP reconstruction.

principle in assessing solitary nodules is in patients older than 40 years, in whom the incidence of malignancy increases markedly. In a study of individuals in this older age group, almost every solitary nodule whose doubling time was less than 37 days was benign.[14]

Attenuation: Calcification

Benign patterns of calcification within a solitary pulmonary nodule are one of the most reliable signs that a lesion is benign.[15–17] Four patterns of calcification are characteristically associated with benign lesions: diffuse, laminated, central, and popcorn

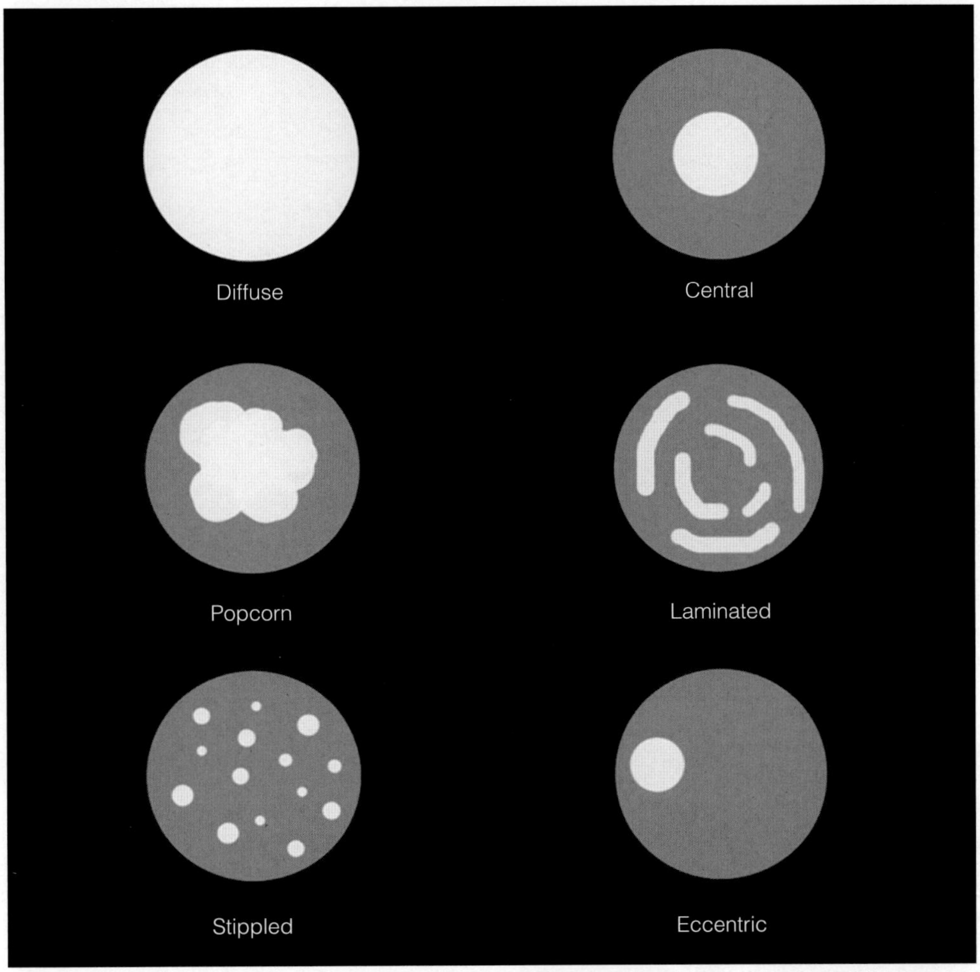

Fig. 4.3 Patterns of calcification. A schematic drawing shows the characteristic patterns of pulmonary nodule calcification. Diffuse calcification, central calcification in nodules 2 cm or less in diameter, popcorn calcification, and laminated calcification are virtually diagnostic of a benign nodule. Diffuse, central, and laminated types of calcification are seen most commonly in calcified granulomas as a result of previous infection by tuberculosis or *Histoplasma* species, and popcorn calcification, albeit rare, is virtually diagnostic of hamartoma. Stippled calcification, particularly when seen in large masses, and eccentric calcification are worrisome for malignancy. They occur most commonly in pulmonary carcinoma.

(Fig. 4.3). The diffuse (Fig. 4.4) and laminated (synonym: concentric or laminar) types of calcification are virtually diagnostic of a granuloma, although this cannot be applied to pulmonary masses (>3 cm in size).[10,16,18] A small central nidus of calcification is seen most commonly with granulomatous lesions (typically tuberculosis and histoplasmosis), although it also occurs in some hamartomas. Popcorn calcification is characteristic of hamartoma (Fig. 4.5). By contrast, the presence of an eccentric calcification in a nodule or mass may represent incorporation of a calcified granuloma within the substance of a carcinoma.

Calcification within a pulmonary nodule is more readily seen on low-kilovoltage than on high-kilovoltage radiographs and much better characterized on CT than on a radiograph. Consequently, CT is the study of choice in assessing pulmonary nodules. In a study of 634 nodules assessed with CT, 153 were diagnosed correctly as benign based on the presence of central or diffuse calcification; although focal areas of calcification were identified in 13% of the primary lung tumors, only 1 carcinoid tumor had a benign pattern of calcification.[16] The other malignant tumors had neither central nor diffuse calcification.

Calcification in malignant tumors may be seen in several circumstances: (1) most important from a differential diagnosis point of view, the isolated instance of a peripheral primary carcinoma engulfing a calcified granuloma, in which case the calcification is usually eccentric; (2) a solitary metastasis of osteogenic sarcoma or chondrosarcoma with bone formation in the osteoid or calcification of the malignant cartilage; (3) occasional primary pulmonary carcinoid tumors; and (4) calcification in large pulmonary carcinomas (Fig. 4.6), particularly in tumors larger than 3 cm in diameter.[19] The calcification in these large tumors may be punctate, chunky, or amorphous in appearance and central, peripheral, or diffuse in distribution. It is related to psammoma bodies, dystrophic calcification of necrotic carcinoma, or incorporation of a focus of previous granulomatous inflammation or calcified bronchial cartilage within the tumor.

Optimal assessment of lung nodules for the presence of calcification by CT requires the use of thin sections (1- to 2-mm collimation) through the nodule so as to minimize volume averaging and errors in nodule classification based on imaging appearance (e.g., solid vs. subsolid).[20] Foci of calcification that are visible on thin-section CT usually have attenuation values

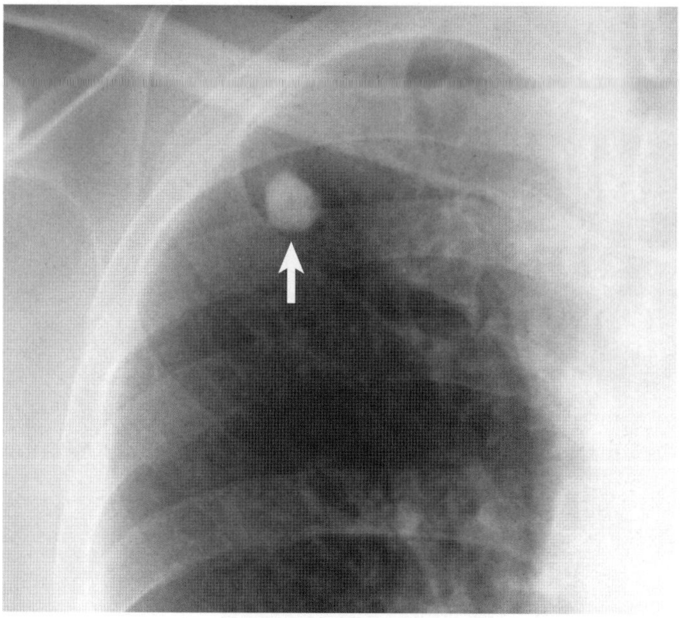

Fig. 4.4 Diffuse calcification from previous tuberculosis. Frontal chest radiograph shows a diffusely calcified right upper lobe nodule *(arrow)*.

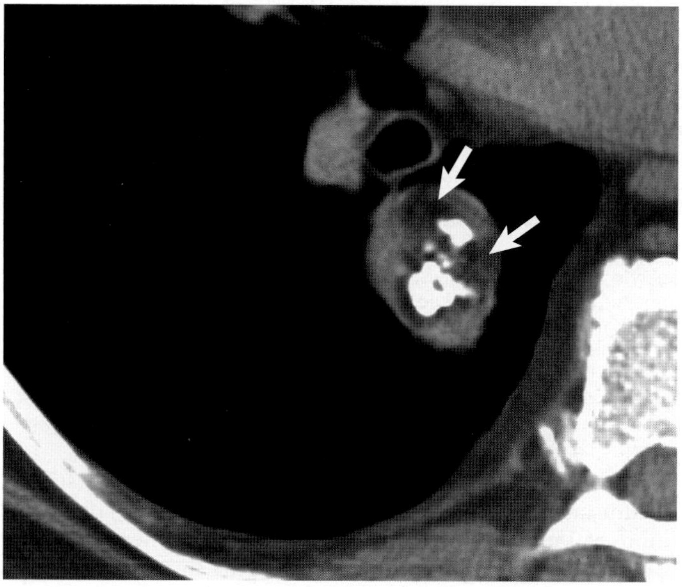

Fig. 4.5 Popcorn calcification in pulmonary hamartoma. Axial CT scan shows a right lower lobe smoothly marginated nodule with several coarse foci of calcification (popcorn calcification). Also note the presence of foci of fat attenuation *(arrows)*. The findings are virtually pathognomonic of hamartoma.

of 400 Hounsfield units (HU) or higher; in the absence of such foci, attenuation values of 200 HU or higher can be considered to represent calcification.[21]

Attenuation: Fat Density

Demonstration of the presence of fat (−30 to −120 HU) attenuation values on thin-section CT within a smoothly marginated lung nodule is virtually diagnostic of hamartoma; however, this should be interpreted with caution as volume-averaging or necrosis can also result in similar attenuation values. In a study of 47 hamartomas, 18 (38%) showed areas of fat, and 10 (21%) showed foci of calcium and fat (see Fig. 4.5).[22] Fat within a spiculated lesion is most suggestive of lipoid pneumonia (Fig. 4.7). The radiographic and CT findings of lipoid pneumonia include single or multiple nodules or masses and localized or confluent areas of consolidation.[23,24] In approximately 80% of patients, focal areas of fat attenuation can be seen on CT using soft tissue windows.[23,24]

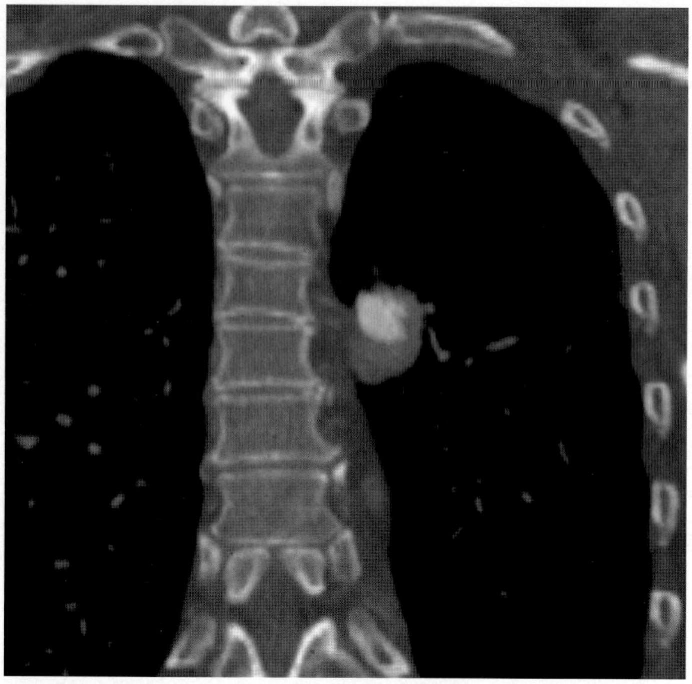

Fig. 4.6 Calcified metastasis from breast cancer. Coronal CT scan shows a calcified nodule in the left lung. Note the eccentric distribution of the calcification. The patient also had calcified liver metastases.

Attenuation: Water Density

Water density (0 HU) on CT plus a thin or invisible wall is diagnostic of a cystic lesion. The differential diagnosis includes bronchogenic cyst, congenital pulmonary airway malformation, hydatid cyst, and fluid-filled bulla (Fig. 4.8). Only 50% of bronchogenic cysts have water density on CT; however, virtually all have characteristic high signal intensity similar to that of cerebrospinal fluid on T2-weighted MR images.[25] Of note, air-fluid levels may occur in lung abscesses or infected cavitary lesions, which require follow-up to ensure resolution.

Attenuation: Air Bronchogram

On thin-section CT, air bronchograms and bronchiolograms occur more commonly with pulmonary carcinomas than with benign nodules.[26] For example, in a review of 132 patients, these features were identified in 33 (29%) of 115 carcinomas and in only 1 (6%) of 17 benign nodules.[27] The patent airways are frequently tortuous and ectatic.

Attenuation: Bubble Lucencies (Pseudocavitation)

Nodules containing round or oval foci of air attenuation are highly suspicious for malignancy, particularly lung adenocarcinoma (Fig. 4.9). These *bubble lucencies* (synonym: pseudocavitations) are rarely identified in benign lesions. Correlation with

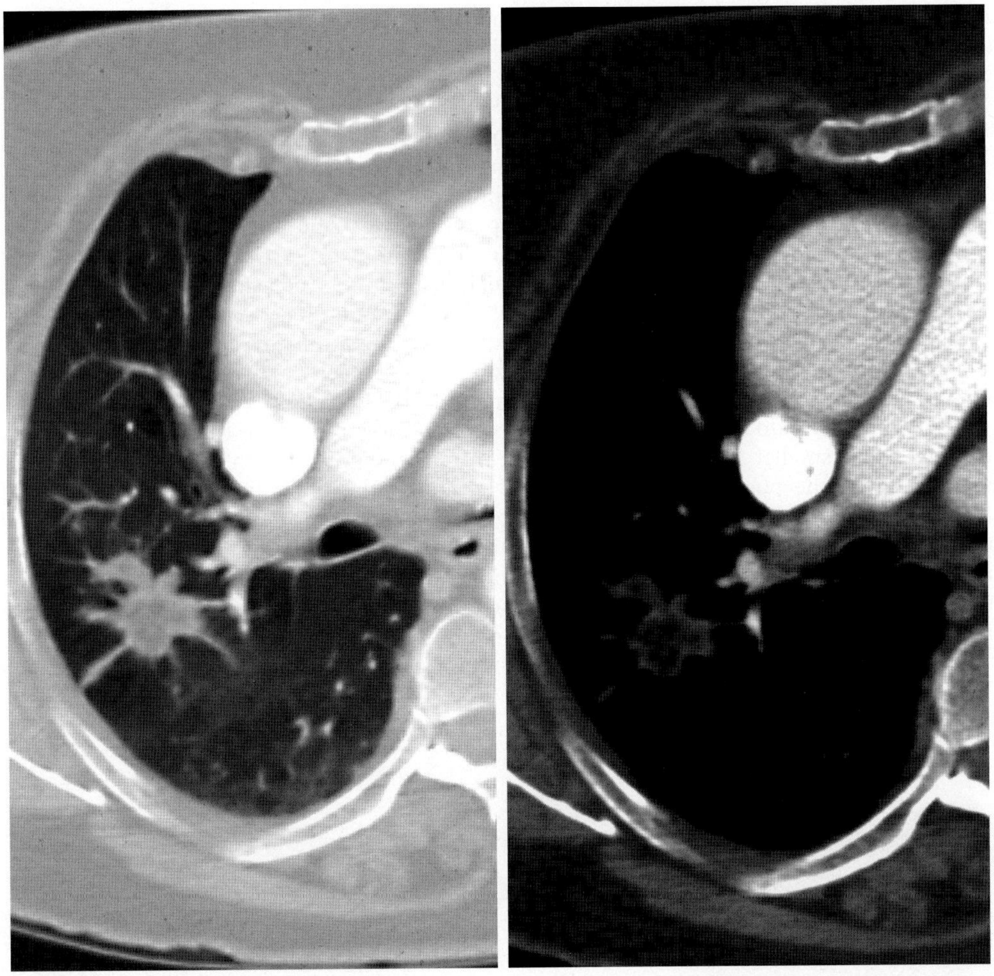

Fig. 4.7 Foci of fat attenuation in lipoid pneumonia. Composite image of the right lung in lung window *(left image)* and soft tissue window *(right image)* shows a right upper lobe spiculated nodule with ill-defined margins containing foci of central fat density that is best appreciated on the soft tissue window.

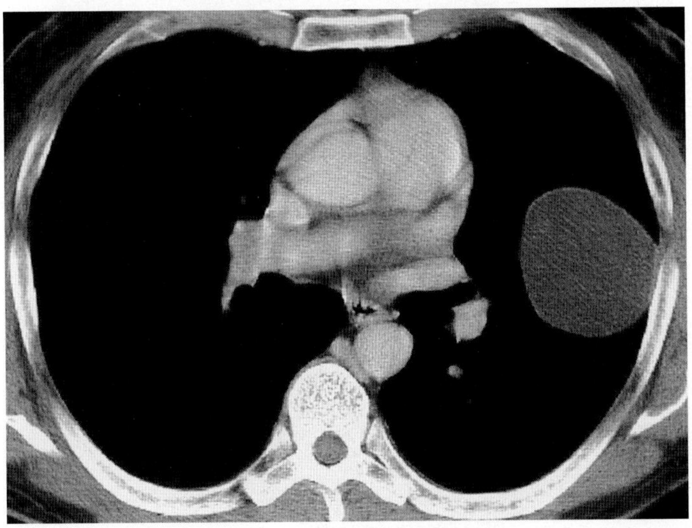

Fig. 4.8 Hydatid cyst caused by *Echinococcus granulosus*. Axial CT scan shows a homogeneous water-density thin-walled cyst in the left upper lobe.

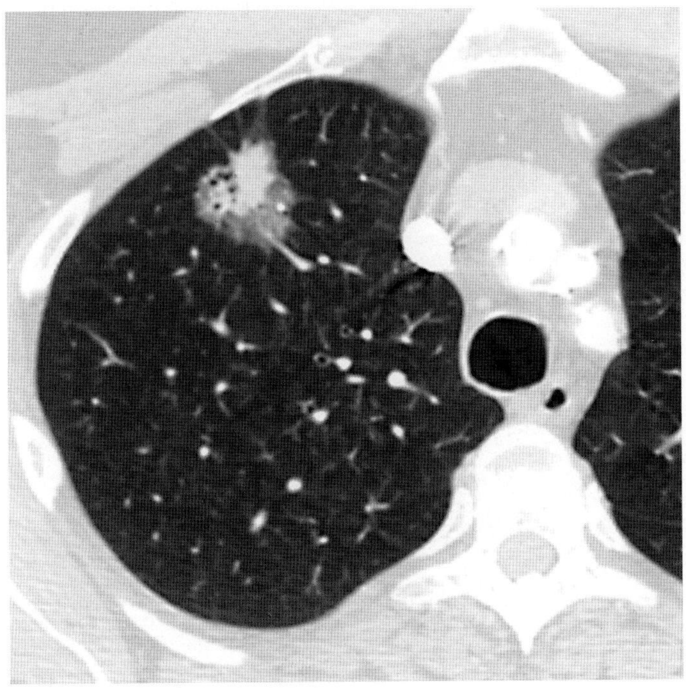

Fig. 4.9 Bubble-like lucencies in lung cancer. Axial CT scan shows a right upper lobe spiculated nodule with small round areas of low attenuation ("bubble lucencies or pseudocavitation").

pathologic findings has shown that the lucencies usually represent patent airways, often ectatic, or foci of emphysema surrounded by carcinoma.[28]

Attenuation: Focal Nodular Ground-Glass Opacity

Ground-glass opacity is a term used to describe increased lung attenuation through which pulmonary vessels can still be seen. The differential diagnosis of a focal area of ground-glass opacity or consolidation is broad and includes focal bacterial, fungal, or viral pneumonia; organizing pneumonia; focal fibrosis; lipoid pneumonia; atypical adenomatous hyperplasia; adenocarcinoma (primary and metastatic); and primary lymphoma of the lung (MALToma). Given this broad differential and the likelihood that infectious/inflammatory lesions will regress or resolve quickly, ground-glass nodules 6 mm and larger should be followed with a 6- to 12-month CT; whereas those smaller than 6 mm can generally be ignored. However, given the possibility of slow-growing cancers (Fig. 4.10), if such nodules persist the revised Fleischner criteria recommend CT follow-up for 5 years rather than 3 years as previously recommended[11,29] (see Tables 4.2 and 4.3). Nodules with mixed ground-glass opacity and a solid component on CT (part-solid nodule) are more likely to be malignant than purely soft tissue nodules (see Fig. 4.10).[30] These nodules often represent adenocarcinoma and require close follow-up or resection.

Attenuation: Computed Tomography Halo Sign

The CT halo sign refers to the presence of ground-glass opacity surrounding a pulmonary nodule (Fig. 4.11). This finding, first reported in immunocompromised patients with angioinvasive aspergillosis, can be seen in various infections (aspergillosis, candidiasis, mucormycosis, cytomegalovirus, herpes), neoplasms (adenocarcinoma, metastatic angiosarcoma, Kaposi sarcoma), vasculitis (granulomatosis with polyangiitis, formerly Wegener granulomatosis), and organizing pneumonia.[31,32] The halo of ground-glass opacity may result from hemorrhage (e.g., invasive aspergillosis), from less dense spread of inflammatory cells (e.g., organizing pneumonia) or tumor (e.g., pulmonary lymphoma), or from the lepidic growth of adenocarcinoma.[31,32]

Although the differential diagnosis is broad, the CT halo sign can be highly suggestive of a specific diagnosis in the proper clinical context (Table 4.4). For example, in an asymptomatic smoker, the presence of a nodule with ground-glass opacity surrounding a solid component is suggestive of bronchogenic carcinoma, most commonly adenocarcinoma.[30,33] In an immunocompromised patient with neutropenic fever, the presence of one

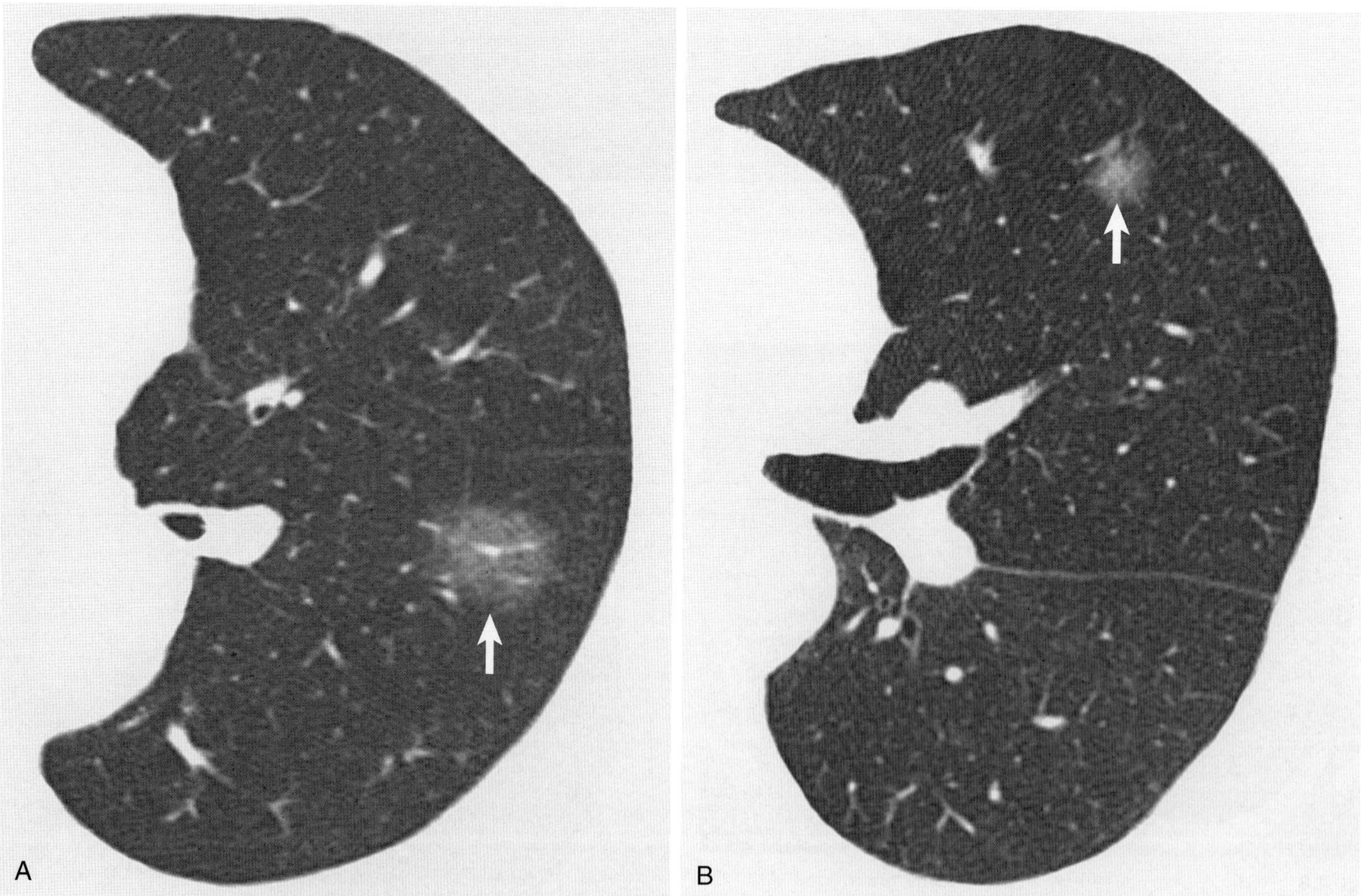

Fig. 4.10 Nodules with ground-glass and part-solid attenuation. (A) High-resolution CT scan shows a solitary left lower lobe nodule composed only of ground-glass opacity *(arrow)*, pathologically proven to represent adenocarcinoma in situ. (B) High-resolution CT scan shows a left upper lobe nodule with predominantly ground-glass opacity but also with central soft tissue opacity *(arrow)* pathologically proven to represent a minimally invasive adenocarcinoma.

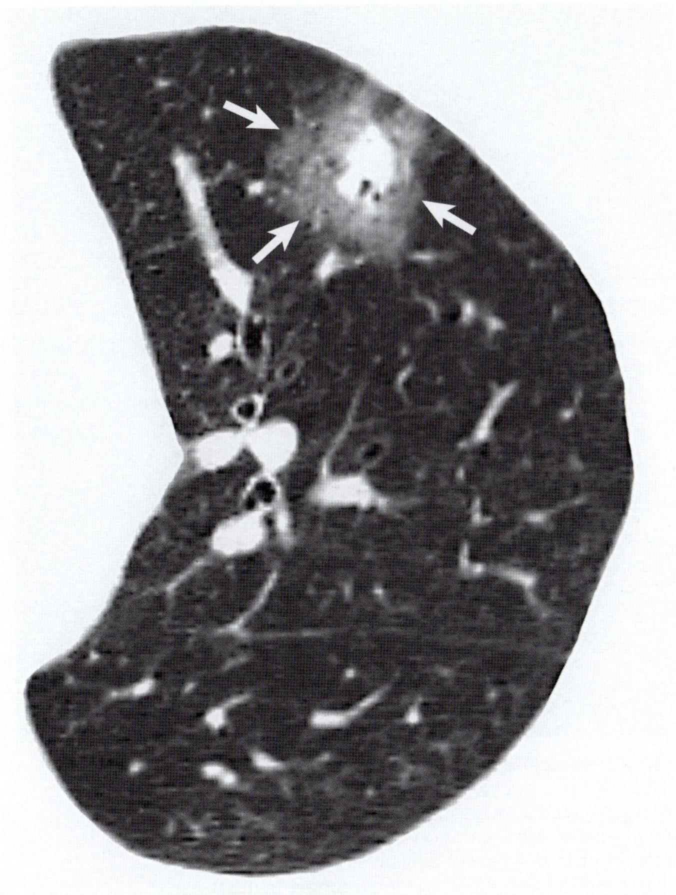

Fig. 4.11 CT halo sign in angioinvasive pulmonary aspergillosis in a man with neutropenic fever and acute leukemia. High-resolution CT scan shows a left upper lobe nodule with surrounding ground-glass opacity (*arrows;* CT halo sign).

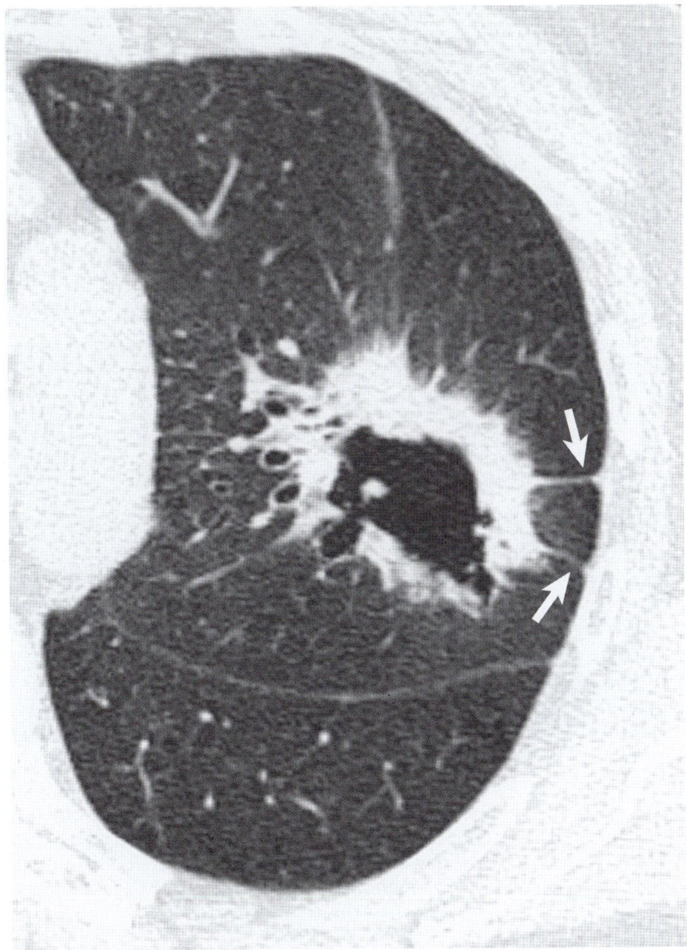

Fig. 4.12 Pleural tags in pulmonary adenocarcinoma. Axial CT scan of the left lung shows a cavitating left upper lobe mass with spiculated margins. Linear opacities can be seen extending from the mass to the visceral pleura (pleural tag) (*arrows*). Note the slight tenting of the visceral pleura at the site of the pleural tag.

TABLE 4.4 COMPUTED TOMOGRAPHY HALO SIGN: DIFFERENTIAL DIAGNOSIS

Differential	Helpful Clinical Features
COMMON	
Invasive aspergillosis	Febrile neutropenic patient
Candidiasis	Severely immunocompromised patient
Cytomegalovirus	Most commonly 1 mo or longer after transplantation
Adenocarcinoma	Patient older than 50 yr, not immunocompromised
LESS COMMON	
Herpesvirus infection	Immunocompromised patient
Metastatic hemorrhagic tumor	Primary angiosarcoma
Metastatic mucus-producing tumor	Primary adenocarcinoma of the colon
Kaposi sarcoma	Male patient with AIDS
Septic embolism	Intravenous drug user; central venous line
Granulomatosis with polyangiitis	Multiple nodules or masses; sinusitis
Organizing pneumonia	Bilateral focal consolidation or nodules; peripheral or peribronchial

or more nodules with a halo sign is suggestive of angioinvasive aspergillosis.[34]

Character of the Nodule-Lung Interface

The interface between a solitary pulmonary nodule and the adjacent lung can be spiculated or smooth. A spiculated appearance is suggestive of malignancy; for example, in a study of 283 tumors, 184 (65%) had focal or diffuse spiculation of their margins (Fig. 4.12), 91 (32%) had smooth but lobulated margins, and only 8 (3%) had smooth nonlobulated margins.[16] The likelihood ratio for malignancy of a nodule that has irregular or spiculated margins has been estimated to be approximately 5.5; the corresponding figures for lobulated and smoothly marginated nodules are about 0.75 and 0.30, respectively.[35] Radiologic-pathologic correlation has shown that spiculation may reflect the presence of fibrosis in the surrounding parenchyma, direct spread of carcinoma into the adjacent parenchyma, or localized lymphangitic spread.[28]

The tail sign (pleural tag) consists of a linear opacity that extends from a peripheral nodule or mass to the visceral pleura (see Fig. 4.12). The tag can represent fibrous tissue that extends from the nodule to the visceral pleura or can result from inward

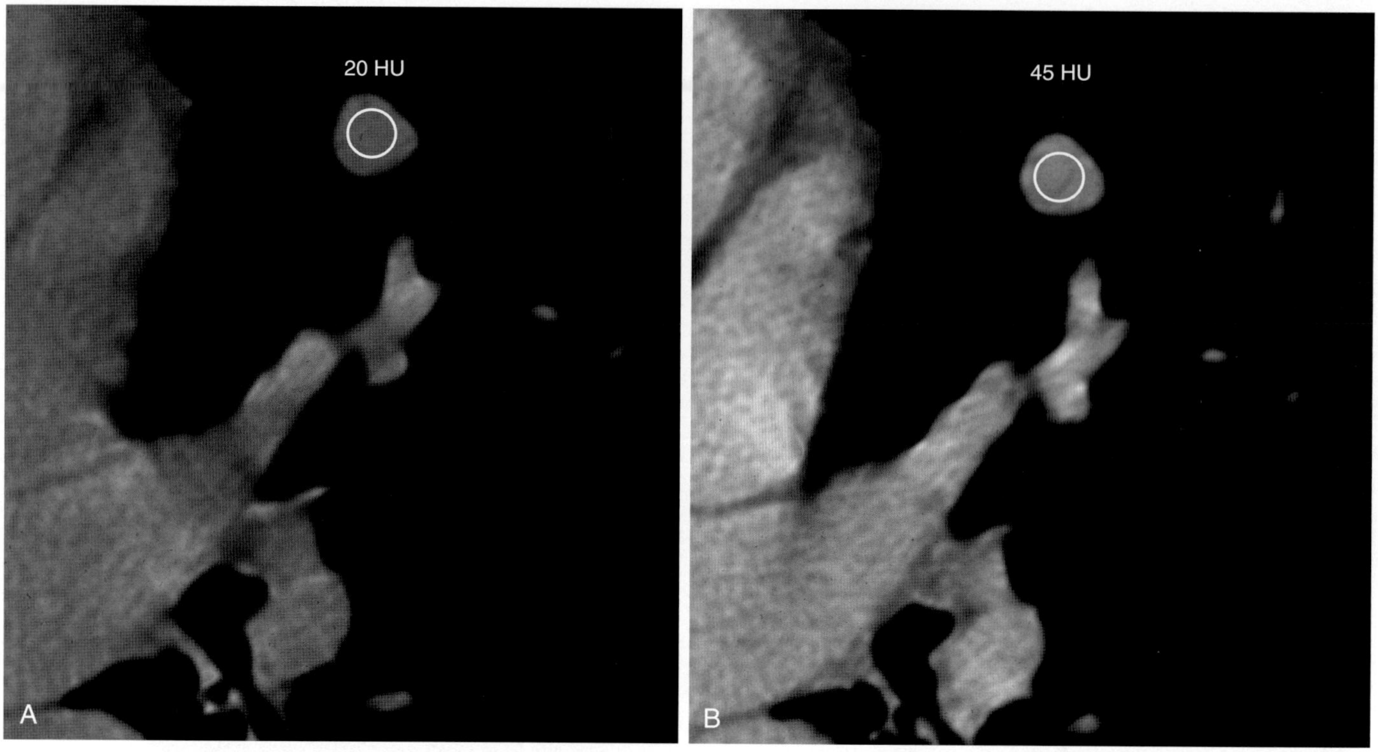

Fig. 4.13 Nodule enhancement on CT in pathologically proven pulmonary carcinoma. (A) Magnified view of the left lung from a CT scan before the injection of intravenous contrast material shows a roughly spherical, smoothly marginated nodule with homogeneous attenuation. The mean attenuation of the nodule was 20 Hounsfield units (HU). (B) CT scan after the administration of contrast material shows enhancement of the nodule. The mean attenuation was 45 HU. Because of difficulties in performing this technique and the advent of PET/CT imaging, CT evaluation for nodule enhancement is almost never performed in daily practice.

retraction and apposition of a thickened visceral pleura.[28] As the visceral pleura invaginates, a small quantity of extrapleural fat is drawn into the area and creates the opacity.[36] Pleural tags have been reported on thin-section CT in 60% to 80% of cases of peripheral pulmonary carcinoma[28]; however, they can also be seen in association with metastases and granulomas, and the sign is therefore of limited value in the differential diagnosis.

Nodule Enhancement: Computed Tomography

Pulmonary nodule enhancement as a means of distinguishing between benign and malignant nodules has been investigated by several groups (Fig. 4.13).[37,38] The results of these studies indicate that lack of enhancement or enhancement less than 15 HU after the intravenous administration of contrast material is virtually diagnostic of a benign lesion. This technique, however, requires meticulous attention to detail and is subject to artifacts from beam-hardening, volume-averaging, and motion.[39] It is also limited to the evaluation of spherical nodules with uniform attenuation (i.e., no calcification, fat, necrosis, or cavitation). Because of the number of false-positive examinations and the difficulties in performance, the presence of contrast enhancement is less helpful in diagnosis and is almost never used in current clinical practice.

Additional studies have assessed the washout characteristics of benign versus malignant pulmonary nodules, akin to adrenal lesions.[40,41] Overall, however, given the increased radiation dose to the patient, meticulous technique required, and superior assessment allowed by positron emission tomography (PET)/CT, these techniques are not routinely used. Perhaps with advances in dual-energy CT technology, such enhancement patterns might be further studied and used.[42]

Nodule Metabolism: Positron Emission Tomography

PET/CT is helpful to distinguish benign from malignant lung nodules and relies on the premise that malignant nodules demonstrate high metabolic activity. Metabolically active cells have increased use of FDG, a glucose analogue labeled with the positron emitter ^{18}F, which gets trapped within these cells. Localizing such uptake with concurrent CT allows the radiologist to diagnose metabolically active lung nodules or masses (Fig. 4.14). Of note, neoplasms with indolent growth such as carcinoid tumor, adenocarcinoma manifesting as a part-solid or ground-glass nodule, and pulmonary carcinoma measuring less than 10 mm in diameter can be falsely negative.[43] False-positive scans can occur with inflammatory conditions, such as tuberculosis, histoplasmosis, organizing pneumonia, and rheumatoid nodules.

SOLITARY PULMONARY MASS

As discussed previously, the division of solitary opacities within the lung into nodules (measuring ≤3 cm in diameter) and masses (measuring >3 cm in diameter) serves one useful purpose—a mass is much more likely than a nodule to be malignant (Fig. 4.15).

Calcification in a mass does not exclude malignancy as it does in the case of a solitary nodule. For example, in a study of 353 carcinomas, 20 (6%) had calcification evident on CT; 17 of the 20 lesions containing calcification (85%) were larger than

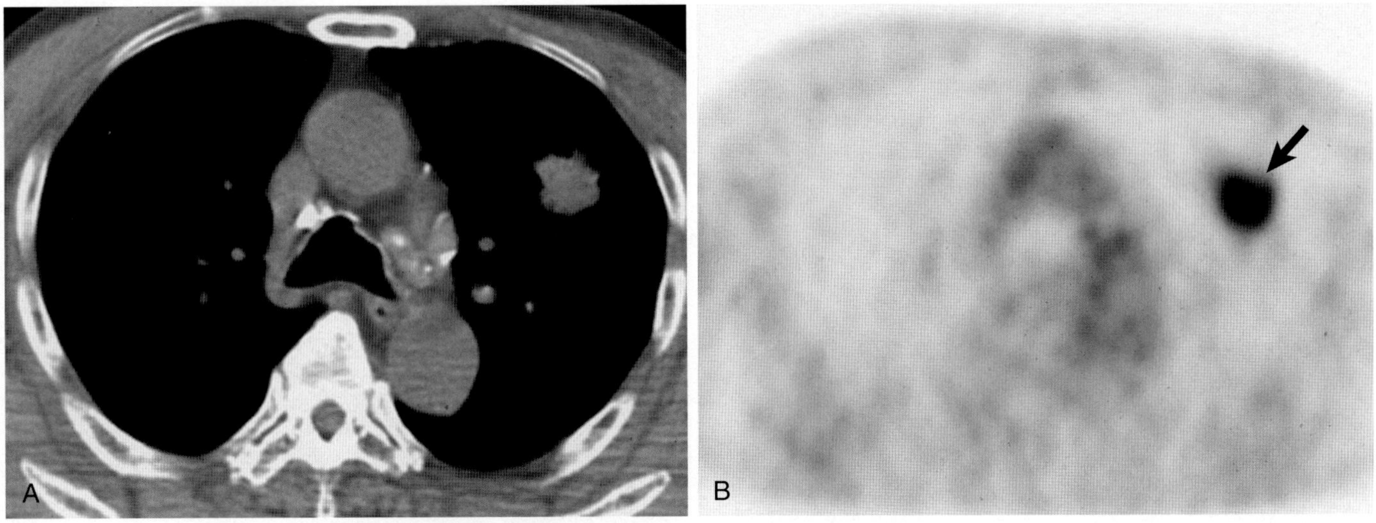

Fig. 4.14 ^{18}F-fluorodeoxyglucose (FDG) uptake in pulmonary adenocarcinoma. (A) CT scan shows a spiculated left upper lobe nodule. (B) PET scan at the same level shows elevated FDG uptake *(arrow)* in the nodule suggesting malignancy.

3 cm in diameter.[44] The calcification in these tumors may be punctate, chunky, or amorphous in appearance and central, peripheral, or diffuse in distribution (Fig. 4.16).[19] Calcification is related to psammoma bodies, dystrophic calcification of necrotic carcinoma, or incorporation of a focus of previous granulomatous inflammation or calcified bronchial cartilage within the tumor.[19,44]

The incidence of cavitation in pulmonary carcinoma is about 10%. Although the complication can occur in tumors of any size, most are larger than 3 cm in diameter.[45] A cavity is defined radiologically as a gas-containing space within a pulmonary consolidation, mass, or nodule (Fig. 4.17).[2] In most cases it is formed by necrosis of the central portion of a lesion and drainage of the resultant, partially liquefied material via communicating airways.

The most common histologic type of primary lung malignancy to cavitate is squamous cell carcinoma; in a review of the radiographic findings in 600 cases, cavitation was seen in 22% of 263 squamous cell carcinomas, 6% of 97 large cell carcinomas, 2% of 126 adenocarcinomas, and none of 114 small cell carcinomas.[46] Most neoplastic cavities have an irregular inner surface as a result of variably sized nodules of neoplastic tissue projecting into the cavity and the patchy nature of necrosis within most tumors. The cavities may be central or eccentric and 1 to 10 cm in diameter.

In many cases the radiologic appearance of the cavity gives some indication of its cause, particularly whether it is benign or malignant. Features to note include the thickness of the cavity wall, the character of its inner lining (whether nodular, shaggy, or smooth), the presence and nature of its contents, the number of lesions, and when multiple, the number of lesions that have cavitated.

The cavity wall is usually thick in an acute lung abscess, primary and metastatic carcinoma, and granulomatosis with polyangiitis, and often thin in chronic infection such as coccidioidomycosis. Assessment of cavity wall thickness is quite useful in distinguishing between a benign and a malignant lesion. In a study of 65 solitary cavities in the lung, all lesions in which the thickest part of the cavity wall was 1 mm or less were benign; of the lesions whose thickest measurement was 4 mm or less, 92% were benign; of those that were 5 to 15 mm in their thickest part, benign and malignant lesions were equally divided; and 92% of lesions whose cavity wall was greater than 15 mm in thickness were malignant.[47] In addition, one recent study showed cavity thickness to be an independent prognostic factor in patients with known lung adenocarcinoma.[48] Patients in this study with a cavity wall thickness greater than 4 mm had a higher frequency of solid-predominant tumor, vascular invasion, lymphatic invasion, necrosis, obstructive pneumonia, intracavity abscess, and bronchiolar obstruction.

The inner lining of the cavity is usually nodular in carcinoma (see Fig. 4.17), shaggy in acute lung abscess, and smooth in most other cavitary lesions. When material is identified within a cavity, it generally represents pus or partially liquefied necrotic neoplasm and appears as a flat, smooth air-fluid level without specific radiologic features. Occasionally, intracavitary material has characteristics that are strongly suggestive of a specific disease. Examples include an intracavitary fungus ball (Fig. 4.18), which may form a mobile mass, and the collapsed membranes of a ruptured *Echinococcus* cyst, which float on top of the fluid within the cyst and create the characteristic water lily sign.[49]

Some cavitary disease is characteristically solitary (e.g., primary pulmonary carcinoma, acute lung abscess, and posttraumatic lung cyst). Other diseases are characteristically multiple (e.g., metastatic carcinoma, granulomatosis with polyangiitis, and septic emboli).

KEY POINTS: PULMONARY NODULE OR MASS

- Discrete focal opacity 3 cm or less in diameter (nodule) or >3 cm (mass)
- Likelihood for malignancy based on size (approximate percentages):
  - 0.6- to 0.8-cm-diameter nodule: 0.5%–2%
  - 2-cm-diameter nodule: 50%
  - 2- to 3-cm-diameter nodule: 80%
  - 3-cm- or greater diameter mass: 95%
- A nodule with diffuse or central calcification is almost always a granuloma
- A solid nodule stable in size for 2 years is usually benign
- Ground-glass and part-solid nodules often represent indolent lung cancer and therefore are followed over a longer time frame than solid pulmonary nodules.

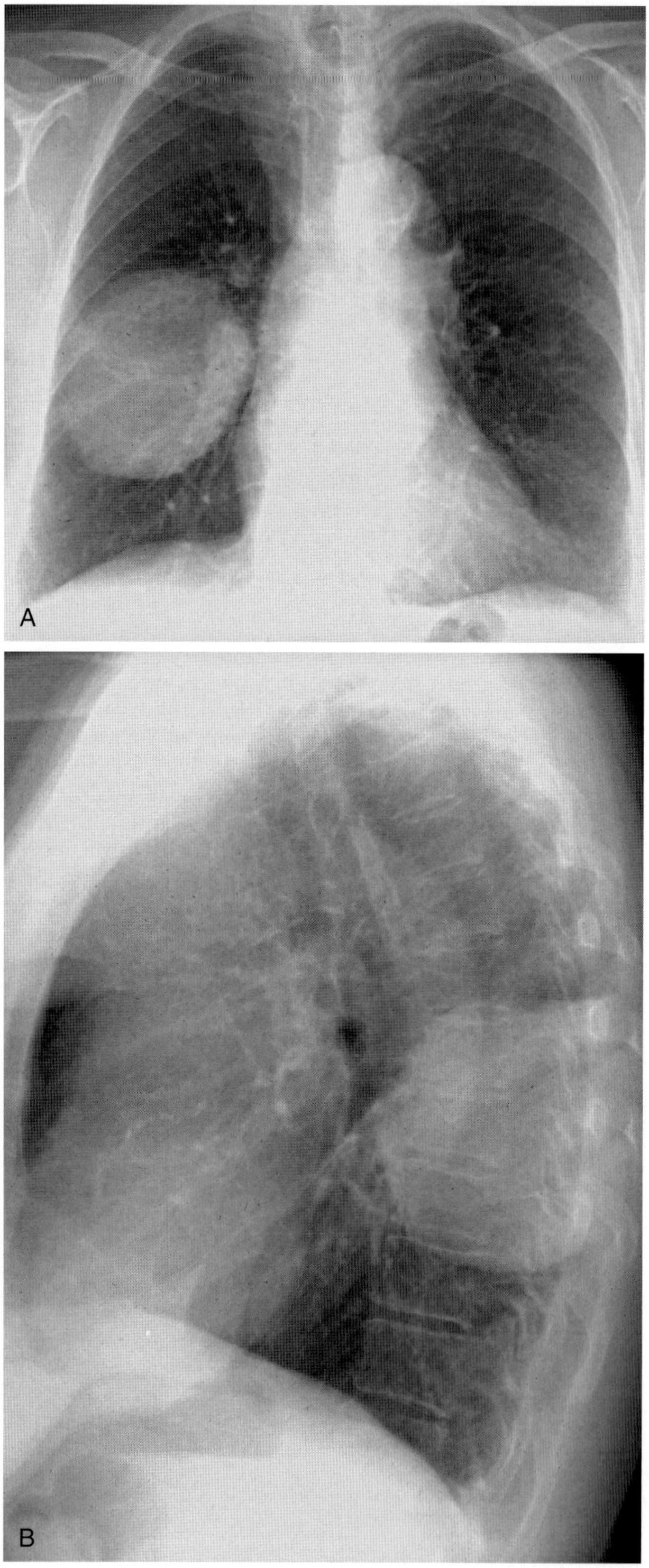

Fig. 4.15 Large pulmonary carcinoma. (A) Posteroanterior and (B) lateral chest radiographs show a large mass in the right lower lobe.

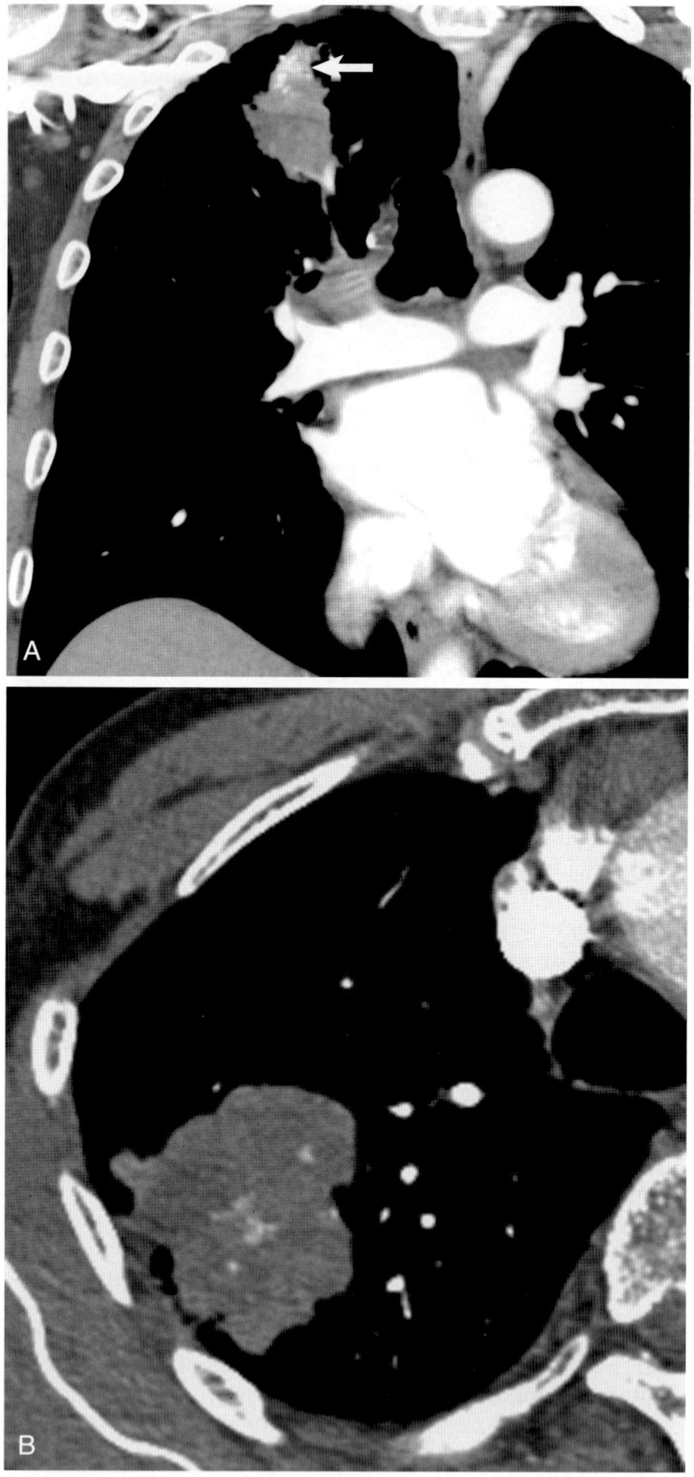

Fig. 4.16 Calcification in malignancy. (A) Coronal CT scan shows an elongated right upper lobe mass with eccentric punctate and amorphous calcification *(arrow)* in a patient with primary lung adenocarcinoma. (B) Axial CT scan from a different patient with metastatic adenocarcinoma of the colon demonstrates foci of amorphous calcification within a lobulated mass.

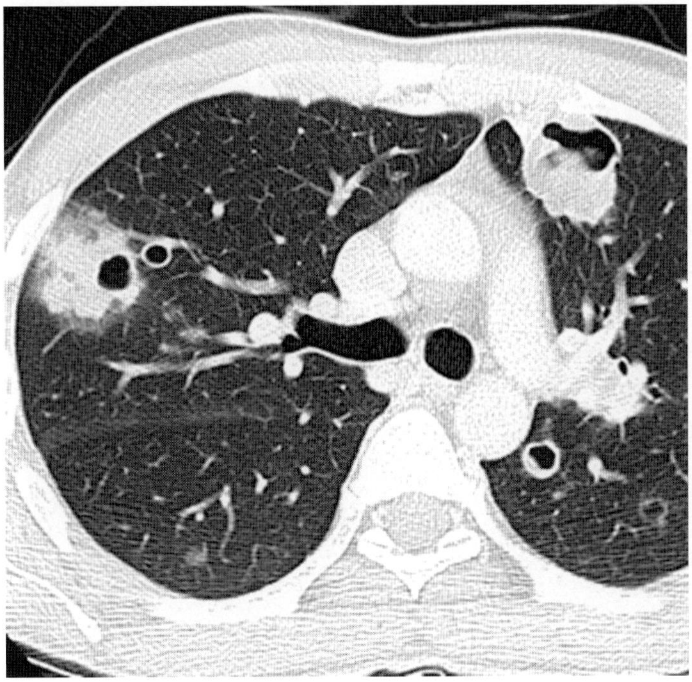

Fig. 4.17 Cavitation in metastatic transitional cell carcinoma. Axial CT scan shows bilateral pulmonary nodules and masses with cavitation. The walls of the cavities are thick and nodular, suggesting malignancy.

ALGORITHM FOR EVALUATION OF PULMONARY NODULES

In many cases lung nodules are initially identified on a chest radiograph. It is important to note, however, that there are several pitfalls in the radiologic diagnosis of pulmonary nodules. Pleural and chest wall abnormalities such as healing rib fractures, a bone island in a rib, and pleural plaques, as well as normal structures (e.g., nipple, conspicuous costochondral junction), may mimic lung nodules (Figs. 4.19 and 4.20). Lung nodules are also often missed on radiographs, and the presence of calcification is difficult to reliably identify. For these reasons, thin-section CT is recommended for further evaluation of indeterminate nodules identified by radiographs. CT may allow confident diagnosis of granuloma by demonstrating central or diffuse calcification not apparent on the chest radiograph. A smoothly marginated nodule containing fat density can be confidently diagnosed as a hamartoma. Pulmonary arteriovenous malformations can readily be recognized by the presence of a feeding artery and a draining vein. The Fleischner Society recommendations for the management of incidental small pulmonary nodules detected on nonscreening CT are routinely used to guide evaluation for pulmonary nodules and were recently revised as outlined in Tables 4.2 and 4.3.[11] Patients continue to be stratified as low or high risk based on smoking history, exposure to known carcinogens (e.g., asbestos), personal history of cancer, or first-degree relative with lung cancer.

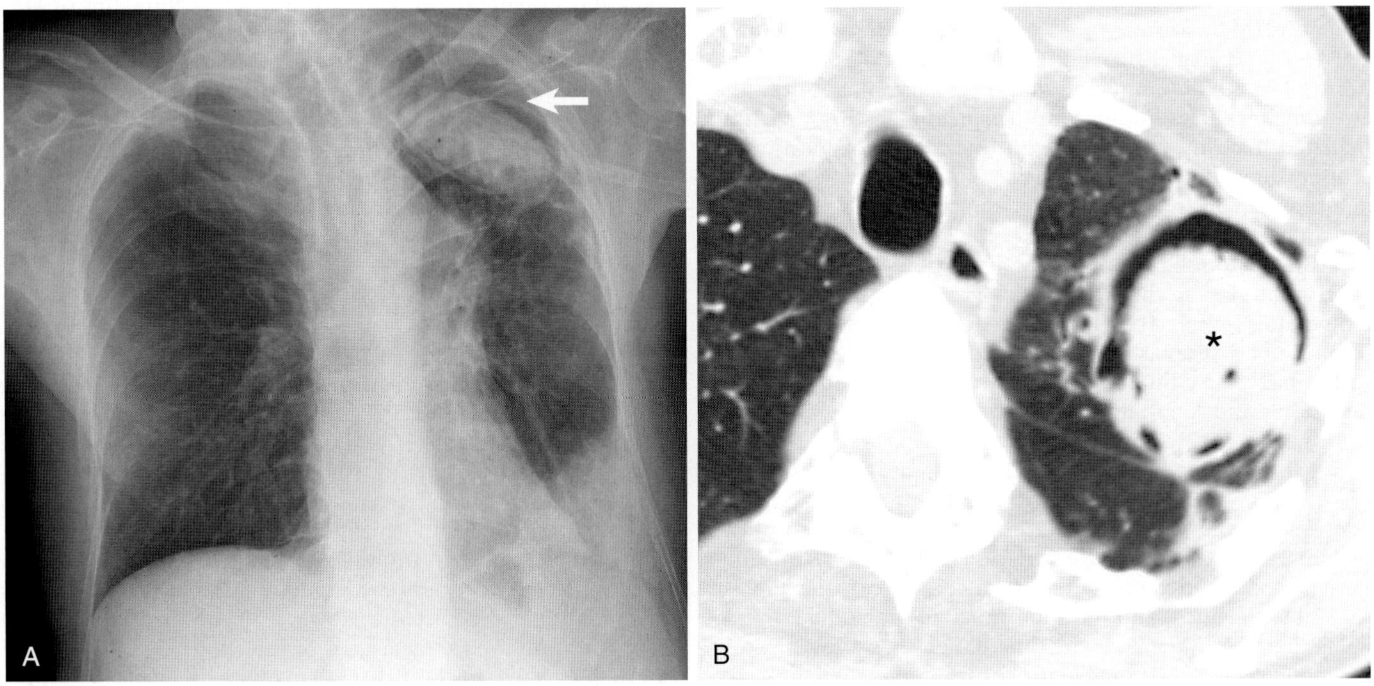

Fig. 4.18 Aspergilloma in a left upper lobe cavity. (A) Frontal chest radiograph shows an air crescent *(arrows)* surrounding a dependent intracavitary left upper lobe mass. (B) Axial CT scan demonstrates a large cavity in the left upper lobe containing a homogeneous soft tissue mass *(asterisk)*. The mass lies in the dependent portion of the cavity, suggesting that it is mobile. The findings are characteristic of an intracavitary mycetoma. Note scarring and bronchiectasis in the left upper lobe and extensive pleural thickening adjacent to the cavity.

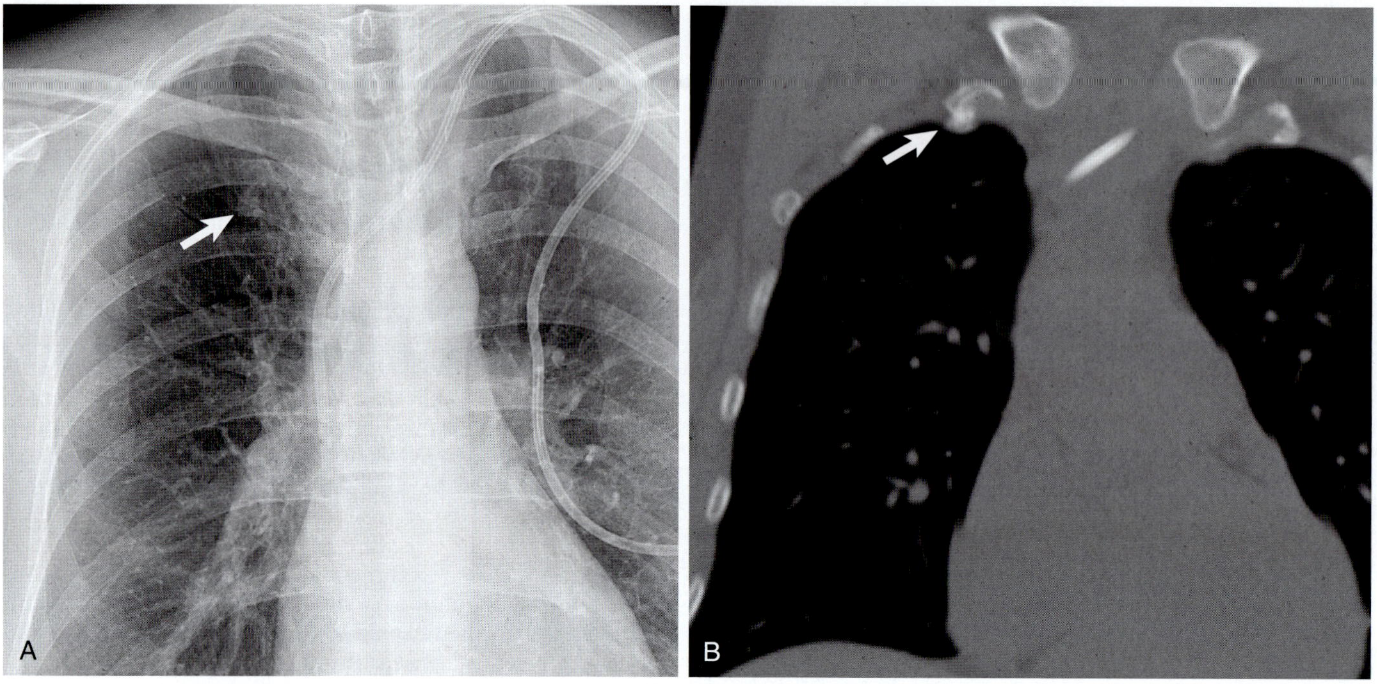

Fig. 4.19 Pseudonodule from first rib. (A) Frontal chest radiograph shows a spiculated nodule *(arrow)* projecting over the right upper lung zone intimately associated with the anterior right first rib. (B) Coronal CT scan shows the nodule seen on chest radiography represents an osteophyte *(arrow)* extending from the anterior right first rib.

In the revised classification nodules must also be differentiated as either single or multiple and as solid or subsolid (includes both part-solid and ground-glass nodules). Solid nodules are further divided by size into three categories: those less than 6 mm, 6 to 8 mm, and greater than 8 mm. Subsolid nodules are divided by size as less than 6 mm or 6 mm or greater. In addition, the new guidelines take into account suspicious features, such as spiculated margins, cavitation with thick walls, or location in an upper lobe. As before, nodules in high-risk patients more often require continued follow-up, especially nodule(s) having suspicious morphology or an upper lobe location.

In contrast to solid nodules, subsolid nodules (both part-solid and ground-glass nodules) 6 mm or greater in size should be followed for 5 years (see Tables 4.2 and 4.3) rather than the minimum of 3 years as previously recommended.[11,29]

MRI has a very limited role in the evaluation of a solitary lung nodule and is not indicated in the routine workup of these patients.[50]

In patients in whom the CT findings are indeterminate or worrisome for malignancy, further workup depends on the pretest probability of cancer and the risk for surgical complications. In patients with average surgical risk, FDG-PET imaging is warranted when there is discordance between the pretest probability of cancer and the appearance of the nodule on CT. PET is therefore indicated when the patient has a low risk for cancer and CT suggests malignancy or when there is a high risk for cancer and CT suggests a benign lesion. FDG-PET imaging has a sensitivity of approximately 97% and a specificity of 78% for the diagnosis of malignancy in nodules 10 mm or larger.[43] The high accuracy of PET is limited to nodules that are solid and 10 mm or greater in diameter.[51]

Transthoracic needle aspiration or biopsy is indicated in patients with solitary lung nodules who decline surgical intervention and in patients who are not operable candidates or are at high risk. In these patients needle aspiration or biopsy is often helpful in establishing a tissue diagnosis. Patients with solitary nodules consistent with malignancy on CT or PET/CT and a high pretest probability of cancer should undergo proper staging and, if they are operable candidates, proceed to thoracotomy. Inoperable patients (because of advanced disease or patient characteristics) are often treated with radiation therapy and/or chemotherapy.

Multiple Lung Nodules and Masses

This section briefly reviews the differential diagnosis of multiple nodules 1 cm or greater in diameter. The nodular pattern of diffuse lung disease, characterized by the presence of innumerable nodules less than 1 cm in diameter, is discussed in the section on interstitial lung disease (see Chapter 5). The differential diagnosis of multiple nodules greater than 1 cm in diameter is broad (Table 4.5) and includes congenital abnormalities (e.g., arteriovenous malformations), infection (e.g., multiple granulomas, septic embolism), inflammatory processes (e.g., granulomatosis with polyangiitis), and pulmonary metastases. However, more than 95% of cases represent pulmonary metastases or infection.

At least 80% to 90% of patients with multiple pulmonary metastases have a previously diagnosed extrathoracic neoplasm or clinical findings directly referable to a synchronous primary. The radiologic manifestations of multiple pulmonary metastases may range from a diffuse micronodular pattern resembling miliary disease to large, well-defined cannonball masses (Fig. 4.21). The

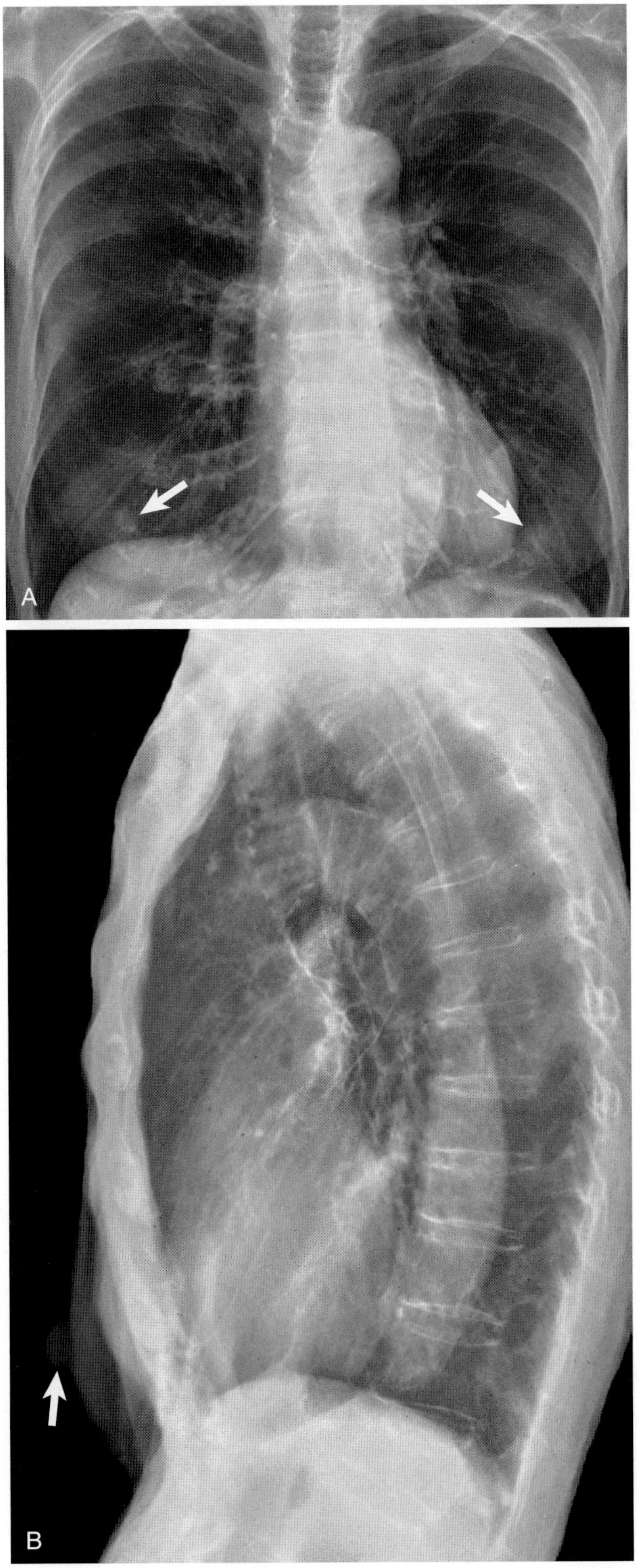

Fig. 4.20 Nipple shadows mimicking pulmonary nodules on chest radiography. (A) Frontal chest radiograph shows small nodular opacities *(arrows)* projecting over the lower lung zones bilaterally, typical of nipple shadows. The left nipple shadow has ill-defined margins. Note the scarring in the right apex. (B) Lateral view demonstrates the right nipple *(arrow)*. Nipple shadows can usually be confidently identified on a posteroanterior chest radiograph because the medial or lateral margin is generally well defined because it is outlined by air, whereas the contralateral margin tends to be poorly defined (i.e., incomplete border sign).

nodules may be of uniform size, indicative of a simultaneous origin in one shower of emboli, or may differ, suggestive of embolic events of different ages. On CT pulmonary metastases are most commonly seen in the outer third of the lungs, particularly the subpleural regions of the lower zones, presumably because of a richer blood supply.[52] Although nodules less than 2 cm in diameter are frequently round and have smooth margins, they may have various shapes; larger nodules are often lobulated and have irregular margins.[53] Irregular margins appear to be particularly common in cases of metastatic adenocarcinoma.[54] Occasionally, a halo of ground-glass opacity can be seen surrounding the nodules. This finding is most common in highly vascular or hemorrhagic tumors, such as angiosarcoma, but may also be seen in metastatic mucinous carcinoma of the colon or metastatic adenocarcinoma.[31,32,55]

Cavitation occurs in approximately 4% of pulmonary metastases.[56] It is seen most often in squamous cell carcinoma, the primary sites usually being in the head and neck in men and the cervix in women (Fig. 4.22).[56] Less commonly, cavitation occurs in metastatic adenocarcinoma and metastatic sarcoma.[56] Calcification of metastatic lesions is rare and almost invariably indicates that the primary neoplasm is osteogenic sarcoma, chondrosarcoma, or synovial sarcoma.[56]

Another common cause of multiple nodules is pulmonary infection. Multiple nodules may be seen in septic embolism, tuberculosis, histoplasmosis, coccidioidomycosis, and cryptococcosis. Multiple nodules in tuberculosis or endemic fungal infection result from endobronchial or miliary spread, and they are usually less than 1 cm in diameter (Fig. 4.23). Similarly, histoplasmosis and coccidioidomycosis generally have a single nodule measuring up to 3 cm in diameter or multiple nodules less than 1 cm in diameter, especially in the immunocompromised patient. Often these smaller nodules cluster around a larger nodule in a "satellite" configuration, although this is not specific to fungal infections and may occur in other granulomatous processes such as sarcoidosis.

Septic embolism occurs most commonly in intravenous drug users and in immunocompromised patients with central venous lines. Septic embolism is characterized by the presence of multiple nodules and wedge-shaped peripheral opacities that measure approximately 1 to 3 cm in diameter and are frequently cavitated (Fig. 4.24). The nodules tend to be most numerous in the peripheral lung regions and the lower lobes.[57,58] On CT scan the nodules often appear to have a vessel leading into them. This has been called the "feeding vessel" sign (Fig. 4.25).[57,59] Multiplanar and MIP reformatted images have shown, however, that in the majority of patients the pulmonary arteries course around the nodule and that vessels appearing to enter the nodule are usually pulmonary veins draining from the nodule.[60]

TABLE 4.5 DIFFERENTIAL DIAGNOSIS OF MULTIPLE NODULES LARGER THAN 1 CM IN DIAMETER

Etiology	Features
CONGENITAL	
Pulmonary arteriovenous malformation	CT shows a feeding artery and a draining vein
INFECTIOUS	
Septic embolism	Mainly lower lobes. Frequently cavitate
Lung abscesses	Cavitation or low-attenuation center on CT
Invasive aspergillosis	Immunocompromised patient. CT halo sign
Candidiasis	Immunocompromised patient. CT halo sign
NEOPLASTIC	
Pulmonary metastases	Smooth margins. Variable size. Mainly lower lobes
Multicentric adenocarcinoma	Nodules have spiculated margins; part solid or ground-glass nodules
Lymphoma	Nodules may have smooth or spiculated margins
Kaposi sarcoma	Patient with AIDS. Peribronchovascular distribution. Nodules have spiculated margins
VASCULITIC	
Granulomatosis with polyangiitis	Multiple nodules and masses. Frequently cavitate
Eosinophilic granulomatosis with polyangiitis	Uncommon. Seldom cavitate
Rheumatoid nodules	Uncommon. Usually associated with subcutaneous nodules
TRAUMATIC	
Hematomas	History of trauma. Slow but progressive decrease in size

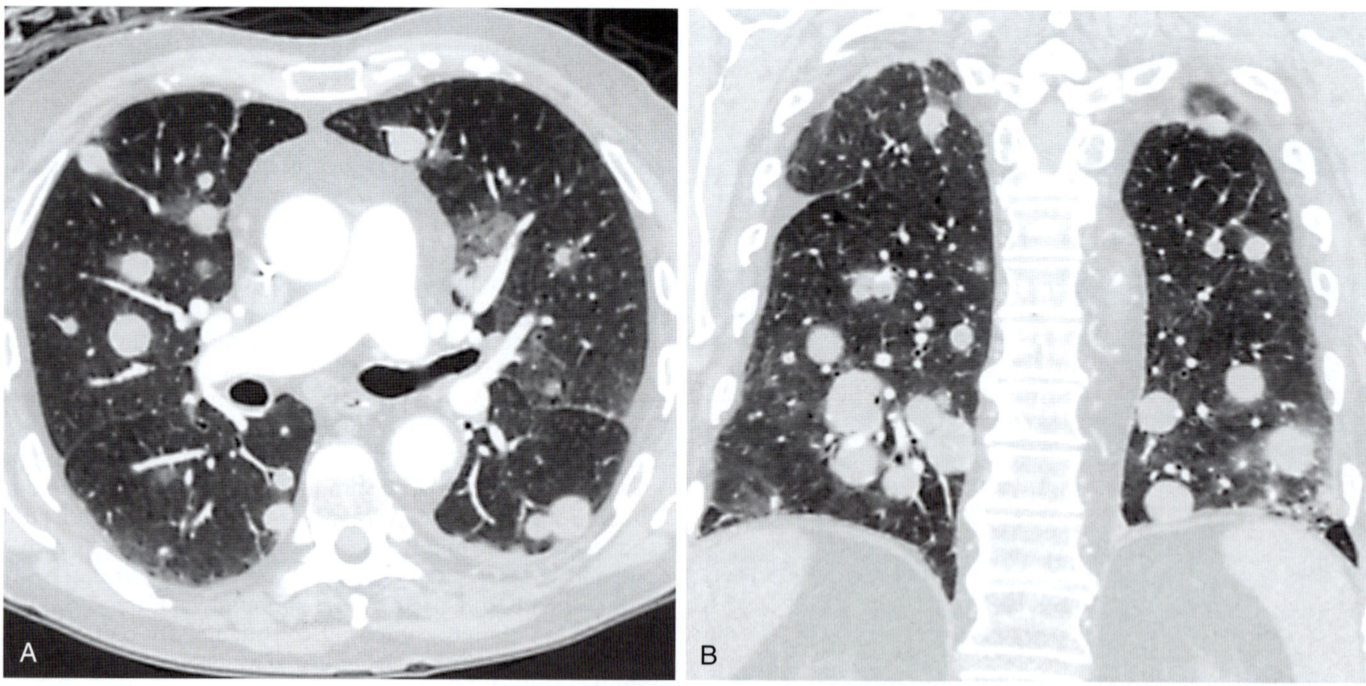

Fig. 4.21 Small and large lung metastases from melanoma. (A) Axial CT scan shows numerous randomly distributed pulmonary nodules of varying sizes. (B) Coronal CT scan better demonstrates the middle and lower lung zone distribution of the nodules reflecting pulmonary blood flow. Many of the nodules have smooth margins, but many have spiculated margins.

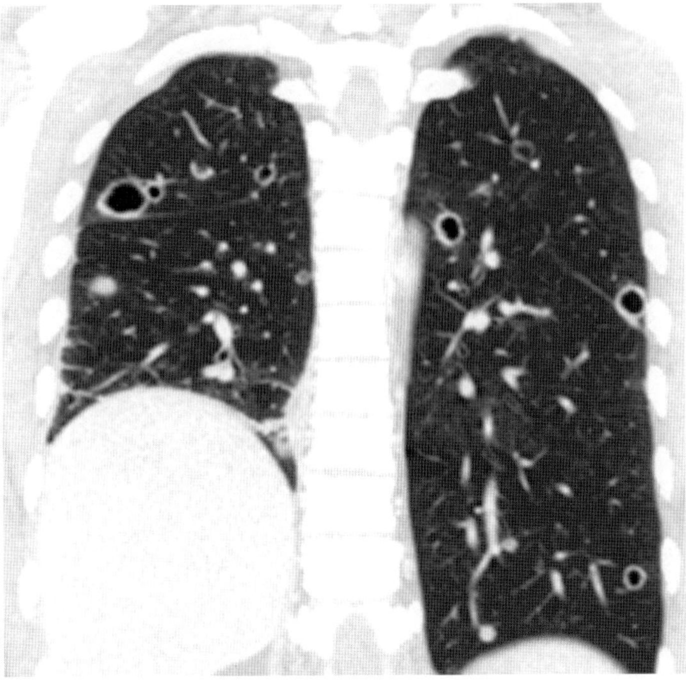

Fig. 4.22 Cavitating metastases from transitional cell carcinoma. Coronal CT scan shows numerous cavitary and solid nodules, many with irregular or ill-defined margins.

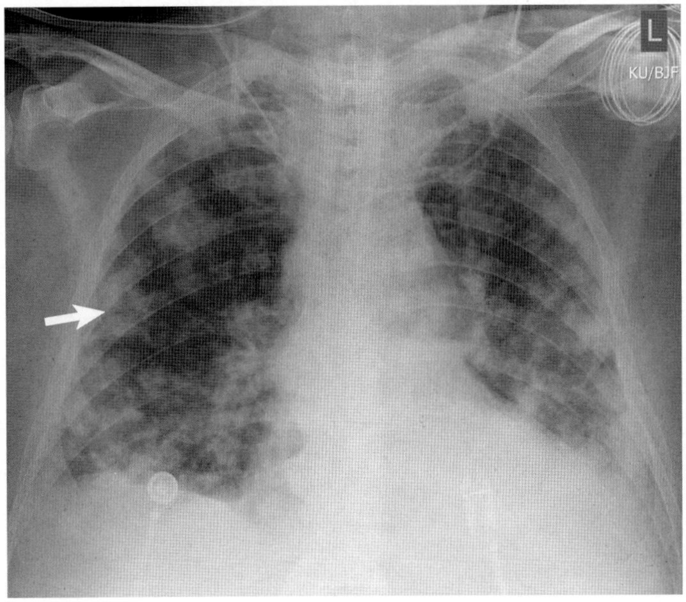

Fig. 4.24 Septic emboli. A frontal chest radiograph shows bilateral nodules, some of which are cavitated *(arrow)*. Note the irregular nodule contours, peripheral location, and random distribution. *(Reproduced with permission from Walker CM. Pulmonary infections. In: Digumarthy S, Abbara S, Chung J, eds.* Problem-Solving in Chest Imaging. *Philadelphia: Elsevier; 2017.)*

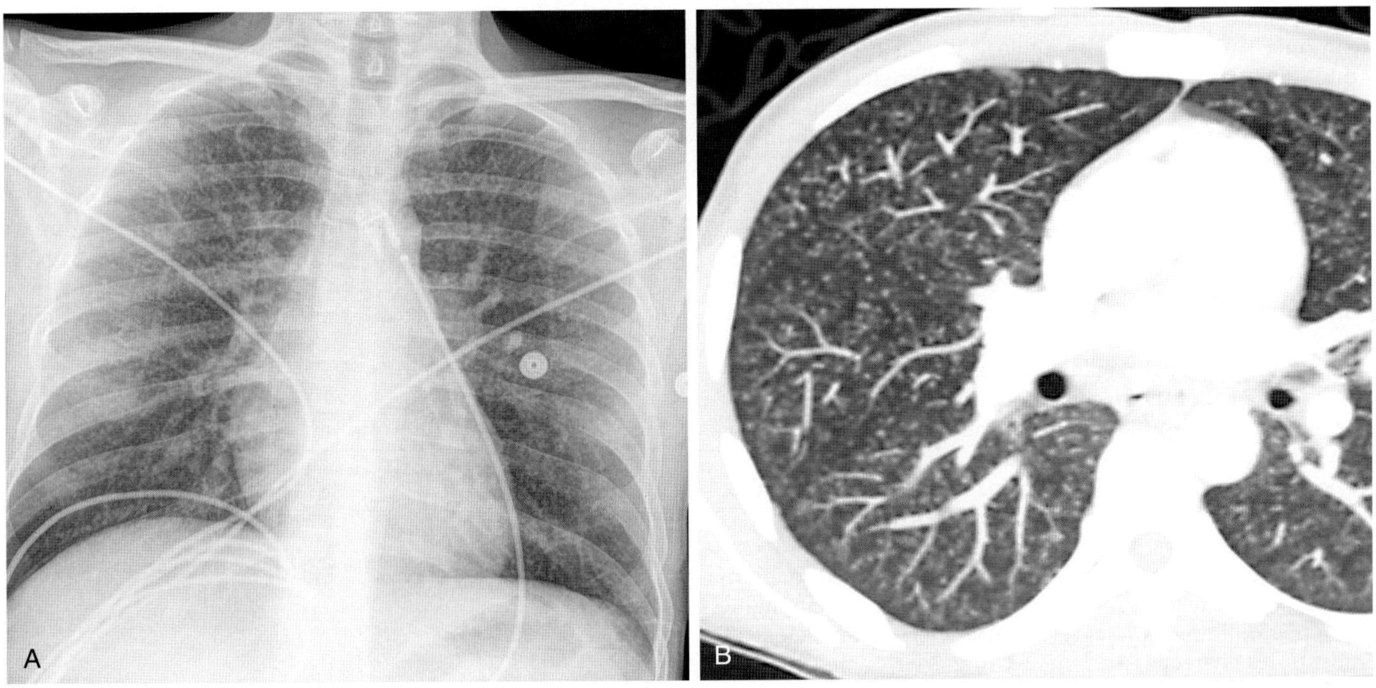

Fig. 4.23 Miliary histoplasmosis in the setting of AIDS. (A) Posteroanterior chest radiograph and (B) axial CT scan show diffuse small nodules in a random distribution. *(Reproduced with permission from Walker CM. Pulmonary infections. In: Digumarthy S, Abbara S, Chung J, eds.* Problem-Solving in Chest Imaging. *Philadelphia: Elsevier; 2019.)*

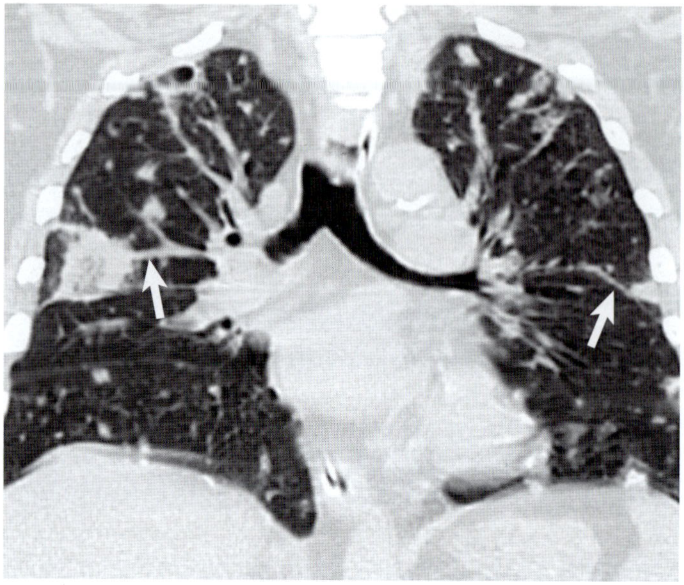

Fig. 4.25 Septic emboli with feeding vessel sign. Coronal CT scan shows bilateral peripheral pulmonary nodules with several feeding vessels *(arrows)*. On close inspection the feeding vessel is actually a pulmonary vein, whereas the pulmonary artery usually courses around the nodule. *(Reproduced with permission from Walker CM, Abbott GF, Greene RE, et al. Imaging pulmonary infection: classic signs and patterns.* AJR Am J Roentgenol. *2014;202:1396.)*

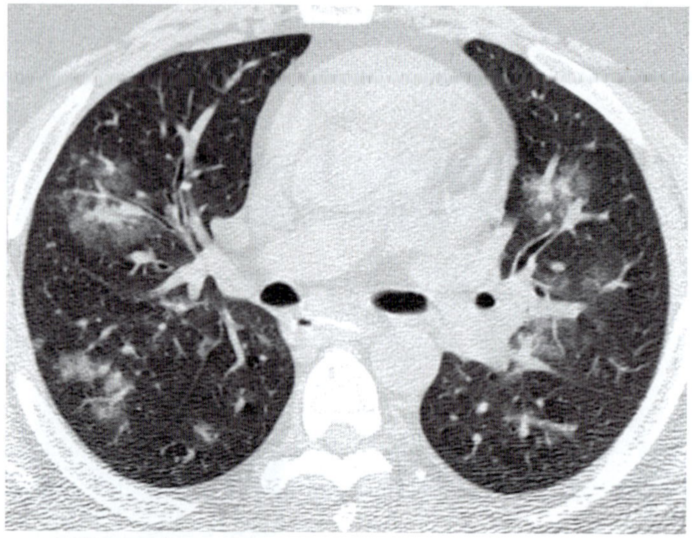

Fig. 4.26 Candidiasis. Axial CT scan shows bilateral pulmonary nodules, many with a surrounding halo of ground-glass opacity (CT halo sign). *(Reproduced with permission from Walker CM, Abbott GF, Greene RE, et al. Imaging pulmonary infection: classic signs and patterns.* AJR Am J Roentgenol. *2014;202:1396.)*

In an immunocompromised host, multiple nodules may result from invasive aspergillosis, candidiasis, and cytomegalovirus pneumonia. Angioinvasive aspergillosis is usually characterized by multiple nodules ranging from a few millimeters to approximately 3 cm in diameter. These nodules tend to have ill-defined margins on a chest radiograph and to be surrounded by a rim of ground-glass opacity on CT scans, known as the CT halo sign (see Fig. 4.11). This rim is due to pulmonary hemorrhage.[61] In the appropriate clinical setting, such as a neutropenic patient with fever, this finding is highly suggestive of angioinvasive aspergillosis.[34] The sign, however, is not pathognomonic. Other causes of multiple nodules with a CT halo sign include candidiasis (Fig. 4.26), cytomegalovirus pneumonia, Kaposi sarcoma, granulomatosis with polyangiitis, and metastatic angiosarcoma.[31,32] The findings of candidiasis may be identical to those of invasive aspergillosis.[62] The nodules in cytomegalovirus and herpesvirus pneumonia usually measure less than 1 cm in diameter.[62]

The most common vascular abnormalities resulting in multiple nodules are congenital arteriovenous malformations, often in patients with hereditary hemorrhagic telangiectasia (Osler-Weber-Rendu syndrome). On radiography, arteriovenous malformations appear as well-defined, lobulated, round or oval opacities ranging from a few millimeters to several centimeters in diameter. CT demonstrates characteristic large feeding arteries and draining veins.[63]

Multiple nodules and masses may also be a manifestation of inflammatory processes, including granulomatosis with polyangiitis, eosinophilic granulomatosis with polyangiitis, and necrobiotic pulmonary nodules in patients with rheumatoid arthritis. Granulomatosis with polyangiitis is typically accompanied by multiple nodules and masses ranging from a few millimeters up to 10 cm in diameter.[64] Usually, fewer than 10 nodules are seen on the radiograph, although more may be evident on CT.[65] The nodules have no predilection for any lung zone, and about 50% cavitate. The most common manifestation of eosinophilic granulomatosis with polyangiitis (formerly Churg-Strauss syndrome) consists of transient patchy bilateral ground-glass opacities or areas of consolidation.[66] Occasionally, it may result in multiple ill-defined unilateral or bilateral nodules that seldom cavitate.[67] Rheumatoid nodules are an uncommon manifestation of rheumatoid arthritis.[68] They may be single or multiple and range from a few millimeters to 5 cm in diameter. They are well defined and tend to predominate in the lung periphery. Rheumatoid lung nodules are typically seen in patients with subcutaneous nodules and tend to wax and wane in proportion to the activity of the arthritis.

SUGGESTED READINGS

Bruzzi JF, Munden RF. PET/CT imaging of lung cancer. *J Thorac Imaging.* 2006;21:123–136.

Bunyaviroch T, Coleman RE. PET evaluation of lung cancer. *J Nucl Med.* 2006;47:451–469.

Ko JP. Lung nodule detection and characterization with multi-slice CT. *J Thorac Imaging.* 2005;20:196–209.

MacMahon H, Naiditch NP, Goo JM, et al. Guidelines for management of incidental pulmonary nodules detected on CT images: from the Fleischner Society 2017. *Radiology.* 2017;284:228–243.

Tan BB, Flaherty KR, Kazerooni EA, et al. The solitary pulmonary nodule. *Chest.* 2003;123(suppl 1):89S–96S.

Truong MT, et al. Update in the evaluation of the solitary pulmonary nodule. *Radiographics.* 2014;34:1658–1679.

The full reference list for this chapter is available at ExpertConsult.com.

5 Interstitial Patterns*

JONATHAN H. CHUNG | CHRISTOPHER M. WALKER

Many diseases involve predominantly or exclusively the pulmonary interstitium. The differential diagnosis of the various entities on the chest radiograph and computed tomography (CT) is based on the pattern and distribution of abnormalities and on the presence of associated findings, such as lymph node enlargement or pleural effusion. Interstitial lung disease results in six distinct radiologic patterns of abnormality: septal, reticular, cystic, nodular, and ground-glass opacities and consolidation. Although each of these patterns can be seen on high-resolution CT and correlated with specific histopathologic findings, the appearances on the chest radiograph are frequently nonspecific and sometimes misleading.[1,2] A reticular pattern on the radiograph may result from summation of smooth or irregular linear opacities, cystic spaces, or both. In approximately 10% of patients with interstitial lung disease, the chest radiograph is normal.[3] Numerous studies have shown that CT, particularly high-resolution CT, is superior to chest radiography in the detection of parenchymal abnormalities and is more accurate in the differential diagnosis.[1,2,4] High-resolution CT is performed almost routinely in the evaluation of patients with suspected or proven interstitial lung disease.

Because of its low cost and low radiation dose, the chest radiograph remains the initial imaging modality of choice in the evaluation of patients with suspected interstitial lung disease and in the follow-up of these patients. Serial chest radiographs often provide a clue to the correct diagnosis by showing the course of the disease process. In this chapter we include the radiographic and the high-resolution CT patterns of abnormality, recognizing that in a high percentage of cases accurate assessment of presence, pattern, and extent of interstitial disease can be made only on high-resolution CT. Consolidation may occur in interstitial lung disease but more commonly reflects the presence of airspace disease. Consolidation is discussed separately in Chapter 2.

Septal Pattern

A septal pattern results from thickening of the interlobular septa (i.e., the tissue that separates the secondary pulmonary lobules) (Fig. 5.1). Normally, no septal lines can be identified on the radiograph, and only a few can be seen on high-resolution CT, mostly in the anterior and lower aspects of the lower lobes. When thickened, interlobular septa (septal lines) are seen on the radiograph as short (1–2 cm) lines perpendicular to and continuous with the pleura (Kerley B lines) or as longer (2–6 cm) lines oriented toward the hila (Kerley A lines) (Fig. 5.2). On high-resolution CT scan septal lines can be seen as short lines that extend to the pleura in the lung periphery and as polygonal arcades outlining one or more pulmonary lobules in more central lung regions (see Fig. 5.2).[5] Thickening of the interlobular septa may be caused by edema, cellular infiltration, or fibrosis. Septal thickening can be smooth, nodular, or irregular in contour.

The most common cause of a septal pattern as the predominant or only pattern is hydrostatic pulmonary edema (Figs. 5.3 and 5.4).[6] Less common causes of smooth septal thickening include lymphangitic spread of carcinoma (see Fig. 5.2),[7] lymphoma (Fig. 5.5),[8] leukemia,[9] Churg-Strauss syndrome,[10] acute lung rejection (Fig. 5.6),[11] congenital lymphangiectasia,[12] and Niemann-Pick syndrome (Fig. 5.7).[13] These various conditions tend to result in extensive septal thickening that is usually bilateral and often symmetric. Localized smooth septal thickening is frequently seen adjacent to pleural inflammation (Fig. 5.8), particularly in patients with empyema or after pleurodesis,[14] lymphoid interstitial pneumonia,[15] and idiopathic bronchiectasis.[16] The interlobular septal thickening in patients with bronchiectasis is presumably due to impaired lymphatic drainage, and the extent of septal lines correlates with the extent and severity of bronchiectasis.[16] Nodular septal thickening occurs most commonly in patients with lymphangitic carcinomatosis (Figs. 5.9 and 5.10),[7] sarcoidosis (Fig. 5.11), Kaposi sarcoma,[20] leukemia,[9] and amyloidosis.[21]

Patients with lymphangitic spread of tumor may have smooth or nodular septal thickening (see Figs. 5.2 and 5.10).[7] In most cases septal thickening is the main abnormality seen in these patients. Other common findings include unilateral or asymmetric hilar lymph node enlargement and pleural effusion. Although septal thickening may be seen in sarcoidosis, it is seldom the main finding. The nodules in sarcoidosis are typically most numerous along the bronchoarterial and pleural interstitium and along the interlobar fissures (see Fig. 5.11).[17,22]

Irregular septal thickening is seen most commonly in patients with interstitial fibrosis, particularly idiopathic pulmonary fibrosis, asbestosis, and sarcoidosis (Fig. 5.12).[23,24] It is usually associated with other findings of fibrosis, such as reticulation, traction bronchiectasis, and traction bronchiolectasis, and is seldom the predominant pattern. The main abnormalities in idiopathic pulmonary fibrosis typically consist of predominantly peripheral and basal reticulation and, commonly, honeycombing.

Reticular Pattern

A reticular pattern is characterized by innumerable interlacing line shadows that suggest a mesh (Fig. 5.13).[25] On the chest radiograph the pattern may be the result of summation of smooth or irregular linear opacities, cystic spaces, or both (Fig. 5.14). Although distinction between these abnormalities often is difficult on the radiograph, it can be made readily on high-resolution CT. The reticular pattern on high-resolution CT results from

Text continued on p. 115

*The editors and the publisher would like to thank Drs. Nestor L. Müller and C. Isabela Silva Müller for contributing material on this topic to the prior edition of this work. It has served as the foundation for the current chapter.

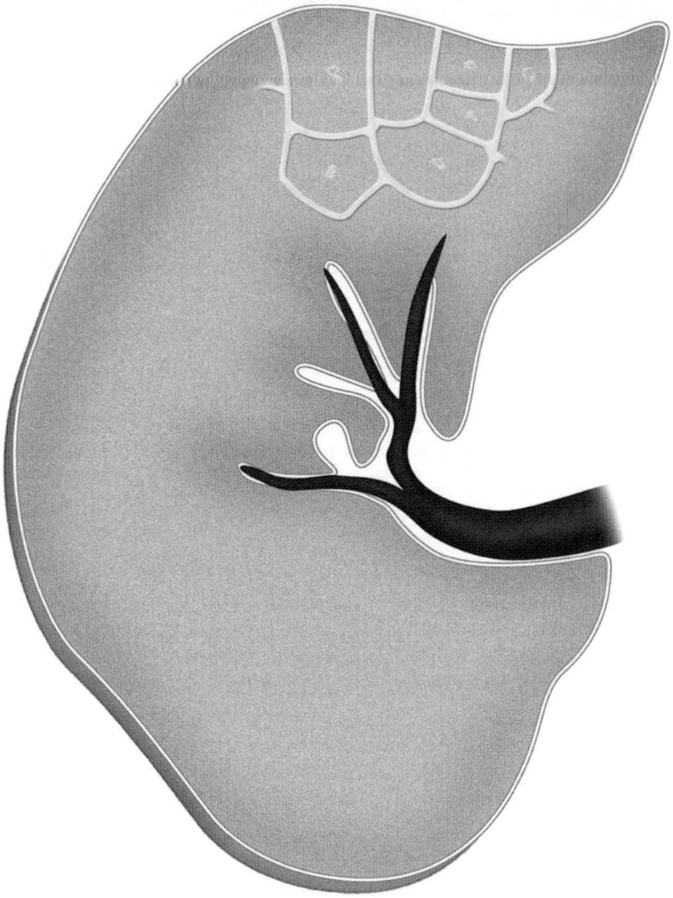

Fig. 5.1 Schematic drawing of septal pattern. Drawing of the right lung shows thin lines separated by 1–2 cm that correspond to thickened interlobular septa.

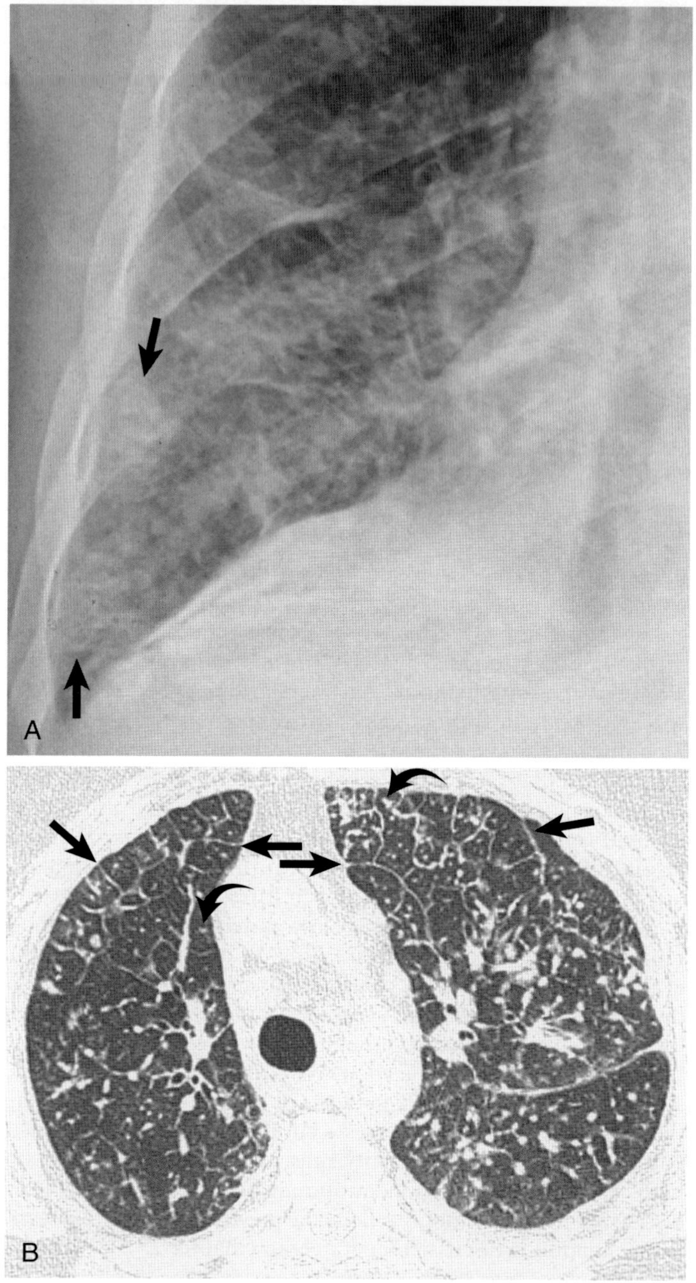

Fig. 5.2 Septal pattern in a patient with lymphangitic carcinomatosis. (A) Magnified view of right lower lung zone shows linear opacities *(arrows)* measuring 1–2 cm in length and perpendicular to the pleura. These represent septal lines (Kerley B lines). (B) High-resolution CT scan shows 0.5- to 2-cm-long lines *(straight arrows)* and polygonal arcades outlining one or more pulmonary lobules. These linear opacities (septal lines) reflect the presence of thickening of the interlobular septa. Prominent centrilobular dots *(curved arrows)*, which represent thickening of the interstitium along the centrilobular bronchiole, and small left pleural effusion also are noted.

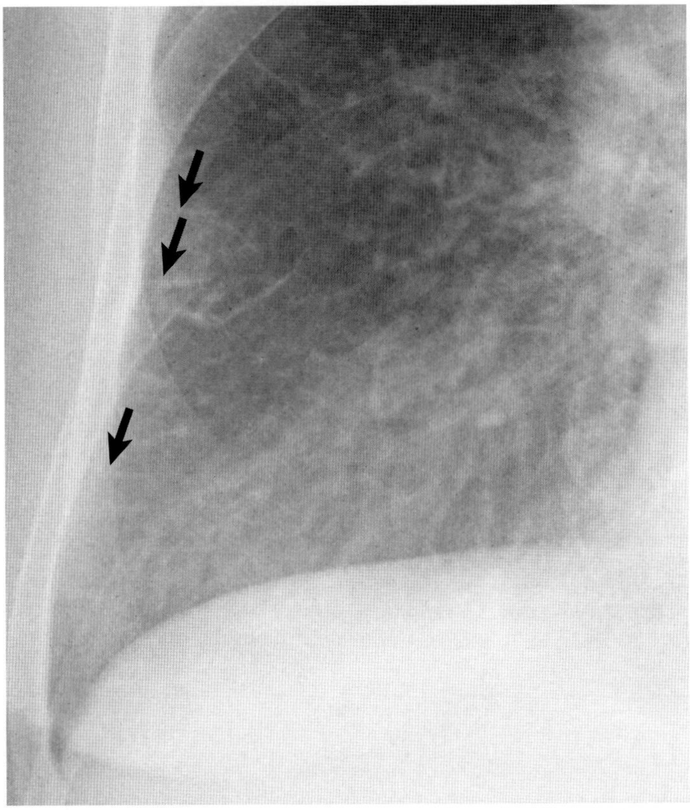

Fig. 5.3 Septal pattern in a patient with interstitial pulmonary edema from left heart failure. Magnified view of right lower lung zone shows linear opacities *(arrows)* measuring 1–2 cm in length and perpendicular to the pleura. These represent septal (Kerley B) lines. Prominence of the pulmonary vessels is also noted.

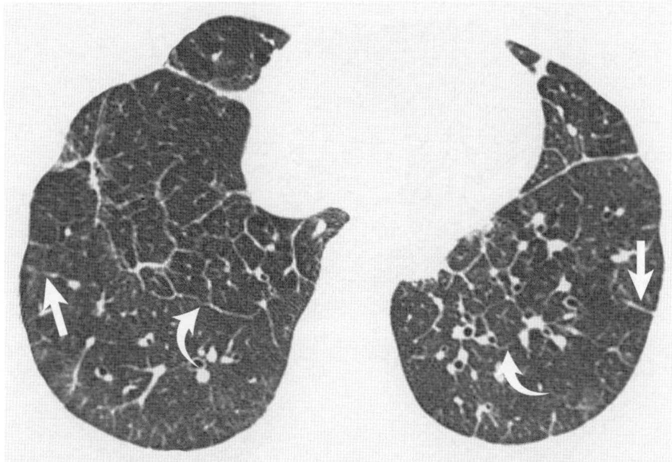

Fig. 5.4 Smooth septal thickening in a patient with interstitial pulmonary edema from left heart failure. High-resolution CT scan at the level of the lower lung zones shows smooth septal lines perpendicular to the pleura *(straight arrows)* and more centrally as polygonal arcades *(curved arrows)*.

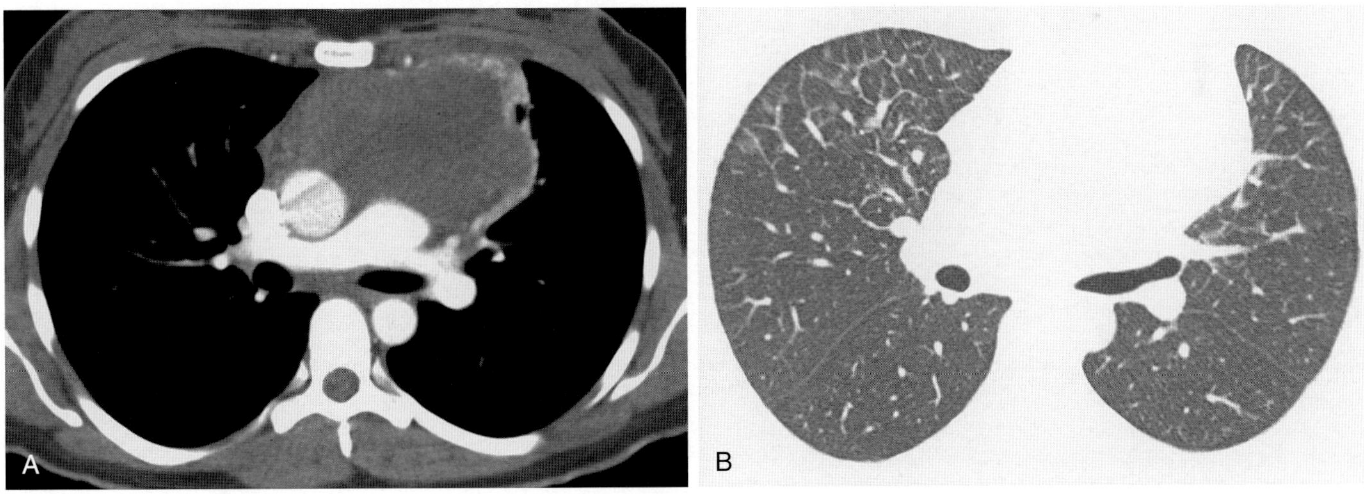

Fig. 5.5 Septal thickening in non-Hodgkin lymphoma. (A) Contrast-enhanced CT scan shows large anterior (prevascular) mediastinal mass. (B) Lung windows show bilateral thickening of the interlobular septa.

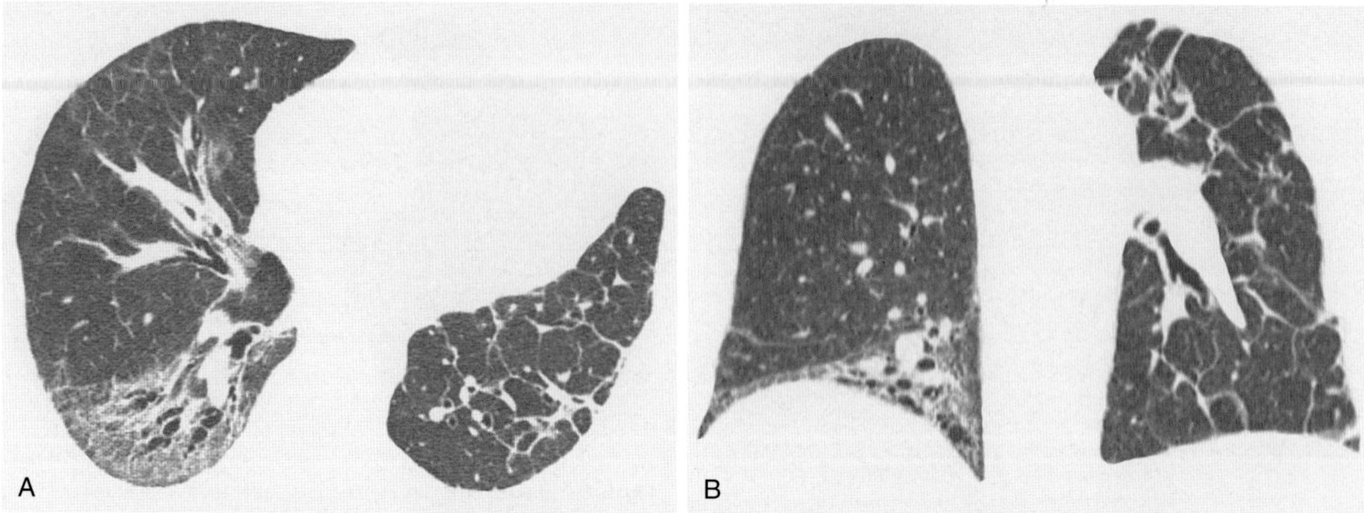

Fig. 5.6 Smooth septal thickening in acute lung rejection. (A) High-resolution CT scan performed in a 41-year-old man with unilateral left lung transplant shows thickening of several interlobular septa in the transplanted lung. Interstitial fibrosis, which was proven to be nonspecific interstitial pneumonia, is evident in the native right lung. (B) Coronal reformation shows extensive septal thickening in the transplanted left lung and lower lung zone fibrosis in the native right lung. Transbronchial biopsy specimens of the left lung showed acute rejection.

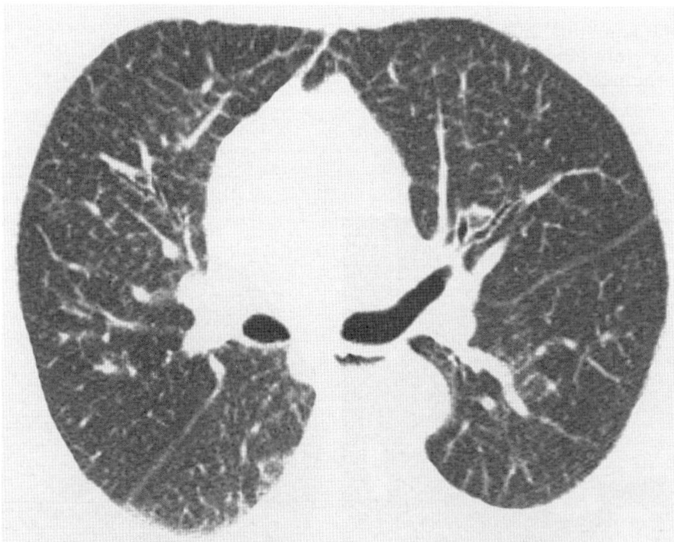

Fig. 5.7 Septal thickening in Niemann-Pick disease. High-resolution CT scan at the level of the bronchus intermedius shows mild bilateral interlobular septal thickening.

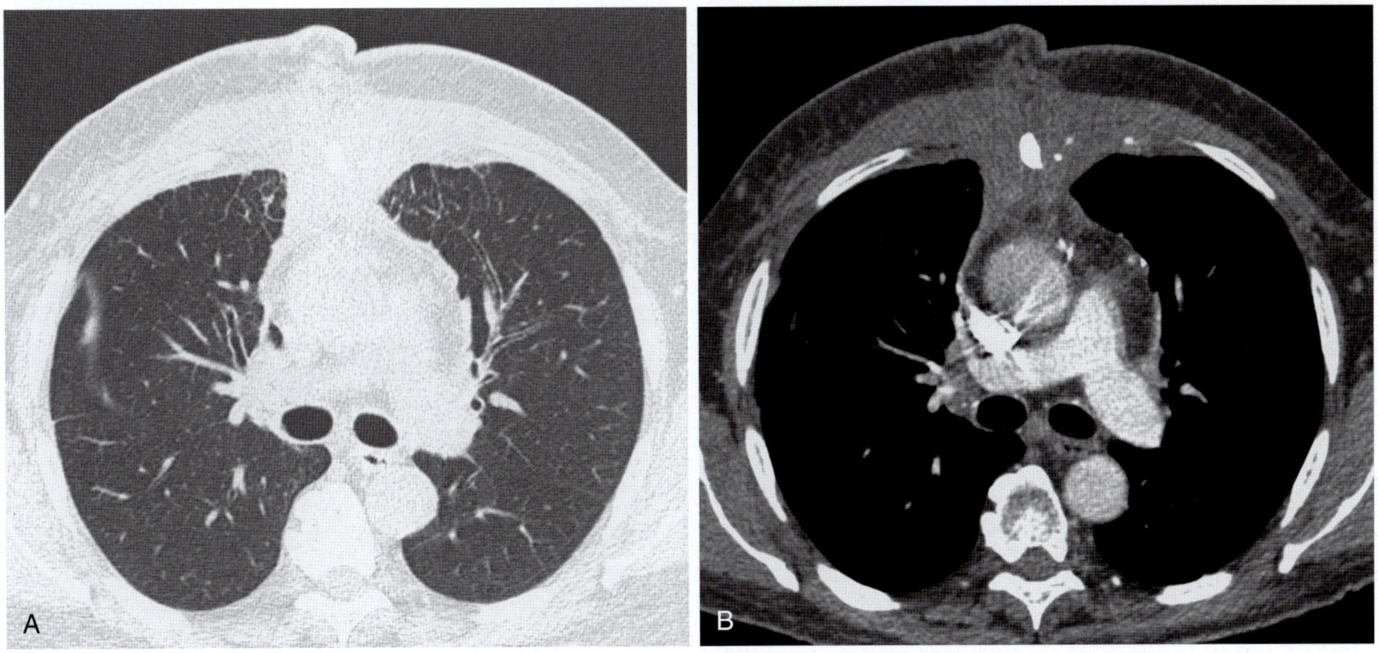

Fig. 5.8 Septal thickening as a result of pleural inflammation in the setting of sternal osteomyelitis after coronary artery bypass graft surgery. (A) High-resolution CT scan shows interlobular septal thickening in the anterior region of the upper lobes. (B) Contrast-enhanced CT scan shows increased soft tissue in the parasternal region and bilateral chest wall and mediastinal pleural thickening. Sternal wound culture grew methicillin-resistant *Staphylococcus aureus.*

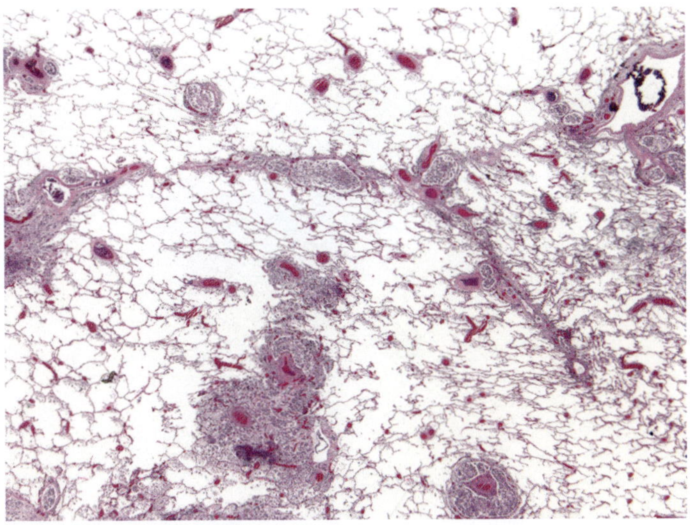

Fig. 5.9 Septal thickening as a result of lymphangitic carcinomatosis. Histologic specimen shows nodular thickening of the interlobular septa by tumor cells. *(Courtesy Dr. Julia Flint, Department of Pathology, Vancouver General Hospital, Vancouver, Canada.)*

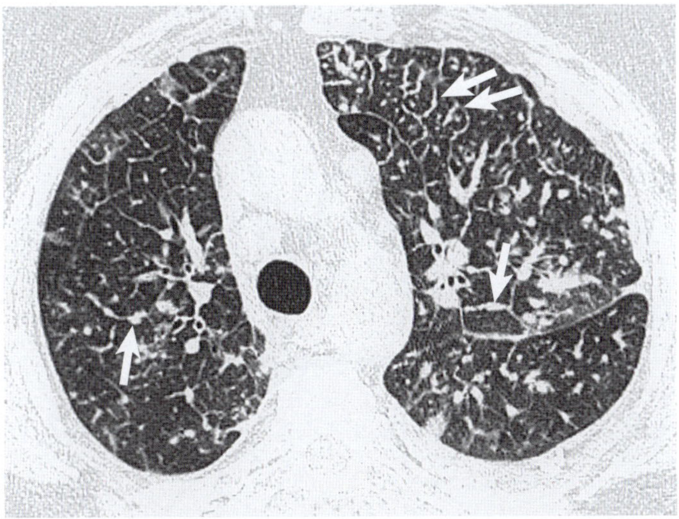

Fig. 5.10 Nodular septal thickening in lymphangitic carcinomatosis. High-resolution CT scan shows extensive bilateral septal thickening and small left pleural effusion. Several of the thickened septa have a beaded nodular appearance *(arrows).* Also evident are enlarged mediastinal lymph nodes.

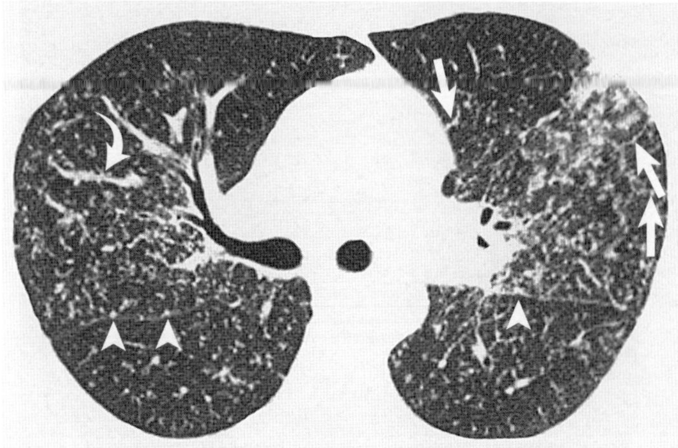

Fig. 5.11 Nodular septal thickening in sarcoidosis. High-resolution CT scan shows nodular thickening of the interlobular septa *(straight arrows)*. Other characteristic features of sarcoidosis also are noted, including nodules along the vessels *(curved arrows)* and interlobar fissures *(arrowheads)*.

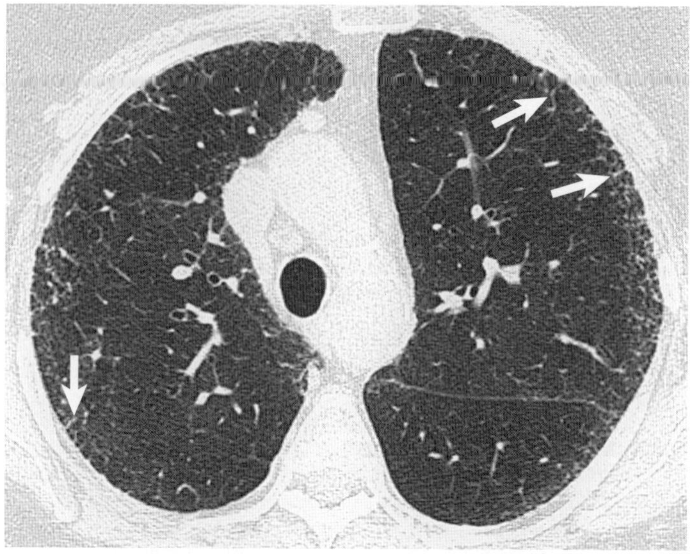

Fig. 5.12 Irregular septal thickening in idiopathic pulmonary fibrosis. High-resolution CT scan shows a few bilateral irregularly thickened septa *(arrows)*. Note also the presence of smaller intralobular lines resulting in a fine reticular pattern, architectural distortion, and subpleural distribution of findings characteristic of idiopathic pulmonary fibrosis.

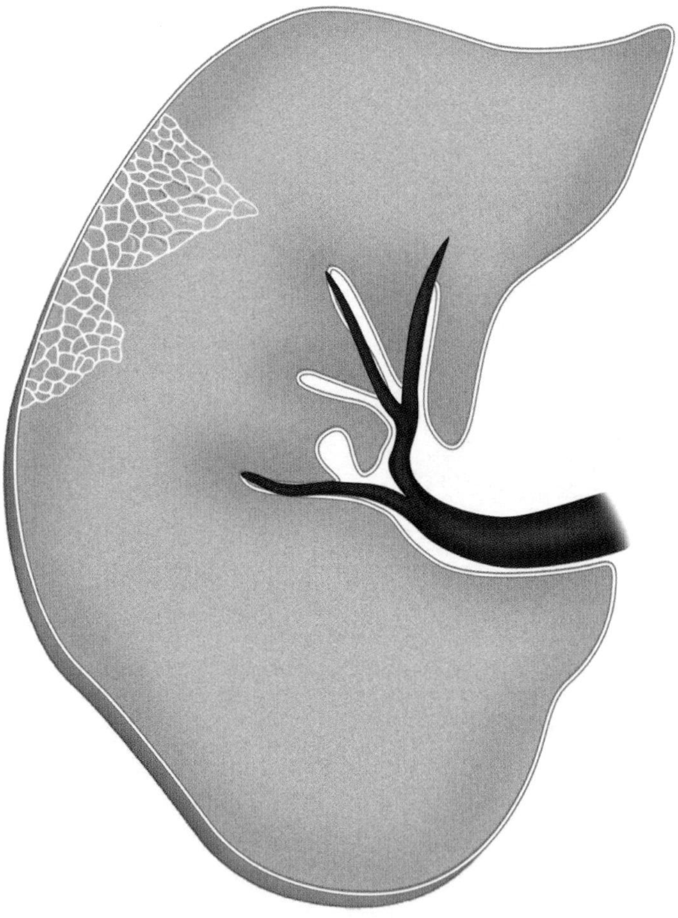

Fig. 5.13 Schematic drawing of reticular pattern. Drawing of the right lung illustrates reticular pattern. A reticular pattern on high-resolution CT typically results from intralobular lines (i.e., fine linear opacities visible within a secondary pulmonary lobule as a result of thickening of the intralobular interstitial tissue).

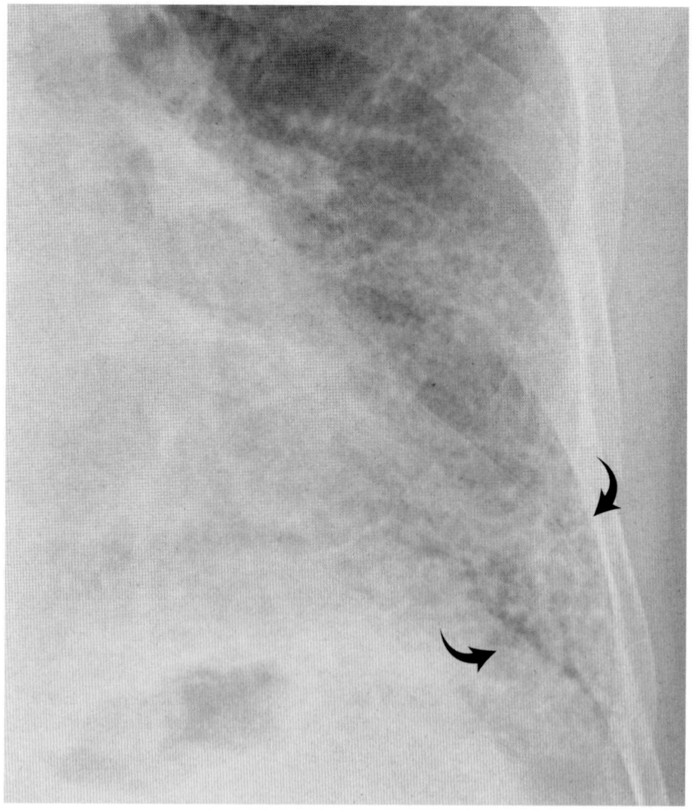

Fig. 5.14 Reticular pattern on chest radiography in idiopathic pulmonary fibrosis. Magnified view of the left lower lung zone shows extensive reticular pattern *(arrows)*. The reticular pattern in this patient was caused by summation of irregular linear opacities and honeycombing.

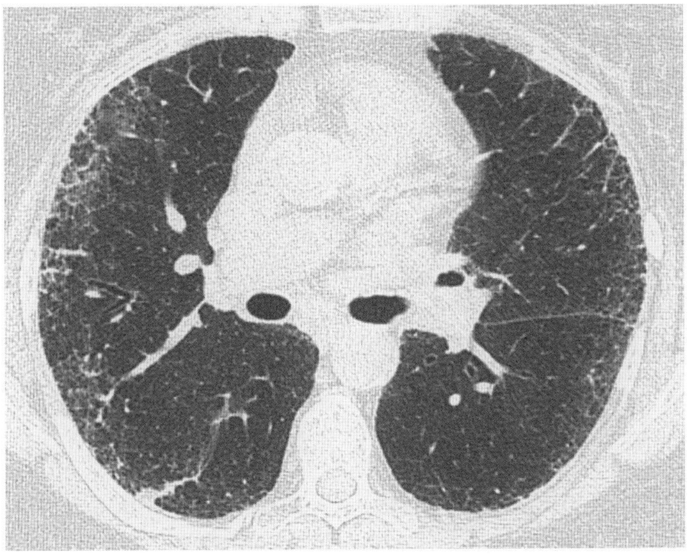

Fig. 5.15 Reticular pattern on high-resolution CT in idiopathic pulmonary fibrosis. High-resolution CT scan at the level of bronchus intermedius shows bilateral subpleural irregular intralobular linear opacities and irregular septal thickening resulting in a fine reticular pattern.

small irregular intralobular linear opacities separated by only a few millimeters (Figs. 5.15 and 5.16). Intralobular linear opacities reflect thickening of the interstitium within the secondary pulmonary lobule and are most commonly caused by fibrosis. Fibrosis also typically results in distortion of the parenchymal architecture, traction bronchiectasis, traction bronchiolectasis, and honeycombing (Fig. 5.17; see also Fig. 5.16).[26,27] Common causes of a reticular pattern include usual interstitial pneumonia, nonspecific interstitial pneumonia, fibrosis associated with collagen vascular disease, chronic hypersensitivity pneumonitis, sarcoidosis, and asbestosis.

Idiopathic pulmonary fibrosis is a chronic interstitial fibrosis limited to the lung and associated with the imaging and histologic pattern of usual interstitial pneumonia.[28] The radiographic findings consist of a symmetric, bilateral reticular pattern that may be diffuse but tend to involve predominantly the lower lung zones (see Fig. 5.14).[29,30] In 60% of patients a predominant peripheral distribution is apparent on the radiograph.[22] As the disease progresses, the reticular pattern becomes coarser and is associated with progressive loss of volume.

The characteristic high-resolution CT findings of idiopathic pulmonary fibrosis consist of a reticular pattern in a patchy distribution and involving all lobes but being most severe in the subpleural lung regions and in the lung bases (see Figs. 5.16 and 5.17).[31,32] The reticular pattern is usually associated with irregular pleural, vascular, and bronchial interfaces; evidence of architectural distortion; and dilation of bronchi and bronchioles (traction bronchiectasis and bronchiolectasis) (see Figs. 5.16 and 5.17).[26,33] Subpleural air-containing cysts measuring 2 to 20 mm in diameter (honeycombing) lining up in rows or stacks are present in 80% to 90% of patients at diagnosis.[34,35]

A reticular pattern also frequently is seen in patients with nonspecific interstitial pneumonia.[31] Nonspecific interstitial pneumonia is a chronic interstitial lung disease characterized histologically by a combination of interstitial fibrosis and inflammation that resembles idiopathic pulmonary fibrosis clinically but has a considerably better prognosis. Nonspecific interstitial

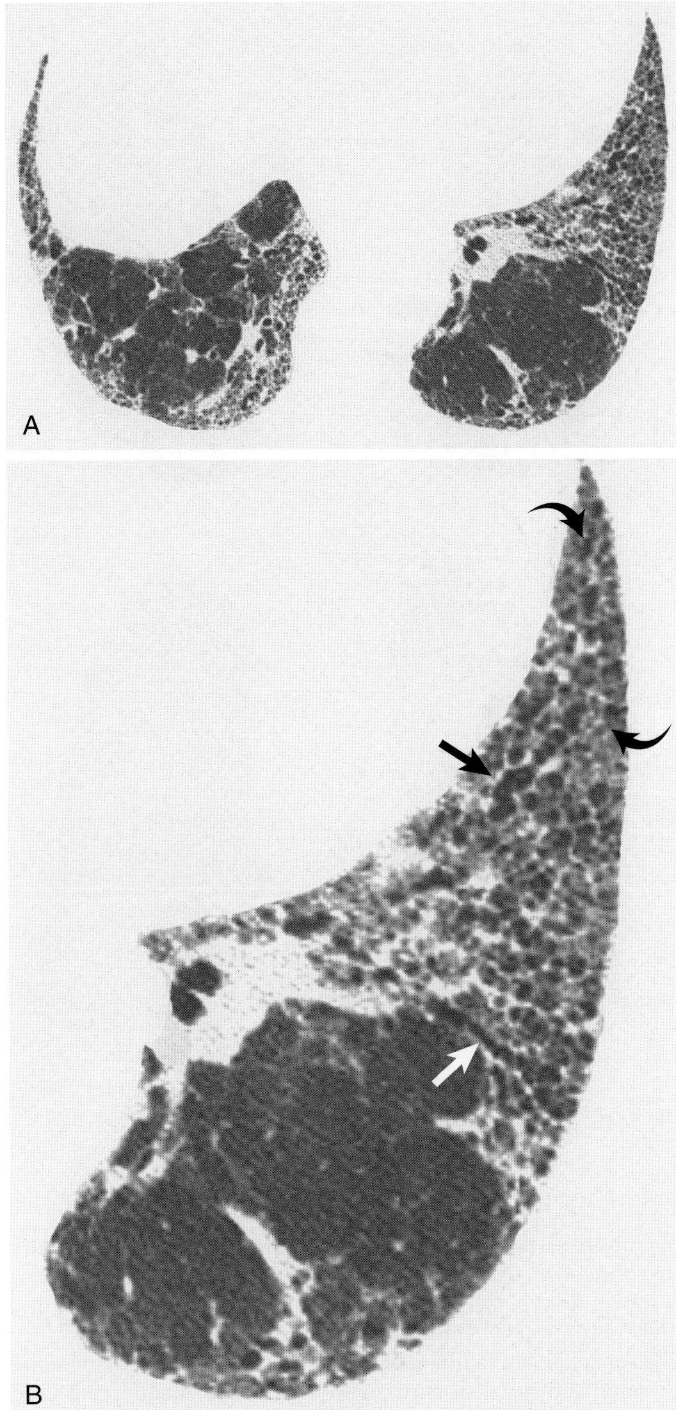

Fig. 5.16 Severe reticular pattern with traction bronchiectasis and bronchiolectasis in idiopathic pulmonary fibrosis. (A) High-resolution CT scan at the level of the lung bases shows reticular pattern in the peripheral regions of the lower lobes and diffusely in the middle lobe and lingula. (B) Magnified view of the left lower lung zone shows reticular pattern. Also noted is dilation and beading of bronchi (traction bronchiectasis) *(straight arrows)*. Dilated airways within approximately 0.5–1 cm from the pleura represent ectatic bronchioles (traction bronchiolectasis) *(curved arrows)*.

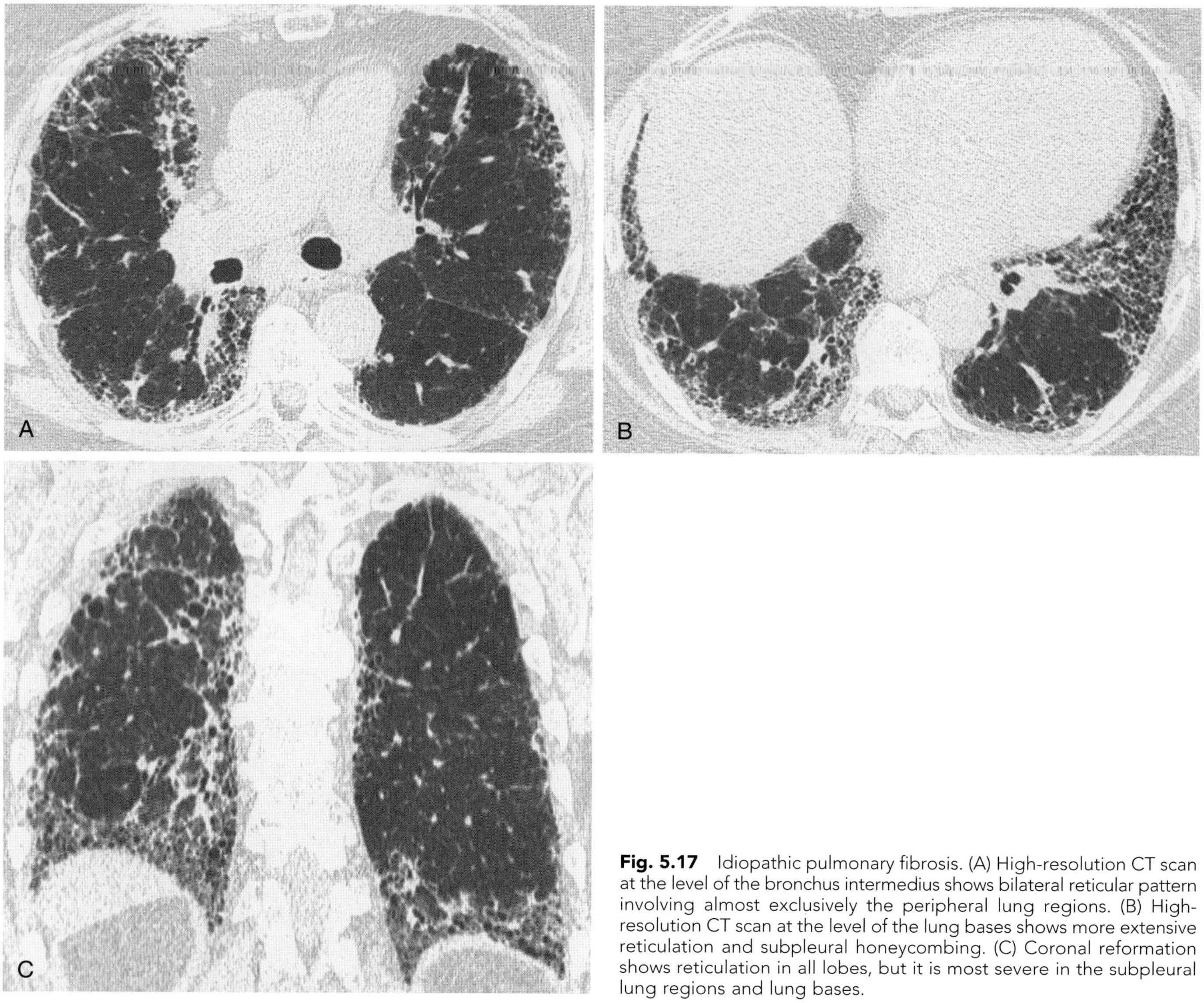

Fig. 5.17 Idiopathic pulmonary fibrosis. (A) High-resolution CT scan at the level of the bronchus intermedius shows bilateral reticular pattern involving almost exclusively the peripheral lung regions. (B) High-resolution CT scan at the level of the lung bases shows more extensive reticulation and subpleural honeycombing. (C) Coronal reformation shows reticulation in all lobes, but it is most severe in the subpleural lung regions and lung bases.

pneumonia is rarely idiopathic and is more commonly secondary to connective tissue disease (particularly scleroderma), drug reaction, or hypersensitivity pneumonitis. The radiographic and high-resolution CT findings most commonly consist of ground-glass opacities and a fine reticular pattern (Fig. 5.18).[36,37] Evidence of architectural distortion with traction bronchiectasis and bronchiolectasis is commonly seen on high-resolution CT, but honeycombing is uncommon at presentation. The abnormalities may be diffuse, but they involve mainly the lower lung zones in 60% to 90% of cases and predominantly the lung periphery in 50% to 70%.[36,38] Although the fibrosis in nonspecific interstitial pneumonia is often predominantly peripheral and basal, in approximately 50% of patients there is relative sparing of the immediate subpleural lung in the dorsal regions of the lower lobes (Fig. 5.19).[39] The presence of predominantly ground-glass opacities, relatively mild reticulation, absence of honeycombing, and relative sparing of the subpleural regions allow distinction of nonspecific interstitial pneumonia from usual interstitial pneumonia in most cases.[36,39] It may be impossible, however, to distinguish fibrotic nonspecific interstitial pneumonia with a predominantly reticular pattern from usual interstitial pneumonia.

The most common collagen vascular diseases associated with a reticular pattern on the chest radiograph and high-resolution CT are scleroderma and rheumatoid arthritis. The histologic, radiographic, and high-resolution CT manifestations of scleroderma are usually those of nonspecific interstitial pneumonia[40,41]; rheumatoid arthritis tends to result in findings of usual interstitial pneumonia and, less commonly, nonspecific interstitial pneumonia.[42]

In chronic hypersensitivity pneumonitis, the fibrosis is situated predominantly in the middle lung zones or shows no zonal predominance (Fig. 5.20).[43] Lung apices and bases are relatively spared. The distribution of fibrosis on high-resolution CT is commonly random but may be predominantly subpleural or peribronchovascular.[43] In most cases there are superimposed findings of subacute disease, typically poorly defined centrilobular nodules, extensive bilateral ground-glass opacities, and lobular areas with decreased attenuation and vascularity (i.e., mosaic attenuation) with air trapping on expiratory images (see Fig.

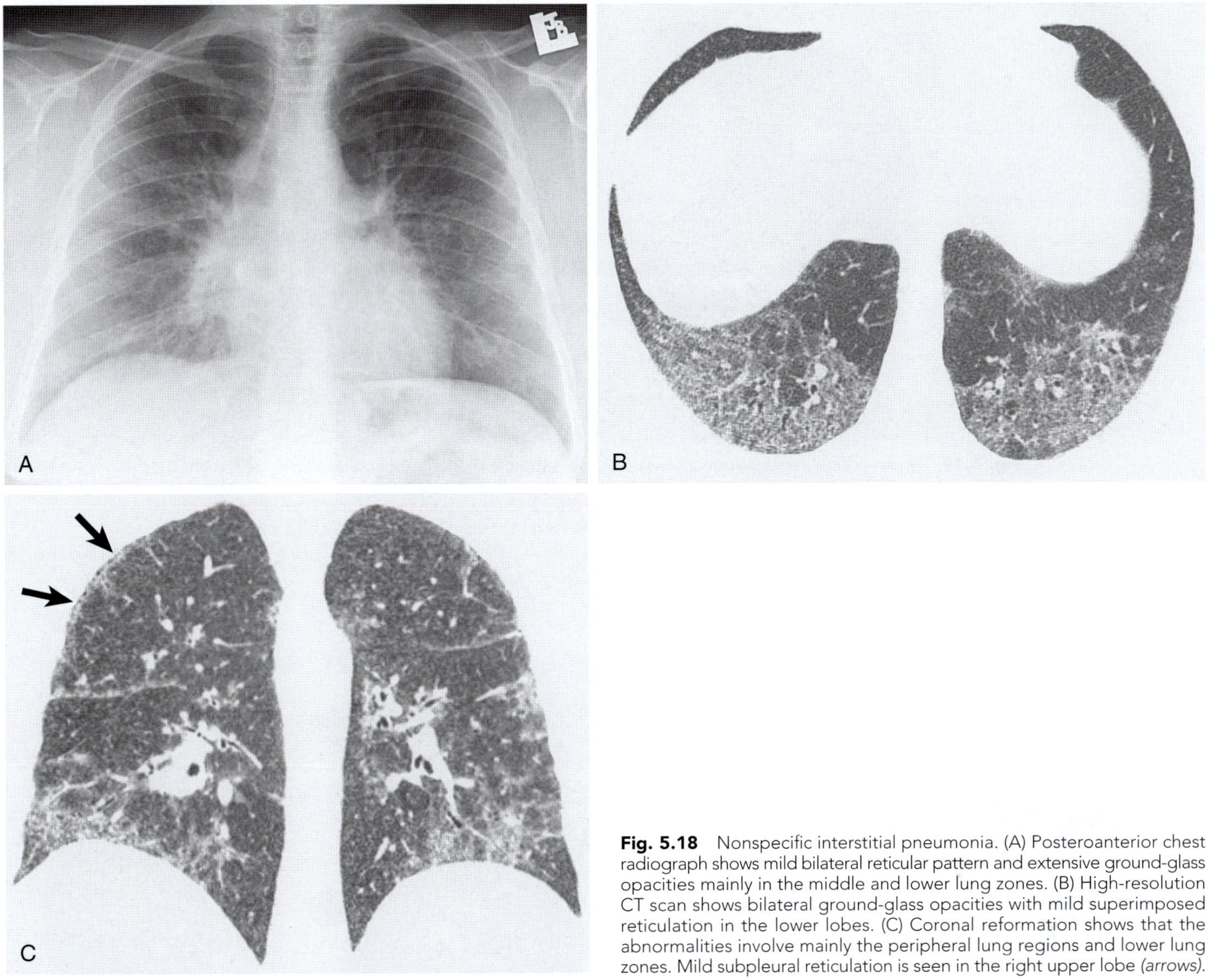

Fig. 5.18 Nonspecific interstitial pneumonia. (A) Posteroanterior chest radiograph shows mild bilateral reticular pattern and extensive ground-glass opacities mainly in the middle and lower lung zones. (B) High-resolution CT scan shows bilateral ground-glass opacities with mild superimposed reticulation in the lower lobes. (C) Coronal reformation shows that the abnormalities involve mainly the peripheral lung regions and lower lung zones. Mild subpleural reticulation is seen in the right upper lobe *(arrows)*.

5.20).[39,44] The predominantly middle lung zone distribution of fibrosis and the presence of centrilobular nodules and lobular areas of air trapping allow recognition of hypersensitivity pneumonitis in most cases. In some patients the findings may mimic those of usual interstitial pneumonia or nonspecific interstitial pneumonia.[39,44]

A reticular pattern is seen in 15% to 20% of patients who have sarcoidosis and radiographically evident parenchymal abnormalities.[17] The fibrosis in sarcoidosis typically involves mainly the upper and middle lung zones. It is typically associated with superior retraction of the hila, traction bronchiectasis of the central bronchi, and compensatory overinflation of the lower lobes (Fig. 5.21).[24,45]

The reticular pattern in asbestosis is usually mild and involves predominantly or exclusively the lower lung zones. High-resolution CT typically shows subpleural reticulation, subpleural curvilinear opacities, and small rounded or branching subpleural opacities involving mainly the dorsal regions of the lower lung zones.[46,47] Most patients have associated pleural plaques or diffuse pleural thickening.[46]

Cystic Pattern

Cystic airspaces are round, air-containing parenchymal spaces with a well-defined wall.[25] The term is used to describe multiple diffusely enlarged airspaces (diffuse cystic lung disease) seen in Langerhans cell histiocytosis, lymphangioleiomyomatosis, and lymphoid interstitial pneumonia (although rarely, Birt-Hogg-Dubé syndrome, amyloidosis, and light-chain deposition disease can also manifest with this imaging appearance); in end-stage fibrosis (honeycombing) as may be seen in idiopathic pulmonary fibrosis; and, less commonly, in chronic hypersensitivity pneumonitis, nonspecific interstitial pneumonia, asbestosis, and sarcoidosis. Among the conditions that cause diffuse cystic lung disease, Langerhans cell histiocytosis and lymphangioleiomyomatosis are the most commonly encountered diagnostic considerations.

Pulmonary Langerhans cell histiocytosis is a disease characterized histologically by infiltration of the lung by Langerhans cells that typically manifests in young adults and is seen almost exclusively in smokers.[48] The parenchymal abnormalities are

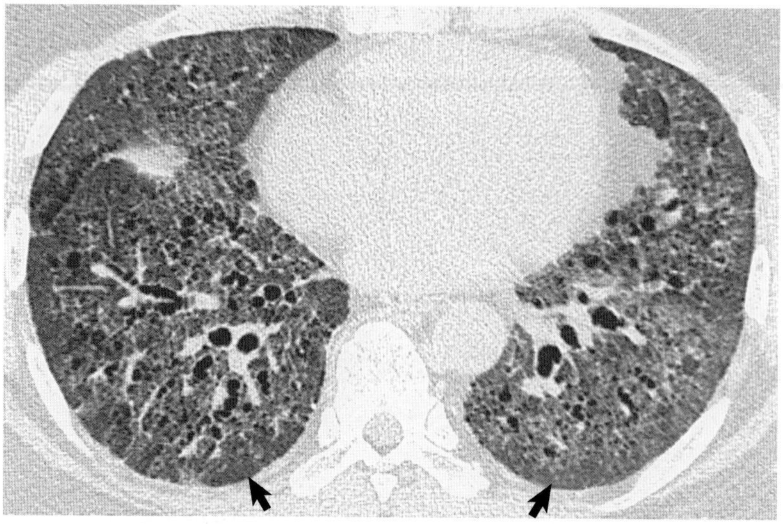

Fig. 5.19 Nonspecific interstitial pneumonia: relative subpleural sparing. High-resolution CT scan shows extensive bilateral ground-glass opacities, traction bronchiectasis, and reticulation. The reticulation is less severe in the lung immediately adjacent to the pleura *(arrows)* than in the lung 1 cm away from the pleura (relative subpleural sparing), a characteristic finding seen in approximately 50% of patients with nonspecific interstitial pneumonia.

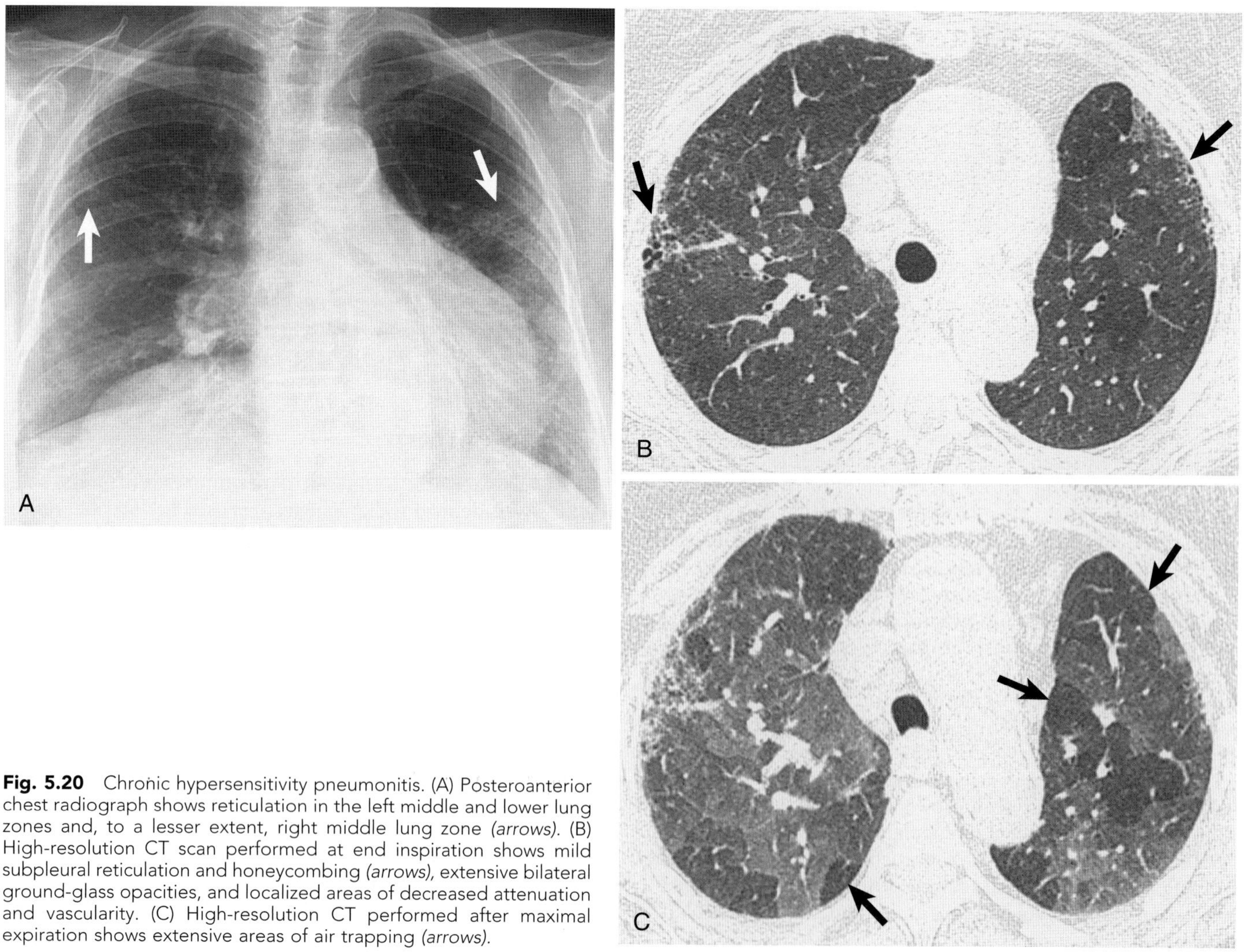

Fig. 5.20 Chronic hypersensitivity pneumonitis. (A) Posteroanterior chest radiograph shows reticulation in the left middle and lower lung zones and, to a lesser extent, right middle lung zone *(arrows)*. (B) High-resolution CT scan performed at end inspiration shows mild subpleural reticulation and honeycombing *(arrows)*, extensive bilateral ground-glass opacities, and localized areas of decreased attenuation and vascularity. (C) High-resolution CT performed after maximal expiration shows extensive areas of air trapping *(arrows)*.

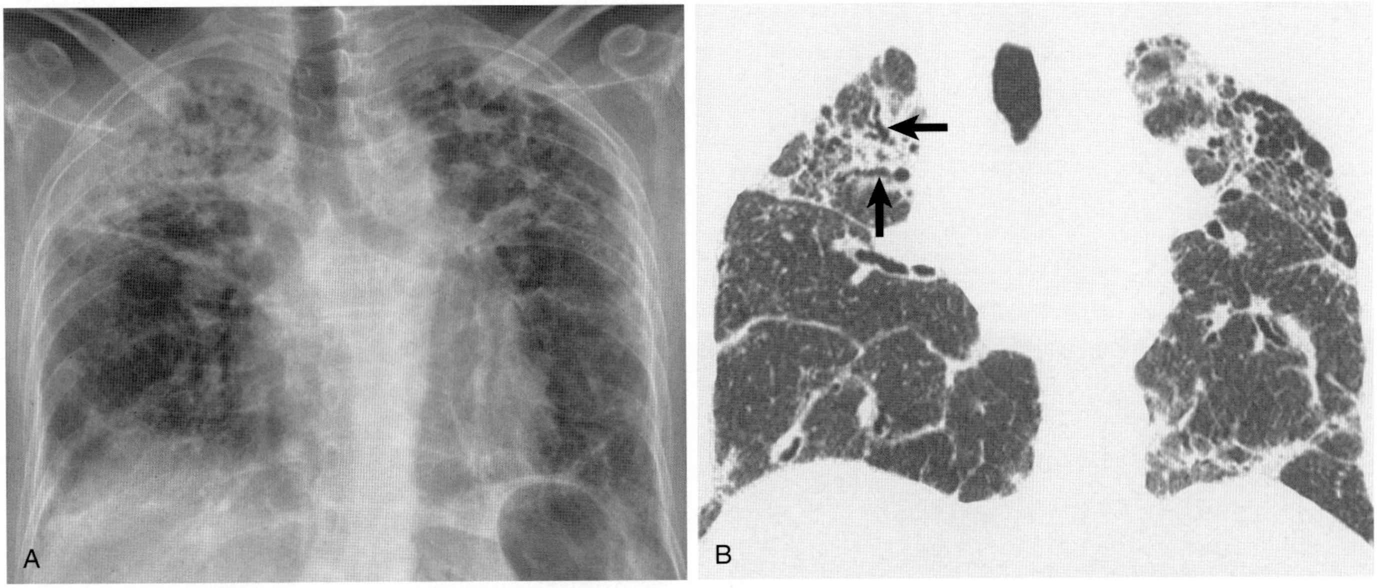

Fig. 5.21 Pulmonary fibrosis in sarcoidosis. (A) Chest radiograph shows extensive bilateral reticulonodular pattern involving mainly the upper lobes with associated volume loss. (B) Coronal reformation CT scan shows upper lobe distribution of the reticulation and traction bronchiectasis *(arrows)*. Note superior retraction of the hila and compensatory overinflation of the lower lobes. Small perilymphatic nodules in the upper and middle lung zones typical of sarcoidosis also are evident.

typically bilateral, symmetric, and diffuse throughout the upper and middle lung zones, with sparing of the costophrenic angles.[49] The chest radiograph tends to show a reticular or reticulonodular pattern (Fig. 5.22).[50] The characteristic findings on high-resolution CT consist of cysts (present in ≈80% of patients) and nodules (present in 60%–80%).[51,52] The nodules predominate in the early phases, and the cysts predominate in the late stages of the disease.[53] The nodules range from 1 to 10 mm in diameter, and the cysts range from a few millimeters to several centimeters in diameter and may be round or oval or have bizarre shapes with bilobed, cloverleaf, and branching configuration.[48] Regardless of the stage of the disease, the abnormalities are diffuse throughout the middle and upper lung zones, with relative sparing of the lung bases (see Fig. 5.22).[49]

Lymphangioleiomyomatosis is a rare disease limited almost exclusively to women and characterized by cyst formation and an interstitial proliferation of smooth muscle–like cells.[54] The radiographic manifestations consist of a diffuse bilateral reticular pattern and, commonly, evidence of hyperinflation manifested by an increase in the retrosternal clear space or flattening of the diaphragm (Fig. 5.23). Cysts can be identified on the radiograph in 50% to 60% of cases.[55,56] The characteristic high-resolution CT finding consists of numerous thin-walled, air-filled cysts surrounded by normal lung parenchyma (see Fig. 5.23).[57] The cysts can be seen on high-resolution CT in patients who have normal radiographs or radiographs showing only reticular opacities. They usually measure 0.2 to 2 cm in diameter and, unlike pulmonary Langerhans cell histiocytosis, are distributed diffusely throughout the lungs without any zonal predominance.[56,57]

Cystic spaces are seen in approximately 30% of patients with *Pneumocystis jirovecii* pneumonia.[58] These may be single or multiple, occur mainly in the upper lobes, and are typically superimposed on ground-glass opacities (Fig. 5.24). The cysts in *Pneumocystis* pneumonia may represent pneumatoceles, premature emphysema, or occasionally cavitated nodules.

Single or multiple cysts typically superimposed on ground-glass opacities also are seen in approximately 60% of patients with lymphoid interstitial pneumonia[15] and 13% of patients with subacute hypersensitivity pneumonitis.[59] The cysts in lymphoid interstitial pneumonia are usually few in number and tend to involve mainly the lower lung zones (Fig. 5.25); lymphoid interstitial pneumonia may also result in extensive cyst formation.[60] The cysts in subacute hypersensitivity pneumonitis may be single or multiple and have a random distribution. In a study of 36 patients with chronic hypersensitivity pneumonitis, Silva and colleagues[39] showed the presence of a few cysts in 14 patients (39%).[39] In most cases the predominant abnormalities of *Pneumocystis* pneumonia, lymphoid interstitial pneumonia, and subacute hypersensitivity pneumonitis are ground-glass opacities.

Honeycombing refers to the presence of cystic spaces, usually measuring 0.3 to 1 cm in diameter, whose walls consist of a variable amount of fibrous tissue (Fig. 5.26). Honeycombing typically tends to be most severe in the subpleural regions and along the interlobar fissures. The most common diseases in which the abnormality is identified are idiopathic pulmonary fibrosis (Fig. 5.27), connective tissue disease, and sarcoidosis; however, the process can be seen in the advanced stage of pulmonary fibrosis of any cause.[24] The spaces represent mainly respiratory bronchioles and alveolar ducts that have become dilated as a result of traction by the adjacent fibrous tissue.[61] The presence, distribution, and extent of honeycombing are assessed much more readily on high-resolution CT scan than on chest radiography. The differential diagnosis of conditions associated with honeycombing is similar to that of reticulation.

In most patients with cystic abnormalities, a confident diagnosis can be made on high-resolution CT based on the appearance and distribution of the cystic changes and the presence of associated findings, such as nodules and ground-glass opacities

Text continued on p. 124

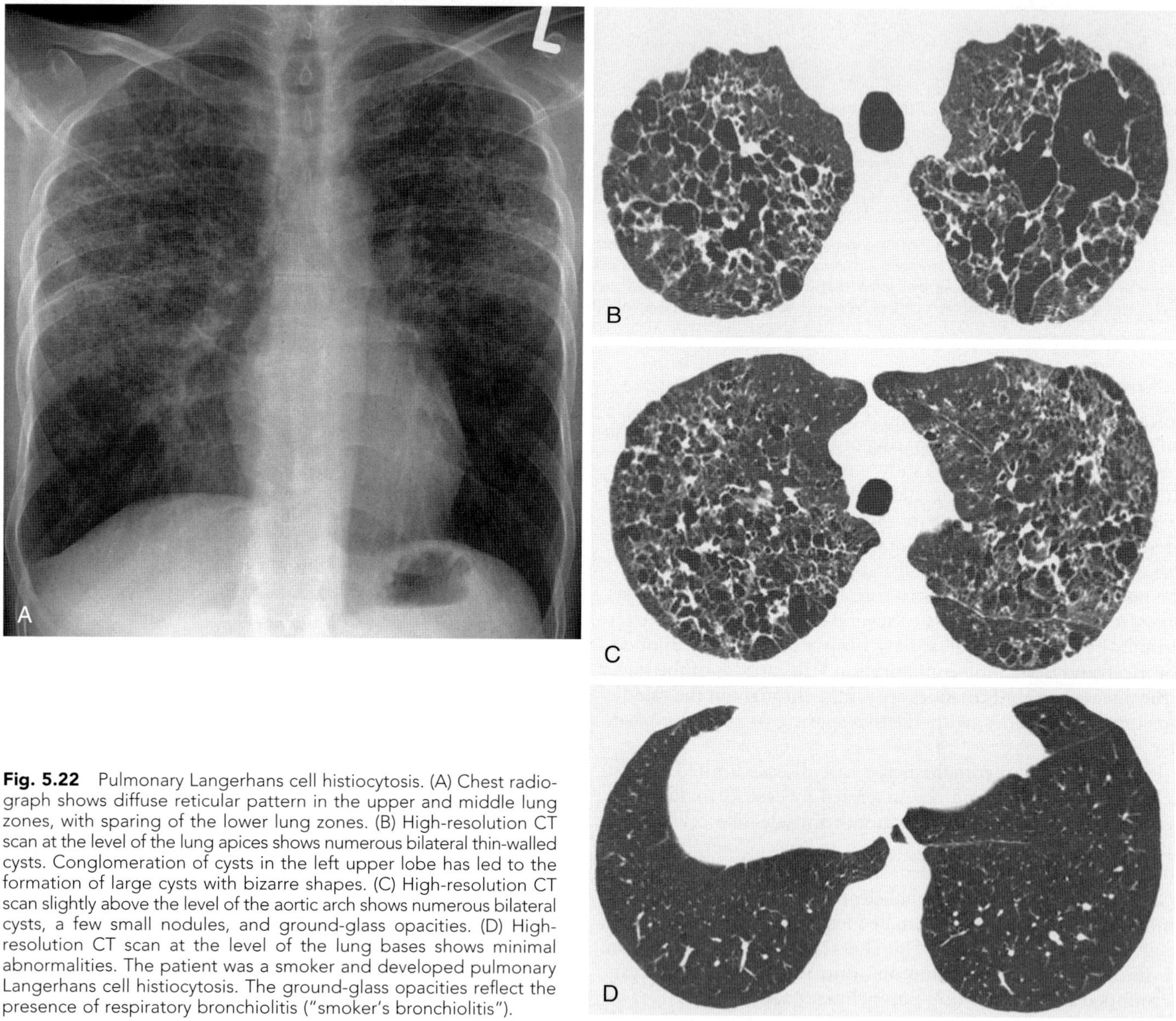

Fig. 5.22 Pulmonary Langerhans cell histiocytosis. (A) Chest radiograph shows diffuse reticular pattern in the upper and middle lung zones, with sparing of the lower lung zones. (B) High-resolution CT scan at the level of the lung apices shows numerous bilateral thin-walled cysts. Conglomeration of cysts in the left upper lobe has led to the formation of large cysts with bizarre shapes. (C) High-resolution CT scan slightly above the level of the aortic arch shows numerous bilateral cysts, a few small nodules, and ground-glass opacities. (D) High-resolution CT scan at the level of the lung bases shows minimal abnormalities. The patient was a smoker and developed pulmonary Langerhans cell histiocytosis. The ground-glass opacities reflect the presence of respiratory bronchiolitis ("smoker's bronchiolitis").

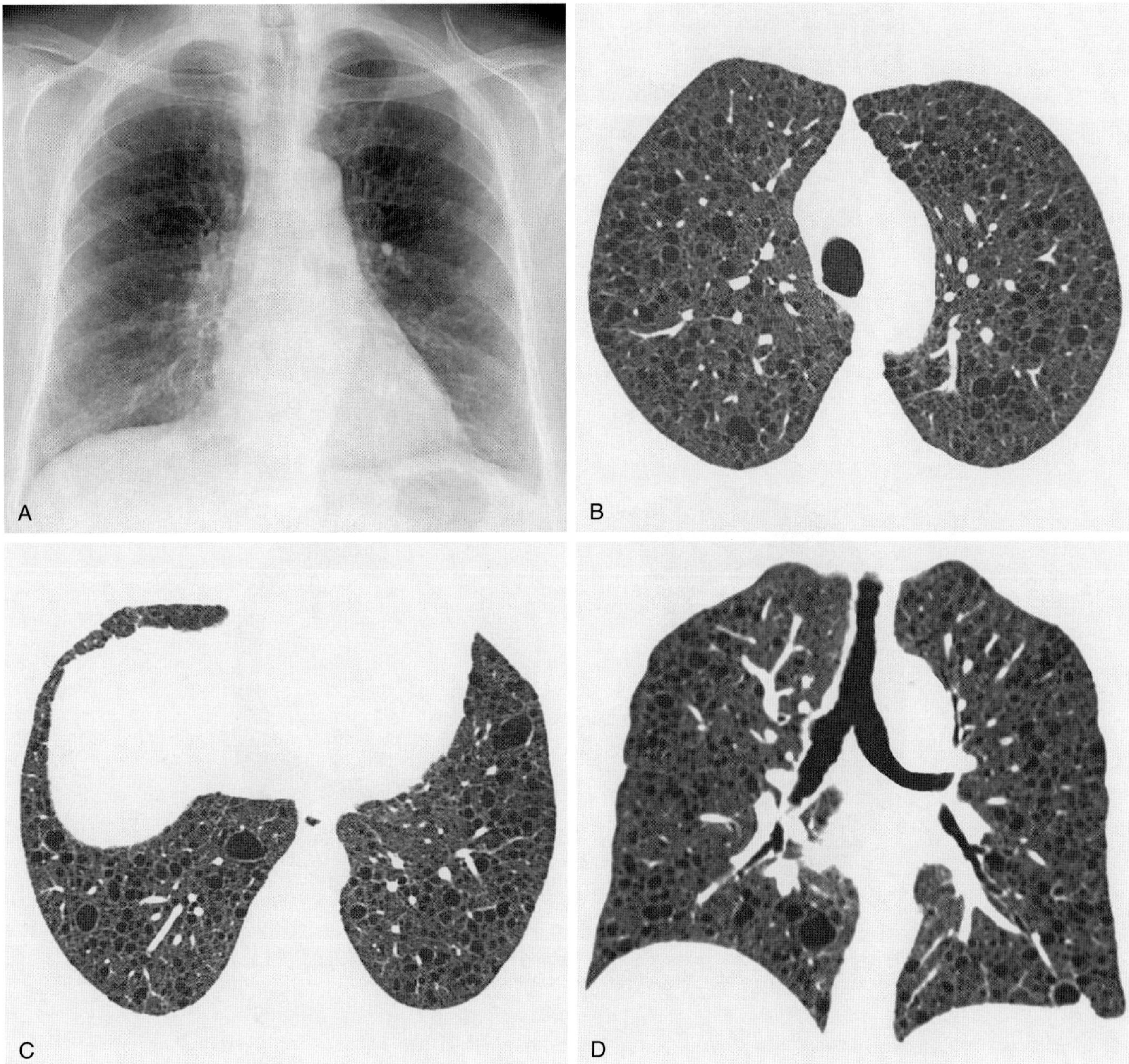

Fig. 5.23 Lymphangioleiomyomatosis. (A) Posteroanterior chest radiograph shows diffuse fine reticular pattern with distortion of the pulmonary vasculature and small areas of lucency. (B) High-resolution CT scan at the level of the upper lobes shows numerous bilateral thin-walled cysts. (C) High-resolution CT scan at the level of the lung bases shows diffuse involvement similar to that in the upper lobes. (D) Coronal reformation shows diffuse distribution of cysts and large lung volumes.

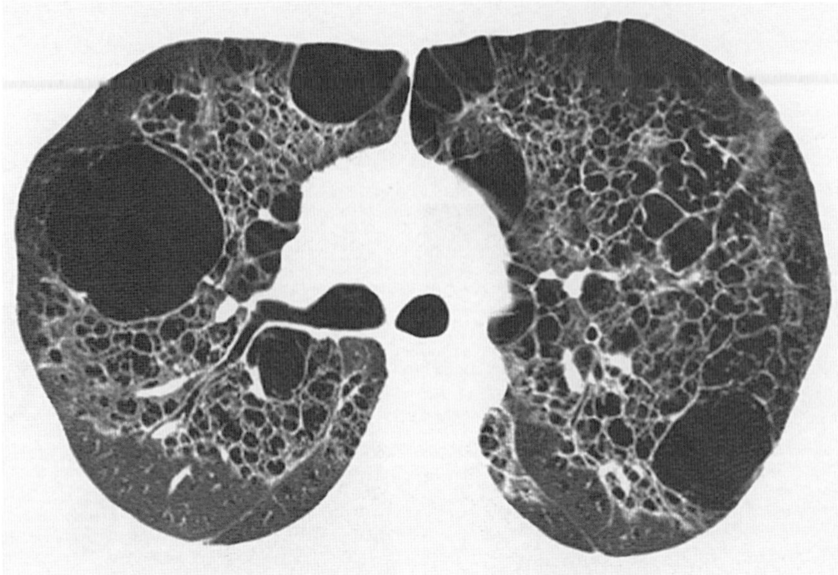

Fig. 5.24 *Pneumocystis* pneumonia in a patient with AIDS. High-resolution CT scan at the level of the upper lobes shows numerous bilateral cysts of various sizes and evidence of paraseptal and centrilobular emphysema. Ground-glass opacities adjacent to the cystic spaces also are noted.

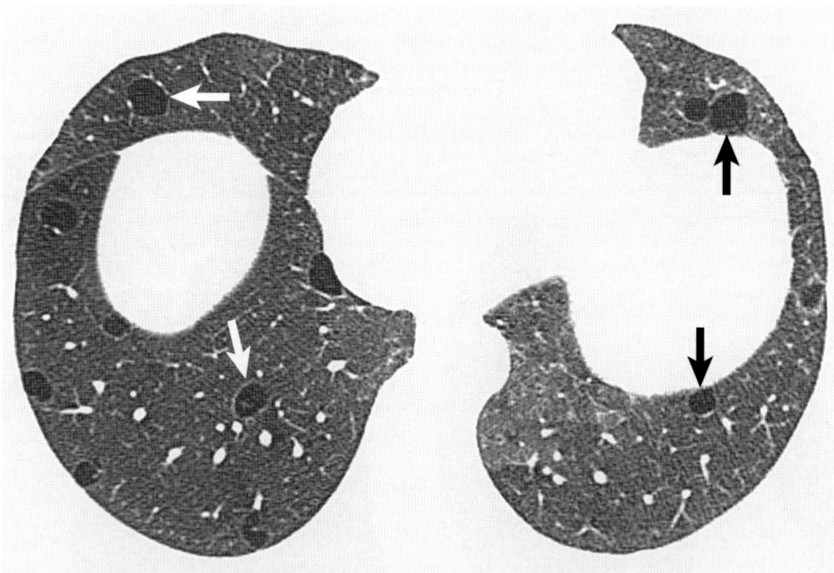

Fig. 5.25 Lymphoid interstitial pneumonia in a lifelong nonsmoker. High-resolution CT scan shows patchy bilateral ground-glass opacities and several thin-walled cysts *(arrows)*.

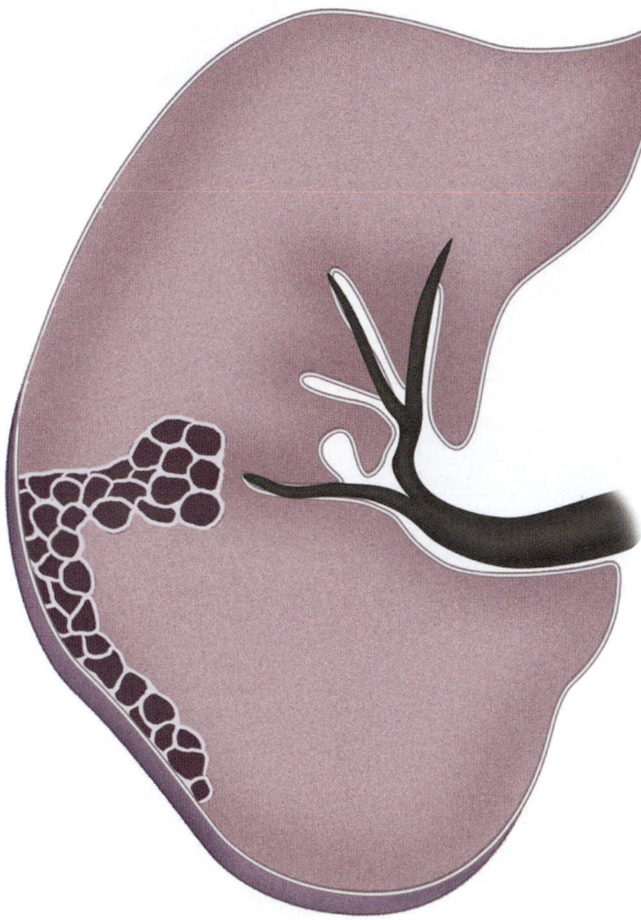

Fig. 5.26 Schematic drawing of the right lung illustrates honeycombing. Honeycombing is characterized on high-resolution CT scan by the presence of clustered cystic airspaces with well-defined walls and typically measuring 3–10 mm in diameter. Honeycombing is a CT feature of end-stage pulmonary fibrosis.

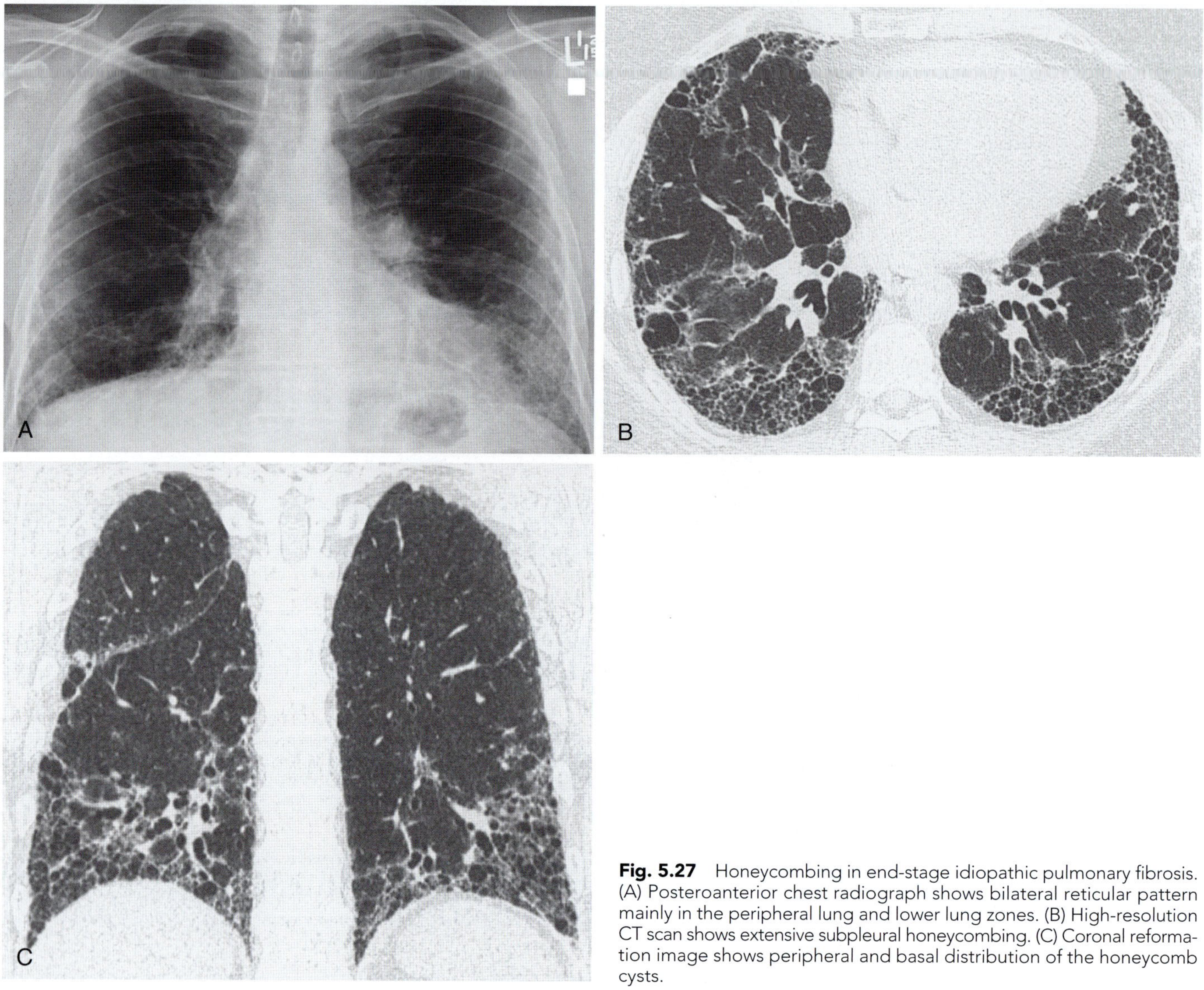

Fig. 5.27 Honeycombing in end-stage idiopathic pulmonary fibrosis. (A) Posteroanterior chest radiograph shows bilateral reticular pattern mainly in the peripheral lung and lower lung zones. (B) High-resolution CT scan shows extensive subpleural honeycombing. (C) Coronal reformation image shows peripheral and basal distribution of the honeycomb cysts.

(Fig. 5.28).[62,63] Similar to other interstitial findings, the final diagnosis requires integration of the high-resolution CT findings with the clinical information and laboratory data. Some patients may require lung biopsy for a definitive diagnosis.

Nodular Pattern

A nodular pattern is characterized by the presence of numerous round opacities measuring less than 1 cm in diameter. The pattern results from expansion of the parenchymal interstitium by a roughly spherical cellular infiltrate, fibrous tissue, or both. The differential diagnosis is based on the pattern and distribution of the nodules, the presence of associated findings such as lymph node enlargement, and the clinical setting. A diffuse small nodular pattern in a febrile patient with acute disease is most suggestive of hematogenous infection, particularly miliary tuberculosis. A similar pattern in a patient with chronic symptoms may result from silicosis, coal workers' pneumoconiosis, intravenous talcosis, metastatic carcinoma (particularly from the thyroid), and adenocarcinoma. The overall distribution of nodules on the radiograph often helps to narrow the differential diagnosis. The nodules in silicosis and coal workers' pneumoconiosis may be diffuse but most commonly involve mainly the middle and upper lung zones, whereas the nodules resulting from hematogenous processes, such as miliary tuberculosis and metastatic carcinoma, are diffuse or involve mainly the lower lung zones (where blood flow is greater).[29,64] The various diseases resulting in multiple nodules typically result in three main patterns of distribution on high-resolution CT: perilymphatic, centrilobular, and random (Fig. 5.29).

PERILYMPHATIC NODULAR PATTERN

A perilymphatic distribution along the bronchovascular interstitium, interlobular septa, and subpleural lung regions is characteristically seen in patients with sarcoidosis[65] and lymphangitic carcinomatosis[7] although the nodular imaging pattern of silicosis and coal workers' pneumoconiosis can also mimic the perilymphatic pattern.[18,19] Perilymphatic nodules tend to be well defined and usually measure 2 to 5 mm in diameter. Nodules in a perilymphatic distribution frequently are associated with nodular thickening of the bronchovascular bundles. Another

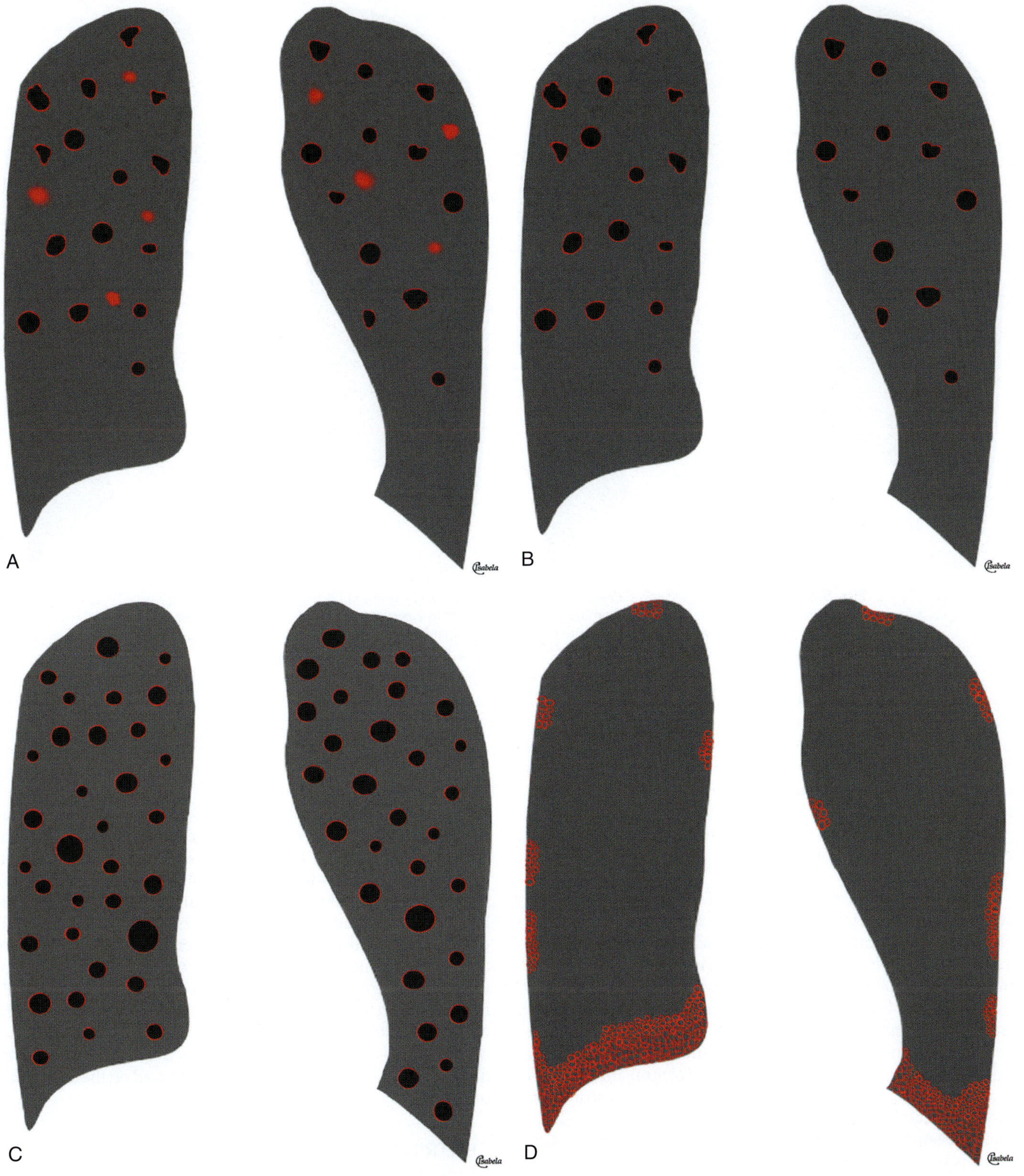

Fig. 5.28 Schematic drawing of cystic pattern and distribution. (A) and (B) Pulmonary Langerhans histiocytosis is characterized by the presence of nodules and cysts (A) or, in the late stage, only cysts in the middle and upper lung zones with relative sparing of the lung bases (B). (C) The cysts in lymphangioleiomyomatosis have a random distribution throughout both lungs. (D) Honeycombing typically involves mainly the peripheral and basal lung regions.

Continued

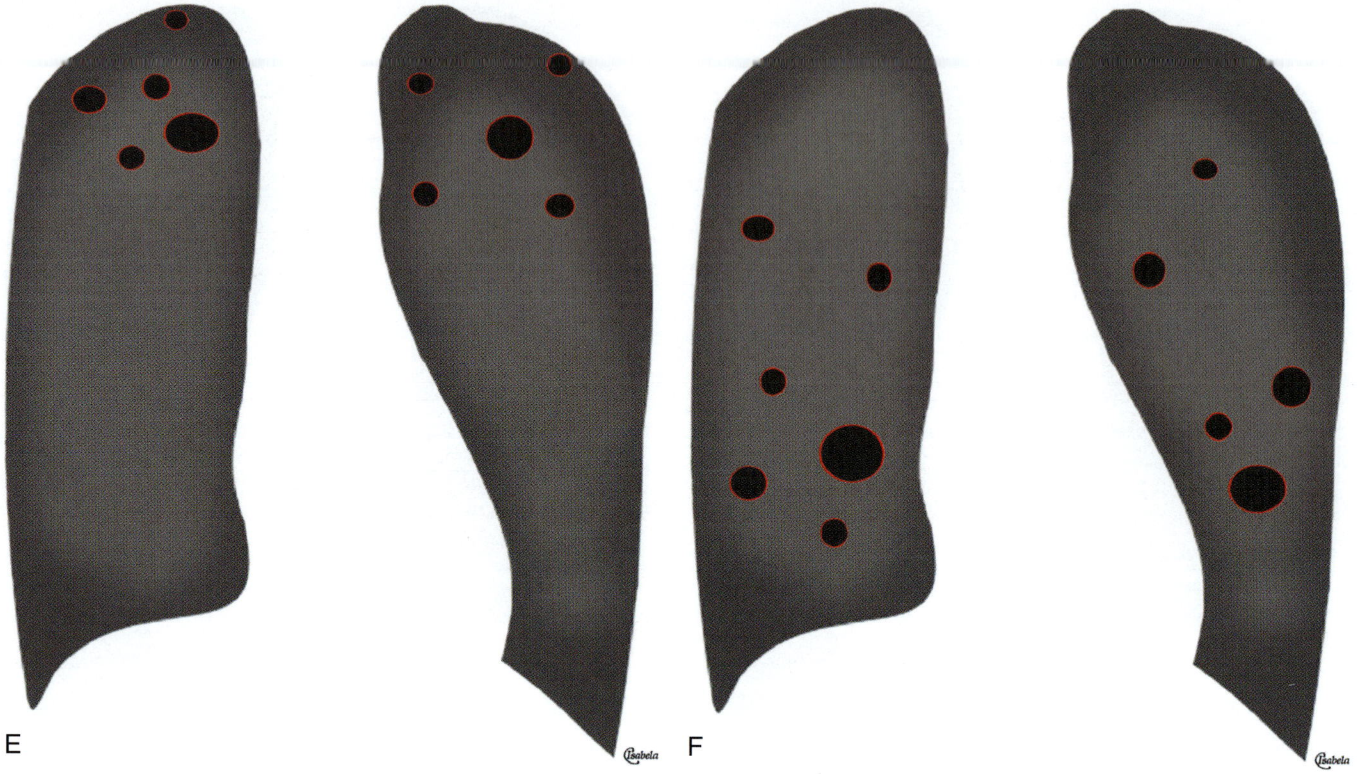

Fig. 5.28, cont'd (E) The cysts in *Pneumocystis* pneumonia typically are superimposed on ground-glass opacities and have upper lobe predominance. (F) The cysts in lymphocytic interstitial pneumonia and subacute hypersensitivity pneumonitis have a random distribution but usually occur in areas with ground-glass opacity and tend to involve mainly the middle and lower lung zones.

sign helpful in assessing the perilymphatic distribution is the presence of subpleural nodules in relation to the interlobar fissures (see Fig. 5.29). The various diseases associated with a perilymphatic distribution of nodules usually can be distinguished on high-resolution CT by the different patterns of involvement of the perilymphatic interstitium and the presence of associated findings.

The most common radiologic manifestation of sarcoidosis is symmetric bilateral hilar and mediastinal lymph node enlargement with or without associated parenchymal abnormalities. Parenchymal involvement typically results in a nodular or reticulonodular pattern involving mainly the upper and middle lung zones (Fig. 5.30).[17,22] On high-resolution CT nodules are seen at initial evaluation in 90% to 100% of patients who have parenchymal abnormalities.[45,65] The nodules are typically most numerous along the bronchoarterial and pleural interstitium and adjacent to the interlobar fissures (Fig. 5.31). This distribution of nodules is highly suggestive of sarcoidosis. Although nodular septal thickening is often evident on high-resolution CT, this seldom is the predominant finding.

In most patients with lymphangitic spread of tumor, the main finding is interlobular septal thickening (see Fig. 5.2). The septal thickening may be smooth or, less commonly, nodular. Peribronchovascular and subpleural nodules may be seen, but they are typically not as profuse as in patients with sarcoidosis.[66] Other common findings seen in patients with lymphatic spread of tumor are unilateral or asymmetric hilar lymph node enlargement and pleural effusion.

Silicosis and coal workers' pneumoconiosis are associated with the presence of small, well-defined nodules, usually measuring 2 to 5 mm in diameter, which are slightly larger than nodules typically seen in sarcoidosis. Similar to sarcoidosis, silicosis and coal workers' pneumoconiosis can be quite extensive but usually involve mainly the middle and upper long zones and frequently are associated with hilar and mediastinal lymph node enlargement. Calcification of lymph nodes and pulmonary nodules often occurs in silicosis but is much less common in coal workers' pneumoconiosis. Similar to sarcoidosis, nodules are frequently seen in the subpleural regions and along the interlobar fissures. However, the nodules in silicosis and coal workers' pneumoconiosis are predominantly centrilobular in distribution and typically are most numerous in the dorsal half of the upper lobes (Fig. 5.32).[18,19] Fine nodularity commonly seen in sarcoidosis is uncommon in silicosis and coal workers' pneumoconiosis. The diagnosis is readily made based on the radiographic or CT findings and exposure history.

CENTRILOBULAR NODULAR PATTERN

Centrilobular nodules are characterized on high-resolution CT by their location several millimeters away from the pleural surfaces, interlobar fissures, and interlobular septa. They reflect the presence of bronchiolocentric interstitial lung disease or bronchiolitis. Centrilobular nodules are typically seen in hypersensitivity pneumonitis,[39,44] various forms of bronchiolitis, including respiratory bronchiolitis,[67] respiratory bronchiolitis–interstitial lung disease (RB-ILD),[67] diffuse panbronchiolitis,[68]

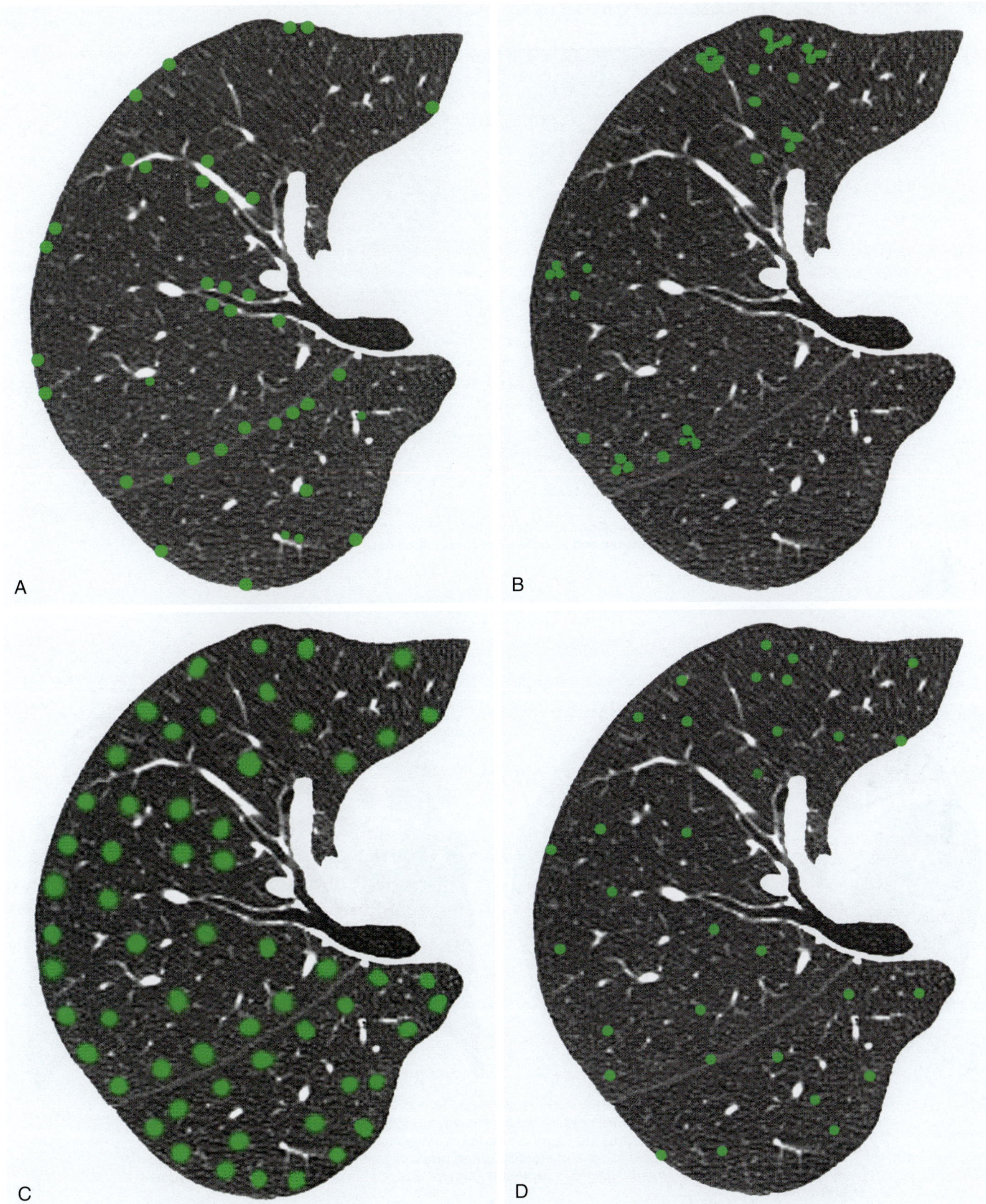

Fig. 5.29 Schematic drawing of nodular pattern and distribution. (A) Perilymphatic distribution is characterized by the presence of nodules along the bronchovascular interstitium, interlobular septa, and subpleural lung regions. (B) and (C) Centrilobular distribution is characterized by the presence of nodules a few millimeters away from the interlobular septa, visceral pleura, interlobar fissures, large vessels, and bronchi. Centrilobular nodules that are well defined with a tree-in-bud appearance and in a patchy distribution (B) are seen most commonly in infectious bronchiolitis. Poorly defined centrilobular nodular opacities (C) are seen most commonly in bronchiolocentric alveolitis as occurs in hypersensitivity pneumonitis and respiratory bronchiolitis. (D) Random distribution is characterized by nodules located throughout the secondary pulmonary lobule without any particular predominance. Some nodules may appear to be centrilobular, whereas others may appear to be perilymphatic.

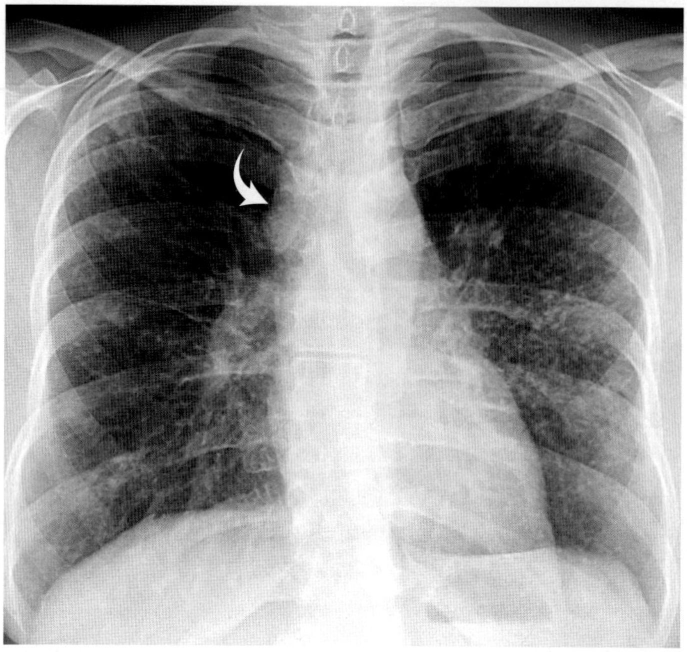

Fig. 5.30 Nodular pattern in sarcoidosis. Posteroanterior chest radiograph shows numerous bilateral nodules involving mainly the upper and middle lung zones. Also note right paratracheal lymph node enlargement *(arrow)*.

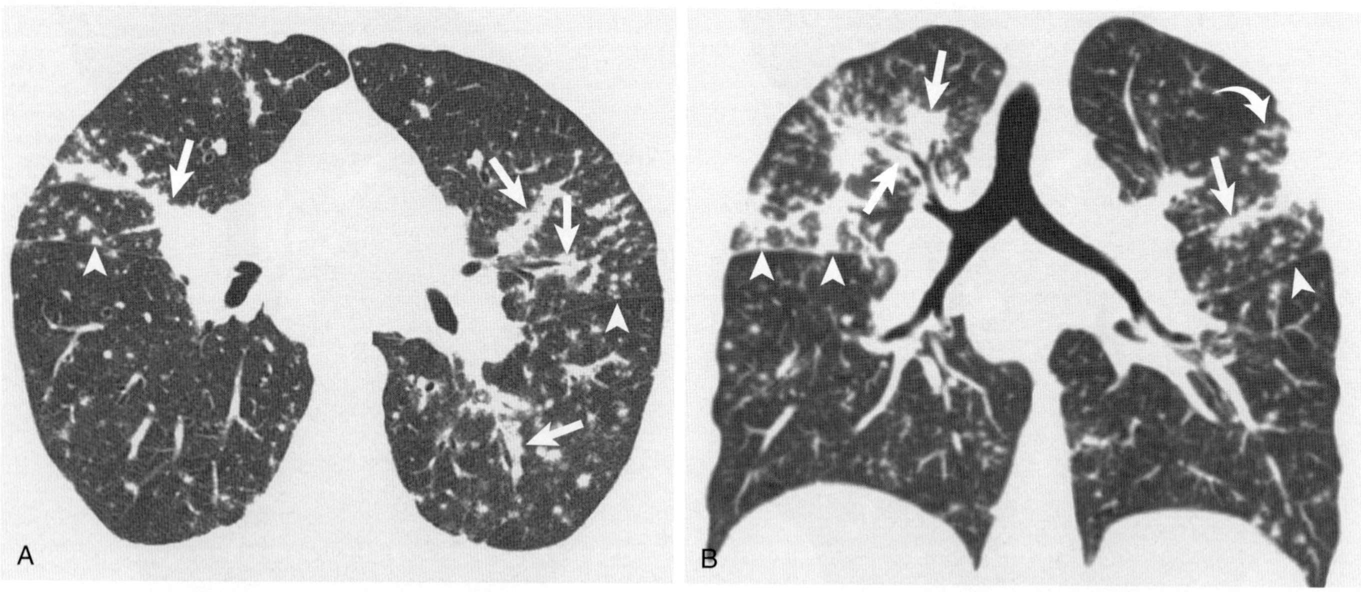

Fig. 5.31 Perilymphatic nodules in sarcoidosis. (A) High-resolution CT scan at the level of the middle lobe bronchus shows numerous small nodules located mainly along the bronchi *(arrows)*, vessels *(arrow)*, and interlobar fissures *(arrowheads)*. (B) Coronal maximum intensity projection image shows that the nodules involve mainly the upper lobes and are distributed predominantly along bronchi *(broad straight arrows)*, vessels *(narrow straight arrow)*, subpleural regions *(curved arrow)*, and interlobar fissures *(arrowheads)*.

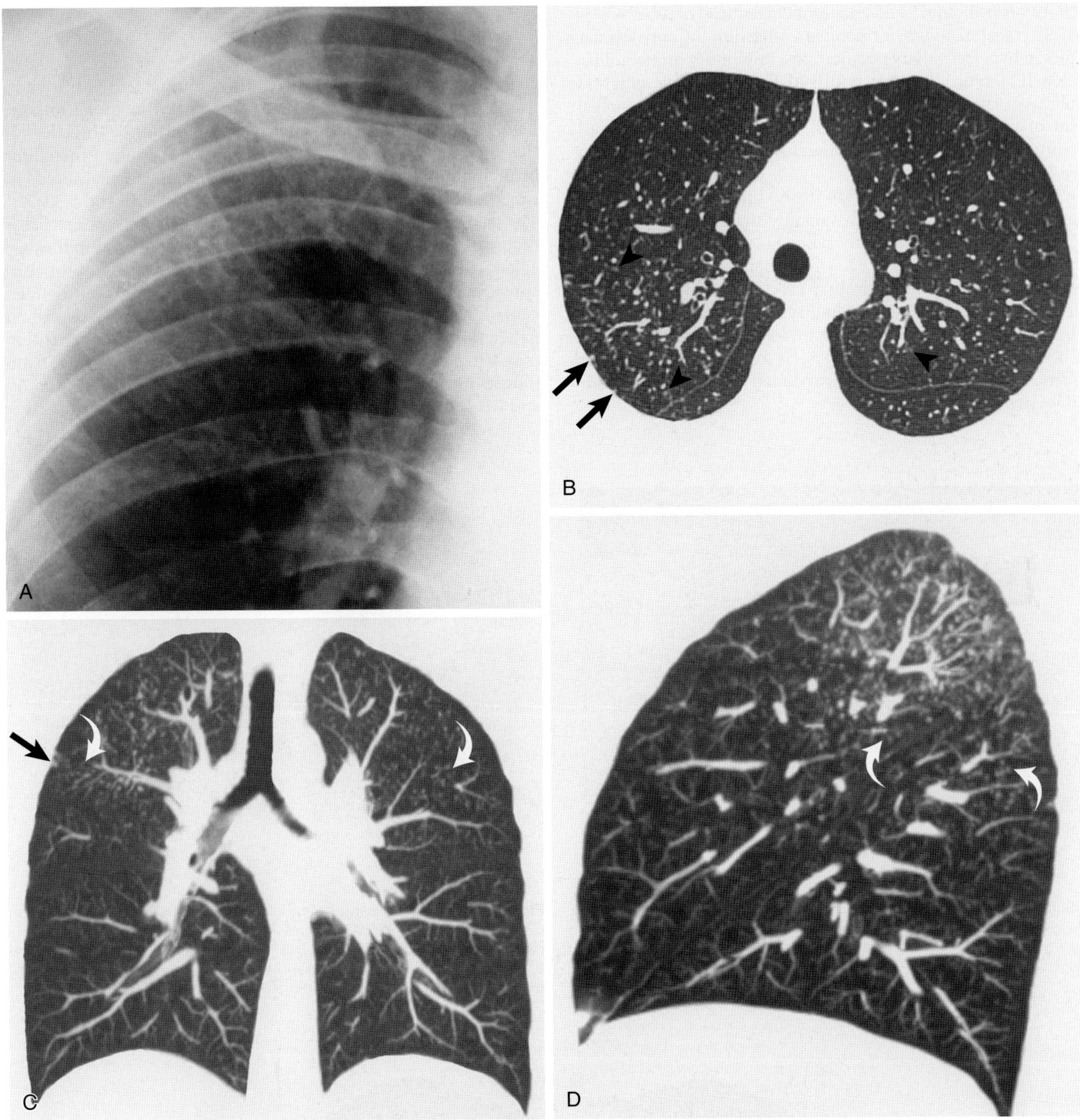

Fig. 5.32 Silicosis. (A) View of the right upper lobe from a posteroanterior chest radiograph shows small nodules. (B) High-resolution CT scan shows small well-defined nodules mainly in the dorsal half of the upper lobes. Some of the nodules can be seen to be in a subpleural *(straight arrows)* and centrilobular *(arrowheads)* distribution. (C) Coronal maximum intensity projection image better shows the nodules and their predominantly centrilobular *(curved arrows)* distribution. Also seen are a few subpleural nodules *(straight arrow)*. (D) Sagittal maximum intensity projection image shows the characteristic predominance of nodules in the dorsal lung regions and the predominant centrilobular distribution *(curved arrows)*. *(Case courtesy Dr. Ericson Bagatin, Department of Occupational Health, State University of Campinas [UNICAMP], Campinas, São Paulo, Brazil.)*

infectious bronchiolitis,[69] and endobronchial spread of tuberculosis or *Mycobacterium avium-intracellulare* infection.[70] Centrilobular nodules in hypersensitivity pneumonitis, respiratory bronchiolitis, and RB-ILD typically have poorly defined margins, whereas nodules associated with infectious bronchiolitis and endobronchial spread of tuberculosis usually have well-defined margins and are commonly associated with branching opacities resulting in a tree-in-bud appearance.

In hypersensitivity pneumonitis the nodules are usually diffuse throughout the lungs or involve mainly the middle and lower lung zones and are frequently associated with ground-glass opacities and lobular areas of decreased attenuation and vascularity with air trapping on expiratory CT (Figs. 5.33 and 5.34).[44] The centrilobular nodules in respiratory bronchiolitis and RB-ILD tend to involve predominantly or exclusively the upper lobes, and because these conditions are seen exclusively in cigarette smokers, they are frequently associated with centrilobular emphysema (Fig. 5.35).[67,71]

Tree-in-Bud Pattern

The tree-in-bud pattern usually reflects the presence of dilated centrilobular bronchioles, their lumina impacted with mucus, fluid, or pus, and often associated with peribronchiolar inflammation. It usually is associated with aspiration or infection of the small airways, the most common causes being infectious bronchiolitis, bronchopneumonia, and endobronchial spread of tuberculosis or *M. avium-intracellulare* (Figs. 5.36 and 5.37).[69,72] The tree-in-bud pattern also can be seen distal to bronchiectasis of any cause[72] and in allergic bronchopulmonary aspergillosis.[73] The various forms of infectious bronchiolitis and endobronchial spread of mycobacterial infection tend to result in well-defined centrilobular nodules and branching opacities (tree-in-bud pattern) in a focal or multifocal unilateral or bilateral distribution (see Fig. 5.37). They usually can be readily distinguished from diffuse interstitial processes, such as hypersensitivity pneumonitis, and RB-ILD that typically result in centrilobular nodular opacities

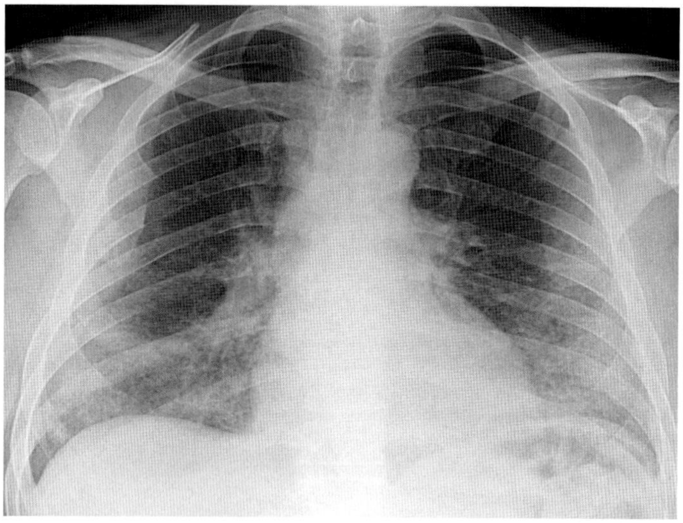

Fig. 5.33 Hypersensitivity pneumonitis. Chest radiograph shows hazy increased opacity (ground-glass opacity) in the middle and lower lung zones and poorly defined nodular opacities.

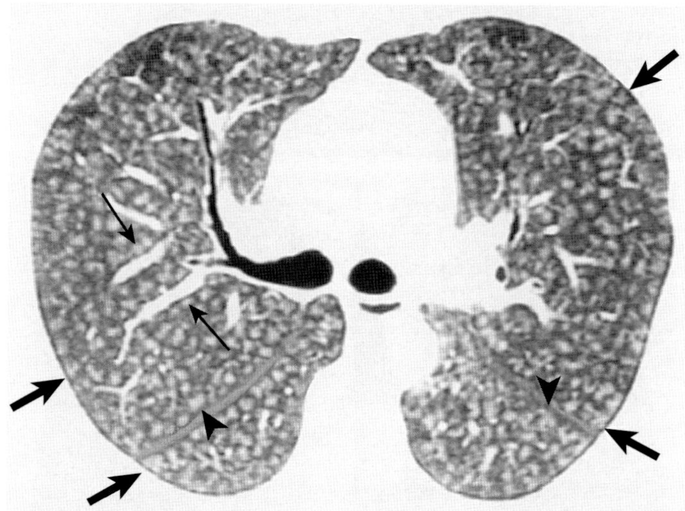

Fig. 5.34 Hypersensitivity pneumonitis in a bird breeder. High-resolution CT scan shows diffuse parenchymal abnormalities consisting of poorly defined centrilobular nodules. The centrilobular opacities typically are a few millimeters away from the pleura *(thick arrows)*, interlobular septa *(arrowheads)*, large vessels *(thin arrows)*, and bronchi.

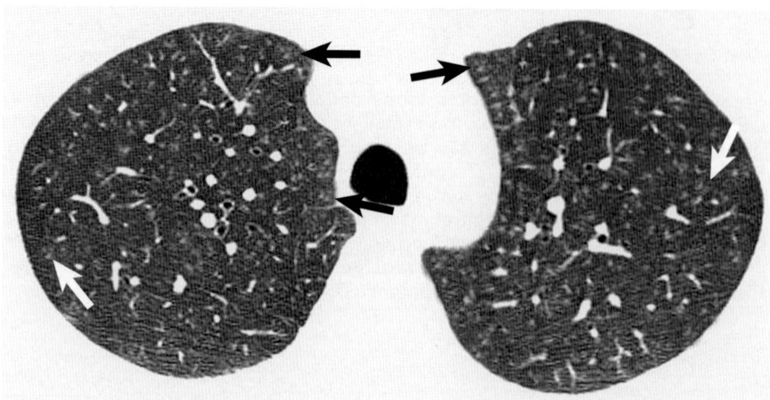

Fig. 5.35 Respiratory bronchiolitis. High-resolution CT scan shows poorly defined centrilobular nodules *(arrows)* in the upper lobes.

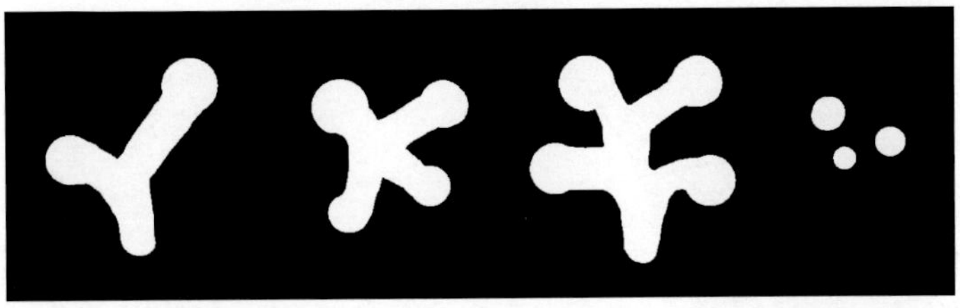

Fig. 5.36 Schematic drawing of tree-in-bud pattern. A tree-in-bud pattern is characterized by centrilobular branching linear and nodular opacities. It is most suggestive of infectious bronchiolitis or sequelae of aspiration.

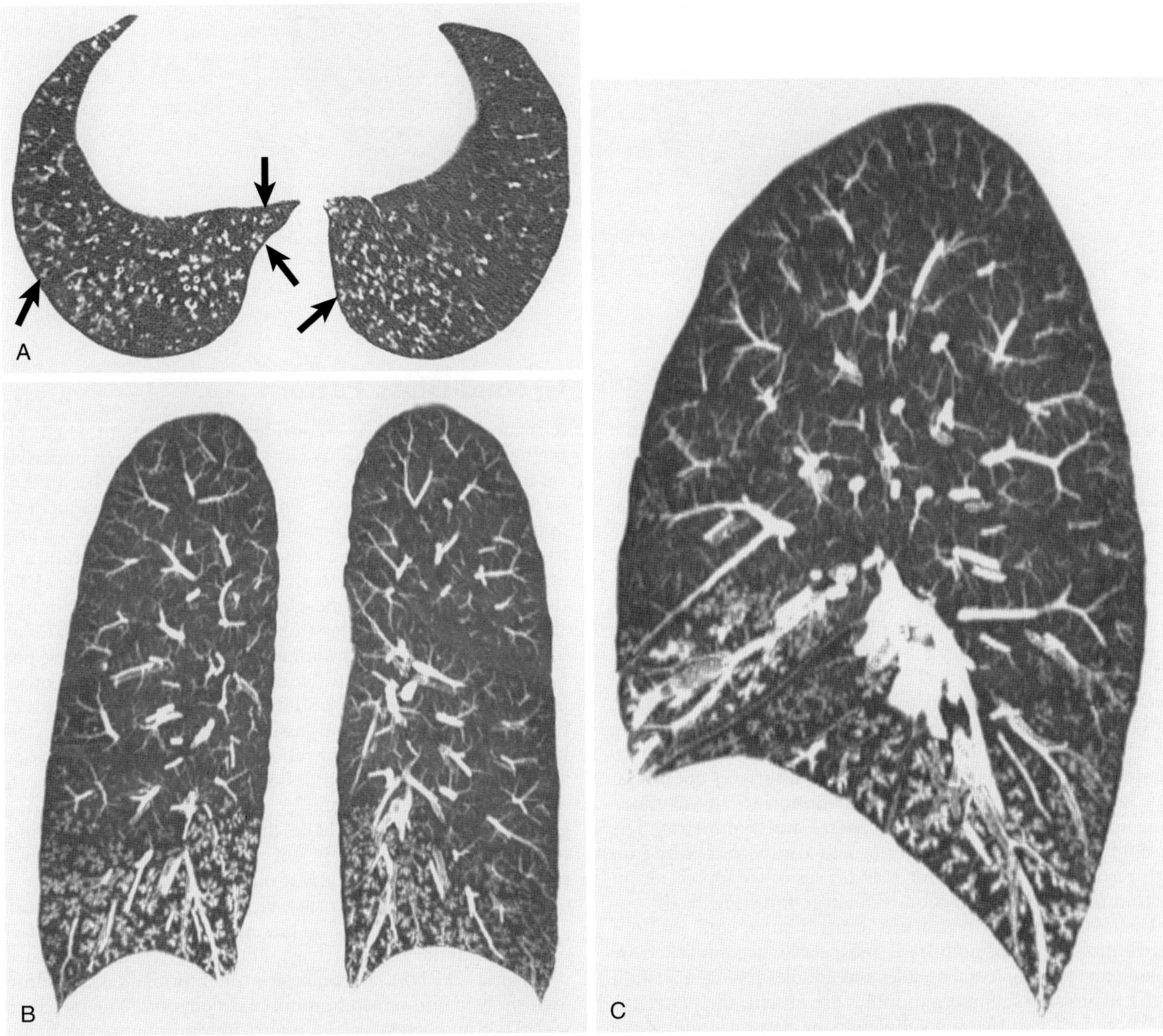

Fig. 5.37 Tree-in-bud pattern in infectious bronchiolitis. (A) High-resolution CT scan shows centrilobular branching nodular and linear opacities resulting in a tree-in-bud appearance *(arrows)*. (B) Coronal maximum intensity projection image shows tree-in-bud pattern in the lower lobes. (C) Sagittal maximum intensity projection image of the right lung shows extensive tree-in-bud pattern in the lower lobe and mild involvement of the middle and right upper lobes.

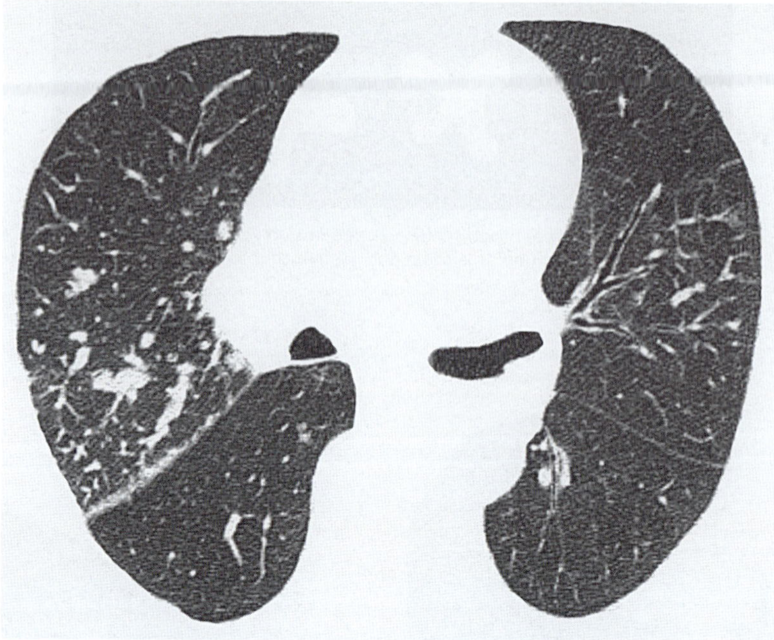

Fig. 5.38 Tree-in-bud pattern as a result of intravascular metastases from renal cell carcinoma. High-resolution CT scan shows centrilobular nodular and branching opacities (tree-in-bud pattern) in the periphery of the upper lobe. Also noted is nodular thickening of the pulmonary vessels.

that are poorly defined (i.e., ground-glass opacity), have a bilateral and symmetric distribution, and are seldom associated with a tree-in-bud pattern. Occasionally, centrilobular nodules and a tree-in-bud pattern may result from abnormalities related to the centrilobular pulmonary arteries, such as may occur in intravascular metastases (Fig. 5.38) or after injection of crushed oral tablets.[74]

RANDOM DISTRIBUTION

Small nodules in a random distribution in relation to structures of the lung and secondary lobule are seen most commonly in miliary tuberculosis (Fig. 5.39),[75] miliary fungal infections,[76] and metastases.[77] Hematogenous miliary infections and metastases tend to be most numerous in the lung periphery and at the lung bases. Randomly distributed nodules can be seen in relation to interlobular septa, small vessels, and pleural surfaces but do not have consistent or predominant distribution to any of these. Lung involvement tends to be bilateral and symmetric. The random distribution of nodules usually can be recognized on high-resolution CT scans but may be easier to appreciate on maximum intensity projection reconstructions (Fig. 5. 40).

Distinction of perilymphatic, centrilobular, and random distribution of small nodules is most easily accomplished by looking first for subpleural nodules and nodules arising in relation to the fissures. If subpleural nodules are absent, the pattern is centrilobular. If numerous subpleural or fissural nodules are present, the pattern is either perilymphatic or random. These two patterns are distinguished by looking at the distribution of other nodules. If they are patchy in distribution, and particularly if a distinct predominance is noted relative to the peribronchovascular interstitium, interlobular septa, or subpleural regions, the nodules are perilymphatic. If the nodules are distributed in a diffuse and uniform manner, the pattern is random.

Ground-Glass Pattern

A ground-glass pattern is considered to be present when there is a hazy increase in opacity without obscuration of underlying vascular markings (Fig. 5.41).[25] If the vessels are obscured, the term *consolidation* is used.[78] The abnormality is a frequent and important finding on high-resolution CT scan but often is difficult to recognize on the chest radiograph. On high-resolution CT ground-glass opacity reflects the presence of abnormalities below the resolution limit. Ground-glass opacities may be seen in many situations, including interstitial disease, airspace disease, and increased capillary blood volume resulting from congestive heart failure or blood flow redistribution. Although ground-glass opacity is a relatively nonspecific finding, the differential diagnosis can be narrowed considerably by assessing the presence of associated findings, such as nodules or reticulation. In patients with associated findings, such as nodules or reticulation, considering the distribution of these findings, rather than the presence of ground-glass opacities, facilitates the differential diagnosis. Clinical information is essential in the assessment of patients with predominantly or exclusively ground-glass opacities.[79]

Acute lung diseases characteristically associated with a ground-glass pattern include atypical pneumonia (e.g., *Pneumocystis* or viral), pulmonary hemorrhage, and acute respiratory distress syndrome (ARDS). *Pneumocystis* pneumonia occurs almost exclusively in immunocompromised patients, particularly patients with AIDS and patients on long-term immunosuppressive therapy (Fig. 5.42).[80] The earliest radiographic manifestations consist of a granular or hazy opacity (ground-glass pattern) typically involving mainly the perihilar areas.[81,82] As the disease progresses, the hazy ground-glass opacities progress to consolidation, and the pulmonary involvement becomes diffuse. The characteristic high-resolution CT finding in *Pneumocystis* pneumonia consists of bilateral ground-glass opacities, which may be diffuse or have

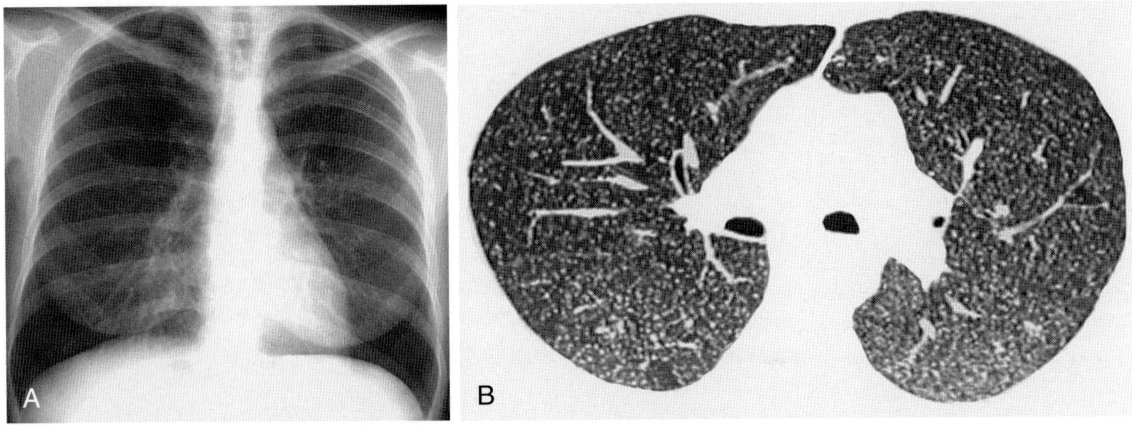

Fig. 5.39 Miliary tuberculosis. (A) Chest radiograph shows numerous 1- to 2-mm diameter nodules throughout both lungs (miliary pattern). (B) High-resolution CT scan shows random distribution of numerous nodules.

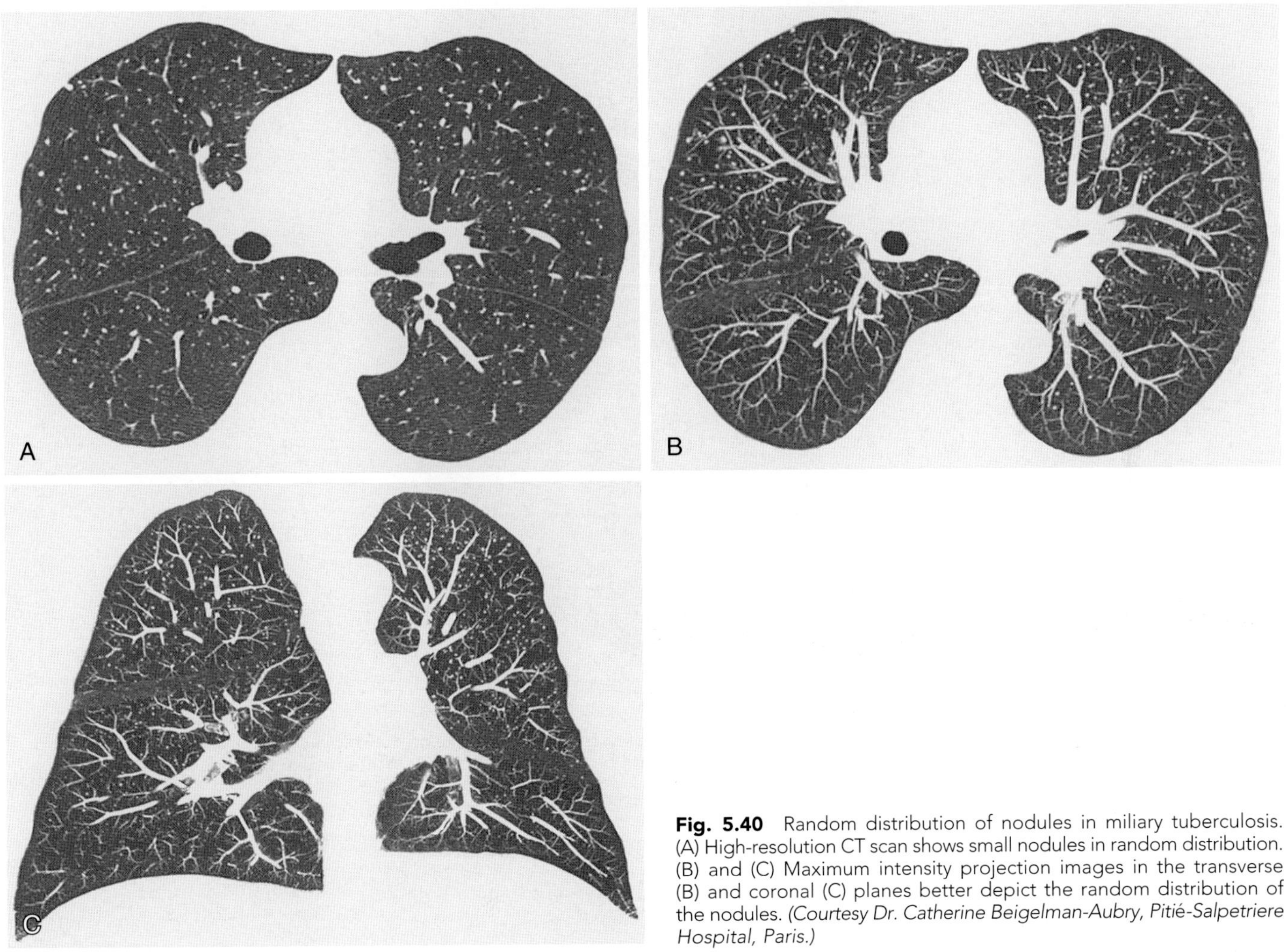

Fig. 5.40 Random distribution of nodules in miliary tuberculosis. (A) High-resolution CT scan shows small nodules in random distribution. (B) and (C) Maximum intensity projection images in the transverse (B) and coronal (C) planes better depict the random distribution of the nodules. *(Courtesy Dr. Catherine Beigelman-Aubry, Pitié-Salpetriere Hospital, Paris.)*

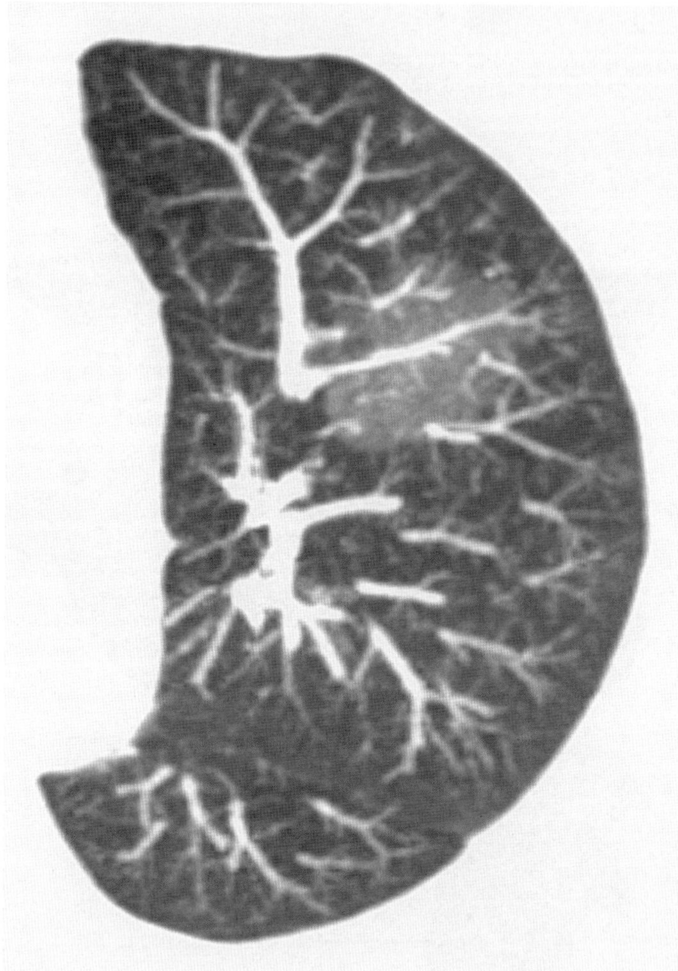

Fig. 5.41 Ground-glass opacity. Maximum intensity projection image of the left lung illustrates characteristic appearance of ground-glass opacity with homogeneous increase in attenuation that does not result in obscuration of underlying vessels.

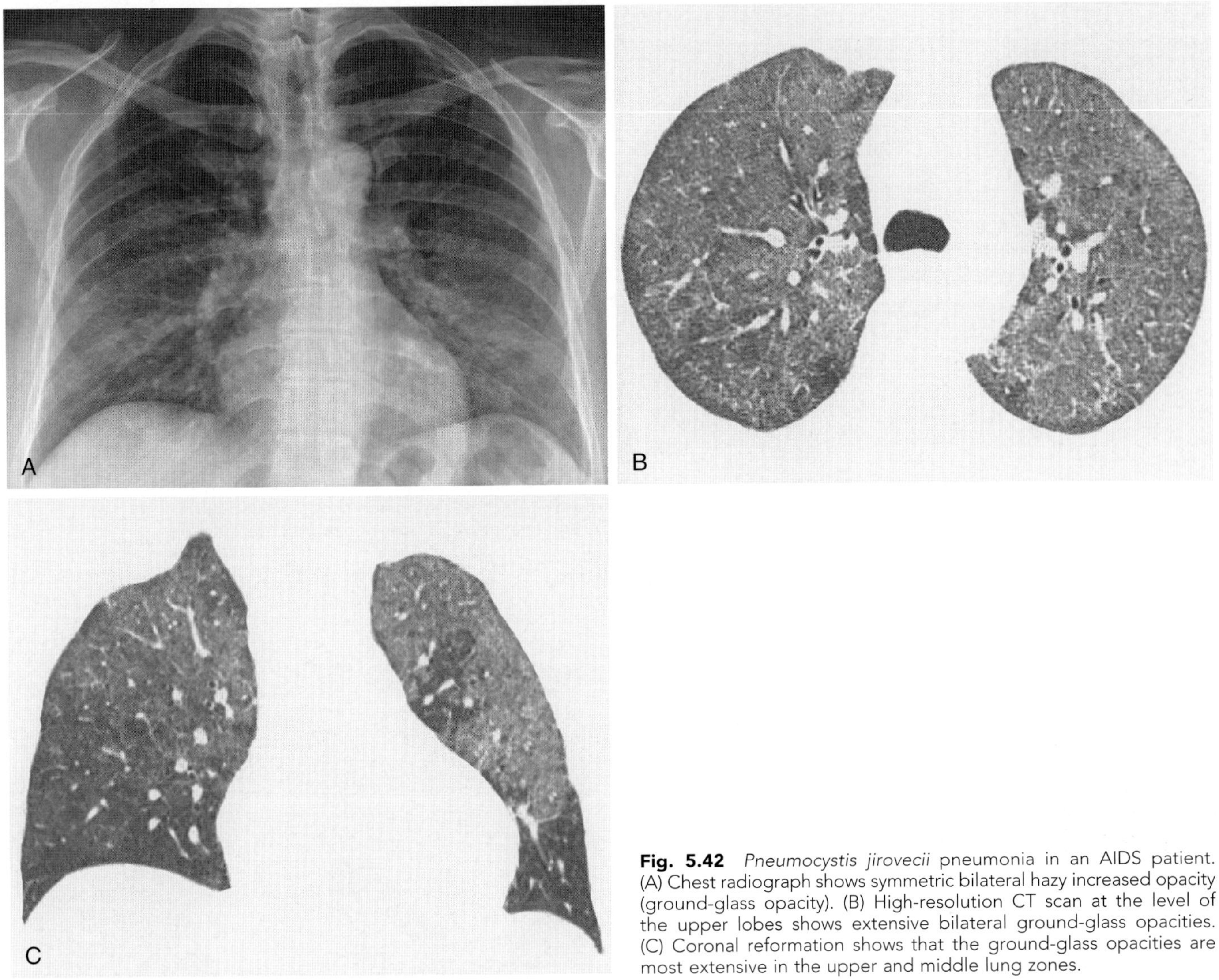

Fig. 5.42 *Pneumocystis jirovecii* pneumonia in an AIDS patient. (A) Chest radiograph shows symmetric bilateral hazy increased opacity (ground-glass opacity). (B) High-resolution CT scan at the level of the upper lobes shows extensive bilateral ground-glass opacities. (C) Coronal reformation shows that the ground-glass opacities are most extensive in the upper and middle lung zones.

a distinct mosaic pattern with areas of normal lung intervening between the ground-glass opacities (see Fig. 5.42).[58] With time, the areas of ground-glass opacity progress to consolidation. Common ancillary findings include cyst formation, seen in approximately 30% of patients, and reticulation.[58] Pleural effusions and lymphadenopathy are generally absent.

The radiographic manifestations of diffuse pulmonary hemorrhage consist of patchy ground-glass opacities or areas of consolidation scattered fairly evenly throughout the lungs (Fig. 5.43). The opacities may be diffuse or more prominent in the perihilar regions and the middle and lower lung zones.[83] The apices and costophrenic angles are almost invariably spared.[83] The high-resolution CT manifestations consist of areas of ground-glass opacity or, less commonly, consolidation; they may be patchy or diffuse but tend to involve mainly the dependent lung regions (see Fig. 5.43).[83,84]

The earliest radiographic manifestations of ARDS consist of bilateral poorly defined hazy (ground-glass) opacities and patchy areas of consolidation.[85,86] The characteristic high-resolution CT findings consist of symmetric bilateral ground-glass opacities and gravity-dependent consolidation.[85,87] On high-resolution CT the lung involvement is typically heterogeneous, with up to one-third of the lung appearing to be normally aerated.[85,88]

The differential diagnosis in patients with chronic respiratory symptoms and exclusively ground-glass opacities includes hypersensitivity pneumonitis, nonspecific interstitial pneumonia, desquamative interstitial pneumonia, RB-ILD, and lymphoid interstitial pneumonia. Hypersensitivity pneumonitis is probably the most common cause of diffuse ground-glass opacities in normal hosts.[79] The areas of ground-glass opacity in hypersensitivity pneumonitis may be diffuse but frequently involve mainly the middle and lower lung zones.[44,89] Localized areas of decreased attenuation and perfusion are often present in conjunction with areas of ground-glass attenuation (Fig. 5.44). The areas of low attenuation in hypersensitivity pneumonitis often have a lobular distribution and show air trapping on CT scans performed at end expiration.[90] Ground-glass opacities also may be seen in conjunction with centrilobular nodules.[44,89] The centrilobular nodules are typically poorly defined, measure less than 5 mm in diameter, and are most numerous in the middle and lower lung zones. Approximately 13% of patients with subacute hypersensitivity pneumonitis have thin-walled lung cysts ranging

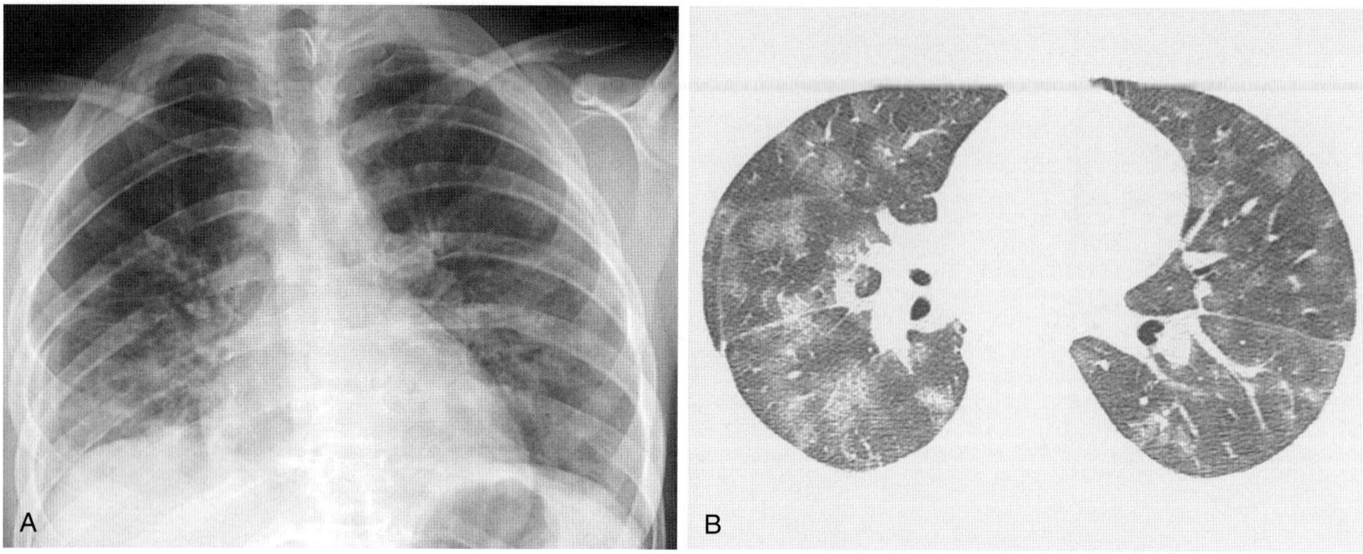

Fig. 5.43 Diffuse pulmonary hemorrhage from vasculitis. (A) Chest radiograph shows ground-glass opacities involving mainly the lower lung zones. (B) High-resolution CT scan shows patchy bilateral ground-glass opacities.

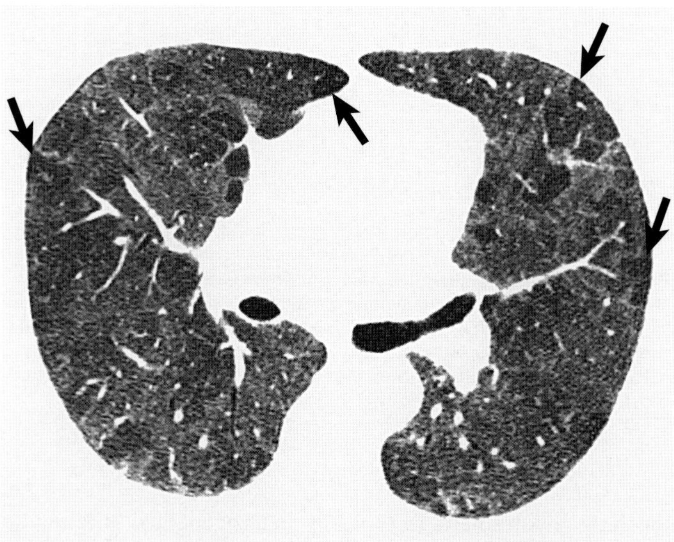

Fig. 5.44 Hypersensitivity pneumonitis. High-resolution CT scan shows extensive bilateral ground-glass opacities, a few centrilobular nodules, and lobular areas of decreased attenuation and vascularity *(arrows).*

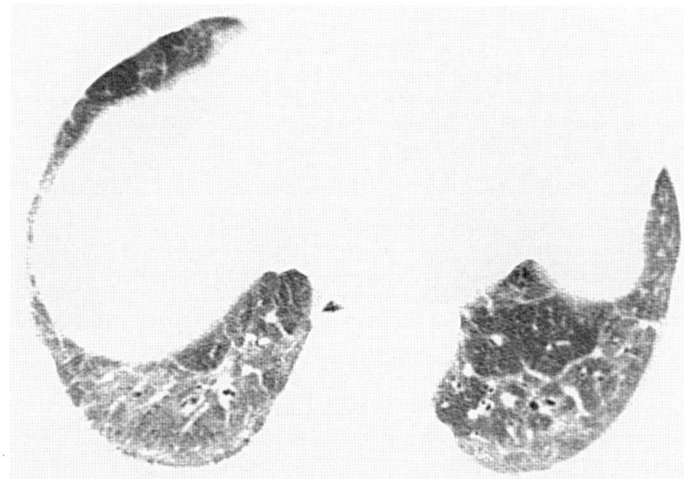

Fig. 5.45 Nonspecific interstitial pneumonia. High-resolution CT scan at the level of the lung bases shows extensive bilateral ground-glass opacities.

from 3 to 25 mm in maximal diameter and 1 to 15 in number in a random distribution.[59]

The most common high-resolution CT manifestation of nonspecific interstitial pneumonia consists of bilateral symmetric ground-glass opacities.[36,37] Most patients have a fine reticular pattern superimposed on the ground-glass opacities, traction bronchiectasis, and architectural distortion.[36,37] The abnormalities in nonspecific interstitial pneumonia tend to involve mainly the lower lung zones; a peripheral predominance is seen in 50% to 70% of patients (Fig. 5.45).[36,37]

Patients who have RB-ILD are typically current smokers with more than 30 pack-years of cigarette smoking.[91] The chest radiograph is often normal or shows nonspecific findings related to chronic obstructive pulmonary disease. The high-resolution CT manifestations of RB-ILD typically consist of ground-glass opacities and poorly defined centrilobular nodules.[67,92] The abnormalities can be diffuse or involve mainly the upper lung zones. Most patients have associated centrilobular emphysema.

Desquamative interstitial pneumonia is an uncommon condition, characterized histologically by the presence of numerous macrophages filling the alveolar airspaces, mild inflammation of the alveolar walls, and mild fibrosis.[91] Approximately 90% of patients who have desquamative interstitial pneumonia are current cigarette smokers.[93] The most common radiographic and high-resolution CT finding consists of symmetric bilateral ground-glass opacities.[93,94] The ground-glass opacities may be patchy or diffuse but in approximately 60% involve mainly the lower lung zones.[94] A fine reticular pattern in a predominantly subpleural and basal distribution is seen in 60% to 80% of patients.[94,95]

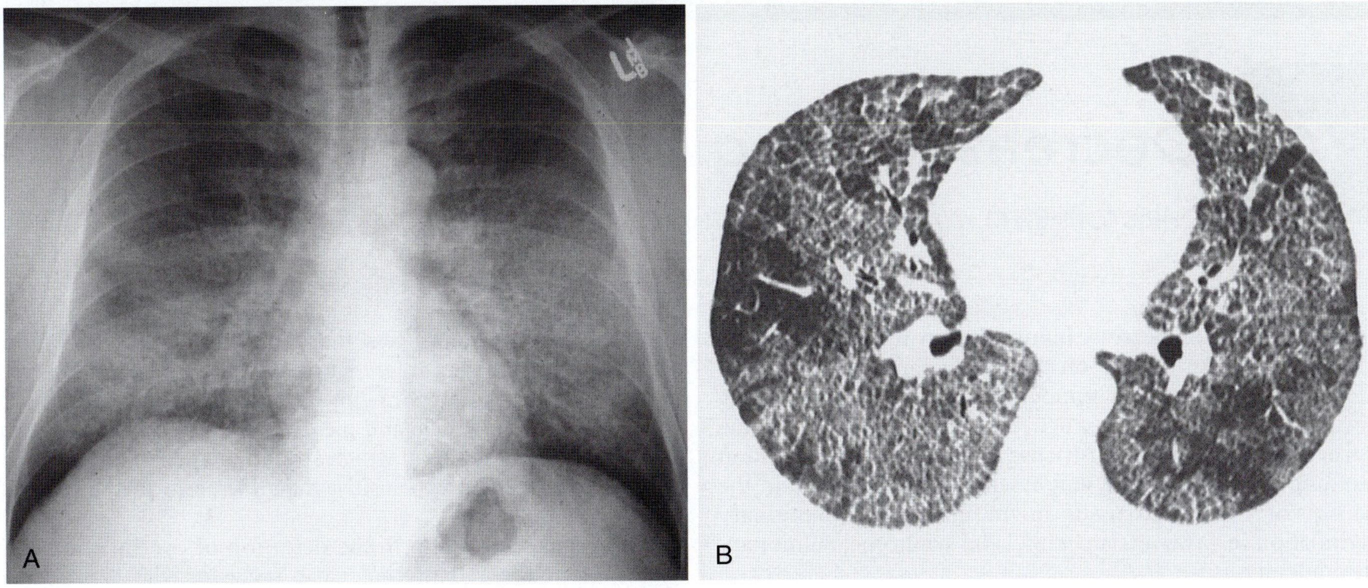

Fig. 5.46 "Crazy paving" pattern in alveolar proteinosis. (A) Chest radiograph shows extensive bilateral ground-glass opacities and areas of consolidation with relative sparing of the lung apices and bases. (B) High-resolution CT scan shows bilateral ground-glass opacities with superimposed smooth septal lines and intralobular lines resulting in a pattern known as "crazy paving."

"CRAZY PAVING" PATTERN

The "crazy paving" pattern consists of patchy or diffuse ground-glass opacities with superimposed interlobular septal thickening and intralobular lines.[96,97] This pattern was first described in patients with pulmonary alveolar proteinosis (Fig. 5.46)[97] and is typical of pulmonary alveolar proteinosis but also may be seen in patients with a variety of other diseases, including ARDS,[96] acute interstitial pneumonia,[96] pulmonary edema,[6] pulmonary hemorrhage,[83] bacterial pneumonia,[96] *Pneumocystis* pneumonia,[98] acute eosinophilic pneumonia,[99] eosinophilic granulomatosis with polyangiitis (Churg-Strauss syndrome),[100] radiation pneumonitis,[101] mucinous adenocarcinoma,[102] and lipoid pneumonia.[103] The differential diagnosis is broad and similar to the differential diagnosis of ground-glass opacities is based largely on the presence and distribution of associated findings, such as consolidation and knowledge of whether symptoms are acute or chronic. In the chronic setting this pattern remains highly suggestive of pulmonary alveolar proteinosis, especially if bilaterally diffuse rather than basilar or posterior preponderant, which increases the likelihood of lipoid pneumonia.

Limitations of the Pattern Approach

The pattern of parenchymal abnormality seen on the chest radiograph and high-resolution CT scan may be modified by associated underlying parenchymal lung disease, particularly emphysema, and by the secondary effects sometimes produced by the diffuse interstitial disease itself. On the radiograph, airspace consolidation superimposed on emphysema may simulate interstitial lung disease, whereas conglomerate interstitial fibrosis may simulate airspace disease.

SUGGESTED READINGS

Boitsios G, Bankier AA, Eisenberg RL. Diffuse pulmonary nodules. *AJR Am J Roentgenol*. 2010;194:W354–W366.

Chong S, Lee KS, Chung MJ, et al. Pneumoconiosis: comparison of imaging and pathologic findings. *Radiographics*. 2006;26:59–77.

Hobbs S, Lynch D. The idiopathic interstitial pneumonias: an update and review. *Radiol Clin North Am*. 2014;52:105–120.

Miller WT Jr. Chest radiographic evaluation of diffuse infiltrative lung disease: review of a dying art. *Eur J Radiol*. 2002;44:182–197.

Miller WT Jr, Shah RM. Isolated diffuse ground-glass opacity in thoracic CT: causes and clinical presentations. *AJR Am J Roentgenol*. 2005;184:613–622.

Raoof S, Bondalapati P, Vydyula R, Ryu JH, Gupta N, Raoof S, Galvin J, Rosen MJ, Lynch D, Travis W, Mehta S, Lazzaro R, Naidich D. Cystic lung diseases: algorithmic approach. *Chest*. 2016;150(4):945–965.

Webb WR. Thin-section CT of the secondary pulmonary lobule: anatomy and the image—the 2004 Fleischner lecture. *Radiology*. 2006;239:322–338.

The full reference list for this chapter is available at ExpertConsult.com.

6 Decreased Lung Density*

CHRISTOPHER M. WALKER | JONATHAN H. CHUNG

Diseases that cause a decrease in lung density result in increased radiolucency (hyperlucency) on chest radiography and decreased attenuation on computed tomography (CT). Decreased lung density may result from obstructive overinflation without lung destruction (e.g., asthma, constrictive bronchiolitis), overinflation with lung destruction (e.g., emphysema), or a reduction in the quantity of blood and tissue in the absence of pulmonary overinflation (e.g., Swyer-James-McLeod syndrome, pulmonary thromboembolism).

It is important to keep in mind that unilateral hyperlucency on a chest radiograph may also result from pneumothorax, patient rotation, and congenital and acquired abnormalities of the chest wall (e.g., congenital absence of the pectoral muscles and mastectomy). In fact, patient rotation and chest wall abnormalities, in particular, mastectomy, are the most common causes of unilateral hyperlucent lung on chest radiography (Fig. 6.1). Patient rotation is observed in up to 1% of all chest radiographs and may cause an apparent unilateral hyperlucent lung. The hyperlucency always occurs on the side to which the patient rotates and is secondary to asymmetric absorption of the x-ray beam by the chest wall.[1]

Alteration in Pulmonary Volume

GENERAL EXCESS OF AIR

Lung diseases that cause decreased density are characterized by overinflation, with the exception of proximal interruption (absence) of the pulmonary artery, unilateral hyperlucent lung (Swyer-James-McLeod syndrome), partly obstructing endobronchial lesions, and pulmonary thromboembolism without infarction.

Radiologic signs that may be observed in association with a general increase in intrapulmonary air relate to the diaphragm, the retrosternal space, and the cardiovascular silhouette, the most important of which are signs related to the diaphragm. In patients who have severe emphysema, the diaphragm is depressed, often to the level of the 7th rib anteriorly and the 11th interspace or 12th rib posteriorly; the normal dome configuration is flattened, and there may be blunting of the posterior costophrenic angle as seen on the lateral chest radiograph (Fig. 6.2). Although such flattening is often evaluated subjectively, direct measurement is more accurate. Flattening of the diaphragm is best assessed on a lateral chest radiograph by drawing a straight line from the sternophrenic junction to the posterior costophrenic junction. The dome of the hemidiaphragm should be 2.6 cm or more above this line; values less than this indicate overinflation.[2] Flattening of the diaphragm can also be assessed on a posteroanterior radiograph by drawing a line from the costophrenic to the costovertebral angle and measuring the height of the dome of each hemidiaphragm, which should be greater than 1.5 cm; this measurement is less sensitive than that performed on a lateral radiograph.[2,3]

Another helpful sign in the detection of overinflation is an increase in the retrosternal clear space on the lateral chest radiograph. Direct measurement is preferred to subjective assessment; a distance greater than 2.5 cm between the posterior sternum and the most anterior margin of the ascending aorta is indicative of overinflation.[4,5]

The most common cause of generalized overinflation of both lungs is emphysema. Less common causes include asthma, constrictive bronchiolitis, pulmonary Langerhans cell histiocytosis, and lymphangioleiomyomatosis.

Radiographic manifestations of emphysema include irregular areas of radiolucency, local avascular areas, distortion of vessels, bullae, and hyperinflation (see Fig. 6.2).[6] The parenchymal abnormalities can be subtle and difficult to detect on radiographs but are usually readily seen on CT, particularly high-resolution CT. On CT emphysema is characterized by the presence of areas of abnormally low attenuation. The areas of low attenuation generally have no visible walls; occasionally, however, walls 1 mm or less are seen, particularly in patients with paraseptal emphysema and bulla formation (Fig. 6.3).[6] On CT vessels can frequently be seen centered within the areas of low attenuation termed the *centrilobular dot sign*.[7]

The most common radiographic abnormalities of asthma are bronchial wall thickening and hyperinflation. Hyperinflation in asthma is more common in children than in adults. High-resolution CT may demonstrate bronchial wall thickening, endobronchial mucous plugging, and areas of decreased attenuation and vascularity (mosaic attenuation); expiratory CT commonly shows multifocal air trapping (Fig. 6.4).[8]

The radiographic manifestations of severe constrictive bronchiolitis (synonym: obliterative bronchiolitis and bronchiolitis obliterans) consist of hyperinflation and a decrease in peripheral vascular markings. In the majority of cases, however, constrictive bronchiolitis results in no definite abnormality on the chest radiograph. Inspiratory and expiratory high-resolution CT scans are the best imaging techniques for the assessment of patients with clinical and functional features suggestive of constrictive bronchiolitis.[9–11] The CT findings consist of areas of decreased attenuation and vascularity on inspiratory CT scans and air trapping on expiratory scans (Fig. 6.5).[10,11] Redistribution of blood flow to uninvolved lung results in a heterogeneous pattern of attenuation and vascularity (mosaic attenuation). Common associated findings include bronchial dilation and bronchial wall thickening.

*The editors and the publisher would like to thank Drs. Nestor L. Müller and C. Isabela Silva Müller for contributing material on this topic to the prior edition of this work. It has served as the foundation for the current chapter.

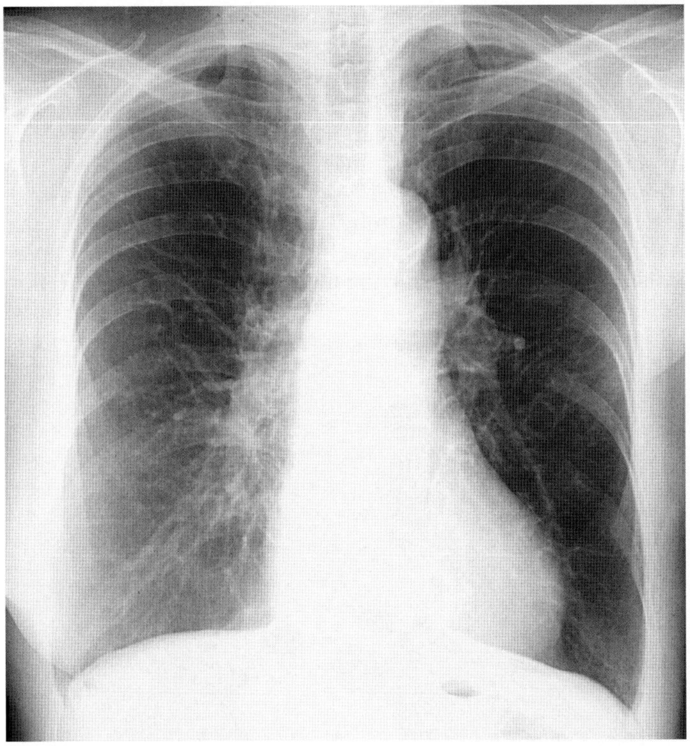

Fig. 6.1 Unilateral hyperlucency secondary to left mastectomy. Posteroanterior chest radiograph shows increased lucency of the left hemithorax.

LOCAL EXCESS OF AIR

Isolated overinflation of a lobe or segment or of one or more lobes occurs in two different sets of circumstances: with and without air trapping. Distinction between the two is of major diagnostic importance.

Overinflation *with air trapping* results from obstruction of the egress of air from affected lung parenchyma. It is seen most commonly in bronchial atresia or congenital lobar overinflation or distal to an endobronchial foreign body as a result of check-valve obstruction in children. Obstructive hyperinflation distal to an endobronchial foreign body or tumor is rarely seen in adults. In a review of the radiographic patterns of 600 cases of bronchogenic carcinoma, overinflation distal to a partly obstructing endobronchial lesion was not seen in any case.[12,13] The volume of lung behind a partly obstructing endobronchial lesion in adults is almost invariably reduced at total lung capacity. Despite this smaller volume, the density of affected parenchyma is typically less than that of the opposite lung as a result of decreased perfusion (oligemia) secondary to hypoventilation-mediated hypoxic vasoconstriction. The overall effect is an increase in radiolucency despite the reduction in volume.

Congenital bronchial atresia is a rare anomaly that results from congenital focal obliteration of a proximal segmental or subsegmental bronchus with the normal development of distal structures. It usually involves a segmental bronchus, most commonly the apicoposterior segmental bronchus of the left upper lobe. The characteristic radiologic manifestations consist of an area of pulmonary hyperlucency and a perihilar opacity (Fig. 6.6).[14,15] The hyperlucency results from oligemia and an increase in the volume of air within the affected segment because of collateral air drift via interalveolar, bronchioloalveolar, and

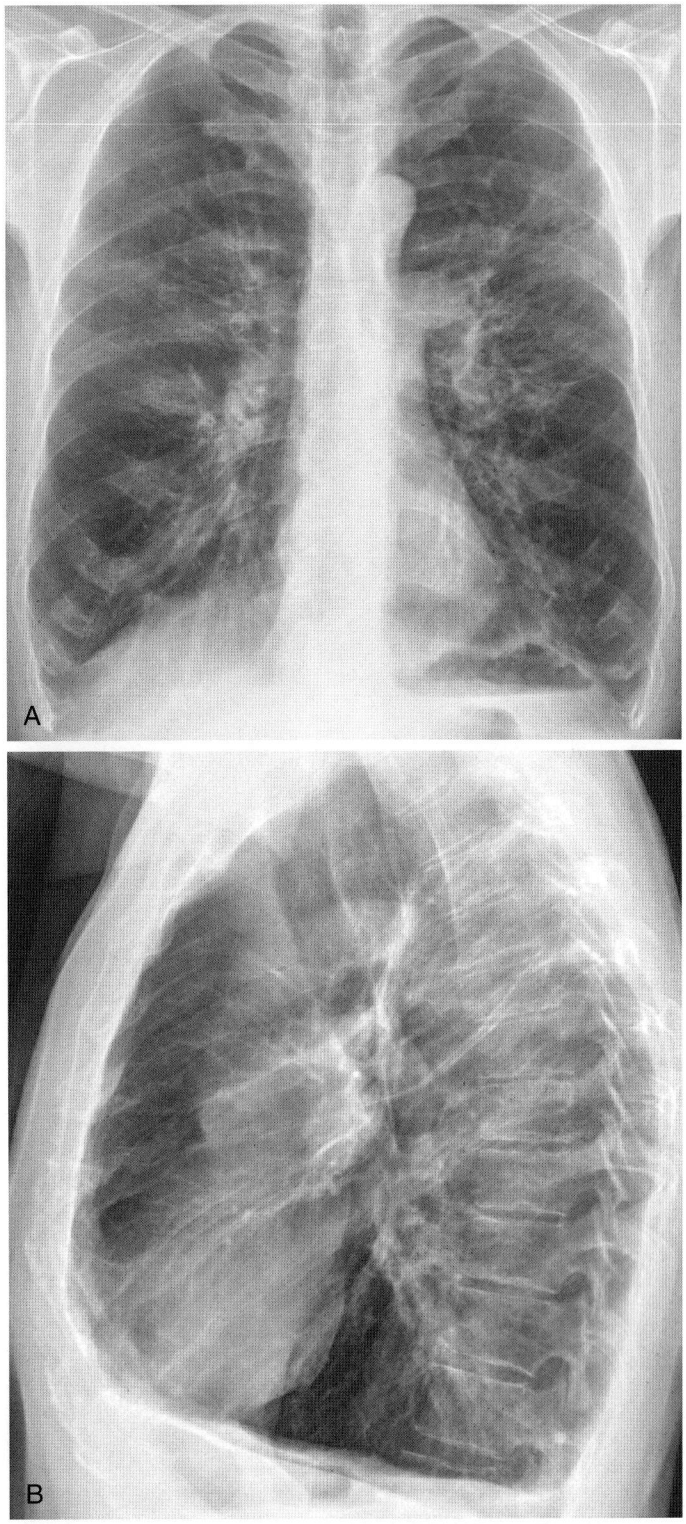

Fig. 6.2 Hyperinflation from panlobular emphysema associated with α1-antitrypsin deficiency. (A) Posteroanterior chest radiograph shows that the dome of the right hemidiaphragm is below the level of the anterior right seventh rib, consistent with increased lung volumes. Note a decrease in peripheral vascular markings. (B) Lateral view demonstrates increased retrosternal clear space (>2.5-cm distance between the posterior sternum and the most anterior margin of the ascending aorta) and flattening of the hemidiaphragms.

interbronchiolar connections (pores of Kohn, canals of Lambert, and channels of Martin, respectively). The perihilar opacity may be round, oval, or branching and is due to the accumulation of secretions and mucoid impaction distal to the bronchial atresia. The abnormalities can be recognized on a chest radiograph but are more clearly defined by CT. CT demonstrates bronchial dilation immediately distal to the atresia; mucoid impaction within the ectatic bronchus (bronchocele); occlusion of the bronchus central to the bronchocele; and overinflation, decreased attenuation, and decreased vascularity distal to the bronchial atresia.[14,15] Mucoid impaction typically has very high signal intensity on T2-weighted MR images.[14] Fiberoptic bronchoscopy may be required to exclude acquired proximal bronchial obstruction by tumor, a foreign body, or an inflammatory stricture.

Congenital lobar overinflation (synonym: congenital lobar hyperinflation), formerly congenital lobar emphysema, is a condition characterized by progressive overdistention of a lobe. It is believed to result from bronchial obstruction or a check-valve mechanism at the bronchial level that causes progressive hyperinflation of the lobe by allowing more air to enter on inspiration

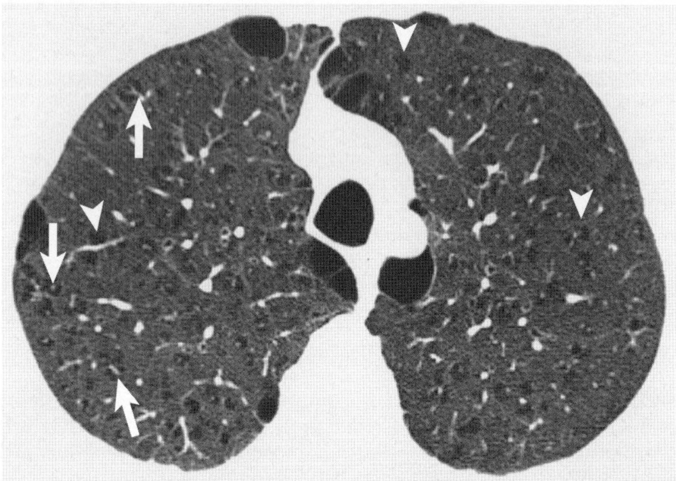

Fig. 6.3 Centrilobular and paraseptal emphysema. High-resolution CT at the level of the upper lobes shows foci of low attenuation *(arrowheads)* characteristic of centrilobular emphysema. Vessels *(arrows)* can be seen within some of the areas of emphysema and is termed the centrilobular dot sign. Note foci of emphysema greater than 1 cm in diameter (bullae) in the subpleural regions, characteristic of paraseptal emphysema. Some of the bullae have thin walls.

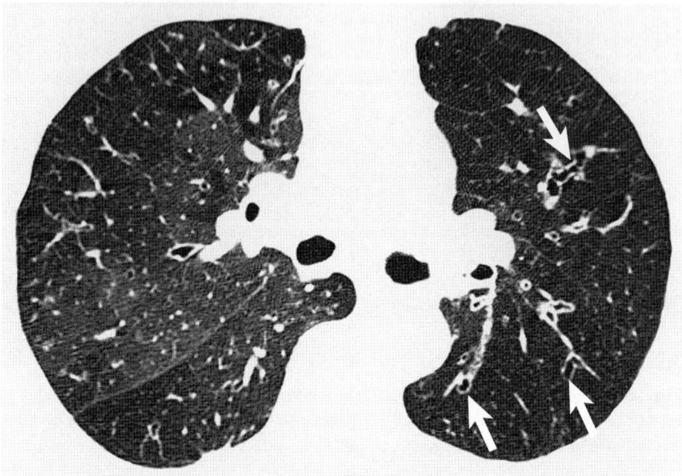

Fig. 6.5 Constrictive bronchiolitis associated with rheumatoid arthritis. High-resolution CT shows decreased attenuation and vascularity in most of the left lung, the anterior aspect of the right upper lobe, and the superior segment of the right lower lobe. Also noted is bronchiectasis *(arrows)*. The findings are characteristic of constrictive bronchiolitis. The uninvolved portions of the right upper lobe have increased vascularity and attenuation because of redistribution of blood flow. The heterogeneous pattern of attenuation and vascularity is known as mosaic attenuation.

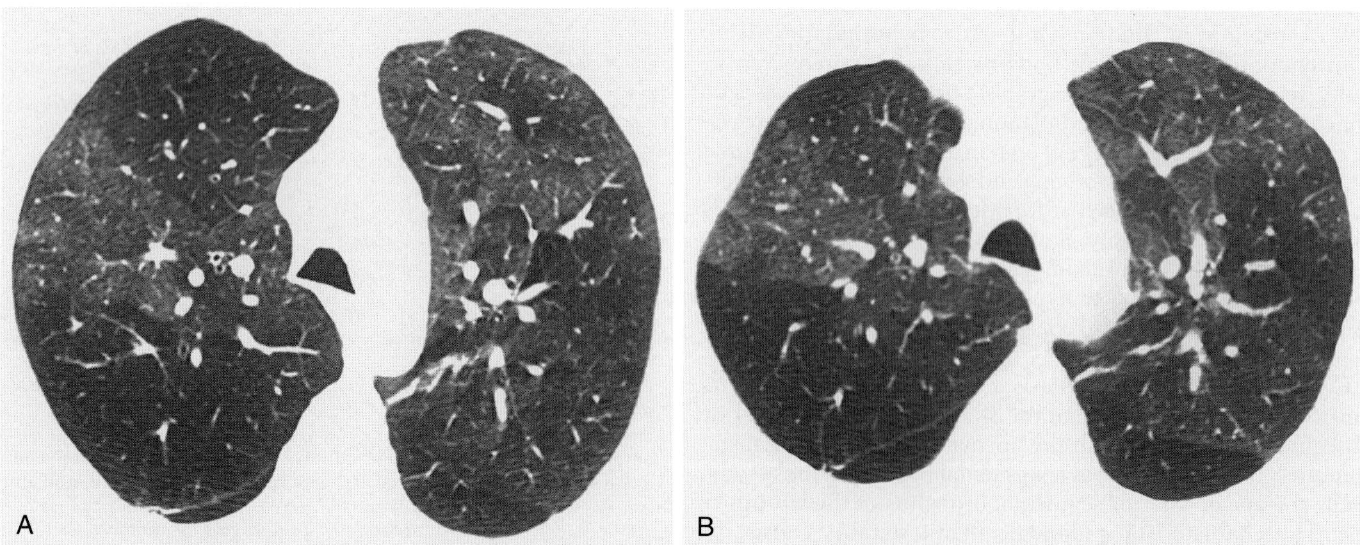

Fig. 6.4 Mosaic attenuation in asthma. (A) High-resolution CT performed at end inspiration shows extensive areas of decreased attenuation and vascularity, with redistribution of blood flow to normal lung resulting in a mosaic attenuation pattern. (B) High-resolution CT performed after maximal expiration demonstrates extensive bilateral air trapping.

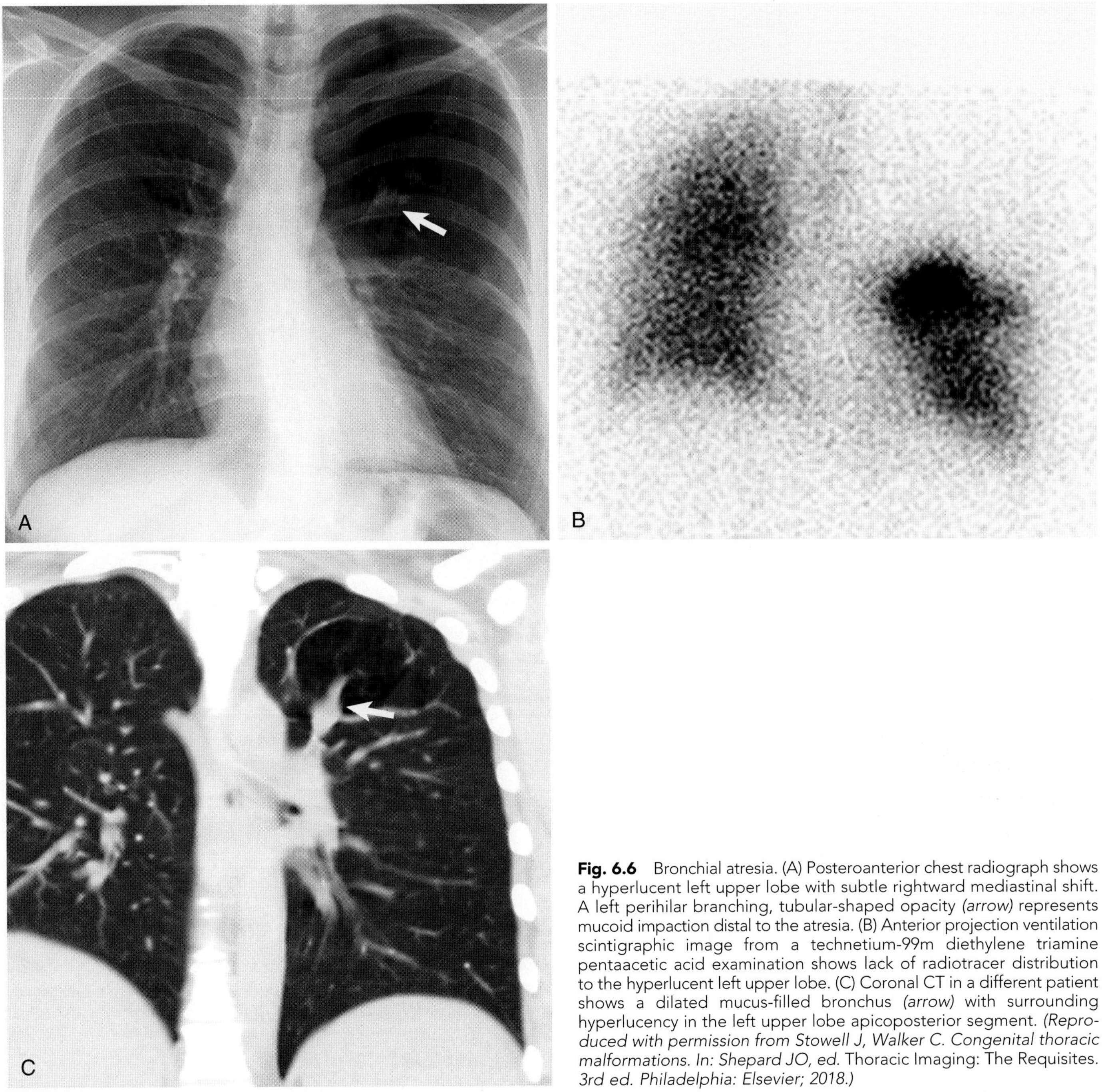

Fig. 6.6 Bronchial atresia. (A) Posteroanterior chest radiograph shows a hyperlucent left upper lobe with subtle rightward mediastinal shift. A left perihilar branching, tubular-shaped opacity *(arrow)* represents mucoid impaction distal to the atresia. (B) Anterior projection ventilation scintigraphic image from a technetium-99m diethylene triamine pentaacetic acid examination shows lack of radiotracer distribution to the hyperlucent left upper lobe. (C) Coronal CT in a different patient shows a dilated mucus-filled bronchus *(arrow)* with surrounding hyperlucency in the left upper lobe apicoposterior segment. *(Reproduced with permission from Stowell J, Walker C. Congenital thoracic malformations. In: Shepard JO, ed.* Thoracic Imaging: The Requisites. *3rd ed. Philadelphia: Elsevier; 2018.)*

than leaves on expiration. It most commonly affects the left upper lobe and less commonly the right middle or right upper lobe.[16] In congenital lobar overinflation the alveoli are overdistended but are not destroyed. Therefore the term *congenital lobar emphysema* is considered less accurate. Most patients become symptomatic before 6 months of age. Occasionally, it may be first seen in older children or be an incidental finding in asymptomatic adults. The chest radiograph and CT show hyperinflation and hyperlucency of the affected lobe and compressive atelectasis of the adjacent lung (Fig. 6.7).[17,18]

Overinflation *without air trapping* is a compensatory process: parts of the lung assume a larger volume than normal in response to loss of volume elsewhere in the thorax. This process may occur after surgical removal of lung tissue or as a result of atelectasis (Fig. 6.8) or parenchymal scarring. The remaining lung contains more than its normal complement of air.

Bulla

A bulla is a sharply demarcated, air-containing space measuring 1 cm or greater in diameter with a smooth wall 1 mm or less in

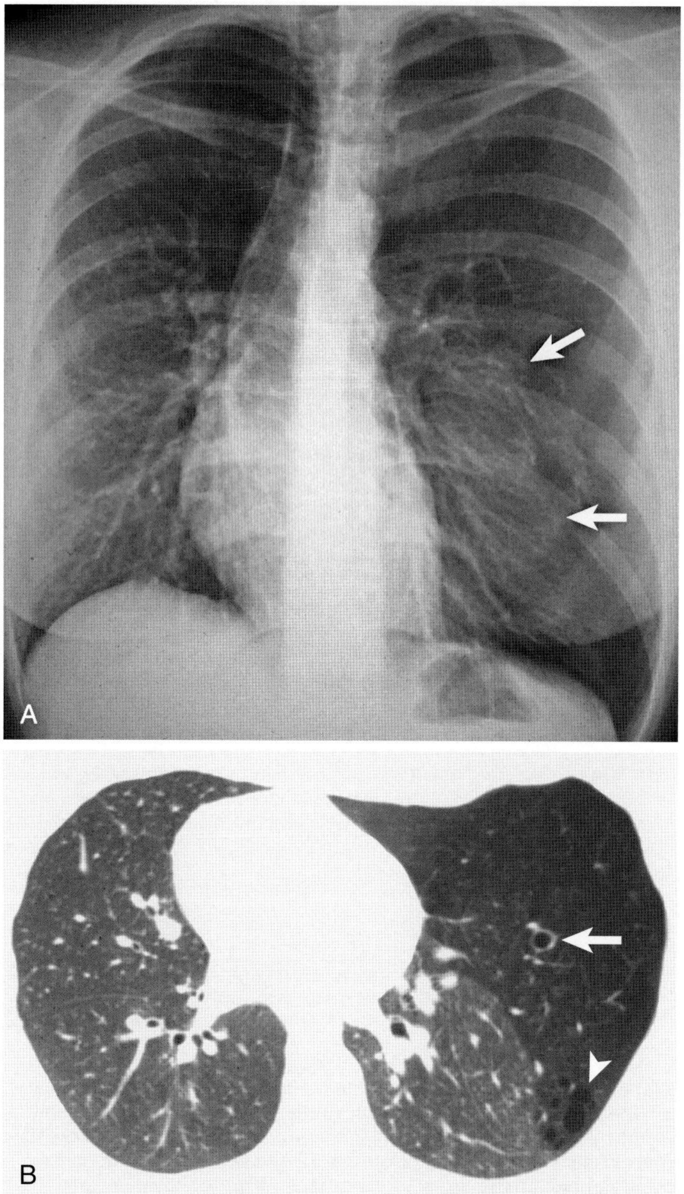

Fig. 6.7 Congenital lobar overinflation. (A) Posteroanterior chest radiograph shows overinflation of the left upper lobe and lingula with compression of the left lower lobe *(arrows)* and rightward shift of the heart and mediastinum. (B) Axial CT shows hyperinflation and decreased attenuation of the left upper lobe with associated compression of the left lower lobe. Note dilated bronchi *(arrow)* and focal cysts *(arrowhead)* posteriorly in the left upper lobe. *(Courtesy Dr. Marie-Pierre Cordeau, Department of Radiology, Hôtel-Dieu de Montréal, Canada.)*

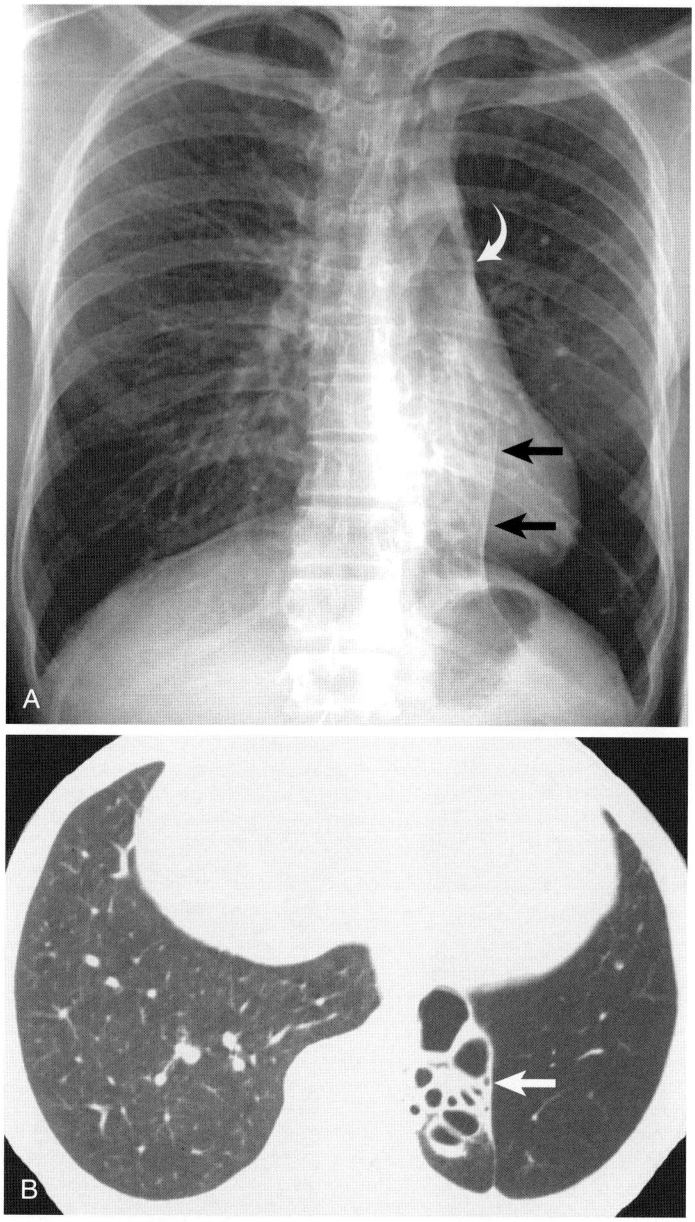

Fig. 6.8 Compensatory overinflation in chronic left lower lobe atelectasis after childhood viral pneumonia. (A) Posteroanterior chest radiograph shows inferior and medial displacement of the left major fissure *(straight arrows)*, characteristic of left lower lobe atelectasis. Note compensatory overinflation of the left upper lobe and, to a lesser extent, the right upper lobe with leftward displacement of the anterior junction line *(curved arrow)*. (B) High-resolution CT shows inferior and medial displacement of the left major fissure *(arrow)*, left lower lobe bronchiectasis, and compensatory overinflation of the left upper lobe.

thickness (see Fig. 6.3).[19] The space may be unilocular or separated into several compartments by thin septa.

Bleb

A bleb was originally defined as a gas-containing space within the visceral pleura.[19] It develops most frequently over the lung apices and now by definition measures less than 1 cm in diameter.[20] Its pathogenesis has been hypothesized to be dissection of gas from ruptured alveoli into adjacent interstitial tissue and the interstitial layer of the visceral pleura, where it accumulates in the form of a cyst.

Pneumatocele

A pneumatocele is a thin-walled, gas-filled space within the lung that characteristically increases in size over a period of days to weeks and almost invariably resolves; it typically occurs in association with infection. The pathogenesis is believed to relate to check-valve obstruction of an airway lumen or local necrosis of

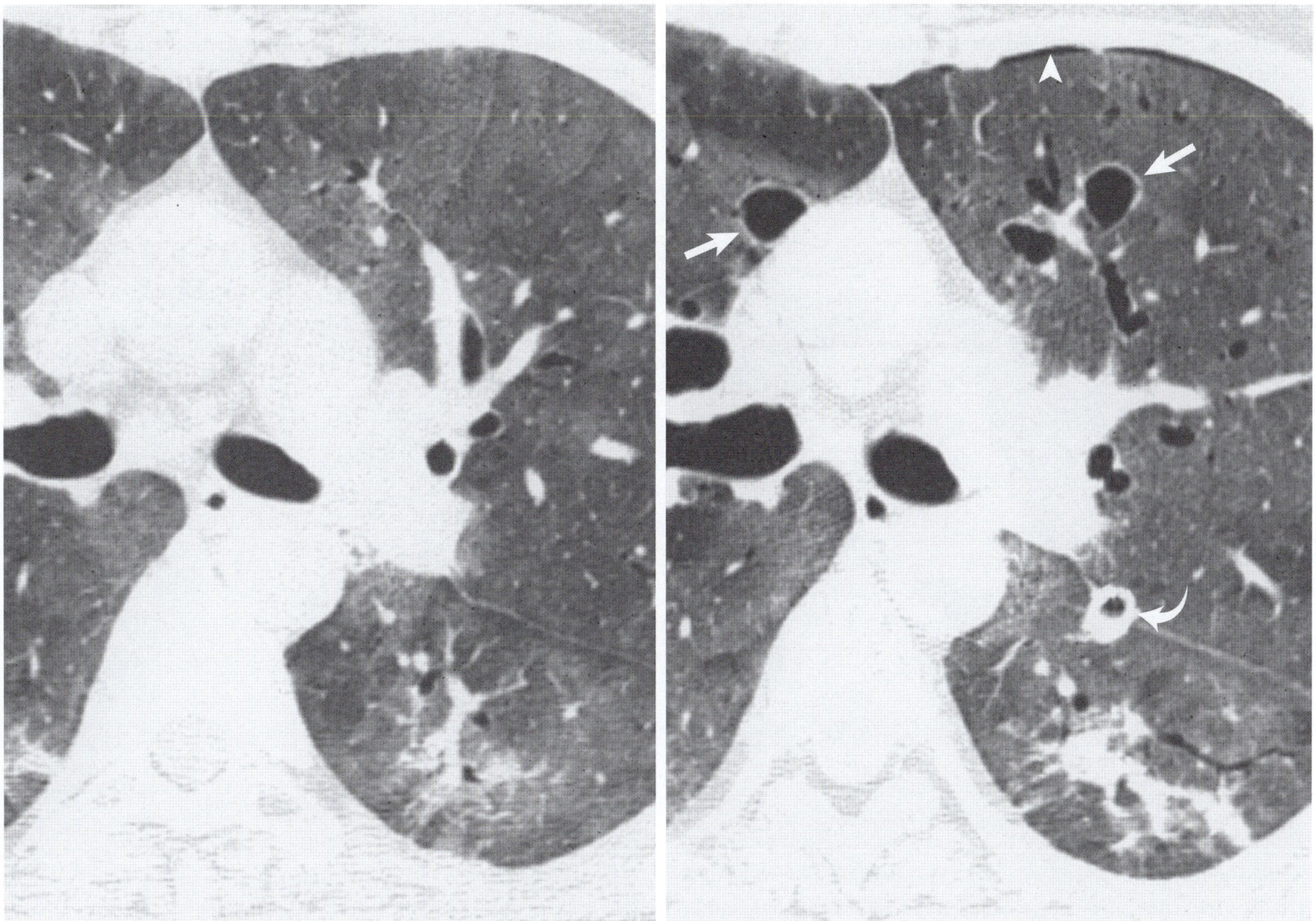

Fig. 6.9 Pneumatoceles secondary to *Pneumocystis* pneumonia. Composite image with axial CT at time of initial pneumonia *(left image)* shows extensive bilateral ground-glass opacities and focal consolidation. Axial CT at the same level 1 month later *(right image)* shows several pneumatoceles *(straight arrows)*. Note a small left pneumothorax *(arrowhead)* and a left chest tube in the major fissure *(curved arrow)*. Follow-up CT (not shown) documented resolution of the pneumatoceles.

a bronchial wall with dissection of air into the adjacent bronchovascular interstitial tissue.[21] It is usually caused by *Staphylococcus aureus* infection in infants and children or *Pneumocystis jirovecii* in immunocompromised patients (Fig. 6.9).[22] Pneumatoceles can also occur after trauma and are referred to as lacerations in this setting (Fig. 6.10). Pneumatoceles typically resolve in a few weeks or months.

Alteration in Pulmonary Vasculature

Oligemia secondary to decreased vascularity may result from vascular obstruction (e.g., pulmonary thromboembolism) or obliteration of small peripheral vessels (e.g., emphysema). Other vascular causes include proximal interruption (absence) of the pulmonary artery, congenital cardiac malformations (e.g., tetralogy of Fallot), and diseases that affect the peripheral pulmonary vasculature (e.g., primary pulmonary hypertension). Nonvascular causes of decreased lung density without overinflation include Swyer-James-McLeod syndrome and partly obstructing endobronchial lesions.

Occlusion of a central, lobar, or segmental artery by acute pulmonary thromboembolism may result in oligemia distal to the obstruction (Westermark sign). Although sometimes helpful, this finding is seldom apparent on radiographs or CT.[23] Areas of oligemia, however, are commonly seen in chronic pulmonary thromboembolic disease, particularly when severe enough to result in pulmonary arterial hypertension.[24,25] The characteristic findings on CT consist of areas of decreased vascularity and attenuation. Redistribution of blood flow to normal lung results in areas of increased attenuation and vascularity (mosaic attenuation). In patients with pulmonary arterial hypertension, the presence of a mosaic pattern on CT is highly suggestive of chronic pulmonary thromboembolic disease (Fig. 6.11). Occasionally, however, a similar pattern may be seen in primary pulmonary hypertension.[26] The diagnosis of acute and chronic pulmonary embolism can usually be readily confirmed by demonstration of characteristic filling defects in the pulmonary arteries on CT angiography (see Fig. 6.11).

Swyer-James-McLeod syndrome is a condition characterized radiographically by a hyperlucent lung or lobe and normal or reduced volume during inspiration and air trapping during expiration (Fig. 6.12). It is generally a sequelum of childhood respiratory infections, most often viral. The hyperlucency of the affected lung or lobe is mainly the result of decreased pulmonary blood volume secondary to constrictive bronchiolitis. High-resolution CT shows decreased attenuation and vascularity of the affected lung on inspiration and air trapping on expiration (Fig. 6.13).[27,28] Most patients have bronchiectasis.

Partial bronchial obstruction by a foreign body or tumor results in decreased perfusion (oligemia) of the affected parenchyma secondary to hypoxic vasoconstriction in response to alveolar hypoventilation. In children the lung distal to the partial obstruction is often hyperinflated. In adults, however, lung volume is almost always reduced at total lung capacity (Fig. 6.14). The overall effect is an increase in radiolucency despite a reduction in volume.

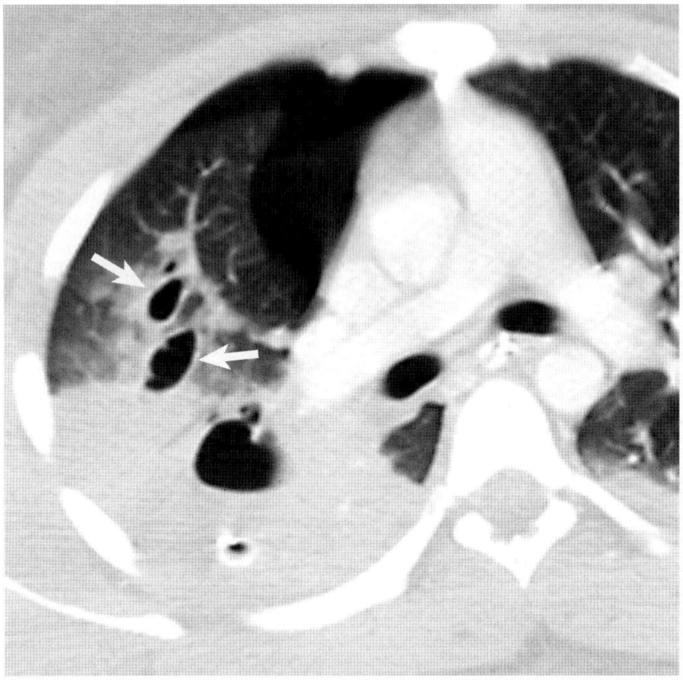

Fig. 6.10 Traumatic pneumatoceles (pulmonary lacerations) after motor vehicle collision. Axial contrast-enhanced CT shows several right lung thin-walled cystic spaces representing pulmonary lacerations *(arrows)*, right pneumothorax, and small bilateral hemothoraces. Dependent right lung consolidation and ground-glass opacities represent pulmonary contusion and hemorrhage.

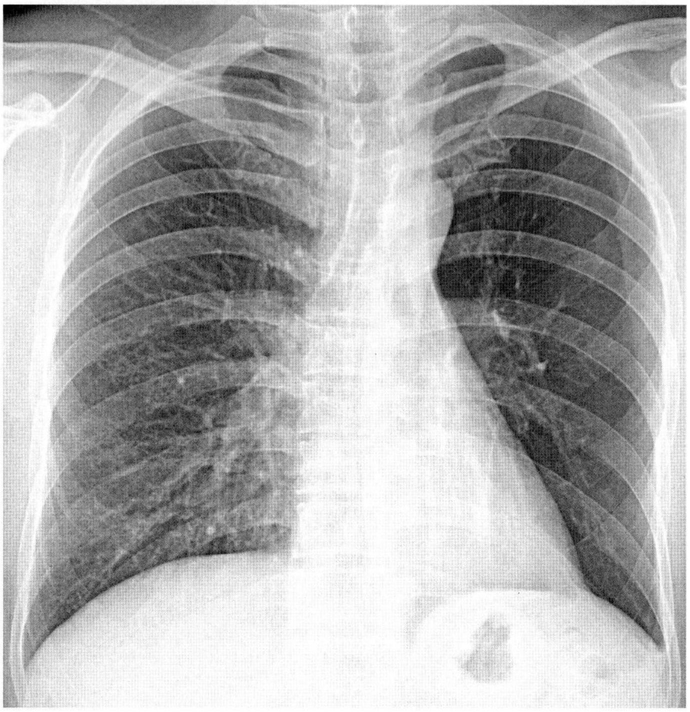

Fig. 6.12 Swyer-James-McLeod syndrome. Posteroanterior chest radiograph shows hyperlucency and decreased vascularity of the left lung. The mediastinum is shifted to the left, consistent with decreased left lung volume.

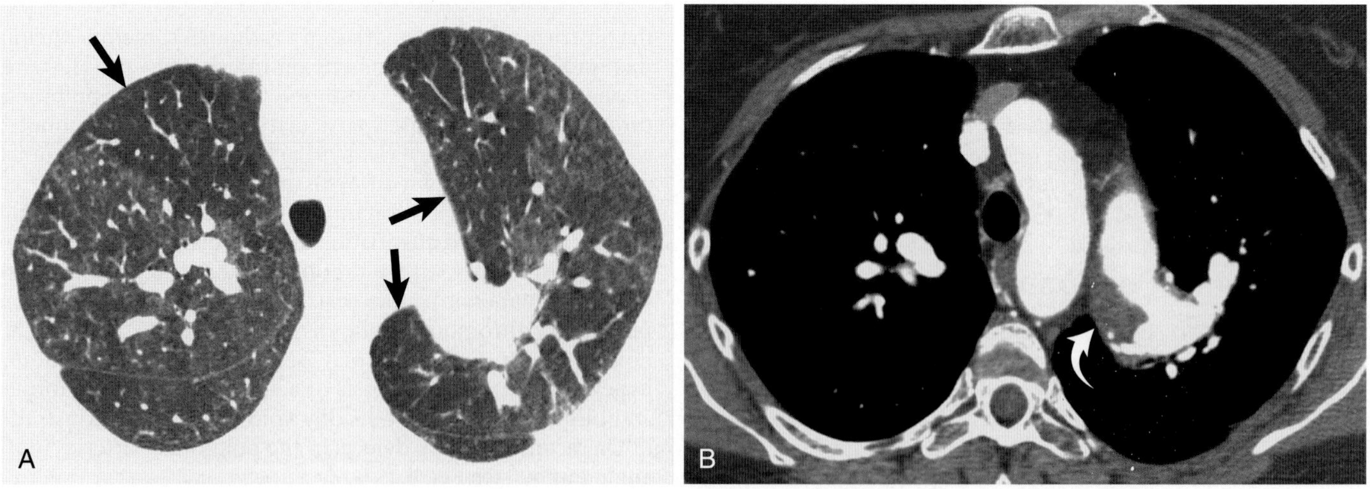

Fig. 6.11 Mosaic attenuation in chronic thromboembolic pulmonary hypertension. (A) High-resolution CT at the level of the upper lobes shows areas with decreased attenuation and vascularity *(arrows)* and areas with increased attenuation and vascularity (mosaic attenuation pattern). Note marked enlargement of the pulmonary arteries in regions of higher lung attenuation compared with the adjacent normal-sized bronchi. (B) CT pulmonary angiogram demonstrates an eccentric filling defect in the left pulmonary artery *(curved arrow)* and an irregular arterial lumen, consistent with chronic pulmonary thromboembolic disease.

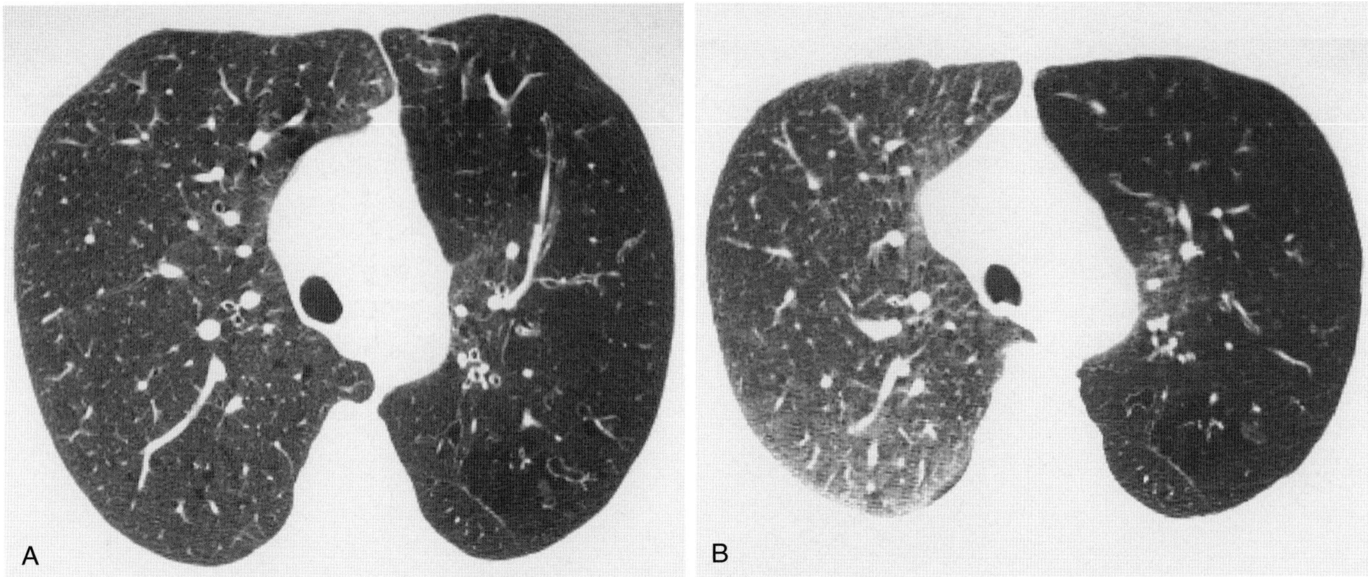

Fig. 6.13 Swyer-James-McLeod syndrome. (A) High-resolution CT shows decreased attenuation and vascularity of the left lung, with associated bronchiectasis and mild volume loss leading to ipsilateral shift of the mediastinum and anterior junction line. (B) Expiratory CT at the same level shows air trapping in the left lung. The mediastinum and anterior junction line are now in the midline.

KEY POINTS: HYPERLUCENT LUNG ON THE CHEST RADIOGRAPH

- **Technical Factors**
  - Rotation: hyperlucency always occurs on the side to which the patient rotates
- **Chest Wall Abnormality**
  - Congenital absence of the pectoral muscles: often associated with Poland syndrome
  - Mastectomy: history of surgery
- **Pleural Abnormality**
  - Pneumothorax: usually readily recognized on radiographs
- **Decreased Lung Density**
  - Bronchial atresia: most commonly the apicoposterior segment of the left upper lobe. Overinflation of the affected segment. Perihilar opacity (bronchocele)
  - Lobar overinflation: overinflation of the affected lobe, most commonly the left upper lobe
  - Proximal interruption of the pulmonary artery: affected lung or lobe often smaller than normal. Aortic arch opposite side of interrupted pulmonary artery. CT or MRI diagnostic
  - Swyer-James-McLeod syndrome: unilateral hyperlucent lung with decreased or normal size of the affected lung. Air trapping. Bronchiectasis on CT
  - Bronchial obstruction by a tumor or foreign body: overinflation common in children, but lung volume always reduced in adults
  - Severe emphysema: diffuse hyperlucency, may be asymmetric

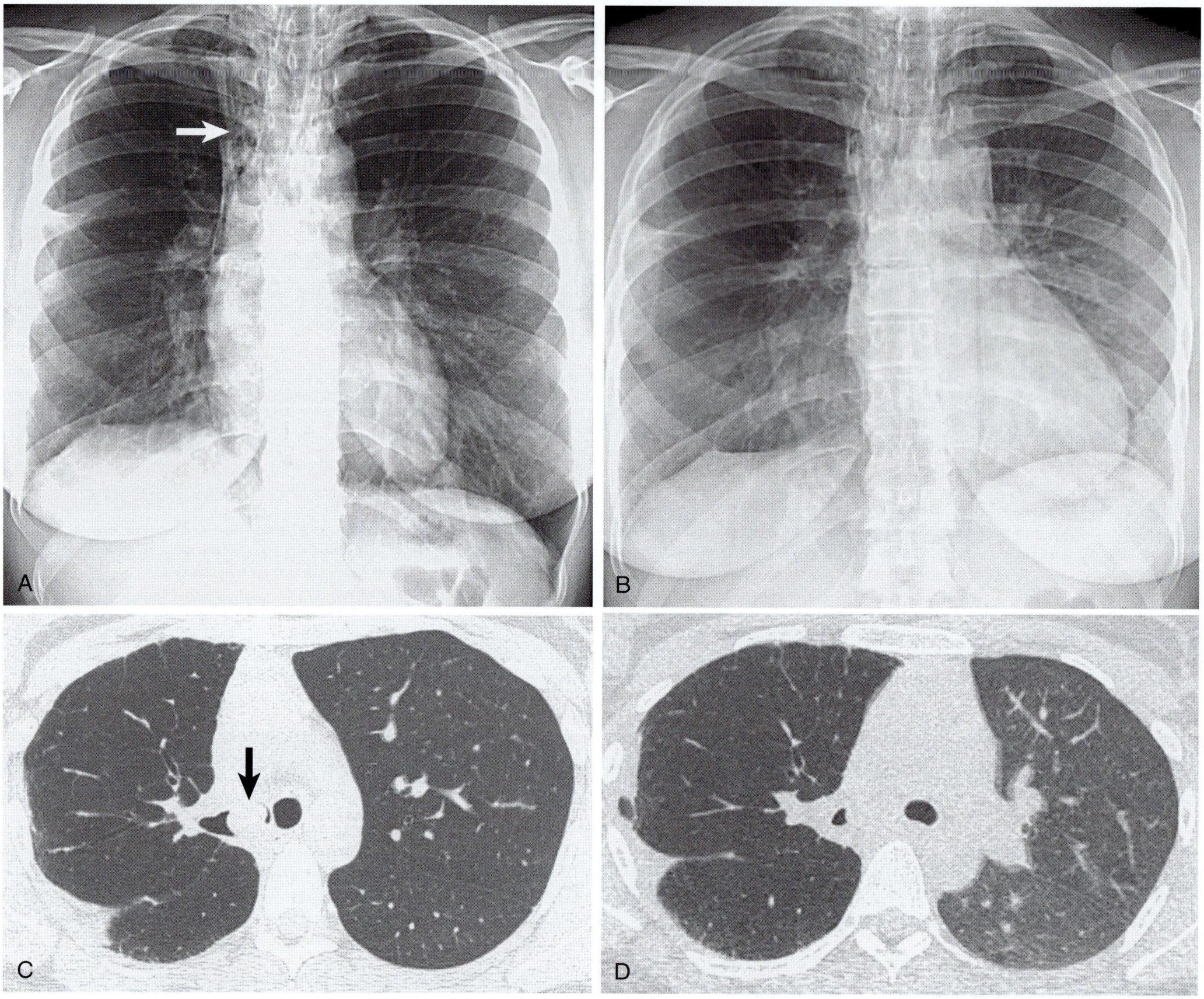

Fig. 6.14 Increased lucency as a result of endobronchial carcinoid. (A) Chest radiograph shows mild hyperlucency and a decrease in volume of the right lung with ipsilateral mediastinal shift. Note pneumomediastinum *(arrow)* and right pleural thickening. (B) Expiratory chest radiograph shows air trapping of the right lung with a contralateral shift of the mediastinum. (C) High-resolution CT demonstrates tumor *(arrow)* in the right main bronchus and an associated decrease in attenuation, vascularity, and volume of the right lung. The pneumomediastinum has resolved. (D) Expiratory high-resolution CT shows extensive right lung air trapping.

SUGGESTED READINGS

Biyyam DR, Chapman T, Ferguson MR, Deutsch G, Dighe MK. Congenital lung abnormalities: embryologic features, prenatal diagnosis, and postnatal radiologic-pathologic correlation. *Radiographics*. 2010;30(6):1721–1738.

Dillman JR, Sanchez R, Ladino-Torres MF, Yarram SG, Strouse PJ, Lucaya J. Expanding upon the unilateral hyperlucent hemithorax in children. *Radiographics*. 2011;31(3):723–741.

Franquet T, Müller NL. Disorders of the small airways: high-resolution computed tomographic features. *Semin Respir Crit Care Med*. 2003;24:437–544.

Silva CI, Colby TV, Müller NL. Asthma and associated conditions: high-resolution CT and pathologic findings. *AJR Am J Roentgenol*. 2004;183:817–824.

The full reference list for this chapter is available at ExpertConsult.com.

7 Airway and Parenchymal Anomalies*

JUSTIN T. STOWELL | CHRISTOPHER M. WALKER | JONATHAN H. CHUNG

Congenital lung disease remains a confusing topic owing to ever-changing histopathologic understanding of the various entities and frequent updates to antiquated clinical and pathologic classification schemes. Past classifications have been based on thoracic anatomic structures, dividing lesions into congenital malformations of the trachea, bronchi, lung, and pulmonary vasculature. Such divisions are controversial because the embryologic basis of these malformations is not clearly understood, as more recent investigations have demonstrated significant overlap or coexistence of histopathologic features among these entities. The current literature points instead to a spectrum of congenital bronchopulmonary malformations (CBM) rather than separate individual entities, which classically included congenital pulmonary airway malformation (CPAM) (formerly congenital cystic adenomatoid malformation [CCAM]), intralobar and extralobar sequestration, and foregut cysts. All exhibit some failure of budding, differentiation, or separation from the primitive foregut between the 3rd and 24th weeks of gestation, with or without superimposed airway obstruction.

Most of these entities are now diagnosed with prenatal imaging and regress prior to birth. However, some can remain asymptomatic during childhood and are diagnosed in the adolescent or adult. This leads to controversy over perinatal management. In select cases, in utero or early postnatal surgery may be required for large lesions that contribute to significant fetal compromise. In this chapter we limit our discussion to developmental abnormalities that are discovered in adults. Diagnosis of most CBMs can be achieved with radiography, prenatal ultrasound, computed tomography (CT), and magnetic resonance imaging (MRI). Management of CBMs is variable, ranging from conservative observation to surgical excision, and is usually dependent on symptomatology or the potential risk of complications.

Anomalous Tracheobronchial Branching

TRACHEAL BRONCHUS

Etiology, Prevalence, and Epidemiology

Variable branching patterns of the tracheobronchial tree have been well described. When an anomalous bronchus arises from the right lateral wall of the trachea (usually <2 cm from the carina) and supplies all or segments of the right upper lobe, it is referred to as a tracheal bronchus.[1–3] However, various other authors have used the term *tracheal* to describe any anomalous bronchus derived from the trachea and main bronchus supplying an upper lobe.[1] The anomalous tracheal bronchus is referred to as supernumerary when the segmental bronchi to the upper lobes exhibit a standard branching pattern—three to the right and four to the left upper lobes. In the absence of one or more of the normal upper lobe segmental bronchi, the tracheal bronchus is considered as displaced. The term *pig bronchus* (bronchus suis) is applied when the entire right upper lobe is supplied by the tracheal bronchus. When a tracheal bronchus ends blindly, it is called a tracheal diverticulum. The territory ventilated by the anomalous bronchus usually has normal vascular supply.

The reported prevalence of a right tracheal bronchus ranges from 0.1% to 2%.[1,3] The reported frequency of a tracheal bronchus supplying the entire right upper lobe (pig bronchus) is approximately 0.2%.[3] Rarely, a similar malformation may be seen on the left side. However, most cases were bilateral tracheal bronchi or associated with bilateral right tracheal bronchi in the setting of right isomerism (described subsequently).[1]

Clinical Presentation

The vast majority of adult patients with a tracheal bronchus are asymptomatic, and the abnormal bronchus is discovered incidentally on CT or at bronchoscopy.[1–3] The anomaly may become clinically significant when the inhibited clearance of the anomalous bronchi leads to conditions such as recurrent right upper lobe pneumonia, air trapping, lobar or segmental postobstructive atelectasis, or bronchiectasis.[1–3]

Manifestations of the Disease

Computed Tomography. Tracheal bronchi, as well as the presence of associated findings such as bronchiectasis or emphysema, are best characterized by CT (Fig. 7.1). Multiplanar reformations, volume-rendered imaging, and virtual bronchoscopy techniques allow reconstruction of CT data to produce three-dimensional images of the tracheobronchial tree (Figs. 7.1 and 7.2).

Synopsis of Treatment Options

Treatment of symptomatic patients is based on the severity of symptoms and ranges from observation to lobectomy.

ACCESSORY CARDIAC BRONCHUS

An accessory cardiac bronchus (ACB) is a mucosa-lined supernumerary bronchus that arises from the medial wall of the right main bronchus or bronchus intermedius.[4] The bronchus courses medially and caudally for 1 to 5 cm. The presence of mural cartilage distinguishes ACB from a diverticulum. ACBs usually end blindly but may be associated with small amounts of abnormal

*The editors and the publisher would like to thank Drs. Nestor L. Müller and C. Isabela Silva Müller for contributing material on this topic to the prior edition of this work. It has served as the foundation for the current chapter.

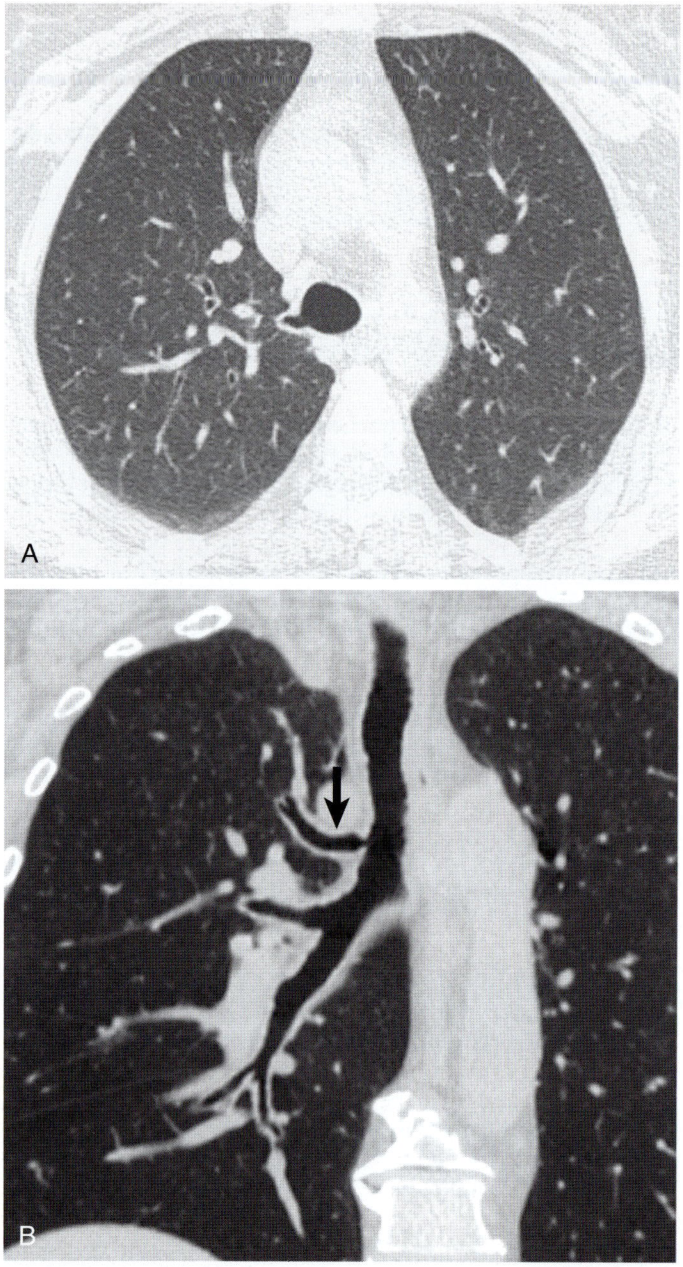

Fig. 7.1 Tracheal bronchus. CT (A) shows a small bronchus originating from the right tracheal wall. Coronal CT from a different patient (B) demonstrates the tracheal bronchus *(arrow)* supplying the apical segment of the right upper lobe. *(Fig. 7.1B reproduced from Stowell J, Walker C. Congenital thoracic malformations. In: Shepard JO, ed.* Thoracic Imaging: The Requisites. *3rd ed. Philadelphia: Elsevier; 2018.)*

pulmonary parenchyma (a so-called cardiac lobe). The anomaly occurs in up to 0.5% of the general population.[3,4]

Clinical Presentation

The vast majority of adult patients are asymptomatic.[3,4] The most common complications are cough and hemoptysis secondary to infection or rarely carcinoma.[2,4] Pneumothorax may result from traumatic injury to the ACB during bronchoscopy.

Manifestations of the Disease

Computed Tomography. The diagnosis of an accessory cardiac bronchus is best accomplished with CT.[2,4] As with other bronchial anomalies, the course of the ACB is best depicted with reformation techniques, such as multiplanar reconstruction, volume rendering, or virtual bronchoscopy (Fig. 7.3).

Synopsis of Treatment Options

Treatment of symptomatic patients is based on the severity of symptoms and ranges from observation to surgical resection.

DISPLACED BRONCHI

Approximately 10% of individuals have displaced segmental or subsegmental bronchi in the same lobe, which are best recognized on CT.[1,3] Less commonly, a segmental or subsegmental bronchus originates from an adjacent lobe. The lung ventilated by the displaced bronchus is normal, but CT often demonstrates an incomplete fissure between the adjacent lobes. Occasionally, segmental bronchi may be absent (bronchial agenesis). Segmental bronchial agenesis occurs most commonly in the right upper lobe.[1,3] Displaced segmental and subsegmental bronchi are asymptomatic and are found incidentally on CT or at bronchoscopy.

Congenital Bronchial Atresia

ETIOLOGY, PREVALENCE, AND EPIDEMIOLOGY

Bronchial atresia occurs when a lobar, segmental, or subsegmental bronchus is congenitally truncated at or near its origin. The bronchi and alveoli distal to the obstruction develop normally. The pathogenesis of bronchial atresia is unknown but proposed to either represent sequelae of an ischemic event to the developing bronchial wall or a developmental error wherein the bronchial lung bud separates from the more distal cell mass of primitive bronchi. Because of its frequent association with other congenital bronchopulmonary malformations (sequestration, CPAM, and congenital lobar overinflation), bronchial atresia is believed to share a common pathogenic mechanism among these entities.[5] Bronchial atresia most commonly occurs in the apicoposterior left upper lobe bronchus, followed in order of frequency by segmental bronchi of the right upper lobe and less commonly the middle lobe and the lower lobes.[2] The estimated population prevalence is approximately 1 case per 100,000 persons and is more common in males.[6]

CLINICAL PRESENTATION

The majority of patients are asymptomatic. Some have recurrent pneumonia.[2,5]

PATHOPHYSIOLOGY

Pathologically, the bronchial tree distal to the point of obliteration is patent and has a normal number of airways and airspaces. A mucocele develops in the distal bronchi, which become dilated and filled with mucus that cannot be cleared through the disconnected larger airway. Because air can enter the affected bronchopulmonary segments only via collateral channels, overinflation and expiratory air trapping within the distal alveoli result.[2,5,6]

MANIFESTATIONS OF THE DISEASE

Radiography

The radiographic findings are usually characteristic and consist of an area of pulmonary hyperlucency, seen in approximately 90%

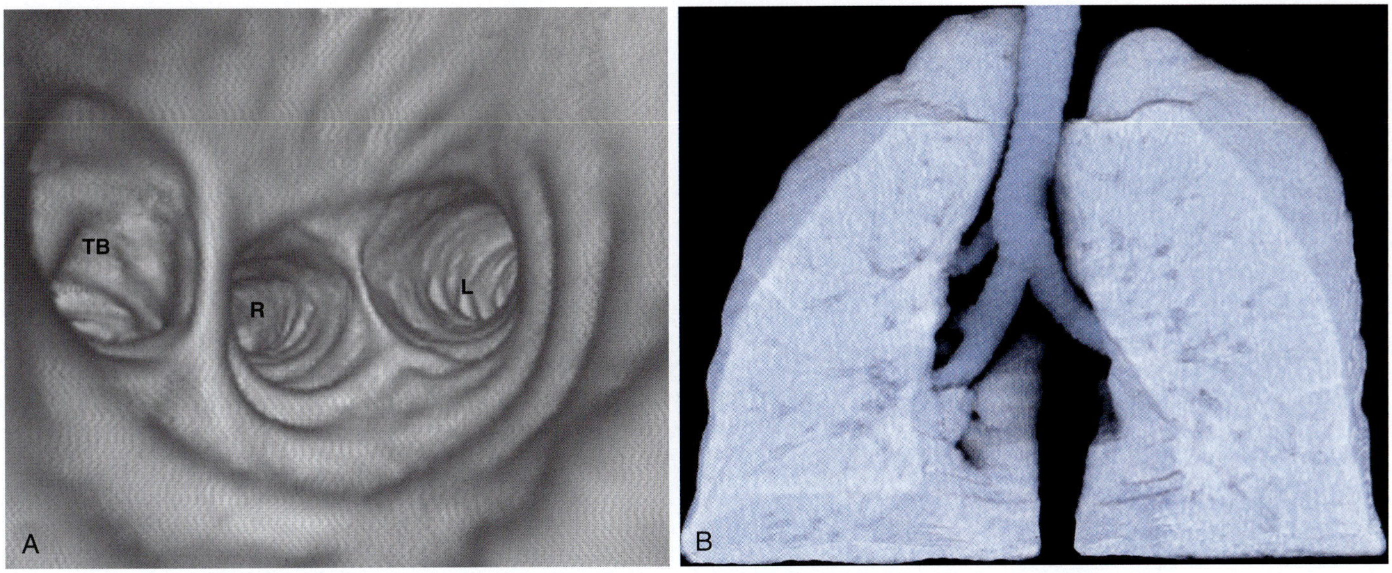

Fig. 7.2 CT bronchoscopy of a tracheal bronchus. (A) CT reformation with volume-rendering ("CT bronchoscopy" or "virtual bronchoscopy") demonstrates a view of the tracheal and bronchial lumina that resembles the view seen at bronchoscopy. The image shows a tracheal bronchus *(TB)*, right main *(R)* bronchus, and left main *(L)* bronchus as "seen" from the level of the lower part of the trachea. (B) A coronal three-dimensional external volume-rendering image shows a tracheal bronchus entering the right lung.

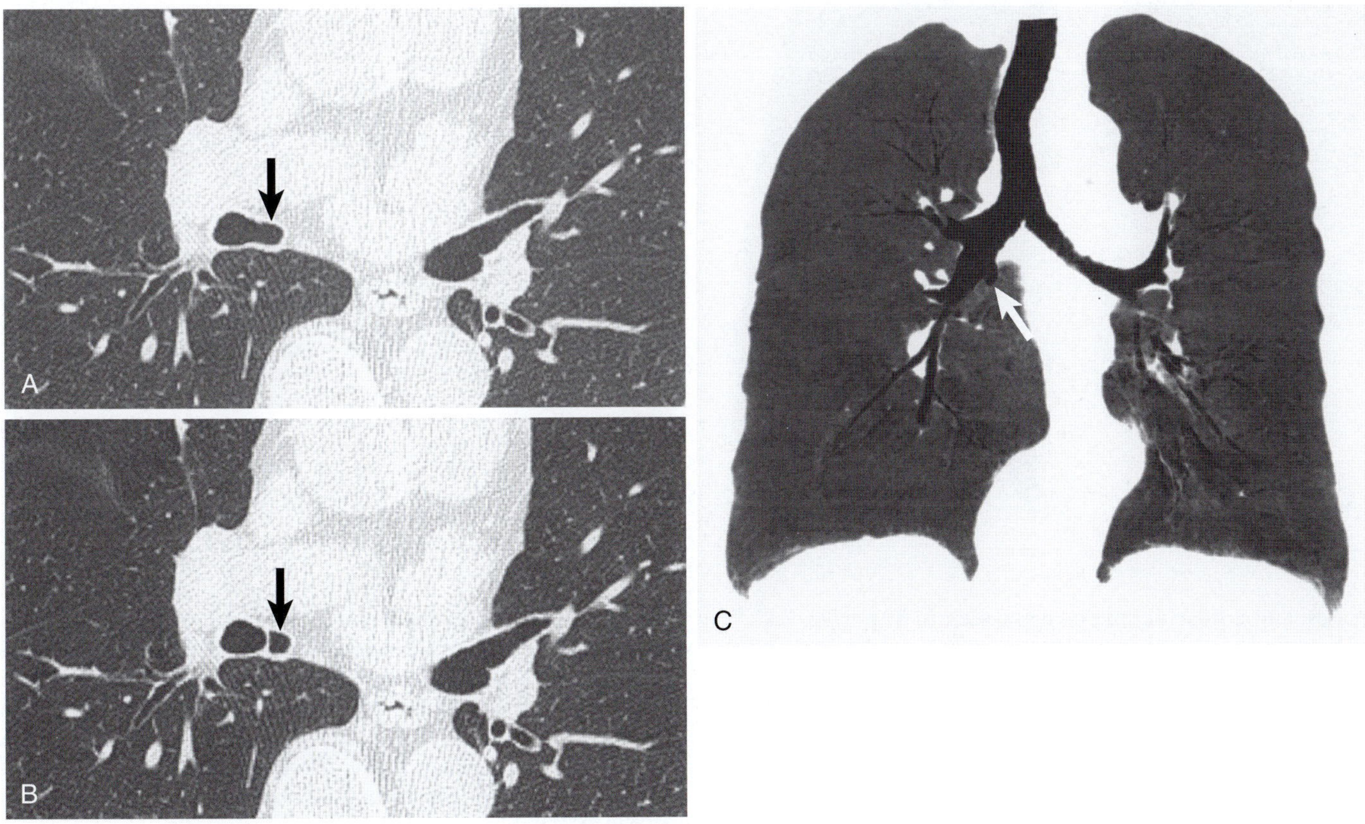

Fig. 7.3 Accessory cardiac bronchus. Axial CT (A and B) shows a cardiac bronchus *(arrow)* originating from the medial wall of the bronchus intermedius, coursing medially, to end in a blind pouch similar to a diverticulum. A minimum-intensity projection coronal reformatted CT (C) of the central airways shows a medial and inferior course of the cardiac bronchus *(arrow)*.

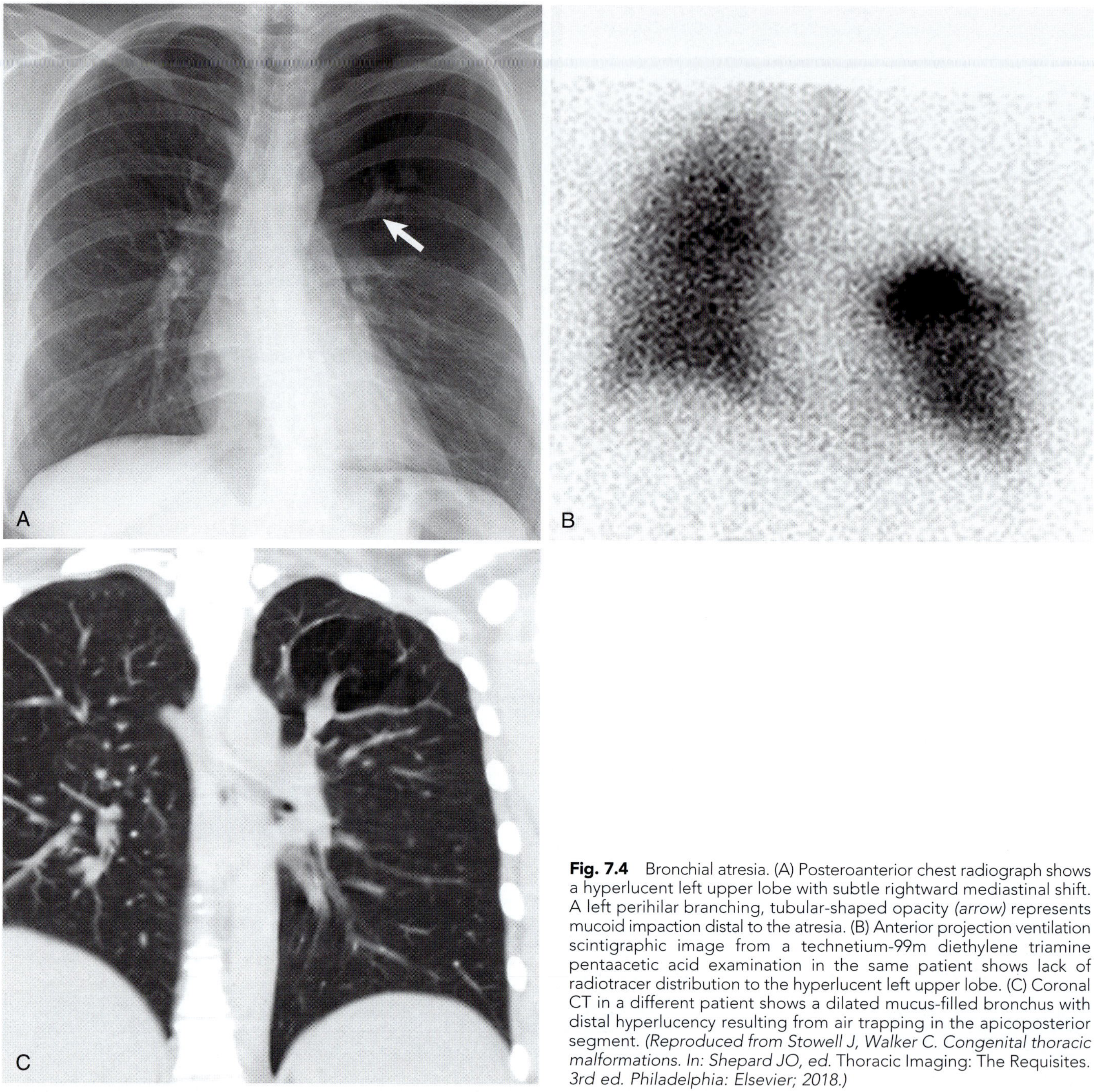

Fig. 7.4 Bronchial atresia. (A) Posteroanterior chest radiograph shows a hyperlucent left upper lobe with subtle rightward mediastinal shift. A left perihilar branching, tubular-shaped opacity *(arrow)* represents mucoid impaction distal to the atresia. (B) Anterior projection ventilation scintigraphic image from a technetium-99m diethylene triamine pentaacetic acid examination in the same patient shows lack of radiotracer distribution to the hyperlucent left upper lobe. (C) Coronal CT in a different patient shows a dilated mucus-filled bronchus with distal hyperlucency resulting from air trapping in the apicoposterior segment. *(Reproduced from Stowell J, Walker C. Congenital thoracic malformations. In: Shepard JO, ed.* Thoracic Imaging: The Requisites. *3rd ed. Philadelphia: Elsevier; 2018.)*

of cases, and a hilar nodule or mass, seen in 80% (Fig. 7.4).[2,5,6] The hyperlucency results from a combination of oligemia and an increase in the volume of air within the affected parenchyma. The adjacent normal lung is compressed and displaced; the mediastinum may or may not show displacement. Accumulation of secretions and mucoid impaction distal to the bronchial atresia result in ovoid, round, or branching opacities near the hilum. Atelectasis may result in adjacent lung segments as a result of compression and mass effect from the hyperinflated lung tissue.

Computed Tomography

Excellent visualization of the mucoid impaction and segmental overinflation and hypovascularity is afforded by CT.[7] Mucoid impaction is readily recognized by the presence of branching soft tissue densities in a bronchial distribution, usually associated with bronchial dilation. Bronchial occlusion, mucoid impaction with bronchial dilation (mucocele) immediately distal to the atretic bronchus, as well as decreased vascularity and attenuation and increased volume of the affected segment are evident on CT (see Fig. 7.4).[7,8] Expiratory CT will demonstrate air trapping in the affected lung segment.

Magnetic Resonance Imaging

The diagnosis of bronchial atresia can be made on MRI.[8] Mucoid impaction has variable signal intensity on T1-weighted images but typically very high signal intensity on T2-weighted images.

Imaging Algorithm

Although the radiographic findings may be characteristic, CT is the most sensitive imaging technique for confirming the diagnosis. It allows excellent visualization of the mucoid impaction, segmental hyperlucency, and decreased vascularity, a combination of findings that is generally considered diagnostic. Mucoid impaction is readily recognized by the presence of branching soft tissue densities in a bronchial distribution, usually associated with bronchial dilation. Although a similar appearance has been reported on MRI, CT is the imaging modality of choice.

DIFFERENTIAL DIAGNOSIS

The main differential diagnosis is partial airway obstruction caused by a foreign body, endobronchial tumor, or acquired bronchocele (e.g., allergic bronchopulmonary aspergillosis or bronchiectasis). Similar to these conditions, the lung distal to bronchial atresia is hyperlucent and shows air trapping. However, endobronchial lesions are rarely, if ever, associated with overinflation of affected bronchopulmonary segments at total lung capacity, an almost invariable finding in bronchial atresia. Therefore the distinction can often be made on a chest radiograph performed at maximal inspiration. A confident diagnosis of mucoid impaction distal to bronchial atresia can generally be made on CT. However, bronchoscopy may be required to rule out other causes of obstruction.

SYNOPSIS OF TREATMENT OPTIONS

Treatment may consist of conservative management in asymptomatic patients. However, some authors advocate for surgical resection of bronchial atresia, even in asymptomatic patients, given the inherent risk for recurrent infection.[5]

KEY POINTS: BRONCHIAL ATRESIA

- Most commonly involves the left upper lobe apicoposterior segmental bronchus
- Common radiologic findings:
  - Chest radiography typically shows hyperlucency (from collateral ventilation and air trapping) of the affected segment, decreased vascularity, and a juxtahilar nodule or mass.
  - CT shows a round, oval, or branching central mucoid impaction, segmental overinflation, and hypovascularity.
  - Impacted mucus exhibits high signal intensity on T2-weighted MRI.

Bronchopulmonary Isomerism and Heterotaxy

Thoracoabdominal visceral relationships are described in terms of situs, depending on the position of the cardiac atria and abdominal viscera relative to the midline. Situs solitus, situs inversus, and situs ambiguous (so-called heterotaxy) have been used to describe the normal, mirror image of normal, and non–mirror-image deviation from the normal left-right viscero-atrial configuration, respectively.[9] Visceroatrial situs should include a description of the position of the upper lobe bronchi to their ipsilateral pulmonary arteries—the most reliable imaging feature of bronchial situs, and thus atrial morphology.[1] The morphologic right lung is defined when the upper lobe bronchus is positioned above the ipsilateral pulmonary artery in the hilum (eparterial). The morphologic left lung is supplied by a hyparterial bronchus, which courses below the ipsilateral pulmonary artery.

Heterotaxy syndromes are frequently associated with bronchopulmonary isomerism—an identical pattern of branching and lobar configuration in each lung.[1] Bilateral eparterial and hyparterial bronchi characterize right and left bronchial isomerism (bilateral right- and left-sidedness), respectively. Right isomerism (bilateral right-sidedness) typically manifests with bilateral trilobed lungs and eparterial bronchi, bilateral right atria, right aortic arch, and asplenia (or some functional loss).[9] Right isomerism is commonly associated with severe congenital heart disease with high mortality rates.[1] Left isomerism typically manifests with bilateral bilobed lungs and hyparterial bronchi, bilateral left atria, and polysplenia (although this feature is variable).[9] Other commonly associated (although variable) findings include midline liver and intestinal malrotation in both forms of heterotaxy. Left isomerism may also manifest with azygos or hemiazygos continuation of the inferior vena cava (IVC) and a truncated pancreas.[10]

ETIOLOGY, PREVALENCE, AND EPIDEMIOLOGY

Heterotaxy syndrome is relatively uncommon, occurring in 1 of 10,000 births.[11] It is difficult to establish the exact prevalence of left isomerism, as patients without symptomatic congenital heart disease may be incidentally diagnosed in adulthood.[1] Situs inversus has a prevalence of 0.01% of the population.[10] Although likely multifactorial, the etiology of isomerism is probably related to defects in various genes (e.g., *ZIC3, Pitx-2, Cited-2, Sonic hedgehog, Lefty-1*) that regulate right- or left-sided patterns during early embryogenesis.[9–13] Furthermore, isomerism is associated with other defects included as part of the spectrum of ciliopathies (e.g., immotile cilia syndrome, sinonasal abnormalities, bronchiectasis, biliary atresia, and brain malformations).[11]

CLINICAL PRESENTATION

Symptoms of bronchopulmonary isomerism are dependent on the severity of associated abnormalities and may range from intractable wheezing and infantile heart murmurs to cyanosis and heart failure.[13] More common in males, right isomerism confers a poorer prognosis and frequent association with asplenia (leading to immune compromise and sepsis) and severe cyanotic congenital heart lesions (e.g., common atrioventricular canal, monoventricle, transposition of the great arteries, and total anomalous pulmonary venous return). Left isomerism (bilateral left-sidedness) is often associated with polysplenia, and although it has an overall better prognosis compared with right isomerism, there is still a 60% mortality in the first year of life.[9,10] Congenital heart defects (most commonly partial anomalous pulmonary venous return, atrial septal defect, and atrioventricular canal) are less frequent or less severe compared with those of right isomerism, but patients may still present with congestive heart failure from left-to-right shunts.[9,10] Patients may also present with midgut volvulus related to intestinal malrotation.

MANIFESTATIONS OF THE DISEASE

Ultrasound

Situs anomalies may be diagnosed on prenatal ultrasound and suggested by the right-sided location of the aorta, cardiac apex, and stomach bubble (inversus) or some deviation thereof, raising suspicion of heterotaxy. Ultrasound can also detect variable venous drainage patterns in the setting of anomalous pulmonary venous return, and the position of the atria may be implied by infradiaphragmatic venous drainage patterns.[10] Abdominal ultrasound in neonates may quickly and safely document polysplenia or asplenia.[12]

Radiography

Historically, chest radiography was used to determine the position of the cardiac apex and stomach bubble but was inconsistent.[10] Furthermore, the presence of bilateral horizontal fissures or eparterial bronchi may be detected on frontal chest radiographs, suggesting right isomerism, or bilateral hyparterial bronchi in the setting of left isomerism.[12] A right-sided aortic arch in the setting of right isomerism and azygos continuation of the IVC in left isomerism can both be detected on chest radiography.[10] Chest radiography may also detect the presence of anomalous pulmonary vessels in the setting of anomalous pulmonary venous return.[12]

Computed Tomography

Today, radiography may identify the presence of situs ambiguous, but cross-sectional imaging is necessary for more detailed categorization of the associated anatomic anomalies.[10] CT of the chest, abdomen, and pelvis readily characterizes and details situs and associated anatomic anomalies (Fig. 7.5). Contrast-enhanced CT allows assessment of cardiac and vascular structures in the setting of complex congenital heart defects and anomalous drainage.[12] CT and fluoroscopy may also detect the site of volvulus in complicated intestinal malrotation.

Magnetic Resonance Imaging

MRI demonstrates exquisite cardiac detail and is frequently used in the evaluation of congenital heart disease, particularly in identifying atrial morphology. In may be the preferred modality for evaluation of children given the risk of radiation exposure from CT.[12]

DIFFERENTIAL DIAGNOSIS

Findings in heterotaxy syndrome are variably present, and thus the differential diagnosis would include situs solitus with congenital heart disease (0.6%–0.8%),[10] right aortic arch, situs solitus with malrotation, hypogenetic lung (scimitar) syndrome, primary ciliary dyskinesia, and Kartagener syndrome.

SYNOPSIS OF TREATMENT OPTIONS

Treatment is determined by the severity and type of malformation present. Typically, early- and often-staged surgical intervention is used for severe cyanotic congenital heart disease.

KEY POINTS: BRONCHOPULMONARY ISOMERISM AND HETEROTAXY

- Situs solitus, situs inversus, and situs ambiguous (so-called heterotaxy) describe the thoracoabdominal visceral relationships, depending on the position of the cardiac atria and abdominal viscera relative to the midline.
- Bilateral eparterial or hyparterial bronchi (bronchial situs) is the most reliable predictor of atrial situs.
- Both right and left isomerisms have a strong association with congenital heart defects and intestinal malrotation, and more severe defects (more common with right isomerism) portend a poor prognosis.
- Common radiologic findings:
  - Radiographs may detect discordant positioning of the cardiac apex and gastric bubble, azygos continuation of the IVC, or anomalies of pulmonary venous drainage, which may raise suspicion for underlying heterotaxy.
  - CT and MR are frequently indicated to better characterize underlying associated visceral anomalies.

Bronchogenic Cyst

ETIOLOGY, PREVALENCE, AND EPIDEMIOLOGY

Bronchogenic cysts result from abnormal separation of localized portions of the tracheobronchial tree from the adjacent airways between the 3rd and 24th weeks of gestation. Most are isolated lesions but may be found in association with other congenital bronchopulmonary malformations, such as sequestration.[14] Approximately 75% to 90% are located in the mediastinum. Other locations include the lung parenchyma, pleura, diaphragm, neck, or abdomen.[5,7,14–16]

CLINICAL PRESENTATION

The majority of bronchogenic cysts are asymptomatic and found incidentally on a chest radiograph or CT. Symptoms are most frequently caused by compression of the trachea or bronchi, producing cough, wheezing, stridor, and pneumonia. Less commonly, bronchogenic cysts may compress the esophagus and lead to dysphagia or compress an adjacent pulmonary vein and result in localized pulmonary edema. Infection occurs in approximately 20% of patients with intraparenchymal cysts.[5] Less common manifestations of intraparenchymal cysts include hemoptysis and pneumothorax.

PATHOPHYSIOLOGY

Bronchogenic cysts are thin walled, unilocular, and roughly spherical in shape. They are filled with serous or mucoid fluid. The cyst wall is lined by respiratory epithelium and contains smooth muscle and cartilage.[14,16] Calcification may occur in the cyst wall or within the mucoid contents. Although bronchogenic cysts do not initially communicate with the tracheobronchial tree, communication may occur secondary to instrumentation or infection.

MANIFESTATIONS OF THE DISEASE

Radiography

Radiographically, mediastinal bronchogenic cysts are usually seen as round or oval mediastinal masses in the subcarinal (Fig. 7.6) or right paratracheal regions. Parenchymal bronchogenic cysts are typically sharply circumscribed, solitary, and round or oval and frequently located in the medial third of the lower lobes.[5,15] Serial radiographs usually show little change in size and shape with time, although slow growth can sometimes be observed over years. Bronchogenic cysts typically do not communicate with the tracheobronchial tree until they become infected. When

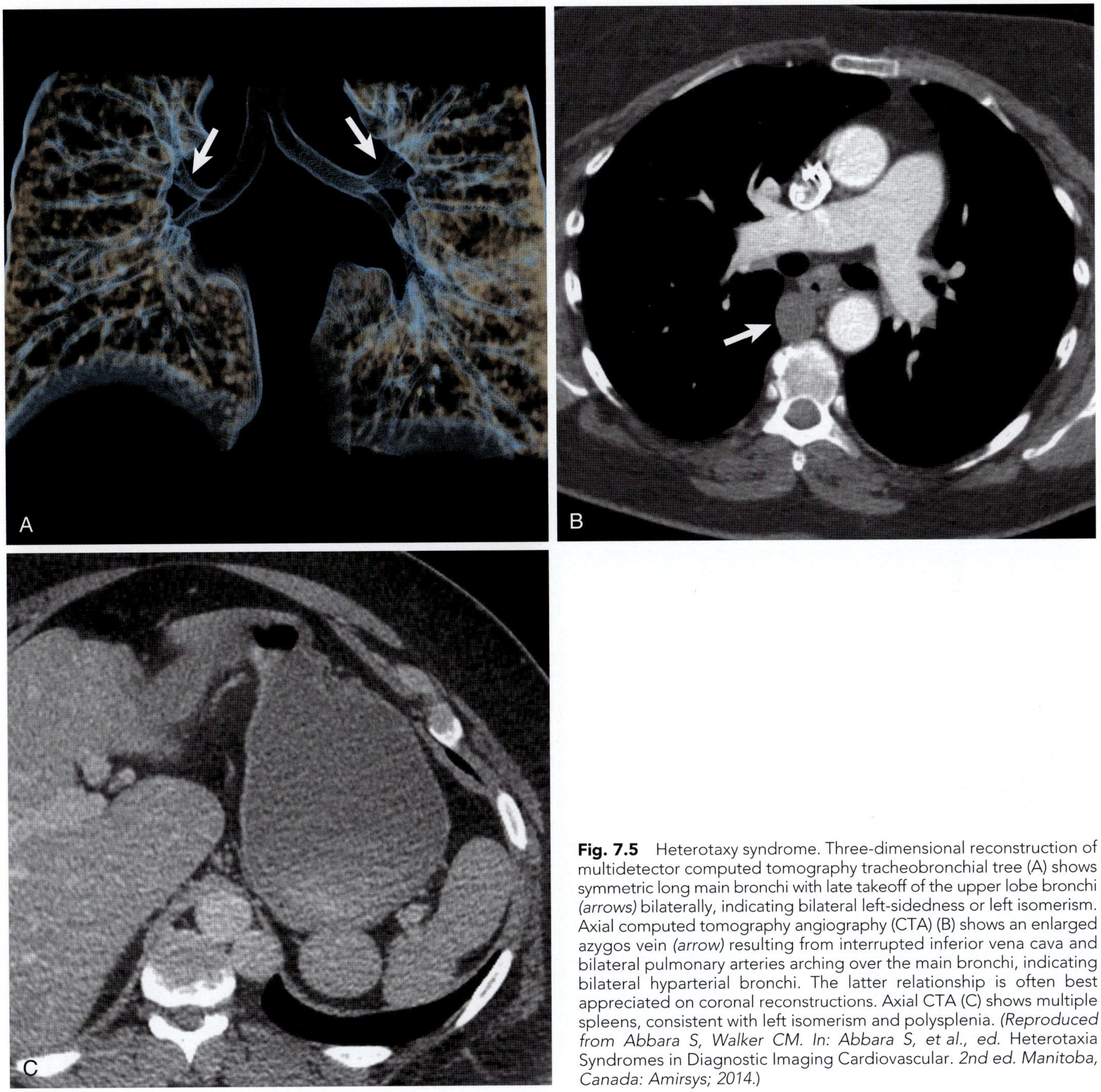

Fig. 7.5 Heterotaxy syndrome. Three-dimensional reconstruction of multidetector computed tomography tracheobronchial tree (A) shows symmetric long main bronchi with late takeoff of the upper lobe bronchi *(arrows)* bilaterally, indicating bilateral left-sidedness or left isomerism. Axial computed tomography angiography (CTA) (B) shows an enlarged azygos vein *(arrow)* resulting from interrupted inferior vena cava and bilateral pulmonary arteries arching over the main bronchi, indicating bilateral hyparterial bronchi. The latter relationship is often best appreciated on coronal reconstructions. Axial CTA (C) shows multiple spleens, consistent with left isomerism and polysplenia. *(Reproduced from Abbara S, Walker CM. In: Abbara S, et al., ed.* Heterotaxia Syndromes in Diagnostic Imaging Cardiovascular. *2nd ed. Manitoba, Canada: Amirsys; 2014.)*

communication is established, the cyst may contain air, with or without fluid.[5,7] Communication between a cyst and the tracheobronchial tree can produce a check-valve mechanism that may result in rapid expansion of the cyst.

Computed Tomography

In approximately 50% of cases the diagnosis of a benign cyst can be made confidently on CT, manifesting as a homogeneous fluid-density (0–20 Hounsfield units [HUs]) nonenhancing mass with a thin, smooth wall (see Fig. 7.6).[5,7,15] Mediastinal cysts tend to conform to the adjacent mediastinal structures, whereas pulmonary cysts displace the adjacent parenchyma. Increased cyst attenuation may result from the presence of protein, hemorrhage, or calcium oxalate within the mucoid cyst contents and may make the cyst indistinguishable from other masses. When infected, the cysts may have inhomogeneous enhancement and resemble an abscess or necrotic lymph node. Occasionally, bronchogenic cysts are air filled and multilocular, mimicking an abscess. The lung adjacent to bronchogenic cysts is frequently abnormal and shows areas of decreased attenuation and scarring.[5]

Magnetic Resonance Imaging

MRI is useful to determine the internal contents of cysts with equivocal CT features. Simple cysts typically manifest with low T1 and high T2 signal properties as cyst contents include predominantly serous fluid, whereas proteinaceous cysts may have higher T1 signal intensity. Regardless of the presence of high protein content, bronchogenic cysts characteristically have

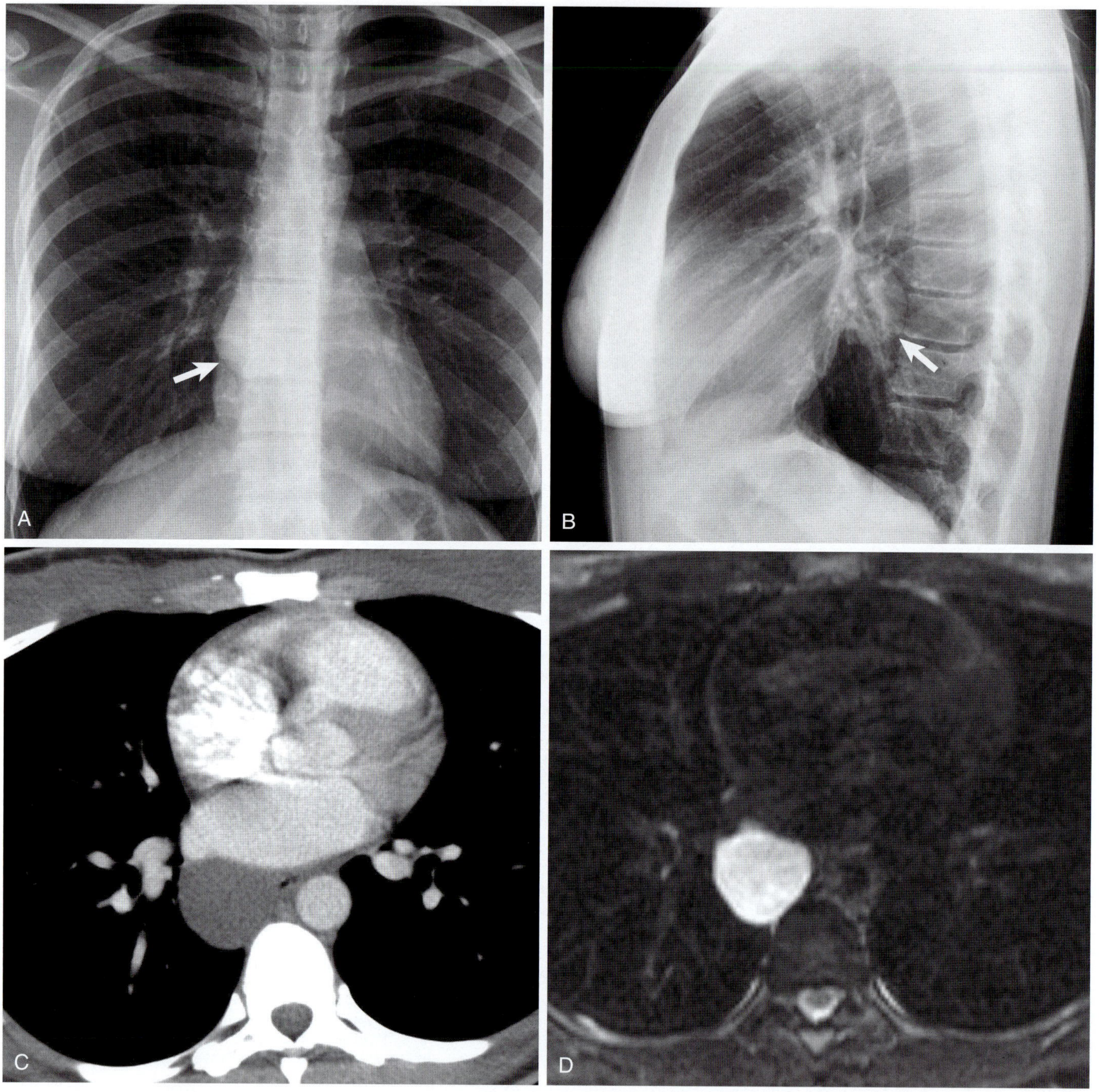

Fig. 7.6 Bronchogenic cyst. Posteroanterior (A) and lateral (B) chest radiographs show a well-circumscribed subcarinal mass *(arrows)*. Axial contrast-enhanced CT (C) shows a round, nonenhancing, homogeneous fluid-attenuating mass, which abuts the esophagus and posterior aspect of the left atrium. (D) T2-weighted MRI demonstrates high signal intensity throughout the lesion, consistent with simple fluid in this bronchogenic cyst.

homogeneous high signal intensity (approximating that of cerebrospinal fluid) on T2-weighted sequences (see Fig. 7.6).[5,14,15] When complicated by infection or hemorrhage, heterogeneous and variable signal intensity on both T1- and T2-weighted images may make the diagnosis less apparent.

Imaging Algorithm

Bronchogenic cysts are often first detected incidentally on routine chest radiography. However, it does not allow a confident diagnosis of bronchogenic cyst. Therefore CT or MRI is recommended for further evaluation. Because of the lack of radiation exposure and higher specificity, MRI is superior to CT in the evaluation of patients with suspected bronchogenic cysts. When neither CT nor MRI is diagnostic, the cystic nature can be confirmed by CT-guided needle aspiration of the cyst contents.

DIFFERENTIAL DIAGNOSIS

The differential diagnosis includes lung tumor, abscess, vascular malformation (e.g., arteriovenous malformation), and congenital pulmonary airway malformation. Bronchogenic cysts can usually be readily distinguished from lung tumor or vascular malformation by the characteristic water density on CT, homogeneous high signal intensity on T2-weighted MR images, and lack of enhancement. In the majority of cases these findings, together with the presence of a thin smooth wall, allow distinction of bronchogenic cysts from lung abscess. However, infected or hemorrhagic cysts may have heterogeneous appearance or signal intensity on CT and MRI, resembling lung abscesses. Bronchogenic cysts can generally be distinguished from congenital pulmonary airway malformations because they consist of a single cystic mass, whereas the latter usually consist of multiple cystic lesions with or without aberrant vascular supply.

SYNOPSIS OF TREATMENT OPTIONS

Despite the presence or absence of symptoms, management of bronchogenic cysts is typically surgical, in children and otherwise healthy young adults who are low risk for surgery. Although endobronchial cyst aspiration may be performed in symptomatic patients, surgical resection is usually necessary to prevent recurrence or rare malignant transformation. Nearly 50% of asymptomatic patients go on to develop symptoms or complications of the cyst, and malignancy has been found in 0.7% of cysts, justifying the aggressive surgical approach to these patients.[17] However, conservative management may also be considered in asymptomatic adult patients in whom a bronchogenic cyst is incidentally detected and close clinical and radiographic follow-up is possible.[14,17]

KEY POINTS: BRONCHOGENIC CYST

- Congenital cyst lined by respiratory epithelium, containing cartilage
- About 75% occur in the mediastinum, although can be found in the lung, or other locations along the primitive foregut
- Typical locations: subcarinal or paratracheal regions and lower lobes
- Common imaging findings:
  - Sharply circumscribed, round or oval mass on chest radiography
  - Water density on CT in about 50%
  - No enhancement after intravenous contrast on CT or MRI
  - Homogeneous high signal intensity on T2-weighted MR images in almost all cases
  - Air-fluid levels, rapid expansion, or enhancement should raise suspicion of superimposed infection or alternative diagnosis

Congenital Pulmonary Airway Malformation

ETIOLOGY, PREVALENCE, AND EPIDEMIOLOGY

CPAM is characterized by a cystic or noncystic mass of abnormal pulmonary tissue that results from early airway malformation. Although the exact pathogenesis is unknown, it has been postulated that CPAMs may represent either localized arrest in development or hamartomatous disorganization of the bronchial tree.[5] Previously referred to as congenital CCAM, the preferred nomenclature of the lesions along this pathologic spectrum is CPAM, as only three of the five entities are truly cystic, and only type III lesions consist of adenomatous tissue on histology.[8] The majority of CPAMs are diagnosed in infants and young children. However, cases have also been detected in adults up to 64 years of age.[18] The incidence of CPAM has been estimated to be 1 in 25,000 to 35,000 pregnancies.

CLINICAL PRESENTATION

The majority of cases are detected in the setting of neonatal respiratory distress. In adults CPAM may be an incidental finding or may be accompanied by symptoms related to recurrent respiratory infections, such as cough and fever.[5,7] Less common complications include pneumothorax and malignant degeneration.[5]

PATHOPHYSIOLOGY

Three main pathologic subtypes of CPAM have been classically described. Less common type 0 and type IV CPAMs have been recently added and highlight a spectrum of airway malformations, each with unique morphology and prognosis.[8,16] Type I CPAMs derive from bronchial or bronchiolar tissue and comprise the majority of adult cases, manifesting as a large (>2 cm) cyst, often multiloculated and sometimes associated with several smaller cysts. Type II lesions contain more uniform small cysts, less than 2 cm in diameter of bronchial origin. Type III lesions are large, solid-appearing lesions and manifest microscopically as tiny cysts and adenomatous elements of bronchiolar and alveolar ducts.[5,8,16] Cyst walls exhibit a bronchiolar-type epithelial lining and contain smooth muscle, usually no cartilage, fluid, air, or both. Type 0 and type IV CPAMs result from dysgenesis of either central large airway (trachea or bronchi) or peripheral acini, respectively. Radiographic features of type 0 and type IV CPAMs are less well defined, as patients with type 0 CPAM are not imaged prior to their early death. Type IV CPAM is composed of a large unlined cyst, differentiating it pathologically from the often radiographically indistinguishable type I CPAM. CPAMs may involve any lobe but are most common in the lower lobes.

MANIFESTATIONS OF THE DISEASE

Radiography

The radiologic manifestations in infants and young children are variable. In older children and adults CPAMs usually appear radiologically as a unilocular or multiloculated cyst or as a complex soft tissue and cystic mass.[5,7] Occasionally, one cyst expands preferentially and creates a single lucent area (Fig. 7.7). Large CPAMs may exhibit mass effect, resulting in compression of adjacent lung tissue or mediastinal shift.[8] Pneumonia in the surrounding parenchyma may lead to obscuration of the malformation or the development of fluid levels (Fig. 7.8). CPAMs usually receive blood from pulmonary arteries and drain via pulmonary veins. However, systemic blood supply has been described in hybrid lesions that share features with sequestration (discussed subsequently).

Computed Tomography

CT manifestations in adults typically consist of a unilocular or multiloculated cyst or a complex soft tissue and cystic mass, ranging from 4 to 12 cm in diameter (see Figs. 7.7 and 7.8).[5,7] Type I lesions have at least one cyst greater than 2 cm in diameter. Type II malformations are characterized by multiple thin-walled cysts, ranging from 2 to 20 mm in diameter (Fig. 7.9).

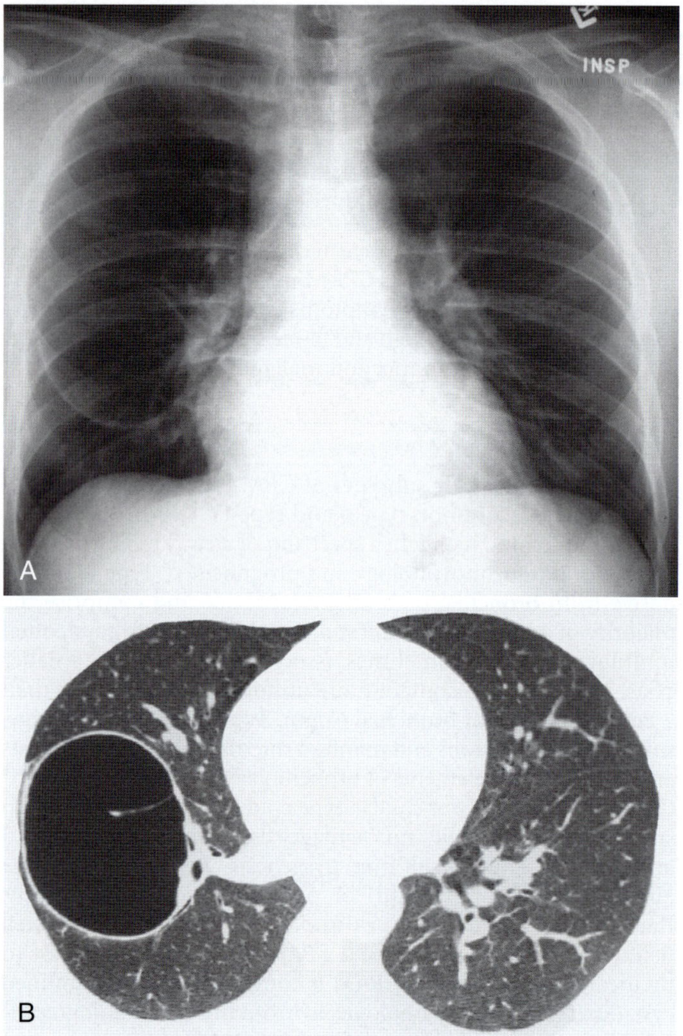

Fig. 7.7 Congenital pulmonary airway malformation, type I. A posteroanterior chest radiograph (A) shows a large cystic lesion in the right lower lobe. CT (B) revealed a thin-walled cyst with septation.

Imaging Algorithm

In some patients the radiographic findings are suggestive of the diagnosis. However, CT is superior to chest radiography in demonstrating both the cystic and the solid components of CPAMs and is performed almost routinely in the evaluation of adults with cystic lung lesions. Contrast-enhanced CT delineates the arterial supply and venous drainage.

DIFFERENTIAL DIAGNOSIS

The main differential diagnoses are lung abscess, bronchogenic cyst, sequestration, and cystic lung cancer. The presence of multiple thin-walled complex cystic masses usually allows reliable distinction from bronchogenic cysts, which are typically isolated. In the presence of air-fluid levels, radiologic findings may mimic those of a lung abscess. Differentiation can often be made by the lack of clinical symptoms of fever and productive cough and the lack of change over a several-week period. However, infected CPAMs may be indistinguishable from lung abscess. Pulmonary arterial supply to these lesions can help differentiate them from sequestration, which typically receive systemic arterial blood supply from the aorta.

SYNOPSIS OF TREATMENT OPTIONS

Because the majority of cases are associated with recurrent infection and risk for the development of carcinoma, CPAMs are usually removed surgically.[5,8,19] Although controversial, others have proposed a conservative management approach in asymptomatic adults diagnosed incidentally.[19]

KEY POINTS: CONGENITAL PULMONARY AIRWAY MALFORMATION

- A heterogeneous, complex congenital malformation, typically cystic, containing smooth muscle but generally no cartilage.
- The vast majority are diagnosed in early childhood and only occasionally are seen in adults.
- Common radiologic findings:
  - Radiographs usually show a cystic or solid mass in the lower lobe that consists of numerous air-containing cysts.
  - CT findings in adults typically consist of multiple thin-walled, complex cystic masses, ranging from 4 to 12 cm in diameter.

Congenital Lobar Overinflation

ETIOLOGY, PREVALENCE, AND EPIDEMIOLOGY

Congenital lobar overinflation (CLO), or congenital lobar hyperinflation, manifests as progressive overdistention of a lobe thought to be a result of partial endoluminal obstruction, creating a one-way ball valve mechanism with resultant air trapping.[5,7] Antiquated nomenclature for this disease included congenital/infantile lobar emphysema, which is inaccurate, as true alveolar destruction is not present. Bronchial obstruction may be the result of an intrinsic cartilage deficiency, luminal web, or extraluminal compression (e.g., bronchogenic cyst or pulmonary vessel). An abnormal increase in the number of alveoli may be identified in a subset of patients with CLO.[5]

CLINICAL PRESENTATION

CLO is typically diagnosed in the neonatal period and infancy, although up to 10% of cases are not discovered until adolescence or adulthood.[5,7] Males are more frequently affected. Patients may present with varying degrees of respiratory compromise, ranging from neonatal respiratory distress to mild dyspnea and wheezing in adults.

MANIFESTATIONS OF THE DISEASE

Radiography

The radiologic findings center around the presence of a hyperinflated lobe, with predilection for the left upper lobe, followed by the right middle and right upper lobes (Fig. 7.10) in decreasing prevalence.[5] The expanded lobe often exerts mass effect within the confines of the chest, leading to varying degrees of mediastinal shift, vascular attenuation, and compressive atelectasis of the adjacent lung. In newborns the affected lobe may initially appear opaque, becoming progressively lucent as retained fetal fluid is reabsorbed. CLO may uncommonly be bilateral or multifocal.[5,7]

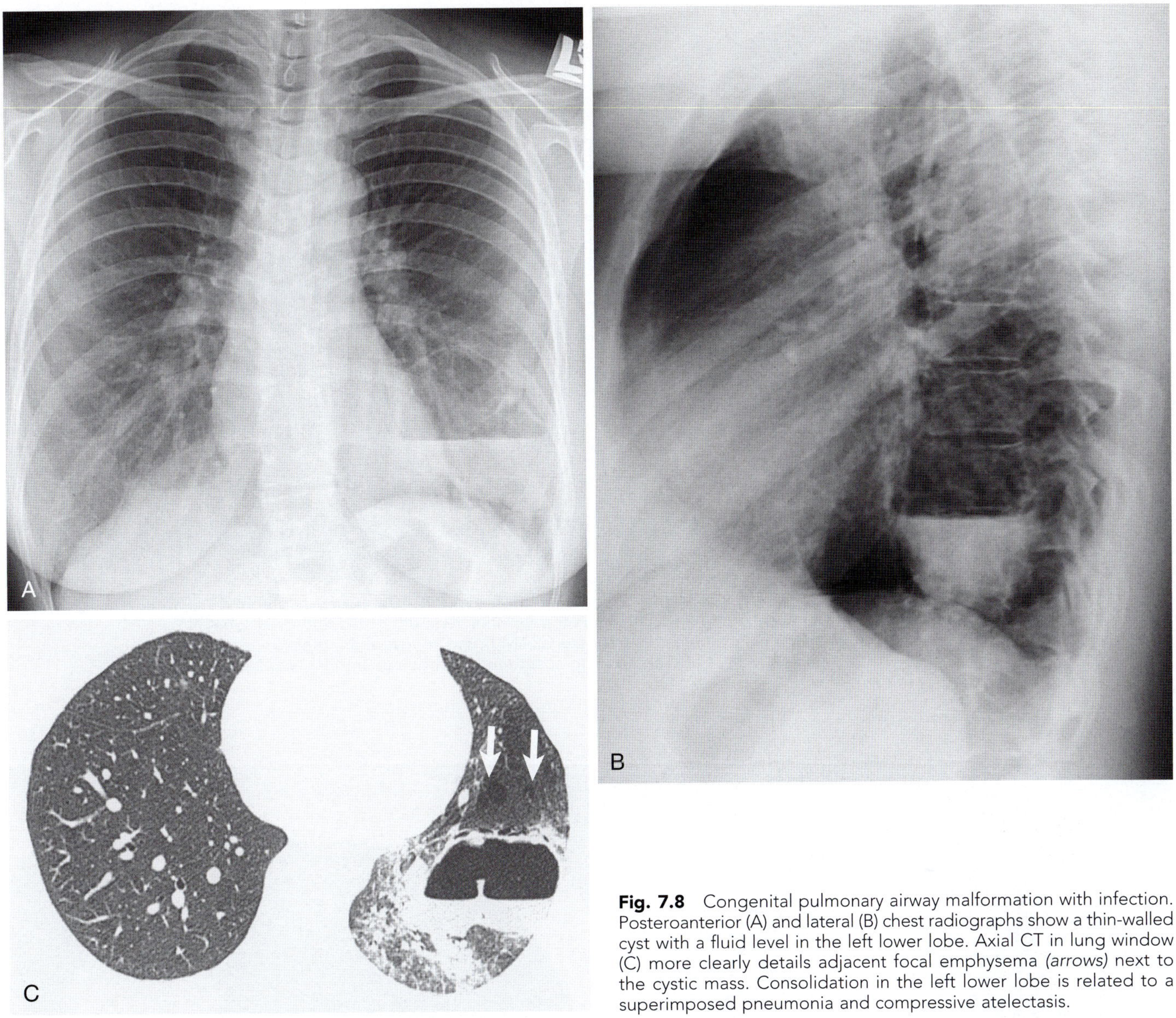

Fig. 7.8 Congenital pulmonary airway malformation with infection. Posteroanterior (A) and lateral (B) chest radiographs show a thin-walled cyst with a fluid level in the left lower lobe. Axial CT in lung window (C) more clearly details adjacent focal emphysema *(arrows)* next to the cystic mass. Consolidation in the left lower lobe is related to a superimposed pneumonia and compressive atelectasis.

Computed Tomography

CT findings of CLO reflect the radiographic abnormalities (see Fig. 7.10). However, CT better defines attenuated vasculature supplying the affected lobe, as well as details structural compromise related to mediastinal shift and compression.[7]

Magnetic Resonance Imaging

CLO may be diagnosed in utero with fetal MR or ultrasound and manifests as a homogeneously hyperintense mass on T2-weighted images on MR and hyperechoic mass on US.[5,8] These modalities are not typically necessary for diagnosis in adults.

DIFFERENTIAL DIAGNOSIS

The differential diagnosis includes endoluminal obstruction from a mass, aspirated foreign body, or mucous plug; extraluminal compression of a bronchus by a mass; bronchial atresia with overinflation from collateral ventilation (not a ball-valve mechanism); CPAM; or Swyer-James-McLeod syndrome.

SYNOPSIS OF TREATMENT OPTIONS

Treatment depends on the clinical manifestations of disease, with lobectomy in cases of acute neonatal respiratory distress. Patients with mild or no symptoms may be managed with conservative, supportive therapy as these lesions may often gradually reduce in size.[5,8]

Sequestration

ETIOLOGY, PREVALENCE, AND EPIDEMIOLOGY

Pulmonary sequestration (intralobar or extralobar) is a malformation in which a portion of nonfunctioning lung tissue (probably

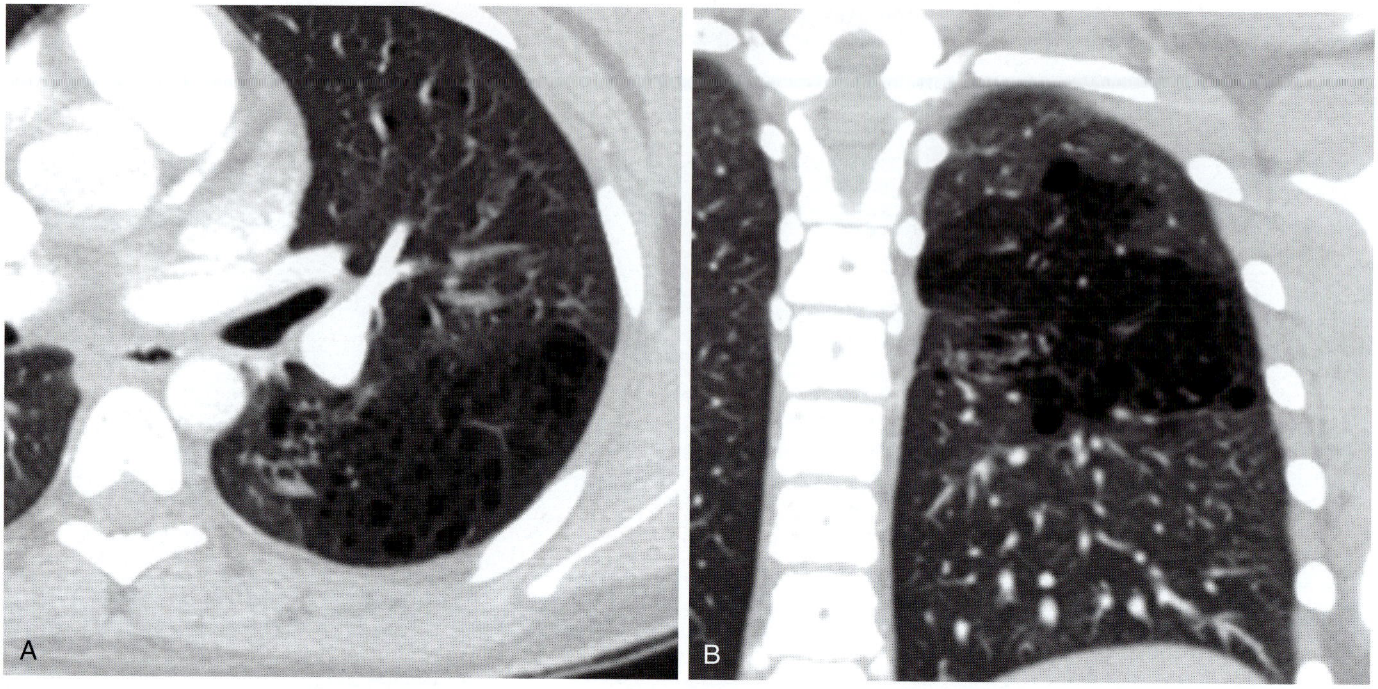

Fig. 7.9 Congenital pulmonary airway malformation (CPAM), type II. Axial (A) and coronal (B) CT show a low-density lesion with multiple small cysts in the superior segment of the left lower lobe. No anomalous artery was found, which helps differentiate CPAM from sequestration. *(Reproduced from Walker CM, Wu CC, Gilman MD, et al. The imaging spectrum of bronchopulmonary sequestration.* Curr Probl Diagn Radiol. *2014;43:100-114.)*

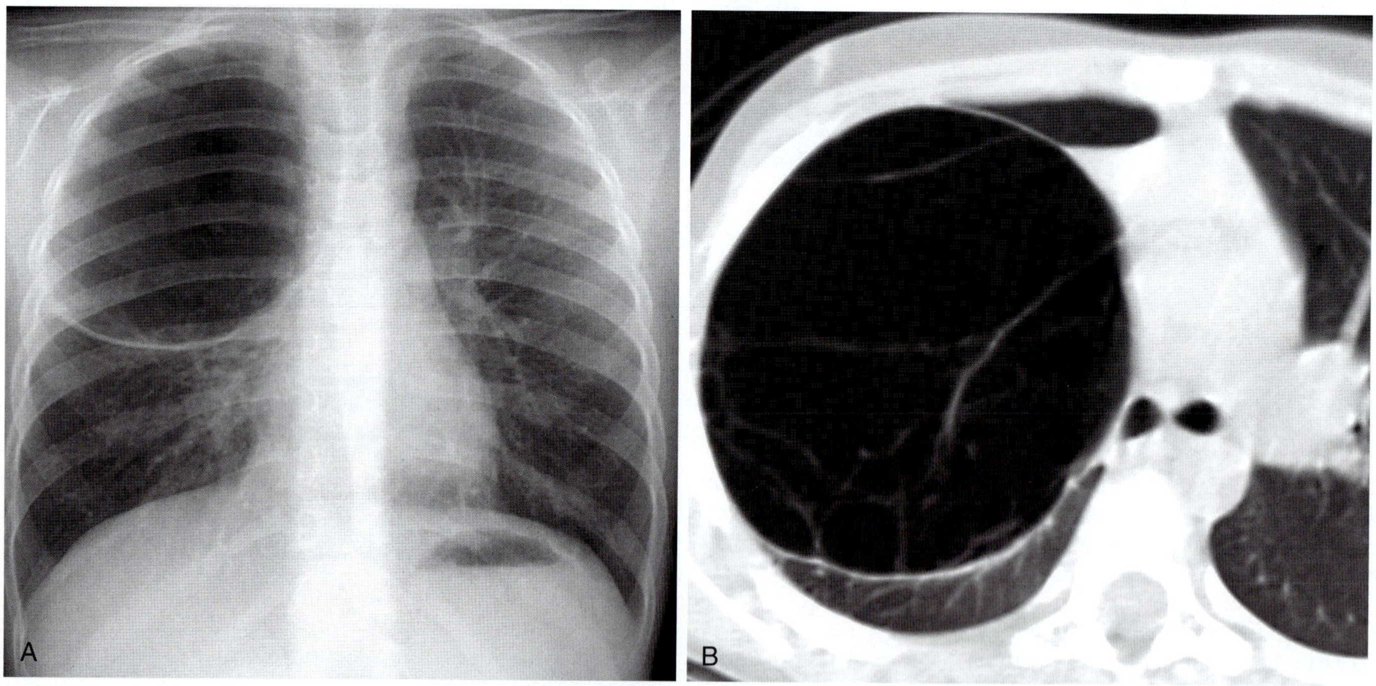

Fig. 7.10 Congenital lobar overinflation (CLO). (A) Chest radiograph shows asymmetric hyperlucency of the right upper lobe and mild left mediastinal shift. (B) Axial image from chest CT in lung window shows severe overinflation of the right upper lobe. CLO occurs most commonly in the left upper lobe but may be seen in any lobe. *(Reproduced from Stowell J, Walker C. Congenital thoracic malformations. In: Shepard JO, ed.* Thoracic Imaging: The Requisites. *3rd ed. Philadelphia: Elsevier; 2018.)*

KEY POINTS: CONGENITAL LOBAR OVERINFLATION

- Most commonly involves the left upper lobe, similar to bronchial atresia
- Common radiologic findings:
  - Chest radiography typically shows hyperlucency, decreased vascularity, and air trapping from a ball-valve effect within the affected segment.
  - CT shows segmental or lobar overinflation and hypovascularity, mediastinal shift, and compressive atelectasis of the adjacent lung.
- Congenital lobar emphysema is a misnomer, as alveolar architecture is preserved.

an accessory lung bud) lacks tracheobronchial continuity with the remaining normal lung and receives its blood supply from a systemic artery, often from primitive foregut vasculature.[5,8,20] In intralobar sequestrations (ILSs) the detached tissue is contained within the same visceral pleural envelope, whereas extralobar sequestrations (ELSs) are enclosed within a unique pleural membrane separate from the native lung.

Although ILSs detected on prenatal imaging are considered as congenital in etiology,[8,20] other authors believe that the majority of ILSs diagnosed in adults are acquired lesions secondary to chronic bronchial obstruction and recurrent infection, in which case arterial supply to these lesions derives from neoangiogenesis and parasitization of systemic vasculature in the infected tissue.[21] ILSs are occasionally associated with other congenital lung anomalies and are usually first recognized in adolescents and young adults. In contradistinction, ELSs are generally regarded by all authors as congenital and are more frequently associated with other congenital abnormalities, such as congenital diaphragmatic anomalies, congenital heart disease, and CPAM.[5,8,21]

Pulmonary sequestrations are rare and account for 0.15% to 6% of pulmonary malformations.[21] Because ELS is commonly associated with other congenital abnormalities, it is usually diagnosed during the neonatal period. ILS is generally diagnosed later in childhood and in young adults but may also be found incidentally in the middle-aged and elderly.

CLINICAL PRESENTATION

Pulmonary sequestrations first recognized in adults are usually asymptomatic, the abnormality being found incidentally on a chest radiograph or CT. The most common clinical manifestations are related to superimposed infection, in which case the signs and symptoms are those of acute lower lobe pneumonia, chest pain, or hemoptysis.[5,21] ILS should be suspected in young adults with nonresolving or recurrent lower lobe pneumonia. Clinically, the main differential diagnosis in these cases is bronchiectasis and lung abscess. Because ELSs do not communicate with the lung, they seldom become infected and are therefore usually asymptomatic.

PATHOPHYSIOLOGY

Pathologically, congenital ILSs are contained within normal lung but do not communicate with the normal bronchi.[5,8,21] Acquired ILSs exhibit connection with the native tracheobronchial tree and thus are not anatomically sequestered. Furthermore, the vessels supplying acquired ILSs are thin and irregular, as opposed to larger, well-defined arteries supplying congenital ILSs. Some clinicians have therefore classified these acquired lesions that mimic sequestration pathologically as "pseudosequestration."[21] ILSs derive arterial supply from the aorta or one of its branches, most commonly the descending thoracic aorta, although generally solitary, multiple tributary vessels may be seen in up to 20% of cases.[21] Typically, the anomalous vessel enters the lung via the lower part of the pulmonary ligament and is much larger than would be expected for the volume of tissue supplied. Venous drainage is almost always via the pulmonary venous system, with a left-to-left shunt usually being produced. The vast majority are situated in the posterior basal segment of a lower lobe, approximately two-thirds being on the left and a third on the right. ILSs usually consist of one or more cystic spaces with a variable amount of intervening solid tissue. The cysts resemble dilated bronchi and are usually filled with mucus or pus.

ELSs are completely enclosed by a pleural membrane.[5,8] Approximately two-thirds abut the left hemidiaphragm and may be subpulmonic, subdiaphragmatic, or, less commonly, contained within the hemidiaphragm. ELSs are composed histologically of immature disorganized lung tissue and a few airways that lack connection with the normal tracheobronchial tree. They derive their arterial supply from the aorta or one of its branches and drain via systemic veins.

MANIFESTATIONS OF THE DISEASE

Radiography

The most common radiographic manifestation of ELS and ILS is a homogeneous opacity in the posterior basal segment of the lower lobes that is often contiguous with the hemidiaphragm (Fig. 7.11).[5,21] Less common findings include a focal area of lucency, bronchiectasis, a solitary or multicystic mass, or prominent vessels in the lower lobe (Fig. 7.12). An air-containing cystic mass, with or without fluid levels, is typically seen when infection has resulted in fistulation with the bronchial tree. When pneumonia occurs, it usually affects the surrounding parenchyma and obscures the sequestration; in fact, the cystic nature of the mass may not become apparent until the pneumonia resolves.

Computed Tomography

The most common CT manifestation of ILS is a focal mass or consolidation, almost always in the posterior basal segment of the left lower lobe (see Fig. 7.11).[21,22] Less common findings include a cyst or cluster of cysts (Fig. 7.13), dilated vessels, mucoid impaction, or foci of calcification. ELS manifests as a homogeneous airless opacity or well-circumscribed soft tissue–density mass on CT (Fig. 7.14); cystic areas are seen occasionally.[21,22] The lung adjacent to sequestrations may have focal areas of hyperlucency and air trapping.

Multiplanar and volumetric reformation of axial thin-section, contrast-enhanced CT or CT angiography (CTA) data allows accurate assessment of the systemic arterial supply in the majority of cases (see Figs. 7.11, 7.13, and 7.14).[21,22] The typical course of the anomalous vessel extends from the lower thoracic or upper abdominal aorta through the inferior pulmonary ligament into the sequestered lung.

Magnetic Resonance Imaging

For differentiating the cystic, solid, hemorrhagic, and mucous components of the mass, MRI is better than CT. MR angiography

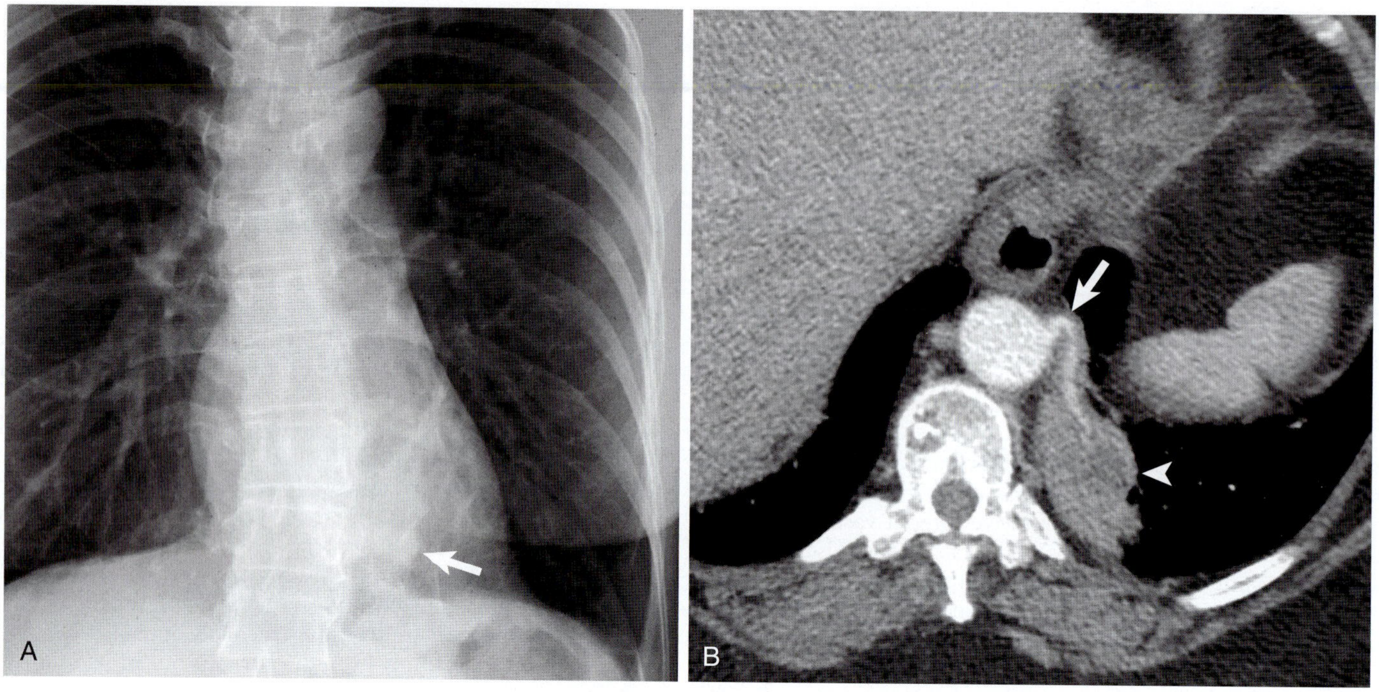

Fig. 7.11 Intralobar sequestration. (A) Chest radiograph shows a mass-like lesion *(arrow)* in the left retrocardiac region, abutting the left hemidiaphragm. (B) Axial contrast-enhanced CT demonstrates an aberrant systemic artery *(arrow)* arising from the descending thoracic aorta supplying the mass of sequestered lung tissue *(arrowhead)*. *(Reproduced from Stowell J, Walker C. Congenital thoracic malformations. In: Shepard JO, ed.* Thoracic Imaging: The Requisites. *3rd ed. Philadelphia: Elsevier; 2018.)*

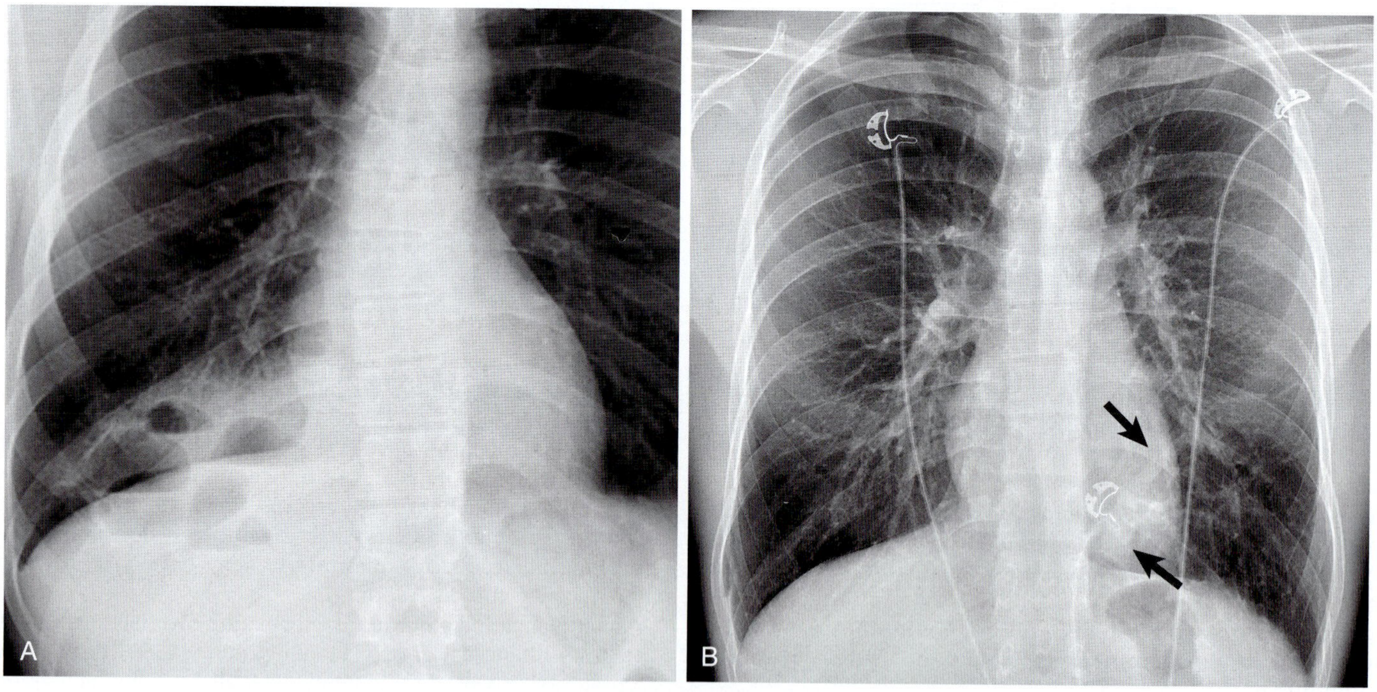

Fig. 7.12 Intralobar sequestration: radiographic manifestations. (A) Posteroanterior chest radiograph shows a multiloculated cystic lesion in the right lower lobe with several air/fluid levels. (B) Posteroanterior chest radiograph from a different patient shows subtle hyperlucency in the left lower lung zone and a large tubular structure *(arrows)* extending from the descending thoracic aorta. Small right pneumothorax is also noted. *(Reproduced from Walker CM, Wu CC, Gilman MD, et al. The imaging spectrum of bronchopulmonary sequestration.* Curr Probl Diagn Radiol. *2014;43:100-114.)*

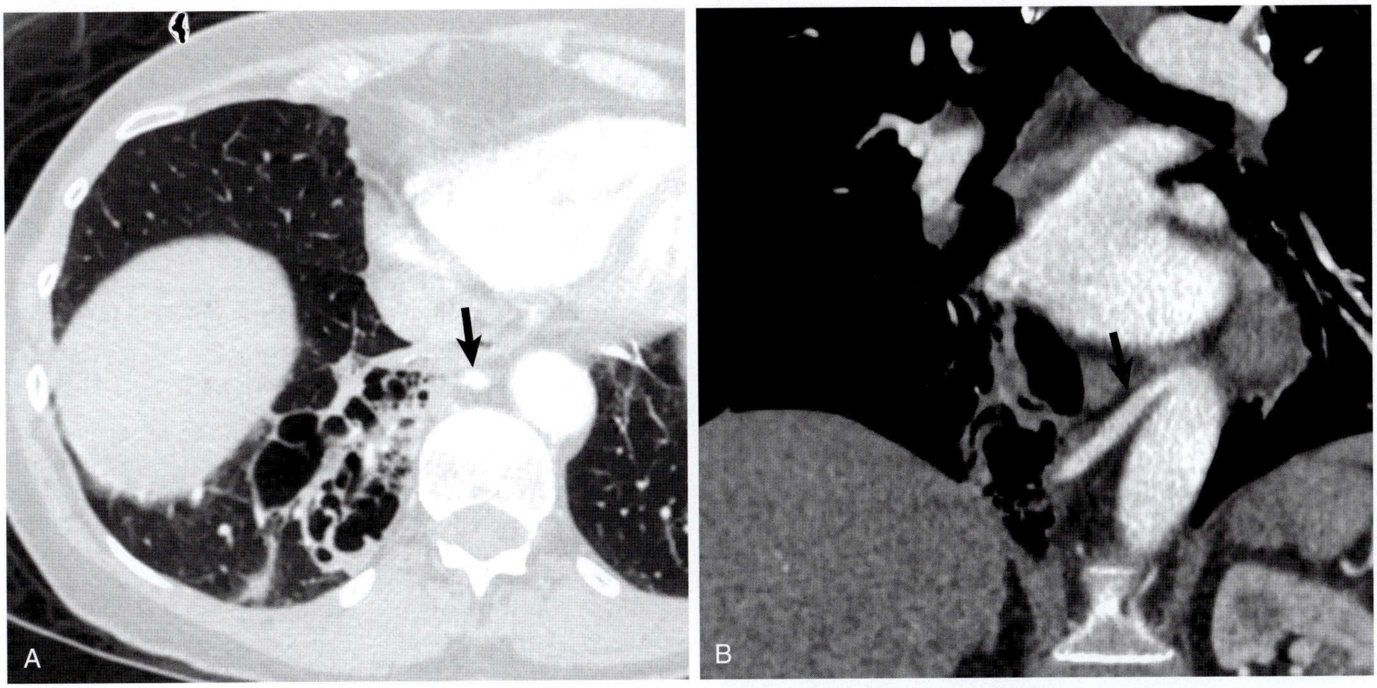

Fig. 7.13 Intralobar sequestration: CT manifestations. Axial (A) and (B) coronal contrast-enhanced CT scans show an aberrant artery *(arrows)* from the descending thoracic aorta supplying a medial right lower lobe mixed cystic and solid mass. *(Reproduced from Stowell J, Walker C. Congenital thoracic malformations. In: Shepard JO, ed.* Thoracic Imaging: The Requisites. *3rd ed. Philadelphia: Elsevier; 2018.)*

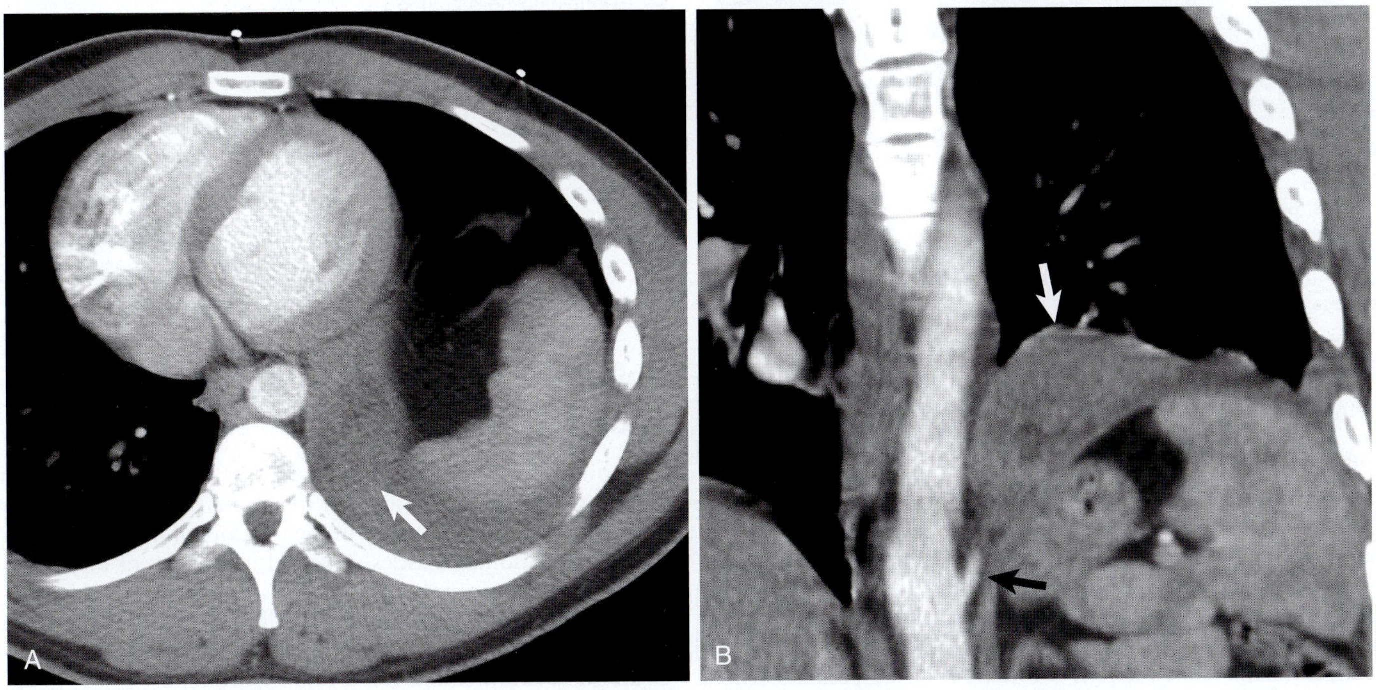

Fig. 7.14 Torsion of extralobar sequestration. Axial (A) and coronal (B) contrast-enhanced CT shows an extrapleural mass *(white arrow)* adjacent to the left hemidiaphragm, supplied by an aberrant artery from the descending thoracic aorta. Abrupt truncation of the anomalous artery *(black arrow)* raised suspicion of torsion of the sequestration, which was confirmed at surgery and on pathology.

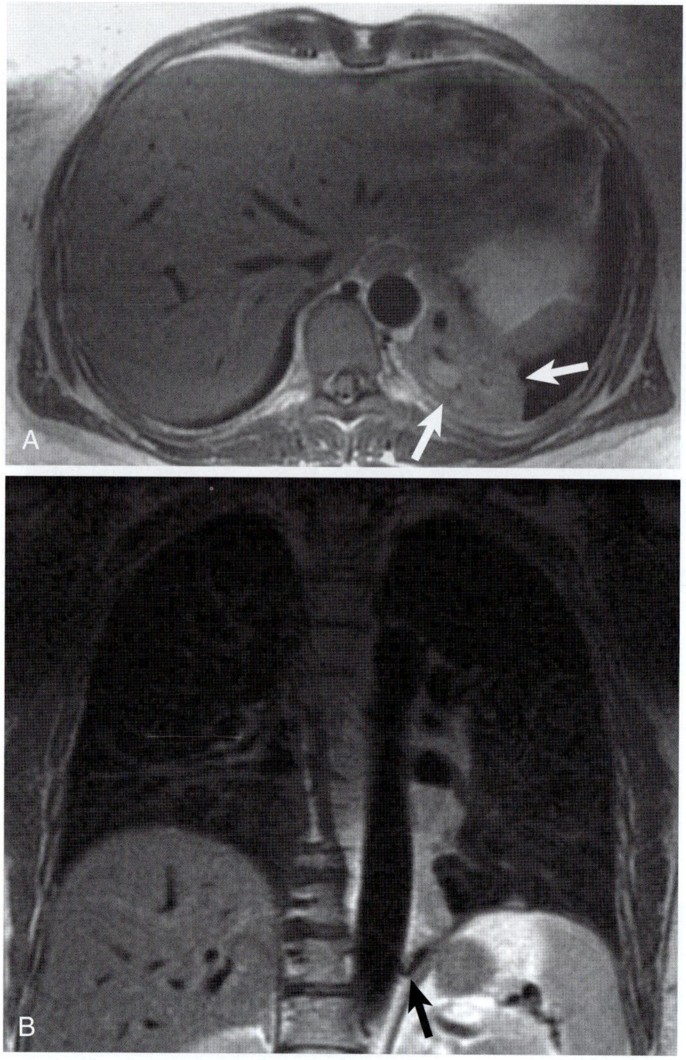

Fig. 7.15 Intralobar sequestration: MRI findings. (A) Axial T1-weighted image shows a left lower lobe medial basal segmental consolidation with intermediate signal intensity *(arrows)*. A coronal T1-weighted image (B) demonstrates an abnormal vessel *(arrow)* from the descending thoracic aorta, supplying the area of consolidation, consistent with intralobar sequestration.

(MRA) can also accurately demonstrate the vascular supply and drainage to the azygos or hemiazygos veins or IVC (Fig. 7.15).[23,24]

Imaging Algorithm

In the majority of patients, pulmonary sequestration is first suspected by the presence of a homogeneous opacity or cystic mass in a lower lobe that abuts the diaphragm. Because of the radiation risk associated with CT in children and young adults and because MRA provides excellent visualization of the anomalous vessels supplying the sequestered lung, MRA is recommended as the modality of choice in the evaluation of patients with suspected lobar sequestration.[21,23] In clinical practice, however, the differential diagnosis often includes abnormalities that are better seen on CT, such as bronchiectasis.

DIFFERENTIAL DIAGNOSIS

The differential diagnosis of pulmonary sequestration includes recurrent pneumonia, bronchial obstruction secondary to a neoplasm or foreign body, recurrent atelectasis, lung abscess, bronchogenic cyst, and CPAM. The essential feature in the differential diagnosis is demonstration of the systemic arterial supply to the abnormal lung. More than one bronchopulmonary malformation may coexist (so-called hybrid lesions), most commonly described with ELS and type 2 CPAM,[5,21] although bronchial atresia, bronchogenic cysts, and CLO are occasionally detected.[5] Sequestration should be differentiated from other conditions that exhibit anomalous systemic arterial supply, such as hypogenetic lung syndrome (scimitar or pulmonary venolobar syndrome) or isolated systemic arterial supply to normal lung.[21]

SYNOPSIS OF TREATMENT OPTIONS

Surgical resection is the treatment of choice for patients with infection or symptoms resulting from compression of normal lung tissue. The majority of investigators also recommend surgical resection (typically lobectomy) of asymptomatic ILS because of the risk of recurrent infection, hemoptysis, and the potential need for more extensive resection if the sequestration becomes chronically infected. However, controversy exists as to the management of asymptomatic, incidentally discovered ELS. In these cases some advocate serial imaging surveillance in 5- to 10-year intervals with CT or MR.[21]

KEY POINTS: INTRALOBAR AND EXTRALOBAR SEQUESTRATION

- By definition, a portion of lung is detached from the remaining normal lung.
- ILS is contiguous with the adjacent lung, whereas ELS is invested by a unique pleural envelope.
- ILS and ELS derive their arterial supply from the aorta; venous drainage of intralobar sequestrations is via pulmonary veins, and drainage of extralobar sequestrations is via systemic veins.
- ILS accounts for about 80% of cases.
- Both types of sequestration occur most frequently in the left lower lobe, adjacent to the hemidiaphragm.
- Anomalous vasculature to and from sequestrations can be better characterized and delineated with CTA or MRA.

Pulmonary Underdevelopment

ETIOLOGY, PREVALENCE, AND EPIDEMIOLOGY

Pulmonary underdevelopment (lung agenesis-hypoplasia complex) refers to a spectrum of incomplete lung development, thought to occur from insults to the developing tracheobronchial tree and pulmonary tissues. Arrested development of the lung can be classified into three types: (1) *agenesis,* in which there is complete absence of one lung, including all bronchial, vascular, and parenchymal tissue; (2) *aplasia,* in which there is suppression of all but a rudimentary blind-ending bronchus; and (3) *hypoplasia,* in which there is a reduction in the number or size of airways, vessels, and alveoli.[2,5,8]

Unilateral agenesis or aplasia occurs in approximately 1 in 10,000 individuals and unilateral hypoplasia in 1 to 2 per 10,000 births. Pulmonary hypoplasia is often associated with anomalies of the ipsilateral pulmonary artery and anomalous pulmonary venous drainage (hypogenetic lung syndrome) and is therefore discussed in Chapter 8.

CLINICAL PRESENTATION

The majority of patients with pulmonary agenesis or aplasia die of associated congenital malformations in the neonatal period. However, patients may occasionally survive to adulthood with minimal or no symptoms. Patients with pulmonary hypoplasia not associated with vascular anomalies may be asymptomatic or exhibit pneumothorax, shortness of breath, or respiratory failure. Affected patients are predisposed to recurrent respiratory infections during childhood.

MANIFESTATIONS OF THE DISEASE

Radiography

The radiographic findings in cases of agenesis, aplasia, or severe hypoplasia are characterized by total or almost total absence of aerated lung in one hemithorax (Fig. 7.16).[5] The markedly reduced volume results in elevation of the ipsilateral hemidiaphragm, ipsilateral shift of the mediastinum, and approximation of the ribs. In most cases the contralateral lung is greatly overinflated and displaced, along with the anterior mediastinum, across the midline into the involved hemithorax.

Computed Tomography

Pulmonary agenesis, aplasia, and hypoplasia can be diagnosed by CT (see Fig. 7.16). In patients with aplasia, CT can demonstrate the rudimentary bronchus, as well as absence of the ipsilateral pulmonary artery; in those with hypoplasia, it can demonstrate the patent bronchus, the pulmonary artery, and the hypoplastic lung.[5,7]

Magnetic Resonance Imaging

Pulmonary underdevelopment can be diagnosed by MRI, particularly gadolinium-enhanced three-dimensional MRA, revealing the absence of lung parenchyma, bronchial tree, and pulmonary vessels on the affected side.[25]

DIFFERENTIAL DIAGNOSIS

The main differential diagnosis of pulmonary underdevelopment is pneumonectomy performed during early childhood, as radiologic findings may be identical. Other considerations include total atelectasis from any cause, severe bronchiectasis with collapse, and advanced fibrothorax—all easily differentiated with CT. The main differential diagnosis of hypoplastic lung is Swyer-James-McLeod syndrome. Although both conditions are associated with unilateral low lung volume, patients with Swyer-James-McLeod syndrome demonstrate air trapping on expiratory CT.

SYNOPSIS OF TREATMENT OPTIONS

As most cases of pulmonary underdevelopment are diagnosed incidentally in asymptomatic adults, no treatment is necessary. However, in the setting of recurrent infection or associated congenital anomalies, corrective surgery may be considered.[26]

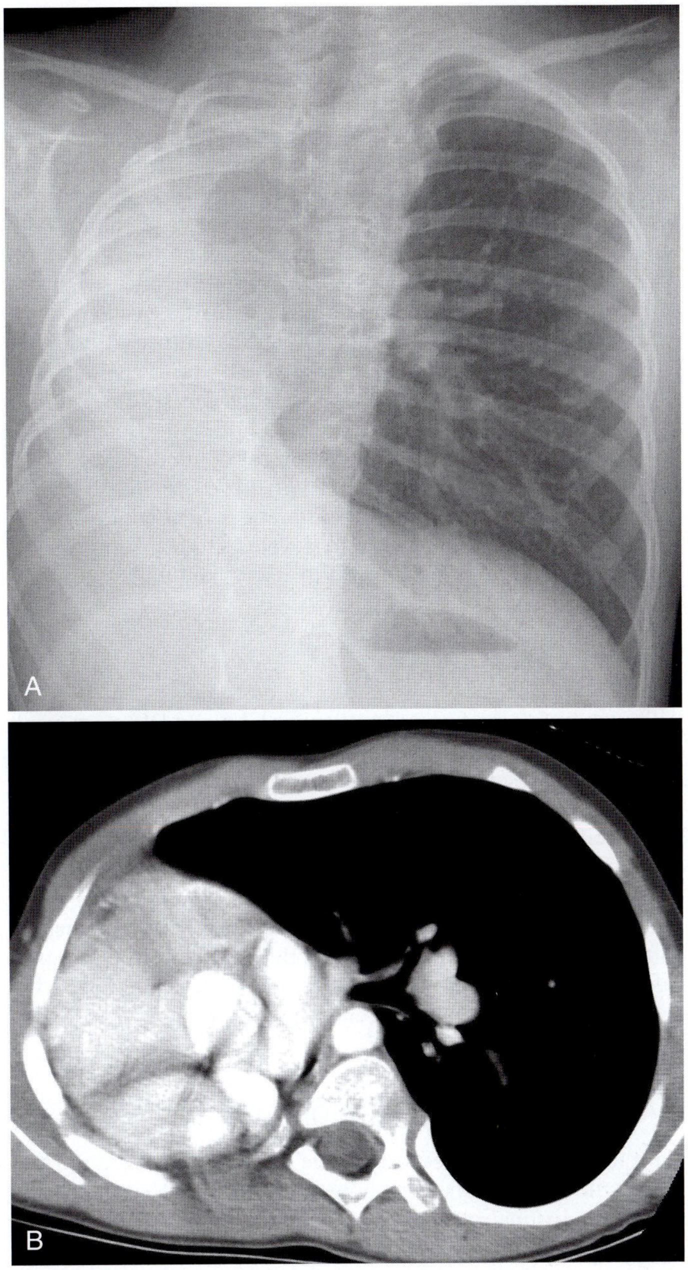

Fig. 7.16 Pulmonary agenesis. (A) Posteroanterior chest radiograph shows complete absence of the right lung, pronounced rightward mediastinal shift, and compensatory left lung hyperinflation. (B) Axial contrast-enhanced chest CT shows complete absence of pulmonary tissue, bronchi, and pulmonary vessels in the right hemithorax, consistent with pulmonary agenesis. *(Reproduced from Stowell J, Walker C. Congenital thoracic malformations. In: Shepard JO, ed.* Thoracic Imaging: The Requisites. *3rd ed. Philadelphia: Elsevier; 2018.)*

Congenital Lymphatic Malformation

Primary lymphatic disorders are rare, resulting from developmental errors of the lymphatic system during early embryogenesis.[27] Although uncertainty of their exact pathogenesis complicates classification and nomenclature, most are considered under the spectrum of lymphatic malformations.[28] However, distinct entities have been historically recognized, including lymphangioma, lymphangiectasis, lymphangiomatosis, lymphatic dysplasia syndrome, and other primary lymphatic disorders (e.g., lymphangioleiomyomatosis). Here we emphasize thoracic lymphangiomatosis, as lymphangioma is discussed in Chapter 77, and primary pulmonary lymphangiectasis occurs in the neonatal period and is rapidly fatal.

ETIOLOGY, PREVALENCE, AND EPIDEMIOLOGY

Lymphangiomatosis has been recently renamed generalized lymphatic anomaly (GLA) by the International Society for the Study of Vascular Anomalies.[28] Although a lymphangioma is defined as a focal multicystic proliferation of mature, expanded anastomosing lymphatic tissue, GLA is more widespread, often involving multiple organ systems to variable extents. Both lymphangioma and GLA likely represent sequestered remnant lymphatic tissues that failed to connect with or arose from primordial lymphatic channels and sacs during early embryogenesis.[27] The condition is subclassified as diffuse pulmonary lymphangiomatosis (DPL) when isolated to the lung, an exquisitely rare condition with fewer than 60 reported cases.[29,30] Patients with GLA may present in childhood or adulthood (usually before 20 years of age), without gender or racial predilection.[27,29–31] Later age of onset of symptoms is believed to be related to hormonally influenced growth differences or a subtler defect requiring a longer time frame to develop clinical symptoms,[27] which explains the higher mortality associated with a younger age at diagnosis.[29]

CLINICAL PRESENTATION

Although histologically benign, thoracic GLA and DPL may result in a slowly progressive respiratory failure and ultimately death.[29–31] The clinical presentation varies depending on which organs are involved, which often delays diagnosis.[27,29–32] Patients exhibit nonspecific symptoms, ranging from mild wheeze to severe dyspnea and respiratory insufficiency. Some patients frequently have nonproductive cough, hemoptysis, or chyloptysis. Symptoms may be the result of associated pleural or pericardial effusions (often chylous). Fever may be seen in the setting of superimposed infection.[29,30] Rare clinical manifestations have included disseminated intravascular coagulation, lymphopenia, and hypoalbuminemia, among others.[29]

MANIFESTATIONS OF THE DISEASE

Thoracic GLA may affect any tissue of the chest where normal lymphatic tissue exists, with lung and bone involved in 75% of cases.[27] Mediastinal, pleural, cardiac, and chest wall lymphangiomas may also be found.

Radiography

Radiographic features are nonspecific and usually include bilateral lower lobe–predominant interstitial opacities, mediastinal widening, pleural effusions, and cardiomegaly (from pericardial effusion).[30] Lytic lesions of the vertebral bodies, ribs, sternum, and scapulae are seen with osseous involvement, but any bone may be affected and is at risk for pathologic fracture.[28] The presence of a chylothorax and lytic bone lesions should raise suspicion for GLA.[27,29] Nonspecific widening of the paraspinal stripes may also be present in GLA.[31]

Computed Tomography

CT features of pulmonary involvement include smooth interlobular septal thickening and peribronchovascular thickening (Fig. 7.17), corresponding to the increased number and volume of lymphatic channels.[27,29,32] Ground-glass opacities have been described and are thought to represent volume averaging of an increased number of hemosiderin-laden macrophages within alveoli.[29] Extensive haziness of the mediastinum and perihilar regions may be seen, as well as characteristic pleural and pericardial effusions (see Fig. 7.17). Increased paraspinal soft tissue on CT has been described in thoracic GLA.[31] Lymphadenopathy is uncommonly present. CT further defines the extent of skeletal disease in GLA (see Fig. 7.17) and characterizes lymphangiomas as low-attenuation, nonenhancing septated, multilobulated masses.[32]

Magnetic Resonance Imaging

In thoracic GLA, MRI readily characterizes the cystic nature of the dilated lymphatic tissue, frequently manifesting as heterogeneous high signal within the mediastinum and within the longitudinal paraspinal soft tissues on fluid-sensitive (T2 and short time inversion recovery) sequence images.[31] Pleural and pericardial effusions may be readily detected with MRI.

Nuclear Medicine

Lymphoscintigraphy may be used to help guide therapy, determine abnormal lymph flow, and confirm the lymphatic nature of the process.[27,29]

DIFFERENTIAL DIAGNOSIS

The diagnosis is often delayed as imaging findings in DPL are nonspecific and overlap with those of pulmonary edema, lymphangitic carcinomatosis, interstitial lung diseases, pulmonary fibrosis (related to amyloidosis, lupus, or other causes), as well as other rare diseases, including pulmonary venooclusive disease, pulmonary capillary hemangiomatosis, or Erdheim-Chester disease. Lymphangioleiomyomatosis is distinct from DPL in that affected patients are overwhelmingly female and cystic lung change occurs in the former. Differentiating among these entities is often not possible by imaging and requires consideration of the patient's age, risk factors, and clinical course. In certain cases the patient's lack of response to diuretics can exclude pulmonary edema, whereas marked worsening of respiratory status after vasodilator therapy may suggest either pulmonary venoocclusive disease or pulmonary capillary hemangiomatosis.

SYNOPSIS OF TREATMENT OPTIONS

Current treatment options have achieved variable success in the palliation of this unrelenting progressive disease. In general, patients are placed on low-fat, high-protein diets containing medium-chain triglycerides to reduce lymphatic flow.[29,30] Occasionally, surgical resection of solitary pulmonary or mediastinal lesions that cause significant mass effect on adjacent structures is indicated. Yet, there is often a high rate of recurrence. Other surgical options include pleurectomy, pleurodesis, ligation of the thoracic duct, or lung transplantation.[29] Serial thoracentesis is typically used to remove reaccumulating chylothoraces. Percutaneous sclerotherapy with various agents (typically doxycycline) may be used for unresectable disease. Systemic treatments with various agents (propranolol, bevacizumab, sirolimus) have resulted in variable outcomes.[29]

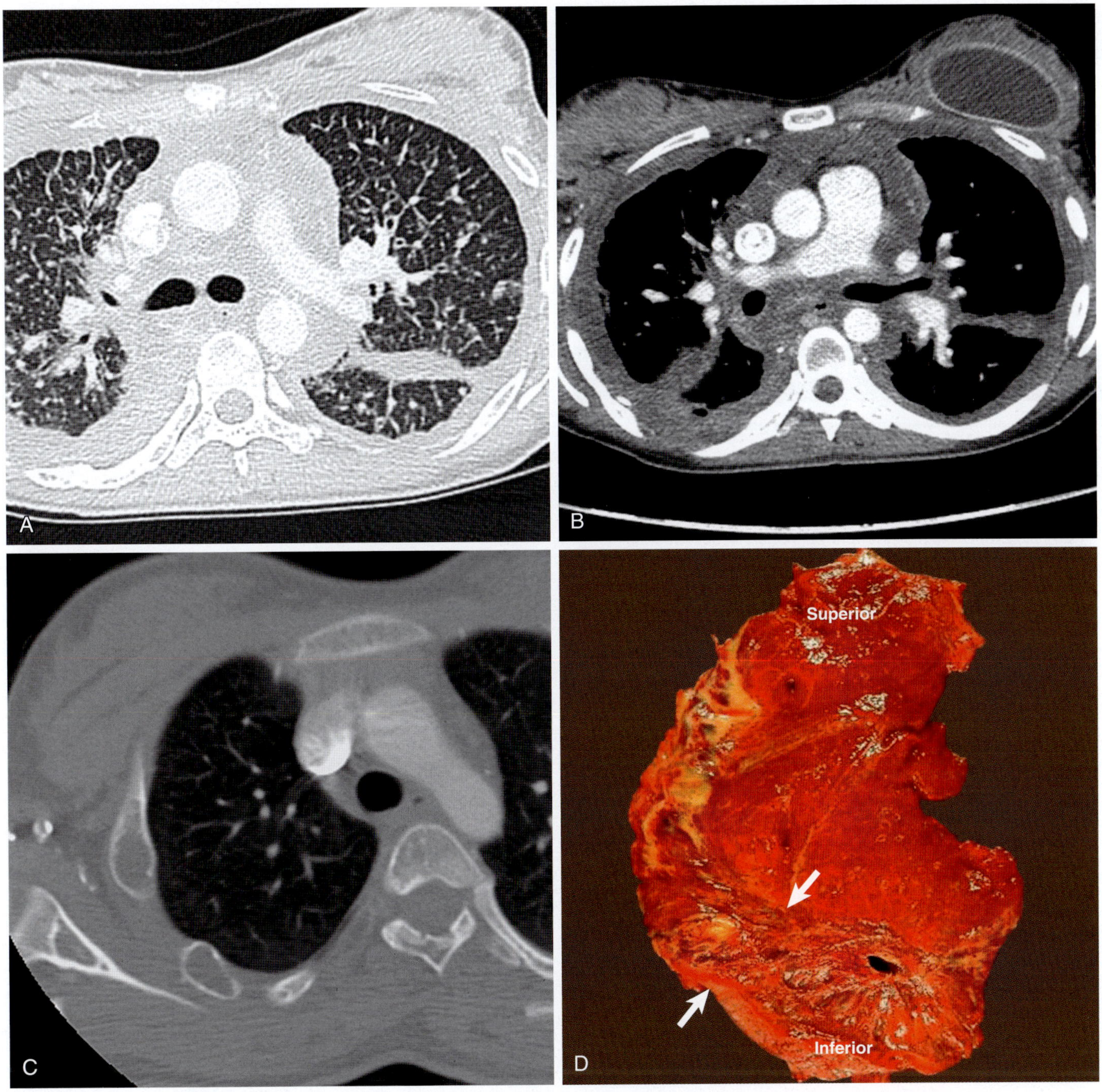

Fig. 7.17 Diffuse lymphangiomatosis. (A) Axial CT in lung and (B) mediastinal windows shows diffuse smooth thickening involving the interlobular and peribronchovascular interstitium, pleural and pericardial thickening and effusions, and mediastinal lymphatic infiltration in diffuse pulmonary lymphangiomatosis. (C) Axial chest CT in a different patient shows expansile lytic lesions throughout the osseous structures, representing skeletal involvement of diffuse lymphangiomatosis. (D) Photograph of a right lung specimen from autopsy in a different patient with diffuse pulmonary lymphangiomatosis shows complex proliferation of dilated lymphatic channels (between *arrows*) at the periphery, with normal lung seen centrally. *(Fig. 7.17A–C reproduced from Stowell J, Walker C. Congenital thoracic malformations. In: Shepard JO, ed.* Thoracic Imaging: The Requisites. *3rd ed. Philadelphia: Elsevier; 2018; Fig. 7.17D reproduced from Walker CM, Takasugi JE, Chung JH, et al. Tumorlike conditions of the pleura.* Radiographics. *2012;32:971-985.)*

KEY POINTS: CONGENITAL LYMPHATIC MALFORMATIONS

- Spectrum of rare disorders of lymphatic development related to early errors in embryogenesis with variable prognosis.
- Symptomatology is determined by the location and extent of thoracic involvement.
- Common radiologic findings:
  - Nonspecific radiographic findings include interstitial opacities, pleural effusion, and mediastinal widening.
  - CT and MR better define the extent of intrathoracic involvement and assist in treatment planning.
  - The presence of chylous pleural effusions and lytic bone lesions should raise suspicion for GLA.

KEY POINTS: CONGENITAL BRONCHOPULMONARY ANOMALIES

- Bronchopulmonary anomalies in adults are usually asymptomatic.
- Symptoms may be due to superimposed infection or compression of an adjacent airway, vessel, or lung.
- The most common bronchopulmonary anomalies seen in adults are anomalous tracheobronchial branching, bronchial atresia, bronchogenic cyst, and pulmonary sequestration.
- Chest radiography seldom allows a specific diagnosis, which is improved with use of contrast-enhanced CT or MRI.

SUGGESTED READINGS

Chassagnon G, et al. Tracheobronchial branching abnormalities: lobe-based classification scheme. *Radiographics.* 2016;36:358–373.

Desir A, Ghaye B. Congenital abnormalities of intrathoracic airways. *Radiol Clin North Am.* 2009;47:203–225.

Lee EY, Dorkin H, Vargas SO. Congenital pulmonary malformations in pediatric patients: review and update on etiology, classification, and imaging findings. *Radiol Clin North Am.* 2011;49:921–948.

Walker CM, Wu CC, Gilman MD, et al. The imaging spectrum of bronchopulmonary sequestration. *Curr Probl Diagn Radiol.* 2014;43:100–114.

The full reference list for this chapter is available at ExpertConsult.com.

8 Congenital Malformations of the Pulmonary Vessels in Adults*

BRENT P. LITTLE

Congenital malformations of the pulmonary vessels include absence or interruption, abnormal sizes, origins, or courses, and abnormal connections of the pulmonary arteries or veins. These abnormalities commonly accompany other congenital pulmonary or cardiac disorders but can occur in isolation. Although some malformations have no clinical significance and may be an incidental finding at imaging, others may have important consequences. For example, pulmonary hypertension may occur in congenital pulmonary artery abnormalities or in anomalies with a left-to-right shunt, such as anomalous pulmonary venous return. In cases in which clinical consequences are absent or mild, recognition and accurate description of congenital abnormalities of the pulmonary vessels are still critical for avoiding misdiagnosis. For example, dysmorphic lung typically seen in interruption of the pulmonary artery can be mistaken for fibrosis or postinfectious scarring.

Radiography may identify a congenital malformation of the pulmonary vessels in a limited number of cases. However, most abnormalities are either first detected or confirmed at computed tomography (CT) or magnetic resonance imaging (MRI), modalities that characterize morphology and identify coexisting abnormalities. An understanding of the typical imaging appearances, associated abnormalities, and clinical manifestations of congenital malformations of the pulmonary vessels is essential in accurate diagnosis of these entities.

Proximal Interruption of the Pulmonary Artery

EMBRYOLOGY, PREVALENCE, AND EPIDEMIOLOGY

This malformation has many names in the literature: unilateral agenesis, atresia, or absence of the pulmonary artery; occult pulmonary artery; and proximal interruption of the pulmonary artery. Interruption of the pulmonary artery is the most appropriate because it describes a break in continuity of the pulmonary arterial tree, beyond which the pulmonary arteries are still present but small because of the reduction in blood flow. Because pulmonary blood flow influences development of the lungs, an interruption in the blood supply in utero results in hypoplasia of the lung. This defect is frequently associated with congenital heart defects, the most common of which are ventricular septal defects and the tetralogy of Fallot. However, other cardiac malformations are also seen, such as coarctation of the aorta, subvalvular aortic stenosis, dextrotransposition or levotransposition of the great arteries, stenosis or aneurysm of the main pulmonary artery, scimitar syndrome,[1] patent ductus arteriosus, and aortopulmonary fistula.

CLINICAL PRESENTATION

This malformation is usually diagnosed in children with associated congenital heart defects, but isolated cases may not be diagnosed until adulthood. In adults it is usually an isolated phenomenon, occurs more frequently on the right than on the left, and is associated with a contralateral aortic arch in the vast majority of cases. Symptoms may result either from pulmonary arterial hypertension, which is present in 19% to 25% of cases,[2] or from pulmonary infections, which frequently occur in the hypoplastic lung.

MANIFESTATIONS OF THE DISEASE

Radiography

Chest radiography shows the expected findings of a small lung (Fig. 8.1). The degree of lucency of the abnormal side is usually similar to that of the contralateral lung, as air trapping is absent. The hilum on the side of interruption is diminutive, and the contralateral hilum is often enlarged, a finding often best detected on the lateral view (see Fig. 8.1). There may be signs of collateral systemic circulation supplying the abnormal lung, such as subpleural reticular opacities, smooth pleural thickening, and unilateral rib notching from enlargement of intercostal arteries. Similar to congenital cardiac diseases associated with pulmonary arterial outflow tract obstruction, there may be parenchymal abnormalities on the side of the interruption that mimic pulmonary fibrosis or scarring from prior infection, such as tuberculosis. Reticulonodular opacities and architectural distortion are common, thought to represent chronic parenchymal damage caused by oligemia.

Ventilation-Perfusion (VQ) Nuclear Imaging

VQ scintigraphy demonstrates complete absence of perfusion and decreased ventilation on the affected side. Delayed washout xenon-133 ventilation scans, which are used to diagnose air trapping, are normal; this contrasts with conditions such as Swyer-James syndrome, in which air trapping is present.

Computed Tomography

Proximal interruption of the pulmonary artery and associated findings can be definitively diagnosed with CT (Fig. 8.2).[3] CT should be performed in all cases, both to establish a diagnosis and for thorough and precise evaluation of the anomaly, particularly because surgical repair may be contemplated, even in young adults. It is therefore necessary to search for a patent pulmonary artery in the hilum beyond the proximal interruption and to demonstrate its anatomic continuity with smaller proximal and distal pulmonary artery branches. Reduced pulmonary blood

*The editors and the publisher would like to thank Drs. Jacques Remy, John F. Bruzzi, and Martine Remy-Jardin for contributing material on this topic to the prior edition of this work. It has served as the foundation for the current chapter.

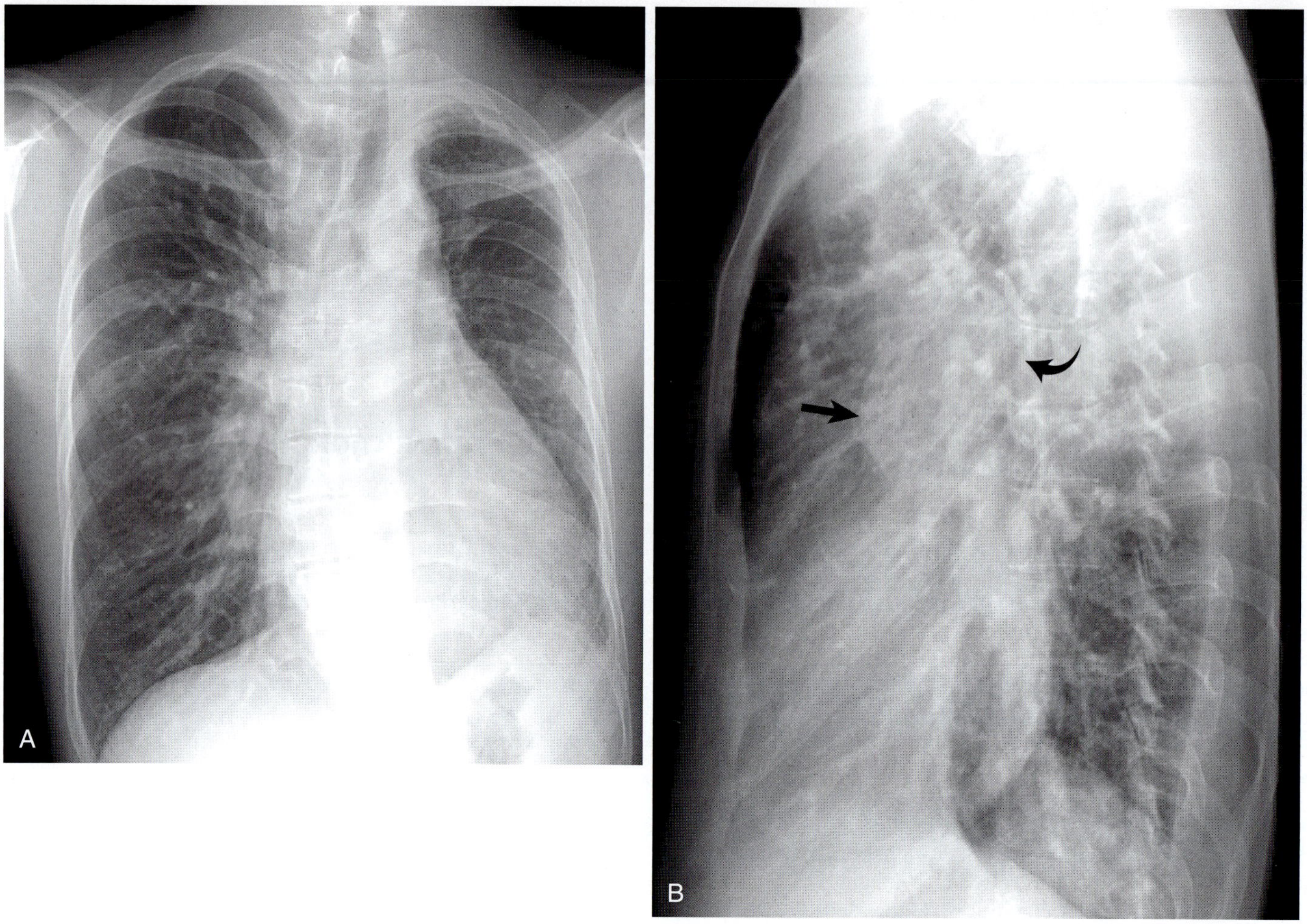

Fig. 8.1 Proximal interruption of the left pulmonary artery. (A) A frontal chest radiograph demonstrates a reduction in left lung volume accompanied by leftward displacement of the trachea and heart. The left pulmonary artery contour is absent, and the left lung shows decreased vascularity and subtle peripheral reticulation. (B) A lateral chest radiograph shows absence of the curvilinear opacity in the left hilum that normally corresponds to the left pulmonary artery *(curved arrow);* in the right hilum the right hilar vascular opacity is clearly seen *(straight arrow).*

flow results in small ipsilateral pulmonary arteries and veins. The systemic arterial system must also be assessed, including the bronchial, phrenic, intercostal, internal mammary, and external mammary arteries, as well as arteries of the pulmonary ligaments. Because embolotherapy of these vessels may be attempted in the event of major hemoptysis, the origin of each artery needs to be carefully analyzed. Systemic anastomoses between the coronary and bronchial arteries may also develop in association with this malformation, for the same reasons that they are seen in chronic thromboembolic disease and other conditions with decreased pulmonary blood flow.[4] The lung parenchyma of the hypoplastic lung or both lungs can demonstrate mosaic attenuation, which may be due to increased collateral perfusion to the abnormal lung, pulmonary hypertension, redistribution of blood flow within the normal lung, or compensatory hyperinflation of the contralateral lung.[2]

On CT indirect signs of systemic collateral circulation include mosaic attenuation, thickened interlobular septa, subpleural reticular opacities or honeycombing, subpleural parenchymal bands, and irregular pleural thickening (Fig. 8.3). All of these findings explain the radiographic appearance of "pseudofibrosis" or "pseudotuberculosis."

Bronchial thickening is frequent; it is usually from dilated bronchial arteries or recurrent bronchial infections. Cylindrical dilation of proximal segmental or subsegmental bronchi may be a result of the decreased caliber of the accompanying pulmonary arteries, which, because they are enclosed within the same bronchovascular connective tissue sheath, allow greater space for the bronchi to expand. Ischemia of the bronchial walls has also been invoked as an explanation for proximal bronchial dilation, in which the vascular supply of affected bronchi is redistributed toward the peripheral pulmonary arterial circulation.[5] This proximal bronchial dilation is identical to that observed in chronic thromboembolic disease but is completely different from the bronchial dilation in varicose and cystic bronchiectasis.[2]

Magnetic Resonance Imaging

MR angiography accurately depicts this condition and is increasingly used for diagnosis and follow-up imaging. Cardiac MR sequences can also be obtained as part of the same study, allowing characterization of pulmonary artery flow, ventricular function, and associated congenital cardiac abnormalities. Because the condition is most often detected or monitored in childhood or

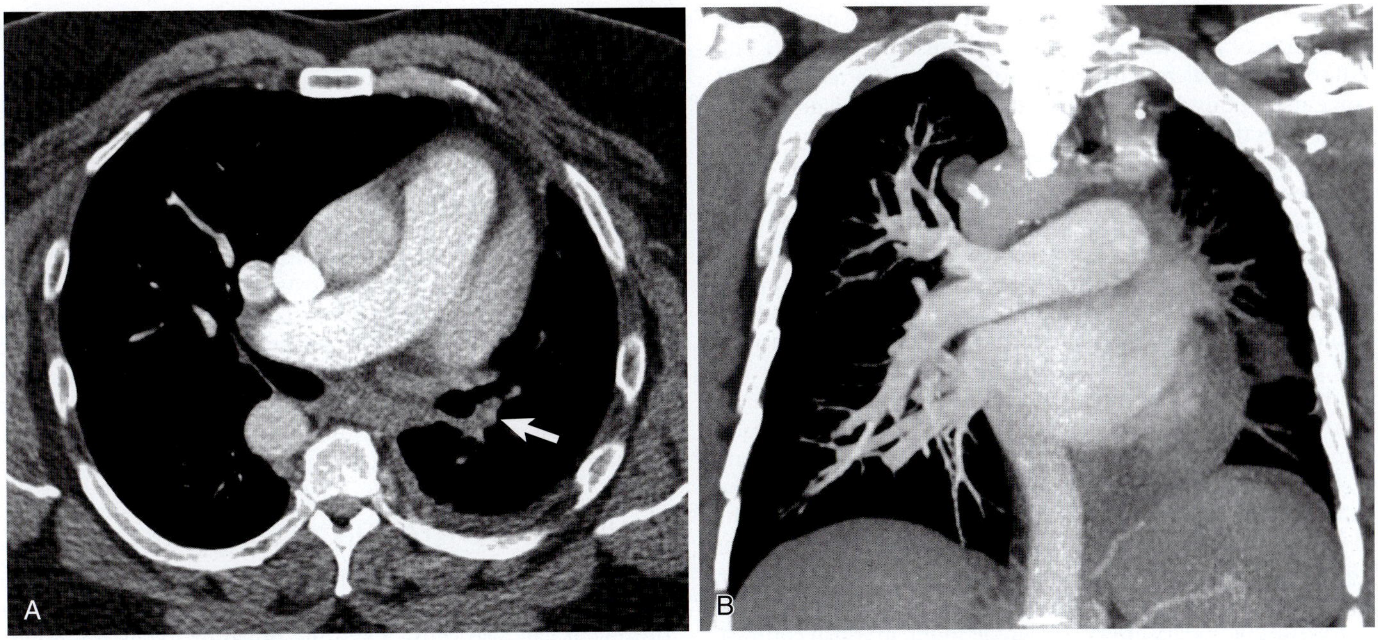

Fig. 8.2 Proximal interruption of the left pulmonary artery. (A) Axial CT image shows absence of the left pulmonary artery, with diminutive left lower lobar pulmonary artery and branches *(arrow)*. A right aortic arch is present, after the expectation that the aortic arch is contralateral to the side of the interruption. The left lung is small, and the pleura is mildly thickened. (B) Coronal reformatted maximum-intensity projection image shows interruption of the left pulmonary artery, with enlargement of the right pulmonary artery and its branches.

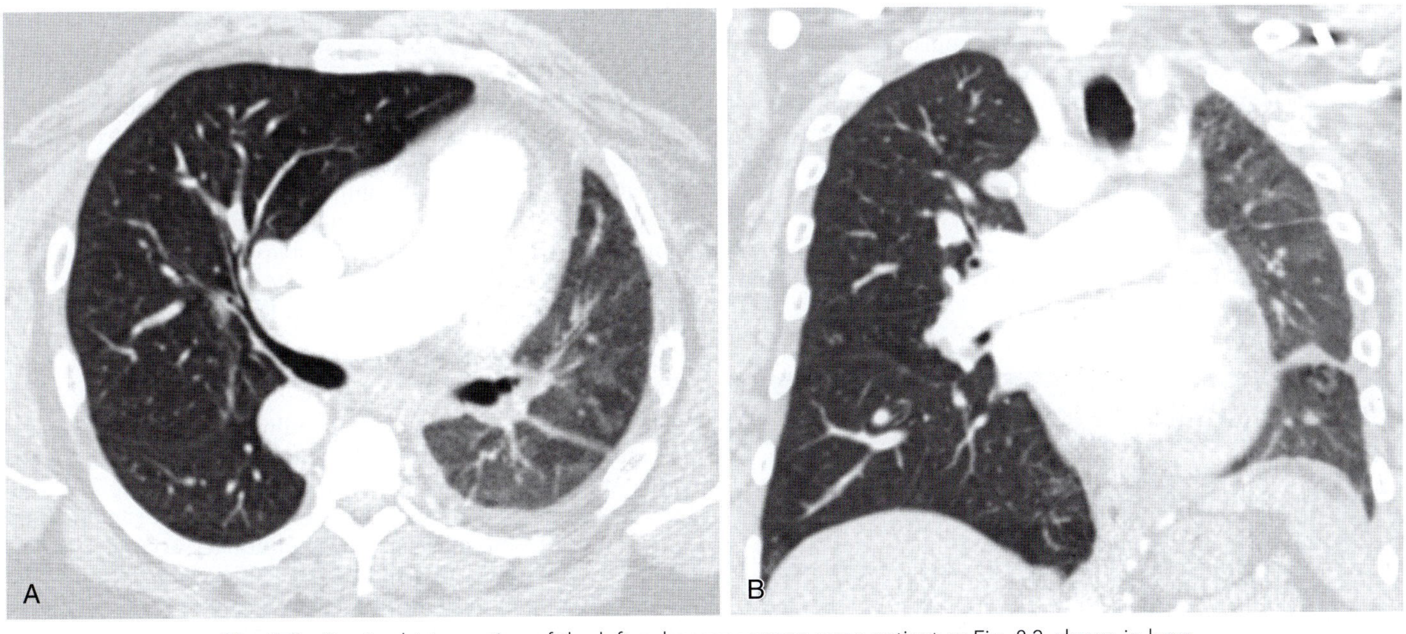

Fig. 8.3 Proximal interruption of the left pulmonary artery; same patient as Fig. 8.2, shown in lung windows. (A) and (B) Axial and coronal reformatted CT images show a small left lung with leftward mediastinal shift. Note left lung mosaic attenuation, peripheral reticulation, and pleural thickening, a common appearance on the side of the interrupted pulmonary artery resulting from chronic pulmonary arterial malperfusion and the abnormal systemic collateral circulation.

early adulthood, MR angiography has the distinct advantage over CT of avoiding radiation exposure.

DIFFERENTIAL DIAGNOSIS

The rarity of this malformation leads to discussion of other possible differential diagnoses, including (1) *unilateral postembolic obstruction of a pulmonary artery.* Even in the absence of a history of thromboembolism, it is necessary to look for the sequelae of chronic thromboembolic disease at the site of arterial interruption and in the contralateral lung. A purely unilateral manifestation of chronic thromboembolic disease is rare. (2) In *Swyer-James-McLeod syndrome,* the ipsilateral pulmonary artery is present but small because of decreased perfusion of the affected lung.

Findings on VQ scintigraphy are different from those of proximal interruption of a pulmonary artery as discussed earlier. (3) The pulmonary arterial manifestations of *Takayasu arteritis* could be included in this discussion, but they are usually bilateral, and in most cases the systemic arteries are also involved. The presence of morphologic abnormalities of the pulmonary and systemic arteries evolving at the same time is strongly suggestive of this diagnosis. Takayasu arteritis is more often confused with chronic thromboembolic disease than with proximal interruption of a pulmonary artery. (4) *Primary neoplasms of the pulmonary artery* and *bronchogenic carcinoma* are two causes of acquired unilateral obstruction of a pulmonary artery, but both are characterized by the presence of a hilar mass. (5) *Fibrosing mediastinitis* involving the hilum can also cause unilateral obstruction of a pulmonary artery. This diagnosis should be suspected when there is a pertinent clinical history or other signs of previous granulomatous infection, including a partially calcified mediastinal mass, or stenosis or interruption of other hilar structures, such as bronchi and pulmonary veins. (6) In cases of *unilateral stenosis or atresia of the pulmonary veins,* the hilar pulmonary artery may appear small and enhanced only in a delayed manner by means of a systemic-to-pulmonary artery retrograde shunt, in which contrast medium reaches the hilar pulmonary artery via retrograde flow. Such a phenomenon can be detected by obtaining a second delayed acquisition focused on the hilum.

SYNOPSIS OF TREATMENT OPTIONS

In children and young adults, revascularization of the interrupted pulmonary artery can be attempted by reimplantation or bypass of the affected segment but only when the hilar or proximal intraparenchymal pulmonary artery is patent and suitable for anastomosis. If the caliber of the artery is too narrow, a temporary palliative anastomosis can be attempted to encourage further development of the vessel. When the malformation is not detected until later adulthood, treatment is purely symptomatic. Such treatment may involve embolotherapy of systemic arteries in cases of recurrent hemoptysis or even pneumonectomy to achieve definitive control of hemorrhage.

KEY POINTS: PROXIMAL INTERRUPTION OF A PULMONARY ARTERY

- Rarely discovered in adulthood
- Usually occurs as an isolated malformation when first seen in an adult
- More common on the right
- Clinical findings: pulmonary hypertension, recurrent infection, hemoptysis
- Common imaging findings:
  - Small lung with peripheral reticulation and architectural distortion
  - Absent or small pulmonary artery at the hilum
  - Normal pulmonary venous return
  - Aortic arch usually contralateral to the anomaly
  - Systemic collateral blood supply

Valvular Pulmonary Stenosis

EMBRYOLOGY, PREVALENCE, AND EPIDEMIOLOGY

Valvular pulmonary stenosis may remain asymptomatic for a long time, depending on the degree of the stenosis, and may not be diagnosed until adulthood, when it may be detected incidentally on chest radiography. Causes of valvular pulmonary stenosis include stenosis secondary to commissural fusion of the pulmonary cusps causing a thickened, dome-like pulmonary valve; a bicuspid pulmonary valve; and valvular dysplasia.

PATHOPHYSIOLOGY

Valvular pulmonary stenosis causes a poststenotic systolic jet in the pulmonary trunk. Elevated postsystolic pressure in the right ventricle leads to muscular hypertrophy of the right ventricle, most marked in the outflow tract. In addition, hypertrophy of the right ventricle leads to elongation and reorientation of the right ventricle. These changes in orientation of the infundibulum and pulmonary trunk cause the poststenotic jet to be directed primarily toward the left pulmonary artery.

CLINICAL PRESENTATION

Valvular pulmonary stenosis may be asymptomatic. It can be associated with fatigue on effort secondary to decreased cardiac output. It can also cause a systolic murmur in the pulmonary outflow tract, as well as electrocardiogram signs of right ventricular hypertrophy.

MANIFESTATIONS OF THE DISEASE

Radiography

The most common radiographic signs are poststenotic dilation of the pulmonary trunk and isolated enlargement of the left pulmonary artery and its proximal branches, with a normal or small right pulmonary artery (Fig. 8.4).[6] These findings can simulate a mediastinal mass or enlarged left hilar lymph nodes. The counterclockwise rotation of the heart can simulate left ventricular hypertrophy. Proximal dilation of the left pulmonary artery may be limited to its upper lobe branches or may extend to involve the left interlobar pulmonary artery, which is easily visible on a lateral view (see Fig. 8.4). The repetitive trauma caused by the poststenotic jet can result in focal calcification of the wall of the left pulmonary artery.

Computed Tomography or Magnetic Resonance Imaging

Selective enlargement of the left pulmonary artery is usually present (see Fig. 8.4), and right ventricular hypertrophy can be seen. At MRI, cine imaging can show a spin-dephasing flow-void artifact from turbulent blood flow arising from the stenotic valve extending into the main and left pulmonary arteries (see Fig. 8.4). The pulmonic valve is moderately thickened, irregular, and dome shaped, and leaflet fusion may be present (see Fig. 8.4). In exceptional cases the leaflets may be calcified. In cases of valvular dysplasia the valvular annulus and the main pulmonary artery itself are moderately hypoplastic.

DIFFERENTIAL DIAGNOSIS

The differential diagnosis includes other causes of dilation of the main pulmonary artery, such as pulmonary hypertension, idiopathic dilation of the main pulmonary artery, incompetence of the pulmonary valve, intravascular malignancy, and aneurysm. It is also important to use CT to exclude tumors and lymphadenopathy involving the mediastinum or left hilum that may mimic this abnormality on radiography.

SYNOPSIS OF TREATMENT OPTIONS

The need for treatment depends on the pressure gradient across the stenosis and its effects on cardiac function. Balloon valvuloplasty has become a primary approach, followed by commissurotomy or "shaving" of thickened leaflets.[7] It may be enough to correct the transvalvular pressure gradient without eliminating the stenosis, thereby effectively exchanging a dome-shaped valve for a bicuspid leaflet. Surgical replacement is used for selected cases, including those refractory to balloon valvuloplasty. Transcatheter bioprosthetic pulmonic valve implantation is now an alternative to surgical replacement at some centers, especially for high-risk patients.

KEY POINTS: VALVULAR PULMONARY STENOSIS

- May be detected incidentally in asymptomatic patients
- Systolic murmur or abnormal chest radiograph
- Common imaging findings:
  - Dilation of the left pulmonary artery and its proximal branches
  - Thickening of the pulmonic valve leaflets
  - Right ventricular hypertrophy

Aberrant Retrotracheal Left Pulmonary Artery (Pulmonary Artery Sling)

EMBRYOLOGY, PREVALENCE, AND EPIDEMIOLOGY

Pulmonary artery sling is thought to be secondary to absence of development, underdevelopment, or resorption of the ventral portion of the sixth left aortic arch or its premature obliteration. As a result, the left pulmonary vascular plexus connects to the sixth right aortic arch. The left pulmonary artery thus develops as a collateral vessel of the right pulmonary artery, from which is derived its anatomic description: anomalous origin of the left pulmonary artery from the right. The great majority of cases are detected in childhood and are associated with other congenital malformations, most commonly involving the tracheobronchial tree and the heart. It is a very rare anomaly in adults, in whom it is often an isolated malformation.

CLINICAL PRESENTATION

The abnormality is asymptomatic unless associated with congenital tracheal or bronchial stenosis, which may give rise to symptoms of dyspnea or recurrent pulmonary infections.[8]

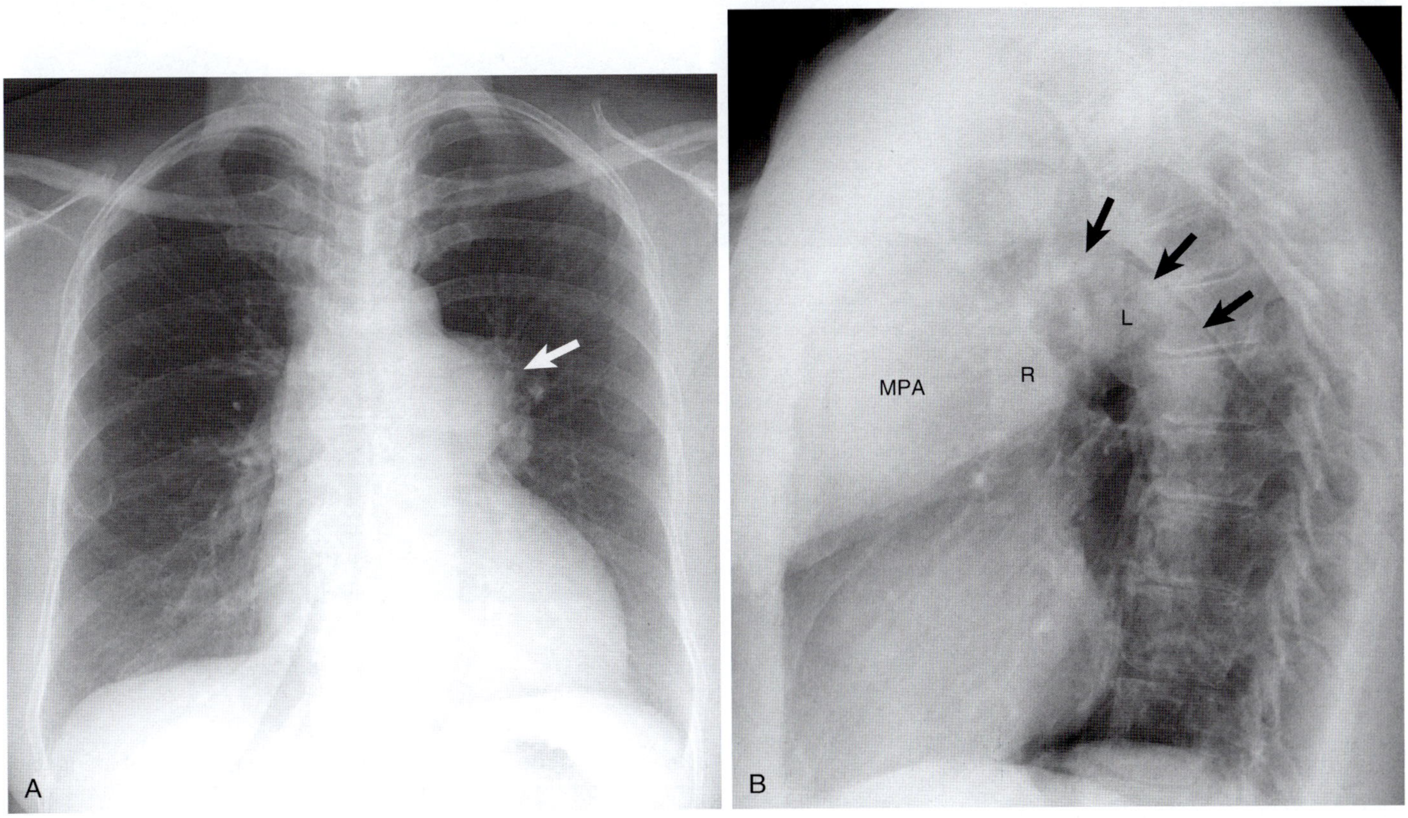

Fig. 8.4 Pulmonary valvular stenosis. (A) Frontal chest radiograph shows enlargement of the main and left pulmonary arteries *(arrow)*; the right pulmonary artery is of normal size. (B) Lateral chest radiograph shows an enlarged main pulmonary artery *(MPA)*, an enlarged left pulmonary artery (*L* and *arrows*), and a normal size of the right hilar vascular opacity *(R)*.

Continued

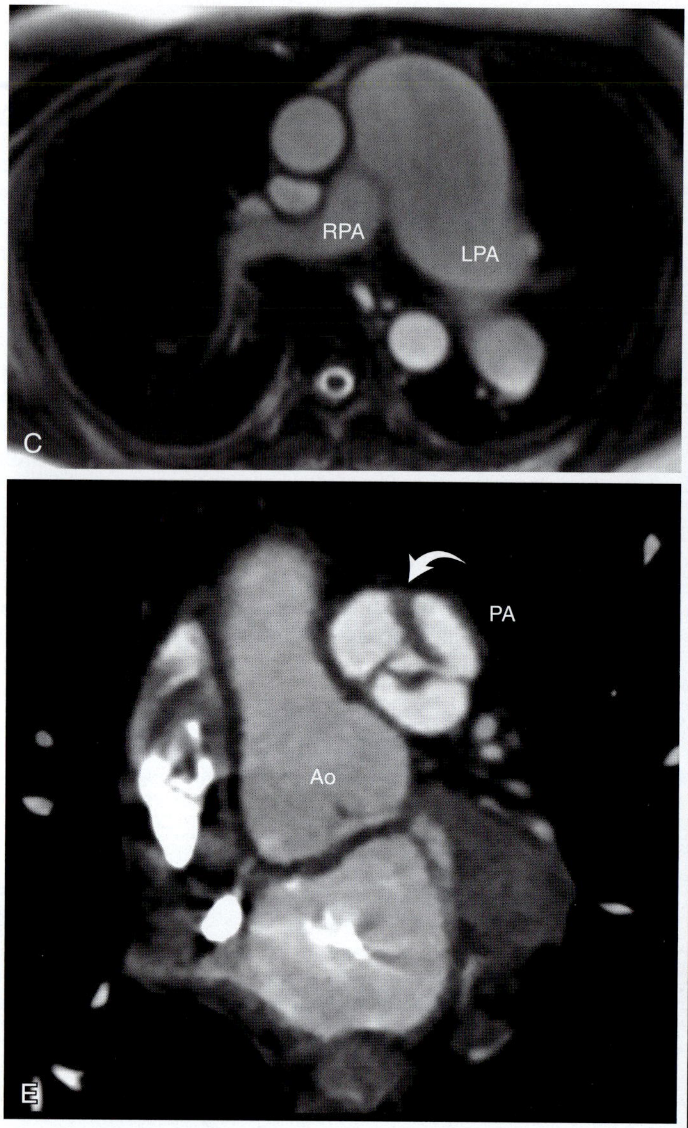

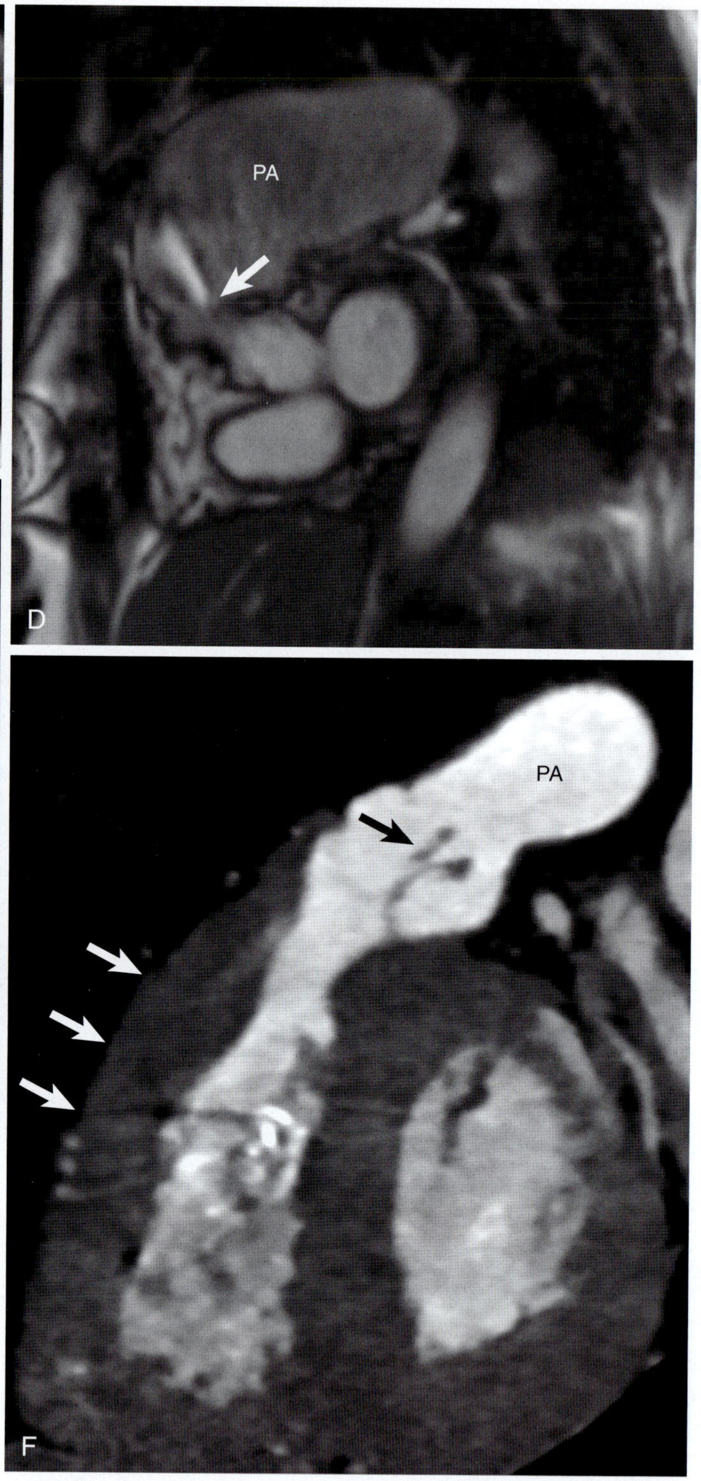

Fig. 8.4, cont'd (C) Steady-state–free precession (SSFP) image through the central pulmonary arteries shows selective enlargement of the main pulmonary artery and the proximal left pulmonary artery (LPA); the right pulmonary artery (RPA) is normal in size. (D) Sagittal SSFP cine MR image through the right ventricular outflow tract shows a severely enlarged main pulmonary artery (PA) and a spin-dephasing jet *(arrow)* corresponding to flow acceleration from pulmonic valve stenosis. (E) Oblique reformatted CT image shows thickened leaflets of the pulmonic valve in keeping with pulmonic stenosis *(curved arrow)*. An aneurysmal aortic root (Ao) is also noted. (F) Sagittal reformatted CT image shows thickening of the pulmonic valve leaflets *(black arrow)*, with a domed appearance of the basal leaflets. Right ventricular hypertrophy is present *(white arrows)*.

MANIFESTATIONS OF THE DISEASE

Radiography

The left pulmonary artery originates from the posterior aspect of the right pulmonary artery, courses above the right mainstem bronchus at its origin, and then takes a pathway to the left between the trachea and esophagus before reaching the left hilum. It may be suspected on chest radiographs by the presence of an opacity measuring approximately 2 cm in diameter in the right tracheobronchial angle (Fig. 8.5). Detection of this opacity should prompt consideration of four possible diagnoses: lymphadenopathy, dilation of the azygos arch, partial anomalous pulmonary venous return to the superior vena cava, and a retrotracheal left pulmonary artery. The aberrant vessel can be detected on lateral radiographs when located in the lower retrotracheal region, on which it appears as a round opacity, 10 to 15 mm in diameter, that is indenting the posterior aspect of the trachea. An esophagram demonstrates a smooth extrinsic impression on the anterior esophageal wall.

Computed Tomography

An aberrant left pulmonary artery is well depicted in the transverse plane. The diagnosis is therefore easily made on a CT examination,[8,9] even without intravenous contrast. The left pulmonary artery passes around the inferior portion of the right and posterior tracheal walls, from which it gets its descriptive name: "pulmonary sling" (Fig. 8.6). Once it reaches the left hilum, the left pulmonary artery adopts a normal intrapulmonary course. Diagnosis by conventional angiography may be difficult because there is almost complete superimposition of the left pulmonary artery on the right pulmonary artery on frontal projections. The aberrant left pulmonary artery may be abnormally small or stenosed. In some cases it may reach the left hilum at a lower position than normal.

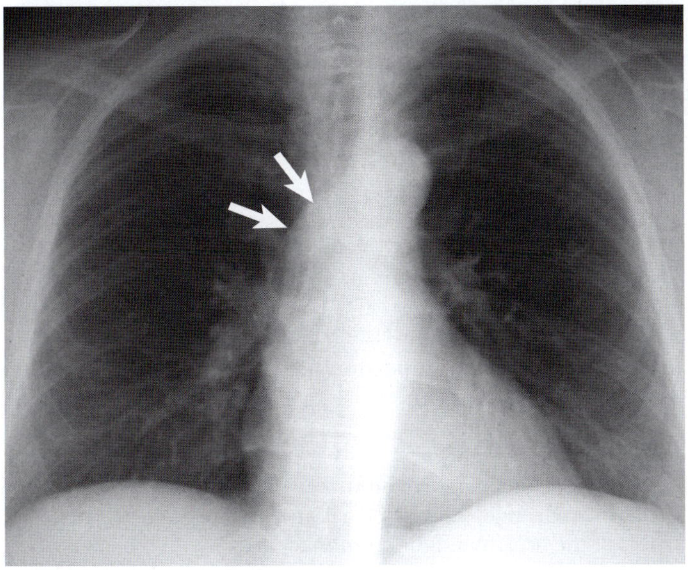

Fig. 8.5 Aberrant retrotracheal left pulmonary artery (pulmonary artery sling). A chest radiograph performed for evaluation of moderate dyspnea shows an abnormal opacity in the right tracheobronchial angle *(arrows)*, proven to represent a pulmonary artery sling.

Associated tracheobronchial malformations include a tracheal bronchus to the right upper lobe, hypoplasia of the distal trachea (Fig. 8.7), stenosis of the right mainstem bronchus, and complete tracheal cartilaginous rings (napkin rings). Reformatted images are useful for identifying moderate tracheal stenosis (Fig. 8.8). This last malformation has been called the "ring-sling" syndrome; it is characterized by a lack of variation in form and diameter of the cartilaginous tracheal rings between inspiration and expiration. In adults partial calcification of the cartilaginous rings may reveal their abnormal complete character.

Magnetic Resonance Imaging

Although MRI is a very valuable diagnostic examination for arterial malformations,[10] it is inferior to CT for identifying abnormalities of the lung parenchyma and tracheobronchial tree.

SYNOPSIS OF TREATMENT OPTIONS

Treatment depends on associated anomalies, particularly of the tracheobronchial tree. A congenital tracheal stenosis can be treated by dilation, stenting, tracheoplasty, or bronchial transplantation. Reimplantation of the left pulmonary artery is not usually attempted in adults.

Right Pulmonary Artery–to–Left Atrium Communication

EMBRYOLOGY, PREVALENCE, AND EPIDEMIOLOGY

There is no known embryologic explanation for this malformation. It is almost always located on the right, but it has also been described on the left.[11] More often congenital than posttraumatic,

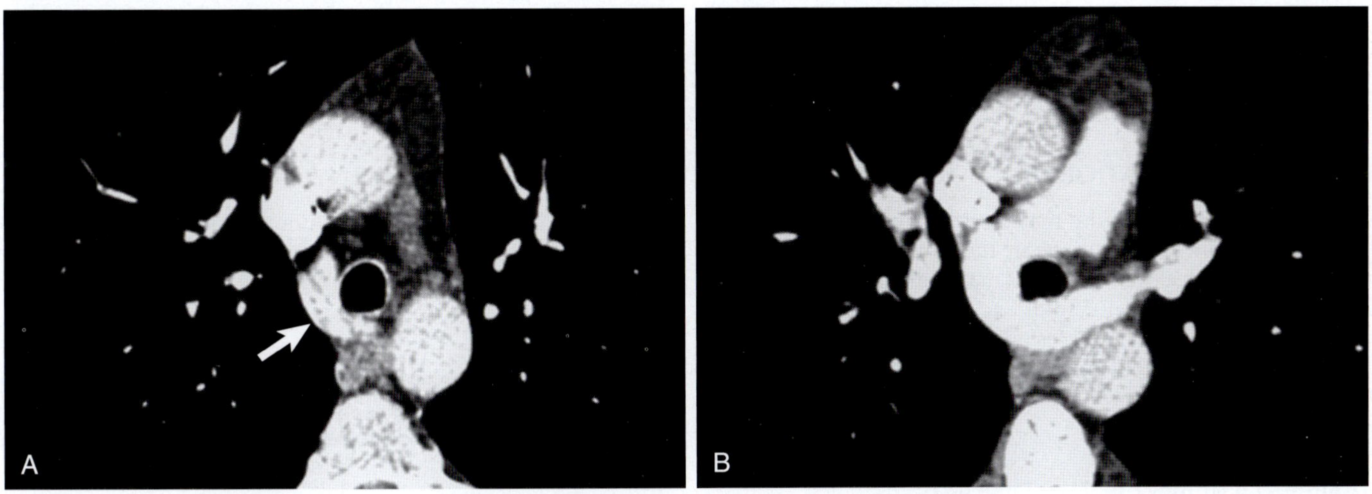

Fig. 8.6 Aberrant retrotracheal left pulmonary artery (pulmonary artery sling): CT findings. (A) CT image at the level of the upper left pulmonary artery *(arrow)*, which courses around the right lateral and posterior aspects of the morphologically normal trachea. (B) CT image at a slightly more caudal level demonstrating the entire course of the left pulmonary artery. It arises from the posterior, proximal right pulmonary artery, passes between the trachea and esophagus, and then courses toward the left hilum. A comparison of tracheal sizes shows that the trachea has a slightly smaller diameter in (B) than at the higher level (A).

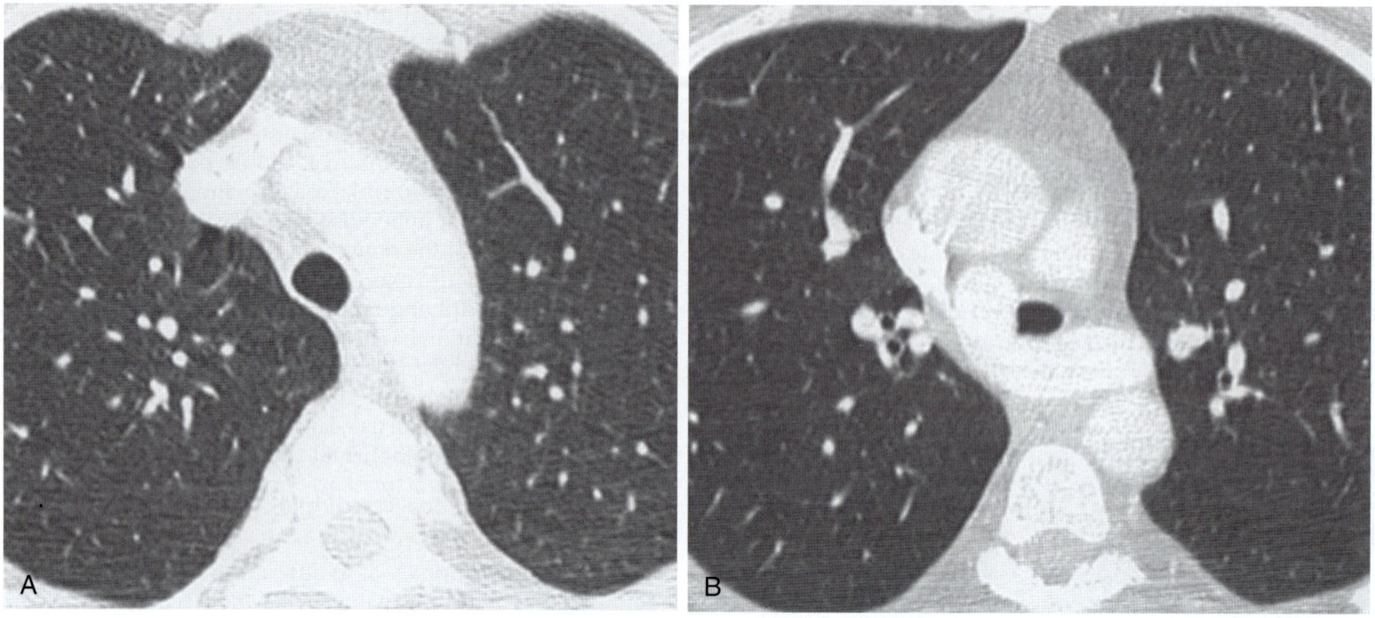

Fig. 8.7 Aberrant retrotracheal left pulmonary artery (pulmonary artery sling): CT findings. CT images at the level of the aortic arch (A) and at the level of the aberrant pulmonary artery (B) again demonstrate the reduction in diameter of the trachea at the level of the ectopic pulmonary artery. Both cases (see Figs. 8.6 and 8.7) represent "ring-sling" syndromes.

KEY POINTS: RETROTRACHEAL LEFT PULMONARY ARTERY (PULMONARY ARTERY SLING)

- May be an incidental finding on radiography or CT
- May be associated with or result in tracheal or bronchial stenosis
- Characteristic imaging findings:
  - Opacity in the right tracheobronchial angle
  - Left pulmonary artery arising from the posterior right pulmonary artery
  - Left pulmonary artery coursing toward the left hilum between the trachea and esophagus

it is extremely rare and may be associated with other malformations, including congenital cardiac malformations and right-sided lobar agenesis.

CLINICAL PRESENTATION

Besides a right-to-left shunt that may be quite severe, other clinically important complications are the same as those associated with pulmonary arteriovenous malformations: paradoxical emboli and rupture of the aneurysmal sac. On contrast-enhanced echocardiography, microbubbles appear in the left atrium later than occurs with a patent foramen ovale and earlier than seen with pulmonary arteriovenous malformations, generally after two to three cardiac cycles.

MANIFESTATIONS OF THE DISEASE

Radiography

This malformation may be suspected on chest radiography by the association of a right-to-left shunt with a right retrocardiac pseudomass,[12] which corresponds to the aneurysmal sac that forms the direct communication between the right pulmonary artery and the left atrium.

Computed Tomography

Four types of this malformation are recognized. In type I venous return from the right lung is normal, and a vessel unites the posterior aspect of the proximal right pulmonary artery with the left atrium. In type II the supernumerary branch of the right pulmonary artery communicates with adjacent venous structures: the left atrium, the right superior pulmonary vein, or both. The right inferior pulmonary vein is absent. In type III both right pulmonary veins drain into a vascular pocket uniting the right pulmonary artery and the left atrium. In type IV the right inferior pulmonary vein is replaced by three small veins connected to an aneurysmal sac. The aneurysmal sac is adjacent to the right posterolateral aspect of the left atrium. The interlobar right pulmonary artery is dilated and located adjacent to the sac, without interpositioning of the afferent arterial vessels.

SYNOPSIS OF TREATMENT OPTIONS

Gianturco coils, Amplatzer occluder devices, ligation, ligation and division, excision, intracardiac repair, and pneumonectomy are all possible options, depending on the angioarchitecture of the malformation.[11]

KEY POINTS: RIGHT PULMONARY ARTERY–TO–LEFT ATRIUM COMMUNICATION

- Very rare
- Right-to-left shunt
- Major complication is rupture of the aneurysmal sac
- Common imaging findings:
  - Right retrocardiac opacity
  - Large proximal communication of the right pulmonary artery with the left atrium

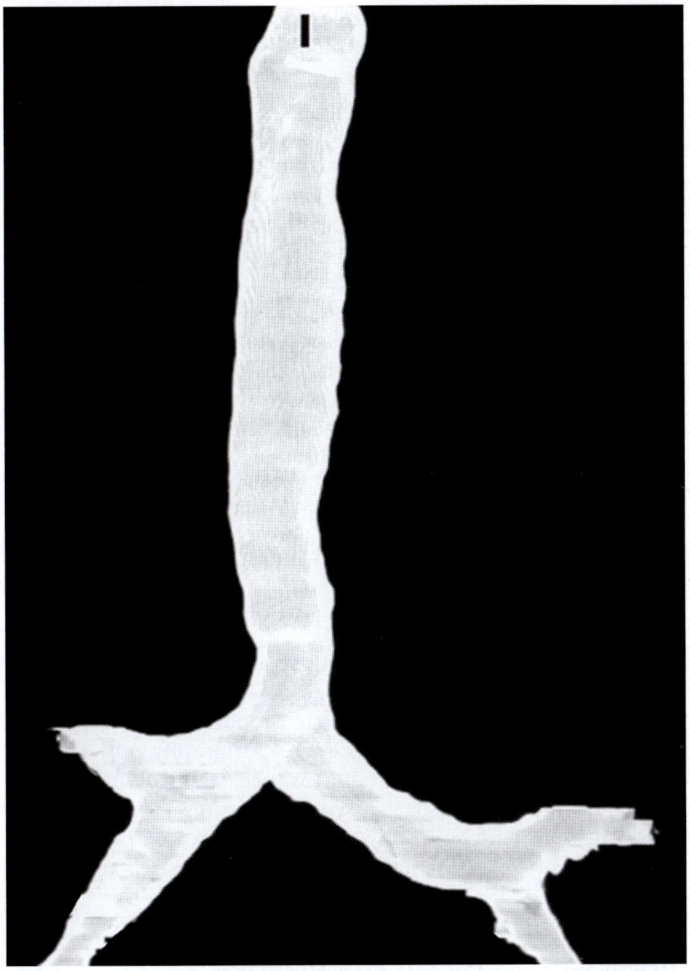

Fig. 8.8 Tracheal stenosis caused by an aberrant retrotracheal left pulmonary artery (pulmonary artery sling). Volumetric reconstruction of the tracheal bifurcation demonstrates moderate stenosis of the distal trachea. This type of stenosis, which is smoothly tapered with respect to the proximal trachea, can easily go undetected during bronchoscopy.

Congenital Pulmonary Artery Stenosis

EMBRYOLOGY, PREVALENCE, AND EPIDEMIOLOGY

The embryology of this congenital malformation is unknown. Congenital pulmonary artery stenosis is classified into four types: (1) stenosis of the main pulmonary artery, (2) stenosis of the bifurcation of the main pulmonary artery involving the origin of the left or right pulmonary arteries, (3) multiple peripheral pulmonary arterial stenoses, and (4) stenoses involving both the proximal and peripheral pulmonary arteries.

PATHOPHYSIOLOGY

Stenoses that involve short segments and that are proximal in location usually cause poststenotic flow acceleration (a poststenotic "jet"). Stenoses of longer segments are not associated with poststenotic jets. The effects of pulmonary arterial stenosis on the right side of the heart are variable.

CLINICAL PRESENTATION

Congenital pulmonary artery stenoses are almost always associated with syndromes.[6] Williams-Beuren syndrome, or idiopathic hypercalcemia of infancy, consists of mental retardation, recognizable facial traits, peripheral pulmonary arterial or venous stenoses, and supravalvular aortic stenosis. Other syndromes include Noonan syndrome, Down syndrome, Alagille syndrome, Ehlers-Danlos syndrome, and sequelae of congenital rubella infection. Supravalvular pulmonary arterial stenoses may also be associated with cardiac anomalies, such as the tetralogy of Fallot, transposition of the great vessels, and atrial and ventricular septal defects. In exceptional cases pulmonary arterial stenosis may be isolated.

MANIFESTATIONS OF THE DISEASE

Radiography and Computed Tomography

The radiologic appearance depends on the location of the stenosis, its hemodynamic consequences, and the existence of poststenotic dilation. It is dominated by heterogeneous pulmonary vascularization with hypovascular areas and fusiform poststenotic vascular dilations. Proximal stenoses (Fig. 8.9) of the main pulmonary artery and its bifurcation cause bilateral symmetric hypovascularization. Their effect on the right side of the heart is the same as for valvular pulmonary stenosis.

DIFFERENTIAL DIAGNOSIS

The differential diagnosis includes chronic thromboembolic disease, fibrosing mediastinitis, and vasculitides, such as Takayasu arteritis, which may result in similar short-segment stenoses with poststenotic jets, as well as longer-segment stenoses.

SYNOPSIS OF TREATMENT OPTIONS

Treatment depends on the hemodynamic consequences of the stenosis. It may involve surgical resection of the stenosis with end-to-end anastomosis or endovascular angioplasty with stenting.

KEY POINTS: CONGENITAL PULMONARY ARTERY STENOSIS

- Most commonly occurring in the setting of a syndrome, most frequently Williams-Beuren syndrome
- Can be associated with cardiac malformations
- Common imaging findings:
  - Poststenotic dilatation of the pulmonary artery branches
  - Mosaic attenuation in the lungs
  - Right ventricular dysfunction

Congenital Stenosis and Atresia of Pulmonary Veins

EMBRYOLOGY, PREVALENCE, AND EPIDEMIOLOGY

This malformation affects one or several pulmonary veins in their extraparenchymal courses, unilaterally or bilaterally. Most often it is discovered during infancy or childhood, rarely in adulthood. There are two types: a localized occlusion secondary to a fibrous ring or a diaphragm, which can be totally obstructive and is located at the venous–left atrial junction, and a more extensive stenosis located at a greater distance from the left atrium, which corresponds to hypoplasia or atresia of the pulmonary vein. Although most investigators agree that stenosis, atresia, and hypoplasia of the pulmonary veins are generally congenital

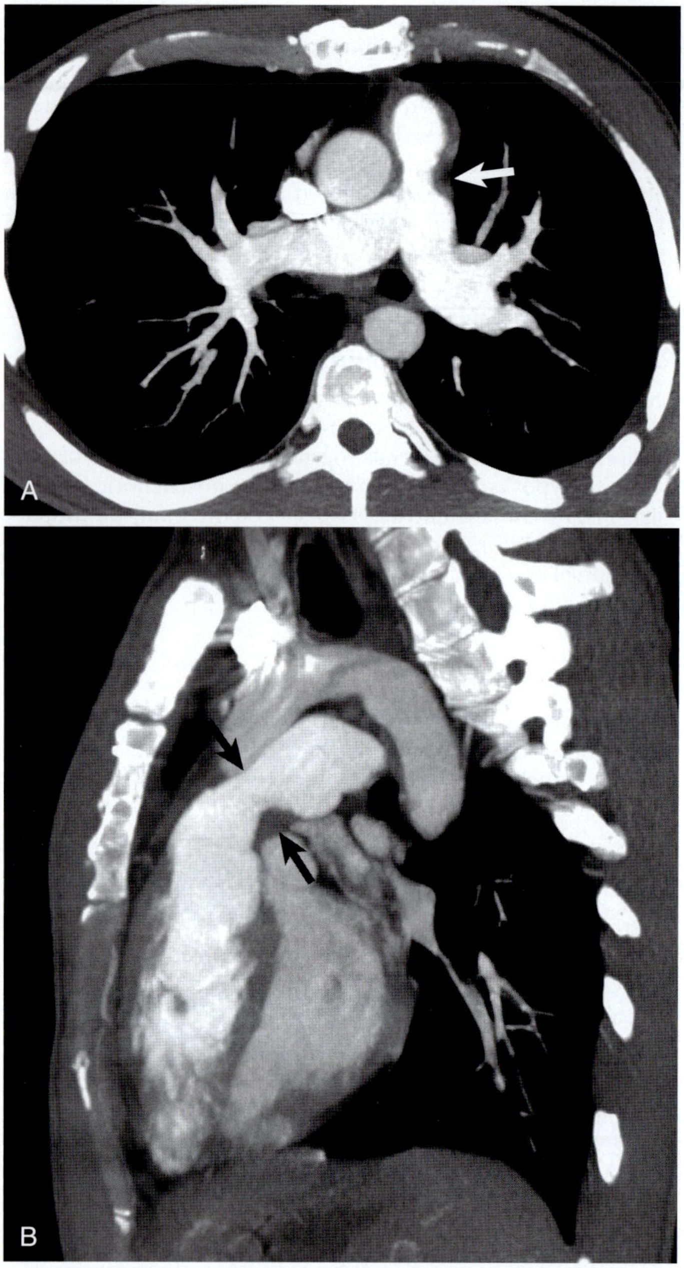

Fig. 8.9 Pulmonary artery stenosis. (A) and (B) Axial and sagittal reformatted CT images show a focal stenosis *(arrows)* of the main pulmonary artery superior to the pulmonic valve, with mildly dilated proximal left and right pulmonary arteries.

in origin, some have suggested venous thrombosis as an additional possible cause.

PATHOPHYSIOLOGY

An understanding of the pathophysiology of a pulmonary venoocclusive syndrome makes it easier to recognize the resultant radiologic signs. This syndrome is associated with an increase in pulmonary vascular resistance in the territory drained by the abnormal veins and redistribution of pulmonary arterial flow to other areas of the lung. The pulmonary artery supplying the venoocclusive territory adapts its caliber according to the reduced blood flow and appears "hypoplastic" yet patent. The resultant oligemia stimulates the development of a collateral systemic-to-pulmonary arterial supply arising from the bronchial and nonbronchial systemic arteries, resulting in a functional systemic-to-pulmonary arterial shunt with retrograde flow within the pulmonary artery. The venous obstruction can cause rerouting of venous blood into the systemic veins, such as the bronchial veins (accounting for the hyperemia of the bronchial walls), transpleural veins, mediastinal veins, periesophageal veins, and the portal venous system. This pulmonary-to-systemic venous shunt explains the "arterialization" and oxygenation of blood in the efferent vessels—namely, the superior or inferior vena cava. The pulmonary venoocclusive syndrome leads to chronic alveolar and interstitial pulmonary edema with thickening of the interlobular septa and peribronchovascular sheets. The chronicity of this edema may lead to pulmonary fibrosis. The lymphatics within the territory of venous occlusion are ectatic, and resorption of alveolar and interstitial fluid via the lymphatics can result in enlargement of the hilar and mediastinal lymph nodes.

CLINICAL PRESENTATION

The clinical manifestations of stenosis or atresia of the pulmonary veins may be those of an associated congenital cardiac anomaly, pulmonary arterial hypertension, recurrent respiratory tract infections, or hemoptysis. VQ scintigraphy may reveal a "pseudopulmonary emboli" appearance with an unmatched reduction in perfusion or a "pseudopneumonia" appearance if the decrease in perfusion is matched by a decrease in ventilation. Hyperemia of the bronchial walls may be a cause of ventilatory obstruction.

MANIFESTATIONS OF THE DISEASE

Radiography

In cases of unilateral obstruction to pulmonary venous return, the chest radiograph shows a small lung with a small hilum without evidence of bronchial obstruction or air trapping. The absence of air trapping must nevertheless be verified by CT because the venoocclusive syndrome can cause subtle bronchial obstruction secondary to edema and engorgement of the veins and lymphatics within the bronchial walls. In addition, pleural thickening may occur.[13] In cases of bilateral venous obstruction, the radiographic findings are those of postcapillary pulmonary hypertension.

Computed Tomography

The presence of a small lung with a small pulmonary hilum and absence of proximal bronchial obstruction can be verified by CT. The pleura may be thickened, with the formation of transpleural adhesions that facilitate the development of transpleural venous anastomoses. In the lung parenchyma there may be patchy ground-glass opacities and interlobular septal thickening in the venooccluded parts of the lung. The bronchial walls are thickened; at bronchoscopy there is often a "pseudoangiomatous" appearance of the bronchial mucosa. The ipsilateral pulmonary artery is small or may be mistakenly thought to be absent if there is retrograde flow of blood within the artery, creating a hemodynamic obstruction to contrast-enhanced blood flow. Its opacification at CT therefore depends on the timing of image acquisition; it is not opacified in the early arterial phase of contrast administration but enhances later secondary to

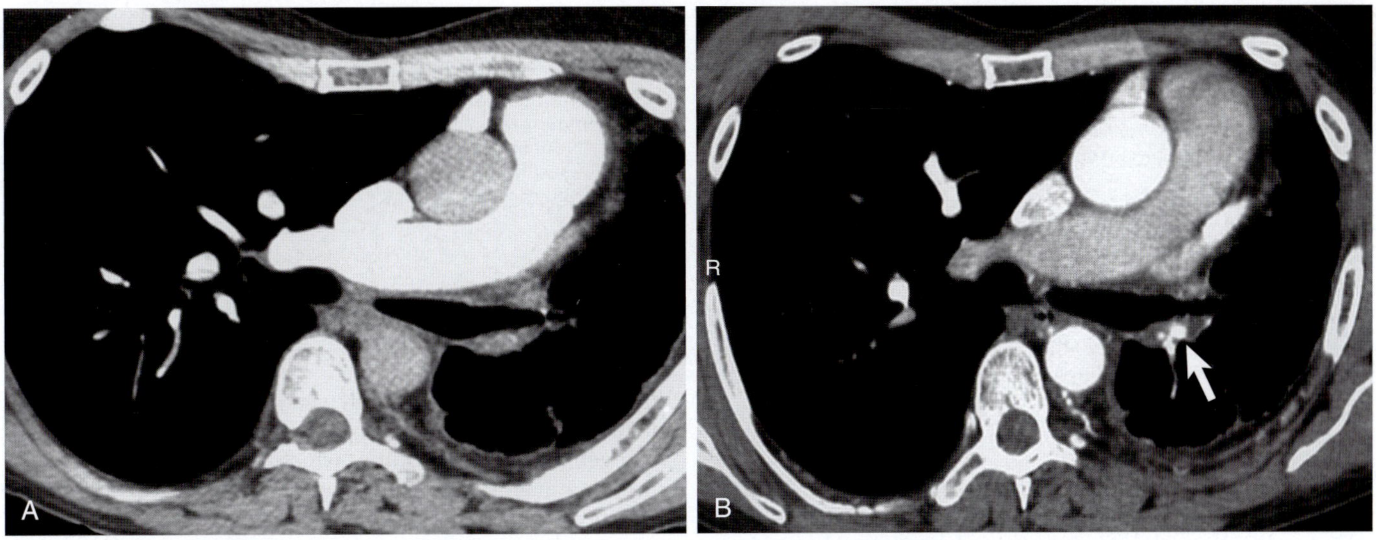

Fig. 8.10 Unilateral atresia of the left pulmonary veins. (A) The first image was performed during a pulmonary arterial enhancement phase. It demonstrates almost complete absence of opacification of the left pulmonary artery, which has a very small caliber. This image slice also demonstrates a reduction in volume of the left lung, associated with increased extrapleural fat in the posterior portion of the lung. The same image level is shown during the phase of systemic arterial enhancement in (B). It demonstrates excellent opacification of the left interlobar pulmonary artery *(arrow)* and simultaneous opacification of the bronchial and intercostal arteries. This delayed opacification of the left pulmonary artery results from a systemic-to-pulmonary arterial shunt flowing retrograde within the left pulmonary artery up to the level of the hilum. Depending on the moment of image acquisition, this pulmonary artery may appear absent, hypoplastic, or thrombosed at the point where the nonopacified pulmonary arterial blood flow meets the retrograde systemic arterial flow within the pulmonary artery.

retrograde flow of contrast medium via collateral systemic-to-pulmonary artery shunts (Fig. 8.10). CT angiography of the hilar region with an early systemic arterial phase, as well as a delayed systemic venous phase, thus provides optimal characterization. The intrapulmonary veins are identifiable, but their juxtaatrial portions are absent. At these sites the left atrial wall appears smooth and does not show the characteristic prominences formed by the pulmonary venous confluence in normal patients. Soft tissue thickening in the ipsilateral hilum and mediastinum may represent the development of a collateral venous circulation bypassing the pulmonary venous occlusion. There may be lymphadenopathy and lymphangiectasia in the ipsilateral hilum and mediastinum secondary to lymphatic engorgement from the pulmonary edema fluid. Signs of venous infarction may also be seen.

Angiography

If the imaging studies just described are not sufficient for a confident diagnosis, nonselective[14] or selective angiography with the tip of the catheter wedged into the occluded capillaries on the venooccluded side[15] can show the stump of the atretic venous sac and can opacify the collateral veins. The development of a collateral arterial circulation can lead to recurrent hemoptysis, necessitating embolization therapy.[13]

Magnetic Resonance Imaging

Although spin-echo, steady-state free precession, and gradient-echo MRI may be useful for the study of pulmonary venous malformations,[16] this modality does not provide optimal characterization of the lung parenchyma, the bronchi, and the collateral venous and arterial circulations.

DIFFERENTIAL DIAGNOSIS

Suspicion of unilateral pulmonary venoocclusive syndrome leads to consideration of a differential diagnosis: proximal interruption of a pulmonary artery, congenital or acquired and anatomic or hemodynamic in nature; infiltration of the hilum or mediastinum by malignancy or fibrosing mediastinitis; and obstruction of pulmonary venous return secondary to acquired rather than congenital causes.

In cases of congenital occlusion a collateral venous system may develop that reroutes venous flow toward the ipsilateral nonobstructed vein.[17] The resulting aberrant, very tortuous intraparenchymal vein can be confused with partial anomalous venous return or with a pulmonary arteriovenous malformation. Axial and multiplanar reformatted images can confirm that the anomalous vessel is venous, that one of the pulmonary veins is stenosed or atretic, and that the other is dilated. The lung parenchyma drained by the aberrant vein appears normal when the collateral venous system compensates sufficiently for the venous obstruction (see the section on aberrant or meandering pulmonary veins).

Pulmonary Varices

EMBRYOLOGY, PREVALENCE, AND EPIDEMIOLOGY

Formation of normal pulmonary venous return involves the development of a primitive venous plexus from the common pulmonary vein that arises from the superior wall of the left atrium and connects the two immature lungs. The common pulmonary vein forms the proximal portion of the left atrium, and the four pulmonary veins form upstream. Stenosis or atresia

KEY POINTS: STENOSIS-ATRESIA OF PULMONARY VEINS

- One or several veins affected, unilateral or bilateral
- Signs of pulmonary venous hypertension
- Symptoms include recurrent bronchopulmonary infections and hemoptysis
- Common imaging findings:
  - Reduced volume of affected lung
  - Mosaic attenuation and septal lines
  - Small corresponding pulmonary arteries with late opacification
  - Bronchial wall thickening
  - Systemic-to-pulmonary artery shunting
  - Juxtaatrial atresia/stenosis of the pulmonary veins

of one of them results in varicose dilation of another. Although they are still called varicosities, these phlebectasias consist of both a localized saccular dilation of a pulmonary vein (or a true varix) and a more tubular dilation of one or several pulmonary veins. In the latter case they can be regarded as the consequence of chronic pulmonary venous hypertension or as an aberrant intrapulmonary collateral venous pathway bypassing a congenital stenosis or atresia of a pulmonary vein. Such anomalies can be isolated or may be associated with other congenital malformations, particularly those involving the pulmonary veins.

CLINICAL PRESENTATION

Pulmonary varices are usually asymptomatic, but rare complications such as hemoptysis or systemic thromboembolism can occur.

MANIFESTATIONS OF THE DISEASE

Radiography

On a chest radiograph, pulmonary varices are seen as tubular or round opacities whose diameter can vary with the Valsalva and Müller maneuvers.[18] They may be confused with true pulmonary nodules or, more rarely, with mediastinal masses.

Computed Tomography

The diagnosis can easily be made with CT, which shows saccular or tubular dilation of the affected vein.[19] CT is also useful for searching for the presence of a thrombus within saccular varices.

DIFFERENTIAL DIAGNOSIS

The differential diagnosis is that of tubular bronchial and vascular opacities. Not all dilated pulmonary veins represent tubular or saccular varices; other diagnoses that must be considered include pulmonary arteriovenous malformations, aberrant intraparenchymal venous pathways, and partial anomalous pulmonary venous return.

SYNOPSIS OF TREATMENT OPTIONS

Surgery is rarely indicated for the treatment of a pulmonary varix unless it is the cause of recurrent hemoptysis or it changes significantly in size or form.[20] Surgery may also be indicated for the treatment of a cardiac disease, such as mitral stenosis, that causes a varix caused by pulmonary venous hypertension.

KEY POINTS: PULMONARY VARICES

- Usually asymptomatic, may result in hemoptysis or systemic thromboembolism
- Common radiologic findings:
  - Nodular or tubular opacity on a chest radiograph
  - Saccular or tubular dilation of a pulmonary vein on CT, MRI, or angiography

Partial Anomalous Pulmonary Venous Return

Partial anomalous pulmonary venous return (PAPVR) can be divided into two broad groups. The first is scimitar syndrome, or hypogenetic lung syndrome, which is often asymptomatic. It involves a malformation of the right lung and an anomalous right pulmonary vein that can be easily identified on chest radiographs as resembling a scimitar, a type of curved sword. This is the most common form of PAPVR detected by radiography. The second group consists of other forms of PAPVR that do not have associated lung abnormalities and are usually asymptomatic.

SCIMITAR SYNDROME (HYPOGENETIC LUNG SYNDROME)

Scimitar syndrome is characterized by partial or total anomalous pulmonary venous return from the right lung, most often to the inferior vena cava and at other times to a suprahepatic vein, the superior vena cava, or the right atrium. In its classic configuration it takes the form of a Turkish sword, from which its name is derived. It is very frequently associated with malformations of the right lung. To underline its complexity, it is preferable to use the term *hypogenetic lung syndrome* or *congenital venolobar syndrome.*

Embryology, Prevalence, and Epidemiology

This syndrome affects both sexes. It is usually sporadic, but familial cases have been reported. The age at detection depends on associated malformations and may vary from the neonatal period to adulthood. There is no known embryologic explanation for the constellation of malformations common to congenital hypogenetic lung syndrome.

Clinical Presentation

Scimitar syndrome may be asymptomatic or may result in symptoms related to associated congenital pulmonary or cardiac malformations or pulmonary arterial hypertension. In order of decreasing frequency, clinical symptoms include recurrent respiratory tract infections, dyspnea on effort, chronic cough, chest pain, wheezing, and recurrent hemoptysis. In 10% of cases there are no symptoms, and the anomaly is discovered incidentally on a routine chest radiograph. Symptoms depend on the magnitude of the left-to-right shunt associated with the anomaly.

Pathophysiology

The term *congenital venolobar syndrome* derives from the fact that the pulmonary malformation is often accompanied by agenesis, aplasia, or hypoplasia of the right upper lobe. The "hypoplasia" of the right pulmonary artery is proportional to the volume of absent lung. A so-called absent right pulmonary artery may in fact be a patent pulmonary artery subjected to retrograde systemic-to-pulmonary arterial shunting. This complex malformation is associated with a number of other anomalies,[21] including arterial or venous, bronchial, and pleural anomalies; cardiac anomalies are seen in approximately 20%.

Moderate dilation of the scimitar vein can occur secondary to the lower vascular resistance in the territory of the left-to-right shunt or be due to increased venous return resulting from perfusion of the lung by systemic arteries. Dilatation of the inferior vena cava is common but is variable and depends on the size of the shunt. The magnitude of the left-to-right shunt as a percentage of cardiac output can be approximately 50% when isolated, may increase to 75% after contralateral lobectomy, and may reach 100% after contralateral pneumonectomy.

Rarely, the abnormal vein may be stenosed at its confluence with the inferior vena cava or in its transdiaphragmatic course and result in a venoocclusive syndrome involving the anomalous venous return. The "scimitar vein" may rarely drain into the supradiaphragmatic portion of the inferior vena cava, the suprahepatic veins, the portal vein, the azygos vein, the coronary sinus, or the right atrium.[22]

Manifestations of the Disease

Radiography. A scimitar vein is often easily visualized and diagnosed on radiography, particularly if the right lung is not too underdeveloped and if the abnormal venous drainage is significant. The classic appearance is a vertically oriented curvilinear vein, convex inferolaterally, and increasing in diameter from superior to inferior (Fig. 8.11). In some cases the volume of the affected lung may be low enough to cause dextrocardia that obscures the abnormal vein, compromising radiographic detection.

A radiopaque stripe is often observed in the retrosternal region on lateral chest radiographs, explained by the fact that the anterior aspect of the right lung is situated more posteriorly than the left. The degree of dextrocardia and dextrorotation is proportional to the degree of hypoplasia of the right lung. A "horseshoe lung" is a rare association, characterized by a portion of the right lung herniating into the left hemithorax behind the heart and coming into contact with the mediastinal aspect of the left lower lobe. It is ventilated by a bronchus arising from the right bronchial tree that crosses the mediastinum. Contact of the two lungs posteriorly is seen as a vertical fissure-like line in the left paramedian retrocardiac region. The two pleural cavities are separate or may communicate.

Computed Tomography. The scimitar vein and the various associated anomalies of the right hemithorax that may be seen in association with hypogenetic lung syndrome can be visualized by multiplanar CT (see Fig. 8.11). Such anomalies include the following:

1. Bronchial abnormalities:
   - Bronchiectasis
   - Rudimentary blind-ending bronchi
   - Bronchial diverticula
2. Pulmonary:
   - Lobar agenesis, aplasia, hypoplasia
   - Horseshoe lung
3. Pulmonary arteries:
   - Hypoplastic right pulmonary artery
   - Proximal interruption of the right pulmonary artery
4. Pleural:
   - Anomalies of the fissures (accessory, incomplete)
   - Absence of the pleura
5. Diaphragmatic:
   - Congenital defects
   - Cysts
   - Duplication (accessory diaphragm)

Hypogenetic lung syndrome can be associated with various cardiovascular malformations that can usually also be recognized on CT, including the following:

1. Malformations of the vena cava:
   - Intrapulmonary course of the right superior vena cava
   - Persistent left superior vena cava
   - Azygos continuation of the inferior vena cava
2. Cardiac malformations:
   - Atrial septal defect
   - Patent ductus arteriosus
   - Tetralogy of Fallot
3. Pulmonary arteriovenous malformations
4. Pericardial defect

Abnormal systemic arteries may originate from branches of the thoracic or abdominal aorta, in particular the internal mammary artery or the right inferior phrenic artery. They may be responsible for symptoms such as hemoptysis or pulmonary hypertension because they participate in left-to-right shunting from the abnormal venous return. They can be successfully treated by embolotherapy. Their intraparenchymal angioarchitecture conforms to that of the peripheral branches of the pulmonary arteries. One variety of abnormal systemic arterialization is represented by a purely vascular intralobar sequestration in which bronchi at the right lung base are moderately dilated and not accompanied by pulmonary arteries.

CT has largely replaced aortography, pulmonary angiography, and bronchography.[23] Because of the tubular nature of the abnormal vein and the frequent associated multiorgan anomalies, multiplanar and three-dimensional image reconstructions are helpful for optimal depiction of the findings.[24]

Magnetic Resonance Imaging. Preoperative hemodynamic assessment of the contributions from the heart and from the pulmonary and systemic vascular systems can be performed by CT, MRI,[25] and echocardiography.[26]

Differential Diagnosis

A scimitar vein most commonly drains into the inferior vena cava. This course should be differentiated from a "pseudoscimitar" vein draining normally into the left atrium (Fig. 8.12) and from anomalous simultaneous drainage into the left atrium and the inferior vena cava. "Pseudoscimitar syndrome" specifically corresponds to an abnormal pathway of a scimitar-like vein that terminates in the left atrium. This latter anomaly may be associated with azygos continuation of the inferior vena cava, systemic arterial supply to the right lung, and a hypogenetic right lung. The most complex malformation of all is characterized by the association in the right lung of a scimitar vein draining into the inferior vena cava, a second scimitar vein draining into the left atrium, and anastomoses between these two veins. Rarely, an intrathoracic rib may resemble an abnormal vein on radiographs.

Synopsis of Treatment Options

Treatment in an adult is rarely indicated for the malformed right lung but depends instead on the associated congenital cardiac diseases. Most often, treatment involves reimplantation of the abnormal pulmonary vein into the left atrium[27] or interruption of the systemic arterial supply to the lung.

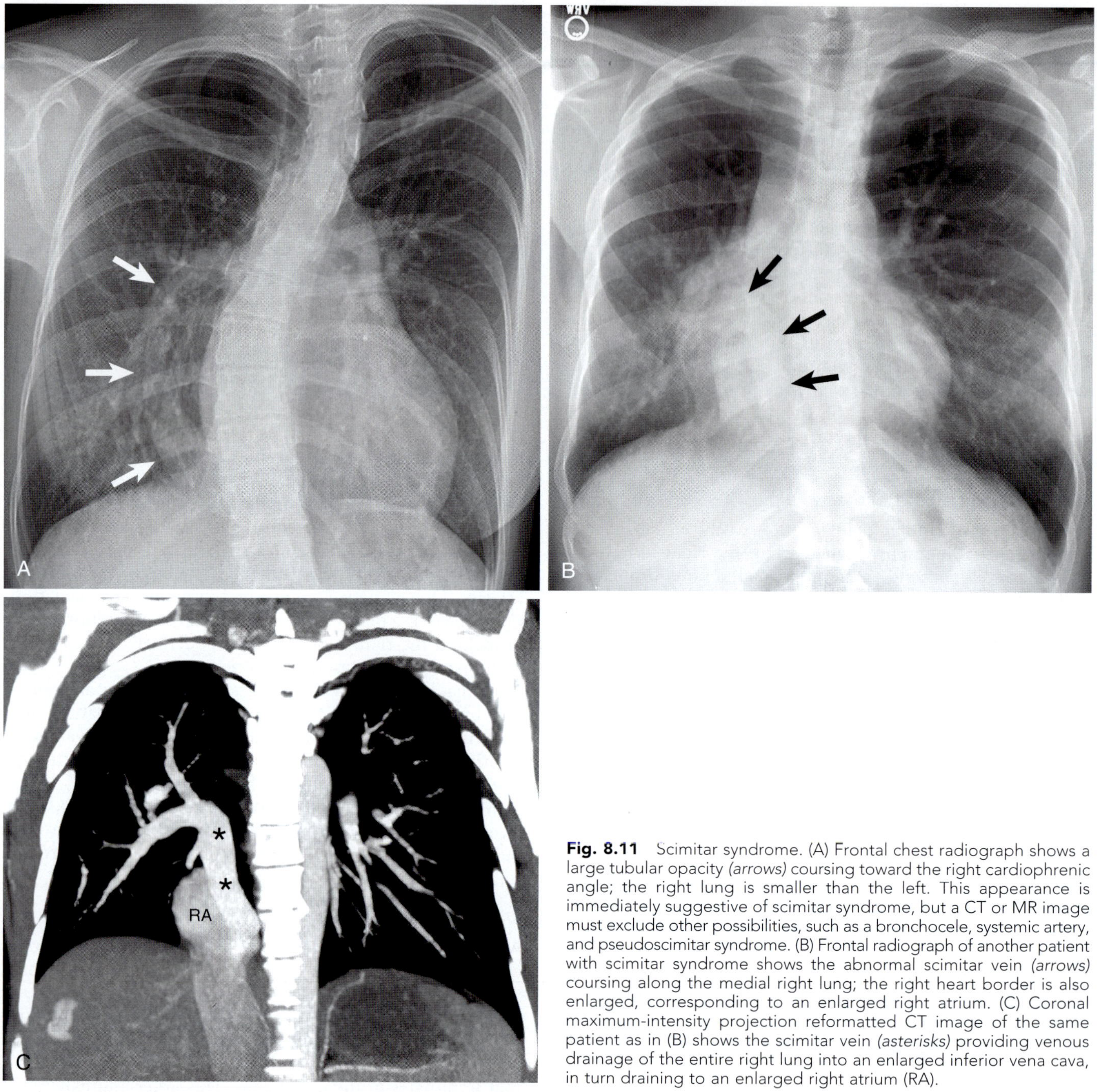

Fig. 8.11 Scimitar syndrome. (A) Frontal chest radiograph shows a large tubular opacity *(arrows)* coursing toward the right cardiophrenic angle; the right lung is smaller than the left. This appearance is immediately suggestive of scimitar syndrome, but a CT or MR image must exclude other possibilities, such as a bronchocele, systemic artery, and pseudoscimitar syndrome. (B) Frontal radiograph of another patient with scimitar syndrome shows the abnormal scimitar vein *(arrows)* coursing along the medial right lung; the right heart border is also enlarged, corresponding to an enlarged right atrium. (C) Coronal maximum-intensity projection reformatted CT image of the same patient as in (B) shows the scimitar vein *(asterisks)* providing venous drainage of the entire right lung into an enlarged inferior vena cava, in turn draining to an enlarged right atrium (RA).

KEY POINTS: SCIMITAR (HYPOGENETIC LUNG) SYNDROME

- May be asymptomatic
- Common clinical findings:
  - Recurrent infections of the right lung
  - Hemoptysis
  - Signs of pulmonary hypertension
- Common radiologic findings:
  - Small right lung with decreased right upper lobe volume
  - Scimitar vein with left-to-right shunt
  - Partial systemic arterialization of the right lung
  - Numerous associated anomalies

OTHER FORMS OF PARTIAL ANOMALOUS PULMONARY VENOUS RETURN

Embryology, Prevalence, and Epidemiology

PAPVR may occur in association with congenital heart disease or as an isolated finding. Isolated PAPVR in the absence of congenital cardiac disease or other malformations is seen in 0.4% to 0.7% of adults, usually as an incidental finding on CT.

The persistence of a connection between the pulmonary and systemic venous return systems toward the right side of the heart can be explained by the embryologic development of these two venous networks.[28] A PAPVR normally drains into an ipsilateral systemic vein: Therefore a right PAPVR drains into the azygos

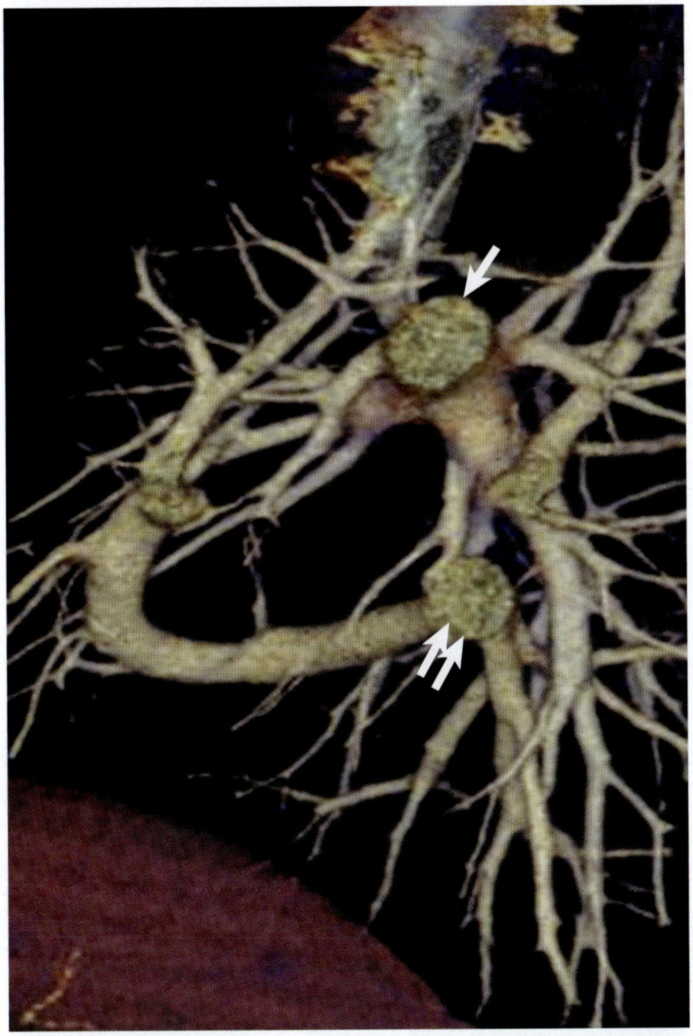

Fig. 8.12 Pseudoscimitar syndrome discovered incidentally in an asymptomatic young adult. A volumetric reconstruction of the right lung shows a long vein with an abnormal trajectory descending from the lung apex toward the anteroinferior portion of the lung and then coursing almost horizontally before terminating in the right inferior pulmonary vein *(double arrow).* The first portion of this aberrant pulmonary vein passes in front of the hilum and corresponds to the section of the right pulmonary artery *(single arrow).* This is the classic appearance of pseudoscimitar syndrome, in which the abnormal vein has a scimitar-like trajectory but terminates normally within the left atrium.

vein, superior vena cava, right atrium, inferior vena cava, or suprahepatic veins, and a left PAPVR drains into a vertical vein (draining to the left brachiocephalic vein), the hemiazygos system, or the coronary sinus. A "vertical vein" probably represents persistence of the left precardinal vein and can be distinguished from a persistent left superior vena cava by drainage of the former into the left brachiocephalic vein, and the latter to either the coronary sinus or left atrium.[29,30] Except in the case of scimitar syndrome, the pulmonary venous return usually drains into the closest ipsilateral systemic vein, although rarely, an anomalous vein can drain directly into the right atrium.[31] Right-sided PAPVRs are twice as common as left-sided ones.

Pathophysiology

The efferent vessels receiving the anomalous vein become dilated because pulmonary venous return toward the right side of the heart has lower vascular resistance than venous return to the left atrium, leading to a redistribution of pulmonary arterial blood flow toward the territory of the PAPVR.

A PAPVR results in a left-to-right shunt that typically represents no more than 25% of cardiac output. However, in adults, an asymptomatic PAPVR can become symptomatic after pneumonectomy of the contralateral lung. The surgery unmasks and increases the magnitude of the previously silent left-to-right shunt.[32] Before surgery, therefore, interpretation of a preoperative CT scan of the thorax should include an assessment of the possible hemodynamic consequences of the PAPVR that might result from the planned resection. In certain cases a two-stage procedure involving initial reimplantation of the PAPVR into the left atrium may be required to avoid postpneumonectomy right-sided heart failure.[33] In other situations, patients with PAPVR in whom congestive heart failure develops may demonstrate asymmetric cardiogenic pulmonary edema because the abnormal vein that drains into the right side of the heart is protected from the effects of pulmonary venous hypertension. Conversely, obstruction of the superior vena cava can cause pulmonary edema in the territory drained by the ectopic vein.

Clinical Presentation

Isolated PAPVR in adulthood is nearly always asymptomatic.

Manifestations of the Disease

Radiography. When sufficiently dilated, anomalous veins in PAPVR may be detected at radiography, with the appearance dependent on the type and course of the anomalous venous drainage:

PAPVR draining into the lower superior vena cava. This malformation consists of partial or total venous drainage of the right upper lobe into the lower superior vena cava, just above the right atrium. This anomaly frequently goes unrecognized at radiography. It may be suspected by the presence of one or several tubular opacities in the right upper lobe (Fig. 8.13) or by an opacity in the right tracheobronchial angle.

PAPVR of the left upper lobe draining into a vertical vein. One or two dilated tubular opacities may be visible in the left upper lobe. This abnormal venous return drains into the vertical vein that unites the upper portion of the left hilum with the left brachiocephalic vein at the point of confluence of the left subclavian and internal jugular veins (confluence of Pirogoff). It has a small diameter and can be identified on chest radiographs as a left mediastinal interface at the level of the aortopulmonary window and the aortic arch.

PAPVR draining into the right atrium. In this malformation the right-to-left shunt is of greater severity than in the preceding cases, on the order of 50% of cardiac output, thus explaining the frequent discovery of this malformation in adults with pulmonary arterial hypertension. There is no intraparenchymal component to the aberrant venous pathway. A heterotaxy syndrome (levoisomerism or polysplenia) and a persistent left superior vena cava are frequent associations.

PAPVR of the right lung draining into the azygos vein or its arch (rare). In these cases it can be difficult to differentiate this ectopic drainage from drainage into the lower superior vena cava. Drainage from the right lower lobe into the superior vena cava has also been described.

Computed Tomography

PAPVR draining into the superior vena cava. The anomalous vein is best depicted at contrast-enhanced CT and can be seen

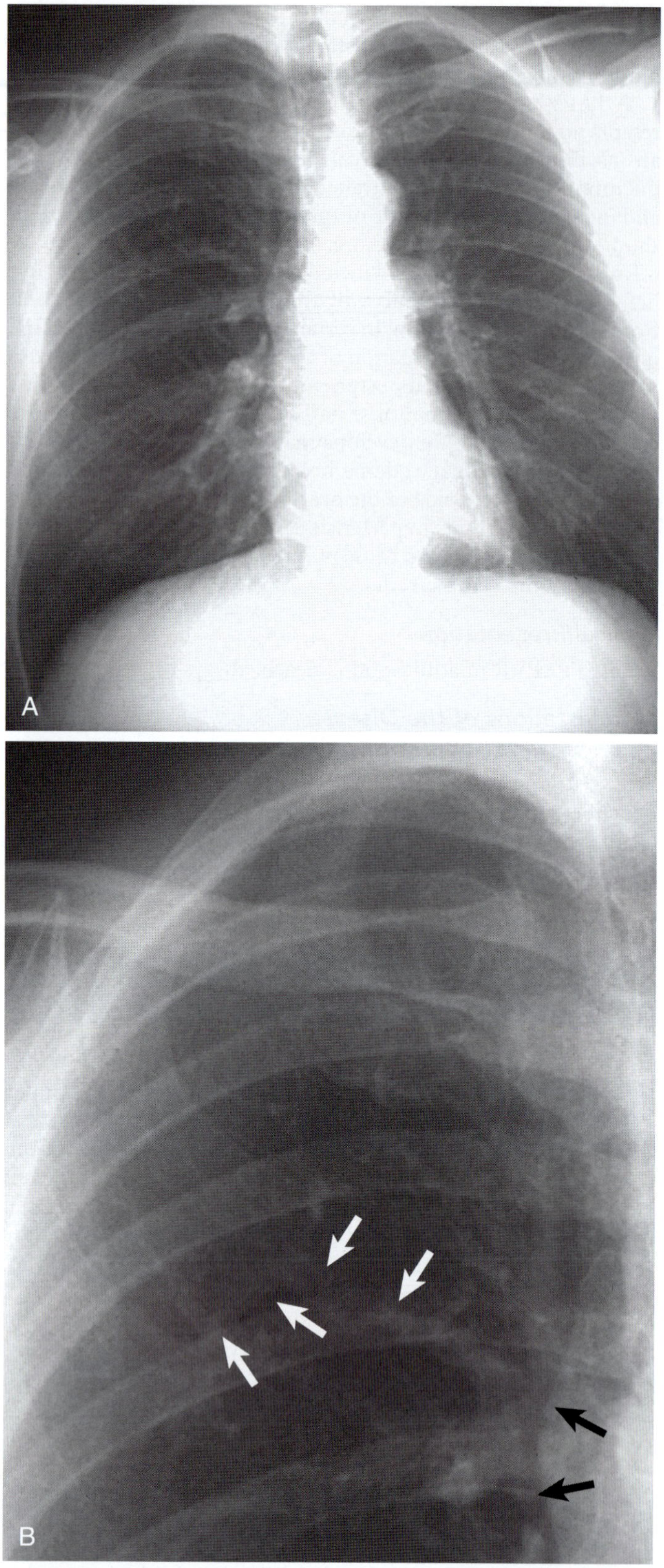

Fig. 8.13 Partial anomalous pulmonary venous return. (A) A frontal chest radiograph and a magnified view of the right upper lobe (B) show a tubular opacity coursing in a lateral-to-medial direction with a trajectory that is initially oblique in a superior direction and then oblique in an inferior direction *(white arrows)*. The second anomaly is a bump on the lower part of the superior vena cava *(black arrows)*. These two associated anomalies are consistent with partial anomalous pulmonary venous return from the right upper lobe into the lower portion of the superior vena cava.

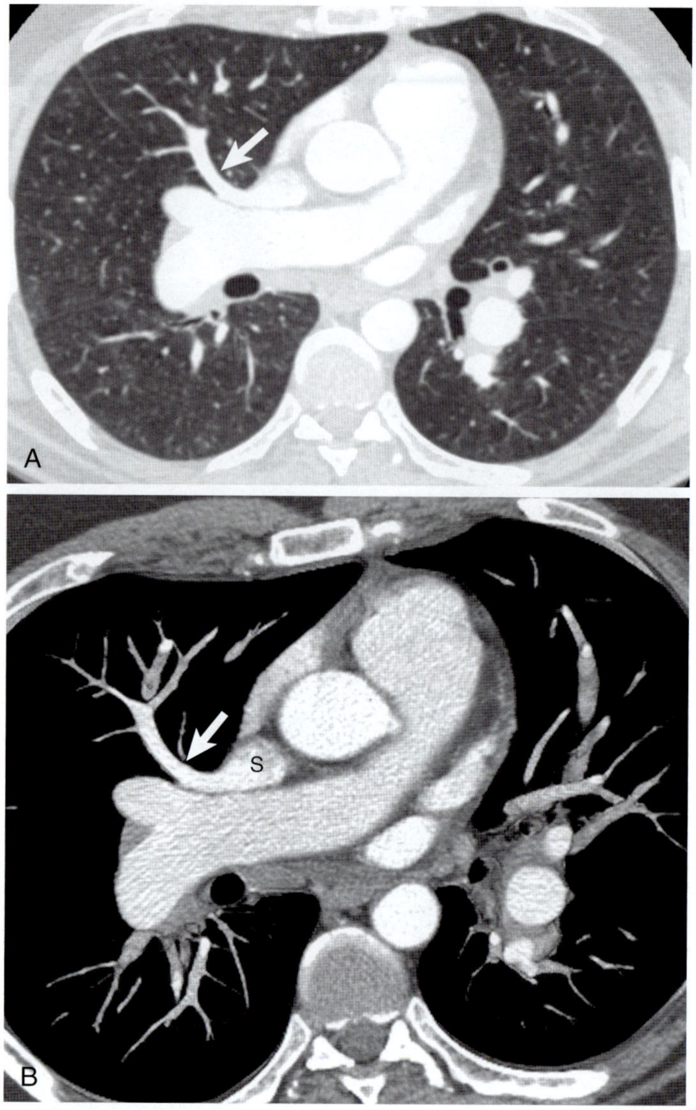

Fig. 8.14 Partial anomalous pulmonary venous return. (A) Axial CT image on lung windows shows an abnormal tubular structure *(arrow)* connecting to the superior vena cava. (B) Axial CT maximum-intensity projection image in soft tissue windows shows anomalous pulmonary venous drainage *(arrow)* from the right upper lobe to the superior vena cava (S).

entering the superior vena cava (Figs. 8.14 and 8.15). An associated sinus venosus atrial septal defect may be present. If surgical intervention is planned, the anatomic anomalies must be meticulously described with respect to drainage of the PAPVR into the lower superior vena cava, the cavoatrial junction, or the upper superior vena cava because such details determine the surgical approach.[34,35]

PAPVR draining into the vertical vein. CT depicts intrapulmonary veins from the left upper lobe draining into the lower part of the vertical vein at the level of the aortopulmonary window. The vertical vein then passes superiorly adjacent to the lateral aspect of the aortic arch (Fig. 8.16).

PAPVR draining into the right atrium. CT angiography can depict abnormal alignment of the interatrial septum with drainage of the right pulmonary veins into the right atrium (Fig. 8.17).[31] Situs abnormalities may be associated, including a persistent left superior vena cava and heterotaxy syndrome (polysplenia or, more rarely, asplenia or even a normal spleen).[36]

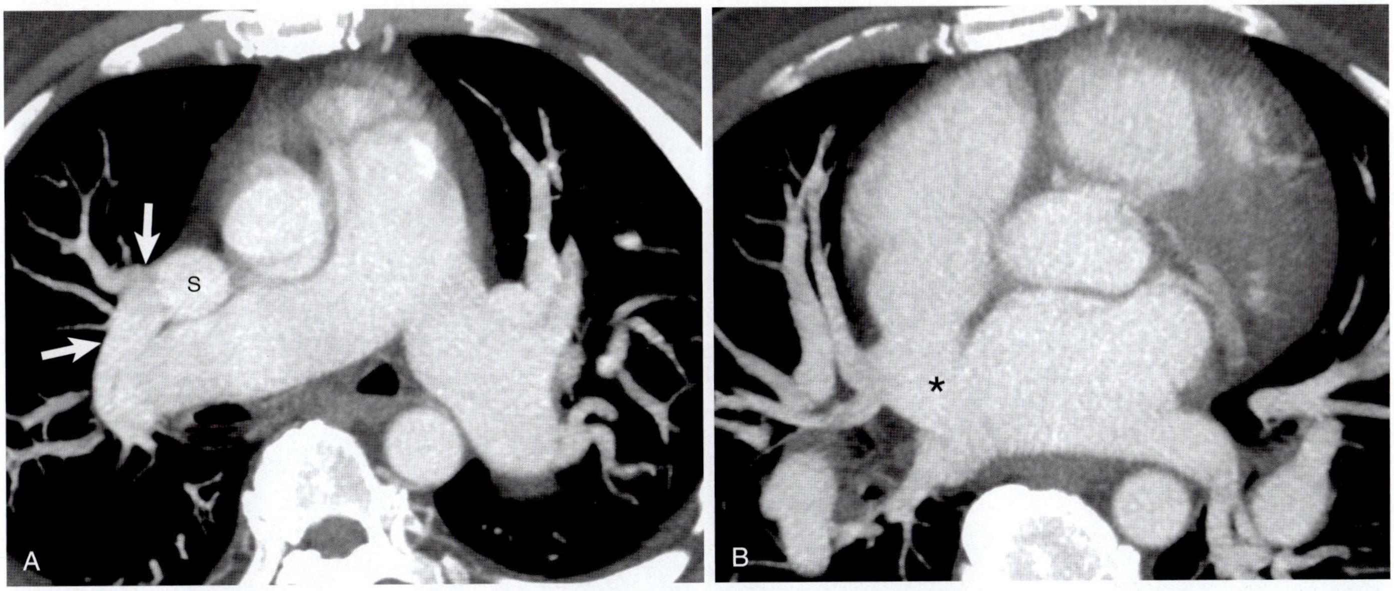

Fig. 8.15 Partial anomalous pulmonary venous return. (A) Axial CT maximum-intensity projection image shows anomalous pulmonary venous drainage from the right upper lobe *(arrows)* to the superior vena cava (S). (B) Image from the same study through the level of the heart shows an associated sinus venosus atrial septal defect *(asterisk)*.

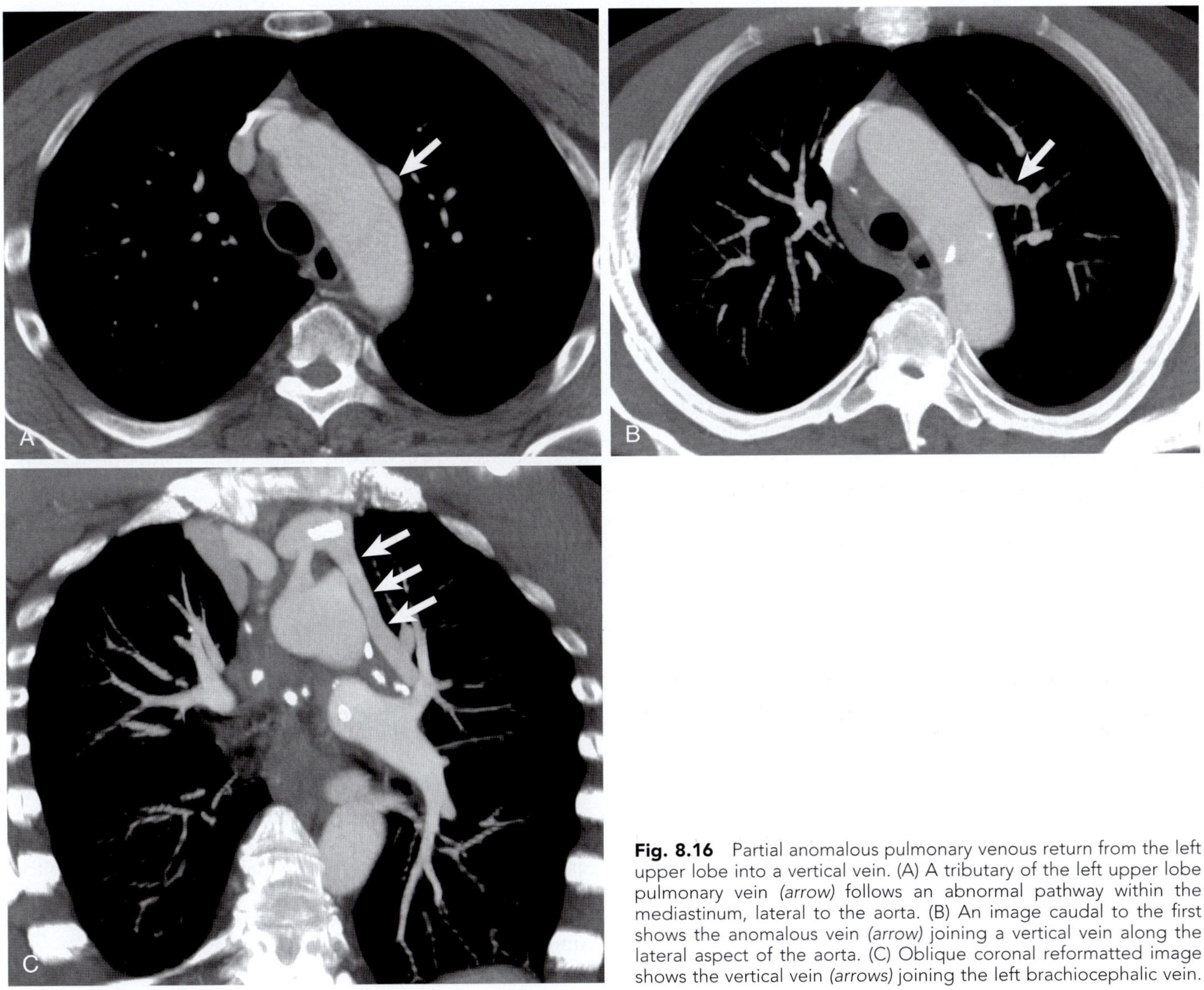

Fig. 8.16 Partial anomalous pulmonary venous return from the left upper lobe into a vertical vein. (A) A tributary of the left upper lobe pulmonary vein *(arrow)* follows an abnormal pathway within the mediastinum, lateral to the aorta. (B) An image caudal to the first shows the anomalous vein *(arrow)* joining a vertical vein along the lateral aspect of the aorta. (C) Oblique coronal reformatted image shows the vertical vein *(arrows)* joining the left brachiocephalic vein.

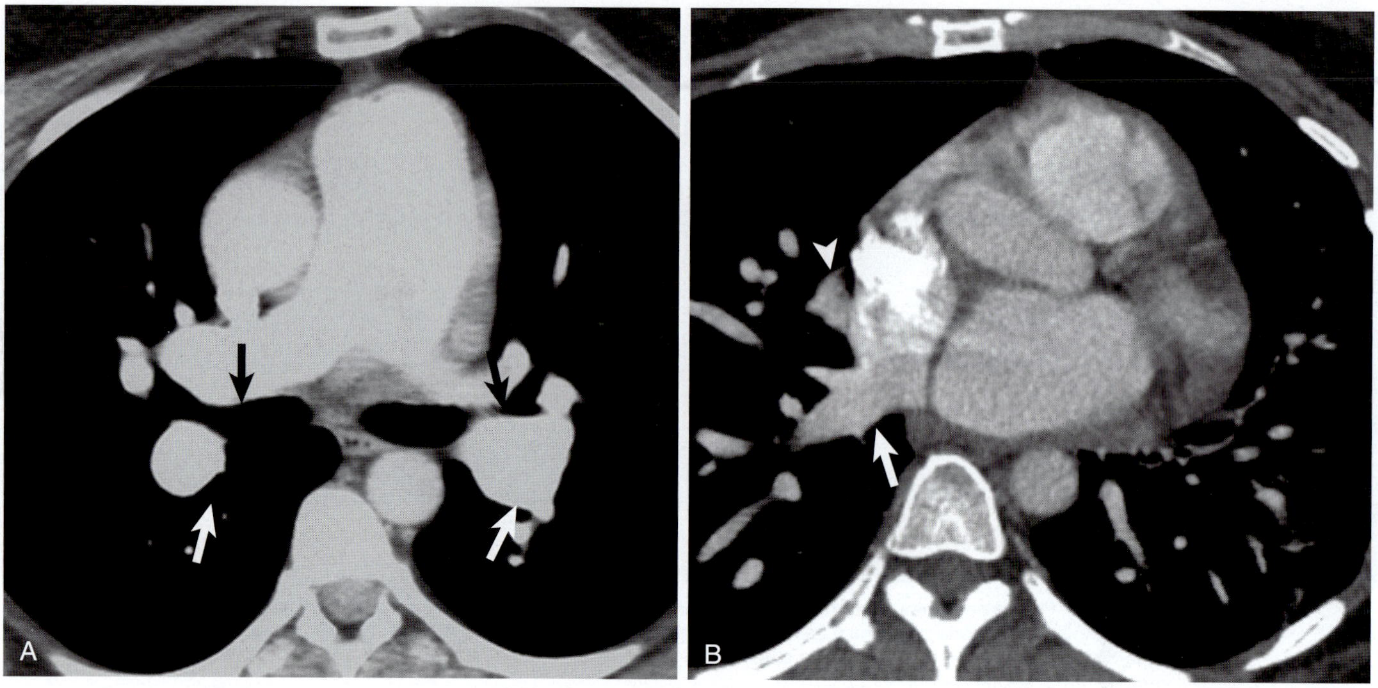

Fig. 8.17 Partial anomalous pulmonary venous return draining into the right atrium in a young woman with pulmonary arterial hypertension. (A) CT scan shows dilation of the main pulmonary artery, whose transverse diameter is greater than that of the ascending aorta. There is also a symmetric position of the upper lobe bronchi *(black arrows)*, representing bronchial isomerism. The abnormally dilated lower lobe pulmonary arteries are both situated posterior to the upper lobe bronchi *(white arrows)*, indicative of bilateral left-sidedness or heterotaxy. (B) A CT scan at the level of the right atrium shows malposition of the interatrial septum, which is directing pulmonary venous return from the right lung toward the right atrium. Right inferior pulmonary vein *(arrow)* and right superior pulmonary vein *(arrowhead)*. *(Part A reprinted with permission of Grenier P.* Imagerie Thoracique de l'Adulte. *Paris: Flammarion; 2006.)*

Magnetic Resonance Imaging. MRI can accurately depict PAPVR and is especially helpful for evaluating associated congenital cardiac disease and for quantification of the magnitude of the left-to-right shunt.

Differential Diagnosis

Other tubular structures within the lung may mimic PAPVR at chest radiography, including bronchoceles and dilated collateral veins. Contrast-enhanced CT can easily differentiate among these possibilities.

Synopsis of Treatment Options

A PAPVR that is isolated and asymptomatic does not require treatment. It may be reimplanted during repair of congenital cardiac disease or before surgical resection of a portion of lung that might be postoperatively expected to cause an increase in the severity of a left-to-right shunt.

KEY POINTS: PARTIAL ANOMALOUS PULMONARY VENOUS RETURN

- Often an isolated, asymptomatic abnormality in adults
- Signs of pulmonary hypertension manifest when the left-to-right shunt is greater than 25%
- Focal pulmonary edema when obstructed
- Risk of cardiac failure after lobectomy or pneumonectomy
- Common radiologic findings:
  - More often detected on CT than on chest radiographs
  - Tubular and/or pseudonodular opacities in the lung
  - Minimal dilation of the draining systemic vein

Aberrant or Meandering Pulmonary Veins

EMBRYOLOGY, PREVALENCE, AND EPIDEMIOLOGY

An aberrant or meandering pulmonary vein is a rare congenital malformation characterized by an abnormal course of the vein, which eventually drains normally into the left atrium and is not associated with a shunt. The abnormal venous pathway is characterized by a sinuous rather than a smooth curvilinear course.

CLINICAL PRESENTATION

Aberrant or meandering pulmonary veins are asymptomatic and almost always discovered incidentally on a chest radiograph or CT but may be confused with other pathologies such as arteriovenous malformations.[37,38]

MANIFESTATIONS OF THE DISEASE

Radiography

Aberrant pulmonary veins are almost always associated with abnormalities in the caliber and number of pulmonary veins within the same territory or elsewhere. They form tubular opacities that are tortuous in configuration. Frequently, they follow a "bucket-handle" course, either in the axial or in the sagittal plane. When the two branches of the "bucket" approach each other, they can simulate a pulmonary arteriovenous malformation.[39]

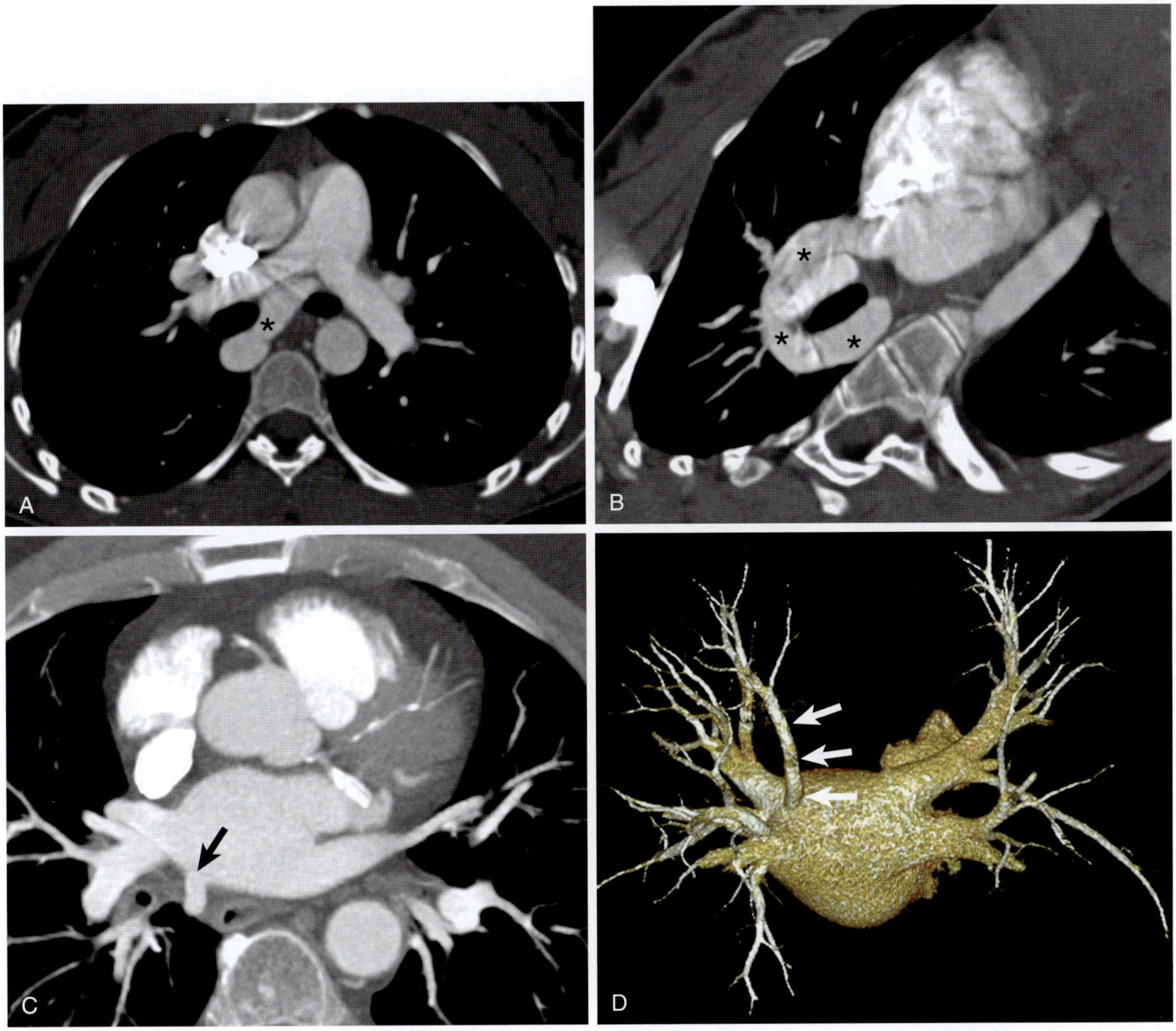

Fig. 8.18 Aberrant pulmonary veins. (A) Axial CT image shows an aberrant pulmonary vein *(asterisk)*, which drained the left upper lobe, crossed the mediastinum, and entered the left atrium. (B) Oblique reformatted image shows the vein *(*)* taking a meandering course within the right lung. (C) "Top" pulmonary vein in another patient. A small vein from the posterior segment of the right upper lobe *(arrow)* enters the roof of the left atrium separate from the ostia of the other right pulmonary veins. (D) The same top pulmonary vein *(arrows)* is shown in a three-dimensional volume-rendered image entering the superior aspect of the left atrium.

Computed Tomography

The diagnosis can readily be made on CT (Figs. 8.18 and 8.19). The venous nature of the abnormality can be recognized by the absence of an accompanying bronchus and by its drainage into the left atrium. In addition, it is useful to describe other anomalies that may be associated: pulmonary arterial hypoplasia, a dilated or tortuous pulmonary artery, bronchopulmonary malformations as part of a hypogenetic lung syndrome, abnormal systemic arteries, and partial anomalous pulmonary venous return in a different lung zone.[40]

Some variations in pulmonary venous return involve intraparenchymal pathways that are only slightly aberrant and are not considered malformations because they are not pathologic. The most common variant is a pulmonary vein draining the posterior segment of the right upper lobe, which, instead of terminating in the right superior pulmonary vein, takes a vertical course posterior to the bronchus intermedius and terminates in the juxtaatrial portion of the right superior pulmonary vein or directly in the left atrium itself. This is often called a "top" pulmonary vein (see Figs. 8.18C and 8.18D) and can be seen uncommonly on the left. Other venous drainage variants can also occur. The normal venous return from the right middle lobe consists of one or two—and sometimes three—intersegmental veins that terminate in the right upper lobe pulmonary vein below the level of the right middle lobe bronchus; however, in

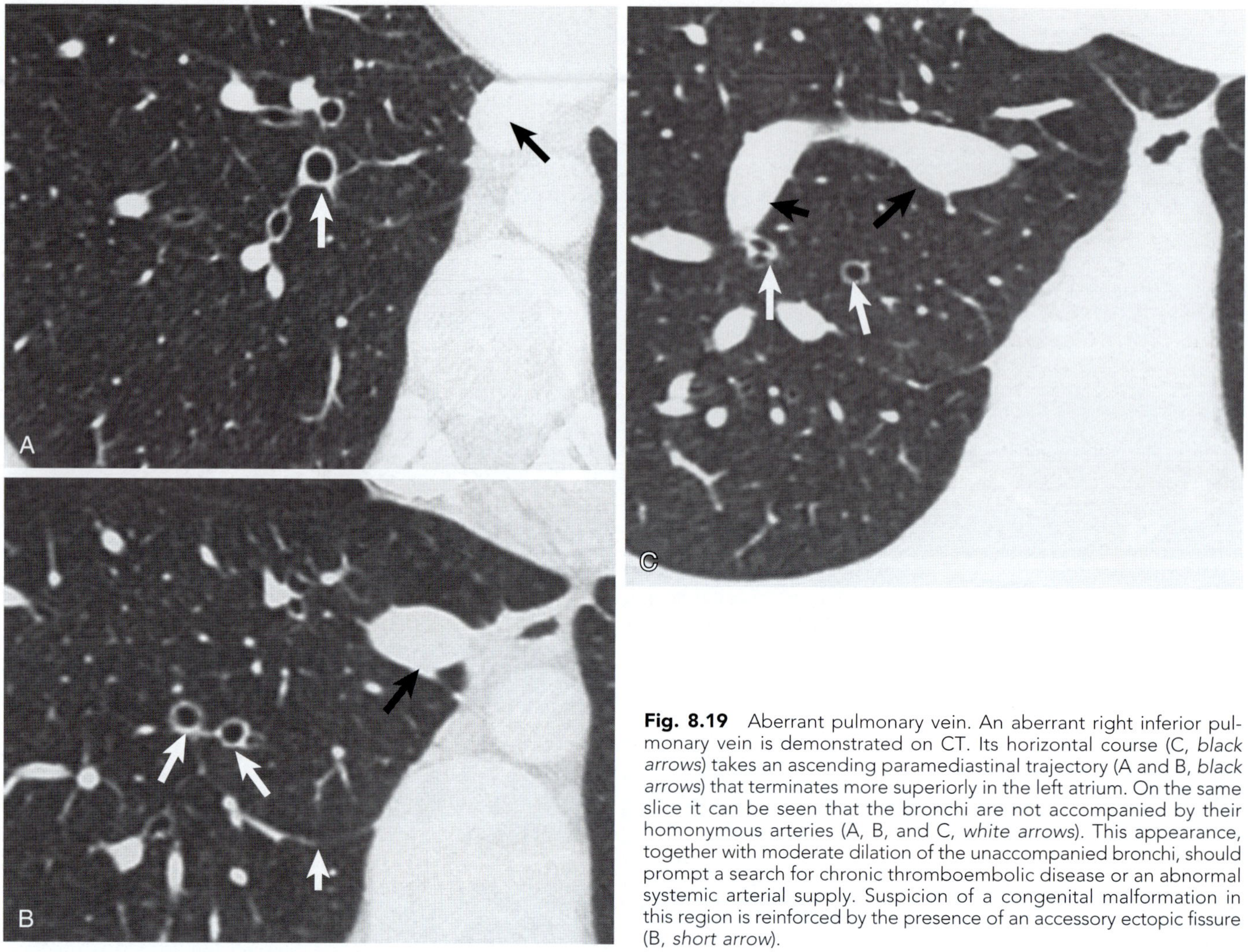

Fig. 8.19 Aberrant pulmonary vein. An aberrant right inferior pulmonary vein is demonstrated on CT. Its horizontal course (C, *black arrows*) takes an ascending paramediastinal trajectory (A and B, *black arrows*) that terminates more superiorly in the left atrium. On the same slice it can be seen that the bronchi are not accompanied by their homonymous arteries (A, B, and C, *white arrows*). This appearance, together with moderate dilation of the unaccompanied bronchi, should prompt a search for chronic thromboembolic disease or an abnormal systemic arterial supply. Suspicion of a congenital malformation in this region is reinforced by the presence of an accessory ectopic fissure (B, *short arrow*).

4.8% of individuals the venous return from the right middle lobe drains into the right inferior pulmonary vein.[19] Venous return from a lung may also drain via a single vein rather than two or more veins.[37]

DIFFERENTIAL DIAGNOSIS

Aberrant venous pathways can simulate the scimitar syndrome,[41] from which the term *pseudoscimitar syndrome* is derived, a condition attributed to an abnormal, vertically oriented right paracardiac vein that terminates normally in the left atrium. A pseudo–pseudoscimitar syndrome has also been described, in which an abnormal scimitar-like vein is directed inferiorly and drains simultaneously into the inferior vena cava and the left atrium. These scimitar-mimicking syndromes may be associated with other anomalies classically encountered in the hypogenetic lung syndrome. Anomalous veins may also simulate pulmonary nodules on chest radiographs.

There is some overlap between aberrant pulmonary veins, pulmonary varices, and pulmonary venous atresia: Atresia of a pulmonary vein can cause rerouting of venous blood toward the other ipsilateral vein by venous anastomoses, which may form aberrant intrapulmonary pathways that can be dilated and are therefore varicose. A single isolated pulmonary vein draining an entire lung can also simulate a varix.[42]

KEY POINTS: ABERRANT PULMONARY VEINS

- Usually asymptomatic; also called meandering pulmonary vein
- Common radiologic findings:
  - Tubular and/or pseudonodular opacities on radiographs
  - Abnormal course of the vein but normal drainage into the left atrium evident on CT

Pulmonary Arteriovenous Malformations

EMBRYOLOGY, PREVALENCE, AND EPIDEMIOLOGY

The embryology of pulmonary arteriovenous malformations (PAVMs) is not precisely known. PAVMs have at times been described as angiodysplastic lesions, and their etiology has also been attributed to hemodynamic, hormonal, and genetic factors. The majority of PAVMs are seen in the context of Rendu-Osler-Weber syndrome, where they are often multiple. For this reason, discovery of a single malformation necessitates exclusion of this genetic syndrome, which is associated with autosomal-dominant transmission.

PATHOPHYSIOLOGY

When an arteriovenous communication is established, it becomes a site of decreased pulmonary vascular resistance and therefore leads to increased blood flow through the malformation. An increase in the overall volume of the body's blood pool, such as during the last 4 months of pregnancy, is also a cause of enlargement of these malformations, and there is an attendant increased risk for complications such as rupture. These hemodynamic factors also explain why PAVMs are most frequent in the lower lobes.

CLINICAL PRESENTATION

Pulmonary arteriovenous malformations may be discovered in one of the following situations[43–45]: (1) incidentally on chest radiography performed for other reasons; (2) secondary to complications, such as a right-to-left shunt with orthopnea, paradoxic septic or thrombotic emboli, and rupture into bronchi or the pleural cavity; (3) in the course of family screening for Rendu-Osler-Weber syndrome; and (4) because of extrathoracic manifestations of Rendu-Osler-Weber syndrome. In Rendu-Osler-Weber syndrome evaluation of the liver should be performed before undertaking treatment of the PAVMs. Hepatic arteriovenous fistulas create a left-to-right shunt effect between the hepatic artery and the suprahepatic veins.[46] They also increase the magnitude of the intrapulmonary right-to-left shunt. One method of reducing the intrapulmonary right-to-left shunt therefore consists of treating the intrahepatic shunt surgically or by embolotherapy.[47] In addition, coexisting pulmonary arterial hypertension and its causes should be searched for before intervention; pulmonary arterial hypertension should be treated before embolotherapy of the PAVMs, and if the hypertension cannot be adequately corrected, it represents a contraindication to embolotherapy.

MANIFESTATIONS OF THE DISEASE

Radiography

Chest radiographs are of limited value in the detection of small- to moderate-sized PAVMs (Fig. 8.20). For this reason, it is difficult to validate its use as a tool for the family screening of Rendu-Osler-Weber syndrome because normal or otherwise, it is likely to be followed by a CT scan. The problems inherent in chest radiography for the detection of PAVMs is made a little easier in some cases by the identification of feeding and draining vessels resulting in a "comet-tail" appearance, which is virtually diagnostic, especially in certain clinical contexts.[48]

Computed Tomography

Detection of PAVMs by CT allows identification of the malformation and its feeding and draining vessels, even when less than a millimeter in size and very peripheral in location. CT is more sensitive than conventional angiography and is currently considered the most diagnostically accurate and least invasive examination for detection of PAVMs (see Fig. 8.20).[49] Its three main indications are for screening, for pretherapeutic evaluation of the angioarchitecture of PAVMs, and for postsurgical and postembolotherapy follow-up.[50,51] Screening CT examinations can be performed at low milliamperage and without intravenous contrast medium, similar to the scanning parameters used for lung cancer screening. For preembolotherapy evaluation, CT angiography is recommended not only for studying the pulmonary vascular malformation itself but also to be able to map the systemic circulation, which can uncommonly be a second source of perfusion of the malformation and may develop further after embolization of the pulmonary arterial feeders. For each malformation it is necessary to describe each arterial pedicle—specifically, its origin, pathway (straight or tortuous), orientation, length, and diameter—in anticipation of endovascular treatment, as well as identify the pulmonary arterial branches that are not involved in perfusion of the aneurysmal sac (and which should be spared during embolotherapy, if possible). In fact, having all this information available provides great reassurance to the interventional radiologist at the beginning of a planned embolotherapy procedure; such details can simplify endovascular manipulations and reduce the amount of contrast medium and radiation dose required. A simple PAVM is most common and is supplied by a single afferent vascular pedicle. Its diameter should be measured, and vasoocclusive material of appropriate diameter should be selected accordingly. A complex PAVM is uncommon and is supplied by more than one vascular pedicle. A diffuse form of this malformation consists of PAVMs involving each subsegmental artery in at least one lobe. Three-dimensional reformatted images are very useful for providing a synthesis of all the available information concerning the angioarchitecture of the malformation.[51]

Magnetic Resonance Imaging

Magnetic resonance angiography is also a valuable examination for screening and pretherapeutic evaluation of these malformations, as long as the aneurysmal sac is greater than 3 to 5 mm in diameter.[52–54] It is not optimal for providing detailed information on small malformations, and it is of limited value in assessing the potential role of the systemic circulation.

DIFFERENTIAL DIAGNOSIS

Opacities that can simulate PAVMs include bronchoceles, aberrant intrapulmonary venous pathways, and shunts between pulmonary arteries or veins and systemic arteries.

SYNOPSIS OF TREATMENT OPTIONS

Intervention is indicated both for prophylactic and for therapeutic reasons. Even asymptomatic malformations are considered for therapy to prevent potential paradoxic embolism. Prophylactic intervention is also aimed at reducing the consequences of a right-to-left shunt and the risk of rupture of the aneurysmal sac. Two types of intervention are possible: surgical and endovascular. CT plays an important role in deciding between these two possible therapeutic approaches by establishing the angioarchitecture of the malformation. Endovascular embolotherapy can be used even in malformations with feeding vessels less than 3 mm in diameter when technically feasible.[55] PAVMs that are best treated surgically include those in which previous embolotherapy has been unsuccessful, those with afferent feeding vessels that are too large in diameter for embolotherapy, those that receive an additional afferent arterial supply from systemic arteries that cannot be embolized safely, and possibly PAVMs that are too numerous for endovascular treatment. In cases that are not suitable for any form of intervention, continued surveillance is

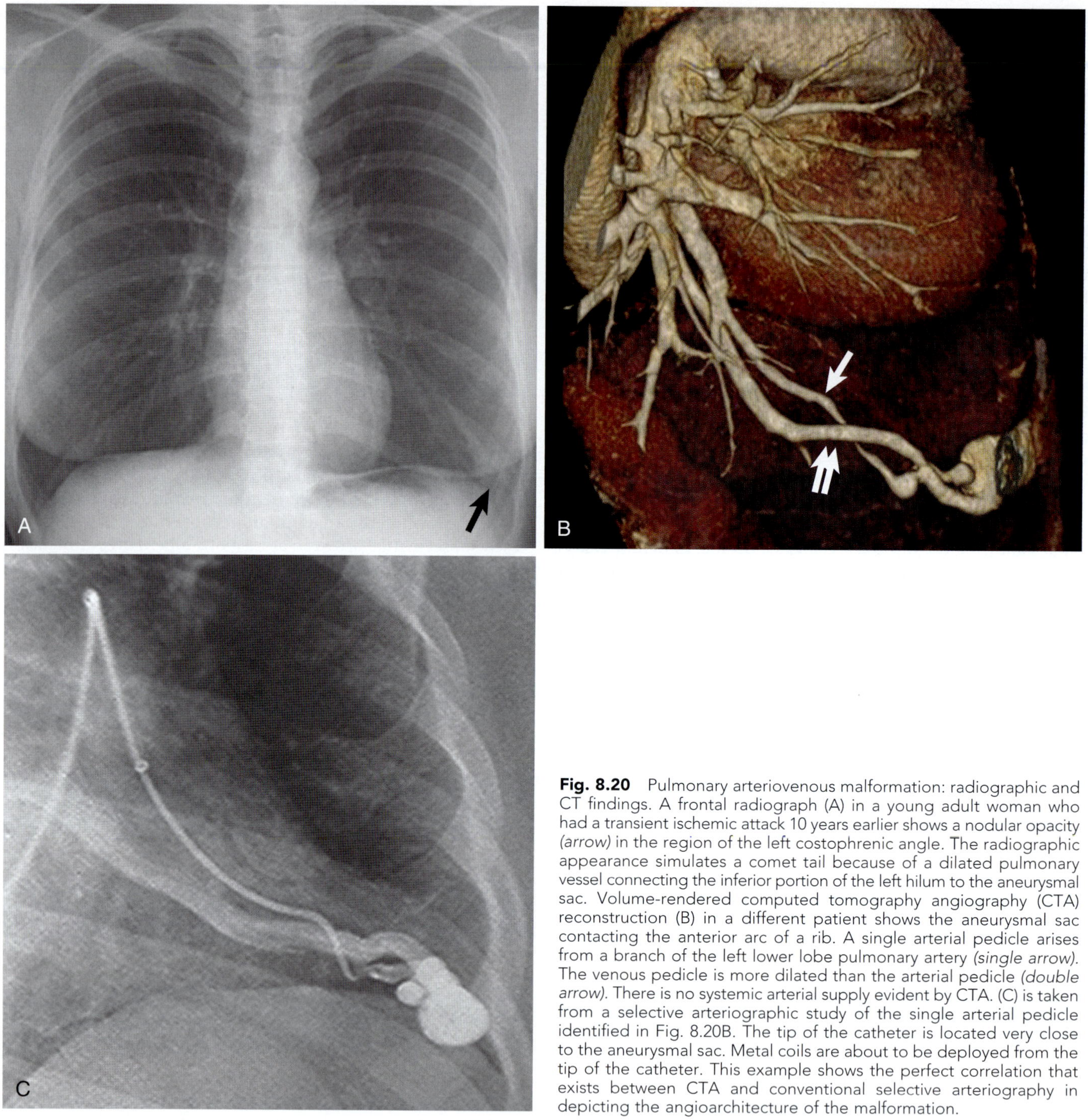

Fig. 8.20 Pulmonary arteriovenous malformation: radiographic and CT findings. A frontal radiograph (A) in a young adult woman who had a transient ischemic attack 10 years earlier shows a nodular opacity *(arrow)* in the region of the left costophrenic angle. The radiographic appearance simulates a comet tail because of a dilated pulmonary vessel connecting the inferior portion of the left hilum to the aneurysmal sac. Volume-rendered computed tomography angiography (CTA) reconstruction (B) in a different patient shows the aneurysmal sac contacting the anterior arc of a rib. A single arterial pedicle arises from a branch of the left lower lobe pulmonary artery *(single arrow)*. The venous pedicle is more dilated than the arterial pedicle *(double arrow)*. There is no systemic arterial supply evident by CTA. (C) is taken from a selective arteriographic study of the single arterial pedicle identified in Fig. 8.20B. The tip of the catheter is located very close to the aneurysmal sac. Metal coils are about to be deployed from the tip of the catheter. This example shows the perfect correlation that exists between CTA and conventional selective arteriography in depicting the angioarchitecture of the malformation.

advised, particularly in pregnant patients, who in the last 4 months of pregnancy may experience a rapid increase in size of the malformations with the attendant risk of rupture and hemoptysis.

Endovascular Treatment

Technique. Materials used for embolotherapy include occlusive balloons, nonferromagnetic metallic coils, and occasionally, microcatheter-delivered microcoils. Metallic coils are most commonly deployed, with coil size selected based on the size and geometry of the AVM.

Results. The overall initial success rate is on the order of 98%, with practically no mortality. Because pulmonary arterial blood flows preferentially toward regions of low vascular resistance, after embolotherapy there is a redistribution of flow toward apparently healthy areas of the lung, in which small malformations can subsequently develop. Surveillance by CT is useful for detecting this complication.

Postembolotherapy follow-up is best performed by CT. The natural history of the aneurysmal sac is one of progressive retraction over a several-month period, which occurs in 85% of occluded malformations. When the sac is very large, it may become filled with fibrous tissue or calcified thrombus. Persistence of a visible sac requires further evaluation with contrast-enhanced CT to exclude residual perfusion of the sac and to search for the presence of systemic feeding arteries that may not have been recognized at the time of the initial vasoocclusion. In a large series that reported imaging findings after vasoocclusion of PAVMs, the frequency of delayed recanalization of a successfully embolized afferent artery varied between 10% and 19% (Fig. 8.21). Factors associated with delayed recanalization include coexisting arteriovenous fistulas within the liver or gastrointestinal tract (or both), presence of pulmonary hypertension, or development of afferent pulmonary arteries that were not detected at the time of initial endovascular treatment. These vessels are amenable to treatment by repeat embolotherapy, thereby leading to definitive treatment of the malformation. The development of clinical or radiologic signs of pulmonary infarction after vasoocclusion should lead to a search for the development of abnormal systemic arteries adjacent to the malformation during long-term follow-up of these patients, developing in 41% of treated cases in one series.[56] The arteries most frequently implicated were the musculophrenic arteries and the inferior phrenic arteries in close contact with the occluded malformations.

KEY POINTS: PULMONARY ARTERIOVENOUS MALFORMATIONS

- May be asymptomatic
- Clinical symptoms:
  - Dyspnea, orthopnea, cyanosis, paradoxic septic or thrombotic emboli
  - Bronchial or pleural bleeding
  - Family context of Rendu-Osler-Weber disease
- Common radiologic findings:
  - Tubular and/or pseudonodular opacities on radiographs
  - CT demonstrates the malformation and the feeding and draining vessels

Isolated Systemic Arterial Supply of the Lung

EMBRYOLOGY, PREVALENCE, AND EPIDEMIOLOGY

This malformation used to be called a Pryce type I sequestration. It is now described by the term *systemic arterialization of normal basal pulmonary segments* or *systemic arterial supply of a lung without sequestration.*[57] In this anomaly the only malformation involves a systemic artery because the lung has developed normally and has normal bronchopulmonary anatomy. The basal segments of the lower lobes are most commonly affected, the left more frequently than the right.

CLINICAL PRESENTATION

Symptoms are due exclusively to the abnormal systemic artery and include cardiac impairment secondary to the left-to-left shunt between the abnormal artery and the pulmonary venous return, aneurysm formation, spontaneous thrombosis, and dissection or rupture of the artery leading to hemoptysis or hemothorax as a result of premature atheromatous disease within the vessel.[58]

MANIFESTATIONS OF THE DISEASE

Radiography

Chest radiographs are frequently normal, except in cases in which the anomalous artery is very large or aneurysmal, in which case a tubular opacity may correspond to the abnormal artery.

Computed Tomography

The abnormal systemic artery arises from the descending thoracic or abdominal aorta and normally reaches the lower lobe via the inferior pulmonary ligament. It often follows a sigmoid course toward the left side, first descending then ascending, after which it divides into several branches that descend toward the basal segments and adopt the course and distribution of the pulmonary arteries. On the left the abnormal artery arises from the descending aorta, whereas on the right it arises from the abdominal aorta, often adopting the origin and pathway of the inferior phrenic artery. Atheromatous lesions, such as calcified plaques and abnormalities in diameter, can be found within this vessel, even in young adults.[59]

Complete evaluation includes analysis of the pulmonary and systemic vessels and bronchi supplying the affected lobe; contrary to pulmonary sequestration, the lung of the affected regions should be normal.[58,60] Bronchi in the affected segments may be dilated, with absence of the expected adjacent homonymous pulmonary arteries (see Fig. 8.19).[58,61] The parenchyma perfused by the systemic artery may exhibit ground-glass opacities secondary to increased vascular perfusion or hemoptysis. The abnormal systemic artery (Fig. 8.22) can at times be regarded as a source of accessory perfusion[62–64] in conjunction with pulmonary artery perfusion.

Magnetic Resonance Imaging

The same information acquired by CT can be obtained with MRI. However, MRI is less precise in obtaining information regarding the bronchial tree, lung parenchyma, and pleura, which is imperative for deciding on treatment.

DIFFERENTIAL DIAGNOSIS

A confident diagnosis requires confirmation that the lung parenchyma, bronchi, and pleura are all normal, thus excluding intralobar sequestration, and exclusion of a systemic artery supply that is acquired secondary to bronchopulmonary and pleural disease ("pseudosequestration"). This malformation is rarely confused with chronic thromboembolic disease, in which the pulmonary artery branches are present but small, whereas in the case of an isolated systemic arterial supply of the lung, the pulmonary artery branches are usually absent, and the anomalies are limited to a single segment.

SYNOPSIS OF TREATMENT OPTIONS

Until recently, all vascular malformations of this type were treated by thoracotomy with ligation of the abnormal artery and resection of the affected pulmonary segment[65] and, in exceptional cases, by reimplantation of the systemic artery into the pulmonary artery. Embolotherapy of the abnormal artery can be performed

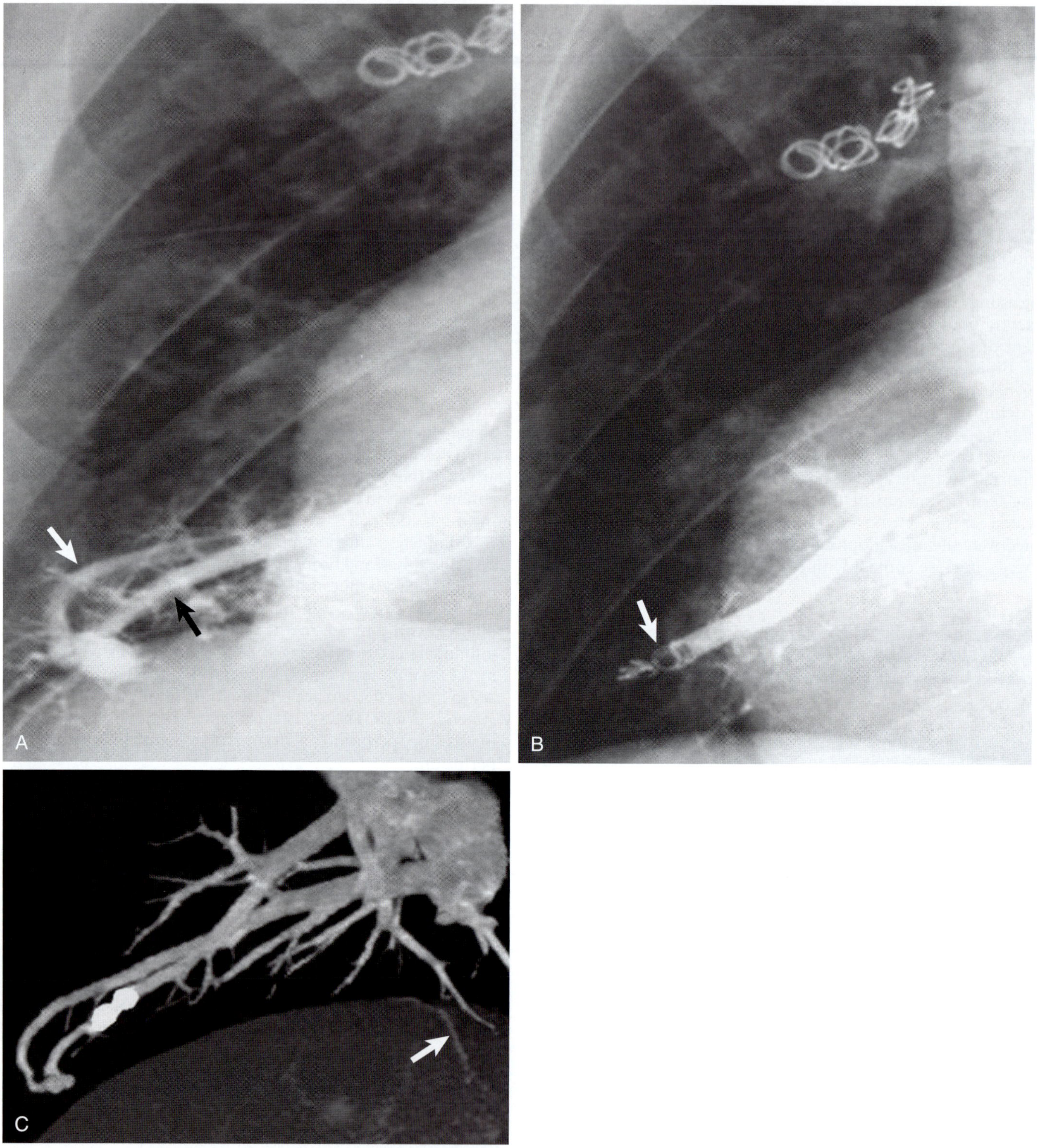

Fig. 8.21 Embolotherapy for a pulmonary arteriovenous malformation. The arterial pedicle (A, *black arrow*) is well opacified with contrast, whereas venous return from the aneurysmal sac (A, *white arrow*) is less well opacified. Several metal coils (B) have been deposited in the arterial pedicle close to the neck of the aneurysmal sac *(arrow)*. A follow-up CT angiographic study (C, maximum-intensity projection reconstruction), performed 2 years after embolotherapy, shows recanalization of the arterial pedicle and perfusion of the aneurysmal sac beyond the metal coils. The small diameter of this pedicle does not necessitate repeat embolotherapy, but continued surveillance is advised. Follow-up examinations should include evaluation of the right inferior phrenic artery (C, *arrow*), which appears to be moderately dilated.

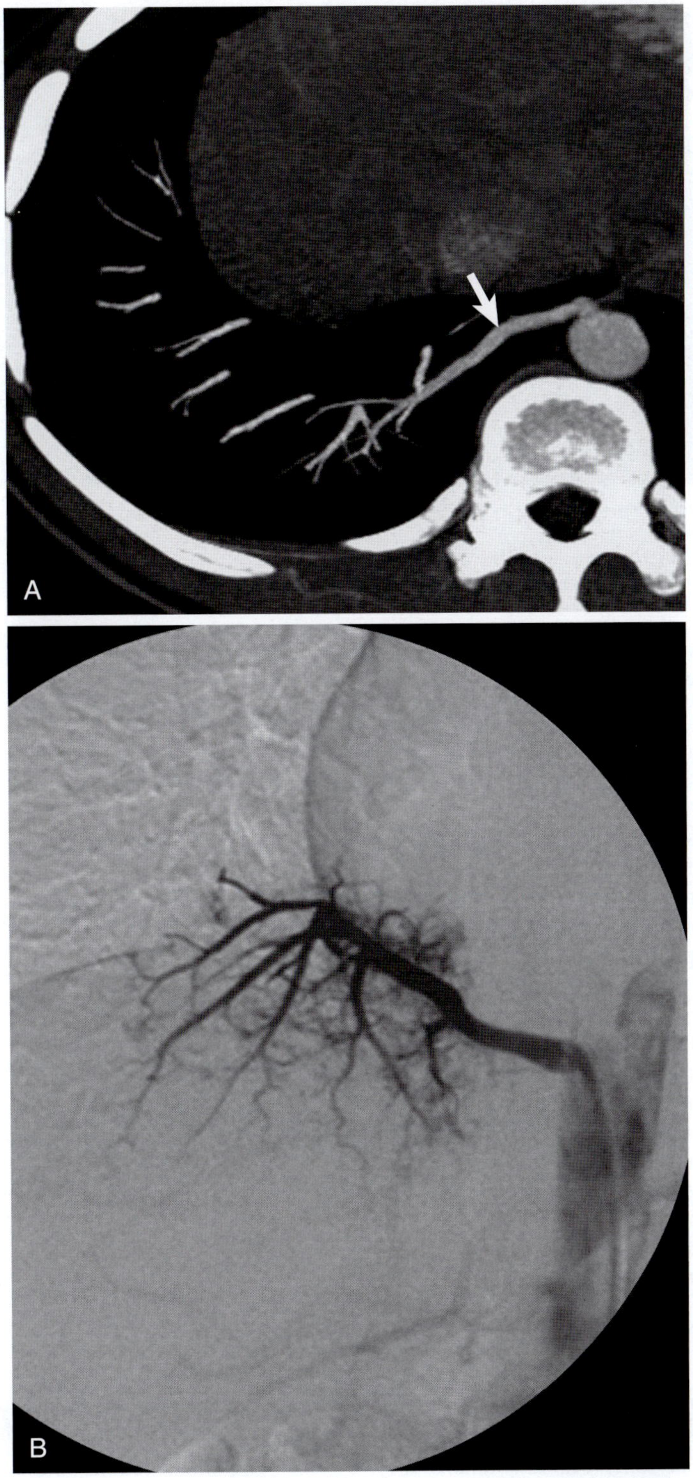

Fig. 8.22 Isolated systemic arterial supply of the lung detected during workup for hemoptysis. A maximum-intensity projection reconstructed image (A) from a CT angiogram shows an abnormal systemic artery *(arrow)* and its origin from the descending thoracic aorta. There are no other abnormal systemic arteries present. Selective angiography (B) of the anomalous vessel shows that the branches of the systemic artery have a distribution similar to that of the peripheral pulmonary arteries. *(Reprinted with permission of Grenier P.* Imagerie Thoracique de l'Adulte. *Paris: Flammarion; 2006.)*

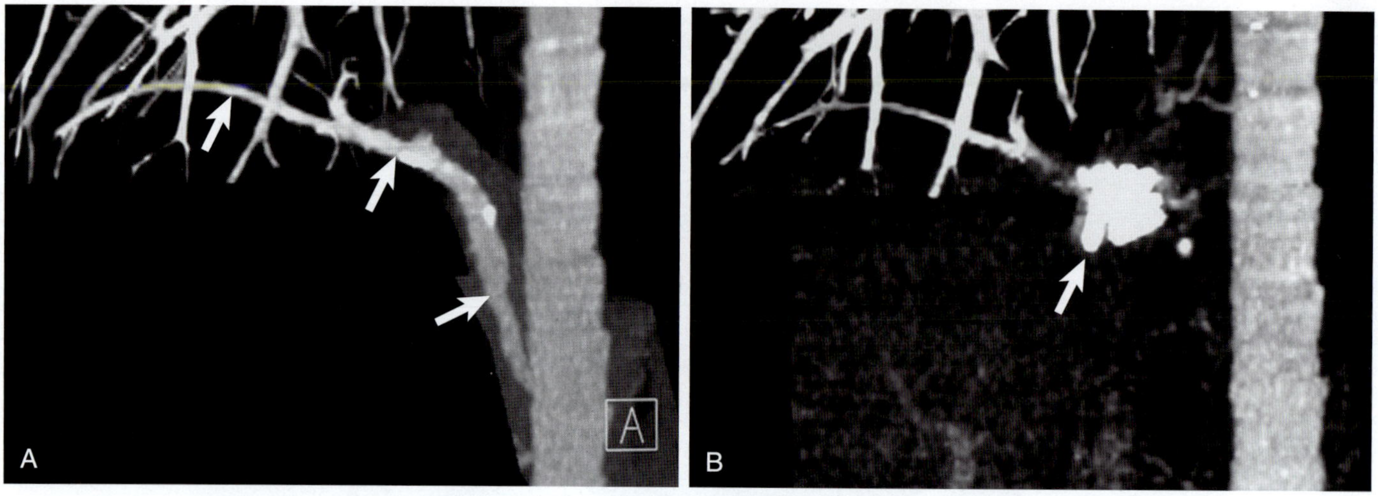

Fig. 8.23 Systemic arterial supply of the lung. A volumetric reformatted image (A) from a CT scan shows an abnormal isolated systemic artery *(arrows)* coursing in the region of the right inferior phrenic artery. There is decreased pulmonary arterial vascularization of the medial basal segment of the right lower lobe. A volumetric reformatted image from a CT scan performed after ligation with surgical clips (B, *arrow*) shows that the oblique ascending portion of the abnormal systemic artery is no longer opacified. The portion distal to the surgical clips is of small diameter and is opacified by anastomoses between the abnormal systemic artery and pulmonary arterial branches. The existence of these anastomoses explains the absence of pulmonary infarction after occlusion of the systemic artery. *(Reprinted with permission of Grenier P.* Imagerie Thoracique de l'Adulte. *Paris: Flammarion; 2006.)*

with metallic coils, although there is a risk of pulmonary infarction when the affected segment is supplied exclusively by the abnormal systemic vessel (Fig. 8.23).[66–68] If pulmonary resection does not seem warranted because of the small volume of affected lung and because the involved lung parenchyma appears normal, surgical ligation of the abnormal artery by video-assisted thoracoscopy remains an alternative to embolotherapy, especially when the origin of the abnormal artery is located close to the artery of Adamkiewicz and there is a risk of paraplegia secondary to iatrogenic embolization of this vessel. Short-term follow-up after endovascular treatment has been favorable in all reported studies, but no series have yet reported long-term outcomes. It is possible that systemic revascularization may occur via other systemic arteries not identified at the time of initial evaluation or because of the development of other systemic arteries after postembolization infarction. When alveolar hemorrhage follows multiple episodes of hemoptysis, video-assisted thoracoscopic lobectomy can be contemplated.[69]

SUGGESTED READINGS

Chowdhury UK, Kothary SS, Airan B, et al. Right pulmonary artery to left atrium communication. *Ann Thorac Surg*. 2005;80:365–370.

Do KH, Goo JM, Im JG, et al. Systemic arterial supply to the lung in adults: spiral CT findings. *Radiographics*. 2001;21:387–402.

Porres DV, Morenza OP, Pallisa E, et al. Learning from the pulmonary veins. *Radiographics*. 2013;33:999–1022.

Konen E, Raviv-Zilka L, Cohen RA, et al. Congenital pulmonary venolobar syndrome: spectrum of helical CT findings with emphasis on computed reformatting. *Radiographics*. 2003;23:1175–1184.

Winer-Muram HT. Adult presentation of heterotaxic syndromes and related complexes. *J Thorac Imaging*. 1995;10:43–57.

Zylak CJ, Eyler WR, Spizarny DL, Stone CH. Developmental lung anomalies in the adult: radiologic-pathologic correlation. *Radiographics*. 2002;22:S25–S43.

The full reference list for this chapter is available at ExpertConsult.com.

KEY POINTS: ISOLATED SYSTEMIC ARTERIAL SUPPLY OF THE LUNG

- Often asymptomatic and found incidentally on radiographs or CT
- Clinical symptoms: hemoptysis, cardiac failure, thrombosis or aneurysm of a systemic artery
- Common radiologic findings:
  - Posterobasal tubular shadow on the radiograph
- Abnormal systemic arterial supply to the lung evident on CT
- Abnormal vessel originating from the thoracic or abdominal aorta
- Normal lung and bronchial tree
- Early atheromatous changes in abnormal vessel

9 Bacterial Pneumonia*

STEPHANE L. DESOUCHES | CHRISTOPHER M. WALKER | JONATHAN H. CHUNG

Etiology, Prevalence, and Epidemiology

Pneumonia and influenza represent the eighth leading cause of mortality in the United States,[1] with an estimated 1.3 million hospital admissions yearly attributable to pneumonia in patients older than 65 years.[2,3] Although pneumonia affects all ages, increased morbidity and mortality are seen at the extremes of age (very young and very old).

Pneumonia is broadly divided into infection acquired in the community versus acquired in health care settings, including hospitals and nursing homes. Multidrug-resistant (MDR) bacteria are more commonly encountered in hospital or health care–associated pneumonia.

Community-acquired pneumonia (CAP) manifests in a patient who has not been recently hospitalized and who has had no regular exposure to the health care system. Incidence in the general population is approximately 5 to 6 per 1000 person years, with about 5.6 million cases of CAP encountered per year, representing one of the most commonly treated infectious diseases.[4,5] *Pneumococcus* remains the most common bacterial pathogen responsible for CAP, although its incidence has declined with the widespread use of the pneumococcal vaccination and with decreased rates of cigarette smoking.[6] In the late 1930s a separate clinical course was described for pneumonia with a longer more indolent onset that progressed to the more typical clinical presentation. This form was termed *atypical*, and the causative agents were termed *atypical* infections. In addition, atypical pneumonia often is associated with more systemic manifestations of disease, including gastrointestinal abnormalities, hepatitis, and meningoencephalitis. With patients surviving longer, this atypical presentation is now seen with both the traditional atypical organisms as well as other infectious agents, making the distinction imprecise and anachronistic. However, given its widespread use in clinical practice, the grouping of typical and atypical causes of pneumonia has persisted. Typical organisms causing CAP include *Streptococcus pneumoniae*, *Haemophilus influenzae*, *Staphylococcus aureus*, group A streptococci, *Moraxella catarrhalis*, anaerobes, and aerobic gram-negative bacteria. Among the atypical infections are *Legionella* spp., *Mycoplasma pneumoniae*, and *Chlamydia pneumoniae*.

Health care–associated pneumonia (HCAP) occurs in patients who have recently been hospitalized for 2 or more days in the 90 days preceding infection; resided in a nursing home or other long-term–care facility; or received recent intravenous antibiotic therapy, chemotherapy, hemodialysis, or wound care within the 30 days preceding infection. Patients with HCAP are more commonly infected with antibiotic-resistant bacteria, such as methicillin-resistant *S. aureus* (MRSA), *Pseudomonas aeruginosa*, and *Acinetobacter* spp.

Hospital-acquired pneumonia (HAP) is defined as pneumonia occurring 48 hours or more after a hospital admission. Ventilator-associated pneumonia (VAP) manifests 48 to 72 hours after endotracheal intubation. HAP and VAP combine to represent the most common cause of death among all hospital-acquired infections, with mortality rates ranging from 20% to 50%.[7–9] Common pathogens for both HAP and VAP include gram-negative bacilli (e.g., *Escherichia coli*, *Klebsiella pneumoniae*, *Enterobacter* spp., *Pseudomonas aeruginosa*, *Acinetobacter* spp.), and gram-positive cocci (e.g., *S. aureus*, including MRSA, and *Streptococcus* spp.). Specifically, with VAP, patients are also commonly found to be infected with oral anaerobic bacteria.

Clinical Presentation

Bacterial pneumonia may have a rapid onset with classic clinical symptoms consisting of high fever, productive cough, sweats, and chills. Some patient groups, particularly the elderly, may demonstrate a more gradual course with less severe symptoms.[10] With infection by some atypical organisms, such as *Legionella* and *Mycoplasma*, systemic symptoms are common. These can include diarrhea, myalgias, headache and confusion, anemia, or skin rash.

Pathologic Findings and Pathophysiology

Particulate material and microbes within the upper respiratory tree, either aerosolized particles or oral secretions, may enter the lower respiratory tract through microaspiration. Even so, lower respiratory tract defenses can typically maintain a sterile environment unless there is a defect in the host defenses, exposure to a particularly virulent organism or overwhelming inoculum.[11] Less commonly, infection can occur via hematogenous spread from bacteremia, infective endocarditis, or infected catheters. Direct spread of infection is uncommon but can arise from infections of the mediastinum or from adjacent organs, such as a liver abscess or esophageal perforation.

Pathologic findings depend upon the pattern of infection; lobar pneumonia, bronchopneumonia, interstitial pneumonia and bronchiolitis, or hematogenous spread of infection.

Lobar pneumonia is characterized histologically with filling of the alveoli by exudative fluid and neutrophils.[10] The consolidation typically starts at the periphery of the lung and spreads

*The editors and the publisher would like to thank Drs. Nestor L. Müller and C. Isabela Silva Müller for contributing material on this topic to the prior edition of this work. It has served as the foundation for the current chapter.

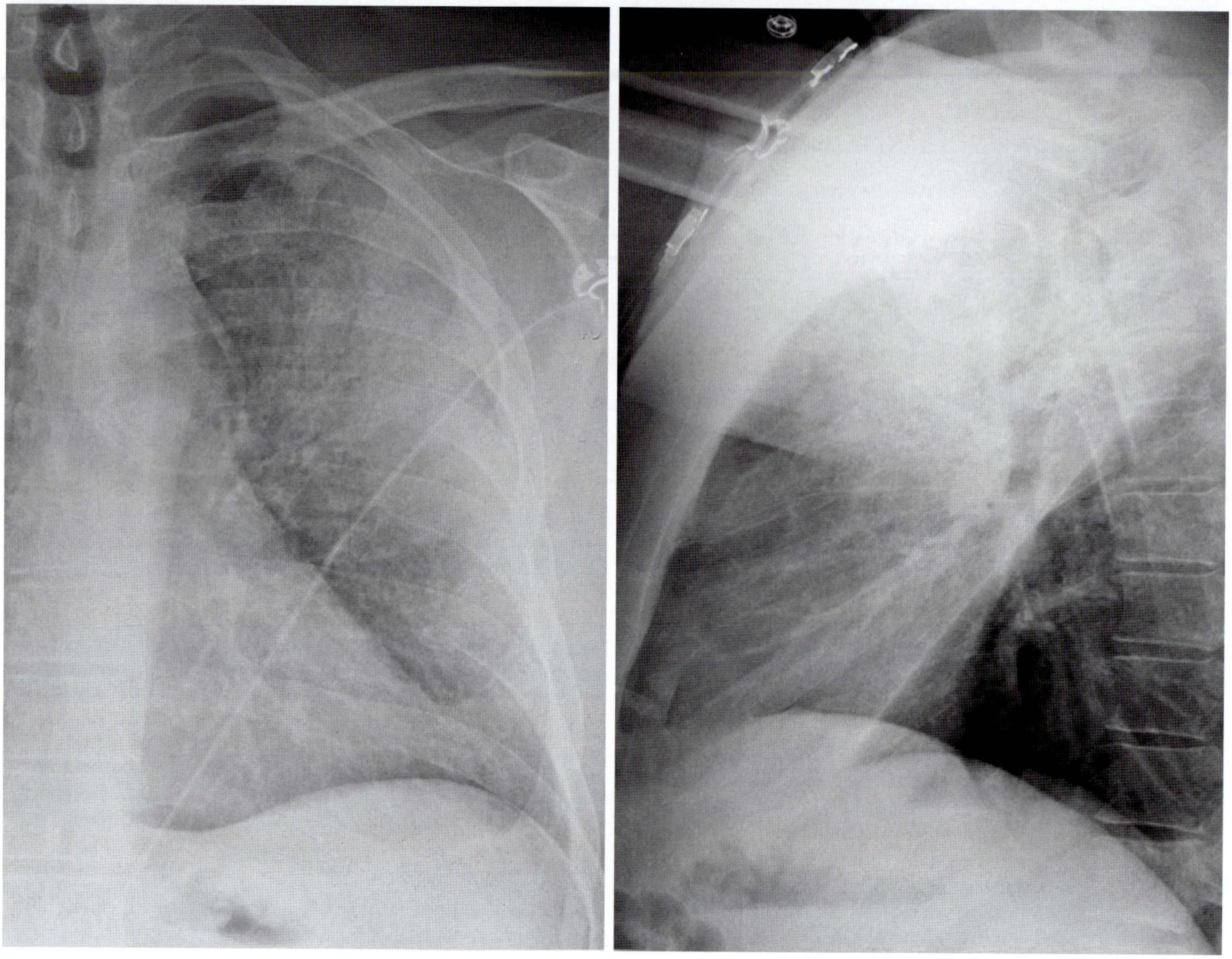

Fig. 9.1 Lobar pneumonia. Composite image with frontal *(left image)* and lateral *(right image)* chest radiographs shows an area of consolidation involving the left upper lobe abutting the major fissure. Patent bronchi (air bronchograms) can be seen within the consolidation.

centripetally via the pores of Kohn and small airways. This airspace filling will extend across pulmonary segments, sometimes involving the entire lobe (Fig. 9.1).

Bronchopneumonia typically shows inflammatory exudate of polymorphonuclear leukocytes within the respiratory bronchioles. This exudate and the associated terminal bronchiolitis likely limits spread of infection initially, resulting in the characteristic patchy appearance seen on radiography (Fig. 9.2). Bronchopneumonia may be associated with areas of parenchymal destruction or necrosis.[12]

Interstitial pneumonia and bronchiolitis are characterized by inflammatory infiltrate within the bronchiolar wall with associated neutrophil-rich intraluminal exudate.[13,14] Extension into the lung parenchyma results in segmental areas of consolidation. Interstitial pneumonia is more commonly associated with atypical organisms, such as *Mycoplasma*, viruses, or *Pneumocystis jirovecii*.

Hematogenous spread of infection (septic emboli) occurs secondary to friable thrombus either along a cardiac valve, bacteremia, or infected catheter or pacemaker wire that breaks off because of turbulent flow and lodges in a pulmonary capillary bed. This form of infection is most commonly associated with *S. aureus*.[15] An uncommon source of septic emboli is thrombophlebitis of the internal or external jugular vein secondary to oropharyngeal infection with *Fusobacterium necrophorum*, referred to as Lemierre syndrome.[16]

Inflammatory changes from pneumonia may irritate the adjacent pleural lining, resulting in increased capillary permeability and an exudative pleural effusion (Fig. 9.3). Histochemically, this "simple" parapneumonic effusion has normal pH and glucose. If this is left untreated, the effusion may progress to a fibropurulent empyema.

Imaging Findings

RADIOGRAPHY AND COMPUTED TOMOGRAPHY

Imaging findings of bacterial pneumonia depend upon the pattern of infection, with certain organisms favoring certain patterns, which may suggest a class of organism, although no sign or pattern is specific.

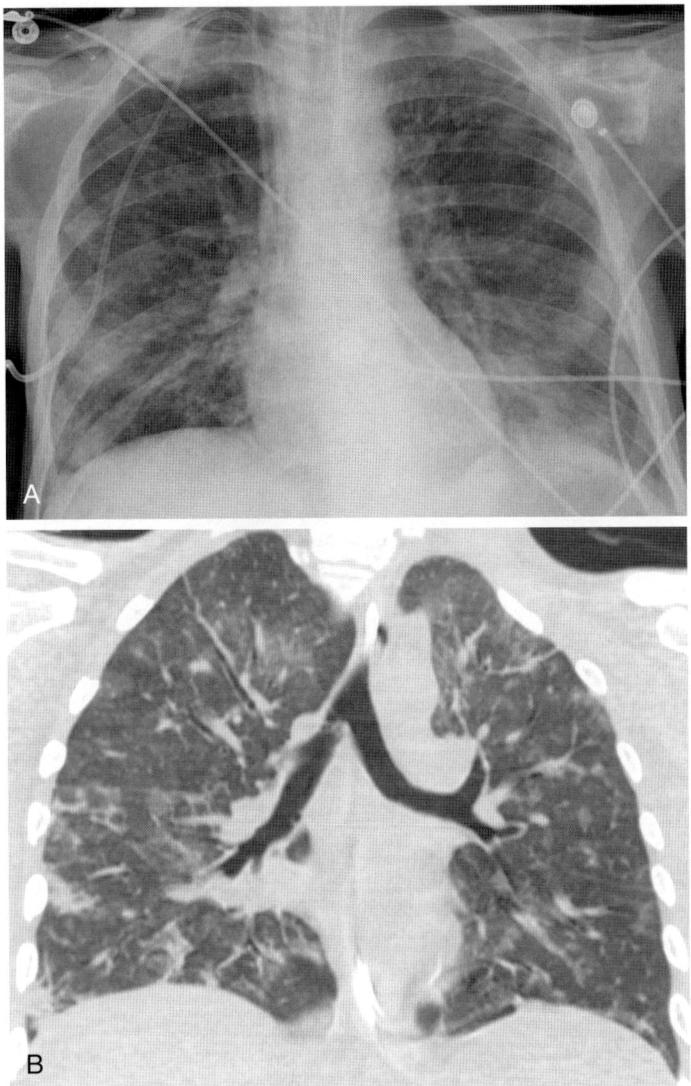

Fig. 9.2 Bronchopneumonia. (A) Frontal chest radiograph shows patchy bilateral areas of consolidation predominantly involving the lower lobes. (B) Coronal reformatted CT image shows patchy consolidation and ground-glass opacities bilaterally.

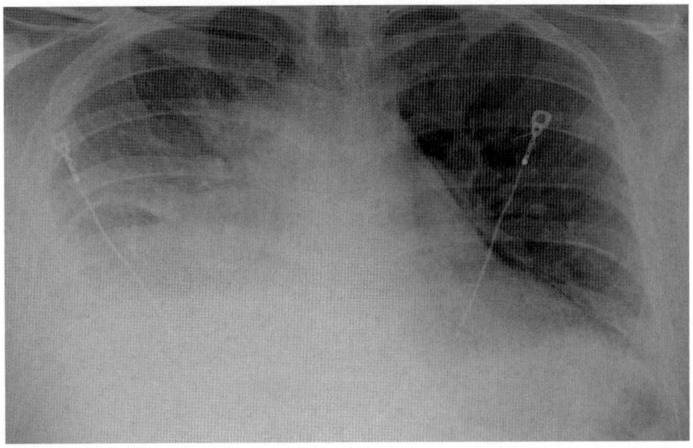

Fig. 9.3 Pleural effusion associated with *Streptococcus pneumoniae* infection. Frontal chest radiograph shows right greater than left lower lobe consolidation with a moderate right pleural effusion. Pleural effusions associated with pneumonia typically are exudative due to increased capillary permeability from irritation.

Lobar Pneumonia

Lobar pneumonia is characterized by homogeneous airspace consolidation involving adjacent segments of a lobe (Fig. 9.4; see Fig. 9.1), often bounded by an interlobar fissure (Fig. 9.5) or the hemidiaphragm.[17] The consolidation tends to occur initially in the peripheral subpleural lung and spreads centrally and may eventually involve the entire lobe, although this is uncommon with early initiation of antibiotics. Air bronchograms are nearly universally present within the consolidation because of the exudative process involving the alveoli rather than the bronchioles (Fig. 9.6). On computed tomography (CT) ground-glass opacities adjacent to the consolidation represent incomplete alveolar filling (Fig. 9.7).[17]

Classic signs associated with lobar pneumonia include the "spine sign" with paradoxical increased density of the lower thoracic spine on the lateral radiograph resulting from the overlying lower lobe consolidation (Fig. 9.8). Uncommonly encountered, the "bulging fissure sign" is due to copious amounts of exudative material within the consolidation, resulting in bulging or displacement of the fissures (Fig. 9.9).[18] Although classically described with *K. pneumoniae*, the bulging fissure sign is more commonly seen with *S. pneumoniae* given its greater prevalence.

Lobar pneumonia is most commonly seen with infection by *S. pneumoniae*, *K. pneumoniae*, and *L. pneumophila*.

Bronchopneumonia and Bronchiolitis

Bronchopneumonia begins with infection of the respiratory bronchioles, eventually extending into the adjacent alveoli. This typically manifests as poorly defined centrilobular or airspace nodules measuring 5 to 10 mm in diameter, tree-in-bud opacities reflecting the alveolar and bronchiole involvement (Fig. 9.10; see Fig. 9.2), and patchy areas of consolidation often involving multiple segments of multiple lobes (Fig. 9.11). Confluence of these areas of pneumonia in adjacent lobar segments may mimic a lobar pneumonia pattern.[19] Distinction may be inferred by noting the segmental distribution of abnormalities in other areas.

Because of the tissue destruction and necrosis often associated with bronchopneumonia, areas of cavitation are commonly encountered, especially in patients with extensive consolidation.[19] The airway involvement can result in volume loss within the affected segments or lobes. Air bronchograms are rarely seen secondary to the intraluminal inflammatory exudate within the bronchi and bronchioles.

With widespread bronchial wall inflammation manifesting as bronchial wall thickening and resultant luminal narrowing, mosaic attenuation of the lung parenchyma can often be seen representing air-trapping.[20]

Bronchopneumonia is most common with infection by *S. aureus*, gram-negative organisms, anaerobic bacteria, and *L. pneumophila*. When only the interstitial manifestations of infection are encountered, including bronchiolitis, bronchial wall thickening, and endoluminal mucous plugging, atypical organisms such as *Mycoplasma*, viruses, or *Pneumocystis jirovecii* are more commonly the infectious agents.

Hematogenous Spread of Infection

Hematogenous spread of bacterial infection (septic emboli) most commonly occurs in intravenous drug users or in patients with

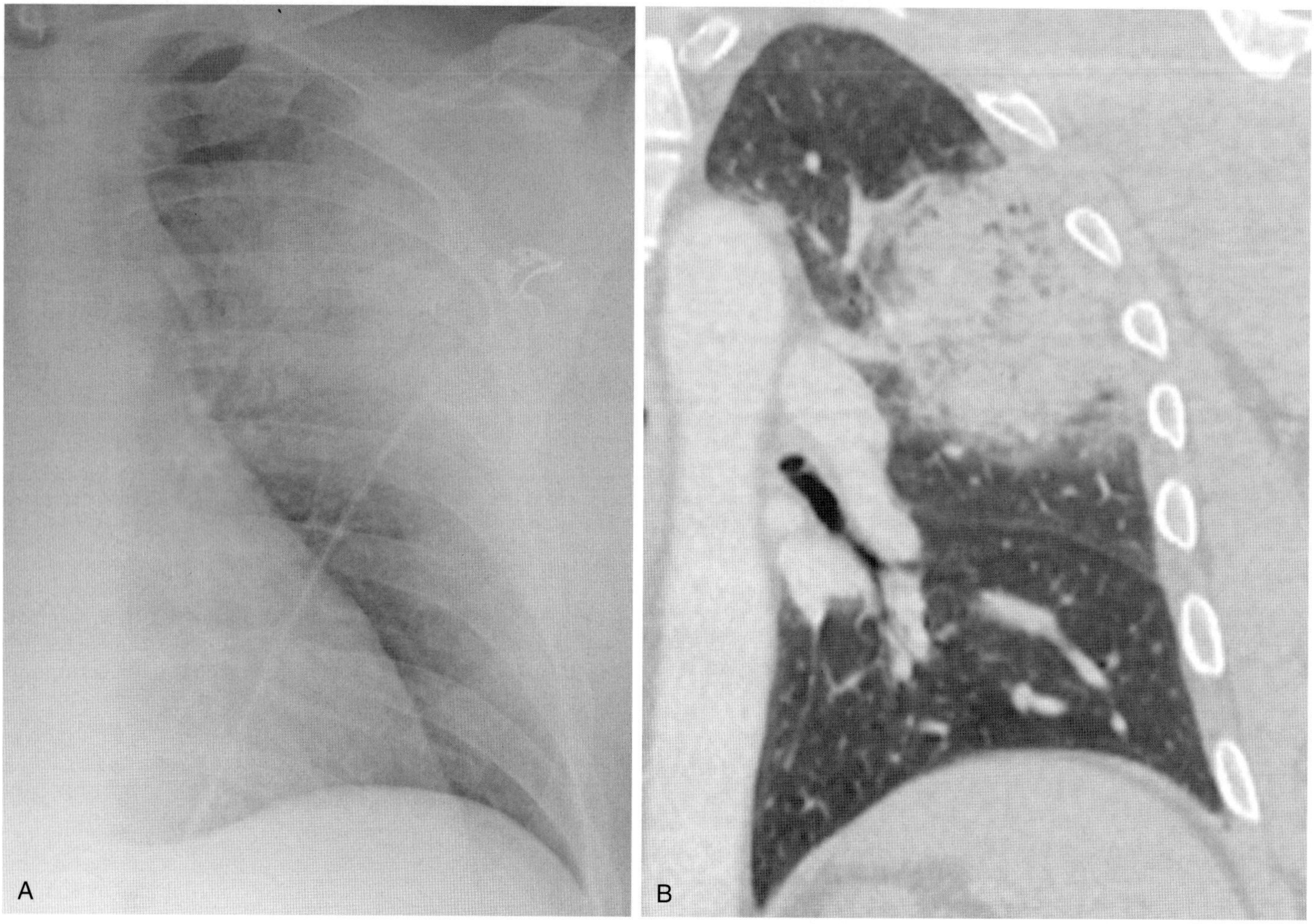

Fig. 9.4 Lobar pneumonia from *Legionella*. (A) Frontal chest radiograph shows left upper lobe consolidation with internal foci of air. (B) Coronal reformatted CT image shows the area of consolidation. Low-attenuation foci within the consolidation represented early cavitation.

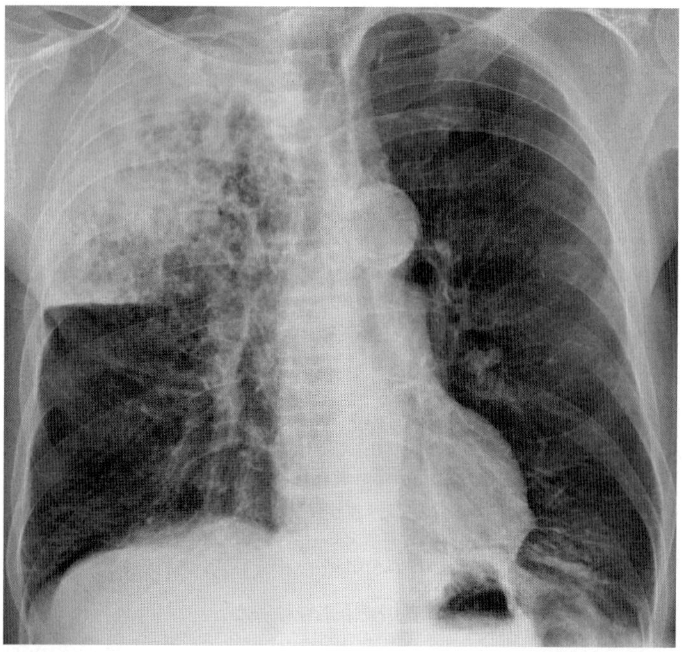

Fig. 9.5 Fissure demarcation in *Klebsiella* pneumonia. Frontal chest radiograph demonstrates extension of the right upper lobe consolidation to the minor fissure without involvement of adjacent lobes.

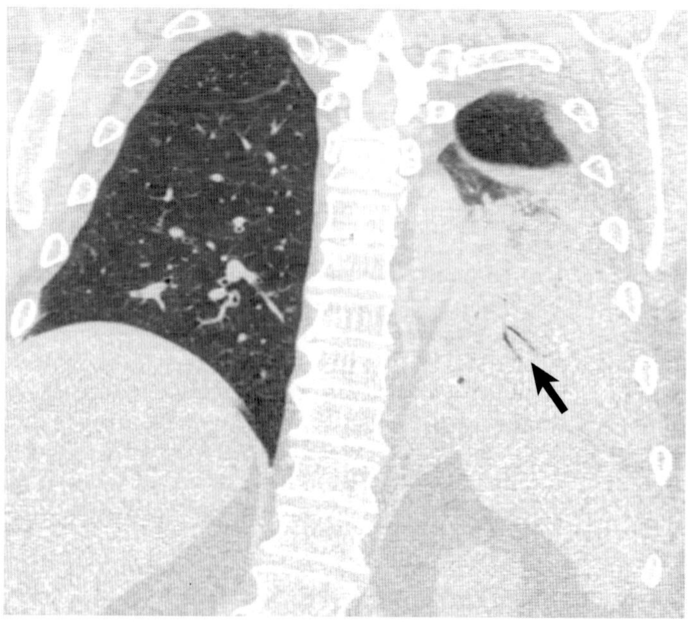

Fig. 9.6 Air bronchogram in *Haemophilus influenzae* pneumonia. Coronal reformatted CT image shows left lower lobe consolidation. Linear areas of hypoattenuation *(arrow)* represent patent bronchi within the consolidation (air bronchograms).

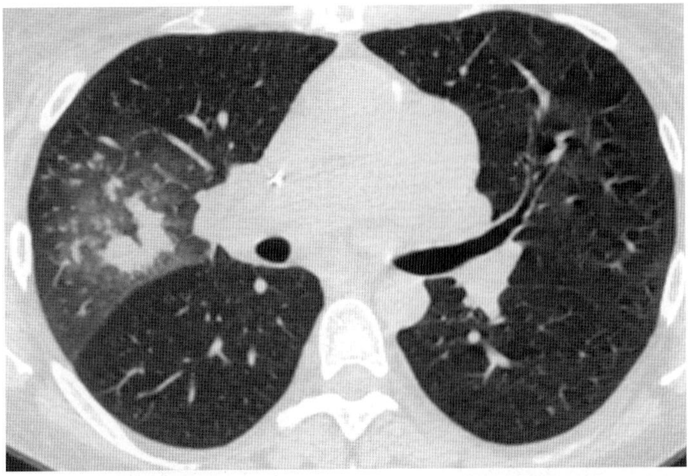

Fig. 9.7 Incomplete alveolar filling in methicillin-sensitive *Staphylococcus aureus* pneumonia. Axial CT image shows a central area of consolidation with surrounding ground-glass opacities. The ground-glass opacities represent areas of incomplete alveolar filling with exudative material.

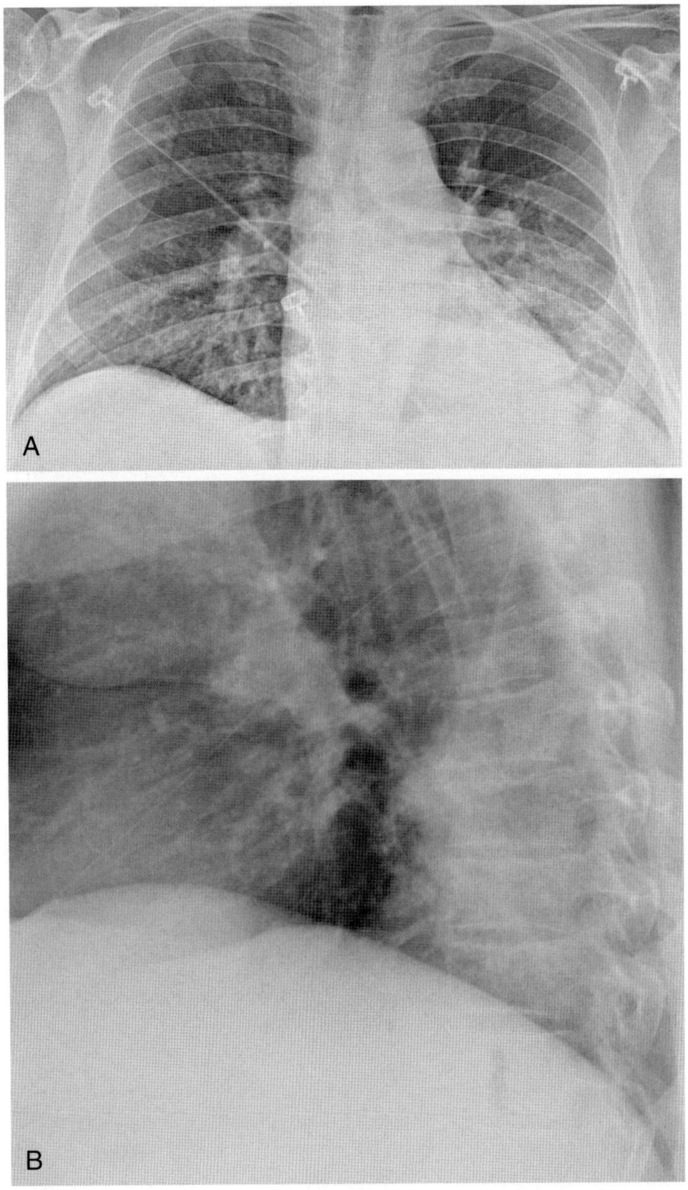

Fig. 9.8 Spine sign in pneumonia. Frontal (A) and lateral (B) chest radiographs demonstrate a left lower lobe consolidation that results in a paradoxical increased density of the lower thoracic spine on the lateral view (density of the lower spine should normally decrease relative to the upper thoracic spine).

infected central catheters. The most common manifestation is multiple middle and lower lung zone poorly defined nodules and wedge-shaped consolidations, frequently demonstrating cavitation on both radiography and CT (Figs. 9.12 and 9.13). This apicobasal gradient reflects the preferential blood flow within the lower, dependent portions of the lungs.[21,22]

These nodules often have closely associated pulmonary vasculature termed the *feeding vessel sign*.[23] Although these vessels may appear to lead to the nodule, thin-section CT imaging has shown that the feeding vessel is actually a pulmonary vein coursing from the nodule, whereas the pulmonary artery actually courses around the nodule (Fig. 9.14). Occlusion of the pulmonary arteries with septic emboli may result in hemorrhage and/or infarction, resulting in ill-defined wedge-shaped areas of consolidation or ground-glass opacities (see Fig. 9.13).[22]

Hematogenous spread of infection is most commonly seen with infections caused by *Staphylococcus* spp., usually *S. aureus*. As mentioned earlier, multiple septic emboli may be encountered less commonly in patients with thrombophlebitis of either the internal or external jugular vein termed *Lemierre syndrome* (Fig. 9.15).[16]

Complications

Especially with long-standing untreated pneumonia, complications including lung abscess formation or lung necrosis, empyema, or chest wall invasion can be seen and must be recognized as they can affect treatment and prognosis.

On contrast-enhanced CT in a patient with pneumonia, areas of inhomogeneous enhancement or cavitation are suggestive of lung necrosis. Lung abscesses usually manifest as thick-walled, peripherally enhancing fluid collections, commonly associated with an air-fluid level (Fig. 9.16).[24] This air-fluid level is similar in length on both posteroanterior and lateral projections owing to the spherical shape of the abscess (Fig. 9.17). This is in contradistinction to empyema, which is lenticular in shape and therefore shows different lengths of the air-fluid level on orthogonal projections (Fig. 9.18). The internal margin of the abscess wall is predominantly smooth (approximately 90% of cases),[25] and the abscess has adjacent parenchymal consolidation in 50% of cases.

Usually manifesting as a small to moderate pleural effusion, a parapneumonic effusion represents free-flowing exudative fluid secondary to increased capillary permeability from irritation by the adjacent pneumonia. As this effusion progresses, internal fibrous septa develop, resulting in loculation and empyema formation. The "split pleura sign" is specific for an exudative effusion and is seen in 50% of all empyemas. This sign represents thickening and enhancement of the visceral and parietal pleura, separated by the loculated fluid (Fig. 9.19). Presence of air within

Text continued on p. 203

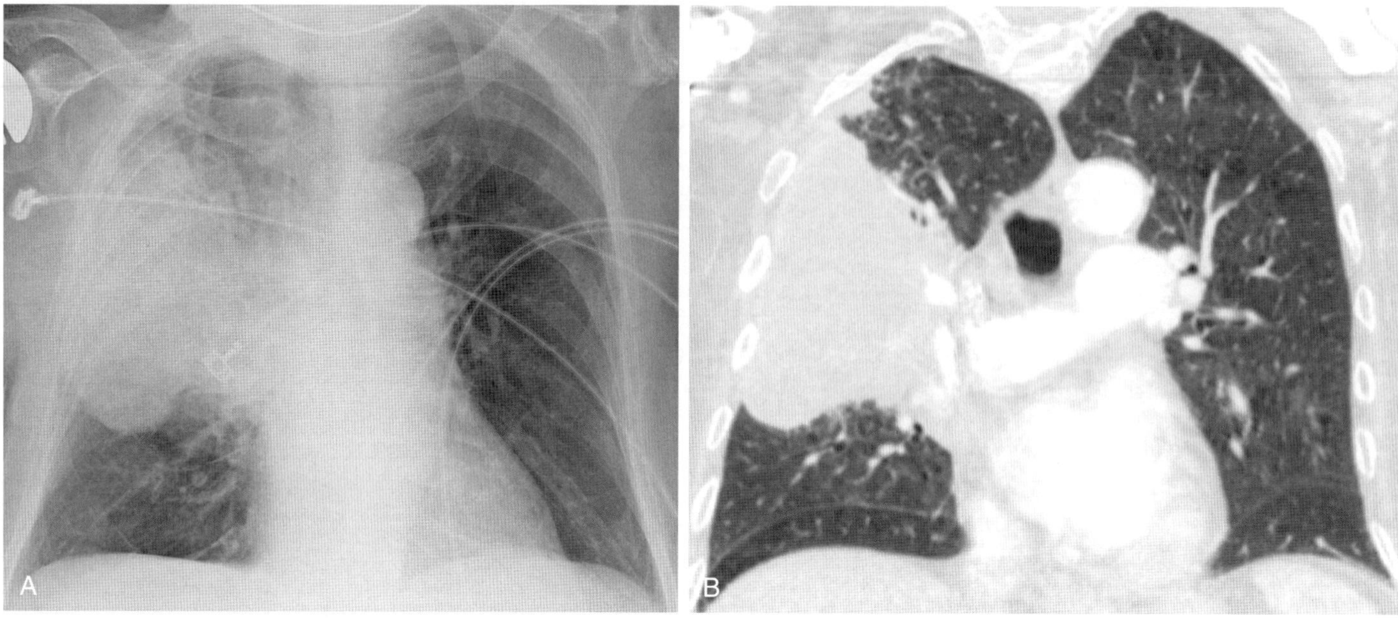

Fig. 9.9 Bulging fissure in *Klebsiella* pneumonia. (A) Frontal chest radiograph shows a right upper lobe consolidation inferiorly displacing the minor fissure. (B) Coronal reformatted CT image shows the bulging and inferiorly displaced minor fissure. Copious exudative material produced by the organism and the host immune system results in "bulging" or displacement of the fissure.

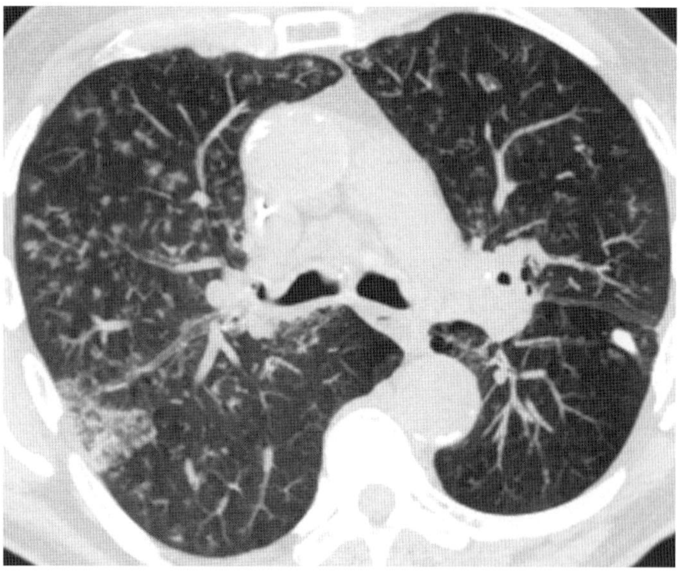

Fig. 9.10 Tree-in-bud sign in bronchopneumonia from *Mycoplasma.* Axial maximal-intensity projection CT image demonstrates bilateral tree-in-bud opacities with consolidation and ground-glass opacities in the right upper lobe. These findings are typical of a bronchopneumonia pattern on CT.

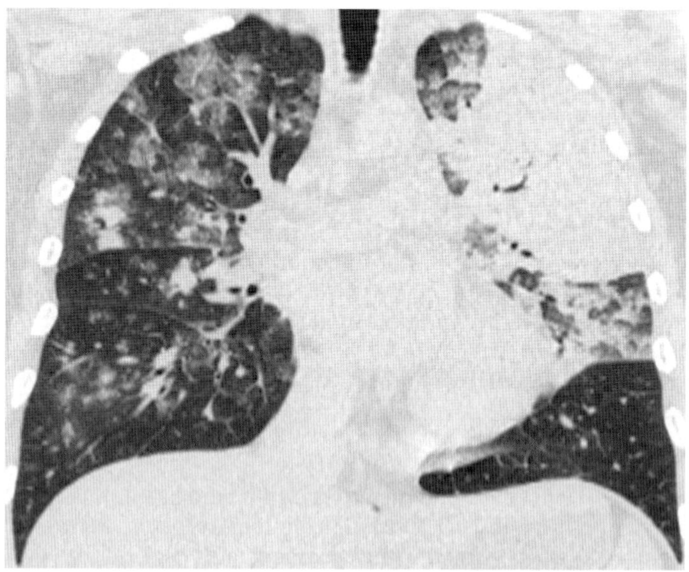

Fig. 9.11 Bronchopneumonia from *Staphylococcus aureus.* Coronal reformatted CT image shows patchy bilateral consolidation and ground-glass opacity consistent with bronchopneumonia pattern. The more homogeneous consolidation in the left upper lobe is due to confluence of segmental lobar involvement.

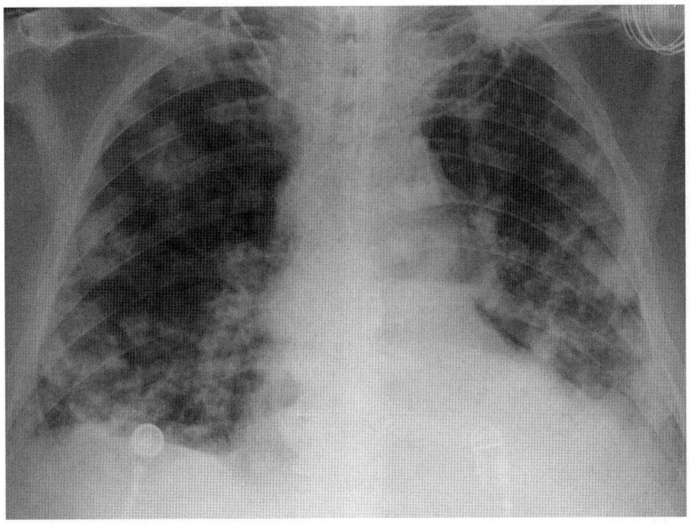

Fig. 9.12 Septic emboli. Frontal chest radiograph shows multiple ill-defined bilateral pulmonary opacities consistent with septic emboli. This patient was an intravenous drug user with tricuspid valve endocarditis on echocardiography.

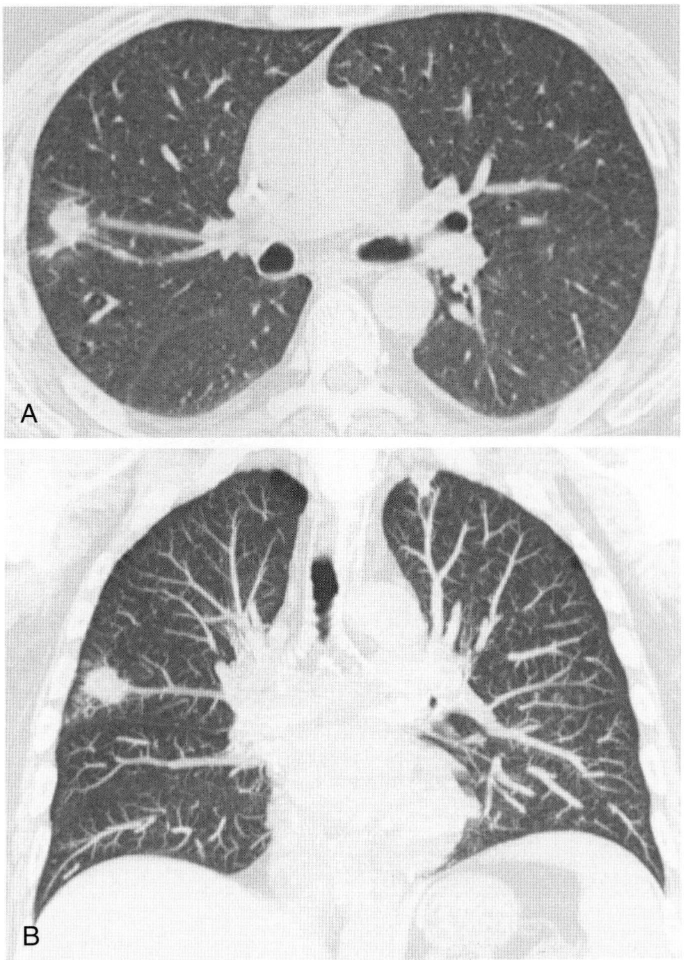

Fig. 9.14 Septic embolism with apparent "feeding vessel" sign. (A) Axial CT scan shows two vessels apparently coursing into a nodule ("feeding vessel sign"). (B) Coronal maximum-intensity projection image shows that the only vessel in close contact with the nodule is a draining vein. Another nodule also drained by a vein is present in the left lung apex.

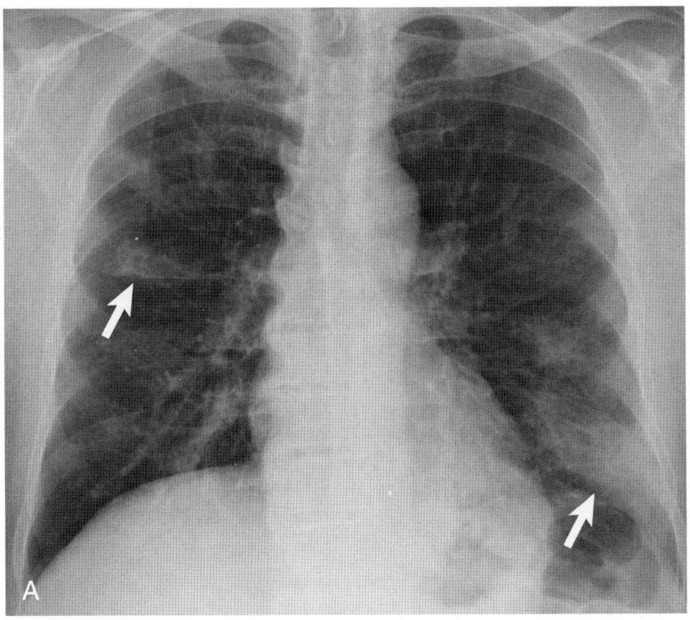

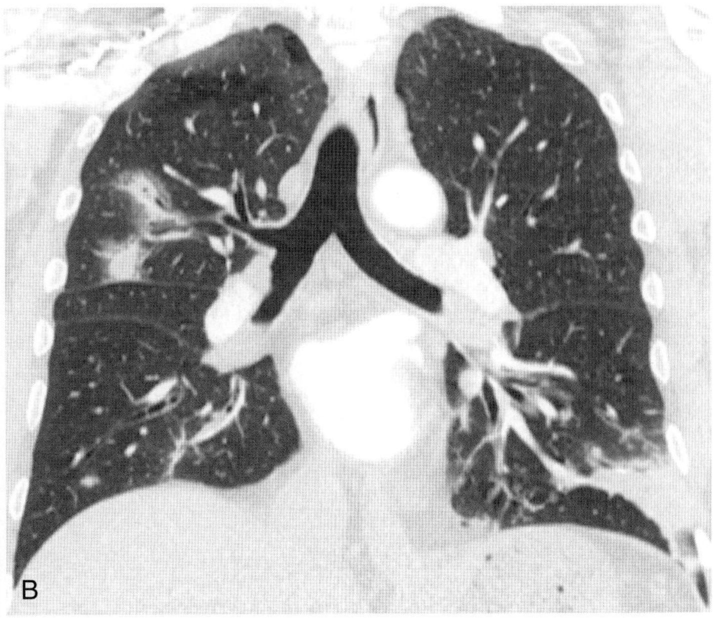

Fig. 9.13 Septic emboli. Frontal chest radiograph (A) and coronal reformatted CT image (B) show bilateral peripheral wedge-shaped opacities secondary to septic emboli (*arrows* in A). The wedge shape is due to obstruction of the distal pulmonary arterioles by emboli, resulting in infarction and hemorrhage into the surrounding lung parenchyma.

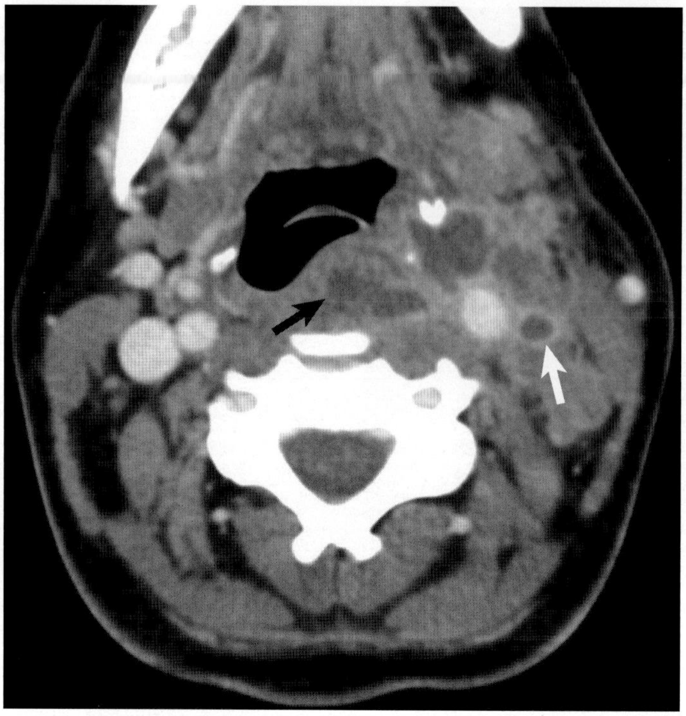

Fig. 9.15 Lemierre syndrome. Axial contrast-enhanced CT image shows a peripherally enhancing retropharyngeal abscess with central low attenuation *(black arrow)*. The abscess extends through fascial layers into the deep soft tissue of the left neck. The left internal jugular vein is occluded *(white arrow)*. This constellation of findings is consistent with Lemierre syndrome, most commonly caused by *Fusobacterium necrophorum*. *(Reproduced with permission from Gutschow SE, Walker CM. Acute thoracic conditions in the intensive care unit. In: Shepard JO, ed.* Thoracic Imaging: The Requisites. *Philadelphia: Elsevier; 2018.)*

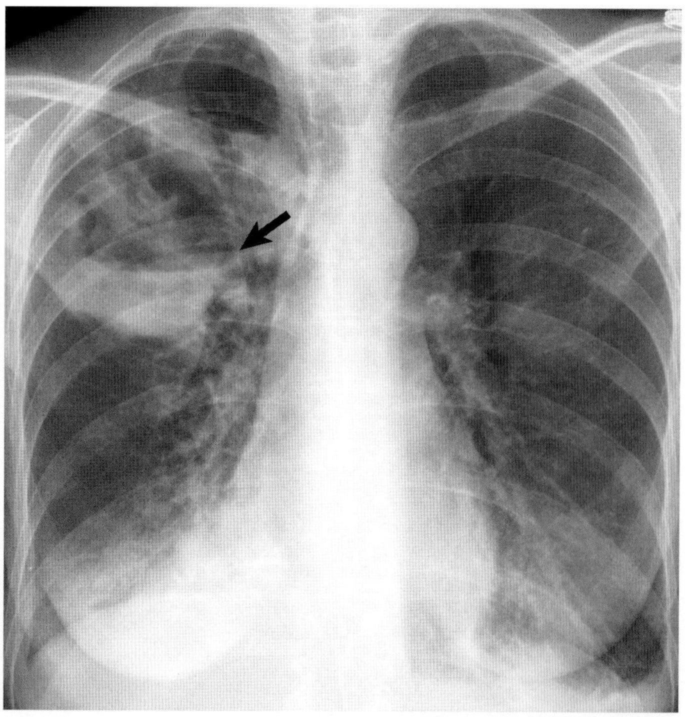

Fig. 9.16 Abscess. Frontal chest radiograph shows a large cavitary mass in the right upper lobe with associated air-fluid level *(arrow)*. Although this could represent a cavitating malignancy, the air-fluid level along with a clinical history supportive of infection makes abscess more likely.

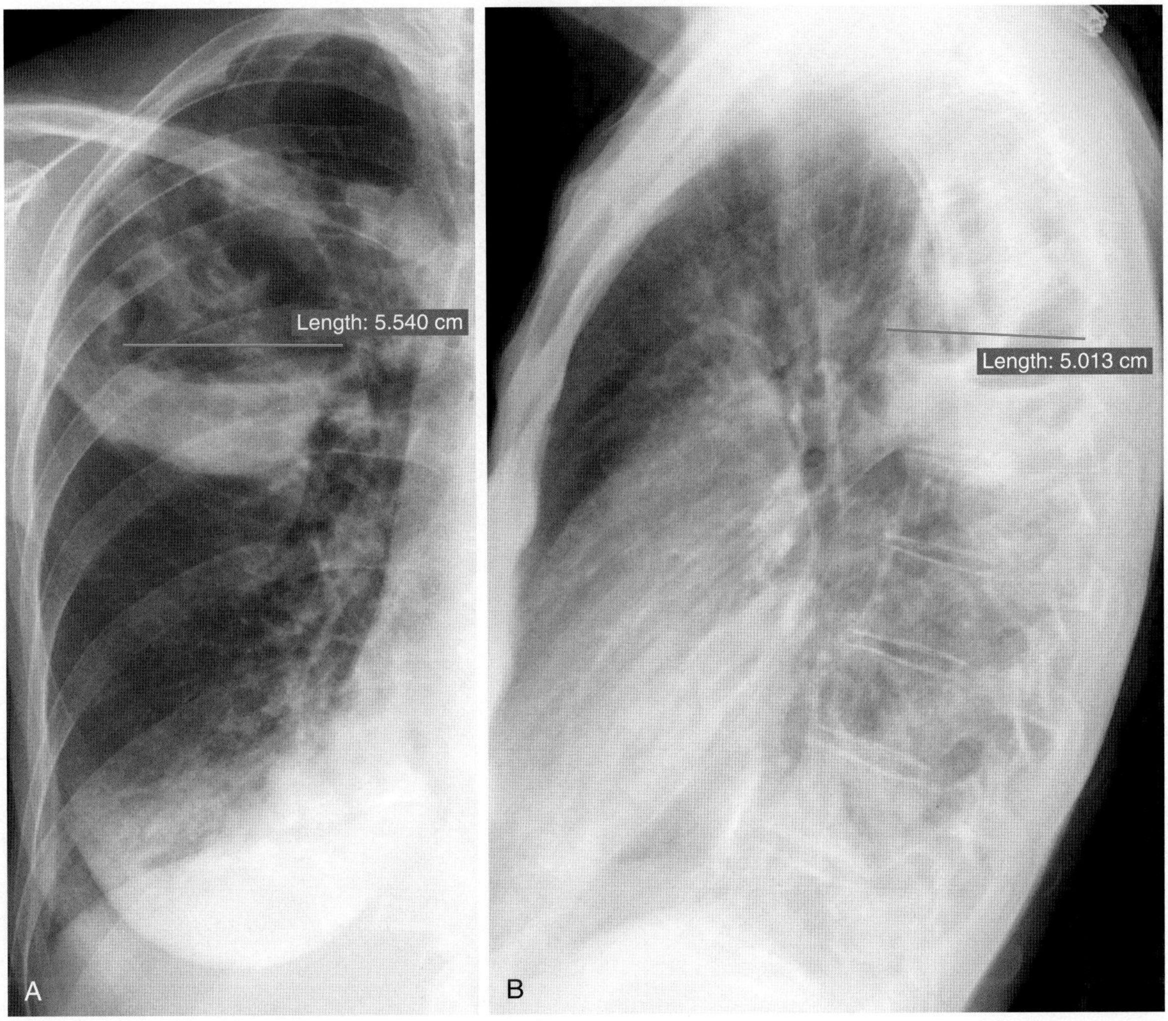

Fig. 9.17 Pulmonary abscess. Coned in frontal (A) and lateral (B) chest radiographs from the same patient as Fig. 9.16 shows pulmonary abscess with transverse and anteroposterior measurements that are similar. Unlike empyema, which is lenticular, a pulmonary abscess is generally round and therefore should have similar anteroposterior and transverse measurements.

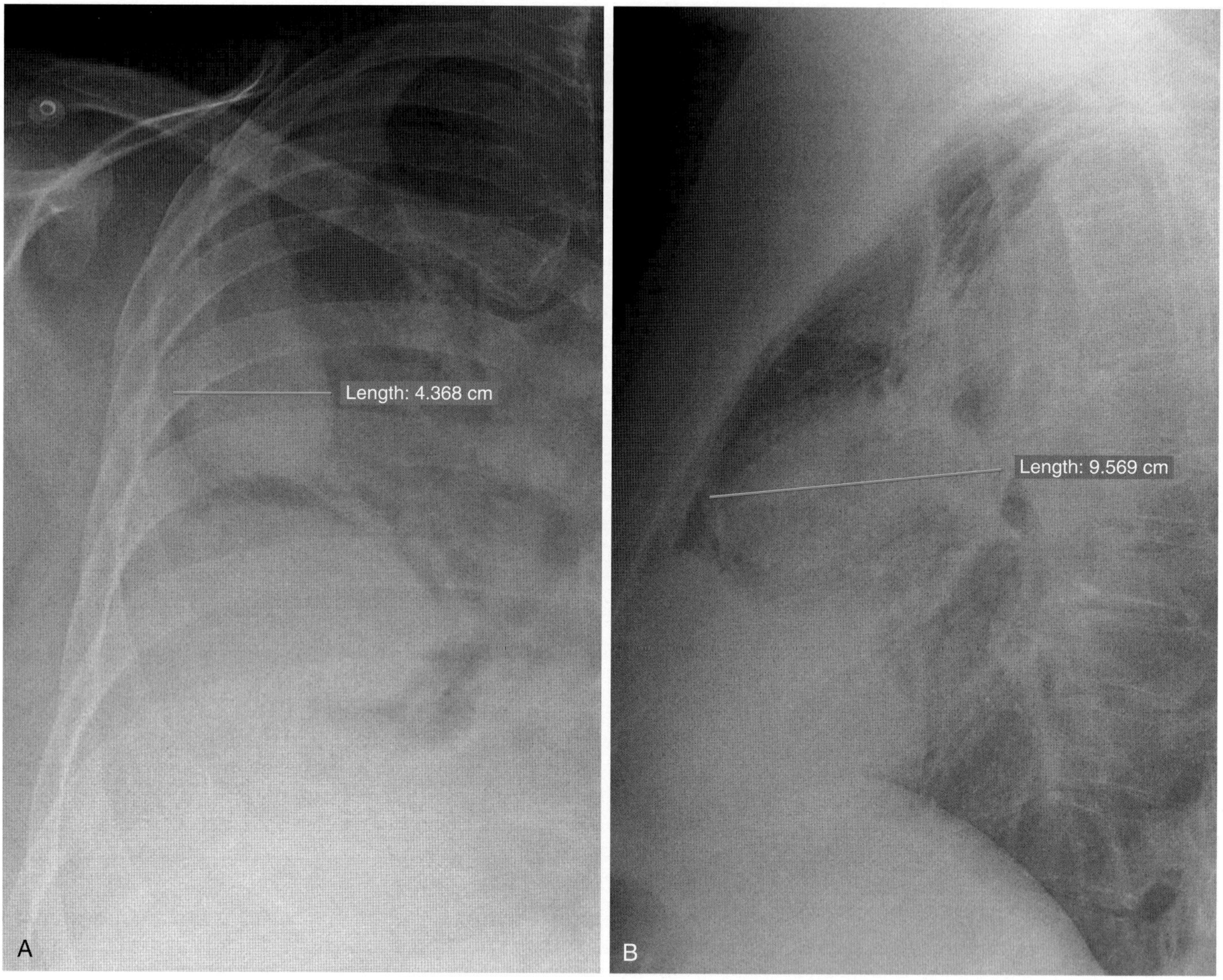

Fig. 9.18 Empyema. Frontal (A) and lateral (B) chest radiographs show a large discrepancy in anteroposterior and transverse diameter consistent with a lenticular shape that is more commonly seen with empyema. Empyema is constrained by the pleura, resulting in the oval shape.

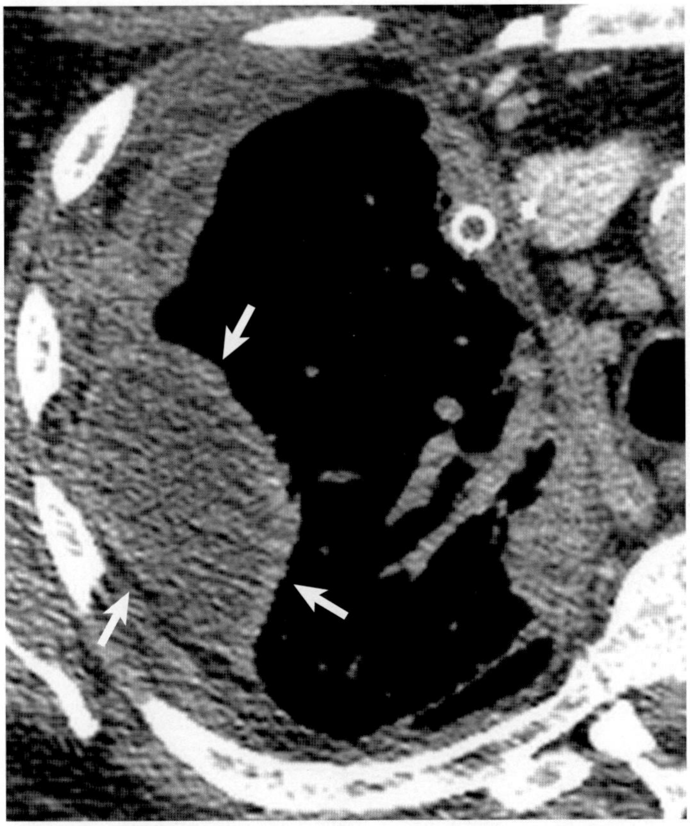

Fig. 9.19 Empyema with "split pleura" sign. Contrast-enhanced axial CT image shows thickening and enhancement of the visceral and parietal pleural layers *(arrows)* separated by loculated fluid. In the appropriate clinical setting of suspected infection, these imaging findings are consistent with a fibropurulent empyema, which will likely require drainage.

the pleural fluid collection in the absence of recent intervention should be regarded as diagnostic of a bronchopleural fistula until proven otherwise (Fig. 9.20).

Although more commonly associated with certain fungal infections, such as blastomycosis, aspergillosis, and mucormycosis, direct invasion of the chest wall or hemidiaphragm may be seen with aggressive bacterial infections from actinomycosis, *Nocardia,* and mycobacterial organisms.

Pneumatoceles manifest as thin-walled, gas-filled spaces within areas of consolidation or ground-glass opacities (Fig. 9.21). A clearly defined thin wall differentiates pneumatoceles from cavitation and lung abscesses. Pneumatoceles demonstrate a typical course with enlargement over days to weeks with resolution over weeks to months.[26] Occasionally, pneumatoceles may rupture, causing a pneumothorax (Fig. 9.22) or pneumomediastinum. Pneumatoceles occur most commonly in *S. aureus* and *P. jirovecii* pneumonia but also may be seen in other infections, including pneumococcal pneumonia.[27]

SPECIFIC ORGANISMS

Despite in-depth evaluation, including cultures and polymerase chain reaction testing, only 20% to 50% of cases of pneumonia in adults have a causative organism identified. This is likely due to early administration of antibiotic therapy and the less severe symptoms in the elderly.

COMMUNITY-ACQUIRED PNEUMONIA

Streptococcus pneumoniae

S. pneumoniae is a gram-positive bacterium, commonly associated with CAP. Currently, *S. pneumoniae* is detected in about 6% of cases of CAP overall, although it accounts for 20% to 60% of cases in older adults. Historically, pneumococcal pneumonia was determined to be the causative organism in 80% of cases of CAP, with the decrease likely due to widespread use of the pneumococcal vaccine in both children and older adults.[28] Infection with *S. pneumoniae* is associated with chronic heart or lung disease, alcoholism, institutionalization, and prior splenectomy.

S. pneumoniae characteristically manifests as a lobar consolidation, involving the peripheral lung and abutting the visceral pleura (Fig. 9.23).[17] Occasionally, infection may manifest as a spherical focus of consolidation that simulates a mass (round pneumonia), although this pattern is seen more commonly in children than in adults (Fig. 9.24).[29] Although a lobar pneumonia pattern is the most frequent manifestation, given how common it is as an infectious agent, other patterns of infection, such as bronchopneumonia, will also be seen.

Pleural effusion is evident in about 10% of patients overall[30]; it affects 30% of patients who have severe pneumonia requiring treatment in the intensive care unit and 50% of patients with bacteremia.[31] Lymphadenopathy is seldom apparent on the radiograph but is evident on CT in 50% of cases.[32]

Most patients respond rapidly to antibiotic therapy. If, despite therapy, patients with clinical signs of pneumococcal pneumonia develop complications, such as lung abscess or necrosis, microaerophilic streptococcal infection, representing aspiration of oral flora, should be considered.

Haemophilus influenzae

H. influenzae is a gram-negative coccobacillus, accounting for 5% to 20% of CAP in patients in whom an organism can be identified successfully.[33] Widespread administration of *H. influenzae* type B vaccine in children has nearly eliminated this subtype as an infectious agent in pneumonia. Nontypeable *H. influenzae* is the most common bacterial cause of acute exacerbation of chronic obstructive pulmonary disease (COPD).[34]

Clinically, pneumonia caused by *H. influenzae* is indistinguishable from other bacterial pneumonias. Radiographically, *H. influenzae* pneumonia may manifest with either a lobar or bronchopneumonia pattern (Fig. 9.25). Nodular opacities, by themselves or in combination with airspace consolidation, can also be seen, reflecting the presence of cellular bronchiolitis.[30,35,36] On CT *H. influenzae* may occasionally demonstrate a diffuse micronodular pattern with bilateral centrilobular nodules measuring less than 5 mm in diameter.[36] Pleural effusion may be seen in up to 50% of patients, although empyema is rare.

Moraxella catarrhalis

M. catarrhalis is an intracellular gram-negative diplococcus, previously classified within the *Neisseria* genus, then the *Branhamella* genus. *M. catarrhalis* is a common upper respiratory tract colonizer seen in 1% to 5% of healthy adults with nasopharyngeal colonization common throughout infancy. It is currently considered the third most common cause of community-acquired bacterial pneumonia (after *S. pneumoniae* and *H. influenzae*).[37] Seldom causing pneumonia in previously healthy individuals, *M. catarrhalis* is a common cause of exacerbation of COPD and is identified in approximately 10% of pneumonias in the elderly.[37]

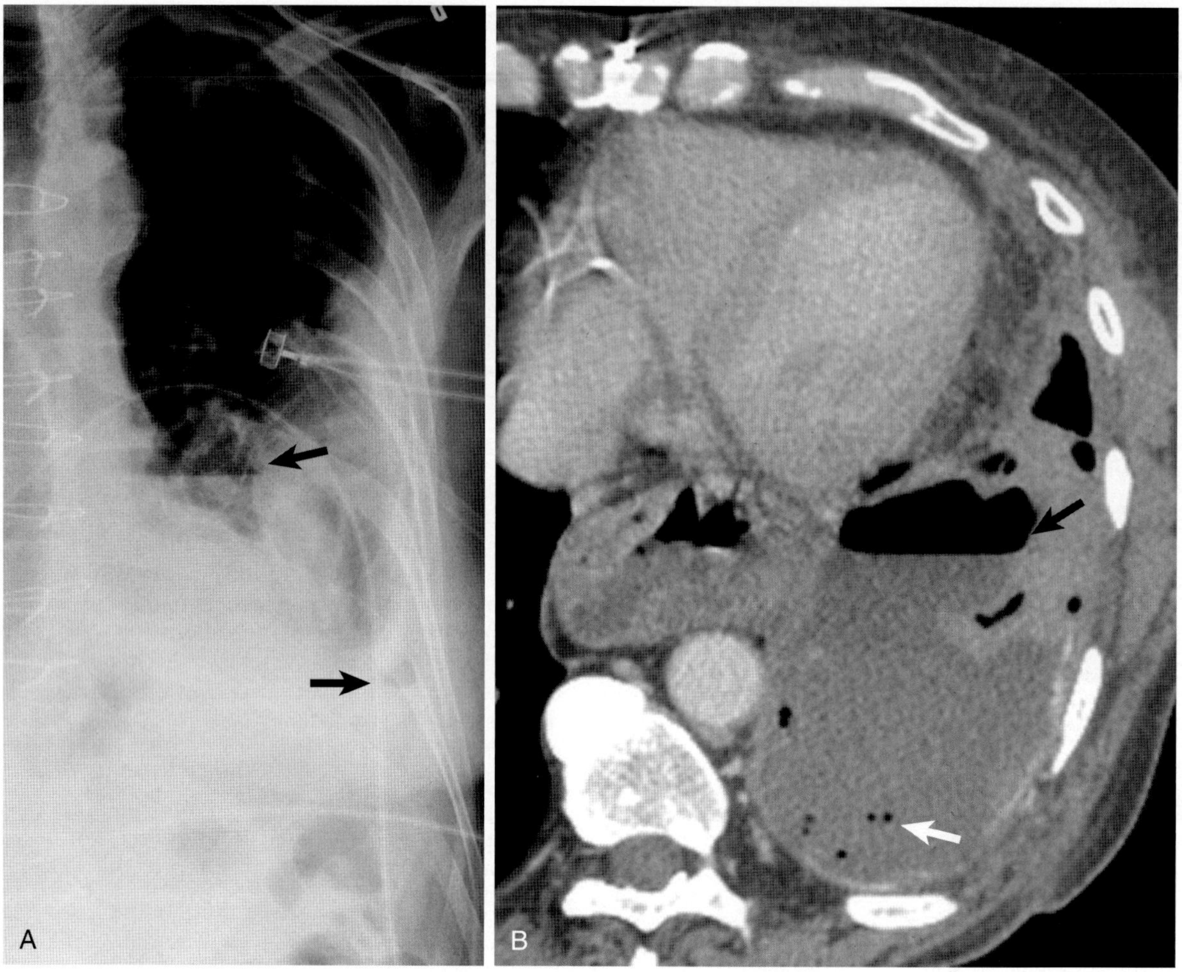

Fig. 9.20 Bronchopleural fistula with empyema. (A) Frontal chest radiograph shows multiple air-fluid levels *(arrows)* within the left hemithorax. (B) Contrast-enhanced axial CT image shows a large air-fluid level *(black arrow)* and multiple foci of air *(white arrow)* within the pleural fluid collection. Air within the empyema (if no percutaneous intervention has occurred) is diagnostic of a bronchopleural fistula. Note thickening and enhancement of the parietal pleural lining posteriorly indicating the presence of an exudative effusion.

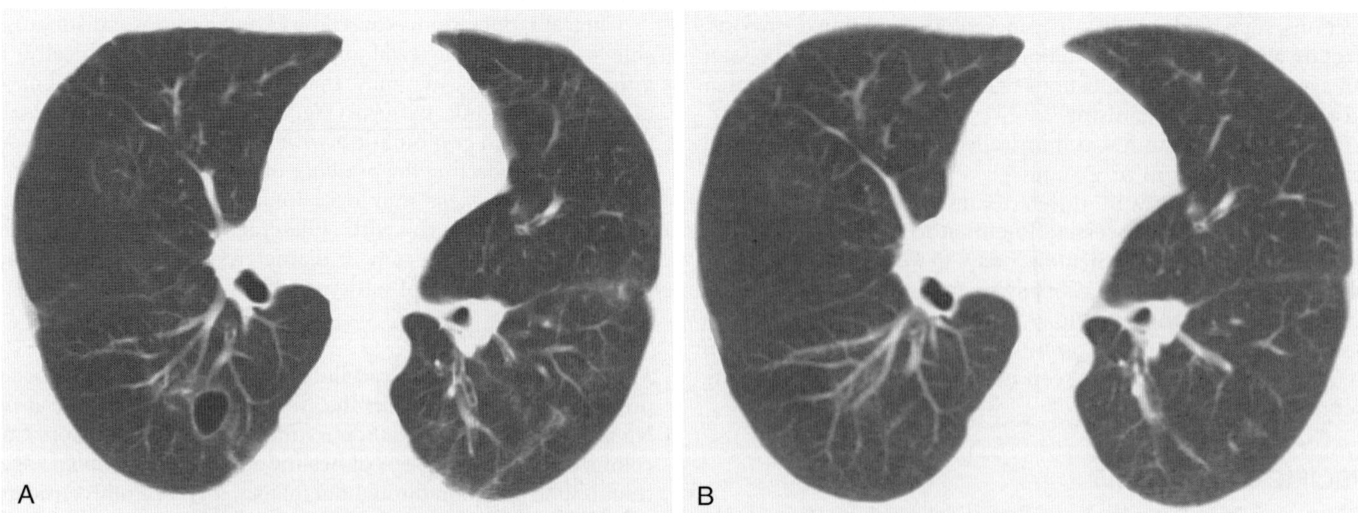

Fig. 9.21 Pneumatocele after *Streptococcus pneumoniae* pneumonia. (A) CT scan in a patient with resolving bronchopneumonia shows a thin-walled cystic lesion (pneumatocele) in the right lower lobe, patchy bilateral ground-glass opacities, and a few poorly defined centrilobular nodules. (B) CT scan 3 months later shows resolution of the pneumatocele in the right lower lobe and residual bilateral scarring.

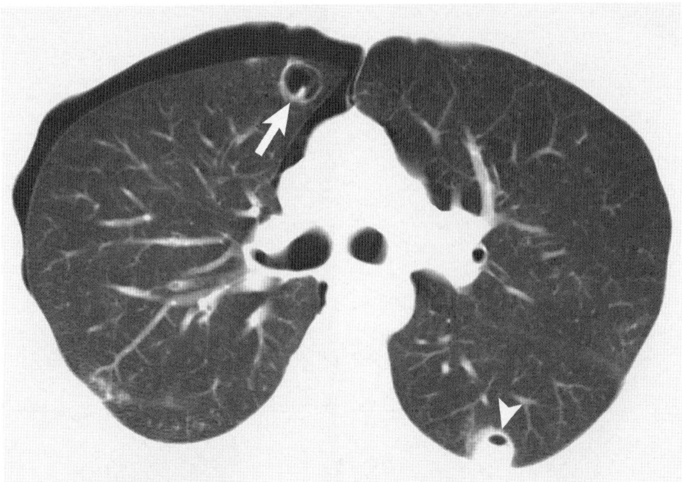

Fig. 9.22 Pneumothorax from septic embolism. CT scan at the level of the right upper lobe bronchus shows a thin-walled cavity *(arrow)* in the right upper lobe and a cavitary nodule *(arrowhead)* in the left lower lobe. Also noted are a right pneumothorax and a few centrilobular nodules in the posterior segment of the right upper lobe.

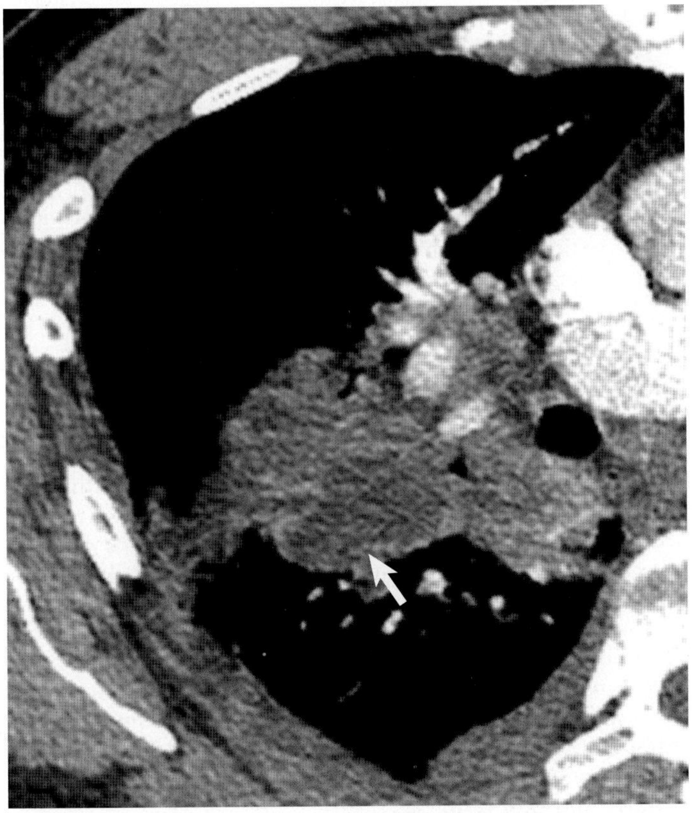

Fig. 9.23 *Streptococcus pneumoniae* with pulmonary necrosis. Contrast-enhanced axial CT image at the level of the bronchus intermedius shows a right lower lobe consolidation with a focal area of hypoattenuation *(arrow)* consistent with pulmonary necrosis.

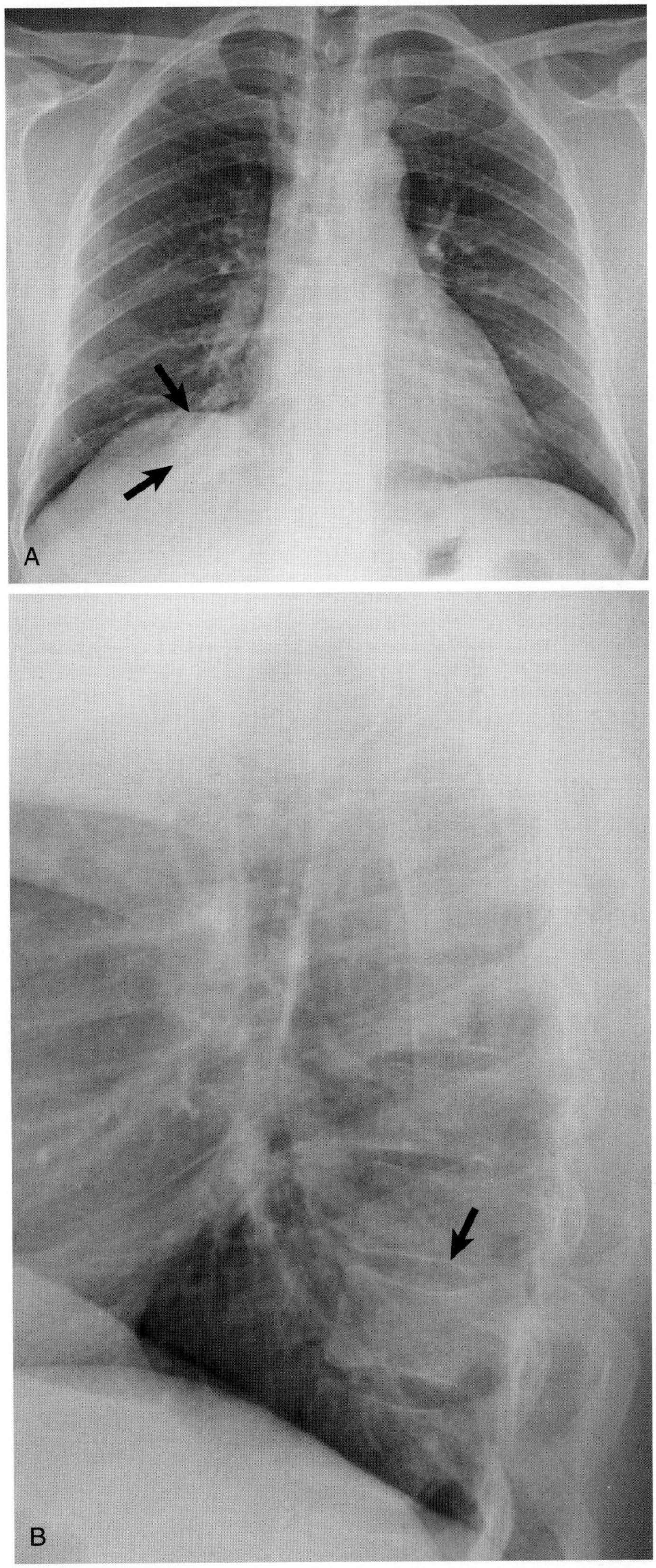

Fig. 9.24 Round pneumonia. Frontal (A) and lateral (B) chest radiographs show a rounded opacity in the right lower lobe *(arrows)*, overlying the spine on the lateral view. This resolved on follow-up imaging (not shown), confirming round pneumonia. Round pneumonia can frequently be confused with malignancy and requires additional imaging and follow-up to ensure resolution.

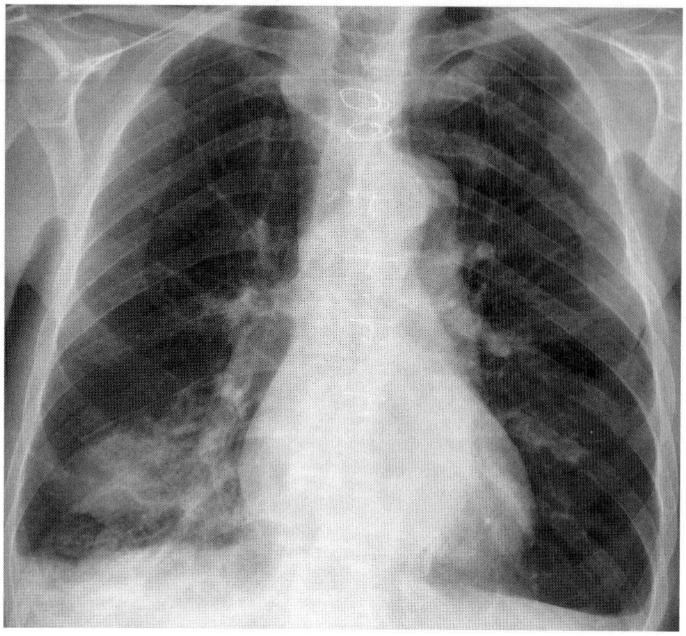

Fig. 9.25 *Haemophilus influenzae* pneumonia with lobar consolidation. Frontal chest radiograph demonstrates right lower lobe consolidation. *H. influenzae* pneumonia may manifest with either a lobar pattern or a bronchopneumonia pattern.

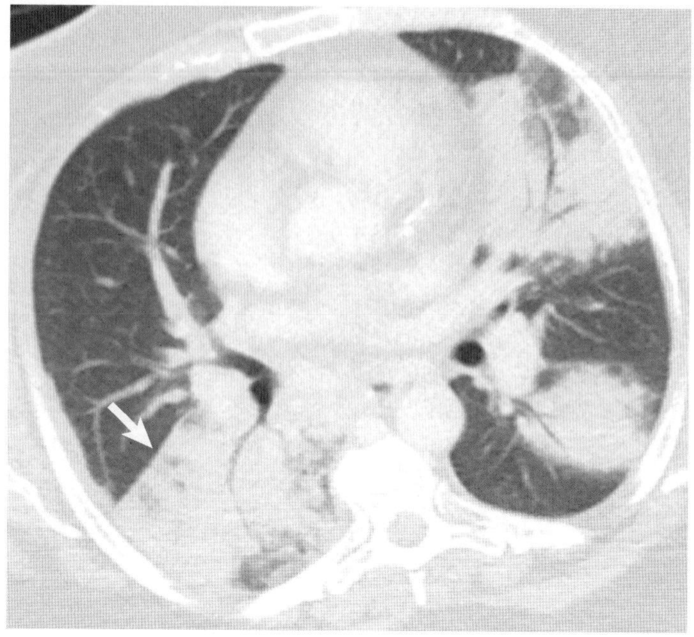

Fig. 9.26 *Legionella pneumophila* pneumonia. Axial CT image shows bilateral consolidation with ground-glass opacity. Presence of air bronchograms suggests multifocal lobar consolidation rather than a bronchopneumonia pattern. Note the fissural demarcation *(arrow)* of the right lower lobe consolidation.

The radiographic findings of *M. catarrhalis* pneumonia typically consist of a bronchopneumonia pattern with patchy unilateral or bilateral consolidation involving mainly the lower lobes.[37]

ATYPICAL INFECTIONS

Atypical pneumonia comprises up to 50% of all cases of CAP, with patients showing slower onset of symptoms and prolonged illness despite treatment.[38,39] Patients also commonly present with systemic manifestations of disease. The three nonzoonotic bacterial atypical infections are *Legionella pneumophila, M. pneumoniae,* and *C. pneumoniae.*

Legionella pneumophila

L. pneumophila, a gram-negative coccobacillus, is the causative organism of legionnaire disease. It results in a rapidly progressive pneumonia, often in older men, most with preexisting conditions such as COPD, renal failure, or malignancy.[40–43] The bacteria reside in biofilms within water, such as air conditioners, showers, and evaporative condensers, with the presumed mechanism of infection being aerosolization of infected water particles.[44] There is a large geographic discrepancy in the incidence of *L. pneumophila* pneumonia, ranging from 0.6% to 23%, with higher rates of infection seen in western Pennsylvania and Ohio compared to other parts of the United States.[45]

Legionella infection frequently exhibits extrapulmonary manifestations as well, including renal insufficiency and electrolyte abnormalities, diarrhea, myalgias, headaches and confusion, and relative bradycardia (i.e., heart rate less than expected given fever).[43]

Initially, infection with *L. pneumophila* can manifest with airspace consolidation (lobar pneumonia pattern), which rapidly progresses to bilateral patchy areas of consolidation more suggestive of bronchopneumonia (Fig. 9.26).[46] As the infection progresses and despite adequate antibiotic therapy, bilateral multifocal lobar consolidation often develops.[42,47]

Complications such as cavitation and abscess formation are uncommon in immunocompetent patients, occurring in 1% to 6% of patients.[47,48] Similar to *S. pneumoniae, L. pneumophila* pneumonia may manifest as a round consolidation simulating a mass (round pneumonia).[49]

Mycoplasma pneumoniae

M. pneumoniae is a bacterium lacking a cell wall, although it grows extracellularly. They are the smallest free-living organisms that can be cultured on artificial media.[50] *M. pneumoniae* infection typically manifests in children and adolescents, with peak incidence between 5 and 15 years of age, but may cause about 15% to 20% of pneumonias in patients older than 40 years.[51,52] Infections occur throughout the year, with a peak during the autumn and early winter in temperate regions. Transmission is person to person via aerosolized respiratory droplets from coughing.

As an organism responsible for atypical pneumonia, onset of symptoms is usually slower and less severe. Like *L. pneumophila,* extrapulmonary manifestations are common, including myringitis, meningoencephalitis, hemolytic anemia, pericarditis and myocarditis, and skin rash.

The predominant histologic and radiographic finding of *M. pneumoniae* infection in adults is bronchiolitis, which progresses to a bronchopneumonia pattern (Fig. 9.27).[50,53,54] Pediatric infection with *M. pneumoniae* more commonly manifests with segmental or lobar consolidation. Lymphadenopathy is more commonly seen in pediatric patients. Bronchial wall thickening, centrilobular nodules, and tree-in-bud opacities are frequently observed on CT imaging and manifest as reticulonodular opacities on chest radiography. Pleural effusion, when present, is usually small and unilateral.[55,56]

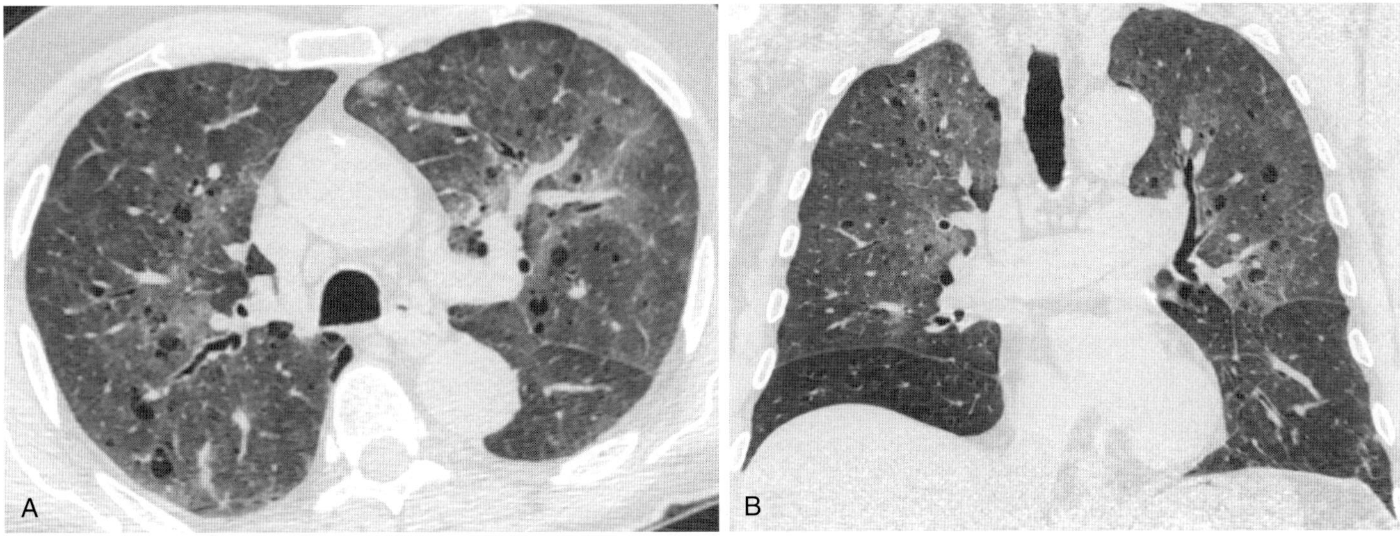

Fig. 9.27 Mycoplasma pneumonia with pneumatoceles. Axial (A) and coronal (B) reformatted CT images shows bilateral ground-glass opacity, mosaic attenuation and scattered pneumatoceles, and centrilobular emphysema. The mosaic attenuation is due to bronchiolitis from infection.

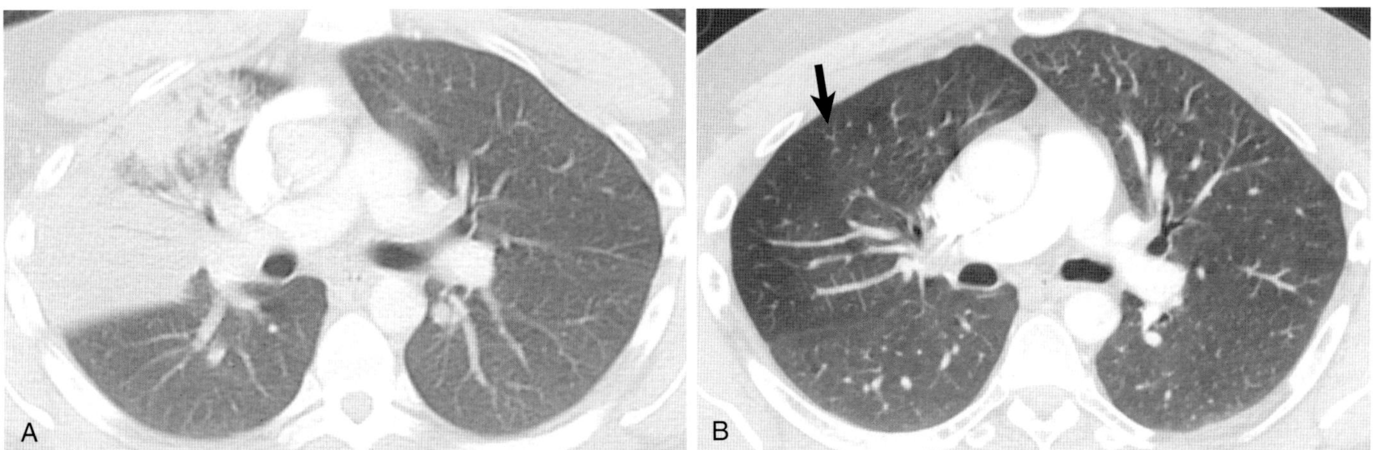

Fig. 9.28 Swyer-James-McLeod syndrome (constrictive bronchiolitis). (A) Axial CT image shows a right upper lobe consolidation with areas of incomplete alveolar filling (ground-glass opacity) and air bronchograms. (B) Follow-up chest CT shows resolution of the consolidation with residual hyperlucent lung *(arrow)* resulting from constrictive bronchiolitis consistent with Swyer-James-McLeod syndrome.

Most patients with *Mycoplasma* pneumonia recover completely; however, a small percentage, particularly children, develop bronchiectasis and constrictive bronchiolitis.[14,57] If extensive involvement occurs, unilateral hyperlucent lung (Swyer-James-McLeod syndrome) may develop (Fig. 9.28).[58] Expiratory CT imaging will show bronchiectasis with patchy air-trapping.[14]

Chlamydia pneumoniae

Another cause of atypical pneumonia, such as *M. pneumoniae* and *L. pneumophila*, *C. pneumoniae* is an obligate intracellular bacterium that can grow only in host cells and not in artificial culture media.[24] *C. pneumoniae* is a common cause of CAP, accounting for 12% to 20% of cases.[59,60] Patients with underlying chronic airway disease, such as chronic obstructive pulmonary disease or cystic fibrosis, are most commonly affected. The mode of transmission is unknown.

Extrapulmonary manifestations of disease are less common with *C. pneumoniae* than other atypical organisms, and respiratory symptoms are more likely to be less severe and longer lasting. Persistent subclinical infection is not uncommon.

The radiographic findings of *C. pneumoniae* pneumonia are indistinguishable from those of *M. pneumoniae* and include bronchiolitis progressing to a bronchopneumonia pattern. When areas of consolidation are seen on radiography, they may be patchy unilateral or bilateral consistent with bronchopneumonia or, less commonly, sublobar or lobar.[61] Evaluation with CT typically shows a more lobar pattern of consolidation, although it may also show patchy and poorly defined areas of consolidation and ground-glass opacities consistent with a bronchopneumonia pattern.[62] Pleural effusions, usually small, are seen in about 25% of patients.[60]

It is difficult to suggest a specific pathogen with imaging alone. *C. pneumoniae* is more likely to affect older patients,

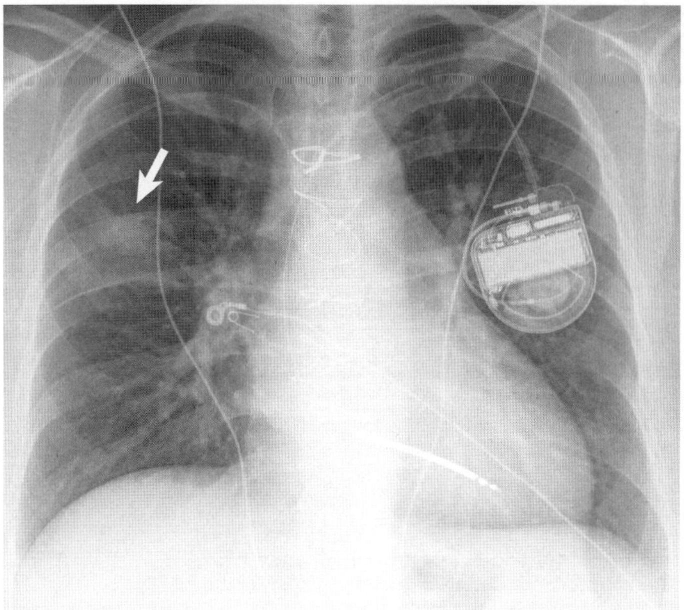

Fig. 9.29 Methicillin-sensitive *Staphylococcus aureus* (MSSA) pneumonia. Frontal chest radiograph in an immunocompromised patient with remote heart transplant shows a focal area of consolidation *(arrow)* in the right upper lobe. Blood cultures grew MSSA.

whereas *M. pneumoniae* tends to affect people younger than 40 years.

HEALTH CARE–ASSOCIATED, HOSPITAL-ACQUIRED, AND VENTILATOR-ACQUIRED PNEUMONIA

Staphylococcus aureus

S. aureus is a gram-positive coccus that is distinguished from other staphylococcal species by its production of coagulase, a plasma clotting enzyme. *S. aureus*, particularly methicillin-resistant *S. aureus* (MRSA), is a common pathogen in hospital-acquired pneumonia, accounting for 20% to 30% of cases. *S. aureus* is a less common cause of CAP, accounting for 10% of microbiologically confirmed cases, usually involving methicillin-sensitive *S. aureus* (Fig. 9.29).[63]

S. aureus is a frequent colonizer of asymptomatic individuals, often seen as a cause of CAP in postinfluenza patients. In the hospital setting, *S. aureus* pneumonia is commonly encountered in patients after intubation or respiratory tract instrumentation. This suggests a breakdown in the host defenses as a mechanism of pathogenesis.

When acquired through the respiratory tree, *S. aureus* pneumonia typically manifests with a bronchopneumonia pattern with poorly defined nodular opacities measuring less than 10 mm in diameter and patchy or confluent areas of consolidation involving one or more segments of a single lobe or multiple lobes.[20] Central bronchial obstruction with inflammatory exudate often results in segmental atelectasis associated with areas of consolidation. Air bronchograms are seldom evident on radiography.[64] The pneumonia is bilateral in approximately 40% of patients.

S. aureus pneumonia commonly cavitates, leading to a necrotizing pneumonia with abscess formation (Fig. 9.30), which places the patient at risk for air-leak phenomena, including pneumomediastinum and pneumothorax with bronchopleural fistula. Pleural effusions occur in 30% to 50% of patients; of these, approximately half represent empyemas.[65]

In patients with *S. aureus* bacteremia or infected central venous catheters, hematogenous spread of infection is common. This manifests as multiple bilateral nodules, usually measuring 1 to 3 cm in diameter. The nodules tend to occur in the periphery of the lower lobes, often with associated cavitation. Occlusion of pulmonary arteries by septic emboli or thrombus may result in hemorrhage or infarction or both and in less well-defined or wedge-shaped foci of consolidation.

Pseudomonas aeruginosa

P. aeruginosa is a gram-negative bacillus found ubiquitously throughout our environment. *P. aeruginosa* is the most commonly implicated gram-negative bacterium in hospital-acquired pneumonia. *P. aeruginosa* is the second most common identified pathogen in ventilator-associated pneumonia, after *S. aureus*.[66] Multiple virulence factors result in high associated mortality rates, ranging from 42% to 87%.[67] Antimicrobial resistance is common.[66] *P. aeruginosa* is such a common pathogen in all of the health care–related pneumonias that the American Thoracic Society and the Infectious Diseases Society of America recommend empiric treatment of these pneumonias to include multiple antipseudomonal antimicrobial agents.

In addition, *P. aeruginosa* is an important cause of chronic airway colonization and pneumonia in patients who have cystic fibrosis or bronchiectasis (Fig. 9.31).

The radiographic and CT manifestations of *P. aeruginosa* pneumonia usually are those of bronchopneumonia, consisting of multifocal bilateral areas of consolidation.[68,69] Less common radiographic manifestations include lobar consolidation with or without bulging fissure or multiple nodular opacities.[68] Pleural effusion and abscess formation are common.[68]

ENTEROBACTERIACEAE

The Enterobacteriaceae are a family of gram-negative bacilli containing many harmless organisms but also containing multiple well-known human pathogens, including *Escherichia coli*, *K. pneumoniae*, *Enterobacter* spp., *Acinetobacter* spp., and *Serratia marcescens*. The most commonly identified organisms within this group are *K. pneumoniae* and *E. coli*.

K. pneumoniae accounts for 1% to 5% of all cases of CAP and approximately 15% of cases of nosocomial pneumonia.[70] Acute pneumonia caused by *K. pneumoniae* occurs predominantly in men, many of whom are chronic alcoholics[71] or have underlying chronic bronchopulmonary disease (Fig. 9.32).[72] *E. coli* accounts for approximately 4% of cases of CAP and 5% to 20% of cases of pneumonia acquired in a hospital or a nursing home.[17] It occurs most commonly in debilitated patients.[73]

K. pneumoniae typically manifests as a lobar pneumonia pattern, beginning peripherally adjacent to the pleura and spreading centripetally via the interalveolar pores of Kohn and small airways.[74] Air bronchograms are frequently present because of lack of central bronchial involvement. Compared with pneumococcal pneumonia, *Klebsiella* pneumonia tends to produce larger amounts of inflammatory exudate, leading to lobar expansion with resultant bulging of interlobar fissures (bulging fissure sign).[18,75] However, because of the greater prevalence of pneumococcal pneumonia, lobar expansion is more likely due

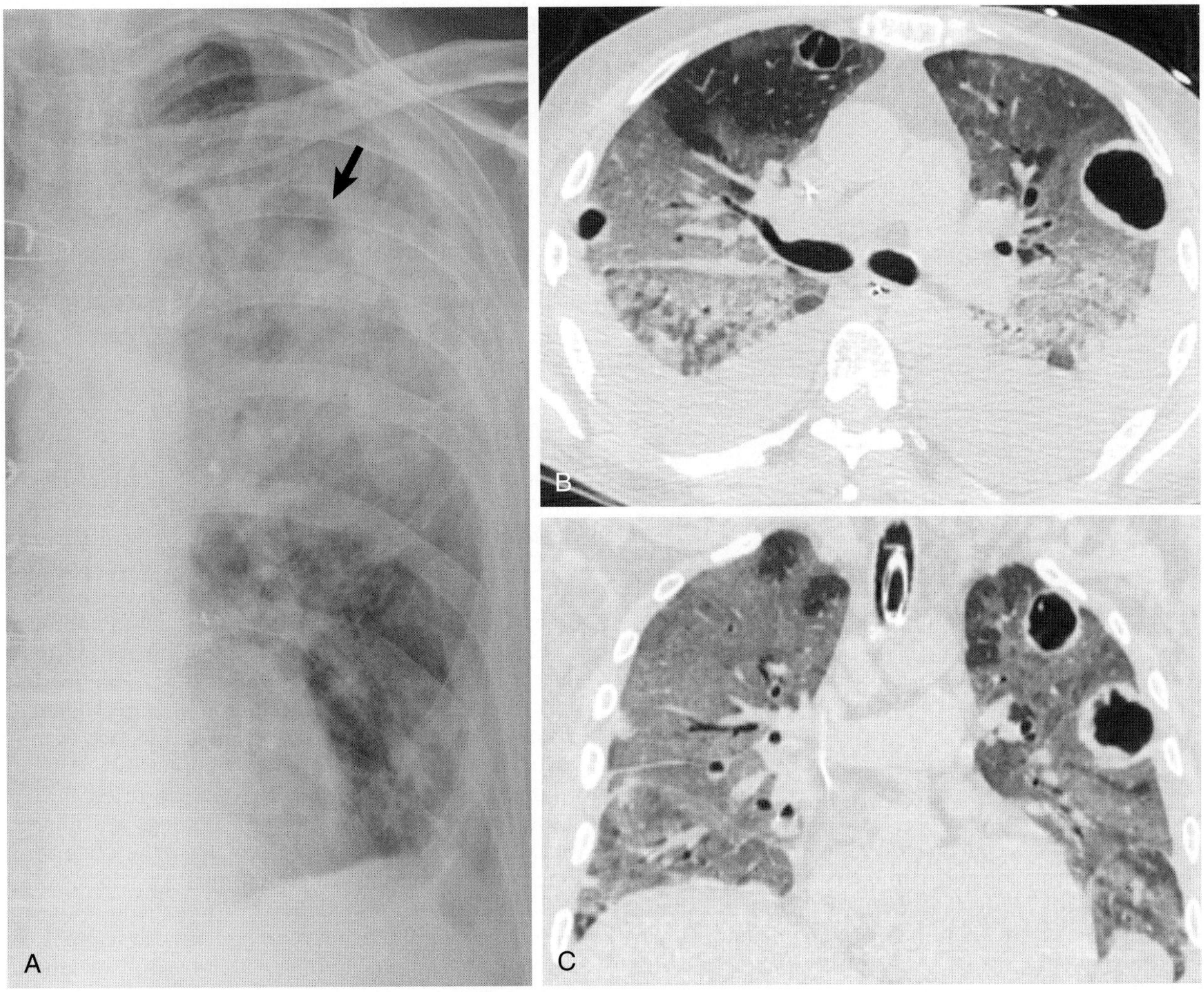

Fig. 9.30 Pulmonary abscesses in *Staphylococcus aureus* pneumonia. (A) Frontal chest radiograph shows a left upper lobe consolidation with rounded lucency *(arrow).* The lucency represents cavitation and abscess within the consolidation. Axial (B) and coronal reformatted (C) CT images from a separate patient also infected with *S. aureus* show bilateral thick-walled cavities within areas of ground-glass opacity consistent with pulmonary abscesses. Moderate bilateral pleural effusions are also noted. The multifocal peripheral involvement in this case is often seen in the setting of septic embolism with abscess formation.

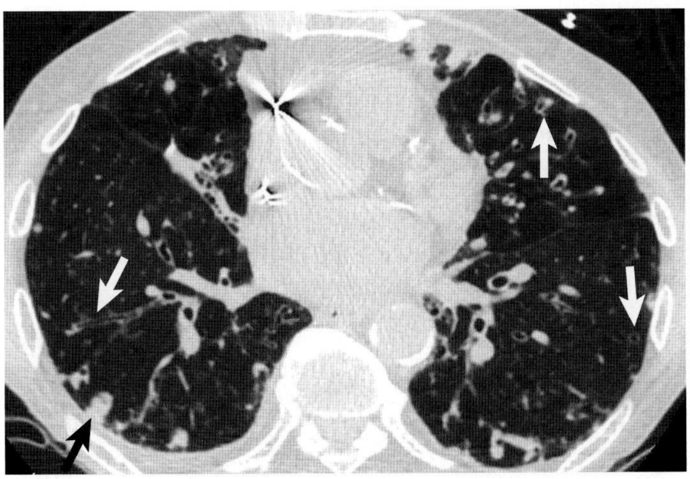

Fig. 9.31 *Pseudomonas aeruginosa* pneumonia. Axial CT image shows bronchiectasis *(white arrows)* and nodules *(black arrow). Pseudomonas aeruginosa* commonly infects or colonizes patients with cystic fibrosis or bronchiectasis. This is a less common manifestation with peripheral nodular opacities *(black arrow).*

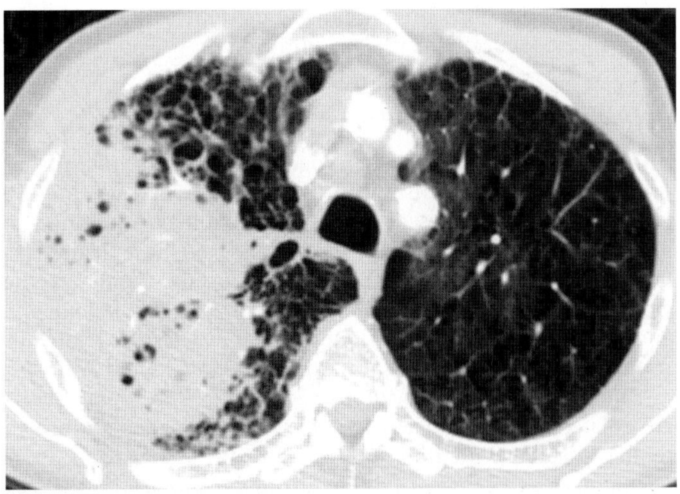

Fig. 9.32 *Klebsiella pneumoniae* in chronic obstructive pulmonary disease (COPD). Axial CT image demonstrates a large consolidation in the right upper lobe with intrinsic lucencies, which may represent emphysematous lung or areas of cavitation. Note severe centrilobular emphysema, particularly in the left upper lobe. *Klebsiella pneumoniae* is a common cause of both community-acquired and nosocomial pneumonia, particularly in patients with underlying chronic bronchopulmonary disease such as COPD.

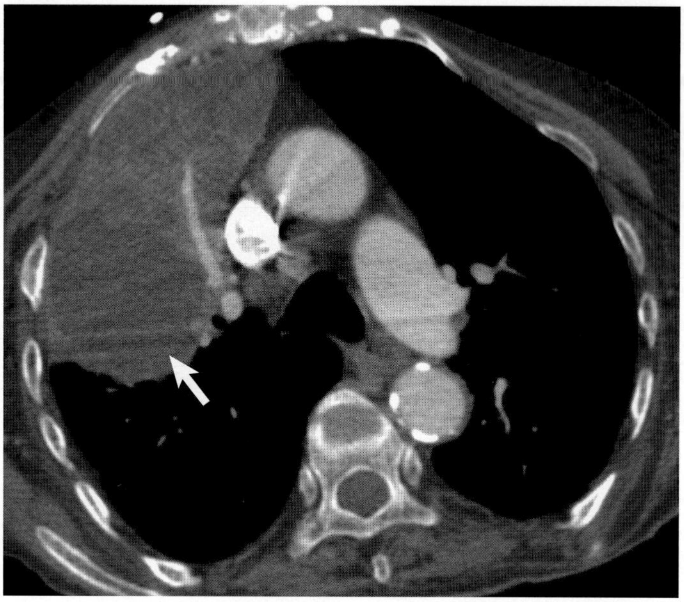

Fig. 9.33 *Klebsiella pneumoniae* with pulmonary necrosis. Contrast-enhanced axial CT image shows right upper lobe consolidation with a nonenhancing portion posteriorly *(arrow)* indicating pulmonary necrosis. *Klebsiella* has a higher propensity for pulmonary necrosis and abscess formation than many other bacterial pathogens.

to *S. pneumoniae* than to *K. pneumoniae*. There is also a greater tendency for abscess formation and pulmonary necrosis in patients with *K. pneumoniae* infection (Fig. 9.33).[18,75] Pleural effusion is seen in 60% to 70% of cases.[74] Rarely, *Klebsiella* pneumonia may result in a bronchopleural fistula. Occasionally, *Klebsiella* pneumonia undergoes only partial resolution and progresses to a chronic phase with cavitation and persistent positive cultures. In this circumstance the radiographic picture simulates that seen in tuberculosis.

The radiographic manifestations of *E. coli* pneumonia usually are those of bronchopneumonia, consisting of multifocal bilateral areas of consolidation, similar to *P. aeruginosa* pneumonia.[68,69] Involvement usually is multilobar and predominantly affects the lower lobes. Pleural effusion is common.

ANAEROBIC BACTERIA

Anaerobic bacteria are a heterogeneous mix of organisms, predominantly representing normal oral flora. More than 30 genera and 200 species of anaerobes have been identified in human infection; as such, infection of the lung usually is polymicrobial.[76–79] Among the most important agents are the gram-negative bacilli *Bacteroides, Fusobacterium, Porphyromonas,* and *Prevotella;* the gram-positive bacilli *Eubacterium* and *Clostridium;* the gram-positive cocci *Peptostreptococcus* and *Peptococcus;* and the gram-negative cocci *Veillonella.*[80,81] Anaerobic bacteria are isolated in approximately 20% to 35% of all patients admitted to the hospital with pneumonia[17] and are second only to *S. pneumoniae* as a cause of CAP requiring hospitalization.[82] They also are an important cause of nosocomial pneumonia.[83,84]

Clinically, anaerobic bacterial pneumonia manifests similarly to other community-acquired and nosocomial infections, with fever, cough, and pleuritic chest pain. The cough is typically nonproductive until cavitation occurs, usually 7 to 10 days or more after the onset of pneumonia.[84,85] In 40% to 75% of cases, the expectoration is putrid.[17] Foul smelling sputum indicates the presence of anaerobic organisms.[17,85,86]

Radiographic manifestations of infection are that of bronchopneumonia, typically involving the posterior segments of the upper lobes or superior segments of the lower lobes in supine patients and the basal segments of the lower lobes in erect patients, reflecting gravitational flow secondary to aspiration (Fig. 9.34).

Cavitation and necrosis occur in approximately 50% of cases (Fig. 9.35). Occasionally, hilar or mediastinal lymph node enlargement is associated with an abscess, a combination of findings that may resemble lung cancer.[24,87]

ZOONOTIC INFECTIONS

Most of the emerging infections recognized in the past decade have been zoonoses. Zoonoses are infectious agents with the capacity to jump between species, from domestic animals and wildlife to humans. Among the zoonotic causes of CAP, *Chlamydia psittaci* (psittacosis), *Coxiella burnetii* (Q fever), and *Francisella tularensis* (tularemia) represent the bacterial pathogens.

C. psittaci is the causative agent of psittacosis and primarily infects birds. Historically, infection was thought to arise from infected parrots (psittacosis arises from the Greek word for parrot), although any bird may be a carrier, and in fact, even mammals, including humans, are rare sources of psittacosis.[67] Humans usually acquire the infection when they inhale dried bird excrement containing the bacteria. Imaging findings are nonspecific and include reticular opacities radiating from the hila or involving the lung bases, homogeneous ground-glass opacities, and segmental or lobar areas of consolidation.[88–90] In patients with severe pneumonia, the clinical and radiologic findings may resemble the findings of pneumococcal pneumonia with lobar consolidation.[91]

C. burnetii is the pathogen responsible for Q fever, an acute self-limited febrile illness. Domesticated livestock, including cattle, sheep, and goats, are common animal reservoirs, shedding the bacteria in urine, feces, milk, and birth products (up to 10^9 organisms per gram of infected sheep placenta).[67] Occasionally, the organism can be transferred via ticks, although this is a less common vector for infection. Radiographically, Q fever manifests similarly to the atypical pneumonia organisms, with bronchopneumonia and bronchiolitis.[67] Segmental areas of consolidation in the subpleural lung are common.[92–94] Pleural effusion is found in up to 35% of patients.[93] Like other atypical infections, extrapulmonary manifestations are common and include headache, myalgia, fatigue, nausea and vomiting, and diarrhea.

F. tularensis is a gram-negative bacteria occurring primarily in small animals such as rabbits and is the causative organism of tularemia. Major vectors of transmission include ticks and biting flies in the United States and mosquitoes in Europe.[67] Ulceroglandular tularemia with enlarged, tender lymphadenopathy is the most common manifestation. Pneumonic tularemia, likely resulting from inhalation of aerosolized particles, was the primary clinical form in 39% of adults and 24% of patients, overall, among reported cases in Missouri between 2000 and 2007.[95]

Pneumonic tularemia typically manifests with bilateral airspace consolidation, either lobar or segmental, often with radiographically visible hilar lymphadenopathy and pleural effusion. Cavitation and bronchopleural fistula formation, although uncommon, may complicate the pneumonia.[67]

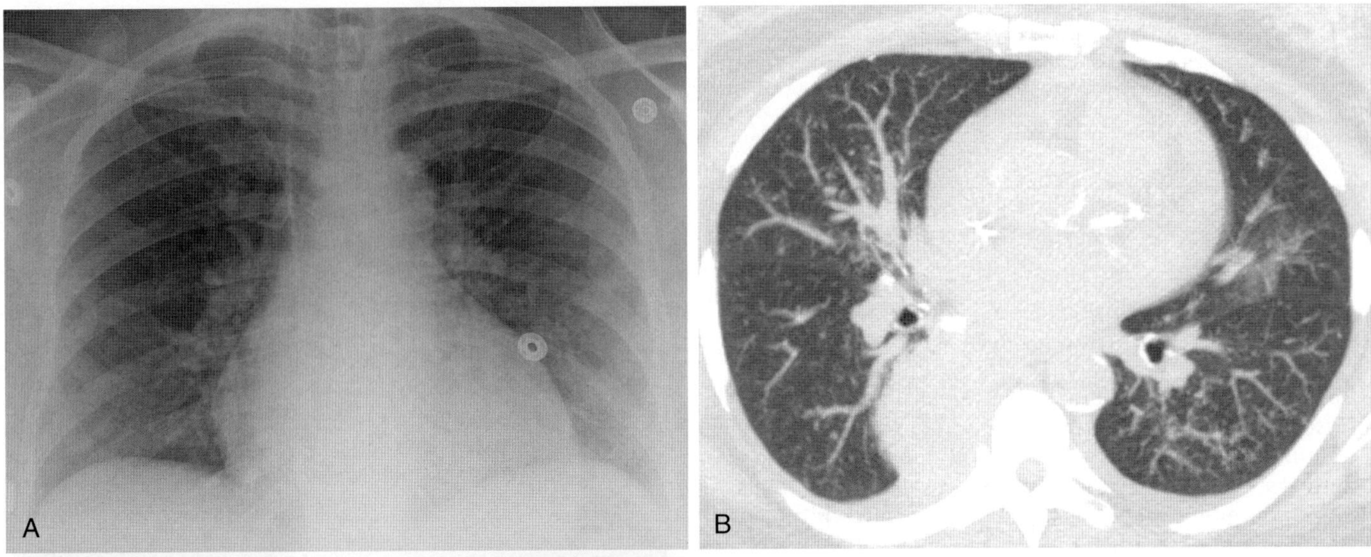

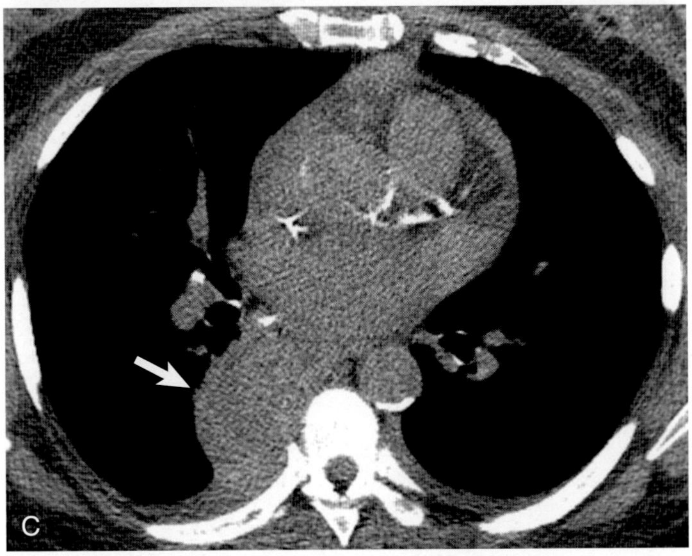

Fig. 9.34 Anaerobic bacterial pneumonia from aspiration. (A) Frontal chest radiograph in a patient presenting with symptoms of pneumonia, shows bibasilar heterogeneous opacities. The patient has a history of achalasia, which predisposes to aspiration. (B) Axial maximal-intensity projection image shows bilateral tree-in-bud opacities most pronounced in the left lower lobe. Aspiration pneumonia can manifest in different areas of the lungs, depending on the position of the patient at time of aspiration. (C) Axial CT image with soft tissue window demonstrates a fluid-filled, dilated esophagus *(arrow)* consistent with known achalasia.

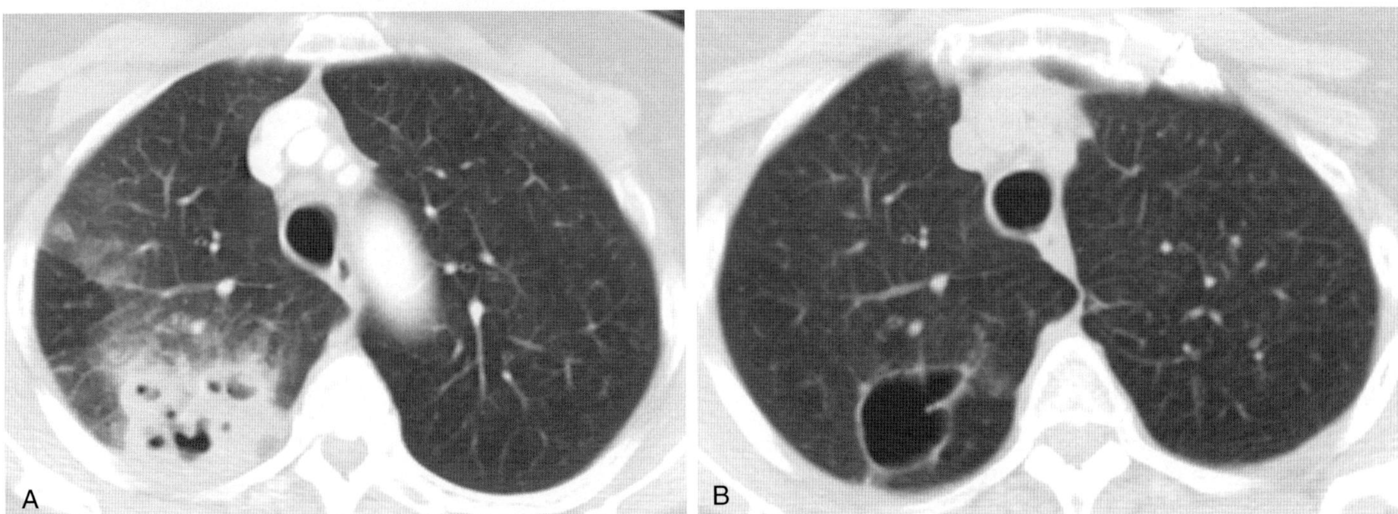

Fig. 9.35 Anaerobic bacterial pneumonia with abscesses. (A) Axial CT image from a patient with aspiration pneumonia shows a superior segment right lower lobe consolidation with multiple air-filled pulmonary abscesses. (B) After treatment, a residual pneumatocele has developed at the site of infection. The pneumatocele will likely resolve over time though can result in areas of pulmonary scarring and fibrosis. Anaerobic bacteria have a high propensity for developing abscesses, occurring in approximately 50% of cases.

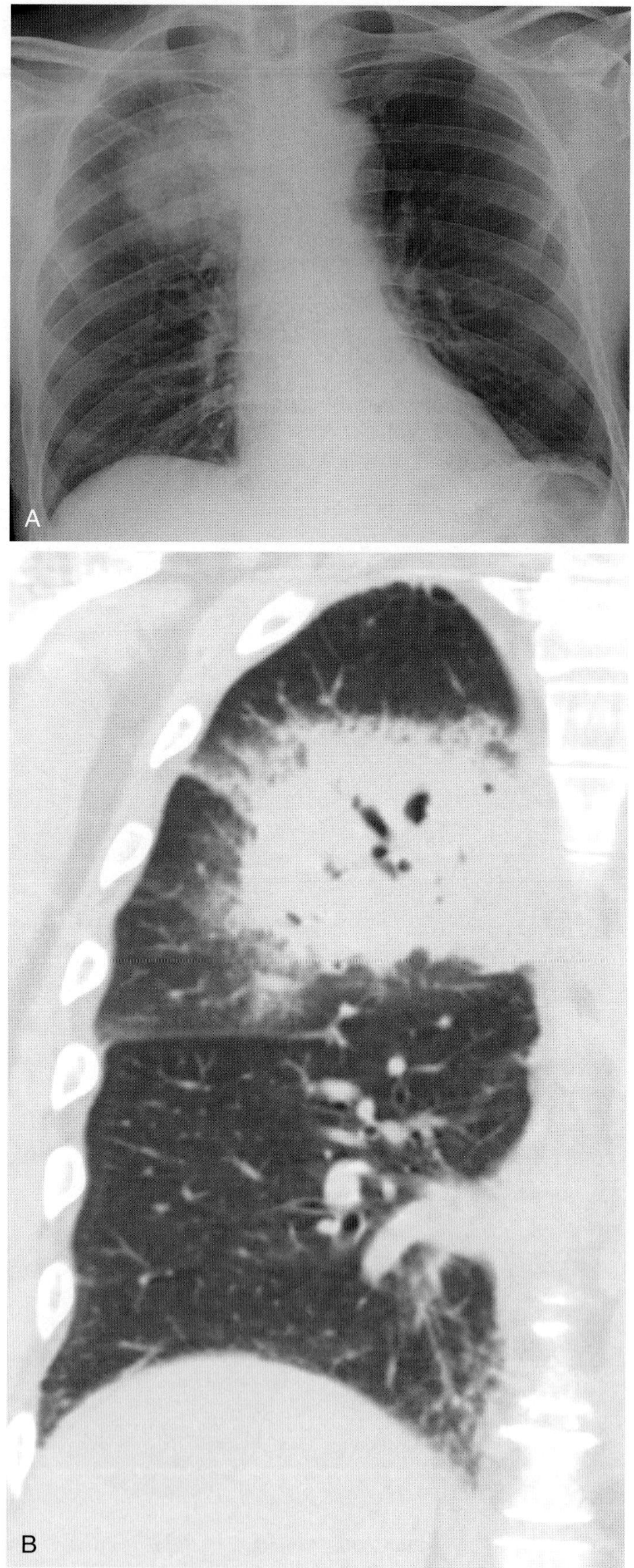

Fig. 9.36 *Nocardia asteroides* pneumonia. (A) Frontal chest radiograph demonstrates a right upper lobe consolidation with intrinsic linear lucencies suggesting air bronchograms or cavitation. (B) Coronal reformatted CT image shows the right upper lobe consolidation with intrinsic lucencies, which represent both air bronchograms and areas of cavitation. Cavitation is common in *Nocardia* infection, occurring in up to a third of patients.

HIGHER-FORM BACTERIA

Nocardia asteroides

N. asteroides is an aerobic gram-positive bacillus found in soil and distributed throughout the world.[24] Although more common in immunocompromised individuals, *N. asteroides* is also an uncommon cause of CAP in otherwise healthy individuals.[24] Infection commonly manifests with low-grade fever, productive cough, and weight loss, often following an intermittent course.[96]

The most common radiographic manifestation of disease is multifocal homogeneous consolidation, usually peripheral and abutting the pleura. Nodules and masses may also be seen. Cavitation is common, occurring in up to one-third of patients (Fig. 9.36). Nodules may demonstrate a rim of ground-glass opacity, the so-called CT halo sign, classically observed in neutropenic patients with angioinvasive aspergillosis.[67] Multiple virulence factors allow invasion into the chest wall, also seen with blastomycosis, aspergillosis, mucormycosis, tuberculosis, and actinomycosis.

Actinomyces israelii

A. israelii is an anaerobic gram-positive filamentous bacterium and the most common pathogen causing actinomycosis. The organism is part of the normal human oral flora and is frequently found in dental caries and at gingival margins of individuals with poor oral hygiene.[17] Approximately 15% of cases of actinomycosis have thoracic involvement.[67] Infection is often caused by frank aspiration or microaspiration, although it may also directly extend from cervicofacial or abdominal infections.[67]

The most common radiographic manifestation of thoracic actinomycosis is unilateral, peripheral, and patchy areas of consolidation, demonstrating a lower lobe predominance. Multiple peripherally enhancing, centrally low-attenuation areas representing necrosis and abscess are frequently seen. Pleural effusion is occasionally the only radiographic manifestation, usually representing empyema.[97] Chronic infection may lead to extensive pulmonary parenchymal fibrosis.[74]

Chest wall involvement, frequently seen in the past, is now uncommon (Fig. 9.37).[98,99] The manifestations of chest wall involvement include a soft tissue mass and rib abnormalities and are better seen on CT than on radiography.[98,100]

IMAGING ALGORITHMS

The main role of radiography in the diagnosis of pneumonia is in the confirmation of presence of parenchymal abnormalities consistent with the clinical diagnosis. Imaging is of limited value in establishing the specific cause of bacterial pneumonia. The cause can be determined from sputum, bronchoscopy specimens, blood culture, urine assays, or fine-needle aspiration. The chest radiograph has a high sensitivity and specificity in the detection and exclusion of CAP.[101] With nosocomial infections, imaging

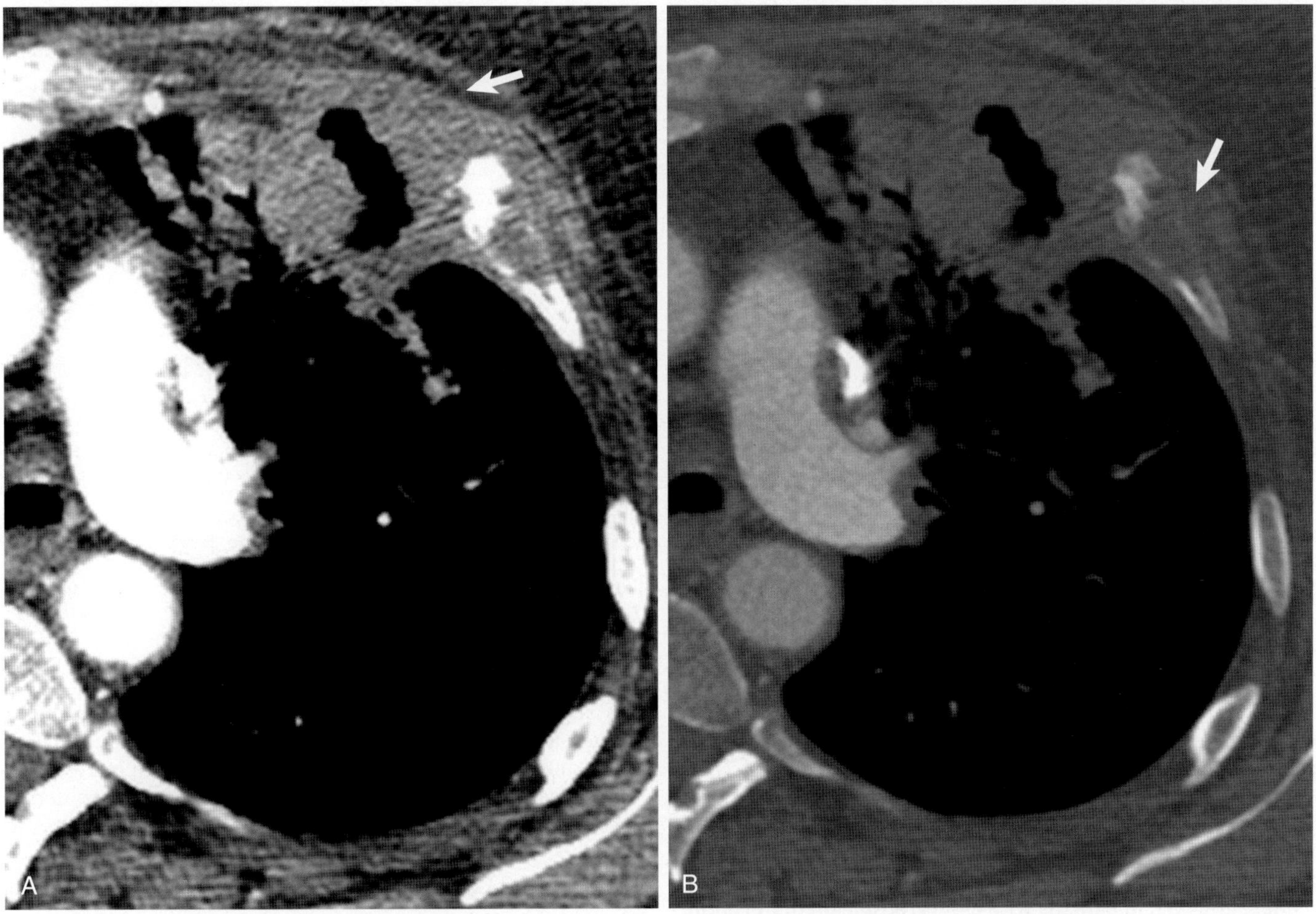

Fig. 9.37 *Actinomyces* infection with chest wall invasion. (A) Contrast-enhanced axial CT image shows direct extension of the infection through the pleura into the anterior chest wall *(arrow)*. (B) Axial CT at the same level with bone window shows a lytic area *(arrow)* within the rib related to osteomyelitis from direct extension of infection.

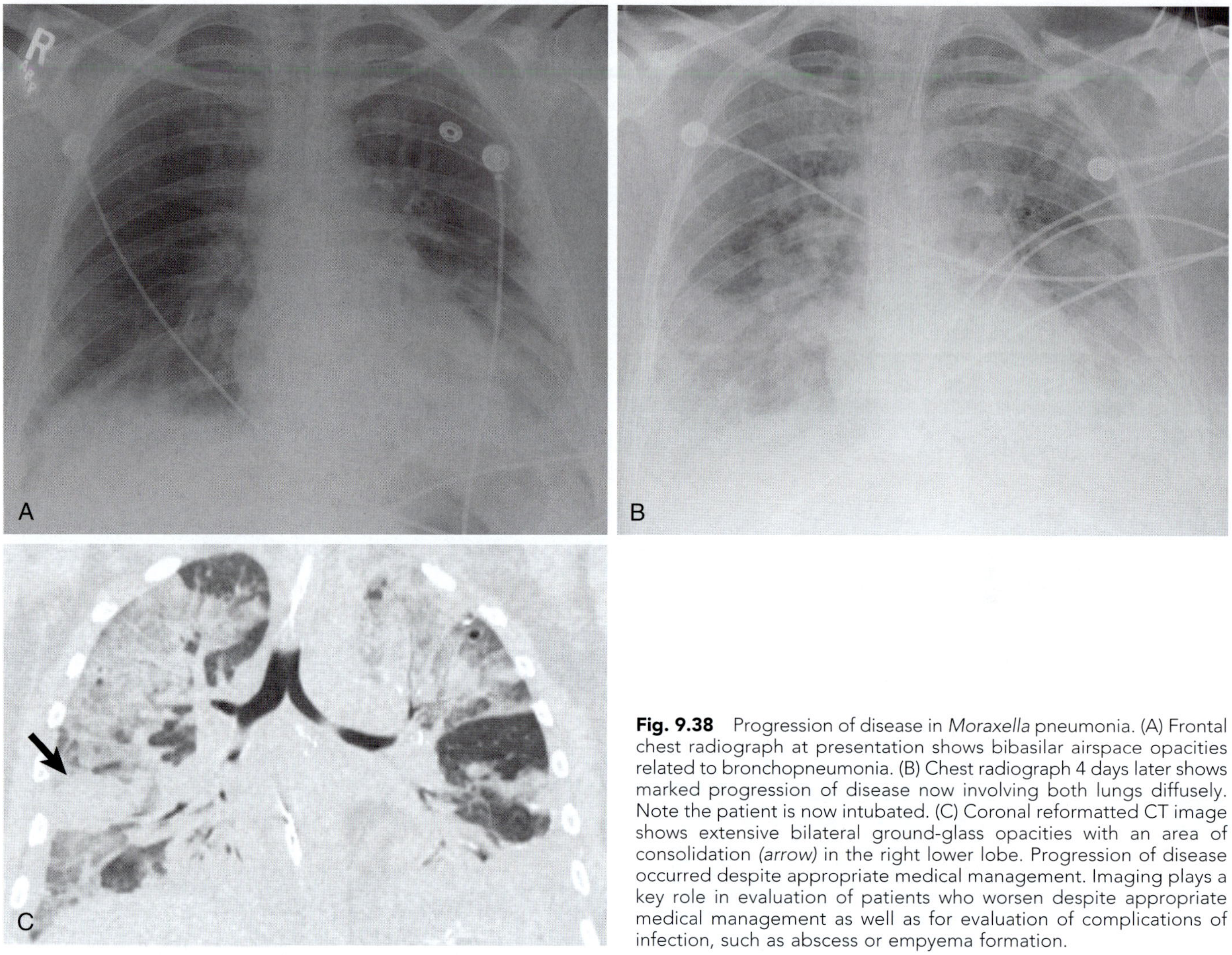

Fig. 9.38 Progression of disease in *Moraxella* pneumonia. (A) Frontal chest radiograph at presentation shows bibasilar airspace opacities related to bronchopneumonia. (B) Chest radiograph 4 days later shows marked progression of disease now involving both lungs diffusely. Note the patient is now intubated. (C) Coronal reformatted CT image shows extensive bilateral ground-glass opacities with an area of consolidation *(arrow)* in the right lower lobe. Progression of disease occurred despite appropriate medical management. Imaging plays a key role in evaluation of patients who worsen despite appropriate medical management as well as for evaluation of complications of infection, such as abscess or empyema formation.

is often obtained within hours of onset of symptoms; chest radiographs may be normal, and management should be based upon clinical and laboratory findings. In one large study of 2706 adults diagnosed with pneumonia, almost one-third initially had a normal chest radiograph.[102]

CT may demonstrate signs suggestive of a particular organism more than radiography but remains nonspecific. CT is recommended, however, in patients with clinical suspicion of infection and normal or nonspecific radiographic findings to assess suspected complications of pneumonia, such as abscess or empyema, or in patients with a suspected underlying lesion, such as pulmonary carcinoma.[101] CT also is indicated in patients with pneumonia and persistent or recurrent pulmonary opacities (Fig. 9.38).[100,103]

Procalcitonin is a peptide precursor produced by cells in the lungs and is useful to differentiate bacterial from nonbacterial infections and other noninfectious causes of inflammation. A procalcitonin level does not generally rise in patients with viral or noninfectious causes of inflammation.

Traditionally, all adults (>40 years of age or in suspicious cases <40 years of age) with consolidation secondary to pneumonia are recommended to have follow-up chest radiographs in 6 to 8 weeks to ensure resolution of the pulmonary opacities and exclude an underlying malignancy (Fig. 9.39). Recent research has suggested that the incidence of a new diagnosis of lung cancer in patients with pneumonia is rare, although certain characteristics were independently associated with increased risk of lung cancer, including age 50 years or older, male gender, and smoking history (Fig. 9.40).[104]

Differential Diagnosis

Although certain radiologic patterns are highly suggestive of pneumonia, chest radiography is of limited value in determining the specific etiology.[105,106] The radiologic pattern is influenced by the presence of underlying disease, such as emphysema, and age and immunologic status of the patient.[105]

Aside from other infections, including viruses, parasites, and other bacteria, the main differential of pneumonia is malignancy. Other causes of a newly discovered pulmonary opacity include mediastinal fat (Fig. 9.41), organizing pneumonia, or pneumonitis either from radiation (Fig. 9.42) or other causes of injury.

Synopsis of Treatment Options

The treatment of pneumonia depends on the organism causing the infection, the immune status of the patient, and the severity of symptoms. Most cases respond to oral antibiotics.

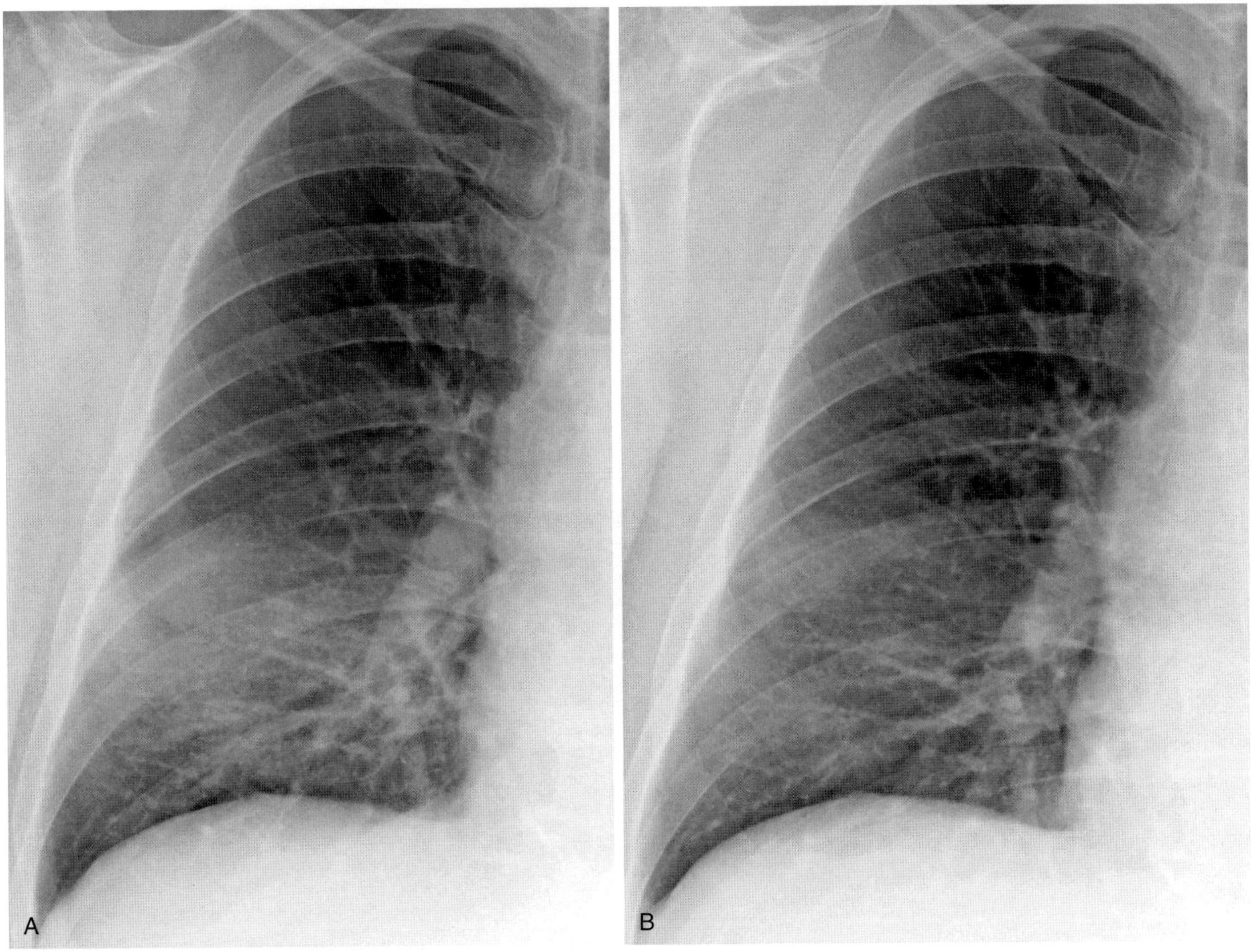

Fig. 9.39 Lobar pneumonia with resolution. (A) Frontal chest radiograph demonstrates a lobar consolidation in the right lung base, with a rounded configuration. In the setting of typical symptoms of pneumonia, follow-up imaging should be obtained in 6–8 weeks to confirm resolution. (B) Follow-up chest radiograph 4 weeks later shows near complete resolution of the pulmonary opacity. Radiographic findings of pneumonia are delayed compared with clinical signs, sometimes by up to 2 weeks at disease onset or during resolution.

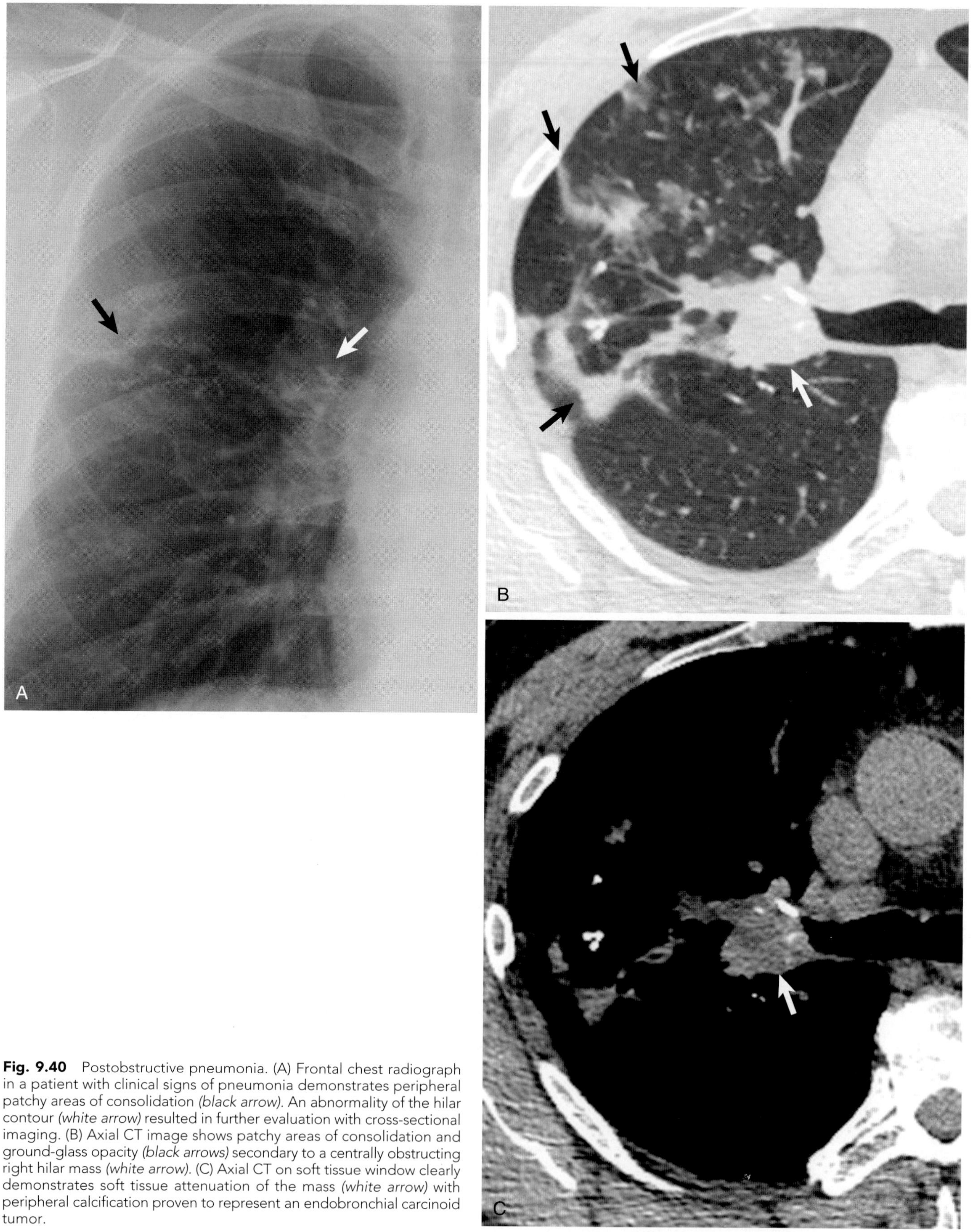

Fig. 9.40 Postobstructive pneumonia. (A) Frontal chest radiograph in a patient with clinical signs of pneumonia demonstrates peripheral patchy areas of consolidation *(black arrow)*. An abnormality of the hilar contour *(white arrow)* resulted in further evaluation with cross-sectional imaging. (B) Axial CT image shows patchy areas of consolidation and ground-glass opacity *(black arrows)* secondary to a centrally obstructing right hilar mass *(white arrow)*. (C) Axial CT on soft tissue window clearly demonstrates soft tissue attenuation of the mass *(white arrow)* with peripheral calcification proven to represent an endobronchial carcinoid tumor.

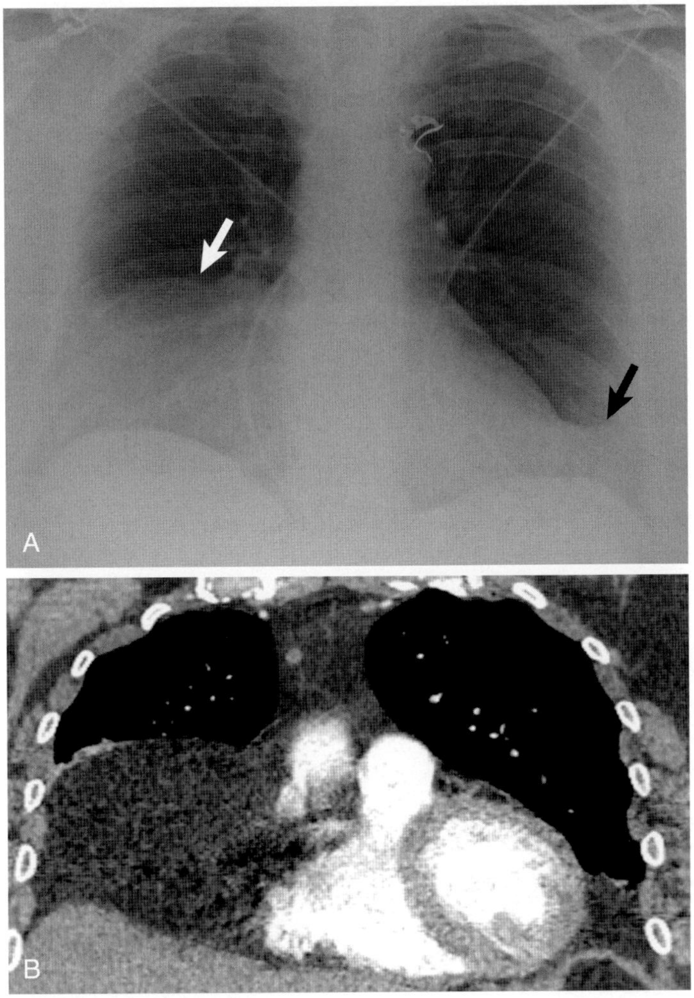

Fig. 9.41 Morgagni hernia and mediastinal fat mimicking pneumonia. (A) Frontal chest radiograph shows bilateral lower lung zone opacities *(arrows)* obscuring the heart borders. (B) Coronal reformatted CT image shows the fat attenuation of the bilateral opacities. The right cardiophrenic angle opacity represents a Morgagni hernia with peritoneal fat, whereas the left cardiophrenic angle opacity represents mediastinal fat.

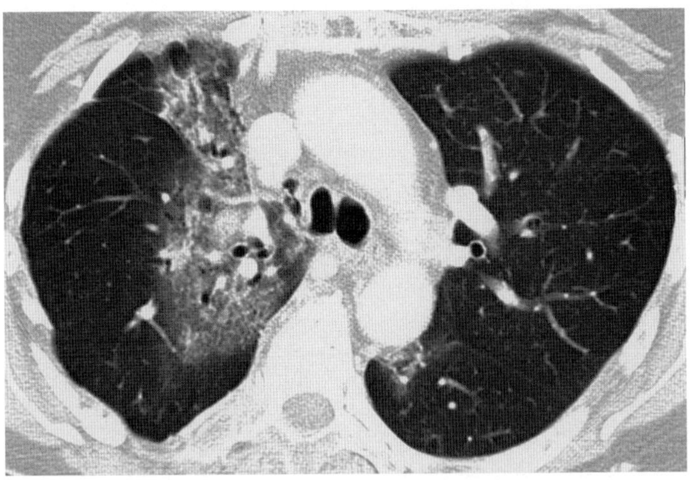

Fig. 9.42 Pneumonitis mimicking pneumonia. Axial CT image shows areas of consolidation and ground-glass opacity involving the right upper lobe. In the appropriate clinical setting, this could represent infection. This patient had a history of prior radiation, and these changes represent postradiation pneumonitis. A well-demarcated lateral border related to the radiation field is a useful sign to suggest radiation-induced lung damage.

KEY POINTS: BACTERIAL PNEUMONIA

- Pneumonia is broadly divided into infection acquired in the community versus acquired in health care settings, including hospitals and nursing homes. Multidrug-resistant bacteria are more commonly encountered in hospital or health care–associated pneumonia.
- Most common organisms responsible for community-acquired pneumonia: *Streptococcus pneumoniae* and *Haemophilus influenzae*, atypical organisms (*Legionella* spp., *Mycoplasma pneumoniae*, *Chlamydia pneumoniae*)
- Most common organisms associated with nosocomial pneumonia: *Pseudomonas aeruginosa*, gram-negative rods, anaerobes, *Klebsiella pneumoniae*, *Staphylococcus aureus*
- Three main imaging patterns of bacterial pneumonia are seen: lobar consolidation, bronchopneumonia, and hematogenous spread of infection
- Lobar pneumonia is a homogeneous consolidation predominantly or exclusively affecting one lobe
  - Air bronchograms are common
  - Most common organisms
    - *S. pneumoniae*
    - *K. pneumoniae*
    - *Legionella pneumophila*
- Bronchopneumonia manifests with patchy, inhomogeneous consolidation and ground-glass opacities, commonly affecting several lobes
  - Centrilobular nodules and tree-in-bud pattern seen on CT
  - Most common organisms
    - *S. aureus*
    - *Escherichia coli*
    - *P. aeruginosa*
    - Anaerobes
    - *H. influenzae*
- Hematogenous spread of infection radiographically demonstrates middle and lower lung zone, poorly defined nodules, and wedge-shaped consolidations.
  - Frequently demonstrates cavitation
  - Most commonly associated with *S. aureus* from endocarditis or infected central venous lines
- Complications of bacterial pneumonia include lung necrosis and abscess, pneumatocele, and bronchopleural fistula.
- The main role of the chest radiograph is in confirming the presence of parenchymal disease in patients with clinically suspected pneumonia.
- Although certain radiologic patterns may be suggestive of certain organisms, chest radiography is of limited value in determining the specific etiology.
- The main role of CT is in the evaluation of suspected pneumonia in immunocompetent patients with normal or nonspecific radiographic findings and in patients with pneumonia and suspected complications, such as empyema.

SUGGESTED READINGS

Apisarnthanarak A, Mundy LM. Etiology of community-acquired pneumonia. *Clin Chest Med*. 2005;26:47–55.

Blasi F, Tarsia P, Aliberti S, et al. Chlamydia pneumoniae and Mycoplasma pneumoniae. *Semin Respir Crit Care Med*. 2005;26:617–624.

Cunha BA. The atypical pneumonias: clinical diagnosis and importance. *Clin Microbiol Infect*. 2006;12(suppl 3):12–24.

Herold CJ, Sailer JG. Community-acquired and nosocomial pneumonia. *Eur Radiol*. 2004;14(suppl 3):E2–E20.

Khawaja A, Zubairi AB, Durrani FK, et al. Etiology and outcome of severe community acquired pneumonia in immunocompetent adults. *BMC Infect Dis*. 2013;13:94.

Lutfiyya MN, Henley E, Chang LF, et al. Diagnosis and treatment of community-acquired pneumonia. *Am Fam Physician*. 2006;73:442–450.

Marrie TJ, Peeling RW, Fine MJ, et al. Ambulatory patients with community-acquired pneumonia: the frequency of atypical agents and clinical course. *Am J Med*. 1996;101:508–515.

Moine P, Vercken JB, Chevret S, et al. Severe community-acquired pneumonia: etiology, epidemiology, and prognosis factors. French Study Group for Community-Acquired Pneumonia in the Intensive Care Unit. *Chest*. 1994;105:1487–1495.

Okada F, Ando Y, Wakisaka M, et al. *Chlamydia pneumoniae* pneumonia and *Mycoplasma pneumoniae* pneumonia: comparison of clinical findings and CT findings. *J Comput Assist Tomogr*. 2005;29:626–632.

The full reference list for this chapter is available at ExpertConsult.com.

10 Pulmonary Tuberculosis

KYUNG SOO LEE | YEON JOO JEONG

Overview

ETIOLOGY, PREVALENCE, AND EPIDEMIOLOGY

Tuberculosis (TB) is a chronic recurrent contagious infection caused by *Mycobacterium tuberculosis. M. tuberculosis* is an aerobic, nonmotile, non–spore-forming rod that is highly resistant to drying, acid, and alcohol. It is transmitted person to person via droplet nuclei containing the organism and spread mainly by coughing. The contagiousness of a patient with TB increases with greater extent of disease, the presence of cavitation, the frequency of coughing, and the virulence of the organism.[1] The risk of developing active TB is the greatest in patients with altered host cellular immunity. These include extremes of age, malnutrition, cancer, immunosuppressive therapy (including steroids and anti–tumor necrosis factor drugs), human immunodeficiency virus (HIV) infection, end-stage renal disease, and diabetes.

In 2014 9.6 million people were estimated to develop TB, and 1.5 million died of the disease, 0.4 million of whom were HIV positive.[2] Of the estimated 9.6 million new cases in 2014, 58% were in Southeast Asia and Western Pacific regions and 28% in the Africa region.[2] During 2014 a total of 9407 confirmed TB cases (3.1 cases per 100,000 population) were reported in the United States. Slightly more than half (54%) of US cases were in foreign-born persons.[3] It is estimated that 43 million lives were saved between 2000 and 2014 through effective diagnosis and treatment. To keep the efforts for global elimination of TB, from 2016 the World Health Organization hopes to end the global TB epidemic by implementing the End TB Strategy, which serves to reduce the number of TB deaths by 90% by 2030, cut new cases by 80%, and ensure that no family is burdened with catastrophic costs resulting from TB.

HIV infection is the strongest known risk factor for progression from latent to active TB. Globally, 12% of the 9.6 million new TB cases in 2014 were HIV positive, and TB killed 0.4 million HIV-positive people.[2] The majority of these patients live in countries with limited health care resources—Africa and Asia. The incidence of TB in these countries is increasing.[4] Immune restoration induced by highly active antiretroviral therapy (HAART) in developed countries has considerably improved the outcome of HIV-positive patients and reduced the prevalence of opportunistic infection and TB in these patients. However, HIV-associated TB continues to occur in countries where HAART is widely used and is seen in patients on antiretroviral treatment.[5] Furthermore, HAART may result in paradoxical worsening of TB manifestations in patients with immune reconstitution inflammatory syndrome (IRIS)[4,6] (see Chapter 15).

CLINICAL PRESENTATION

Patients with active pulmonary TB may be asymptomatic, have mild or progressive dry cough, or present with multiple symptoms, including fever, fatigue, weight loss, night sweats, and productive cough. Elderly patients with pulmonary TB may have different clinical presentations, including more frequent dyspnea and comorbid medical conditions, such as cardiovascular disease, diabetes, and chronic obstructive pulmonary disease.[7]

Pathologic Findings and Pathophysiology

Inhaled mycobacteria are phagocytized by alveolar macrophages, where the organisms multiply and eventually kill the cells. Interaction of macrophages with T lymphocytes results in differentiation of macrophages into epithelioid histiocytes. The epithelioid histiocytes aggregate into small clusters resulting in granulomas. After several weeks granulomas are well formed, and their central portions undergo necrosis.[1] As the disease progresses, individual necrotic foci tend to enlarge and coalesce. The rapid bacillary growth phase is arrested with the development of cell-mediated immunity and delayed-type hypersensitivity at 2 to 10 weeks after the initial infection.[8,9] The initial focus of parenchymal disease is termed the *Ghon focus*. The Ghon focus may be microscopic or large enough to be visible radiologically. It either enlarges as disease progresses or, much more commonly, undergoes healing. Healing may result in a visible scar that may be dense and contain foci of calcification. However, commonly there is residual central necrotic material. Although the disease at this stage is inactive, the encapsulated necrotic areas contain viable organisms and are a potential focus for reactivation in later life.[1] Latent TB (LTB) or latent TB infection (LTBI) means that, even though a patient is infected with *M. tuberculosis*, that the patient does not have active TB (imaging study is normal or seen as scar with dense or calcific lesion); LTBI is not contagious.

During the early stage of infection, organisms commonly spread via lymphatic channels to regional hilar and mediastinal lymph nodes and via the bloodstream to more distant sites in the body. The combination of the Ghon focus and affected lymph nodes is known as the Ranke complex.[1] The course of the disease in lymph nodes is similar to that in the parenchyma, consisting initially of granulomatous inflammation and necrosis followed by fibrosis and calcification. However, the inflammatory reaction is usually much greater in lymph nodes, resulting in lymph node enlargement. Hematogenous dissemination in primary TB is probably common but seldom results in miliary disease.[1]

The initial infection is usually clinically silent. Development of specific immunity is usually adequate to limit further multiplication of the bacilli.[10] Some of the bacilli remain dormant and viable for many years. This condition, known as LTBI, may be detectable only by means of a positive purified protein derivative tuberculin skin test or immunoglobulin-γ release assay, or by the presence of radiologically identifiable calcification at the site of the primary lung infection or in regional lymph nodes.[11]

In about 5% of infected individuals immunity is inadequate, and clinically active disease develops within 1 year of infection, a condition known as progressive primary TB.[8] Risk factors for progressive primary disease include immunosuppression (especially HIV infection), extremes of age, or a large inoculation of mycobacteria. In most infected individuals, however, TB remains clinically and microbiologically latent for many years.

In approximately 5% of the infected population (eventually 10%, 5% plus 0.1% per year thereafter), endogenous reactivation of latent infection or reinfection by new strains develops many years after the initial infection.[12] Such postprimary TB frequently is associated with malnutrition, debilitation, or immunosuppression. Pulmonary TB in immunocompetent hosts tends to involve predominantly the apical and posterior segments of the upper lobes and the superior segments of the lower lobes. This localization is likely due to a combination of relatively higher oxygen tension and impaired lymphatic drainage in these regions.[1,11] As distinct from primary TB, in which healing is the rule, postprimary TB tends to progress. The main abnormalities are progressive extension of inflammation and necrosis, frequently with development of communication with the airways and cavity formation.[1] Endobronchial spread of necrotic material from a cavity may result in tuberculous infection in the same or in other lobes. Hematogenous dissemination may result in miliary TB.

New Concept of Manifestations of the Disease

Patients who develop disease after initial exposure are considered to have primary TB. Patients who develop disease as a result of reactivation of a previous focus of TB or reinfection by new strains are considered to have postprimary TB. Traditionally, it was believed that the clinical, pathologic, and radiologic manifestations of postprimary TB were quite distinct from those of primary TB. However, more recent studies based on DNA fingerprinting suggest that the radiographic features are often similar in patients who apparently have primary disease and those who have postprimary TB.[13] In addition, a recent study revealed that the most common radiographic findings in primary pulmonary TB by recent infection in previously healthy adolescents were consolidation, nodules, and cavities in the upper lung, which were thought to be radiographic findings of reactivation pulmonary TB by remote infection[14] (Fig. 10.1). Time from acquisition of infection to development of clinical disease does not reliably predict the radiographic appearance of TB. The only independent predictor of radiographic appearance is integrity of the host immune response.[13] Patients with normal response tend to show parenchymal granulomatous inflammation with slowly progressive nodularity and cavitation, whereas patients with immunodeficiency tend to develop lymphadenopathy, lower lobe parenchymal consolidation, miliary dissemination, and pleural effusion. Therefore the traditional concept of differences in imaging findings between primary and postprimary TB should be changed, and new radiologic classifications by lesion sites—namely, parenchymal, lymph node, airway, and pleural TB—are proposed in this textbook.

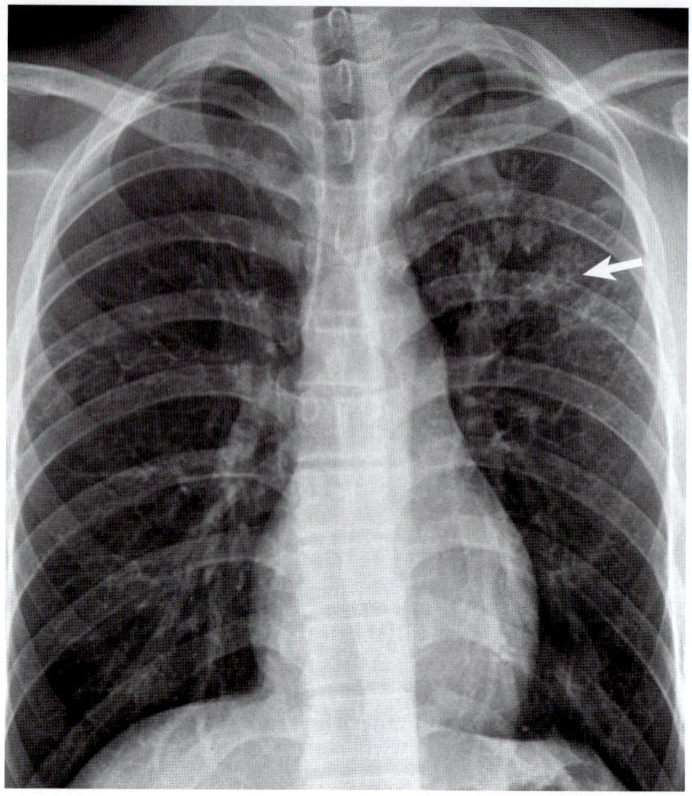

Fig. 10.1 Primary pulmonary tuberculosis by recent infection in an 18-year-old boy with typical radiographic findings. Chest radiograph shows a cavitary nodule *(arrow)* with multiple small nodules and patchy consolidation in left upper lung zone.

KEY POINTS: PULMONARY TUBERCULOSIS

- Conditions associated with increased risk of tuberculosis
  - Old age (>70 years), malnutrition, cancer, immunosuppressive therapy, HIV infection, end-stage renal disease, and diabetes
- Characteristic manifestations
  - Granulomatous inflammation—that is, necrotic focus with surrounding epithelioid histiocytes and multinucleated giant cells
- Primary infection
  - Initial parenchymal lesion (Ghon focus) and lymph node inflammation (Ranke complex), usually heal but remain as a dormant infection (latent tuberculosis infection)
- Postprimary tuberculosis
  - Eventually, 10% of patients with primary infection develop reactivation or reinfection by new strains.
- New concept
  - The only independent predictor of radiographic appearance of tuberculous lung infection is integrity of the host immune response, not time from acquisition of infection to development of clinical disease.

RADIOGRAPHIC FINDINGS

The typical radiographic manifestation of parenchymal TB in immunocompetent hosts consists of focal or patchy heterogeneous consolidation involving the apical and posterior segments of the upper lobes and the superior segments of the lower lobes (Fig. 10.2; see Fig. 10.1).[15,16] Another common finding is the presence of poorly defined nodules and linear opacities (fibronodular pattern of TB). In one review of the radiographic features of 158 patients with postprimary TB, approximately 55% presented with consolidation, 25% with a fibronodular pattern, and 5% with a mixed pattern.[16] Single or multiple cavities

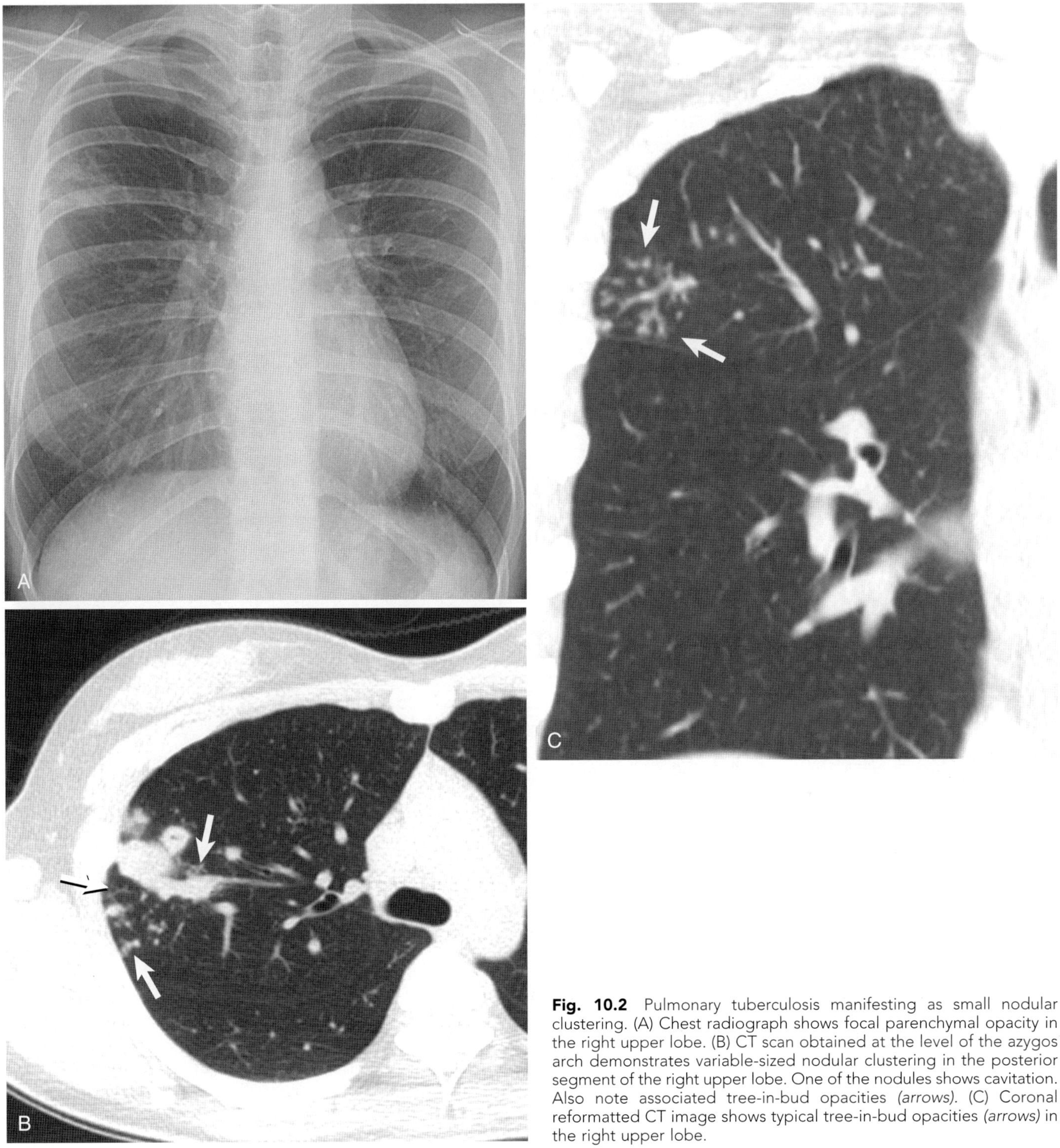

Fig. 10.2 Pulmonary tuberculosis manifesting as small nodular clustering. (A) Chest radiograph shows focal parenchymal opacity in the right upper lobe. (B) CT scan obtained at the level of the azygos arch demonstrates variable-sized nodular clustering in the posterior segment of the right upper lobe. One of the nodules shows cavitation. Also note associated tree-in-bud opacities *(arrows)*. (C) Coronal reformatted CT image shows typical tree-in-bud opacities *(arrows)* in the right upper lobe.

are evident radiographically in 20% to 45% of patients[15–17] (Figs. 10.3 and 10.4). Air-fluid levels are seen in 10% to 20% of tuberculous cavities.[16,17] In approximately 85% of patients the cavities involve the apical or posterior segments of the upper lobes and, in approximately 10%, the superior segments of the lower lobes.[15] Endobronchial spread, manifested as 4- to 10-mm-diameter nodules distant from the site of the cavity, is evident radiographically in 10% to 20% of cases[16,18] (see Fig. 10.3).

In approximately 5% of patients with postprimary TB, the main manifestation is a tuberculoma, defined as a sharply marginated round or oval lesion measuring 0.5 to 4.0 cm in diameter (Fig. 10.5).[16,17] Histologically, the central part of the tuberculoma consists of caseous material and the periphery of epithelioid histiocytes and multinucleated giant cells and a variable amount of collagen. Tuberculomas usually occur in the upper lobes; approximately 80% are single and 20% are multiple. Satellite

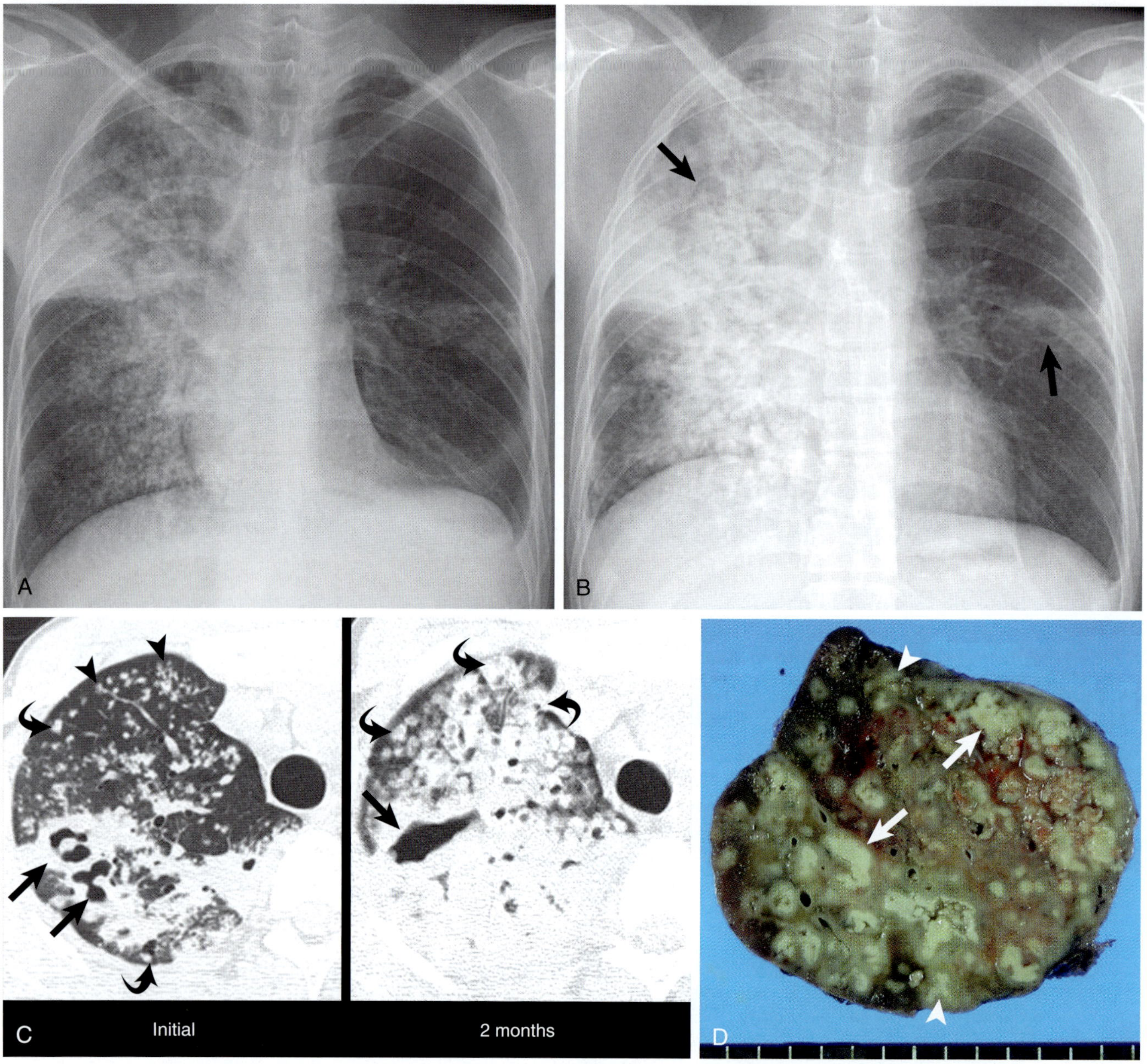

Fig. 10.3 Cavitary multidrug-resistant pulmonary tuberculosis demonstrating progressive disease over 2 months. (A) Initial chest radiograph shows patchy opacities and extensive small nodular clustering in both lungs. Also note segmental consolidation in the right upper lobe and a small left pleural effusion. (B) Follow-up radiograph obtained 2 months later shows increased extent of disease with main pattern of airspace consolidation in both lungs. Also note cavitating lesions *(arrows)*. (C) Composite image with CT scan obtained at the time of initial presentation and the first chest radiograph *(left image)*, and 2 months later at the same time as the second chest radiograph *(right image)* shows progressive right upper lobe cavitating *(arrows)* and noncavitating consolidation, tree-in-bud opacities *(arrowheads)*, and variable-sized nodular lesions *(curved arrows)*. (D) Photomicrography of right pneumonectomy pathologic specimen demonstrates abscess *(arrows)* containing yellowish creamy necrotic materials, nodules, small nodules of centrilobular location, and nodular branching lesions *(arrowheads)*. Branching means that lesions are airway centered.

nodules histologically identical to the larger focus of disease and measuring 1 to 5 mm in diameter are present in most cases (see Fig. 10.5).

In immunocompromised hosts, pulmonary TB manifests as miliary TB, hilar or mediastinal lymphadenopathy, and pleural effusion. Hilar or mediastinal lymphadenopathy is uncommon in postprimary TB, being seen in approximately 5% to 10% of patients.[16,17] Pleural effusion, typically unilateral, occurs in 15% to 20% of patients.[19] Although pleural effusion is usually associated with parenchymal abnormalities (Fig. 10.6), it may be the only radiologic manifestation of TB (Fig. 10.7). Pleural effusion can be caused by rupture of a tuberculous cavity into the pleural space. This may result in the formation of tuberculous empyema and, occasionally, a bronchopleural fistula with pleural air-fluid level.[20]

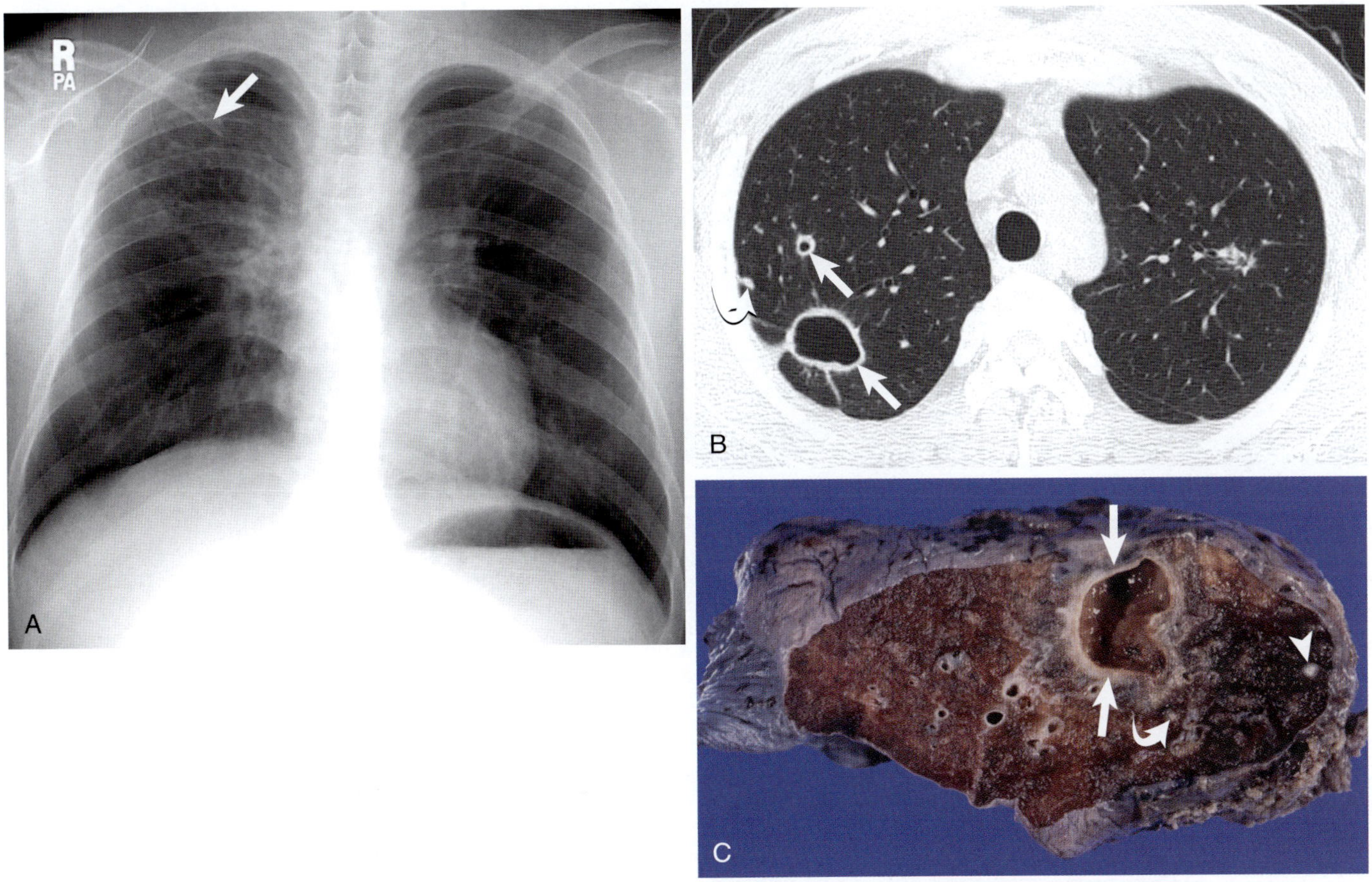

Fig. 10.4 Cavitary multidrug-resistant pulmonary tuberculosis. (A) Chest radiograph shows nodular and cavitary *(arrow)* lesions in both lungs. (B) CT scan obtained at the level of the aortic arch demonstrates thin-walled cavitary lesions *(arrows)* and small centrilobular nodules *(curved arrows)*. Images of the lower lobes (not shown) demonstrated tree-in-bud opacities indicating endobronchial spread of infection. (C) Sagittal section of a right upper lobectomy pathologic specimen demonstrates a cavity *(arrows)* and calcified *(arrowhead)* and noncalcified *(curved arrow)* small nodules in right upper lobe.

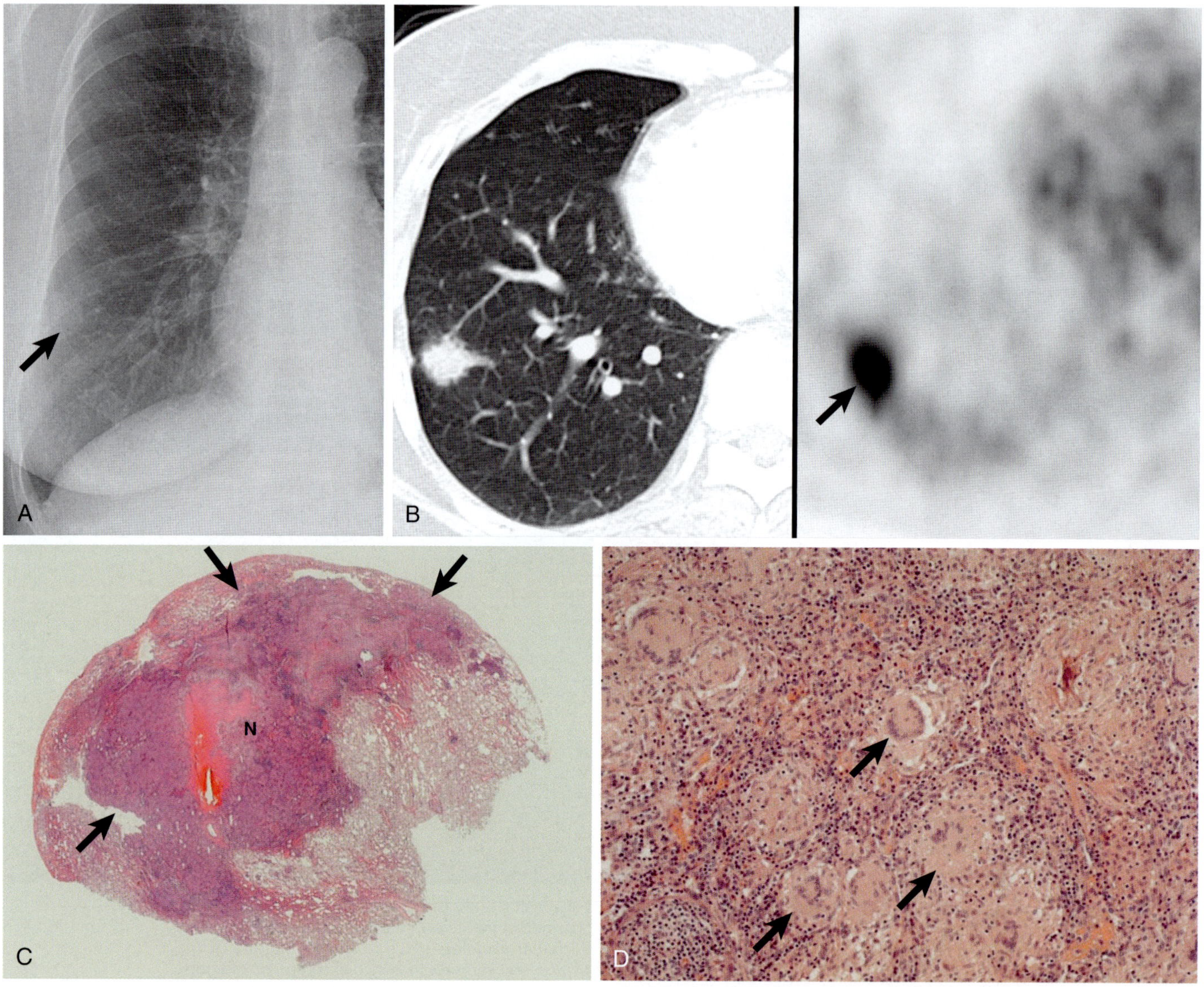

Fig. 10.5 Tuberculoma. (A) Chest radiograph shows a poorly defined nodule *(arrow)* in the right lower lung zone. (B) Composite image with CT scan obtained at the level of the basal segmental bronchi *(left image)*, and a ^{18}F-fluorodeoxyglucose (FDG) positron emission tomography (PET) scan *(right image)* shows an FDG-avid nodule *(arrow)* in the lateral basal segment of the right lower lobe. (C) Photomicrography of a wedge resection pathologic specimen shows a tuberculoma *(arrows)* containing areas of caseation necrosis (N). (D) Magnified view of granulomas demonstrates epithelioid histiocytic infiltration and multinucleated giant cells *(arrows)*.

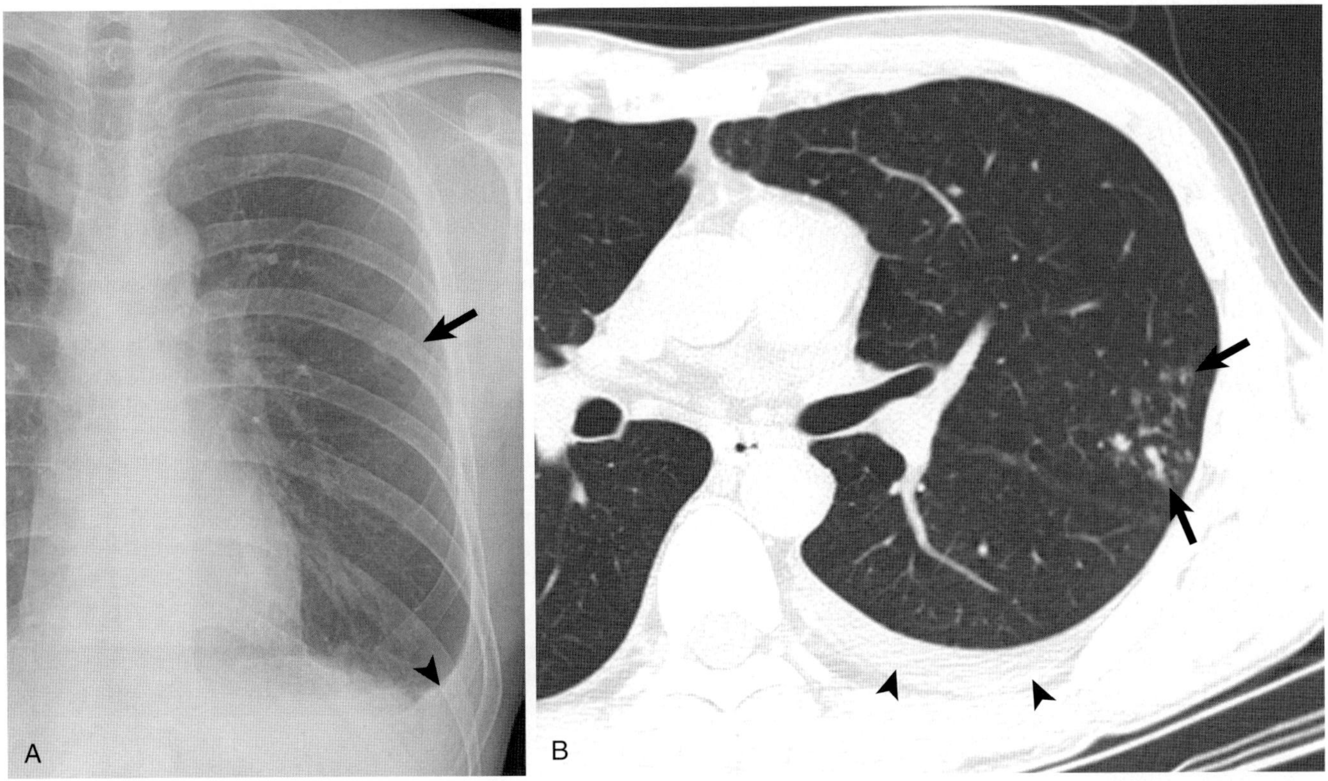

Fig. 10.6 Tuberculous pleurisy and pulmonary tuberculosis. (A) Chest radiograph shows a small left pleural effusion *(arrowhead)* and left middle lung zone nodular densities *(arrow)*. (B) CT scan obtained at the level of the left upper lobar bronchus demonstrates tree-in-bud opacities *(arrows)* in the left upper lobe. Also note the left pleural effusion *(arrowheads)*.

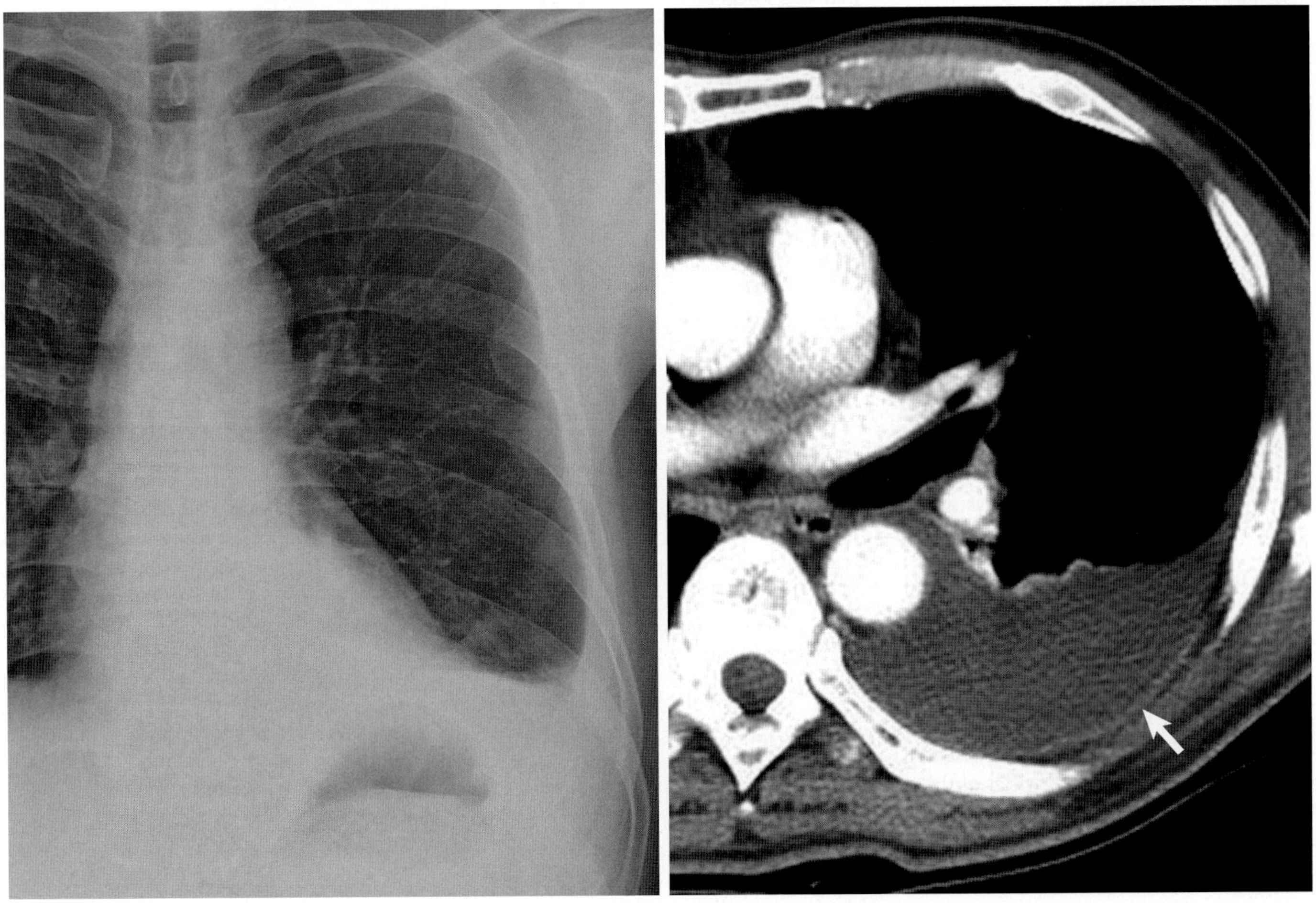

Fig. 10.7 Tuberculous pleurisy. Composite image with chest radiograph *(left image)* and axial CT scan *(right image)* shows a left pleural effusion with homogeneous parietal pleural enhancement *(arrow)*.

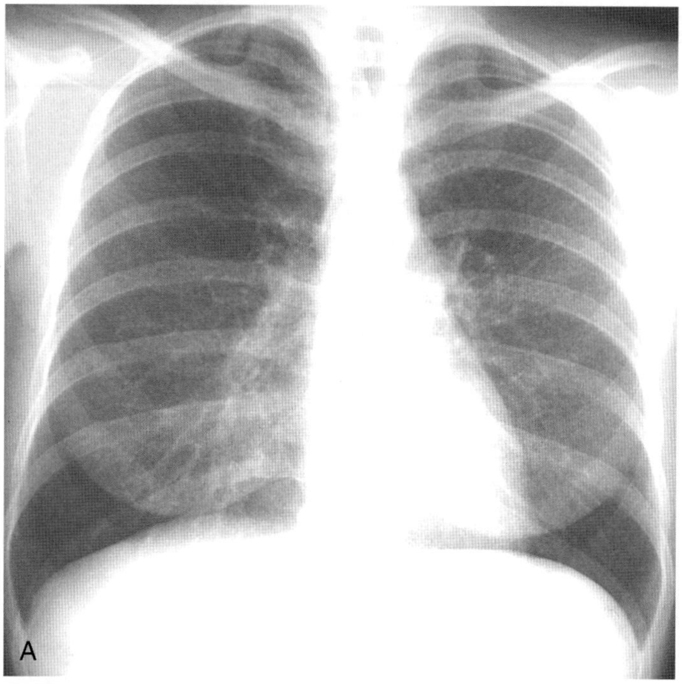

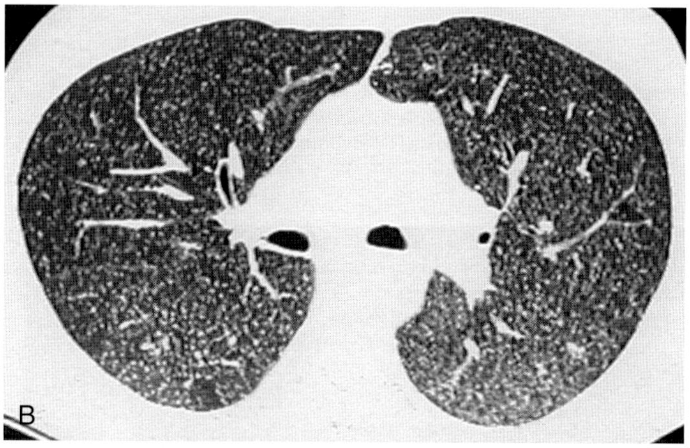

Fig. 10.8 Miliary tuberculosis. (A) Chest radiograph shows numerous 1- to 2-mm-diameter nodules throughout both lungs (miliary pattern). (B) CT scan obtained at the level of the main bronchi demonstrates random distribution of numerous small nodules.

Miliary spread of TB can occur in both primary and recurrent disease[21] (Figs. 10.8 and 10.9). In the latter situation it may be seen in association with typical parenchymal changes as described previously or may be the sole pulmonary abnormality. Each focus of miliary infection results in local granulomas, which when well developed consist of a region of central necrosis surrounded by a relatively well-delimited rim of epithelioid histiocytes and fibrous tissue (see Fig. 10.9).

Pulmonary TB may result in a number of complications and sequelae.[20,22,23] Parenchymal and airway complications include acute respiratory distress syndrome (ARDS),[24–26] extensive lung destruction and cicatrization, multiple cystic lung lesions (Fig. 10.10), aspergilloma, bronchiectasis, tracheobronchial stenosis (Fig. 10.11), and broncholithiasis.[20,23] The radiologic manifestations of ARDS secondary to TB include extensive bilateral ground-glass opacities or consolidation superimposed on findings of miliary or endobronchial spread of TB. Multiple cystic lesions may develop in patients recovering from ARDS or in patients with extensive consolidation resulting from TB.[27] The cystic lesions may resemble pneumatoceles or bullae. They may resolve over several months or persist[27] (see Fig. 10.10).

Vascular complications of pulmonary TB include pulmonary and bronchial arteritis and thrombosis, bronchial artery pseudoaneurysm, and Rasmussen aneurysm (Fig. 10.12).[20] Rasmussen aneurysm is a pseudoaneurysm that results from weakening of the pulmonary artery wall by adjacent cavitary TB. Mediastinal complications include esophagomediastinal or esophagobronchial fistula, constrictive pericarditis (Fig. 10.13), and fibrosing mediastinitis.[20] Pleural complications include tuberculous pleurisy and empyema, empyema necessitatis, fibrothorax, pneumothorax, and bronchopleural fistula.[20,22] Empyema necessitatis (Fig. 10.14) results from leakage of tuberculous empyema through the parietal pleura with discharge of its contents into the subcutaneous tissues of the chest wall or, less commonly, pericardium, vertebral column, or esophagus.[22] The main chest wall complications are tuberculous osteomyelitis and chondritis, tuberculous spondylitis (Fig. 10.15), and empyema necessitatis.[20,22]

KEY POINTS: RADIOGRAPHIC FINDINGS OF PULMONARY TUBERCULOSIS

- Immunocompromised hosts
  - Lymph node enlargement, pleural effusion, miliary dissemination, lower lobe consolidation
- Immunocompetent hosts
  - Focal or patchy consolidation in apical and posterior segments of upper lobes and superior segments of lower lobes
  - Cavitation (20%–45%)
  - Small nodules away from primary lesion (20%–25%)

MULTIDETECTOR OR HIGH-RESOLUTION COMPUTED TOMOGRAPHY

The most common CT findings of parenchymal pulmonary TB are centrilobular nodules and branching linear and nodular opacities (tree-in-bud pattern), patchy or lobular areas of consolidation, and cavitation (see Figs. 10.2 to 10.4).[28–30] The centrilobular nodules and tree-in-bud pattern are due to the presence of caseation necrosis and granulomatous inflammation filling and surrounding terminal and respiratory bronchioles and alveolar ducts.[29,31] Clusters of small nodules or tree-in-bud pattern may result in localized CT galaxy sign(s) on thin-section CT[32] (Fig. 10.16). Multilobar and widespread involvement of small centrilobular nodules and tree-in-bud opacities reflects the presence of endobronchial spread of TB. Coalescence of small nodules or clustering of small nodules leads to formation of a large nodule (Fig. 10.17). The majority of tuberculous cavities are thick walled, but thin-walled cavities are also common, particularly in patients undergoing treatment.

According to a report[30] in which CT findings were assessed in 29 patients with newly diagnosed pulmonary TB and 12 patients with recent reactivation, the most common abnormality on CT was the presence of 2- to 4-mm-diameter centrilobular nodules and/or branching linear structures (tree-in-bud pattern) seen in 95% of patients. Other common findings included cavitary nodules (69% of patients), lobular consolidation (52% of patients), interlobular septal thickening (34% of patients), and

Text continued on p. 233

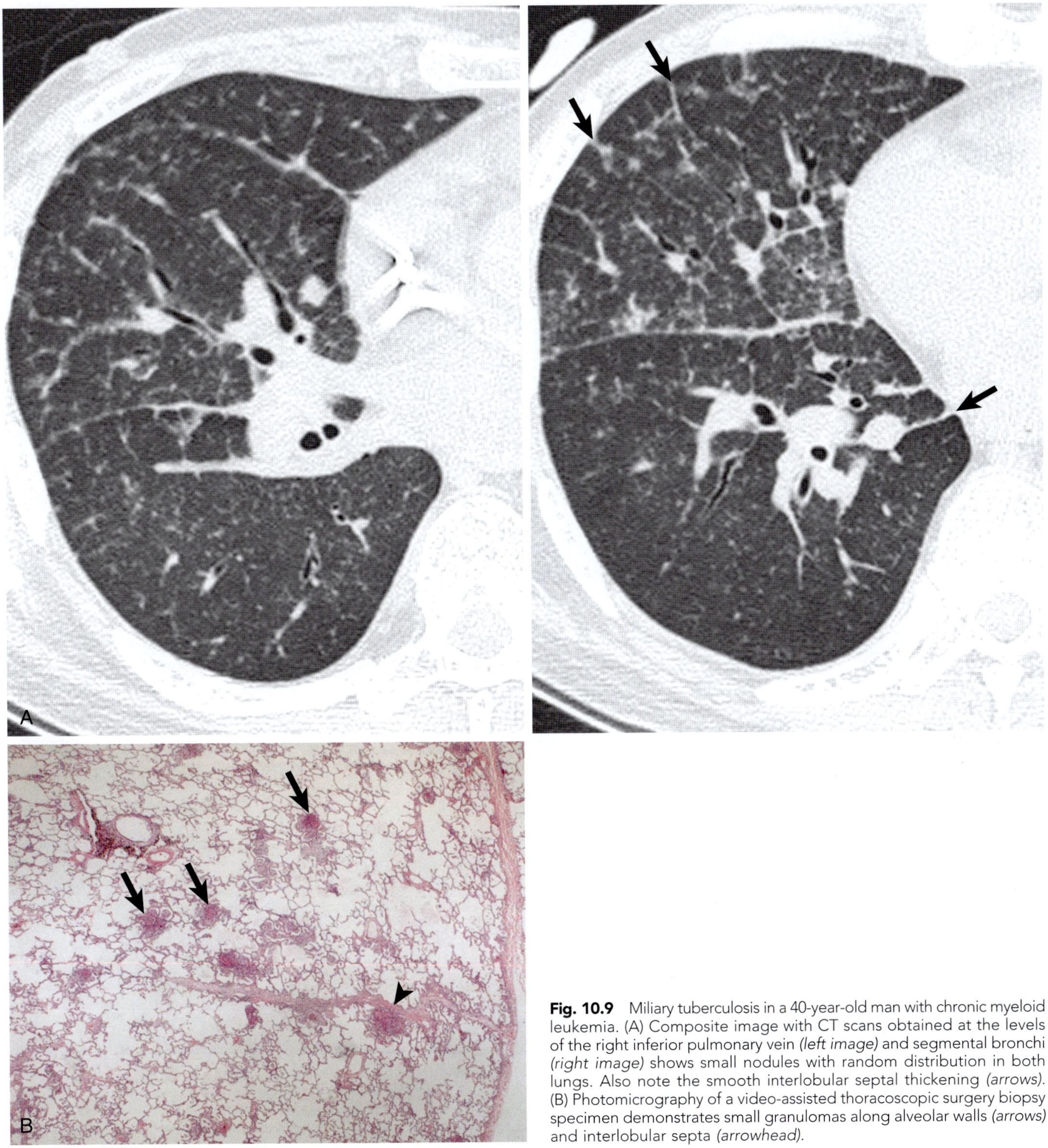

Fig. 10.9 Miliary tuberculosis in a 40-year-old man with chronic myeloid leukemia. (A) Composite image with CT scans obtained at the levels of the right inferior pulmonary vein *(left image)* and segmental bronchi *(right image)* shows small nodules with random distribution in both lungs. Also note the smooth interlobular septal thickening *(arrows)*. (B) Photomicrography of a video-assisted thoracoscopic surgery biopsy specimen demonstrates small granulomas along alveolar walls *(arrows)* and interlobular septa *(arrowhead)*.

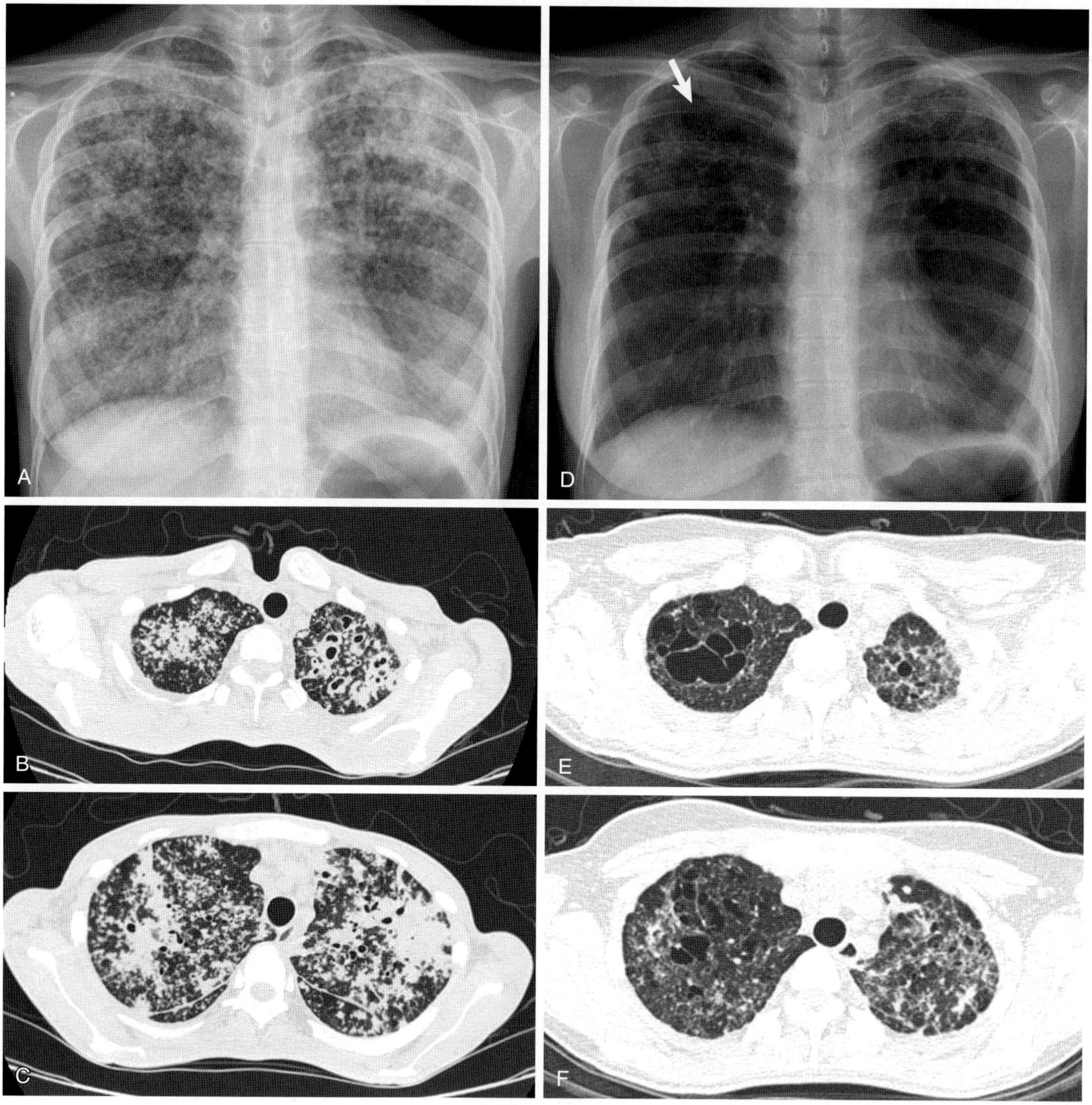

Fig. 10.10 Pulmonary tuberculosis manifesting as extensive parenchymal consolidation and subsequently as cystic lung disease. (A) Initial chest radiograph shows multiple nodules in both lungs with airspace consolidation in both upper lobes. Note small left pleural effusion. (B) and (C) Initial CT scans obtained at the levels of the sternal notch (B) and manubrium (C) show upper lobe centrilobular nodules, tree-in-bud opacities, cavitary nodules, and airspace consolidation. (D) A follow-up chest radiograph obtained 4 months after (A) with antituberculous therapy demonstrates a decreased extent of parenchymal opacities in both lungs but new cystic lesions *(arrow)* in the right upper lung zone. (E) and (F) Follow-up CT scans obtained at the same levels of (B) and (C) and at the same time as (D) show multiple cystic lesions in the right upper lobe. The extent of airspace consolidation and centrilobular nodules decreased.

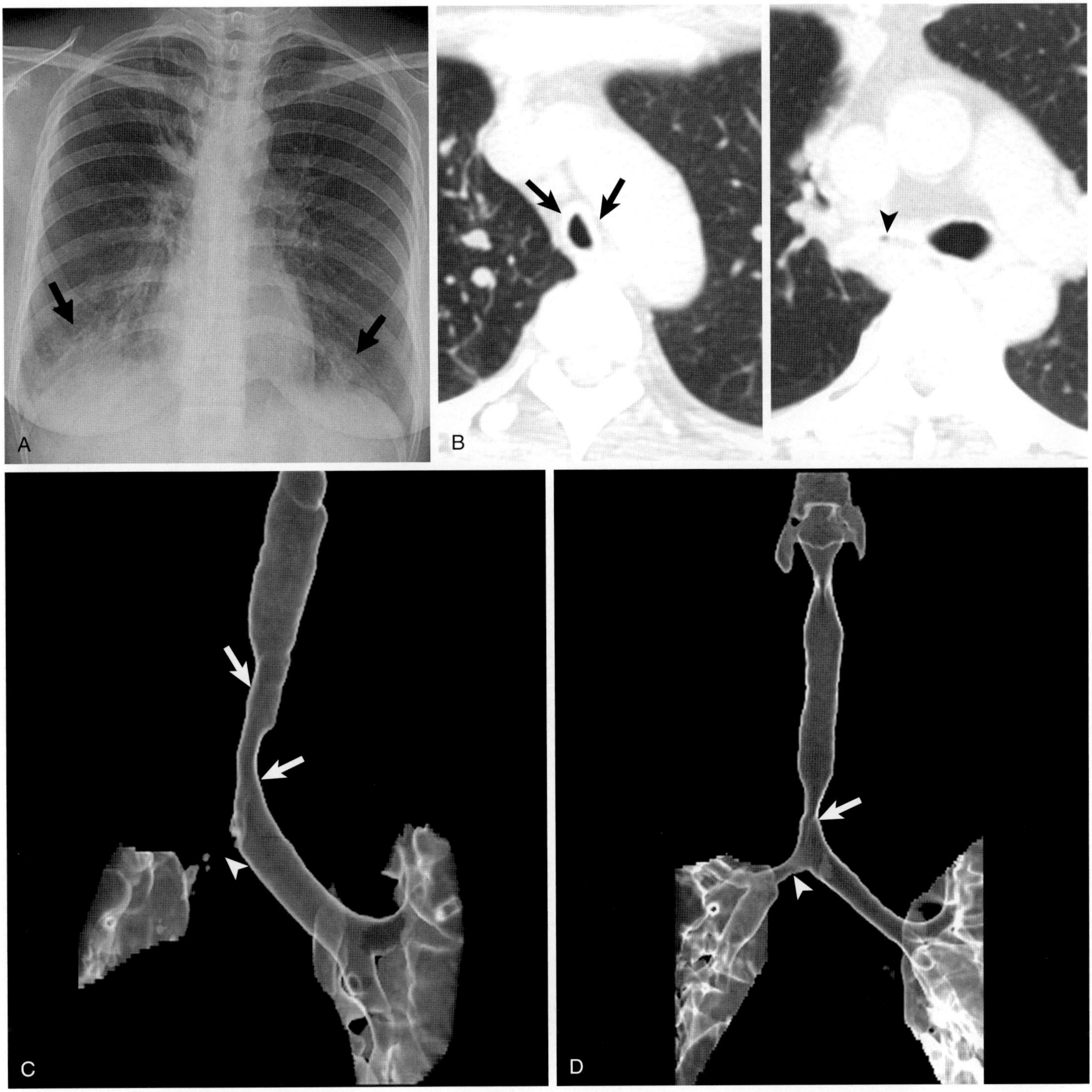

Fig. 10.11 Serial follow-up of bronchial tuberculosis in a 31-year-old woman. (A) Initial chest radiograph shows right upper lobe volume loss and bilateral lower lung zone parenchymal opacities *(arrows)*. (B) Composite image with CT scans obtained at the levels of the aortic arch *(left image)* and main bronchi *(right image)* demonstrates luminal narrowing and wall thickening in the distal trachea *(arrows)* and nearly completely obliterated right main bronchus lumen *(arrowhead)* with marked wall thickening. (C) Volume-rendering image shows luminal narrowing of the intrathoracic trachea *(arrows)* and obliterated lumen of the right main bronchus *(arrowhead)*. (D) Volume-rendering image of a 6-month follow-up CT study with antituberculous chemotherapy demonstrates improvement of airway disease with reconstitution of the right main bronchus. However, findings of smooth luminal narrowing in the distal trachea *(arrow)* and right main bronchus *(arrowhead)* (fibrotic stage of airway tuberculosis) remain.

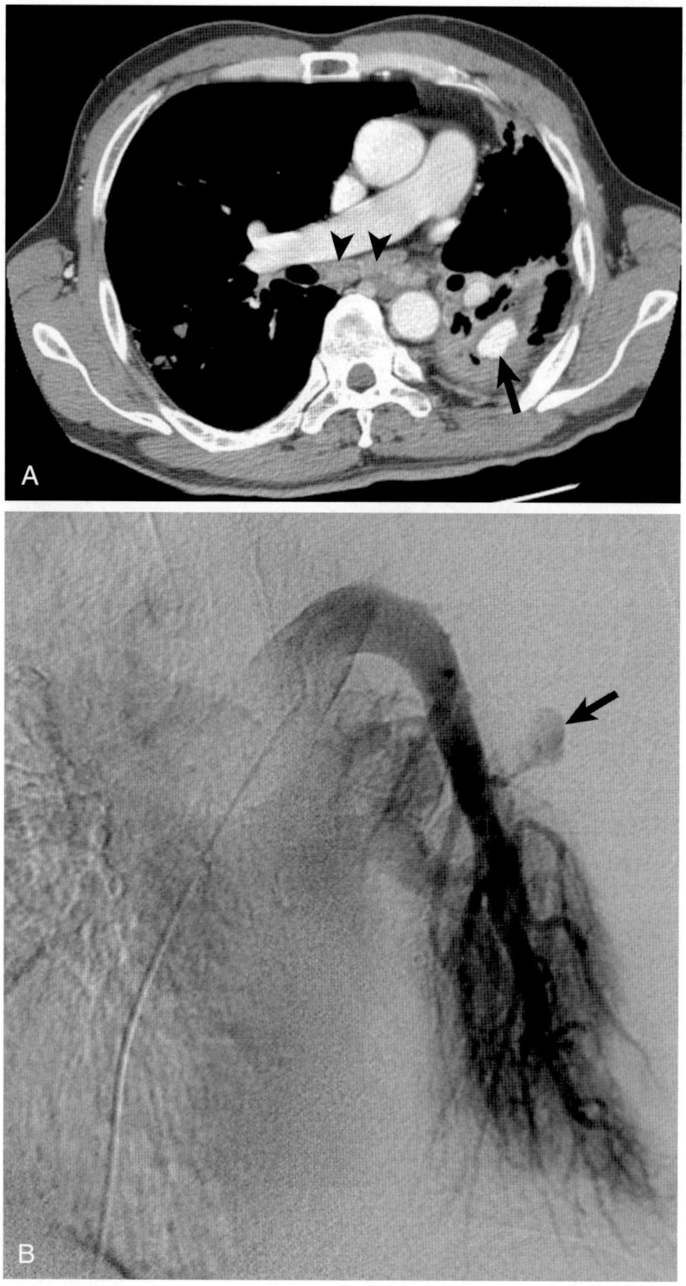

Fig. 10.12 Rasmussen aneurysm in chronic destructive pulmonary tuberculosis. (A) Contrast-enhanced CT image obtained at the level of the bronchus intermedius shows a contrast-filling aneurysm *(arrow)* within parenchymal consolidation in the superior segment of the left lower lobe. Also note the enlarged lymph nodes *(arrowheads)* in the subcarinal station. (B) Nonselective left pulmonary angiography shows a contrast-filling aneurysm *(arrow)* from a branch of the left pulmonary artery.

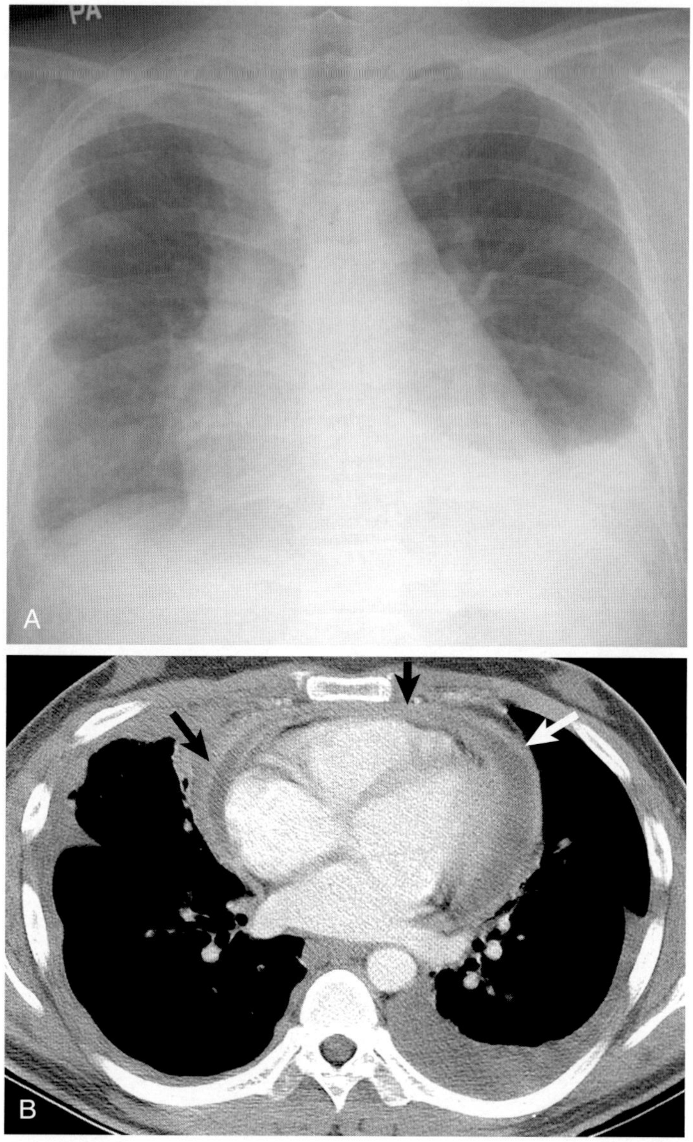

Fig. 10.13 Tuberculous constrictive pericarditis. (A) Chest radiograph shows cardiomegaly and bilateral pleural thickening/effusions. (B) CT scan obtained at the left atrial level shows pericardial effusion and bilateral pleural effusions. Also note the markedly enhancing and thickened parietal pericardium *(arrows)*.

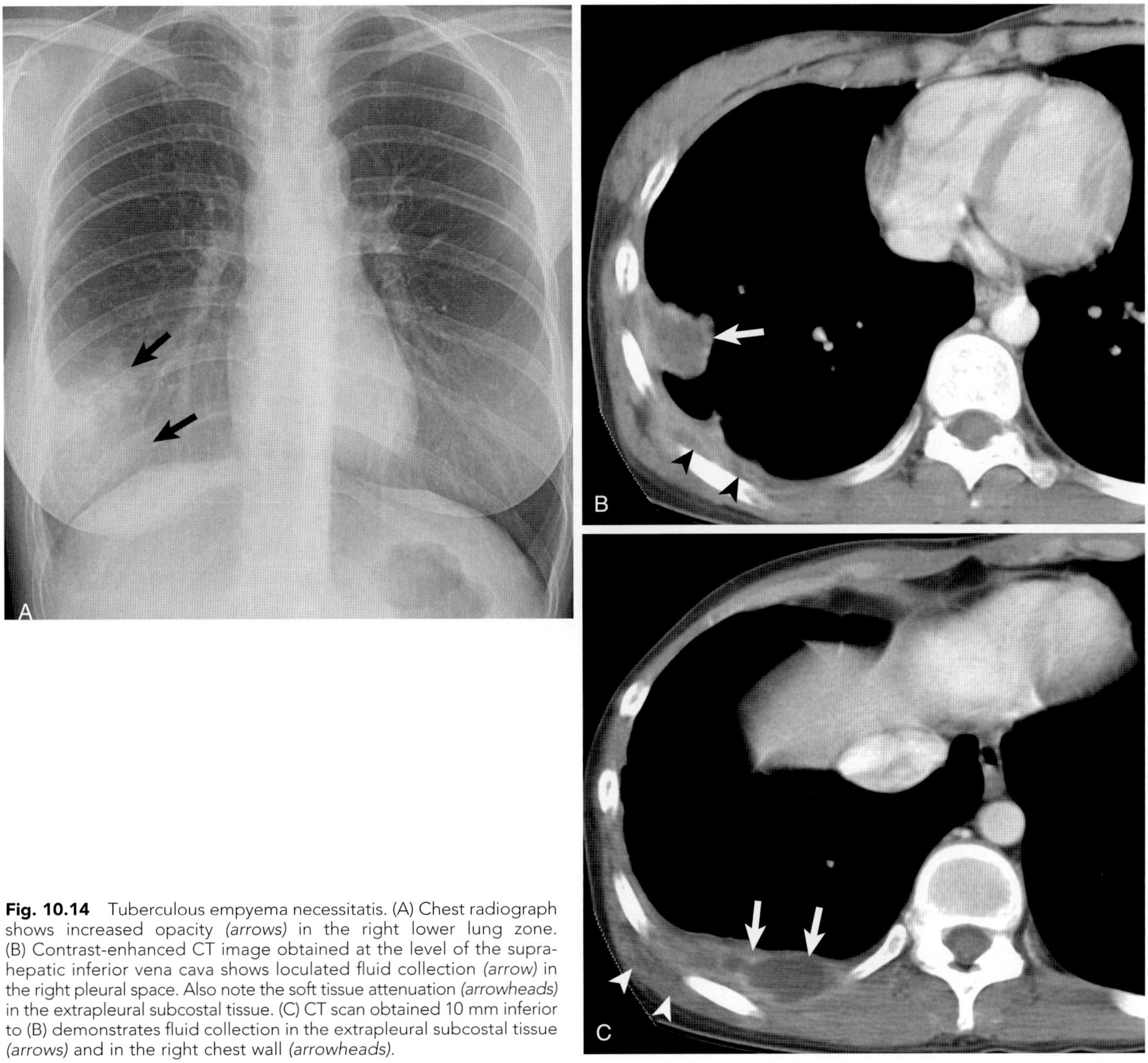

Fig. 10.14 Tuberculous empyema necessitatis. (A) Chest radiograph shows increased opacity *(arrows)* in the right lower lung zone. (B) Contrast-enhanced CT image obtained at the level of the suprahepatic inferior vena cava shows loculated fluid collection *(arrow)* in the right pleural space. Also note the soft tissue attenuation *(arrowheads)* in the extrapleural subcostal tissue. (C) CT scan obtained 10 mm inferior to (B) demonstrates fluid collection in the extrapleural subcostal tissue *(arrows)* and in the right chest wall *(arrowheads)*.

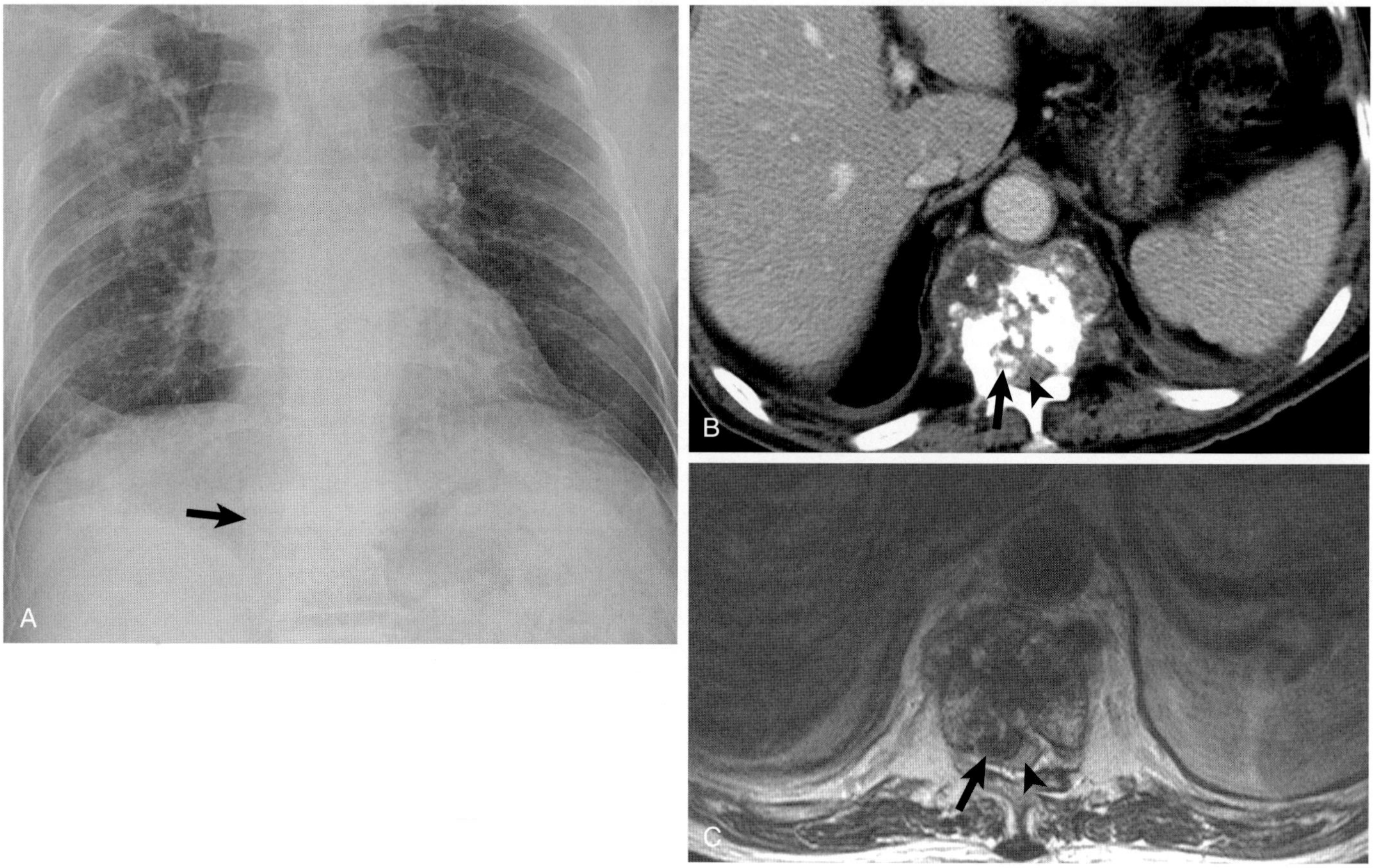

Fig. 10.15 Tuberculous spondylitis. (A) Chest radiograph shows patchy distribution of small nodular and tubular densities in both lungs. Also note the laterally displaced right paraspinal interface *(arrow)*. (B) Contrast-enhanced CT scan obtained at the level of the liver caudate lobe shows a calcified, heterogeneous, and low-attenuation soft tissue lesion in the paraspinal region, bilaterally. Note the vertebral body osseous destruction and intraspinal extension *(arrow)* of the soft tissue lesion with cord compression *(arrowhead)*. (C) T2-weighted MR image obtained at a similar level to (B) demonstrates intraspinal extension of the lesion *(arrow)* with cord compression *(arrowhead)*.

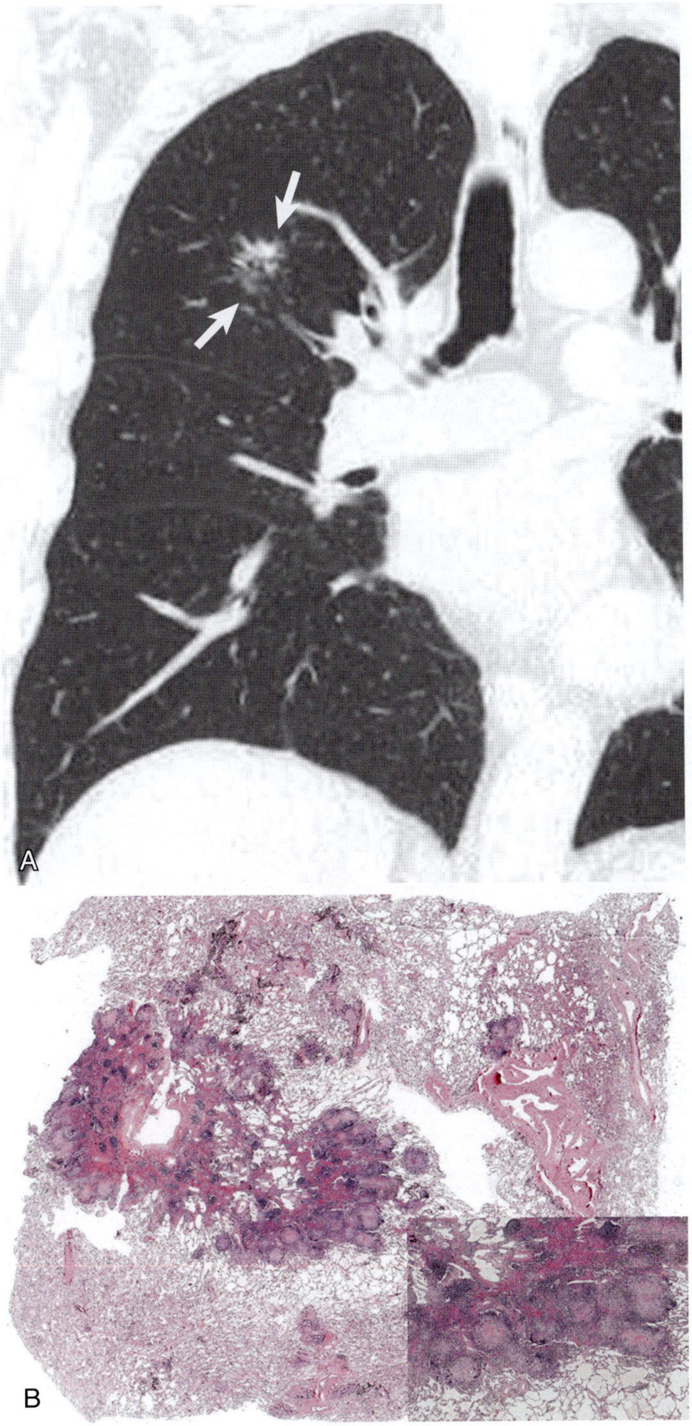

Fig. 10.16 Active pulmonary tuberculosis manifesting the CT galaxy sign. (A) Coronal CT image depicts the galaxy sign *(arrows)* in the right upper lobe with a larger nodule and smaller peripheral nodules. (B) Low-magnification photomicrograph shows aggregation of small granulomas, which forms the galaxy sign on the CT scan. Inset: multiple TB granulomas on high-magnification photomicrograph.

bronchovascular distortion (17% of patients). Findings of endobronchial spread of TB were often present in the absence of cavitation. In 11 of 12 patients with recent reactivation TB, CT clearly differentiated old fibrotic lesions from new active lesions by demonstrating centrilobular nodules or a tree-in-bud

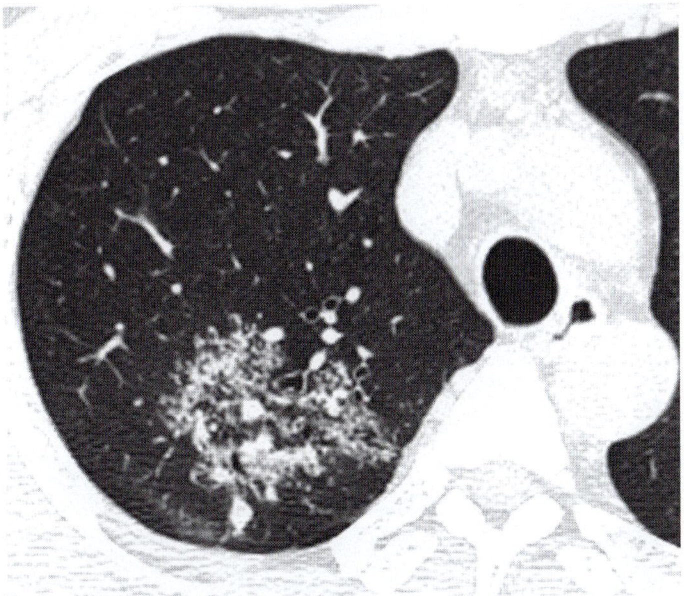

Fig. 10.17 Pulmonary tuberculosis showing coalescence of small nodules and tree-in-bud opacities. CT scan obtained at the level of the aortic arch shows a parenchymal lesion composed of coalescence of tree-in-bud opacities, suggestive of active pulmonary tuberculosis.

pattern. Patients having follow-up high-resolution CT during treatment showed a gradual decrease in lobular consolidation. Most of centrilobular nodular and branching opacities disappeared within 5 months after the start of treatment. On the other hand, bronchovascular distortion, fibrosis, emphysema and bronchiectasis increased on follow-up scans.[30]

Hatipoglu and coworkers[33] compared the high-resolution CT findings in 32 patients who had newly diagnosed active pulmonary TB and 34 patients who had inactive disease. Findings seen only in patients who had active TB included centrilobular nodules (91% of patients), tree-in-bud pattern (71% of patients), nodules 5 to 8 mm in diameter (69% of patients), and consolidation (44% of patients). Cavitation was present in 50% of patients who had active TB and 12% of patients who had inactive disease.[33] Poey coworkers[34] performed high-resolution CT before and after 6 months of antituberculosis treatment in 27 patients with postprimary pulmonary TB. Centrilobular nodules and poorly marginated nodules were present only before treatment. Reticular pattern (intralobular and septal thickening) and fibrosis were seen both before and after treatment.[34]

Tuberculomas are most commonly smoothly marginated on CT (Fig. 10.18); however, fibrosis related to vessels, interlobular septa or lung parenchyma adjacent to the nodule may result in a spiculated margin.[13,28,35] Calcification within the nodule or satellite nodules around the periphery of the dominant nodule is present in 20% to 30% of cases (see Fig. 10.5). Cavitation within the dominant nodule or the surrounding satellite nodules may be also seen. After intravenous administration of contrast, tuberculomas often show no enhancement or ring-like or curvilinear enhancement on CT (see Fig. 10.18). The latter corresponds histologically to the fibrous tissue/granulomatous inflammatory tissue capsule, whereas the nonenhancing area corresponds to the central necrotic material (see Fig. 10.18).[35]

In miliary TB the characteristic high-resolution CT findings consist of 1- to 3-mm-diameter nodules randomly distributed

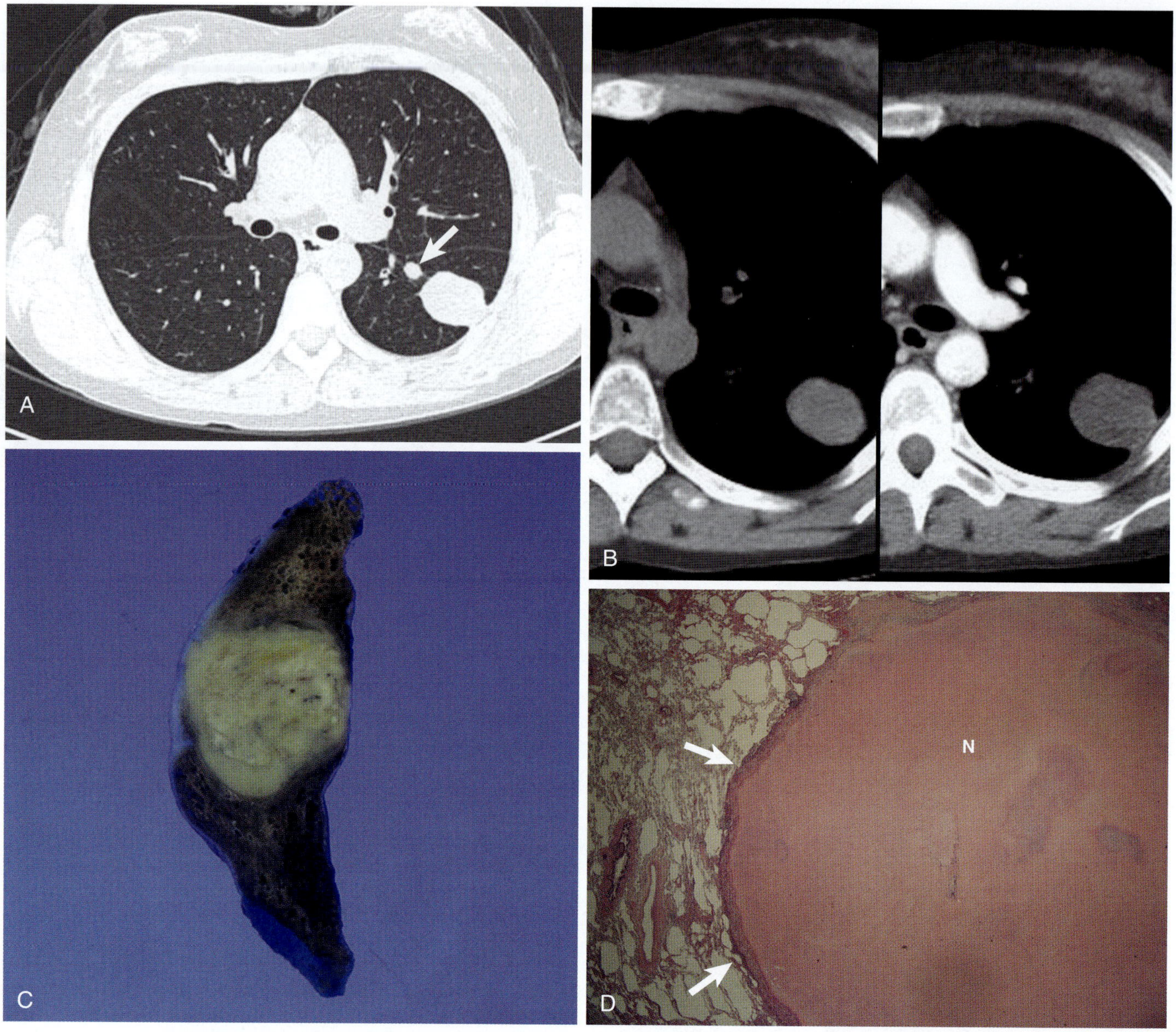

Fig. 10.18 Tuberculoma. (A) CT scan obtained at the level of the right bronchus intermedius shows a well-margined mass with a satellite nodule *(arrow)* in the left lower lobe. (B) Composite image with nonenhanced *(left image)* and contrast-enhanced *(right image)* CT scans demonstrates this mass does not show any enhancement. (C) Photography of a wedge resection pathologic specimen shows a mass containing a granular and cheese-like substance. (D) Photomicrograph (hematoxylin and eosin, ×12.5) of a wedge resection pathologic specimen shows a tuberculoma *(arrows)* containing areas of caseation necrosis (N).

throughout both lungs (see Figs. 10.8 and 10.9).[21,36] Thickening of interlobular septa and fine intralobular linear opacities are frequently evident.[30]

Hilar and mediastinal lymph node enlargement is commonly seen on CT in patients who have active TB.[37,38] In the study by Im and coworkers,[30] mediastinal lymph node enlargement was seen on high-resolution CT in 9 of 29 (31%) patients who had newly diagnosed disease and in 2 of 12 (17%) patients who had reactivation. Enlarged lymph nodes in patients with active TB typically showed central areas of low attenuation on contrast-enhanced CT, with peripheral rim enhancement[39] (Fig. 10.19). Moon and coworkers[40] assessed the role of CT in the diagnosis of tuberculous mediastinal lymphadenitis in 37 patients who had active disease and 12 patients who had inactive disease. In the 37 patients who had active disease, mediastinal lymph nodes ranged in size from 1.5 to 6.7 cm (mean, 2.8 ± 1.0 cm), and all had central low-attenuation and peripheral rim enhancement. Foci of calcification were seen within the lymph nodes in 7 patients (19%). In the 12 patients who had inactive disease, the nodes were usually smaller than nodes in patients who had active disease, and they appeared homogeneous without low-attenuation areas. Calcifications within the nodes were seen in 10 of the 12 (83%) patients who had inactive disease. Low-attenuation areas within the lymph nodes in patients who had active TB corresponded pathologically to caseous necrosis. In all 25 patients followed after treatment, enlarged mediastinal

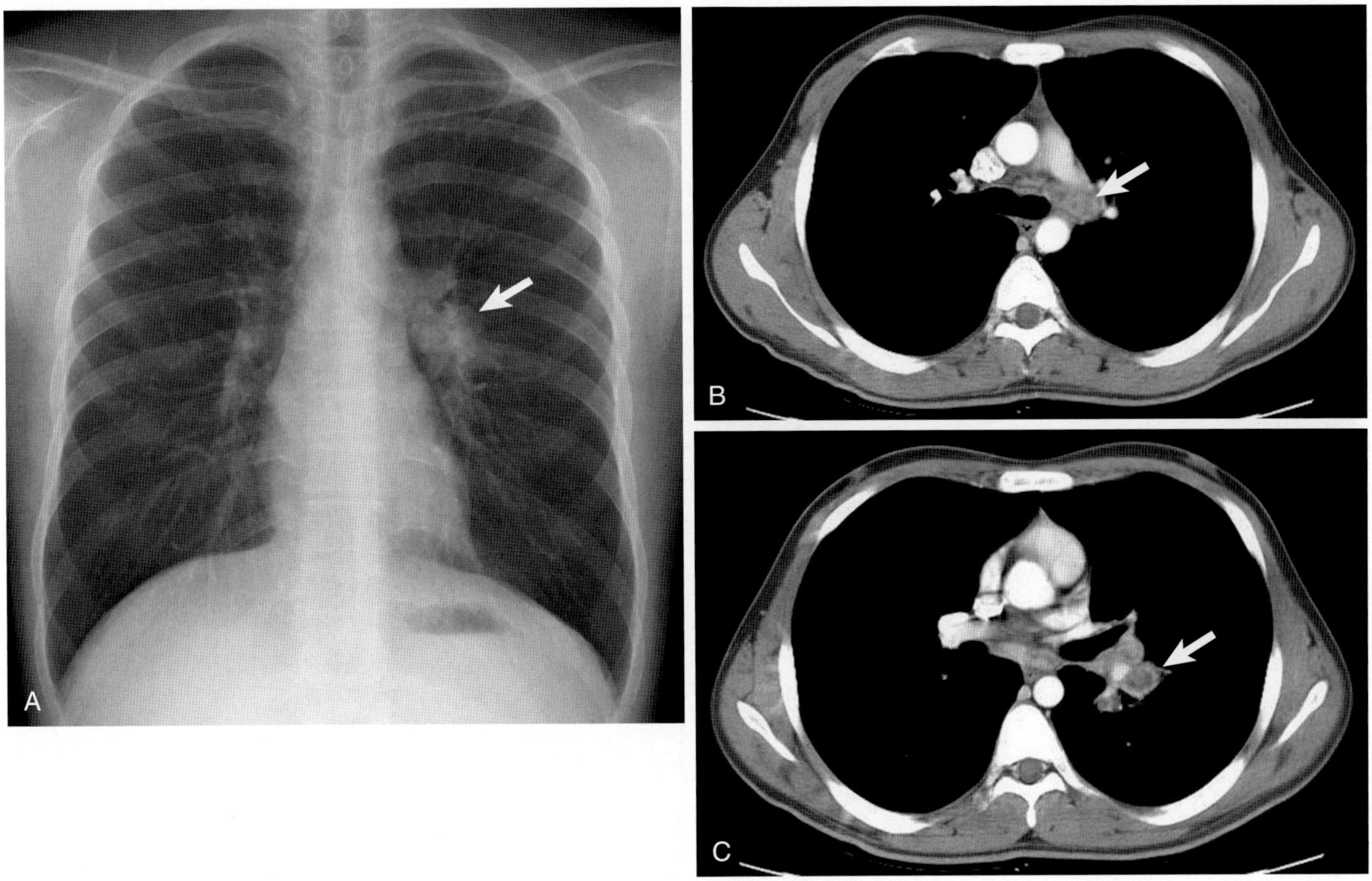

Fig. 10.19 Tuberculous lymphadenitis. (A) Chest radiograph shows a left hilar enlargement *(arrow)*. (B) and (C) CT scans obtained at the levels of the carina (B) and left upper lobar bronchus (C) show enlarged left hilar and peribronchial lymph nodes *(arrows)* with central low attenuation and peripheral rim enhancement.

nodes decreased in size, and low-attenuation areas within the nodes disappeared.[40]

Airway TB has been reported in 10% to 20% of all patients with pulmonary TB.[41] The characteristic CT findings of airway TB are circumferential wall thickening and luminal narrowing, with involvement of a long segment of the bronchi.[41] In active disease the airways are irregularly narrowed and have thick walls, whereas in fibrotic disease the airways are smoothly narrowed and have thin walls (Fig. 10.20).

In tuberculous pleural effusion CT usually shows homogeneous fluid in the pleural space. After contrast administration, pleural layers enhance and are revealed as a smooth thickening of the visceral and parietal pleural surfaces separated by a variable amount of fluid (split pleura sign).[42] New subpleural lung nodules may develop after 3 to 12 weeks after taking medication for TB pleural effusion (Fig. 10.21). It should not be regarded as treatment failure. These paradoxical subpleural nodules will eventually show improvement with continued medication.[43]

The manifestations of TB in acquired immune deficiency syndrome (AIDS) patients are influenced by the degree of immunosuppression and whether or not the patient is receiving HAART.[44] In mildly immunosuppressed (>200 CD4 cells/μL) patients, the radiologic manifestations are similar to those in the normal host, with focal consolidation and nodular opacities involving mainly the upper lobes. Patients with moderate or severe immunosuppression (<200 CD4 cells/μL) have the predominant abnormalities consisting of hilar or mediastinal lymph node enlargement and airspace consolidation. Enlarged hilar or mediastinal nodes are evident on the radiograph in 30% to 60% of patients and on CT in 70% to 90%.[4,44] The enlarged nodes usually show decreased attenuation and often show rim enhancement after intravenous administration of contrast.[44] The TB lymphadenitis in moderate or severe immunosuppression is usually combined with extensive lung parenchymal, extrathoracic lymph node, and extrathoracic organ TB involvement.[45] Markedly immunosuppressed individuals have a greater prevalence of miliary TB or pleural effusion. However, 10% to 20% of severely immunocompromised AIDS patients with TB have normal radiographs.[4,44] In AIDS and TB patients no significant differences in clinical and radiologic manifestations of TB are recorded according to antiretroviral therapy status.[5] However, paradoxical exacerbations of pulmonary and central nervous system TB infection may occur in patients with HAART. This condition is called IRIS and is related to an increase in the CD4 counts and a decrease in the viral loads.[46] Typical imaging findings of IRIS include intrathoracic or cervical lymphadenopathy in 70% of patients, new or increasing parenchymal consolidation, and pleural effusion (Fig. 10.22). Intraabdominal manifestations or tuberculous meningitis may also complicate IRIS. Treatment of this condition includes continuation of antituberculous chemotherapy to decrease the antigenic load, continuation of effective HAART, and judicious use of antiinflammatory agents.[6]

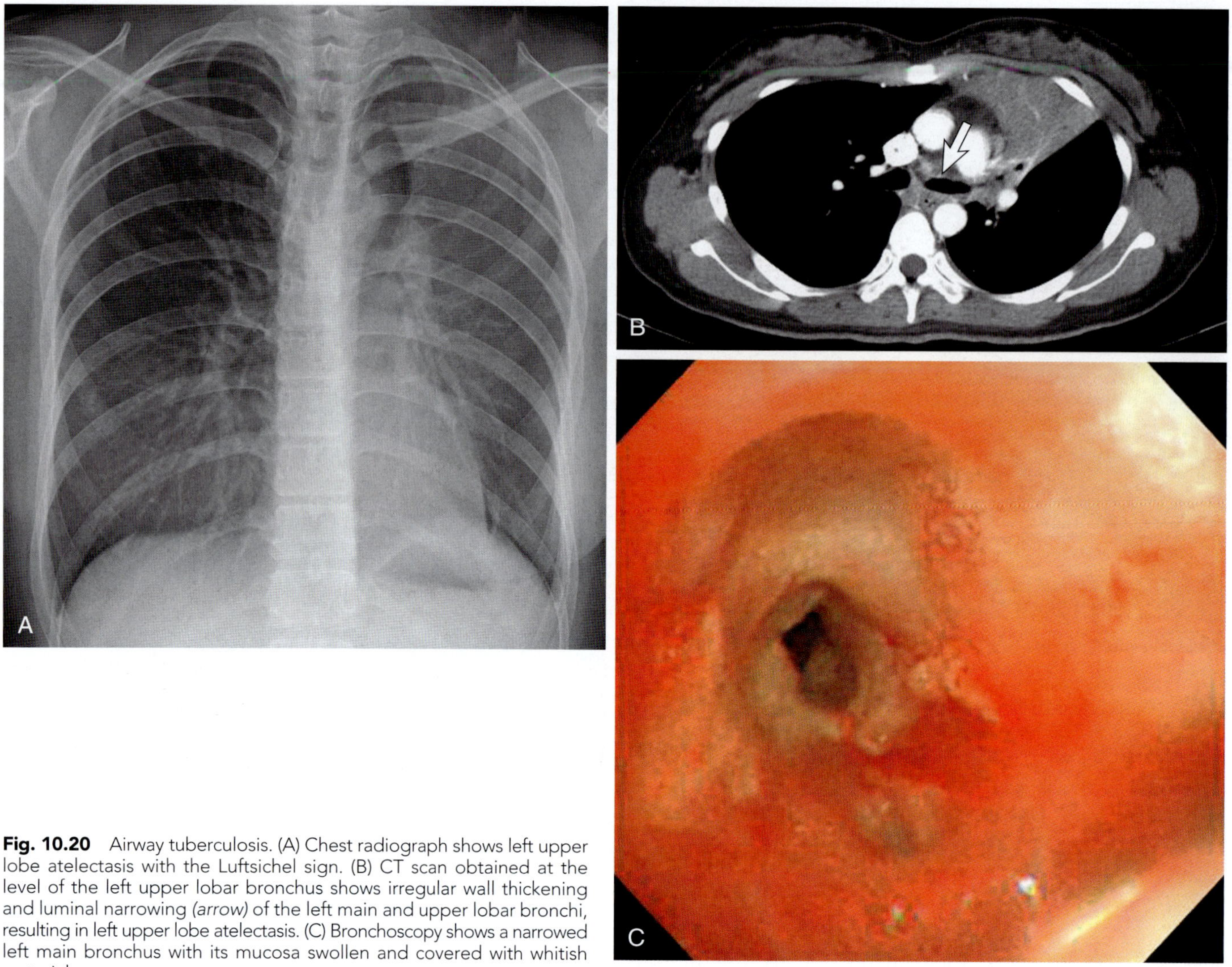

Fig. 10.20 Airway tuberculosis. (A) Chest radiograph shows left upper lobe atelectasis with the Luftsichel sign. (B) CT scan obtained at the level of the left upper lobar bronchus shows irregular wall thickening and luminal narrowing *(arrow)* of the left main and upper lobar bronchi, resulting in left upper lobe atelectasis. (C) Bronchoscopy shows a narrowed left main bronchus with its mucosa swollen and covered with whitish materials.

Multidrug-resistant (MDR) TB is defined as a strain of *M. tuberculosis* resistant to at least isoniazid and rifampin. Extensively drug-resistant (XDR) TB is defined as a strain of *M. tuberculosis* resistant to any type of fluoroquinolone and at least one of the three following injectable drugs: amikacin, capreomycin, or kanamycin, in addition to isoniazid and rifampin. Although the imaging findings of MDR TB are similar to those of drug-sensitive TB, prior studies have shown that bronchiectasis, lung destruction, a calcified granuloma, and cavities are more frequent in MDR TB.[47] In primary MDR TB patients who have no history of treatment or treatment history within 1 month, bilateral involvement, segmental or lobar consolidation, and multiple cavities are more frequent than in acquired MDR TB[48] (Fig. 10.23). Therefore it should be kept in mind that the presence of multiple cavities on CT is suggestive of MDR TB; however, MDR TB can appear as ordinary TB lesions with tree-in-bud pattern, small nodules, or lobular consolidation without a cavity.[49] Imaging findings of XDR TB are similar to those of MDR TB; the extent of consolidation and tree-in-bud opacities is more extensive in XDR TB.[50]

KEY POINTS: COMPUTED TOMOGRAPHY FINDINGS OF PULMONARY TUBERCULOSIS

- Typical parenchymal tuberculosis
  - 2- to 4-mm-diameter centrilobular nodules in apical and posterior segments of upper lobes and superior segments of lower lobes
  - Tree-in-bud opacities (70%–80%)
  - 5- to 10-mm-diameter airspace nodules (60%–70%)
  - Cavitation (60%–70%)
  - Lobular consolidation (50%–60%)
  - Multiple cavitary lesions should raise the possibility of multidrug-resistant TB
- Miliary tuberculosis
  - 1- to 3-mm-diameter nodules randomly distributed throughout both lungs
- Lymph node tuberculosis
  - Central low attenuation with peripheral rim enhancement
- Airway tuberculosis
  - Circumferential wall thickening and luminal narrowing, with involvement of a long segment of bronchi
- Pleural tuberculosis
  - Smooth thickening of visceral and parietal pleural surfaces separated by variable amount of fluid

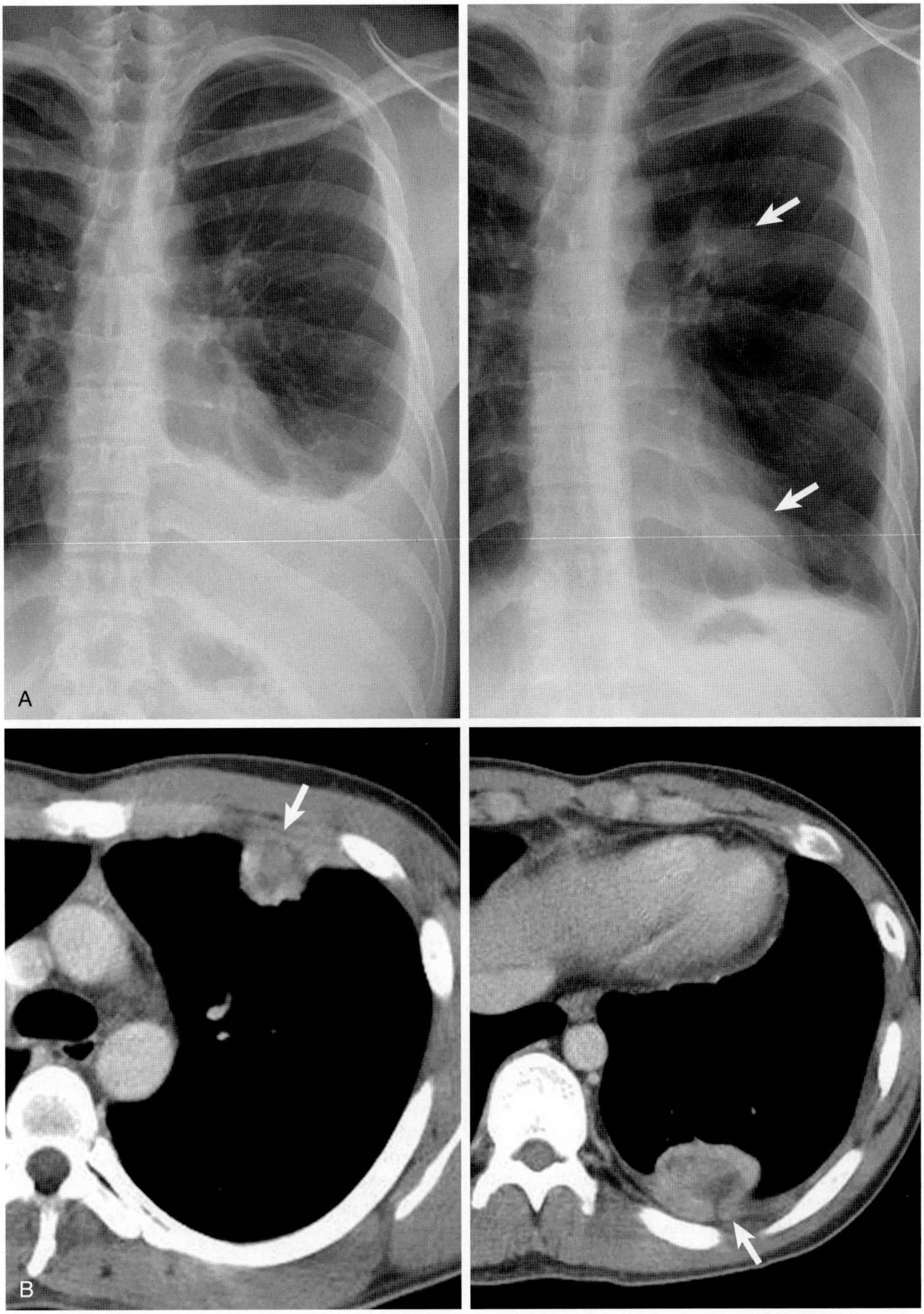

Fig. 10.21 Paradoxical subpleural nodules in tuberculous pleurisy. (A) Composite image with an initial chest radiograph *(left image)* and a chest radiograph obtained 4 months after starting treatment with antituberculous medication *(right image)* shows a decreased amount of left pleural effusion with new pleural nodularity *(arrows)*. (B) Composite image of a CT scan obtained at time of follow-up chest radiograph shows pleural nodules *(arrows)* with peripheral enhancement. These nodules disappeared with continued medication (not shown).

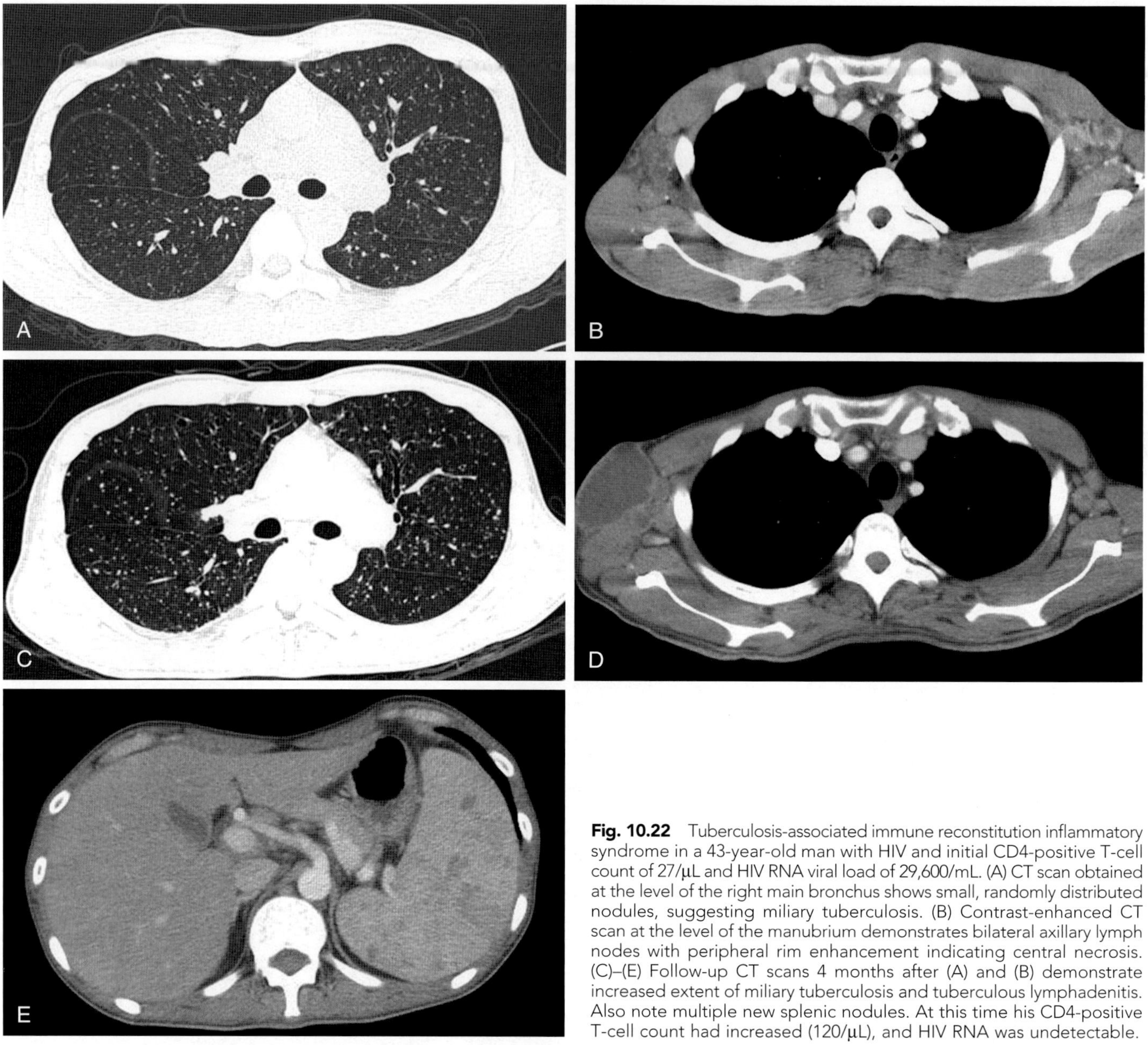

Fig. 10.22 Tuberculosis-associated immune reconstitution inflammatory syndrome in a 43-year-old man with HIV and initial CD4-positive T-cell count of 27/μL and HIV RNA viral load of 29,600/mL. (A) CT scan obtained at the level of the right main bronchus shows small, randomly distributed nodules, suggesting miliary tuberculosis. (B) Contrast-enhanced CT scan at the level of the manubrium demonstrates bilateral axillary lymph nodes with peripheral rim enhancement indicating central necrosis. (C)–(E) Follow-up CT scans 4 months after (A) and (B) demonstrate increased extent of miliary tuberculosis and tuberculous lymphadenitis. Also note multiple new splenic nodules. At this time his CD4-positive T-cell count had increased (120/μL), and HIV RNA was undetectable.

IMAGING ALGORITHM BASED ON PROS AND CONS OF VARIOUS MODALITIES

Chest radiography is the primary imaging tool for the evaluation of pulmonary TB. It plays a major role in the diagnosis and management of patients with TB. However, the radiographs may be normal or show only mild or nonspecific findings in patients with active disease.[17,38] Common causes of a missed diagnosis of TB on chest radiograph are failure to recognize the presence of mild parenchymal abnormalities, hilar or mediastinal lymphadenopathy, and failure to recognize that an upper lobe nodule or mass surrounded by small nodular opacities or scarring may represent TB.[17] The sensitivity of radiography is particularly low in patients with disseminated disease. For instance, in one study that included the chest radiographs of 71 patients with miliary TB, three independent observers recognized the presence of miliary disease in only 42 to 49 of the 71 patients (sensitivity, 59% to 69%).[21]

CT is more sensitive than chest radiography in the detection and characterization of subtle parenchymal disease and mediastinal lymphadenopathy.[30,36,51,52] In patients clinically suspected of having TB with normal or equivocal radiographic abnormalities, the increased sensitivity of CT may allow prompt diagnosis before results of culture. In one study of 41 consecutive children with confirmed TB, 8 (20%) had the diagnosis suggested only on CT. The findings on CT in these 8 patients with no apparent abnormalities on chest radiographs included low-attenuation lymph nodes with rim enhancement, calcifications, and nodules of bronchogenic spread or miliary disease in patients with no abnormalities evident on the radiograph.[51] In 15 patients (37%) CT scans provided information that altered clinical management.

Thin-section CT is particularly helpful in the detection of small foci of cavitation in areas of confluent pneumonia and in areas of dense nodularity and scarring.[33,53] For example, in one study of 41 patients who had active TB, CT showed cavities in 58%, whereas chest radiographs showed cavities in only 22%.[30]

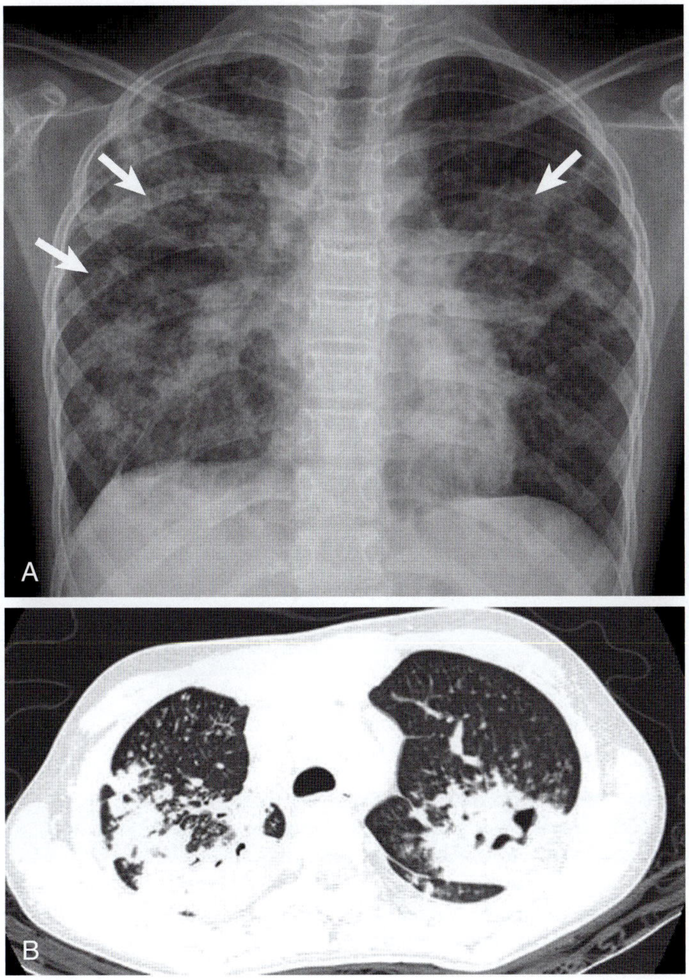

Fig. 10.23 Primary multidrug-resistant tuberculosis. (A) Chest radiograph shows multiple patchy consolidations and small nodules in both lungs. Also note multiple cavitary nodules *(arrows)* in both lungs. (B) CT scan at the level of the distal trachea demonstrates bilateral consolidation with cavitation, large nodules, centrilobular nodules, and tree-in-bud opacities in both lungs.

Thin-section CT is also helpful in detecting the presence of diffuse lung involvement when the chest radiographs are normal or show only questionable or minimal abnormalities.[28,30,54] Moreover, CT is more sensitive than radiography in demonstrating the presence of miliary disease and evidence of endobronchial spread of TB, a finding that is highly suggestive of active disease.[40,51] Endobronchial spread of TB is characterized by the presence of centrilobular nodules and tree-in-bud pattern distant from the primary site of infection. Lee and coworkers[53] assessed the utility of CT in the evaluation of pulmonary TB in 188 patients. A tentative diagnosis of active TB on CT was based on the pattern of parenchymal abnormalities and the presence of cavitation or evidence of endobronchial spread. A total of 133 of 146 patients (91%) with TB were correctly identified on CT as having pulmonary TB, whereas 32 of 42 patients (76%) without TB were correctly excluded. The main causes of misdiagnosis of TB were lung cancer and bacterial pneumonia. Active TB was correctly identified on CT in 71 of 89 (80%) patients and inactive disease in 51 of 57 (89%) patients.[54]

CT is also helpful in the evaluation of pleural complications, including tuberculous effusion, empyema, and bronchopleural fistula, and may demonstrate pleural disease not evident on chest radiography.[54,55] However, both radiation dose and cost of CT remain the limiting factors of CT in the diagnosis of TB. New imaging modalities, such as dual energy subtraction digital radiography and digital tomosynthesis, give better diagnostic performance than chest radiography, particularly in the detection of cavity and centrilobular nodules, while reducing radiation hazards associated with repeated CT examinations (Fig. 10.24).[56]

Differential Diagnosis

Pulmonary TB manifesting as lobar or segmental consolidation should be differentiated from bacterial pneumonia. In TB consolidation usually appears in association with mediastinal or hilar lymph node enlargement. Findings of sequelae of previous TB (including Ghon focus) or bronchogenic spread of TB may also be helpful as a clue in reaching a diagnosis of tuberculous pneumonia. Multiple cavities on CT also suggest tuberculous pneumonia (Fig. 10.25). Kim and coworkers[57] evaluated CT findings of 52 patients with lobar consolidation, including 24 with tuberculous pneumonia, 21 with obstructive pneumonia resulting from central lung cancer, and 7 with necrotizing lung abscess. They found that areas of consolidation containing three or more cavities were usually caused by TB. In addition, lack of clinical response to antibiotics for the common bacterial pneumonias may suggest TB. Mediastinal or hilar lymph node enlargement with central areas of low attenuation and peripheral rim enhancement after intravenous administration of contrast may also occur in lymphoma,[53] metastases particularly from testicular carcinoma,[58] small cell lung cancer, and benign conditions such as Whipple and Crohn diseases.[59]

Upper lobe cavitary TB should be differentiated from nontuberculous mycobacterial pulmonary disease, fungal infection, cavitary squamous cell carcinoma, and other pyogenic bacterial pneumonias caused by *Staphylococcus aureus*, *Klebsiella pneumoniae*, and anaerobic organisms.

Multiple nodules (10–30 mm in diameter, tuberculomas) may simulate the findings of pulmonary metastases, lymphoreticular malignancy, or angiitis and granulomatosis, such as granulomatosis with polyangiitis (formerly Wegener granulomatosis) and lymphomatoid granulomatosis.[53]

Small (<10 mm in diameter) centrilobular nodules and/or tree-in-bud opacities are the most important findings in making a diagnosis of active pulmonary TB. However, these findings may be also observed in cases of bacterial, fungal or viral bronchiolitis, aspiration, diffuse panbronchiolitis, and nontuberculous mycobacterial pulmonary diseases. Bilateral symmetric subpleural involvement with lower lung zone predominance, particularly when they are associated with bronchiectasis, favors the diagnosis of diffuse panbronchiolitis.[60] The presence of positive findings of chronic paranasal sinusitis also favors the diagnosis of diffuse panbronchiolitis. The presence of bilateral asymmetric multilobar involvement of bronchiolitis and bronchiectasis, when the right middle lobe and lingular division of the left upper lobe are most severely involved, suggests nontuberculous mycobacterial pulmonary disease.[61]

Long-standing military TB with coarse small nodules, especially when it is associated with pericardial effusion, may be confused with pulmonary metastases. Transbronchial lung biopsy may help differentiate these two conditions.[53]

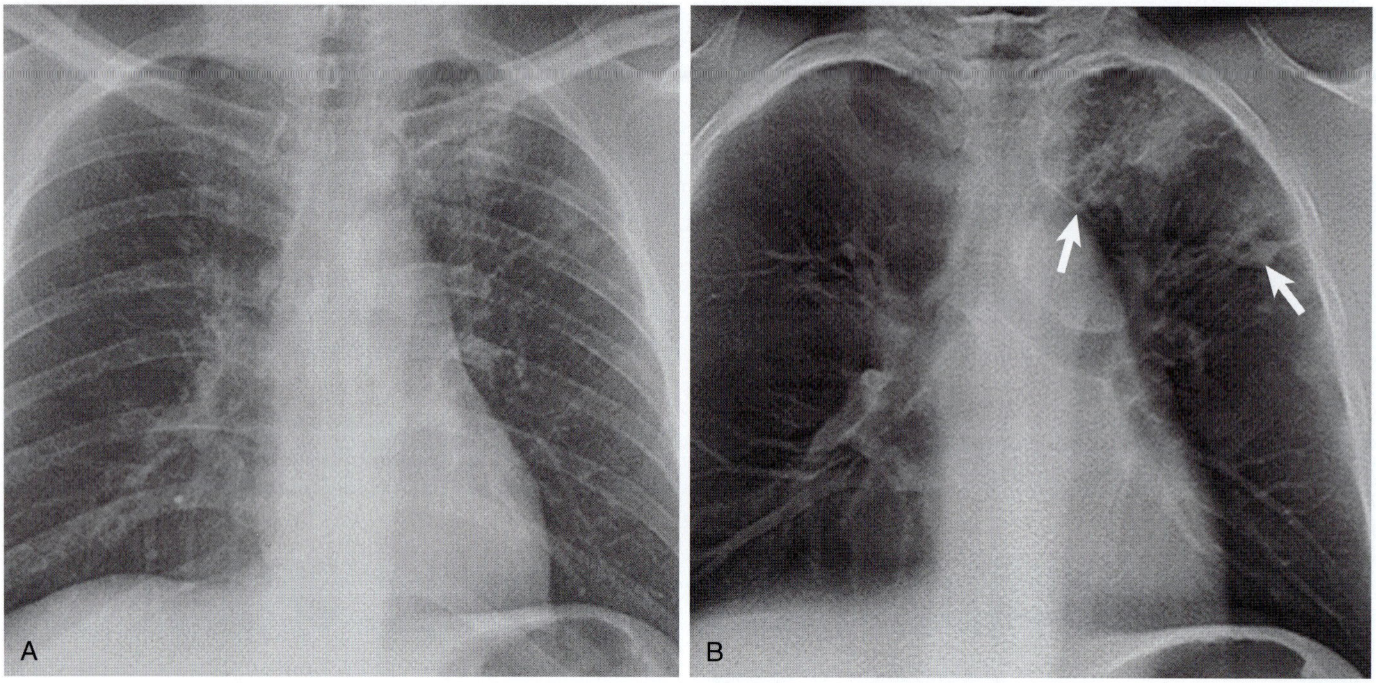

Fig. 10.24 Cavitary pulmonary tuberculosis. (A) Chest radiograph shows opacity in the left upper lung zone. (B) Chest digital tomosynthesis demonstrates opacity in the same left upper lobe with identifiable cavitary lesions *(arrows)*.

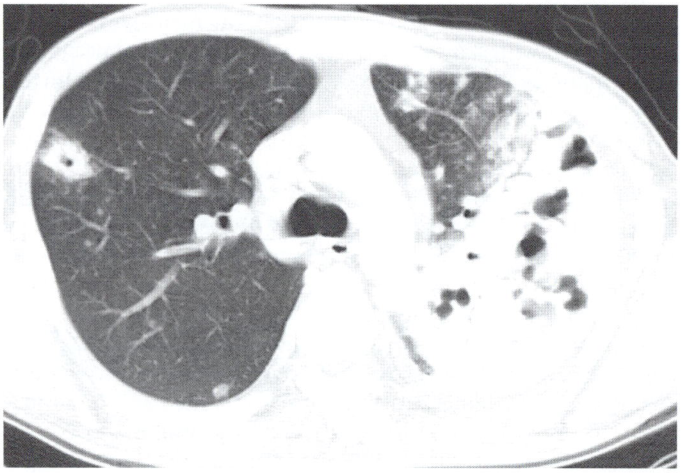

Fig. 10.25 Tuberculosis manifesting as consolidation containing multiple cavities. CT scan obtained at the level of the main bronchi shows large consolidation containing multiple cavities in the left lung. Also note the cavitating nodule in the right upper lobe and noncavitating variable-sized nodular lesions in both lungs.

KEY POINTS: DIFFERENTIAL DIAGNOSIS OF INTRATHORACIC TUBERCULOSIS

- Lobar or segmental tuberculous pneumonia
  - Bacterial pneumonia
- Tuberculous lymphadenitis
  - Lymphoma
  - Metastasis
  - Small cell lung cancer
  - Benign reactive nodes associated with Whipple and Crohn disease
- Nodules
  - Lymphoproliferative malignancy
  - Granulomatosis with polyangiitis
  - Pulmonary metastases
- Centrilobular small nodules and tree-in-bud opacities
  - Infectious bronchiolitis
  - Nontuberculous mycobacterial infection
  - Diffuse panbronchiolitis
  - Aspiration
- Miliary tuberculosis
  - Miliary metastases
  - Miliary endemic fungal infection

Synopsis of Treatment Options

The basic treatment regimen for previously untreated patients with pulmonary TB consists of an initial phase of isoniazid, rifampin, and pyrazinamide given daily for 2 months, followed by 4 months of isoniazid and rifampin. Ethambutol should be added in the initial 2 months if there is any suspicion of resistance to isoniazid or if the patient is known to be or is suspected of being HIV infected. In other words, patients from countries of a high prevalence of resistance to isoniazid and patients currently living in communities of high resistance rates should be given four drugs from the onset.[62,63] There are several caveats in pulmonary tuberculosis treatment that should be kept in mind. First, the organisms must be susceptible to the drugs used. Second, patients must take all or nearly all of the prescribed treatment. Third, the bacteriologic response should be documented to be successful using sputum cultures (should be negative by the end of 3-month treatment).

SUGGESTED READINGS

Restrepo CS, Katre R, Mumbower A. Imaging manifestations of thoracic tuberculosis. *Radiol Clin North Am*. 2016;54(3):453–473.

Rozenshtein A, Hao F, Starc MT, Pearson GD. Radiographic appearance of pulmonary tuberculosis: dogma disproved. *AJR Am J Roentgenol*. 2015;204(5):974–978.

The full reference list for this chapter is available at ExpertConsult.com.

11 Nontuberculous (Atypical) Mycobacterial Infection*

BRENT P. LITTLE

A variety of nontuberculous mycobacteria (NTMB) can cause pulmonary infections, with important differences in epidemiology, microbiology, host response, and treatment options across the various species. The severity of an infection caused by NTMB is largely determined by the immune status of the individual and whether coexisting disease is present. More complex manifestations of NTMB are now recognized, such as the overlapping pathology of hypersensitivity pneumonitis and infection seen in patients with so-called hot tub lung.

Prevalence and Epidemiology

NTMB can be classified as "environmental opportunistic" mycobacteria because they are ubiquitous, not transmitted from person to person, and occur in water (natural sources such as rivers and domestic drinking water), dust, and soil. The *Mycobacterium avium* complex is the most readily recovered from the natural environment and from patients with NTMB disease. There are also differences in prevalence of individual NTMB species among geographic regions; for example, *Mycobacterium malmoense* is more common in Europe than in North America.

In some parts of the world, water supplies have been investigated as a potential source of NTMB; even when water appears to be sterile, a "biofilm" (layering on the internal surfaces of water pipes) may be positive for NTMB. A biofilm deposit of NTMB may also be present on dental drilling equipment or bronchoscopes,[1] creating resistance to disinfection. NTMB occur both in natural bodies of water and in artificial sources, including swimming pools and whirlpool baths. Inhalation of droplets containing NTMB may result in a hypersensitivity pneumonitis (see later section Hot Tub Lung). Environmental exposure to NTMB may occur in water-damaged buildings, in which high concentrations of NTMB may be generated, particularly during building demolition.

The relatively low incidence of clinically significant infection caused by NTMB (on the order of 0.5 to 10 per 100,000 population, depending on the geographic location), despite an undoubtedly high level of environmental exposure, indicates that NTMB are of relatively low pathogenicity. Nevertheless, the reported incidence of NTMB infections continues to rise, in part as a consequence of the increasing awareness and identification of NTMB as human pathogens.

*The editors and the publisher would like to thank Dr. David M. Hansell for contributing material on this topic to the prior edition of this work. It has served as the foundation for the current chapter.

Classification of Nontuberculous Mycobacteria

Decades ago the genus *Mycobacterium* consisted of approximately 30 species; today, more than 150 species are recognized.[2] Many of these species, some of which have exotic names (e.g., *M. conspicuum, M. heckeshornense,* and *M. mucogenicum*), can cause pulmonary disease.[3] A wide variety of other diseases can be caused by NTMB; for example, *M. avium* can be responsible for conditions ranging from tenosynovitis to bacteremia in AIDS patients, as well as the more widely recognized pulmonary manifestations.

NTMB can be divided into slowly growing or rapidly growing groups. Of the many slow-growing NTMB, the species most frequently associated with human lung disease are *M. avium* and *M. intracellulare,* nearly identical organisms that are usually referred to as the *M. avium* complex (MAC). *M. chelonae, M. fortuitum,* and *M. abscessus* comprise the three important rapidly growing species, all of which can cause pulmonary disease. The NTMB can be further subdivided on the basis of colony characteristics, including pigment production.[4] A prolonged period needs to elapse before the culture characteristics of slow-growing NTMB become evident. By contrast, polymerase chain reaction assays are rapid and highly specific for some NTMB species, although false-positive results can arise in the presence of clinically nonsignificant NTMB.

Clinical Presentation: Colonization Versus Infection

Because NTMB are so widespread in the environment, respiratory secretions (sputum specimens or bronchoalveolar lavage samples) will occasionally contain NTMB, which may represent a contaminant as opposed to a clinically significant infection. Colonization can also occur, with NTMB recovered from an individual on more than one occasion without accompanying features of pulmonary infection. A diagnosis of clinically significant NTMB infection depends on supportive clinical findings. American Thoracic Society (ATS) guidelines specify three criteria for establishing a diagnosis of NTMB disease: (1) the clinical manifestations and time course must be compatible with NTMB-related pulmonary infection, (2) the radiographic findings must be compatible, and (3) the organism should be recovered in sufficient number (either from sputum or as a positive culture from bronchial washings).[5] There are difficulties with these criteria; for example, patients with radiographically progressive MAC infection may be asymptomatic, and conversely, symptoms may be a reflection of the underlying pulmonary disease that predisposes an individual to colonization/infection by NTMB rather than being caused by the NTMB itself. Radiographic findings of MAC infection may be subtle, and high-resolution computed tomography (HRCT) findings may be nonspecific. Integration of all available information from the clinical features, imaging (particularly HRCT), and microbiology is needed to make the sometimes very difficult distinction between colonization and clinically important infection.

Pathology

Pathogenic mechanisms differ among the various NTMB species, and an understanding of these differences helps explain the clinical situations in which NTMB cause important infection. The slow-growing NTMB generally breach the host's mucosal surface, the gastrointestinal or the respiratory tract in the case of MAC.[6] Organisms introduce themselves into alveolar epithelial cells and replicate without causing a major inflammatory response. Once across the "host barrier," the more virulent mycobacteria are able to replicate within monocytes and macrophages.[7–9] A granulomatous host response eventually occurs.[10] In one of the histopathologic studies of pulmonary NTMB infection, Fujita and colleagues[11] identified extensive peribronchial granulomas (Fig. 11.1) and associated ulceration of bronchial walls; from these features they concluded that MAC caused, rather than colonized, preexisting bronchiectasis.

The immune status of the host has a profound effect on the potential expression of disease caused by NTMB. The predisposition to disseminated NTMB disease in HIV-infected patients has been recognized for many years. The development of NTMB infection, notably MAC, in apparently otherwise healthy individuals may be due to defects in interferon production or specific interferon receptors.[12] More obvious perturbations of the host's immune state, such as steroid treatment and coexisting disease, are discussed in a later section.

The rapidly growing NTMB (*M. fortuitum, M. chelonae,* and *M. abscessus*) most frequently cause infections of soft tissues, particularly wounds. Pulmonary infections are often part of a disseminated picture in which there is multiorgan involvement. In this situation the degree of host immunity is a crucial determinant in the severity of the illness and prognosis. In addition, *M. fortuitum* and *M. chelonae* may cause diffuse pulmonary infection in patients with esophageal motility disorders, such as achalasia, hiatal hernia, dysmotility after stroke, or colonic interposition.

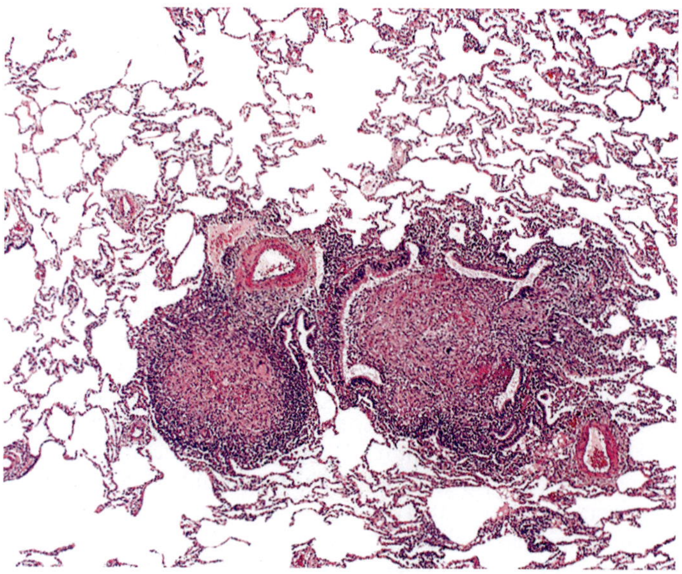

Fig. 11.1 Peribronchial granulomas. A low-power photomicrograph of a lung biopsy specimen shows granulomas centered on a bronchovascular bundle in a patient with *Mycobacterium avium-intracellulare* infection. The granuloma on the right occupies and is occluding the bronchiolar lumen. *(Courtesy Dr. Thomas V. Colby, Mayo Clinic, Scottsdale, AZ.)*

MYCOBACTERIUM AVIUM-INTRACELLULARE COMPLEX

Pulmonary infection by MAC is quite common in clinical practice but frequently overlooked. The radiologist is in a good position to raise the possibility of the diagnosis, especially because the clinical manifestations tend to be nonspecific. The radiographic manifestations of MAC are modulated by the immune status of the host and the presence or absence of preexisting lung disease; thus the spectrum can range from a few inconspicuous nodules to destructive cavitary disease on a background of emphysema. Chest radiography has a valuable role in monitoring patients with a confirmed diagnosis of MAC infection, whereas HRCT may detect earlier disease and suggest the diagnosis.

Manifestations of Mycobacterium avium-intracellulare *Complex Infection*

Radiography. Many of the early radiographic studies of NTMB did not attempt to distinguish among the various species, so it is difficult to determine whether there are definite differences in radiographic manifestations among the species. Any putative differences may, in fact, reflect the characteristics of the host rather than the specific NTMB species; in addition, more than one species of NTMB may be present.

The more florid cavitary form of disease (called the "classic" form for its resemblance to cavitary tuberculosis), reported in the earlier literature, probably reflects the use of sputum culture as the primary tool for confirming the diagnosis,[13,14] which means that only those with a relatively high burden of NTMB in their sputum would have been included in these series. This type of disease is most commonly encountered in elderly men, frequently with a background of pulmonary disease, especially chronic obstructive pulmonary disease (COPD) (Fig. 11.2).[15,16] At the other end of the radiographic spectrum are the normal or nearly normal radiographic findings in patients with confirmed MAC infection. In one of the largest series, Christensen and coauthors[15] reported that 7 of 114 patients with sputum culture–positive MAC infection had normal chest radiographs, and 7 had a reticulonodular pattern. The majority of individuals in early radiographic series had focal pulmonary abnormalities ranging from small nodules to large cavities.[13,15,16] The high frequency of radiographically evident cavities (in the study by Christensen and colleagues,[15] nearly 98% of individuals had identifiable cavities) has probably declined with the trend toward earlier diagnosis. There is a tendency for cavities caused by NTMB to be smaller and thinner walled (average diameter, 2.5 cm) than those caused by *M. tuberculosis* (average diameter, 6 cm),[13] although the overlap in size is so great that differentiation cannot be made on the basis of these size criteria.

The less florid form of MAC infection, called the "nonclassic" form, is now more frequently recognized than the "classic" form and is seen most often in elderly women with no obvious preexisting lung disease or clearly characterized immune defect. In such individuals the radiographic manifestations of MAC infection include normal radiographs, small inconspicuous nodules

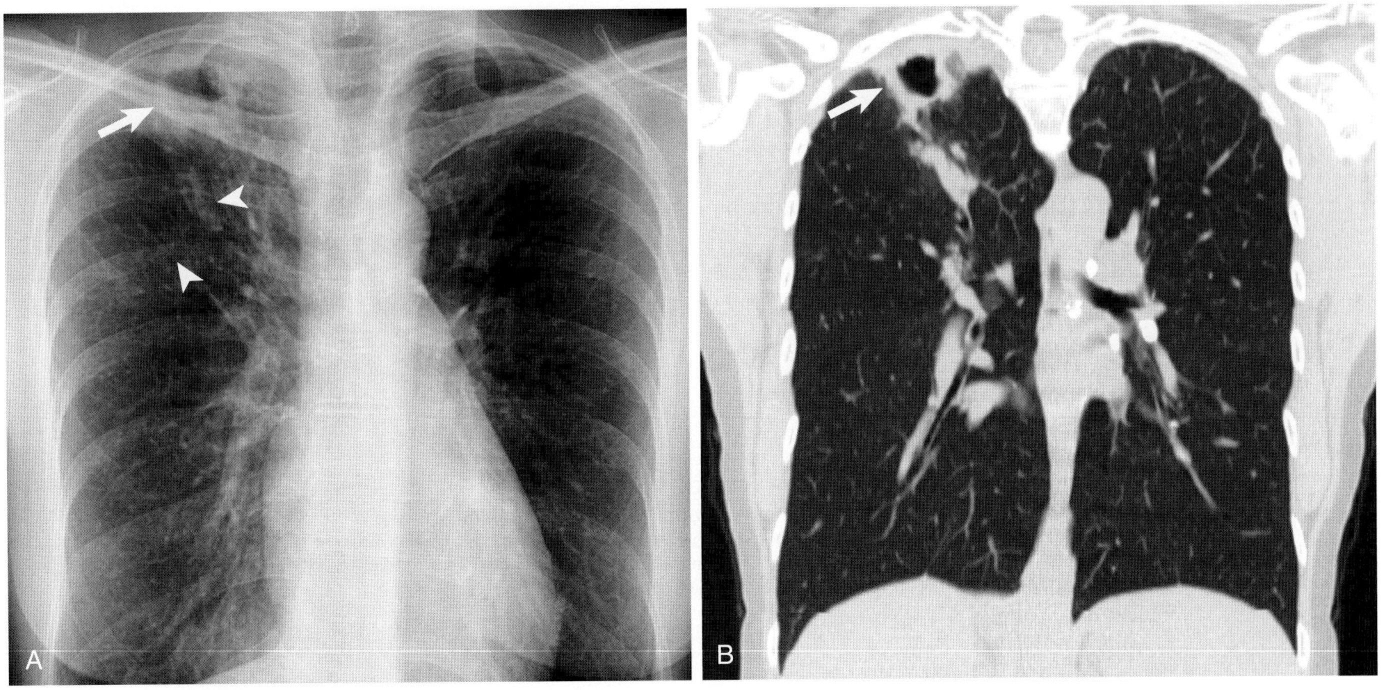

Fig. 11.2 Nontuberculous mycobacteria (NTMB) infection in chronic obstructive pulmonary disease (COPD). A chest radiograph (A) and coronal noncontrast CT scan (B) show hyperinflated lung volumes with a cavitary right upper lobe nodule *(arrows)* with adjacent nodular opacities *(arrowheads)*. This appearance represents reactivation tuberculosis infection until proven otherwise. NTMB infection may appear similar and is most common in alcoholic patients or in those with COPD. *(From Walker CM, Digumarthy S. Pulmonary infections. In: Digumarthy S, Abbara S, Chung J, eds.* Problem-Solving in Chest Imaging. *Philadelphia: Elsevier; 2019.)*

(ranging from a few millimeters to approximately 1.5 cm), and patchy foci of consolidation with bronchiectasis, often with a right middle lobe and lingular predominance (Fig. 11.3). Small nodules often represent endobronchial spread (corresponding to the HRCT finding of a tree-in-bud pattern [Fig. 11.4]). Indolent disease usually associated with elderly women may wax and wane without treatment, and some nodules may disappear spontaneously, only to reappear at different locations months or years later. In the series of Woodring and associates,[16] the average time over which there was definite radiographic progression in patients with MAC infection was 6.4 years, and in one particular case, 12 years elapsed after diagnosis before radiographic progression occurred. In the same study the authors remarked on the delay (1–16 years) between initial evaluation and the diagnosis of MAC infection, again highlighting the nonspecific nature of the clinical and radiographic findings.[16] An uncommon manifestation of MAC infection is as a single focal pulmonary mass or solitary nodule on a chest radiograph.[17] Such nodules and masses range in size from 1 to 5 cm, and whether they represent a truly solitary lesion, in the absence of CT corroboration, is uncertain.

Bronchiectasis in the right middle lobe and lingula (Fig. 11.5) may be particularly prominent in some elderly women with the nonclassic form of disease, and the term *Lady Windermere syndrome* has been coined for this pattern.[18]

Computed Tomography. CT is sensitive for detection of pulmonary MAC infection and may show relatively widespread involvement even when radiographs are unimpressive.[14] Although individual CT features of MAC are nonspecific, the combination of CT signs (see the next box), particularly when seen in an

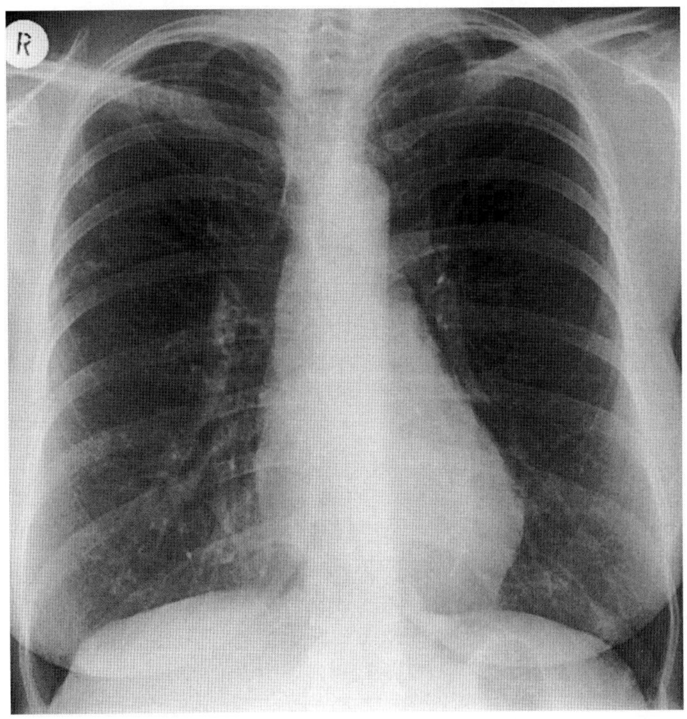

Fig. 11.3 Radiographic findings of *Mycobacterium avium-intracellulare* infection. A chest radiograph shows subtle nodular shadowing in the periphery of the right upper lobe caused by *M. avium-intracellulare*. A chest radiograph obtained 9 months later showed resolution (the patient was not undergoing treatment).

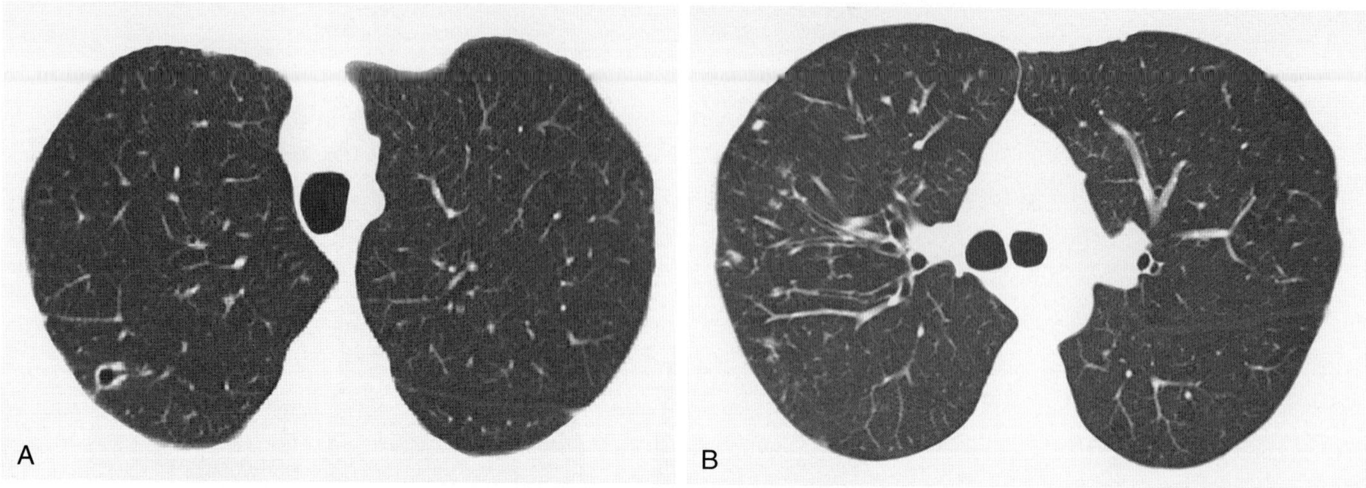

Fig. 11.4 CT findings of *Mycobacterium avium-intracellulare* infection in the same patient as in Fig. 11.3. A CT image at the level of the trachea (A) shows a small right upper lobe cavitary lesion. A CT section at the level of the main bronchi (B) demonstrates tree-in-bud and nodular opacities typical of *M. avium-intracellulare* infection. Also noted is thickening and mild dilation of the right upper lobe bronchi.

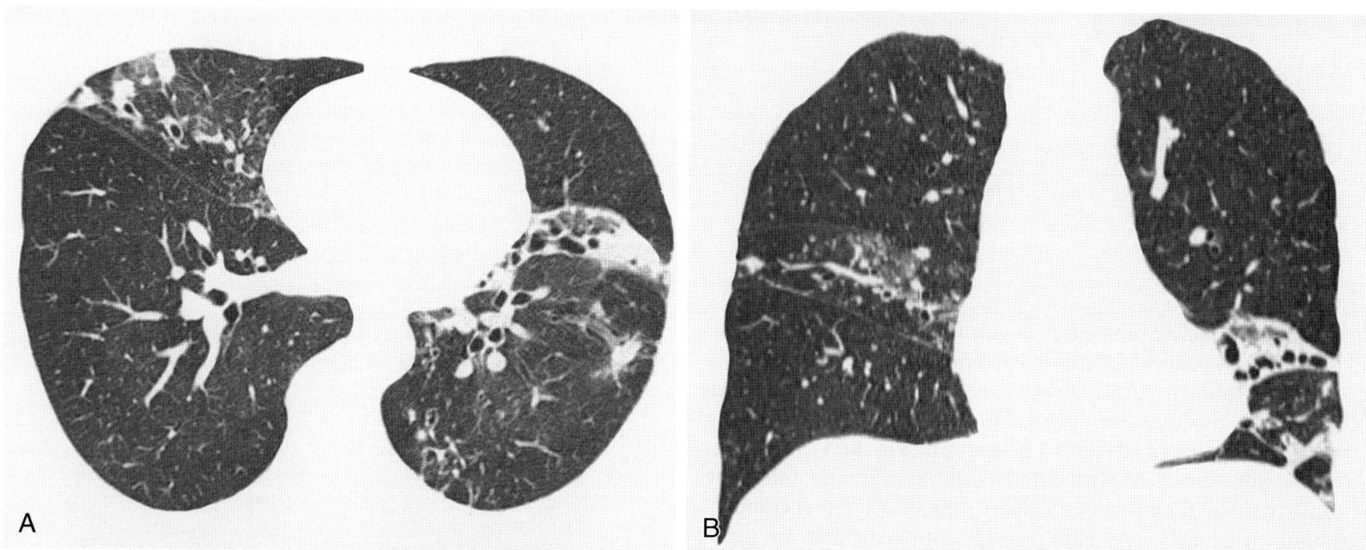

Fig. 11.5 CT findings of *Mycobacterium avium-intracellulare* infection in a 67-year-old woman with a "Lady Windermere" distribution. A CT image at the level of the right inferior pulmonary vein (A) shows bilateral bronchiectasis. Ground-glass opacities and mild consolidation are present in the right middle lobe, lingula, and left lower lobe. Also evident are small nodular opacities and a few tree-in-bud opacities. A coronal reformatted CT image (B) better demonstrates the predominant distribution of the abnormalities in the right middle lobe and lingula.

elderly woman, is highly suggestive of the diagnosis (Fig. 11.6; also see Figs. 11.4 and 11.5). Indeed, the CT appearance may be sufficiently characteristic of MAC infection even in the absence of any overt clinical features.

CT findings vary in predictive ability for MAC infection. In a study by Tanaka and coworkers,[10] 26 patients with HRCT appearances suggestive of MAC infection were monitored for 4 years. Half of these individuals subsequently proved to be culture positive for MAC. Similarly, a study by Swensen and colleagues,[19] using the criterion of bronchiectasis with coexistent nodules in the same lobe, found that just greater than 50% of individuals had culture-positive MAC (as opposed to 4% of individuals with CT evidence of bronchiectasis but no lung nodules), thus suggesting a relatively high specificity of 87% and a sensitivity of 80%. In another study the combination of bronchiectasis and nodules in the same lobe, particularly when the middle lobe/lingula was the predominant site of involvement, was highly suggestive of MAC infection.[20] The pathologic correlate of the tree-in-bud pattern in the context of MAC infection is likely to represent exudate in and around the small airways; when present, additional scattered randomly distributed nodules likely represent infective consolidation. Cavitation can be seen in a subset of nodules, with an occasional connection between a terminal or lobular bronchus and the cavity.[21]

CT sometimes reveals mosaic attenuation, reflecting obliterative small airways disease (Fig. 11.7). Whether this is associated with preexisting bronchiectasis or is a direct consequence of MAC infection, as suggested by Kubo and coworkers,[22] is unclear.

KEY POINTS: HIGH-RESOLUTION COMPUTED TOMOGRAPHY FINDINGS IN *MYCOBACTERIUM AVIUM-INTRACELLULARE* PULMONARY INFECTION

DOMINANT FEATURES

- Bronchiectasis
  - Usually multilobar with a right middle lobe and lingular predominance
  - Usually cylindrical and mild to moderate in severity; rarely cystic or end-stage bronchiectasis
- Nodules
  - Small centrilobular branching nodules (tree-in-bud pattern)
  - Occasional random nodules up to approximately 2 cm in diameter, occasionally cavitary

RARE FEATURES

- Fibrosis associated with bronchiectasis, pleural thickening or pleural effusion, mediastinal lymphadenopathy

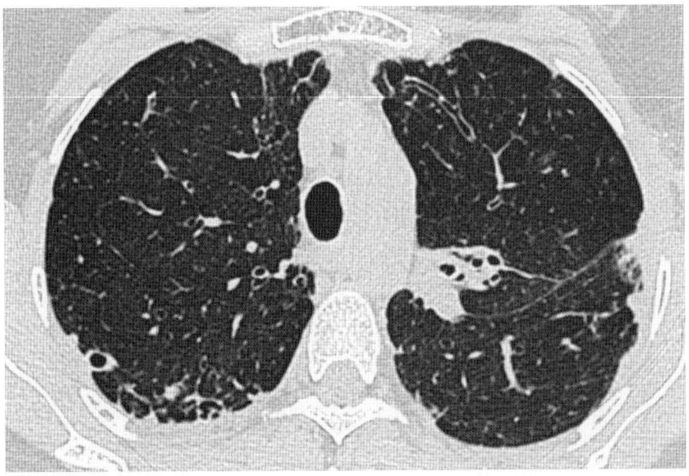

Fig. 11.6 CT findings of *Mycobacterium avium-intracellulare* infection. An elderly woman with no known predisposing cause shows the typical features of *M. avium-intracellulare* infection on CT through the lung apices: mild cylindrical bronchiectasis, a few bilateral centrilobular nodules, a small cavitary lesion in the periphery of the right apex, and small foci of consolidation. Note the loss of volume in the left upper lobe.

Other occasional features include patchy ground-glass opacification and hilar lymphadenopathy, but these ancillary signs are nonspecific and usually do not occur without the more classic CT findings of MAC infection. Extensive mediastinal lymphadenopathy as a sole manifestation of MAC infection in the absence of HIV infection is extremely rare.[23]

MYCOBACTERIUM KANSASII

Of all the NTMB, *M. kansasii* most closely resembles *M. tuberculosis*,[24] particularly in its responsiveness to conventional antituberculous drugs and its imaging appearances. The exact incidence of *M. kansasii* infection is unknown, but after MAC it is one of the most common NTMB responsible for pulmonary disease. *M. kansasii* is particularly prevalent in the southern states of North America[25] and in HIV-positive individuals.[26,27] Of interest, *M. kansasii* infection was thought to be relatively uncommon in Korea,[28] but its incidence is now increasing.[29] *M. kansasii* typically infects middle-aged men rather than elderly women (as in MAC infection). Important risk factors for *M. kansasii* infection include COPD, alcoholism, pneumoconiosis, neoplasia, previous mycobacterial disease, and other debilitating disease.[30]

The radiographic appearances of *M. kansasii* infection are almost always cavitary and involve the upper lobes with coexisting fibrosis and consolidation. The cavities found in *M. kansasii* infection vary widely in size and wall characteristics, with appearances similar to postprimary pattern of tuberculosis (TB) infection (Fig. 11.8).[31,32] A CT study by Hollings and colleagues[33] documented that cavities were present in just less than half the patients with *M. kansasii* infection—the cavities, when present, were confined to the upper lobes; predominantly lower lobe involvement makes *M. kansasii* infection unlikely.[34] Bronchiectasis, as shown on HRCT, was an invariable feature in the small series ($n = 9$) of *M. kansasii* infection included in the comparative study by Hollings and colleagues.[33] However, of all the NTMB, *M. kansasii* is the least likely to be responsible for an HRCT appearance characterized by bronchiectasis and bronchiolitis (tree-in-bud pattern) alone.[35] The pattern of *M. kansasii* infection will be modified by any preexisting pulmonary disease, notably centrilobular emphysema or pulmonary fibrosis (Fig. 11.9).

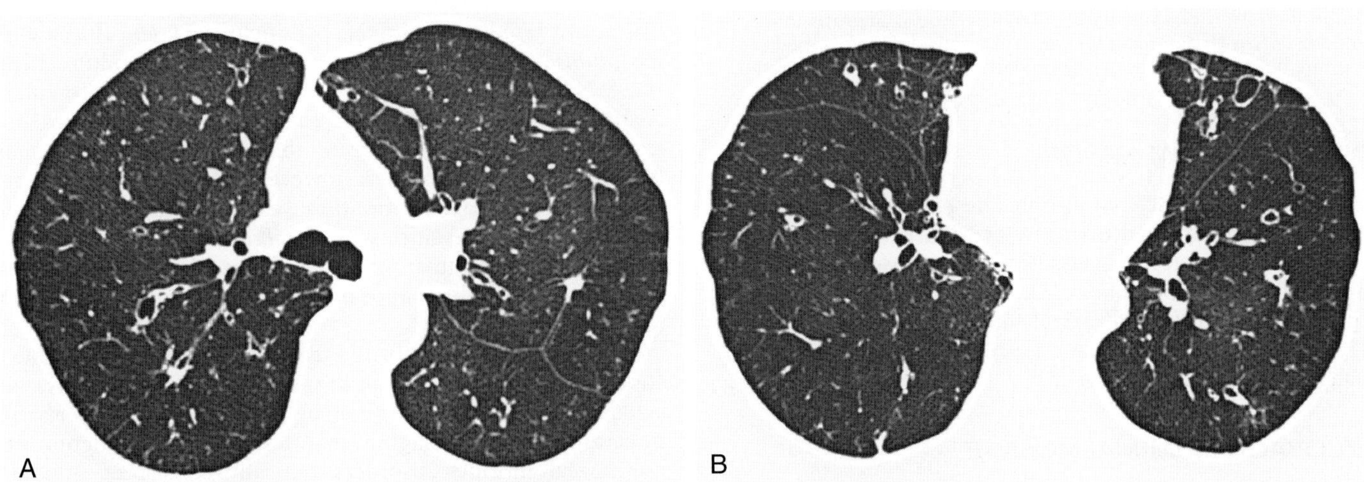

Fig. 11.7 *Mycobacterium avium-intracellulare* infection with associated small airways disease. CT images at the level of the upper (A) and lower lung zones (B) show widespread bronchiectasis, more severe in the right middle lobe and lingula (B), and mosaic attenuation reflecting obliterative small airways disease in a patient with severe airflow limitation.

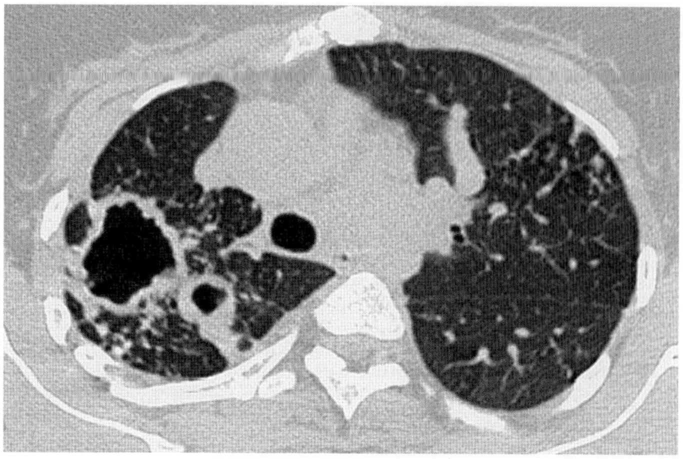

Fig. 11.8 CT findings of *Mycobacterium kansasii* infection. A CT image through the upper lobes of a patient with background centrilobular emphysema and *M. kansasii* infection demonstrates thick-walled cavities at the right lung apex and bilateral centrilobular nodular opacities. The appearance is similar to the reactivation pattern of tuberculosis.

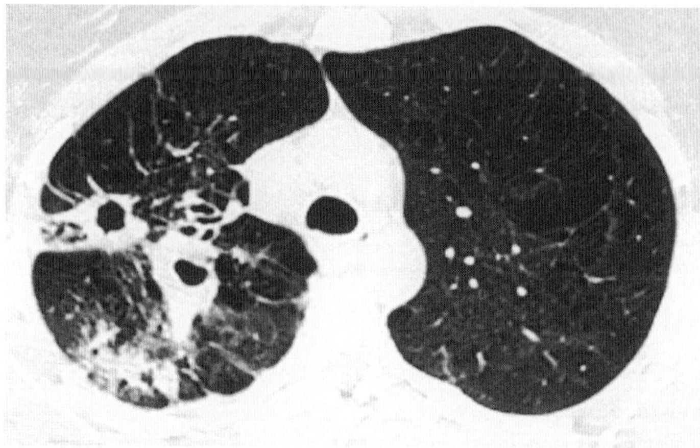

Fig. 11.10 CT findings of *Mycobacterium xenopi* infection. A CT image through the upper lung zone shows cavitary lesions on a background of severe centrilobular emphysema. These appearances of *M. xenopi* are indistinguishable from those of *Mycobacterium kansasii* (see Fig. 11.8) and *Mycobacterium tuberculosis*.

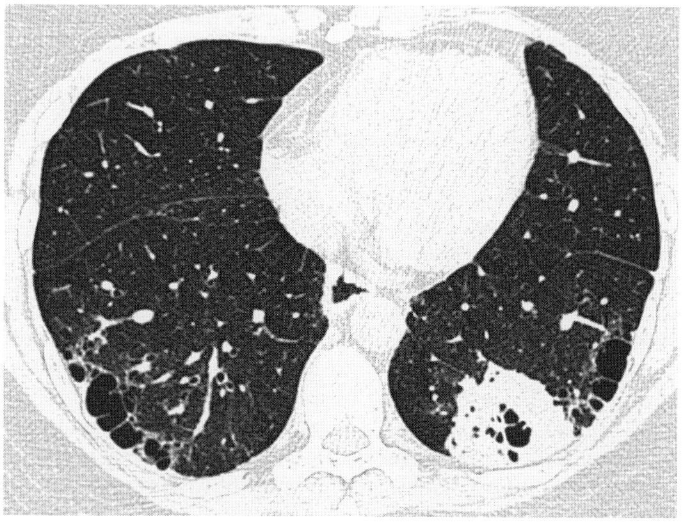

Fig. 11.9 CT findings of *Mycobacterium kansasii* infection. A CT image through the lower lobes of a patient with systemic sclerosis (note the dilated esophagus) demonstrates mass like consolidation in the fibrotic peripheral lung that subsequently proved to be *M. kansasii* infection.

MYCOBACTERIUM XENOPI

M. xenopi is often clustered in time and place with *M. kansasii*, a common source being drinking water.[36] Furthermore, *M. xenopi* has imaging characteristics very similar to those of *M. kansasii* (Fig. 11.10). The upper lobes are usually involved, with findings of cavitation, fibrosis, and variable degrees of nodular and tree-in-bud patterns; bronchiectasis is an inconstant feature in the small series reported to date.[33,37,38]

MYCOBACTERIUM MALMOENSE

M. malmoense appears to have a greater prevalence in mainland Europe than in North America. Few studies investigate the imaging features of *M. malmoense*.[33,39] In the comparative study by Evans and associates,[39] the presence of cavities larger than 6 cm and air-fluid levels within cavities favored *M. malmoense* rather than *M. tuberculosis* infection; conversely, consolidation involving more than one bronchopulmonary segment was more frequent in TB.

MYCOBACTERIUM GORDONAE

M. gordonae is usually a nonpathogenic contaminant. In a study of 19 cases of sputum-positive patients with *M. gordonae* infection, the authors concluded that there were no characteristic radiographic findings associated with this particular NTMB[40] and that in each case there was an alternative cause for the chest findings, including community-acquired pneumonia, TB, *Pneumocystis jirovecii* pneumonia, lung cancer, and emphysema.

MYCOBACTERIA CHELONAE AND OTHER RAPIDLY GROWING NONTUBERCULOUS MYCOBACTERIA

M. chelonae is one of the so-called rapidly growing NTMB (other important rapidly growing NTMB include *M. abscessus* and *M. fortuitum*) because of its relatively rapid growth on culture media; these NTMB are somewhat resistant to drug treatment.[41,42] A study of 14 patients with *M. chelonae* infection documented a pattern of disease similar to that of MAC, with frequent bronchiectasis and nodules; however, there was no lobar predominance, and cavity formation was more common than with MAC.[43] CT manifestations of *M. abscessus* lung infection are bilateral small nodular opacities, bronchiectasis, and cavity formation,[44] and these appearances overlap with those seen in MAC infection.[45]

Patients with cystic fibrosis seem to be particularly prone to superinfection with *M. abscessus*,[46,47] whereas patients with achalasia of the esophagus may be predisposed to *M. fortuitum* infection.[48,49] The imaging manifestations in patients with esophageal motility disorders typically consist of unilateral or bilateral reticulonodular or airspace opacitie without lobar predominance. Pleural effusion and cavitary disease are uncommon, occurring in 20% and 15% of reported cases, respectively.[50]

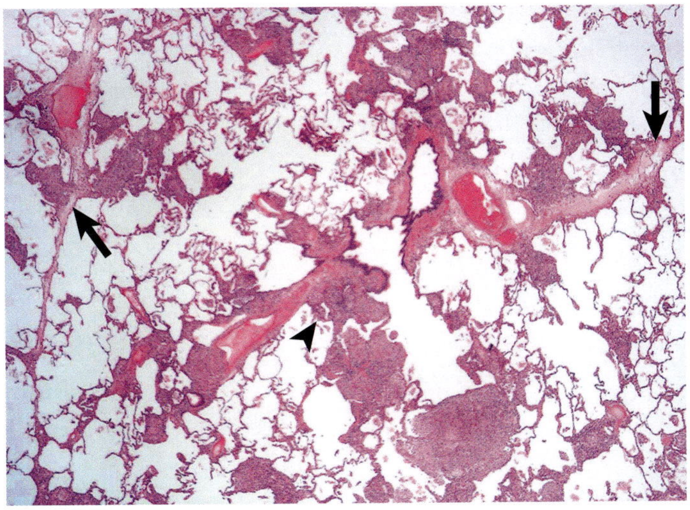

Fig. 11.11 Pathologic findings of hot tub lung. A surgical lung biopsy specimen demonstrates numerous nonnecrotizing, well-formed granulomas accompanied by a moderate chronic interstitial inflammatory infiltrate. Note the lack of a definite predilection for any anatomic distribution of the nonnecrotizing granulomas. They are seen along the interlobular septa *(arrows)* and bronchovascular bundles *(arrowhead)*. *(Courtesy Dr. Andrew Churg, University of British Columbia, Vancouver, Canada.)*

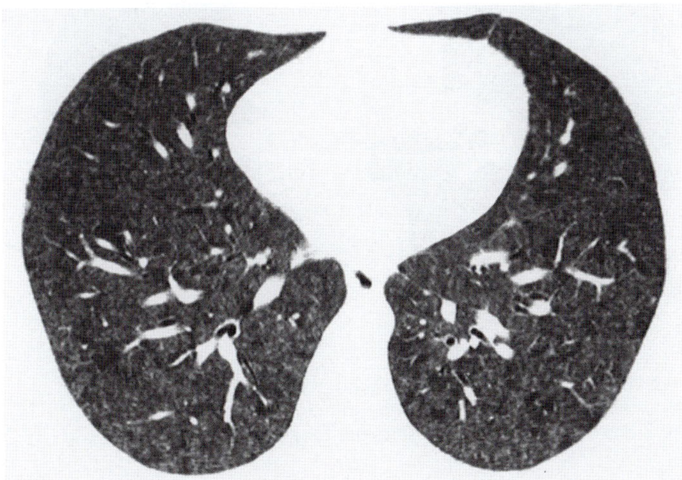

Fig. 11.12 CT findings of hot tub lung. A CT scan through the lower lobes of a patient with biopsy-proven hot tub lung (same patient as in Fig. 11.11) demonstrates diffuse ground-glass opacity and indistinct small nodules measuring approximately 1 to 2 mm in diameter, findings resembling those of subacute hypersensitivity pneumonitis.

HOT TUB LUNG

NTMB disease can uncommonly be caused by hot tubs, with users exposed to aerosolized droplets containing MAC. Most of the cases reported have occurred in otherwise fit and relatively young individuals who were using indoor hot tubs. The ensuing host response may represent a hypersensitivity reaction or a granulomatous response to infection (Fig. 11.11).[51] The reported HRCT appearances more closely resemble subacute hypersensitivity pneumonitis (Fig. 11.12).[52] This, coupled with the fact that symptomatic improvement typically occurs with cessation of hot tub use and antituberculous drug therapy is not invariably needed, suggests that a hypersensitivity response is the dominant pathologic process.

Individuals with hot tub lung usually have a subacute presentation consisting of a dry cough and some degree of hypoxemia. HRCT studies suggest a resemblance to subacute hypersensitivity pneumonitis, with poorly defined, relatively low-attenuation centrilobular nodules, patchy ground-glass opacification, and air-trapping on expiratory CT indicative of an element of small airways obstruction (Fig. 11.13).[52,53] A tree-in-bud pattern may occasionally be present, unusual in hypersensitivity pneumonitis from other causes.[54]

COEXISTING DISEASE AND INFECTION WITH NONTUBERCULOUS MYCOBACTERIA

Numerous risk factors related to generalized or localized (pulmonary) host immunity influence the susceptibility of an individual to clinically significant NTMB infection. The exact increase in risk conferred by individual factors has not been fully worked out, and only the more important ones are shown in the box that follows.

KEY POINTS: RISK FACTORS FOR INFECTION WITH NONTUBERCULOUS MYCOBACTERIA

- Environmental
  - Warm climate
  - Mining industry
- Host factors
  - Increasing age (>40 years)
  - Male (with preexisting lung disease)
  - "Elderly women" otherwise normal
  - Esophageal dysmotility disorders
- Preexisting systemic disease
  - HIV infection/AIDS
  - Diabetes mellitus
  - Alcohol abuse
- Preexisting pulmonary disease
  - Smoking-related COPD
  - Bronchiectasis of any cause (notably cystic fibrosis)
  - Localized pulmonary fibrosis (e.g., radiation fibrosis, previous TB)
  - Silicosis/pneumoconiosis
  - Chronic aspiration
  - Causes of chronic lung destruction (e.g., chronic necrotizing aspergillosis)

Although patients with MAC infection without preexisting pulmonary or systemic disease are usually women older than 50 years, MAC infection in COPD tends to occur in younger men between 40 and 50 years of age. The nonspecific nature of symptoms related to COPD with occasional non-NTMB infective exacerbations makes recognition of NTMB infection, superimposed on a background of COPD, particularly challenging. CT may occasionally suggest the diagnosis, particularly when nodular opacities, focal bronchiectasis, and cavitary lesions appear in a patient with "uncomplicated" emphysema. Although unexpected clinical deterioration in a patient with COPD and supportive CT findings are helpful, microbiologic evidence of NTMB is considered necessary in this situation before treatment is instituted.[55]

The majority of patients with NTMB infection, of whatever species, have some degree of bronchial damage, and most have bronchiectasis by HRCT criteria.[33] The question of the degree to which an active NTMB infection causes progression of

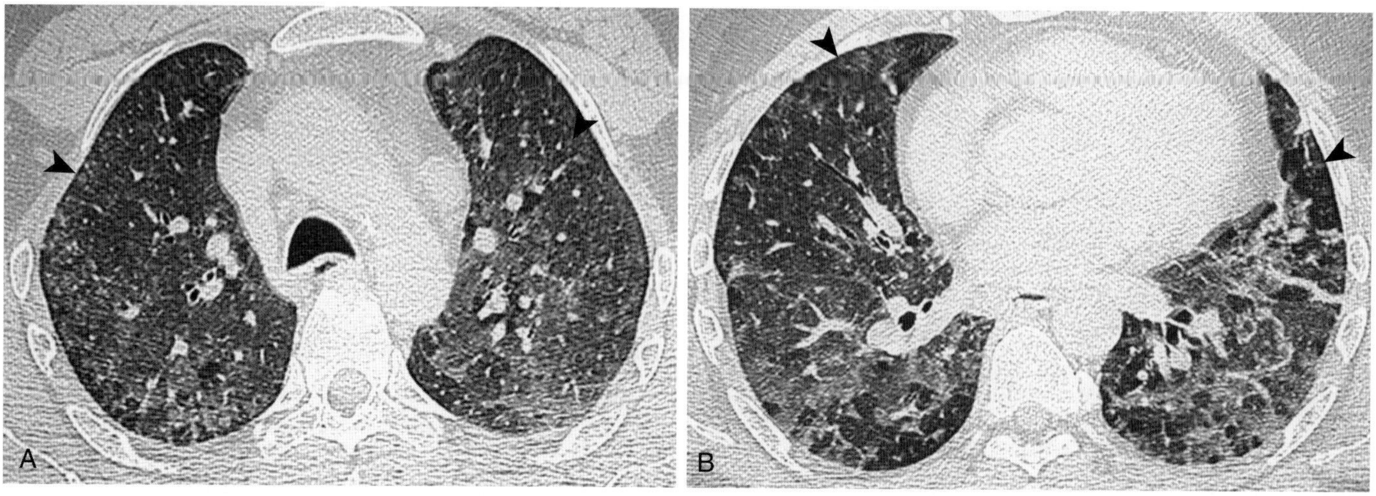

Fig. 11.13 CT findings of hot tub lung. Two representative expiratory CT images at the level of the upper (A) and lower (B) lung zones show lobular air trapping in addition to ground-glass opacity and centrilobular nodules *(arrowheads). (Courtesy Dr. Thomas V. Colby, Mayo Clinic, Scottsdale, AZ.)*

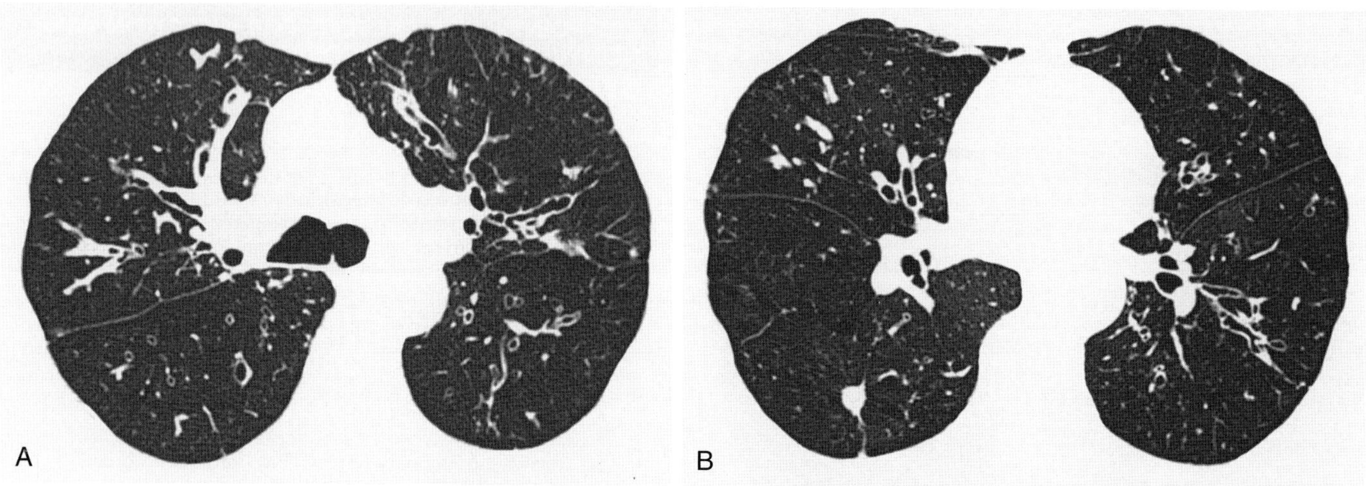

Fig. 11.14 Cystic fibrosis and *Mycobacterium chelonae* infection. CT images were taken at the level of the upper lungs (A) and inferior pulmonary veins (B) in a patient with *M. chelonae* infection on a background of features typical of cystic fibrosis; there are no signs of a significant coexisting nontuberculous mycobacterial infection.

bronchiectasis, as opposed to colonizing (but not necessarily damaging) previously existing bronchiectasis, is unresolved. Patients with cystic fibrosis are at risk for the development of NTMB infections, especially by *M. abscessus*, MAC, *M. fortuitum*, and *M. kansasii*.[47,56] However, CT findings of such infections are similar to those resulting from cystic fibrosis alone, and cystic fibrosis patients can also develop chronic pulmonary NTMB infection (Fig. 11.14). Nevertheless, HRCT appearances may deteriorate more rapidly in patients with cystic fibrosis and NTMB infection than in those without NTMB infection.[57]

An archetypal cause of predisposing impaired immunity is HIV, although the precise defect that predisposes HIV patients to NTMB disease is unknown (Fig. 11.15).[58] The considerable immunosuppression that may be present in HIV-infected individuals makes disseminated NTMB infections more likely, especially when the CD4 cell count falls to less than 50 cells/mm^3. In severely immunosuppressed patients, the radiographic manifestation of NTMB is often atypical and includes diffuse nodular patterns and mediastinal lymphadenopathy; central low attenuation can be seen in a subset of cases.[59,60] Mediastinal lymphadenopathy may also appear centrally necrotic in the setting of the immune reconstitution inflammatory syndrome.

IMAGING ALGORITHM

Chest radiography is the mainstay of imaging in patients with known or suspected NTMB infection and can show nodules, consolidation, cavities, and occasionally bronchiectasis. However, the relative insensitivity of chest radiography for the detection of "active" NTMB infection, particularly MAC, is recognized in the ATS guidelines,[5] which emphasize the use of CT in cases of noncavitary disease. Nevertheless, in individuals with a positive chest radiograph at initial evaluation, follow-up radiographs remain a satisfactory means of monitoring the disease and response to treatment.

In sputum-negative patients, imaging findings, particularly on CT, may be suggestive enough to initiate a more thorough search for NTMB organisms.[10] In addition, CT may reveal

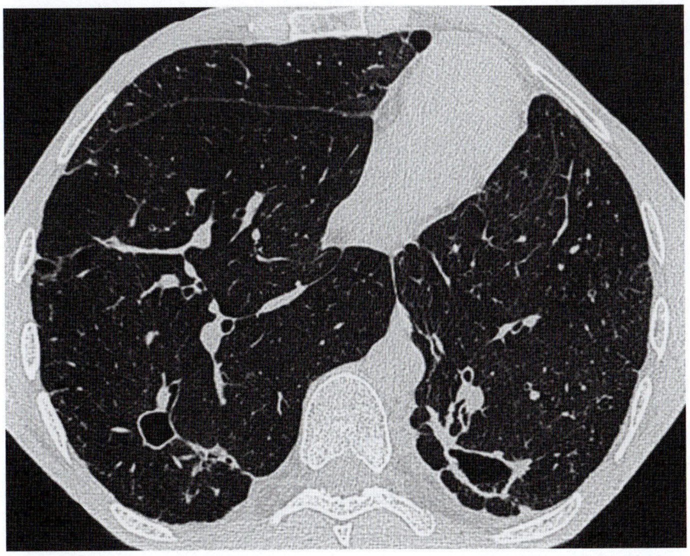

Fig. 11.15 *Mycobacterium szulgai* infection in an HIV-infected patient. A CT image shows multiple cavitating lesions in an HIV patient from whom *M. szulgai* was cultured from sputum samples.

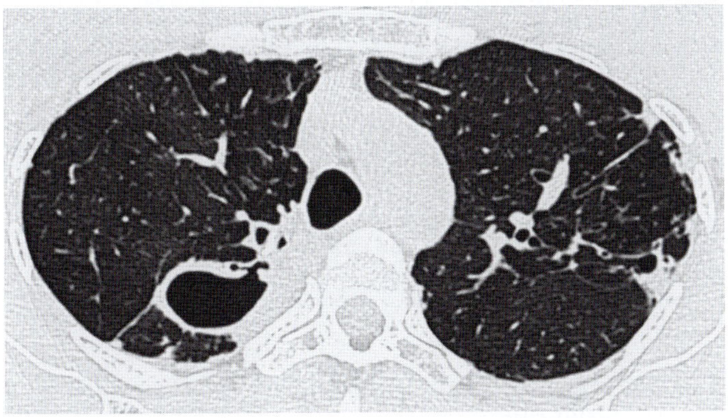

Fig. 11.16 *Mycobacterium kansasii* infection and chronic necrotizing aspergillosis. A CT image at the level of the aortic arch demonstrates a thick-walled cavity and adjacent pleural thickening in the superior segment of the right lower lobe. Also evident are mild bronchiectasis and scarring in the left upper lobe. In addition to *M. kansasii, Aspergillus* was isolated from bronchoscopic samples. The patient responded to a combination of appropriate antituberculous and antifungal drugs.

background parenchymal lung disease, which can be helpful in elucidating the complex and sometimes severe pulmonary function deficits in these patients. CT may be used to investigate patients in whom there is clinical decline in the absence of an obvious explanation on chest radiography. In such circumstances, CT may reveal progression of the NTMB infection itself (e.g., increasing nodular and tree-in-bud patterns) or supervening *Aspergillus* involvement, including chronic necrotizing aspergillosis, which is also referred to as semiinvasive *Aspergillus* infection (Fig. 11.16).[61]

Chronic pulmonary NTMB infection often has a waxing and waning course. New nodules often appear at follow-up CT, whereas others may decrease in size or resolve. Although clusters of small tree-in-bud nodules are easily attributed to NTMB infection, larger nodules may pose more of a diagnostic challenge, as they are not easily distinguished from malignancy by morphology alone. Although a short-term follow-up CT at 3 months is often performed for incidentally detected new pulmonary nodules according to the Fleischner Society guidelines, this practice may lead to an overuse of CT in chronic infections such as *M. avium-intracellulare*. Although no consensus guidelines have been published addressing this topic, knowledge of the often waxing and waning course of *M. avium-intracellulare* may encourage the judicious use of CT. More aggressive follow-up may be reserved for nodules with concerning features or growth disproportionate to that of the background of other infectious nodules.

Synopsis of Treatment Options

MEDICAL TREATMENT

The decision to treat NTMB infection and the drug regimen chosen are largely empirical and based on a clinician's judgment, the patient's symptoms, and patient preference. Drug treatment, with its potentially serious side effects, is more likely to be started in patients with symptomatic and progressive (e.g., cavitary) disease. By comparison, individuals with mild bronchiectasis and few respiratory symptoms may not obviously benefit from a protracted and arduous regimen of drug treatment, particularly in the absence of evidence that there is long-term benefit with such a stratagem.[62]

Several of the NTMB cannot be successfully treated by standard antimycobacterial drugs, and there is some uncertainty about which agents and combinations are appropriate for a given NTMB species. Nevertheless, guidelines such as those from the ATS[5] have recommended specific drug regimens for infections with individual NTMB species. A case has been made for in vitro susceptibility testing to enable even more selective use of these drugs.[63,64]

Despite the complex nature of the drug treatment of NTMB infection, there is some consensus that an uncomplicated first manifestation of MAC infection should be treated with a standard three- or possibly four-drug combination, in line with the ATS guidelines.[5] The most commonly used drugs in such combinations include a macrolide (e.g., clarithromycin or azithromycin), a rifamycin, and ethambutol.[62] Treatment is usually continued for 1 year after sputum conversion (three consecutive negative sputum cultures). Close monitoring of patients for side effects from these relatively toxic drugs, as well as for subtle clinical indicators of response to treatment, is mandatory.

Serial HRCT examinations may be helpful in assessing the regression of exudative changes (e.g., nodules and tree-in-bud pattern) with treatment. However, serial chest radiographs may be sufficient to determine whether there is a response to treatment, simply by monitoring the resolution or persistence of poorly defined nodular opacities. In individuals in whom standard treatment has failed or when there is subsequent relapse, susceptibility testing of the NTMB, recovered from sputum, may be necessary and additional drugs substituted or added.

After MAC, *M. kansasii* is probably the most frequently encountered NTMB requiring drug treatment, and for this organism, inclusion of a rifamycin is a key element in multidrug combinations; sputum conversion rates (or sterilization of *M. kansasii*) approach 100% when a rifamycin is included. The clinical and radiographic manifestations of *M. kansasii*, as described in earlier sections, are very similar to conventional postprimary pattern TB infection, and such patients are often

KEY POINTS: NONTUBERCULOUS MYCOBACTERIA

- Prevalence and epidemiology
  - NTMB organisms are omnipresent in the environment, particularly in water and soil, with geographic variations in the prevalence of NTMB species.
  - In a hospital setting, NTMB infection may originate from biofilm sources, particularly on bronchoscopes.
  - The range of species and the incidence of clinically significant NTMB pulmonary infections continue to rise.
  - In addition to differences between the NTMB species, differences in host defense may modify the manifestations of NTMB disease.
- Classification
  - NTMB species can be broadly divided into fast- and slow-growing types.
  - The most common and most important slow-growing species is *M. avium* complex (MAC) (increasing incidence worldwide). A wide variety of other species are recognized, many of which do not cause clinically significant infection.
  - Fast-growing types include *M. chelonae*, *M. fortuitum*, and *M. abscessus*, all of which can cause pulmonary disease.
- Clinical presentation
  - The level of host immunity has a profound effect on the severity of infection caused by NTMB.
  - The slow-growing NTMB (e.g., MAC) cause a variable immune (granulomatous) response once across the bronchial mucosa surface.
  - A secure diagnosis of pulmonary NTMB infection can be made only when microbiologic, clinical, and imaging findings are considered. A normal chest radiograph does not preclude the diagnosis of NTMB infection.
- Treatment
  - The decision to treat NTMB infection is complex and often influenced by patient factors and the NTMB species.
  - Surgical resection is an option in localized disease, particularly for drug-resistant species (e.g., *M. abscessus*).

treated with a regular anti-TB combination, which usually includes a rifamycin.

Experience in the treatment of infections caused by rapidly growing mycobacteria (e.g., *M. abscessus* and *M. fortuitum*) is less extensive,[41] but treatment of this form of NTMB infection includes clarithromycin. Of importance, there are differences in the chance of successful antimicrobial treatment between these species. In general, *M. abscessus* is relatively resistant to treatment, with little obvious response and a poor outcome.

SURGICAL TREATMENT

In some individuals with intractable NTMB infections, particularly when the disease appears to be severe and localized on CT, surgical resection is an important therapeutic option. Patients with fibrotic and cavitary disease may respond dramatically to surgery and become sputum negative despite having already received "adequate" drug treatment.[65] A surgical approach may be more readily considered for NTMB infections that are not responsive to drug treatment, such as *M. abscessus*.

SUGGESTED READINGS

Chalermskulrat W, Gilbey JG, Donohue JF. Nontuberculous mycobacteria in women, young and old. *Clin Chest Med*. 2002;23:675–686.

Ellis SM, Hansell DM. Imaging of non-tuberculous (atypical) mycobacterial pulmonary infection. *Clin Radiol*. 2002;57:661–669.

Erasmus JJ, McAdams HP, Farrell MA, Patz EF. Pulmonary nontuberculous mycobacterial infection: radiologic manifestations. *Radiographics*. 1999;19:1487–1503.

Griffith DE, Aksamit T, Brown-Elliott BA, Catanzaro A, Daley C, Gordin F, et al. An official ATS/IDSA statement: diagnosis, treatment, and prevention of nontuberculous mycobacterial diseases. *Am J Respir Crit Care Med*. 2007;175:367–416.

Heifets L. Mycobacterial infections caused by nontuberculous mycobacteria. *Semin Respir Crit Care Med*. 2004;25:283–295.

Henry MT, Inamdar L, O'Riordain D, et al. Nontuberculous mycobacteria in non-HIV patients: epidemiology, treatment and response. *Eur Respir J*. 2004;23:741–746.

The full reference list for this chapter is available at ExpertConsult.com.

12 Fungal Infections

SUZANNE C. BYRNE | REBECCA M. LINDELL | THOMAS E. HARTMAN

Etiology

Fungal infections of the chest can be divided into two groups based on pathogenesis. The first group is composed of endemic fungi, including *Histoplasma capsulatum, Coccidioides immitis, Blastomyces dermatitidis,* and *Cryptococcus gattii,* and the second group is composed of opportunistic fungi, including *Aspergillus, Candida, Cryptococcus neoformans,* and *Zygomycetes.*

Prevalence and Epidemiology

The endemic fungi typically reside in the soil of certain regions, which is discussed in more detail in subsequent subsections. Infection primarily occurs when an otherwise healthy individual lives in or visits an endemic area and inhales microconidia (spores) of the fungus. In contrast, opportunistic fungi are ubiquitous and are found worldwide. These fungi tend to infect individuals with underlying lung disease or suppressed immune systems.

Clinical Presentation

In most individuals respiratory infection with endemic fungi is mild or subclinical and self-limited. In a few patients the infection is more severe, may disseminate, and can be fatal. Infection tends to be more severe after heavy microconidial exposure.[1] The infection may manifest after the patient has left the endemic area, so clinical familiarity with the disease is important even outside the endemic regions.

Opportunistic fungal infections, especially *Aspergillus* infection, have a variety of clinical manifestations that will be described in detail. Immunocompromised individuals and individuals with underlying lung disease are at increased risk of more serious disease with either endemic or opportunistic fungal infections.

Pathophysiology

PATHOLOGY

Immunocompetent patients with endemic fungal chest infection most often develop bronchopneumonia with regional lymph node involvement. These patients rarely progress to chronic forms of the disease or dissemination. Patients with underlying lung disease or immunocompromised patients are at risk for more serious forms of infection, such as dissemination, chronic infection, angioinvasion, or extension into the pleura or chest wall. Asthmatics may develop a hypersensitivity reaction to *Aspergillus* infection, resulting in dilated segmental and proximal subsegmental bronchi that often contain mucus plugs.

Manifestations of the Disease

HISTOPLASMOSIS

Acute Histoplasmosis

General. Histoplasmosis is caused by inhalation of the microconidia of the dimorphic fungus *H. capsulatum.* Endemic regions include central and eastern North America, especially in the Ohio, Mississippi, and St. Lawrence River valleys. Bird and bat droppings enhance its growth by accelerating sporulation.[1] More than half of adults living in endemic areas have been infected with *H. capsulatum.*[1] Acute histoplasmosis may be asymptomatic or may result in a flu-like illness, including a fever, dry cough, and fatigue. The severity of the illness may vary with level of exposure or immune status or both.

Radiography. The chest radiograph in most patients is normal.[2] In asymptomatic individuals the most common finding is a solitary pulmonary nodule of variable size.[3] Nodules in asymptomatic individuals may enlarge, may be multiple, and are often associated with lymphadenopathy.[3] Nodule cavitation is rare.[3] Symptomatic patients most commonly show single or multiple areas of patchy airspace consolidation with a lower lung predominance (Fig. 12.1).[3] Mediastinal and hilar lymphadenopathy is common and may be the only finding.[2] Pleural effusions are rare.[3] More severe cases, such as cases occurring after heavy exposure, may show multiple small nodules or patchy airspace consolidation in both lungs (see Fig. 12.1). The former may resemble metastatic disease.[3] Airspace consolidation may form a nodule while clearing.[3]

A nodule may persist despite resolution of the acute infection. It may subsequently calcify, forming a calcified granuloma. Infected lymph nodes also may calcify (Fig. 12.2). The presence of central, laminar, or diffuse calcification within a nodule, calcification within an associated lymph node, or both helps identify a nodule as a calcified granuloma. This also helps to distinguish a nodule from a primary lung cancer.

Computed Tomography. Computed tomography (CT) may reveal unilateral or bilateral nodules or areas of consolidation and lymphadenopathy that often mimic primary lung cancer (see Fig. 12.1).[4] Satellite nodules and centrilobular nodules (sometimes with a tree-in-bud pattern) also may be seen. As the findings of acute histoplasmosis resolve, a nodule may persist and develop central, laminated, or diffuse calcification (see Fig. 12.2). CT without intravenous (IV) contrast administration is helpful to detect these benign patterns of calcification and identify them as a calcified granuloma, with histoplasmosis being one possible cause. CT without IV contrast administration also improves detection of calcification of associated lymph nodes. Calcified granulomas also may be seen in the liver and spleen.

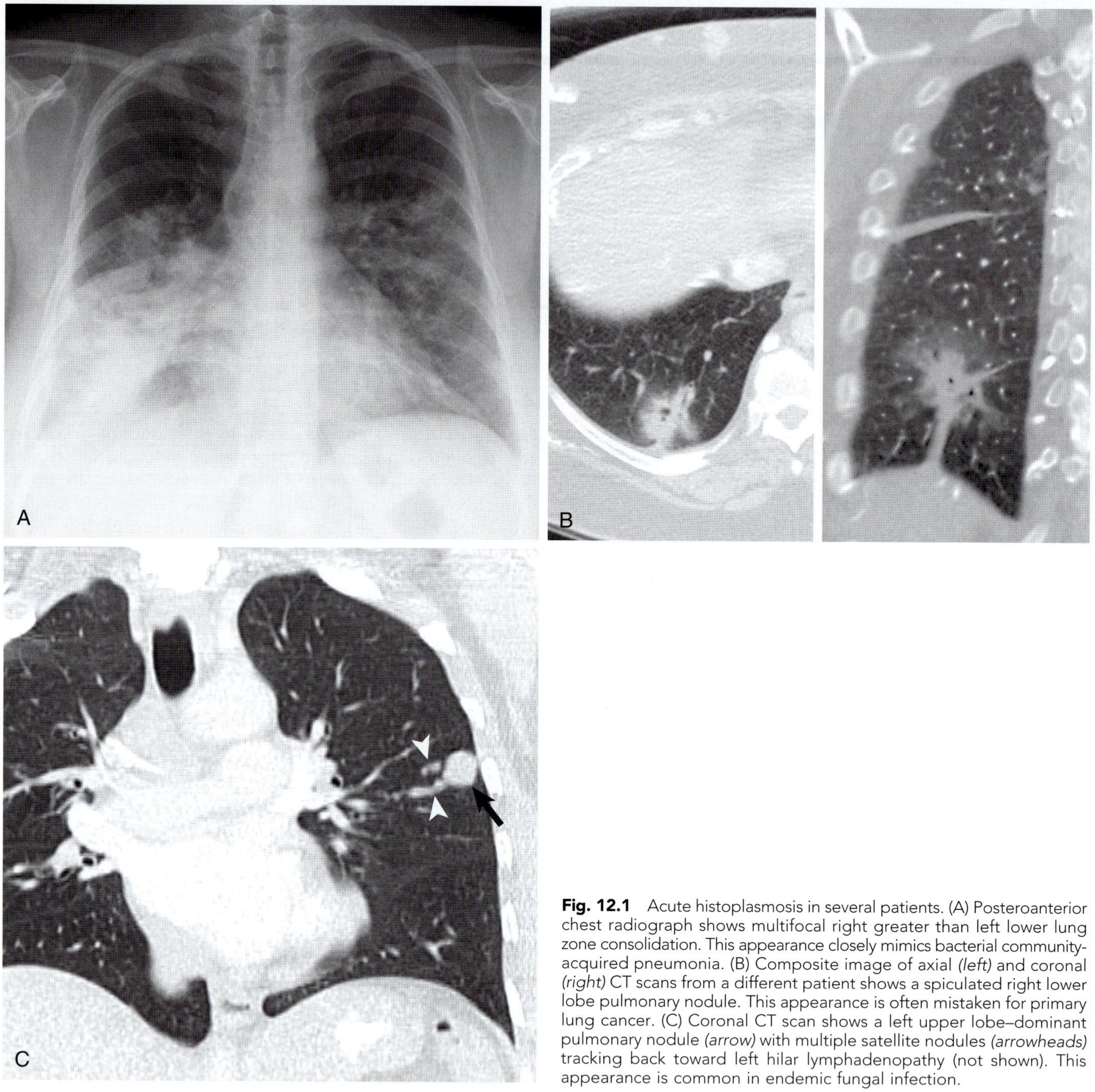

Fig. 12.1 Acute histoplasmosis in several patients. (A) Posteroanterior chest radiograph shows multifocal right greater than left lower lung zone consolidation. This appearance closely mimics bacterial community-acquired pneumonia. (B) Composite image of axial *(left)* and coronal *(right)* CT scans from a different patient shows a spiculated right lower lobe pulmonary nodule. This appearance is often mistaken for primary lung cancer. (C) Coronal CT scan shows a left upper lobe–dominant pulmonary nodule *(arrow)* with multiple satellite nodules *(arrowheads)* tracking back toward left hilar lymphadenopathy (not shown). This appearance is common in endemic fungal infection.

Positron Emission Tomography/Computed Tomography. In general, infection may have increased glucose metabolism and cause a false-positive positron emission tomography (PET)/CT scan. This may be a confounding factor when PET/CT is used in the workup of histoplasmosis or any fungal infection.

Imaging Algorithms. Initially, the patient would likely have a posteroanterior and lateral chest radiograph. A routine chest CT would not typically be obtained unless there was clinical uncertainty about the diagnosis (i.e., concern for malignancy) or if the patient's clinical course was not progressing as expected. CT without IV contrast administration is suggested because it helps detect and characterize calcification in nodules and lymph nodes.

CLASSIC SIGNS

- Normal chest radiograph
- Solitary or multiple nodules
- Single or patchy areas of airspace consolidation
- Mediastinal or hilar lymphadenopathy
- Possible satellite nodules on CT
- Nodules and lymphadenopathy often calcify with time

Chronic Histoplasmosis

General. Chronic pulmonary histoplasmosis is rare and occurs almost exclusively in middle-aged men with emphysema.[3,5] The infection can mimic post–primary tuberculosis, but symptoms

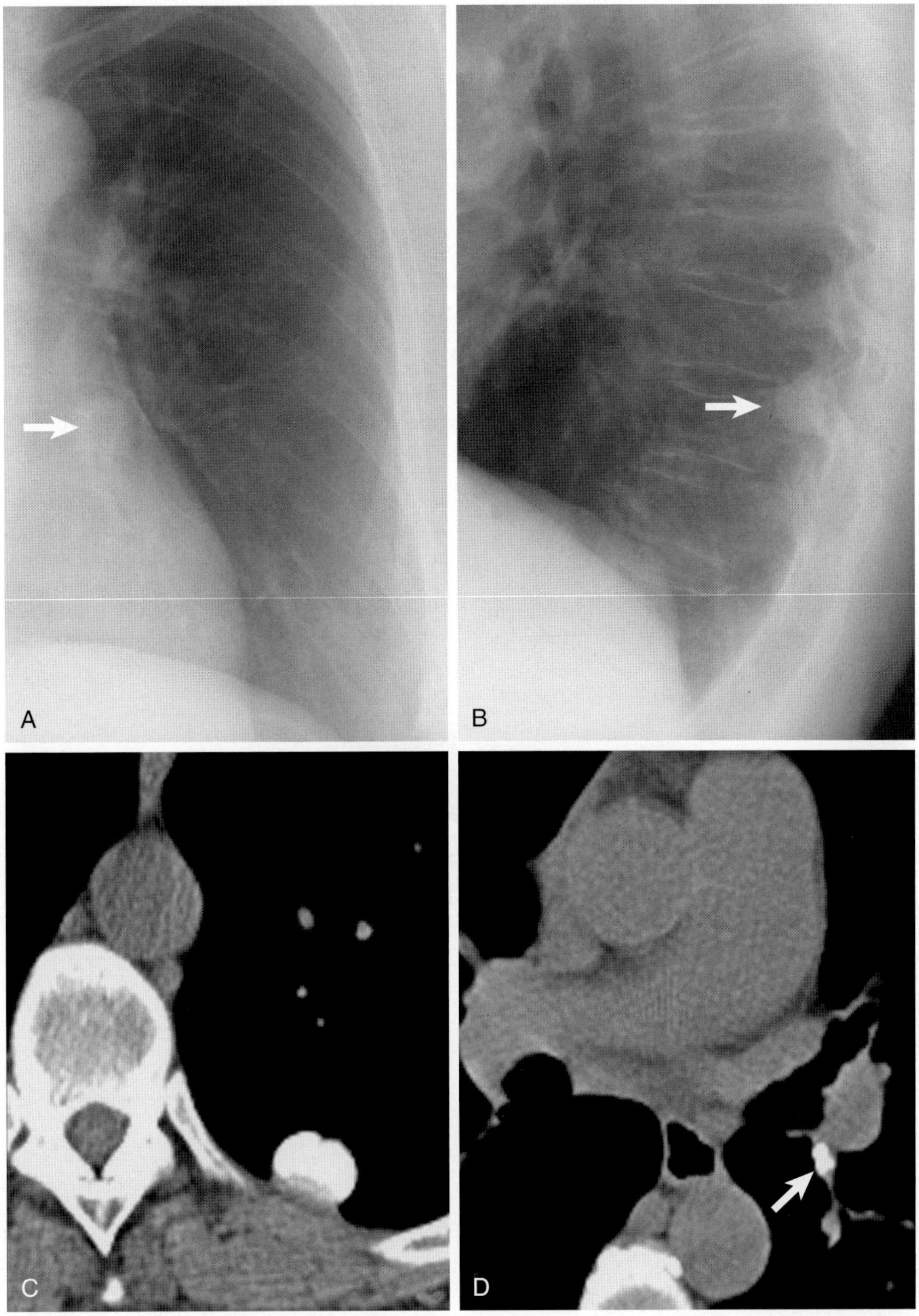

Fig. 12.2 Calcified granuloma secondary to histoplasmosis. Posteroanterior (A) and lateral (B) chest radiographs show an indeterminate nodule *(arrows)* in the left lower lobe. (C) and (D) CT scans show that the nodule is densely calcified and is associated with a calcified left hilar lymph node (D, *arrow*).

are not as severe, and the course is usually self-limited and nonfatal.[5] Pathogenesis is thought to be caused by spore inhalation into upper lobe bullae resulting in fluid formation within the bullae.[3] The antigen-filled fluid may spread via spillage into the bronchial tree, resulting in pneumonitis in other areas of the lungs.[3] Symptoms include productive cough, fever, dyspnea, fatigue, weight loss, and hemoptysis.[1]

Radiography. Radiographs show unilateral or bilateral upper lobe airspace opacities that usually extend to the pleura.[3] There are usually changes of emphysema. If a bulla is surrounded by airspace opacity, it may resemble a cavitary lesion, mimicking tuberculosis. The "cavity" may develop wall thickening, change size, or develop an air-fluid level.[3,5] The thickness of the wall roughly reflects the activity level of the infection.[3] There may be adjacent pleural thickening. Adjacent lung parenchyma may be destroyed as the cavity enlarges. The cavity may become secondarily infected by an aspergilloma (see subsequent section). In contrast to acute histoplasmosis, lymphadenopathy is usually absent.[5]

Computed Tomography. CT may be used to show the aforementioned radiographic findings in more detail.

Imaging Algorithms. Chronic histoplasmosis would likely be imaged using a chest radiograph, followed by chest CT for further evaluation. Either modality could be used to follow the response to treatment.

CLASSIC SIGNS

- Unilateral or bilateral upper lobe airspace opacities with emphysema
- Bulla with surrounding airspace opacity, mimicking a cavitary lesion
- No lymphadenopathy

Histoplasmoma

General. When a nodule resulting from histoplasmosis slowly enlarges over time, it is referred to as a histoplasmoma.[5] Histologic sections show that a histoplasmoma is a small necrotic focus surrounded by a massive fibrous capsule.[6] Increasing fibrosis at the periphery of the lesion results in its growth.[5,7] Histoplasmomas are typically asymptomatic.

Radiography. The most common finding is a discrete nodule measuring less than 30 mm in diameter that is most often located peripherally and in a lower lobe.[2,5] The nodule may be uncalcified or may have central, diffuse, or laminated calcification.[6] In one study,[6] the growth rate varied from 0.5 to 2.8 mm per year, averaging 1.7 mm per year. Satellite nodules and calcified hilar lymph nodes are common.[2]

Computed Tomography. CT without IV contrast administration is more sensitive than radiographs in detecting benign patterns of calcification and can help distinguish a histoplasmoma from a bronchogenic carcinoma. Growth rates can be measured more accurately on CT, which may be helpful because histoplasmomas tend to grow more slowly than typical bronchogenic carcinomas (Fig. 12.3).

Imaging Algorithms. Histoplasmomas likely would be detected first as a nodule on a chest radiograph. A thin-section chest CT scan without IV contrast administration would be helpful to detect and characterize possible internal calcification. Follow-up using unenhanced CT would be helpful to assess for change in calcification or size over time.

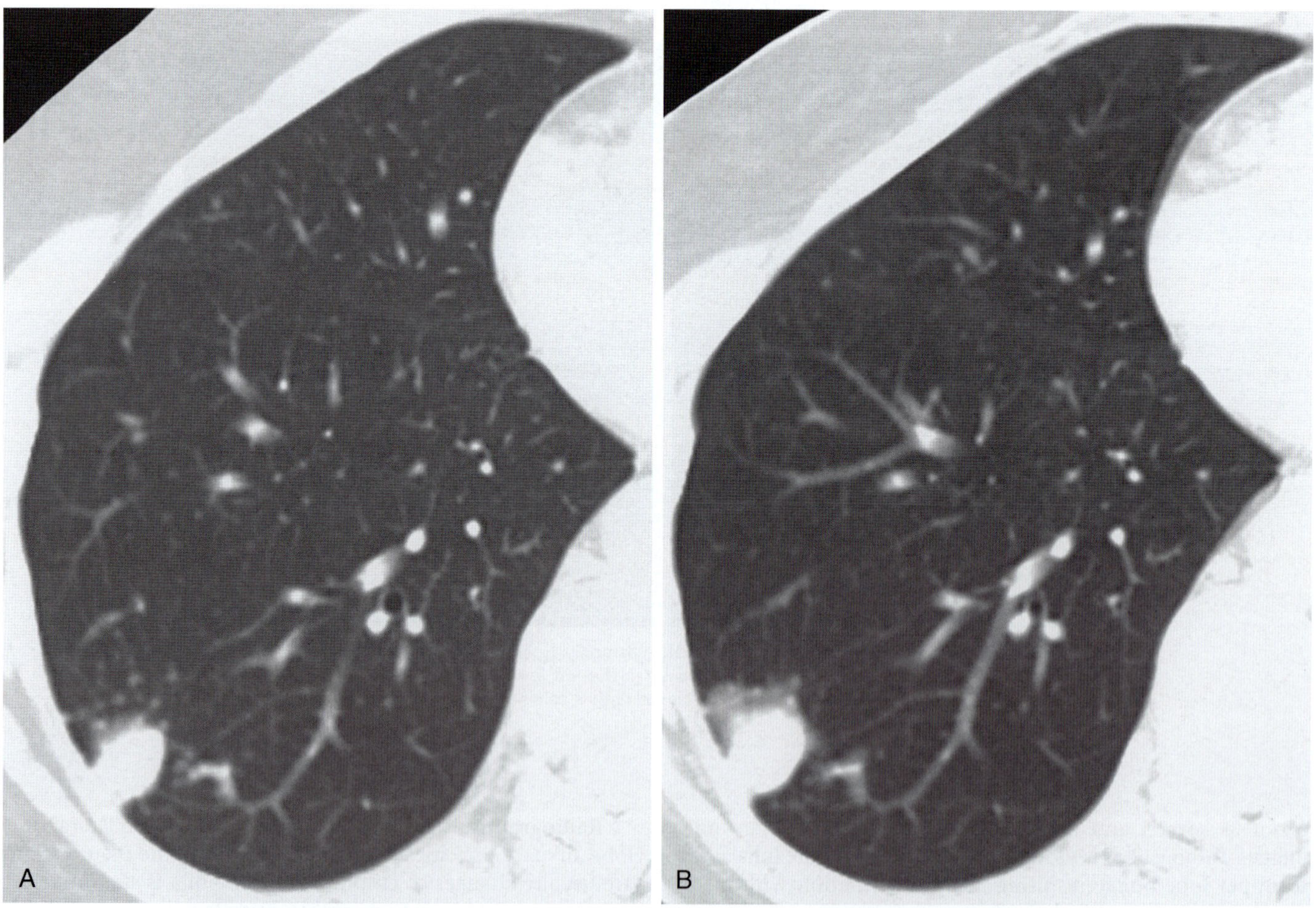

Fig. 12.3 Histoplasmoma incidentally discovered on routine chest radiograph. (A) CT scan shows a peripheral right lower lobe nodule with tiny surrounding satellite nodules. (B) CT scan 13 months later shows that the nodule is larger, and satellite nodules have improved. The nodule was noncalcified on both scans. It was surgically removed and was compatible with a histoplasmoma.

CLASSIC SIGNS

- Discrete nodule enlarging slowly over time
- May have central, diffuse, or laminated calcification
- Associated satellite nodules or calcified lymphadenopathy

Disseminated Histoplasmosis

General. Disseminated histoplasmosis, a rare form of histoplasmosis infection, is an opportunistic infection that affects immunocompromised individuals, such as organ transplant recipients or acquired immune deficiency syndrome (AIDS) patients, infants, or adults older than 54 years, especially men.[2,3,5] Human immunodeficiency virus-1 infection is a major risk factor.[1] Dissemination may result from progression of a primary infection or from reactivation of a prior infection. Severely immunocompromised patients and infants may present with respiratory distress, hepatic and renal failure, shock, and coagulopathy and are at risk of a rapidly fatal course.[1] Other patients experience chronic progressive symptoms of fever, cough, weight loss, dyspnea, night sweats, and fatigue. Decreased mental status and headaches occur in 40% of patients.[3]

Radiography. Chest radiographs may be normal.[3] Normal chest radiographs occur in approximately 50% of AIDS patients compared with 30% of patients with immunodeficiency from other causes.[3] When abnormal, radiographs most commonly show multiple diffuse bilateral nodules, usually measuring 3 mm in size (Fig. 12.4).[3,5] The second most common finding is the presence of linear or irregular opacities, which are often diffuse.[3] Nodules or linear opacities may progress to diffuse airspace disease.[5] Focal airspace opacities occur in approximately 10% of cases.[3] Lymphadenopathy and pleural effusions are uncommon.[3,5]

Computed Tomography. Miliary nodules may be seen on CT, measuring 1 to 3 mm in diameter with poorly or sharply defined margins (see Fig. 12.4). The nodules are randomly distributed and can be seen along interlobular septa, vessels, and fissures and within the secondary pulmonary lobule. There is frequently mild hilar and mediastinal lymphadenopathy.[8]

Imaging Algorithms. Chest radiographs may be obtained initially, but thin-section chest CT without IV contrast would be more sensitive to detect disease.

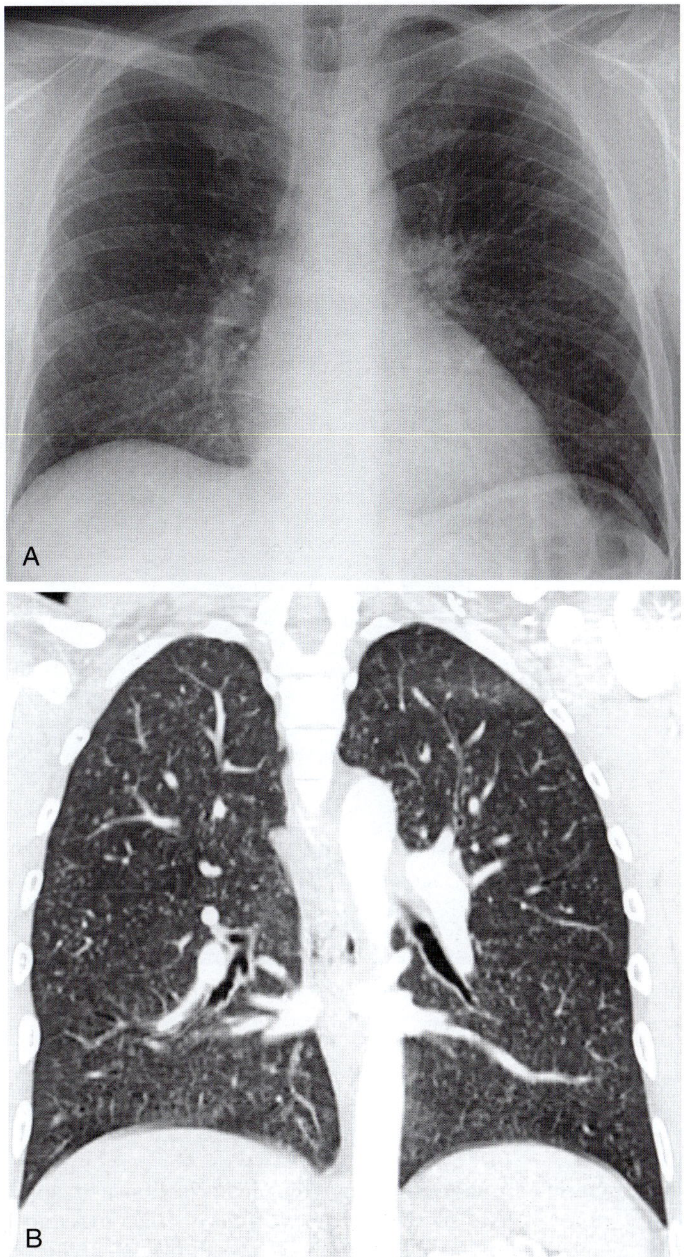

Fig. 12.4 Disseminated histoplasmosis in man with AIDS. (A) Chest radiograph shows diffuse bilateral tiny pulmonary nodules. (B) Coronal CT scan shows randomly distributed miliary nodules throughout both lungs.

CLASSIC SIGNS

- Chest radiograph may be normal
- Multiple diffuse bilateral 1- to 3-mm nodules that may progress to airspace disease

Mediastinal Granuloma and Fibrosing Mediastinitis

General. As a sequela to histoplasmosis infection, a chronic fibrotic process may develop in the mediastinum either diffusely (fibrosing mediastinitis) or locally (mediastinal granuloma).[5] The latter process is more common and is composed of enlarged lymph nodes that have become matted together and surrounded by a fibrous capsule.[3,5] Mediastinal granuloma or fibrosis may lead to obstruction of the superior vena cava, pulmonary vessels, central airways, or esophagus.[1]

Radiography. Chest radiographs may show mediastinal widening (from the granuloma or distended collateral vessels or both), atelectasis or consolidation (from central airway obstruction), signs of pulmonary infarct (from vascular obstruction), or nodal calcification.[3,5,9]

Computed Tomography. CT is essential to reveal the specific details of mediastinal fibrosis or granuloma. The most common finding is a localized calcified mediastinal or hilar soft tissue mass, which in the appropriate clinical setting is highly suggestive of histoplasmosis-induced fibrosing granuloma or mediastinitis (Fig. 12.5).[9,10] There may be associated lymph nodes that may be calcified. With IV contrast, CT can demonstrate vascular involvement, including superior vena cava obstruction and pulmonary venous or arterial narrowing (see Fig. 12.5). Tracheal and/or bronchial narrowing may also be seen, depending on the location and extent of involvement.[9,10]

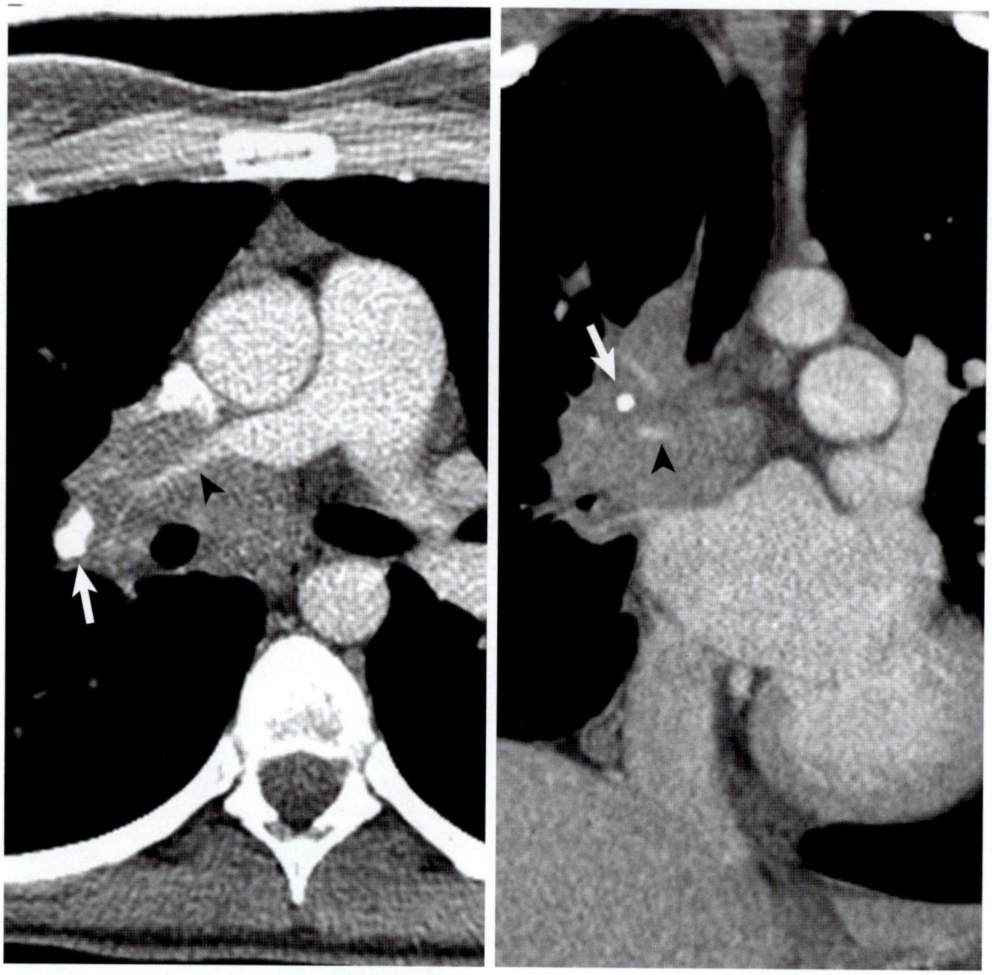

Fig. 12.5 Fibrosing mediastinitis. Composite image with axial *(left)* and coronal *(right)* contrast-enhanced CT scans shows a partially calcified *(arrows)* right hilar and mediastinal mass that encases and narrows the right pulmonary artery *(arrowhead)* and occludes the right superior pulmonary vein.

Magnetic Resonance Imaging. Magnetic resonance imaging (MRI) may be used to show a mediastinal or hilar mass and vascular narrowing or obstruction. There is typically a heterogeneous, infiltrating mass of intermediate signal intensity on T1-weighted images and variable signal intensity on T2-weighted images.[11] Fibrosis and calcification are typically responsible for decreased signal intensity on T2-weighted images, whereas areas of active inflammation can cause increased T2 signal intensity.[11] The presence of decreased signal intensity within a mediastinal mass on MRI may help distinguish it from neoplasm.[11] MRI may be an alternative to CT in patients who cannot receive IV CT contrast agents.[11]

Positron Emission Tomography/Computed Tomography. Fibrosing mediastinitis or mediastinal granuloma may cause a false-positive PET/CT scan, and this modality is not routinely used for evaluation of this condition.[12,13]

Imaging Algorithms. Routine chest CT without and with IV contrast administration is helpful to detect and define the fibrosis or granuloma, associated calcifications, and vascular or central airway narrowing. In cases of esophageal involvement, an esophagogram may be helpful to evaluate motility and patency and to detect possible traction diverticula.

CLASSIC SIGNS

- Widened mediastinum on chest radiograph
- Mediastinal or hilar soft tissue mass with calcifications
- Secondary narrowing of airways, superior vena cava, pulmonary vessels, or esophagus

Broncholithiasis

General. A calcified peribronchial lymph node caused by histoplasmosis occasionally may erode into an airway, causing broncholithiasis.[14] Symptoms most commonly include a nonproductive cough and hemoptysis. Less commonly, patients may have fever, chills, and pain from post–obstructive pneumonitis. Expectoration of a broncholith (lithoptysis) also may occur.

Radiography. The calcified lymph node may be seen on chest radiograph and may be associated with post–obstructive atelectasis, pneumonitis, or bronchiectasis. However, it may be difficult to see that the calcified lymph node is endoluminal.

Computed Tomography. Broncholithiasis may be diagnosed on CT as a calcified endobronchial or peribronchial nodule that has associated signs of obstruction, such as atelectasis, pneumonitis, and bronchiectasis (Fig. 12.6).[14] Unenhanced CT, using

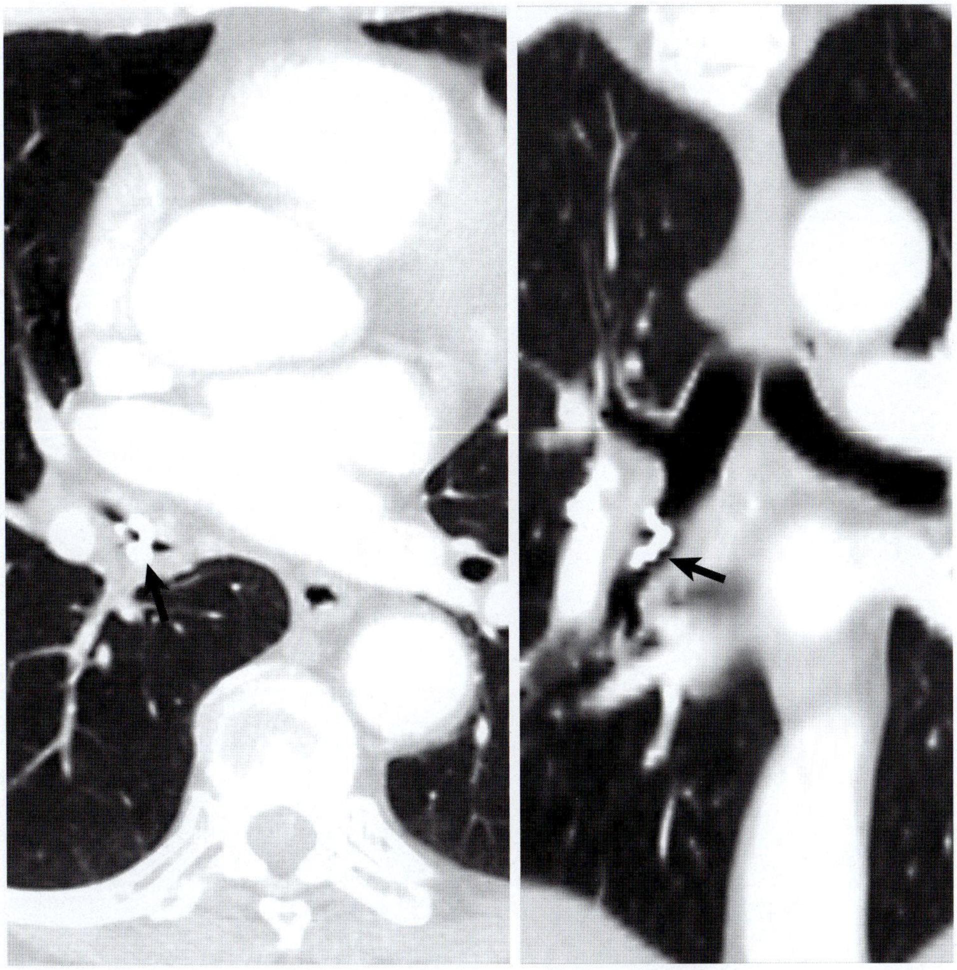

Fig. 12.6 Broncholithiasis. Composite image of axial *(left)* and coronal *(right)* contrast-enhanced CT scans shows a calcified broncholith *(arrows)* in the bronchus intermedius. Broncholiths are most common with previous histoplasmosis or tuberculosis infection.

thin collimation and multiplanar reconstruction, may be necessary to localize the broncholith accurately within the lumen and may aid bronchoscopic removal.

Imaging Algorithms. Routine chest CT is recommended without IV contrast administration. Thin-section imaging and multiplanar reconstruction may be necessary to localize the broncholith. Virtual bronchoscopy may aid in bronchoscopic removal.

CLASSIC SIGNS

- Calcified nodule in a bronchus
- Signs of prior granulomatous infection
- Post–obstructive atelectasis or consolidation or both

COCCIDIOIDOMYCOSIS

Coccidioidomycosis (San Joaquin Valley fever) is caused by the dimorphic fungus *C. immitis.*[15] This fungus is found in soil and is endemic in the southwestern United States, northern Mexico, and, to a lesser degree, regions of Central and South America.[15,16] Specific endemic areas of the United States include south-central Arizona, southern California (notably the San Joaquin Valley), western Texas, and parts of New Mexico.[15,16] The incidence of pulmonary coccidioidomycosis is highest in the late summer and early fall, when the soil is driest.[15] Infection is caused by inhalation of the fungal arthrospores or arthroconidia.[15–17]

Primary Coccidioidomycosis or Acute Pulmonary Coccidioidomycosis

General. Similar to histoplasmosis, most cases of primary coccidioidomycosis are asymptomatic or mild, although symptoms occur more frequently than in histoplasmosis.[15] Symptoms typically develop 1 to 4 weeks after exposure and comprise flu-like symptoms such as cough, fever, chest pain, fatigue, anorexia, and headache.[15–17] Skin rashes also may occur. The most common skin rash is a diffuse erythematous rash called toxic erythema, occurring in 10% to 30% of patients. Approximately 5% of patients develop erythema nodosum or erythema multiforme. These rashes may be associated with arthralgias and mild conjunctivitis, termed *Valley fever complex.*[15] The infection is usually self-limited, resolving over 3 to 6 weeks.[17]

Radiography. Various nonspecific findings are observed on chest radiographs.[16] The most common finding consists of single or multiple foci of airspace consolidation.[18] Single or multiple nodules also may occur,[19] which may cavitate and develop air-fluid

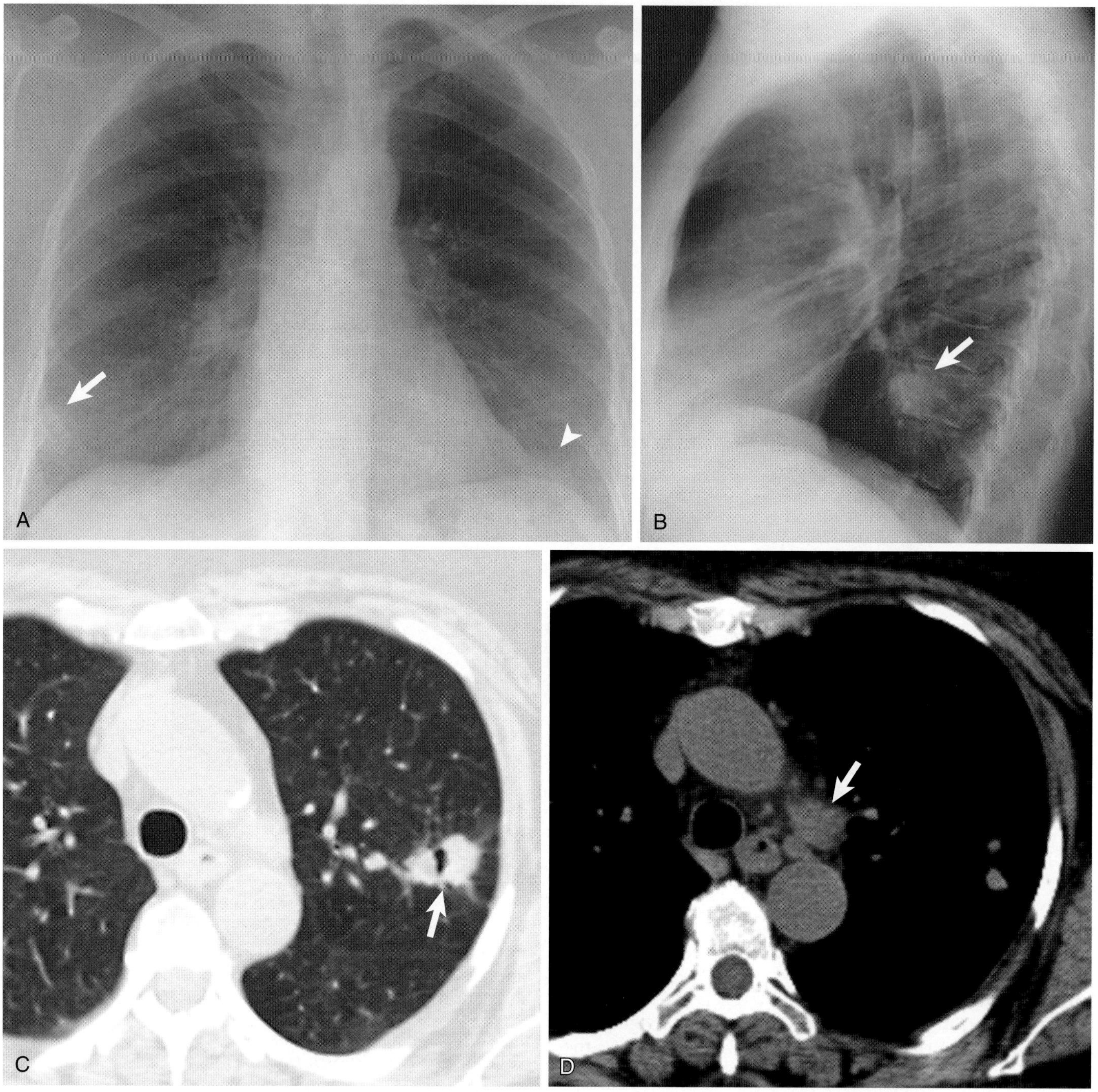

Fig. 12.7 Disseminated coccidioidomycosis acquired while vacationing in Arizona. Posteroanterior (A) and lateral (B) chest radiographs show a 3-cm mass *(arrow)* in the right lower lobe with associated right hilar lymphadenopathy and a small nodule (A, *arrowhead*) in the left lower lung. (C) Axial CT scan from a different patient shows a polylobulated cavitary left upper lobe pulmonary nodule *(arrow)* with small adjacent satellite nodules. (D) Axial CT scan in soft tissue window shows an enlarged aorticopulmonary window lymph node *(arrow)*. This CT appearance closely mimics primary lung cancer.

levels.[16] Hilar or mediastinal lymphadenopathy occurs in approximately 20% of cases, usually in association with lung parenchymal findings (Fig. 12.7).[19] Pleural effusions, most commonly small, may occur in 10% to 20% of patients as a result of contiguous spread from a subpleural focus.[16] Radiographic findings usually resolve completely.[16] Endobronchial or endotracheal involvement is rare.[20]

Computed Tomography. Chest CT may be used to show the morphology of small pulmonary lesions that are poorly seen on chest radiography.[17] Nodules (see Fig. 12.7) or consolidation may be seen. There may be associated satellite nodules (Fig. 12.8).

Imaging Algorithms. Chest radiographs are most commonly obtained. Chest CT may be helpful if the diagnosis is uncertain,

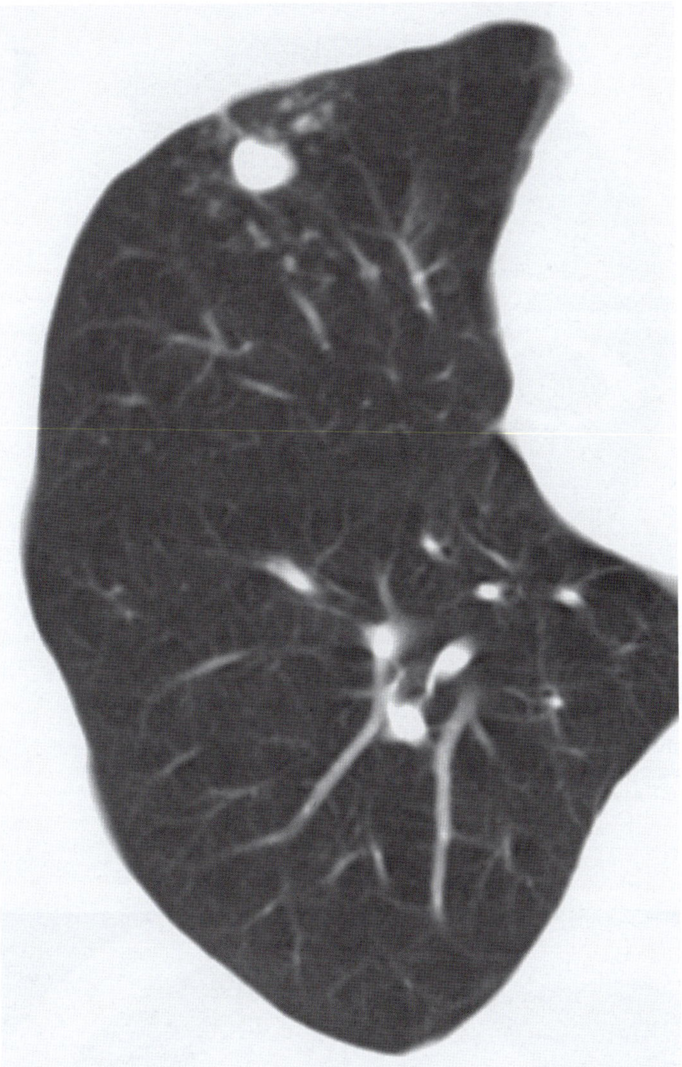

Fig. 12.8 Coccidioidomycosis in an asymptomatic man from Arizona. A chest radiograph (not shown) 1 year before was negative. Chest CT image shows a right middle lobe nodule surrounded by tiny satellite nodules. Surgical resection revealed caseating granulomas and coccidioidomycosis.

or if the patient does not improve as expected or develops a complication. Chest CT also may show satellite nodules not apparent on the radiograph.

CLASSIC SIGNS

- Single or multiple foci of consolidation or nodules
- May cavitate
- May have satellite nodules on CT

Chronic or Persistent Pulmonary Coccidioidomycosis

General. Approximately 5% of cases of primary coccidioidomycosis become chronic.[15] The infection commonly continues to be asymptomatic or mild but may develop into a severe pneumonia with fever, productive cough, night sweats, and hemoptysis.[16]

Radiography. The most common radiographic finding is cavitation, which is usually thin-walled, solitary, and in the upper lobes and is said to resemble a grape skin (Fig. 12.9).[16,21] Cavitations may become secondarily infected or may rupture into the pleural space and may cause pleural effusion, empyema, or pneumothorax.[16] Another radiographic finding consists of single or, less commonly, multiple pulmonary nodules.[16,18] Nodules or masses are 5 to 50 mm in diameter and are usually peripheral.[18] These can be difficult to distinguish from bronchogenic carcinoma or metastatic disease.

Computed Tomography. A retrospective analysis of 18 patients with chronic coccidioidomycosis showed that the most common CT finding was a solitary nodule measuring 10 to 20 mm in diameter in the periphery of the lungs.[22] Focal areas of ground-glass opacity and consolidation were less common. Nodules were most commonly homogeneous in attenuation, but central low attenuation, cavitation, or calcification also occurred (see Fig. 12.9). A few of these nodules had surrounding ground-glass opacity (CT halo sign), likely resulting from granulomatous inflammation or hemorrhage.

Imaging Algorithms. Chest radiographs are routinely obtained, but chest CT is more sensitive in depicting the findings and complications of chronic coccidioidomycosis.

CLASSIC SIGNS

- Solitary nodule or cavitation, usually thin-walled (grape skin sign)
- Upper lobe, peripheral

NORTH AMERICAN BLASTOMYCOSIS

General

North American blastomycosis is caused by the inhalation of asexually produced spores or conidia of the thermally dimorphic fungus *Blastomyces dermatitidis.*[23] The disease has endemic regions in Africa, Central America, and South America, but it is most common in North America. In North America endemic areas include the south-central and southeastern United States along the Ohio and Mississippi River valleys, midwestern states and Canadian provinces along the Great Lakes, and a small area in New York and Canada along the St. Lawrence River.[23] The fungus proliferates in the warm, moist soil of wooded areas rich in organic debris.[23]

Similar to histoplasmosis and coccidioidomycosis, blastomycosis may be asymptomatic or cause mild flu-like symptoms. More commonly, it manifests as acute pneumonia with fever, productive cough, pleuritic chest pain, arthralgias, and myalgias. Diagnosis is often delayed because its clinical and radiographic findings are nonspecific and variable and often mimic more common diseases.[23–26] Cutaneous lesions may occur and improve diagnostic accuracy.[24] These include a verrucous lesion with a raised, irregular border with crusting and drainage or an ulcerative lesion with a sharp, heaped-up border and exudate at its base.[23]

Radiography

Radiographic findings are varied and nonspecific and include consolidation, masses, nodules, cavitation, and interstitial changes. There is often an upper lobe predominance.[27,28] Findings often resemble community-acquired pneumonia, but granulomatous infection should be suspected if the findings progress or are slow

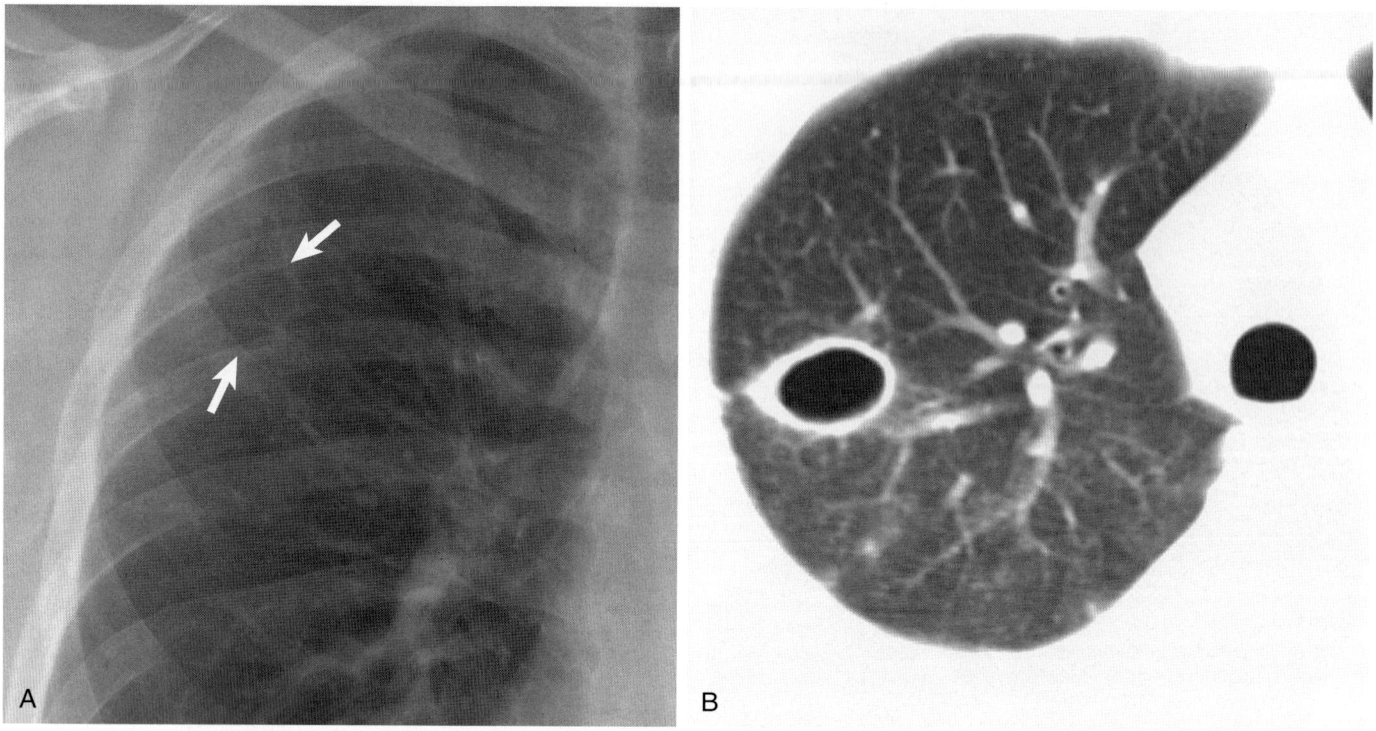

Fig. 12.9 Chronic coccidioidomycosis in a man with a chronic productive cough who developed acute chest pain while on vacation in Arizona. Chest radiograph (A) showed a subtle thin-walled cavity *(arrows)* in the right upper lobe that was confirmed on CT scan (B). Cultures from sputum and bronchial washings grew *Coccidioides immitis.*

to resolve.[25] The most common appearance is patchy or confluent airspace consolidation, which often has ill-defined margins and air bronchograms and is more commonly segmental or subsegmental than lobar.[27–30] The second most common appearance is a pulmonary mass or masses, which are typically well circumscribed, with smooth or irregular margins and 3 to 10 cm in diameter.[28–30] These may be confused with bronchogenic carcinoma.[29,31] Cavitation occurs in 11% to 37% of cases.[27,28,30,31] Interstitial changes, usually diffuse and bilateral, and nodules are less common.[28–30] Lymphadenopathy is uncommon.[29,30] Pleural effusions, usually very small, may occur in 21% of cases.[30] Pleural thickening without pleural effusion may occur.[28] Rarely, blastomycosis may aggressively cross tissue planes to cause pleural effusions, is chest wall masses, rib erosions, and cutaneous fistulae.[29]

Computed Tomography

In a study of CT findings in 16 patients with pulmonary blastomycosis, the most common finding was pulmonary masses (88%), which frequently contained air bronchograms.[26] Other common findings included nodules less than 2 cm in diameter (75%), perihilar location of parenchymal disease (75%), satellite lesions (69%), and consolidation (56%) (Figs. 12.10 and 12.11). Less common findings included lymphadenopathy (25%), pleural thickening (25%), pleural effusion (13%), and cavitation (13%). Parenchymal findings or lymphadenopathy is occasionally calcified (25% and 44%, respectively).

Imaging Algorithms

Chest radiography is helpful to detect disease, but chest CT is more sensitive and depicts the findings and possible complications. Both modalities are helpful in monitoring treatment response.

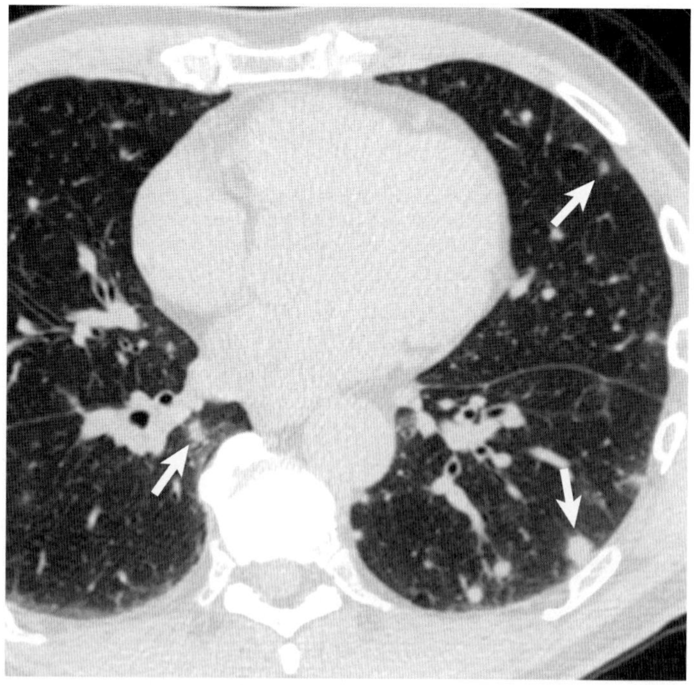

Fig. 12.10 Blastomycosis in a man with myalgias, fever, and fatigue. Axial CT scan shows multiple bilateral pulmonary nodules *(arrows)* of varying sizes. Bronchial washings grew *Blastomyces dermatitidis.*

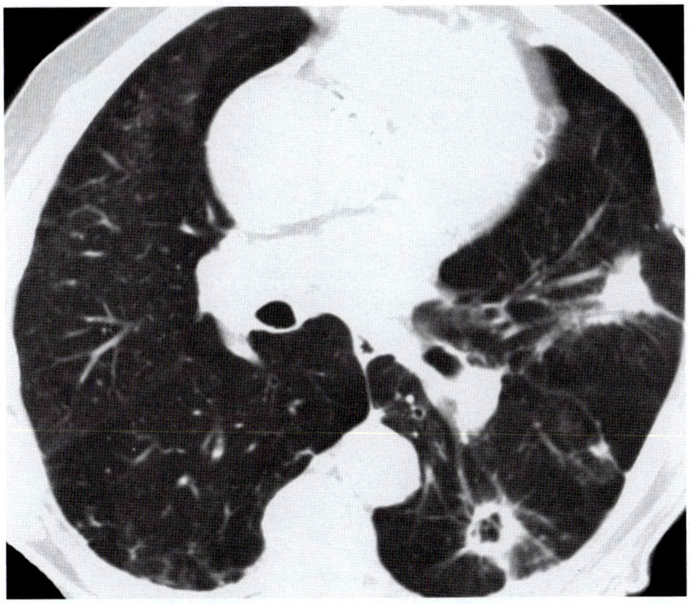

Fig. 12.11 Blastomycosis in a diabetic man with worsening chronic cough with blood-streaked sputum. CT scan shows an irregular cavitary nodule in the left lower lobe and an adjacent smaller nodule. Note additional spiculated nodule in the lingula. Serology was positive for *Blastomyces*.

CLASSIC SIGNS

- Radiologic findings are varied and nonspecific
- Consolidation, masses, nodules, cavitation, or interstitial changes
- May mimic community-acquired pneumonia or bronchogenic carcinoma

ASPERGILLOSIS

Aspergillus is a ubiquitous opportunistic fungus that has been found in soil, in decaying organic matter, and even in the sand of the Sahara Desert.[32] There are approximately 200 species of *Aspergillus,* but only a few cause aspergillosis in humans.[33] The most common of these is *Aspergillus fumigatus,* followed by *Aspergillus flavus* and *Aspergillus niger. Aspergillus* infection may manifest in clinically and radiologically distinct patterns: (1) saprophytic aspergillosis (aspergilloma), (2) allergic bronchopulmonary aspergillosis, (3) semiinvasive aspergillosis, (4) airway invasive aspergillosis, and (5) angioinvasive aspergillosis.[34]

Saprophytic Aspergillosis (Aspergilloma)

General. The most common form of *Aspergillus* infection is an aspergilloma, also known as fungus ball or mycetoma.[33] It is composed of fungal mycelia, inflammatory cells, fibrin, mucus, and tissue debris and usually develops in a preexisting lung cavity.[33] Other fungi may cause a mycetoma, but *Aspergillus* is the most common cause.[32,33] Preexisting lung cavities may result from numerous causes, such as tuberculosis, sarcoidosis, emphysematous bulla, bronchiectasis, ankylosing spondylitis, bronchial cysts, neoplasm, infarction, or cavitary infections.[33] Clinically, the patient may be asymptomatic or may have mild hemoptysis. Severe hemoptysis also may occur.

Radiography. The classic radiographic finding is an upper lobe rounded or oval mass within a cavity with a crescent of air around the mass (air crescent sign) (Figs. 12.12 and 12.13).[32,33]

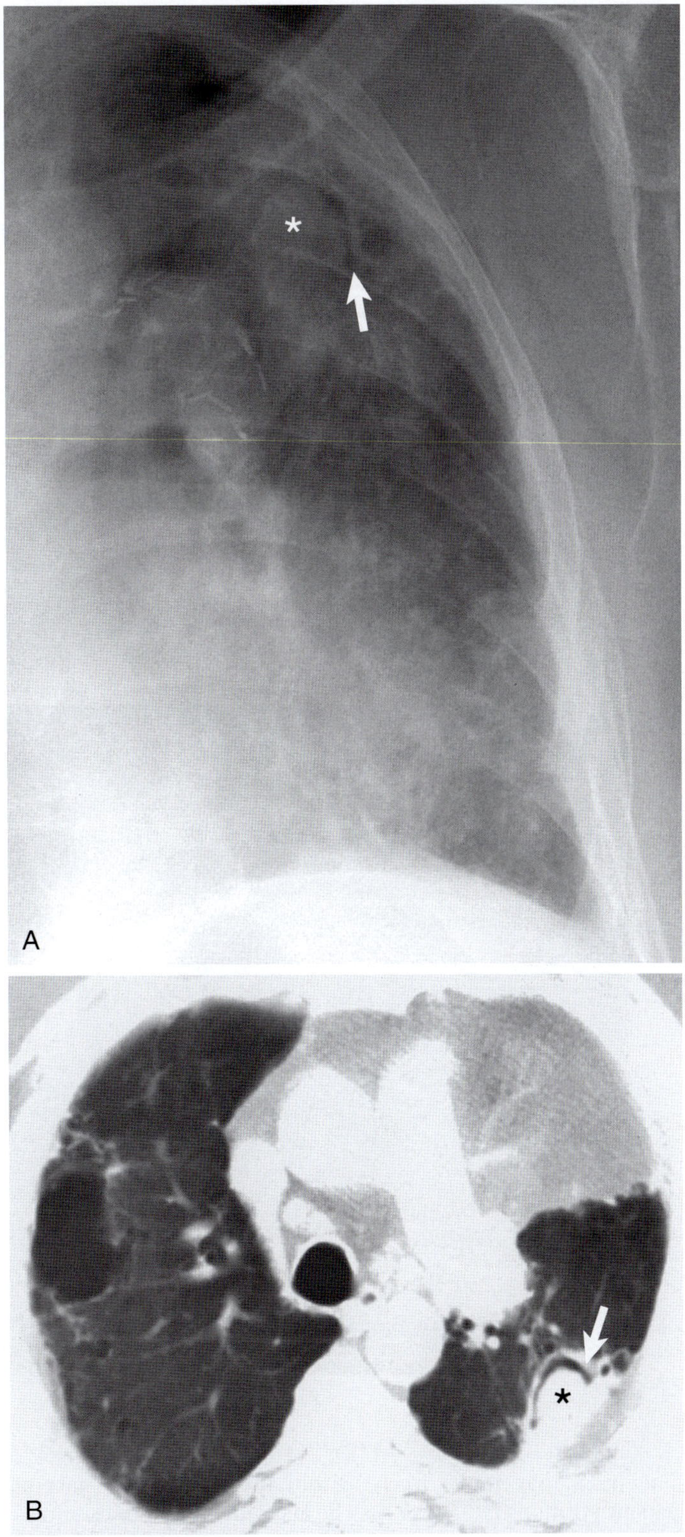

Fig. 12.12 Aspergilloma in a man with bullous emphysema and hemoptysis status post left upper lobectomy 6 years previously for an aspergilloma. (A) Close-up view on chest radiograph shows the nodular opacity *(asterisk)* in the left upper lung with a crescent of air surrounding the nodule *(arrow)*, known as the air crescent sign. (B) Axial CT scan shows a soft tissue nodule *(asterisk)* with air crescent sign *(arrow)* within a cavity in the left upper lung and emphysema in the right lung.

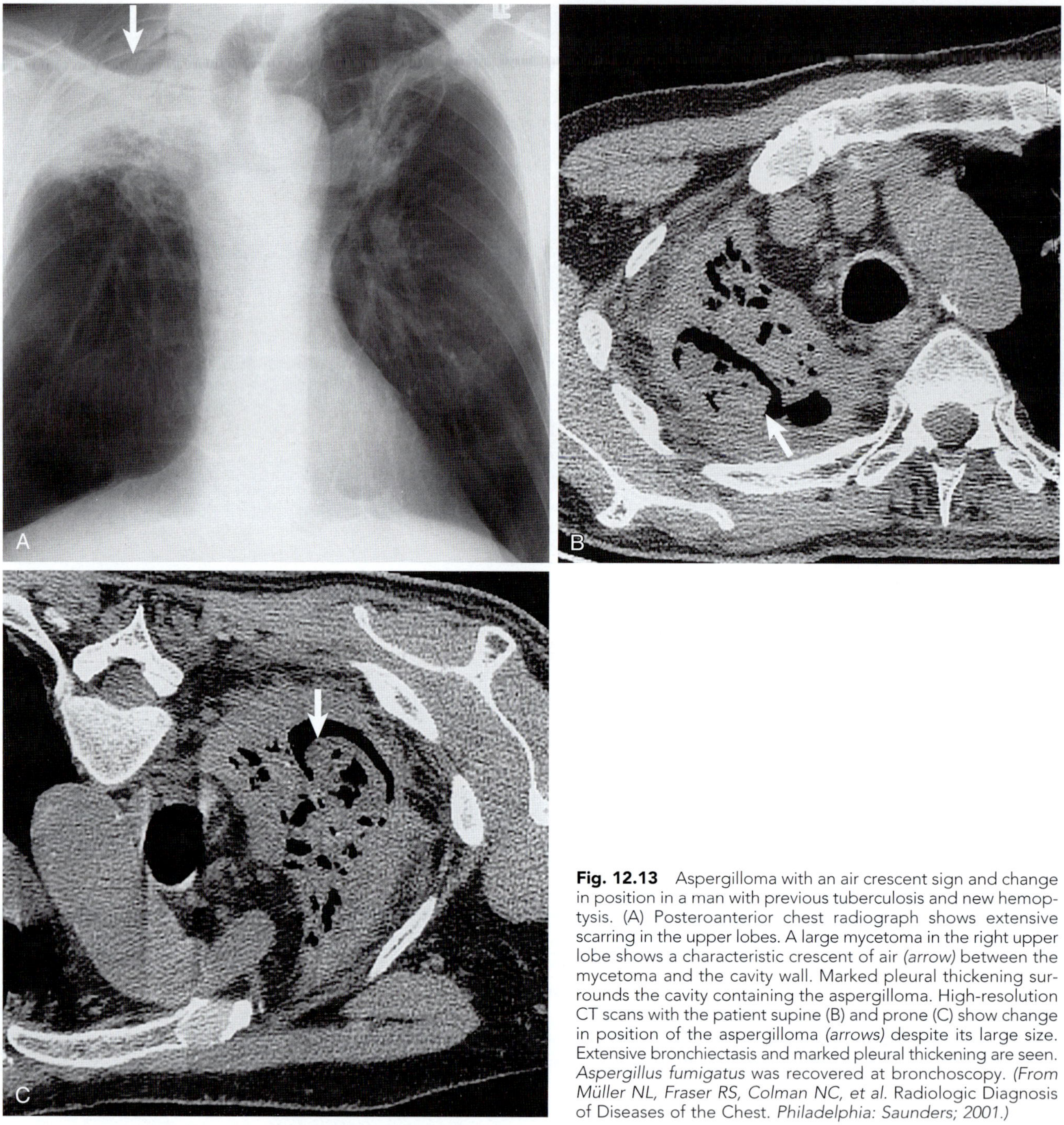

Fig. 12.13 Aspergilloma with an air crescent sign and change in position in a man with previous tuberculosis and new hemoptysis. (A) Posteroanterior chest radiograph shows extensive scarring in the upper lobes. A large mycetoma in the right upper lobe shows a characteristic crescent of air *(arrow)* between the mycetoma and the cavity wall. Marked pleural thickening surrounds the cavity containing the aspergilloma. High-resolution CT scans with the patient supine (B) and prone (C) show change in position of the aspergilloma *(arrows)* despite its large size. Extensive bronchiectasis and marked pleural thickening are seen. *Aspergillus fumigatus* was recovered at bronchoscopy. *(From Müller NL, Fraser RS, Colman NC, et al.* Radiologic Diagnosis of Diseases of the Chest. *Philadelphia: Saunders; 2001.)*

The mass may move freely within the cavity with varying patient positions.[33,35] There may be adjacent pleural thickening.[33] Pleural thickening may precede the development of the fungus ball within the cavity by up to 3 years.[36] Occasionally, the air crescent sign is not seen because it may be too small to be detected by radiography or the aspergilloma completely fills in the cavity.

Computed Tomography. Areas of increased attenuation, likely as a result of calcification, may be seen within the aspergilloma on CT.[35] CT may depict an air crescent sign that was too small to be seen on the chest radiograph. CT also may show signs of a developing aspergilloma, such as the fungal fronds developing on cavity walls or intersecting with each other to form a sponge-like irregular mass within the cavity (Fig. 12.14).[35]

Imaging Algorithms. Chest CT may show signs of an aspergilloma that are not detectable on chest radiography. For this reason, chest CT is preferred for diagnosis and monitoring treatment.

CLASSIC SIGNS

- Upper lobe rounded mass within a cavity
- Crescent of air around the mass (air crescent sign)
- Mass may be mobile
- Fronds or sponge-like appearance on CT

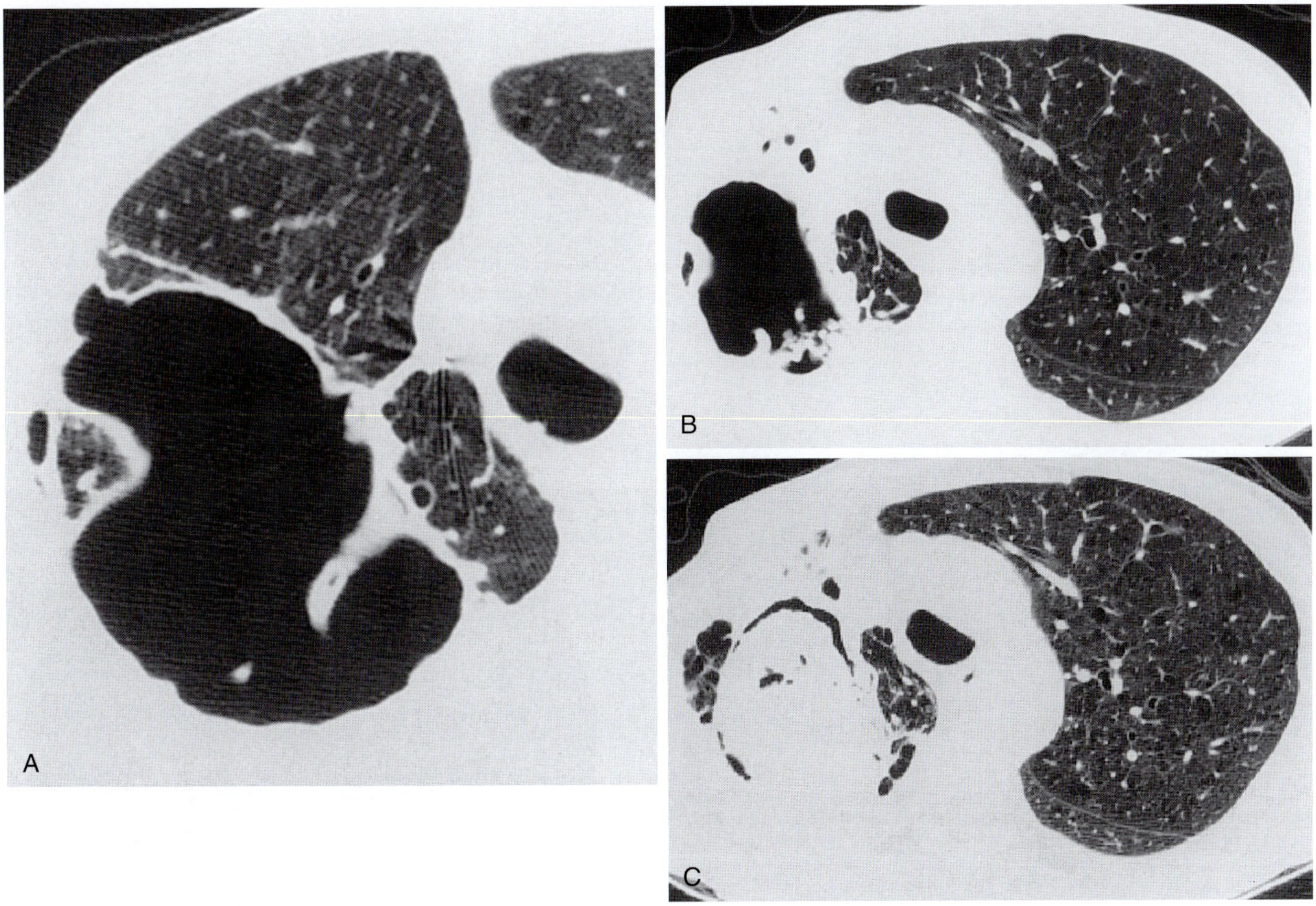

Fig. 12.14 Aspergilloma: development and growth over time in a woman with previous right mastectomy and right upper lobectomy who presented with cough and weight loss. (A) High-resolution CT scan targeted to the right lung showed a large cystic lesion in the superior segment of the right lower lobe. There is evidence of bronchiectasis. No other abnormality was found. All cultures were negative. (B) High-resolution CT scan 18 months later shows a small amount of soft tissue in the dependent portion of the cystic lesion. There is increased thickness of the wall of the cyst. The patient also has evidence of extensive bronchiectasis and scarring in the right lung. Four years later, the patient developed hemoptysis. (C) High-resolution CT scan shows a large mycetoma within the cavity. *Aspergillus fumigatus* was recovered at bronchoscopy. *(From Müller NL, Fraser RS, Colman NC, et al.* Radiologic Diagnosis of Diseases of the Chest. *Philadelphia: Saunders; 2001.)*

Allergic Bronchopulmonary Aspergillosis

General. Allergic bronchopulmonary aspergillosis is the result of a hypersensitivity reaction to *Aspergillus* antigens. It is estimated to occur in 7% to 14% of corticosteroid-dependent asthmatics and 6% of patients with cystic fibrosis.[33] Airway colonization by *Aspergillus* causes persistent inflammation and fibrosis, leading to segmental and subsegmental bronchiectasis, mucoid impaction, and parenchymal scarring.[37] Allergic bronchopulmonary aspergillosis usually is suspected clinically by the presence of wheezing, expectoration of brown mucus plugs, pleuritic chest pain, and fever. Radiologic and serologic tests can confirm the diagnosis.[33]

Radiography. Radiographs show findings of central bronchiectasis and tubular, homogeneous, finger-like opacities of soft tissue density in a central segmental bronchial distribution, most marked in the upper lobes representing mucoid impactions in dilated central bronchi (Fig. 12.15).[38] Mucoid impactions may be transient or may persist for months.[38] In the acute setting, areas of consolidation and volume loss may be seen.[39]

Computed Tomography. CT more clearly shows the central bronchiectasis with impaction of dilated bronchi by mucus and hyphal masses (Fig. 12.16). In approximately 30% of patients, the impacted mucus may be increased in attenuation because of the presence of calcium salts, metals, and dessicated mucus (see Fig. 12.15).[34] Mucoid impaction may cause bronchial obstruction, resulting in distal atelectasis or collapse on radiographs or CT, although collateral air flow most often prevents this.[38]

Imaging Algorithms. Chest radiographs or chest CT may be used to evaluate allergic bronchopulmonary aspergillosis. Unenhanced chest CT shows more detail, such as increased attenuation of a mucus plug, which may be helpful in diagnosis. Thin-section CT images may be helpful to assess for bronchiectasis.

CLASSIC SIGNS

- Central bronchiectasis
- Finger-in-glove or tube-like opacities corresponding to mucus or hyphal plugs
- Increased attenuation or calcification of mucus plugs on CT

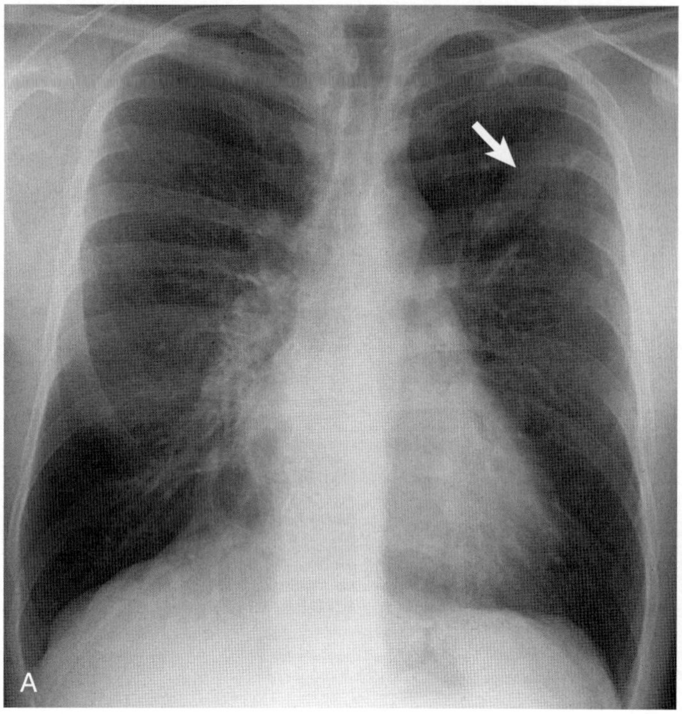

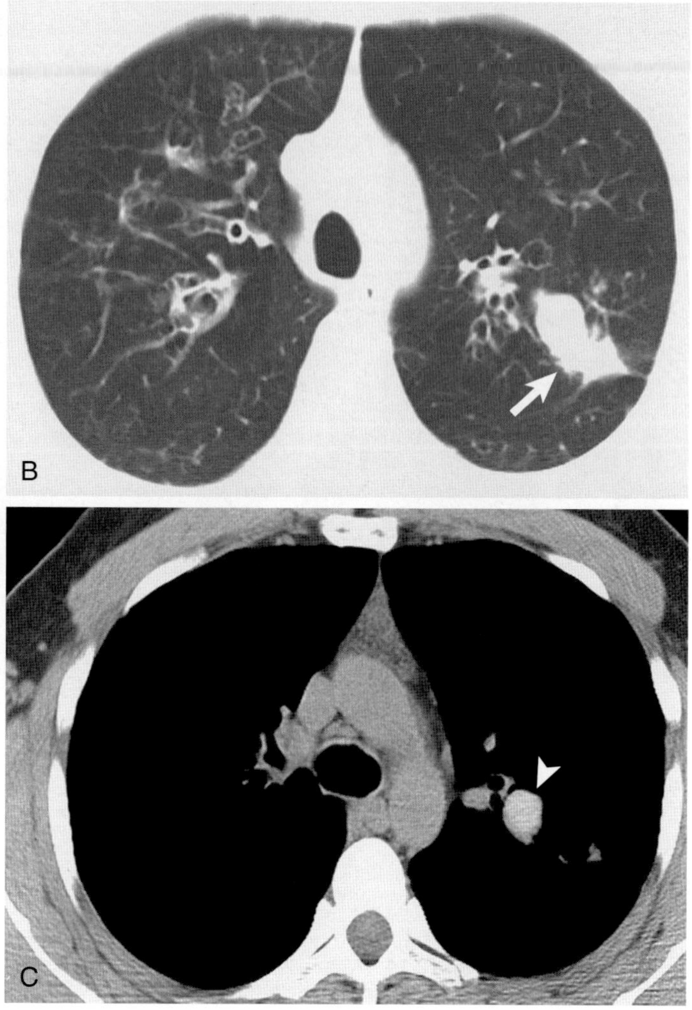

Fig. 12.15 Allergic bronchopulmonary aspergillosis in a man with a history of asthma, recurrent pneumonias, and expectoration of brownish mucus plugs. (A) Chest radiograph shows centrally predominant bronchiectasis in both lungs and a tubular soft tissue opacity *(arrow)* in the left upper lung. (B) CT scan confirms bilateral central bronchiectasis and a left upper lobe mucus plug *(arrow)*. (C) Soft tissue windows show that the mucoid impaction has mildly increased attenuation owing to calcification *(arrowhead)*.

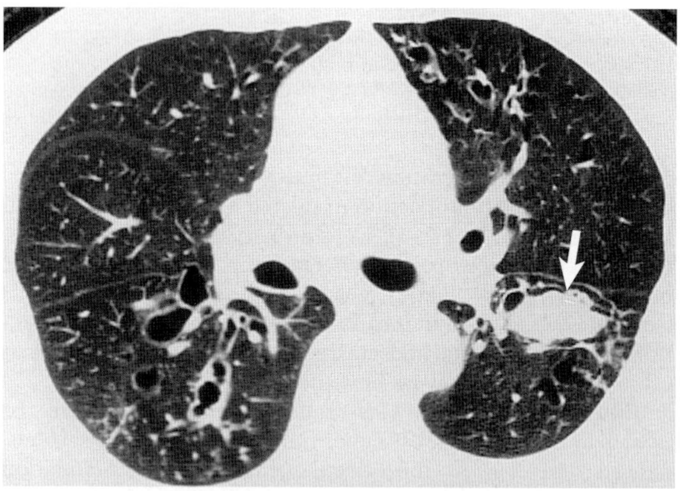

Fig. 12.16 Allergic bronchopulmonary aspergillosis. High-resolution CT scan shows extensive bronchiectasis involving mainly the central bronchi. Mucoid impaction *(arrow)* is present in an ectatic bronchus within the superior segment of the left lower lobe. *(From Müller NL, Fraser RS, Colman NC, et al.* Radiologic Diagnosis of Diseases of the Chest. *Philadelphia: Saunders; 2001.)*

Semiinvasive or Chronic Necrotizing Aspergillosis

General. Semiinvasive or chronic necrotizing aspergillosis primarily occurs in patients with underlying chronic lung disease, such as chronic obstructive pulmonary disease; patients with mildly depressed immune systems, such as a chronic debilitating illness, diabetes, malnutrition, alcoholism, advanced age, or prolonged corticosteroid therapy; or patients with both types of conditions.[34] Symptoms include a chronic productive cough, fever, fatigue, dyspnea, and hemoptysis.[34,40,41]

Radiography. Radiographs most commonly show segmental or lobar consolidation and, less often, nodules or masses.[40,42] There is often upper lung predominance, and the findings may be multiple and bilateral.[40] Cavitation may develop over several weeks to months, mimicking the appearance of tuberculosis. The cavity may contain soft tissue, such as a mycetoma, and may have associated pleural thickening.[38] The infection may extend into the chest wall or mediastinum.[38]

Computed Tomography. CT most often shows consolidation, whereas nodules or masses are less common. On CT nodules most often have ill-defined margins, and cavities often have irregular walls and measure 1 to 4 cm in diameter.[40]

Imaging Algorithms. Chest radiographs are helpful, but findings are better depicted on CT, and CT is often preferred in monitoring treatment and assessing for possible complications, such as mediastinal or chest wall invasion.

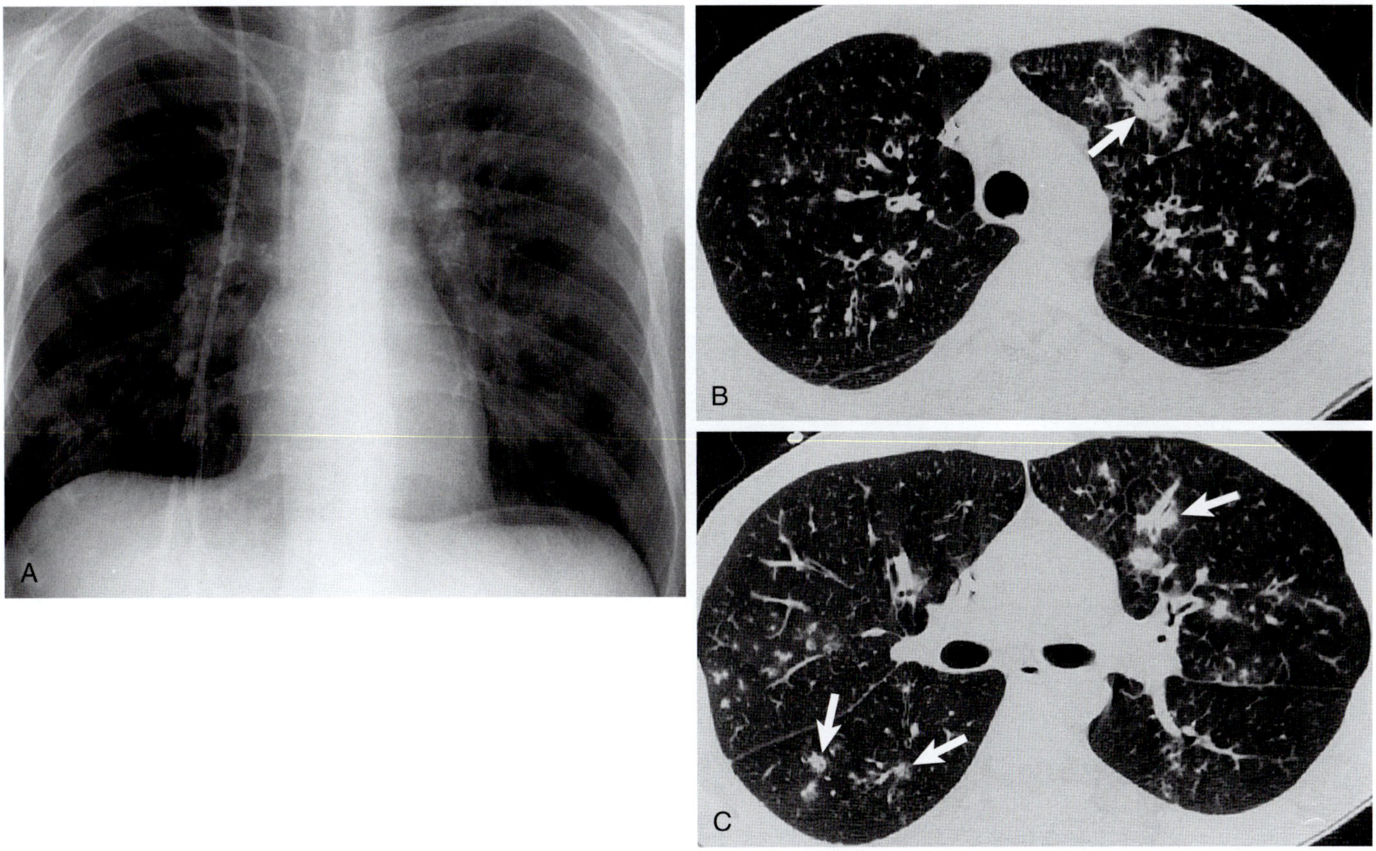

Fig. 12.17 *Aspergillus* bronchopneumonia in a man with fever and cough after allogeneic bone marrow transplantation. (A) Anteroposterior chest radiograph shows poorly defined bilateral nodular opacities. (B) and (C) High-resolution CT scans show focal areas of consolidation in a predominantly peribronchial distribution *(arrows)* and centrilobular nodules. The appearance is characteristic of a bronchopneumonia. Transbronchial biopsy showed *Aspergillus fumigatus* and pneumonia. *(From Müller NL, Fraser RS, Colman NC, et al.* Radiologic Diagnosis of Diseases of the Chest. *Philadelphia: Saunders; 2001.)*

CLASSIC SIGNS

- Patient who is chronically ill or on prolonged corticosteroid treatment
- Consolidation, mass, or nodule in an upper lobe that develops cavitation over several weeks to months

Airway Invasive Aspergillosis

General. Airway invasive aspergillosis is characterized by the presence of *Aspergillus* deep to the airway basement membrane.[43] It occurs most commonly in neutropenic and AIDS patients.[34] It causes a spectrum of diseases, including acute tracheobronchitis, bronchiolitis, and bronchopneumonia.[32,34]

Radiography. The radiologic appearance of tracheobronchitis may be normal, or there may be wall thickening of the trachea or bronchi.[34] Bronchiolitis may cause small, ill-defined nodules, whereas bronchopneumonia may result in consolidation (Fig. 12.17).[43] Findings are often bilateral.[43]

Computed Tomography. Centrilobular nodules and branching linear or nodular areas with a tree-in-bud appearance may be seen on CT in patients with bronchiolitis (Fig. 12.18).[34] Bronchopneumonia may result in areas of consolidation in a peribronchial distribution (see Fig. 12.17).[43] Bronchiectasis may be seen. Findings are often bilateral.[43] Wall thickening of trachea or bronchi often occurs with tracheobronchitis.

Imaging Algorithms. Chest radiographs are helpful in detecting disease and monitoring treatment response, but thin-section CT may be needed for subtle findings, such as centrilobular nodules, bronchiectasis, and tracheobronchial wall thickening.

CLASSIC SIGNS

- Usually neutropenic or AIDS patient
- Nonspecific findings of airway wall thickening, centrilobular nodules, or consolidation
- Often bilateral

Angioinvasive Aspergillosis

General. Angioinvasive aspergillosis primarily affects severely immunocompromised patients, such as patients with AIDS, hematologic malignancies (especially leukemia), and bone marrow transplants.[32,44,45] It is caused by hyphal invasion of blood vessels, resulting in infarction and necrosis.[46] Clinically, it is characterized by a hemorrhagic bronchopneumonia with fever, cough, dyspnea, and chest pain.[32]

Radiography. Chest radiographs show nonspecific patchy, subsegmental, segmental, or lobar areas of consolidation or

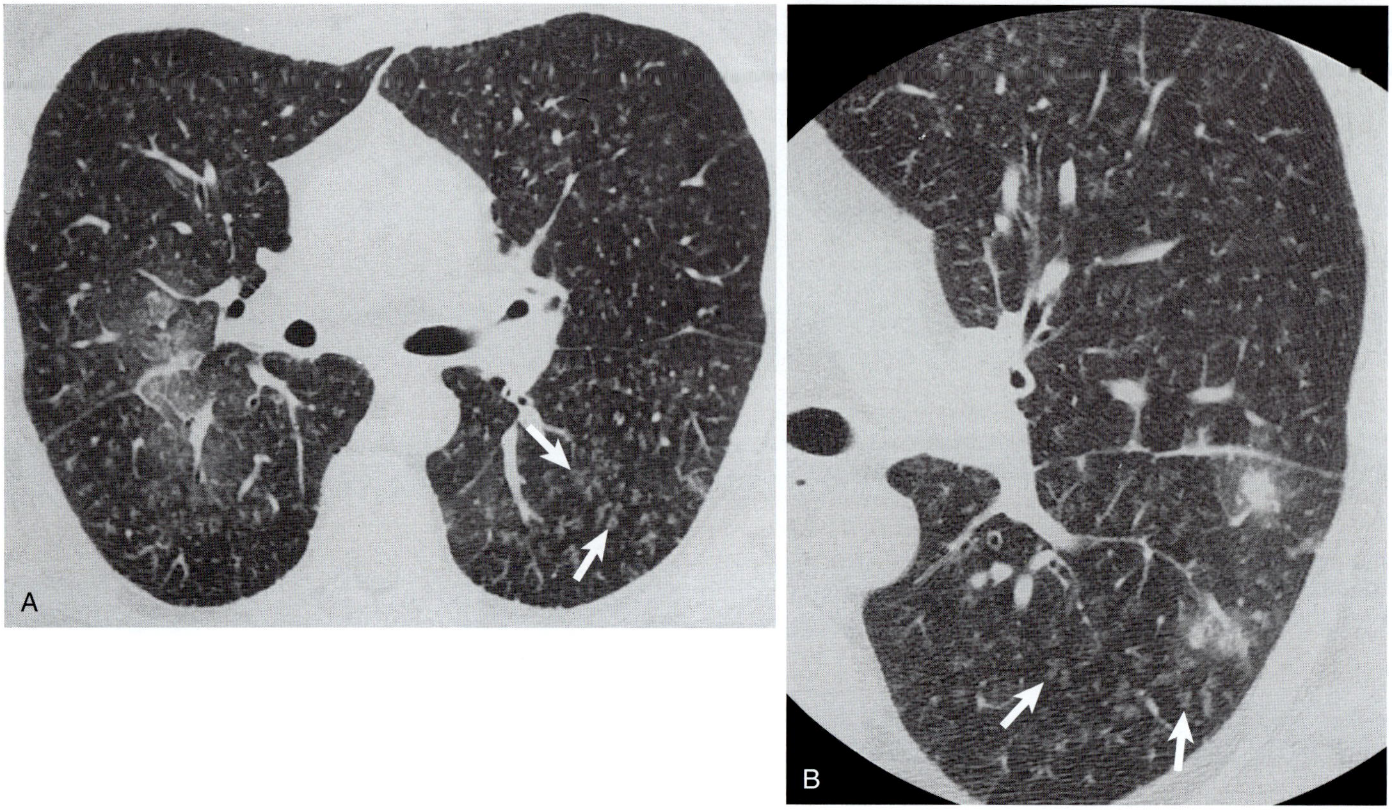

Fig. 12.18 *Aspergillus* bronchiolitis and bronchopneumonia in a man after bone marrow transplantation. (A) High-resolution CT scan shows localized area of ground-glass opacity in the right lung and bilateral, poorly defined small nodular opacities *(arrows).* (B) High-resolution CT scan targeted to the left lung delineates better the small nodular and branching opacities *(arrows)* and shows them to have a centrilobular distribution characteristic of bronchiolitis. Focal areas of consolidation are visible in the left lower lobe. Open-lung biopsy showed *Aspergillus* bronchiolitis and bronchopneumonia. *(From Müller NL, Fraser RS, Colman NC, et al.* Radiologic Diagnosis of Diseases of the Chest. *Philadelphia: Saunders; 2001.)*

multiple ill-defined nodular opacities (Fig. 12.19).[2] Cavitation commonly occurs, and an air crescent sign can be seen.[47]

Computed Tomography. CT typically shows nodules or masses that may be surrounded by a halo of ground-glass opacity (CT halo sign) (Fig. 12.20) or subpleural, wedge-shaped areas of consolidation.[48,49] The halo sign is caused by hemorrhage surrounding the nodule or mass of necrotic fungal-infected lung tissue.[48] The halo sign is generally seen early in the course of infection, affecting 96% of patients at day 0 and only 19% of patients at day 14 in a group of 25 patients with proven invasive pulmonary aspergillosis.[50] Numerous disease processes, such as *Candida* infection, granulomatosis with polyangiitis (formerly Wegener granulomatosis), Kaposi sarcoma, and hemorrhagic metastases, may cause a halo sign, but it is highly suggestive of angioinvasive aspergillosis in a patient with febrile neutropenia.[34] The nodules or masses subsequently develop cavitation or an air crescent sign that coincides with the return of neutrophil function (Fig. 12.21).[49] Less commonly, angioinvasive aspergillosis will manifest the reverse halo sign representing peripheral consolidation with central ground-glass opacities.[51]

Imaging Algorithms. In the appropriate clinical setting an abnormal chest radiograph is likely to be followed by a chest CT scan. The latter is more sensitive in detecting signs of angioinvasive aspergillosis, such as the halo or reverse halo signs.

CLASSIC SIGNS

- Severely immunocompromised
- Nonspecific patchy or lobar consolidation or multiple ill-defined nodular opacities
- CT halo sign or less commonly reverse halo sign
- Cavitation commonly occurs with return of neutrophil function

CANDIDIASIS

General

Pulmonary candidiasis is a rare opportunistic infection typically caused by *Candida albicans* and, less commonly, by *Candida tropicalis* or *Candida krusei.*[52] *Candida* is a ubiquitous human saprophyte that is normally present in the gastrointestinal tract, oropharynx, vagina, and skin.[53,54] Respiratory infection usually is the result of overgrowth of endogenous *Candida,* but nosocomial transmission may occur.[53] Symptoms include fever, tachypnea, chest pain, cough, and sputum production.[54]

Radiography

Radiographs most commonly show nonsegmental, segmental, or lobar consolidation that is more commonly bilateral than

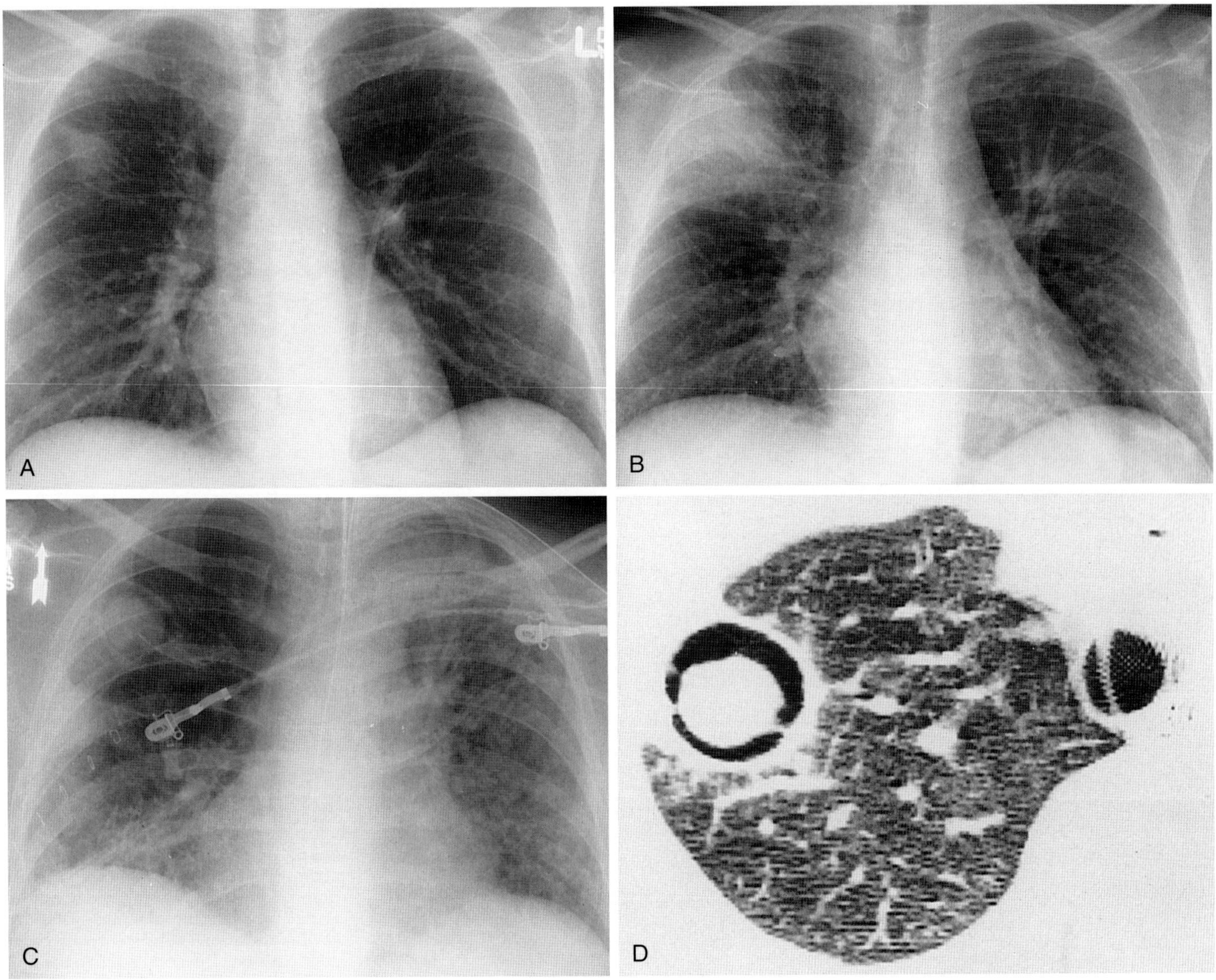

Fig. 12.19 Angioinvasive aspergillosis: progression of radiographic findings in a patient with acute leukemia who presented with fever and cough. Anteroposterior chest radiograph (A) shows a rounded area of consolidation in the right upper lobe, which 1 week later (B) has shown considerable progression. The next day, the patient underwent open-lung biopsy, which showed pulmonary hemorrhage but failed to identify any organisms. Anteroposterior chest radiograph 2 weeks after biopsy (C) and high-resolution CT scan (D) show a smoothly marginated cavity in the right upper lobe containing a soft tissue mass. Repeat biopsy performed under CT guidance confirmed the diagnosis of invasive aspergillosis; the soft tissue mass within the cavity, in this case, represented necrotic lung (sequestrum). *(From Müller NL, Fraser RS, Colman NC, et al.* Radiologic Diagnosis of Diseases of the Chest. *Philadelphia: Saunders; 2001.)*

unilateral.[55] There may be superimposed interstitial and nodular opacities (Figs. 12.22 and 12.23). Pleural effusions have been reported in 18% to 25% of radiographs or CT scans.[55,56]

Computed Tomography

The most common CT finding is nodules, followed by consolidation and ground-glass opacities (see Fig. 12.23).[56,57] The abnormalities do not typically have a zonal (i.e., upper, middle, or lower) lung predominance,[57] although Franquet and colleagues[56] reported that nodules were most commonly in the lower lungs, ranged from 3 to 30 mm, and had irregular or, less commonly, well-defined borders. The distribution of the nodules may be centrilobular or random and may have a tree-in-bud appearance.[56,57] A halo of ground-glass opacification surrounding a nodule (halo sign) may occur in approximately 30% of cases.[56,57] *Candida* is an uncommon cause of a mycetoma.[58]

Imaging Algorithms

Chest radiograph and chest CT scan can be used to detect pulmonary candidiasis and monitor treatment response. Chest CT with thin-section imaging is more sensitive in detecting and defining small nodules and ground-glass opacities.

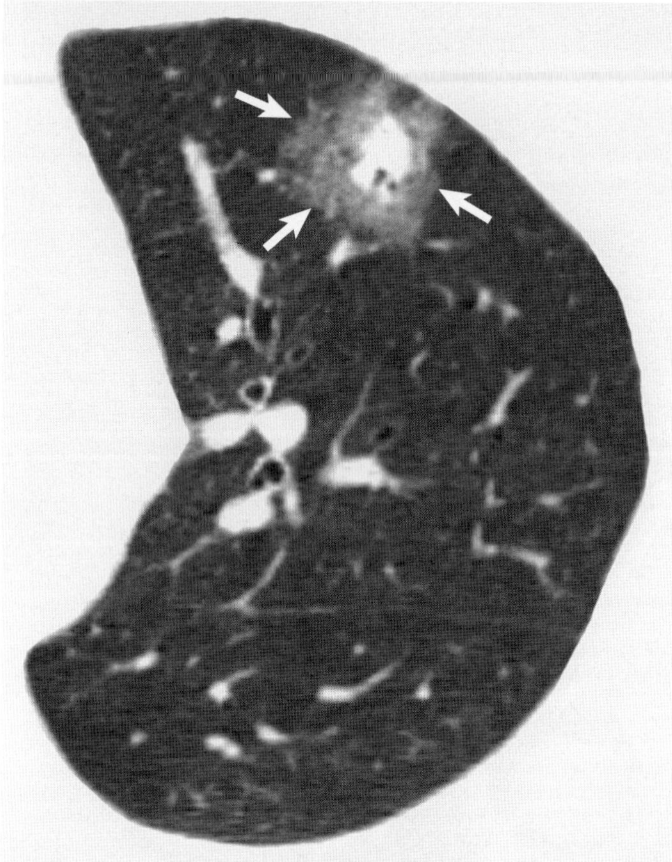

Fig. 12.20 CT halo sign in invasive pulmonary aspergillosis in a man with acute leukemia and febrile neutropenia. Magnified view of the left lung from high-resolution CT scan shows nodule with surrounding ground-glass opacity (CT halo sign, *arrows*).

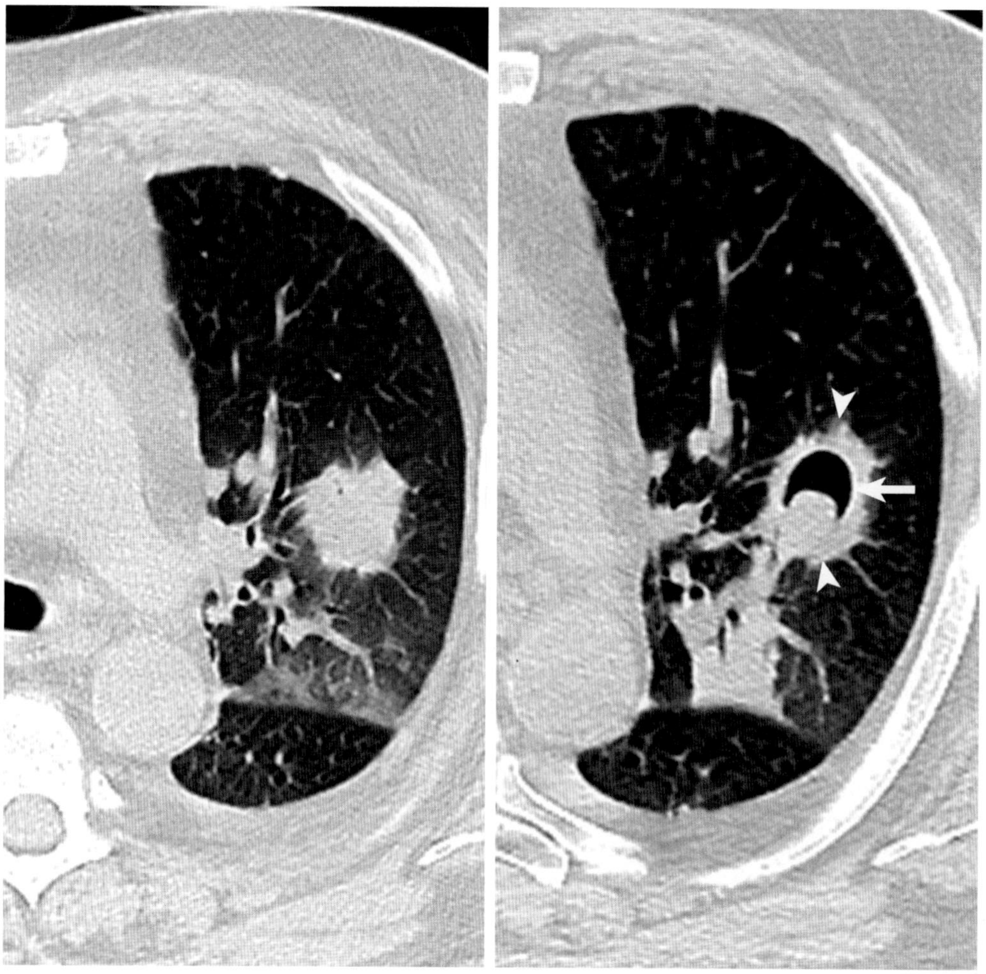

Fig. 12.21 Angioinvasive *Aspergillus* infection with air crescent sign. Composite image of two axial CT images obtained at time of neutropenic fever *(left)* and after granulocyte recovery *(right)* show a left upper lobe nodule that has undergone cavitation *(arrow)* consistent with the air crescent sign. The nodule within the cavity represents infarcted lung tissue that is separated from hemorrhagic but viable lung tissue *(arrowheads)*. *(Reproduced from Walker CM, Digumarthy S. Pulmonary infections. In: Digumarthy S, Abbara S, Chung JH, eds.* Problem Solving in Chest Imaging. *Philadelphia; Elsevier; 2019.)*

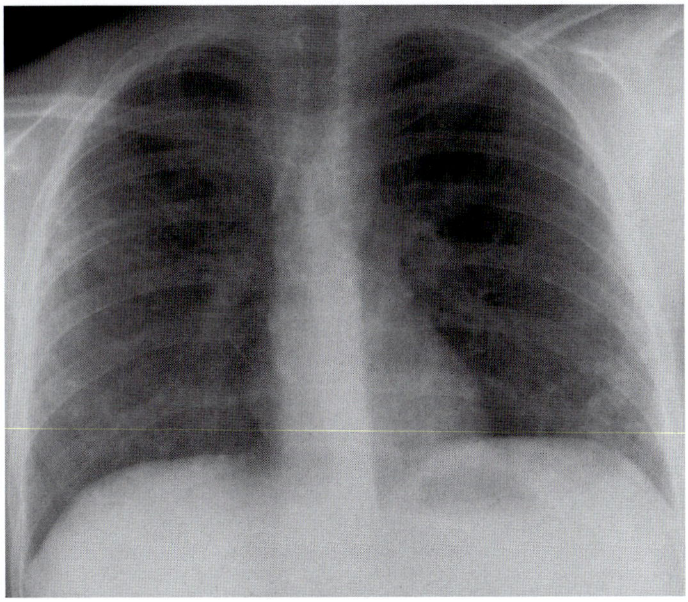

Fig. 12.22 Candidiasis in a boy on chemotherapy with fever. Chest radiograph shows multiple nodules in both lungs with a cluster of nodules in the right upper lung.

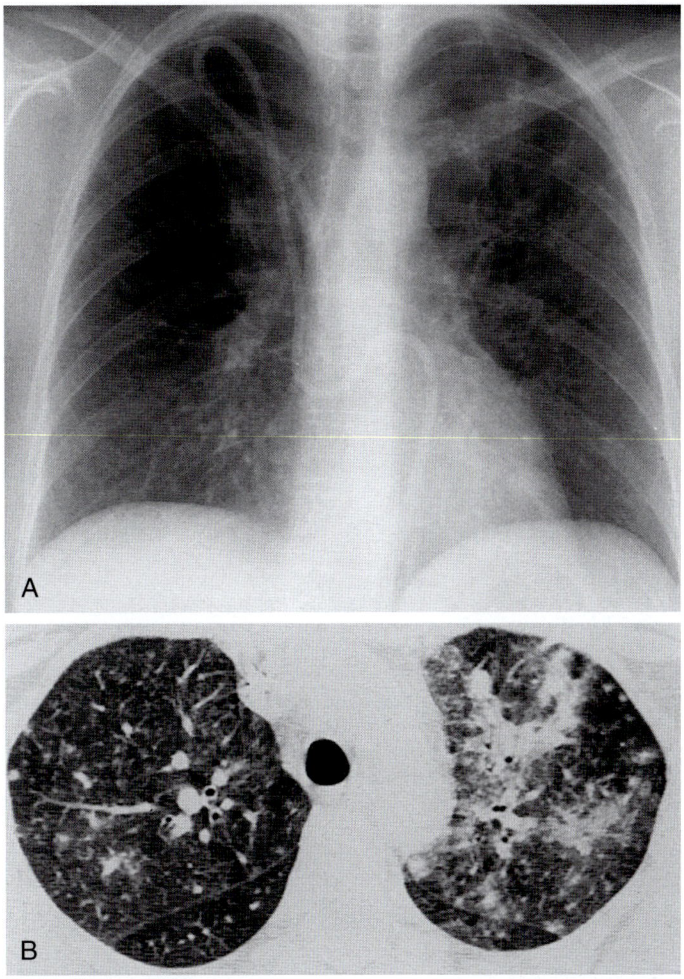

Fig. 12.23 *Candida* pneumonia in a woman status post bone marrow transplantation. (A) Posteroanterior chest radiograph shows poorly defined areas of consolidation and a few nodular opacities in the upper lobes. (B) High-resolution CT scan shows nodules of various sizes, focal areas of consolidation, and ground-glass opacity. *From Müller NL, Fraser RS, Colman NC, et al.* Radiologic Diagnosis of Diseases of the Chest. *Philadelphia: Saunders; 2001.)*

CLASSIC SIGNS

- Nodules or consolidation or both
- Possible ground-glass opacities
- Centrilobular or random nodule distribution on thin-section CT
- CT halo sign

CRYPTOCOCCOSIS

General

Cryptococcosis is a thin-walled, nonmycelial, budding encapsulated yeast.[59] Infection occurs via inhalation of cryptococcal particles. *C. neoformans* is the most recognized species of this pathogen. It is found worldwide in association with excreta of certain birds, including pigeons, canaries, and cockatoos.[60] *C. neoformans* typically infects immunocompromised patients, such as those with AIDS, hematologic malignancy, steroid therapy, or organ transplant.[60] Immunocompetent individuals are uncommonly infected by *C. neoformans.*[61] Recently, *C. gattii* has emerged as a pathogen affecting both immunocompromised as well as immunocompetent individuals. This species was first recognized on Vancouver Island, British Columbia, Canada, but now involves the Pacific Northwest.[62]

Patients infected with *C. neoformans* may be asymptomatic or may have signs of pneumonia, such as fever, chest pain, cough, sputum production, and weight loss.[60] *C. gattii* infection usually results in pneumonia or dissemination in distant tissues and is more often associated with serious neurologic sequelae or death.[62]

Radiography

Radiographs most commonly show solitary or multiple nodules or masses measuring 5 to 40 mm in diameter with well-defined or ill-defined margins (Fig. 12.24).[63–65] Nodules may cavitate. Areas of consolidation, most often segmental or lobar, may be seen. Lymphadenopathy or pleural effusions may occur. Miliary nodules may be seen in hematogenous dissemination.[65] Immunocompetent patients also most commonly show single or multiple nodules but rarely have consolidation, cavitation, lymphadenopathy, or pleural effusions.[63,65]

Computed Tomography

One study looked at CT findings in seven immunocompromised and four immunocompetent patients but did not distinguish between the two.[66] The study found that the most common CT finding was single or multiple pulmonary nodules with varied margins, ranging from 6 to 20 mm in diameter (Fig. 12.25; see also Fig. 12.24). Masses occurred in 36% of the patients in the study. *C. gattii* causes cryptococcomas in the lung and brain (often multifocal, large lesions) more often than *C. neoformans.*[62] Consolidation, pleural effusions, lymphadenopathy, and areas of ground-glass opacity were uncommon. Studies reviewing only immunocompetent patients have shown that single or multiple nodules are most common.[67,68]

Imaging Algorithms

Chest radiographs and chest CT are helpful in detecting disease and monitoring response to treatment.

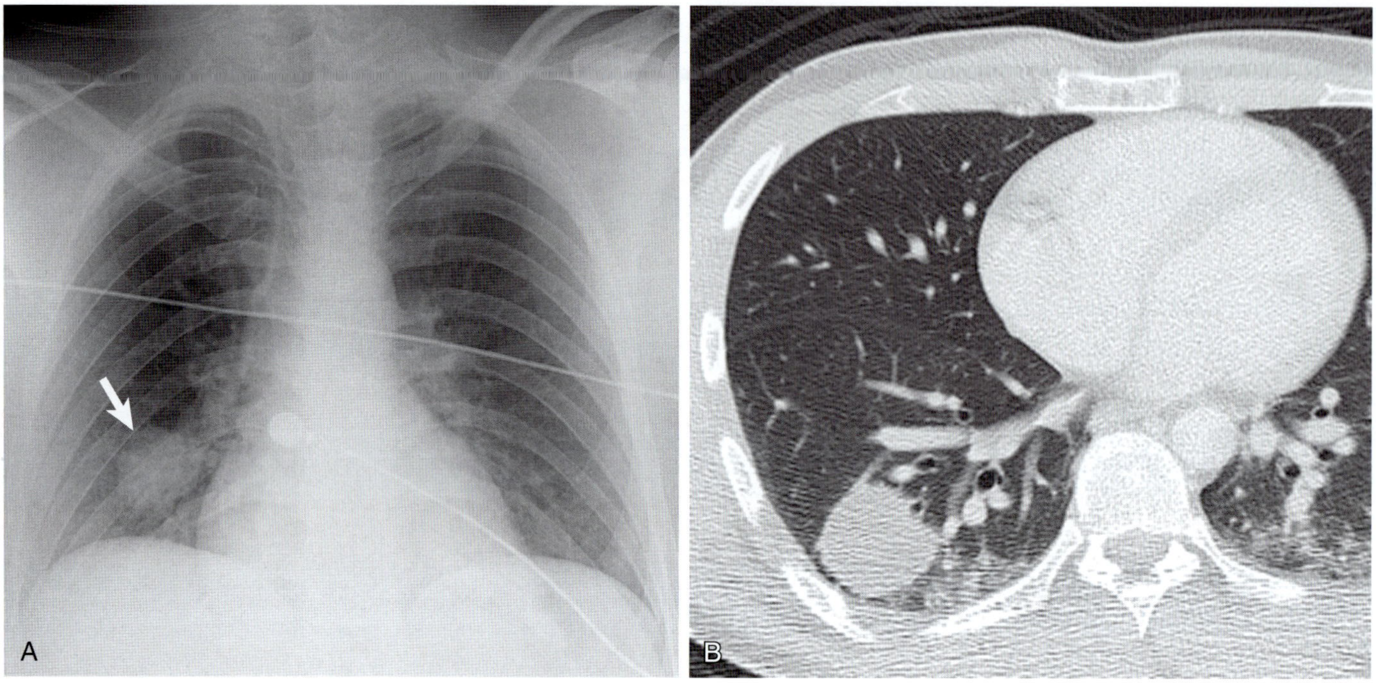

Fig. 12.24 Cryptococcosis. (A) Anteroposterior chest radiograph shows a right lower lung zone mass *(arrow)*. (B) Axial CT scan shows a right lower lobe mass. A solitary nodule or mass is the most common manifestation of cryptococcosis in the lungs.

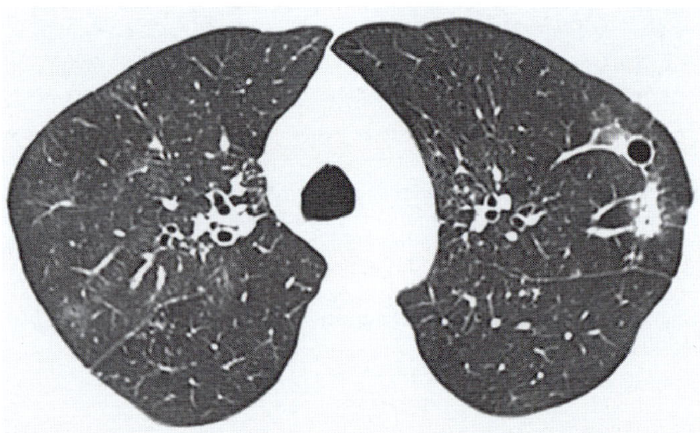

Fig. 12.25 Cryptococcosis in a woman with cough, fatigue, and weakness. Chest CT scan shows nodules with cavitations in the left upper lobe and patchy ground-glass opacities in the right lung. Note bilateral small nodules. *Cryptococcus neoformans* was revealed on bronchoscopy.

CLASSIC SIGNS

- Single or multiple nodules or masses with varied margins that may cavitate
- May have consolidation, lymphadenopathy, or pleural effusions

ZYGOMYCOSIS

General

Zygomycosis (mucormycosis, phycomycosis) is an often fatal opportunistic fungal infection. Although relatively uncommon, zygomycosis infection has become more common with increased use of prophylactic antifungals in those prone to aspergillosis. Poorly controlled diabetes is a known risk factor. It is caused by a variety of species of the fungal subclass Zygomycetes and orders Mucorales and Entomophthorales.[69,70] Pulmonary infection most often results in pneumonia, pulmonary infarction, or hemorrhage secondary to large vessel thrombosis or, less commonly, cavitation or abscess.[70]

Radiography

Chest radiographs most often show unilateral or bilateral airspace consolidation, which may rapidly progress.[69] Consolidations may be round and may evolve into abscesses (Fig. 12.26). Solitary or multiple pulmonary nodules often occur and may be small or large.[71] Diffuse bilateral hazy opacities or pleural effusions may occur.[69]

Computed Tomography

Nodules or consolidation or both are most commonly seen on CT.[72] Consolidations are most commonly posterior, abutting the pleura. Consolidations may be wedge shaped and may have air bronchograms. Nodules and masses may have central low attenuation and may cavitate. Nodules may have a halo of ground-glass opacity surrounding them (halo sign) or may manifest as a peripheral consolidation with central ground-glass opacities or irregular lines (reverse halo and bird's nest signs, respectively) (Fig. 12.27). Mediastinal and hilar lymphadenopathy and pleural effusions may occur. Imaging features that favor a diagnosis of mucormycosis over angioinvasive *Aspergillus* infection in a febrile neutropenic patient include a reverse halo or bird's nest sign, more than 10 pulmonary nodules, and development of infection despite prophylaxis with voriconazole.[51,73,74]

Imaging Algorithms

A chest radiograph and CT are usually both obtained and are complementary in monitoring response to therapy.

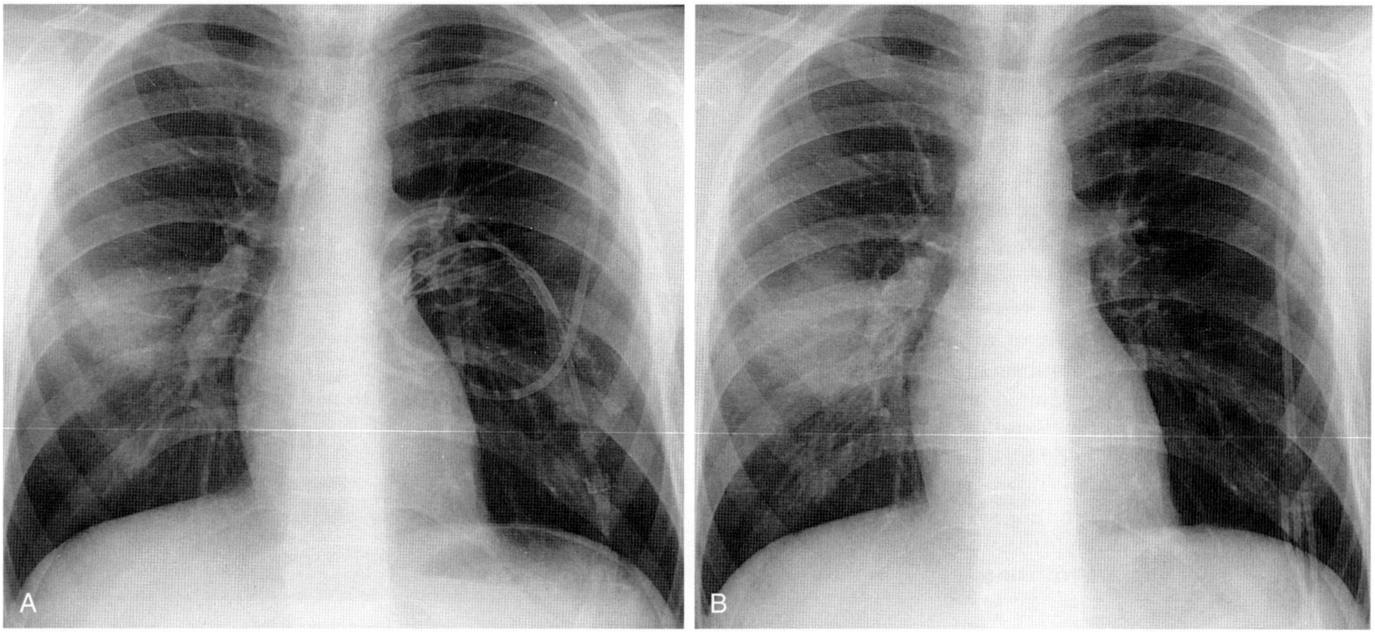

Fig. 12.26 Zygomycosis (mucormycosis) in a boy who had severe neutropenia secondary to chemotherapy for acute leukemia. (A) Posteroanterior chest radiograph shows a rounded area of consolidation in the superior segment of the right lower lobe. (B) Follow-up radiograph obtained the next day shows considerable increase in size of the consolidation. Because of the patient's severe clinical findings, a right lower lobectomy was performed. Hemorrhagic necrosis with extensive angioinvasive mucormycosis was found. *(Case courtesy Dr. James Barrie, University of Alberta Hospital, Edmonton, Canada. From Müller NL, Fraser RS, Colman NC, et al.* Radiologic Diagnosis of Diseases of the Chest. *Philadelphia: Saunders; 2001.)*

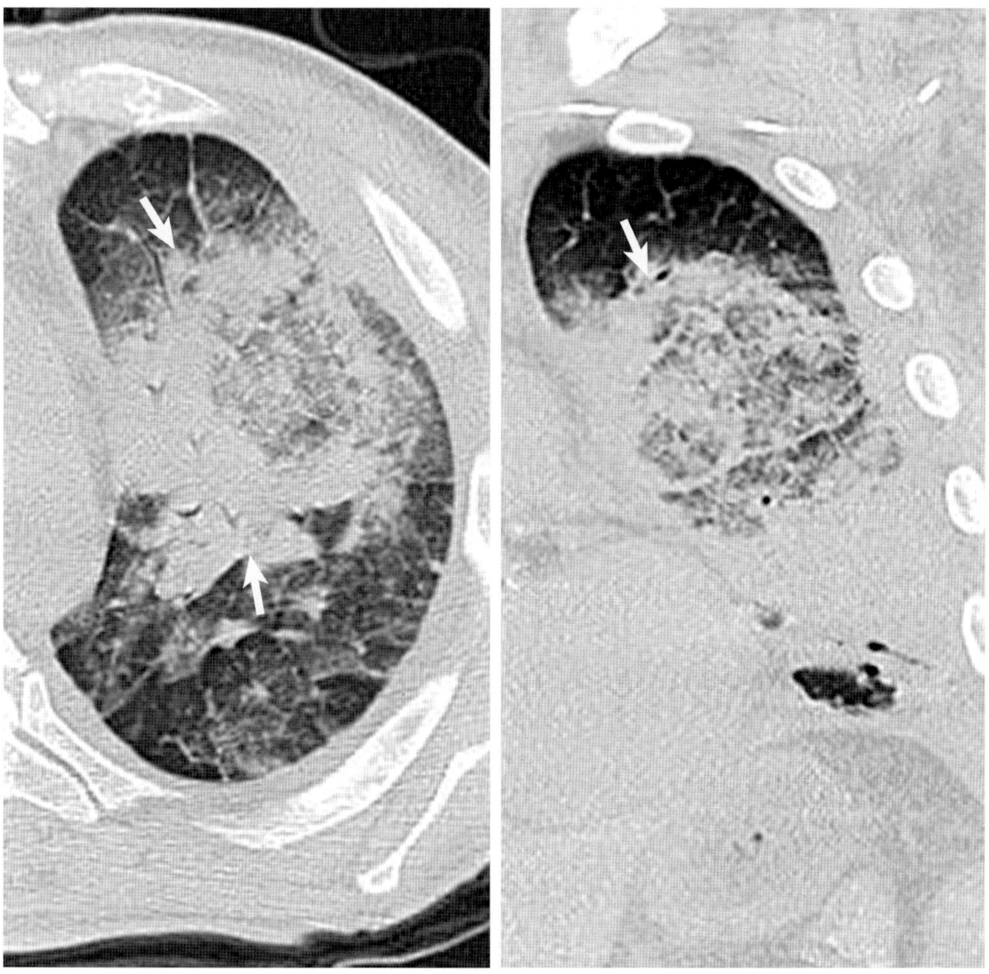

Fig. 12.27 Mucormycosis infection with reverse halo and bird's nest sign in a patient with febrile neutropenia. Composite image with axial *(left image)* and coronal *(right image)* CT scans shows a peripheral rim of consolidation surrounding central ground-glass opacities with associated reticulation and nodularity. This appearance has been called both the reverse halo sign and bird's nest sign *(arrows)*. Early diagnosis of mucormycosis is necessary because standard voriconazole therapy is not effective for treatment. *(Courtesy Chou S, University of Washington, Seattle, WA.)*

CLASSIC SIGNS

- Rapidly progressive pneumonia in an immunocompromised patient
- Nodules or consolidation
- Possible cavitation, reverse halo sign, or halo sign

Differential Diagnosis

FROM CLINICAL DATA

The main differential diagnosis of a patient presenting with clinical signs and symptoms of fungal bronchopneumonia is the more common community-acquired bronchopneumonia, such as that caused by *Streptococcus pneumoniae.* Lack of response to typical antibiotic therapy should raise clinical suspicion, as should a clinical history of travel to an endemic region, underlying lung disease, or a compromised immune system. Lymphadenopathy or the presence of cutaneous lesions (coccidioidomycosis, blastomycosis) may help differentiate from community-acquired pneumonia.

FROM SUPPORTIVE DIAGNOSTIC TECHNIQUES

The radiographic and CT findings of the various fungal infections have considerable overlap, which is why clinical history is helpful. To distinguish among the fungal organisms diagnostically, direct visualization or culture of the fungus from sputum, tissues, or other infected material (i.e., bronchial washings); serodiagnosis; or enzyme immunoassays may be helpful.[75]

Synopsis of Treatment Options

MEDICAL

- *Prevention:* mask or respirator use in high-risk situations in endemic areas; avoidance of exposures in high-risk patients; antifungal prophylaxis in immunocompromised patients; use of formalin spray to inactivate conidia before construction work[1]
- *No treatment:* most endemic infections are asymptomatic and self-limited
- *Antifungal medication:* if symptoms of endemic infection are not improved after 3 to 4 weeks or in less severe opportunistic infections (i.e., itraconazole, fluconazole); in severely ill patients (i.e., amphotericin B); possibly helpful in mediastinal granulomatosis or fibrosing mediastinitis (histoplasmosis)
- *Corticosteroids:* may be helpful in cases of severe infection with hypoxia

SURGICAL

- *Intravascular stent placement:* may be helpful in superior vena cava or pulmonary arterial obstruction from fibrosing mediastinitis (histoplasmosis)
- *Angiographic embolization of bronchial arteries:* may relieve pulmonary hemorrhage (angioinvasive aspergillosis, mycetoma)
- *Surgical resection:* may be helpful in granulomatous mediastinitis not responding to antifungal medication (histoplasmosis); controversial in fibrosing mediastinitis owing to low benefit and high mortality rates[1]; mycetoma resection (i.e., aspergilloma, zygomycosis)

KEY POINTS

- Endemic fungal infections typically affect otherwise healthy individuals.
- Opportunistic fungal infections tend to affect patients who are immunosuppressed, are chronically ill, or have underlying lung disease.
- Infection may manifest after the patient has left the endemic region. Travel and residence history is important in the diagnosis.
- Endemic fungal infections are typically asymptomatic or mild and self-limited.
- Endemic fungal infections can have a variety of radiologic appearances and may mimic community-acquired pneumonia, metastases, or bronchogenic carcinoma.
- *Aspergillus* infection has a variety of clinical and radiologic manifestations, depending on the immune status of the host.

SUGGESTED READINGS

Chong S, Lee KS, Yi CA, et al. Pulmonary fungal infection: imaging findings in immunocompetent and immunocompromised patients. *Eur J Radiol.* 2006;59(3):371–383.

Waite S, Jeudy J, White CS. Acute lung infections in normal and immunocompromised hosts. *Radiol Clin North Am.* 2006;44(2):295–315, ix.

Wheat LJ, Goldman M, Sarosi G. State-of-the-art review of pulmonary fungal infections. *Semin Respir Infect.* 2002;17(2):158–181.

The full reference list for this chapter is available at ExpertConsult.com.

13 Viruses*

CHRISTOPHER M. WALKER | JONATHAN H. CHUNG

Viruses are the most common cause of respiratory infection and may result in rhinitis, pharyngitis, laryngotracheitis, bronchitis, bronchiolitis, and, less commonly, pneumonia. Most viral pneumonias in immunocompetent adults are due to influenza viruses; other common viral etiologies include respiratory syncytial virus (RSV) and adenovirus. Immunocompromised hosts are particularly susceptible to pneumonias caused by cytomegalovirus (CMV) and herpesviruses. Risk factors associated with increased incidence and severity of viral infections include very young and old age, crowding, malnutrition, and immunologic disorders.[1] Respiratory viral infections are a much greater problem in developing countries than in developed countries and are one of the leading causes of death in children younger than 5 years.[1] In addition to these acute complications, viral-induced childhood bronchiolitis is well recognized as a precursor of adult bronchiectasis and constrictive bronchiolitis. Airway infection can also induce symptoms of asthma in patients who have this disease, and there is evidence that such infection in childhood is involved in the pathogenesis of asthma in later life.[2] Finally, several viruses, such as Epstein-Barr virus (EBV), herpesvirus 8, and papillomavirus, are implicated in the development of some pulmonary and pleural neoplasms.

The diagnosis of viral pneumonia is often one of exclusion and is based on an absence of sputum production, a failure to culture pathogenic bacteria, a relatively benign clinical presentation, a white blood cell count or procalcitonin level that is normal or only slightly elevated, a chest radiograph that reveals bronchopneumonia or localized interstitial disease, and a lack of response to antibiotic therapy. Confirmation of the diagnosis and identification of the specific causative virus can be accomplished by a variety of means, including culture, serology, detection of viral antigens within respiratory tract secretions or blood by monoclonal antibodies, detection of virus-associated molecules by in situ hybridization or polymerase chain reaction (PCR), and observation of virus-induced changes cytologically or histologically.[3,4] The sensitivity and specificity of these tests vary and are related to some extent to the underlying organism.

Patterns of Disease

The radiographic manifestations of viral infection are protean and cannot be reliably differentiated from other infections caused by bacterial organisms. Chest radiographs may be normal or often show unilateral or bilateral foci of consolidation, ground-glass opacities, nodular opacities, and bronchial wall thickening (Figs. 13.1 and 13.2). Lobar consolidation, lymphadenopathy, and pleural effusions are uncommon and are not seen in most cases of viral pneumonia.[5]

A retrospective study compared the computed tomography (CT) appearances of 93 viral pneumonias and 22 bacterial pneumonias in both immunocompetent and immunocompromised hosts to determine CT patterns that may allow a specific diagnosis.[6] Viral or bacterial pneumonia was determined to be present if a patient had lower respiratory tract symptoms and laboratory evidence of infection. Viral pneumonias manifested with one of five different CT patterns:

1. A normal CT or a CT with abnormalities unrelated to infection (e.g., linear scar, emphysema, etc.) was the most common CT appearance observed in 35% of patients with viral pneumonia.
2. Airway centric disease was the second most common CT appearance observed in 33% of patients (Fig. 13.3). Typical features include bronchial wall thickening, bronchiolitis with centrilobular nodules or tree-in-bud opacities, and peribronchial consolidation or ground-glass opacities. Centrilobular nodules typically measure less than 10 mm. Other frequent CT abnormalities that often coexist with airway centric disease include mosaic attenuation, lung hyperinflation, and expiratory air trapping.
3. Multifocal airspace pattern was the third most common CT appearance observed in 24% of patients (Fig. 13.4). Typical features include multifocal ground-glass opacities and/or consolidation with intervening normal portions of lung. Of importance, bronchial abnormalities, including tree-in-bud opacities, are generally minimal or absent.
4. Unifocal airspace pattern was uncommon, affecting 6% of patients (Fig. 13.5). Typical features include focal consolidation, ground-glass opacities, or tree-in-bud opacities.
5. Diffuse airspace pattern was rare, affecting 2% of patients (Fig. 13.6). Typical features include diffuse, relatively uniform bilateral ground-glass opacities, or consolidation.

When these patterns were compared with patients with bacterial pneumonia, the diffuse disease pattern and the presence of a pleural effusion were more commonly associated with bacterial pneumonia, and only the normal CT pattern was more commonly associated with viral pneumonia.[6–9] Otherwise, the imaging appearances overlapped considerably, and other methods, including patient presentation and laboratory analysis, were used in conjunction with the imaging findings to make a specific diagnosis.

Interlobular septal thickening (Fig. 13.7) is an uncommon manifestation that is usually seen only in certain infections, such as hantavirus or in viral infection that progresses to acute respiratory distress syndrome (ARDS). Significant lymphadenopathy and moderate or large pleural effusions are uncommon in viral infection and should prompt search for an alternative etiology.

*The editors and the publisher would like to thank Drs. Nestor L. Müller and C. Isabela Silva Müller for contributing material on this topic to the prior edition of this work. It has served as the foundation for the current chapter.

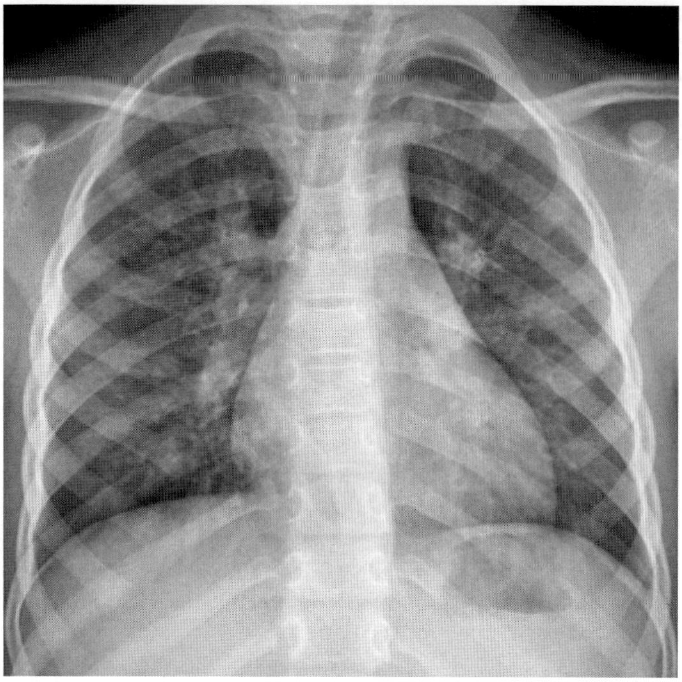

Fig. 13.1 Viral bronchiolitis secondary to respiratory syncytial virus infection. Anteroposterior chest radiograph shows bilateral perihilar bronchial thickening typical of a viral infection or reactive airways disease. *(From Walker CM, Digumarthy S. Pulmonary infections. In: Digumarthy S, Abbara S, Chung JH, eds.* Problem Solving in Chest Imaging. *Philadelphia: Elsevier; 2019.)*

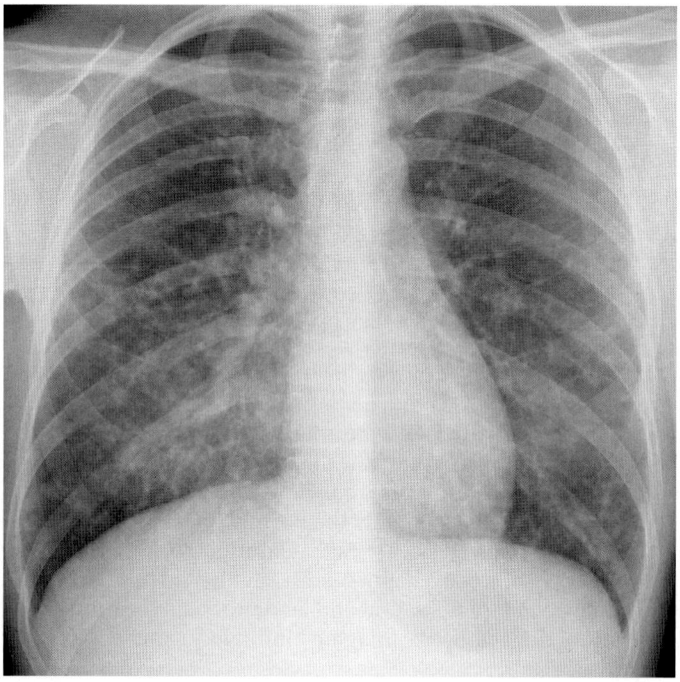

Fig. 13.2 Varicella pneumonia. Posteroanterior chest radiograph shows multiple bilateral nodular opacities and bronchial wall thickening typical of interstitial pneumonia. An interstitial pattern of pneumonia is most common with atypical organisms, including viruses, mycoplasma, or pneumocystis. *(From Walker CM, Digumarthy S. Pulmonary infections. In: Digumarthy S, Abbara S, Chung JH, eds.* Problem Solving in Chest Imaging. *Philadelphia: Elsevier; 2019.)*

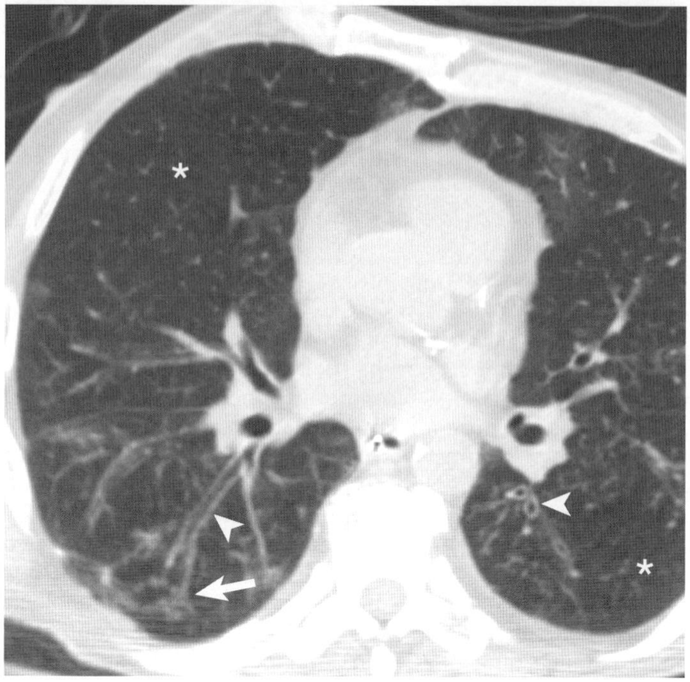

Fig. 13.3 Airway centric pattern with parainfluenza pneumonia. Axial CT shows bilateral bronchial wall thickening *(arrowheads)*, patchy ground-glass opacities, and tree-in-bud opacities *(arrow)*. Note focal areas of decreased lung attenuation *(asterisks)* representing mosaic attenuation caused by small airways infection and secondary air trapping. *(From Walker CM, Digumarthy S. Pulmonary infections. In: Digumarthy S, Abbara S, Chung JH, eds.* Problem Solving in Chest Imaging. *Philadelphia: Elsevier; 2019.)*

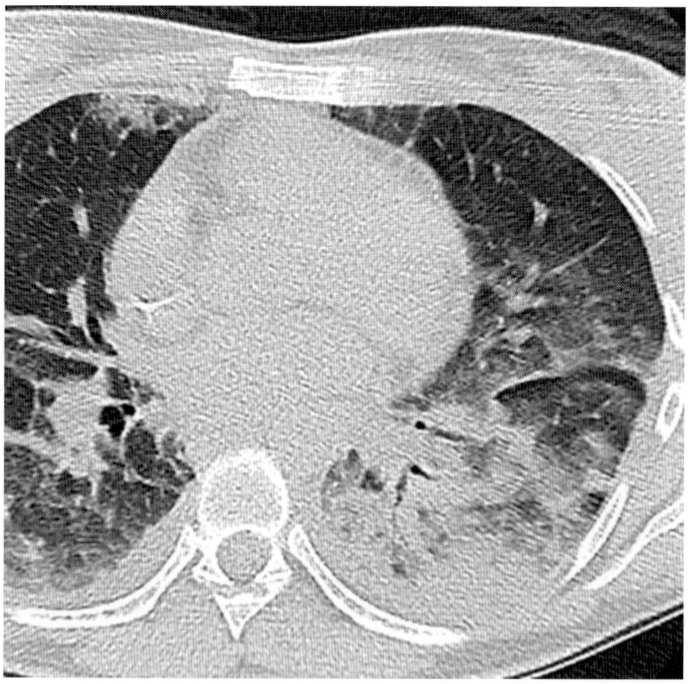

Fig. 13.4 Multifocal airspace pattern with adenovirus pneumonia. Axial CT shows multifocal consolidation and ground-glass opacities.

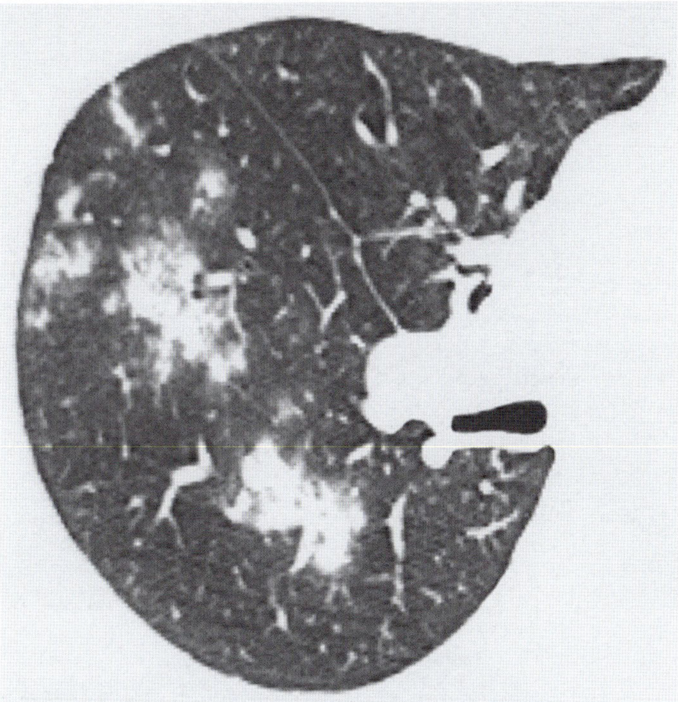

Fig. 13.5 Unifocal airspace pattern with influenza pneumonia. Axial CT at the level of the right upper lobe bronchus shows focal peribronchial consolidation and small nodular opacities.

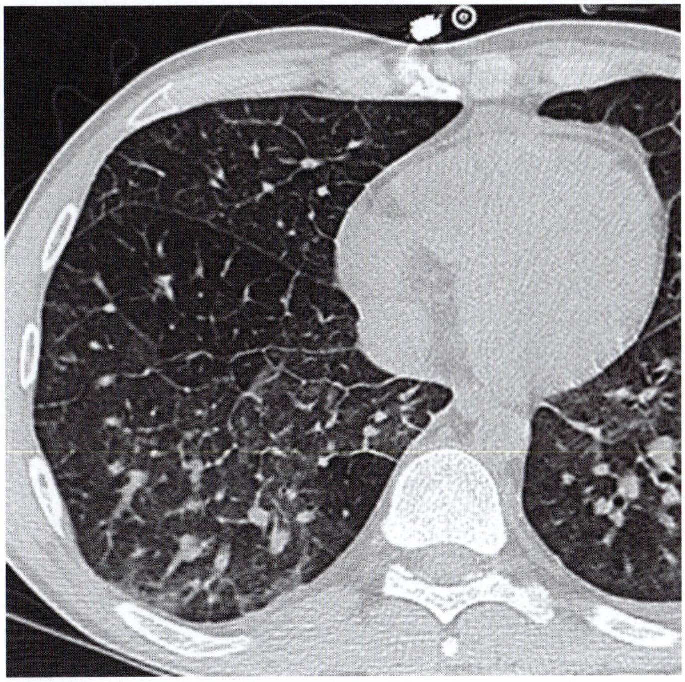

Fig. 13.7 Interlobular septal thickening in cytomegalovirus pneumonia in a bone marrow transplant recipient. Axial CT shows extensive smooth interlobular septal thickening and ground-glass opacities, an appearance that closely mimics interstitial pulmonary edema.

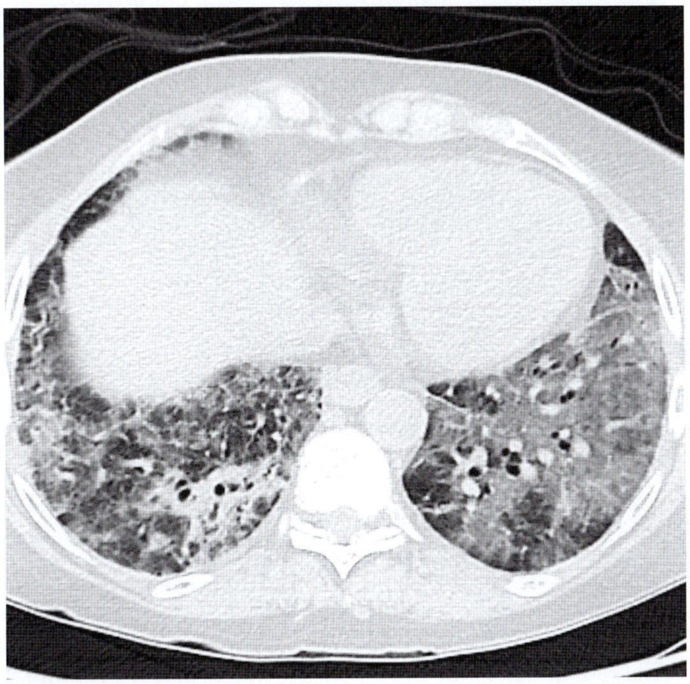

Fig. 13.6 Diffuse airspace pattern with influenza A pneumonia. Axial CT shows bilateral ground-glass opacities with peribronchial consolidation in the right lower lobe. The findings affected both lungs diffusely.

Specific Viruses

Influenza Viruses

ETIOLOGY, PREVALENCE, AND EPIDEMIOLOGY

Influenza viruses are single-stranded ribonucleic acid (RNA) viruses found worldwide. They are subdivided into three antigenic types A, B, and C. Influenza can occur in pandemics, epidemics, or sporadically in individuals or small clusters of patients. Type A viruses cause almost all severe epidemics and all pandemics. These organisms have the ability to change their structural and antigenic nature, the variant forms possessing different virulence from that of their progenitors.

Although the type A virus is generally transmitted from person to person by droplet infection, antigenically similar viruses also infect swine, horses, and wild and domesticated birds, and human disease is occasionally derived from these sources.[4] It is believed that these animals serve as a milieu for genetic recombination whereby new and sometimes more virulent strains capable of causing human disease are created.[10] Influenza is an important infection worldwide, being estimated to result in symptomatic disease in approximately 20% of children and 5% of adults each year.[11]

Influenza outbreaks tend to occur on an annual basis, typically during the winter in temperate climates; in tropical and subtropical areas, they occur either during the rainy season or throughout the year, depending on the particular location.[11] Attack rates are especially high in schoolchildren; complications and hospitalization also are more likely in these individuals and in the elderly.

The 24- to 48-hour incubation period allows rapid spread of the disease. It is highly contagious, and a large proportion of individuals may contract the disease to some degree in closed environments, such as on cruise ships and airplanes.[12] Nosocomial transmission of disease is well documented.[13]

Pneumonia is an uncommon but serious complication of influenza infection that is usually caused by type A and occasionally type B organisms.[14] Although it is often mild, it can be overwhelming and rapidly fatal, with most cases recognized during epidemics or pandemics. In approximately one-third of cases of severe pneumonia, the illness develops abruptly in apparently healthy individuals.[4] Most of the remainder have a predisposing condition, such as cardiac disease, pregnancy, cystic fibrosis, or immunodeficiency.[4,14] Infants and the elderly are at particular risk for serious disease.[4,14,15] Death can result from severe influenza pneumonia or from superinfection by bacteria, such as *Staphylococcus aureus, Streptococcus pneumoniae, Haemophilus influenzae,* and *Moraxella catarrhalis.*[14]

CLINICAL PRESENTATION

The most common manifestations of influenza infection consist of rapid onset of dry cough, myalgia, chills, headache, conjunctivitis, and fever of greater than 38°C.[4,16] In older patients and patients with underlying cardiopulmonary disease, there is a tendency for involvement of the lower respiratory tract, with development of bronchitis, bronchiolitis, and pneumonia. Patients who have pneumonia tend to have more severe cough and may develop severe dyspnea, cyanosis, and hypoxemia.[4]

Bacterial superinfection usually develops within a few days after the initial viral infection.[4] Superimposed bacterial infection occurs most commonly in the elderly and in patients with underlying pulmonary disease. Clinically, these patients initially present with typical influenza symptoms. The symptoms seem to be improving when the clinical course is complicated by recrudescence of fever and development of chills, pleuritic chest pain, and productive cough.[4] The symptoms in these patients tend to be milder than in patients with primary influenza pneumonia, and the mortality is lower.

PATHOPHYSIOLOGY

Transmission of influenza viruses is by airborne droplets and may result in rhinitis, pharyngitis, laryngitis, tracheobronchitis, bronchiolitis, and bronchopneumonia. The histologic appearance of fatal influenza pneumonia is diffuse alveolar damage, the parenchyma showing a variably severe interstitial mononuclear inflammatory infiltrate; consolidation of airspaces by edema, hemorrhage, and fibrin; and hyaline membranes.[4,17] Less severe cases of pneumonia may result in findings of mild acute lung injury and organizing pneumonia.[17] The virus can be cultured or seen by immunofluorescence in a large proportion of cases.[4]

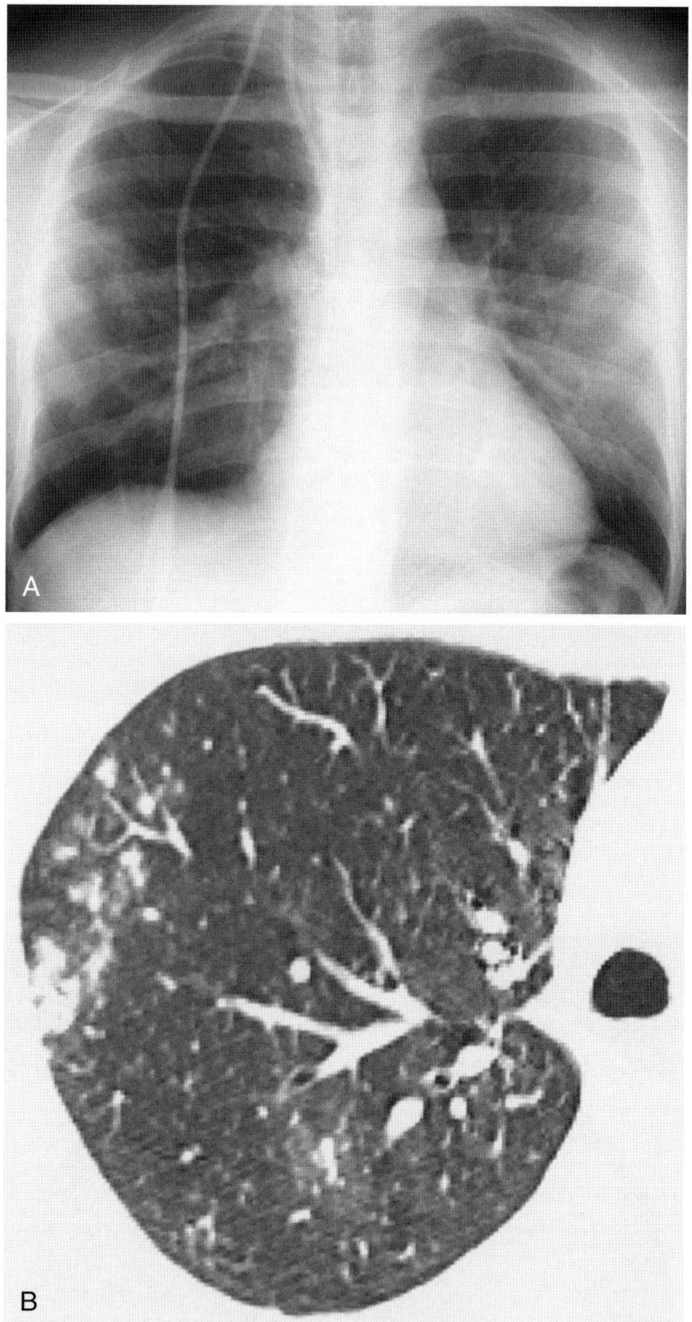

Fig. 13.8 Influenza pneumonia. (A) Chest radiograph shows poorly defined reticulonodular opacities in the right middle lung zone. Also noted is a central venous line. (B) View of the right upper lobe from a high-resolution CT shows centrilobular nodules and small foci of consolidation in the right upper lobe.

MANIFESTATIONS OF THE DISEASE

Radiography

The most common radiographic manifestations of influenza pneumonia consist of bilateral reticulonodular opacities with or without superimposed areas of consolidation (Fig. 13.8).[18,19] Less commonly, patients with primary influenza pneumonia may present with focal areas of consolidation, usually in the lower lobes, without apparent reticular or reticulonodular opacities. Serial radiographs may show poorly defined, patchy or nodular areas of consolidation, 1 to 2 cm in diameter, which become rapidly confluent (Fig. 13.9).[4,19] Pleural effusion is uncommon. The radiologic abnormalities usually resolve in approximately 3 weeks.[19] The manifestations of secondary bacterial pneumonia are the same as bronchopneumonia and consist of lobular, subsegmental, or segmental unilateral or bilateral areas of consolidation.[14,18]

Computed Tomography

Miller and associates[6] described the CT findings of influenza infection in 60 patients. Influenza had a myriad of imaging appearances comprising a normal CT (43%), an airway centric pattern manifesting with bronchial wall thickening, centrilobular nodules, and tree-in-bud opacities (27%), a multifocal airspace pattern with multifocal consolidation and/or ground-glass opacities (20%) (see Fig. 13.8), a focal airspace pattern with focal ground-glass opacity or consolidation (8%), and a diffuse airspace pattern with bilateral ground-glass opacities or consolidation (2%) (Fig. 13.10). The centrilobular nodules seen with influenza often measure 2 to 9 mm in diameter and are usually bilateral and asymmetric in distribution (see Fig. 13.8).[20]

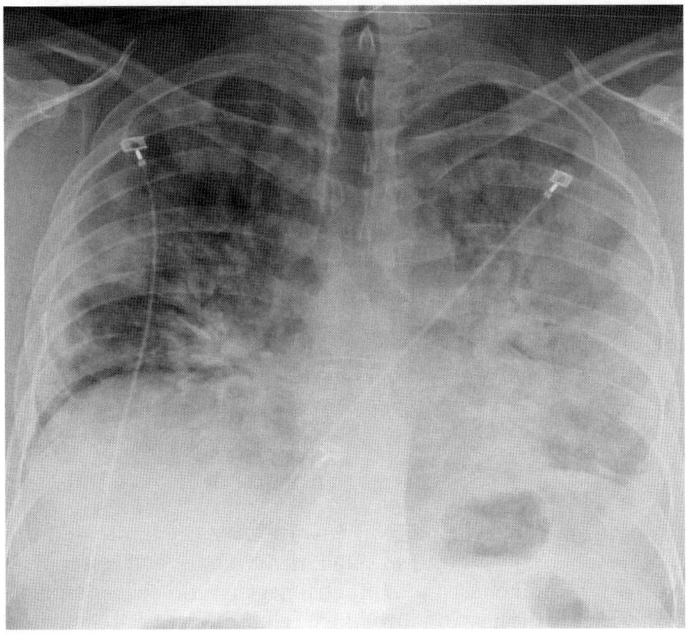

Fig. 13.9 Influenza A pneumonia. Chest radiograph shows diffuse left greater than right consolidation. Influenza was the only virus detected at bronchoscopy.

Avian influenza strain H5N1, swine influenza strain H1N1, and most recently a new avian influenza strain H7N9 have emerged with periodic outbreaks related to cross-species transmission after humans acquire the virus after being in close contact with infected birds or pigs or their products. Infection by these influenza viruses preferentially affects younger, previously healthy individuals, and transmission of the H1N1 strain was declared to be in a worldwide pandemic state by the World Health Organization in 2009. The case fatality rate is usually high and has approached 60% in patients infected by certain strains. The CT appearance of avian influenza consists of focal, multifocal, or diffuse ground-glass opacities or consolidation. Pleural effusions, lymphadenopathy, centrilobular nodules, pseudocavitation, and pneumatocele formation are often also noted.[5] Swine influenza (H1N1) often resembles organizing pneumonia, manifesting as peribronchial or peripheral predominant consolidation and ground-glass opacities (Fig. 13.11).[21] Of importance, patients with H1N1 infection also have an elevated risk of pulmonary thromboembolic disease.

KEY POINTS: INFLUENZA VIRUSES

- Symptomatic disease (influenza) occurs in 20% of children and 5% of adults per year.
- Risk factors for primary influenza virus pneumonia include old age and cardiopulmonary disease.
- The most common imaging manifestations of primary influenza virus pneumonia follow:
  - Reticulonodular pattern
  - Focal areas of consolidation that may become confluent
  - Peripheral or peribronchial consolidation that resembles organizing pneumonia in some infected with H1N1 strain
- Secondary bacterial pneumonia is relatively common and most commonly affects the elderly and those with underlying cardiopulmonary disease.
- The most common radiologic manifestation of secondary bacterial pneumonia is patchy or confluent unilateral or bilateral consolidation.

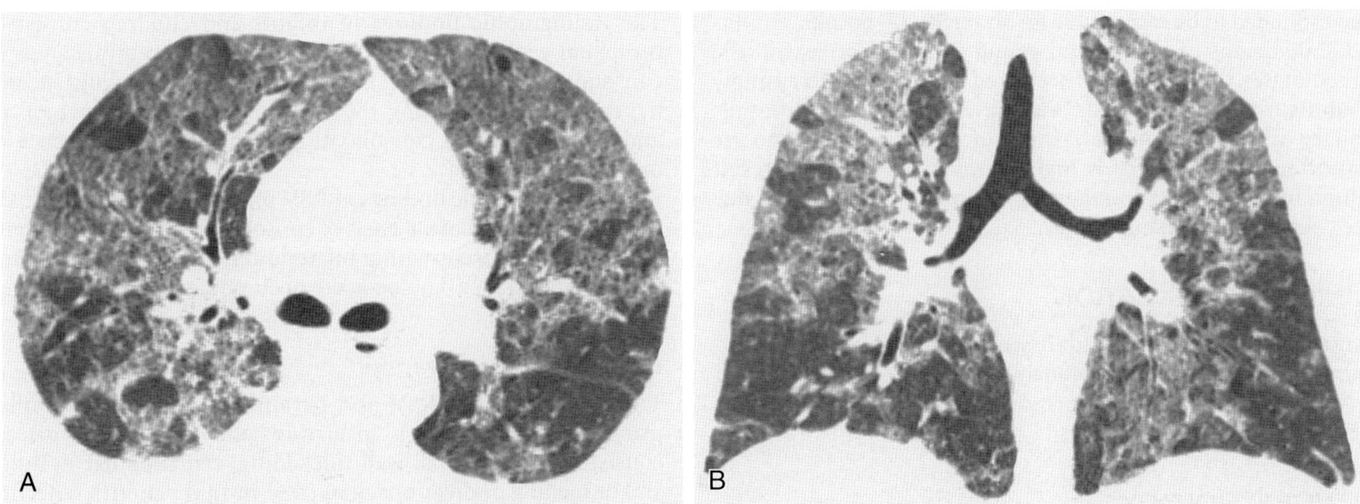

Fig. 13.10 Influenza pneumonia. (A) Axial CT shows extensive bilateral ground-glass opacities with superimposed fine linear opacities ("crazy-paving" pattern) and small bilateral pleural effusions. (B) Coronal reformation shows overall extent of the parenchymal abnormalities.

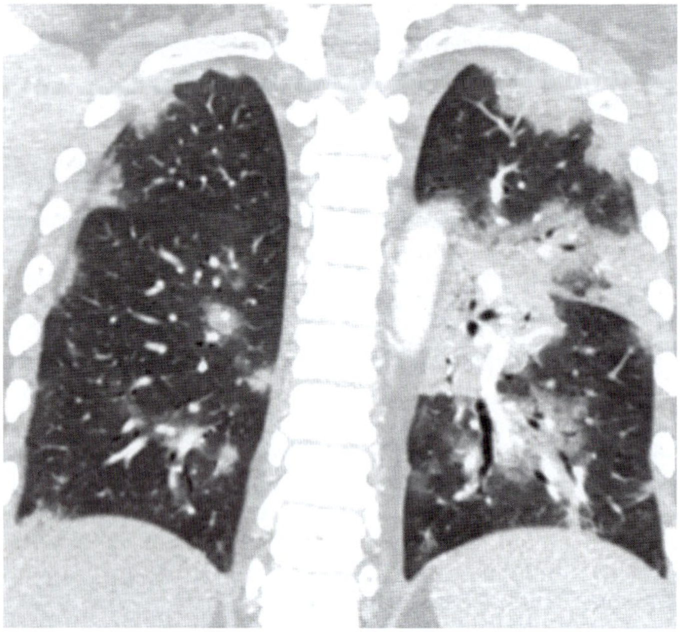

Fig. 13.11 H1N1 influenza infection with organizing pneumonia-like pattern. Coronal CT shows bilateral peripheral and peribronchial predominant consolidation. Differential considerations include organizing pneumonia, eosinophilic pneumonia, and infection such as influenza.

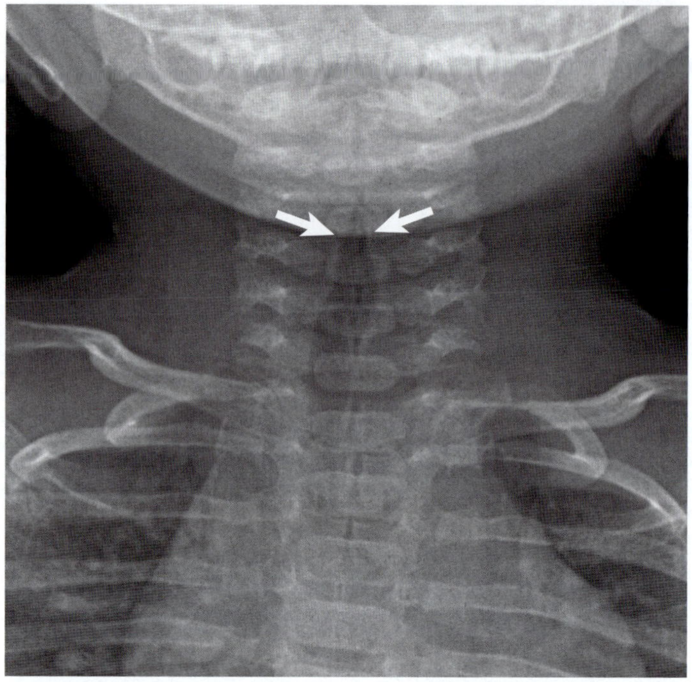

Fig. 13.12 Viral croup with steeple sign. Anteroposterior radiograph of the upper airway shows subglottic tracheal narrowing with an inverted V configuration *(arrows)*. *(Courtesy Sherwin Chan, MD, PhD, Kansas City, Missouri. From Walker CM, Digumarthy S. Pulmonary infections. In: Digumarthy S, Abbara S, Chung JH, eds.* Problem Solving in Chest Imaging. *Philadelphia: Elsevier; 2019.)*

Respiratory Syncytial Virus and Parainfluenza Virus

ETIOLOGY, PREVALENCE, AND EPIDEMIOLOGY

Respiratory syncytial virus (RSV) and parainfluenza virus account for a high proportion of cases of pneumonia, acute bronchiolitis, and tracheobronchitis (croup) in young children (Fig. 13.12) and occasionally cause lower respiratory tract infection in adults. Both are single-stranded RNA viruses and members of the Paramyxoviridae family.

RSV infects virtually all children in the first few years of life and is the most common cause of bronchiolitis and one of the most common causes of pneumonia in these patients.[22] It has been estimated to be responsible for about 90,000 hospitalizations and 4500 deaths of infants and young children per year in the United States.[23] Both viruses are being recognized increasingly in adults, particularly adults who have underlying cardiopulmonary disease, malignancy, or immunodeficiency or who are institutionalized.[24,25] RSV is highly contagious and may result in high infection rates in relatively enclosed places, such as day care centers and nursing homes.

CLINICAL PRESENTATION

Symptoms of infection in adults are usually those of a "cold" (rhinitis, pharyngitis, and conjunctivitis). Manifestations of lower respiratory tract involvement (most often cough) are seen in a significant number of patients.[4]

PATHOPHYSIOLOGY

Transmission is by airborne droplets or hand-to-surface contact. Viral infection may involve mainly the airways or less commonly the parenchyma. When airway involvement predominates, the most severe changes occur in small membranous and respiratory bronchioles and consist of epithelial degeneration accompanied by a variably intense inflammatory cell infiltrate.[4] Parenchymal involvement results in interstitial pneumonitis or diffuse alveolar damage.[4]

MANIFESTATIONS OF THE DISEASE

Radiography

The radiographic findings in infants and children consist of bronchial wall thickening and peribronchial (central) areas of consolidation (see Fig. 13.1).[26,27] Other common findings include hyperinflation (reflecting the presence of acute bronchiolitis) and patchy bilateral consolidation (reflecting the presence of bronchopneumonia).[27]

The radiographic findings of RSV pneumonia in adults usually consist of patchy bilateral areas of consolidation.[28] Less commonly, patients may present with a bilateral reticulonodular pattern.[28] Rarely, patients may develop acute pneumonia with rapid progression to ARDS.[29]

Computed Tomography

The CT findings of RSV and parainfluenza virus are similar, usually manifesting with an airway centric pattern of disease consisting of bronchial wall thickening, centrilobular nodules, and branching nodular opacities (tree-in-bud pattern), reflecting the presence of bronchiolitis (see Fig. 13.3). There are often peribronchiolar ground-glass opacities or areas of consolidation, owing to bronchopneumonia (Fig. 13.13). Inspiratory CT may

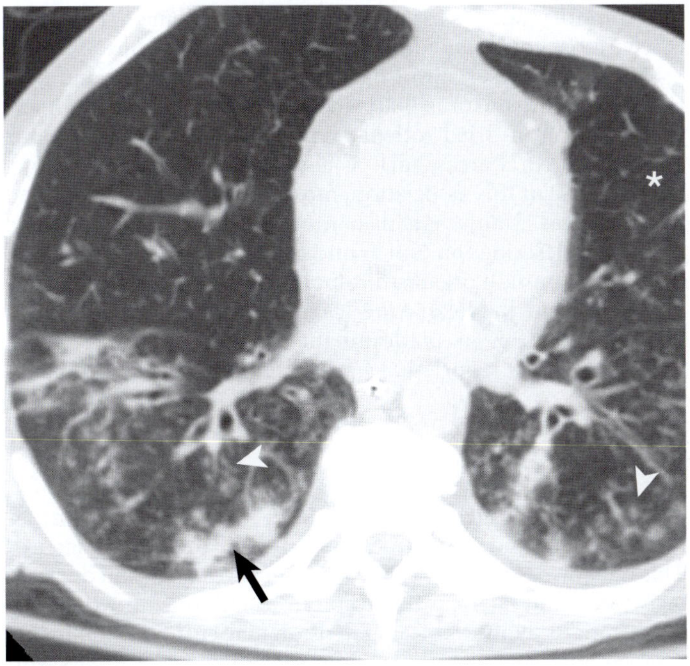

Fig. 13.13 Parainfluenza pneumonia. Axial CT shows bronchial wall thickening, mosaic lung attenuation *(asterisk)*, centrilobular micronodules with tree-in-bud opacities *(arrowheads)*, and peribronchial consolidation *(arrow)*.

show mosaic attenuation, and expiratory CT may show air trapping. Less common manifestations include multifocal airspace or focal airspace patterns without appreciable bronchial or small airways involvement.[6,7,30]

KEY POINTS: RESPIRATORY SYNCYTIAL VIRUS AND PARAINFLUENZA VIRUS

- Infection with RSV and parainfluenza virus is common in infants and children; infection is less common in adults.
- Risk factors for RSV bronchiolitis include young age (infants and young children).
- The most common radiologic manifestations include:
  - Hyperinflation
  - Bronchial wall thickening and peribronchial opacities
  - Steeple sign in croup
- Risk factors for pneumonia include the extremes of age (infants, young children, the elderly) and chronic illness.
- The most common CT manifestations include:
  - Airway centric pattern of disease with bronchial wall thickening, centrilobular nodules, and tree-in-bud opacities
  - Patchy peribronchial consolidation or ground-glass opacities

Severe Acute Respiratory Syndrome Coronavirus

ETIOLOGY, PREVALENCE, AND EPIDEMIOLOGY

The SARS coronavirus is the cause of severe acute respiratory syndrome (SARS), an infectious disease that first emerged in southern China in 2002. When it reached Hong Kong, the disease spread rapidly to other parts of the world by international air travel.[31] Within approximately 8 months, SARS affected 8422 patients in numerous countries and resulted in 916 deaths (case-fatality rate of 11%).[31] Most of the infections occurred in hospitals,

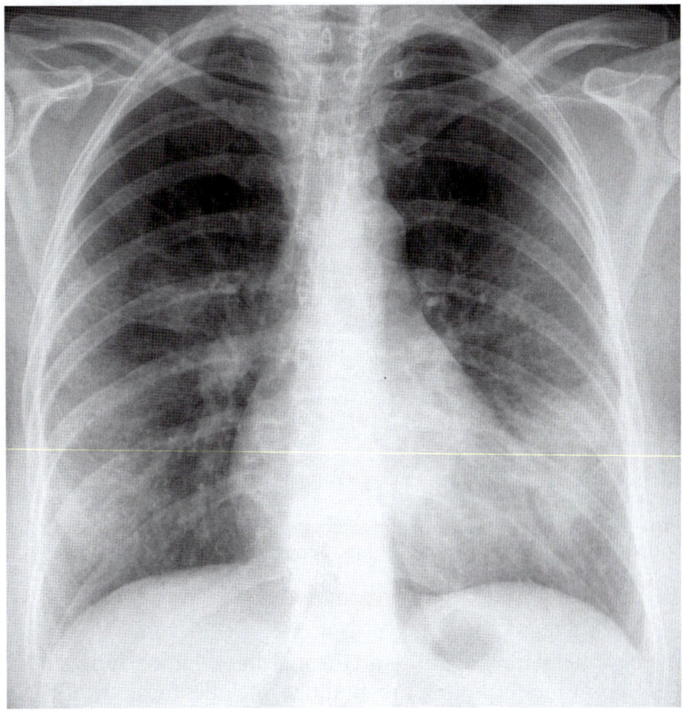

Fig. 13.14 Severe acute respiratory syndrome. Chest radiograph shows patchy bilateral consolidation. *(From Müller NL, Ooi GC, Khong PL, et al. Severe acute respiratory syndrome: radiographic and CT findings. AJR Am J Roentgenol. 2003;181:3–8.)*

laboratories involved in diagnosis or research on the organism, and nursing homes. Only a few sporadic cases of SARS have been reported since 2003.[32]

The natural reservoir of the organism is believed to be wild animals, such as raccoon-dogs, ferrets, and civets.[33] The disease is transmitted by droplets or direct inoculation from contact with infected surfaces.[31] The mean incubation period is 6 days (range, 2–10 days).[31]

CLINICAL PRESENTATION

Presenting symptoms include fever, chills, dry cough, myalgia, and headache.[34] These can progress to clinical, radiologic, and pathologic features of ARDS. Laboratory findings include lymphopenia, evidence of disseminated intravascular coagulation, and elevated blood levels of lactate dehydrogenase and creatine kinase.[34]

PATHOPHYSIOLOGY

The predominant pattern of lung injury in autopsy specimens was diffuse alveolar damage.[35] Cases of 10 or fewer days of duration showed acute-phase diffuse alveolar damage. Cases of more than 10 days of duration exhibited organizing-phase diffuse alveolar damage and, frequently, superimposed bacterial bronchopneumonia.[35]

MANIFESTATIONS OF THE DISEASE

Radiography

The most common radiologic manifestations consist of focal unilateral or multifocal unilateral or bilateral areas of consolidation (Fig. 13.14).[36–38] The consolidation tends to involve predominantly

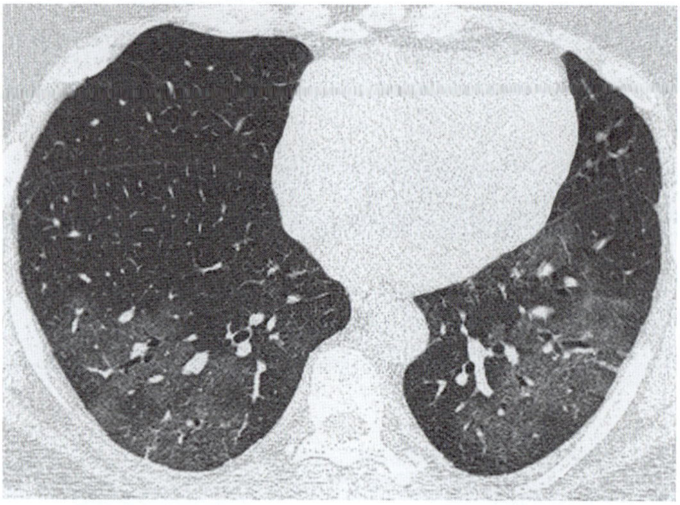

Fig. 13.15 Severe acute respiratory syndrome. High-resolution CT shows patchy bilateral ground-glass opacities in the lower lobes.

the peripheral lung regions and the middle and lower lung zones. Less common radiographic findings include focal or diffuse ground-glass opacities and, rarely, lobar consolidation. Approximately 20% to 40% of patients with SARS have normal radiographs at presentation.[36,38]

Computed Tomography

The most common high-resolution CT findings consist of focal, multifocal, or diffuse ground-glass opacities or areas of consolidation (Fig. 13.15).[37,39,40] Interlobular septal and intralobular interstitial thickening are often seen superimposed on the ground-glass opacities ("crazy-paving" pattern).[37,39,40] High-resolution CT findings commonly seen in other pneumonias, such as branching nodular and linear opacities (tree-in-bud pattern), hilar and mediastinal lymphadenopathy, and pleural effusion, are uncommon in patients with SARS.[39]

KEY POINTS: SEVERE ACUTE RESPIRATORY SYNDROME CORONAVIRUS

- SARS infection is transmitted by droplets or direct inoculation.
- A pandemic occurred in 2003; sporadic cases have occurred since.
- The most common radiologic manifestations include:
  - Focal or multifocal unilateral or bilateral consolidation affecting peripheral lung regions and middle and lower lung zones
  - Chest radiograph initially normal in 20%–40% of cases
  - Thin-section CT usually abnormal when radiograph normal

Hantaviruses

ETIOLOGY, PREVALENCE, AND EPIDEMIOLOGY

Hantaviruses are single-stranded RNA viruses that result in two distinct symptom complexes: hemorrhagic fever with renal syndrome and hantavirus pulmonary syndrome. Hemorrhagic fever with renal syndrome is characterized by fever, hypotension, and renal failure and is seen most commonly in Southeast Asia.[41,42] Hantavirus pulmonary syndrome is characterized by the presence of respiratory distress from noncardiogenic edema.[43] This form is seen most commonly in North and South America.[41]

The natural reservoir of hantavirus is wild rodents and deer mice.[44] The organism is believed to be transmitted to humans by inhalation of dried rodent excreta associated with outdoor activities in rural areas, such as cleaning barns and harvesting rice. Because of this association, most cases have been identified in rural areas. Many cases of hantavirus pulmonary syndrome have been described in North and South America and in Asia. The most common organism responsible for hantavirus pulmonary syndrome in North America is the Sin Nombre virus, and the deer mouse is its predominant reservoir.[45] An increase in human cases was reported in several regions of the United States in 2006.[45]

CLINICAL PRESENTATION

The disease typically begins with a 2- to 3-day prodrome of fever, myalgia, and, sometimes, abdominal pain and headache.[44] This is followed after 3 to 6 days by progressive cough and dyspnea, tachypnea, and tachycardia. Respiratory failure with worsening hypoxemia and intractable hypotension may ensue. Disseminated intravascular coagulation develops in some cases. Patients who survive these acute events enter a convalescent phase, which may be remarkably rapid. The case-fatality rate is about 30% to 40%.[45]

PATHOPHYSIOLOGY

Pathologic examination of the lungs of patients dying of hantavirus pulmonary syndrome show interstitial and airspace edema with a mild to moderate interstitial infiltrate of cytologically mature and activated lymphocytes.[46] Evidence of virus-induced tissue damage, such as epithelial necrosis, vascular thrombosis, or hyaline membranes, is typically sparse or absent.

MANIFESTATIONS OF THE DISEASE

Radiography and Computed Tomography

The chest radiograph may be initially normal or show findings consistent with interstitial pulmonary edema, including septal (Kerley B) lines, perihilar haze, and peribronchial cuffing.[47,48] Patients with normal radiographs at presentation usually develop interstitial pulmonary edema within 48 hours. The edema may gradually resolve or, in patients with severe disease, progress to bibasilar, perihilar, or diffuse consolidation.[47,48] Pleural effusions, which may be small or large, are present in approximately 50% of cases. The time to resolution of the radiographic findings ranges from about 1 to 3 weeks in most cases (Fig. 13.16). The CT appearance is not well described. A report of one patient demonstrated bilateral ground-glass opacities, interlobular septal thickening, a few poorly defined nodules, bronchial wall thickening, and small pleural effusions.[49]

KEY POINTS: HANTAVIRUS

- Hantavirus infection results from exposure to wild rodents.
- Risk factors include outdoor activities in rural areas.
- The most common radiologic manifestations include:
  - Findings of interstitial edema, including septal lines, perihilar haze, and peribronchial cuffing
  - Rapid progression to perihilar or lower lung zone–predominant airspace consolidation with pleural effusions

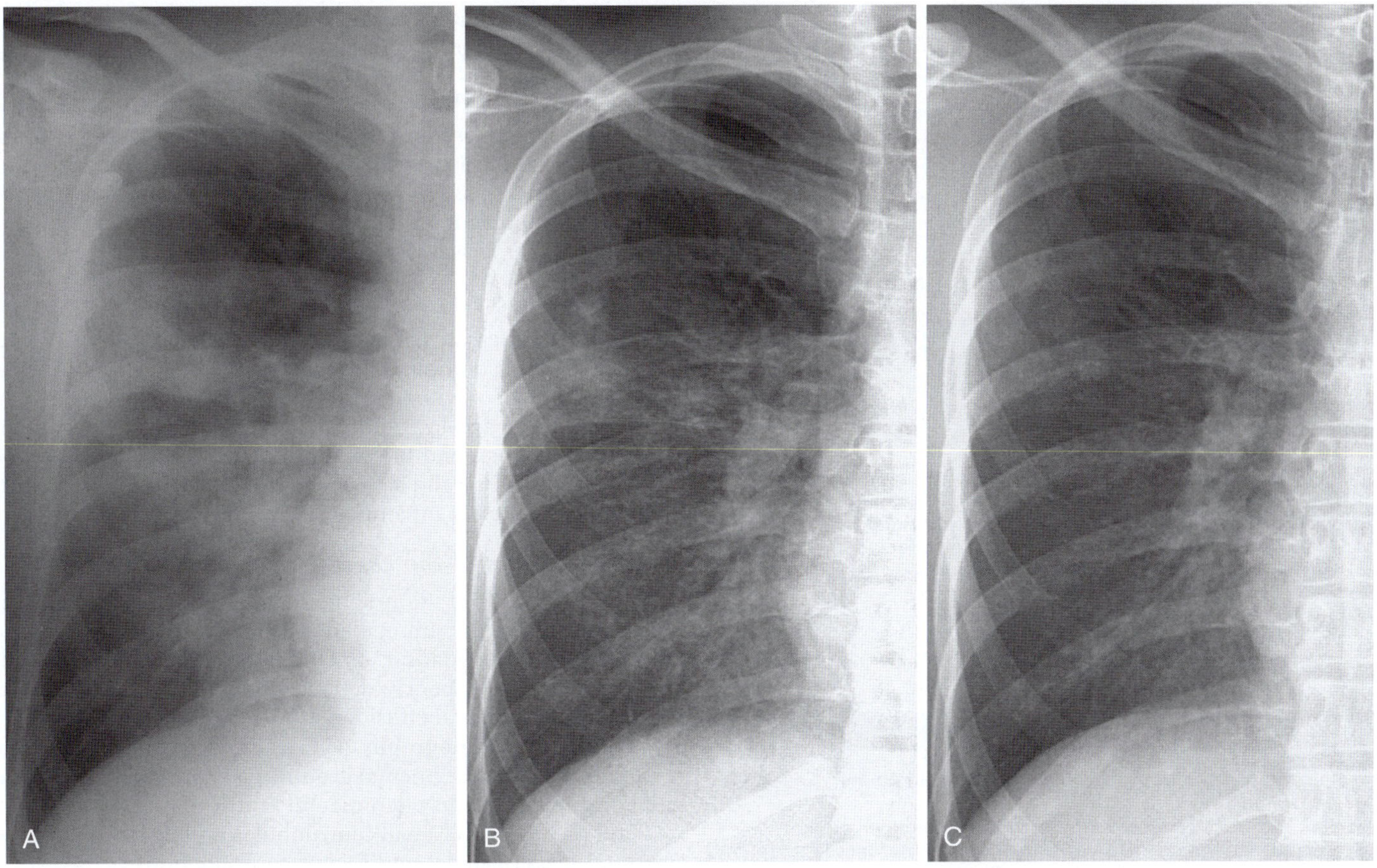

Fig. 13.16 Hantavirus hemorrhagic fever with renal syndrome. (A) View of the right lung from a chest radiograph shows extensive airspace consolidation. (B) View of the right lung from a chest radiograph 1 week later, when the patient was on hemodialysis for renal failure, shows considerable improvement but residual interstitial pulmonary edema. (C) View of the right lung from a chest radiograph made 3 days after (B) shows further improvement in the interstitial pulmonary edema. *(Courtesy Dr. Kyung Soo Lee, Samsung Medical Center, Seoul, South Korea.)*

Adenoviruses

ETIOLOGY, PREVALENCE, AND EPIDEMIOLOGY

Adenoviruses account for 5% to 10% of all respiratory illnesses in children[50,51] and may result in pharyngitis, laryngotracheobronchitis, bronchiolitis, and occasionally bronchopneumonia.[52] Although less common than during childhood, adenovirus may result in lower respiratory tract infection and pneumonia in immunocompetent[53,54] and immunocompromised adults.[55,56] Adenovirus infection in immunocompromised patients is often severe and can be fatal.[55] Infections may occur sporadically or as outbreaks in specific groups, such as military populations or individuals in geriatric care centers.

CLINICAL PRESENTATION

The most common clinical symptoms include fever, pharyngitis, cough, and hoarseness. The pneumonia when it occurs is generally mild and associated with upper respiratory symptoms.[4]

PATHOPHYSIOLOGY

Histologic findings include necrotizing bronchitis and bronchiolitis and interstitial inflammation.[4] Severe pneumonia is characterized by the presence of patchy areas of hemorrhagic consolidation, necrotic changes with diffuse alveolar damage, and areas of overinflation or atelectasis.[57]

MANIFESTATIONS OF THE DISEASE

Radiography

The radiographic manifestations of adenovirus bronchopneumonia in children and adults consist of patchy bilateral areas of consolidation in a lobular or segmental distribution.[19,58] Other common findings in children include hyperinflation and lobar atelectasis.[58] Long-term sequelae of adenovirus bronchiolitis and bronchopneumonia in children include bronchiectasis, constrictive bronchiolitis, and unilateral hyperlucent lung (Swyer-James-McLeod) syndrome.[59,60]

Computed Tomography

The CT findings of adenoviral pneumonia consist of multifocal ground-glass opacities or consolidation usually without airway inflammatory abnormalities, such as bronchial wall thickening or tree-in-bud opacities (Fig. 13.17; see Fig. 13.4).[6]

Herpesviruses

Herpesviruses are double-stranded deoxyribonucleic acid viruses that are able to remain dormant within infected cells, without

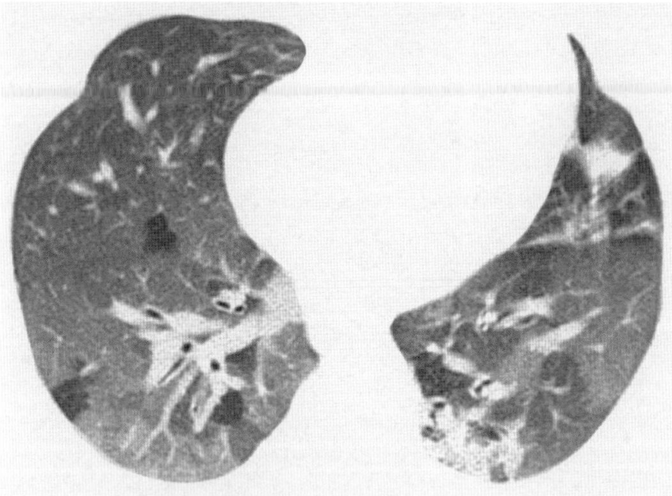

Fig. 13.17 Adenovirus bronchopneumonia. High-resolution CT shows focal areas of consolidation in the lingula and left lower lobe, ground-glass opacities, and small foci of decreased attenuation and vascularity compatible with mosaic attenuation. *(Courtesy Dr. Kyung Soo Lee, Samsung Medical Center, Seoul, South Korea.)*

KEY POINTS: ADENOVIRUSES

- Infection with adenovirus is common in children and uncommon in adults.
- Risk factors for adenovirus pneumonia include young age (infants and young children) and immunocompromised state.
- The most common radiologic manifestations of adenovirus pneumonia include:
  - Patchy bilateral consolidation in a lobular, segmental, or subsegmental distribution
  - Hyperinflation common in infants and young children
  - Airway inflammatory abnormalities often minimal or absent
- Sequelae of adenovirus bronchopneumonia in childhood include:
  - Bronchiectasis
  - Constrictive bronchiolitis and Swyer-James-McLeod syndrome

causing recognizable disease. In certain circumstances, often of an immunocompromising nature, but sometimes without obvious clinical correlate, reactivation occurs, and clinically evident disease ensues. Such disease usually is localized and well tolerated in otherwise healthy individuals; however, in an immunocompromised patient, it is frequently disseminated and severe. The most common pathogens are herpes simplex virus, varicella virus (varicella-zoster virus), CMV, and EBV.

HERPES SIMPLEX VIRUS

Etiology, Prevalence, and Epidemiology

Herpes simplex virus is transmitted in situations of close personal contact through saliva or vesicle fluid. The most common manifestations are acute gingivostomatitis in children and recurrent cold sores (herpes labialis) in adults. The virus may spread to the lung by aspiration or extension of oropharyngeal infection into the lower respiratory system or by hematogenous spread in patients with sepsis.[61] Most patients with herpes simplex pneumonia have an underlying predisposing condition, such as severe burn, acquired immune deficiency syndrome (AIDS), malignancy, or organ transplant.[62,63]

Clinical Presentation

The clinical manifestations of herpes simplex virus tracheobronchitis and pneumonia include fever; productive cough; and, in some patients, signs of bronchospasm and shortness of breath.[4] Pseudomembranes related to tracheal ulcers may be large enough to cause upper airway obstruction.

Pathophysiology

The histologic features of herpes simplex lower respiratory tract infection consist of focal or diffuse ulcers in the tracheobronchial epithelium with or without associated necrotizing bronchopneumonia.[19,64] The airway lesion is characterized histologically by epithelial necrosis and ulceration. Pneumonia is characterized by alveolar necrosis and a proteinaceous exudate with a variable polymorphonuclear inflammatory response.[19,65]

Manifestations of the Disease

Radiography. The radiographic manifestations usually consist of patchy bilateral subsegmental or segmental ground-glass opacities or consolidation.[19,66] Other common findings include reticular opacities, poorly defined nodular opacities (airspace nodules), and pleural effusions.[67,68]

Computed Tomography. CT findings include multifocal subsegmental and segmental ground-glass opacities, focal areas of consolidation, and often pleural effusion.[66] High-resolution CT frequently shows small centrilobular nodules in addition to ground-glass opacities and foci of consolidation.[69]

KEY POINTS: HERPES SIMPLEX VIRUS

- Herpes simplex pneumonia is seen almost exclusively in immunocompromised patients.
- The most common radiographic manifestations of herpes simplex pneumonia include:
  - Patchy bilateral consolidation in a lobular, subsegmental, or segmental distribution
  - Reticular opacities
  - Pleural effusion
- Thin-section CT findings follow:
  - Lobular, subsegmental or segmental consolidation or ground-glass opacities
  - Centrilobular nodules and tree-in-bud pattern

VARICELLA VIRUS

Etiology, Prevalence, and Epidemiology

Varicella virus (varicella-zoster virus) infection is seen in two clinical forms: varicella (chickenpox), representing primary and usually disseminated disease in previously uninfected individuals, and zoster (shingles), representing reactivation of latent virus, typically as a unilateral dermatomal skin eruption.[4] Although either form may be associated with pneumonia, most cases occur after chickenpox. In addition, varicella-zoster virus infection may be complicated by unilateral diaphragmatic paralysis, presumably as a result of extension of infection from the dorsal root to the adjacent posterior and lateral spinal cord and anterior horn cells.[70]

Varicella is a highly contagious, predominantly mucocutaneous disease that tends to occur during the colder months in temperate climates. It is believed to be transmitted by droplet infection. Varicella typically affects children 2 to 8 years old but is decreasing

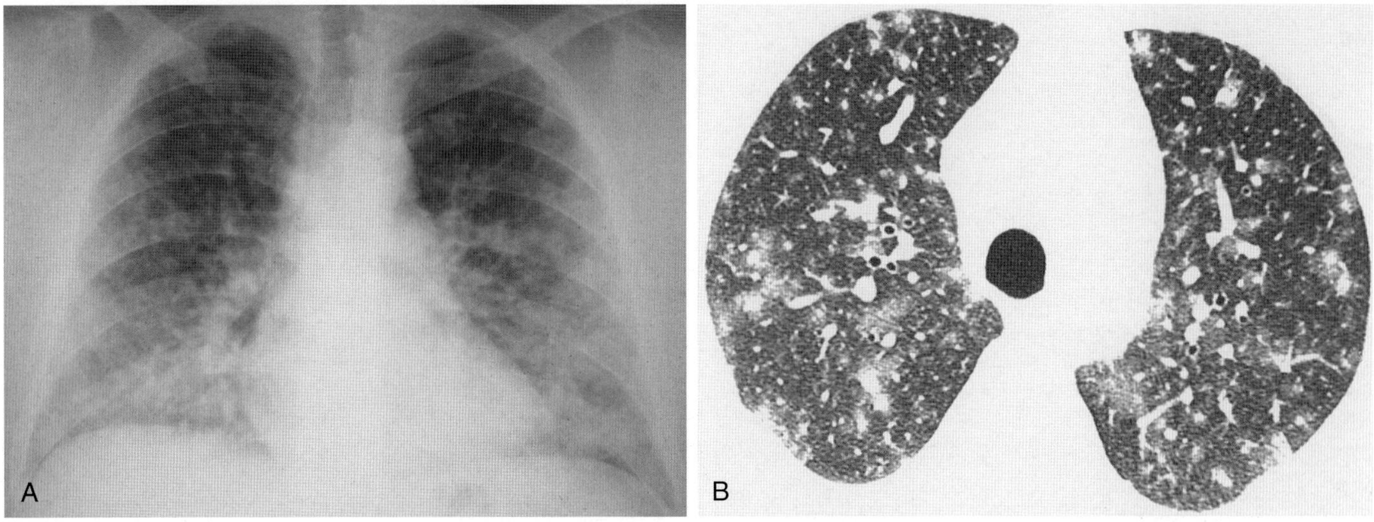

Fig. 13.18 Acute varicella-zoster pneumonia. (A) Chest radiograph shows multiple, poorly defined nodular opacities. (B) High-resolution CT shows bilateral nodular opacities and patchy ground-glass opacities. Many of the nodules have a halo of ground-glass attenuation (CT halo sign). *(Courtesy Dr. Jaime Barbosa, Presidente Prudente, São Paulo, Brazil.)*

in incidence because of vaccination.[71] Data from Europe and North America have shown that the incidence of chickenpox in adults has doubled in the past 2 decades and that approximately 7% of adults are susceptible to the disease.[71] Most cases of varicella pneumonia occur in very young children or adults. Predisposing conditions include underlying malignancy, particularly leukemia and lymphoma, and other causes of immunodeficiency.[72] Overall, approximately 1 in 400 children with varicella develop pneumonia.[71] Adults who develop chickenpox are at much greater risk of developing pneumonia, with the reported incidence ranging from 5% to 50%.[71,73]

Clinical Presentation

The onset of chickenpox is often marked by high fever, which may precede the rash by 2 to 3 days. The rash itself may be scarlatiniform in its early stages but rapidly becomes maculopapular, vesicular, and pustular. Most patients have a history of contact with an affected child 3 to 21 days before onset of the acute illness. Symptoms and signs of pneumonia usually develop 2 to 3 days after appearance of the skin eruption and consist of cough, dyspnea, tachypnea, pleuritic chest pain, and, in severe cases, hemoptysis and cyanosis.[4] The temperature may be elevated. Expectorant is not purulent, unless there is secondary bacterial infection.

Pathophysiology

Vesicles similar to those on the skin and mucous membranes may be seen in the trachea and larger bronchi and on the pleural and peritoneal surfaces. Histologic findings in more severe cases of pneumonia consist of diffuse alveolar damage.[4] With recovery from the initial disease, spherical nodules are often seen, scattered randomly throughout the lungs.[19] Histologically, the nodules are composed of an outer fibrous capsule enclosing areas of hyalinized collagen or necrotic tissue.[19]

Manifestations of the Disease

Radiography. The characteristic radiographic pattern of acute varicella pneumonia consists of multiple 5- to 10-mm-diameter nodular opacities (Fig. 13.18; see Fig. 13.2).[19,71,74] With progressive disease, the nodules enlarge and coalesce, forming extensive areas of consolidation, especially near the hila and in the lung bases.[74] Other findings include ill-defined reticular or reticulonodular opacities and patchy or confluent areas of consolidation.[74] Hilar lymphadenopathy and pleural effusion may be seen.

Occasionally, varicella lung lesions may calcify and persist as numerous well-defined, randomly scattered, 2- to 3-mm densely calcified nodules (Fig. 13.19).[75] The hilar lymph nodes do not calcify.[4]

Computed Tomography. Thin-section CT usually shows 1- to 10-mm well-defined or ill-defined nodules diffusely throughout both lungs.[74,76] Other findings include nodules with a surrounding halo of ground-glass attenuation, patchy ground-glass opacities, and coalescence of nodules (see Fig. 13.18). These findings disappear concurrently with healing of skin lesions after antiviral chemotherapy.[76]

KEY POINTS: VARICELLA VIRUS

- Varicella pneumonia occurs in a small percentage of young children and adults with varicella.
- Risk factors include leukemia, lymphoma, and immunodeficiency.
- The most common imaging manifestations of varicella pneumonia include:
  - Multiple ill-defined, 5- to 10-mm-diameter nodules, many with halo of ground-glass opacity
  - Multifocal areas of consolidation or ground-glass opacities
  - Healed lesions may manifest as multiple small calcified nodules

CYTOMEGALOVIRUS

Cytomegalovirus (CMV) is a common human pathogen, with seropositivity rates varying from 40% to 100% in different adult populations around the world. Most infections are not associated with symptoms, the only significant effect being the presence of latent virus as a potential source of reinfection. CMV is the most

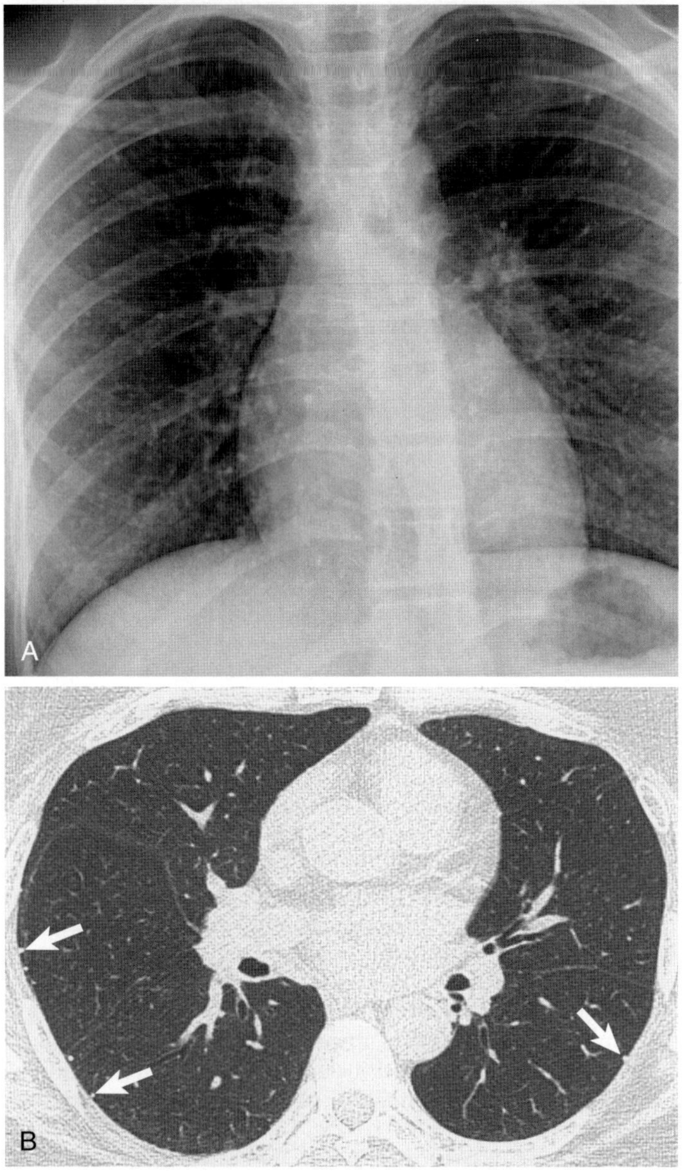

Fig. 13.19 Healed varicella-zoster lesions. (A) Chest radiograph shows numerous bilateral small calcified nodules. The differential considerations include old miliary histoplasmosis infection or varicella infection. (B) High-resolution CT at the level of the lower lobes in a different patient shows multiple small, well-defined bilateral calcified nodules *(arrows)*.

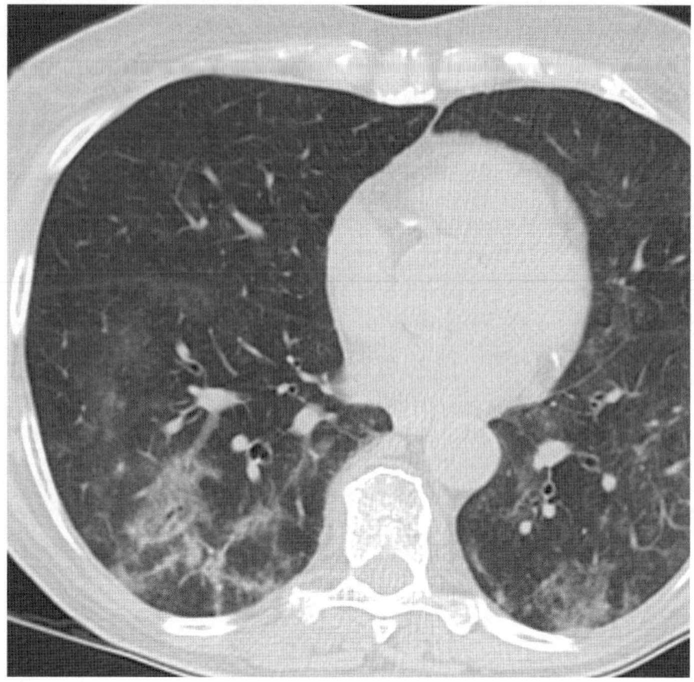

Fig. 13.20 Cytomegalovirus pneumonia in renal transplant recipient. Axial CT shows peribronchial consolidation and ground-glass opacities with bronchial wall thickening.

common viral pathogen associated with life-threatening pulmonary infection in the immunocompromised host. Risk factors include transplantation, AIDS, and long-term corticosteroid therapy. In solid-organ and hematopoietic stem cell transplant patients, the infection typically arises 30 to 100 days after transplantation in the postengraftment period. Delayed onset of infection may occur in patients who have received cytomegalovirus prophylaxis.[77]

Manifestations of the Disease

Radiography and Computed Tomography. The radiographic manifestations of CMV pneumonia consist of bilateral opacities with nodules measuring less than 5 mm in diameter. On CT there is usually lobar or bilateral consolidation, ground-glass opacities (Fig. 13.20), crazy-paving pattern (see Fig. 13.7), irregular reticular opacities, and nodules measuring less than 10 mm; nodules may have a random, subpleural, or centrilobular distribution and sometimes are associated with a halo of ground-glass opacity (CT halo sign).[78,79] The CT appearance of CMV associated with AIDS may be different and includes ground-glass opacity, consolidation, and nodular or mass-like opacities measuring up to 3 cm.[5]

KEY POINTS: CYTOMEGALOVIRUS PNEUMONIA

- CMV pneumonia generally only affects immunosuppressed patients and is most common after stem cell transplant or AIDS patients with a very low CD4 level.
- The most common imaging manifestations of CMV pneumonia include:
  - Lobar or bilateral consolidation or ground-glass opacities
  - Nodules measuring less than 10 mm

EPSTEIN-BARR VIRUS

EBV infects B lymphocytes and pharyngeal epithelial cells, in which it can remain dormant for prolonged periods. Infection usually occurs by direct person-to-person spread. The virus is best known as the cause of infectious mononucleosis, a syndrome that affects predominantly young adults and consists of pharyngitis; fever; more or less diffuse lymph node enlargement; splenomegaly; and an increase in lymphocytes, often cytologically atypical, in peripheral blood. Intrathoracic disease is uncommon and is manifested most often by lymph node enlargement, interstitial pneumonitis, or both. Patients typically complain of the insidious onset of weakness, malaise, fever, and sore throat. Spasmodic cough productive of small amounts of sputum and dyspnea are manifestations of lower respiratory tract involvement.

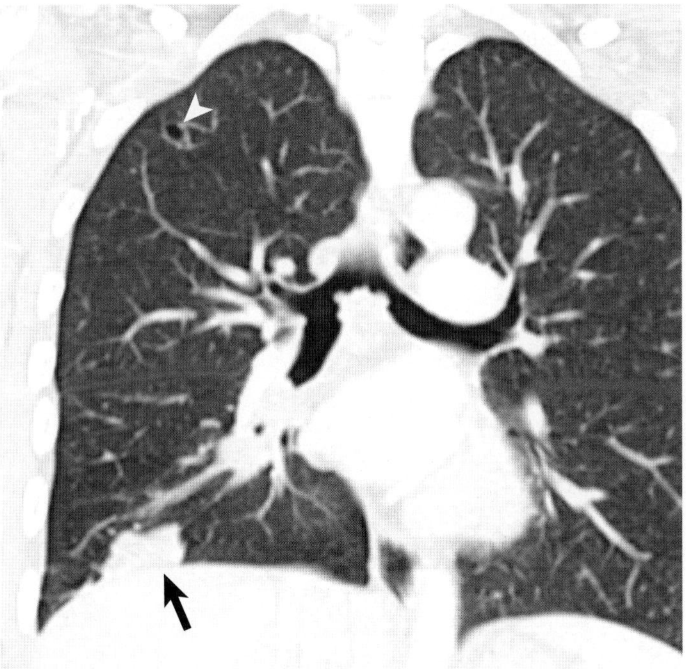

Fig. 13.21 Tracheobronchial papillomatosis with right lower lobe squamous cell carcinoma. Coronal CT shows a right lower lobe mass *(arrow)* and a right upper lobe cavitary nodule *(arrowhead)*. Note nodules involving the tracheal carina and proximal main bronchi compatible with tracheobronchial papillomatosis. The right lower lobe mass was fluorodeoxyglucose avid (not shown) and represented a squamous cell carcinoma at surgical resection.

EBV has been implicated in the development of several lymphoproliferative disorders, particularly high-grade lymphoma in association with AIDS or organ transplants (posttransplant lymphoproliferative disorders).[80] There also is evidence that it has a role in the pathogenesis of lymphocytic interstitial pneumonia.[81]

PAPILLOMA VIRUSES

Papilloma viruses are the cause of squamous papillomas in the larynx and, less commonly, in the lower respiratory tract. The papillomas may be multiple (tracheobronchial papillomatosis) and involve the lung parenchyma. The most common imaging appearance consists of multiple pulmonary cysts and nodules in conjunction with tracheobronchial nodularity (Fig. 13.21). The cysts are round or irregular in shape with smooth but asymmetric thick walls measuring 2 to 3 mm. The majority of intraparenchymal papillomas are lobular in contour and measure less than 3 cm in diameter.[5] There is evidence that the viruses are responsible for the development of pulmonary carcinoma in some patients who have this condition (see Fig. 13.21).[82]

IMAGING ALGORITHM

The chest radiograph is the initial imaging modality used to assess patients with suspected or proven viral pneumonia. In certain viral infections that are highly contagious, including from SARS and hantavirus, further imaging with CT is generally discouraged. CT may be helpful in patients with clinically suspected pneumonia and normal or nonspecific radiographic findings. CT is also helpful in assessing complications, particularly related to superimposed infection, including abscess formation or empyema.

DIFFERENTIAL DIAGNOSIS

The clinical and radiologic manifestations of viral pneumonia are nonspecific. The differential diagnosis for the airway centric, multifocal airspace, and unifocal airspace patterns includes bacterial and fungal respiratory pathogens, aspiration, and asthmatic bronchitis.[16] Initially, hantavirus infection has identical radiographic manifestations as interstitial pulmonary edema but may progress rapidly to diffuse consolidation secondary to noncardiogenic pulmonary edema. The differential diagnosis includes other causes of interstitial pulmonary edema and ARDS. The diagnosis of varicella pneumonia should be suspected in all patients with symptoms of pneumonia developing within a few days after the appearance of the characteristic varicella skin rash. The characteristic radiologic manifestations consist of numerous bilateral 5- to 10-mm-diameter nodular opacities.

The diagnosis of a specific viral infection can be confirmed by clinical, epidemiologic, and laboratory criteria, such as direct immunofluorescence, enzyme-linked immunosorbent assay, viral culture, PCR, serologic testing, biopsy, and acute and convalescent antibody titers.[16,22] Viral culture and PCR often have the highest sensitivity and specificity in the diagnosis.[16]

TREATMENT

The treatment of viral pneumonia is usually supportive care. For several decades, the adamantine drugs, amantidine and rimantadine, were the only drugs available as prophylactic and therapeutic agents for influenza. Several influenza A strains have become resistant to these drugs, however.[83] More recently, neuraminidase inhibitors, such as oseltamivir and zanamivir, have been shown to be effective in the prevention and treatment of influenza A.[83,84] Patients with RSV or parainfluenza viral pneumonia are often treated supportively but may also receive ribavirin in complicated cases. Patients with varicella or herpes simplex pneumonia usually are treated with intravenous acyclovir.[74] Cytomegalovirus pneumonia may be treated with ganciclovir, foscarnet, or less commonly, cidofovir.[85]

KEY POINTS: VIRAL PNEUMONIA

- Most viral pneumonias in immunocompetent adults are due to influenza viruses; other common viral etiologies include RSV and adenovirus. Immunocompromised hosts are particularly susceptible to pneumonias caused by CMV and herpesviruses.
- The imaging findings of viral pneumonia are nonspecific and are often mistaken for a bacterial pneumonia. Viral pneumonia should be considered in the following situations:
  - Airway centric disease with bronchial wall thickening, centrilobular nodules, and tree-in-bud opacities
  - Multifocal consolidation or ground-glass opacities that may predominantly affect the peribronchial areas
- Uncommon imaging manifestations of viral pneumonia include:
  - Unifocal consolidation or ground-glass opacities
  - Diffuse consolidation or ground-glass opacities
  - Pleural effusion
  - Lymphadenopathy
  - Interstitial edema pattern with interlobular septal thickening
- Influenza may manifest with any of the CT patterns of infection.
- RSV and parainfluenza virus usually manifest with an airway centric pattern of disease.
- Adenovirus usually manifests with a multifocal airspace pattern consisting of multifocal consolidation or ground-glass opacities without bronchial involvement.

SUGGESTED READINGS

Franquet T. Imaging of pulmonary viral pneumonia. *Radiology*. 2011;260:18–39.

Kim EA, Lee KS, Primack SL, et al. Viral pneumonias in adults: radiologic and pathologic findings. *Radiographics*. 2002;22:S137–S149.

Miller WT Jr, Mickus TJ, Barbosa E Jr, Mullin C, Van Deerlin VM, Shiley KT. CT of viral lower respiratory tract infections in adults: comparison among viral organisms and between viral and bacterial infections. *AJR Am J Roentgenol*. 2011;197(5):1088–1095.

The full reference list for this chapter is available at ExpertConsult.com.

14 Parasites*

CHRISTOPHER M. WALKER | JONATHAN H. CHUNG

Parasites are defined as organisms that live in or on another living organism, obtain part or all of their organic nutriment from that organism, and cause some degree of damage to their host. Parasitic infestations occur mainly in tropical and subtropical regions. Pulmonary disease secondary to parasites in North America and Europe is seen in individuals who traveled to endemic areas and in recent immigrants. Parasites that most commonly result in pulmonary disease include protozoa (amebiasis), nematodes (ascariasis and strongyloides), cestodes (echinococcosis), and trematodes (schistosomiasis and paragonimiasis). Although rare in the United States and in other developed countries, parasitic diseases should at least be considered in the following situations:

1. Peripheral blood eosinophilia
2. Recent travel to or emigration from endemic areas
3. Migratory pulmonary opacities or nodules without obvious cause
4. Exacerbation of pulmonary disease after administration of corticosteroids
5. Development of peripheral blood eosinophilia after administration of corticosteroids

Amebiasis

ETIOLOGY, PREVALENCE, AND EPIDEMIOLOGY

Amebiasis is a protozoan infection caused by *Entamoeba histolytica,* a species usually associated with colonic disease (amebic dysentery). It is estimated to affect about 1% of the world population and to result in 40,000 to 110,000 deaths annually.[1] The infestation is acquired by ingestion of cysts that become trophozoites in the colon. The prevalence of infection is highest in areas of crowding, areas of poor sanitation, and the tropics. Most cases in the United States develop in immigrants from endemic regions who have been in the country for less than 2 years.[2]

The most common extraintestinal manifestations of amebiasis are liver abscess and pleuropulmonary involvement.[3] Pleuropulmonary extension occurs in 6% to 40% of patients with amebic liver abscess.[3] Less commonly, it may result from aspiration or hematogenous dissemination.

CLINICAL PRESENTATION

Patients with amebic liver abscesses are usually febrile and typically present with right upper quadrant pain.[3] Gastrointestinal symptoms, mainly diarrhea, may or may not be present. Extension into the pleural space usually is associated with acute onset of sharp lower thoracic pain that frequently radiates to the ipsilateral shoulder, cough, progressive dyspnea, and evidence of sepsis.

PATHOPHYSIOLOGY

The cysts are passed in the feces of affected individuals (who are frequently asymptomatic) and are ingested by the new host in contaminated water or food.[4] The ingested cysts of *E. histolytica* travel to the small intestine, where the trophozoites excyst. They later migrate to the colon, where they multiply and, in some cases, pass through the epithelium into the submucosa. Penetration of the mucosa is associated with necrosis, ulceration, and characteristic symptoms of amebic dysentery. The organism subsequently may enter the colonic venous circulation and pass via the portal veins to the liver, where abscesses may develop. Amebic liver abscesses are usually solitary and affect the right lobe in 80% of cases. The abscesses contain sterile pus and reddish brown ("anchovy-paste") liquefied necrotic liver tissue.

Pleuropulmonary manifestations of amebiasis usually occur by direct extension of disease from a hepatic abscess.[5] Such abscesses may extend into the subphrenic space and form a separate subdiaphragmatic abscess, resulting in elevation of the diaphragm and pleural effusion. The abscesses may also extend through the diaphragm and involve the pleura and lung. Greater than 95% of amebic lung abscesses develop in parenchyma contiguous to the diaphragm.

MANIFESTATIONS OF THE DISEASE

Radiography

The most common radiographic manifestations in the chest consist of elevation of the right hemidiaphragm (Fig. 14.1), pleural effusion, and atelectasis or consolidation in the right lower lobe.[1,3] The effusion can be sterile, reflecting the presence of inflammatory pleural reaction, or represent an empyema if the hepatic abscess ruptures and traverses the diaphragm. Pulmonary involvement results in airspace consolidation and cavitation. The pulmonary abnormalities are typically adjacent to the diaphragm.

Drainage of the liver abscess into a bronchus may result in hepatobronchial or bronchobiliary fistula.[1] Invasion of the inferior vena cava occurs occasionally and may result in pulmonary thromboembolism.

Computed Tomography

Contrast-enhanced computed tomography (CT) allows assessment of the liver abscess (see Fig. 14.1) and its extension into the subphrenic space or across the diaphragm into the pleura or lung.[6,7] It also is superior to the radiograph in showing the presence of amebic lung abscess. Liver abscesses typically are round and have smooth margins and a low-attenuation center surrounded by a contrast-enhancing rim. Uncommonly, the

*The editors and the publisher would like to thank Drs. Nestor L. Müller and C. Isabela Silva Müller for contributing material on this topic to the prior edition of this work. It has served as the foundation for the current chapter.

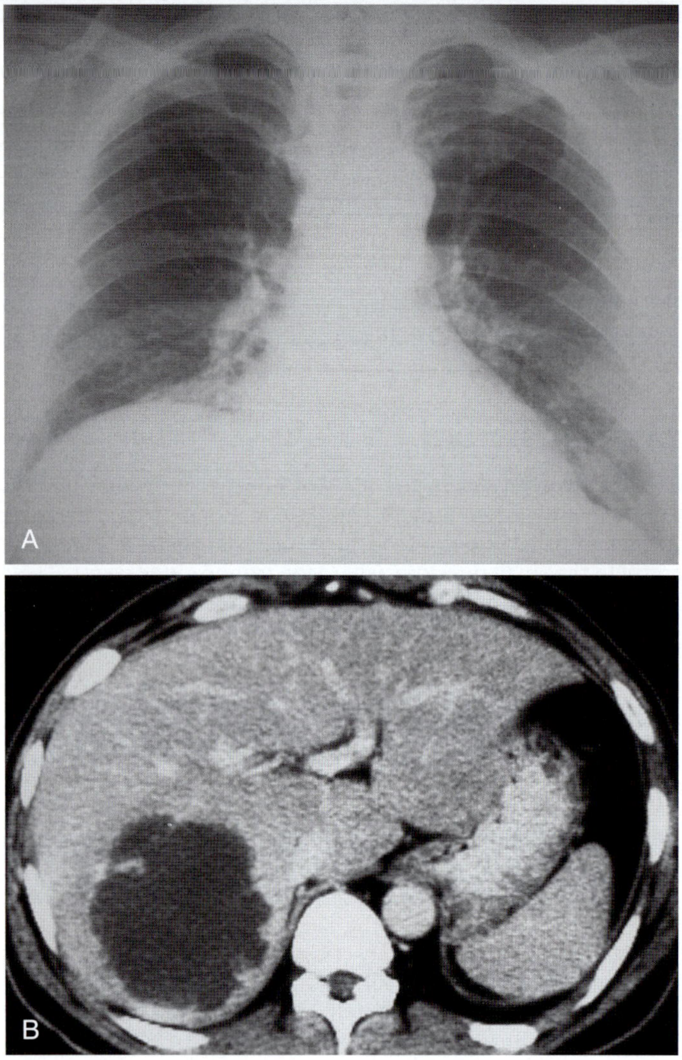

Fig. 14.1 Amebiasis in a patient with a 1-week history of fever and chills; physical examination showed tenderness in the right upper quadrant. (A) Posteroanterior chest radiograph shows elevation of the right hemidiaphragm. (B) Contrast-enhanced CT shows a large cystic lesion in the right lobe of the liver. The diagnosis of amebiasis was proved by fine-needle aspiration under ultrasound guidance. *(Courtesy Dr. Soon Ju Cha, Inje University Hospital, Seoul, South Korea.)*

hepatic abscess may communicate with the pericardial space, leading to pericardial effusion, tamponade, or pericarditis.

Magnetic Resonance Imaging

Amebic liver abscesses, similar to abscesses of other etiology, usually appear as sharply circumscribed, heterogeneous, low–signal intensity masses on T1-weighted images.[8] T2-weighted images typically show the abscess cavity as a hyperintense region, often surrounded by a rim of increased signal intensity extending from the cavity margins to the liver surface, corresponding to edematous but morphologically normal liver tissue.

Ultrasonography

Ultrasonography shows the size and position of the liver abscess.[6] Aspiration of the abscess contents may be performed under ultrasound guidance but is indicated only if rupture of the abscess is considered to be imminent. Amebae are seldom recovered from the aspirate.

Imaging Algorithm

The clinical manifestations are mainly related to the amebic liver abscess. The initial diagnostic modality is usually ultrasound or CT of the liver. Ultrasonography is the recommended examination because of its low cost and lack of radiation. The thoracic manifestations are typically assessed on the chest radiograph. Contrast-enhanced CT scans of the chest and abdomen are recommended in patients with suspected intrathoracic extension of liver abscess.

DIFFERENTIAL DIAGNOSIS

Amebic liver abscesses resemble pyogenic abscesses on ultrasound and CT. Suspicion of amebic abscess is based on clinical history. A positive diagnosis can be made by showing organisms in sputum, pleural fluid, or material obtained by needle aspiration. A presumptive diagnosis can be made if trophozoites or cysts are identified in stool.

SYNOPSIS OF TREATMENT OPTIONS

Most uncomplicated amebic abscesses resolve after treatment with metronidazole.[9] Patients who do not respond to medical therapy may require percutaneous catheter drainage of the liver abscesses.[9] Drainage can be performed under ultrasound or CT guidance.

KEY POINTS: AMEBIASIS

- Amebiasis is caused by *E. histolytica*.
- Endemic areas include tropical regions and areas of poor sanitation.
- The most common extraintestinal manifestation of amebiasis is liver abscess.
- The most common radiologic manifestations of amebiasis include:
  - Elevation of right hemidiaphragm
  - Pleural effusion
  - Consolidation and atelectasis of right lower lobe
- CT and ultrasonography are helpful to diagnose liver abscess

Ascariasis

ETIOLOGY, PREVALENCE, AND EPIDEMIOLOGY

The nematodes *Ascaris lumbricoides* and, less commonly, *Ascaris suum* are acquired by ingesting food or fluids contaminated with feces. The infection is distributed worldwide and is one of the most common parasitic infections, affecting 1.3 billion people and causing about 1550 deaths per year.[1] Parasites migrate from the small intestine to the pulmonary circulation, where they mature and destroy capillaries and alveolar walls with subsequent edema, hemorrhage, and epithelial cell desquamation, causing chemotaxis of neutrophils and eosinophils.[1]

CLINICAL PRESENTATION

Clinical manifestations of pulmonary involvement include low-grade fever, cough, and expectoration. Leukocytosis of 20,000 to 25,000 cells/mm^3 is common, with an eosinophilia of 30% to 70%.[10] Pulmonary disease is usually self-limited.

PATHOPHYSIOLOGY

The adult worm lives in the small intestine. The eggs are passed in the feces. When ingested the ovum hatches in the small intestine, and the larvae enter the portal veins or intestinal lymphatics. From there they pass to the lungs, where they are trapped by the alveolar capillaries, and exit into the airspaces. At this point they develop into third-stage larvae that migrate up the airways to the larynx, where they are swallowed to complete their cycle by developing into mature worms in the small intestine.

Pulmonary disease usually results from passage of the larvae through the lungs. The histologic findings include patchy interstitial thickening, an inflammatory exudate composed largely of eosinophils, and alveolar hemorrhage and edema.[1,10]

MANIFESTATIONS OF THE DISEASE

Radiography

The chest radiograph shows migratory, patchy airspace opacities that characteristically clear within 10 days. Lobar consolidation and alveolar hemorrhage have also been described.[1,10,11] The *Ascaris* worms sometimes may be seen on radiographs of the abdomen outlined against intestinal gas.

Computed Tomography

The chest CT findings consist of patchy bilateral ground-glass opacities, subpleural nodules with or without a halo of ground-glass opacity (CT halo sign), and focal areas of consolidation without any zonal predominance, typical of eosinophilic pneumonia. CT of the abdomen shows the *Ascaris* as cylindrical filling defects within contrast-filled bowel loops.[12] The intestinal tract of the roundworm itself is often seen as a thin thread of oral contrast material within the tubular filling defect.

Imaging Algorithm

In most cases chest radiography is the only imaging modality performed in patients with suspected eosinophilic lung disease secondary to *Ascaris* infestation.

DIFFERENTIAL DIAGNOSIS

The radiologic manifestations in the lungs are similar to the manifestations seen in strongyloidiasis: simple pulmonary eosinophilia and eosinophilic reaction to drugs. The diagnosis is confirmed by identifying larvae in the sputum or eggs in the stool.[1]

SYNOPSIS OF TREATMENT OPTIONS

Acceptable treatments include albendazole or mebendazole.[13]

KEY POINTS: ASCARIASIS

- Ascariasis is caused by *A. lumbricoides*.
- Infestation is common in Southeast Asia, South America, Africa, and the United States.
- The most common pulmonary manifestation is eosinophilic lung disease.
- The most common radiologic manifestations include:
  - Patchy bilateral areas of consolidation or ground-glass opacities
  - Typically migratory and transient opacities

Strongyloidiasis

ETIOLOGY, PREVALENCE, AND EPIDEMIOLOGY

Humans are the primary host of *Strongyloides stercoralis,* a microscopic nematode with infective larvae that invade the lungs and small intestine by migrating from the soil through the skin.[1] The parasite is found in all tropical and subtropical regions. About 35 million people are infected worldwide.[1] The highest infection rates in the United States are in the Southeast and Puerto Rico.

CLINICAL PRESENTATION

Clinical manifestations include cough, shortness of breath, and bronchospasm.[10] Abdominal symptoms, including diarrhea, weight loss, and midepigastric pain, are commonly present. The patients usually have peripheral eosinophilia. Severely immunocompromised patients may develop disseminated *Strongyloides* infection that manifests as fever, cough, and rapidly progressive and severe shortness of breath. Abdominal pain and diarrhea are present in most patients.

PATHOPHYSIOLOGY

The infective larvae migrate from the soil through the skin, eventually reaching the small intestine, where the adult worm resides. Pulmonary disease is caused mainly by the migration of larvae through alveolar capillaries into airspaces. Normal migration results in eosinophilic lung disease or mild intraalveolar hemorrhage.

Disseminated *Strongyloides* infection (hyperinfection syndrome) is an uncommon complication that may occur in immunocompromised patients. In these patients larvae may disseminate and involve multiple organs, including the brain. The most common manifestation of *Strongyloides* hyperinfection syndrome is extensive alveolar injury and pulmonary hemorrhage. The mortality in these patients can exceed 70%.[14]

MANIFESTATIONS OF THE DISEASE

Radiography

Radiographic manifestations consist of ill-defined, patchy areas of consolidation, presumably caused by an allergic reaction to migration of the filariform larvae through the lungs.[1] The areas of consolidation may be migratory and typically resolve within 1 to 2 weeks.

Hyperinfection may result in extensive bilateral consolidation or diffuse reticulonodular or nodular pattern (Fig. 14.2).[1,15] The nodules may have poorly defined or well-defined margins. Occasionally, the findings may resemble miliary tuberculosis.[16] Pleural effusion and secondary superimposed bacterial infection with cavitation and abscess formation may also be seen.[14]

Computed Tomography

The chest CT findings in eosinophilic reaction to the passage of larvae through the lungs consist of migratory patchy bilateral ground-glass opacities and focal areas of consolidation without any zonal predominance.

Imaging Algorithm

In most cases chest radiography is the only imaging modality performed in patients with suspected eosinophilic lung disease secondary to *Strongyloides.*

DIFFERENTIAL DIAGNOSIS

The radiologic manifestations of strongyloidiasis, similar to those of ascariasis, usually result from eosinophilic lung disease secondary to normal passage of larvae through the lungs and are similar

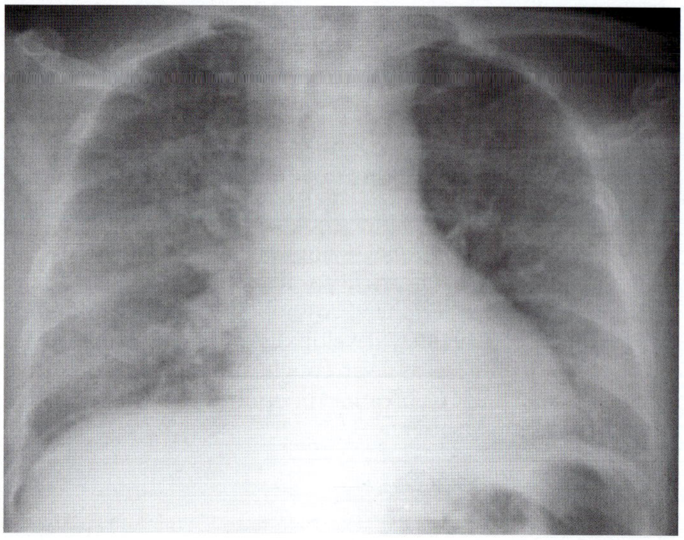

Fig. 14.2 *Strongyloides* hyperinfection in a patient undergoing chemotherapy for pancreatic lymphoma. Anteroposterior chest radiograph shows bilateral poorly defined hazy opacities, areas of consolidation, and poorly defined small nodular opacities. Fiberoptic bronchoscopy and bronchoalveolar lavage showed pulmonary hemorrhage and numerous filariform larvae of *Strongyloides stercoralis.*

to the radiologic manifestations of simple pulmonary eosinophilia and eosinophilic reaction to drugs. The diagnosis is usually confirmed by detection of larvae in the stool.

The differential diagnosis of hyperinfection includes opportunistic infection, diffuse pulmonary hemorrhage, and acute respiratory distress syndrome from any cause. Definitive diagnosis is made by identifying the larvae in the sputum.[17]

SYNOPSIS OF TREATMENT OPTIONS

Treatment is with antiparasitic drugs such as ivermectin.

KEY POINTS: STRONGYLOIDIASIS

- Strongyloidiasis is caused by *S. stercoralis.*
- Infestation occurs in tropical and subtropical countries and the southeastern United States.
- The most common pulmonary manifestation is eosinophilic lung disease.
- The most common radiologic manifestations include:
  - Patchy bilateral areas of consolidation or ground-glass opacities
  - Typically migratory and transient opacities
  - Occasionally, hyperinfection in immunocompromised patient may result in extensive consolidation and a diffuse reticulonodular or nodular pattern

Echinococcosis (Hydatid Disease)

ETIOLOGY, PREVALENCE, AND EPIDEMIOLOGY

Hydatid disease is caused by small larvae of *Echinococcus,* usually *Echinococcus granulosus.* It occurs in two forms: pastoral and sylvatic.[10] The pastoral form is more common and is seen mainly in the Mediterranean region, eastern Europe, South America, the Middle East, Australia, and New Zealand. The intermediate hosts are usually sheep, cows, or pigs, and the definite hosts are dogs. The sylvatic form is more common in Alaska and northern Canada. The intermediate hosts of the sylvatic variety are usually moose, deer, or caribou, and the definite hosts are dogs, wolves, and coyotes.[18]

CLINICAL PRESENTATION

Most patients are asymptomatic. Cyst rupture, either spontaneous or as a result of secondary infection, may result in abrupt onset of cough, expectoration, and fever.[10] Occasionally, cyst rupture results in acute hypersensitivity reaction, with urticaria, pruritus, and in some cases hypotension.

PATHOPHYSIOLOGY

Humans acquire the disease by direct contact with definite hosts or by ingestion of eggs present in water, food, or soil.[10] The eggs hatch in the duodenum into larvae that pass via the portal system to the liver, where most are trapped. Most larvae that escape are trapped in pulmonary alveolar capillaries. In the pastoral variety, approximately 65% to 70% of cysts occur in the liver and 15% to 30% in the lungs. For reasons that are unclear, lung cysts seem to be more common than liver cysts in the sylvatic variety of hydatid disease.[19]

In liver and lung the larvae develop into cysts that are typically spherical or oval in shape. The cysts are surrounded by an outer protective layer termed the *pericyst,* which consists of fibrous tissue containing a nonspecific chronic inflammatory infiltrate.[10] The surrounding lung usually shows compressive atelectasis. The cyst itself consists of a laminated, acellular layer (the ectocyst) and a thin inner germinal layer (the endocyst) that contains intracystic fluid, daughter vesicles, daughter cysts, and larval protoscoleces. A multicystic structure may result from serial cyst formation over several generations.

MANIFESTATIONS OF THE DISEASE

Radiography

Hydatid cysts manifest as sharply circumscribed spherical or oval masses surrounded by normal lung (Fig. 14.3).[20,21] They are most commonly single but may be multiple in 30% of patients. Their size ranges from 1 cm to greater than 20 cm in diameter.[22] Most are located in the lower lobes. Although usually spherical or oval, hydatid cysts may have an irregular shape, attributed by some to the fact that they impinge on relatively rigid structures, such as bronchovascular bundles, as they grow and become indented and lobulated.[20] When communication develops between the cyst and the bronchial tree, air may enter the space between the pericyst and exocyst and produce a thin crescent around the periphery of the cyst—the meniscus or crescent sign. After the cyst has ruptured into an airway, its membrane may float on residual fluid within the cyst and give rise to the classic water lily sign (Figs. 14.4 and 14.5).

Occasionally, hydatid cysts may involve the mediastinum, heart, bronchus, pulmonary artery, chest wall, or diaphragm (Fig. 14.6).[23] The radiographic findings of transdiaphragmatic extension of hydatid liver cysts include elevation of the hemidiaphragm, pleural effusion, and lower lobe atelectasis or consolidation.

Computed Tomography

The typical CT manifestations consist of round or oval fluid-filled cysts (see Figs. 14.3 and 14.5). The fluid has attenuation values

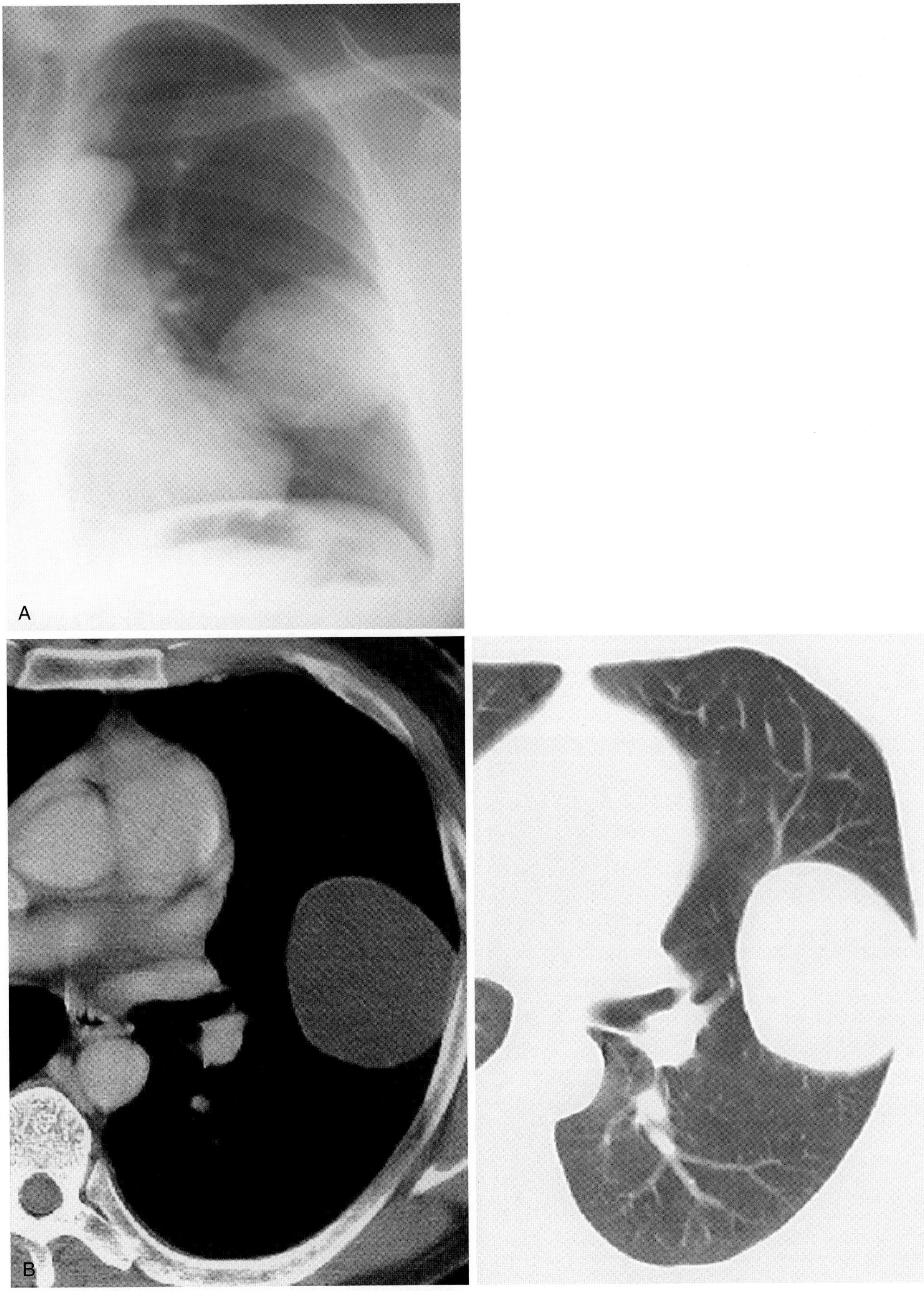

Fig. 14.3 Hydatid cyst in an asymptomatic man who hunted for several years in northern Canada. (A) Posteroanterior chest radiograph shows a smoothly marginated mass in the left lung. (B) Composite image with CT in soft tissue window *(left image)* and in lung window *(right image)* shows a smoothly marginated lingular cyst containing fluid with an attenuation value similar to water (0 Hounsfield units).

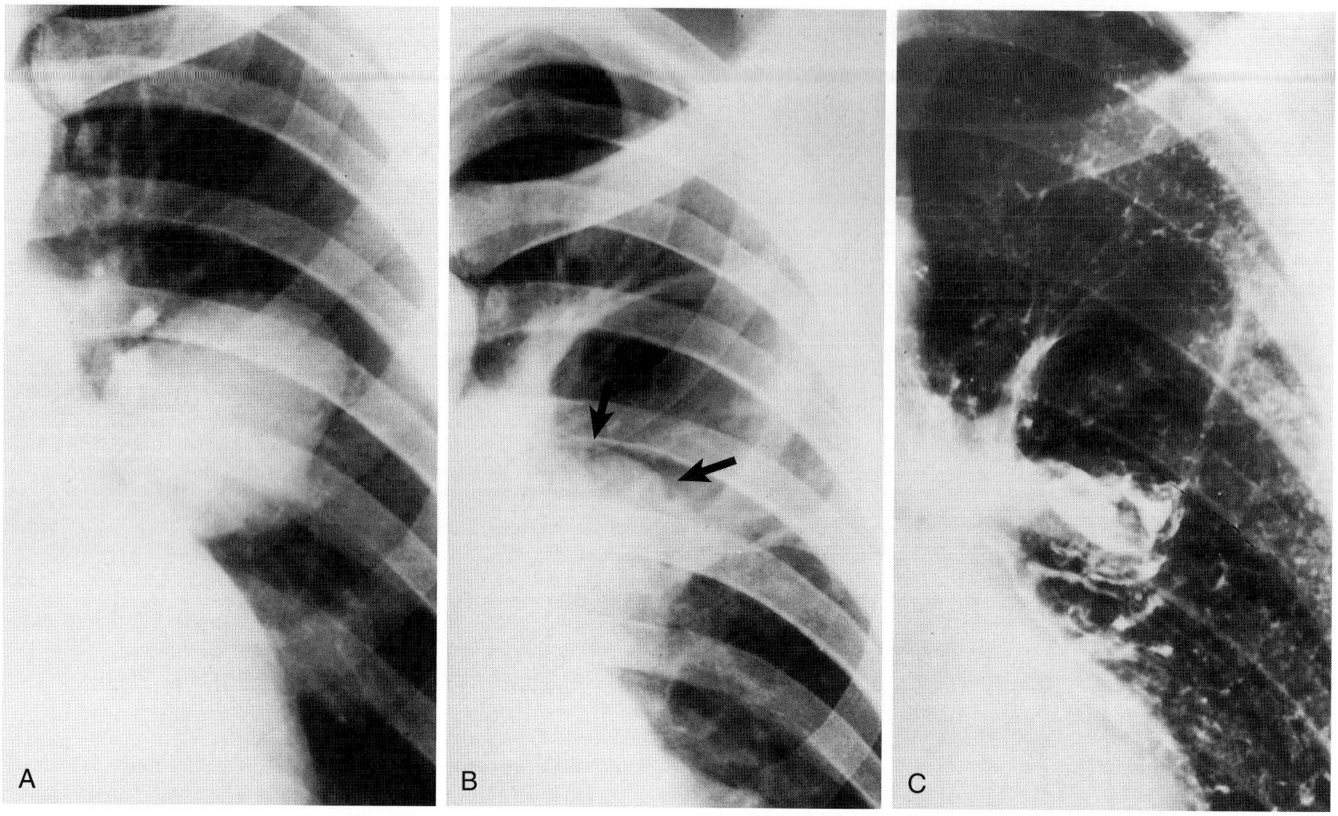

Fig. 14.4 Hydatid cyst with rupture. (A) Sharply circumscribed homogeneous mass visible in the left midlung has a smooth but lobulated contour. (B) Four years later the cyst has expelled all of its liquid contents into the tracheobronchial tree and now contains air; an irregular mass present at the bottom of the cyst *(arrows)* represents collapsed membranes. (C) Bronchogram shows contrast material within the cyst, outlining the membranes. *(Courtesy Alfred Hospital, Melbourne, Australia. From Müller NL, Fraser RS, Colman NC, et al., eds.* Radiologic Diagnosis of Diseases of the Chest. *Philadelphia: Saunders; 2001.)*

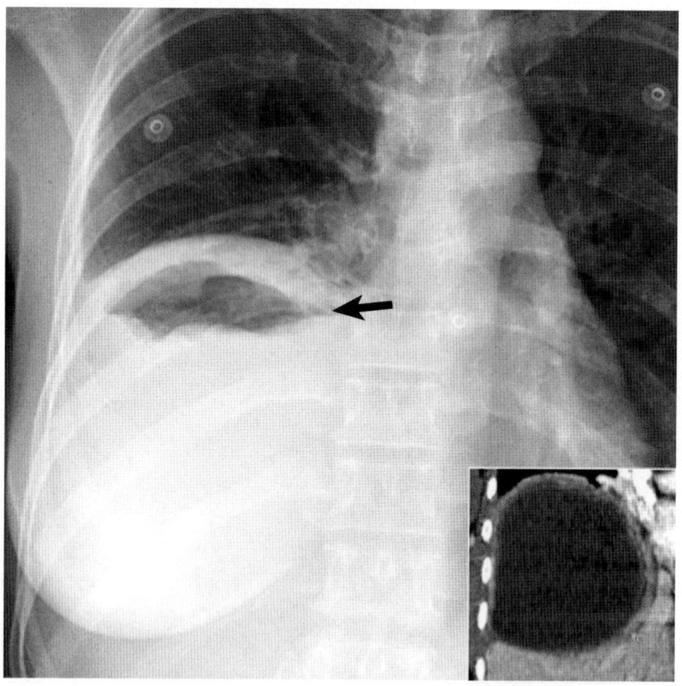

Fig. 14.5 Pulmonary hydatid disease with water lily sign. Posteroanterior chest radiograph shows a large right lower lobe thick-walled cavity with lobulated air–soft tissue interface representing a floating endocyst *(arrow)*. Coronal CT inset from years prior shows the unruptured cyst. *(From Walker CM, Abbott GF, Greene RE, et al. Imaging pulmonary infection: classic signs and patterns.* AJR Am J Roentgenol *2014;202:479–492.)*

close to 0 Hounsfield units.[1,24] The cysts have smooth, thin walls that enhance after contrast material injection. Calcification of lung cyst walls, common in liver disease, is not usually seen.

The meniscus, cumbo, and water lily signs occur when air dissects between the various cyst layers (Fig. 14.7). As cysts enlarge, they may erode adjacent bronchioles, allowing air to dissect between the pericyst and ectocyst and causing the meniscus or air crescent sign. The meniscus sign is thought by some authors to be indicative of impending cyst rupture. With progression, air penetrates through the ectocyst, leading to an air crescent and air-fluid level within the endocyst, termed the *Cumbo sign* or *onion peel sign* by some authors. With further accumulation of air, the cyst layers collapse and float on top of the fluid, resulting in the water lily sign.[21] Rupture can be associated with consolidation adjacent to the cyst and poor definition of the margins of the cyst.

CT scans of the chest and abdomen may show coexistence of liver and lung cysts, which occurs in about 6% of patients. CT findings in transdiaphragmatic extension of liver cysts include elevation of the hemidiaphragm, pleural effusion, pleural cysts, and pulmonary invasion.

Magnetic Resonance Imaging

Magnetic resonance imaging (MRI), similar to CT, allows reliable differentiation of fluid-filled hydatid cysts from solid tumors.[25] The cysts have low signal intensity on T1-weighted images and homogeneous high signal intensity on T2-weighted images (see Fig. 14.6).

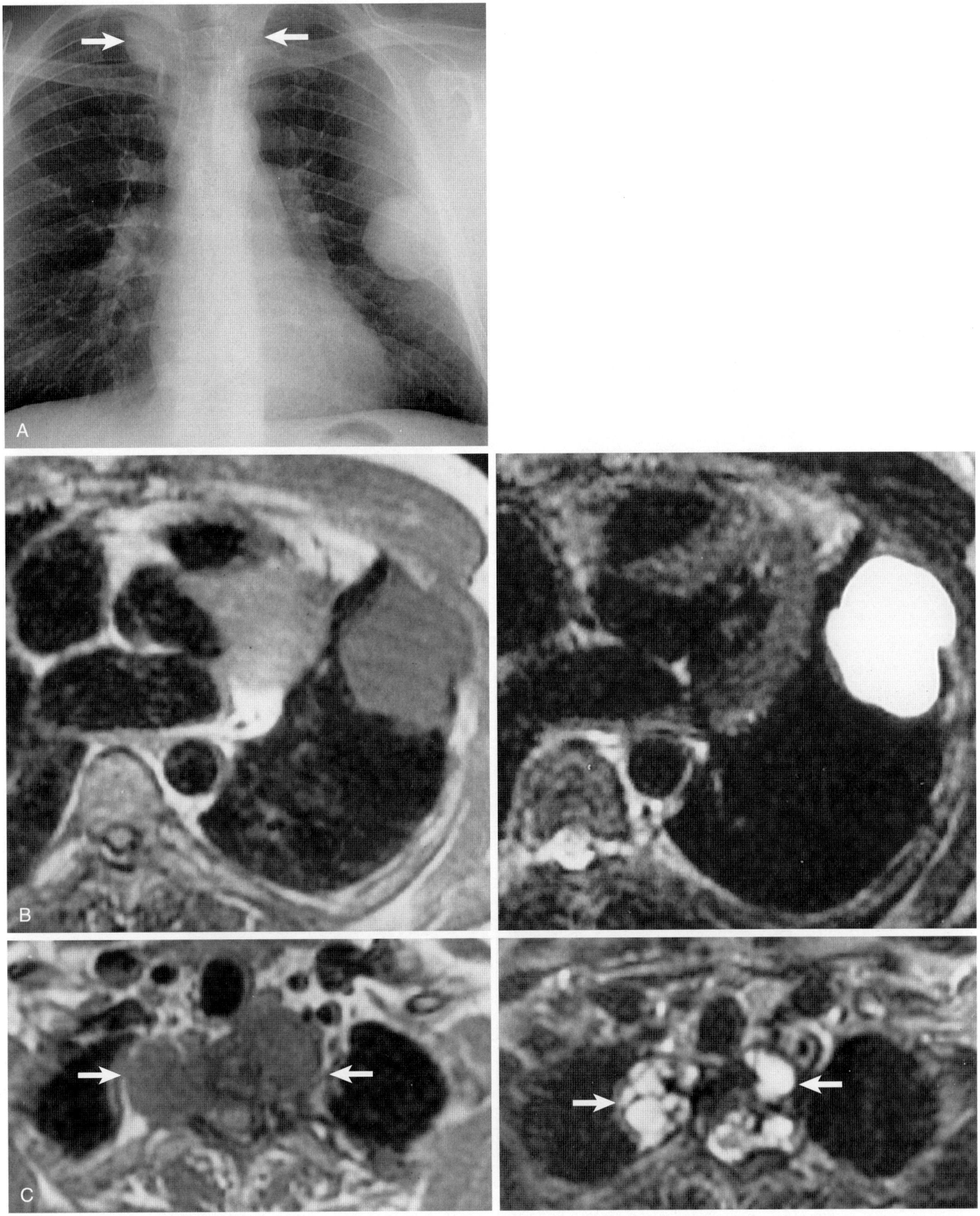

Fig. 14.6 Hydatid disease with chest wall and vertebral involvement in a man who had been a sheep herder in Iraq. (A) Chest radiograph shows a smoothly marginated mass in the left lung and widening of the paravertebral soft tissues *(arrows)*. (B) Composite image with T1-weighted *(left image)* and T2-weighted *(right image)* MR shows a cystic lesion with focal extension into the chest wall. The relatively low signal intensity on the T1-weighted image and the very high signal intensity on the T2-weighted image reflect the fluid content of the cyst. (C) Composite image with T1-weighted *(left image)* and T2-weighted *(right image)* MR at the level of the lung apices show paravertebral cysts *(arrows)* with associated destruction of the adjacent vertebral body. *(From Fraser RS, Müller NL, Colman N, et al. eds.* Fraser and Paré's Diagnosis of Diseases of the Chest. *Philadelphia: Saunders; 1999.)*

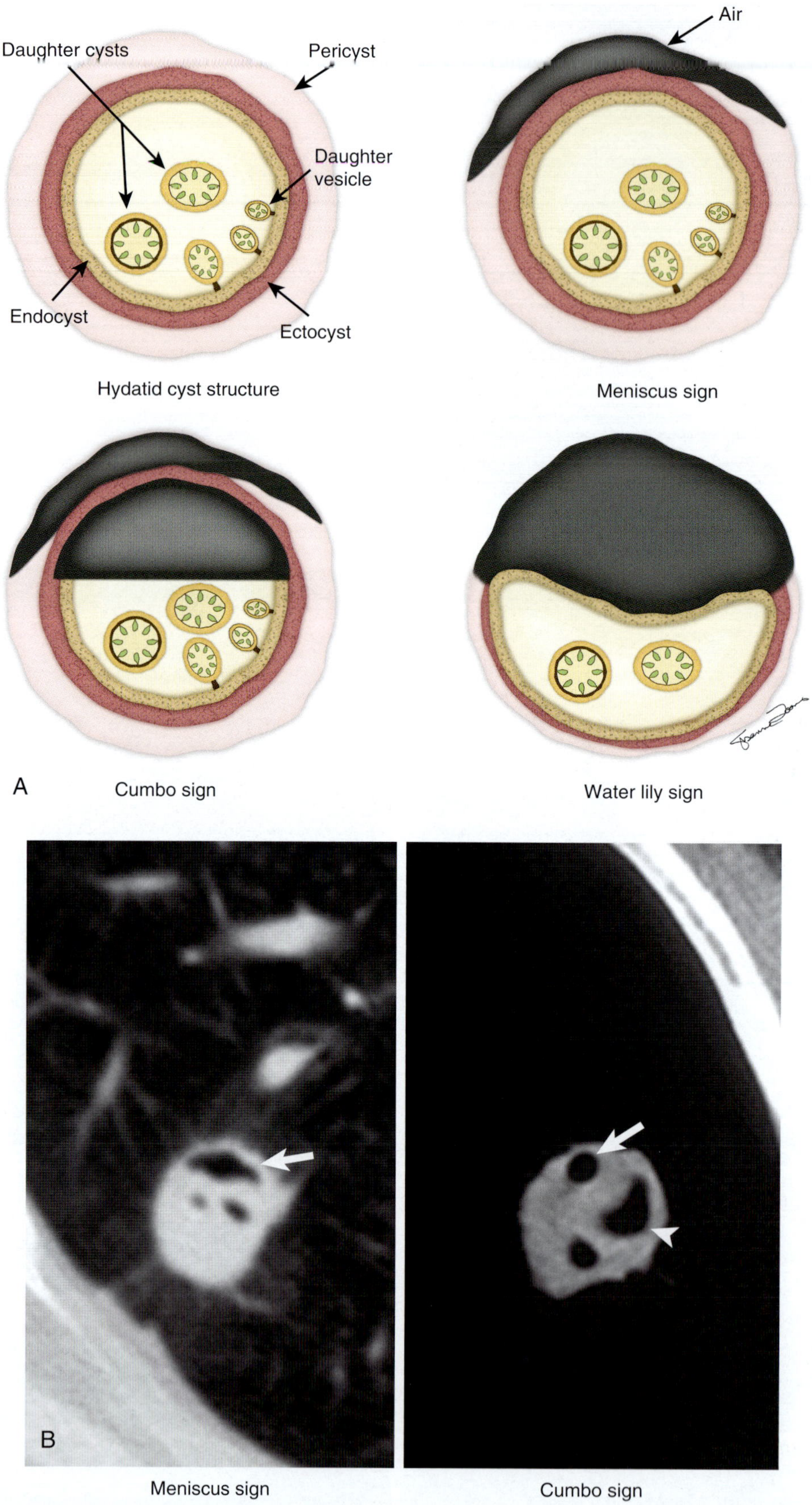

Fig. 14.7 Pulmonary hydatid disease imaging signs. (A) Drawings show normal hydatid cyst and meniscus, cumbo, and water lily signs. (B) Composite image with air between the pericyst and ectocyst layers *(arrows)* consistent with the meniscus sign. Air-fluid level in the endocyst (arrowhead in *right image)* in combination with the meniscus sign *(arrow in right image)* forms the Cumbo sign. *(A courtesy S. Loomis, REMS Media Services, Mass General Imaging, Boston, MA; B courtesy S. Rossi, Buenos Aires, Argentina. From Walker CM, Abbott GF, Greene RE, et al. Imaging pulmonary infection: classic signs and patterns.* AJR Am J Roentgenol. *2014;202:479–492.)*

Imaging Algorithm

The chest radiograph is usually the first imaging modality performed in these patients, but CT or MRI is required to identify the cystic nature of the lesions. In patients with suspected hydatid cysts and in young patients with lung nodules or masses, MRI is the imaging modality of choice because of the lack of radiation exposure.

DIFFERENTIAL DIAGNOSIS

The differential diagnosis mainly includes other conditions that may result in fluid-filled lung lesions, particularly bronchogenic cysts and fluid-filled bullae. Distinguishing features include blood eosinophilia, usually mild, present in 25% to 50% of cases.[26] Laboratory aids in diagnosis include indirect hemagglutination, latex agglutination, complement fixation, and enzyme-linked immunosorbent assay; these tests have a sensitivity ranging from 80% to 100% and a specificity of 88% to 98% for hepatic cysts; however, their sensitivity for the detection of pulmonary cysts is only 50% to 55%.[18] In addition, their specificity is limited by cross-reactions with antigens of other parasites.

SYNOPSIS OF TREATMENT OPTIONS

Hydatid cysts, particularly cysts measuring less than 6 cm in diameter, frequently resolve after treatment with albendazole or mebendazole. Larger cysts may require surgical resection.[27] Video-assisted thoracoscopic surgery has been reported as a reliable option in the treatment of superficial, small to moderate-sized pulmonary hydatid cysts.[28]

KEY POINTS: ECHINOCOCCOSIS (HYDATID DISEASE)

- Echinococcosis is caused by *E. granulosus*.
- In the pastoral variety, the intermediate host is mainly sheep, and endemic areas include southeastern Europe, the Middle East, South America, and Australia.
- In the sylvatic variety, the intermediate host is mainly moose, deer, and elk, and endemic areas include northern Canada and Alaska.
- The most common radiologic findings include:
  - Single or multiple nodules or masses
  - Smoothly marginated
  - Water density on CT
- Other manifestations include:
  - Air crescent sign (when cyst communicates with bronchus)
  - Cumbo sign (air crescent sign and air-fluid level)
  - Water lily sign (when cyst membrane floats in residual fluid)

Schistosomiasis

ETIOLOGY, PREVALENCE, AND EPIDEMIOLOGY

Schistosomiasis is caused by flukes of the class Trematoda, including *Schistosoma mansoni, Schistosoma japonicum,* and *Schistosoma haematobium.* The disease occurs in areas inhabited by the intermediate host, the snail. Infestation by *S. mansoni* and *S. haematobium* is endemic in the Middle East (Egypt and parts of Saudi Arabia) and in large areas of central and southern Africa. *S. mansoni* is found in the Caribbean islands and in South America, particularly in Brazil, whereas *S. japonicum* is seen mainly in China, Japan, and the Philippines.[10] Schistosomiasis is a common parasitic infection, affecting 150 to 200 million people and causing 500,000 deaths each year.[1] Although the disease is most commonly identified in endemic regions, increased emigration from these regions has resulted in increased prevalence in nonendemic regions. It has been estimated that approximately 400,000 infected immigrants reside in the United States.[29] Acute schistosomiasis (Katayama fever), which can be seen during migration of larvae through the lungs, also is increasingly being recognized in travelers to regions where the disease is endemic.[30]

CLINICAL PRESENTATION

Migration of the schistosomula through the pulmonary circulation may be associated with an acute syndrome consisting of fever, cough, diarrhea, and hives; leukocytosis and eosinophilia are almost invariable.[10] The most important pulmonary manifestation of schistosomiasis is pulmonary arterial hypertension, which develops after years of persistent infestation and continuous exposure and manifests with progressive shortness of breath, chest pain, fatigue, palpitations, and cough.[1] Signs of extrathoracic disease are almost invariably present in these patients. The eggs of *S. mansoni* and *S. japonicum* are deposited mainly in the liver and result in symptoms and signs of cirrhosis and hepatosplenomegaly. *S. haematobium* infestation is associated with dysuria and hematuria.[10]

PATHOPHYSIOLOGY

Humans acquire the infestation by drinking, swimming, working, or washing in fresh water containing infective cercariae.[10] The latter penetrate the skin, pass via the venous circulation to the pulmonary capillaries, and through these vessels to the systemic circulation. Histologic findings in transbronchial biopsy specimens from patients with acute symptoms related to migration of the schistosomula through the pulmonary circulation (Katayama fever) have been consistent with eosinophilic pneumonia.[31]

The worms migrate to the superior mesenteric *(S. japonicum)*, inferior mesenteric *(S. mansoni)*, or vesical *(S. haematobium)* veins. Tissue damage results from the release of eggs into host tissues, with subsequent immunologic reaction, inflammation, and fibrosis.[10] Eggs may reach the lungs directly through the inferior vena cava or, when the liver has become cirrhotic as a result of *Schistosoma*-related fibrosis, via anastomotic channels between the portal and systemic venous systems. When they reach the lungs, most embolized eggs become impacted in pulmonary arterioles. The host reaction to the eggs may result in obliterative arteriolitis and, eventually, pulmonary arterial hypertension and cor pulmonale. In the chronic infection the *Schistosoma* eggs are typically surrounded by granulomatous inflammation.

MANIFESTATIONS OF THE DISEASE

Radiography

Migration of larvae through the lungs may result in patchy, migratory areas of consolidation, small nodular lesions with poorly defined borders or, less commonly, a reticulonodular pattern or bilateral ground-glass opacities.[1] Granulomatous reaction to eggs deposited in the pulmonary vasculature may result in radiologic findings of pulmonary hypertension and cor pulmonale.[1] Findings include enlarged central pulmonary arteries; rapid tapering; and, in severe cases, cardiomegaly.

Computed Tomography

The findings of eosinophilic lung disease secondary to schistosomiasis are similar to the findings of simple pulmonary eosinophilia and consist of patchy bilateral areas of consolidation and ground-glass opacities. Although usually the ground-glass opacities surround areas of consolidation, the reverse also may occur, resulting in a reverse halo sign (Fig. 14.8). Acute schistosomiasis (Katayama fever) may manifest with multiple pulmonary nodules (Fig. 14.9). In patients with pulmonary hypertension secondary to schistosomiasis, CT shows enlarged central pulmonary arteries but is otherwise nonspecific (Fig. 14.10). Additional findings in chronic infection include portal hypertension and cirrhosis.

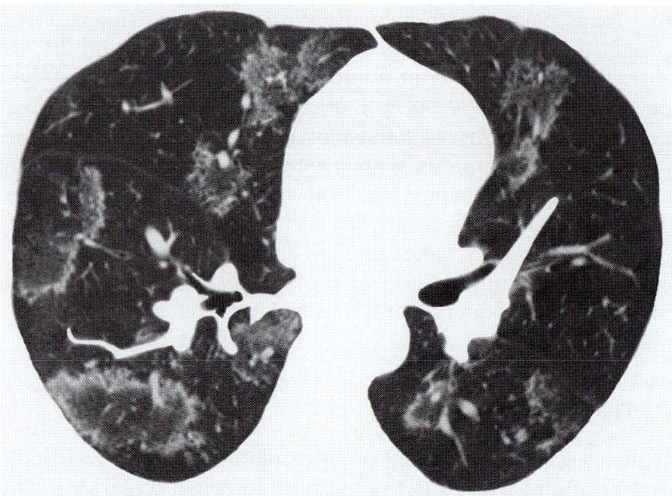

Fig. 14.8 Schistosomiasis: parenchymal abnormalities. High-resolution CT shows patchy bilateral ground-glass opacities. Ring-like areas of consolidation outline some of the ground-glass opacities (reverse halo sign). The diagnosis of schistosomiasis was confirmed by open-lung biopsy, which showed granulomatous inflammation surrounding *Schistosoma* eggs. *(Courtesy Dr. Gustavo Meirelles, São Paulo, Brazil.)*

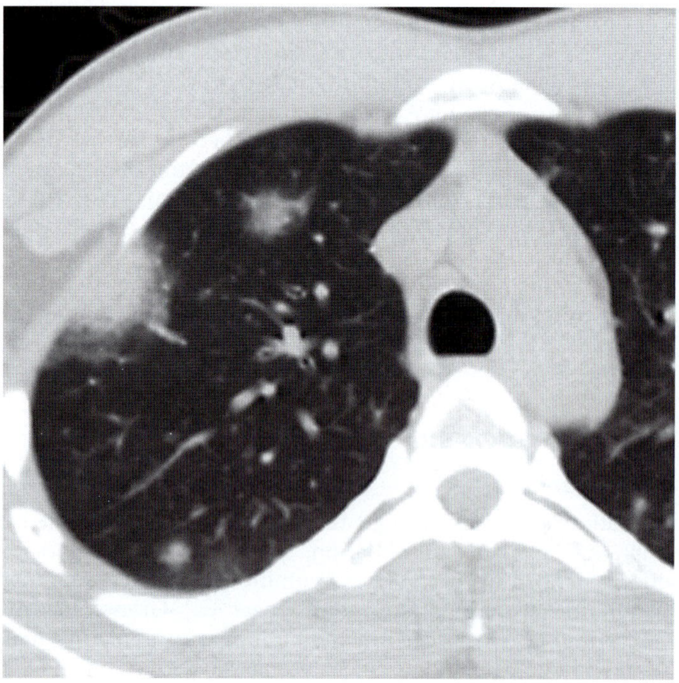

Fig. 14.9 Acute schistosomiasis. Axial CT shows multiple pulmonary nodules, many with surrounding ground-glass opacity (CT halo sign).

Imaging Algorithm

The diagnosis of pulmonary arterial hypertension usually is suggested by the clinical findings or chest radiograph and confirmed at echocardiography or right heart catheterization.

DIFFERENTIAL DIAGNOSIS

Pulmonary arterial hypertension caused by schistosomiasis is usually radiologically indistinguishable from pulmonary arterial hypertension resulting from any other cause. The diagnosis of schistosomiasis usually is confirmed by showing ova in stool or urine specimens or on rectal biopsy specimen. Serologic tests are of limited value because they are unable to differentiate a former infection from current disease.[30]

SYNOPSIS OF TREATMENT OPTIONS

Treatment for several years has been based on the use of praziquantel. More recent studies have shown resistance to the praziquantel-based therapy in some cases, however.[32]

KEY POINTS: SCHISTOSOMIASIS

- Main endemic areas for schistosomiasis follow:
  - *S. mansoni*: Caribbean islands, South America
  - *S. japonicum*: China, Japan, and the Philippines
  - *S. haematobium*: Middle East and Africa
- The most common radiologic findings include:
  - Patchy, migratory areas of consolidation
  - Lung nodules in acute schistosomiasis (Katayama fever)
  - Findings of pulmonary arterial hypertension and cirrhosis

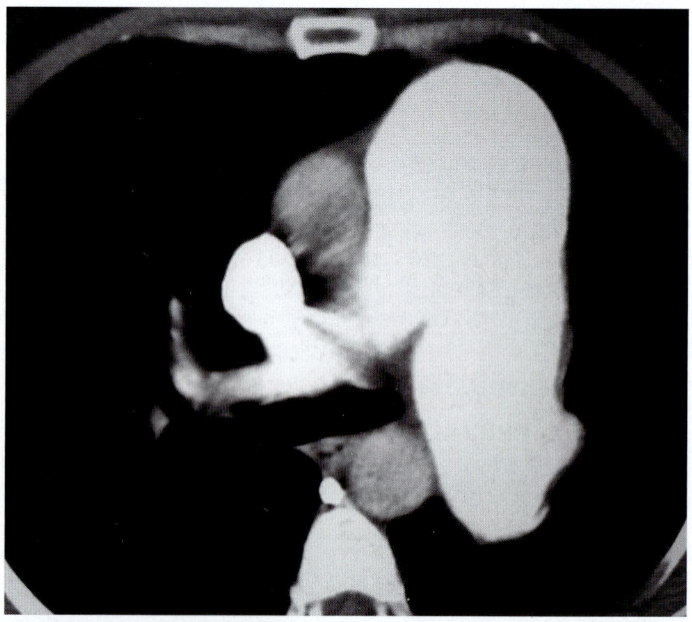

Fig. 14.10 Pulmonary arterial hypertension secondary to schistosomiasis. Contrast-enhanced CT in a patient with long-standing schistosomiasis shows markedly enlarged central pulmonary arteries. *(Courtesy Dr. Claudia Figueiredo, São Paulo, Brazil.)*

Paragonimiasis

ETIOLOGY, PREVALENCE, AND EPIDEMIOLOGY

Paragonimiasis is caused by flukes of the genus *Paragonimus;* the most frequent etiologic agents are *Paragonimus westermani* and *Paragonimus kellicotti,* which are endemic to Asia and North America, respectively.[33] Humans typically acquire the disease by ingesting raw or undercooked crabs or crayfish infected with the metacercariae or by drinking contaminated water. The main endemic areas are East Asia, Southeast Asia, Latin America, and Africa. It affects approximately 20 million people in endemic areas.[1] Numerous cases also have been reported in the United States among Indo-Chinese and Latin American immigrants as well as campers who had ingested raw crawfish during camping trips involving alcohol.[33–35]

CLINICAL PRESENTATION

The most common symptoms are intermittent hemoptysis or blood-tinged sputum and cough.[36] Less common symptoms include episodic chest pain owing to pleurisy, pneumothorax, and fever. The hemoptysis tends to occur sporadically for months or years in the absence of other signs of illness.

PATHOPHYSIOLOGY

The imaging manifestations of disease parallel the life cycle of the parasite. The organism is ingested by humans, and it penetrates through small bowel mucosa to gain access to the peritoneal cavity, where it incites an inflammatory reaction. Several weeks later, the organism travels through the diaphragm on its way to the pleural space. After finding a mate the organisms burrow through the visceral pleura into the lung, where they produce cysts that contain eggs. The eggs are then expectorated through bronchioles to complete the life cycle. Paragonimiasis typically results in single or multiple 1- to 4-cm cystic spaces containing reddish brown mucinous fluid and usually a single adult parasite.[10] The cysts frequently are located near larger bronchioles or bronchi; although predominantly subpleural, they can occur anywhere within the lung parenchyma. When erosion occurs into a draining airway, the contents of the cyst may be coughed up or may spread to other portions of the lung parenchyma and result in exudative or hemorrhagic pneumonia.

MANIFESTATIONS OF THE DISEASE

Radiography

The radiographic manifestations may consist of a nodule, focal areas of consolidation, or cystic lesions (Fig. 14.11).[36,37] The cystic lesions may be single or multiple, measure 0.5 to 4 cm in diameter, and are usually thin walled. They may be seen in areas of consolidation or as isolated thin-walled ring shadows. They often have a crescent-shaped or oval opacity along one aspect of the inner lining; this opacity has soft tissue attenuation on CT and presumably represents the worm. Irregular tracks or burrows measuring 5 mm in diameter and connecting adjacent cysts may be seen in a few patients. Pleural abnormalities occur in approximately 60% of patients and include unilateral or bilateral effusion, hydropneumothorax, and, less commonly, pleural thickening.[37]

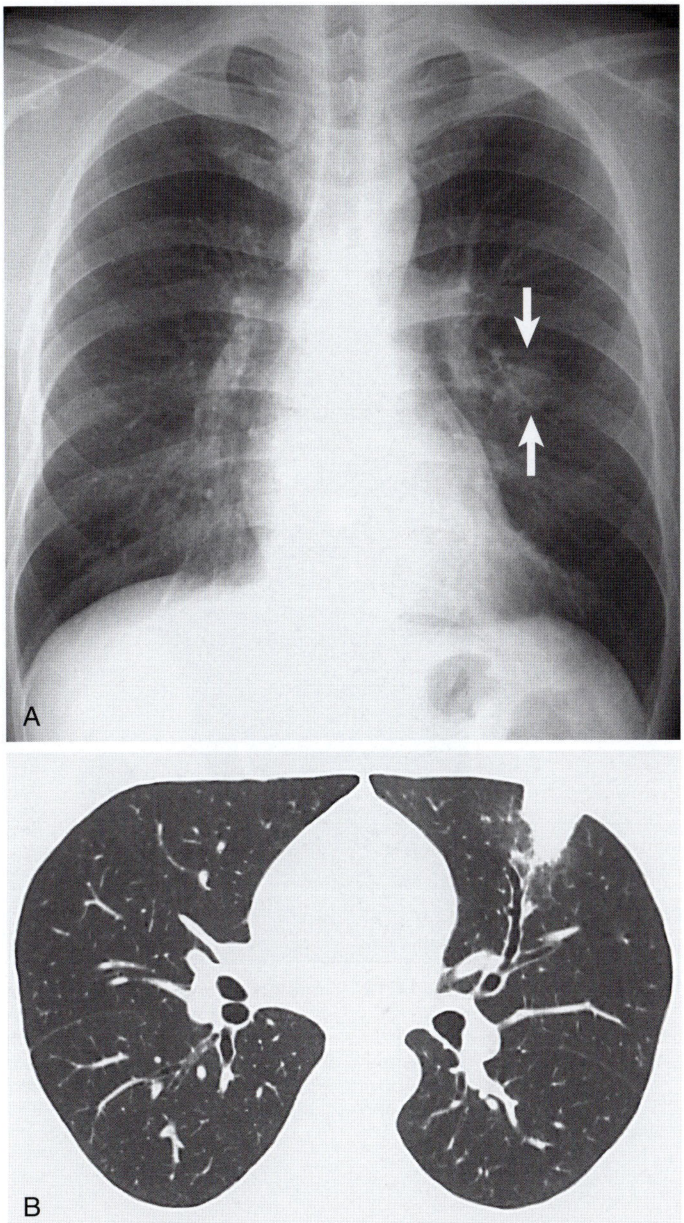

Fig. 14.11 Paragonimiasis: single opacity. (A) Posteroanterior chest radiograph shows a poorly defined nodular opacity in the lingula *(arrows).* (B) CT shows this opacity to represent subpleural consolidation surrounded by a halo of ground-glass opacity. The appearance is consistent with a pulmonary infarct. The diagnosis of paragonimiasis was confirmed by open-lung biopsy in this South Korean man who presented with left chest pain. *(Courtesy Dr. Kyung Soo Lee, Samsung Medical Center, Seoul, South Korea.)*

Computed Tomography

The most common imaging manifestations include a subpleural nodule or nodules, often with a linear tract directed toward the pleural surface (burrow sign) (Fig. 14.12).[38] The nodules measure 1 to 4 cm in diameter and frequently contain a low-attenuation area or cavitation. There is often consolidation, pleural thickening, or ground-glass opacity surrounding the nodule (Fig. 14.13; see Fig. 14.11).[37,39] The total number of nodules is usually fewer than five, and the nodules may involve a single lobe or multiple lobes.[37] Pleural effusion or hydropneumothorax is seen in approximately 30% of patients, and hilar or mediastinal lymphadenopathy, including anterior diaphragmatic and internal mammary lymph

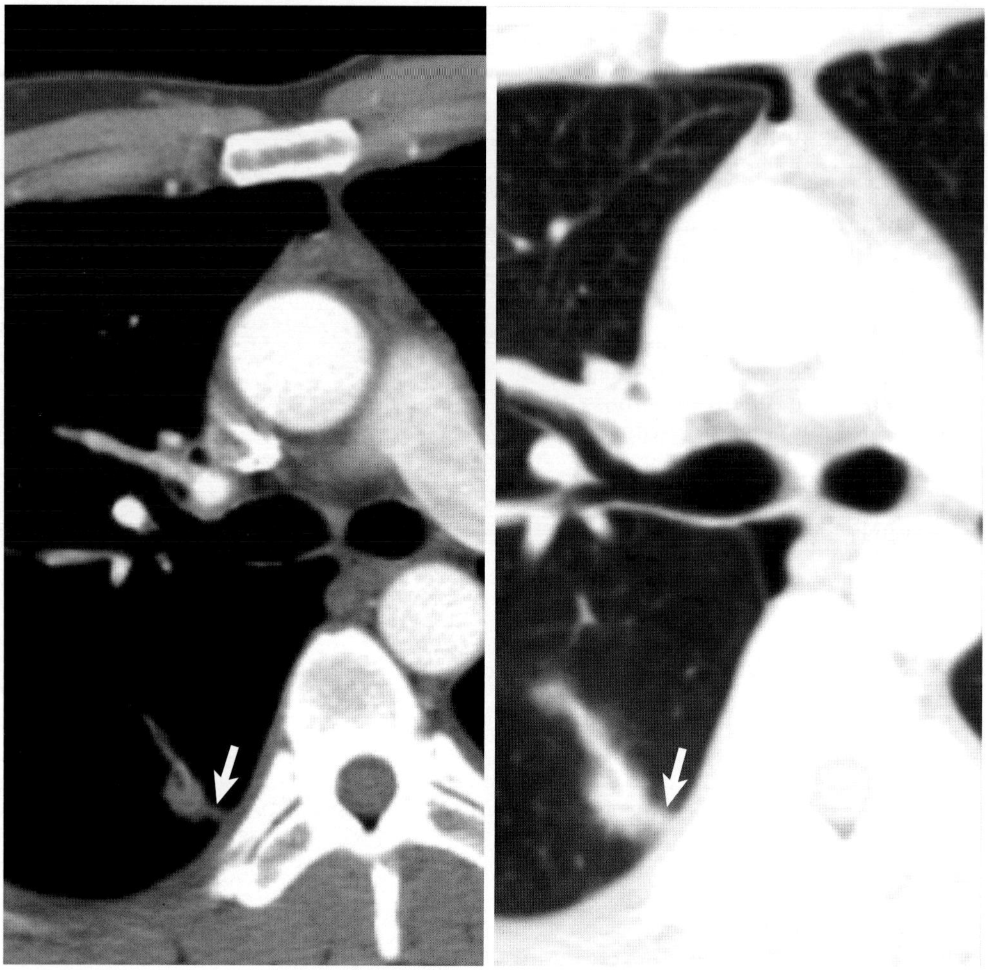

Fig. 14.12 North American paragonimiasis occurring after raw crawfish ingestion. Composite image with axial CT in soft tissue window *(left image)* and lung window *(right image)* shows linear burrow track *(arrows)* extending from thickened pleura to the pulmonary nodule. Note trace right hydropneumothorax. *(Courtesy T. Henry, University of California-San Francisco, San Francisco, CA. From Walker CM, Abbott GF, Greene RE, et al. Imaging pulmonary infection: classic signs and patterns.* AJR Am J Roentgenol. *2014;202:479–492.)*

node enlargement, is seen in up to 10% of patients. Omental fat stranding has been described in the early stages of infection.[33]

The appearance of pulmonary lesions is influenced by the stage of the infection and the surrounding tissue reaction. Early findings are caused by the migration of juvenile worms and consist of focal airspace consolidation, linear opacities, pleural effusion, pneumothorax, or hydropneumothorax. Later findings result from worm cysts and include thin-walled cysts, mass-like consolidation, nodules, and bronchiectasis.

CT also may show a subpleural streaky opacity, 2- to 7-mm thick and 5- to 60-mm long, connecting the pleura and the nodule, which represents the worm migration track (burrow sign) (see Fig. 14.12).[37,40] CT also may show irregular tracks or burrows connecting adjacent cysts or communicating between the cysts and a bronchus.[37]

Positron Emission Tomography

Pulmonary paragonimiasis may show positive uptake on positron emission tomography with fluorodeoxyglucose imaging, mimicking lung cancer.[41]

Imaging Algorithm

The chest radiograph is usually the first and often the only imaging modality used in the assessment of these patients. CT is recommended in selected cases, however, for further characterization of pattern and extent of abnormalities.

DIFFERENTIAL DIAGNOSIS

Recognizing the linear burrow sign is the key differentiating feature of this entity from other diagnoses, such as tuberculosis, other parasitic infections, malignancy, or fungal infections.[36,38,42] The diagnosis of paragonimiasis is confirmed by detecting the parasite eggs in sputum samples, bronchial washing fluid, or lung biopsy specimens or by serologic tests, most commonly enzyme-linked immunosorbent assay.[36]

SYNOPSIS OF TREATMENT OPTIONS

Praziquantel and triclabendazole have been shown to be effective in the treatment of paragonimiasis.[43]

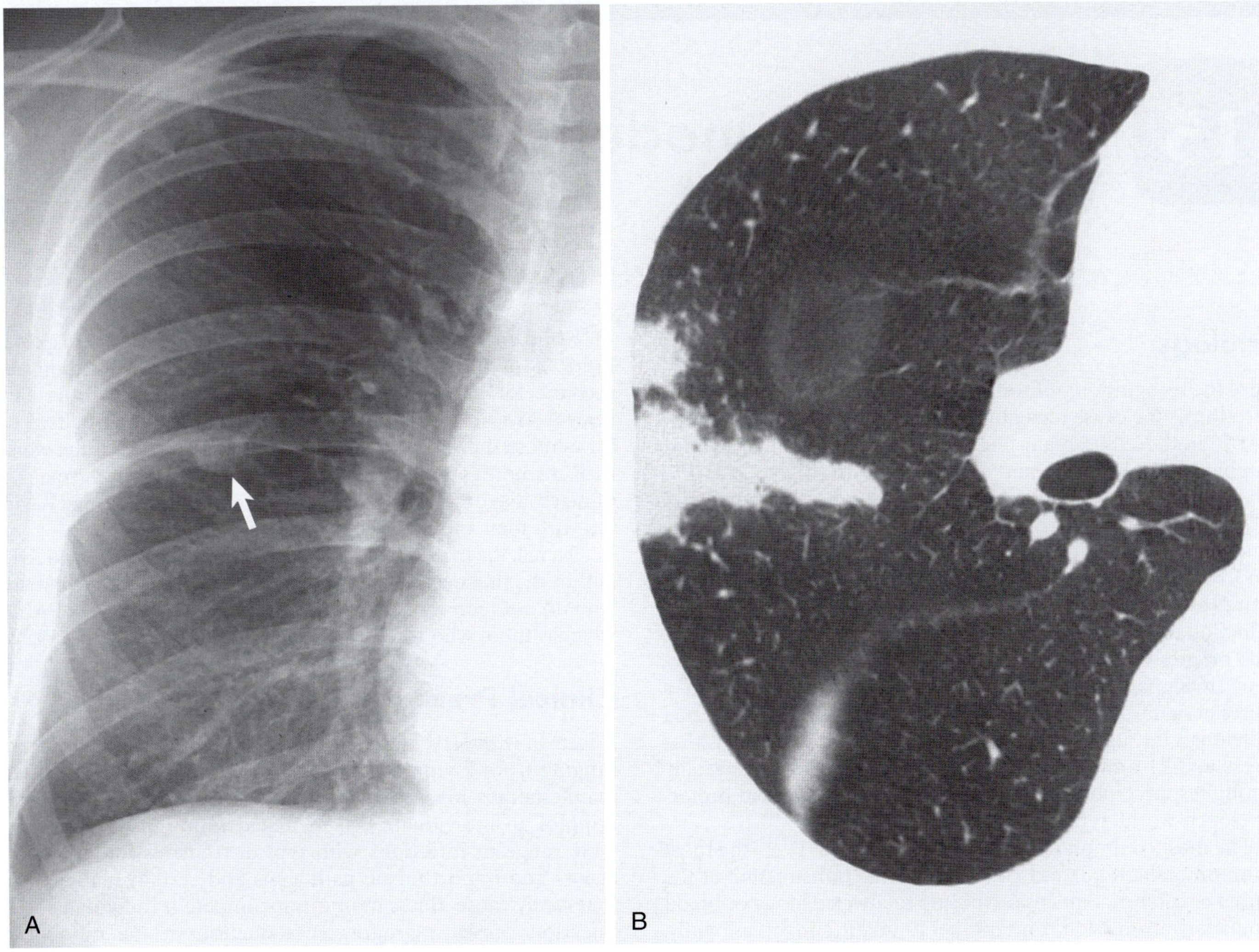

Fig. 14.13 Paragonimiasis: multiple opacities in a man with vague chest pain and cough. (A) Posteroanterior chest radiograph shows poorly defined nodular opacities in the right midlung zone *(arrow)*. (B) CT shows subpleural nodular opacities and focal consolidation. The diagnosis was confirmed by enzyme-linked immunosorbent assay and transthoracic needle aspiration, which showed characteristic ova. *(Case courtesy Dr. Kyung Soo Lee, Samsung Medical Center, Seoul, South Korea.)*

KEY POINTS: PARAGONIMIASIS

- Paragonimiasis is caused by *P. westermani*.
- Endemic areas include Southeast Asia, South America, and western Africa.
- Episodic cases have been described in the Midwestern United States, associated with camping trips involving alcohol after the ingestion of raw crawfish.
- The most common radiologic findings include:
  - Single or multiple nodules with burrow sign connecting the nodule to the pleural surface
  - Single or multiple 1- to 4-cm diameter cystic lesions
  - Focal areas of consolidation
  - Fluid-filled or air-filled cystic lesions on CT
  - Pleural effusion or hydropneumothorax in about 60% of cases

SUGGESTED READINGS

Martinez S, Restrepo CS, Carrillo JA, et al. Thoracic manifestations of tropical parasitic infections: a pictorial review. *Radiographics*. 2005;25:135–155.

Shamsuzzaman SM, Hashiguchi Y. Thoracic amebiasis. *Clin Chest Med*. 2002;23:479–492.

Walker CM, et al. Imaging pulmonary infection: classic signs and patterns. *AJR Am J Roentgenol*. 2014;202:479–492.

The full reference list for this chapter is available at ExpertConsult.com.

15 Human Immunodeficiency Virus Infection*

CAROL C. WU | JOHN P. LICHTENBERGER | KIRAN BATRA

Etiology

Since the recognition of human immunodeficiency virus (HIV) infection as the cause of acquired immune deficiency syndrome (AIDS) in the 1980s, many changes have occurred in the demographics, complications, and treatment of this disease. AIDS is the most advanced stage of HIV infection, where patients have a CD4 count of less than 200 cells/mm^3 or an AIDS-defining condition, such as recurrent bacterial pneumonia, Kaposi sarcoma (KS), or *Pneumocystis jirovecii*. Pneumonia. The introduction of antiretroviral therapy (ART) has been associated with a dramatic reduction in HIV-associated morbidity and mortality.[1,2] Despite such progress, pulmonary disorders, including respiratory infections, malignancies, and inflammatory conditions, remain a source of significant morbidity and mortality among HIV-infected individuals throughout the world. Compounding this fact is that access to ART and treatment for specific conditions, especially among resource-poor individuals in the developed and underdeveloped world, remains a problem.

The most common modes of infection with HIV-1 (the most common phenotype) and HIV-2 are sexual transmission at the genital or colorectal mucosa, exposure to infected blood or blood products, transmission from mother to infant, and, occasionally, accidental occupational exposure. Infection is initiated by the binding of the virion gp120Env protein to the CD4 molecule found on some T cells, macrophages, and microglial cells. Reverse transcription occurs, yielding a strand of deoxyribonucleic acid (DNA) from the viral ribonucleic acid (RNA). Double-stranded DNA forms and integrates into the genome of the cell, enabling virus production. Genes on the newly formed DNA direct production of protease, reverse transcriptase, and other proteins that are variably targeted by ARTs.[3]

Prevalence and Epidemiology

According to the United Nations AIDS fact sheet, the number of people living with HIV or AIDS worldwide was estimated to be 36.7 million in 2016, with about 1.8 million people becoming newly infected. New HIV infections among children and adults have decreased worldwide by 47% and 11%, respectively, since 2010 and have declined in most regions except Eastern Europe and Central Asia. Around half of all people living with HIV have access to treatment.[4] AIDS-related deaths have decreased by 48% around the globe since 2005 with improved therapies. There are significant differences in the epidemiology of HIV infection around the world. In eastern and southern Africa, women and girls account for 59% of those living with HIV infection. This region also accounts for 43% of new worldwide HIV infections. Western and central African women also account for more than half of the HIV-infected population, whereas in other regions of the world, men are more commonly affected. In the United States the majority of newly diagnosed HIV infections were attributed to men having sex with men and intravenous (IV) drug use.[5,6]

Overall, the majority of HIV-infected patients progress to AIDS within the first decade of diagnosis. The majority of the patients who do not receive ART die within 2 years of the onset of AIDS, whereas those who receive ART survive more than 10 years.[7]

Clinical Presentation

Infection with HIV may result in varied clinical manifestations, ranging from asymptomatic carriage, to various organ system manifestations, to severe opportunistic disease. HIV most severely cripples an individual's cell-mediated immunity, leading to a wide range of infections with typical transmissible infectious agents and opportunistic pathogens and certain malignancies that rarely cause illness in immunocompetent individuals. HIV infection causes a progressive reduction in the number of functioning CD4 helper T-cell lymphocytes; in addition, it causes deficiencies in other humoral, cell-mediated, and phagocytic functions.[8] The incidence of specific opportunistic infections varies greatly with local factors (i.e., the prevalence of certain diseases in certain geographic regions).

The World Health Organization (WHO) specifies four clinical stages of HIV infection, which range from asymptomatic individuals (stage 1) to individuals who have experienced at least one opportunistic infection or malignancy (stage 4).[9] The CD4 count is the most widely used indicator of the degree of immunosuppression and relates directly to the complications that occur.[10,12–14] An important threshold is a CD4 count less than 200 cells/mm^3, which is considered an AIDS-defining event for an HIV-infected individual, even in the absence of an AIDS-defining illness, and places the patient at risk for opportunistic infections and certain malignancies. Patients with a CD4 count greater than 200 cells/mm^3 may develop bacterial pneumonia, tuberculosis (TB), and lung cancer, but most of the classic complications of AIDS (e.g., *Pneumocystis* pneumonia, disseminated fungemia, KS, and AIDS-related lymphoma) occur with CD4 counts less than 200 cells/mm^3 and usually less than 100 cells/mm^3. There are few generalities regarding clinical presentation to indicate the etiology of complications in HIV patients. In contrast to most malignancies, except lymphoma, pulmonary infections typically manifest with fever. Among various infections, bacterial pneumonia often is associated with an acute onset of fever, pleuritic chest pain, productive cough, and purulent sputum. In contrast, *Pneumocystis*

*The editors and the publisher would like to thank Drs. Joel E. Fishman, Galit Aviram, and Ahuva Grubstein for contributing material on this topic to the prior edition of this work. It has served as the foundation for the current chapter.

pneumonia typically has a more insidious onset, with symptoms present for more than 1 week before the individual presents to medical attention with symptoms of dyspnea and dry cough. In contrast to bacterial pneumonia, pleuritic chest pain is usually absent in patients with *Pneumocystis* pneumonia, unless it has been complicated by a pneumothorax.[14]

Manifestations of the Disease

INFECTION

Bacterial Respiratory Infection

General. Bacterial respiratory infections, including infectious airways disease and pneumonia, are currently the most common respiratory diseases in HIV-infected individuals in developed countries.[15–17] HIV infection is associated with a 10-fold to 25-fold increased incidence of bacterial pneumonia over that in the general community.[18] The significance of bacterial pneumonia in HIV infection is underscored by the inclusion of severe bacterial pneumonia as a stage 3 disease by the WHO[9] and recurrent bacterial pneumonia as an AIDS-defining illness for an HIV-infected individual, regardless of the CD4 cell count.[19]

Although HIV infection is most closely associated with alterations in cell-mediated immunity, humoral immunity is also impaired, particularly in advanced stages.[20] Altered B-cell function and defects in neutrophil function, which are especially prevalent among HIV-infected children, place HIV-infected individuals at high risk for frequent infections with encapsulated bacteria. A specific causative agent can be identified in approximately 40% to 75% of HIV-infected adults with bacterial pneumonia.[21] *Streptococcus pneumoniae* is the most common bacterial cause of community-acquired pneumonia (CAP) among HIV-infected adults,[17] causing approximately 20% of all bacterial pneumonias.[20] Other common infectious agents include *Haemophilus influenzae, Staphylococcus aureus, Legionella pneumophila,* and *Klebsiella pneumoniae.* HIV-infected patients are at increased risk for developing infectious airways disease, such as bacterial tracheobronchitis and bronchiolitis. The most common bacterial organisms responsible for infectious airways disease in AIDS are the same ones that cause frank pneumonia, and the clinical presentation is similar.[22]

AIDS patients with advanced immunosuppression also are vulnerable to unusual pulmonary infections, including *Nocardia asteroides, Rhodococcus equi, Bartonella henselae,* and *Bartonella quintana.* The lung is the most commonly involved organ in HIV-related nocardiosis. Patients with nocardial pulmonary infection are typically in an advanced stage of immunosuppression, with CD4 counts usually less than 100 cells/mm^3. A severely immunosuppressed patient may succumb to, or with, *Nocardia* infection. *R. equi,* an endemic infection in horses, manifests in AIDS patients with an indolent course of cough, fever, and dyspnea. Bacillary angiomatosis, an infection caused by *B. henselae* and *B. quintana,* is characterized by a neovascular proliferation involving multiple sites in the body, including skin, liver, spleen, lymph nodes, and lung. Exposure to cats, cat fleas, and lice is the main risk factor for this infection. Affected patients typically present with angiomatous skin lesions that mimic KS. Clinical symptoms include fever, night sweats, cough, and occasional hemoptysis.

Although bacterial pneumonia often occurs earlier in the course of HIV than do other opportunistic infections, the most consistent risk factor for bacterial pneumonia is the stage of HIV disease. HIV-infected individuals with CD4 counts less than 200 cells/mm^3 have a fivefold increase in prevalence of bacterial pneumonia, compared with HIV-infected individuals with CD4 counts greater than 500 cells/mm^3.[20] HIV-infected IV drug users and individuals who smoke illicit drugs (e.g., cocaine, crack, marijuana) have an increased risk of bacterial pneumonia.[23]

HIV-infected individuals with bacterial pneumonia usually have the same signs and symptoms as HIV-free patients. Typically, such patients present with a relatively rapid onset of clinical symptoms, such as productive cough, fever, chills, pleuritic chest pain, and dyspnea. Symptoms are usually present for less than 1 week before a patient seeks medical attention.[20] In contrast, HIV patients with most other pulmonary infections, including *Pneumocystis* pneumonia and tuberculosis, typically present after having symptoms for more than 1 week to a month or longer.[24] Laboratory evaluation of HIV patients with bacterial pneumonia usually shows leukocytosis, but leukopenia can occur. Serum lactate dehydrogenase (LDH) levels are typically normal or only mildly elevated. The treatment of HIV/AIDS patients with bacterial pneumonia has the same spectrum of antibiotics used in non-HIV populations. HIV-infected individuals with uncomplicated bacterial pneumonia caused by typical pathogens usually have a clinical and radiographic response to antibiotic therapy, with a time course similar to that of normal hosts undergoing treatment for CAP. Lower CD4 cell counts have been associated with increased mortality and rate of intubation.[17]

Radiography. Chest radiographs in HIV patients with bacterial pneumonia commonly show focal consolidation, in either a segmental or a lobar distribution, similar to non–HIV-infected patients.[25] HIV patients have a distinctly higher propensity, however, for multilobar and bilateral disease than immunocompetent patients (Fig. 15.1).[12,25] In almost half of cases of bacterial pneumonia, a radiographic pattern other than focal consolidation is observed.[25,26] Bacterial infections also may manifest as solitary (Fig. 15.2) or multiple lung nodules or masses. A study on the etiology of pulmonary nodules in HIV-infected patients found bacterial pneumonia to be the most common etiology, followed by tuberculosis.[27] Cavitation is common in HIV-related bacterial lung infection.[28] In most patients with cavitation, more than one pathogen was identified. *S. aureus* is frequently associated with septic emboli among IV drug abusers and usually manifests as multiple cavitary nodules. *S. aureus* CAP in non-IV drug users can also manifest as cavitary nodules or consolidation (Fig. 15.3).[17] Parapneumonic pleural effusions are seen in a significant minority of cases of bacterial pneumonia and are usually small in size.[26] Intrathoracic lymph node enlargement is not usually evident on chest radiographs.

Chest radiographs of patients with acute bacterial bronchitis are usually normal but may show bronchial wall thickening.[22] Extensive bronchiolitis may create reticulonodular opacities, which represent impacted bronchioles.[10] This pattern may be symmetrically distributed, with lower lobe predominance, resembling *Pneumocystis* pneumonia. Radiographic manifestations of *Nocardia* include nodules and consolidation, which may be mass-like (Fig. 15.4). There is a tendency toward upper lobe predominance. Cavitation, lymphadenopathy, and pleural effusions also may be present.

Computed Tomography. Computed tomography (CT) may be useful in some patients with suspected bacterial pneumonia, especially when the chest radiographic findings are atypical, and when culture or serology has failed to identify an organism. CT can identify the presence of mild or subtle disease suggesting

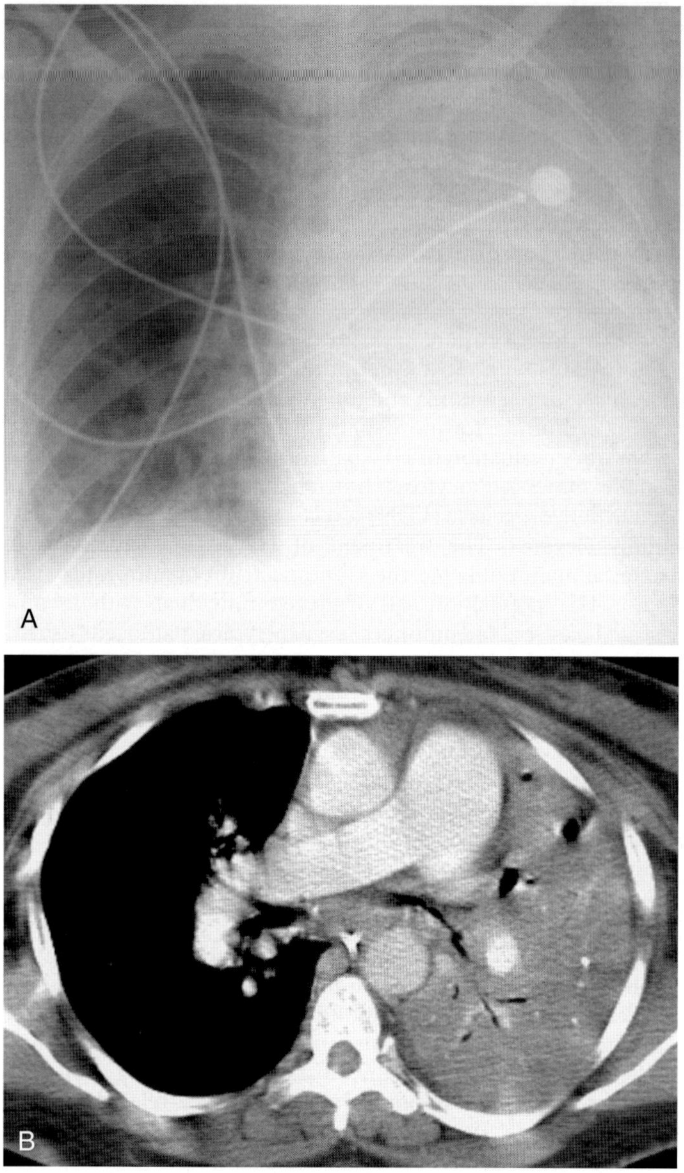

Fig. 15.1 Pneumococcal pneumonia. (A) Chest radiograph shows complete opacification of the left hemithorax. (B) Contrast-enhanced CT scan shows diffuse left lung consolidation without pleural effusion.

bacterial or other etiologies; characterize the distribution of that disease for further testing or therapy, such as bronchoscopy or drainage; and identify lymphadenopathy, cavitation, pleural fluid or empyema, and other differential features that may be occult on the chest radiograph. Mildly enlarged mediastinal and hilar lymph nodes are frequently seen on CT scans of patients with bacterial pneumonia, but they rarely achieve sizes of greater than 2 cm.[26] Nodular disease may be subtle on chest radiographs and better seen by CT. CT is more sensitive and specific than radiographs in detecting bronchitis and bronchiolitis.[22] In a patient with suspicious symptoms but a normal chest radiograph, CT may show findings of small airways disease despite the absence of radiographic findings.[10] The characteristic findings of infectious bronchiolitis on CT consist of centrilobular and tree-in-bud opacities. Pyogenic airway infections lead to inflammatory changes involving the walls of the bronchi and bronchioles, resulting in airway wall thickening and dilation. These changes may be

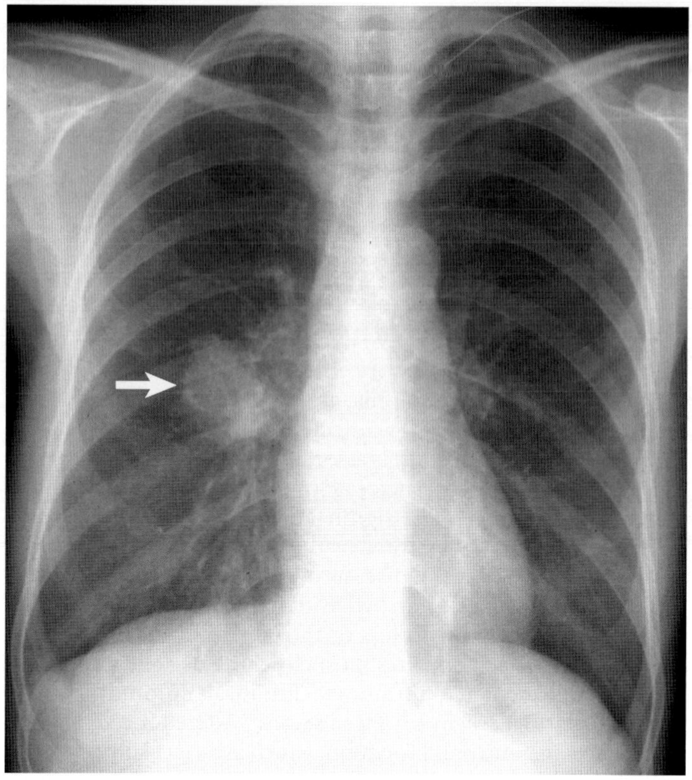

Fig. 15.2 *Pseudomonas* pneumonia. Chest radiograph shows a mass-like consolidation *(arrow)* in the right hilar region.

irreversible if not treated early with antimicrobial agents. *R. equi* pneumonia usually manifests with one or more foci of cavitary consolidation, often with an upper lobe predominance; additional features may include empyema and lymphadenopathy.[29] Bacillary angiomatosis manifests as endobronchial lesions, pulmonary nodules, pleural effusions, and densely enhancing lymphadenopathy and chest wall masses.

Pneumocystis *Pneumonia*

General. *Pneumocystis* is an opportunistic fungal pulmonary pathogen; the pathogenic form in humans is named *Pneumocystis jirovecii.* Since the first descriptions of profound immunodeficiency occurring in previously healthy homosexual men in 1981, the histories of AIDS and *Pneumocystis* pneumonia have been closely associated.[30] It is considered an AIDS-defining condition[19] and a WHO clinical stage 4 disease.[9] The introduction of ART and widespread *Pneumocystis* pneumonia prophylaxis in industrialized nations has brought about dramatic declines in the incidence of *Pneumocystis* pneumonia.[31] Despite such progress, *Pneumocystis* pneumonia remains one of the most common AIDS-defining opportunistic infections in the United States and Western Europe.[32] Twenty-five percent to 33% of cases of *Pneumocystis* pneumonia occur in patients unaware of their HIV infection.[32] Patients who develop *Pneumocystis* pneumonia almost always have CD4 counts less than 200 cells/mm^3 and often less than 100 cells/mm^3.[3,31,33]

Affected patients present with an insidious onset of fever, dry cough, and dyspnea.[33,34] On average, symptoms are present for about 1 month before patients seek medical attention. Physical findings include tachypnea, tachycardia, and cyanosis, but lung auscultation reveals few abnormalities. Reduced arterial oxygen

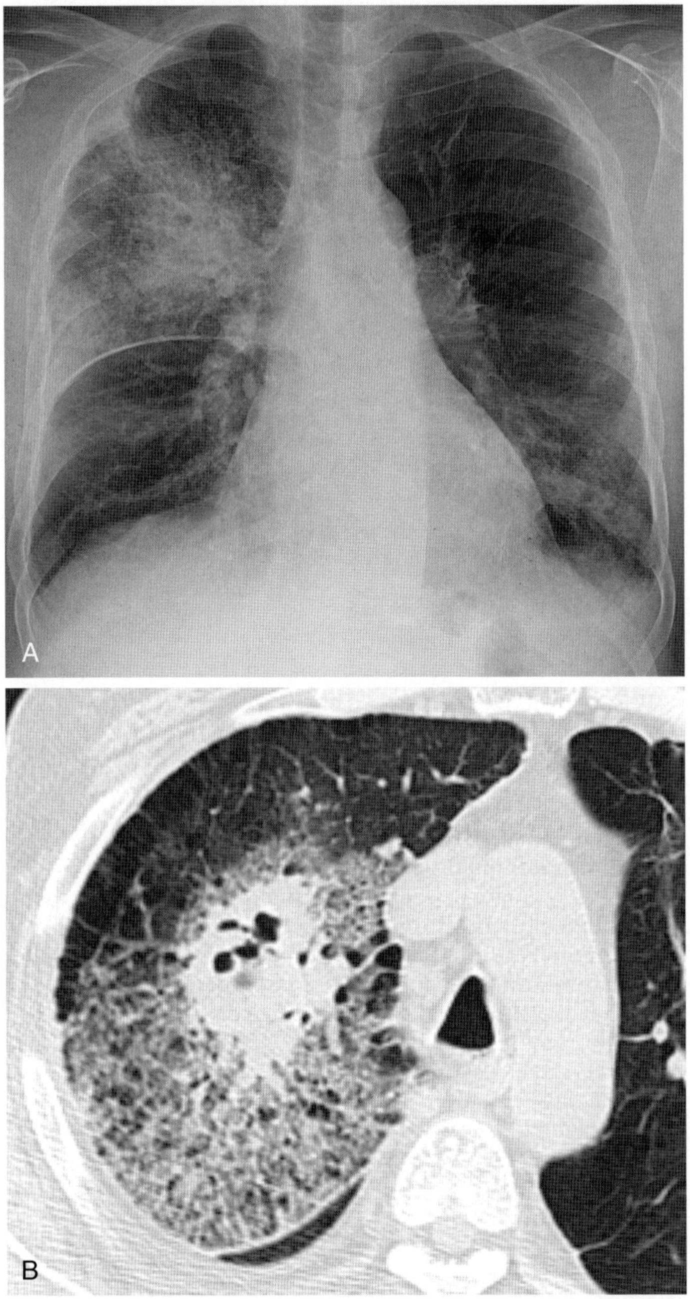

Fig. 15.3 Staphylococcal pneumonia. (A) Chest radiograph shows patchy opacities in the right upper and left lower lung zones and bilateral pleural effusions. (B) Axial CT image from the same date shows cavitation within the right upper lobe opacity. Respiratory culture was positive for methicillin-resistant *Staphylococcus aureus* in this man with a CD4 count of 132.

pressure, increased alveolar-arterial oxygen gradient, and respiratory alkalosis are evident. Decreased diffusing capacity of carbon dioxide is generally present as well. An elevated serum LDH level is highly sensitive for *Pneumocystis* pneumonia but is not highly specific. Serum β-D-glucan, a component of the fungal cell wall, is elevated in many patients with *Pneumocystis* pneumonia, in addition to other fungal processes.[32] Because *P. jirovecii* cannot be grown in culture, a diagnosis is made by morphologic identification of the organism through histopathologic staining. Currently, direct fluorescent antibody stain, which detects both the cystic and trophic forms, is frequently used.[32] Polymerase chain reaction (PCR) testing of respiratory samples for *P. jirovecii* is also used where a negative result has high specificity for excluding the diagnosis.[32] Specimens usually are obtained from induced sputum or fiberoptic bronchoscopy with bronchoalveolar lavage.[33]

Trimethoprim-sulfamethoxazole, which acts by inhibiting folic acid synthesis, is the drug of choice for *Pneumocystis* pneumonia infection and prophylaxis. Pentamidine, associated with more severe toxicities, is less frequently used. Additional medications include atovaquone and dapsone. In those with moderate to severe disease, corticosteroids are given to prevent respiratory deterioration resulting from inflammatory response. Mortality ranges from 4% to 10% in recent years.[32]

Radiography. The classic appearance of *Pneumocystis* pneumonia on chest radiography is bilateral perihilar or diffuse symmetric opacities, which may be finely granular, reticular, or ground-glass in appearance (Fig. 15.5).[33–35] If left untreated, the parenchymal opacities may progress to airspace consolidation.[33] Radiographic improvement usually lags at least a few days behind clinical improvement; frequent chest radiographs may be unnecessary during treatment for patients who show clinical signs of response to therapy.[36] Advances in the prevention and treatment of *Pneumocystis* pneumonia have been associated with an increased frequency of unusual manifestations and a trend toward more subtle radiographic manifestations.[33,35,37] *Pneumocystis* pneumonia is extremely dyspnogenic, with patients often profoundly hypoxic or symptomatic despite minimal radiographic abnormalities. A normal chest radiograph has been reported in up to 39% of cases at the time of presentation, especially in patients with severe impairment in immune status. The true frequency of normal chest radiographs in *Pneumocystis* pneumonia is probably closer to 10%, however.[34]

Computed Tomography. CT is more sensitive than chest radiographs for detecting *Pneumocystis* pneumonia and may be helpful in evaluating symptomatic patients with normal or equivocal radiographic findings.[33–35,37] The classic CT finding in *Pneumocystis* pneumonia is extensive ground-glass opacity, which corresponds to the presence of intraalveolar exudate, consisting of surfactant, fibrin, cellular debris, and organisms (see Fig. 15.5).[33,38] It is often distributed in a patchy or geographic fashion, with a predilection for the central, perihilar, and upper lungs.[33,38,39] Pleural effusions and thoracic lymphadenopathy are rare on CT.[37] When a tree-in-bud appearance is present on CT, *Pneumocystis* pneumonia infection is unlikely.[16]

Cystic lesions are found in approximately 50% of patients (Fig. 15.6). Some cysts have been shown to be secondary to tissue invasion by *P. jirovecii*, followed by necrosis.[38] The presence of cysts may lead to spontaneous pneumothorax (Fig. 15.7). The presence of cysts is not required, however, for pneumothorax to occur. Cysts associated with *Pneumocystis* pneumonia are more common in HIV-infected patients than in patients with other causes of immunosuppression.[40] Occasionally, the cysts may resolve with therapy.

Residual interstitial fibrosis after *Pneumocystis* pneumonia also is common.[33,34,37,38] Interstitial fibrosis also has been reported as the primary radiographic finding in a subset of patients with *Pneumocystis* pneumonia who experienced relatively stable symptoms over months to years. The disease of this subset has been referred to as chronic *Pneumocystis* pneumonia.[41]

Fungal Infections Other Than Pneumocystis *Pneumonia*

General. With the exception of *Pneumocystis* pneumonia, fungal organisms are relatively uncommon causes of pulmonary infection

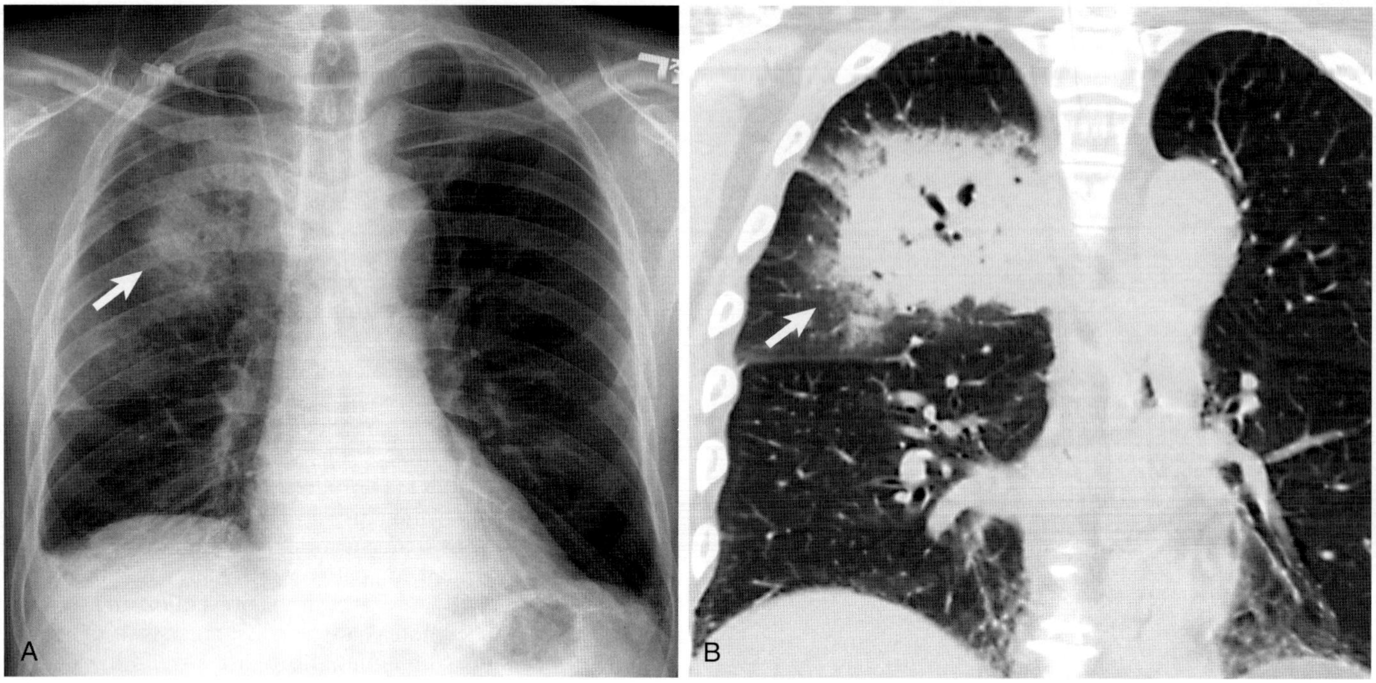

Fig. 15.4 *Nocardia asteroides.* (A) Chest radiograph shows right upper lobe consolidation *(arrow).* (B) Coronal CT image shows a right upper lobe mass-like opacity with surrounding ground-glass opacity *(arrow). (Reproduced from Walker CM, Digumarthy S. Pulmonary infections. In: Digumarthy S, Abbara S, Chung JH, eds.* Problem Solving in Chest Imaging. *Philadelphia; Elsevier; 2020.)*

in HIV-infected patients. Nevertheless, thoracic infection from endemic and opportunistic fungi can occur. Although the most common fungal organism identified in the aerodigestive tract of AIDS patients is *Candida,* its presence is almost always caused by colonization, oral thrush, or esophagitis; true pulmonary infection is rare.

Most thoracic fungal infections occur in the setting of disseminated disease when the degree of immunosuppression is severe (CD4 count < 100 cells/mm^3).[8,10] This is particularly true of the endemic fungi, including histoplasmosis, blastomycosis, and coccidioidomycosis.[42] Of opportunistic fungi, *Cryptococcus neoformans,* ubiquitous in the environment, is the most common fungal pathogen to involve the lungs.[29,43] More than half of patients are fungemic, and most patients have concomitant central nervous system (CNS) infection.[44] Disseminated disease can also involve the skin, bone, and eyes in addition to the lungs.[45] Perhaps because of relatively preserved neutrophil and granulocyte functions in AIDS, the incidence of invasive pulmonary aspergillosis in patients with HIV infection was found to be only 0.1%.[45] Drug-induced neutropenia in HIV-positive individuals, usually acquired from drugs such as zidovudine, ganciclovir, or steroids, increases the risk of disease from *Aspergillus,* however.[29,43,46]

Radiography. Fungal pulmonary infections may have varied appearances. Disseminated histoplasmosis and coccidioidomycosis commonly appear as diffuse miliary pulmonary nodules (Fig. 15.8). The endemic fungal diseases also may manifest as cavities or reticulonodular opacities with or without lymphadenopathy.[47,49] Cryptococcal imaging findings are often nodular or multinodular with areas of conglomeration. Foci of consolidation and reticular or reticulonodular opacities may occur.[50] Parenchymal abnormalities may be accompanied by lymph node enlargement and pleural effusion.[43,50] Patients with angioinvasive aspergillosis may show cavitary disease with an upper lobe predominance or multifocal areas of consolidation or nodules.[43,46,51] The chest radiograph may be normal in AIDS patients with disseminated fungal infection.[34]

Computed Tomography. CT allows detection or better characterization of small pulmonary nodules and intrathoracic lymphadenopathy of disseminated fungal diseases (see Fig. 15.8). The halo sign suggestive of invasive *Aspergillus* infection also requires CT to be detected. Airway invasive aspergillosis manifests as tracheobronchitis, and bronchiolitis usually results in airway wall thickening and tree-in-bud opacities on CT. CT findings of various fungal infections in HIV-infected patients are similar to findings in uninfected patients, and additional details can be found in Chapter 12.

Tuberculosis

General. Worldwide, TB remains the leading cause of death among HIV-infected individuals, accounting for approximately one in three AIDS-related deaths. Of TB cases, 1.2 million (11% of all) occur in patients with HIV infection. TB-related deaths have decreased since 2005, but nearly 60% of TB cases among HIV-infected patients remained undiagnosed or untreated.[4] TB remains the main pulmonary infection of HIV-infected patients in sub-Saharan Africa, Latin America, and Southeast Asia.[17] One in four HIV-infected individuals is estimated to have latent TB infection, and the development of active TB is 26-fold more likely among HIV-infected, compared to non–HIV-infected, patients.[52] Multidrug-resistant strains of tuberculosis (MDR-TB), which originate only sporadically in the developed world,[53] are of persistent concern in resource-poor environments. Ease of international travel is a potential mechanism by which such strains may disseminate.

TB can occur at any stage of HIV infection.[54] Pulmonary TB is considered a WHO stage 3 disease, whereas extrapulmonary

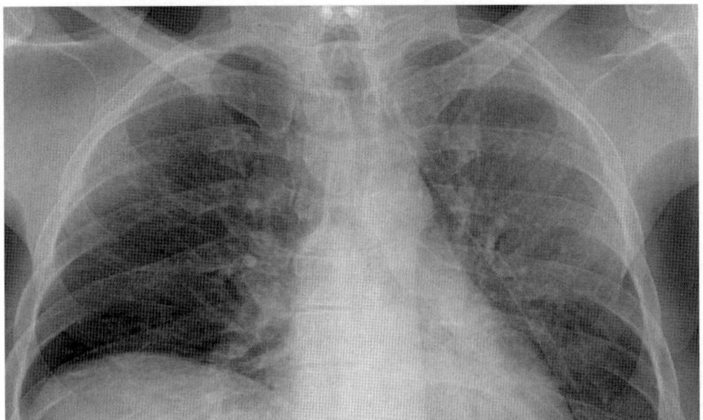

Fig. 15.5 *Pneumocystis* pneumonia. (A) Posteroanterior chest radiograph shows hazy opacities in bilateral lungs. (B) Axial CT image shows bilateral ground-glass opacities in this man with known human immunodeficiency virus infection who presented with low-grade fever and dyspnea.

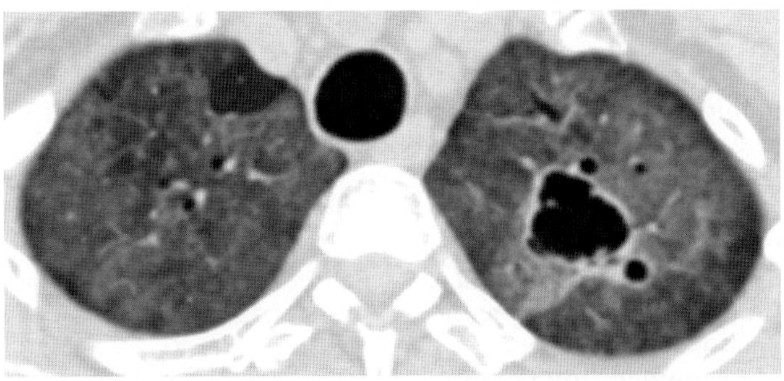

Fig. 15.6 *Pneumocystis* pneumonia. Axial CT image shows diffuse bilateral ground-glass opacities with a thin-walled cyst in this man who presented with weight loss and dyspnea. Bronchoalveolar lavage revealed *Pneumocystis* pneumonia, and subsequently human immunodeficiency virus infection was diagnosed.

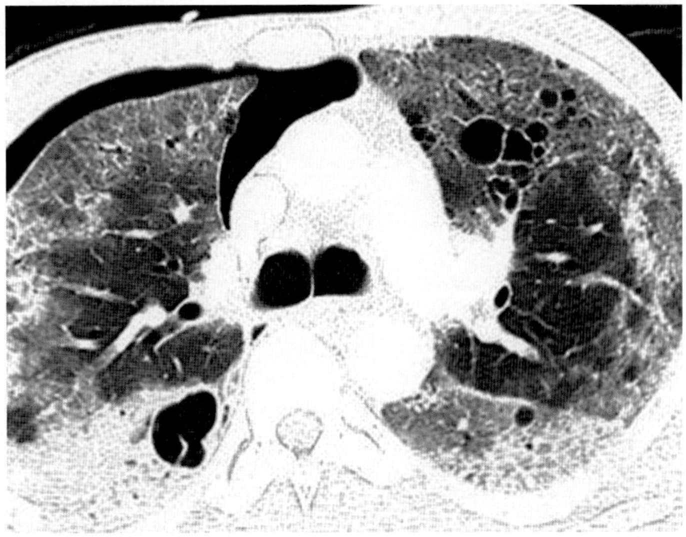

Fig. 15.7 *Pneumocystis* pneumonia. Axial CT image shows bilateral patchy ground-glass opacities and consolidation with multiple thin-walled cysts and right pneumothorax (CD4 count, 140 cells/mm^3).

TB is classified as stage 4 disease.[9] Reactivation (postprimary) pattern TB is often one of the initial manifestations of HIV infection. HIV-infected individuals at particularly high risk for tuberculosis include IV drug abusers and patients from areas where TB is endemic.[54] Classic symptoms include cough, fever, night sweats, and weight loss.[52] Symptoms are often present for more than 7 days before patients seek medical attention.[24] The median CD4 count in HIV patients coinfected with TB is approximately 350 cells/mm^3.[8] In early HIV disease, skin tests are positive, and the infection is confined to the lungs.[8] As the degree of immunosuppression becomes more severe, false-negative skin test results become more prevalent.[52] Interferon gamma release assay blood tests, including T-Spot (Oxford Immunotec, Marlborough, MA) appear to retain sensitivity at lower CD4 counts.[52] Because highly immunosuppressed patients may be infected with a lower colony count of *Mycobacterium tuberculosis*, diagnosis may be more difficult than in immunocompetent patients. The frequency of sputum smear-negative, culture-positive pulmonary TB is higher in patients with advanced immunosuppression, who often also have minimal findings on chest radiography.[52] The WHO recommends the use of the rapid PCR test known as the Xpert MTB/RIF (resistance to rifampicin) assay (Cepheid, Sunnyvale, CA) as an initial diagnostic test in patients suspected to have HIV-associated TB or MDR-TB.[55] The test is reported to be highly specific and can give a diagnosis of TB in less than 2 hours and determine rifampicin resistance.[52] Diagnosis sometimes requires more invasive procedures, such as bronchoscopy, thoracentesis, lymph node aspiration, or pleural biopsy. In patients with miliary disease, blood cultures can be positive.

When TB is diagnosed, treatment with multiple drugs administered under direct observation is started as soon as possible. Regimens usually last longer than 6 months. The initiation of ART in the course of TB treatment is complicated by issues such as drug toxicities and interactions, treatment adherence, and immune reconstitution inflammatory syndrome (IRIS). Patients with low CD4 counts of less than 50 to 100 cells/μL should start ART within 2 weeks of anti-TB therapy unless there

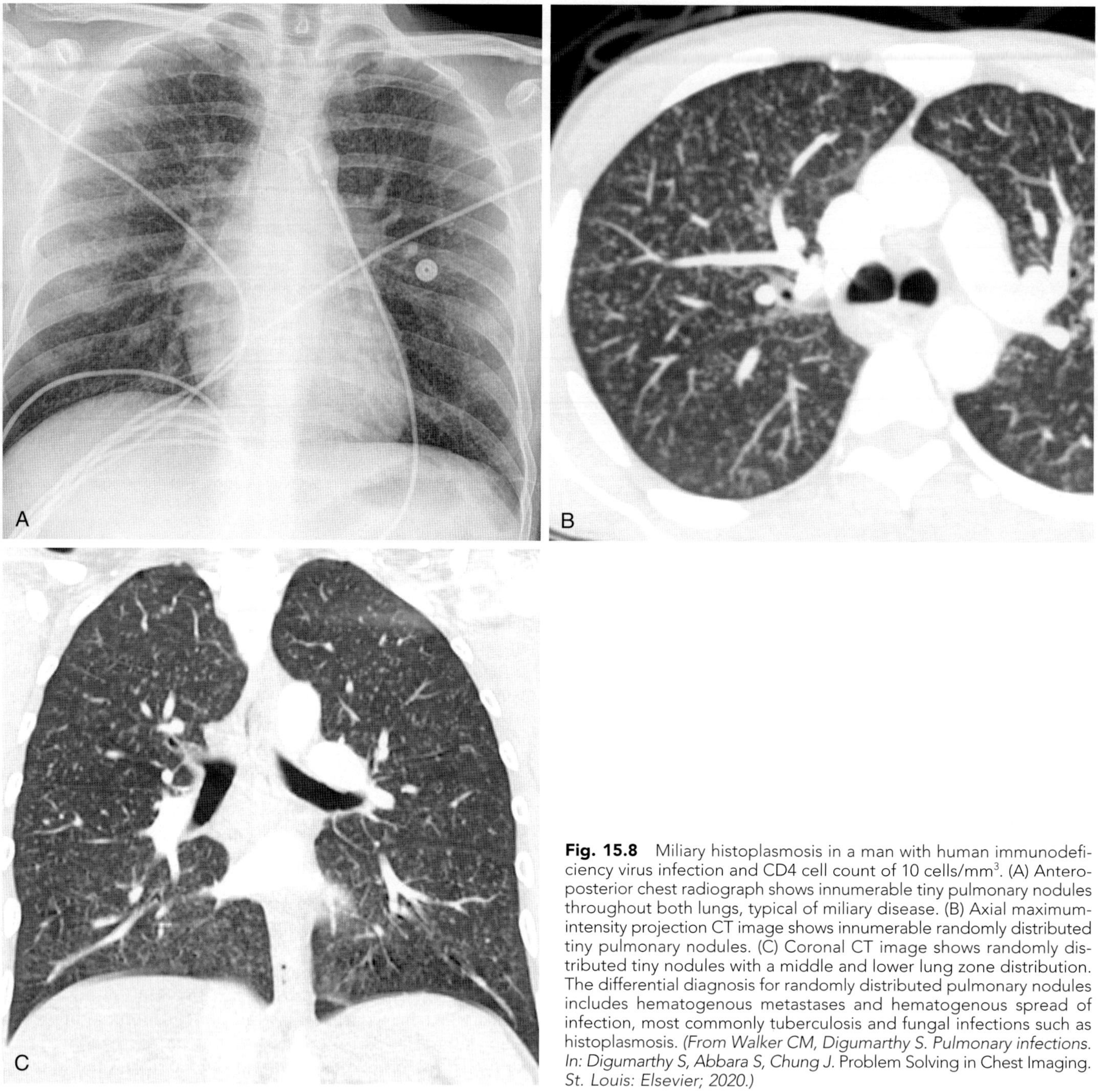

Fig. 15.8 Miliary histoplasmosis in a man with human immunodeficiency virus infection and CD4 cell count of 10 cells/mm^3. (A) Anteroposterior chest radiograph shows innumerable tiny pulmonary nodules throughout both lungs, typical of miliary disease. (B) Axial maximum-intensity projection CT image shows innumerable randomly distributed tiny pulmonary nodules. (C) Coronal CT image shows randomly distributed tiny nodules with a middle and lower lung zone distribution. The differential diagnosis for randomly distributed pulmonary nodules includes hematogenous metastases and hematogenous spread of infection, most commonly tuberculosis and fungal infections such as histoplasmosis. *(From Walker CM, Digumarthy S. Pulmonary infections. In: Digumarthy S, Abbara S, Chung J.* Problem Solving in Chest Imaging. *St. Louis: Elsevier; 2020.)*

is concomitant TB meningitis, whereas those with higher CD4 counts could defer ART for 8 to 12 weeks.[17,52]

Radiography. Early in HIV infection, when the CD4 count is greater than 200 cells/mm^3, the imaging features are typically those associated with postprimary pattern TB and include parenchymal opacities, occasionally cavitary, often located within the apical, posterior, and superior segments of the lungs (Fig. 15.9).[56,57] In patients with decreased CD4 counts (<200 cells/mm^3), findings are more typically those of primary pattern TB (regardless of the actual mechanism of infection), including middle and lower lung zone consolidation, pleural effusion, and lymph node enlargement (Fig. 15.10).[54,56] Progressive primary infection is common in AIDS, with diffuse lung disease, multiple pulmonary nodules, mediastinal lymphadenopathy, or miliary spread, and a lower likelihood of cavitary disease.[56–58] At advanced levels of immunosuppression, 20% of HIV-positive patients with TB have normal chest radiographs.[59] A negative chest radiograph may predict poorer outcome in AIDS patients with TB.[60] The use of ART, with subsequent partial immune restoration, may shift the overall radiographic appearance back toward a postprimary pattern.[61]

Computed Tomography. On CT enlarged lymph nodes secondary to TB are easily identified, are often hypodense, and may show rim enhancement (Fig. 15.11).[62] CT in patients with TB who have a normal or near-normal chest radiograph usually reveals abnormalities, including lymph node enlargement and

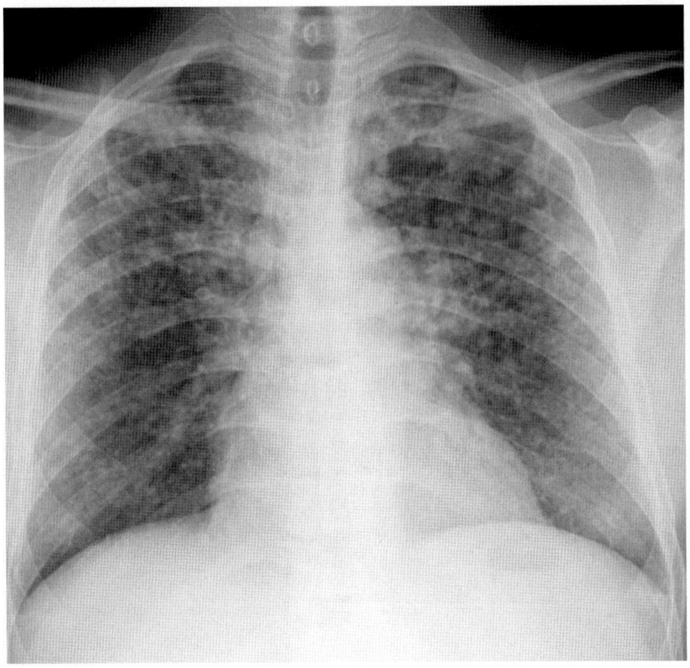

Fig. 15.9 Tuberculosis: reactivation pattern of infection. Chest radiograph shows bilateral nodular opacities with upper lobe predominance (CD4 count, 278 cells/mm^3).

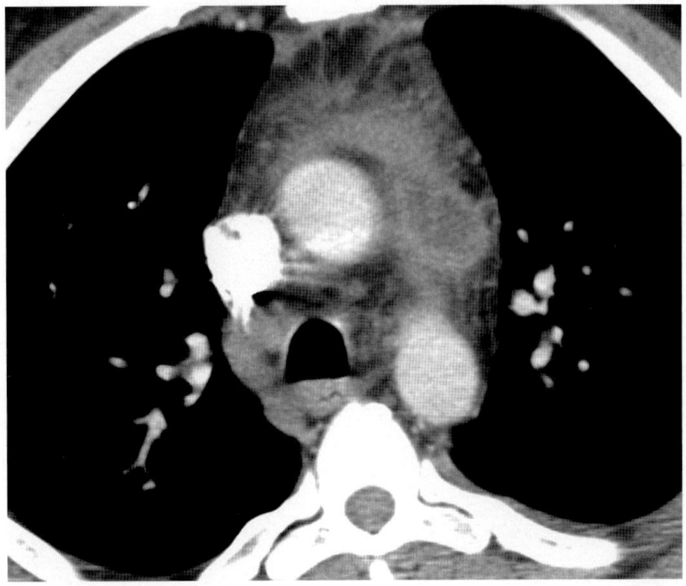

Fig. 15.11 Tuberculosis. CT image shows mediastinal fat stranding with an enlarged prevascular lymph node with peripheral enhancement and central low attenuation characteristic of mycobacterial infection (CD4 count, 55 cells/mm^3). *(Reproduced from Walker CM, Digumarthy S. Pulmonary infections. In: Digumarthy S, Abbara S, Chung JH, eds.* Problem Solving in Chest Imaging. *Philadelphia; Elsevier; 2020.)*

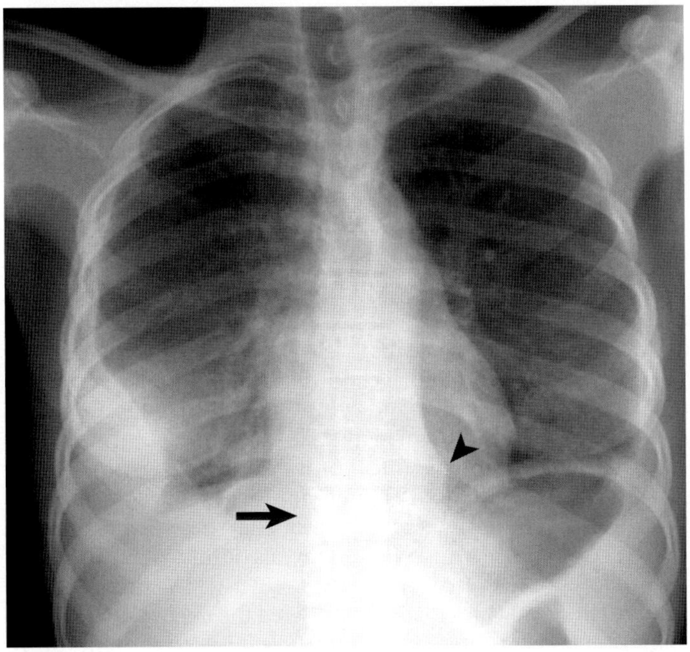

Fig. 15.10 Tuberculosis: primary pattern of infection. Chest radiograph shows bilateral pleural effusions and tuberculous infection of the T10 vertebral body (Pott disease) *(arrow)* with paraspinal widening *(arrowhead)*.

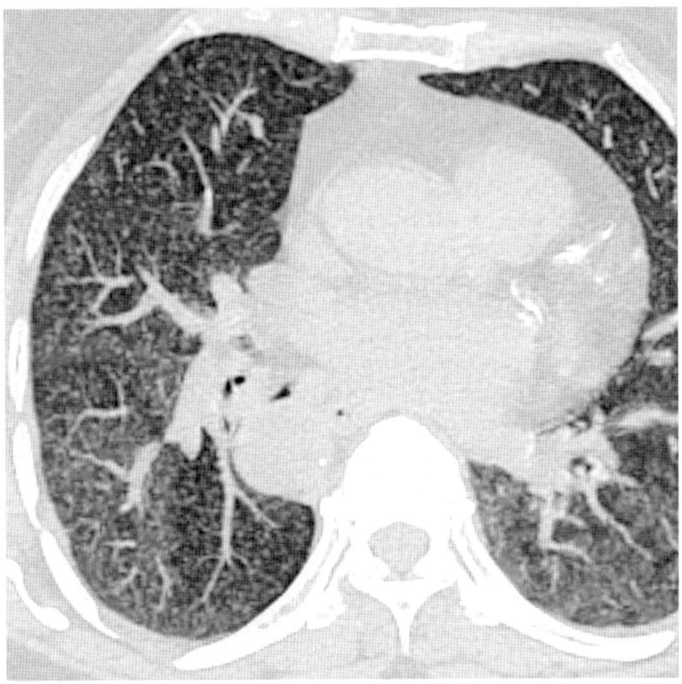

Fig. 15.12 Tuberculosis: miliary pattern. CT images shows innumerable randomly distributed pulmonary nodules bilaterally.

small or miliary nodules (Fig. 15.12).[58] Bronchitis and bronchiolitis frequently occur in HIV-positive and AIDS patients, even in patients without cavitary disease. Endobronchial spread caused by either *M. tuberculosis* or *Mycobacterium avium* complex (MAC) may have identical CT appearances, typically resulting in a tree-in-bud pattern.[39,58] Extrapulmonary findings, such as pleural effusion, lymphadenopathy, and pericardial effusion and thickening, are more common in HIV-infected than non–HIV-infected patients.[63]

Nontuberculous Mycobacterial Infections

General. In addition to TB, a wide range of mycobacterial species have been documented to infect patients with HIV/AIDS. Nontuberculous mycobacterial infections in AIDS patients are

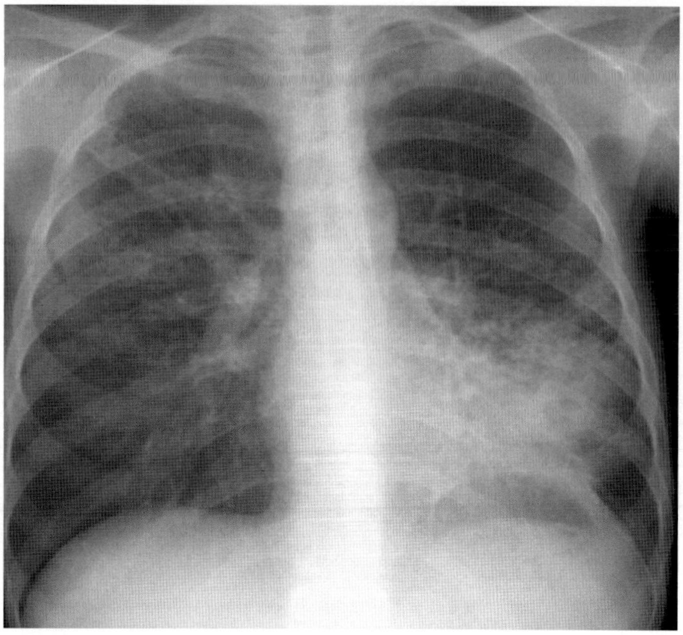

Fig. 15.13 *Mycobacterium kansasii.* Chest radiograph shows predominately lingular consolidation.

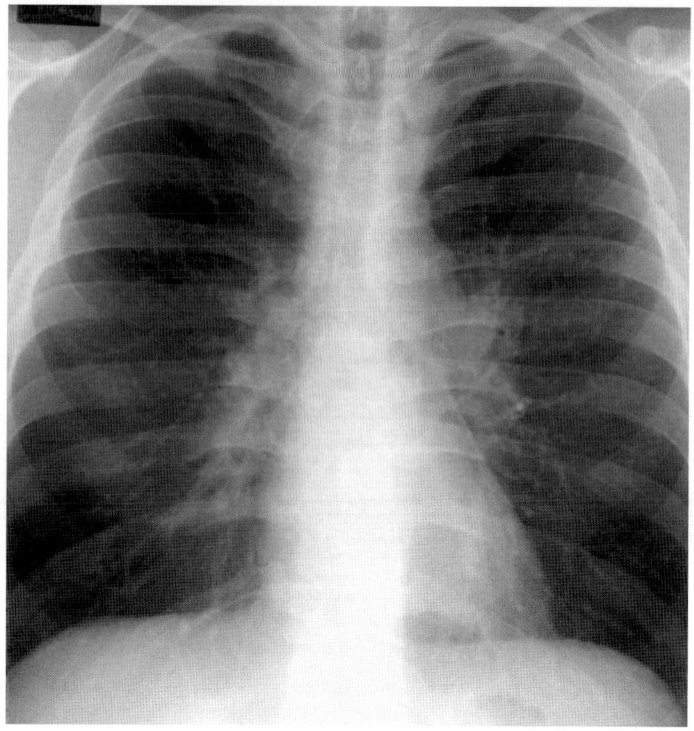

Fig. 15.14 *Mycobacterium avium* complex. Chest radiograph shows bilateral hilar and mediastinal lymphadenopathy.

usually secondary to MAC, but identification of MAC in sputum usually signifies colonization and not true infection.[64] Other mycobacteria that may lead to pulmonary and extrathoracic disease in AIDS include *Mycobacterium kansasii, Mycobacterium fortuitum,* and *Mycobacterium xenopi,* among others.[64–66] Because MAC and other nontuberculous mycobacteria are less virulent than *M. tuberculosis,* they are usually encountered in the setting of more advanced immunosuppression (CD4 < 50 cells/mm^3).[57,66] The incidence has decreased significantly after introduction of ART.[68] In many patients the nontuberculous mycobacterial infection was disseminated, with respiratory tract involvement.[64] However, isolated pulmonary involvement can occur, particularly with *M. kansasii.*[69] Clinical characteristics are similar among AIDS patients with nontuberculous infections, including fever, cough, and weight loss occurring over weeks or months.

Prophylactic treatment with weekly azithromycin is recommended for HIV-positive patients with CD4 counts less than 50 cells/mm^3. Therapy of nontuberculous mycobacterial infections involves prolonged multidrug regimens.[68,70]

Radiography. Imaging findings in the lungs vary if present and may include patchy consolidation (Fig. 15.13), ill-defined nodules, cavities, and lymphadenopathy (Fig. 15.14).[10] Lymphadenopathy is frequently present and similar in occurrence and appearance to lymphadenopathy in AIDS patients with tuberculosis.[71] A normal chest radiograph may be observed in 20% to 25% of patients with pulmonary infection from MAC or *M. kansasii.*[71]

Computed Tomography. As is the situation with tuberculosis, CT findings in nontuberculous mycobacterial infections may include lymphadenopathy (Fig. 15.15), cavitation, and bronchiolar (tree-in-bud) opacities that are invisible on the chest radiograph.

Viral Infections

General. Defects in cellular immunity permit many different viruses to cause pneumonia in HIV-infected patients, including respiratory syncytial virus, varicella, influenza, and human cytomegalovirus (CMV). Of these, CMV, a member of the Herpesviridae family, is the most common viral pulmonary pathogen in AIDS patients.[72,73] Although it is frequently recovered from the respiratory system in vivo and at autopsies, CMV is more often an extrathoracic pathogen than a cause of clinical pneumonia. ART has substantially reduced all manifestations of CMV in AIDS patients. When present, CMV pneumonitis affects patients with advanced levels of immunosuppression (CD4 counts < 100 cells/mm^3).[74] CMV infection occurs most frequently in patients infected with HIV by heterosexual or homosexual contact.[12] CMV pneumonitis is characterized by a mixed neutrophilic and inflammatory cell infiltrate in alveolar septa and airspaces. Typical nuclear and cytoplasmic inclusions are found in cells within the inflamed tissue, the presence of which is required to confirm true infection as opposed to colonization. AIDS patients with CMV pneumonia usually present with nonspecific symptoms, such as fever, shortness of breath, and hypoxia on room air. Auscultation reveals diffuse rales, and blood tests show an elevated LDH level. Anti-CMV therapy with ganciclovir or valganciclovir is considered the treatment of choice. Ganciclovir also is used in maintenance doses to prevent future infection.

Radiography. Chest radiography in patients with pulmonary CMV usually reveals diffuse bilateral opacities.[74] Opacities may be of ground-glass, reticular, or alveolar pattern. These patterns are also seen in other viral pneumonias (Fig. 15.16). Nodules are frequently identified; occasionally, nodules may be mass-like. Additional imaging findings include bronchiectasis and bronchial wall thickening.[38,74]

Computed Tomography. CT is more sensitive than radiography in the identification of parenchymal abnormalities and is useful when infection is suspected despite a negative or equivocal radiograph. CT images better show ground-glass opacity, dense

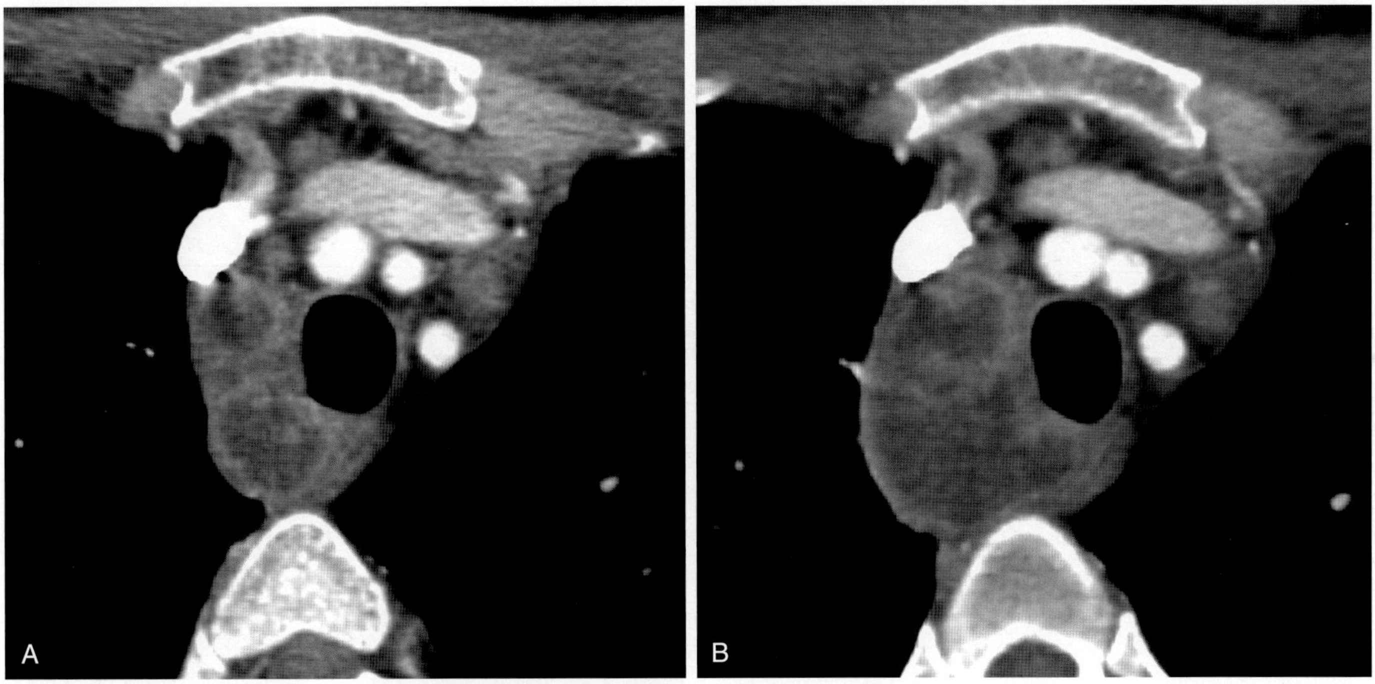

Fig. 15.15 *Mycobacterium avium* complex. (A) Axial CT image shows right paratracheal lymphadenopathy with central low density and peripheral enhancement characteristic of mycobacterial infection. (B) Axial CT 6 weeks after initiation of antiretroviral therapy shows further enlargement of right paratracheal lymphadenopathy thought to be related to immune reconstitution inflammatory syndrome. *(From Wu CC. HIV/AIDS. In: Rosado-de-Christenson ML, Abbott GF, Martinez-Jiménez S.* Diagnostic Imaging: Chest. *2nd ed. Philadelphia: Amirsys; 2012.)*

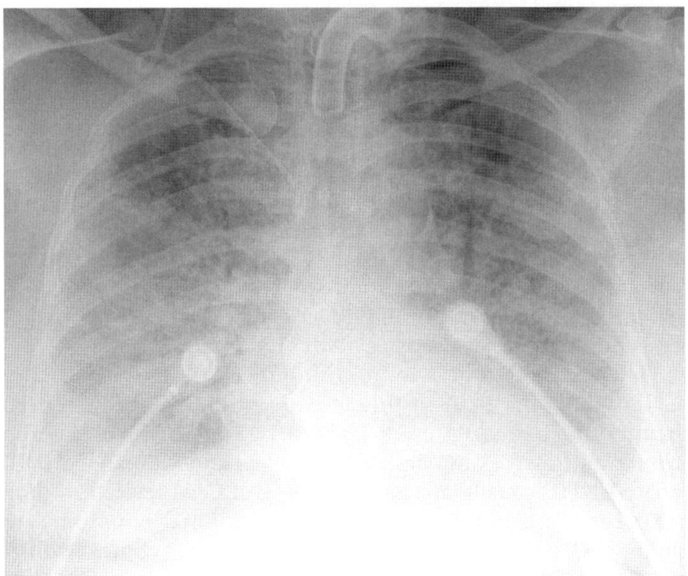

Fig. 15.16 Influenza (H1N1) pneumonia. Chest radiograph shows bilateral diffuse opacities. Imaging findings of viral pneumonia are often nonspecific.

consolidation, bronchial wall thickening or bronchiectasis, and interstitial reticulation.[74]

Neoplasms

Three malignancies—KS, non-Hodgkin lymphoma (NHL), and cervical cancer—are considered AIDS-defining malignancies. After the introduction of ART, the incidence of AIDS-defining malignancies, particularly KS and NHL, has decreased, and non–AIDS-defining cancer (NADC) now comprises 58% of cancer diagnoses. Lung cancer is the most common NADC.[75]

Kaposi Sarcoma

General. KS is a low-grade mesenchymal tumor that involves the blood and lymphatic vessels, affecting primarily the skin and causing disseminated disease in a variety of organs, including lymph nodes, gastrointestinal tract, and lungs. Early in the AIDS era, 40% of homosexual men presented with KS at the time of their initial AIDS diagnosis.[10] ART and other factors have led to a significant decrease in the incidence of KS among HIV-infected individuals, from approximately 10% to 20% in the early 1990s to even lower levels at present.[76] Most KS affect men who have sex with men[77] while being infected with human herpesvirus type 8 (HHV-8). KS is most common in patients with advanced immunosuppression whose CD4 cell count is usually less than 100 cells/mm^3.[78] Thoracic disease is found at autopsy in 45% to 50% of patients with cutaneous AIDS-related KS and is clinically detected in approximately 33%.[79] Pulmonary KS in the absence of cutaneous involvement is uncommon.[79] The most common presenting symptoms of pulmonary KS are dyspnea and cough; hemoptysis and chest pain are less common. Grossly, the surface of the lungs shows disk-shaped red to violaceous plaques confined to the visceral pleura. Parenchymal changes include lymphangitic thickening causing a red-blue discoloration around interlobular septa and bronchovascular bundles. Violaceous plaque lesions may be seen in the mucosal membranes of the bronchial tree.

A variety of treatments exist, including chemotherapy with liposomal anthracycline and ART. Airway lesions often respond

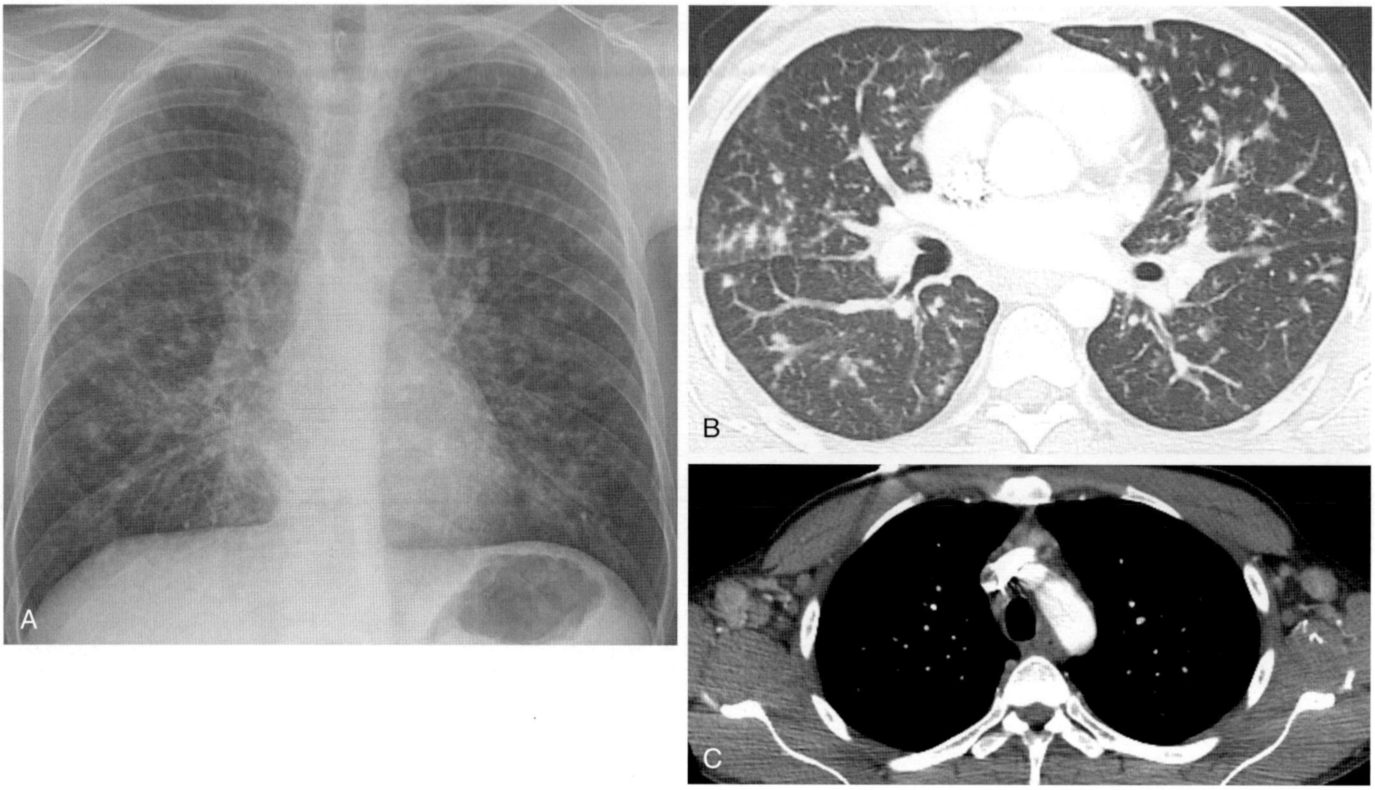

Fig. 15.17 Kaposi sarcoma. (A) Chest radiograph shows bilateral ill-defined nodular opacities and hilar lymphadenopathy. (B) Axial CT image in lung window demonstrates characteristic bilateral peribronchovascular nodules with irregular margin and subtle ground-glass halos. (C) Axial CT in soft window shows enlarged and enhancing prevascular and bilateral axillary lymphadenopathy in this man with human immunodeficiency virus (CD4 count, 130 cells/mm^3) who presented with cough.

to localized radiation therapy. Two-year survival of KS patients has increased to 85% from 30% since the introduction of ART.[75]

Radiography. The earliest chest radiographic findings in KS are interstitial, with thickening of the peribronchovascular bundles, tram track opacities, and peribronchial cuffing typically in the perihilar regions.[78] As the tumor grows, reticulonodular opacities may appear (Fig. 15.17), mainly in the lower lobes. The ill-defined nodular opacities may coalesce to form dense areas of airspace consolidation. Pleural effusions are common, may be unilateral or bilateral, and vary considerably in size.[10,78,80]

Computed Tomography. CT of the chest offers additional benefits over radiography by showing mediastinal lymphadenopathy (50% of cases) and improved characterization of the interlobular septal thickening and peribronchovascular nodules.[80] A characteristic CT finding in AIDS-related KS is the presence of bilateral and symmetric ill-defined nodules in a peribronchovascular distribution (flame-shaped lesions) (see Fig. 15.17), usually 1 cm or larger in diameter.[81] Ground-glass opacities resulting from hemorrhage may surround the nodules (CT halo sign).[82] Extrapulmonary findings, including lytic lesions of the sternum and thoracic spine and soft tissue masses or infiltration of the skin and subcutaneous fat, are found in about half of patients with thoracic KS.[80]

Lymphoma

General. NHL is one of three AIDS-defining malignancies and is the second most common malignancy in AIDS, occurring in 2% to 10% of HIV-infected individuals.[83] Although CNS lymphoma is the most common type, a variety of AIDS-related lymphomas may involve the thorax. Approximately two-thirds of AIDS-related lymphomas are categorized as diffuse B-cell NHL, which are aggressive, high-grade tumors that include poorly differentiated large anaplastic lymphomas.[84] Burkitt lymphomas constitute 25%, and other histologies make up a much smaller proportion. As with primary CNS lymphoma, herpesviruses, particularly Epstein-Barr virus (EBV) and HHV-8, are believed to be the responsible cofactors stimulating overproduction of B cells that results in lymphoma. Coinfections with EBV and HHV-8 have led to primary effusion lymphomas (body cavity lymphoma).

There seems to be a more pronounced decline in primary CNS lymphoma than in thoracic or abdominal AIDS-related lymphoma in the ART era.[85] The disease is twice as common in whites and men as in African Americans and women.[86] AIDS-related NHL usually affects patients with CD4 levels less than 100 cells/mm^3.[87] At presentation, constitutional symptoms are commonly reported. Pulmonary involvement is clinically diagnosed in only 6% to 10% of AIDS patients with NHL.[88] The most common symptoms are cough, dyspnea, and pleuritic chest pain. Pathologically, the chest may be involved in 40% of patients, but chest involvement is clinically diagnosed in only 10%.[88] Extranodal involvement of the CNS, gastrointestinal tract, liver, spleen, kidneys, and bone marrow is frequently observed.[86]

Approximately one-third to one-half of patients are cured with cytotoxic treatment regimens that are used in immunocompetent patients with lymphoma. ART is usually also administered. The survival has improved in recent years.

Imaging. Common imaging findings consist of lymphadenopathy, multiple pulmonary nodules or masses (Fig. 15.18),

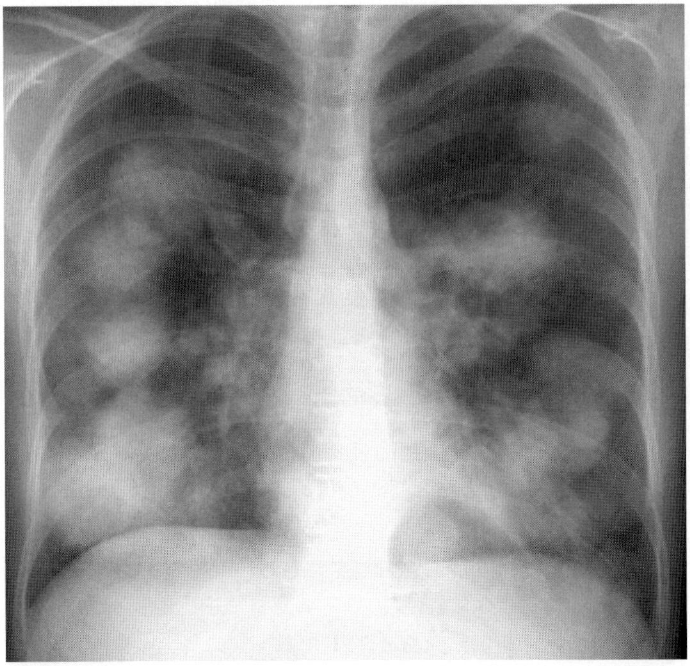

Fig. 15.18 Pulmonary lymphoma. Chest radiograph shows multiple ill-defined pulmonary masses. *(From Boiselle PM, Aviram G, Fishman JE. Update on lung disease in AIDS.* Semin Roentgenol. *2002;37:54–71.)*

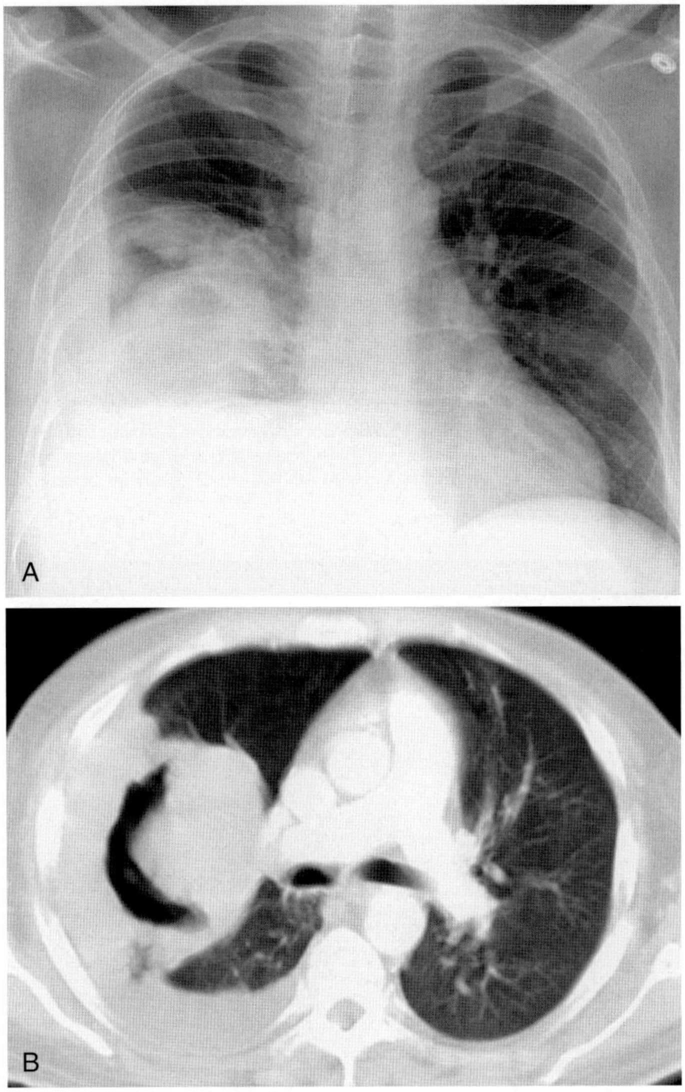

Fig. 15.19 Pulmonary lymphoma. (A) Chest radiograph shows a right lung mass-like opacity with central lucency and right pleural effusion. (B) CT confirms crescentic cavitation within solid mass and right pleural effusion.

areas of consolidation, and pleural effusions (Fig. 15.19).[88] Lung nodules/masses are usually well circumscribed and range in size from 0.5 to 5 cm in diameter; air bronchograms are frequently present. A halo sign may be observed on CT. AIDS-related NHL occasionally may manifest as a mediastinal, chest wall (Fig. 15.20), or pleural mass in the absence of pulmonary parenchymal disease. Lymphomatous involvement of the heart can also be seen (see Fig. 15.20).

Body cavity lymphoma is characterized by pleural, pericardial, or peritoneal effusions without adenopathy or pulmonary lesions.[84]

Lung Cancer

General. Although HIV-infected patients have a higher smoking prevalence than the general population, HIV infection has been found to confer an estimated 2- to 4-fold increased risk of lung cancer after adjusting for smoking and other risk factors.[75] Emerging evidence suggests immunosuppression and inflammatory processes as likely explanations.[89] Adenocarcinoma is the most common cell type.[92,93] HIV patients have clinical presentations of lung cancer similar to non-HIV patients, although HIV-infected patients tend to present at younger ages with more advanced-stage disease. The CD4 counts of most HIV-infected patients at the time of lung cancer diagnosis are greater than 200 cells/mm^3. Treatment for lung cancer is the same for HIV-infected patients as in the general population. Mortality in these patients appears to be primarily driven by lung cancer instead of HIV infection, although mortality is higher than in non–HIV-infected patients,[75] in part resulting from treatment disparities.[89]

Imaging. The most frequent imaging manifestation of lung cancer, similar to HIV-negative individuals, is a central or peripheral nodule or mass (Fig. 15.21).[90] Upper lobe peripheral masses are most common.[92] Ipsilateral hilar and variable mediastinal lymphadenopathy, postobstructive consolidation or atelectasis, and pleural effusion or pleural mass also are common.[90,93] A relatively common scenario in HIV patients is a chest radiograph obtained after treatment of a presumed infection that fails to show complete resolution of a lung opacity. Such persistent opacities are suspicious for malignancy and should be appropriately evaluated.

Although low-dose CT is now used for lung cancer screening in high-risk smokers, it is not clear if HIV-infected smokers will benefit from screening at younger ages.[89]

Multicentric Castleman Disease

General. Multicentric Castleman disease (MCD) is a rare lymphoproliferative disorder associated with HHV-8 and interleukin-6 dysregulation. Plasmablastic MCD, more aggressive than other subtypes, tends to be multifocal and is found with greater frequency in HIV-infected patients. The incidence appears to have increased in the era of ART. The involved lymph nodes contain large abnormal plasma cells. Patients can present with fever, lymphadenopathy, hepatosplenomegaly, weight loss, and

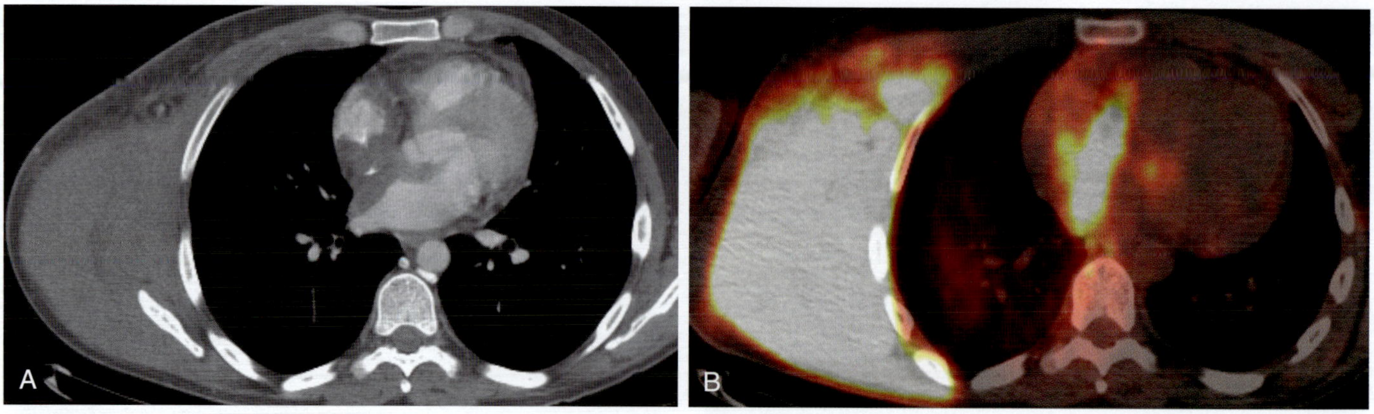

Fig. 15.20 Burkitt lymphoma. Axial contrast-enhanced CT (A) and fused positron emission tomography–CT (B) images show a large and markedly fluorodeoxyglucose-avid right lateral chest wall mass and soft tissue infiltration of the right atrial myocardium and interatrial septum.

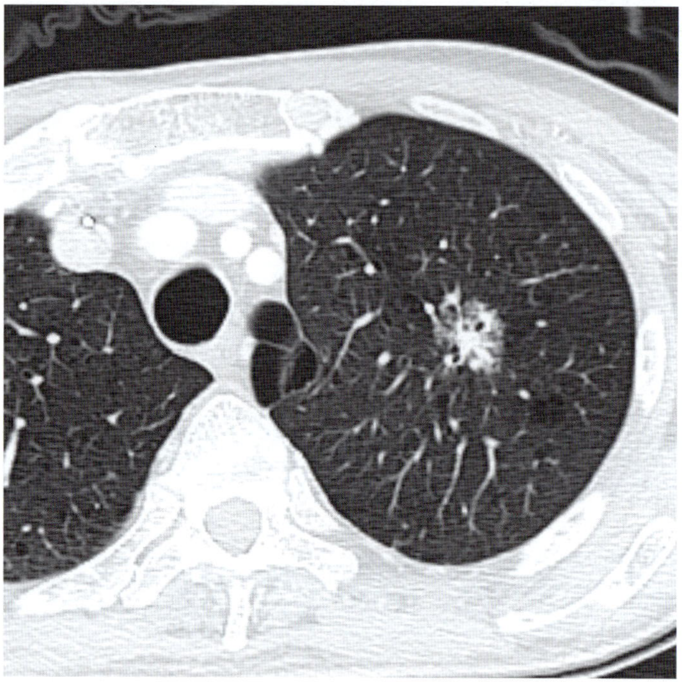

Fig. 15.21 Lung adenocarcinoma. Axial CT image in lung window shows a left upper lobe mix-attenuation spiculated nodule and multiple osseous metastases (not shown) 10 years after diagnosis of human immunodeficiency virus infection. Note associated emphysema.

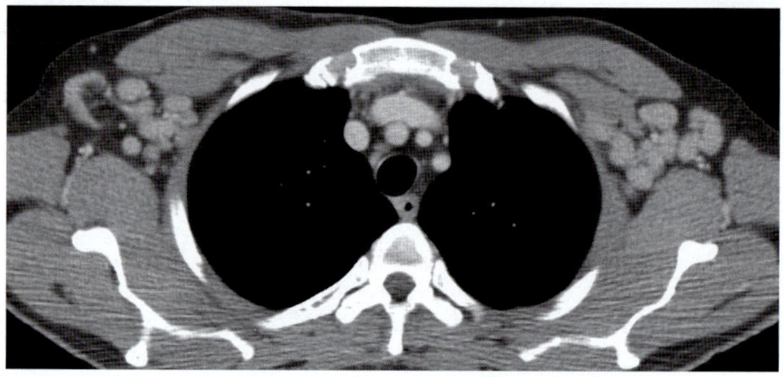

Fig. 15.22 Multicentric Castleman disease. Axial CT image shows avidly enhancing bilateral axillary lymphadenopathy (CD4 count, 349 cells/mm^3). *(From Lichtenberger JP, et al. What a differential a virus makes: a practical approach to thoracic imaging findings in the context of HIV infection—part 2, extrapulmonary findings, chronic lung disease, and immune reconstitution syndrome.* AJR Am J Roentgenol. *2012;198:1305–1312.)*

respiratory symptoms. Patients often also have some manifestations of POEMS syndrome (polyneuropathy, organomegaly, endocrinopathy, monoclonal gammopathy, and skin changes).

Patients with MCD have a higher incidence of KS and lymphoma related to HHV-8 infection. The malignancies may occur before, at the same time, or after the MCD diagnosis.[91] Rituximab is often used with or without chemotherapy for the treatment of MCD.[92]

Imaging. Imaging findings of MCD often consist of enlarged lymph nodes involving the mediastinum, hila, and axilla and/or splenomegaly and are difficult to distinguish from lymphoma. Avid enhancement of lymph nodes (Fig. 15.22) is suggestive of the diagnosis but not always present. Centrilobular nodules and thickening of bronchovascular bundles and interlobular septa similar to those seen in lymphocytic interstitial pneumonia can be seen. Pulmonary nodules, masses, and consolidation are less common findings. Marked radiotracer uptake is usually seen on ^{18}F-fluorodeoxyglucose (FDG)–positron emission tomography (PET).[91]

NONINFECTIOUS, NONNEOPLASTIC ENTITIES

Lymphocytic Interstitial Pneumonia

General. Lymphocytic interstitial pneumonia (LIP) is characterized by interstitial lung infiltration by mature lymphocytes and plasma cells resulting in peribronchovascular nodules without airspace involvement.[93] LIP is seen in 30% to 40% of HIV-infected children with pulmonary disease and is considered an AIDS-defining condition among children younger than 13 years by the Centers for Disease Control and Prevention.[19] It is less frequently seen in adults. Patients may be asymptomatic or show an insidious onset of respiratory distress with cough and mild hypoxemia.

Radiography. Characteristic findings of LIP on chest radiography consist of fine or coarse reticular and nodular opacities (Fig. 15.23).[93]

Computed Tomography. CT of LIP reveals ill-defined 2- to 4-mm nodules, often in a peribronchovascular distribution, and

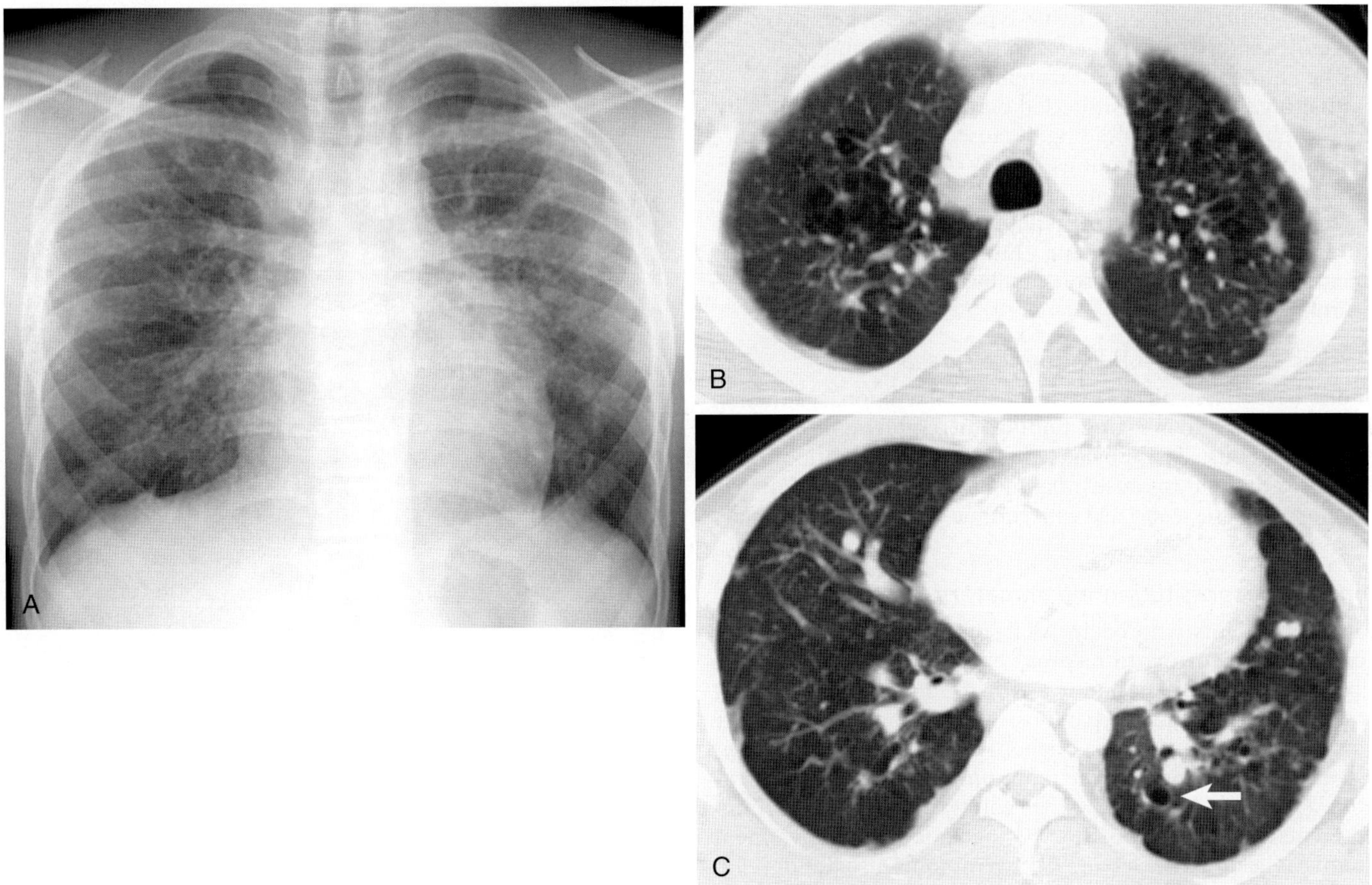

Fig. 15.23 Lymphocytic interstitial pneumonia. (A) Chest radiograph shows coarse perihilar reticulonodular opacities and faint nodules. (B) and (C) CT images reveal multiple ill-defined nodules and occasional cysts (*arrow* in C).

bilateral ground-glass opacities (see Fig. 15.23).[94] Poorly defined centrilobular nodules involving all lung zones can be identified. Thickening of bronchovascular bundles and interlobular septa, small subpleural nodules, and cysts also are observed in most patients. Mediastinal or hilar lymphadenopathy is frequent but not predominant.[94]

Esophagitis

General. Esophageal disease affects one-third of AIDS-infected individuals. Esophagitis is most commonly due to *Candida albicans,* but a variety of organisms, including CMV, *M. tuberculosis,* nontuberculous mycobacteria, and fungi, may be responsible. Symptoms include dysphagia and odynophagia and are usually indolent in nature. *Candida* esophagitis is the presumed etiology in patients with advanced immunosuppression and esophageal symptoms, with or without signs of oral candidiasis. Such individuals should be empirically treated with antifungal therapy, which has a high success rate.

Imaging. Imaging studies are of limited diagnostic value for AIDS-related esophagitis, although barium esophagram often shows focal or confluent plaques or a diffuse "shaggy" appearance.[95] Thickening of the esophageal wall (>5 mm) is the most common CT finding.[96] The target sign with enhancement of the mucosa and a hypodense submucosa[96] is seen in a minority of patients with esophagitis.

Pulmonary Hypertension

General. Several groups of investigators have documented a relationship between HIV infection and pulmonary arterial hypertension (PAH).[97] Chronic exposure to HIV viral proteins and HIV-induced immune dysregulations are thought to have an impact on pulmonary endothelial cells. Substance abuse also plays a role.[98] A recent study reports 3-year survival of 72% in patients treated with ART- and PAH-specific therapy, and the prognosis is mainly related to CD4 count and cardiac function.[99]

Imaging. Imaging findings include cardiomegaly, pulmonary artery dilatation, dilation of the right heart chambers on cross-sectional imaging, and straightening or bowing of the interventricular septum toward the left ventricle.[97]

Thrombosis

General. HIV-infected patients have a 2- to 10-fold increased risk of venous thrombosis, compared with the general population of the same age.[100] Most case reports and series have documented venous thrombosis, particularly deep vein thrombosis of the legs; pulmonary embolism and other venous and arterial thrombi have been described less often.[101,102] Numerous hematologic abnormalities may account for the occurrence of thrombosis, including deficiencies of protein S and protein C; activated protein C resistance; presence of lupus anticoagulant; antiphospholipid antibodies; and increased fibrinogen, D-dimer, plasminogen activator inhibitor-1, and tissue-type plasminogen activator antigen.[102] Another adverse effect of protease inhibitor therapy may be an increased risk of thrombosis.[102]

Imaging. In cases of suspected pulmonary embolism, chest radiography may be misleading because of the high prevalence of abnormal thoracic findings in HIV/AIDS patients. Consequently, CT pulmonary angiography is recommended as the preferred imaging method for pulmonary embolism rather than ventilation-perfusion scanning. Either CT lower extremity venography or Doppler ultrasonography is used to identify venous thrombosis.

Chronic Obstructive Pulmonary Disease

Studies have shown higher rates of dyspnea, pulmonary function abnormalities, and imaging findings of emphysema in HIV-infected patients. The imbalance in CD4:CD8 cell ratio in HIV patients is thought to cause inflammation and release of matrix metalloproteinases associated with chronic obstructive pulmonary disease.[98]

Immune Reconstitution Inflammatory Syndrome

General. Patients who begin ART sometimes show transient clinical decline, owing to recovery of the immune system and subsequent inflammation in response to unmasking of a latent or subclinical infection or paradoxical worsening of previously recognized disease.[103] This phenomenon is termed *immune restoration disease* or *immune reconstitution inflammatory syndrome* (IRIS).[104–106] A baseline CD4 count less than 50 cells/mm^3 represents a risk factor for IRIS.[104] A higher level of pretreatment viremia is also a risk factor. IRIS symptoms usually develop within a week to a few months after initiation of ART. Mycobacteria, including tuberculous and nontuberculous mycobacteria, are the most commonly implicated infectious organisms in IRIS, accounting for almost 40% of the cases reported up to 2002.[107] IRIS is associated with restoration of cutaneous delayed-type hypersensitivity reaction to tuberculin.[104] IRIS has also been reported in patients with *Pneumocystis* pneumonia. Noninfectious diseases, such as KS, have also been reported to worsen after ART. Sarcoidosis can occur or recur after ART. Manifestations of IRIS in an affected HIV-infected patient who is successfully treated with ART may be as subtle as fever, cough, and minor lymph node enlargement or as dramatic as respiratory failure or neurologic deterioration.[107,108]

Several diagnostic criteria have been proposed for establishing the diagnosis of IRIS, including atypical presentation of opportunistic infections in patients responding to ART, decrease in plasma HIV RNA levels, and increased blood CD4 count. The differential diagnosis of IRIS includes progressive disease owing to nonadherence to treatment, single drug–resistant or multidrug-resistant mycobacterial infection, adverse drug reaction, and concurrent opportunistic infection or malignancy. Treatment consists of antimicrobials with or without steroids.[104]

Imaging. Of patients with IRIS, 13% to 45% may show thoracic abnormalities.[105,106,109] The imaging findings of IRIS vary and depend on the underlying disease process. In tuberculosis or nontuberculous-related IRIS, a common radiologic feature is lymph node enlargement, often with central low-attenuation centers (see Fig. 15.15).[108,109] The nodes may be located in abdominal, axillary, and mediastinal locations. Lung parenchymal abnormalities also are frequent, usually manifesting as consolidation, nodules, or micronodules.[108,109] Pleural effusions are less common than nodal or parenchymal disease.[108,109] Findings generally appear 1 to 5 weeks after beginning ART and resolve within months.[109] Although uncommon, AIDS patients on ART may develop thoracic sarcoidosis with characteristic findings of lymphadenopathy (Fig. 15.24) and pulmonary parenchymal disease.[110]

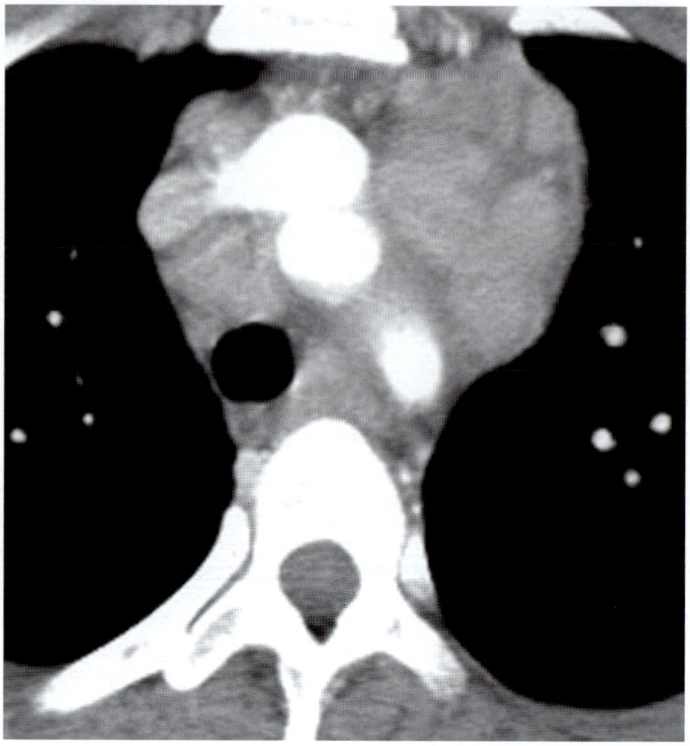

Fig. 15.24 Immune reconstitution inflammatory syndrome. Axial CT image shows bulky mediastinal lymphadenopathy 2 months postinitiation of antiretroviral therapy. Biopsy revealed benign granulomatous inflammation consistent with sarcoidosis.

Differential Diagnosis

CLINICAL DATA

The clinical likelihood of various pulmonary complications of HIV depends on several factors. The most important measure of a patient's immune status is the serum CD4 lymphocyte count. The CD4 count is only one parameter, however, and it does not reflect the activity of the entire immune system. Symptoms may assist further in developing a relevant differential diagnosis. Patients with pulmonary infections typically present with fever. Mild fever may occur in inflammatory disorders but is uncommon in malignancies, except lymphoma. The temporal occurrence of symptoms also is of interest. Bacterial pneumonia is often associated with an acute onset of fever, pleuritic chest pain, productive cough, and purulent sputum. *Pneumocystis* pneumonia typically has a more insidious onset, with patients experiencing dyspnea, dry cough, and shortness of breath for 1 week or more before seeking medical attention. Symptoms of TB, nontuberculous mycobacteria, and fungal disease may be vague and occur over weeks to months before diagnosis.

Patient demographics may direct the workup further because certain groups share a predilection for certain diseases. IV drug abusers with HIV infection experience bacterial pneumonia and abscess formation, septic emboli, and TB more frequently than other AIDS patients.[20] CMV occurs more frequently in patients infected with HIV through sexual contact, whereas KS occurs almost exclusively in homosexual men.[12,77] Finally, geography can be a helpful factor. Bacterial pneumonia is the most common cause of CAP in HIV-infected patients in Europe and the United States, but TB remains the main pulmonary infection in much of Africa, South America, and Southeast Asia.[17]

IMAGING FINDINGS

Tables 15.1 to 15.5 summarize the differential diagnoses for patients with HIV infection based on imaging findings.

TABLE 15.1 DIFFERENTIAL DIAGNOSIS OF PULMONARY CONSOLIDATION IN HUMAN IMMUNODEFICIENCY VIRUS–INFECTED PATIENTS

	CD4 Count (cells/mm^3)
INFECTION	
Bacterial	Any
Mycobacterial	<200
Fungal	<200
NEOPLASM	
Lung cancer	Any
Lymphoma	Any

Adapted from Lichtenberger JP 3rd, Sharma A, Zachary KC, et al. What a differential a virus makes: a practical approach to thoracic imaging findings in the context of HIV infection—part 1, pulmonary findings. *AJR Am J Roentgenol.* 2012;198:1295–1304.

TABLE 15.2 DIFFERENTIAL DIAGNOSIS OF GROUND-GLASS OPACITIES IN HUMAN IMMUNODEFICIENCY VIRUS–INFECTED PATIENTS

	CD4 Count (cells/mm^3)
INFECTION	
Atypical bacterial	Any
Viral	Any
Pneumocystis jirovecii pneumonia	<200
Cytomegalovirus	<100
INTERSTITIAL LUNG DISEASE	
Lymphocytic interstitial pneumonia	Any

Adapted from Lichtenberger JP 3rd, Sharma A, Zachary KC, et al. What a differential a virus makes: a practical approach to thoracic imaging findings in the context of HIV infection—part 1, pulmonary findings. *AJR Am J Roentgenol.* 2012;198:1295–1304.

TABLE 15.3 DIFFERENTIAL DIAGNOSIS OF PULMONARY CYSTIC LESIONS IN HUMAN IMMUNODEFICIENCY VIRUS–INFECTED PATIENTS

Entities	CD4 Count (cells/mm^3)
Pneumocystis pneumonia	<200
Lymphocytic interstitial pneumonia	Any

Adapted from Lichtenberger JP 3rd, Sharma A, Zachary KC, et al. What a differential a virus makes: a practical approach to thoracic imaging findings in the context of HIV infection—part 1, pulmonary findings. *AJR Am J Roentgenol.* 2012;198:1295–1304.

IMAGING ALGORITHM

Chest radiography is usually the first imaging test obtained to assess an HIV-infected individual with respiratory symptoms.[39] In asymptomatic HIV patients, an abnormal chest radiograph usually signifies an active process. In this setting mycobacterial infection is the most likely entity.[111]

CT generally is used to characterize radiographic abnormalities or when the chest radiograph appears normal in the presence of respiratory symptoms. A normal chest radiograph can be seen in a significant minority of HIV-positive patients with active pulmonary infection secondary to a variety of organisms, including *P. jirovecii* and mycobacterial, fungal, and viral organisms. CT is usually positive in such patients.[12] In addition to identifying the presence of infection, CT often reveals characteristic findings that can help to determine the most likely etiologies and guide further workup. Hartman and associates[112] have shown that CT

TABLE 15.4 DIFFERENTIAL DIAGNOSIS OF PERIBRONCHOVASCULAR OPACITIES IN HUMAN IMMUNODEFICIENCY VIRUS–INFECTED PATIENTS

	CD4 Count (cells/mm^3)
NEOPLASTIC	
Kaposi sarcoma	<200
Lymphoma	Any
Lymphangitic carcinomatosis	Any
Castleman disease	Any
OTHER	
Lymphocytic interstitial pneumonia	Any
Sarcoidosis	As CD4 count increases with antiretroviral therapy

Adapted from Lichtenberger JP 3rd, Sharma A, Zachary KC, et al. What a differential a virus makes: a practical approach to thoracic imaging findings in the context of HIV infection—part 1, pulmonary findings. *AJR Am J Roentgenol.* 2012;198:1295–1304.

TABLE 15.5 DIFFERENTIAL DIAGNOSIS OF LYMPHADENOPATHY IN HUMAN IMMUNODEFICIENCY VIRUS–INFECTED PATIENTS

	CD4 Count (cells/mm^3)
LOW-ATTENTUATION CENTER	
Mycobacterial infection	Most commonly <50
Fungal infection	<200
ENHANCING	
Multicentric Castleman disease	Any
Kaposi sarcoma	<200
HOMOGENEOUS SOFT TISSUE DENSITY	
Infection	Any
Lymphoma	Any
Sarcoidosis	As CD4 count increases with antiretroviral therapy

Adapted from Lichtenberger JP 3rd, Sharma A, Zachary KC, et al. What a differential a virus makes: a practical approach to thoracic imaging findings in the context of HIV infection—part 2, extrapulmonary findings, chronic lung disease, and immune reconstitution syndrome. *AJR Am J Roentgenol.* 2012;198:1305–1312.

KEY POINTS

- Thoracic disorders, including respiratory infections, malignancies, and inflammatory conditions, remain a source of significant morbidity and mortality among human immunodeficiency virus (HIV)-infected individuals throughout the world.
- In patients for whom it is available, antiretroviral therapy (ART) has produced a dramatic reduction in HIV-associated morbidity and mortality.
- The CD4 count is the most widely used indicator of the degree of immunosuppression; a CD4 count <200 cells/mm^3 places a patient at risk for opportunistic infections and certain malignancies.
- Bacterial respiratory infections, including infectious airways disease and pneumonia, are the most common respiratory diseases among HIV-infected individuals in developed countries.
- *P. jirovecii* (*Pneumocystis* pneumonia) is the most prevalent opportunistic infection in HIV-infected patients. Imaging features of *Pneumocystis* pneumonia consist mainly of bilateral ground-glass opacities with symptoms often out of proportion to the radiographic findings.
- Thoracic manifestations of tuberculosis are highly variable and dependent on the CD4 count.
- Kaposi sarcoma is the most common acquired immune deficiency syndrome (AIDS)-defining malignancy but has shown a marked decline in incidence owing to ART.
- Thoracic AIDS-related lymphoma often shows parenchymal opacities in the absence of lymphadenopathy, effusions, or extrathoracic disease.
- HIV-infected patients usually present with lung cancer at a younger age than non–HIV-infected individuals.
- AIDS patients who begin ART sometimes show transient clinical worsening, a phenomenon known as immune restoration disease or immune reconstitution inflammatory syndrome.

is highly accurate in diagnosing *Pneumocystis* pneumonia (94%) and KS (90%). CT also has a high negative predictive value for excluding active disease.[112,113] An important aspect of CT findings is that they can be used to direct bronchoscopy or biopsy.[114]

PET with FDG is useful for staging lung cancer and lymphoma.

Synopsis of Treatment Options

MEDICAL

ART is the cornerstone of management of patients with HIV infection and is currently offered to all HIV-infected patients with detectable viremia regardless of CD4 count.[115,116] ART medications inhibit or interfere with various steps of the HIV life cycle, including viral entry, reverse transcription (reverse transcriptase inhibitors), integration (integrase strand transfer inhibitors), and budding (protease inhibitor). For most patients, the recommended initial regimens include two nucleoside reverse transcriptase inhibitors and an integrase strand transfer inhibitor.[116] ART is effective in suppressing viremia and maintaining adequate peripheral blood CD4 counts. Treatment goals are to reduce HIV-related complications and prevent transmission of the virus. Because ART does not clear the viral infection, lifelong treatment is necessary. Therapeutic strategies to achieve a cure are being investigated.[117]

Prophylaxis for *Pneumocystis* infection is recommended for patients with a CD4 count less than 200 cells/mm^3. Prophylaxis against disseminated MAC is recommended for patients with a CD4 count less than 50 cells/mm^3. Because of a high risk of infection with *S. pneumoniae*, pneumococcal vaccination is recommended for all HIV-infected patients regardless of CD4 count.[118]

Specific therapies for infectious, malignant, and other thoracic manifestations of HIV infection are listed earlier in the appropriate sections.

SURGICAL

Few of the thoracic complications of HIV infection are surgically remediable. Exceptions include primary lung cancer and certain fungal infections, such as mucormycosis and *Aspergillus* infection resistant to antifungal therapy.

SUGGESTED READINGS

Almeida A, Boattini M. Community-acquired pneumonia in HIV-positive patients: an update on etiologies, epidemiology and management. *Curr Infect Dis Rep.* 2017;19(1):2.

Chou SH, Prabhu SJ, Crothers K, Stern EJ, Godwin JD, Pipavath SN. Thoracic diseases associated with HIV infection in the era of antiretroviral therapy: clinical and imaging findings. *Radiographics.* 2014;34(4):895–911.

Lichtenberger JP 3rd, Sharma A, Zachary KC, Krishnam MS, Greene RE, Shepard JA, Wu CC. What a differential a virus makes: a practical approach to thoracic imaging findings in the context of HIV infection—part 1, pulmonary findings. *AJR Am J Roentgenol.* 2012;198(6):1295–1304.

Lichtenberger JP 3rd, Sharma A, Zachary KC, et al. What a differential a virus makes: a practical approach to thoracic imaging findings in the context of HIV infection—part 2, extrapulmonary findings, chronic lung disease, and immune reconstitution syndrome. *AJR Am J Roentgenol.* 2012;198(6):1305–1312.

Presti RM, Flores SC, Palmer BE, Atkinson JJ, Lesko CR, Lau B, Fontenot AP, Roman J, McDyer JF, Twigg HL 3rd. Mechanisms underlying HIV-associated noninfectious lung disease. *Chest.* 2017;152:1053–1060.

Sigel K, Makinson A, Thaler J. Lung cancer in persons with HIV. *Curr Opin HIV AIDS.* 2017;12(1):31–38.

The full reference list for this chapter is available at ExpertConsult.com.

16 Screening for Lung Cancer

SUZANNE C. BYRNE | THOMAS E. HARTMAN

Background

Lung cancer is the third most common cancer and the leading cause of cancer-related death in the United States.[1] The most important risk factor for lung cancer is smoking, which results in approximately 85% of all US lung cancer deaths. It is estimated that 224,390 new cases and 158,080 deaths from lung cancer occurred in the United States in 2016. Deaths from lung cancer exceed the combined totals of breast, colorectal, and prostate carcinomas, which are the three next most common causes of cancer death.[1] If mortality rates remain stable, more than 1 million Americans will die of lung cancer in the next 7 years. If there were an effective screening tool for lung cancer that resulted in a 10% mortality reduction, however, an estimated 16,000 lives per year could be saved in the United States alone. There are currently screening programs for breast, colorectal, and prostate carcinomas, all of which have shown a mortality reduction. Recently, screening for lung cancer has begun in the United States based on the findings of the National Lung Screening Trial (NLST).

Conditions for Screening

Numerous conditions must be met to screen effectively for a particular disease. The two primary conditions are (1) an asymptomatic phase of the disease, during which it can be detected, and (2) availability of an effective intervention during the presymptomatic phase that would alter the eventual outcome of the disease.

For the purpose of lung cancer screening, most stage I lung cancers are asymptomatic. It has been estimated that most stage I lung cancers have been present for at least 4 years before diagnosis.[2] Given these estimates, it would seem that lung cancer meets the first criterion for screening.

Previous survival studies after resection of stage I lung cancer have shown survival rates ranging from 62% to 82%.[3–6] In addition, studies of unresected stage I lung cancer have shown a survival rate of only 4%.[2] These studies would seem to support the second criterion in that intervention at an earlier stage may translate into decreased mortality. Survival and mortality are not equivalent terms, however, and the second condition had not previously been conclusively proven.

History of Lung Cancer Screening

During the 1970s, there were three mass screening trials at Johns Hopkins, Memorial Sloan Kettering, and the Mayo Clinic[7–9] that used the chest radiograph as the screening modality. In combination, these studies enrolled more than 30,000 men 45 years old or older who were current smokers. In these studies the screening group had more early-stage cancers and increased 5-year survival; however, a mortality reduction from lung cancer in the screened group versus the control group was not shown. Another study done in Czechoslovakia in the 1980s, which involved more than 6000 participants, also failed to show a mortality reduction.[10] Finally, in 1996 extended follow-up of the participants in the Mayo Clinic study showed no mortality difference between the screened and control groups.[11] The inability of the chest radiograph to show a decrease in lung cancer mortality in these studies is why no current organizations recommend using the chest radiograph for lung cancer screening.

History of Computed Tomography Screening

Because the chest radiograph failed to screen effectively for lung cancer, investigators turned to low-dose CT (LDCT) as a potential screening tool. In a seminal study by Kaneko and colleagues,[12] 3457 low-dose spiral CT scans were performed on 1369 men 50 years old or older who had a greater than 20 pack-year smoking history. Each participant was imaged with a chest radiograph and an LDCT scan. The LDCT scan detected 15 lung cancers. Only 4 of the 15 cancers detected on CT were visible on the chest radiograph. CT also was shown to detect smaller cancers. The average diameter of the cancers detected on CT was 16 mm, whereas the average diameter of the cancers detected on chest radiograph was 30 mm. Finally, it was shown that 93% of the CT-detected cancers were stage I. This was much higher than the historic percentage of 20% to 25% potential resectable cancers and gave the impetus for further evaluation of LDCT as a screening modality for lung cancer.

The second important early study that provided encouraging data about the prospects for LDCT screening was the Early Lung Cancer Action Project (ELCAP).[13] This study enrolled 1000 participants who were 60 years old or older and had at least a 10 pack-year smoking history. Participants were imaged with a chest radiograph and a low-dose spiral CT scan. In this study 27 lung cancers were detected on LDCT, and only 7 of these were visible on the chest radiograph. Of the 27 cancers detected on CT, 85% were stage I cancers. These early studies showed CT could identify more cancers and cancers at an earlier stage than was possible using the chest radiograph, which illustrated the potential for CT to be an effective screening tool.

More recently, Henschke and colleagues[14] reported the results of a large collaborative study. These results showed a high incidence of stage I lung cancers (85%). In addition, the group of participants who had clinical stage I lung cancer had an estimated 10-year disease-specific survival rate of 88%. The improved survival was encouraging; however, this study was limited as it did not focus on mortality.

The largest published study on the effectiveness of LDCT for lung cancer screening was the NLST. This double-blind trial enrolled participants who were between 55 and 74 years of age, had a history of cigarette smoking of at least 30 pack-years and, if former smokers, had quit within the previous 15 years. The study excluded persons who had previously received a diagnosis of lung cancer, had undergone chest CT within 18 months before enrollment, had hemoptysis, or had an unexplained weight loss of more than 6.8 kg (15 lb) in the preceding year.[15] A total of 53,454 persons were enrolled. This trial showed a reduction in lung cancer mortality of 20% and a reduction in all-cause mortality of 6.7% (95% confidence interval [CI], 1.2% to 13.6%).[15] Results of this trial have shown a sensitivity of 93.8% and a specificity of 73.4% for the detection of lung cancer on a screening examination. In the NLST the positive predictive value of finding nodules of 4 mm or larger was 3.8%.[16] Modeling has shown that annual screening with LDCT provides the maximal benefit compared with biennial or triennial screening.[17] Benefits were measured as a percentage of early-stage lung cancer detection, number of lung cancer deaths avoided, and total number of life-years gained. Modeling studies have also illustrated the potential issue of overdiagnosis. One study performed for the US Preventive Services Task Force (USPSTF) estimated that 10% to 12% of screen-detected cancer cases would not have been detected in the patient's lifetime without screening.[18]

In contrast to the NLST, there have been small-scale European trials that have been unable to reproduce the findings of the NLST, concluding that there is no benefit to screening.[19–21] These trials include the DANTE (Detection and Screening of Early Lung Cancer by Novel Imaging Technology and Molecular Essays) trial and the DLCST (Danish Lung Cancer Screening Trial). However, these were smaller trials (n = 2472 and 4104, respectively) that may have been underpowered, preventing the study from finding a benefit to screening, should one exist. In addition, the inclusion criteria in the DLCST resulted in younger and healthier participants than in other trials, which may have resulted in bias.[21] The relative risk for all-cause mortality in the DLCST was 1.46 (95% CI, 0.99 to 2.15). This finding highlights the potential harm of screening a young, healthy population.

In Europe the ongoing Dutch-Belgian Lung Cancer Screening Trial (NELSON [Nederlands-Leuvens Longkanker Screenings ONderzoek]) is investigating whether screening with LDCT can reduce lung cancer mortality by at least 25% compared with no screening at 10 years of follow-up for individuals aged 50 to 75 years who had a smoking history of greater than or equal to 15 cigarettes per day for greater than or equal to 25 years or greater than or equal to 10 cigarettes for greater than or equal to 30 years, and who were still smoking or had quit less than or equal to 10 years ago. Since the start of the NELSON study in 2003, more than 7000 participants were randomized to CT screening. Results from the NELSON Trial are anticipated soon. The findings of this study will be a valuable addition to the current data on LDCT for lung cancer screening.

SCREENING PROGRAMS AND REIMBURSEMENT

Using data from NLST and modeling studies, the USPSTF determined that annual LDCT screening provides net benefit to patients aged 55 to 80 years at high risk for lung cancer. Currently, the USPSTF recommends annual screening for lung cancer with LDCT in adults aged 55 to 80 years who have a 30 pack-year smoking history and are currently smoking or have quit within the past 15 years. Screening should be discontinued once a person has not smoked for 15 years or develops a health problem that substantially limits life expectancy or the ability or willingness to have curative lung surgery. This is a category B recommendation.[18] The implications for this USPSTF recommendation are that insurance companies in the United States are now required to cover lung cancer screening for their enrollees.

More recently, the Centers for Medicare and Medicaid Services (CMS) has approved lung cancer screening for participants enrolled in Medicare. The age group covered by CMS differs slightly from the group covered by the USPSTF recommendations. CMS also has several reporting requirements that must be met in order for the lung cancer screening episode to be reimbursed. These include shared decision making, reporting of the scanning protocol and findings, and the development of a registry that can track patient outcomes after screening.[22] To help with these requirements, the American College of Radiology (ACR) has developed scanning and reporting protocols for lung cancer screening and has also developed a registry that can be used.[23] As specified by the ACR–Society of Thoracic Radiology (STR) Practice Parameter for the Performance and Reporting of Lung Cancer Screening Thoracic Computed Tomography,[24,25] a CT scanner should meet or exceed the following capabilities: (1) gantry rotation times: less than or equal to 0.5 seconds, (2) slice thickness: less than or equal to 2.5 mm (≤1.0 mm is preferred), and (3) preferably greater than or equal to 16 detector rows. In addition, the CT scanner and/or the viewing platform should be capable of generating maximum-intensity projection and multiplanar reconstruction images. The low-dose screening technique should be set to yield a computed tomography dose index volume of less than 3 mGy for a standard-sized patient (typical average radiation dose of 1.5 mSv). It should be reduced for smaller-sized patients and increased for larger-sized patients.[26–30]

LUNG COMPUTED TOMOGRAPHY SCREENING REPORTING AND DATA SYSTEM (LUNG-RADS)

To assist radiologists with reporting the findings from lung cancer screening examinations, the ACR has developed Lung-RADS, which allows standardized impressions and recommendations to be generated based on the findings on the screening CT examination. The most updated version of Lung-RADS can be found on the ACR website. The primary drivers for determination of the impression and recommendation are the size and attenuation of the nodule. This differs slightly from the NLST, which only took into account the size of the nodule when making recommendations.

Studies by Henschke and colleagues[31] and Midthun and colleagues[32] have shown that for nodules less than 5 mm the likelihood of malignancy is less than 1%, even in a high-risk screening population. In addition, even when these tiny nodules were shown to be lung cancer, most of these were still stage I cancers. Although the nodules would still need to be followed, a less aggressive follow-up of these smallest nodules would be possible according to these results. Using these and other studies, Lung-RADS changed the recommended size for a positive study that would require shorter-term follow-up from 4 mm (as in the NLST) for a solid nodule to 6 mm.

The attenuation characteristics of the nodules are broken down into solid, part-solid, and pure ground-glass. If nodules are part-solid, an additional measurement of the solid component of the nodule is required to appropriately guide the recommendation for further workup. The attenuation of the nodule also influences the recommendations for the size of the nodule as solid nodules have different recommendations based on size compared with part-solid and ground-glass nodules. Part-solid nodules also take into consideration the size of the solid component when making recommendations for further workup. Margins of the nodule and associated findings can also be taken into account when making the recommendation for further workup.

There are five main Lung-RADS categories plus additional modifiers (see the most up-to-date version of Lung-RADS at www.acr.org). These include categories 1 (negative; Figs. 16.1 and 16.2) and 2 (benign appearing; Figs. 16.3 and 16.4), which correspond to a negative screening. Categories 3 (probably benign) (Fig. 16.5) and 4 (suspicious) correspond to a positive screening. Category 4 is further divided into 4A (Fig. 16.6), 4B (Fig. 16.7), and 4X (Fig. 16.8).[16] Category 0 is given to an examination that is considered incomplete. All nodules should be measured on lung windows and reported as the average diameter rounded to the nearest whole number. A negative screening result assumes that reevaluation will occur at the next annual screening, whereas a positive screening result means that additional evaluation is recommended before the next annual screening. This evaluation often involves a short-term follow-up diagnostic CT that can be

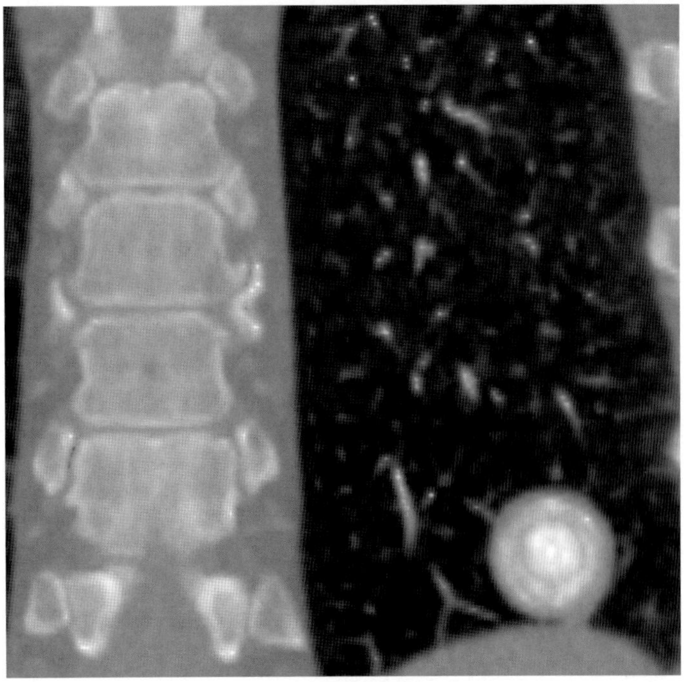

Fig. 16.2 Lung-RADS category 1, calcified granuloma from remote histoplasmosis. Coronal low-dose computed tomography (LDCT) shows a round left lower lobe nodule containing laminar calcification, diagnostic of a benign granuloma. This is considered a negative screen, and the patient will return for LDCT in 1 year. *(Reproduced with permission from Walker CM. Lung cancer screening. In: Rosado-de-Christenson ML, Carter BW, eds.* Specialty Imaging: Thoracic Neoplasms, *Philadelphia: Amirsys; 2016.)*

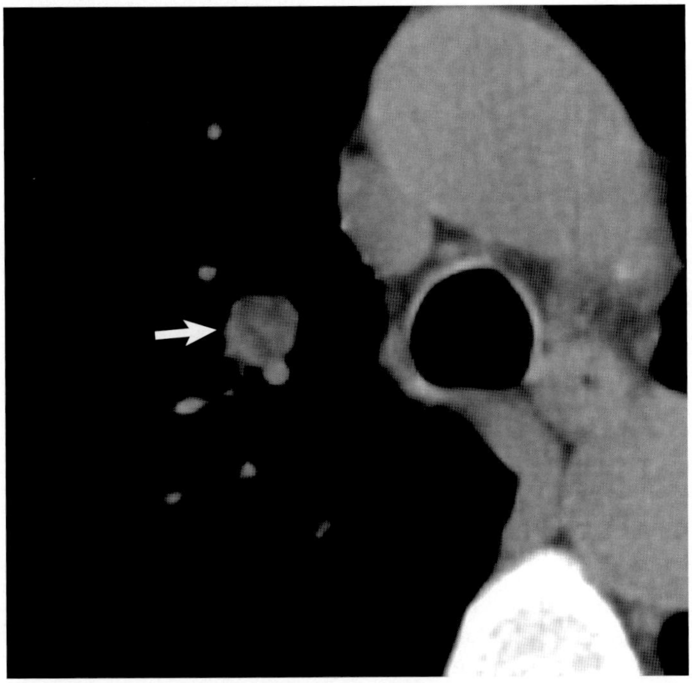

Fig. 16.1 Lung-RADS category 1, pulmonary hamartoma. Axial low-dose computed tomography (LDCT) shows a well-circumscribed, lobular right upper lobe nodule *(arrow)* containing macroscopic fat, diagnostic of pulmonary hamartoma. This is considered a negative screen, and the patient will return for LDCT in 1 year. *(Reproduced with permission from Walker CM. Lung cancer screening. In: Rosado-de-Christenson ML, Carter BW, eds.* Specialty Imaging: Thoracic Neoplasms, *Philadelphia: Amirsys; 2016.)*

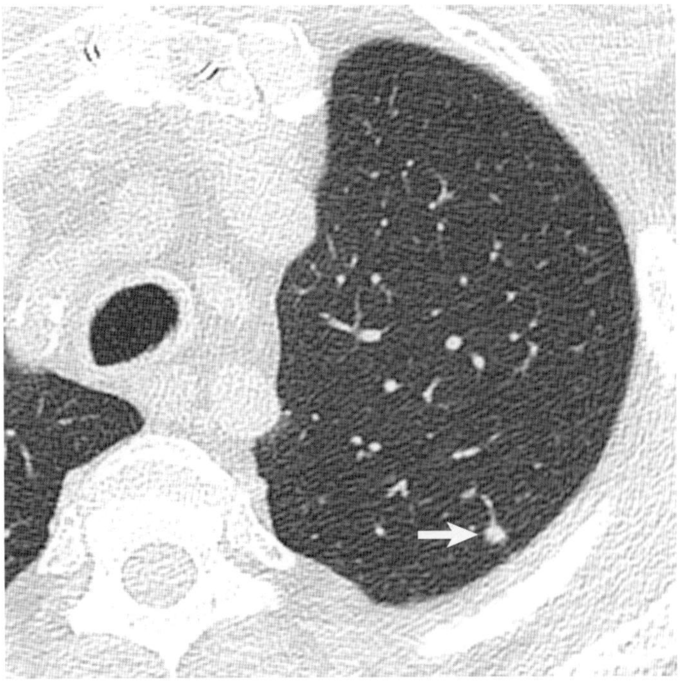

Fig. 16.3 Lung-RADS category 2, less than 6-mm solid pulmonary nodule at baseline CT scan. Axial low-dose computed tomography (LDCT) shows a well-circumscribed round nodule *(arrow)* in the left upper lobe measuring 4 mm. Solid nodules measuring less than 6 mm on the baseline screen are considered a negative screen, and the patient should return for LDCT in 1 year.

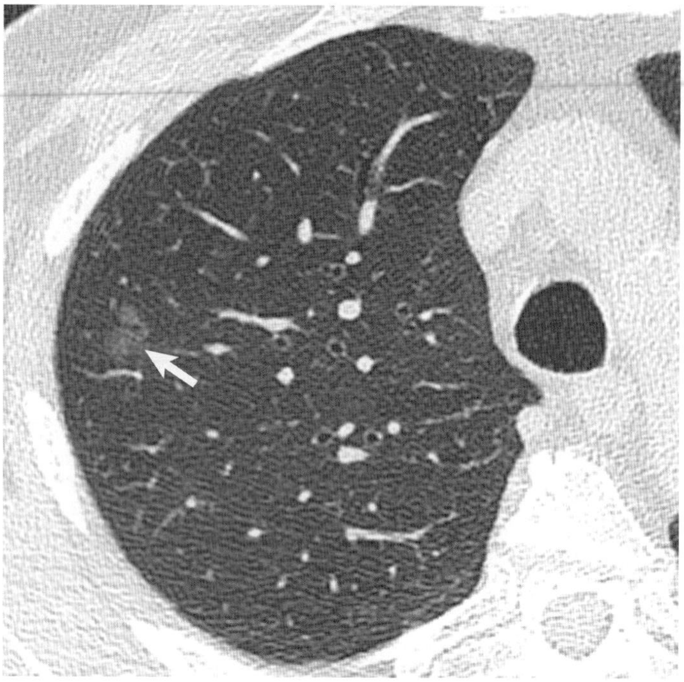

Fig. 16.4 Lung-RADS category 2, less than 20-mm nonsolid nodule (ground-glass nodule) at baseline CT scan. Axial low-dose computed tomography (LDCT) shows a 12-mm right upper lobe ground-glass nodule *(arrow)*. Ground-glass nodules measuring less than 20 mm or slowly growing ground-glass nodules measuring >20 mm are considered a negative screen, and the patient should return for LDCT in 1 year.

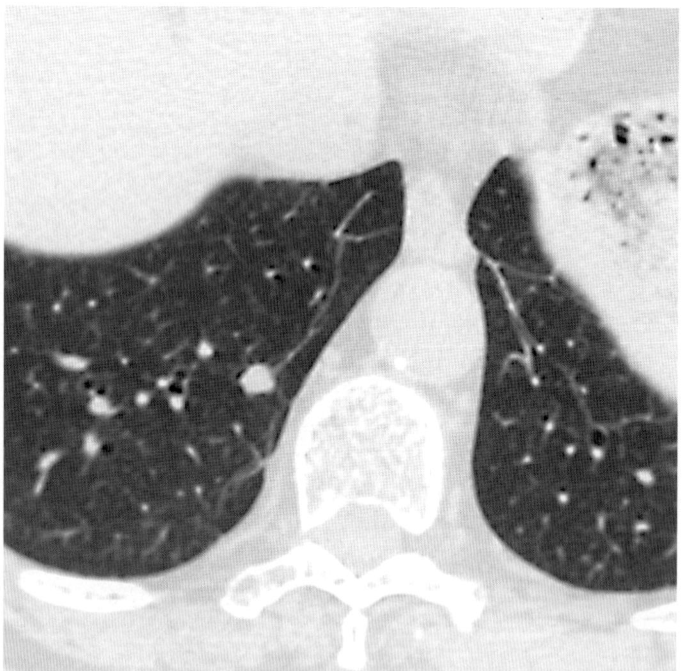

Fig. 16.5 Lung-RADS category 3, solid nodule ≥6 mm and <8 mm at baseline CT scan. Axial low-dose computed tomography (LDCT) shows a 7-mm right lower lobe pulmonary nodule. Solid nodules measuring ≥6 mm and <8 mm are considered a positive screen, and the patient should return for diagnostic CT scan in 6 months that can be performed with low-dose technique. *(Reproduced with permission from Walker CM. Lung cancer screening. In: Rosado-de-Christenson ML, Carter BW, eds.* Specialty Imaging: Thoracic Neoplasms, *Philadelphia: Amirsys; 2016.)*

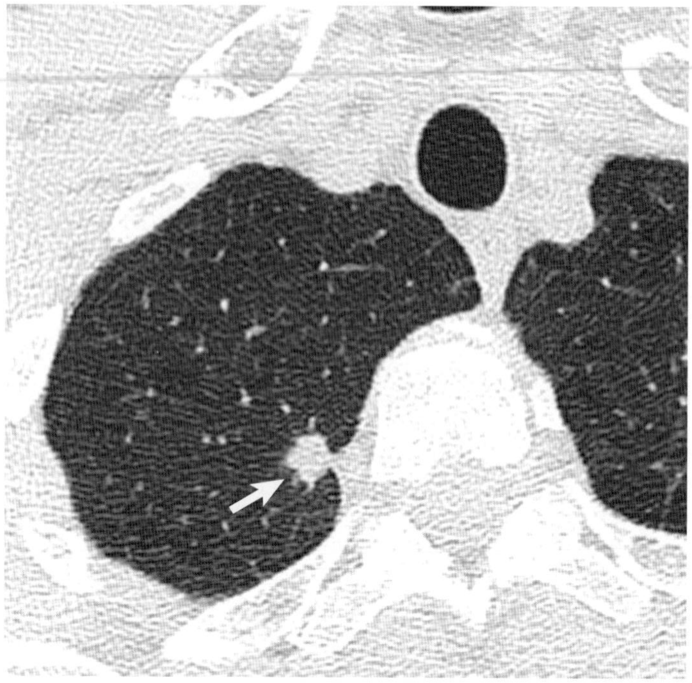

Fig. 16.6 Lung-RADS category 4A, solid nodule ≥8 mm and <15 mm at baseline CT scan. Axial low-dose computed tomography (LDCT) shows a 10-mm right upper lobe pulmonary nodule *(arrow)*. Solid nodules measuring ≥8 mm and <15 mm are considered a positive screen and may be managed with positron emission tomography–CT or a short-term follow-up LDCT scan.

performed with a low dose. Category 3 or 4A nodules that are unchanged on the interval CT scan should be recoded as category 2 and the patient returned to annual screening. Nodules with additional worrisome features (such as spiculation) or imaging findings that increase suspicion for cancer (such as enlarged lymph nodes) can qualify as category 4X (see Fig. 16.8), even if the nodule would have been classified as a category 3 nodule based on size. The overall Lung-RADS screening category is determined by the nodule with the highest individual Lung-RADS score.[24]

Additional modifiers in the Lung-RADS reporting system are categories S (another potentially significant or significant finding; Fig. 16.9) and C (prior personal history of lung cancer).

Lung-RADS criteria distinguish between baseline and subsequent screenings. For baseline screening examinations, the criteria are based on nodule size, as measured by average diameter, and nodule attenuation (solid, part-solid, or nonsolid). For subsequent screenings, the criteria also consider the preexistence and growth of the nodule. For a positive screening result on subsequent examinations, 4 mm is required for new (solid or part-solid) nodules, and preexisting nodules must show growth, defined as an increase in size of greater than 1.5 mm.

Although Lung-RADS provides a structured framework for management of nodules detected on screening, there are situations in which management has not been addressed. Many of these issues surround ground-glass and part-solid nodules. One example would be management of a part-solid nodule with growth of the solid component but no actual increase in overall size, a finding that is worrisome for lung cancer. Another issue is that many ground-glass nodules require comparison to very remote CT scans to document nodule stability or growth. As screening programs become more prevalent, these scenarios will likely

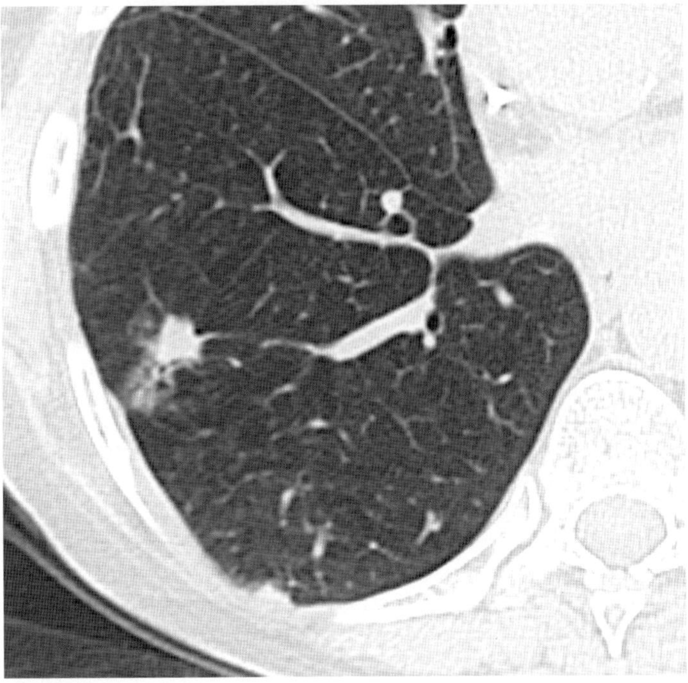

Fig. 16.7 Lung-RADS category 4B, part-solid nodule with solid component measuring ≥8 mm. Axial low-dose computed tomography shows a right lower lobe part-solid nodule with the solid component measuring 10 mm, concerning for primary lung cancer. Part-solid nodules with a solid component measuring ≥8 mm are considered a positive screen and may be managed with contrast-enhanced chest CT, positron emission tomography–CT, and/or tissue sampling. *(Reproduced with permission from Walker CM. Lung cancer screening. In: Rosado-de-Christenson ML, Carter BW, eds.* Specialty Imaging: Thoracic Neoplasms, *Philadelphia: Amirsys; 2016.)*

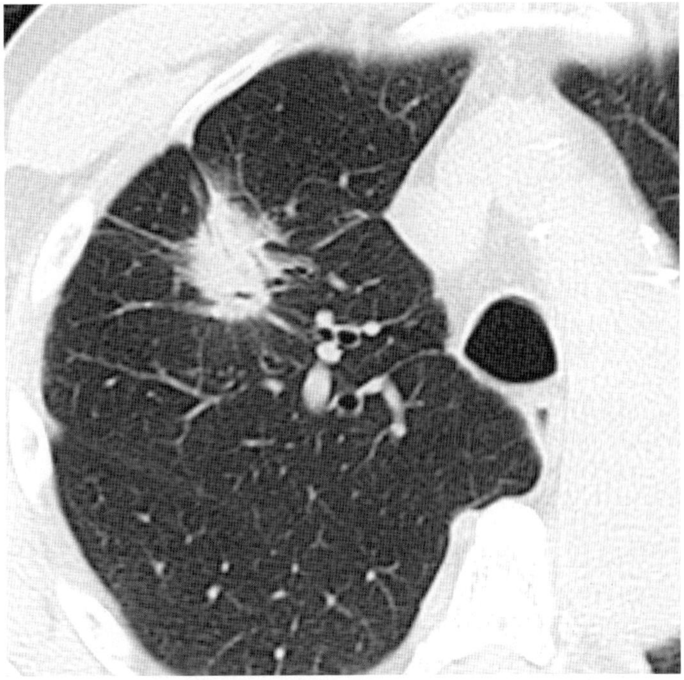

Fig. 16.8 Lung-RADS category 4X, category 3 or 4 nodules with features or imaging findings that strongly suggest lung cancer. Axial low-dose computed tomography shows a spiculated right upper lobe mass, highly concerning for primary lung cancer. Nodules with features strongly suggestive of malignancy (e.g., spiculation, lymph node enlargement, evidence of metastatic disease) are considered a positive screen and should be managed with contrast-enhanced chest CT, positron emission tomography–CT and/or tissue sampling. *(Reproduced with permission from Walker CM. Lung cancer screening. In: Rosado-de-Christenson ML, Carter BW, eds.* Specialty Imaging: Thoracic Neoplasms, *Philadelphia: Amirsys; 2016.)*

become more obvious and may require specific recommendations in future versions of Lung-RADS.

ENRICHING THE SCREENED POPULATION

There are special populations that may yield even greater benefit from lung cancer screening. These subgroups are being identified and evaluated in current studies. The findings from these may assist in future recommendations, especially if future studies suggest that there is no benefit to large-scale lung cancer screening. Of the subjects enrolled in the NLST, those who had additional risk factors, such as a greater cumulative exposure to tobacco smoke, were at the highest risk, and it was this population that experienced the most benefit from screening. A validated multivariate model showed that persons in the highest 60% of risk accounted for 88% of all deaths preventable by screening.[33]

The Pan-Canadian Early Detection of Lung Cancer Study (PanCan) with validation data from the British Columbia Cancer Agency recently examined predictors of nodule malignancy in lung cancer screening participants on first screening CT.[34] Predictors of cancer in the PanCan model included older age, female sex, family history of lung cancer, emphysema, larger nodule size, upper lobe location of the nodule, part-solid nodule type, lower nodule count, and spiculation.[34] These characteristics may be useful in estimating the likelihood that a nodule detected on baseline screening CT is malignant.

Chronic obstructive pulmonary disease (COPD) is an obstructive lung disease common in smokers and it has independently been associated with increased lung cancer risk.[35] The association between COPD and lung cancer was first described in the 1980s by Skillrud and colleagues[36] and Tockman and colleagues.[37] These studies, performed on patients with airflow obstruction, demonstrated a fourfold increase in lung cancer incidence and mortality. Several epidemiologic studies, including lung cancer screening trials, have found a two- to fourfold increase in lung cancer risk in patients with COPD when compared with individuals without airflow obstruction.[35–39,61] Radiographic and clinical evidence of emphysema and chronic bronchitis may be valuable in selecting patients to participate in future lung cancer screening programs.

COMPUTER-AIDED DETECTION ASSESSMENT OF NODULES

Computer-aided detection (CAD) and evaluation of nodules shows promise in assisting with nodule assessment on screening studies. Li and colleagues[40] demonstrated that the use of more than 50 morphologic nodule features improved radiologist discrimination of malignant nodules. Other studies have shown that CAD volumetry results in improved prediction of nodule malignancy.[41,42] The use of nodule volumetric assessment is limited by nodule size and location. Nodules abutting other surfaces, such as the pleura or vasculature, are difficult to assess. Nodule mass is another concept that has been proposed to help identify malignant pulmonary nodules. Nodule mass is a combination of the nodule volume and the nodule attenuation and is most

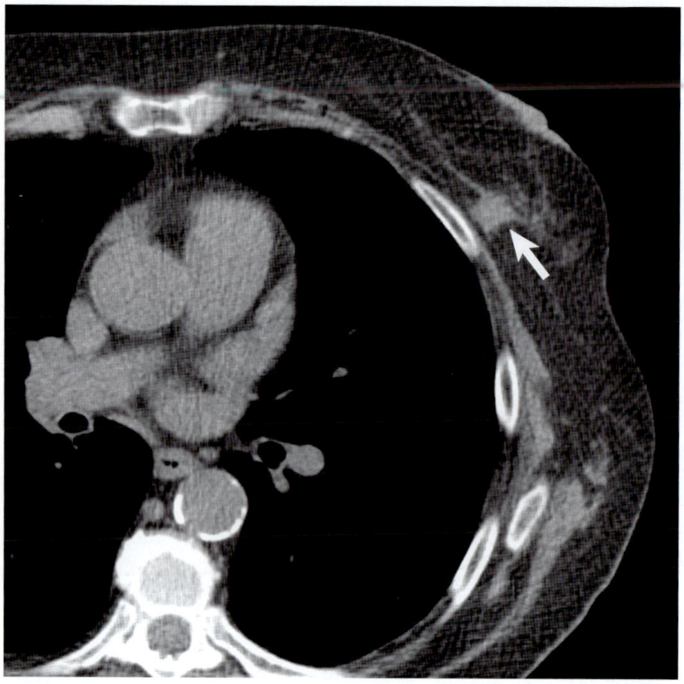

Fig. 16.9 Lung-RADS modifier S, breast cancer. Axial low-dose computed tomography shows a spiculated 12-mm mass in the subareolar location of the left breast concerning for breast cancer *(arrow)*. This requires diagnostic mammography and potentially ultrasound for further evaluation. Clinically significant or potentially clinically significant findings, such as breast masses, thyroid nodules >15 mm, renal masses, and extensive aortic valve leaflet calcifications, should be coded with the modifier S and may require further evaluation. *(Reproduced with permission from Walker CM. Lung cancer screening. In: Rosado-de-Christenson ML, Carter BW, eds.* Specialty Imaging: Thoracic Neoplasms, *Philadelphia: Amirsys; 2016.)*

helpful in identifying ground-glass nodules that are malignant on follow-up examinations when the nodule shows increasing "mass."[43]

Additional tools are being developed that do histogram analysis of nodules to allow discrimination of malignant from benign nodules based on the histogram analysis of the nodule compared with a standardized set of known benign and malignant nodules.[44,45] The advantage of this process is that for nodules with a "malignant" histogram at initial CT, more aggressive interventions could be undertaken regardless of the size of the nodule.

BIOMARKERS

Previous screening studies have identified a target population primarily based on age and pack-years of smoking history. Another novel approach to enriching the population of individuals undergoing lung cancer screening or identifying at-risk patients is through the use of biomarkers. Several studies examine biomarkers in sputum, blood, urine, and exhaled breath to better target the population to be screened for lung cancer.[46–48] The use of complementary biomarkers may become a strategy to help identify an at-risk population. Biomarkers identified in blood have been the most widely studied and show promise as a noninvasive diagnostic tool.[49] A study looked at exhaled breath condensate for the detection of lung cancer[48]; if this is ultimately shown to be effective, it could be incorporated into spirometry. With more effective targeting of the population to be screened, there is the potential to decrease the number of false-positive examinations.

Conclusion

Lung cancer screening using LDCT shows promise; however, results from various screening trials are still contradictory. The NLST trial showed a 20% reduction in lung cancer mortality, but smaller European studies have failed to replicate those results. The results of the NELSON Trial are anticipated soon, and it is hoped that this can provide further clarification regarding the effectiveness of CT screening in lung cancer. In the meantime, lung cancer screening is now a covered examination in the United States for the appropriate population and is currently underway. The registries being compiled with the information on outcomes that will be obtained will provide further evidence regarding the effectiveness of lung cancer screening and will provide data that can be used to improve lung cancer screening.

KEY POINTS

- Lung cancer is the most common fatal malignancy in the United States. It is estimated that 174,000 new cases and 162,000 deaths from lung cancer occurred in the United States in 2016.
- Previous studies using chest radiography as a screening tool showed no mortality difference between the screened and control groups.
- Several studies have shown that CT can detect more cancers and smaller cancers than are visible on the chest radiograph and can detect them at an earlier stage.
- Approximately 80%–90% of cancers detected by CT screening are stage I, which is a considerably higher percentage than the 20%–25% potentially resectable cancers found by conventional methods.
- With effective intervention, the hope is that the earlier detection would lead to decreased lung cancer mortality.
- The main problem with screening is the high number of false-positive examinations resulting from the overall number of nodules detected and the low prevalence of malignancy, even in high-risk patients.
- Most (98%) nodules detected by CT screening are benign (false positives). The workup of these nodules can place a significant burden on health care costs and can decrease the quality of life for the individuals who have an indeterminate nodule.
- For a percentage of indeterminate nodules, surgical biopsy is still necessary to make the diagnosis. Surgical biopsy and resection are associated with morbidity and mortality, albeit relatively low.
- Another limitation of CT screening is that many of the cancers detected are slow growing and may have a mean doubling time of 2 years or more. Because the average life expectancy of a 75-year-old male past smoker is less than 5 years as a result of complications from smoking other than lung cancer, such as chronic obstructive pulmonary disease, vascular diseases, and esophageal carcinoma, the question arises whether these are cancers that the individual would die with instead of from.
- Despite the aforementioned difficulties, the National Lung Screening Trial was able to demonstrate a 20% reduction in lung cancer mortality and a 6.7% reduction in all-cause mortality.
- The US Preventive Services Task Force and Centers for Medicare and Medicaid Services (CMS) recommend lung cancer screening be covered for the appropriate patient groups.
- The CMS requires that certain scanning and reporting protocols are adhered to in the performance of lung cancer screening and that results of lung cancer screening are reported to a registry.
- Further studies are required to prove that CT screening reduces mortality from lung cancer.

SUGGESTED READINGS

MacMahon H, Naidich DP, Goo JM, et al. Guidelines for Management of Incidental Pulmonary Nodules Detected on CT Images: From the Fleischner Society 2017. *Radiology*. 2017;284(1):228–243.

Winer-Muram HT. The solitary pulmonary nodule. *Radiology*. 2006;239: 34–49.

The National Lung Screening Trial Research Team. Reduced lung-cancer mortality with low-dose computed tomographic screening. *N Engl J Med*. 2011;365:395–409.

The full reference list for this chapter is available at ExpertConsult.com.

17 Lung Cancer: Radiologic Manifestations and Diagnosis*

CAROL C. WU | JEFFREY S. KLEIN

Etiology

Lung cancer arises when cells lining the bronchi or peripheral airways undergo neoplastic change in response to an inciting agent or agents. The most common and well-recognized cause of lung cancer is cigarette smoking, which has been unequivocally linked with this disease through case-control studies since the 1950s.[1] A dose-response relationship between cigarette consumption and the development of lung cancer has been well established. Although all forms of lung cancer are associated with cigarette smoking, squamous cell and small cell carcinomas of lung are more closely related to the intensity of smoking than is adenocarcinoma.[2] In addition to the association between active smoking and lung cancer, second-hand smoke exposure is associated with a 20% to 30% increase in the risk of lung cancer among nonsmoking adults.[1]

Although approximately 85% of all cases of lung cancer in North America and Europe can be attributed to cigarette smoking,[3] many additional risk factors have been identified, most of which are environmental or occupational in nature. The most well-recognized occupational exposure associated with lung cancer is asbestos, which itself produces a 7- to 10-fold increase in the risk of lung cancer and has a synergistic effect with cigarette smoke on lung cancer development. Other established exposures associated with an increased risk include silica, radiation (i.e., radon, x-rays, and gamma rays), air pollution, arsenic, cadmium, and chromium. Intrinsic risk factors for the development of lung cancer include the presence of chronic obstructive pulmonary disease (COPD), emphysema, and interstitial fibrosis. In recent years lung cancer susceptibility risk foci have been mapped to various chromosomal regions, such as 15q and 5p, in different ethnic populations in genome-wide association studies.[4–6]

Prevalence and Epidemiology

Lung cancer is the most common non–skin cancer worldwide both in terms of incidence and mortality. It is estimated that globally, in 2012, 1.8 million new cases of lung cancer were diagnosed (12.9% of total cancer incidence), and 1.59 million lung cancer deaths occurred (19.4% of all cancer deaths).[7,8] Lung cancer is responsible for more deaths in the United States than the next three most commonly diagnosed cancers (colon, breast, and prostate) combined.[9] Adenocarcinoma has become the most common subtype of lung cancer both in smokers and nonsmokers.[8]

The incidence and death rates from lung cancer in the United States have declined with increased awareness of hazards associated with smoking and smoking restrictions in public areas. The incidence of lung cancer increases with increasing age.[10] The median age at time of lung cancer diagnosis during the 2008 to 2012 period was 70 years, with a median age at death of 72 years.[10]

There are specific racial, ethnic, geographic, and socioeconomic associations with lung cancer incidence. Central and eastern Europe and eastern Asia have the highest incidence rates of lung cancer in men (50–54 per 100,000), whereas North America and northern Europe have the highest estimated incidence for women (17–34 per 100,000).[8] In the United States, African Americans have higher incidence and mortality rates (68 and 48 per 100,000 in 2012, respectively) compared with Caucasians (54 and 46 per 100,000, respectively). The 5-year survival rate in the United States for 2011 was 18.0%.[10]

Clinical Presentation

ASYMPTOMATIC

It is estimated that 25% of patients with lung cancer are asymptomatic at the time of diagnosis. It is likely that as the indications for the use of computed tomography (CT) in the evaluation of pulmonary and cardiovascular diseases expand, the incidental detection of asymptomatic lung cancers will increase. In particular, with increasing use of low-dose CT to screen for asymptomatic lung cancer, it is likely that more lung cancers will be detected at an asymptomatic point in the natural course of the disease.

SYMPTOMATIC

Because many patients with lung cancer have concomitant chronic obstructive pulmonary disease (COPD), symptoms caused by a developing lung cancer may mimic an exacerbation of COPD or be masked by the chronic cough and shortness of breath commonly associated with this condition. The main symptoms associated with lung cancer depend on the site of origin of the primary tumor and the pattern of spread within the thorax and body. Although there are likely numerous genetic, host immune, and anatomic factors that affect the natural history of lung cancer and determine the presenting symptoms and signs of disease, the clinical presentation of lung cancer is most closely associated with the specific cell type of lung cancer as seen on light microscopy.

Squamous cell carcinoma and small cell carcinoma most often arise from a central (i.e., main, lobar, or segmental) bronchus with early spread to regional hilar and mediastinal lymph nodes. As a result, these tumors most often produce symptoms associated

*The editors and the publisher would like to thank Dr. Anthony Febles for contributing material on this topic to the prior edition of this work. It has served as the foundation for the current chapter.

with central airway involvement, including cough, hemoptysis, shortness of breath, wheezing, and post–obstructive pneumonia or abscess formation. In addition to airway compromise, large central or paramediastinal tumors and lymph node masses can result in symptoms related to local compression or invasion of mediastinal structures, such as hoarseness from medial left upper lobe tumors or aorticopulmonary window lymph node masses invading the left recurrent laryngeal nerve, diaphragmatic dysfunction from phrenic nerve involvement, or dysphagia as a result of esophageal compression or invasion. Locally invasive superior sulcus (Pancoast) tumors can produce Horner syndrome (triad of miosis [constricted pupil], partial ptosis, and hemifacial anhidrosis [loss of sweating]) from sympathetic chain involvement, shoulder pain, and brachial plexopathy. Large medial right upper lobe and paratracheal lymph node masses can produce superior vena cava syndrome. Paracardiac tumors can extend into the heart, most often via the pulmonary vein, or into the pericardium, leading to systemic tumor embolization or pericardial effusion. Peripherally situated tumors can produce chest pain as a result of parietal pleural and chest wall invasion, often with associated pleural effusion. Shortness of breath can result from post–obstructive pneumonitis or atelectasis, lymphangitic spread or tumor in the affected lung or lobe, or malignant pleural effusion. Rarely, a cavitary peripheral tumor, such as a squamous cell carcinoma, can rupture through the visceral pleura and manifest with a spontaneous pneumothorax.

Because approximately 40% to 50% of patients with non–small cell lung cancer and most patients with small cell carcinoma of the lung have metastatic disease at presentation, their clinical symptoms are often manifestations of extrathoracic involvement. Because the most common sites of metastatic lung cancer include the bones, liver, brain, lung, and adrenal glands, common presenting symptoms include headache, seizures, bone pain (often from pathologic fracture), anorexia, weight loss, and rarely adrenal insufficiency.

Of patients with lung cancer, 10% to 15% present with paraneoplastic syndromes.[11] Most paraneoplastic syndromes are associated with small cell carcinoma, with neuromuscular and endocrine syndromes, including Lambert-Eaton syndrome (i.e., muscle weakness that improves with continued contraction of the muscle), syndrome of inappropriate antidiuretic hormone, and Cushing syndrome, the most common. Humoral hypercalcemia of malignancy secondary to lung cancer is most often associated with squamous cell carcinoma and is the result of a parathyroid hormone–related protein secreted by the tumor.[11]

PATHOLOGY

The 2015 World Health Organization (WHO) classification system for lung tumors incorporates recent advances in clinical, radiologic, histologic, and genetic aspects of lung cancer.[12] Exact histopathologic subtyping of lung cancer has become increasingly important in the past decade with the discovery of new therapeutic options that specifically target certain types of lung cancers.

Adenocarcinoma is the most common histologic subtype of lung cancer. Microscopically, adenocarcinoma cells are large and cuboidal, columnar, or polygonal in shape with prominent nucleoli (Fig. 17.1). These malignant tumors usually arise from the cells lining the distal bronchioles and alveoli and are seen grossly as well-circumscribed lobulated solid nodules surrounded by lung, with tumors that vary in size from less than 10 mm in diameter to the size of the entire lung. Scarring often associated with adenocarcinoma produces puckering of adjacent pleural surfaces. Classification of adenocarcinoma has changed significantly based on the 2015 WHO classification (Box 17.1).[12] Invasive adenocarcinomas are further classified based on the predominant growth pattern, such as lepidic, acinar, papillary, solid, or micropapillary. The term *bronchioloalveolar cell carcinoma* is no longer used. Instead, *lepidic pattern* is used to describe neoplastic cell growth along the alveolar septa with no architectural disruption and no evidence of lymphovascular or pleural invasion. Tumors that show a predominant lepidic (i.e., bronchioloalveolar) pattern but do contain invasive components are classified as lepidic adenocarcinoma. The terms *adenocarcinoma in situ* (AIS) and *minimally invasive adenocarcinoma* (MIA) have been introduced to describe small lesions with a pure and predominant lepidic pattern that have a 100% cure rate with resection.[12,13] The pathologic criteria for AIS and MIA are listed, respectively, in Boxes 17.2 and 17.3. Atypical adenomatous hyperplasia (AAH) is considered a precursor or preinvasive lesion in the adenocarcinoma spectrum. Immunocytochemical analysis of lung adenocarcinoma shows positive staining for the presence of thyroid transcription factor-1, a feature that helps to distinguish primary lung adenocarcinoma from metastatic adenocarcinoma of the breast or gastrointestinal tract. Because of the availability of new effective, targeted therapeutic agents, molecular testing for epidermal growth factor receptor mutations and anaplastic lymphoma kinase rearrangements of lung adenocarcinoma is now recommended by various professional societies.[14]

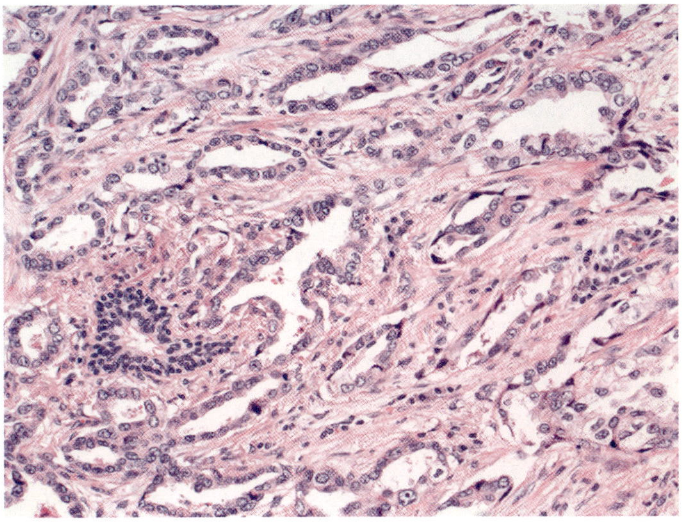

Fig. 17.1 Adenocarcinoma: pathology. Adenocarcinoma characterized by irregularly shaped glands with cytologically malignant cells exhibiting irregular hyperchromatic nuclei in a fibroblastic stroma.

BOX 17.1 2015 WORLD HEALTH ORGANIZATION CLASSIFICATION OF ADENOCARCINOMA[12]

- Lepidic
- Acinar
- Papillary
- Micropapillary
- Solid
- Invasive mucinous
- Colloid
- Fetal
- Enteric
- Minimal invasive
  - Nonmucinous
  - Mucinous
- Preinvasive lesions
  - Atypical adenomatous hyperplasia
  - Adenocarcinoma in situ
    - Nonmucinous
    - Mucinous

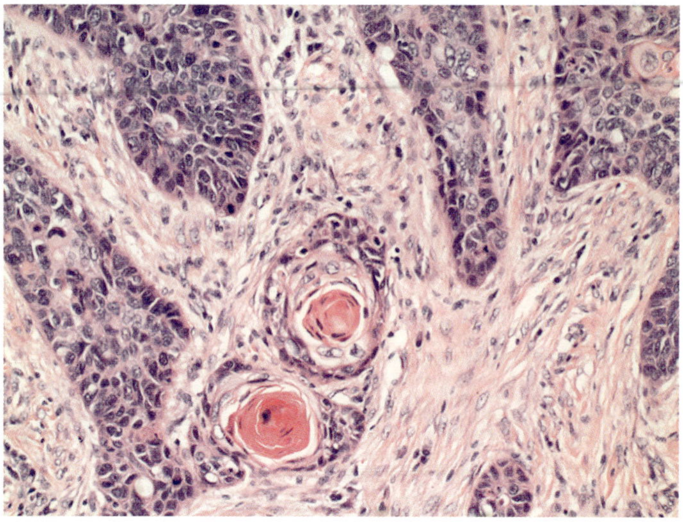

Fig. 17.2 Squamous cell carcinoma: pathology. Squamous cell carcinoma invading fibrous stroma. Squamous cell differentiation is evident by the keratin pearls, and malignancy is indicated by the cytologic atypia with pleomorphic, hyperchromatic nuclei.

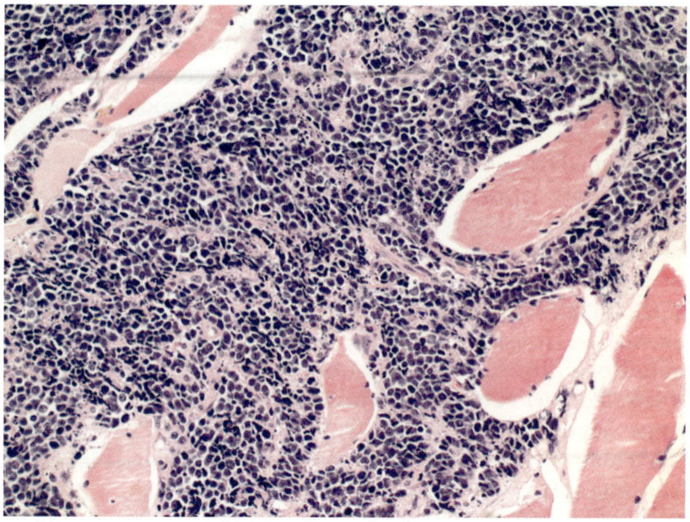

Fig. 17.3 Small cell carcinoma: pathology. Small cell carcinoma seen infiltrating skeletal muscle, characterized by cells that are densely packed, small, with scant cytoplasm, finely granular chromatin, and absence of nucleoli. Nuclear molding is readily identified; also noted are numerous mitotic figures and apoptotic cells.

BOX 17.2 DIAGNOSTIC CRITERIA FOR ADENOCARCINOMA IN SITU[12]

- Solitary tumor ≤3 cm
- Pure lepidic growth
- No stromal, vascular, or pleural invasion
- No pattern of invasive adenocarcinoma (such as acinar, papillary)
- No spread through airspaces
- Cell type mostly nonmucinous
- Nuclear atypia absent or inconspicuous

BOX 17.3 DIAGNOSTIC CRITERIA FOR MINIMALLY INVASIVE ADENOCARCINOMA (MIA)[12]

- Solitary tumor ≤3 cm
- Predominantly lepidic growth
- ≤0.5-cm invasive component in greatest dimension in any one focus
- Invasive component includes any histologic subtype other than a lepidic pattern (such as acinar, papillary, etc.)
- Tumor cells infiltrating myofibroblastic stroma
- Cell type mostly nonmucinous
- MIA diagnosis excluded if the tumor contains necrosis, spreads through airspaces or if the tumor invades lymphatics, blood vessels, airspaces, or pleura

Squamous cell carcinoma (SCC) is recognized pathologically by the presence of nests of malignant cells with associated keratinization and intercellular bridges (Fig. 17.2). In the absence of clear evidence of keratinization, immunohistochemistry with positive squamous markers, such as p40 or p63, is required to diagnose nonkeratinizing SCC. Based on the updated WHO classification, SCC now consists of keratinizing, nonkeratinizing, and basaloid subtypes.[12] Most of these tumors arise within the segmental or subsegmental bronchi and are generally smaller than other lung cancers at the time of presentation because they produce masses in the central regions of the lung that produce symptoms of obstruction or cough. Macroscopically, these tumors manifest as solid masses, commonly associated with necrosis and hemorrhage; cavitation is seen in one-third of lesions.

Small cell lung carcinoma (SCLC) is the most common form of neuroendocrine tumors of the lung and accounts for approximately 15% to 20% of all lung cancers. Other neuroendocrine tumors include carcinoid tumor (discussed in detail in Chapter 19) and large cell neuroendocrine carcinoma (LCNEC). SCLC has distinct microscopic features that include small size cells with a round shape, large nuclei with granular (i.e., salt-and-pepper) appearance, and scant cytoplasm (Fig. 17.3). Regions of necrosis are common, and mitoses are frequent (>10 mitoses per 2 mm^2).[15] These tumors usually arise centrally, infiltrate the peribronchial tissues, and often are associated with regional lymph node metastases at the time of diagnosis. Immunohistochemistry markers for neuroendocrine tumors include chromogranin, synaptophysin, and CD56. Ki-67 is used to separate the high-grade SCLC and LCNEC from low- and intermediate-grade carcinoid tumors.[15]

LCNEC comprises approximately 3% of lung cancers and clinically behaves in an aggressive manner, with poor prognosis similar to SCLC.[16,17] The cytologic features of large cell size and low nuclear to cytoplasmic ratio are similar to non–small cell lung carcinoma; however, LCNEC has high mitotic rate and demonstrates positivity for one or more neuroendocrine markers on immunohistochemical staining.[15]

LUNG FUNCTION

Pulmonary functional abnormalities are common in patients with lung cancer but are nonspecific because they generally reflect the presence of underlying lung disease. Chronic hypoxemia with compensated respiratory acidosis and expiratory airflow limitation in lung cancer patients are common manifestations of underlying COPD. An acute deterioration in blood oxygen saturation levels should suggest the development of obstructive pneumonitis, a malignant pleural effusion, or complicating pulmonary embolism. Less commonly, restrictive lung disease is seen, particularly in patients with lung cancer complicating idiopathic pulmonary fibrosis. The development of diminished diffusing capacity and decreased lung volumes in a patient with lung cancer in concert with developing interstitial changes on chest radiography or CT should suggest the possibility of lymphangitic carcinomatosis. Rarely, the presence of a centrally obstructing tracheal or main bronchial lesion is suggested by characteristic changes on a flow/volume loop.

Patients with potentially resectable lung cancer should routinely undergo pulmonary function testing, including measurement of forced expiratory volume in 1 second (FEV1) obtained by spirometry and diffusing capacity for carbon monoxide (DLCO). The type and volume of lung to be resected factors into the decision of whether resection can be performed safely in patients with lung functional abnormalities, with more strict functional exclusionary criteria for patients requiring pneumonectomy compared with lobectomy, segmentectomy, or localized wedge resection. Patients being considered for lobectomy who have an FEV1 of less than 1.5 L may require cardiopulmonary exercise testing with measurement of maximal oxygen consumption and quantitative ventilation/perfusion scanning to assess more accurately for perioperative risk of complications before potential curative lung resection.[18] An FEV1 or DLCO less than 40% of predicted and a maximal oxygen consumption less than 15 mL/kg/min are associated with an increased risk of perioperative complications.

Manifestations of the Disease

A familiarity with the spectrum of imaging manifestations of lung cancer should facilitate the timely and accurate diagnosis of the disease, directing the appropriate imaging, surgical, and oncologic evaluation to stage the disease and determine the appropriate management.

RADIOGRAPHY

Solitary Pulmonary Nodule or Mass

Important radiographic features in the evaluation of a solitary pulmonary nodule (SPN) or mass include change in size over time, margins, and the presence of calcification (see Chapter 4). The first step in the evaluation of a radiographically detected SPN is to determine if the nodule was present on prior radiographs. The confirmation of a stable SPN 2 years or longer of duration is strong evidence of benign status. In general, any growth in an SPN or an SPN that was not evident on prior radiographic examinations requires CT for further evaluation. Irregularly marginated lesions, particularly lesions with spiculated borders (Fig. 17.4), are viewed with concern and almost invariably warrant further evaluation, whereas a smooth margin generally indicates a benign lesion. The presence of diffuse, central, laminar, or popcorn calcification signals a benign process, such as granuloma or hamartoma, whereas other types of calcification require further evaluation. Occasionally, the radiographic detection of feeding or draining vessels or a comet tail entering the hilar aspect of a subpleural round lesion is evidence of a benign lesion, specifically an arteriovenous malformation and rounded atelectasis, respectively.

Lobar or Segmental Consolidation or Atelectasis

The detection of lobar opacification with or without volume loss in an adult patient should always be viewed with concern

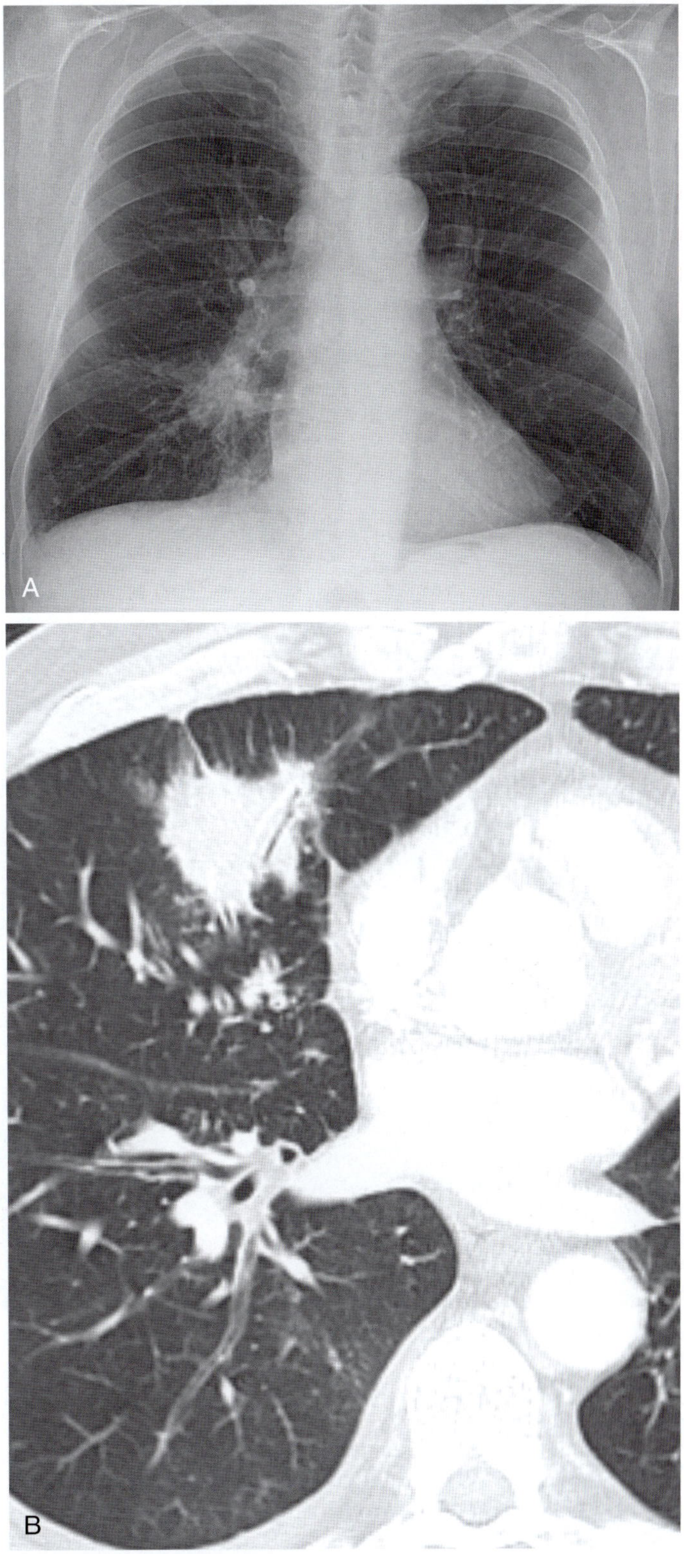

Fig. 17.4 Solitary pulmonary mass. (A) Posteroanterior radiograph shows a solitary mass with spiculated margins in the right infrahilar region. (B) Axial CT image shows a right middle lobe mass with spiculated margins and internal air bronchogram. CT-guided needle biopsy and subsequent resection showed adenocarcinoma.

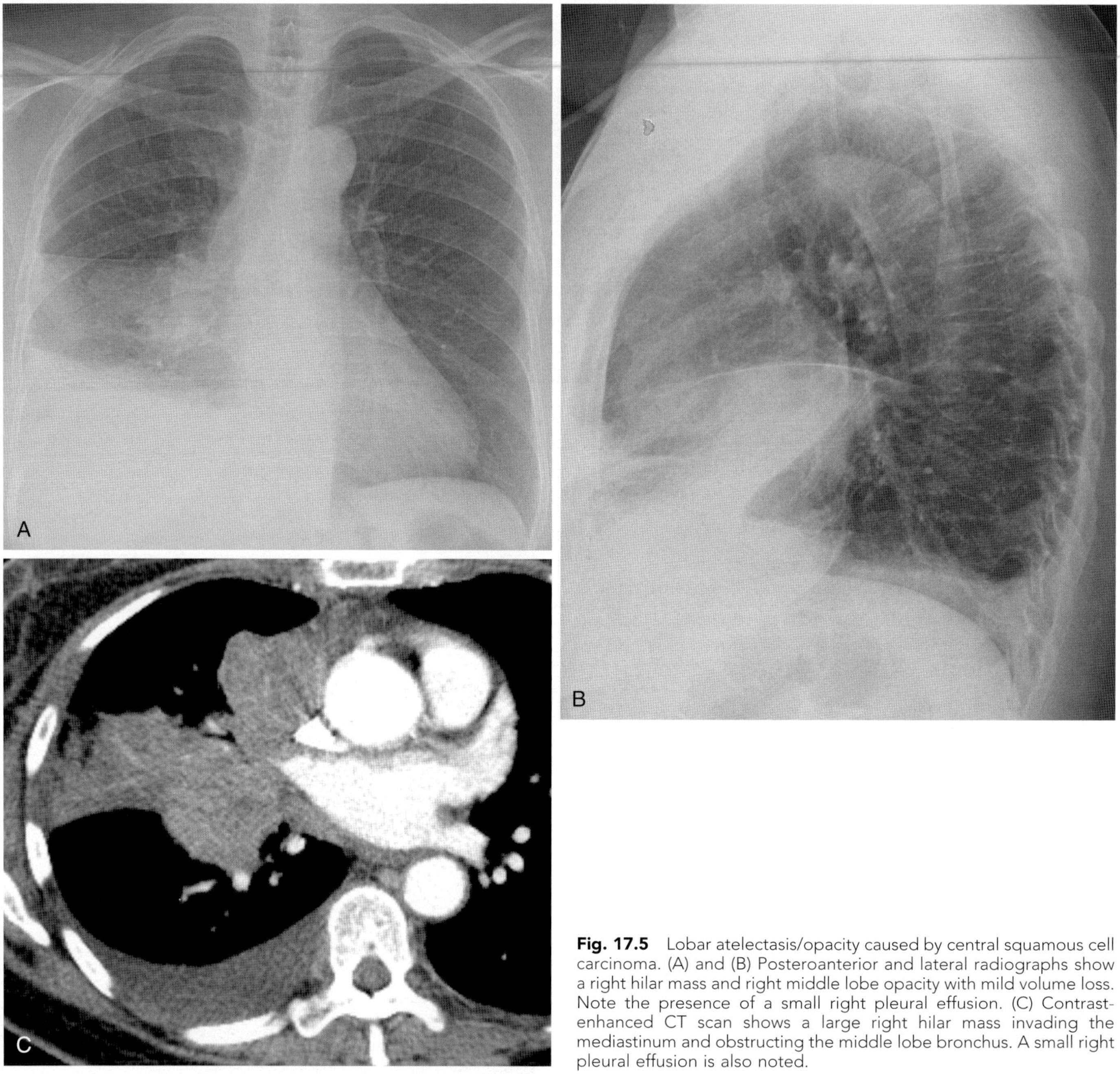

Fig. 17.5 Lobar atelectasis/opacity caused by central squamous cell carcinoma. (A) and (B) Posteroanterior and lateral radiographs show a right hilar mass and right middle lobe opacity with mild volume loss. Note the presence of a small right pleural effusion. (C) Contrast-enhanced CT scan shows a large right hilar mass invading the mediastinum and obstructing the middle lobe bronchus. A small right pleural effusion is also noted.

because pneumonia involving an entire lobe is uncommon in the modern antibiotic era, and lung cancer may manifest in this manner (Fig. 17.5). The mechanism of lobar opacification is usually due to post–obstructive atelectasis (Fig. 17.6) or endogenous lipoid pneumonia distal to a centrally obstructing mass, most typically squamous cell or small cell carcinoma. Rarely, mucinous adenocarcinoma may manifest as segmental or lobar consolidation (Fig. 17.7), often associated with ill-defined nodular opacities. In patients with lobar or segmental opacity, the absence of air bronchograms; a central convexity to the opacified lobe (termed the *S sign of Golden* to signify the contour of the obstructed, atelectatic lobe along with contiguous centrally obstructing mass or regional lymph node involvement, as outlined by adjacent aerated lung); lack of improvement for treated asthma, bronchitis, or pneumonia; and associated hemoptysis or weight loss are clues to the diagnosis and should prompt CT or bronchoscopic evaluation or both.

Hyperlucent Lung

Occasionally, a central tumor may result in partial obstruction of a main or lobar bronchus and hyperlucent lung distal to the mass. Patients who present with hyperlucent lung secondary to lung cancer often have associated cough, hemoptysis, or wheezing owing to the central location of the tumor. This finding is more commonly associated with slow-growing central tumors such as carcinoid tumors, which have intraluminal and extraluminal components.

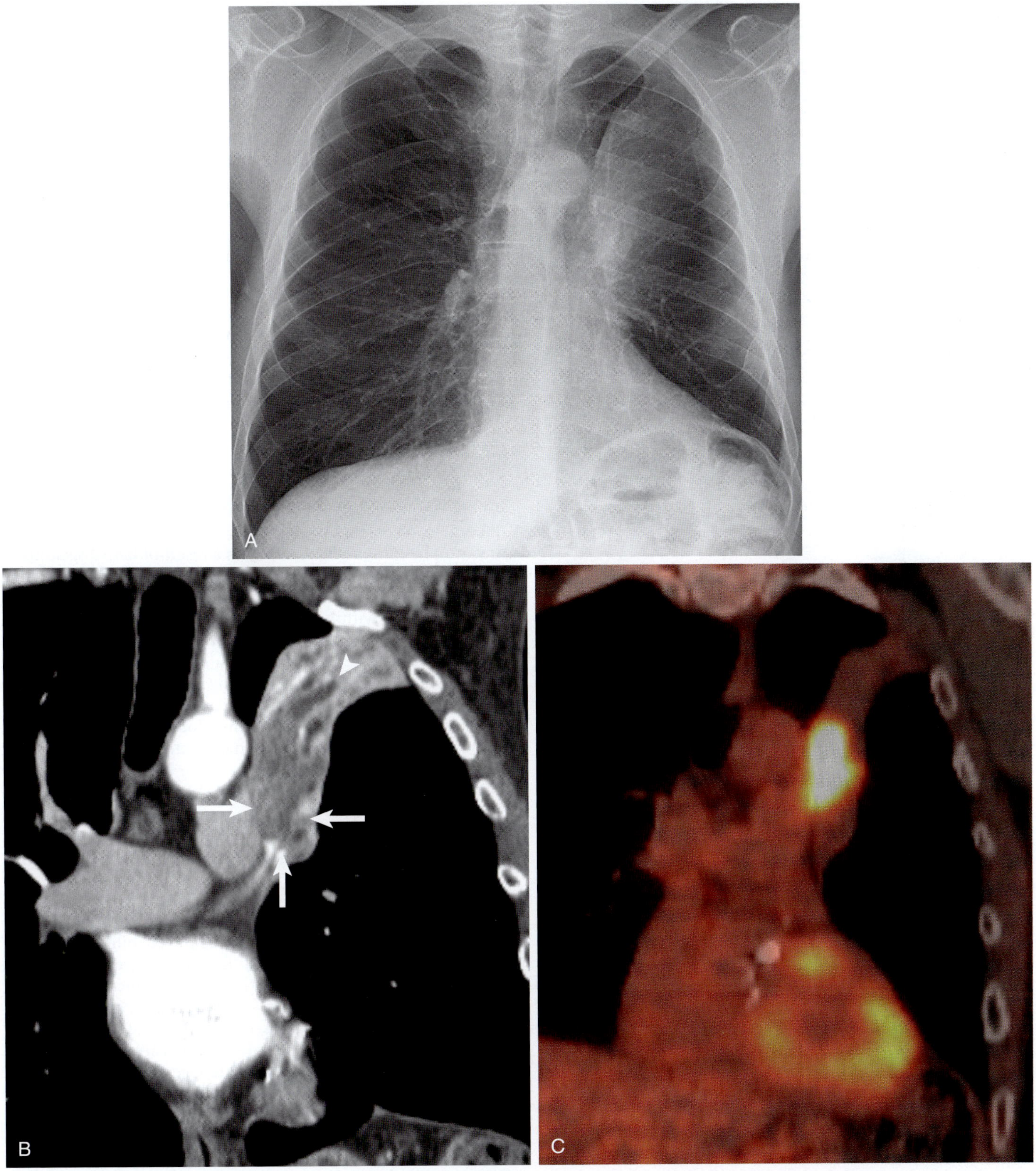

Fig. 17.6 Left upper lobe atelectasis secondary to squamous cell carcinoma. (A) Posteroanterior radiograph shows left upper lobe collapse with relative lucency adjacent to the aortic arch consistent with the Luftsichel sign. (B) Coronal reformatted CT image shows a medial left upper lobe mass *(arrows)* with occlusion of the left upper lobe bronchus and resultant left upper lobe atelectasis. Note the tubular low-attenuation structures *(arrowhead)* within the collapsed lobe because of retained secretion in the distal bronchi. (C) Fused PET-CT image shows marked fluorodeoxyglucose uptake within the mass and minimal uptake in the adjacent atelectatic lung. Bronchoscopy revealed squamous cell carcinoma.

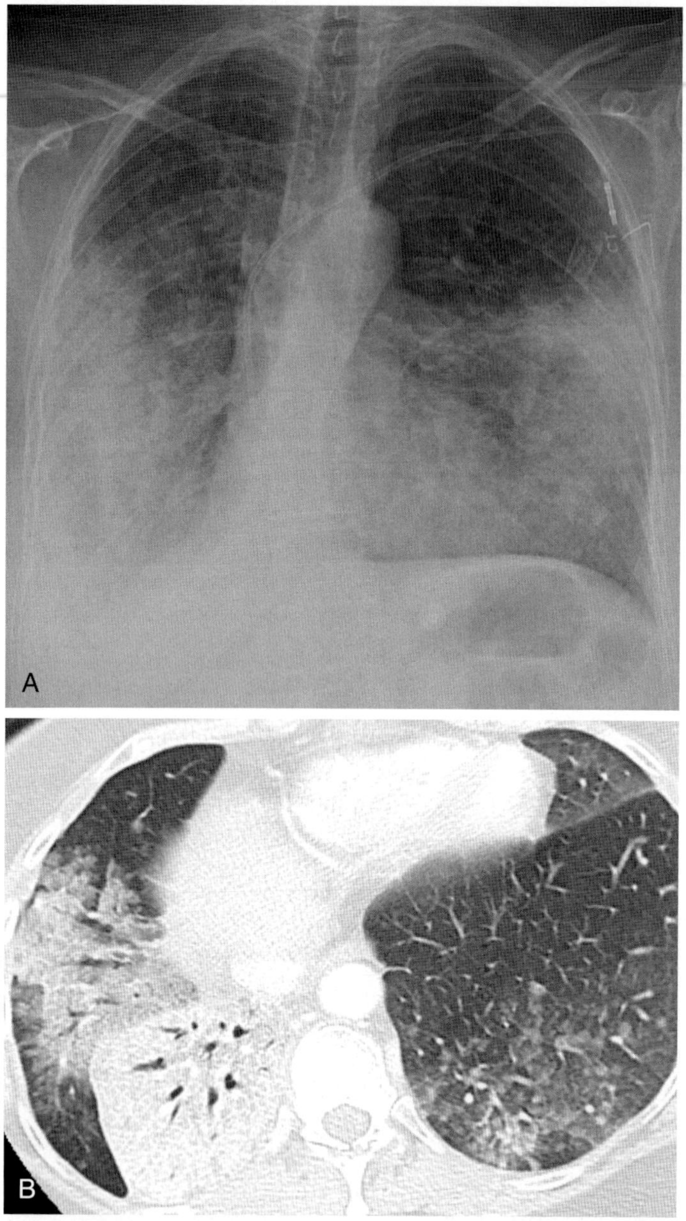

Fig. 17.7 Mucinous adenocarcinoma with multifocal opacities. (A) Posteroanterior radiograph shows bilateral patchy pulmonary opacities. (B) Axial CT image shows right lower lobe consolidation as well as bilateral ground-glass opacities.

Hilar or Mediastinal Mass

The most common cause of a unilateral hilar or middle mediastinal mass in adults is lung cancer, with the mass reflecting central tumor or regional lymph node enlargement (see Fig. 17.5). Squamous cell and small cell carcinoma are the most frequent cell types to produce a mediastinal or hilar mass, although approximately 25% of adenocarcinomas manifest in this manner. These masses are often associated with central airway compromise, producing segmental, lobar, or complete lung atelectasis, or vascular invasion, producing superior vena cava syndrome or lung infarction, the latter resulting from pulmonary arterial or venous invasion by the tumor. Uncommonly, a central lung cancer involves the phrenic nerve, resulting in diaphragmatic paralysis with elevation of the ipsilateral hemidiaphragm, or the recurrent laryngeal nerve, resulting in hoarseness.

Diffuse Interstitial Disease

Rarely, the initial chest radiographic findings in patients with lung cancer are primarily the findings of interstitial lung disease. Diffuse interstitial disease may be seen in patients who present with lung cancer associated with lymphangitic carcinomatosis, which appears as regional or diffuse linear opacities often with associated hilar and mediastinal lymph node enlargement, subpleural edema, and pleural effusions. A less common cause of interstitial disease in lung cancer patients is the presence of underlying chronic interstitial lung disease, most often idiopathic pulmonary fibrosis, which is associated with an increased incidence of lung cancer and can obscure the presence of the underlying malignancy.

Chest Wall and Lung Apex Involvement

Lung cancers that arise peripherally, particularly adenocarcinoma and Pancoast tumors arising in the lung apex (Fig. 17.8), can occur as chest wall masses secondary to local chest wall invasion. Radiographically, these lesions may be difficult to distinguish from primary chest wall lesions, and biopsy is necessary for accurate diagnosis.

Pleural Effusion and Pleural Thickening

Pleural involvement by lung cancer can arise from direct pleural invasion by tumor (Fig. 17.9) or as a result of hematogenous or lymphatic spread to the pleura. Pleural involvement by lung cancer most often results in pleural effusion, which when unilateral and associated with a lung, mediastinal, or hilar mass should suggest the diagnosis. Nodular pleural thickening on chest radiographs with or without associated effusion should suggest malignant pleural involvement by lung cancer, although metastatic adenocarcinoma from extrathoracic malignancy and mesothelioma are additional considerations. Not all pleural effusions in patients with lung cancer reflect malignant pleural involvement because post–obstructive pneumonitis or infectious pneumonia complicating a central lung cancer likewise can produce an exudative effusion.

COMPUTED TOMOGRAPHY

Pulmonary Nodule(s)

CT is the primary imaging modality used to characterize pulmonary nodules. With the widespread availability and use of CT and the use of low-dose CT for lung cancer screening in high-risk individuals, the detection of lung cancer manifesting as small pulmonary nodule(s) with lobulated, spiculated, and ill-defined borders has increased significantly. CT features that are important to analyze include size, density, margins, three-dimensional shape, and growth rate (see Chapters 4 and 16). On CT lung cancer may manifest with pure ground-glass, solid or mixed (both ground-glass and solid) attenuation. AAH and AIS manifest as small pure ground-glass nodules (Fig. 17.10). MIA is usually of ground-glass or mixed attenuation. The soft tissue component of mixed attenuation lesions can represent the invasive component and/or fibrosis and alveolar collapse (Fig. 17.11). The degree of invasion is reported to correlate directly with the size of the soft tissue component on CT. Bubbly internal lucencies termed *pseudocavitation* (Fig. 17.12) or an internal air bronchogram (see Fig. 17.4) may be identified on CT. The solitary nodule is associated with excellent prognosis when it is resected in early-stage disease.

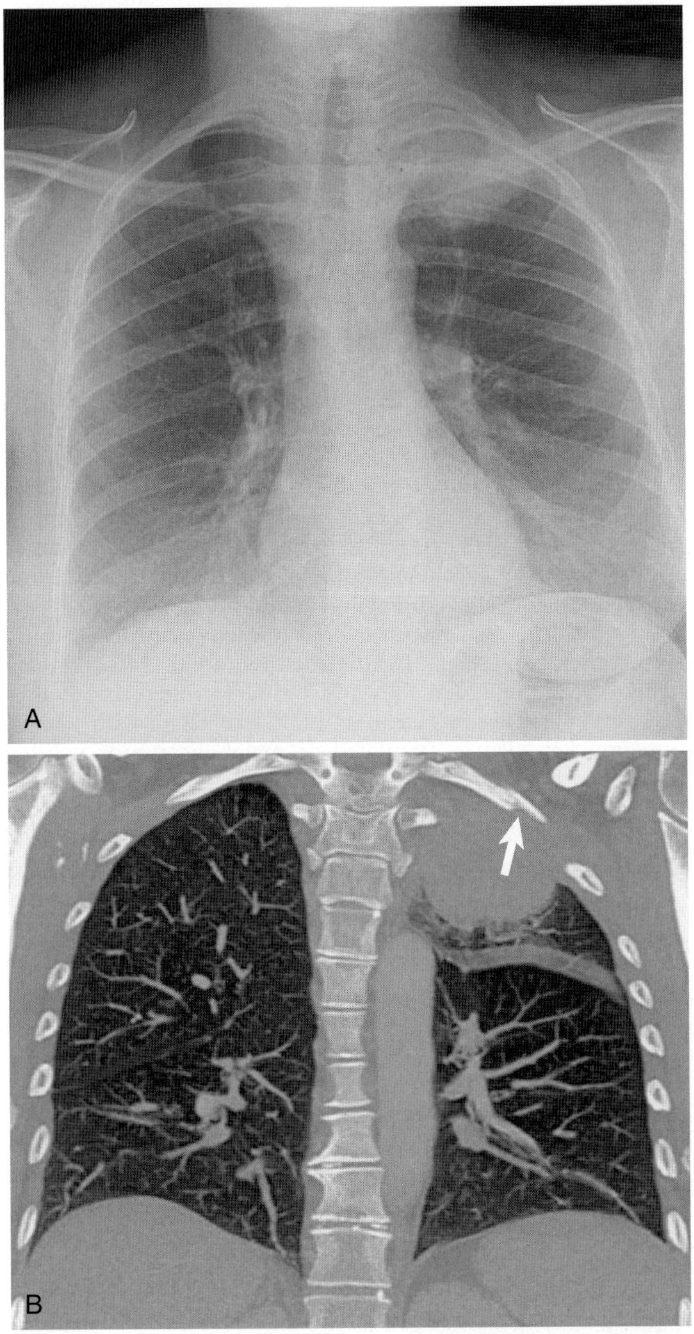

Fig. 17.8 Pancoast tumor. (A) Frontal chest radiograph shows a left apical mass. Note the convex inferior margin. (B) Coronal maximum-intensity projection reconstruction CT image shows a soft tissue mass in the left lung apex with subtle erosion of the undersurface of the left first rib *(arrow)*. Biopsy specimen revealed non–small cell lung carcinoma.

Lobar or Segmental Consolidation or Atelectasis

CT evaluation of patients with lobar or segmental consolidation or lobar atelectasis is done to assess for the presence of a central endobronchial mass, peribronchiolar mass, or adenopathy as an explanation for nonresolving consolidation or to assess a radiographic finding of a hilar or mediastinal mass further before bronchoscopic evaluation. Contrast-enhanced CT typically delineates the low-attenuation central mass as distinct from homogeneous enhancement of post–obstructive atelectasis (see Fig. 17.6) and allows assessment of airway involvement in central lesions. In post–obstructive pneumonia, retained mucus accumulates in and distends the distal airways and can be seen as tubular branching low-attenuation structures within areas of consolidation (see 17.6B). In patients with mucinous adenocarcinoma, the mucoid material produced by the malignant cells fills the bronchi and alveolar spaces, producing opacities that may be nodular (Fig. 17.13) or confluent (see Fig. 17.7). When confluent, this can be seen on contrast-enhanced CT as enhancing pulmonary arteries traversing an area of consolidation. This finding has been termed the *CT angiogram sign* (Fig. 17.14), which can be seen in adenocarcinoma, pneumonia, lymphoma, and other conditions.[19]

Hilar or Mediastinal Disease

The presence of asymmetrically enlarged hilar or mediastinal lymph nodes can be the initial manifestation of lung cancer (see Fig. 17.5), particularly small cell lung cancer (Fig. 17.15). When malignant nodal disease extends beyond the capsule of individual lymph nodes, more conglomerate mediastinal disease develops, which can diffusely infiltrate the mediastinal fat and invade mediastinal structures, particularly the superior vena cava, central airways, esophagus, pulmonary arteries and veins, and left atrium. Central necrosis on contrast-enhanced CT is typically seen in squamous cell carcinoma. De novo calcification is unusual in centrally situated lung cancer and when seen within malignant lymph nodes most often reflects prior granulomatous calcification engulfed by tumor.

Chest Wall and Pleural Involvement

The relationship of peripheral lung cancers to the pleural surface and chest wall is best depicted on CT, although magnetic resonance imaging (MRI) can be valuable in specific situations. Although it is important to determine if a patient with lung cancer has chest wall invasion, this finding alone does not render the patient unresectable; however, it does alter the operative approach to resection. Findings that are suggestive but not specific for pleural or chest wall invasion include a length of contact exceeding 3 cm, obtuse margins between the mass and the adjacent pleural surfaces, and obliteration of the extrapleural fat seen normally in some patients on thin-section CT. The only specific findings of chest wall invasion include visualization of the mass extending through an intercostal space to involve intercostal or subcutaneous tissues or bone destruction (see Fig. 17.8B). In patients with Pancoast tumors, local invasion of the subclavian artery or brachial plexus is well depicted on coronal and sagittal reformatted CT images, although MRI may prove more useful in this assessment.

Because the normal pleura is invisible on CT, pleural invasion can be inferred only when chest wall invasion is evident. The presence of pleural effusion and in particular pleural nodularity in association with a peripherally situated lung cancer suggests pleural involvement but requires cytologic or histologic confirmation (see Fig. 17.9). Rarely, the recognition of spontaneous or iatrogenically introduced air or fluid interposed between a peripheral tumor and the parietal pleura can exclude parietal pleural invasion.

Computed Tomography–Guided Biopsy of Intrathoracic Lesions

CT-guided transthoracic needle biopsy (CT-TNB) of intrathoracic lesions, including subsolid nodules exceeding 10 mm in diameter, has a high diagnostic yield for malignancy, with a sensitivity exceeding 90%.[20] The sensitivity of CT-TNB for subsolid nodules is lower than that reported for solid nodules, but the positive predictive value is high, hence allowing confident diagnosis of malignancy when the result is positive.[21,22] A diagnosis of lung cancer and distinction between small cell and non–small cell lung cancer can be made on light microscopic analysis of cytologic material aspirated from lesions using small-bore 20- to 22-gauge biopsy needles placed using CT or CT-fluoroscopic guidance. Core needle biopsy with coaxial technique is now routinely used to provide tissue samples for immunochemical and molecular testing.[23] Complications of the procedure include pneumothorax in approximately 20% of patients and hemoptysis in less than 5%.[24]

MAGNETIC RESONANCE IMAGING

MRI has a limited role in the initial diagnosis of lung cancer. The sensitivity of MRI for small nodules less than or equal to 8 mm remains inferior to CT,[25,26] although its sensitivity for detection of greater than 8-mm nodules was reported to be 100% in a recent study.[26] However, MRI is useful in the evaluation of superior sulcus (i.e., Pancoast) tumors, where coronal and sagittal MRI allows assessment of local invasion of the subclavian artery and brachial plexus. MRI can also be used in patients with contraindications to iodinated contrast to evaluate for mediastinal or vascular invasion of medially situated tumors.

ULTRASONOGRAPHY

The role of sonography in patients with lung cancer is complementary to that of radiography and CT. In patients with peripherally situated nodules or masses that contact the chest wall, ultrasound-guided needle biopsy can provide material for cytologic or histologic diagnosis. Similarly, pleural effusion and focal areas of pleural thickening associated with lung cancer are well depicted on sonography and can be sampled for diagnostic and staging purposes. In patients with suspected lung cancer and palpable or CT-detected supraclavicular lymphadenopathy, ultrasound-guided biopsy of these nodes can be performed.

Positron Emission Tomography

The utility of positron emission tomography (PET) using the radiopharmaceutical ^{18}F-fluorodeoxyglucose (FDG) in the evaluation of focal lung lesions, including SPNs, is now well established. FDG uptake in focal lesions is measured semiquantitatively by calculating a standardized uptake value (SUV) or subjectively by comparing lesion uptake with background mediastinal activity. When assessing lesions greater than 10 mm in diameter, positive FDG-PET has a sensitivity of 97% and a specificity of 78% in the detection of malignant SPNs (see Fig. 17.6).[27] The low false-negative rate of PET makes this a useful adjunct to CT in excluding malignancy and allows imaging follow-up of non–FDG-avid lesions, particularly in patients with a low to intermediate clinical suspicion of malignancy. In addition to its ability to distinguish benign from malignant SPNs, PET offers prognostic value as SUV and total lesion glycolysis (TLG) correlate with patient outcome.[28–31] TLG is calculated as metabolic tumor volume multiplied by the mean SUV and can be generated by using dedicated PET software.

Although PET has a high negative predictive value for characterizing SPNs as benign, there are malignant lesions that have

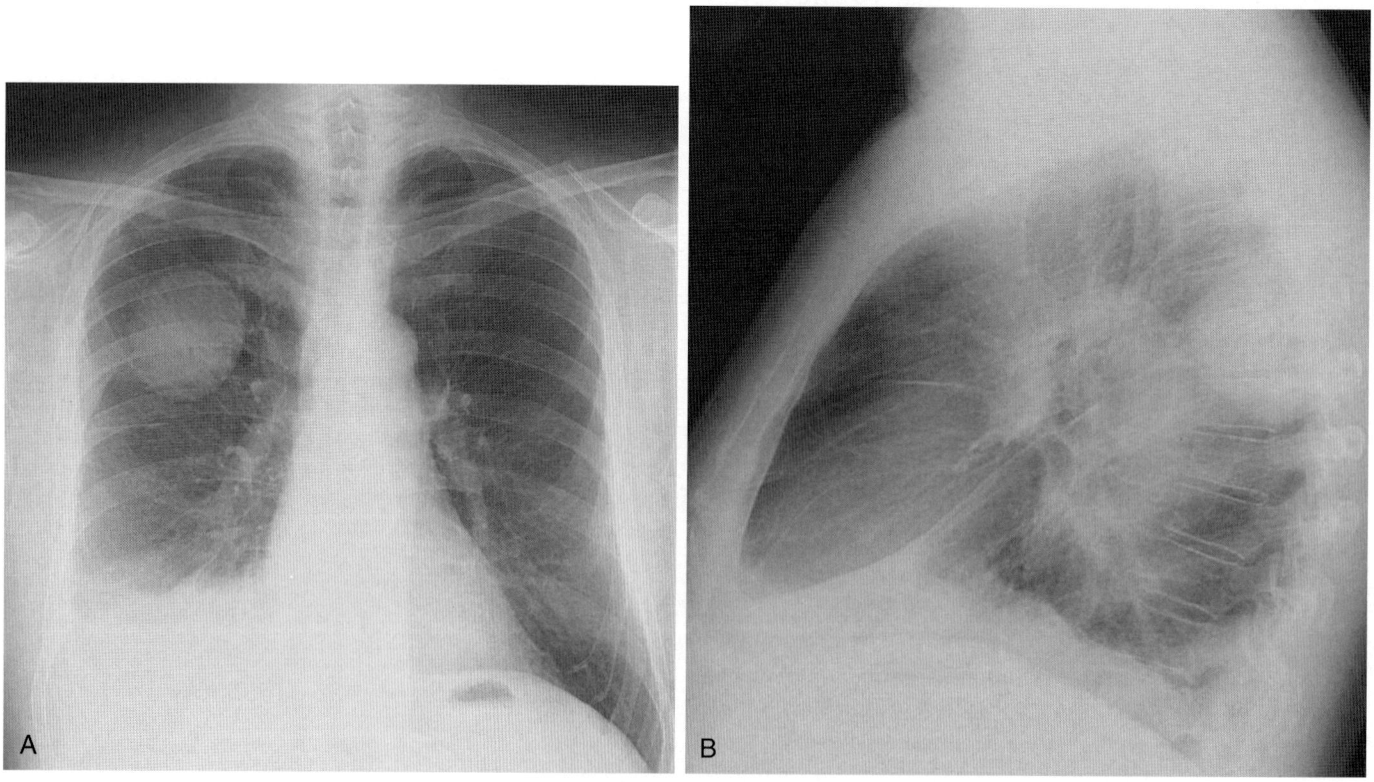

Fig. 17.9 Peripheral lung cancer with pleural invasion. Frontal (A) and lateral (B) chest radiographs show a mass in the superior segment of the right lower lobe with an associated right pleural effusion.

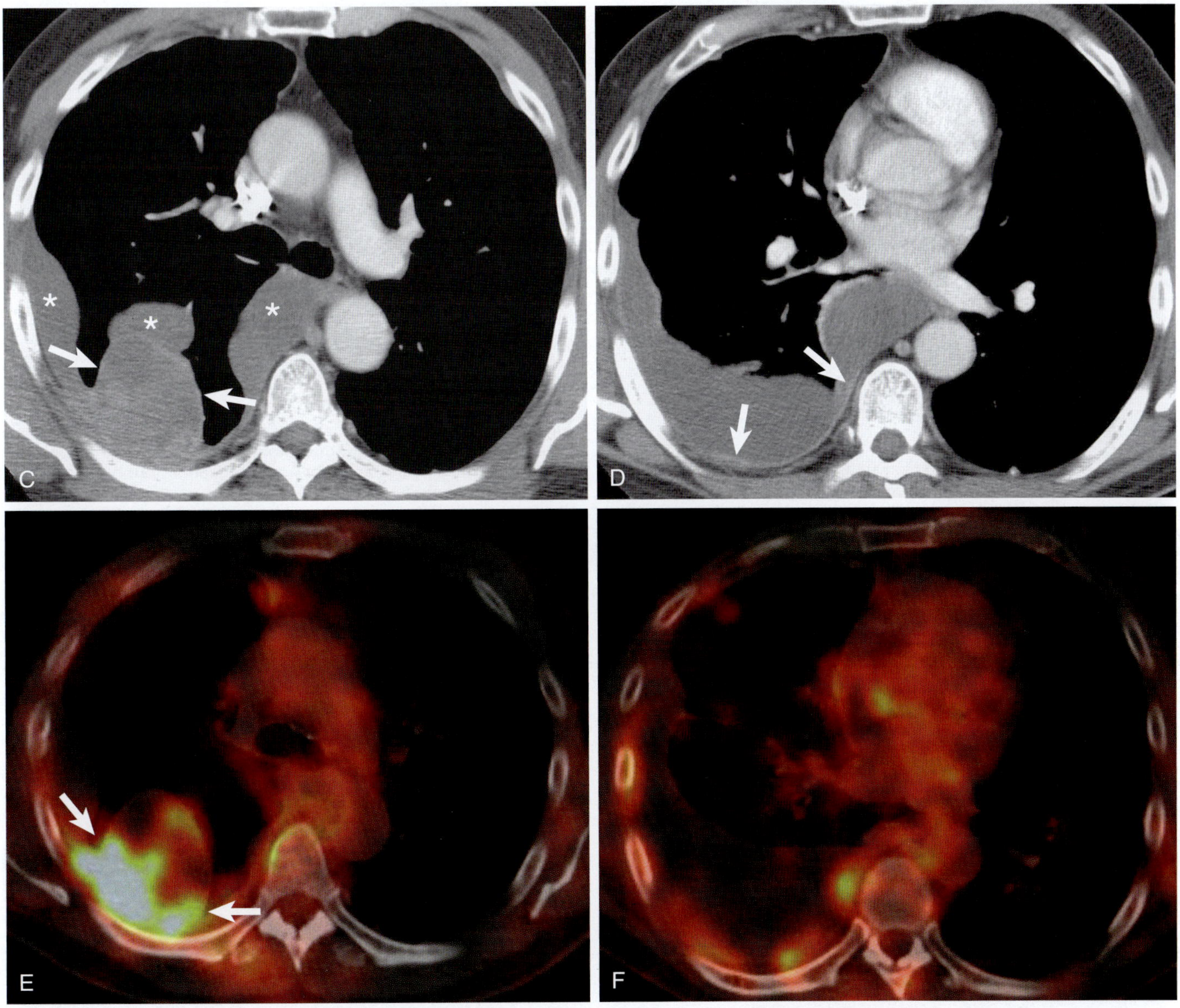

Fig. 17.9, cont'd (C) Contrast-enhanced CT image shows a soft tissue mass *(arrows)* in the superior segment of the right lower lobe with mixed enhancing nodules posteriorly and regions of low attenuation. Note the presence of multiloculated right pleural fluid *(asterisks)*. (D) CT image at the level of the inferior pulmonary veins shows subtle foci of parietal pleural thickening and enhancement *(arrows)* within the more dependent portions of the pleural fluid. (E) Fused PET-CT image at same level as (C) shows increased metabolic activity in the right lower lobe mass *(arrows)*. (F) Fused PET-CT image at approximately the same level as (D) shows multiple foci of increased activity along the pleura corresponding to the findings in (D). Thoracoscopic biopsy specimen revealed non–small cell lung carcinoma with pleural involvement.

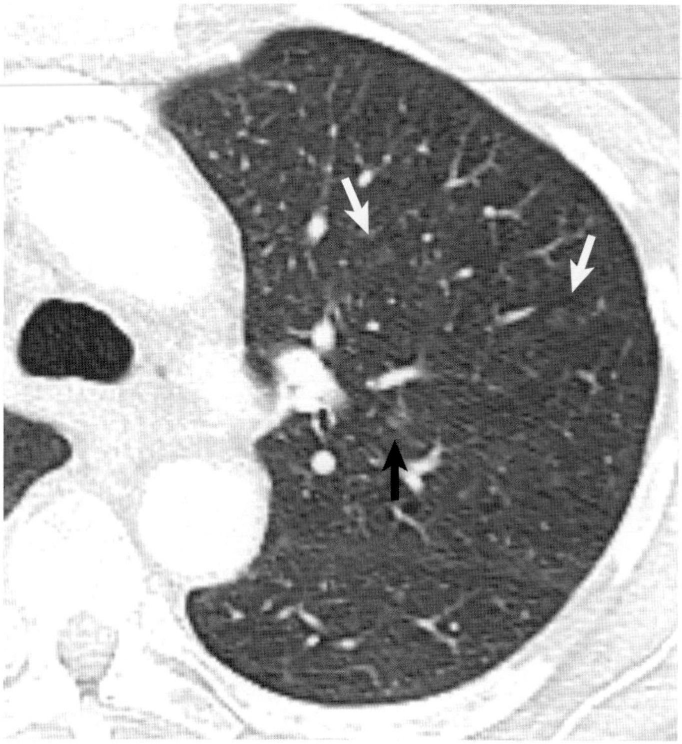

Fig. 17.10 Multifocal atypical adenomatous hyperplasia. Axial CT image shows multiple 4- to 5-mm ground-glass nodules *(arrows)* in the left upper lobe confirmed to represent multifocal atypical adenomatous hyperplasia in the lobectomy specimen (surgery performed for adenocarcinoma, not shown).

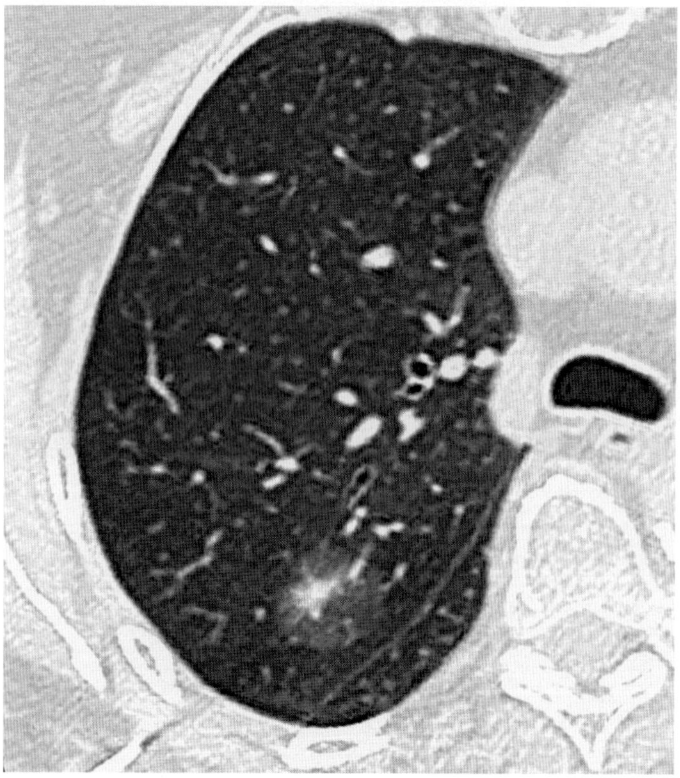

Fig. 17.11 Mixed solid/ground-glass nodule reflecting adenocarcinoma. A mixed-attenuation lesion with central solid component and peripheral ground-glass opacity is evident in the posterior segment of the right upper lobe. Biopsy specimen revealed well-differentiated adenocarcinoma.

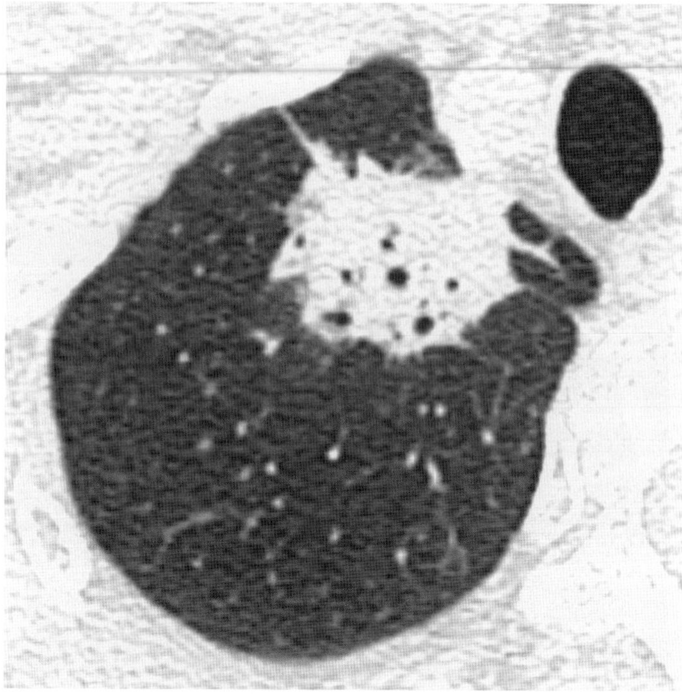

Fig. 17.12 Bubble-like lucencies in adenocarcinoma. Magnified view of right upper lobe from a high-resolution CT scan shows mass containing small round areas of low attenuation (bubble lucencies or pseudocavitation).

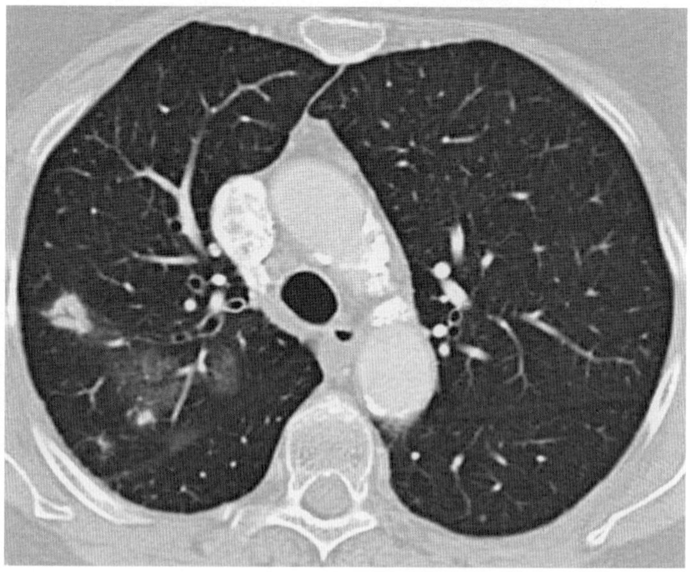

Fig. 17.13 Mucinous adenocarcinoma as nodular airspace opacities. CT scan shows mixed ground-glass and dense nodular opacities in the right upper lobe. Note the presence of an air bronchogram traversing the denser nodule. Right upper lobe resection revealed adenocarcinoma.

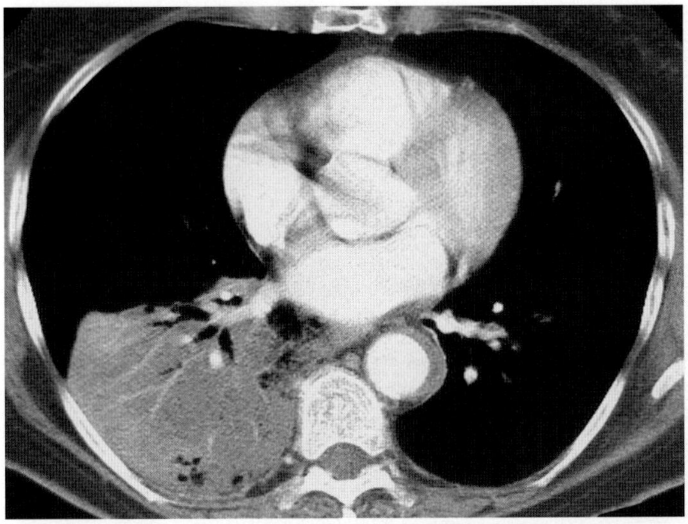

Fig. 17.14 Adenocarcinoma and CT angiogram sign. Contrast-enhanced CT scan shows that some of the areas of right lower lobe consolidation have lower attenuation than the chest wall muscles and that opacified vessels are well seen within the consolidation (CT angiogram sign).

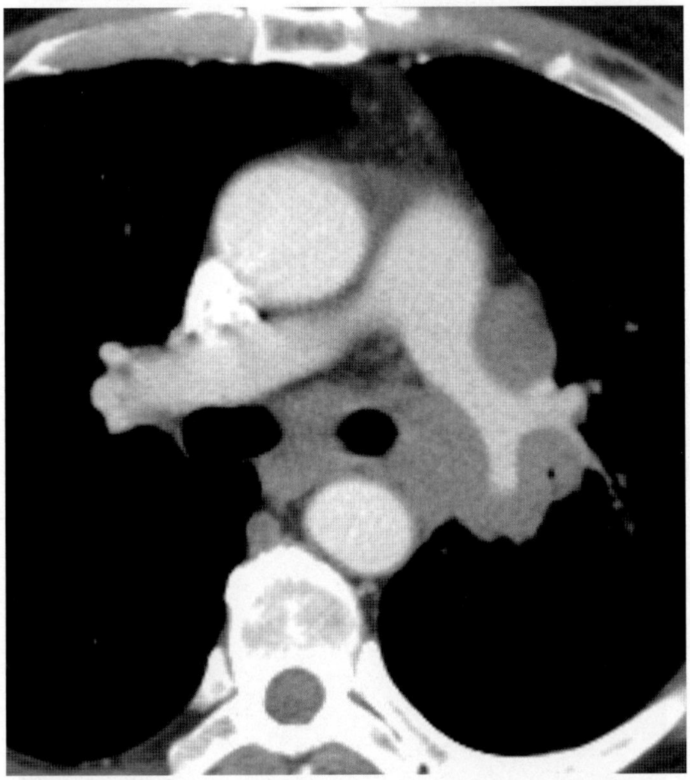

Fig. 17.15 Asymmetric left hilar mass in small cell lung cancer. Contrast-enhanced CT image shows asymmetric left hilar mass and mediastinal lymphadenopathy.

an unacceptably high false-negative rate on PET as a result of their intrinsic low metabolic activity. The most common of these are lesions with little or no solid components, such as AIS, MIA, and well-differentiated adenocarcinoma (Fig. 17.16). A persistent or slowly enlarging subsolid lesion with irregular or lobulated margins or internal cystic lucencies, particularly in a high-risk patient, is suspicious for adenocarcinoma regardless of FDG uptake, and PET is not particularly useful for characterization of the lesion or in detecting metastatic disease.[32,33] Paradoxically, part-solid or ground-glass SPNs with high SUV are more likely to be inflammatory than malignant[34] (Fig. 17.17). Typical carcinoid tumors, with low metabolic activity, also tend to demonstrate little or no uptake on FDG-PET (see Chapter 19).

False-positive PET studies are usually seen in granulomas with active inflammation, foci of organizing pneumonia, and occasionally hamartomas,[35,36] and in these situations needle biopsy or sublobar resection is often necessary for definitive diagnosis.

PET can be useful in assessing central masses when lung cancer is a diagnostic consideration. The absence of uptake in a hilar or mediastinal mass effectively excludes lung cancer as a diagnosis. PET is also helpful in separating the central lung cancer from adjacent post–obstructive atelectasis (Fig. 17.18; see Fig. 17.6). In patients with lung cancer who have nonspecific pleural effusion or thickening on CT, PET can help detect the presence of malignant pleural involvement.[37] The use of PET-CT for nodal staging and the detection of distant metastases in lung cancer is reviewed in Chapter 18.

IMAGING ALGORITHMS

Solitary Pulmonary Nodule

The algorithm for the evaluation of an SPN is dependent on the patient's underlying risk for lung cancer. For SPNs detected on screening low-dose CT of high-risk patients, the American College of Radiology (ACR) Lung CT Screening Reporting and Data System (Lung-RADS) provides an algorithm for classification and further management (see Chapter 16 for further details). For SPNs detected on CT performed outside of screening programs, the recently revised Fleischner Society guidelines provide management recommendations based on a patient's risk for malignancy and nodule features, including size, attenuation, and number.[43] See Chapter 4 for additional details.

Hemoptysis

In a patient with hemoptysis the clinical scenario dictates the imaging evaluation. Bronchoscopy should be considered as the primary technique for the evaluation of massive hemoptysis (>300–400 mL of blood over a 24-h period) because these patients may require prompt endoscopic, surgical, or transcatheter arterial embolization for treatment. In patients with a more insidious onset of hemoptysis, imaging plays a central role in the evaluation, with CT allowing recognition of underlying neoplasm or bronchiectasis as likely causes of hemoptysis. The ACR appropriateness criteria support the use of a CT chest scan with contrast in patients in the following scenarios: (1) massive hemoptysis without cardiopulmonary compromise; (2) persistent/recurrent hemoptysis (<30 mL) *and* age older than 40 years or greater than 30 pack-year smoking history; (3) hemoptysis greater than or equal to 30 mL; and (4) hemoptysis, age older than 40 years, and greater than 30 pack-year smoking history.[44]

Hilar or Mediastinal Mass on Radiography

The first decision when a hilar or mediastinal mass is seen on chest radiography is whether the finding could represent a normal variant, prominent cardiovascular structure, fat, or a true hilar/mediastinal mass. A comparison with prior radiologic studies usually ends the diagnostic workup when a contour abnormality is seen to be unchanged from prior examinations. If a mediastinal or hilar mass is new or associated with obvious clinical or

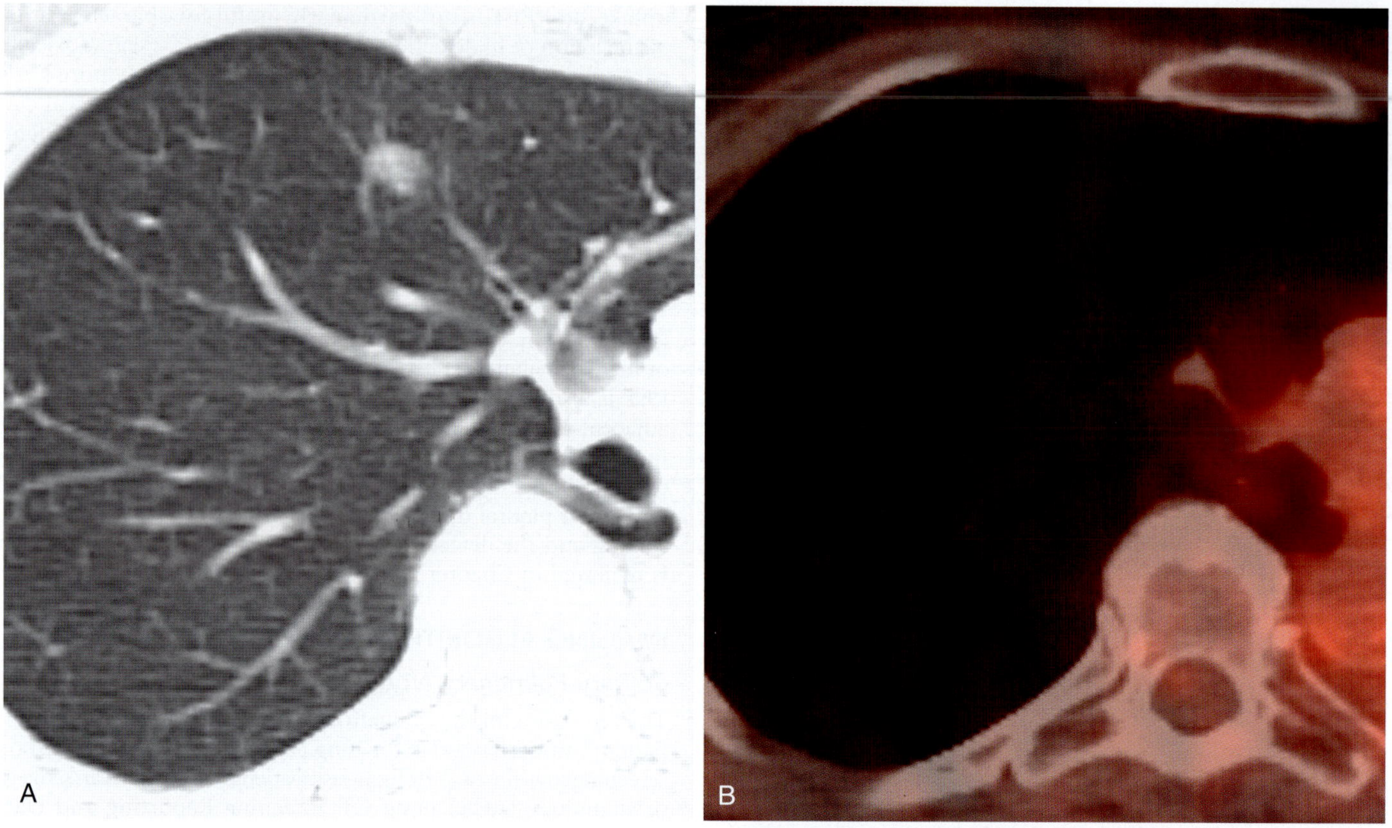

Fig. 17.16 Well-differentiated adenocarcinoma manifesting as a part-solid nodule. (A) Axial CT shows a 1.2-cm right upper lobe enlarging part-solid nodule proven to represent a well-differentiated adenocarcinoma. (B) Corresponding fused PET-CT image shows no significant fluorodeoxyglucose uptake, a common finding in indolent lung cancers.

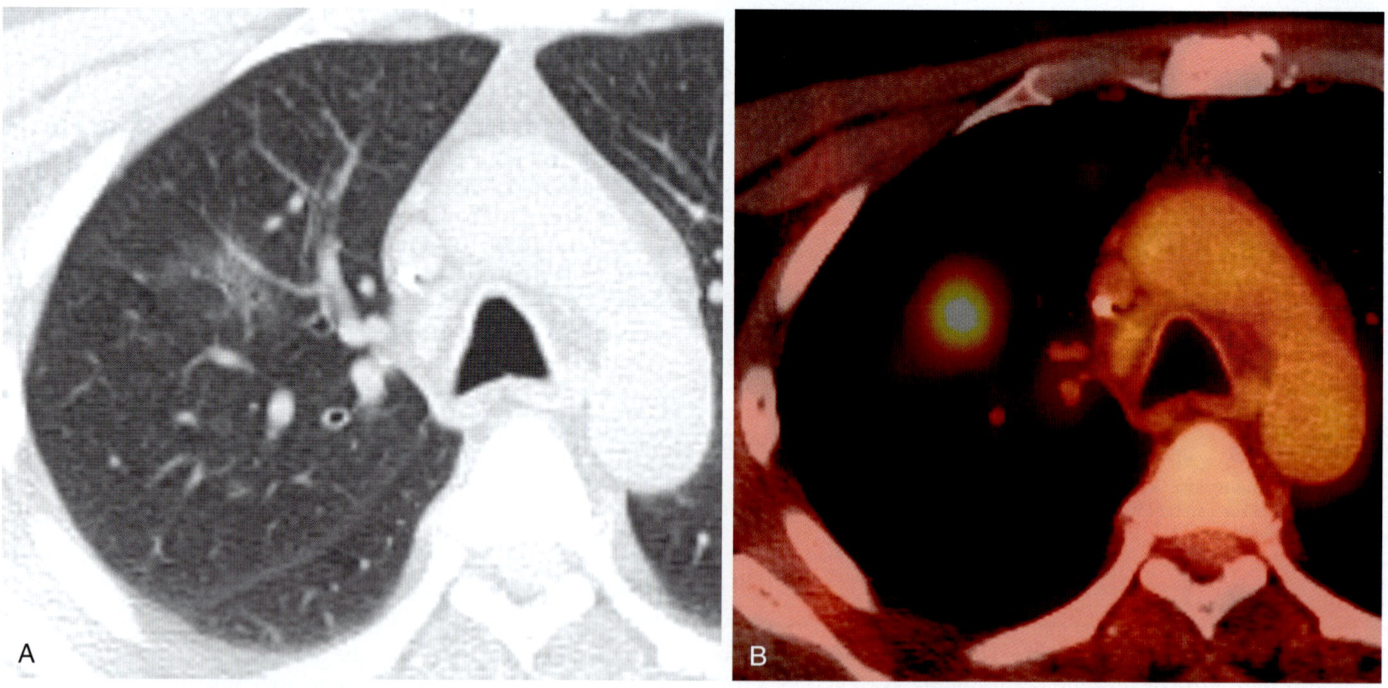

Fig. 17.17 Inflammatory ground-glass opacity with fluorodeoxyglucose (FDG) uptake. (A) Axial CT image demonstrates focal right upper lobe ground-glass opacity that was new since 2 months prior and resolved on subsequent scan, consistent with an infectious or inflammatory process. (B) Corresponding fused PET-CT image shows marked FDG uptake. Marked FDG uptake associated with a ground-glass attenuation lesion usually signals an infectious or inflammatory process instead of malignancy.

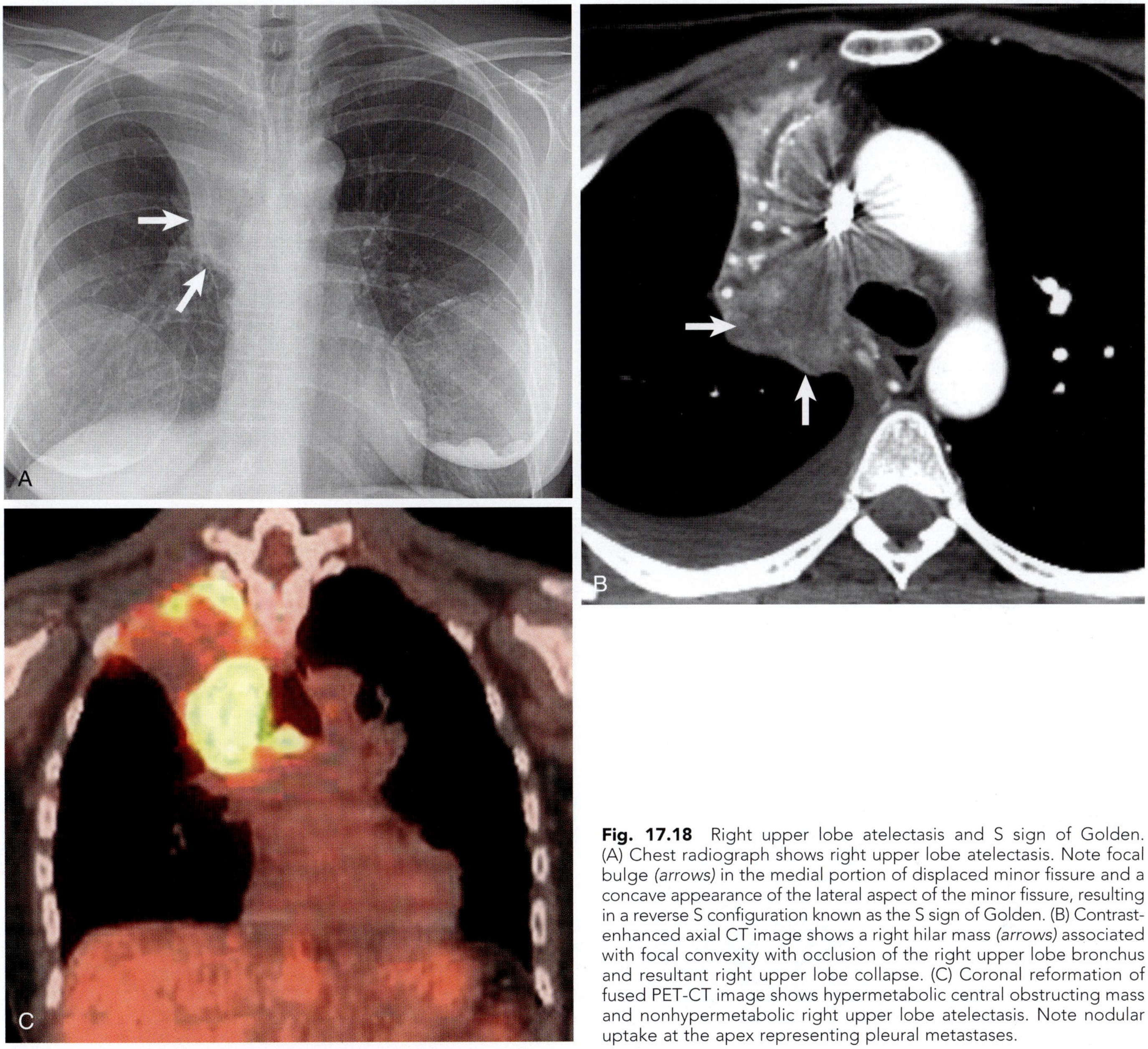

Fig. 17.18 Right upper lobe atelectasis and S sign of Golden. (A) Chest radiograph shows right upper lobe atelectasis. Note focal bulge *(arrows)* in the medial portion of displaced minor fissure and a concave appearance of the lateral aspect of the minor fissure, resulting in a reverse S configuration known as the S sign of Golden. (B) Contrast-enhanced axial CT image shows a right hilar mass *(arrows)* associated with focal convexity with occlusion of the right upper lobe bronchus and resultant right upper lobe collapse. (C) Coronal reformation of fused PET-CT image shows hypermetabolic central obstructing mass and nonhypermetabolic right upper lobe atelectasis. Note nodular uptake at the apex representing pleural metastases.

radiologic evidence of local invasion (i.e., hemoptysis, superior vena cava syndrome, hoarseness owing to left vocal cord paralysis, Horner syndrome), contrast-enhanced CT should be performed for further characterization. For solid lesions the method of cytologic or histologic confirmation of lesions suspected to represent central lung cancer is guided by the clinical and imaging findings.

Lobar Consolidation or Atelectasis

Most patients with lobar or segmental consolidation or lobar atelectasis, in the absence of central mass on radiography, have pneumonia or an exacerbation of asthma or COPD. There are a variety of clinical and imaging factors, however, that may dictate CT or bronchoscopic evaluation of patients presenting with lobar consolidation. These factors include the presence of hemoptysis or bronchorrhea, gradual rather than acute onset of respiratory symptoms, significant weight loss, the detection of a hilar or mediastinal mass or lymph node enlargement on chest radiography, or nonresolving clinical or radiographic abnormalities in a patient after broad-spectrum antibiotic treatment of community-acquired pneumonia.[45]

Peripheral Lesion

The evaluation of a subpleural or pleural lesion detected radiographically is best accomplished with multidetector CT (see Fig. 17.9). Alternatively, if there is suspicion of a loculated fluid collection as the etiology of a peripheral opacity, sonography can be done to determine if the mass is completely anechoic and reflects a pleural effusion. Fat attenuation masses reflect lipomas or hernias and require no further evaluation, whereas soft tissue masses almost invariably require CT-guided or ultrasound-guided biopsy for definitive characterization.

CLASSIC IMAGING FINDINGS

CORONA RADIATA

The spiculated margins of many peripheral lung cancers are produced by the presence of tumor or fibrosis extending radially from the central portion of the tumor. This appearance is termed the *corona radiata* (Fig. 17.19) and when identified in association with an SPN is highly suggestive of primary malignancy.

S SIGN OF GOLDEN

The S sign of Golden describes the outline of the combined atelectatic lobe, which is concave, in association with a centrally obstructing mass that has a convex margin (see Fig. 17.18). This sign is most often due to squamous cell or small cell carcinoma because these types of lung cancers tend to produce hilar masses as they arise within lobar bronchi.

LUFTSICHEL SIGN IN LEFT UPPER LOBE ATELECTASIS

In patients with left upper lobe atelectasis of any cause, but particularly secondary to lung cancer, the atelectatic lobe creates a subtle increase in density as it collapses anteriorly. In some cases the superior segment of the left lower lobe becomes hyperinflated as a compensatory mechanism and expands to outline the aortic arch, producing a crescent of air or Luftsichel sign on frontal radiography (see Fig. 17.6).

PANCOAST TUMOR

Lung cancer that arises in the apical region of the lung has been termed a *Pancoast* or *superior sulcus tumor* (see Fig. 17.8). Malignancy should be suspected when frontal radiographs reveal an asymmetric apical opacity, particularly if the inferior margin is convex, and there is associated rib or vertebral body destruction.

BUBBLE OR CYSTIC LUCENCIES

In patients with adenocarcinomas that pathologically show a component of lepidic growth along alveolar walls, patent bronchi or airspaces within the lesion produce bubble or cystic lucencies that can be appreciated on thin-section CT scans (see Fig. 17.12). In a patient with a persistent lesion larger than 10 mm in diameter and containing these lucencies, the incidence of adenocarcinoma is greater than 25%.[38]

MIXED ATTENUATION (SUBSOLID) LUNG NODULES

The CT findings of SPNs detected on low-dose CT and multidetector CT for lung cancer screening in high-risk patients have shown a relatively high incidence of malignancy in lesions with mixed attenuation (i.e., containing solid and ground-glass attenuation) (see Fig. 17.11).

COMPUTED TOMOGRAPHY ANGIOGRAM SIGN

The CT angiogram sign describes the CT appearance of consolidation in which the contrast-enhanced pulmonary arteries appear as high-attenuation branching structures relative to low-attenuation material filling the surrounding airspaces (see Fig. 17.14). Although initially thought to be relatively specific for mucinous adenocarcinoma, this sign has been reported in association with a variety of other malignant and several nonmalignant conditions, including lymphoma, lipoid pneumonia, infectious pneumonia, and pulmonary edema.[19]

CYST OR BULLA WALL THICKENING

There is increased recognition of the association of lung cancer with cystic airspaces,[39–41] which occasionally is a cause of missed lung cancer.[42] Increased nodularity (Fig. 17.20) or thickness of the cyst or bulla wall, regardless of FDG uptake, should prompt consideration of lung cancer, leading to follow-up imaging or tissue sampling. Other factors such as lesion location in the periphery of the upper lobes and presence of imaging findings such as emphysema, additional cystic lesions or ground-glass nodules, and lymphadenopathy, as well as prior lung cancer should also increase suspicion for lung cancer[39] and prompt additional imaging follow-up.

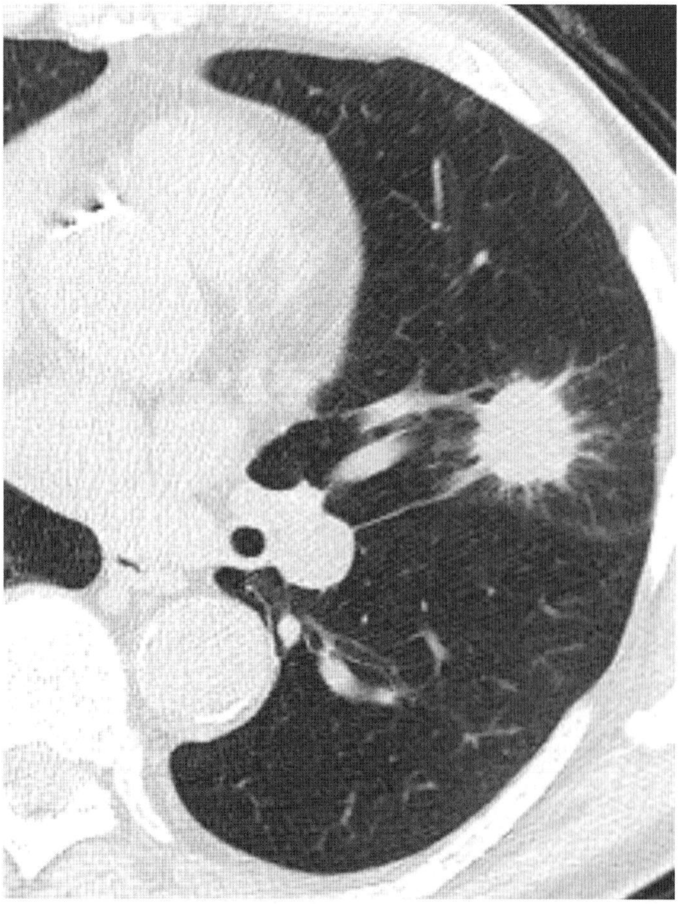

Fig. 17.19 Corona radiata in malignant solitary pulmonary nodule. Axial CT image shows a spiculated lingular nodule. Biopsy specimen showed adenocarcinoma.

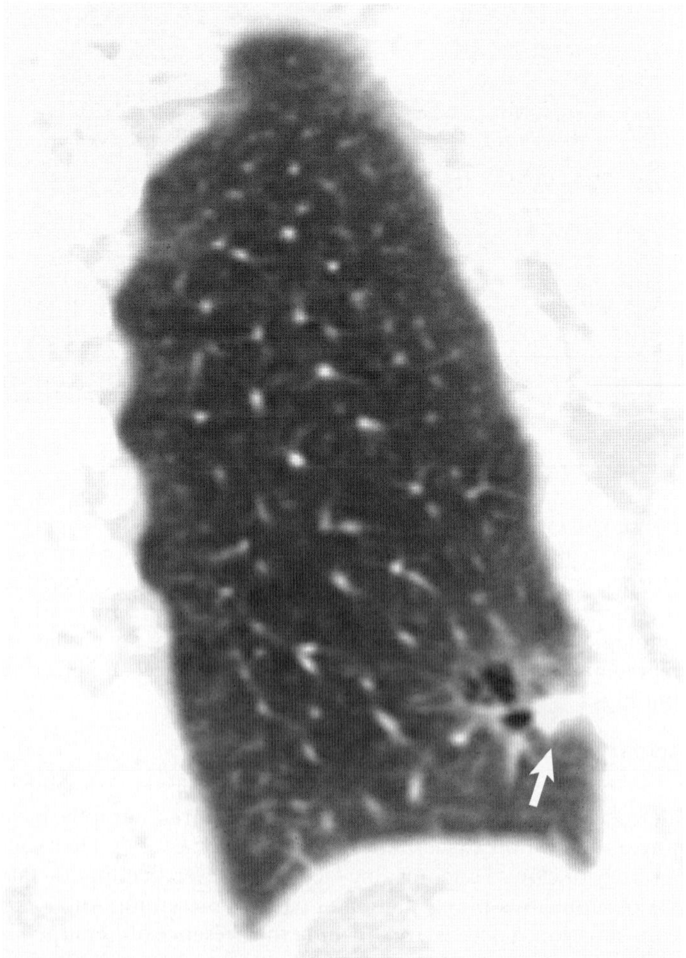

Fig. 17.20 Adenocarcinoma with cystic airspace. Coronal CT image shows an irregular cystic lesion with a mural nodule *(arrow)*. Biopsy showed adenocarcinoma.

Differential Diagnosis

CLINICAL PRESENTATION

Hemoptysis

Although the presence of hemoptysis in a cigarette smoker should prompt concern for an endobronchial mass secondary to lung cancer as the source of bleeding, most patients with hemoptysis have inflammatory airways disease, such as bronchitis or bronchiectasis. Additional causes of hemoptysis include alveolar hemorrhage syndromes, such as Goodpasture syndrome and granulomatosis with polyangiitis; neoplasms other than lung cancer, including carcinoid tumors, pulmonary embolism, pulmonary artery aneurysm or pseudoaneurysm, pulmonary arteriovenous malformation, mycetomas, tuberculosis, and rarely aortobronchial fistula complicating aortic aneurysm.

Cough

Cough is clinically divided into acute and chronic forms, with cough persisting beyond 4 to 8 weeks generally categorized as chronic. The differential diagnosis of chronic cough is broad and in addition to lung cancer includes asthma, gastroesophageal reflux, chronic bronchitis, bronchiectasis, drug-induced side effect, and postnasal drip syndrome. Although most patients with lung cancer have cough during the course of their disease, chronic cough is an uncommon presenting feature of lung cancer because most cancers develop peripherally, where cough receptors are sparse. Nevertheless, a new or worsening cough in a patient with risk factors for lung cancer is best evaluated further with CT to exclude a central mass lesion.

Dyspnea

As with cough, dyspnea is a common manifestation of a variety of infectious, neuromuscular, cardiac, respiratory, autoimmune, and renal diseases, among others. Complicating matters is that patients with lung cancer frequently have COPD and experience dyspnea as a result of their underlying condition. Dyspnea resulting from lung cancer is highly unlikely in the face of a normal chest radiograph, but complications associated with lung cancer that can manifest primarily as dyspnea include malignant pleural disease, pulmonary embolism, lymphangitic spread of tumor, central airway compromise with or without post-obstructive pneumonitis or atelectasis, and rarely progressive consolidation in mucinous adenocarcinoma.

Constitutional and Paraneoplastic Symptoms (Fever, Weakness, Weight Loss)

Most patients with lung cancer have constitutional symptoms, including weight loss, anorexia, and weakness. Many somatic and psychiatric conditions can produce similar symptoms, with extrathoracic malignancies, such as lymphoma, colon cancer, and hematologic malignancies, among the most common. As discussed in the section on clinical presentation, 10% to 15% of lung cancer patients, particularly patients with small cell carcinoma, present with a paraneoplastic syndrome. In patients with muscle weakness, Lambert-Eaton syndrome must be distinguished from myasthenia gravis. Adults with dermatomyositis have a significantly higher incidence of lung cancer and extrathoracic malignancy. Hypertrophic pulmonary osteoarthropathy can be seen in many chronic pulmonary processes, of which lung cancer is the most common. As a cause for hypercalcemia of malignancy, lung cancer is second only to breast cancer in frequency. Although small cell lung cancer is the most common tumor causing Cushing syndrome, the adrenal glands, pituitary, and thymus are additional sources of adrenocorticotropic hormone–producing tumors.

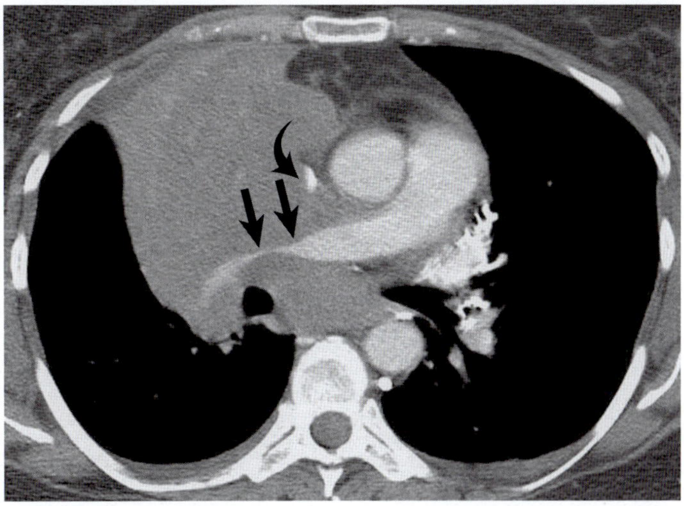

Fig. 17.21 Small cell carcinoma with superior vena cava syndrome. Contrast-enhanced CT scan shows a large mass in the right hilum and mediastinum with marked encasement of the right descending pulmonary artery *(straight arrows)* and near-complete occlusion of the superior vena cava *(curved arrow)*. Note the presence of mediastinal venous collaterals as a result of the superior vena cava obstruction.

Superior Vena Cava Syndrome

Any right-sided mediastinal mass compressing or occluding the superior vena cava or brachiocephalic venous confluence can produce the superior vena cava syndrome. Although small cell lung carcinoma (Fig. 17.21) and lymphoma are the most common neoplasms associated with superior vena cava syndrome, malignant thymic and germ cell tumors, fibrosing mediastinitis, and venous thrombosis from central venous catheterization are additional diagnostic considerations.

Vocal Cord Paralysis

Masses in the aorticopulmonary window or abutting the left upper mediastinal border along the course of the left recurrent laryngeal nerve can invade or compress the nerve and produce left vocal cord paralysis resulting in hoarseness. Involvement of the right recurrent laryngeal nerve occurs less frequently but can be seen in the setting of right mediastinal lymphadenopathy adjacent to the right subclavian artery or a superior sulcus tumor extending into the supraclavicular space.[46] Other major causes of unilateral vocal cord paralysis include surgery, neck trauma, and as an idiopathic condition.[47] An evaluation for malignant involvement of the vagus or recurrent laryngeal nerve within the neck or upper chest with CT is warranted in the absence of a relevant history of recent surgery or trauma.

Horner Syndrome

Horner syndrome results from an interruption of the sympathetic nerve supply to the eye, with resultant ptosis from denervation of the Müller muscle, miosis (a constricted pupil), and hemifacial anhidrosis. It most commonly develops from abnormalities of the sympathetic chain or along the course of the carotid artery. Lung cancer arising in the superior sulcus of the lung (Pancoast tumor) is the most common cause, although trauma, carotid artery aneurysm or dissection, and cervical lymphadenopathy from tuberculosis are additional causes.

IMAGING FINDINGS

Solitary Pulmonary Nodule

The differential diagnosis of an SPN is broad, but four conditions account for 95% of cases: granulomas, intrapulmonary lymph nodes, lung cancer, and hamartomas. In general, most smooth SPNs reflect benign conditions, whereas spiculated or irregular margins suggest malignancy. Please refer to Chapter 4 for additional discussion.

Lobar Consolidation or Atelectasis

The main differential diagnosis in patients with lung cancer resulting in lobar opacification is lobar pneumonia. The distinction is usually a clinical one, although associated clinical findings suggesting malignancy, such as weight loss, may prompt early evaluation with CT or bronchoscopy or both.

Mediastinal or Hilar Mass

Most middle mediastinal or unilateral hilar masses in adults are due to lung cancer, although other lesions can produce similar radiologic findings. The primary considerations in the differential diagnosis include bronchopulmonary foregut cysts, which are readily distinguished from solid masses by CT and/or MRI; lymphoma; granulomatous infections, including tuberculosis and fungal infection; metastatic lymphadenopathy from extrathoracic primary malignancies (primarily head and neck tumors, breast cancer, melanoma, and genitourinary tumors); pulmonary artery aneurysms; and rarely sarcoidosis.

Pleural Effusion

A unilateral exudative pleural effusion is most often a complication of pulmonary infection (parapneumonic effusion). Additional causes of a unilateral effusion include trauma, pulmonary embolism, tuberculosis, cirrhosis, and malignancy, particularly lung cancer. The presence of associated nodular pleural thickening or pleural nodules/masses is suggestive of malignancy. Pleural fluid cytology or pleural biopsy is usually diagnostic.

KEY POINTS

- Lung cancer manifests with variable imaging findings including solitary nodule/mass, consolidation, atelectasis, and ground-glass opacity.
- CT should be obtained to exclude malignancy in patients with nonresolving consolidation or atelectasis, clinical findings worrisome for malignancy (constitutional symptoms, hemoptysis), or radiographic findings of a new or enlarging nodule or mass.
- The high sensitivity of PET for malignant solid SPNs larger than 10 mm allows imaging follow-up when results are negative in patients with a low or intermediate risk for lung cancer. FDG-PET is of limited utility for the evaluation of SPNs with small or no solid component given the high false-negative rate.
- Cyst or bulla wall thickening and/or nodularity is an increasingly recognized manifestation of lung cancer.

SUGGESTED READINGS

Bruzzi JF, Komaki R, Walsh GL, Truong MT, Gladish GW, Munden RF, Erasmus JJ. Imaging of non-small cell lung cancer of the superior sulcus: part 1: anatomy, clinical manifestations, and management. *Radiographics.* 2008;28(2):551–560.

Carter BW, Glisson BS, Truong MT, Erasmus JJ. Small cell lung carcinoma: staging, imaging, and treatment considerations. *Radiographics.* 2014;34(6):1707–1721.

Chi WK. Advanced imaging tools in pulmonary nodule detection and surveillance. *Clin Imaging.* 2016;40(2):296–301.

Madsen PH, Holdgaard PC, Christensen JB, Høilund-Carlsen PF. Clinical utility of F-18 FDG PET-CT in the initial evaluation of lung cancer. *Eur J Nucl Med Mol Imaging.* 2016;43(11):2084–2097.

Rampinelli C, Calloni SF, Minotti M, Bellomi M. Spectrum of early lung cancer presentation in low-dose screening CT: a pictorial review. *Insights Imaging.* 2016;7(3):449-459.

Travis WD, Brambilla E, Noguchi M, et al. International Association for the Study of Lung Cancer/American Thoracic Society/European Respiratory Society international multidisciplinary classification of lung adenocarcinoma. *J Thorac Oncol.* 2011;6(2):174–185.

Truong MT, Ko JP, Rossi SE, et al. Update in the evaluation of the solitary pulmonary nodule. *Radiographics.* 2014;34(6):1658–1679.

Wu CC, Maher MM, Shepard JA. CT-guided percutaneous needle biopsy of the chest: preprocedural evaluation and technique. *AJR Am J Roentgenol.* 2011;196(5):W511–W514.

The full reference list for this chapter is available at ExpertConsult.com.

18 Pulmonary Carcinoma Staging

KYUNG SOO LEE | YEON JOO JEONG

Schemes for Staging

The most widely used scheme for staging non–small cell lung cancer (NSCLC) is the TNM classification. A variety of alterations in this scheme have been made to better group patients with similar prognosis and treatment options. The seventh edition of the TNM classification of lung cancer, published in 2009, was based on the analysis of a retrospective international database collected from 1990 to 2000 by the International Association for the Study of Lung Cancer (IASLC)[1] (Table 18.1). The revision in the seventh edition consisted of changes in the T descriptors that emphasized the prognostic impact of tumor size and redefined the classification of additional tumor nodules and malignant pleural effusion, the subclassification of M1, the validation of the classification for bronchopulmonary carcinoid tumors, and the rearrangement of stage grouping, whereas the N descriptors remained the same. Recently, the IASLC had collected new data of 77,156 patients diagnosed with lung cancer from 1999 to 2010.[2] This new database was used to inform the eighth edition of the TNM classification for lung cancer, due to be published in 2018. In this chapter, all descriptors for T, N, M and TNM stage groups of NSCLC and staging of small cell lung cancer (SCLC) will be based on the eighth edition of the TNM classification for lung cancer.[3–8] Specific properties of each of the T, N, and M subtypes as proposed by this revision are shown in Table 18.2. The various combinations of T, N, and M that define different stages are depicted in Table 18.3.

KEY POINTS: PULMONARY CARCINOMA STAGING

- T (tumor), N (node), and M (metastasis) (TNM) system is used for determining tumor subgrouping and staging for lung cancer.
- The eighth edition of the TNM Classification for Lung Cancer was proposed by the International Association for the Study of Lung Cancer (IASLC).

Methods of Staging

A variety of techniques can be used to investigate T, N, and M parameters to determine the appropriate tumor stage.

T (PRIMARY TUMOR)

Radiography

The presence of pulmonary carcinoma is often first suspected on the chest radiograph. The radiograph also provides information about the T staging by demonstrating the size of the lesion in patients in whom it is circumscribed and the degree of associated atelectasis or obstructive pneumonitis in the presence of airway obstruction in patients in whom it is not circumscribed. It may also show the presence of pleural effusion and, in some cases, evidence of chest wall or mediastinal invasion. Direct extension of a neoplasm into the chest wall may be established by radiographic evidence of destruction of ribs or vertebrae or clinical evidence of a palpable mass. Evidence of invasion into the mediastinum may be suggested by marked elevation of a hemidiaphragm (related to phrenic nerve paralysis). With these few exceptions, however, the chest radiograph is unreliable in detecting invasion of the chest wall, diaphragm, or the mediastinum.[9,10]

Computed Tomography

The seventh edition of the TNM classification for lung cancer emphasized the prognostic impact of the tumor size and subclassified T descriptors according to the tumor size. This finding was also confirmed in the new IASLC database for the eighth edition of the TNM classification.[3] Although the 3-cm cutpoint still remains a landmark to separate T1 from T2 tumors, the survival analyses showed that a progressive degradation of survival was observed for each 1-cm cutpoint. On the basis of the new IASLC database, the following rearrangement of T descriptors was provided: T1 tumors were subdivided into three subgroups at 1-cm cutpoints; T2 tumors were subdivided into two subgroups; T2 tumors greater than 5 cm and less than or equal to 7 cm were reclassified as T3; T3 tumors greater than 7 cm were reclassified as T4 (see Table 18.2). The survival analysis also showed that involvement of the main bronchus either less than 2 cm or more than 2 cm from the carina has a similar prognosis. Therefore the new IASLC database provided that T3 tumors classified by endobronchial location were combined as T2 tumor. Total atelectasis or pneumonitis, a T3 descriptor in the seventh edition, showed better prognosis than other T3 tumors in the new IASLC database; therefore the IASLC project provided grouping of partial and total atelectasis/pneumonitis as a T2 descriptor. It also reclassified diaphragm invasion as a T4 descriptor. Mediastinal pleural invasion without mediastinal tissue invasion is difficult to determine clinically and is rare at pathologic staging; therefore the new IASLC staging deleted mediastinal pleural invasion as a T descriptor.

Other T3 and T4 descriptors were not changed from the seventh edition of TNM staging. It is important to emphasize that if a tumor abuts a pleural surface or when pleural thickening is noted immediately adjacent to a tumor mass, the CT findings must be interpreted as indeterminate or merely as suspicious

TABLE 18.1 TUMOR-NODE-METASTASIS CLINICAL CLASSIFICATION (SEVENTH EDITION)[1]

TX	Primary tumor cannot be assessed, or tumor proven by the presence of malignant cells in sputum or bronchial washings but not visualized by imaging or bronchoscopy
T0	No evidence of primary tumor
Tis	Carcinoma in situ
T1	Tumor ≤ 3 cm in greatest dimension, surrounded by lung or visceral pleura, without bronchoscopic evidence of invasion more proximal than the lobar bronchus[a] (i.e., not in the main bronchus)
	T1a: tumor ≤ 2 cm in greatest dimension
	T1b: tumor > 2 cm, ≤ 3 cm in greatest dimensions
T2	Tumor > 3 cm, ≤ 7 cm; or tumor with any of the following features: involves main bronchus, ≥ 2 cm distal to the carina, invades the visceral pleura, associated with atelectasis or obstructive pneumonitis that extends to the hilar region but does not involve the entire lung
	T2a: tumor > 3 cm, ≤ 5 cm in greatest dimension
	T2b: tumor > 5 cm, ≤ 7 cm in greatest dimension
T3	Tumor > 7 cm or any size that directly invades any of the following: chest wall (including superior sulcus tumor), diaphragm, phrenic nerve, mediastinal pleura, parietal pericardium; or tumor in the main bronchus < 2 cm distal to the carina but without involvement of the carina; or associated atelectasis or obstructive pneumonitis of the entire lung or separate tumor nodule(s) in the same lobe as the primary
T4	Tumor of any size that invades any of the following: mediastinum, heart, great vessels, trachea, recurrent laryngeal nerve, esophagus, vertebral body, carina; separate tumor nodule(s) in a different ipsilateral lobe to that of the primary
NX	Regional lymph node cannot be assessed
N0	No regional lymph node metastasis
N1	Metastasis to ipsilateral peribronchial and/or ipsilateral hilar lymph nodes, and intrapulmonary nodes involved by direct extension of the primary tumor
N2	Metastasis to ipsilateral mediastinal and/or subcarinal lymph node(s)
N3	Metastasis to contralateral mediastinal, contralateral hilar, ipsilateral or contralateral scalene, or supraclavicular lymph node(s)
MX	Presence of distant metastasis cannot be assessed
M0	No distant metastasis
M1	Distant metastasis present
	M1a: separate tumor nodule(s) in a contralateral lobe; tumor with pleural nodules or malignant pleural or pericardial effusion[b]
	M1b: distant metastasis

[a]The uncommon superficial tumor of any size with its invasive component limited to the bronchial wall, which may extend proximal to the main bronchus, is also classified as T1a.

[b]Most pleural (pericardial) effusions with lung cancer are due to tumor. In a few patients, however, multiple microscopic examinations of pleural (pericardial) fluid are negative for tumor, and the fluid is nonbloody and is not an exudate. When these elements and clinical judgment dictate that the effusion is not related to the tumor, the effusion should be excluded as a staging element, and the patient should be classified as M0.

for pleural and chest wall invasion. Chest wall invasion can be diagnosed confidently only when tumor obliterates the fat planes between parietal pleura and chest wall muscle or when there is associated bone destruction (Figs. 18.1 and 18.2). Lung carcinomas are likely to be extensively invasive and unresectable (T4) if they involve the tracheal carina or surround, encase, or abut more than 180 degrees of the circumference of the aorta (Fig. 18.3), main or proximal portion of the right or left pulmonary arteries, or the esophagus.[9,11] Primary pulmonary carcinoma may be unresectable (T4) if it invades the heart, great vessels, or the vertebral body.

Magnetic Resonance Imaging

MRI is superior to CT in the demonstration of the pericardium, cardiac chambers, and mediastinal vessels with the added advantage of not requiring IV contrast medium[12] (see Fig. 18.3). Disruption of the normal 2- to 3-mm-thickness low signal intensity of the pericardium is suggestive of pericardial infiltration, although this does not preclude complete surgical resection. Coronal images are particularly helpful in the assessment of tumor extension into the subcarinal region, aortopulmonary window, and superior vena cava.[10]

MRI may allow better delineation of mediastinal and superior sulcus invasion (Fig. 18.4). MRI is especially useful in the evaluation of brachial plexus, subclavian vessel, or vertebral body invasion in Pancoast tumors. However, there is no significant difference in the overall diagnostic accuracy between CT and MRI. In one large study, the sensitivity of CT and MRI was 63% and 56%, respectively, and the specificity was 84% and 80% for distinguishing T3 and T4 tumors from less extensive pulmonary carcinomas.[10] Similar to CT, the main limitation of MRI is the inability to distinguish tumor invasion of mediastinal fat from inflammatory changes.

Disadvantages of MRI include lower spatial resolution than CT, longer scan time, higher cost, and artifacts as a result of respiratory motion. Recently introduced MRI techniques using fast (T2W half-Fourier acquisition single-shot turbo-spin-echo (HASTE), and T1W fat-saturated three-dimensional gradient-echo sequences with nearly isotropic resolution) and high-quality (breath-hold, electrocardiogram-gated, black-blood techniques on T2W turbo-spin-echo [TSE] and short-T1 inversion recovery [STIR] sequences) scan parameters have greatly improved the image quality and the potential role of MRI in the staging of lung cancer (Figs. 18.5 and 18.6). Moreover, increased spatial resolution can be obtained using parallel acquisition and reconstruction techniques: sensitivity encoding (SENSE) and simultaneous acquisition of spatial harmonics (SMASH).[13,14] Recent analyses of T staging using advanced MRI protocols showed that diagnostic

TABLE 18.2 PROPOSED TUMOR-NODE-METASTASIS CLINICAL CLASSIFICATION (EIGHTH EDITION)[3–5]

TX	Primary tumor cannot be assessed, or tumor proven by the presence of malignant cells in sputum or bronchial washings but not visualized by imaging or bronchoscopy
T0	No evidence of primary tumor
Tis	Carcinoma in situ
T1	Tumor ≤ 3 cm in greatest dimension, surrounded by lung or visceral pleura, without bronchoscopic evidence of invasion more proximal than the lobar bronchus[a] (i.e., not in the main bronchus)
	T1a(mi): minimally invasive adenocarcinoma[b]
	T1a: tumor ≤ 1 cm in greatest dimension
	T1b: tumor > 1 cm, ≤ 2 cm in greatest dimension
	T1c: tumor > 2 cm, ≤ 3 cm in greatest dimension
T2	Tumor > 3 cm, ≤ 5 cm; or tumor with any of the following features: involves main bronchus regardless of distance from the carina without involvement of the carina, invades the visceral pleura, associated with atelectasis or obstructive pneumonitis
	T2a: tumor > 3 cm, ≤ 4 cm in greatest dimension
	T2b: tumor > 4 cm, ≤ 5 cm in greatest dimension
T3	Tumor > 5 cm, ≤ 7 cm in greatest dimension; or directly invades any of the following: chest wall (including parietal pleura and superior sulcus tumor), phrenic nerve, parietal pericardium; separate tumor nodule(s) in the same lobe as the primary
T4	Tumor > 7 cm in greatest dimension or associated with separate tumor nodule(s) in a different ipsilateral lobe to that of the primary or direct invasion of any of the following: diaphragm, mediastinum, heart, great vessels, trachea, recurrent laryngeal nerve, esophagus, vertebral body, carina
NX	Regional lymph node cannot be assessed
N0	No regional lymph node metastasis
N1	Metastasis to ipsilateral peribronchial and/or ipsilateral hilar lymph nodes and intrapulmonary nodes involved by direct extension of the primary tumor
N2	Metastasis to ipsilateral mediastinal and/or subcarinal lymph node(s)
N3	Metastasis to contralateral mediastinal, contralateral hilar, ipsilateral or contralateral scalene, or supraclavicular lymph node(s)
MX	Presence of distant metastasis cannot be assessed
M0	No distant metastasis
M1	Distant metastasis present
	M1a: separate tumor nodule(s) in a contralateral lobe; tumor with pleural nodules or malignant pleural or pericardial effusion[c]
	M1b: single extrathoracic metastasis[d]
	M1c: multiple extrathoracic metastases in one or more organs

[a]The uncommon superficial tumor of any size with its invasive component limited to the bronchial wall, which may extend proximal to the main bronchus, is also classified as T1a.
[b]Solitary adenocarcinoma, ≤3 cm with a predominantly lepidic pattern and ≤5-mm invasion in any one focus.
[c]Most pleural (pericardial) effusions with lung cancer are due to tumor. In a few patients, however, multiple microscopical examinations of pleural (pericardial) fluid are negative for tumor, and the fluid is nonbloody and is not an exudate. When these elements and clinical judgment dictate that the effusion is not related to the tumor, the effusion should be excluded as a staging element, and the patient should be classified as M0.
[d]This includes involvement of a single distant (nonregional) lymph node.

accuracies of MRI were 82% to 94.3%, which were comparable to those of PET-CT (86%–91.4%).[15–17]

Positron Emission Tomography

Integrated PET-CT provides morphologic as well as metabolic data of lung cancer and is widely accepted to be the first-line imaging tool for staging. It has been shown to be more useful than CT alone in determining the T stage of the primary tumor and in assessing chest wall invasion.[18–20] According to a report, although statistically not significant (P =.25), integrated PET-CT accurately staged the primary tumor (T stage) in 86% (91 of 106) of patients, whereas CT accurately staged the primary tumor in only 79% (84 of 106) of patients.[19]

The main limitation of PET-CT in the T staging is false positivity in cases of inflammatory lesions. In this context, the newly introduced PET-MRI system with superior soft tissue contrast and dedicated sequences has the potential to compensate the shortcomings of PET-CT. According to the studies with comparison of PET-MRI and PET-CT in the preoperative staging of NSCLC, the diagnostic accuracy of PET-MRI (65%–94.3%) in the T staging was comparable to that of PET-CT (70%–91.4%).[16,17,21,22]

KEY POINTS: T STAGING

- Chest radiography is generally unreliable in detecting invasion of the chest wall, diaphragm, or mediastinum.
- Computed tomography (CT) can reliably detect invasion of the mediastinum, provided that major mediastinal vessels or bronchi are surrounded by tumor.
- Magnetic resonance imaging (MRI) is superior to CT in the demonstration of the pericardium, cardiac chambers, and mediastinal vessels, with the added advantage of not requiring intravenous (IV) contrast medium. Recent analyses of T staging using advanced MRI protocols showed that diagnostic accuracies of MRI were 82%–94.3%, which were comparable to those of positron emission tomography (PET)-CT (86%–91.4%).

N (LYMPH NODES)

Radiography and Computed Tomography

Lymph node involvement in lung cancer is categorized according to the location of the metastatic lymph nodes as N0 (no nodes involved), N1 (ipsilateral peribronchial, interlobar, or hilar node involvement), N2 (ipsilateral mediastinal or subcarinal node involvement), or N3 (contralateral mediastinal, contralateral

TABLE 18.3 PROPOSED STAGE GROUPINGS FOR THE EIGHTH EDITION OF THE TUMOR-NODE-METASTASIS CLASSIFICATION FOR LUNG CANCER[6]

Stage	TNM Subset
Occult carcinoma	TXN0M0
0	TisN0M0
IA1	T1a(mi)N0M0 T1aN0M0
IA2	T1bN0M0
IA3	T1cN0M0
IB	T2aN0M0
IIA	T2bN0M0
IIB	T1a-cN1M0 T2aN1M0 T2bN1M0 T3N0M0
IIIA	T1a-cN2M0 T2a-bN2M0 T3N1M0 T4N0M0 T4N1M0
IIIB	T1a-cN3M0 T2a-bN3M0 T3N2M0 T4N2M0
IIIC	T3N3M0 T4N3M0
IVA	Any T, Any N M1a Any T, Any N M1b
IVB	Any T, Any N M1c

hilar, or supraclavicular node involvement), regardless of the number of involved lymph nodes.[23] Analysis of the new IASLC database with respect to the N staging has shown that the N categories in the seventh edition of TNM staging for lung cancer are still useful for distinguishing among tumors with significantly different prognoses in both clinical and pathologic staging.[4] However, with regard to pathologic staging, the survival curves for N1 at multiple stations and N2 at a single station with N1 involvement overlapped each other, and N2 at a single station without N1 involvement had a better prognosis than N1 at multiple stations, although the difference was not significant. The following represents the most widely accepted criteria for radiologic assessment.

1. Lymph nodes should be classified according to a standardized lymph node map. The one adopted by the American Joint Committee on Cancer and the International Union Against Cancer in 2009 (Fig. 18.7 and Table 18.4) is the IASLC nodal map and anatomic definitions, and it is still the recommended means of describing regional lymph node involvement for lung cancers in the proposed eighth edition.[4,24]
2. The most reliable and practical measurement of lymph node size on CT is its short-axis diameter (i.e., the shortest diameter on the cross-sectional image); this parameter correlates better than the long-axis diameter with the node volume and is less influenced by the spatial orientation of the node.[25] Although some authors have suggested the use of various nodal size criteria specific for each mediastinal nodal station,[26,27] for practical reasons we and others consider a diameter greater than 10 mm in short axis as abnormal, regardless of nodal station.[28]

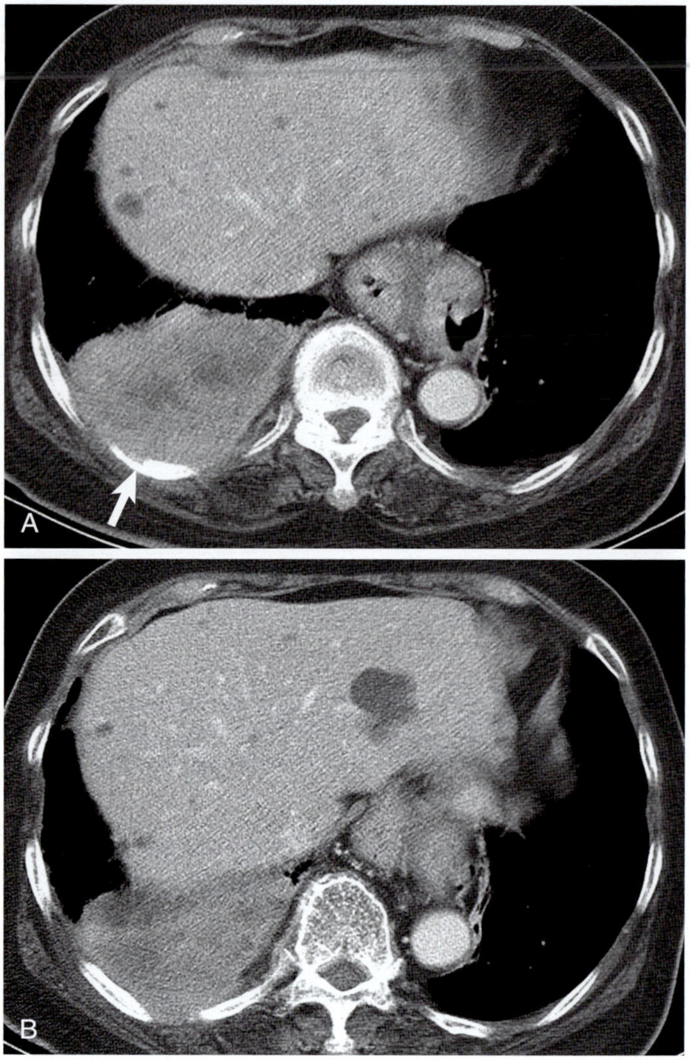

Fig. 18.1 T4 squamous cell carcinoma with surgically proven chest wall and right hemidiaphragmatic invasion. (A) CT scan obtained at level of liver dome shows enhancing, heterogeneous mass in the right lower lobe, abutting the chest wall. Erosion of a posterior right rib *(arrow)* indicates chest wall invasion. (B) CT scan obtained 15 mm caudal to (A) demonstrates overt chest wall and probable right hemidiaphragmatic invasion.

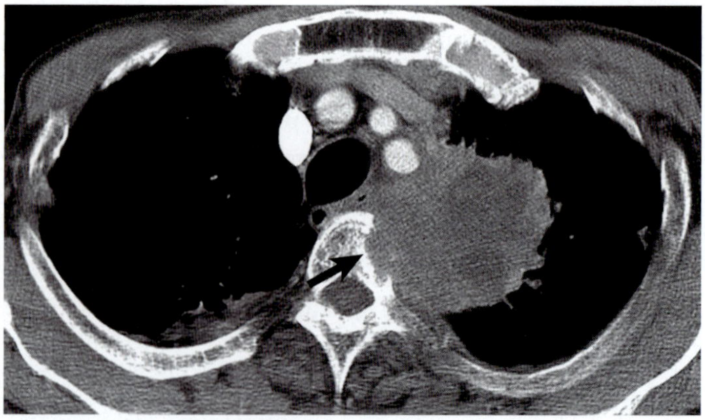

Fig. 18.2 T4 large-cell lung cancer. Contrast-enhanced axial CT scan obtained at the level of the great vessels shows a large left upper lobe heterogeneous mass invading the adjacent vertebral body *(arrow)*.

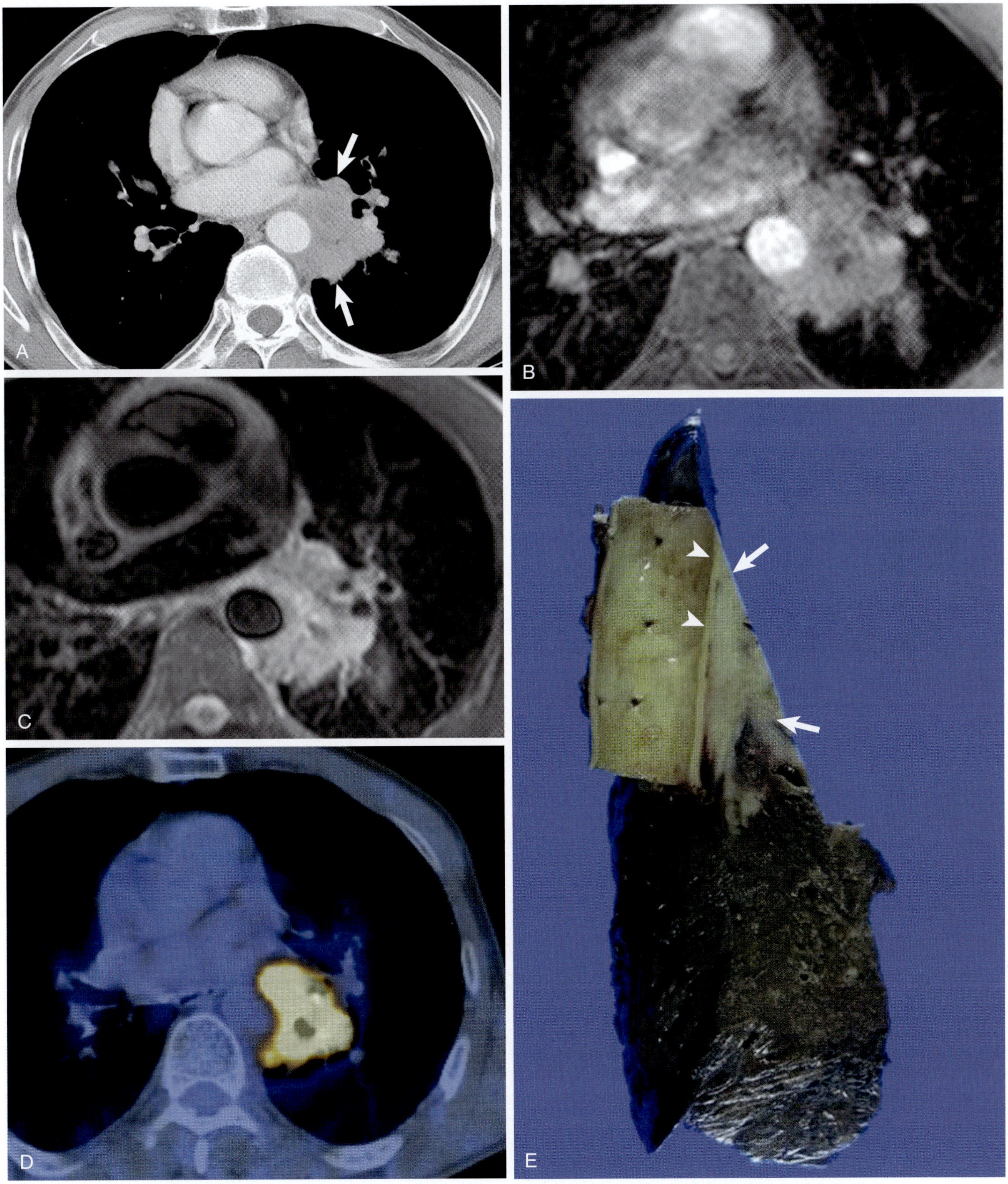

Fig. 18.3 T4 squamous cell lung cancer showing descending thoracic aortic invasion. (A) Contrast-enhanced CT scan obtained at left atrial level shows a mass *(arrows)* in the superior segment of the left lower lobe partially encircling the descending thoracic aorta over about 180 degrees of the aortic circumference. (B) and (C) T1W turbo-field-echo (B) and T2W triple inversion black-blood (C) MR images show the high-signal intensity mass abutting descending thoracic aorta over approximately 180 degrees. (D) Integrated PET-CT shows tumor with high FDG uptake abutting aorta over about 180 degrees. (E) Gross pathologic specimen shows that tumor *(arrows)* has invaded into the aortic adventitia *(arrowheads)*. Microscopic examination (not shown here) confirmed aortic invasion.

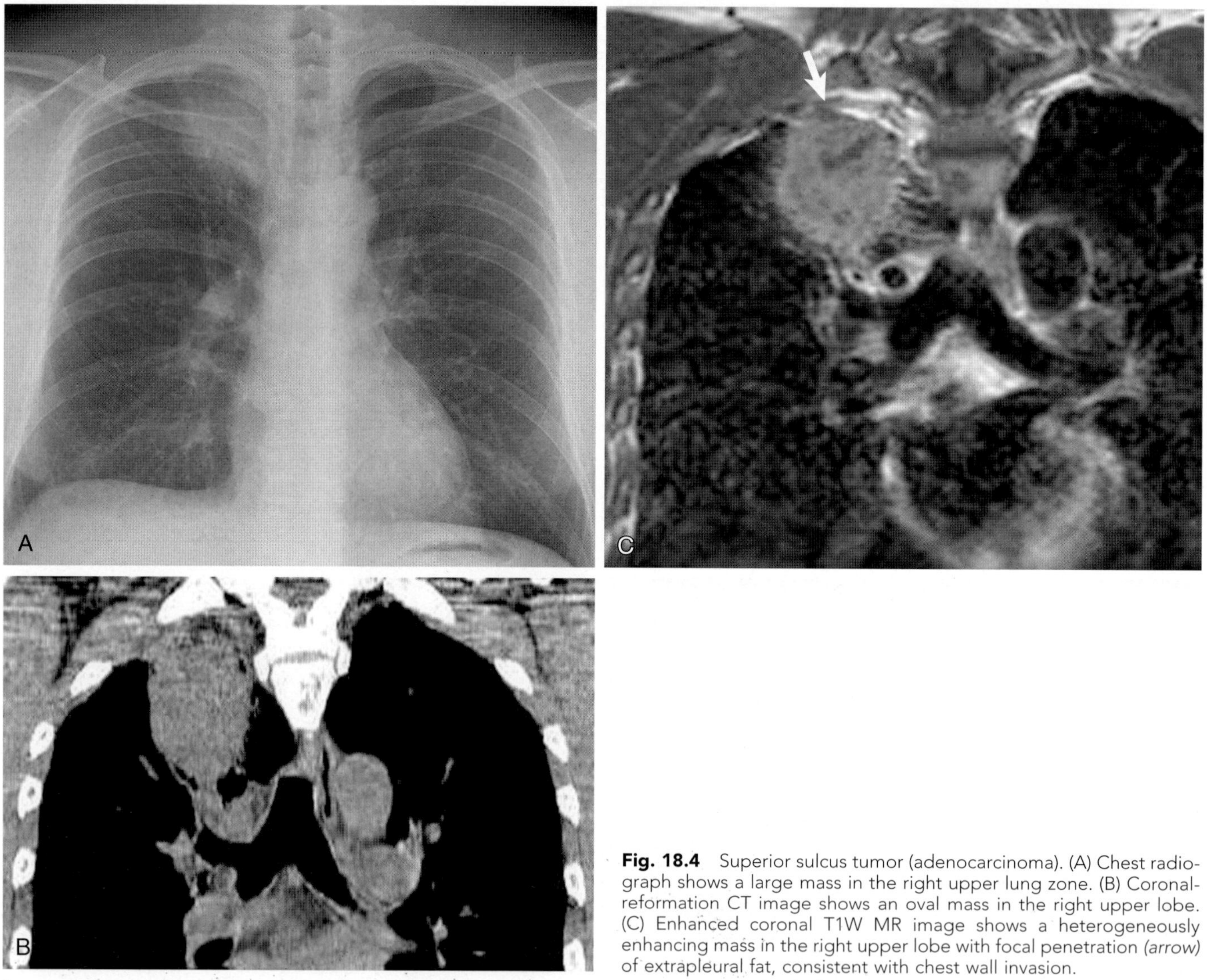

Fig. 18.4 Superior sulcus tumor (adenocarcinoma). (A) Chest radiograph shows a large mass in the right upper lung zone. (B) Coronal-reformation CT image shows an oval mass in the right upper lobe. (C) Enhanced coronal T1W MR image shows a heterogeneously enhancing mass in the right upper lobe with focal penetration *(arrow)* of extrapleural fat, consistent with chest wall invasion.

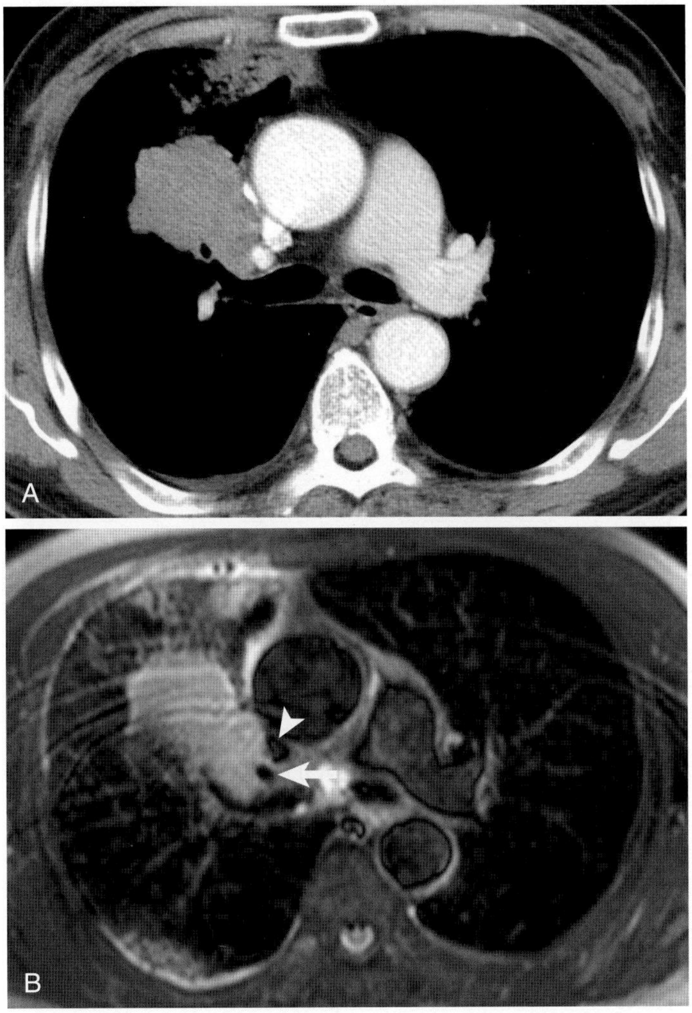

Fig. 18.5 Contrast-enhanced CT image compared with MR image in a 71-year-old man with large cell neuroendocrine carcinoma. (A) Contrast-enhanced axial CT scan obtained at the level of the right upper lobar bronchus shows a mass lesion in the right upper lobe with post–obstructive pneumonia. (B) Axial T2W triple inversion black-blood MR image obtained at similar level to (A) demonstrates a right upper lobe mass and accompanying post–obstructive pneumonia. Tumor encircles the truncus anterior *(arrow)*, but the superior vena cava *(arrowhead)* appears to be intact.

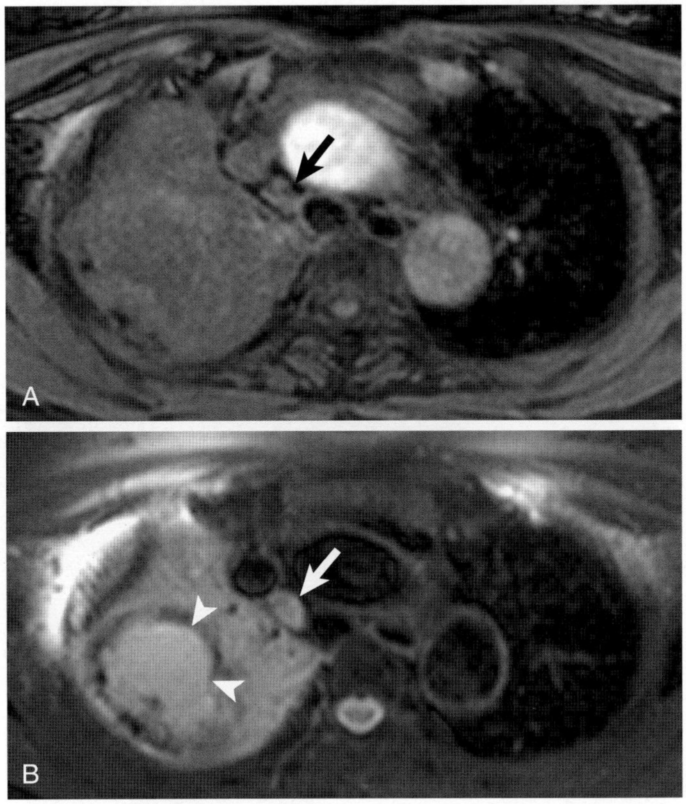

Fig. 18.6 MRI in squamous cell lung carcinoma. (A) T1W turbo-field-echo MR image shows an intermediate signal intensity lesion in the right upper lobe. Also note enlarged lymph node *(arrow)* in the lower right paratracheal station. (B) T2W triple inversion black-blood MR image shows a lung mass *(arrowheads)* and surrounding atelectatic right upper lobe. Also note enlarged right paratracheal lymph node *(arrow)* with high signal intensity. Patient had proven T2N2 lung cancer.

3. Factors that facilitate visualization of mediastinal lymph nodes include the presence of mediastinal fat, use of IV contrast material, and thinner CT section. IV contrast material is particularly helpful in the distinction of the truncus anterior from a right paratracheal lymph node and in the assessment of the aortopulmonary window region, where the superior aspect of the main or left pulmonary artery may be misinterpreted as an enlarged lymph node on scans performed without IV contrast material. Despite these advantages, we believe that IV contrast material is not required routinely for the assessment of mediastinal nodes when using spiral CT technique and collimation of 5 mm or less.[29] Although IV contrast material is not required for the evaluation of mediastinal lymph nodes, assessment of hilar lymph nodes requires the use of IV injection of contrast material and dynamic incremental or spiral CT. IV contrast material is recommended in patients in whom hilar lymph node enlargement is suspected on the radiograph.[30–32]

Although there is no question that CT is superior to chest radiography in the detection of mediastinal lymph node metastases, the specificity for the diagnosis is slightly less. For example, in one study of 418 patients, the sensitivity and specificity of chest radiography for the detection of mediastinal lymph node metastases were 40% and 99%, respectively; CT had sensitivity and specificity of 84.4% and 84.1%, respectively.[33] In another investigation of 170 patients, the sensitivity and specificity of the radiograph were 9% and 92%, respectively, whereas the corresponding figures for CT were 52% and 69%, respectively.[34] Visualization of mediastinal lymph node enlargement on radiography almost invariably indicates the presence of metastatic carcinoma.

A known limitation of CT in staging mediastinal lymph node involvement is that mediastinal lymph node metastases are assessed only on the basis of nodal size (Figs. 18.8 and 18.9). False-negative CT scans are due to the presence of metastases in normal-sized lymph nodes, and false-positive CT findings are due to lymph node enlargement secondary to benign inflammatory processes. As the results of the previous studies suggest, there has been considerable variability in the reported sensitivity and specificity of CT in the assessment of mediastinal nodal metastases. Although several groups have shown a sensitivity greater than 85%,[35,36] others have reported values of 40% to 70%.[34,37] According to the most recently published meta-analysis, CT has 57% sensitivity and 82% specificity for staging the mediastinal lymph nodes.[38] This variability

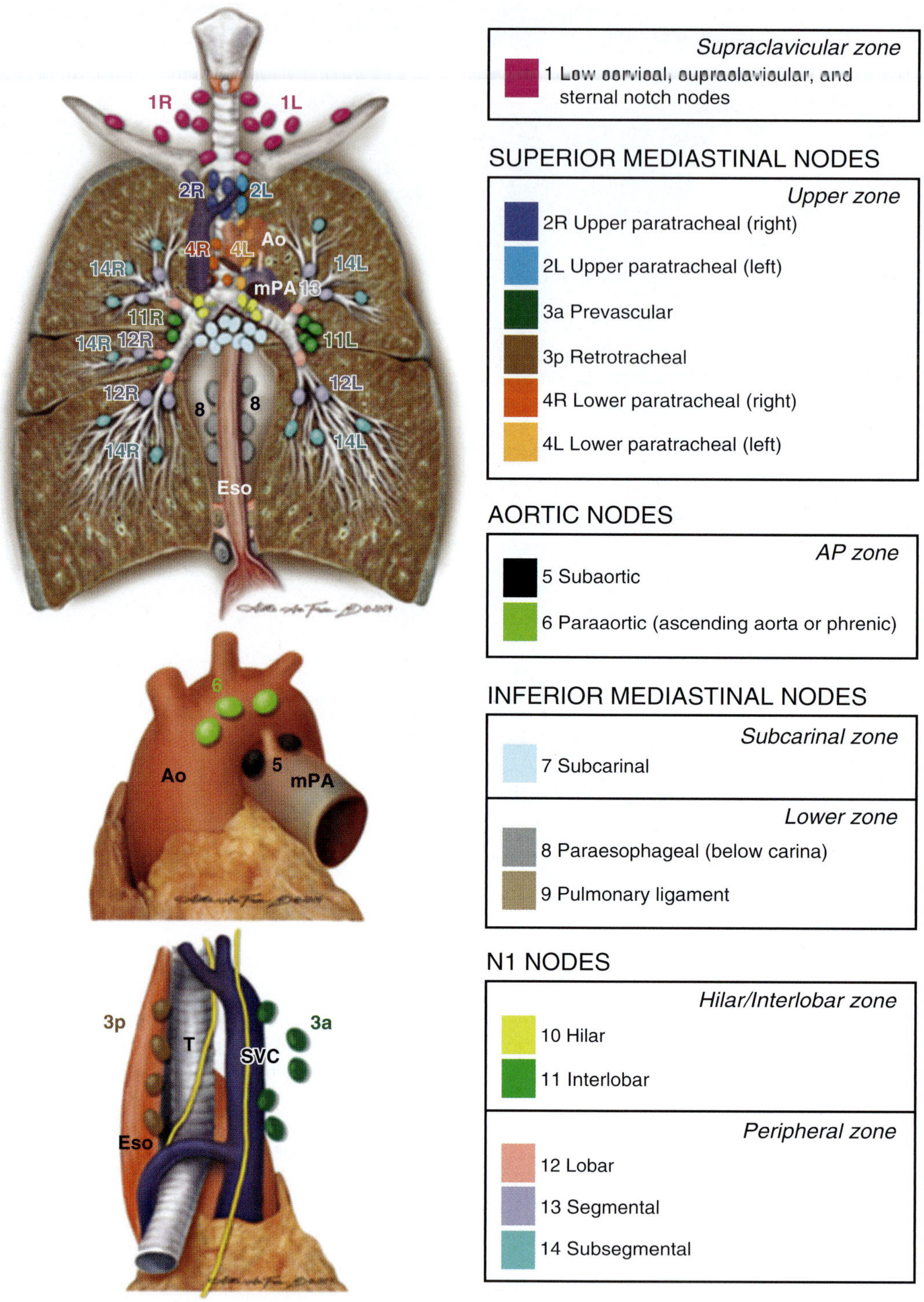

Fig. 18.7 The International Association for the Study of Lung Cancer (IASLC) lymph node map, including the grouping of lymph node stations into "zones" for the purpose of prognostic analyses. *Ao,* Aorta; *AP,* aortopulmonary zone; *Eso,* esophagus; *mPA,* main pulmonary artery; *SVC,* superior vena cava; *T,* trachea. *(Reprinted with permission from the International Association for the Study of Lung Cancer. The IASLC Lung Cancer Project. A proposal for a new international lymph node map in the forthcoming seventh edition of the TNM classification for lung cancer.* J Thoracic Oncol. *2009;4:568–577.)*

is related to several factors, including different size criteria for abnormal lymph nodes, different patient populations studied, and use of a per-patient versus a per-nodal station analysis, interobserver variability, and differences in the diagnostic gold standard. Therefore, given the limitations of mediastinal staging by CT, biopsy is recommended for the confirmation of regional lymph node metastases. Mediastinoscopy and/or ultrasound-guided bronchoscopic or transesophageal endoscopic biopsy of nodes are performed to accurately determine the presence and location of nodal metastasis.[39,40] Guidelines for staging of lung cancer suggest that

TABLE 18.4 LYMPH NODE MAP DESCRIPTION

Nodal Station	Anatomic Landmarks
1. Low cervical, supraclavicular and sternal notch nodes	*Upper border:* lower margin of cricoid cartilage; *lower border:* clavicles bilaterally and, in the midline, the upper border of the manubrium The oncologic midline is the midline of the trachea.
2. Upper paratracheal nodes	2R and 2L: *upper border:* apex of lung and pleural space and, in the midline, the upper border of the manubrium; 2R *lower border:* intersection of caudal margin of innominate vein with the trachea 2L *lower border:* superior border of the aortic arch (the oncologic midline is along the left lateral border of the trachea)
3. Prevascular and retrotracheal nodes	3a: prevascular Right: *upper border:* apex of chest; *lower border:* level of carina; *anterior border:* posterior aspect of sternum; *posterior border:* anterior border of superior vena cava Left: *upper border:* apex of chest; *lower border:* level of carina; *anterior border:* posterior aspect of sternum; *posterior border:* left carotid artery 3p: retrotracheal *Upper border:* apex of chest; *lower border:* carina; *anterior border:* posterior tracheal wall
4. Lower paratracheal nodes	4R: includes right paratracheal nodes, and pretracheal nodes extending to the left lateral border of trachea *Upper border:* intersection of caudal margin of innominate vein with the trachea; *lower border:* lower border of azygos vein 4L: includes nodes to the left of the left lateral border of the trachea, medial to the ligamentum arteriosum *Upper border:* upper margin of the aortic arch; *lower border:* upper rim of the left pulmonary artery
5. Subaortic (aortopulmonary window)	Subaortic nodes lateral to the ligamentum arteriosum *Upper border:* the lower border of the aortic arch; *lower border:* upper rim of the left pulmonary artery
6. Paraaortic nodes (ascending aorta or phrenic)	Nodes lying anterior and lateral to the ascending aorta and the aortic arch *Upper border:* a line tangential to the upper border of the aortic arch; *lower border:* the lower border of the aortic arch
7. Subcarinal nodes	*Upper border:* the carina of the trachea; *lower border:* the upper border of the lower lobe bronchus on the left; the lower border of the bronchus intermedius on the right
8. Paraesophageal nodes (below carina)	Nodes lying adjacent to the wall of the esophagus and to the right or left of the midline, excluding subcarinal nodes *Upper border:* the upper border of the lower lobe bronchus on the left; the lower border of the bronchus intermedius on the right; *lower border:* the diaphragm
9. Pulmonary ligament nodes	Nodes lying within the pulmonary ligament *Upper border:* the inferior pulmonary vein; *lower border:* the diaphragm
10. Hilar nodes	Includes nodes immediately adjacent to the mainstem bronchus and hilar vessels including the proximal portions of the pulmonary veins and main pulmonary artery *Upper border:* the lower rim of the azygos vein on the right; upper rim of the pulmonary artery on the left *Lower border:* interlobar region bilaterally
11. Interlobar nodes	Between the origin of the lobar bronchi
12. Lobar nodes	Nodes lying adjacent to the lobar bronchi
13. Segmental nodes	Nodes lying adjacent to the segmental bronchi
14. Subsegmental nodes	Nodes lying adjacent to the subsegmental bronchi

endobronchial ultrasound-guided transbronchial needle aspiration (EBUS-TBNA) should be considered the best first test of nodal staging for radiologically abnormal lymph nodes that are accessible by EBUS-TBNA.[41]

Positive nodes missed on CT scan are less likely to be associated with extracapsular spread of tumor than nodes larger than 1 cm in diameter. Patients who have metastasis to normal-sized nodes are more likely to have negative results at mediastinoscopy and to have the affected nodes discovered only at subsequent thoracotomy. There is evidence that patients who have microscopic metastases discovered at the time of thoracotomy have an improved survival rate if the primary tumor and the involved mediastinal nodes are resected.[42,43]

Magnetic Resonance Imaging

Similar to CT, MRI relies on size criteria to determine nodal abnormalities and is comparable to CT in the assessment of mediastinal nodal metastasis.[10] According to a recent meta-analysis, MRI has an overall high sensitivity (0.87 [95% confidence interval (CI): 0.78–0.92]) and high specificity (0.88 [95% CI: 0.77–0.94]) on a per-patient basis and 0.88 (95% CI: 0.78–0.94) and 0.95 (95% CI: 0.87–0.98) on a per-node basis, respectively.[44]

Studies of MRI with quantitative diagnostic assessment, such as apparent diffusion coefficients (ADC) or lesion-to-phantom ratios (LPR) of metastatic hilar and mediastinal lymph nodes, showed significantly higher diagnostic performance on a per-node basis than studies with qualitative assessment with visual inspection of lesion size and morphology of individual metastatic regional lymph nodes (relative diagnostic odds ratio, 7.25 [95% CI: 1.75–30.09]; $P = .01$).[44] Hilar and mediastinal lymph node metastases usually show high signal on T2W MR images (Fig. 18.10; see Fig. 18.8). Quantitative assessment of LPR using STIR TSE MRI showed a direct relationship between LPR and the likelihood of a metastatic lymph node.[45–50] Diffusion-weighted images (DWI) can also be used in the quantitative assessment of metastatic lymph nodes. In a prospective study with histopathologic validation, the ADCs of metastatic lymph nodes were reported to be significantly lower than the ADCs of lymph nodes without metastasis.[50,51] However, because DWI is currently obtained with the echo-planar imaging (EPI) sequence without

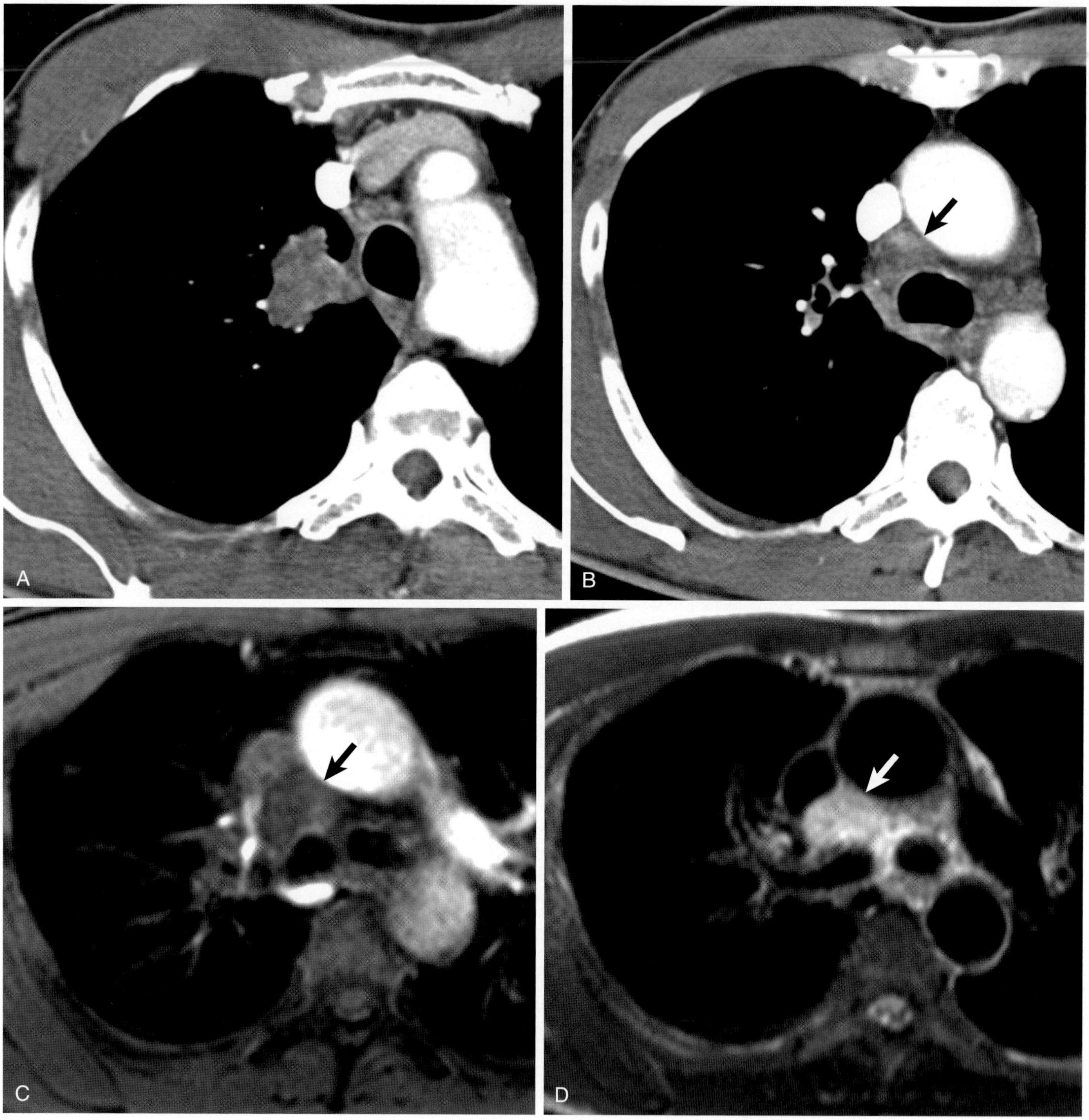

Fig. 18.8 True positive mediastinal nodal metastasis (N2 disease) detected at CT in squamous cell lung carcinoma. (A) Contrast-enhanced axial CT scan obtained at the level of the aortic arch shows 2.3-cm nodule in the right upper lobe. (B) CT scan obtained at level of azygos arch shows an enlarged lymph node with evidence of extracapsular invasion *(arrow)* in the lower right paratracheal station (nodal station 4R). (C) and (D) T1W turbo-field-echo (C) and T2W triple inversion black-blood (D) MR images demonstrate enlarged nodes in right lower paratracheal station. The absent fatty hilum (*arrow* in C) on T1W image and high-signal intensity (*arrow* in D) on T2W image suggest metastasis.

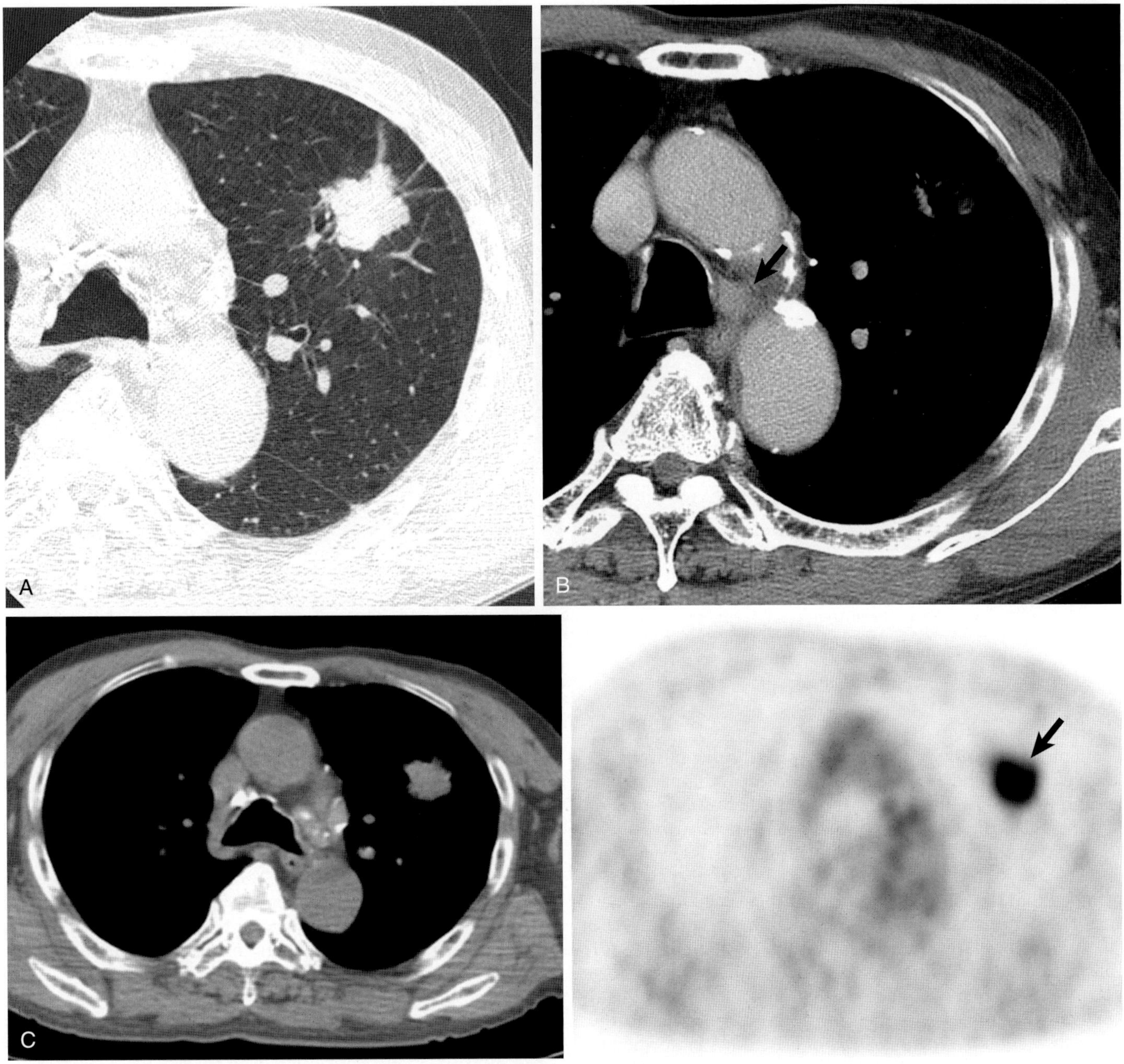

Fig. 18.9 False-positive mediastinal node at CT in pulmonary adenocarcinoma. (A) Axial CT scan obtained at level of azygos arch shows a spiculated 2.4-cm nodule in the left upper lobe. (B) CT scan obtained at carinal level shows a slightly enlarged lymph node *(arrow)* in the lower left paratracheal station (nodal station 4L). (C) CT and corresponding PET images show increased FDG uptake *(arrow)* in the spiculated left upper lobe nodule but not in the lymph node. There was no evidence of lymph node metastasis at surgery.

any motion correction, this may result in relatively lower spatial resolution and less anatomic information than can be obtained with STIR TSE imaging. Recently, advanced DWI based on the fast advanced SE (FASE) sequence has been developed, and the accuracy of N-stage assessment using STIR-FASE imaging (84.2% [80%–95%]) and DWI-FASE (83.2% [79%–95%]) was significantly higher than that using DWI-EPI (76.8% [73%–95%]) and PET-CT(73.7% [70%–95%]).[52]

Positron Emission Tomography

Although CT and MR imaging rely on the anatomic assessment of lymph nodes, PET relies on the increased metabolic rate of neoplastic cells compared with normal cells. Mediastinal nodes containing carcinoma cells have been shown to have increased uptake and accumulation of fluorodeoxyglucose (FDG) (Fig. 18.11). Several groups have shown that PET is superior to CT in the assessment of mediastinal nodal metastases.[53,54] In one study of

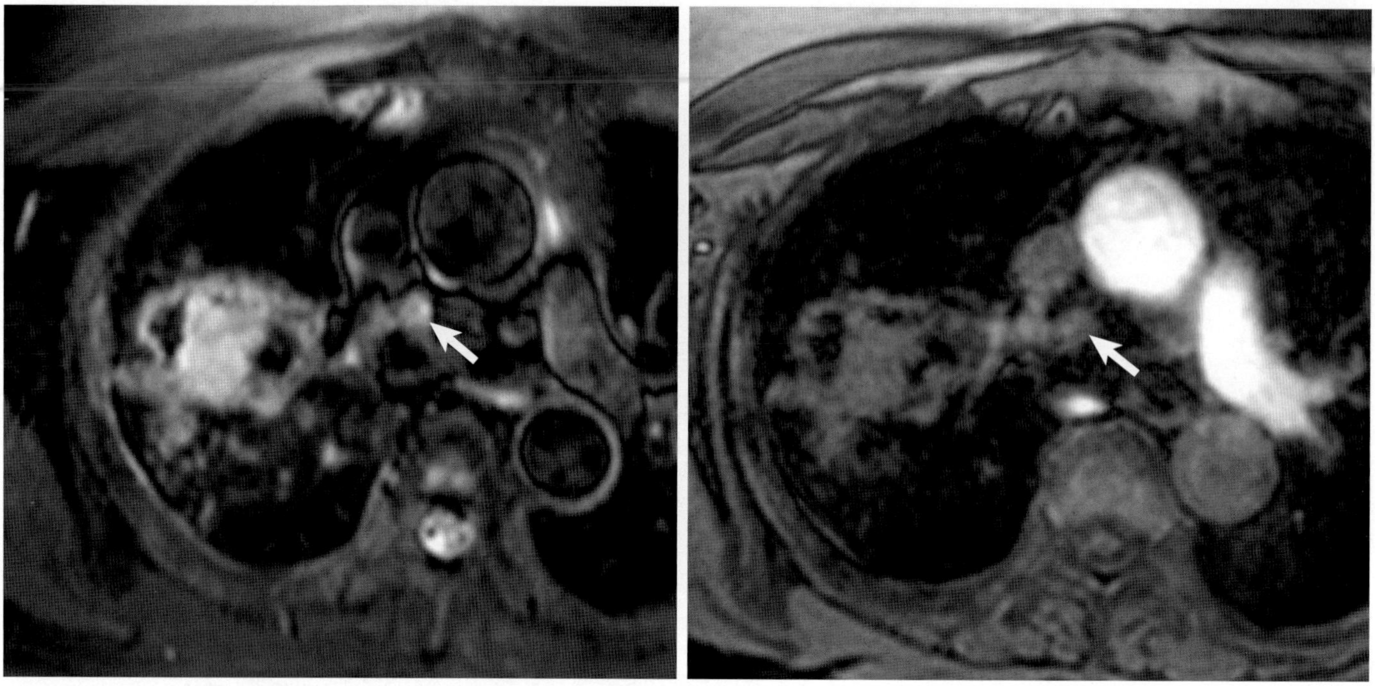

Fig. 18.10 True positive mediastinal nodes on turbo MR images in pulmonary adenocarcinoma. T2-weighted TIBB turbo SE *(left)* and T1-weighted three-dimensional turbo-field-echo *(right)* images show a cavitary mass in the right upper lobe with a small but high signal intensity lymph node in the lower right paratracheal station *(arrows)*. Involvement of the paratracheal nodes was confirmed at surgical biopsy.

99 patients, the sensitivity and specificity for the diagnosis of N2 disease were 83% and 94%, respectively, for PET compared with 63% and 73%, respectively, for CT.[55] In another investigation of 100 patients, mediastinal lymph nodes were staged correctly in 85% of cases with PET compared with 58% on CT.[56] The authors of a meta-analysis of 14 studies published between 1990 and 1998 concluded that the sensitivity of PET for the detection of mediastinal nodal metastases is 79% to 84%, and the specificity is 89% to 91%.[57] By comparison, meta-analysis of 29 studies using CT published during the same period showed a sensitivity of 60% and a specificity of 77%.[57] The sensitivity of PET in the meta-analysis of the studies published in the 1990s is similar to the previously mentioned meta-analysis of CT studies performed in the 1980s,[58] whereas that of CT has become substantially lower.

The main limitation of PET imaging is a low spatial resolution. This limitation has been minimized by the development of integrated PET-CT scanners. PET-CT allows fusion of the PET and CT images and thus combines the functional information from PET with the anatomic information from CT (Fig. 18.12). According to an initial study,[59] integrated PET-CT results in improved sensitivity, specificity, and overall accuracy (78%, 95%, and 89%, respectively) for the detection of malignant lymph nodes, compared with visually correlated PET and CT (67%, 95%, and 86%, respectively). The greater sensitivity and accuracy of integrated PET-CT have since been corroborated by several studies.[19,20,60] According to a recent meta-analysis of nodal staging in NSCLC with integrated PET-CT, sensitivity and specificity on a per-node basis were 0.62 (95% CI: 0.54, 0.70) and 0.92 (95% CI: 0.88, 0.95), respectively, and sensitivity and specificity on a per-patient basis were 0.67 (95% CI: 0.54, 0.79) and 0.87 (95% CI: 0.82, 0.91), respectively.[61] Studies from tuberculosis-endemic countries showed lower sensitivity (0.56 vs. 0.68, $P = .03$) on a node basis and lower specificity (0.83 vs. 0.89, $P < .01$) on a patient basis.

According to the studies with comparison of PET-MRI and PET-CT in the preoperative staging of NSCLC, the diagnostic accuracy of PET-MR (57.1%–77%) in the N staging was comparable to that of PET-CT (52.4%–86%).[21,22,62] However, diagnostic accuracy of PET-MRI with signal intensity assessment (91.4%) in the N staging was significantly higher than that of PET-CT (80.7%).[16]

KEY POINTS: N STAGING

- The most reliable and practical measurement of lymph node size on CT is the short-axis diameter (i.e., the shortest diameter on the cross-sectional image). Nodes are enlarged if they measure >10 mm in short-axis diameter.
- False-negative CT scans are due to the presence of metastasis in normal-sized lymph nodes, and false-positive scans are due to lymph node enlargement secondary to benign inflammatory processes.
- Meta-analysis of studies performed in the 1980s showed 83% sensitivity and 81% specificity for CT in detecting mediastinal nodal metastases; however, meta-analysis in the 1990s showed sensitivity of 60% and specificity of 77%, presumably because of more careful surgical staging.
- MRI with quantitative diagnostic assessment with apparent diffusion coefficients or lesion-to-phantom ratios of metastatic hilar and mediastinal lymph nodes showed significantly higher diagnostic performance.
- Recent meta-analysis showed that MRI has a high sensitivity and specificity on a per-node and a per-patient basis; however, integrated PET-CT has a high specificity but a low sensitivity for detecting lymph node metastasis.

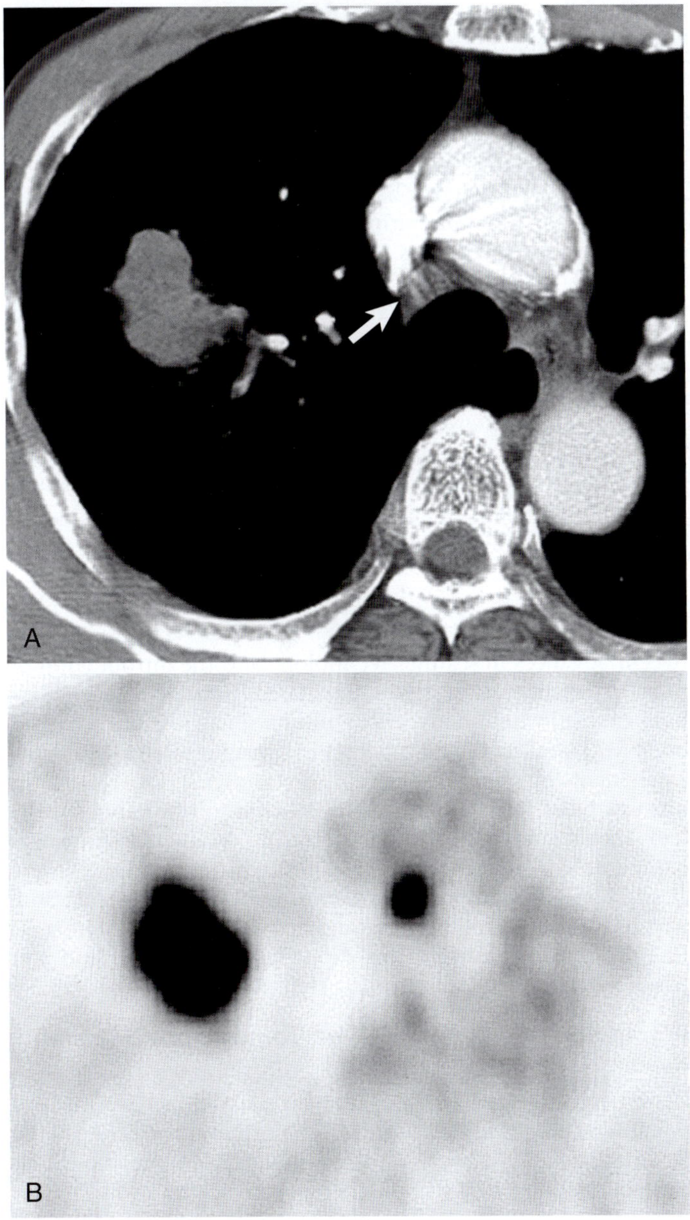

Fig. 18.11 Positive nodes on PET in lung adenocarcinoma. (A) Contrast-enhanced CT scan shows a mass in the right upper lobe and a right paratracheal lymph node measuring less than 10 mm *(arrow)*. This node was interpreted as negative for malignancy. (B) PET scan obtained at same level to (A) demonstrates increased FDG uptake within the right upper lobe mass. The lymph node in the right paratracheal station also shows markedly increased FDG uptake (maximum standardized uptake value, 6.1), which proved to be a metastatic node. *(Reprinted with permission from Shim SS, Lee KS, Kim B-T, et al. Non-small cell lung cancer: prospective comparison of integrated FDG PET-CT and CT alone for preoperative staging.* Radiology. *2005;236:1011–1019.)*

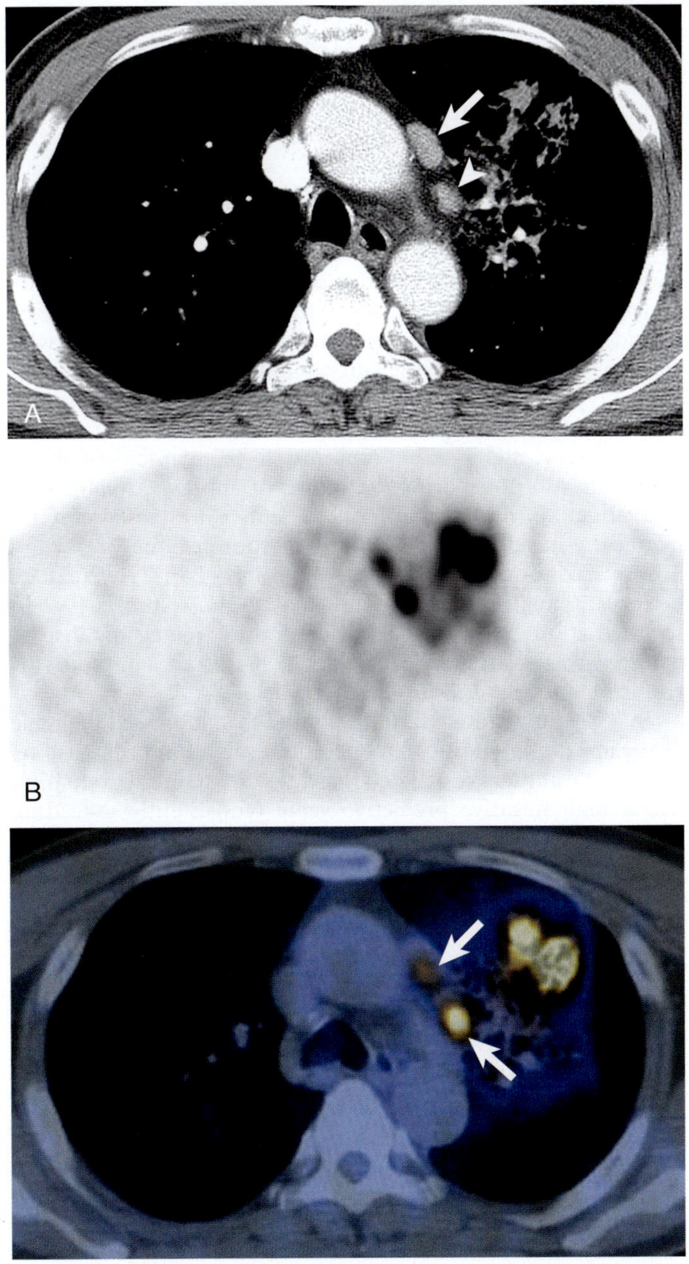

Fig. 18.12 True positive integrated PET-CT in lung adenocarcinoma. (A) Contrast-enhanced CT scan shows enlarged lymph nodes in the paraaortic (station 6, *arrow*) and subaortic (station 5, *arrowhead*) stations. Also note obstructive atelectasis in the left upper lobe. (B) PET and integrated PET-CT show increased FDG uptake (maximum standardized uptake value, 11.5) in enlarged nodes *(arrows)* as well as primary lung cancer. The patient had surgically confirmed lymph node metastases.

M (DISTANT METASTASES)

Since the seventh edition of the TNM staging classification for NSCLC was published in 2009, several developments in diagnosis, imaging, and treatment of NSCLC have been added to lung cancer management. They include common use of PET in diagnostic practice, minimally invasive endoscopic and surgical methods for diagnosing and treating small pleural and pulmonary lesions, precise radiotherapy techniques such as brain or body stereotactic radiotherapy, and molecular-targeted agents. Therefore it is necessary to reanalyze the new IASLC database for the development of proposals for the new M descriptors of the eighth edition of TNM classification. On the basis of analysis of the new database, the prognosis of the former M1a descriptor (including pleural or pericardial effusions, contralateral or bilateral lung nodules, or pleural/pericardial nodules) is similar. Therefore, in the eighth edition of TNM staging classification for NSCLC, the M1a descriptor is maintained as the use of the seventh edition of the M1a category.[5] The new database also showed that the number of metastatic lesions may be more prognostic than the number of organs involved. Therefore the proposed eighth edition of the TNM staging system reclassified M1 categories as M1a, M1b (single metastatic lesion in one organ), and M1c (multiple metastases in either a single organ or multiple organs) (see Table 18.3).

Conventional Staging

The most widely used techniques to investigate patients who have possible extrathoracic metastases are CT (to show metastases to the adrenal glands and liver), MR imaging (to detect brain and adrenal metastases), and radionuclide scans (to identify skeletal metastases). The use of these techniques should be considered in the context of clinical findings. In patients who have an NSCLC, brain MRI and radionuclide scanning of bone generally are indicated only if there is clinical or laboratory evidence of metastatic disease. Such evidence includes not only organ-specific signs and symptoms (liver enlargement, bone pain) but also nonspecific symptoms of anorexia, weight loss, and fatigue. In one study of 309 patients who had an NSCLC in an early stage (T1 or T2, N0 or N1), routine bone, brain, and liver scans or bone scan and abdominal and brain CT were done before anticipated surgery. Only 1 of the 472 studies (0.2%) revealed an unexpected metastasis; all other metastatic disease detected was associated with clinical signs and symptoms or abnormal biochemical profiles.[63]

In a 1995 meta-analysis of 25 studies that addressed the issue of the appropriateness of preoperative evaluation of metastatic disease, the authors concluded that a negative clinical evaluation had a high negative predictive value (consistently exceeding 90%) for finding occult metastases by bone scan and CT evaluation of the brain and abdomen.[64] These values were more impressive (>97%) when an expanded clinical evaluation, which included consideration of constitutional symptoms, was used. Although some investigators have reported occult brain metastases in asymptomatic individuals, especially those who have adenocarcinoma,[65–67] such findings must be balanced against the low cost-effectiveness of the procedure. In the meta-analysis cited previously, the prevalence of brain metastases in asymptomatic patients was only 5%. Because gadolinium-enhanced MRI is more sensitive than CT in the detection of such metastases, it is possible that the prevalence is higher than that suggested by the CT data.

Computed Tomography

Abdominal CT scans have been obtained for the detection of liver or adrenal metastasis (note description on adrenal imaging to follow).

Magnetic Resonance Imaging

Dedicated liver MRI or whole-body MRI (with breath-hold fat-suppressed T2W imaging of the liver and dynamic T1W data acquisition) imaging has been shown to be the most accurate tool for noninvasive detection and characterization of hepatic mass lesions.[68] MRI (gadolinium–diethylene triamine pentaacetic acid [DTPA] T1W sequence) is also more sensitive than CT in the detection of brain metastases, especially for small lesions.[67,69] MRI is comparable to PET in the detection of bone metastases[70]; both modalities are superior to bone scintigraphy.

Bone Scintigraphy

Scintigraphy provides a rapid overview of the skeletal system. It is superior to MRI in the assessment of the ribs, the scapula, and skull (Fig. 18.13). However, MRI is superior to scintigraphy in the detection of osseous metastases located in the spine and pelvis and in the distinction of osseous metastases from primary bone tumors.[71] Overall, bone scintigraphy is inferior to MRI or PET in the detection of osseous metastases.[55]

Whole-Body Positron Emission Tomography

Whole-body PET imaging has the advantage over other imaging modalities of demonstrating not only adrenal metastases but also other metastases that may not be apparent on CT (Fig. 18.14), MRI, or bone scintigraphy. In one investigation of 100 patients with newly diagnosed pulmonary carcinoma, PET correctly indicated the M status in 40 (91%) of 44 patients with metastatic disease compared with 35 (80%) with conventional imaging. PET and CT correctly identified all sizes of adrenal metastases (sensitivity 100%), but PET has a specificity and positive predictive value of 100% compared with 93% and 46%, respectively, for CT. PET correctly identified 11 (91%) of 12 patients with bone metastases compared with 6 (50%) identified on scintigraphy; both modalities had a specificity of 92%[55] (Fig. 18.15).

Whole-Body Magnetic Resonance Imaging

Recent advances in scanner technology and the introduction of moving patient platforms with integrated surface-coil technology have enabled whole-body MRI within a single session.[72] Whole-body MRI similar to whole-body PET imaging allows the overall assessment of the presence of metastases (Fig. 18.16). In one study of 154 patients with NSCLC,[15] whole-body MRI had an accuracy of 86% for detecting M stage, which was comparable to that of PET-CT. Although the differences were not statistically significant, whole-body MR imaging was more useful for detecting brain and hepatic metastases, whereas PET-CT was more useful for detecting lymph node and soft tissue metastases.

Whole-Body Positron Emission Tomography–Magnetic Resonance Imaging

Recent technical advances in image registration have made it possible to combine PET with MRI information as coregistered or integrated PET-MRI. The combination of the molecular component of the PET with MRI's capability for tissue discrimination allows more accurate preoperative staging of NSCLC (Fig. 18.17).[17] For the assessment of the presence of distant metastasis, diagnostic accuracy of coregistered PET-MRI with signal intensity assessment (98.6%) was significantly higher than that of whole-body PET-MRI without signal intensity assessment (91.4%) and integrated PET-CT (90.7%).[16] Another study with integrated PET-MRI showed no significant differences in the accuracy of metastasis staging between PET-CT and PET-MRI.[22]

Adrenal Imaging

Routine contrast-enhanced CT through the liver for the staging of lung cancer rarely changes tumor stage and is therefore not warranted.[64,73] However, because the adrenal glands are common sites for metastatic pulmonary carcinoma and because of the ease of examination, most radiologists extend the chest CT scan to include the adrenal glands in patients who have a pulmonary tumor. In one study of 110 patients who had pulmonary carcinoma (cell type not specified), adrenal masses were identified in 11 (10%); in 5 patients the adrenal glands were the only site of metastasis.[74]

Text continued on p. 359

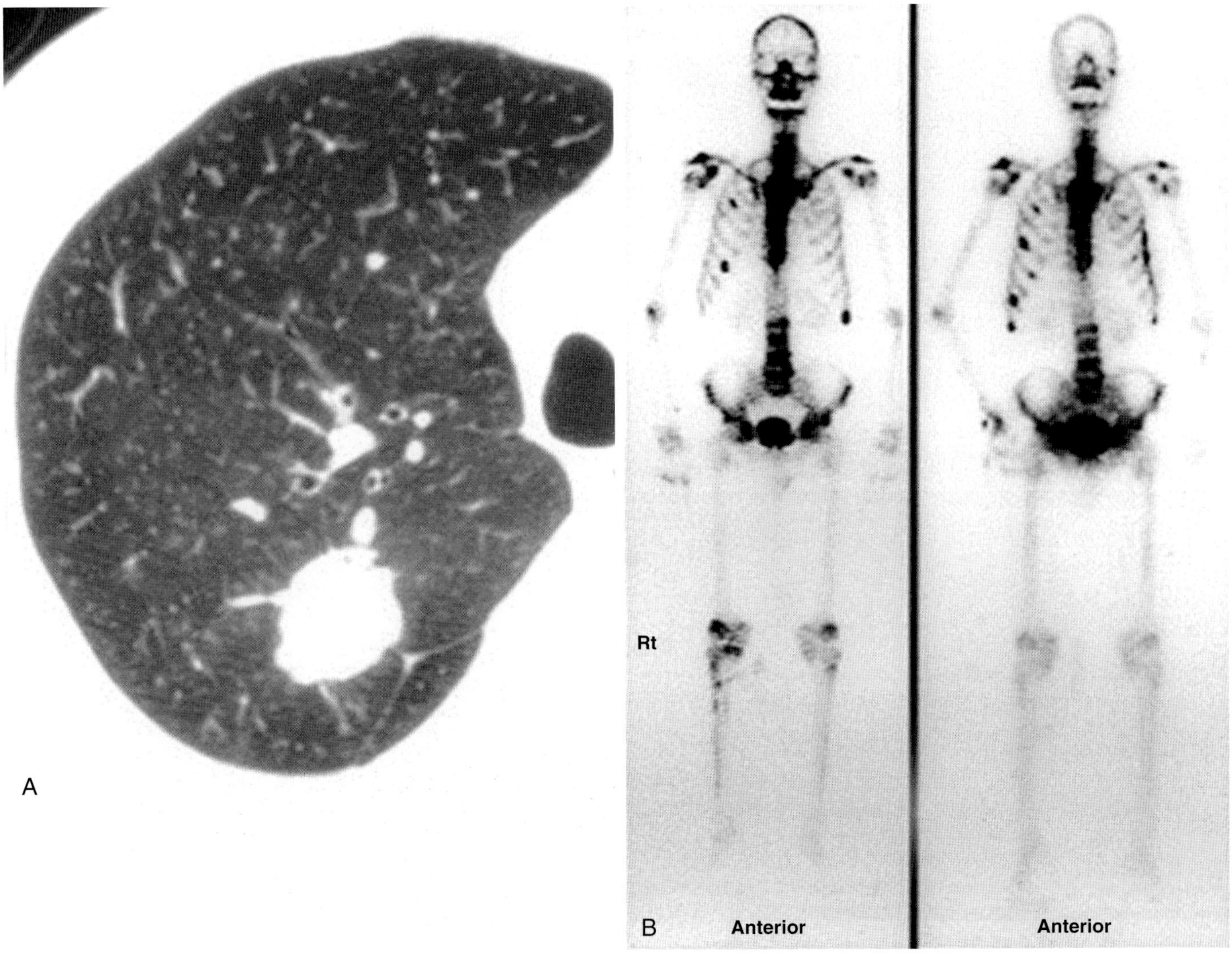

Fig. 18.13 Bone metastasis detected by bone scintigraphy in lung adenocarcinoma. (A) Axial CT scan obtained at level of azygos arch shows a 2.3-cm right upper lobe nodule with fissural retraction. (B) Initial *(left)* and 3-month follow-up *(right)* whole-body bone scintigraphs show progressive osseous metastases, most numerous in the ribs.

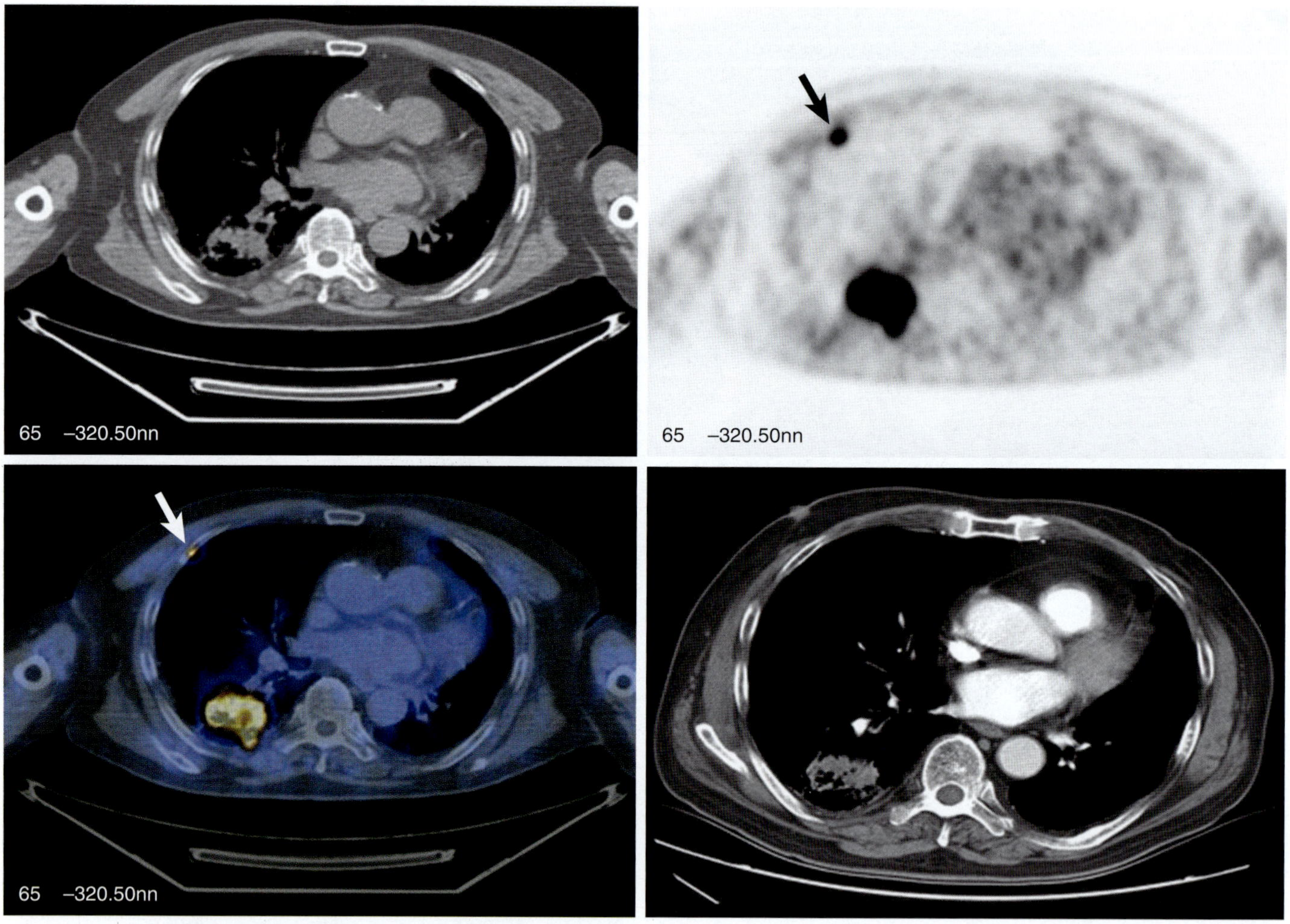

Fig. 18.14 Rib metastasis detected at integrated PET-CT but not at CT in large cell carcinoma. PET and integrated PET-CT images show increased FDG uptake *(arrows)* in an anterior right rib, which is not apparent on the CT image alone.

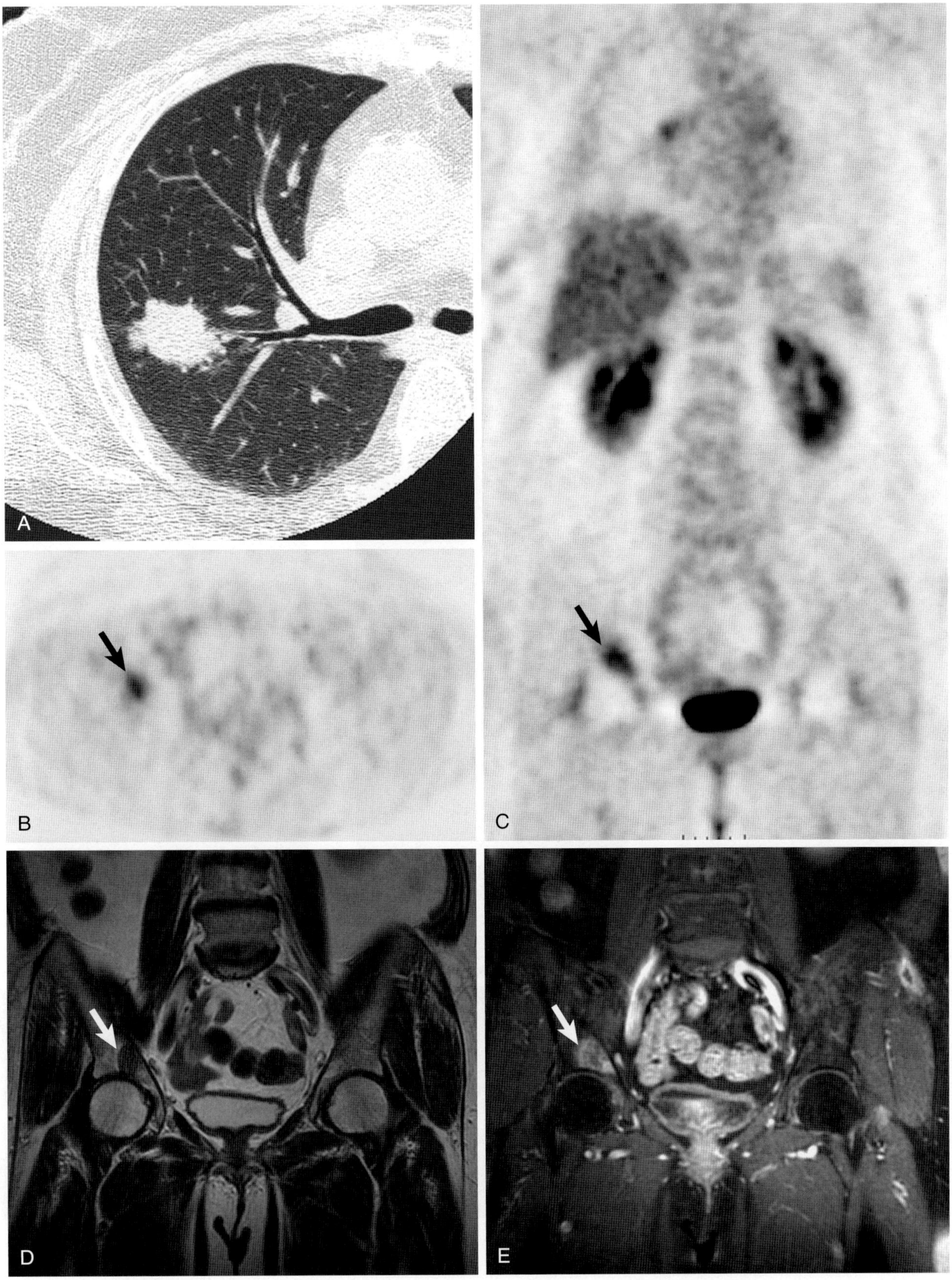

Fig. 18.15 Pelvic bone metastasis detected at integrated PET-CT but not at CT in lung adenocarcinoma. (A) Axial CT scan shows a right upper lobe nodule with lobulated and spiculated margins. Axial (B) and coronal (C) PET images show increased FDG uptake *(arrows)* in the right ilium. (D) Coronal T2W MR image shows a low–signal intensity lesion *(arrow)* in the right ilium. (E) Enhanced T1W MR image shows a high–signal intensity lesion *(arrow)* with trabeculation. MRI suggested the possibility of both metastasis or hemangioma, but bone biopsy demonstrated metastatic adenocarcinoma.

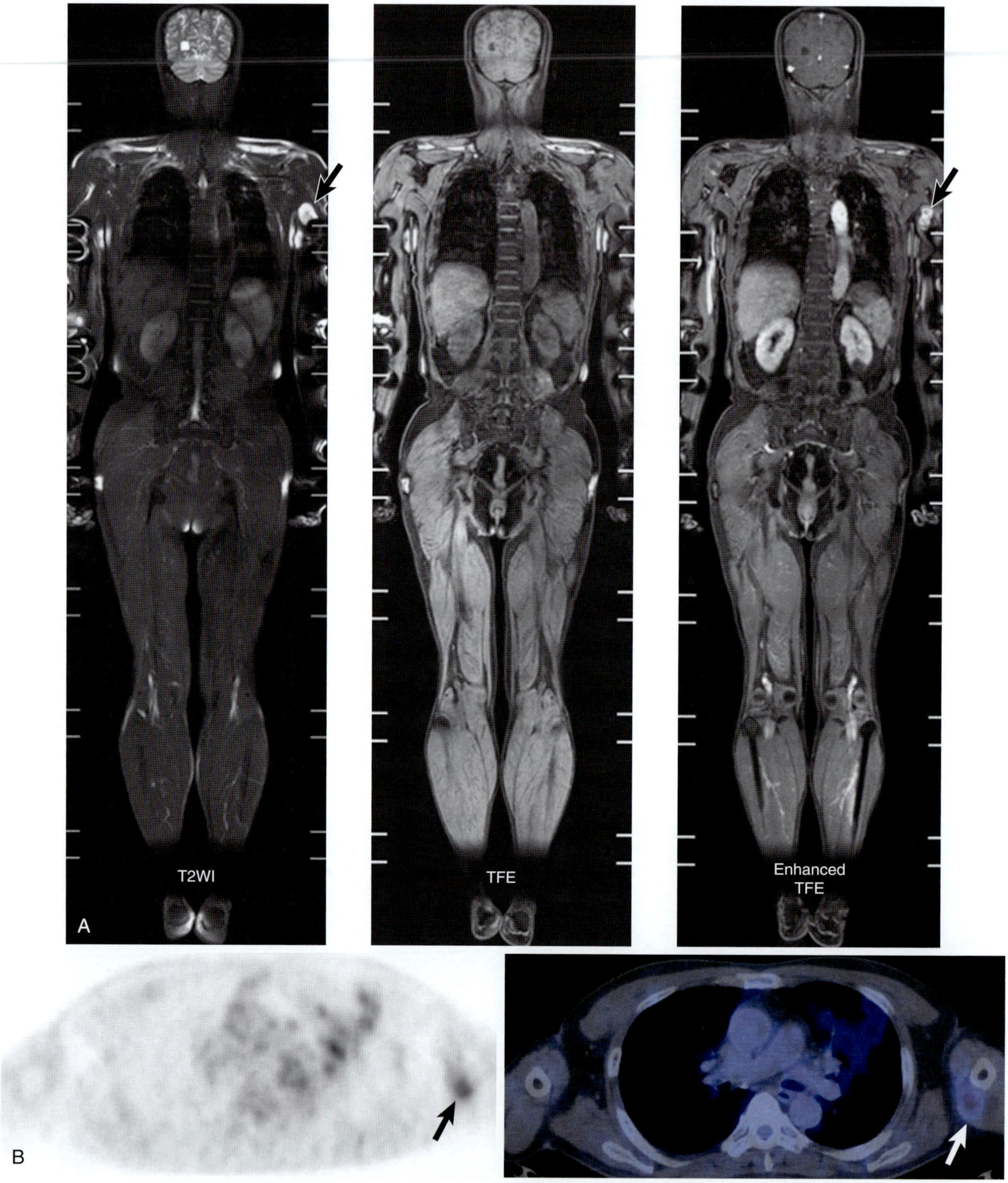

Fig. 18.16 Left arm metastasis in pulmonary adenocarcinoma. (A) Coronal whole-body MR images show metastatic soft tissue lesion (*arrows* in T2WI and enhanced T1W TFE images) in left axillary area. T2W is a T2-weighted image; T1W TFE is a T1-weighted turbo-field-echo image. (B) Whole-body PET-CT image shows increased FDG uptake in the left arm lesion *(arrows)* (maximum standardized uptake value, 3.0) at the same area observed on whole-body MR images.

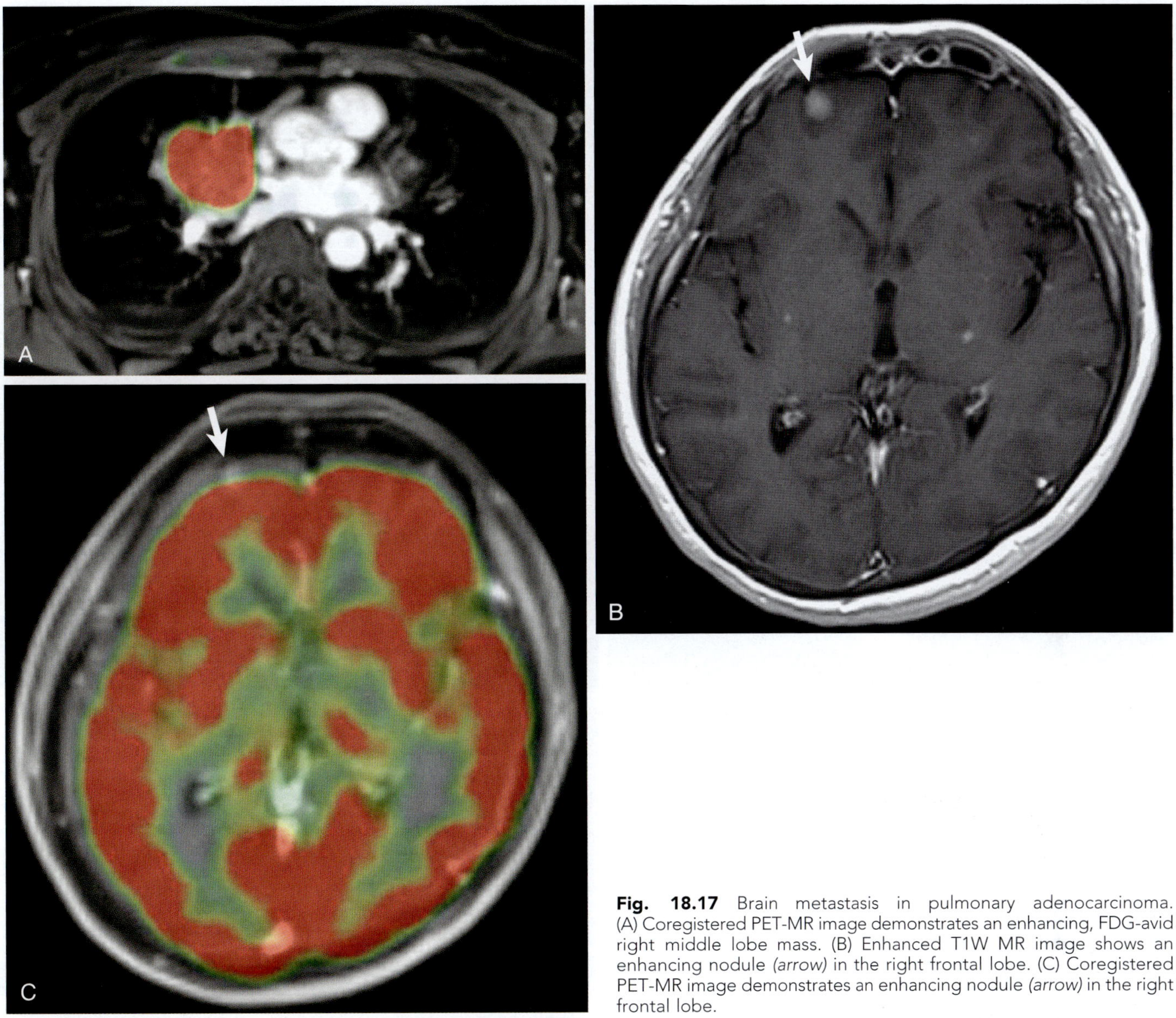

Fig. 18.17 Brain metastasis in pulmonary adenocarcinoma. (A) Coregistered PET-MR image demonstrates an enhancing, FDG-avid right middle lobe mass. (B) Enhanced T1W MR image shows an enhancing nodule *(arrow)* in the right frontal lobe. (C) Coregistered PET-MR image demonstrates an enhancing nodule *(arrow)* in the right frontal lobe.

The other main differential diagnosis of an adrenal mass in a patient who has pulmonary carcinoma is a nonfunctioning adenoma. The most helpful diagnostic features on CT scan for distinguishing between a metastasis and an adenoma are tumor size and attenuation value. Lesions 1 cm or less in diameter are more likely to be adenomas, whereas lesions 3 cm or larger usually are metastases (Fig. 18.18). A more reliable distinction is obtained by measuring the attenuation of the mass on an unenhanced CT scan: Adrenal adenomas typically have homogeneous low attenuation, whereas metastases have high attenuation values. A meta-analysis of 10 studies to determine an optimal threshold for differentiating benign from malignant lesions yielded a sensitivity of 71% and a specificity of 98% for characterizing adrenal masses with a threshold of 10 HUs.[75] Based on the data in the literature prior to 2000, one group of investigators has shown that unenhanced CT with a 10-HU threshold is currently the most cost-effective method for distinguishing adrenal adenoma from metastasis in patients with newly diagnosed pulmonary carcinoma.[76] On adrenal dynamic CT the relative percentage washout value can be calculated, and lesions of greater than 50% relative percentage washout are benign (Fig. 18.19). Ninety-nine (98%) of 101 lesions were correctly characterized as benign or malignant with this technique. Therefore calculation of relative percentage washout on dynamic and delayed enhanced CT scans is a highly specific test for adrenal lesion characterization, thus reducing the need for, and possibly obviating, follow-up imaging or biopsy.[77]

Several groups of investigators have assessed the diagnostic accuracy of MRI in the detection of adrenal metastases and in their distinction from adenomas. The results of the initial studies showed considerable overlap between the MRI signal characteristics of malignant and benign lesions on conventional spin-echo and gradient-recalled echo images. The ability to distinguish metastases from adenomas has improved considerably with the introduction of more sophisticated MRI techniques, such as fat saturation, chemical-shift, and dynamic gadolinium-enhanced MRI.[78–82]

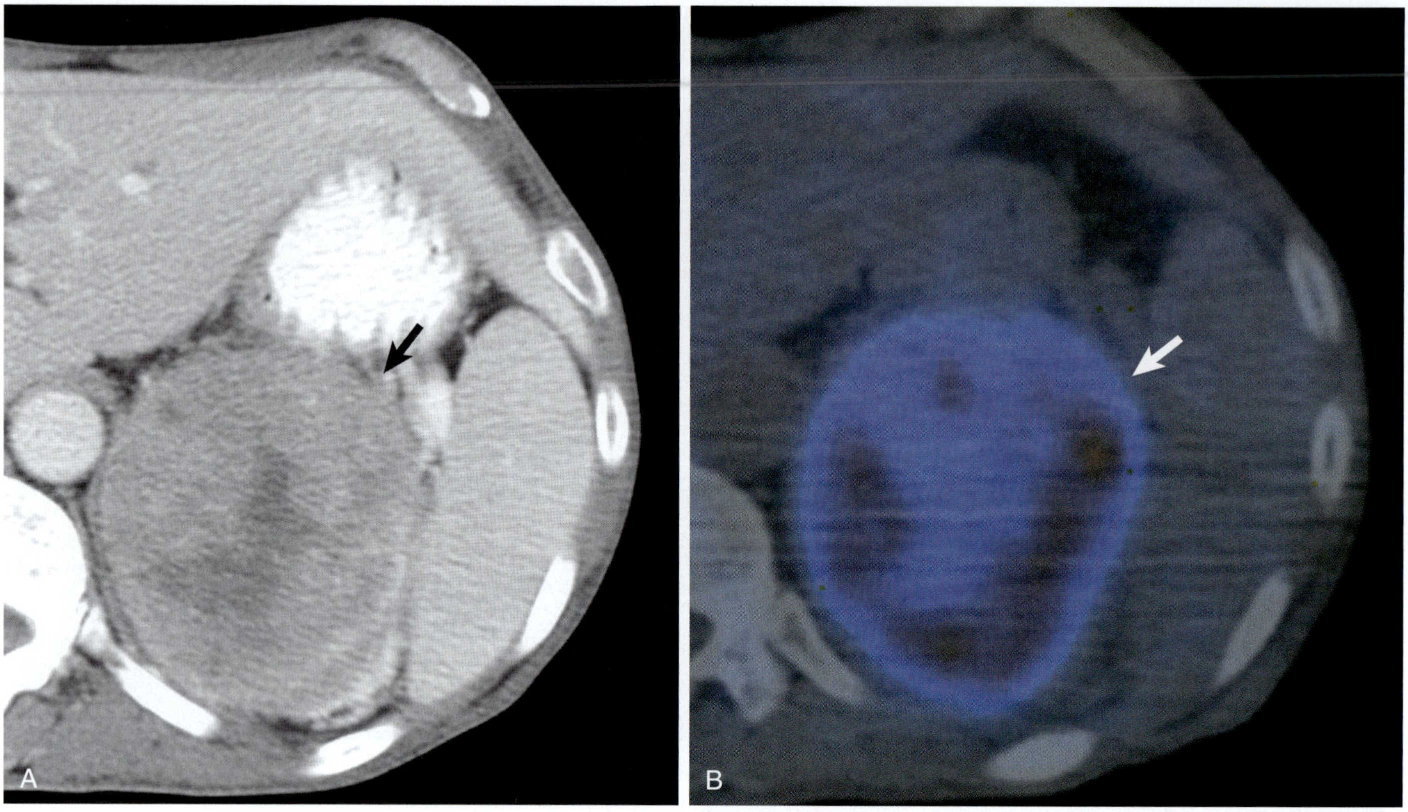

Fig. 18.18 Adrenal metastasis in pulmonary adenocarcinoma. (A) Contrast-enhanced CT scan shows a 10-cm left adrenal mass *(arrow)* with central low attenuation. (B) Integrated FDG–PET-CT scan shows increased uptake (maximum standardized value, 12.8) in the left adrenal mass *(arrow)*.

On spin-echo MRI performed using the fat-saturation technique, adrenal adenomas have a characteristic hyperintense rim; in one study of 48 patients, this sign was seen in 26 of 28 (92%) adenomas and in only 1 of 20 (5%) metastases.[79] One group of investigators correlated the MRI findings with histologic results in 114 patients with 134 adrenal masses. Chemical-shift and dynamic gadolinium-enhanced MRI had a sensitivity of 91% and a specificity of 94% in distinguishing benign and malignant adrenal masses.[82] In chemical-shift MRI the percentage signal intensity decrease is calculated, normalizing signal intensity to the kidney or the spleen parenchyma. All malignant nodules showed less than 20% signal intensity decrease, even if they had high attenuation (>10 HUs) at CT[83] (Fig. 18.20).

According to a recent study,[84] FDG-PET showed excellent diagnostic performance in differentiating 50 adrenal lesions detected on CT or MRI, with a sensitivity of 100%, a specificity of 94%, and an accuracy of 96%. Because FDG-PET has the additional advantage of evaluating the primary lesions as well as metastases, it can be cost effective and the modality of choice for the characterization of adrenal lesions, especially in patients with malignancy. Integrated PET-CT improves the performance of ^{18}F-FDG-PET alone in discriminating benign from malignant adrenal lesions in oncology patients (Fig. 18.21). In one study of 175 adrenal masses in 150 patients,[85] PET data alone using a standardized uptake value cutoff of 3.1 yielded a sensitivity, specificity, and accuracy of 99% (67 of 68 nodules), 92% (98 of 107), and 94% (165 of 175), respectively. For combined PET-CT data, the sensitivity, specificity, and accuracy were 100% (68 of 68 nodules), 98% (105 of 107), and 99% (173 of 175), respectively. Specificity was significantly higher for PET-CT ($P < .01$).

KEY POINTS: M STAGING

- The most widely used imaging techniques to investigate patients who have possible extrathoracic metastases are CT (to assess the adrenal glands and liver), MRI (to assess the brain and adrenals), and radionuclide bone scans (to identify skeletal metastases).
- The most helpful diagnostic features on CT scan for distinguishing between adrenal metastasis and adenoma are tumor size and attenuation value. Lesions 1 cm or less in diameter are more likely to be adenomas, whereas lesions 3 cm or larger are usually metastases. Lesions with attenuation values less than 10 Hounsfield units (HUs) on unenhanced CT are adenomas.
- Dynamic CT (analyzing wash-in and washout characteristics), chemical-shift MRI, and PET imaging have an accuracy of greater than 90% in characterizing adrenal lesions in patients with an NSCLC.
- Whole-body PET imaging has the advantage over other imaging modalities of showing not only adrenal metastases but also other metastases that may not be apparent on CT, MRI, or bone scintigraphy.
- Recent advances in scanner technology and image registration have enabled whole-body MRI and PET-MRI. Diagnostic accuracy of PET-MRI with signal intensity assessment (98.6%) was significantly higher than that of whole-body PET-MRI without signal intensity assessment (91.4%) and integrated PET-CT imaging (90.7%)

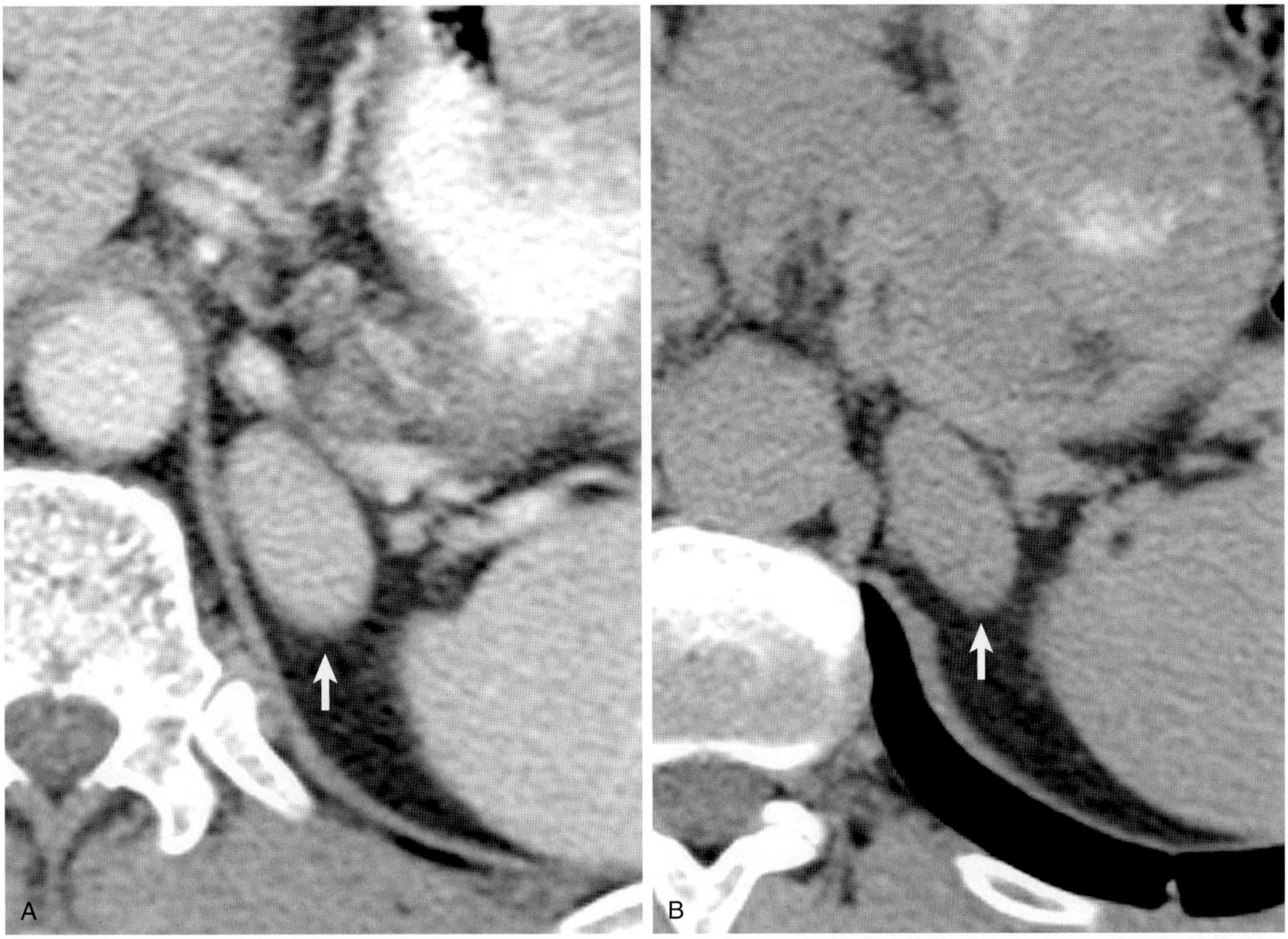

Fig. 18.19 Adrenal adenoma showing high percentage of washout in non–small cell lung carcinoma. Early (A) and delayed (B) contrast-enhanced adrenal CT scans show a 3.4-cm, ovoid mass *(arrows)* in the left adrenal gland. Percentage of washout value is calculated as 68%, suggesting benign adrenal adenoma.

STAGING FOR LUNG CANCERS WITH MULTIPLE PULMONARY SITES OF INVOLVEMENT

The seventh edition of the TNM classification for lung cancer contained some ambiguity with respect to the classification of lung cancer with multiple pulmonary sites of involvement. To provide better clarity for the eighth edition of the TNM classification, the IASLC project defined four patterns associated with multiple pulmonary sites of lung cancer: synchronous primary lung cancers, primary lung cancer with a separate tumor nodule (intrapulmonary metastases), multifocal lung cancer presenting as multiple nodules with ground-glass/lepidic features, and diffuse pneumonic-type adenocarcinoma.[7] Proposed recommendations for TNM classification are as follows: synchronous primary lung cancers are classified with a T, N, and M category for each tumor; separate tumor nodules result in a T3, T4, or M1a category depending on the separate nodule's location relative to the primary tumor; multifocal ground glass/lepidic feature tumors are classified by the highest T lesion, with the number or *m* for multiple in parentheses (number/*m*) and an N and M category for all tumor nodules collectively; and for pneumonic-type adenocarcinoma, the T component is classified by size or as T3 if in one lobe, as T4 if in two ipsilateral lobes, and M1a if in contralateral lobes, with a single N and M category for all sites of pulmonary involvement collectively.[7]

TUMOR-NODE-METASTISIS STAGING FOR SMALL CELL LUNG CANCER

Early staging systems for SCLC divided them into two subgroups: limited and extensive. Limited disease is characterized by tumors confined to one hemithorax, although local extension and ipsilateral or supraclavicular nodes could also be present if they could be encompassed in the same radiation portal as the primary tumor. All other cases are classified as extensive disease. However, when the seventh edition of TNM classification was published in 2009, it was recommended to favor the TNM classification for staging of patients with SCLC.

Analysis of the new database of IASLC suggested that clinical and pathologic TNM staging in patients with SCLC has a prognostic value, and the use of proposed T, N, M descriptors for NSCLC is recommended in patients with SCLC.[8,86] However, for M descriptors, it remains uncertain whether survival differences in patients with single-site metastasis in the brain simply

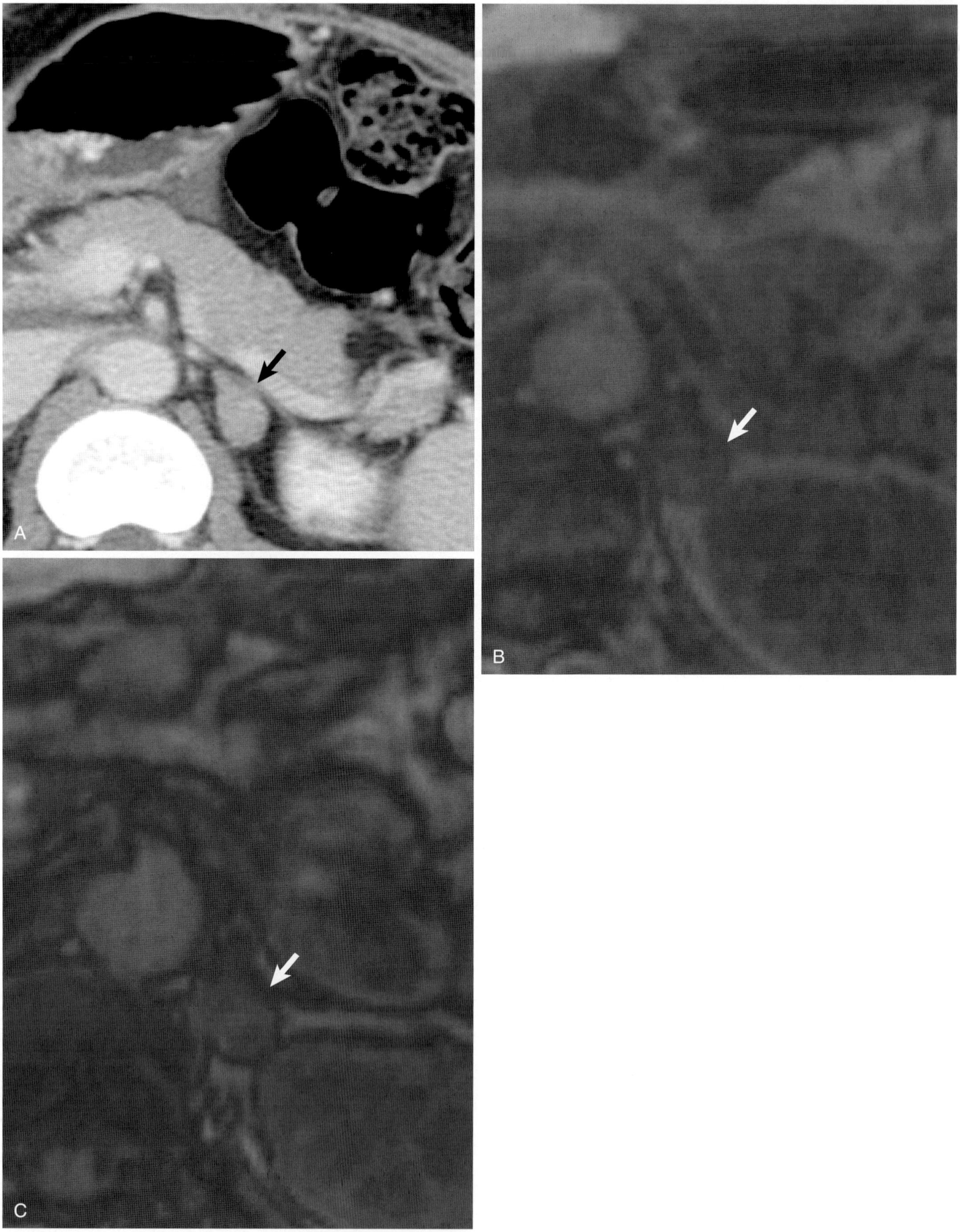

Fig. 18.20 Metastatic adrenal nodule on chemical-shift MRI in lung adenocarcinoma. (A) Enhanced axial CT scan shows a homogeneously enhancing nodule *(arrow)* in the left adrenal gland. (B) and (C) Chemical-shift MR images show no change of signal intensity in the adrenal nodule *(arrows)* between in-phase (B) and out-of-phase (C) images.

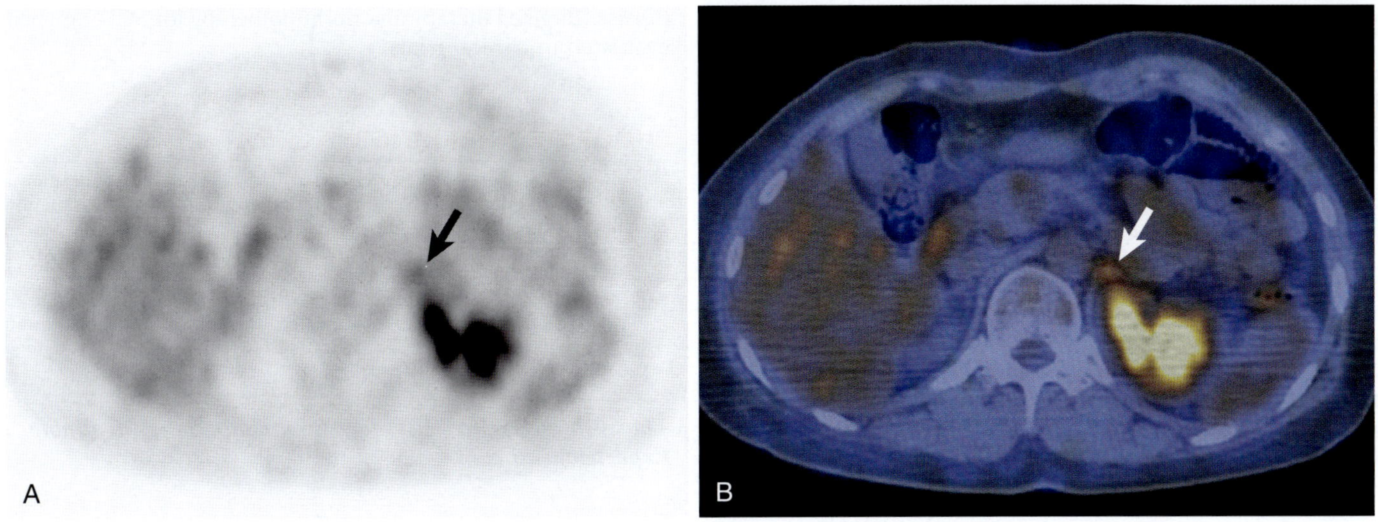

Fig. 18.21 False-negative interpretation PET image, but true positive interpretation with integrated PET-CT in a 33-year-old woman with adrenal metastasis from lung adenocarcinoma. (A) FDG-PET demonstrates increased uptake *(arrow)* in the left adrenal gland area with maximum standardized uptake value of 3.5. Uptake was regarded as benign by PET alone because the uptake was interpreted as being in the left kidney. (B) On integrated PET-CT image, the uptake *(arrow)* corresponds to the left adrenal gland, thus enabling a correct interpretation as positive uptake (uptake intensity is equal to that of liver).

reflect better treatment options rather than better survival based on anatomic extent of disease.

Synopsis of Treatment Options

NON–SMALL CELL LUNG CANCER

For stage I to IIIA disease, complete surgical resection remains the most effective therapy for patients who can tolerate surgery. In many clinical centers, induction chemotherapy with or without radiation therapy is given prior to surgery, particularly for those with stage IIB and IIIA disease, to reduce tumor burden and increase the probability of achieving a tumor-free resection margin.[87] The type of surgical resection is dependent on tumor size and location. Lobectomy or pneumonectomy is usually performed with en bloc resection of locally invaded chest wall structures and sampling or removal of all accessible mediastinal lymph nodes.[33] Sublobar resections (segmentectomy or nonanatomic wedge resection) are sometimes performed for patients with small, peripherally located, incidentally or screen-detected lung cancer, particularly in patients with multiple lesions and/or poor pulmonary reserve. Stereotactic body radiation therapy and image-guided thermal ablation are treatment options for poor surgical candidates with early-stage disease without nodal involvement. In selected stage IV patients with oligometastases in the brain or adrenal glands, resection of metastatic lesions has been shown to improve survival.[87] Cisplatin-based adjuvant chemotherapy is the standard of care for resected stage II and IIIA NSCLC and sometimes also offered to patients with resected stage IB disease. Adjuvant radiation therapy is often given for resected stage III disease. Platinum-based regimens are the first-line therapy for locally advanced (i.e., stage III) or metastatic (i.e., stage IV) NSCLC because they provide modest 5% to 13% improvements in 5-year survival rates.[88]

More recently, molecularly targeted therapy has revolutionized the care of lung cancer patients. Tyrosine kinase inhibitors (such as gefitinib and erlotinib) against the epidermal growth factor receptors (EGFR) that are overexpressed on the cell surface of NSCLCs carrying EFGR mutations have been shown to result in higher response and longer progression-free survival compared with chemotherapy treatment in the setting of advanced-stage disease. The EGFR mutation is more commonly found in women, nonsmokers, and East Asians. Similarly, in patients with tumors harboring translocations of anaplastic lymphoma kinase (ALK), treatment with crizotinib (an ALK inhibitor) has been found to be very effective.[89] Because of the benefits of targeted therapy, it is now recommended that all resected adenocarcinomas and mixed lung cancers with an adenocarcinoma component should undergo EGFR and ALK testing. In addition, EGFR mutation and ALK rearrangement testing should also be performed on biopsy specimens at the time of diagnosis in patients who present with advanced-stage disease and in those with recurrence or progression who were not previously tested.[90]

Immunotherapy modulates the patient's immune system to fight cancer. Programmed death-1 (PD-1) inhibitors disrupt the immune checkpoint interaction to enable the host immune system to destroy tumors. Nivolumab and pembrolizumab are two PD-1 inhibitors approved as second-line treatment of advanced-stage NSCLC.[89] In patients treated with immunotherapy agents, the response to treatment may be delayed. Pseudoprogression or transient enlargement of responding tumor can occur, which is postulated to be due to infiltration of the tumor by immune cells.

In patients with multiple persistent pulmonary nodules suspected to represent multifocal synchronous adenocarcinomas, the timing of follow-up imaging and tissue sampling is usually based on the most suspicious-appearing lesion(s). The designation of the most suspicious lesion is not based purely on size but instead should take into consideration rate of growth and nodule features, such as size, attenuation, and margin. Similarly, the treatment is usually driven by the stage, with the T category determined by the highest level T lesion.[91]

SMALL CELL LUNG CANCER

Small cell lung cancer is generally believed to represent a systemic disease at the time of diagnosis and as such is not considered to be a surgically resectable disease. In a minority of cases where SCLC manifests as a solitary pulmonary nodule without identifiable nodal or distant metastases, surgical resection can be performed.

Limited-stage SCLC can be treated with platinum-based chemotherapy and thoracic and prophylactic cranial radiation with 20% to 25% long-term survival. Extensive stage disease is usually treated with combination chemotherapy to prolong survival and improve quality of life. Thoracic radiation and prophylactic cranial radiation are given to those who respond to chemotherapy. Most patients, particularly patients with extensive disease beyond the thorax, relapse and die of their disease. Targeted therapy and immunotherapy for SCLC are being evaluated in clinical trials.[92]

SUGGESTED READINGS

Nicholson AG, Chansky K, Crowley J, et al. The International Association for the Study of Lung Cancer staging project: proposals for the revision of the clinical and pathologic staging of small cell lung cancer in the forthcoming eighth edition of the TNM classification for lung cancer. *J Thorac Oncol.* 2016;11:300–311.

Rami-Porta R, Bolejack V, Crowley J, et al. The IASLC Lung Cancer Staging Project: proposals for the revisions of the T descriptors in the forthcoming eighth edition of the TNM classification for lung cancer. *J Thorac Oncol.* 2015;10:990–1003.

The full reference list for this chapter is available at ExpertConsult.com.

19 Neuroendocrine Hyperplasia, Pulmonary Tumorlets, and Carcinoid Tumors*

STEPHANE L. DESOUCHES | CHRISTOPHER M. WALKER | JONATHAN H. CHUNG

Neuroendocrine Hyperplasia and Pulmonary Tumorlets

ETIOLOGY, PREVALENCE, AND EPIDEMIOLOGY

Normal lung tissue contains scattered neuroendocrine (Kulchitsky) cells within the bronchial and bronchiolar epithelium. These cells play a role in the detection of hypoxia as well as fetal lung development[1] and may be involved in local epithelial cell growth and regeneration.[2,3] Hyperplasia of these cells can be seen as a response to chronic airway inflammation, such as in patients with emphysema or chronic bronchitis.[4] When no known cause can be identified, this hyperplasia is designated diffuse idiopathic pulmonary neuroendocrine cell hyperplasia (DIPNECH). Extension of hyperplastic neuroendocrine cells beyond the basement membrane is termed a *tumorlet* if the cell mass is less than 5 mm and *carcinoid tumor* if the cell mass is 5 mm or greater in diameter.[5] Neuroendocrine cell hyperplasia and tumorlets may coexist with carcinoid tumors.[2,5–7] In the absence of lung injury (leading to reactive pulmonary neuroendocrine cell hyperplasia), DIPNECH is considered a preinvasive condition that may develop into carcinoid tumors, and imaging follow-up is required.[6]

DIPNECH typically manifests in the fifth to sixth decades of life, with women affected nearly four times as often as men.[4] DIPNECH usually occurs in nonsmokers, but former and current smokers are occasionally affected. Tumorlets also demonstrate a female preponderance (>4 : 1) and are often seen in patients 60 to 70 years old.[4]

In the 2015 update to the World Health Organization (WHO) classification of lung tumors,[8] DIPNECH is classified as a preinvasive lesion. Although the diagnosis remains purely histologic, some authors have proposed the term *DIPNECH syndrome* be used to indicate patients with respiratory symptoms and appropriate imaging findings.[9] Although initially thought to be rare, with few cases described in the literature, DIPNECH is likely an underrecognized condition.

CLINICAL PRESENTATION

Up to half of patients with DIPNECH or tumorlets are asymptomatic, and the diagnosis is made incidentally on chest computed tomography (CT) or surgical lung biopsy performed for other reasons. When patients are symptomatic, they often present with a history of protracted nonproductive cough and/or dyspnea and are often mistakenly diagnosed with asthma.[10,11] Pulmonary function tests may show obstructive or obstructive/restrictive alterations, likely caused by airway obstruction from the hyperplasia as well as constrictive bronchiolitis from peribronchial fibrosis.[2]

PATHOPHYSIOLOGY

Neuroendocrine cell hyperplasia (NECH) is characterized by single, clustered, or linear arrays of Kulchitsky cells confined by the basement membrane.[6] Tumorlets are distinguished by extension beyond the basement membrane. Both of these entities show no mitoses or necrosis per 10 high-power fields on histologic examination.[7] NECH and tumorlets are usually an incidental finding in lung parenchyma scarred by bronchiectasis or other chronic inflammatory processes.

As stated earlier, constrictive bronchiolitis in patients is secondary to submucosal fibrosis of affected airways in regions with and regions without tumorlets and NECH.[2]

IMAGING FINDINGS

Radiography

Chest radiographs of patients with DIPNECH or pulmonary tumorlets may demonstrate pulmonary micronodules (Fig. 19.1)[7] but are more often normal. Secondary signs of constrictive bronchiolitis, including hyperinflation and attenuation of peripheral pulmonary vasculature, can occasionally be seen.

Computed Tomography

High-resolution CT of the chest with inspiratory and expiratory imaging will demonstrate multifocal pulmonary micronodules with or without associated mosaic attenuation or air trapping.[10] These micronodules are typically in a centrilobular distribution and can be ground-glass or solid in attenuation.[4] Nodules less than 5 mm correspond to carcinoid tumorlets, whereas nodules 5 mm or greater represent carcinoid tumors at histopathologic examination. Asymptomatic patients are more likely to demonstrate micronodules without significant mosaic attenuation as the extent of mosaic attenuation often correlates with physiologic airflow obstruction.[4,5] Bronchial wall thickening with or without bronchiectasis is occasionally seen. Nodular bronchial wall thickening is the most direct radiologic-pathologic correlation of NECH, corresponding to the histologic findings of intraluminal protrusion of the proliferating cells. There are no imaging features to distinguish NECH from pulmonary tumorlets. This distinction

*The editors and the publisher would like to thank Drs. Nestor L. Müller and C. Isabela Silva Müller for contributing material on this topic to the prior edition of this work. It has served as the foundation for the current chapter.

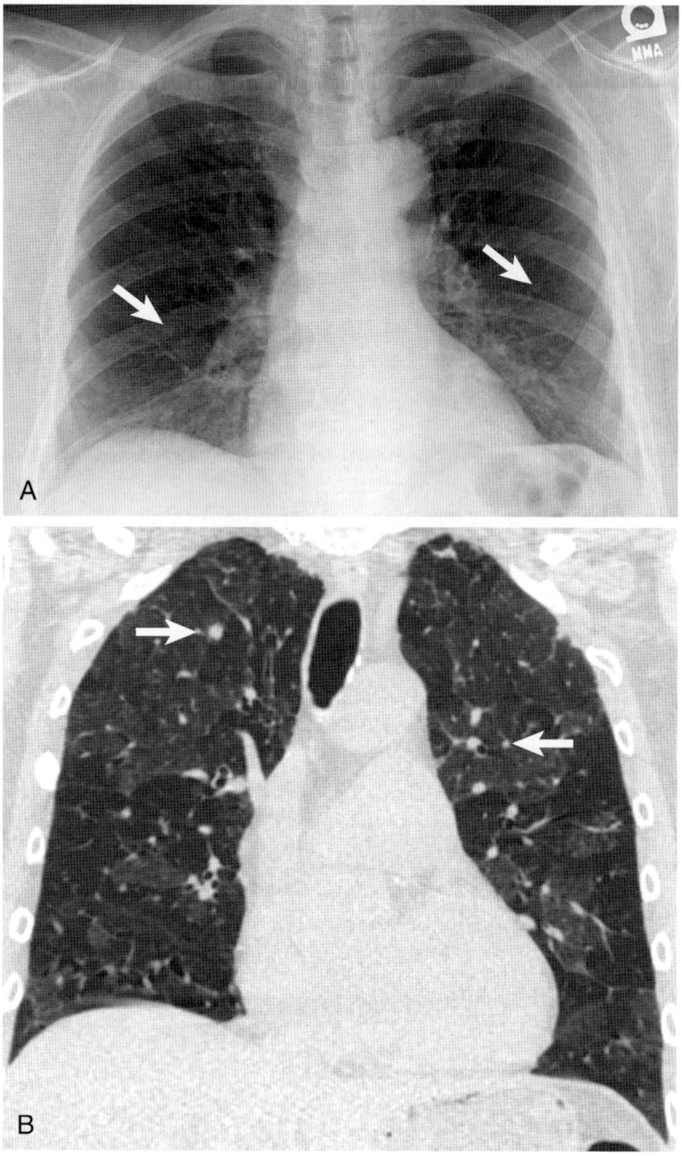

Fig. 19.1 Diffuse idiopathic pulmonary neuroendocrine cell hyperplasia. (A) Posteroanterior chest radiograph shows multiple small nodules *(arrows)*. (B) Coronal CT shows small pulmonary nodules measuring 2–8 mm *(arrows)*. Note mosaic attenuation from associated constrictive bronchiolitis.

can only currently be made on histology.[2] A recent study, evaluating 30 patients with DIPNECH, proposed nonsurgical diagnostic criteria. These included clinical presentation, pulmonary function, imaging findings on high-resolution CT, findings from transbronchial biopsy, and serum markers such as elevated serum chromogranin A levels.[11]

DIFFERENTIAL DIAGNOSIS

Detection of one or more pulmonary nodules is a common diagnostic dilemma on CT. The differential considerations for a single nodule or multiple pulmonary nodules include infectious, inflammatory, and neoplastic etiologies. The diagnosis of DIPNECH may be suggested based upon typical imaging findings, mosaic attenuation of the lung parenchyma on inspiratory imaging (Fig. 19.2), and air trapping on expiratory imaging.

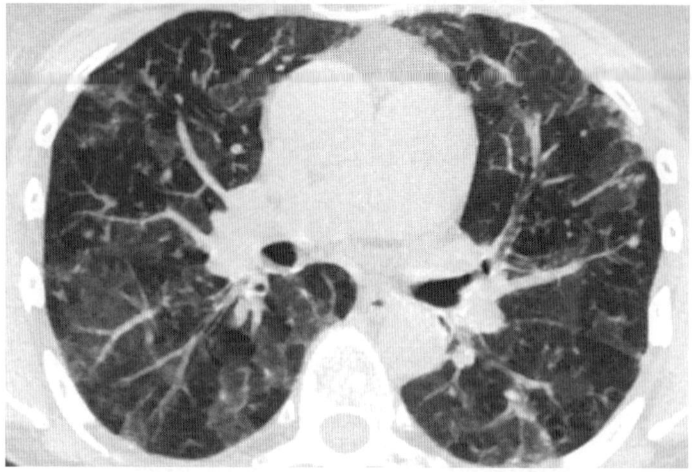

Fig. 19.2 Diffuse idiopathic pulmonary neuroendocrine cell hyperplasia. Maximum-intensity projection (MIP) axial CT accentuates the mosaic attenuation and small pulmonary nodules. MIP imaging can be very useful for evaluating the extent of disease.

Definitive diagnosis, however, requires open lung or thoracoscopic biopsy (Fig. 19.3).[5]

SYNOPSIS OF TREATMENT OPTIONS

Asymptomatic patients are usually managed conservatively, with a good long-term prognosis of 83% survival at 5 years. Long-term imaging follow-up is recommended to exclude nodule growth, development of carcinoid tumors, or metastatic disease.[5] Patients presenting with worsening lung function can be managed more aggressively, with some showing a response to steroids, interferon-α, or chemotherapeutic agents.[10] The use of somatostatin receptor analogues (given the neuroendocrine origin of cells) has shown good results with limited side effects.[11–13]

KEY POINTS: NEUROENDOCRINE HYPERPLASIA AND PULMONARY TUMORLETS

- Neuroendocrine cell hyperplasia represents proliferation of Kulchitsky cells within the bronchial and bronchiolar epithelium.
- Pulmonary tumorlets are nodular proliferations of these same cells with extension beyond the basement membrane. By definition, they measure less than 5 mm in diameter; if 5 mm or greater, they are referred to as carcinoid tumors.
- Most patients are asymptomatic; however, when symptoms are present, they are nonspecific and are most commonly a history of protracted nonproductive cough and/or dyspnea that is often initially mistaken for asthma.
- Chest radiographs are predominantly normal but may show increased lung volumes.
- Inspiratory CT may show mosaic attenuation (usually in symptomatic patients), and expiratory CT may show air trapping.
- New WHO classification categorizes diffuse idiopathic pulmonary neuroendocrine cell hyperplasia as a preinvasive entity, and long-term imaging follow-up is recommended to exclude nodule growth, development of carcinoid tumors, or metastatic disease.

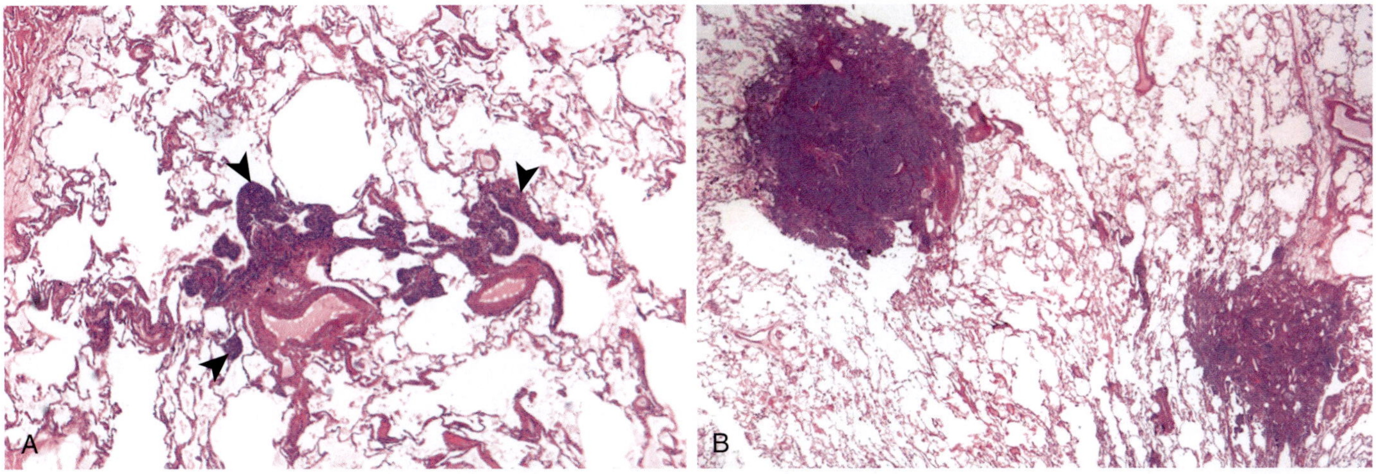

Fig. 19.3 Diffuse idiopathic pulmonary neuroendocrine cell hyperplasia. (A) Lung biopsy specimen shows focal neuroendocrine cell proliferation *(arrowheads)* in the bronchovascular sheath. (B) Histologic specimen from another area shows carcinoid tumorlets. The patient was a 72-year-old woman with diffuse idiopathic pulmonary neuroendocrine cell hyperplasia with multiple pulmonary tumorlets and carcinoid tumors and constrictive bronchiolitis. *(Courtesy Dr. John English, Department of Pathology, Vancouver General Hospital, Vancouver, Canada.)*

Typical and Atypical Carcinoid Tumors

ETIOLOGY, PREVALENCE, AND EPIDEMIOLOGY

The respiratory tract is the second most common location for carcinoid tumors, accounting for 10% to 30% of carcinoids.[14,15] Pulmonary carcinoids have shown an increase in prevalence relative to other primary sources over the past few decades.[15] Carcinoid tumors constitute about 1% to 2% of all primary lung malignancies.[6,16,17] As noted previously, carcinoid tumors represent an extension of the proliferative neuroendocrine cells within the bronchial epithelium beyond the basement membrane, with the cell mass measuring 5 mm or greater in diameter. Carcinoid tumors are further subdivided into typical (84%–90%) and atypical (10%–16%) types. Typical carcinoid tumors demonstrate a nearly 1 : 1 male to female ratio, whereas atypical carcinoid tumors have a 2 : 1 female predominance.[18] Although lung inflammation secondary to smoking has been correlated with atypical carcinoid development, no such association has been seen with the more common typical carcinoid tumor. Typical carcinoid tumors have a mean age of presentation of 46 years,[7,19,20] whereas patients with atypical carcinoid tumors are typically 50 to 60 years old.[14,20] Carcinoid tumors are the most common primary pulmonary neoplasm in children and adolescents.

CLINICAL PRESENTATION

Centrally located carcinoid tumors usually manifest with symptoms, most commonly cough and hemoptysis.[8] Patients present less commonly with wheeze, recurrent infection, chest pain, dyspnea, and constitutional symptoms. Peripheral tumors are usually asymptomatic and are discovered incidentally because of a CT performed for other reasons.[10]

Despite the neuroendocrine cell origin of these neoplasms, paraneoplastic syndromes are rare.[8] Cushing syndrome is reported in approximately 2% of bronchial carcinoids and manifests with hypokalemia and elevation of adrenocorticotropic hormone.[14,21] Although carcinoid syndrome can be seen when gastrointestinal carcinoid tumors metastasize to the liver and release serotonin into the systemic blood system, this is extremely rare with pulmonary carcinoids. When patients develop carcinoid syndrome from a pulmonary primary, it is typically in those with metastatic disease to the liver.[19] The carcinoid syndrome is characterized by skin flushing, severe diarrhea, bronchoconstriction, and right-sided valvular disease.

PATHOPHYSIOLOGY

Typical carcinoid tumors are defined as cell masses 5 mm or greater in size that lack necrosis and demonstrate fewer than 2 mitoses per 10 high-power fields (HPFs). Atypical carcinoid tumors are diagnosed when there is cellular necrosis or 2 to 10 mitoses per 10 HPFs.[8] Although diagnosis of these entities is usually evident on hematoxylin-eosin staining, antibodies directed to CD56 or components of the neurosecretory granules, including chromogranin and synaptophysin, can be used in equivocal cases.[22] Carcinoid tumors are typically composed of polygonal cells with eosinophilic cytoplasm and finely granular chromatin most commonly arranged in an organoid or trabecular pattern.[8,10]

No single staining method is diagnostic for differentiating typical from atypical carcinoid tumors. Differentiation of carcinoid from more aggressive neoplasms, such as small cell lung cancer, may be difficult with crushed biopsy specimens. In these cases staining with Ki-67 may be helpful as it assesses proliferation rate and is elevated in small cell lung cancer and large cell neuroendocrine carcinoma.[8,10]

IMAGING FINDINGS

Radiography

Typical and atypical carcinoids share similar imaging features. Most often this is a centrally located well-defined solitary nodule

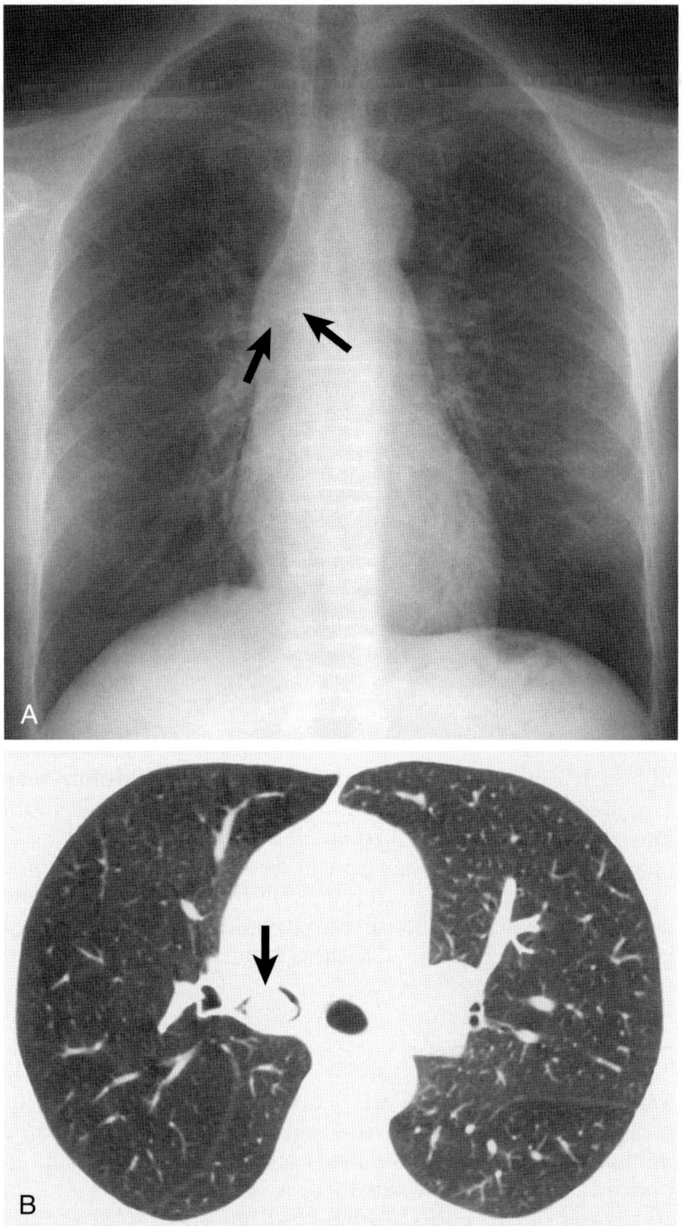

Fig. 19.4 Central typical carcinoid tumor. (A) Posteroanterior chest radiograph shows a tumor in the right main bronchus *(arrows)*. The right lung is slightly smaller than the left and shows decreased vascularity. (B) Axial CT confirms the presence of an intraluminal tumor in the right main bronchus *(arrow)*. Note decreased attenuation and vascularity of the right lung compared with the left lung, as a result of reflex vasoconstriction.

or mass with or without lobular borders in the main (Fig. 19.4), lobar, or segmental bronchi. Tumors range in size from 2 to 5 cm, and calcification within the lesion is infrequently detected on radiography. They frequently cause post–obstructive atelectasis (Fig. 19.5) and/or pneumonia.[7,14,23] Segmental atelectasis or pneumonia may show periodic exacerbations and remissions, likely secondary to the ball-valve mechanism of the central lesion.

Peripheral carcinoid tumors appear as a well-defined solitary nodule or mass with round or oval morphology and possibly slightly lobulated contour (Fig. 19.6).[24] Atypical carcinoid tumors

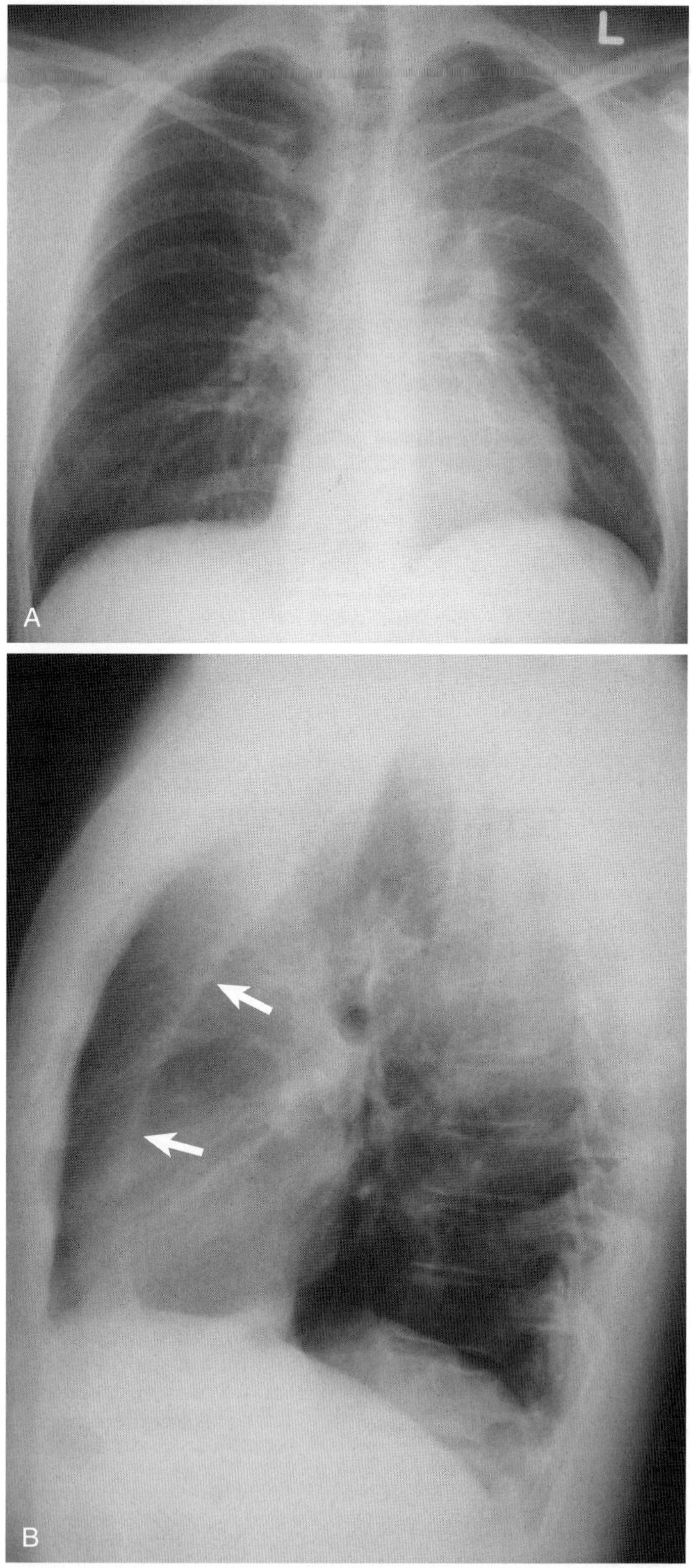

Fig. 19.5 Central carcinoid tumor with obstructive atelectasis of the left upper lobe. (A) Posteroanterior chest radiograph shows poorly defined increased opacity of the left hemithorax associated with superior displacement of the left hilum and elevation of the left hemidiaphragm characteristic of left upper lobe atelectasis. (B) Lateral chest radiograph shows anterior displacement of the left major fissure *(arrows)* and compensatory overinflation of the left lower lobe. The obstructing carcinoid tumor was not visible radiographically.

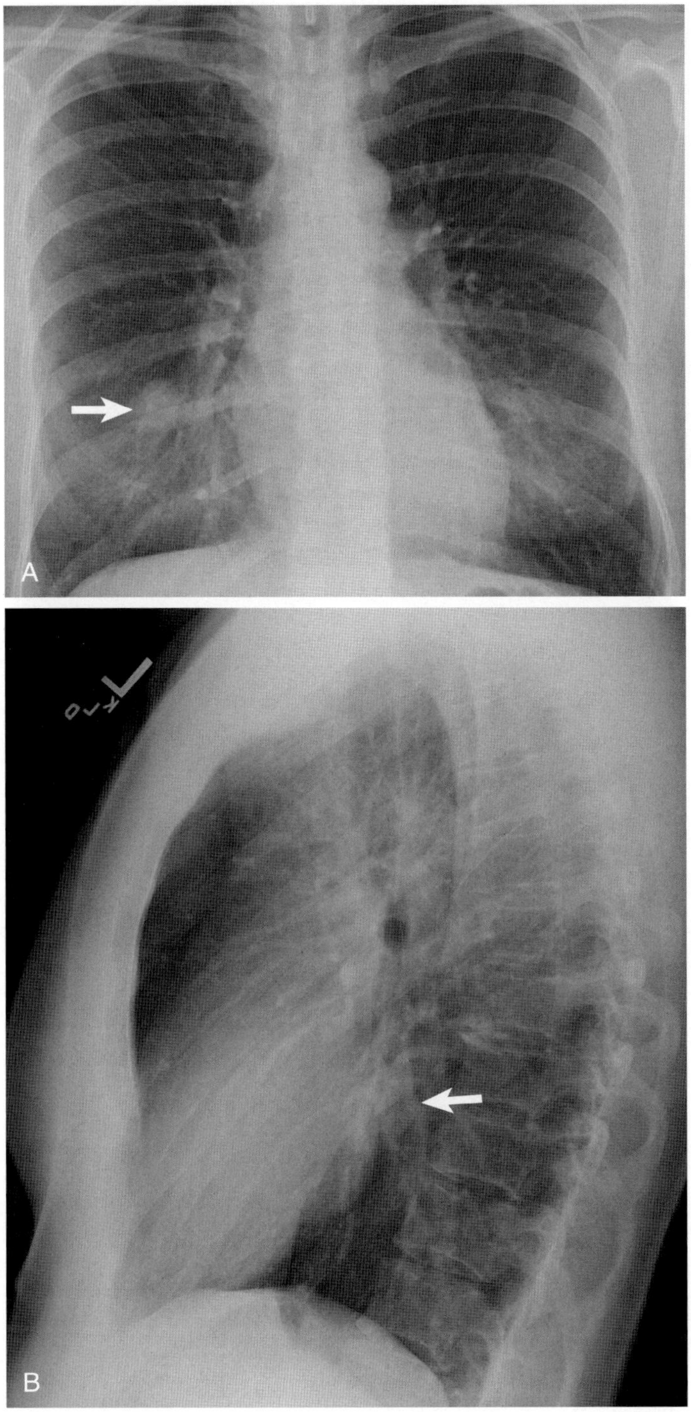

Fig. 19.6 Peripheral typical carcinoid. Posteroanterior (A) and lateral (B) chest radiographs show a 2.5-cm smoothly marginated nodule in the right lower lobe *(arrows)*.

tend to be larger and more peripheral than typical carcinoids. More than 40% of carcinoid tumors are detected incidentally on chest radiography performed for other reasons.[25]

Computed Tomography

Multidetector CT typically demonstrates a central soft tissue nodule with or without distal obstructive atelectasis (Fig. 19.7) or a peripheral solitary nodule (Fig. 19.8). The lesion usually appears as a well-defined slightly lobulated spherical or ovoid nodule or mass. The carcinoid tumor may be completely or partially endoluminal, and CT allows identification of the affected bronchus and any associated signs, such as distal bronchiectasis, mucoid impaction, or air trapping.[10] In some cases carcinoid tumors may demonstrate a "tip of the iceberg" morphology, wherein only a small portion of the carcinoid is intraluminal compared with the bulk of the tumor.[14] Occasionally, the tumor is seen within and surrounding a bronchus, creating the so-called bronchus sign (Fig. 19.9). Transbronchial biopsy is expected to have greater yield in lesions with this sign as a direct path to biopsy is present.[18]

On histology approximately 30% of carcinoids demonstrate internal calcification, which can often be visualized with CT imaging.[14,23] This calcification may be punctate, eccentric (Fig. 19.10), or diffuse.[14,23,26]

Carcinoids are highly vascular and may demonstrate avid homogeneous enhancement on CT after intravenous contrast administration. Atypical carcinoids tend to show more heterogeneous enhancement (Fig. 19.11) compared with typical variants. Additionally, these enhanced studies may help to differentiate the centrally obstructing carcinoid tumor from the adjacent/distal atelectasis or pneumonia.[10]

CT imaging also allows evaluation for mediastinal and hilar lymphadenopathy (seen in 6%–25% of cases) or other evidence of metastatic disease, such as liver, bone (sclerotic metastases) or adrenal gland lesions.[14,27] At presentation regional lymph node metastasis is present in 10% to 15% of typical carcinoids and 40% to 50% of atypical carcinoids.[8] It should be noted that although enlarged thoracic lymph nodes may represent metastatic disease, the enlargement could be secondary to reactive hyperplasia from recurrent or chronic infection.[14]

Magnetic Resonance, Scintigraphy, and Positron Emission Tomography

Magnetic resonance imaging is not typically used in the imaging workup of pulmonary carcinoid. When seen, lesions usually show high T2 signal intensity and intense enhancement during the arterial phase of imaging that is likely secondary to a parasitized blood supply from the bronchial arteries.[28,29]

The neoplastic cells of carcinoid tumors have membrane receptors with high affinity for the neuroregulatory peptide somatostatin.[30] Scintigraphy using a radiolabeled somatostatin analogue (indium-111 [^{111}In]-octreotide) can be used to identify occult primary lesions (Fig. 19.12), although it is more often used for staging and to assess response to therapy.[15,31] Imaging with metaiodobenzylguanidine (MIBG) is considered less sensitive for detection when compared with octreotide.

Typical carcinoid tumors usually do not show increased metabolic activity on fluorodeoxyglucose positron emission tomography (FDG-PET), limiting its usefulness for distinguishing typical carcinoids from benign lesions. Some studies have shown an application of FDG-PET in differentiating typical (Fig. 19.13) from atypical carcinoid tumors (Fig. 19.14). Increased standardized uptake value (SUV) of 6 or greater was shown to have a greater than 95% predictive value for atypical histology.[32]

Recently approved in the United States, ^{68}Ga-Dotatate PET imaging has shown improved spatial resolution and lesion detectability compared with octreotide and MIBG scintigraphy.[33] Specifically in pulmonary imaging, ^{68}gallium-labeled somatostatin

Text continued on p. 374

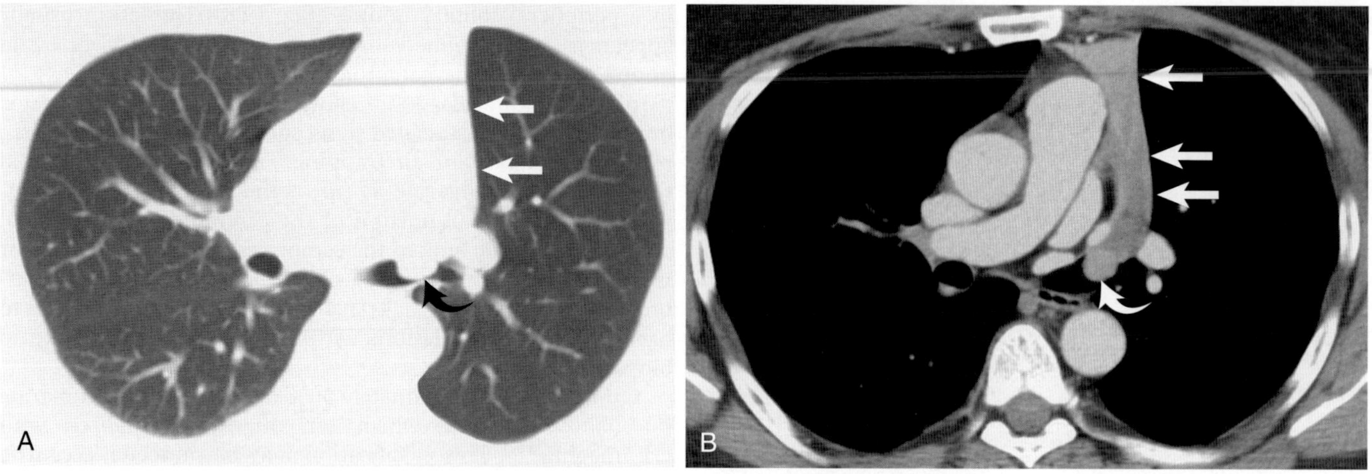

Fig. 19.7 Endobronchial carcinoid tumor with obstructive atelectasis of the left upper lobe. (A) Axial CT shows tumor *(curved arrow)* obstructing the left upper lobe bronchus with associated complete left upper lobe atelectasis *(straight arrows)*. Note anterior and medial shift of the left major fissure *(straight arrows)*, compensatory overinflation of the left lower lobe, and decreased volume and attenuation of the left lung compared with the normal right lung. (B) Contrast-enhanced CT shows enhancing endobronchial tumor *(curved arrow)* and distal atelectasis *(straight arrows)*.

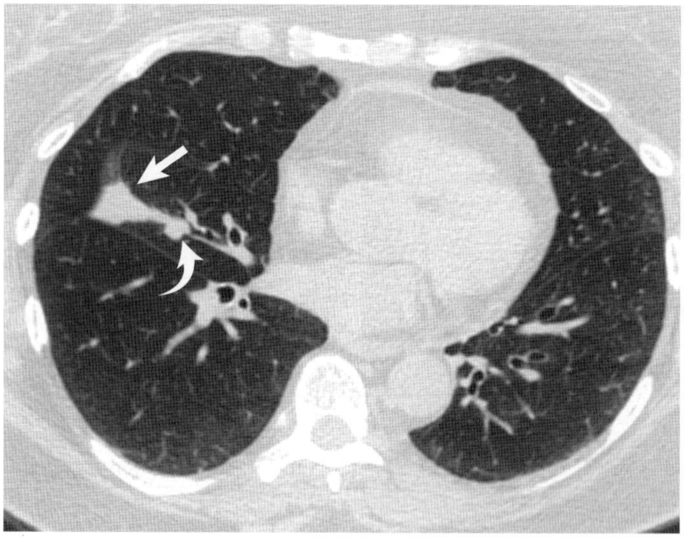

Fig. 19.8 Peripheral endobronchial typical carcinoid. Axial CT shows an endobronchial nodule *(curved arrow)* obstructing a subsegmental bronchus of the right middle lobe, resulting in partial middle lobe atelectasis *(arrow)*.

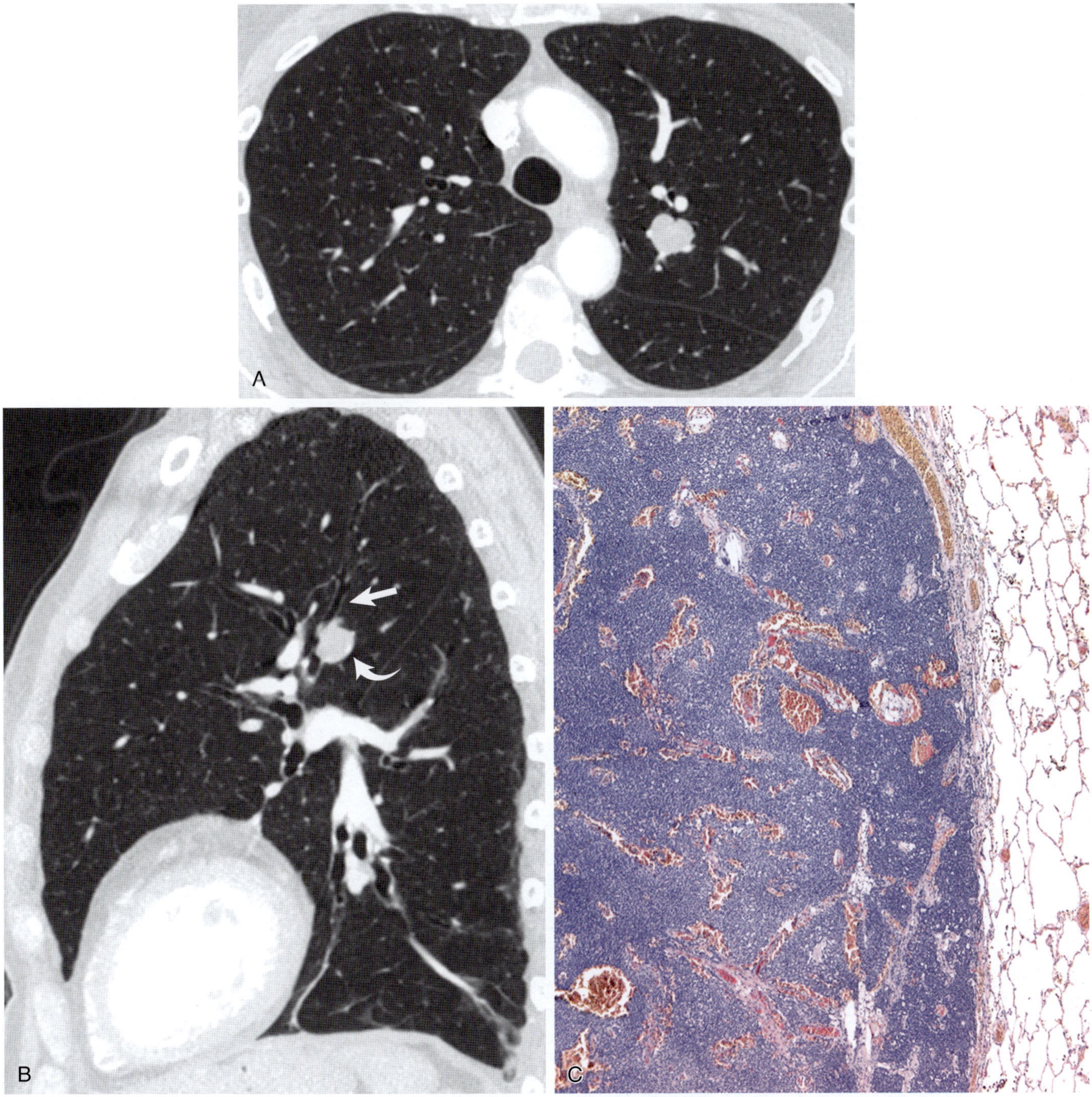

Fig. 19.9 Peripheral carcinoid tumor. Axial (A) and sagittal (B) CT show a small tumor *(curved arrow)* in the left upper lobe and its relationship to a subsegmental bronchus *(arrow)*. (C) Surgical specimen from a different patient shows characteristic features of typical carcinoid: cells with a moderate amount of cytoplasm and nuclei with small nucleoli and scarce mitotic figures. The immunohistochemical panel was positive for the neuroendocrine markers synaptophysin and chromogranin. *(C courtesy Dr. John English, Department of Pathology, Vancouver General Hospital, Vancouver, Canada.)*

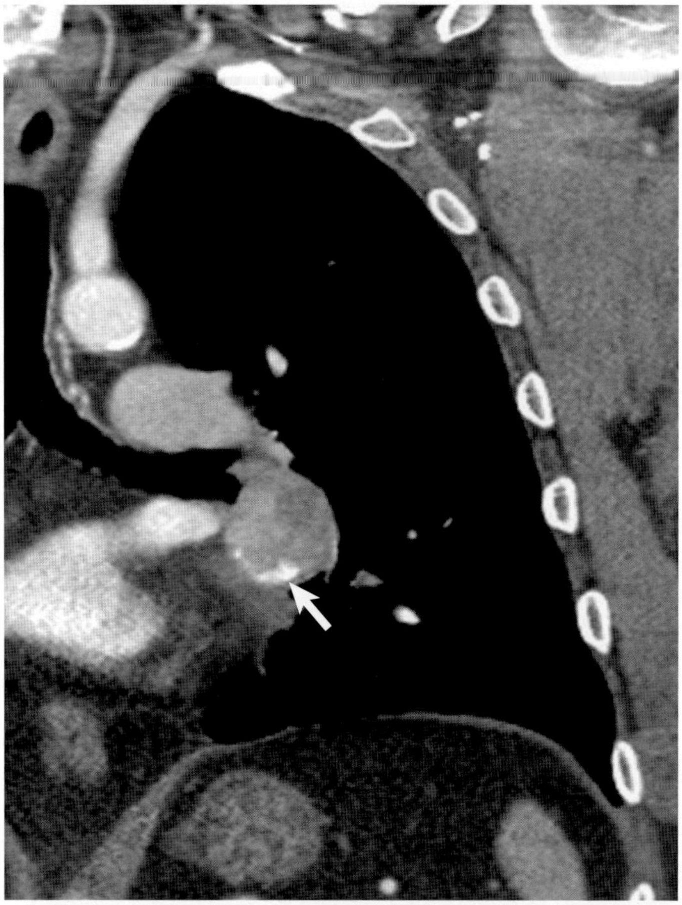

Fig. 19.10 Calcification of carcinoid tumor. Coronal CT shows a well-circumscribed, heterogeneously enhancing mass obliterating the left lower lobe bronchus. Scattered eccentric calcification (arrow) can be seen within the tumor.

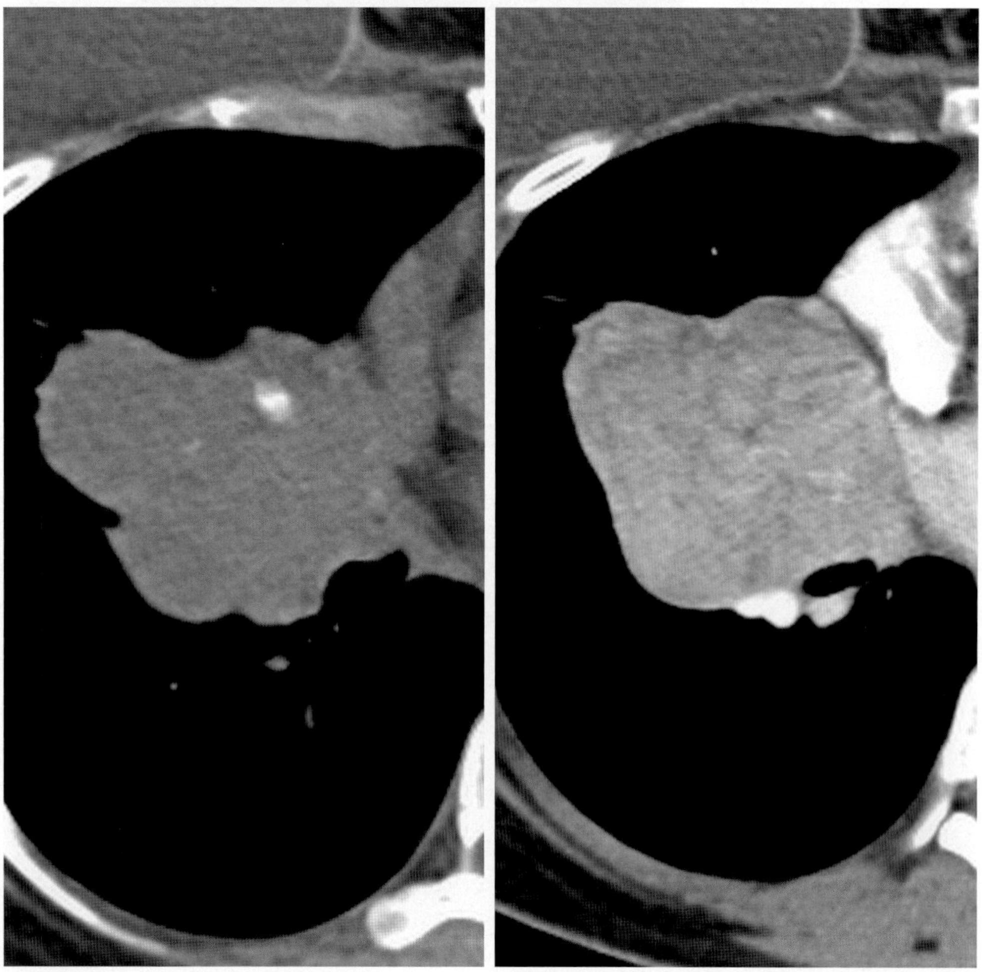

Fig. 19.11 Atypical carcinoid tumor. Composite image with axial precontrast *(left image)* and axial postcontrast *(right image)* CT shows a large heterogeneously enhancing right hilar mass containing coarse eccentric calcification. *(Courtesy Emily Tsai, Carol Wu. Atypical carcinoid. In: Rosado-de-Christenson ML, Carter BW.* Specialty Imaging: Thoracic Neoplasms. *1st ed. Philadelphia: Elsevier; 2015.)*

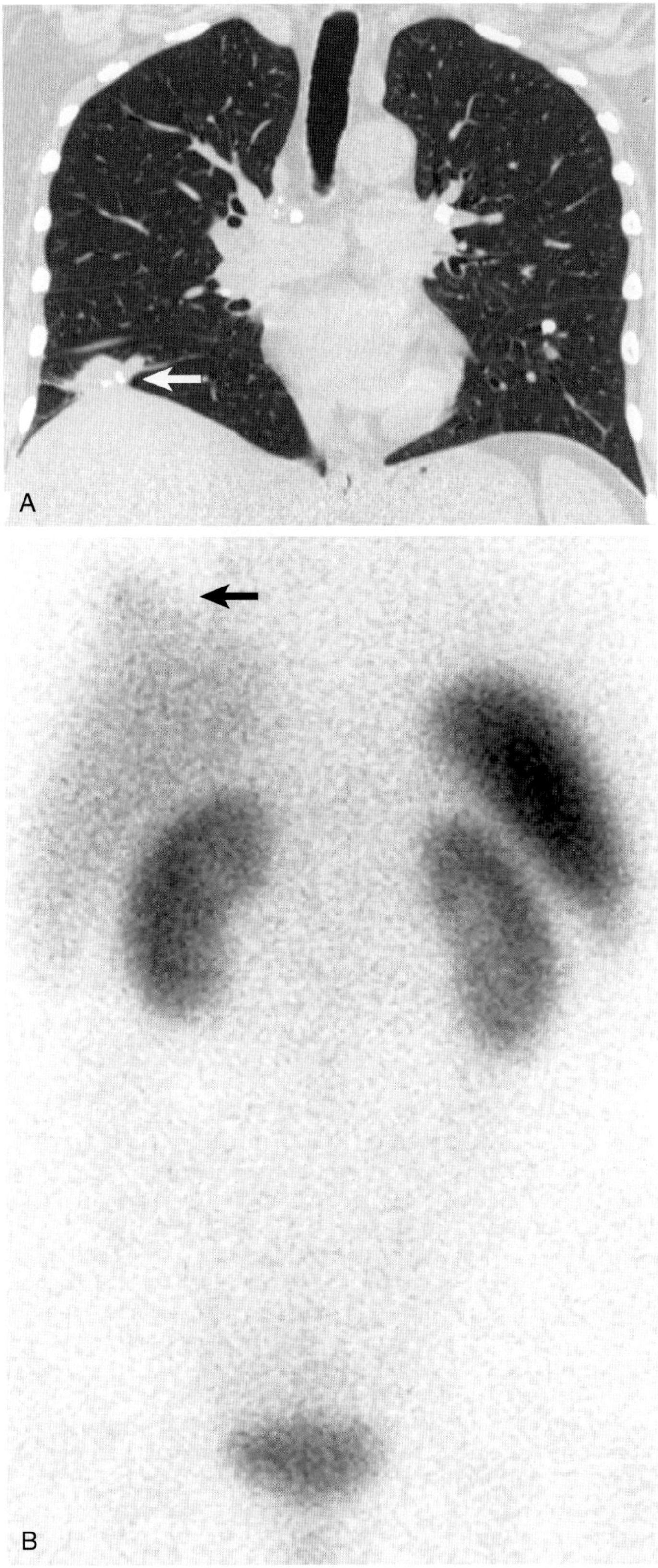

Fig. 19.12 Typical carcinoid tumor on OctreoScan. (A) Coronal CT shows a partially calcified nodule *(arrow)* in the right lower lobe adjacent to the hemidiaphragm. (B) Coned image from whole-body ^{111}In-octreoscan shows a focus of uptake *(arrow)* corresponding to the lesion seen on CT. Carcinoid tumors express somatostatin receptors, allowing visualization with somatostatin analogues.

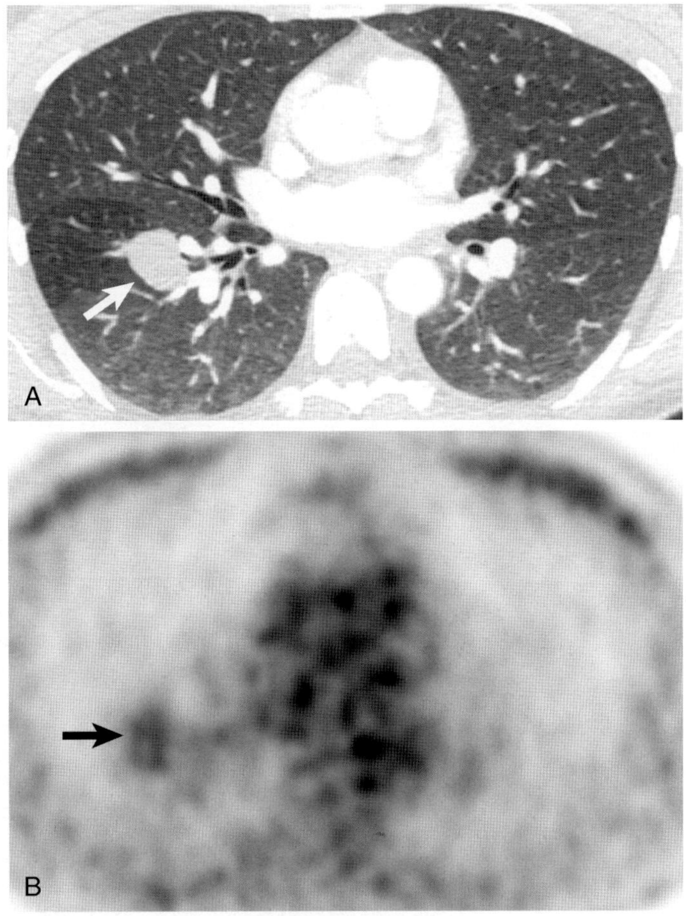

Fig. 19.13 Typical carcinoid tumor on PET-CT. (A) Axial contrast-enhanced CT shows a peripheral lesion *(arrow)* with distal mosaic attenuation of the right lower lobe. (B) Corresponding PET shows mild FDG uptake *(arrow)*, similar to less than mediastinal uptake. The patient had surgically proven typical carcinoid.

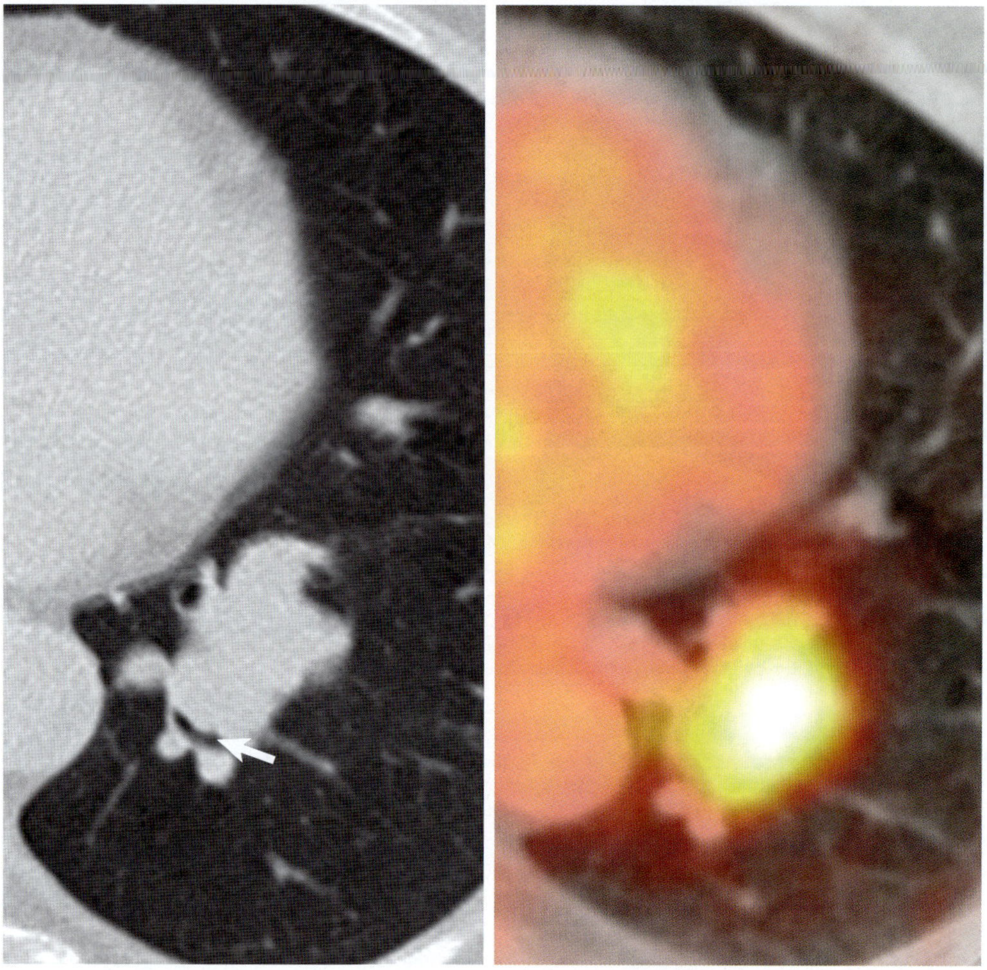

Fig. 19.14 Atypical carcinoid tumor on PET-CT. Composite image with axial CT *(left)* and axial fused FDG–PET-CT *(right)* shows an intensely FDG-avid left lower lobe mass containing an endobronchial component *(arrow)*. *(Courtesy Emily Tsai, Carol Wu. Atypical carcinoid. In: Rosado-de-Christenson ML, Carter BW.* Specialty Imaging: Thoracic Neoplasms. *1st ed. Philadelphia: Elsevier; 2015.)*

analogues have shown improved sensitivity compared with ^{111}In-octreotide scintigraphy (sensitivity 100% vs. 85%).[34]

DIFFERENTIAL DIAGNOSIS

The differential diagnosis of carcinoid tumors includes bronchogenic carcinoma, hamartoma, mucoepidermoid carcinoma, and benign lesions such as papilloma, and distinction cannot be reliably made radiographically. Diagnosis of carcinoid tumor requires microscopic tissue evaluation, which can be obtained through endobronchial biopsy, thoracotomy, or image-guided percutaneous biopsy. Although carcinoid tumors are highly vascular, most investigators have experienced no serious problems with hemorrhage after biopsy.[27,35]

SYNOPSIS OF TREATMENT OPTIONS

Treatment of limited disease depends upon the location of the carcinoid tumor (central or peripheral) and accessibility and degree of invasion (entirely intraluminal vs. local invasion). For peripheral lesions, segmentectomy or lobar resections are the treatment of choice, with or without lymphadenectomy. Central lesions may be amenable to lung-parenchymal–sparing surgery, although given the high rate of lymph node involvement (10%–15% of typical carcinoids and 40%–50% of atypical carcinoids), systematic regional and mediastinal nodal dissection should be performed concurrently. In the case of carcinoid tumors without extraluminal extension, endobronchial laser or cryotherapy can be quite effective in treatment.[25]

After surgical resection of typical carcinoid, CT imaging is carried out at 3 and 6 months posttreatment and then every 12 months for the first 2 years. Subsequently, annual chest radiography and biochemical profile should be obtained with a CT every 3 years. For atypical carcinoid, closer monitoring is recommended. After the initial 3-month follow-up CT, CT should be obtained every 6 months for 5 years, followed by annual CT after 5 years. Scintigraphic octreotide imaging should be obtained at 1 year posttreatment and then on suspicion of recurrence.[25]

In patients with known metastatic disease or known atypical carcinoid tumor, nonsurgical therapy with chemotherapy, immunotherapy, or radiolabeled somatostatin analogues should be considered.[25]

Prognosis is good for patients with typical carcinoid, with 5-, 10-, and 15-year survival rates of 91%, 89%, and 81%, respectively, compared with 76%, 49%, and 35% for patients with atypical carcinoid.[36] The presence or absence of lymph node metastases is the feature most strongly correlated with survival rates.

KEY POINTS: CARCINOID TUMORS

- Carcinoid tumors account for 1%–2% of primary pulmonary neoplasms and are the most common primary pulmonary neoplasm in children and adolescents.
- The two types of tumors are typical carcinoid (80%–90% of cases) and atypical carcinoid (10%–20% of cases).
- Most common presenting symptoms are cough and hemoptysis. Most patients are asymptomatic at diagnosis.
- Paraneoplastic syndromes associated with carcinoid tumors include Cushing syndrome, carcinoid syndrome, and acromegaly.
- Radiological manifestations of carcinoid tumors include:
  - 80%–85% are central in the main, lobar, or segmental bronchi
  - Distal atelectasis or pneumonia
  - Endobronchial nodule or mass on radiography or CT
  - Positive uptake on somatostatin receptor scintigraphy
  - Usually negative uptake on FDG-PET (except in some cases of atypical carcinoid)

SUGGESTED READINGS

Benson RE, Rosado-de-Christenson ML, Martínez-Jiménez S, et al. Spectrum of pulmonary neuroendocrine proliferations and neoplasms. *Radiographics*. 2013;33:1631–1649.

Caplin ME, Baudin E, Ferolla P, et al. Pulmonary neuroendocrine (carcinoid) tumors: European Neuroendocrine Tumor Society expert consensus and recommendations for best practice for typical and atypical pulmonary carcinoids. *Ann Oncol*. 2015;26:1604–1620.

The full reference list for this chapter is available at ExpertConsult.com.

20 Pulmonary Hamartoma*

CHRISTOPHER M. WALKER | JONATHAN H. CHUNG

Etiology, Prevalence, and Epidemiology

Pulmonary hamartomas are benign neoplasms, probably derived from bronchial wall mesenchymal cells.[1] Hamartomas are the most common benign pulmonary neoplasm and account for about 8% of primary lung tumors.[2] Although they may be seen in adolescents and young adults, most cases occur in patients older than 40 years; the peak incidence is in the seventh decade of life.[2,3] Men are affected two to three times more often than women. Endobronchial hamartomas are much less common than parenchymal lesions, accounting for 5% to 20% of pulmonary hamartomas.

Although hamartomas are benign neoplasms, they may rarely coexist with pulmonary carcinoma.[4] Occasionally, they may be multiple.[5] Multiple pulmonary hamartomas may be part of the Carney triad or, rarely, the Cowden syndrome.[6] The Carney triad consists of pulmonary chondroma (often multiple), gastric epithelioid leiomyosarcoma, and functioning extraadrenal paraganglioma.[7,8] This rare disease usually affects women younger than 35 years. It is recommended that patients with multiple pulmonary hamartomas have further examinations to rule out gastric leiomyosarcoma and extraadrenal paragangliomas.[6]

Clinical Presentation

Pulmonary hamartomas usually do not cause symptoms.[3] Occasionally, patients may present with hemoptysis or cough.[9] Endobronchial hamartomas may result in bronchial obstruction, and patients may present with cough, hemoptysis, and recurrent pneumonia.[3]

Pathophysiology

Most hamartomas are solitary, well-circumscribed, slightly lobulated tumors located within the parenchyma, usually in a peripheral location.[10] Most measure 1 to 4 cm in diameter, but tumors 25 cm in diameter have been described.[11] On cut section the tumors consist of lobules of white, cartilaginous-appearing tissue.[10] Histologically, the lobules are often composed of a central area of more or less well-developed cartilage surrounded by loose fibroblastic tissue. Adipose tissue, smooth muscle, and seromucinous bronchial glands also may be seen. Calcification and ossification of the cartilage can be present and are occasionally extensive. Although endobronchial hamartomas can be morphologically identical to the parenchymal variety, more often they appear as fleshy, polypoid tumors attached to the bronchial wall by a narrow stalk.[10] Endobronchial hamartomas typically contain more macroscopic fat than parenchymal hamartomas.

*The editors and the publisher would like to thank Drs. Nestor L. Müller and C. Isabela Silva Müller for contributing material on this topic to the prior edition of this work. It has served as the foundation for the current chapter.

Manifestations of the Disease

RADIOGRAPHY

The radiologic manifestations of parenchymal tumors usually consist of a well-circumscribed, smoothly marginated solitary nodule without lobar predilection (Fig. 20.1).[12,13] Most are smaller than 4 cm in diameter. Although calcification has been identified pathologically in 15% of tumors in some series, it is visible on the chest radiograph in less than 10% of cases. The radiographic pattern of calcification may resemble popcorn; although virtually diagnostic, this appearance is uncommon.[13] Endobronchial hamartomas usually manifest radiographically by the effects of airway obstruction with distal atelectasis and obstructive pneumonitis (Fig. 20.2). The endobronchial lesion is uncommonly visible.

COMPUTED TOMOGRAPHY

The characteristic finding on CT consists of a sharply defined, smoothly marginated nodule. Up to 60% of larger hamartomas have focal areas of fat density (see Fig. 20.1).[14] The presence of fat can be ascertained by comparison of the areas of low density with that of subcutaneous fat or by measurement of attenuation values (fat can be considered present when the CT attenuation values are −40 to −120 Hounsfield units (HUs) in at least eight voxels).[14] In review of the CT findings in 47 hamartomas, CT allowed diagnosis in 28 (60%) cases by identifying the presence of fat or fat alternating with areas of calcification (Fig. 20.3).[14] Of the remaining cases, 17 showed no discernible calcium or fat (the diagnosis being made by other means), and 2 revealed diffuse calcification.[14] Hamartomas also may manifest as nodules with soft tissue attenuation and single or multiple foci of calcification. Multiple coarse foci of calcification are referred to as "popcorn calcification" (see Fig. 20.2). With the increasing use of CT, smaller hamartomas are being detected but often lack diagnostic CT features. In a recent review of 21 cases of pathologically proven hamartomas (median diameter, 10 mm), none had characteristic internal fat or calcification, but all were well circumscribed with a round or lobular shape (Fig. 20.4).[15] Occasionally, pulmonary hamartoma may have the appearance of a collection of multiple tiny nodules.[16] This appearance results when pulmonary alveoli and bronchioles are entrapped within the hamartoma with tumor buds appearing in a multicentric manner.[16] Serial chest radiographs or CT may show slow growth, with a doubling time usually greater than 450 days (Fig. 20.5).[15]

Endotracheal and endobronchial hamartomas may appear on CT to be composed entirely of fat or a mixture of fat and

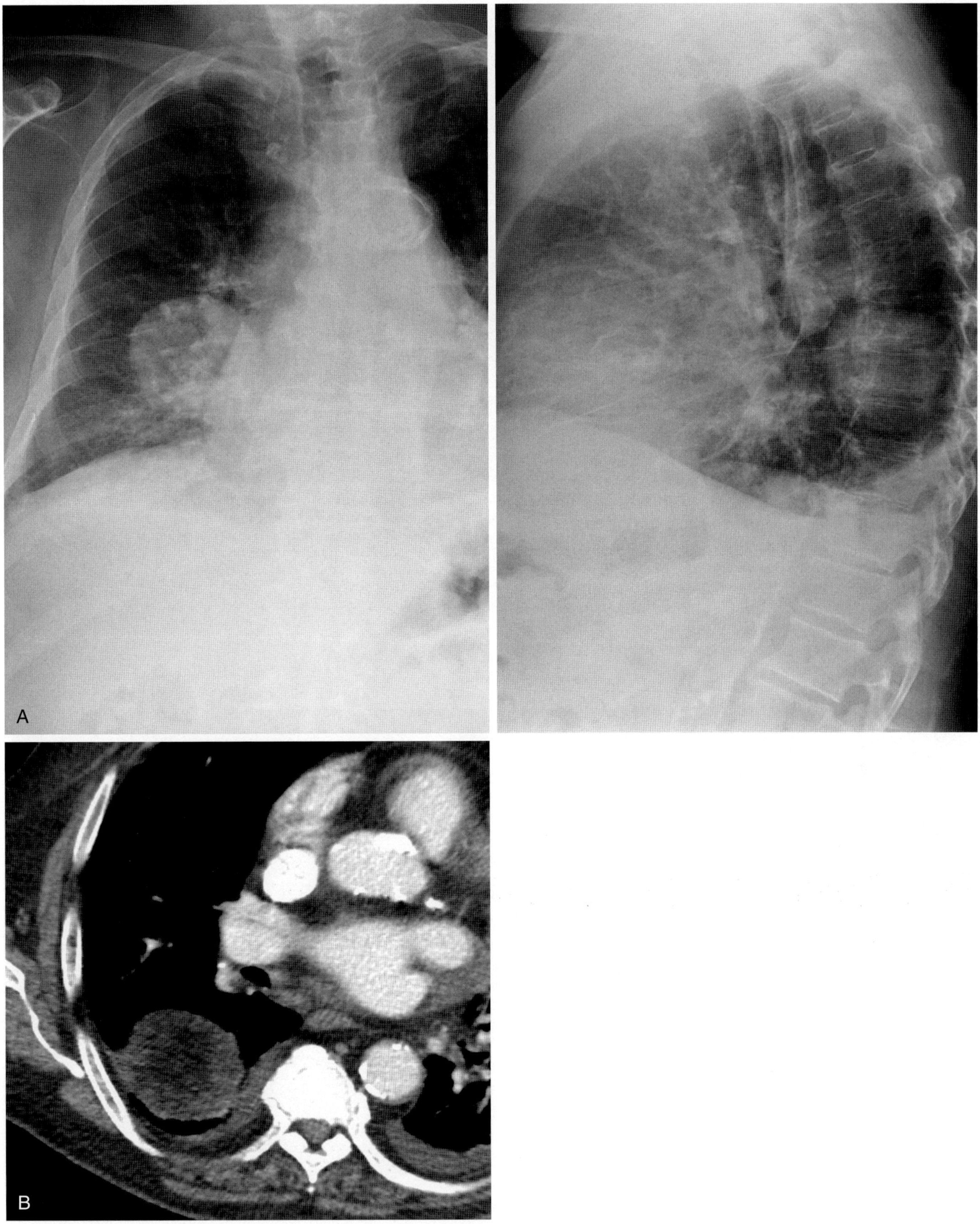

Fig. 20.1 Pulmonary hamartoma: characteristic radiographic and CT findings. (A) Composite image of posteroanterior *(left)* and lateral *(right)* chest radiographs show a well-defined, 5-cm right lower lobe mass. (B) Axial contrast-enhanced CT shows a smoothly marginated mass containing large amounts of central fat. This CT appearance is diagnostic of pulmonary hamartoma despite its large size.

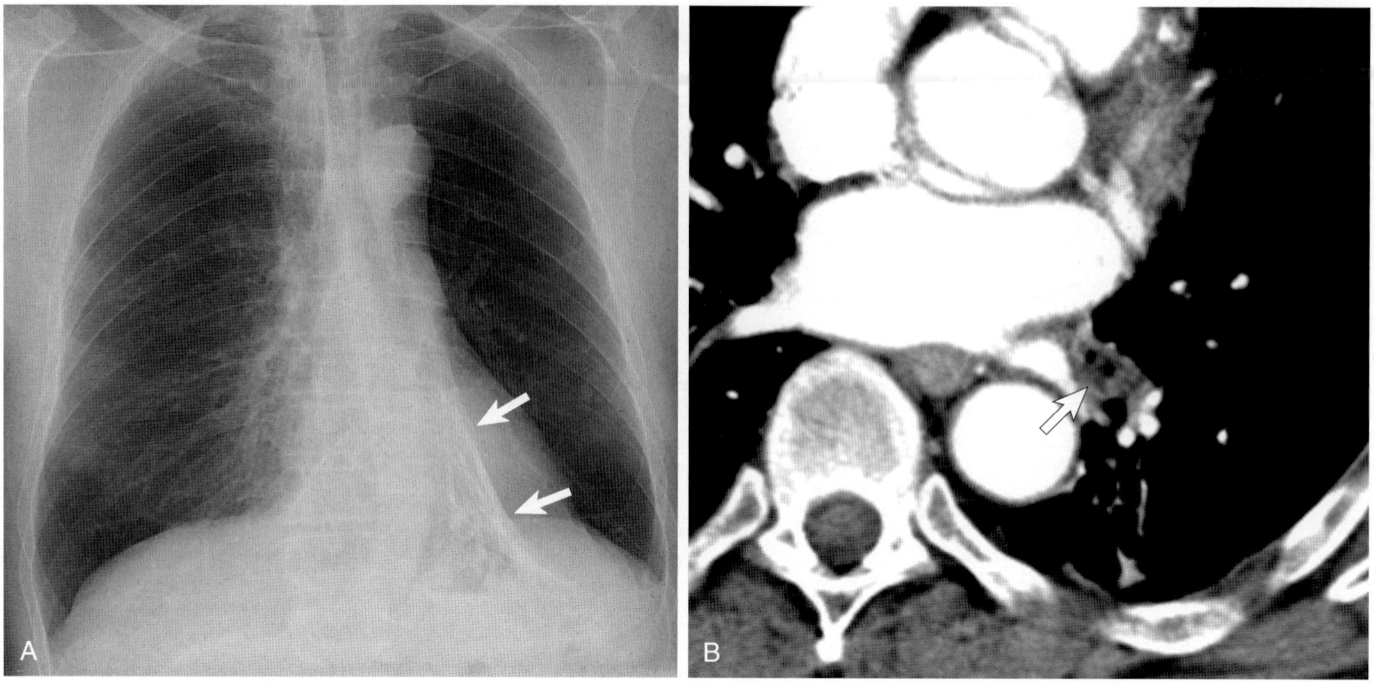

Fig. 20.2 Endobronchial hamartoma. (A) Posteroanterior chest radiograph shows left lung volume loss and left lower lobe atelectasis *(arrows)*. Note bronchiectatic airways in the atelectatic left lower lobe, suggestive of chronic collapse. (B) Axial contrast-enhanced CT shows a hypoattenuating left lower lobe endobronchial nodule with macroscopic fat *(arrow)*, surgically proven to represent an endobronchial hamartoma. Endobronchial lipoma could also be considered in the differential diagnosis but would exhibit only fat attenuation on CT. *(From Walker CM. Tracheobronchial hamartoma. In: Rosado-de-Christenson ML, Carter BW.* Specialty Imaging: Thoracic Neoplasms. *Philadelphia: Elsevier; 2016.)*

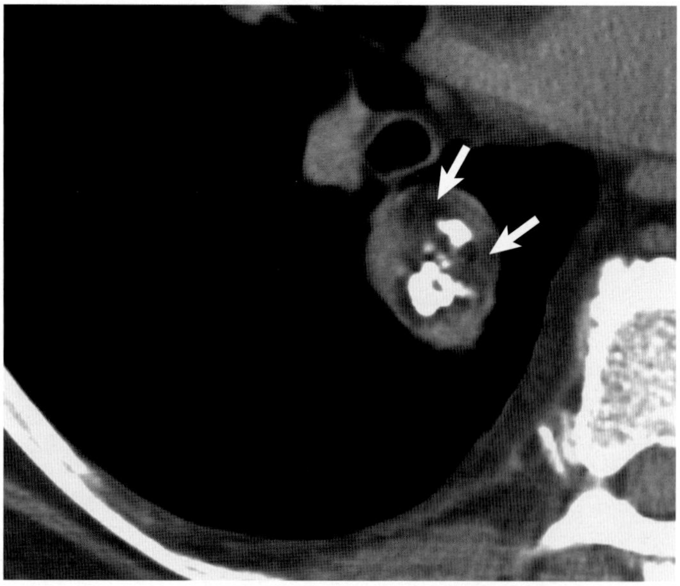

Fig. 20.3 Pulmonary hamartoma. Axial CT shows a smoothly marginated nodule in the right lower lobe containing several coarse foci of calcification (popcorn calcification) and macroscopic fat *(arrows)*.

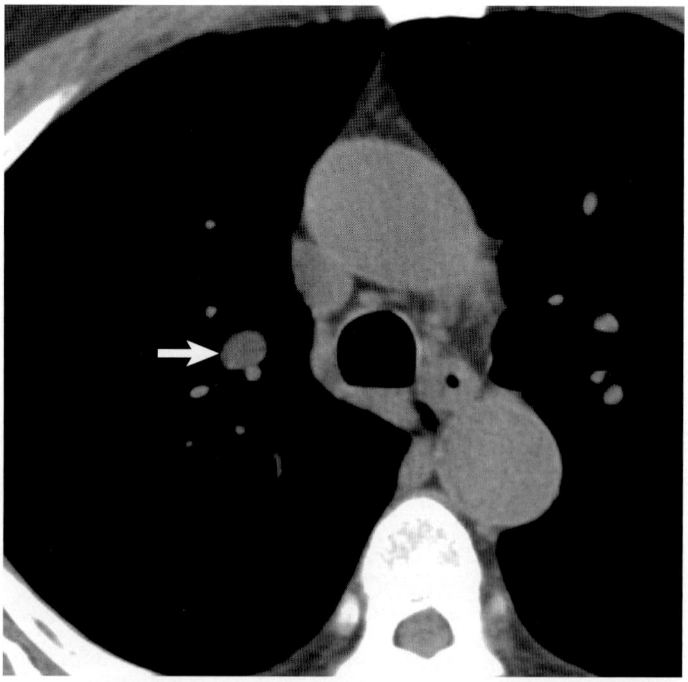

Fig. 20.4 Pulmonary hamartoma. Axial CT shows a well-defined, round nodule *(arrow)* in the medial right upper lobe without macroscopic fat or calcification. Smaller hamartomas often lack internal fat or calcification and must be followed with CT or biopsied to exclude malignancy.

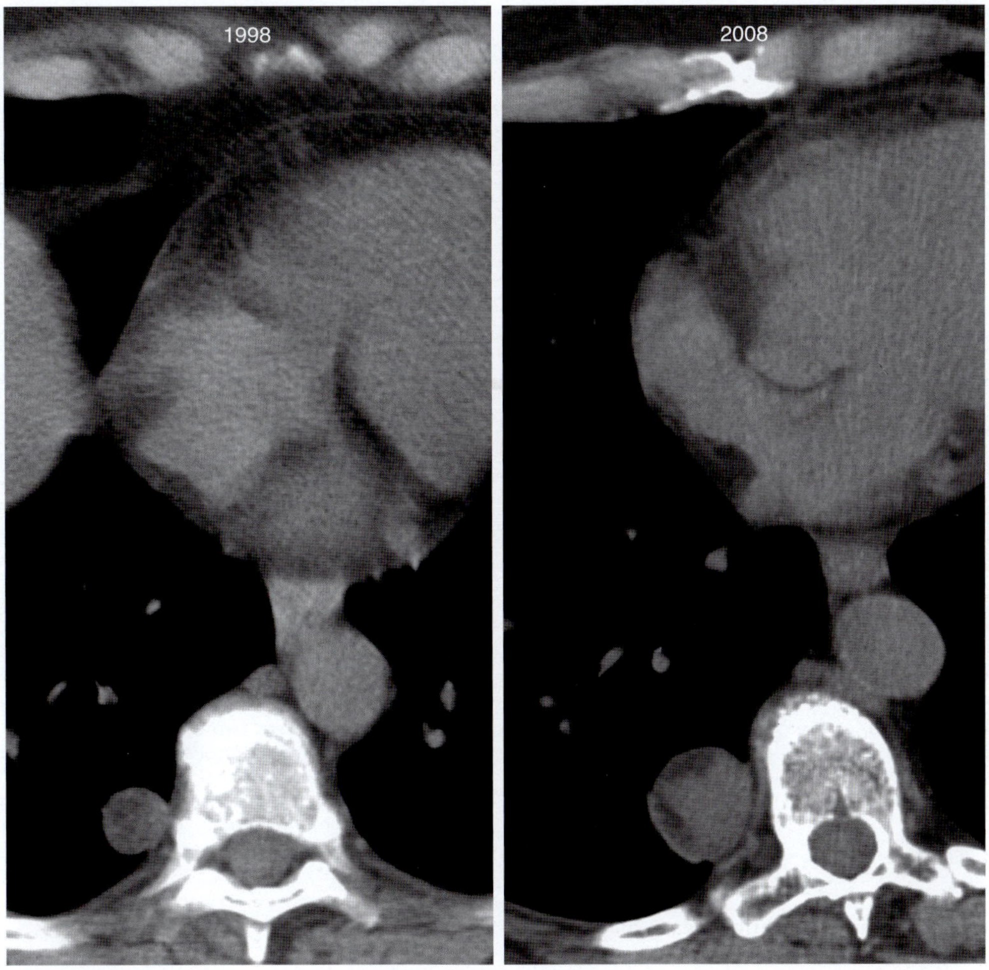

Fig. 20.5 Composite image of two axial CT images obtained 10 years apart shows slow growth of a right lower lobe hamartoma. The doubling time for most hamartomas is greater than 450 days.

soft tissue or calcification, or they may have soft tissue attenuation with or without foci of calcification (Fig. 20.6; see Fig. 20.2).[17,18] Endobronchial hamartomas may be associated with obstructive atelectasis or pneumonitis (see Fig. 20.2).

MAGNETIC RESONANCE IMAGING

Magnetic resonance imaging has a limited role in assessment. In a review of the findings in six patients, fat was not evident in any, and focal areas of calcification caused signal void or were missed.[19] The hamartomas had intermediate signal intensity (higher than that of skeletal muscle but lower than that of fat) on T1-weighted images and high signal intensity on T2-weighted images. They frequently contained septa that had high signal intensity on T1-weighted images and low signal intensity on T2-weighted images. Gadolinium-enhanced T1-weighted images showed marked enhancement of the septa that separated the tumors into less well-enhanced lobules. Restricted diffusion is usually absent.[20]

POSITRON EMISSION TOMOGRAPHY

Pulmonary hamartomas are slow-growing benign tumors, with the majority showing fluorodeoxyglucose (FDG) uptake less than mediastinal blood pool on positron emission tomography (PET). A review of 42 consecutive cases showed suspicious or malignant FDG uptake in about 20% of pathologically proven hamartomas (usually of a large size with a mean diameter of 23 mm). Suspicious FDG uptake was defined as FDG uptake greater than normal lung parenchyma, and malignant FDG uptake was defined as FDG uptake greater than mediastinal blood pool.[21]

IMAGING ALGORITHM

In most cases pulmonary hamartomas are incidental findings on chest radiography or CT. In up to 60% of cases a confident diagnosis can be made on CT by the presence of focal areas of fat density in a smoothly marginated nodule. PET may be helpful in confirming the benign nature of the tumor. In patients with nonspecific CT findings, definitive diagnosis of hamartoma can be made by transthoracic core needle biopsy of peripheral hamartomas and bronchoscopic biopsy of endobronchial hamartomas.

Differential Diagnosis

The presence of focal areas of fat density (−40 to −120 HUs) in a smoothly marginated lung nodule is considered a reliable indicator of a hamartoma.[14] Caution should be exercised when subjective or even quantitative areas of fat attenuation are small

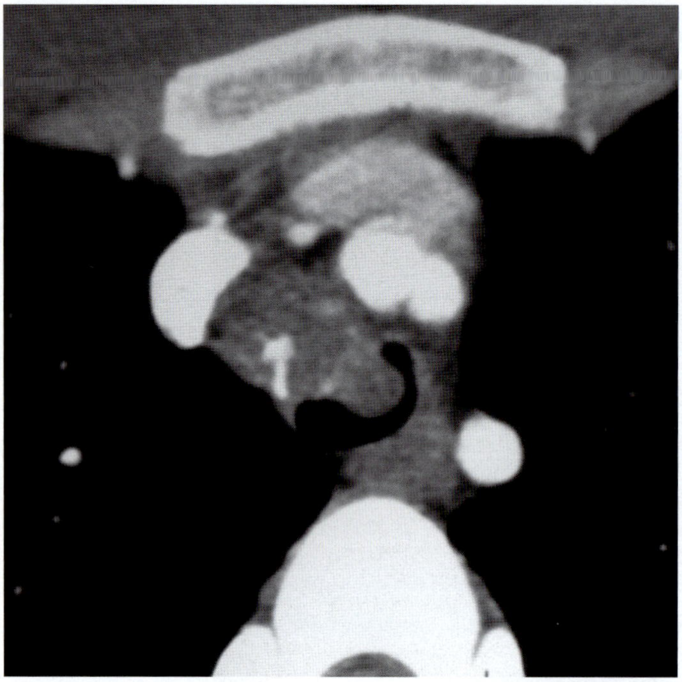

Fig. 20.6 Endotracheal hamartoma with foci of calcification. Axial contrast-enhanced CT at the level of the great vessels shows a large soft tissue mass originating from the tracheal wall and extending into the tracheal lumen and right paratracheal region. Note punctate calcification within the mass.

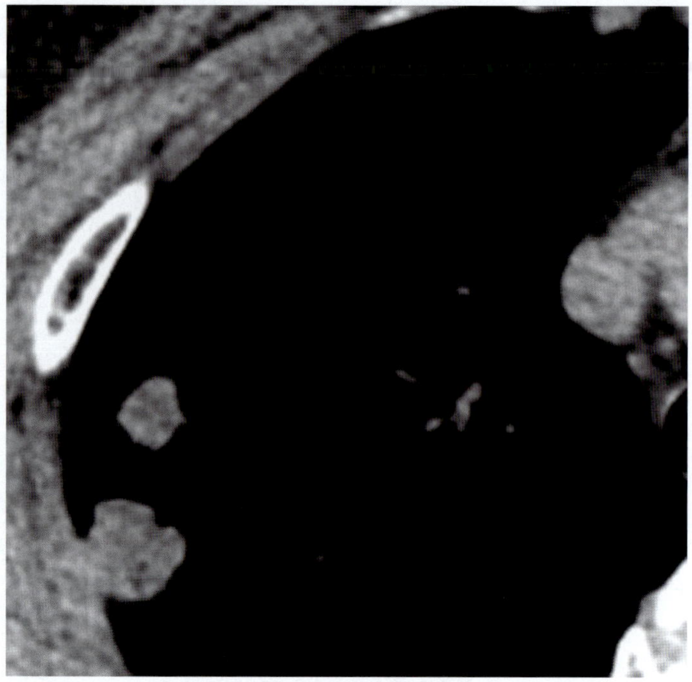

Fig. 20.7 Metastatic breast cancer masquerading as hamartomas. Axial noncontrast CT shows two small nodules in the right upper lobe with central low attenuation, suggesting macroscopic fat. The region of interest (not shown) showed Hounsfield units of –43. These nodules were confirmed to be malignant via transthoracic needle biopsy. *(From Oh JK, Han DH. False-positive multi-detector CT finding for hamartomas.* Ann Thorac Surg. *2010;90:1398; author reply 1398–1399.)*

in size, as other entities such as metastatic disease or primary lung cancer may occasionally manifest similarly, likely related to internal necrosis rather than true macroscopic fat (Fig. 20.7).[22] In the absence of focal areas of fat attenuation on CT, the differential diagnosis of pulmonary hamartomas must include all other solitary pulmonary nodules, particularly carcinoma.

Transthoracic fine-needle aspiration has a low sensitivity in the diagnosis of hamartomas and may lead to misdiagnosis of carcinoma. In one study the specificity of fine-needle aspiration for making the correct general reference interpretation of benign was 78%.[23] The false-positive rate was 22%, with the most common false-positive diagnoses being carcinoid tumor, adenocarcinoma, and small cell carcinoma.[23]

Because of the low yield of needle aspiration in the diagnosis of hamartomas and other benign nodules, an increasing number of centers are performing transthoracic core needle biopsy, a procedure in which a core of tissue is obtained using a cutting needle. This procedure has a sensitivity of 97% for malignant and benign lung nodules.[24]

Synopsis of Treatment Options

Hamartomas are benign, and adequate surgical excision results in cure in most patients. Excision of peripheral lesions can be made by video-assisted thoracoscopic surgery; more central lesions may require thoracotomy and enucleation, wedge resection, or occasionally lobectomy.[25]

Endobronchial hamartoma can often be resected by transbronchial endoscopic surgery to preserve the lung parenchyma.[26] Large lesions may require a combination of bronchoplasty and transbronchial endoscopic surgery or occasionally lobectomy.[26]

KEY POINTS

- Pulmonary hamartoma is the most common benign neoplasm of the lung.
- Pulmonary hamartoma accounts for approximately 8% of lung tumors.
- Most pulmonary hamartomas occur in patients older than 40 years (median age, 50–60 years).
- The most common radiologic findings include:
  - 1- to 4-cm diameter, smooth or slightly lobulated nodule
  - Popcorn calcification characteristic but uncommon
  - 60% of larger hamartomas have foci of fat density (–40 to –120 HUs) on CT and are virtually diagnostic in a smoothly marginated nodule.
  - Small hamartomas (1 cm or less in diameter) often lack internal fat and calcification.
  - FDG uptake on PET is usually less than the mediastinal blood pool.

SUGGESTED READINGS

Gaerte SC, Meyer CA, Winer-Muram HT, et al. Fat-containing lesions of the chest. *Radiographics.* 2002;22:S61–S78.

Ngo AV, Walker CM, Chung JH, et al. Tumors and tumorlike conditions of the large airways. *AJR Am J Roentgenol.* 2013;201(2):301–313.

Siegelman SS, Khouri NF, Scott WW, et al. Pulmonary hamartoma: CT findings. *Radiology.* 1986;160:313–317.

The full reference list for this chapter is available at ExpertConsult.com.

21 Inflammatory Pseudotumor*

JONATHAN H. CHUNG | CHRISTOPHER M. WALKER

Etiology, Prevalence, and Epidemiology

Inflammatory pseudotumor, also known as inflammatory myofibroblastic tumor, is a quasineoplastic lesion that clinically and radiologically tends to mimic a malignant neoplasm and that histologically consists of a mixture of inflammatory cells, myofibroblastic spindle cells, and plasma cells.[1,2] The proportion of the various cells varies considerably from pseudotumor to pseudotumor. Pseudotumors with a predominance of plasma cells are commonly referred to as plasma cell granulomas, and pseudotumors with approximately equal numbers of fibroblasts, and histiocytes are referred to as fibrous histiocytomas.[2]

In most cases the etiology is unknown, although infection, infarcts, and radiation have been implicated as risk factors. Up to a half of pseudotumors demonstrate abnormality at the anaplastic lymphoma kinase receptor tyrosine kinase gene (2p23 locus), suggesting an underlying genetic defect.[3] Organisms found in association with pulmonary inflammatory pseudotumor include various bacteria and *Mycoplasma*.[4]

Inflammatory pseudotumors are rare. They may affect individuals of any age but have a predilection for children and young adults.[5] They are the most common primary lung mass seen in children.[6]

Clinical Presentation

Most patients are asymptomatic, and the pseudotumor is an incidental finding seen on chest radiography or CT. The most common symptoms are cough, fever, dyspnea, and hemoptysis.[7,8]

Pathophysiology

Inflammatory pseudotumors are fibroinflammatory lesions that are believed to result from an exaggerated response to tissue injury.[5] Histologically, they consist of a mixture of inflammatory cells, myofibroblastic spindle cells, and plasma cells.[1,2] The proportion of these cells varies, but it is believed that the progenitor cell of the various pseudotumors is the myofibroblast.[5] These lesions also are commonly referred to as inflammatory myofibroblastic tumors.[5]

On the basis of the predominant histopathologic features, inflammatory pseudotumors can be divided into three histologic types: (1) focal organizing pneumonia pattern, characterized by small airways and adjacent parenchyma filled with fibroblasts and foamy histiocytes; (2) fibrous histiocytic pattern, characterized by spindle-shaped myofibroblasts arranged in whorls; and (3) lymphohistiocytic pattern, characterized by a mixture of lymphocytes and plasma cells with only minimal fibrous connective tissue.[1]

*The editors and the publisher would like to thank Drs. Nestor L. Müller and C. Isabela Silva Müller for contributing material on this topic to the prior edition of this work. It has served as the foundation for the current chapter.

Manifestations of the Disease

RADIOGRAPHY

The most common radiologic manifestation consists of a solitary peripheral sharply circumscribed lobulated nodule or mass.[1,6] The lesion may have smooth or spiculated margins and range from 1 to more than 6 cm in diameter (Fig. 21.1).[8] Calcification is present occasionally, particularly in children, and cavitation is present rarely.[1,6] Endobronchial tumors can cause obstructive pneumonitis and atelectasis.[1,6] Hilar or mediastinal lymph node enlargement and pleural effusion occur occasionally.

COMPUTED TOMOGRAPHY

Inflammatory pseudotumors may have smooth or spiculated margins (Fig. 21.2; see Fig. 21.1), homogeneous or heterogeneous attenuation, and either no enhancement or variable enhancement after intravenous administration of contrast medium.[1,6,9] On computed tomography (CT) the nodules are usually closely associated with a bronchus.[10] Multiple lesions are seen in 5% of cases.[1] Approximately 10% of inflammatory pseudotumors manifest as endobronchial masses.[1] Occasionally, they may be endotracheal.[10]

MAGNETIC RESONANCE IMAGING

Inflammatory pseudotumors tend to have intermediate signal intensity at T1-weighted magnetic resonance imaging (MRI), have high signal intensity on T2-weighted MRI, and enhance after intravenous administration of gadolinium.[6]

POSITRON EMISSION TOMOGRAPHY

Inflammatory pseudotumors tend to have high-intensity uptake on positron emission tomography (PET) with fluorodeoxyglucose (FDG-PET), indicating a high degree of metabolic activity (see Fig. 21.2).[11] They also have high uptake on PET performed with rubidium-82, indicating the presence of increased perfusion.[11]

Differential Diagnosis

The radiologic differential diagnosis for inflammatory pseudotumor occurring as a solitary pulmonary nodule or mass includes primary or secondary neoplasm and granuloma.

Synopsis of Treatment Options

The biological potential of inflammatory pseudotumor varies. Long-term follow-up often shows no change in size or configuration.

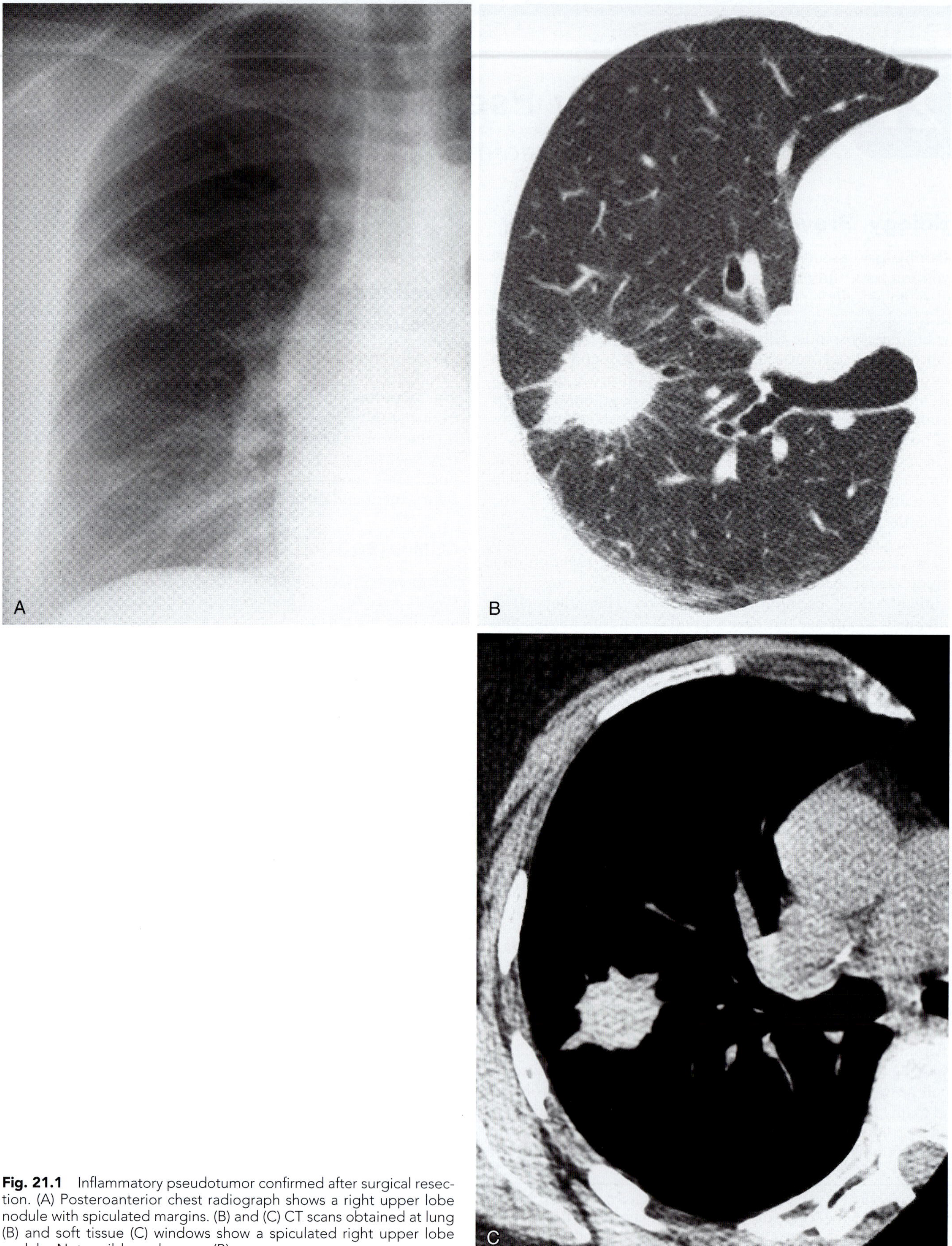

Fig. 21.1 Inflammatory pseudotumor confirmed after surgical resection. (A) Posteroanterior chest radiograph shows a right upper lobe nodule with spiculated margins. (B) and (C) CT scans obtained at lung (B) and soft tissue (C) windows show a spiculated right upper lobe nodule. Note mild emphysema (B).

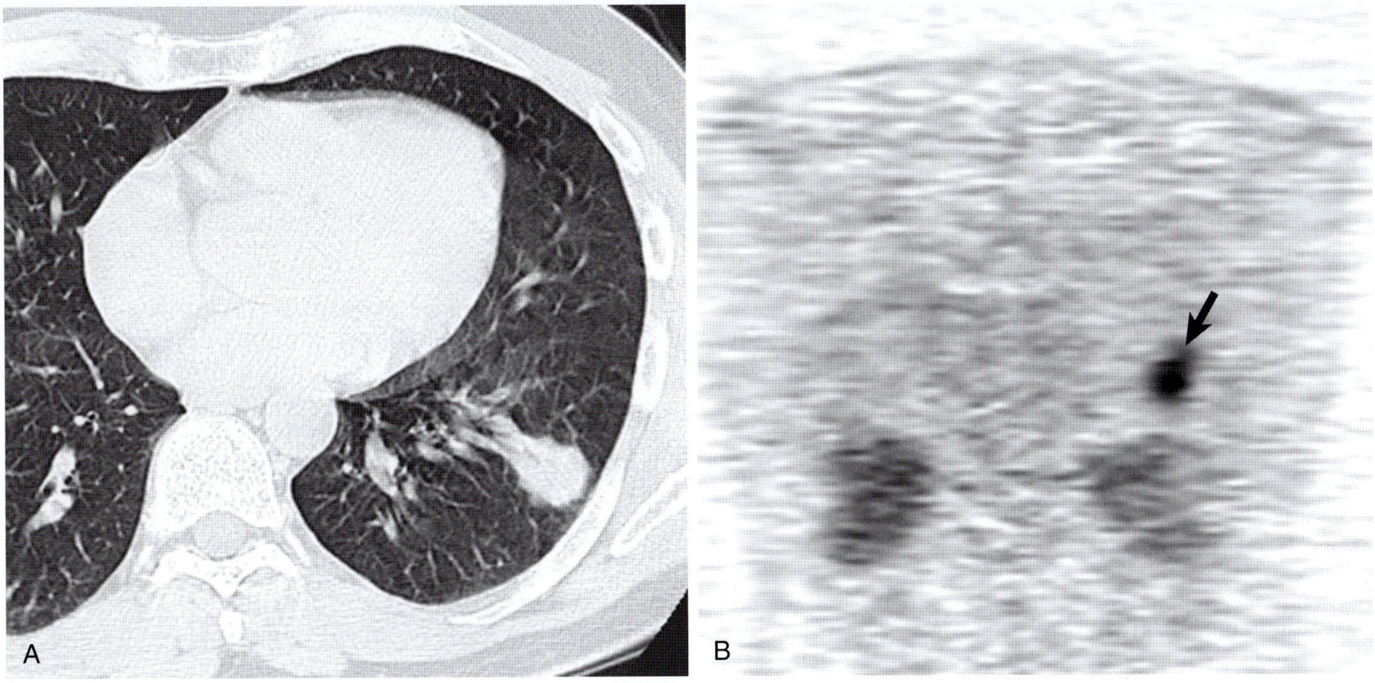

Fig. 21.2 Inflammatory pseudotumor. Axial image from chest CT (A) shows a nodule in the left lower lobe shown to represent an inflammatory pseudotumor. Coronal image from FDG-PET (B) shows high FDG avidity within the nodule *(arrow)*.

Some lesions have been shown to regress with or without steroid therapy.[1,12] Some lesions increase in size, however, and may infiltrate the pulmonary vessels, the chest wall, or mediastinum.[1] Complete surgical resection is the treatment of choice in adults.[1,8] Local recurrence may occur in some cases even after apparent complete surgical resection.[8]

KEY POINTS

- Inflammatory pseudotumors consist of variable proportions of inflammatory cells, myofibroblastic spindle cells, and plasma cells.
- Inflammatory pseudotumors are rare, affecting mainly children and young adults.
- Inflammatory pseudotumors are usually benign but occasionally may be invasive and recur after surgical resection.
- Radiologic manifestations are as follows:
  - Nodules or masses 1–6 cm in diameter (average, 3 cm)
  - May have foci of calcification (more common in children)
  - Smooth, lobulated, or spiculated margins
  - Most commonly peripheral; approximately 10% are endobronchial
  - Homogeneous or heterogeneous attenuation on CT
  - Homogeneous or heterogeneous enhancement with intravenous contrast material
  - High uptake on FDG-PET imaging

SUGGESTED READINGS

Narla LD, Newman B, Spottswood SS, et al. Inflammatory pseudotumor. *Radiographics.* 2003;23:719–729.

Surabhi VR, Chua S, Patel RP, Takahashi N, Lalwani N, Prasad SR. Inflammatory myofibroblastic tumors: current update. *Radiol Clin North Am.* 2016;54:553–563.

The full reference list for this chapter is available at ExpertConsult.com.

22 Pulmonary Metastases*

STEPHANE L. DESOUCHES | CHRISTOPHER M. WALKER | JONATHAN H. CHUNG

Etiology, Prevalence, and Epidemiology

Pulmonary metastases are common—present at autopsy in 20% to 54% of patients with extrapulmonary malignancy.[1] The most common primary sites associated with pulmonary metastases in biopsy series are the breast, colon, kidney, uterus, bladder, melanoma, and head and neck.[2]

Clinical Presentation

Most pulmonary metastases occurring as single or multiple nodules are asymptomatic. When present, symptoms are nonspecific and include cough, hemoptysis, and shortness of breath. The most common clinical manifestation of lymphatic spread of tumor is dyspnea. The dyspnea is typically insidious in onset but tends to progress rapidly.[3] Similarly, the most common symptom of endobronchial metastases is dyspnea; other common symptoms include cough, recurrent infection, and hemoptysis.[4]

Pathophysiology

Pulmonary metastases may occur by hematogenous, lymphatic, or aerogenous spread.

HEMATOGENOUS SPREAD

Most pulmonary metastases spread to the lungs through the arterial system, lodging within small pulmonary arterioles or arteries. In most cases the newly formed tumor extends into the surrounding lung parenchyma, forming a relatively well-defined nodule.[3,5] Hematogenous metastases are usually bilateral and manifest with randomly distributed nodules in the outer third of the lower lung zones.[6]

Occasionally, hematogenous metastases to the lungs may result in tumor growth only in the vessel lumen and wall without extension into the extravascular tissue. This condition is known as tumor embolism and is seen most commonly in metastatic renal cell carcinoma; hepatocellular carcinoma; and carcinomas of the breast, stomach, and prostate.[7]

LYMPHATIC SPREAD

Lymphatic metastases are most often indirect with first hematogenous spread to pulmonary arteries and arterioles with subsequent invasion of the adjacent interstitial space and lymphatics.[8] Less commonly, lymphatic spread of tumor is retrograde from mediastinal and hilar lymph node metastases. Although virtually any metastatic neoplasm can result in lymphatic spread, the most common extrathoracic cell type is adenocarcinoma from breast and gastrointestinal origin, as well as melanoma, lymphoma, and leukemia.[5]

Pathologically, lymphangitic carcinomatosis ranges from a slight accentuation of the interlobular septa and peribronchovascular connective tissue to marked thickening of these structures.[3] Microscopically, neoplastic cells can be present within the lymphatic spaces or in the adjacent peribronchovascular and interlobular interstitial tissue. Edema or a desmoplastic reaction to the tumor can contribute significantly to the interstitial thickening (Fig. 22.1).

AEROGENOUS SPREAD

Airway spread of tumor occurs through direct invasion or seeding of the bronchi by tumor, usually from pulmonary adenocarcinoma or bronchial carcinoid, although upper airway malignancies, such as laryngeal carcinoma, can also progress this way.[3,9] Endobronchial metastases from hematogenous spread are a different entity and are discussed separately.

Manifestations of the Disease

Pulmonary metastases may result in four main types of imaging manifestations: nodules, lymphatic spread, tumor emboli, and endobronchial tumor.

RADIOGRAPHY

Lung Nodules

The most common manifestation of pulmonary metastases consists of multiple nodules, most numerous in the basal portions of the lungs, reflecting the effect of gravity on blood flow.[10] They range in size from barely visible to large masses (Fig. 22.2). The nodules usually are of varying size; although less often, they are approximately equal, suggesting a single shower of tumor emboli. Rarely, nodular deposits are so numerous and of such minute size as to suggest the diagnosis of miliary fungal infection or tuberculosis (Fig. 22.3).

Certain primary neoplasms are more likely than others to produce solitary metastases on radiography, including carcinoma of the kidney, testicle, breast, and rectosigmoid colon; sarcomas (particularly sarcomas originating in bone); and malignant melanoma.[11]

Lymphatic Spread (Lymphangitic Carcinomatosis)

The characteristic radiographic pattern consists of septal lines and thickening of the bronchovascular markings, simulating interstitial pulmonary edema (Fig. 22.4). The linear accentuation sometimes is associated with a nodular component, resulting in a coarse reticulonodular pattern.[12] Hilar and mediastinal lymph node

---

*The editors and the publisher would like to thank Drs. Nestor L. Müller and C. Isabela Silva Müller for contributing material on this topic to the prior edition of this work. It has served as the foundation for the current chapter.

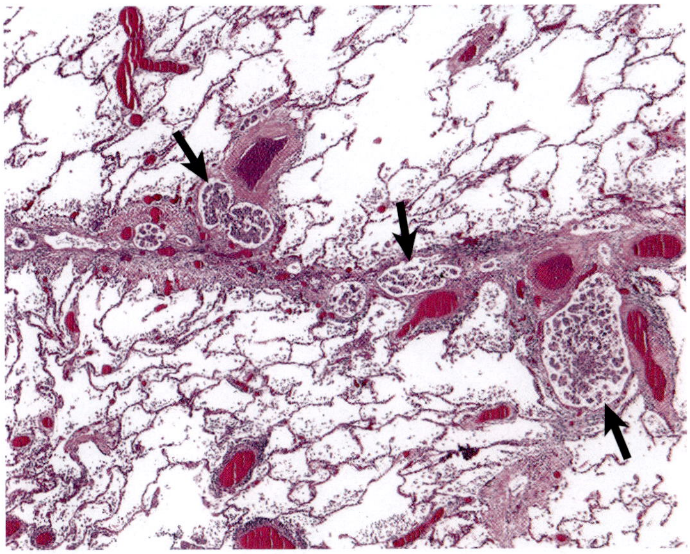

Fig. 22.1 Lymphangitic carcinomatosis: pathologic findings. Pathologic specimen shows thickening of interlobular septum by edema and focal accumulations of tumor cells *(arrows)* within dilated lymphatics. *(Courtesy Dr. John English, Department of Pathology, Vancouver General Hospital, Vancouver, Canada.)*

enlargement is seen radiographically in 20% to 40% of patients, and pleural effusion is seen in 30% to 50%.[12,13] Although characteristic, these findings lack specificity and sensitivity for the diagnosis. The chest radiograph is normal in 30% to 50% of patients who have pathologically proven lymphangitic carcinomatosis.[12]

COMPUTED TOMOGRAPHY

Lung Nodules

On computed tomography (CT), nodular metastases range from a few millimeters to several centimeters in diameter and are usually of varying size with smooth or irregular margins (see Fig. 22.2B). The nodules tend to be most numerous in the outer third of the lungs, particularly the subpleural regions of the lower zones, and have a random distribution within the secondary pulmonary lobules.[5] Surrounding ground-glass opacities may result from airspace disease, lepidic growth of neoplasm, or hemorrhage.[6] Metastatic nodules with hemorrhage often manifest the CT halo sign and are most common with choriocarcinoma, melanoma, renal cell carcinoma, angiosarcoma, and Kaposi sarcoma.[5]

Cavitation occurs most often in metastatic squamous cell carcinoma or transitional cell carcinoma but may also be seen with metastatic adenocarcinoma.[1] The wall of a cavitated metastasis is generally thick and irregular (Fig. 22.5), although thin-walled cavities can be found with metastases from sarcomas and adenocarcinomas.[1] Cavitation may also be induced by chemotherapy.[1]

Calcification of metastatic nodules is uncommon and suggests certain primary neoplasms, such as osteogenic sarcoma, mucinous carcinoma, or papillary thyroid carcinoma (Fig. 22.6). Small calcified nodules may mimic benign lesions, especially if eccentric calcification is difficult to ascertain.[14] Calcification can develop at the site of pulmonary metastases that have vanished after successful chemotherapy.[15] This chemotherapeutic effect may manifest with persistent nodules that, on histologic examination, show only necrosis and fibrosis without residual viable neoplastic tissue.[16,17]

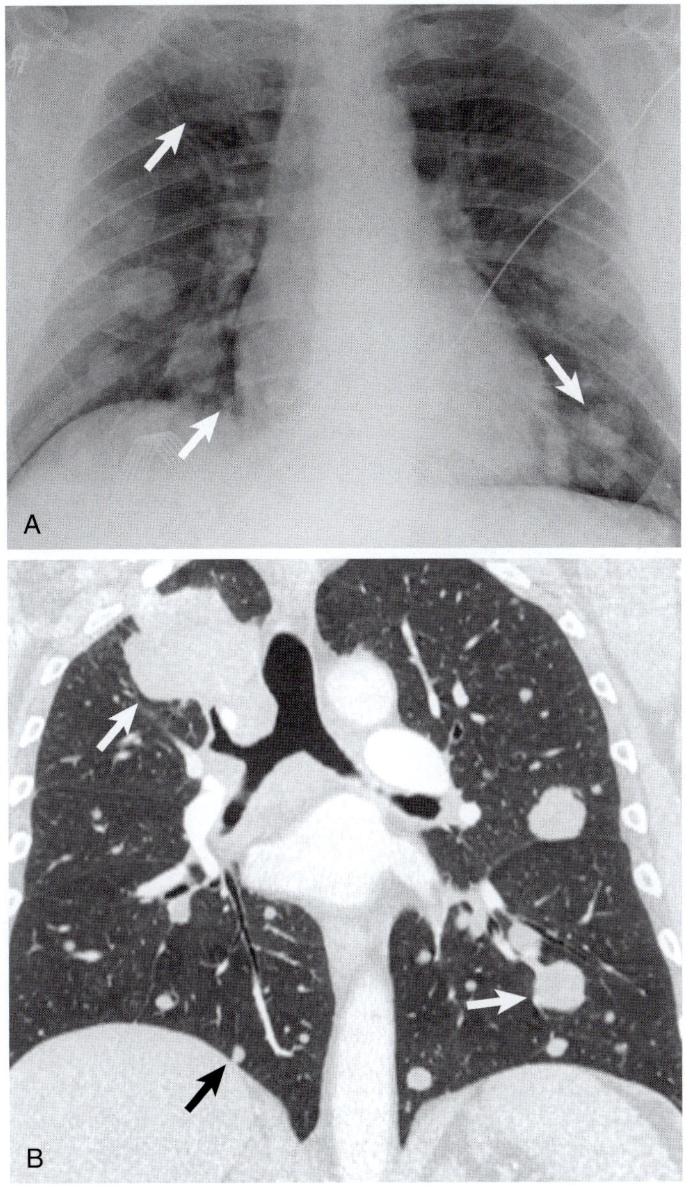

Fig. 22.2 Pulmonary metastases: nodules and masses. (A) Posteroanterior chest radiograph shows multiple pulmonary nodules and masses ranging from a few millimeters to greater than 3 cm in diameter *(arrows)*. The lesions have smooth margin and, while in all five lobes, demonstrate a basilar predominance. (B) Coronal CT shows the dominant right upper lobe mass and multiple bilateral pulmonary nodules *(arrows)*, showing a basilar predominance.

Although hematogenous pulmonary metastases usually result in soft tissue nodules, metastases from adenocarcinoma may spread into the lung along the intact alveolar walls (lepidic growth), in a fashion similar to a primary pulmonary adenocarcinoma.[1,17] The CT findings of metastases from adenocarcinoma include nodules, consolidation, ground-glass opacities, and nodules with CT halo sign (Fig. 22.7).[1,18]

Spontaneous pneumothorax resulting from metastatic disease to the lung is rare and should suggest sarcoma, choriocarcinoma, or cavitary metastasis.[19] It has been suggested that the

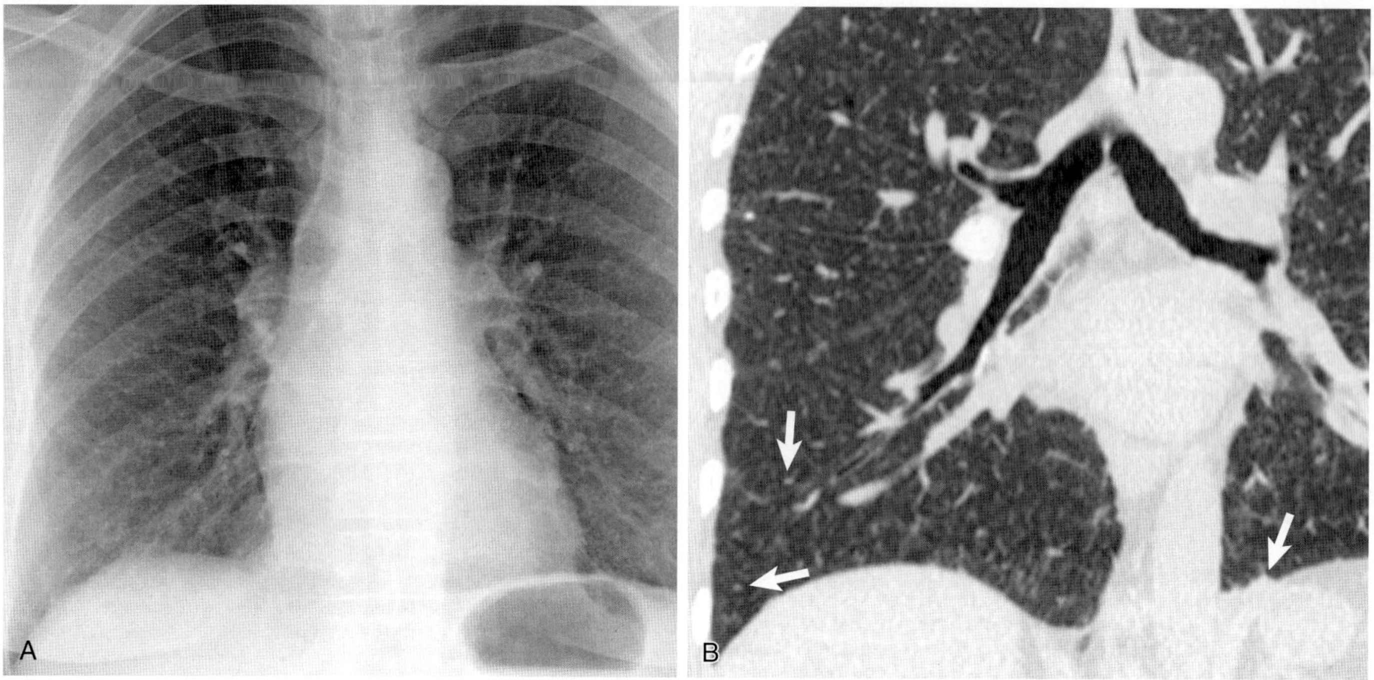

Fig. 22.3 Pulmonary metastases: miliary pattern. (A) Posteroanterior chest radiograph shows subtle small nodules throughout both lungs. (B) Coronal reformatted CT shows that the small nodules *(arrows)* have a random distribution in relation to the secondary pulmonary lobules. Note several conspicuous interlobular septa.

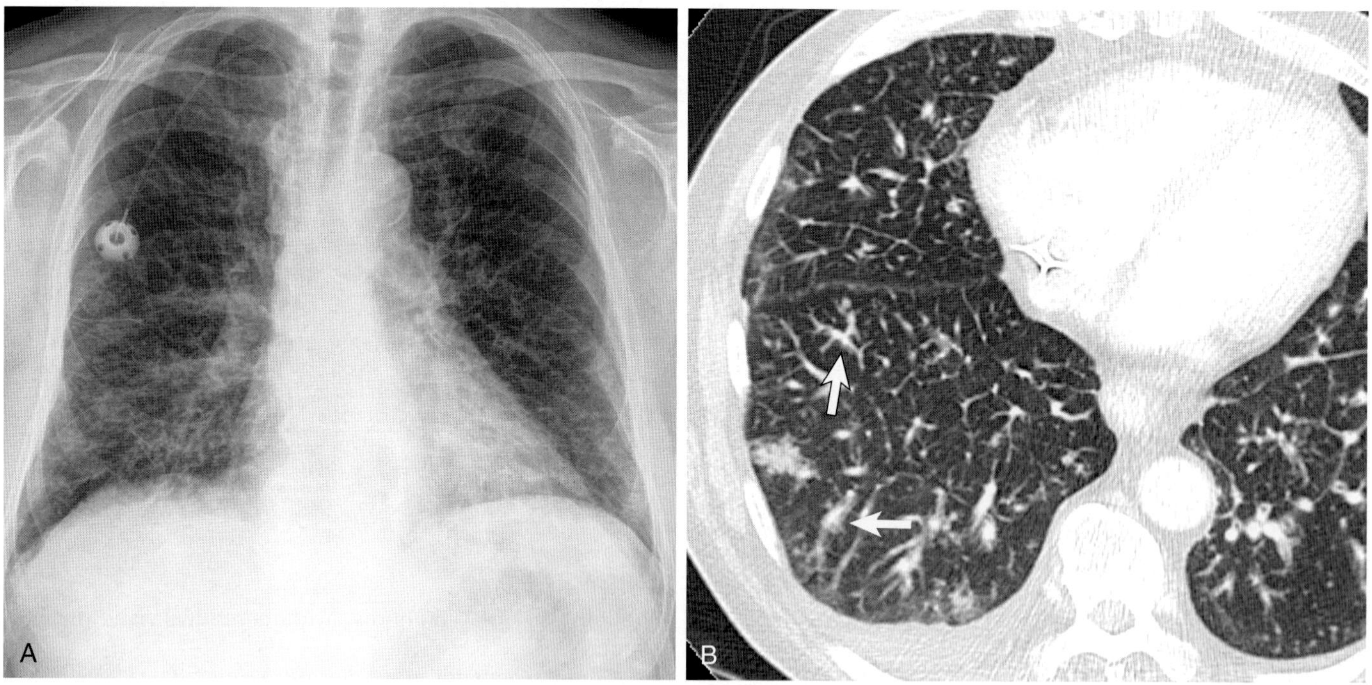

Fig. 22.4 Lymphangitic carcinomatosis from metastatic breast cancer. (A) Posteroanterior chest radiograph shows diffuse interstitial opacities with thickened interlobular septa. (B) Axial CT shows nodular septal thickening in the lower lobes. Note tree-in-bud opacities and a beaded appearance to several peripheral pulmonary arteries *(arrows)* likely representing coexistent intravascular metastases.

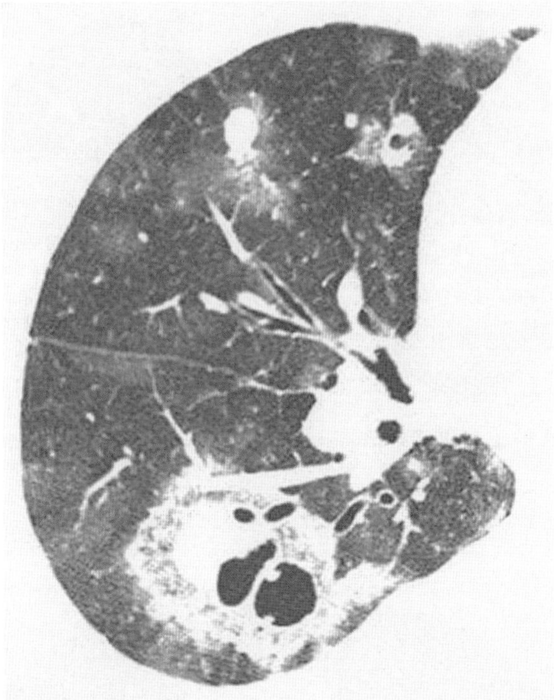

Fig. 22.5 Hemorrhagic and cavitating angiosarcoma metastases. Axial CT of the right lung shows several nodules and masses of various sizes, many surrounded by a halo of ground-glass opacity. Note cavitation of some of the nodules and masses.

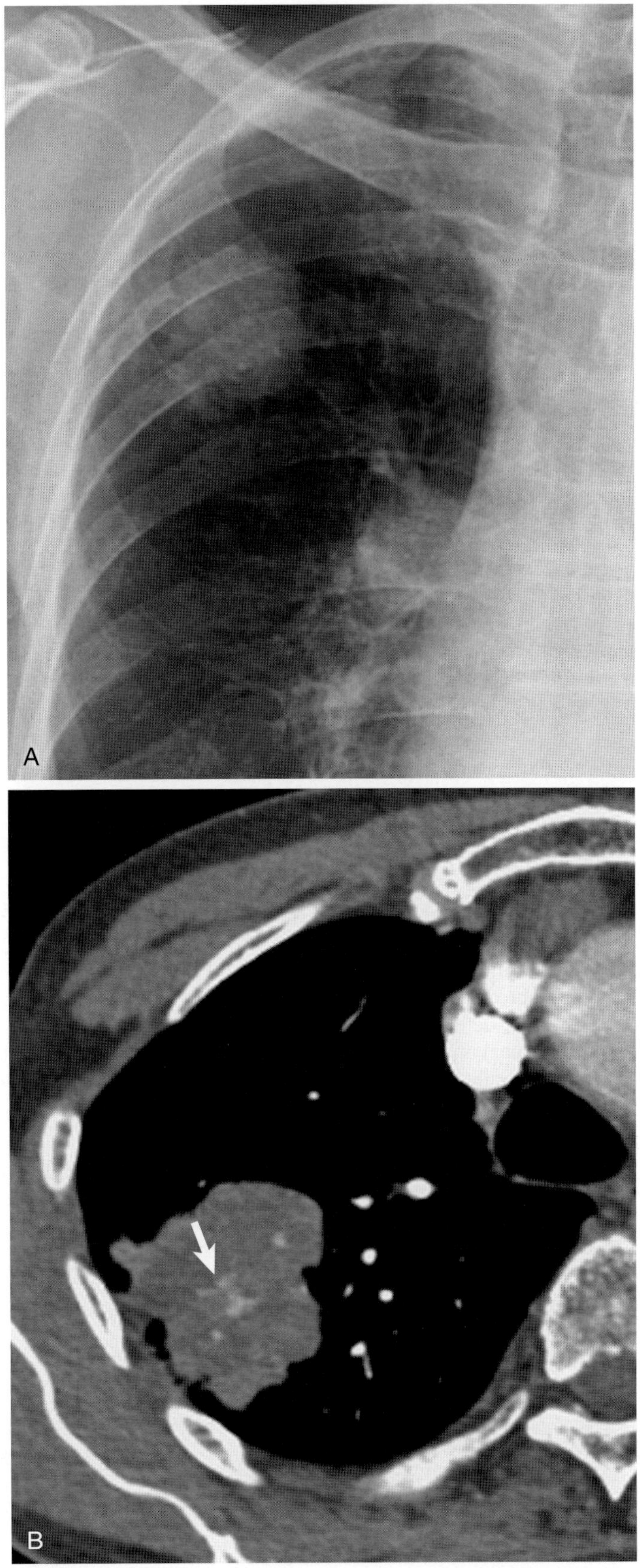

Fig. 22.6 Foci of calcification in metastatic colorectal adenocarcinoma. (A) Posteroanterior chest radiograph shows a right upper lobe mass with foci of increased opacity suggesting underlying calcification. (B) Axial CT confirms the presence of punctate calcification *(arrow)* within the right upper lobe mass. The extent of calcification increased on a subsequent CT (not shown).

complication is more frequent in patients undergoing chemotherapy. It may also occur before radiographic visibility of metastases.[20]

Solitary pulmonary nodules representing metastatic disease from extrathoracic primaries are rare, accounting for 2% to 10% of solitary pulmonary nodules in some studies. This percentage is based on radiographic findings and with the routine use of CT for screening; solitary metastases are much less common. Many of the nodules identified on CT in patients with extrathoracic malignancies represent granulomas or intrapulmonary lymphoid tissue.[21] Munden and associates[22] determined that 3-month follow-up imaging of patients with extrathoracic malignancies and small, less than 5 mm, incidentally detected pulmonary nodules for the first year and every 6 months thereafter effectively determines the malignant potential of the nodules.

Multiple studies have shown greater than 50% of solitary pulmonary nodules in patients with a history of prior extrapulmonary neoplasia turned out to be primary lung malignancies or benign lesions on surgery or autopsy.[23] The distinction between a new primary and a metastasis has important prognostic and therapeutic implications. Although new chemotherapeutic, and even molecular, therapies continue to develop, pulmonary metastasectomy remains the treatment of choice for most solitary pulmonary metastases.[24] With few exceptions, there are no criteria by which a solitary metastasis can be distinguished definitively from a primary pulmonary carcinoma by imaging.[25,26] Despite this lack of criteria, certain features of the pulmonary nodule as well as the particular primary neoplasm are associated with an increased probability of one or the other.[27] A solitary nodule in a patient who has a high-grade sarcoma or deeply invasive melanoma is much more likely to be a metastasis than a new primary. A nodule in a patient who has a squamous cell carcinoma of the

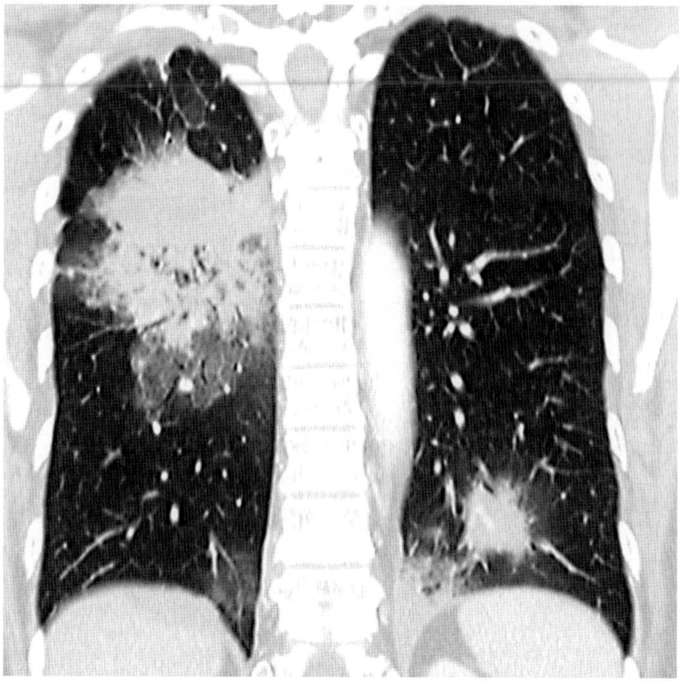

Fig. 22.7 Metastatic mucinous adenocarcinoma. Coronal reformatted CT shows a superior right lower lobe consolidation with surrounding ground-glass opacity. Note the smaller consolidation with surrounding ground-glass opacity in the left lower lobe. This represents airway spread of lung cancer.

head and neck is more likely a primary pulmonary carcinoma. The time interval between the initial tumor and the appearance of the pulmonary lesion is also important with most metastatic lesions occurring within 5 years of the original diagnosis. The major exception to this rule are carcinomas originating in the breast or kidney, in which metastases can occur many years after the original tumor is identified. Older age and a history of cigarette smoking increase the likelihood that the tumor is primary in the lung. Overall, detection of pulmonary nodules in patients with extrapulmonary malignancy is high, although most nodules are benign, especially if they are smaller than 10 mm in diameter or are less than 10 mm from the pleural surface.[28]

KEY POINTS: METASTATIC PULMONARY NODULES

- Metastatic pulmonary nodules are usually multiple.
- A single nodule is most common in carcinoma of the colon or kidneys and osteosarcoma.
- Metastatic pulmonary nodules have smooth or irregular margins and are randomly distributed, with predilection for the peripheral middle and lower lung zones.
- Cavitation occurs in 4% of metastases, most commonly in squamous cell carcinoma of the head and neck or cervix.
- Calcification is uncommon and occurs with osteogenic sarcoma; chondrosarcoma; synovial sarcoma; or carcinoma of the colon, ovary, breast, or thyroid.
- Small, less than 5-mm pulmonary nodules detected in cancer patients are usually benign. Malignant potential can be determined by looking for growth on 3-month follow-up CT examinations.

Lymphatic Spread (Lymphangitic Carcinomatosis)

Lymphangitic carcinomatosis has a characteristic high-resolution CT appearance, consisting of smooth or nodular thickening of

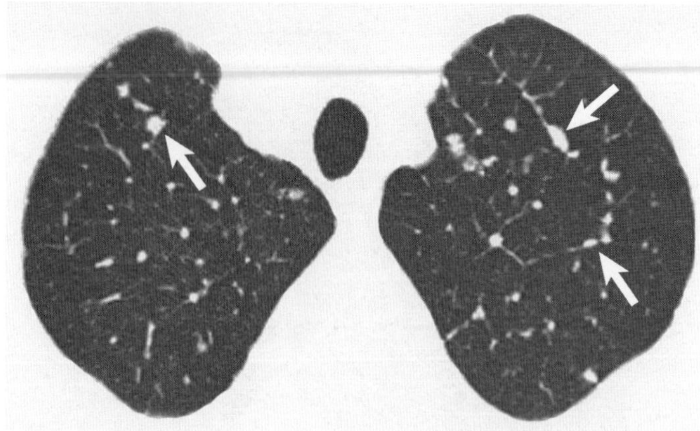

Fig. 22.8 Lymphangitic carcinomatosis: nodular septal thickening. High-resolution CT shows bilateral nodular thickening *(arrows)* of the interlobular septa.

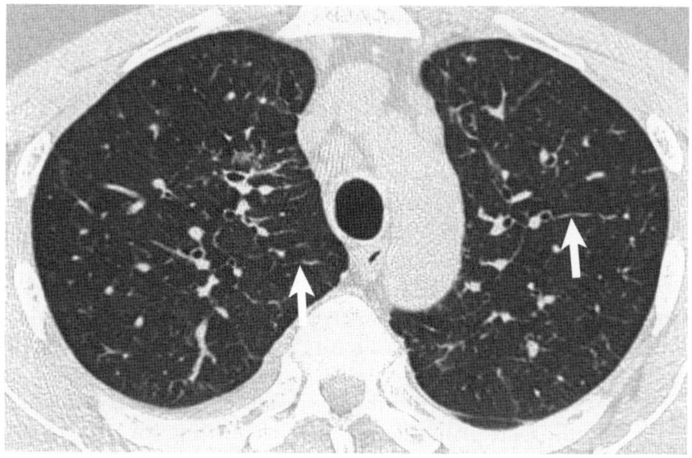

Fig. 22.9 Lymphangitic carcinomatosis: mild abnormalities. High-resolution CT shows mild, smooth, bilateral, interlobular septal thickening *(arrows)*. Lymphangitic carcinomatosis manifests with smooth septal thickening in about half of all cases.

the interlobular septa and peribronchovascular interstitium with preservation of normal lung architecture (Figs. 22.8 to 22.11).[13,29] The abnormalities may be initially subtle but tend to progress to extensive bilateral disease with associated ground-glass opacities. There is a great deal of overlap between the imaging findings of lymphangitic carcinomatosis and pulmonary edema as the conditions often coexist because of the obstruction of normal lymphatic drainage of fluid from the lungs by the tumor. Pleural effusion is seen on CT in about 30% of cases, and hilar or mediastinal lymph node enlargement is seen in 40%.[13]

At the time of diagnosis, the CT findings of lymphangitic carcinomatosis are unilateral or markedly asymmetric in 50% of cases (see Fig. 22.11).[13,30] Unilateral disease is particularly common in patients with lung cancer, whereas bilateral involvement is more common with extrapulmonary metastases. Disease may be obvious on CT in patients who have normal or nonspecific radiographic findings.[29,31]

Intravascular Tumor Emboli

Tumor emboli are visualized histopathologically in many patients who have nodular metastases, but they tend to occur in arterioles

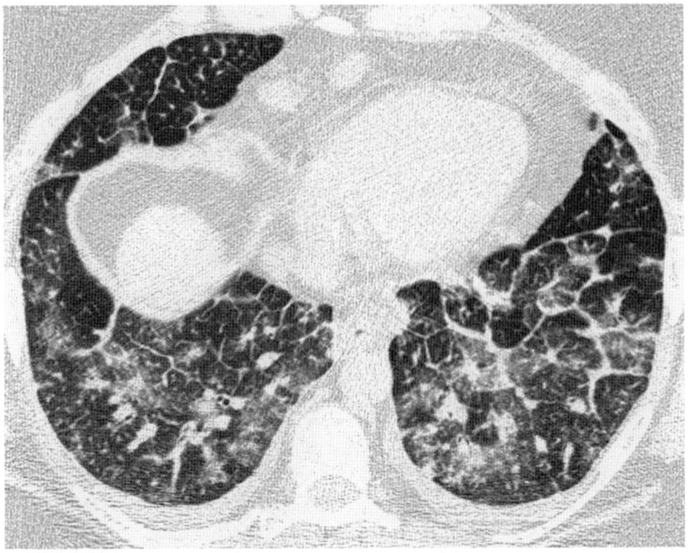

Fig. 22.10 Lymphangitic carcinomatosis: diffuse abnormalities. High-resolution CT shows extensive bilateral septal thickening with multiple polygonal arcades. Also noted are diffuse ground-glass opacities and trace bilateral pleural effusions caused by pulmonary edema.

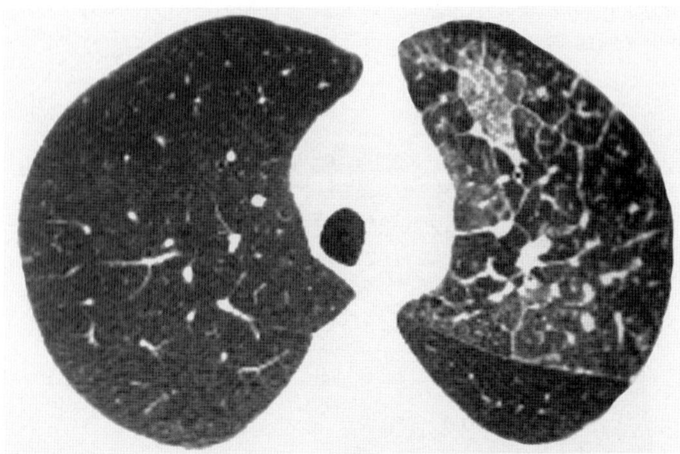

Fig. 22.11 Lymphangitic carcinomatosis: unilateral distribution. High-resolution CT shows septal thickening and ground-glass opacities in the left upper lobe caused by lymphangitic carcinomatosis from adenocarcinoma of the lung.

KEY POINTS: LYMPHANGITIC CARCINOMATOSIS

- Common primaries include carcinomas of the lung, breast, stomach, and pancreas.
- Lymphangitic carcinomatosis usually is bilateral except in pulmonary carcinoma.
- Imaging findings include:
  - Smooth or nodular thickening of interlobular septa and peribronchovascular interstitium
  - Lymphadenopathy in 30%
  - Pleural effusion in 30%–50%

or small arteries and are below the resolution of CT. Tumor emboli occasionally manifest indirectly as pulmonary infarcts with peripheral wedge-shaped opacities.[5] Uncommonly, tumor emboli manifest as filling defects in the central pulmonary arteries (Fig. 22.12), as nodular or beaded thickening of the peripheral pulmonary arteries, or as nodular and branching centrilobular opacities (tree-in-bud pattern) representing enlarged centrilobular arteries (Fig. 22.13).[7,32,33]

Intravascular tumor emboli usually coexist with another pattern of pulmonary involvement, most often lymphangitic carcinomatosis (see Fig. 22.4B). When emboli are the sole manifestation, the chest radiograph may be normal or may show dilation of central pulmonary arteries and the right ventricle, reflecting pulmonary hypertension.

KEY POINTS: INTRAVASCULAR TUMOR EMBOLI

- Intravascular tumor emboli are rarely identified radiographically.
- Common primaries include carcinomas of the breast, stomach, prostate, and kidney.
- Findings on CT include:
  - Wedge-shaped peripheral opacities
  - Intravascular filling defects on contrast-enhanced CT
  - Nodular or beaded thickening of the peripheral pulmonary arteries
  - Nodular and branching centrilobular opacities (tree-in-bud pattern)

Bronchial and Tracheal Metastases

Endobronchial metastases usually are secondary to carcinoma of the breast, colorectum, kidney, and cervix or to melanoma or sarcoma.[4,34] Endobronchial metastases are often radiographically occult. When present, the usual findings are those of bronchial obstruction, either partial (causing oligemia and expiratory air-trapping) or complete (with atelectasis and obstructive pneumonitis).[1,35] Metastases to the trachea are rare (Fig. 22.14). Similar to endobronchial metastases, the most common primary sites are breast, kidney, colon, and melanoma.[35–37]

Endobronchial and endotracheal metastases result in single or, less commonly, multiple endoluminal soft tissue lesions that usually can be readily identified on CT.[37,38] The tumors may be polypoid or have a glove-finger appearance with bronchial dilation. They typically enhance after intravenous administration of contrast material.[38]

KEY POINTS: BRONCHIAL AND TRACHEAL METASTASES

- Bronchial and tracheal metastases are uncommon.
- Common primaries include melanoma and carcinomas of the breast, rectum, and kidney.
- Bronchial and tracheal metastases are seldom evident on chest radiography but may manifest indirectly with distal air-trapping or atelectasis.
- Bronchial and tracheal metastases are usually solitary, manifesting as a soft tissue attenuating nodule.

MAGNETIC RESONANCE IMAGING

Although initial studies showed a low sensitivity of magnetic resonance imaging (MRI) compared with CT in the evaluation of pulmonary nodules,[39] the sensitivity of MRI has increased considerably with the improvement of MRI quality and development of specialized sequences. CT remains more sensitive than MRI for the detection of small (<6 mm) pulmonary nodules (88.5% vs. 71.9%), although each showed similar accuracy in the evaluation of lymph node metastases.[40] MRI is more specific for

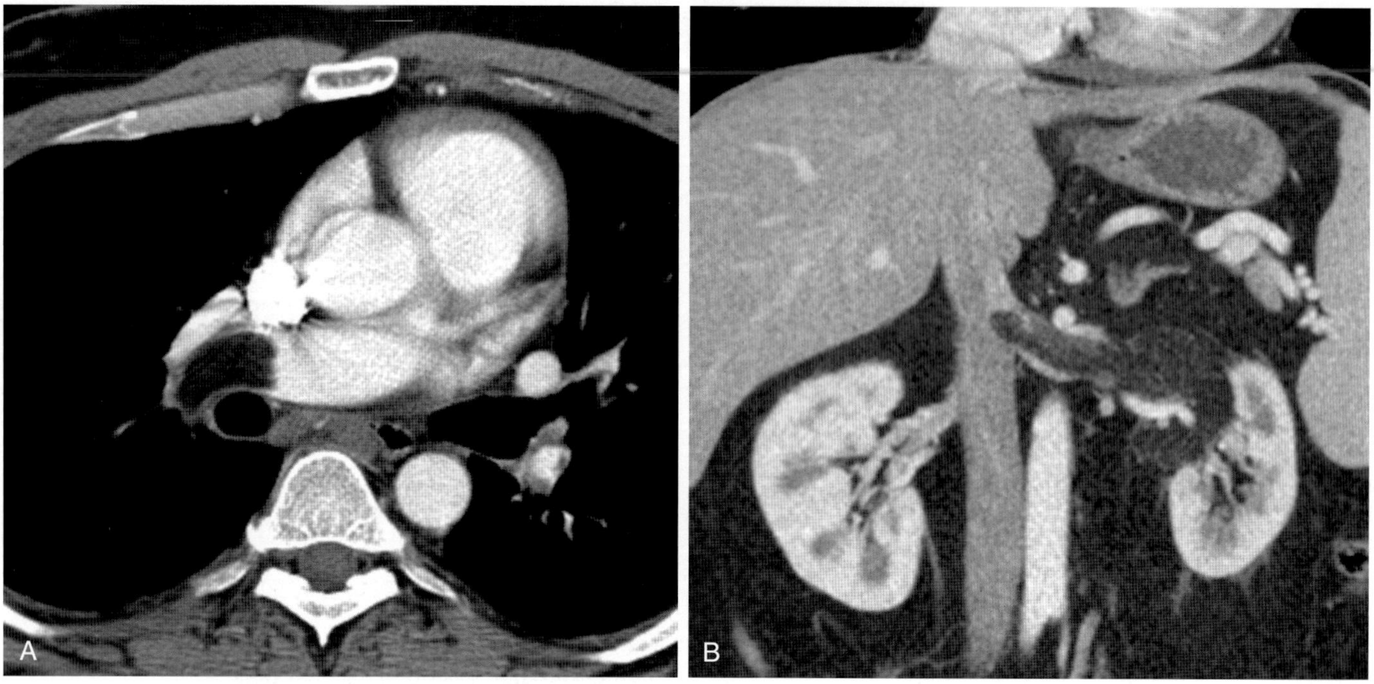

Fig. 22.12 Intravascular metastasis. (A) Axial contrast-enhanced CT shows a large fat attenuation–filling defect in the right pulmonary artery. (B) Coronal CT through the upper abdomen shows the left kidney angiomyolipoma extending into the renal vein and inferior vena cava.

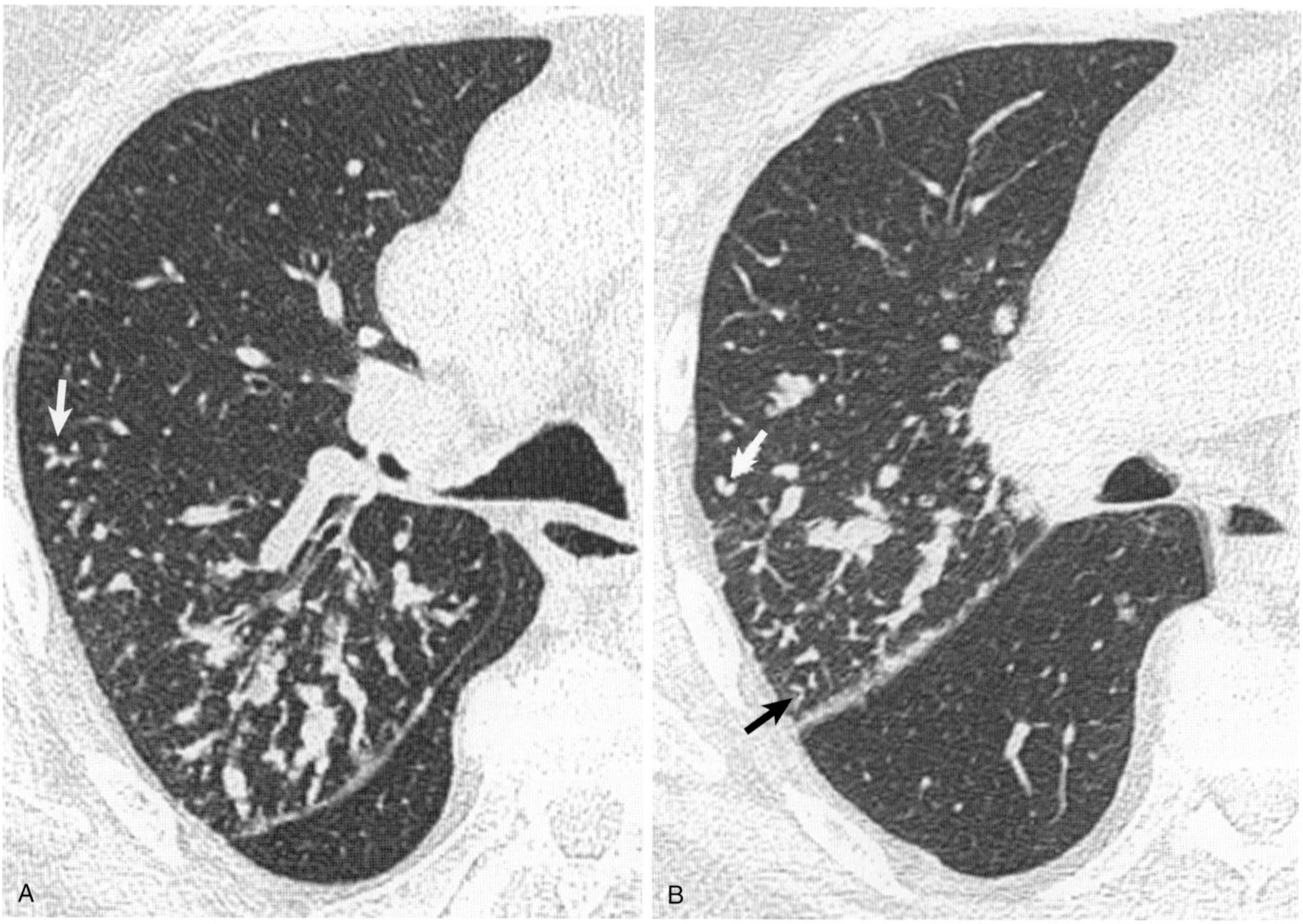

Fig. 22.13 Intravascular metastases from renal cell carcinoma. (A) and (B) Axial CTs of the right lung at the level of the tracheal carina (A) and bronchus intermedius (B) show nodular thickening of the pulmonary vessels and centrilobular nodular and branching opacities *(arrows)*.

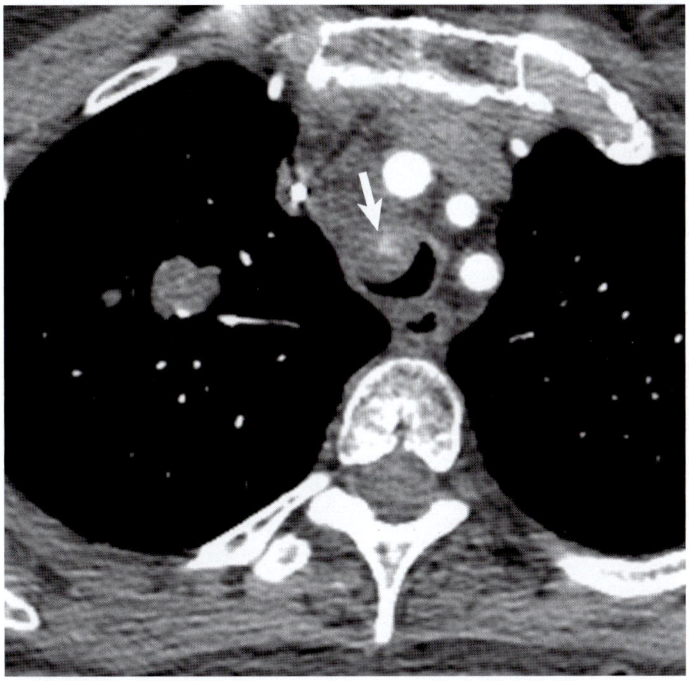

Fig. 22.14 Tracheal metastasis from papillary thyroid carcinoma. Axial CT shows an intraluminal lesion *(arrow)* arising from the anterior wall of the middle trachea. Subtle central densities relate to calcification associated with papillary thyroid cancer. Note additional right lung metastasis.

evaluation of pulmonary metastases from certain primary malignancies, such as melanoma, because of intrinsic signal characteristics of the nodules compared with CT (83.4% vs. 50.4%).[41]

Vogt and associates[42] showed the sensitivity of half-Fourier acquisition single-shot turbo-spin-echo (HASTE) MRI increased with lesion size, ranging from 95% for nodules 5 to 10 mm in diameter to 100% for lesions exceeding 3 cm in diameter.

With the advent of volumetric acquisition images allowing nearly isotropic resolution, image quality comparable to that of conventional two-dimensional images is achievable with much shorter scan times.[43] Diffusion-weighted MR imaging (DWI), although of limited use in evaluation of smaller pulmonary nodules (<1 cm), can help to differentiate benign from malignant nodules on the basis of tissue cellularity.[43]

Lauenstein and colleagues[44] compared whole-body MRI findings with results obtained at skeletal scintigraphy, CT, and dedicated MRI in 51 patients with known malignant tumors. All cerebral, pulmonary, and hepatic metastases greater than 6 mm in diameter could be identified with whole-body MRI. Small pulmonary metastases were missed with MRI, but these misses did not change therapeutic strategies. Additionally, MRI depicted a single hepatic metastasis that was missed with CT. Skeletal scintigraphy depicted osseous metastases in 21 patients, whereas whole-body MRI revealed osseous metastases in 24 patients. The additional osseous metastases seen with MRI were confirmed at follow-up examinations but did not result in a change in therapy. Whole-body MRI demonstrated sensitivity and specificity values of 100%.[44]

POSITRON EMISSION TOMOGRAPHY

Several studies have shown that positron emission tomography (PET) with fluorodeoxyglucose (FDG) can be useful for the detection of intrathoracic metastases.[45,46] Pastorino and coworkers[45] evaluated the role of PET in the preoperative assessment of lung metastases, deemed resectable at CT. In 19 cases (21%), lung surgery was excluded on the basis of PET results showing extrapulmonary metastases, primary site recurrence, mediastinal lymphadenopathy, or benign disease. All mediastinal node metastases (seven cases) were detected by PET (sensitivity, 100%), compared with a sensitivity of 71% for CT. The PET sensitivity for detection of lung metastasis was 87%. Multiple additional studies showed similar sensitivity and specificity of FDG-PET for the detection of pulmonary metastases.[47,48]

Because of the limited sensitivity of PET in detection of small metastases and the limited specificity of CT, it is recommended that combined PET-CT be used in the assessment of pulmonary metastases. Reinhardt and colleagues[46] found that hypermetabolic lesions, particularly those between 5 mm and 13 mm, were better visualized on the non–attenuation-corrected images compared with attenuation-corrected images. This is important because traditionally the corrected images are often used exclusively for interpretation.

FDG-PET has greater sensitivity and specificity than CT in detecting nodal metastases from lung cancer and extrathoracic malignancies. Eubank and colleagues[49] found that PET had an accuracy of 88% in detecting metastatic breast cancer to the mediastinum and internal mammary lymph nodes compared with 73% accuracy of CT.

The emergence of PET-MRI as an integrated hybrid imaging system has allowed simultaneous acquisition and highly accurate coregistration of PET and MRI datasets.[50] A comprehensive study of PET-CT versus PET-MRI in staging of oncology patients showed no statistically significant difference in tumor-node-metastasis staging between the modalities.[50] As MRI continues to advance, use of PET-MRI will likely become more accepted for whole-body imaging, although its use for the evaluation of pulmonary metastases remains limited.

IMAGING ALGORITHMS

Although radiography is often the first-line imaging study for the evaluation of patients with suspected pulmonary metastases, the vast majority of patients will also receive CT. Addition of FDG-PET can be helpful for further assessment, particularly in patients with potentially resectable lesions. A recent study by Altenbernd and colleagues,[51] using dual-energy CT for the creation of virtual noncontrast images, showed that the enhancement characteristics of the lung nodule can be evaluated with arterial and delayed venous-phase imaging and can be used to help delineate the type of primary malignant tumor (e.g., differentiating metastatic lung carcinoma or salivary gland cancer from colorectal carcinoma or malignant melanoma).

Differential Diagnosis

Multiple studies have shown solitary pulmonary nodules in patients with extrathoracic malignancy are more likely to represent lung cancer than metastasis.[52,53] Although multiple nodules of various sizes in a patient with known extrathoracic malignancy or a pattern of lymphangitic carcinomatosis is suggestive of metastatic disease, cytologic or histologic proof or imaging follow-up showing growth usually is required to confirm the diagnosis.

Although bronchoscopic biopsy usually demonstrates lower yields with metastatic disease compared with primary lung malignancies, diagnostic rates of 50% to 60% have been reported.[54,55] The positive yield is highest in tumors with endobronchial extension.

In contrast, transthoracic needle biopsy has much greater diagnostics rates, approaching 85% to 90%. Because a larger portion of tissue is often acquired, when the site of the extrathoracic primary tumor is known, a definitive cytologic diagnosis of metastatic cancer is frequently possible. In some neoplasms, such as renal cell or colorectal carcinoma, cytologic features alone may be sufficiently characteristic to suggest the site of origin.

SUGGESTED READINGS

Hanamiya M, Aoki T, Yamashita Y, et al. Frequency and significance of pulmonary nodules on thin-section CT in patients with extrapulmonary malignant neoplasms. *Eur J Radiol*. 2012;81:152–157.

Seo JB, Im JG, Goo JM, et al. Atypical pulmonary metastases: spectrum of radiologic findings. *Radiographics*. 2001;21:403–417.

The full reference list for this chapter is available at ExpertConsult.com.

23 Pulmonary Lymphoid Hyperplasia and Lymphoid Interstitial Pneumonia (Lymphocytic Interstitial Pneumonia)*

JONATHAN H. CHUNG | CHRISTOPHER M. WALKER

Pulmonary Lymphoid Hyperplasia (Follicular Bronchiolitis)

ETIOLOGY, PREVALENCE, AND EPIDEMIOLOGY

Pulmonary lymphoid hyperplasia, also known as follicular bronchiolitis or hyperplasia of bronchus-associated lymphoid tissue, is a benign condition characterized histologically by the presence of polyclonal lymphoid aggregates along the bifurcation of the bronchioles and along the pulmonary lymphatics and is mainly differentiated from lymphocytic interstitial pneumonia (LIP) by its typical distribution limited mainly to the airways.[1,2] It is seen most commonly in association with connective tissue disease, particularly rheumatoid arthritis; immunodeficiency, particularly acquired immune deficiency syndrome (AIDS) (usually in children); hypersensitivity disorders; and as a nonspecific response in patients with airway infection, airway obstruction, or bronchiectasis.[1,2]

CLINICAL PRESENTATION

Pulmonary lymphoid hyperplasia may occur in children and adults (age range, 1.5–77 years).[2] The most common presenting symptoms are progressive shortness of breath and cough. Other manifestations include fever, recurrent pneumonia, and weight loss.[1,2]

PATHOLOGY

Pulmonary lymphoid hyperplasia is characterized histologically by the presence of discrete foci of hyperplastic lymphoid tissue, often associated with germinal centers, along the bronchovascular bundles (Figs. 23.1 and 23.2).[1,2] Hyperplastic lymphoid tissue also may be present within interlobular septa and visceral pleura.[1,2]

*The editors and the publisher would like to thank Drs. Nestor L. Müller and C. Isabela Silva Müller for contributing material on this topic to the prior edition of this work. It has served as the foundation for the current chapter.

MANIFESTATIONS OF THE DISEASE

Radiography

The chest radiograph may be normal or show bilateral reticular or reticulonodular opacities (Fig. 23.3).[1,2]

Computed Tomography

The main high-resolution computed tomography (CT) findings consist of bilateral centrilobular and peribronchial nodules.[3] Most nodules measure less than 3 mm in diameter. Nodules 3 to 12 mm in diameter are present in approximately 50% of patients, and patchy ground-glass opacities are present in approximately 75% of patients; small foci of consolidation may be seen in some patients (see Fig. 23.3).[3] The nodules may be diffuse or involve mainly the lower lung zones. The nodules reflect the predominant histologic findings of peribronchiolar inflammation and coalescent germinal centers.[3] Less common manifestations include mild interlobular septal thickening and bronchial dilation.

DIFFERENTIAL DIAGNOSIS

Centrilobular nodules are seen in a variety of diseases that affect predominantly the bronchioles or peribronchiolar interstitium. Common causes include hypersensitivity pneumonitis, respiratory bronchiolitis, and infectious bronchiolitis. Pulmonary lymphoid hyperplasia requires lung biopsy for definitive diagnosis.

SYNOPSIS OF TREATMENT OPTIONS

Patients with pulmonary lymphoid hyperplasia usually have a good prognosis. Treatment may be directed at the underlying disease or may consist of steroids or azathioprine.[1]

Lymphoid Interstitial Pneumonia (Lymphocytic Interstitial Pneumonia)

ETIOLOGY, PREVALENCE, AND EPIDEMIOLOGY

LIP is a rare condition limited to the lungs and characterized at histology by diffuse infiltration of the alveolar septa by polyclonal

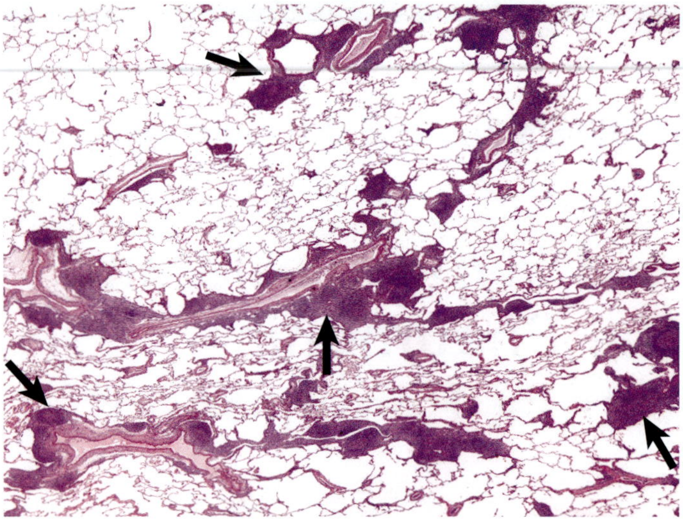

Fig. 23.1 Pulmonary lymphoid hyperplasia in a patient with rheumatoid arthritis: pathologic findings. Low-power view shows hyperplastic lymphoid follicles *(arrows)* along the bronchovascular bundles. *(Courtesy Dr. John English, Department of Pathology, Vancouver General Hospital, Vancouver, Canada.)*

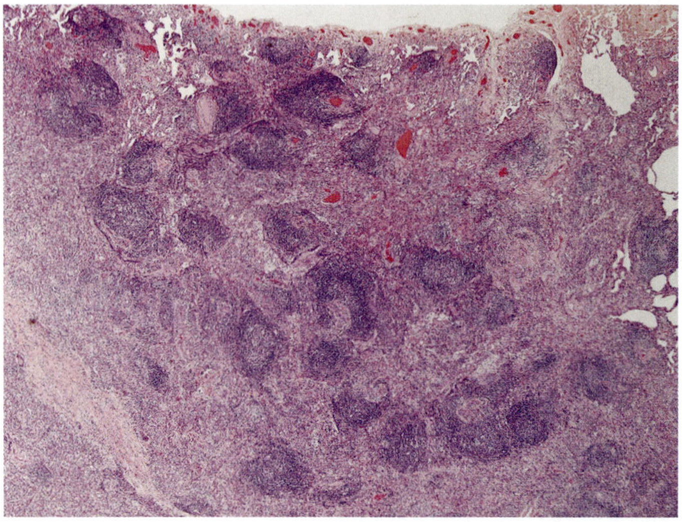

Fig. 23.2 Pulmonary lymphoid hyperplasia: pathologic findings. Histologic specimen shows extensive lymphoid hyperplasia with lymphoid nodules, including lymphoid follicles, adjacent to small airways. *(Courtesy Dr. William D. Travis, Department of Pathology, Memorial Sloan Kettering Cancer Center, New York.)*

KEY POINTS: PULMONARY LYMPHOID HYPERPLASIA

- Pulmonary lymphoid hyperplasia or follicular bronchiolitis is a benign condition characterized by the presence of polyclonal lymphoid aggregates mainly along the bifurcation of the bronchioles.
- Symptomatic pulmonary lymphoid hyperplasia occurs most commonly in patients with rheumatoid arthritis and immunodeficiency.
- The chest radiograph may be normal or show bilateral reticular or reticulonodular opacities.
- The main high-resolution CT finding consists of small bilateral centrilobular and peribronchial nodules.
- Definitive diagnosis requires surgical lung biopsy. Prognosis is usually favorable.

BOX 23.1 CONDITIONS ASSOCIATED WITH LYMPHOID INTERSTITIAL PNEUMONIA

COLLAGEN VASCULAR DISEASE

Sjögren syndrome
Systemic lupus erythematosus
Rheumatoid arthritis
Polymyositis

AUTOIMMUNE DISEASES

Hashimoto thyroiditis
Myasthenia gravis
Hemolytic anemia
Pernicious anemia
Autoerythrocyte sensitization syndrome
Chronic active hepatitis
Celiac sprue
Primary biliary cirrhosis

SYSTEMIC IMMUNODEFICIENCY STATES

HIV/AIDS
Common variable immunodeficiency
Agammaglobulinemia

DRUG INDUCED

Diphenylhydantoin
Captopril

INFECTIONS (OTHER THAN HIV)

Legionella pneumonia
Tuberculosis
Mycoplasma
Chlamydia
Epstein-Barr virus infection
Human herpesvirus 8

MISCELLANEOUS

Complication of allogeneic bone marrow transplantation
Pulmonary alveolar microlithiasis
Pulmonary alveolar proteinosis
Idiopathic

AIDS, Acquired immune deficiency disease syndrome; *HIV*, human immunodeficiency virus.

lymphocytes.[1,4–6] LIP has been considered part of a spectrum of pulmonary lymphoproliferative disorders that range in severity from benign airway-centered cellular aggregates (lymphoid hyperplasia) to malignant lymphomas[4,5]; however, immunohistochemical and molecular analyses indicate that the risk of transformation to pulmonary lymphoma is low.[7] Most cases of LIP occur in patients with underlying autoimmune disease or immunodeficiency, most commonly Sjögren syndrome, autoimmune disorders, dysproteinemia, and AIDS; the last-mentioned is particularly seen in children (Box 23.1).[1,5] When underlying systemic diseases are excluded, a diagnosis of "idiopathic" LIP can be made; however, idiopathic LIP is extremely rare.[1,7] The clinical and radiologic manifestations of LIP often resemble those of other interstitial pneumonias, and the histologic pattern is that of an interstitial pneumonia that can mimic nonspecific interstitial pneumonia and occasionally hypersensitivity pneumonitis.[5] LIP is part of the updated American Thoracic Society/European Respiratory Society international multidisciplinary consensus classification of idiopathic interstitial pneumonias and is one of the "rare" idiopathic interstitial pneumonias.[5]

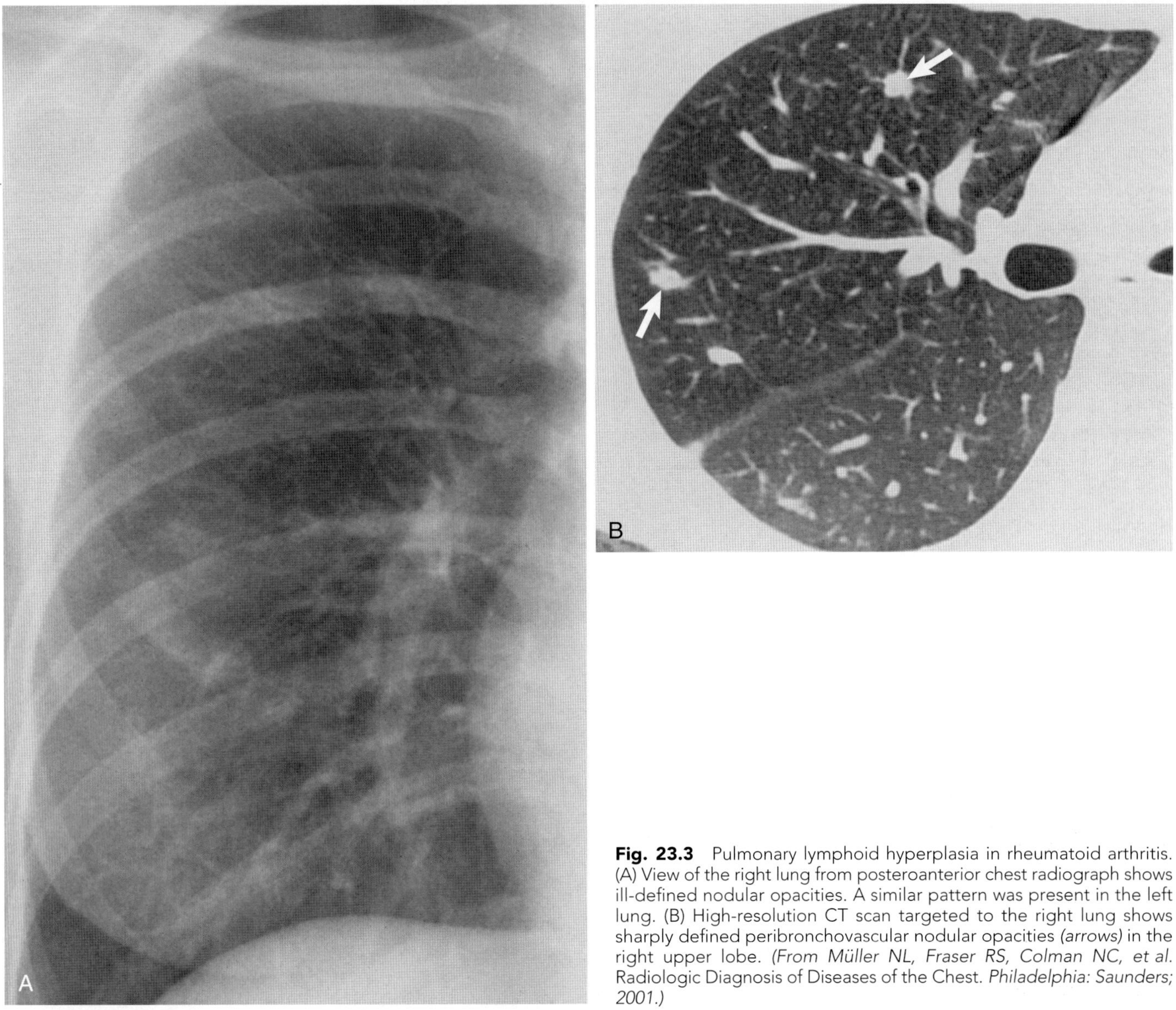

Fig. 23.3 Pulmonary lymphoid hyperplasia in rheumatoid arthritis. (A) View of the right lung from posteroanterior chest radiograph shows ill-defined nodular opacities. A similar pattern was present in the left lung. (B) High-resolution CT scan targeted to the right lung shows sharply defined peribronchovascular nodular opacities *(arrows)* in the right upper lobe. *(From Müller NL, Fraser RS, Colman NC, et al.* Radiologic Diagnosis of Diseases of the Chest. *Philadelphia: Saunders; 2001.)*

CLINICAL PRESENTATION

The average age of presentation is 50 to 60 years; women are affected twice as commonly as men.[1,4,7] The onset is typically insidious over several years.[5,7] The main clinical symptoms are cough, dyspnea, and fatigue.[7] Approximately 80% of patients have serum dysproteinemia, most commonly polyclonal hypergammaglobulinemia.[4] Analysis of bronchoalveolar lavage fluid frequently shows lymphocytosis (30%).[7]

PATHOLOGY

LIP is characterized histologically by extensive infiltration of the alveolar septa with polyclonal lymphocytes and variable numbers of plasma cells (Fig. 23.4).[1] Although usually more or less diffuse within the lobule, small nodular foci may be seen as a result of localized proliferation or the formation of germinal centers. Fibrosis is usually absent or mild in severity; occasionally, it may be associated with remodeling and a honeycomb appearance.[1,8] Airspaces are typically unaffected.

Lung Function

Pulmonary function tests show a restrictive defect with reduction of total lung capacity, forced vital capacity, and forced expiratory volume in 1 second, and increased ratio of forced expiratory volume in 1 second to forced vital capacity.[7]

MANIFESTATIONS OF THE DISEASE

Radiography

Radiographic findings consist of a reticular or reticulonodular pattern involving mainly the lower lung zones.[4,9,10] Less common abnormalities include a nodular pattern, hazy increased opacities (ground-glass opacities), and airspace consolidation (Fig. 23.5). Cystic lesions also may be seen on the chest radiograph (Fig. 23.6).

Computed Tomography

The main findings on high-resolution CT consist of extensive bilateral ground-glass opacities and poorly defined centrilobular

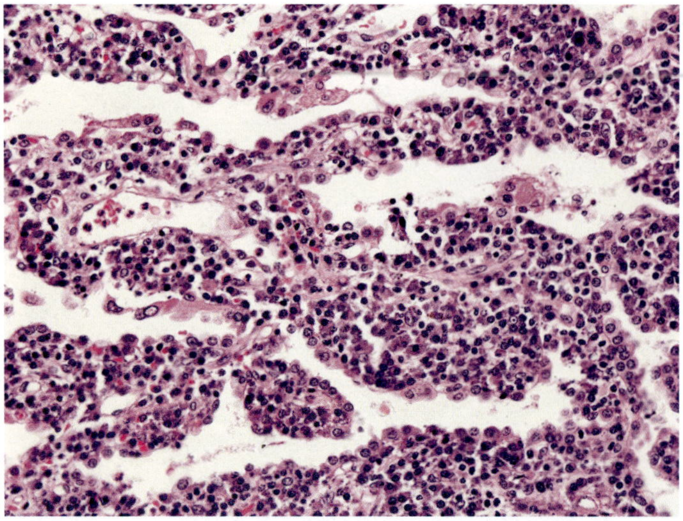

Fig. 23.4 Lymphoid interstitial pneumonia: pathologic findings. Histologic specimen shows diffuse lymphocytic infiltration of the pulmonary interstitium. *(Courtesy Dr. William D. Travis, Department of Pathology, Memorial Sloan Kettering Cancer Center, New York.)*

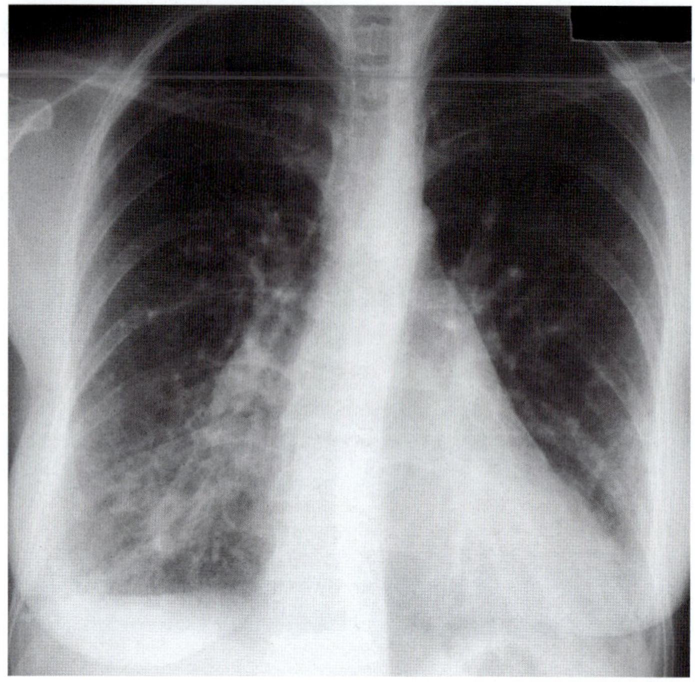

Fig. 23.5 Lymphoid interstitial pneumonia in a woman with Sjögren syndrome and juvenile rheumatoid arthritis. Posteroanterior chest radiograph shows bilateral areas of hazy increased opacity and consolidation involving the lower lung zones.

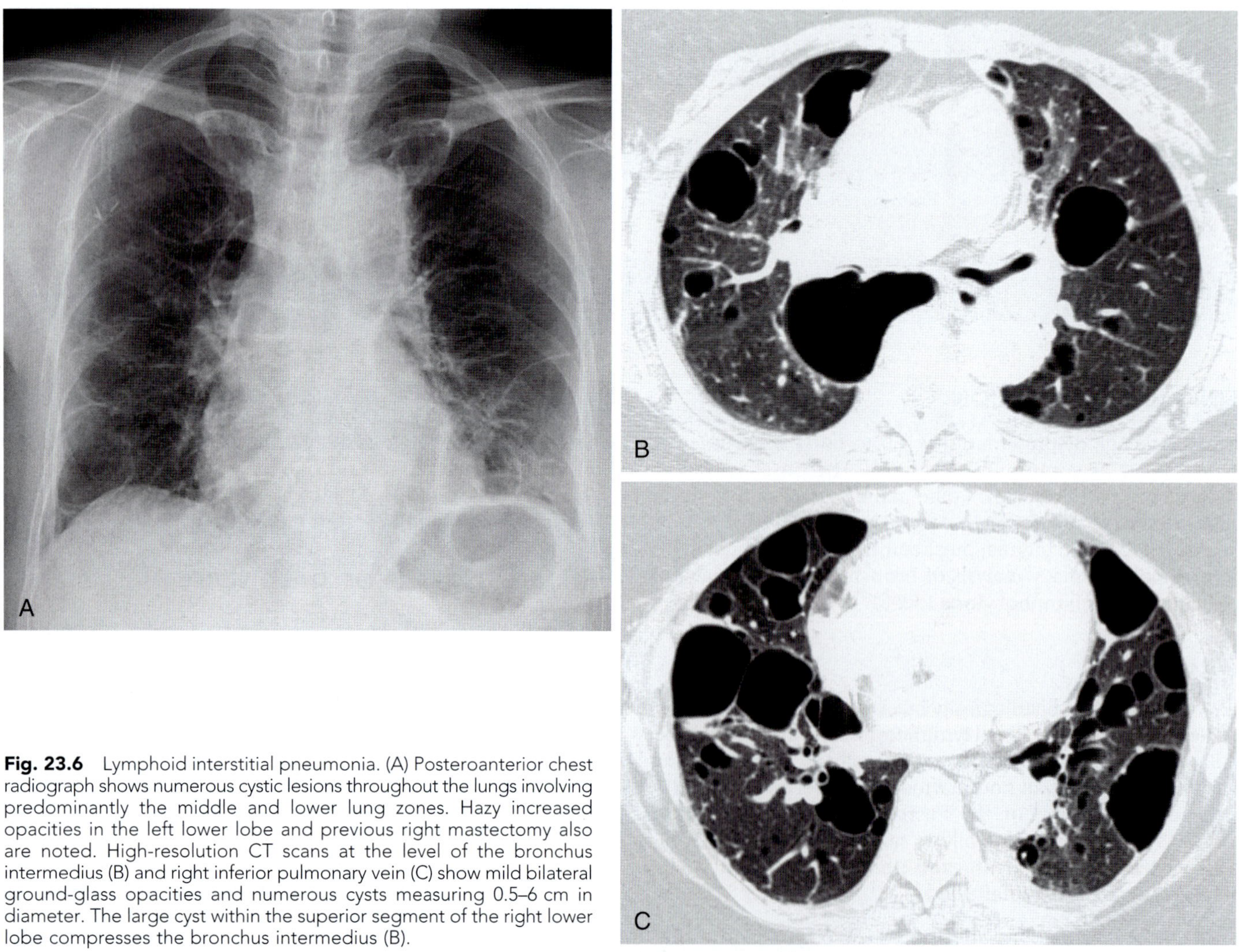

Fig. 23.6 Lymphoid interstitial pneumonia. (A) Posteroanterior chest radiograph shows numerous cystic lesions throughout the lungs involving predominantly the middle and lower lung zones. Hazy increased opacities in the left lower lobe and previous right mastectomy also are noted. High-resolution CT scans at the level of the bronchus intermedius (B) and right inferior pulmonary vein (C) show mild bilateral ground-glass opacities and numerous cysts measuring 0.5–6 cm in diameter. The large cyst within the superior segment of the right lower lobe compresses the bronchus intermedius (B).

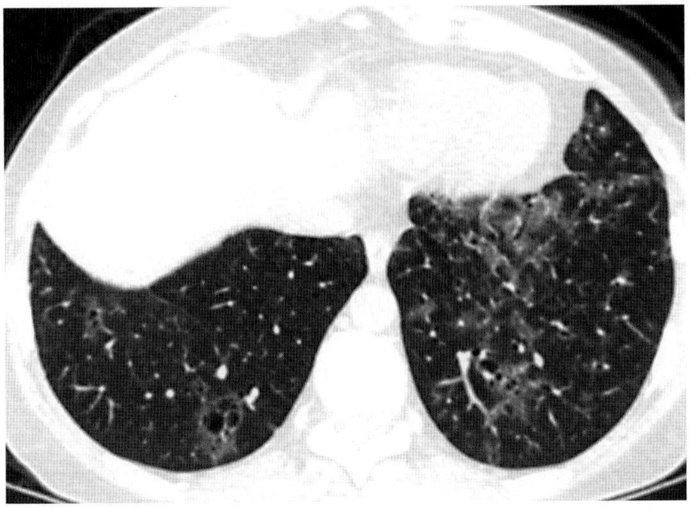

Fig. 23.7 Lymphoid interstitial pneumonia. High-resolution CT scan shows bilateral ground-glass opacities, mild reticulation, and clustered cysts predominantly affecting the lower lobes.

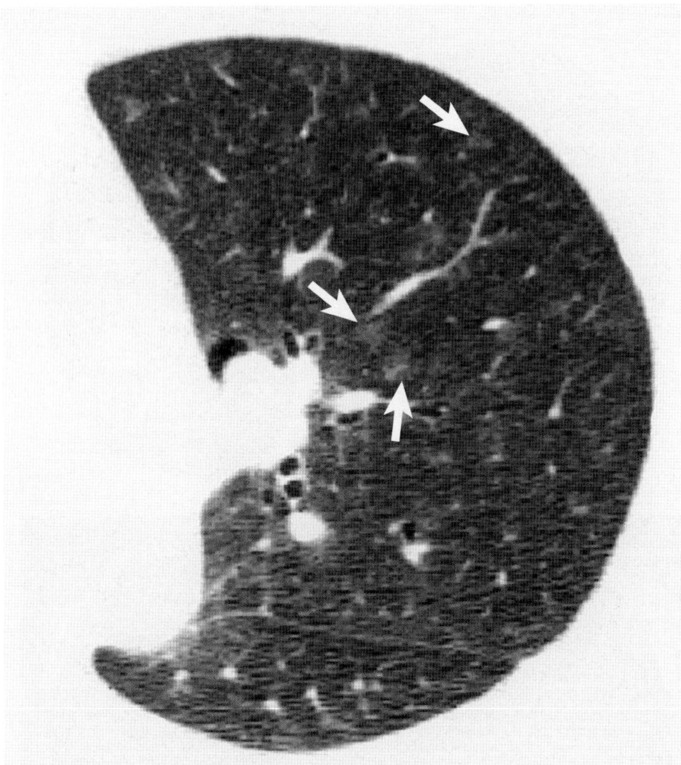

Fig. 23.8 Lymphoid interstitial pneumonia in a woman with mixed connective tissue disease. High-resolution CT scan targeted to the left lung shows mild ground-glass opacities and a few poorly defined centrilobular nodules *(arrows)*.

nodules (Figs. 23.7 and 23.8); other common manifestations include subpleural nodules, thickening of the bronchovascular bundles, and a few cystic airspaces (Fig. 23.9).[8,11,12]

In one review of the high-resolution CT findings in 22 patients who had LIP, all patients had areas of ground-glass opacity and poorly defined centrilobular nodules, 86% had small subpleural nodules, 86% had thickening of the peribronchovascular interstitium, 82% had mild interlobular septal thickening, and approximately 70% had cystic airspaces.[8] The cystic airspaces had thin walls, measured 1 to 30 mm in diameter, and involved less than 10% of the lung parenchyma. The cysts tend to have a predominantly perivascular and subpleural distribution (Fig. 23.10). Less common manifestations include nodules 1 to 2 cm in diameter, airspace consolidation, bronchiectasis, and occasionally honeycombing.[8,13] Although lymph node enlargement is seldom evident on the chest radiograph, slightly enlarged mediastinal lymph nodes are seen on CT in 70% of patients with LIP.[8]

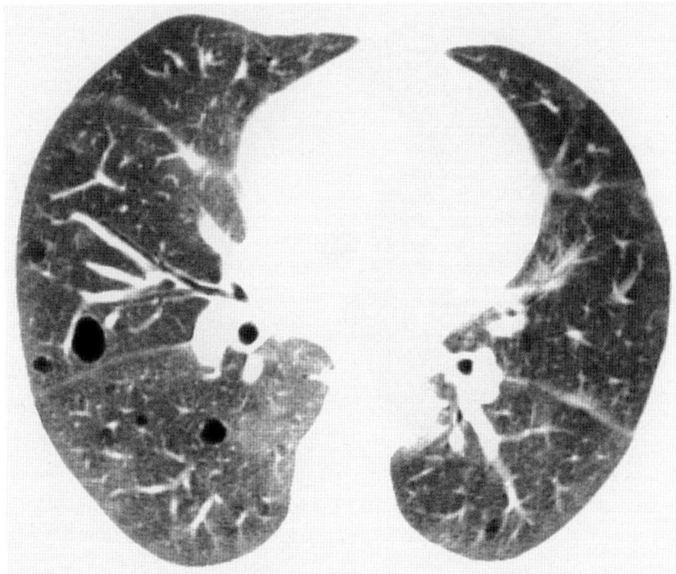

Fig. 23.9 Lymphoid interstitial pneumonia associated with Sjögren syndrome: classic CT findings. High-resolution CT scan shows extensive ground-glass opacities and a few bilateral cysts.

The cystic changes in LIP are usually mild and are associated with ground-glass opacities. Occasionally, the cysts may be an isolated finding or may be extensive. Silva and colleagues[14] reported the findings in one patient who had idiopathic LIP and diffuse lung cysts as the predominant high-resolution CT findings and who underwent unilateral lung transplantation. The cysts measured 0.5 to 10 cm in diameter (see Fig. 23.6) and resembled severe bullous emphysema and lymphangioleiomyomatosis. The cysts in the native lung remained unchanged on follow-up high-resolution CT 4 years later. Histologic correlation has shown the cystic airspaces to be due to partial airway obstruction by the peribronchiolar cellular infiltration.[11] In one patient who underwent lung transplant, the lung explant showed several markedly ectatic bronchioles and small peripheral bronchi that directly communicated with the large cystic spaces.[14] The cysts were identified within the lung parenchyma mostly in areas with lymphocytic infiltration. The centrilobular nodules seen on high-resolution CT are due to peribronchiolar infiltration with lymphocytes and plasma cells, whereas the ground-glass opacities reflect a diffuse interstitial infiltration. Nodules occasionally seen in association with the cysts or within the cystic changes in patients with LIP should raise the possibility of coexistent pulmonary amyloidosis; the nodules may calcify (Fig. 23.11).[13]

Ground-glass opacities and small nodular opacities in patients with LIP tend to improve on follow-up, but the cysts usually persist and may increase in size over time (Fig. 23.12).[15] In one study the authors performed serial high-resolution CT scans 4 to 82 months (median, 13 months) apart in 14 patients with

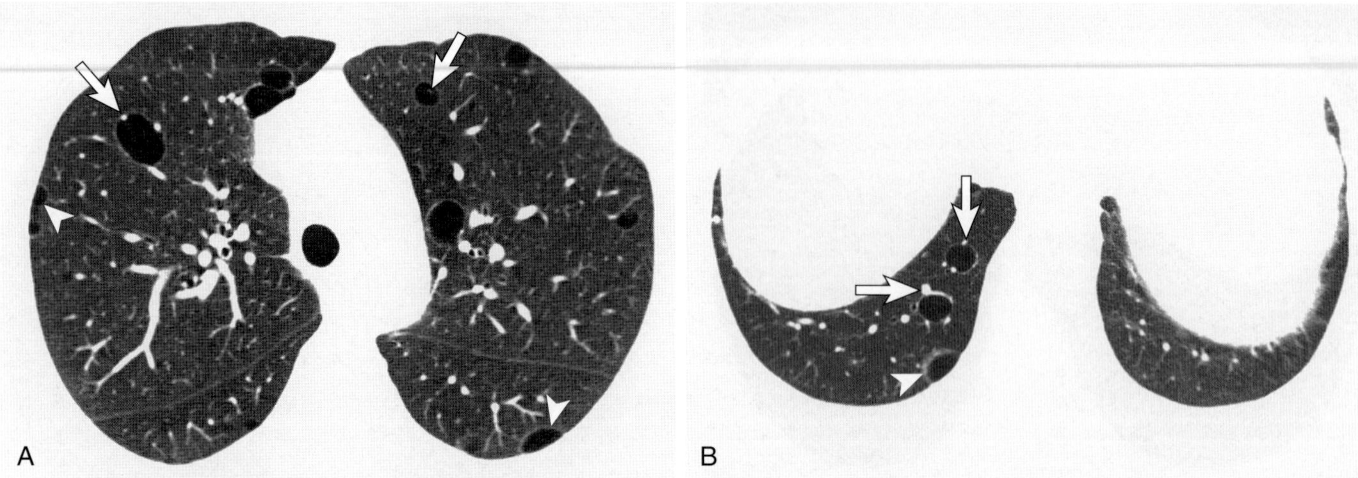

Fig. 23.10 Lymphoid interstitial pneumonia: cystic changes. High-resolution CT scans at the level of the aortic arch (A) and lung bases (B) show bilateral thin-walled cysts. Some of the cysts have a perivascular *(arrows)* or subpleural *(arrowheads)* distribution.

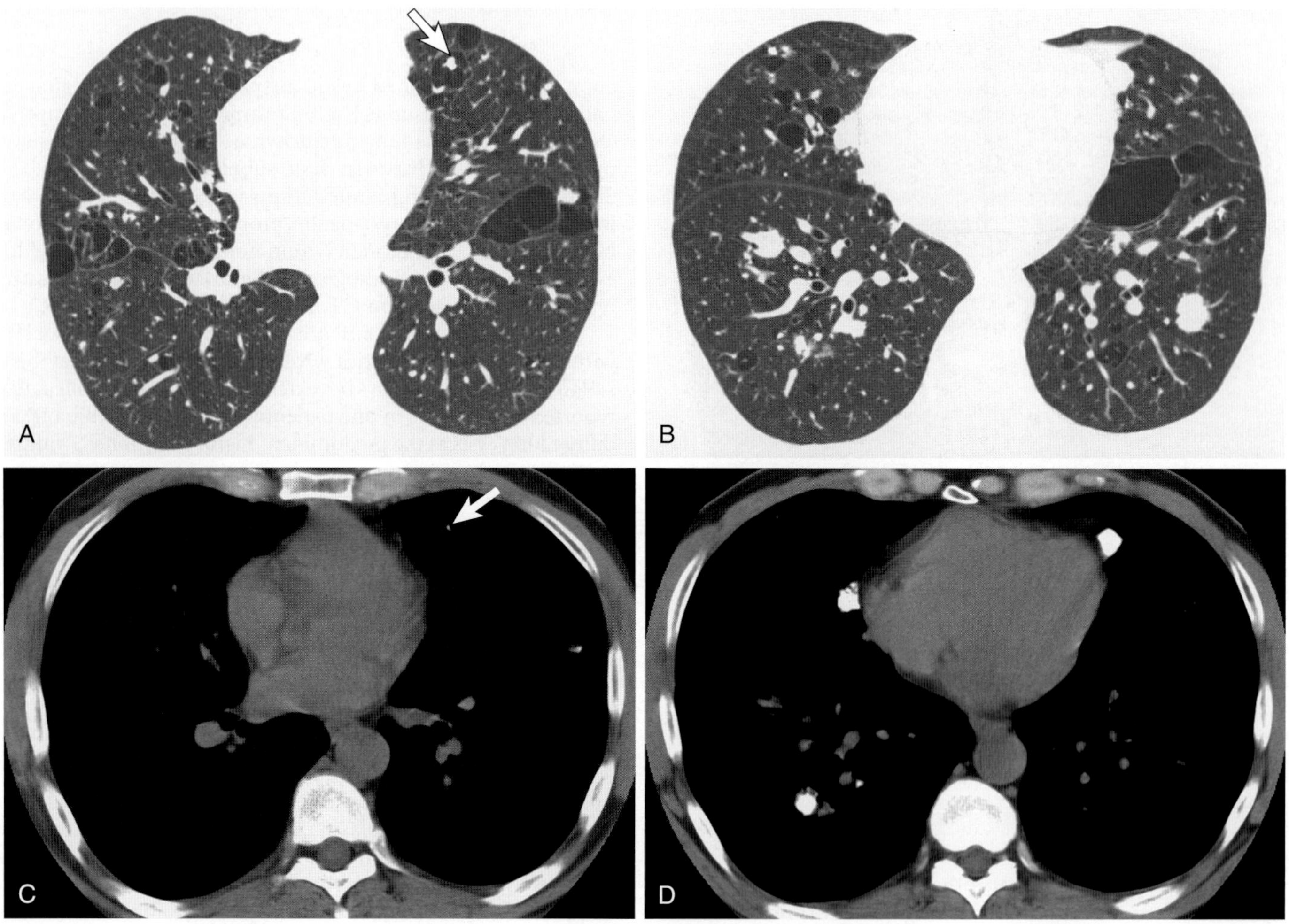

Fig. 23.11 Lymphoid interstitial pneumonia and amyloid in a patient with Sjögren syndrome. High-resolution CT scans at the level of inferior pulmonary veins (A) and slightly more caudal (B) show irregular nodules and multiple cysts. Note subpleural distribution (along the fissures) of some cysts and nodule within the central region of the cyst in the lingula (*arrow* in A). (C) and (D) CT scans at soft tissue windows show that some of the nodules are calcified, including the nodule within the cyst (*arrow* in C), consistent with amyloid. *(Courtesy Dr. Neil Colman, McGill University Healthy Centre, Montreal General Hospital, Montreal, Quebec, Canada.)*

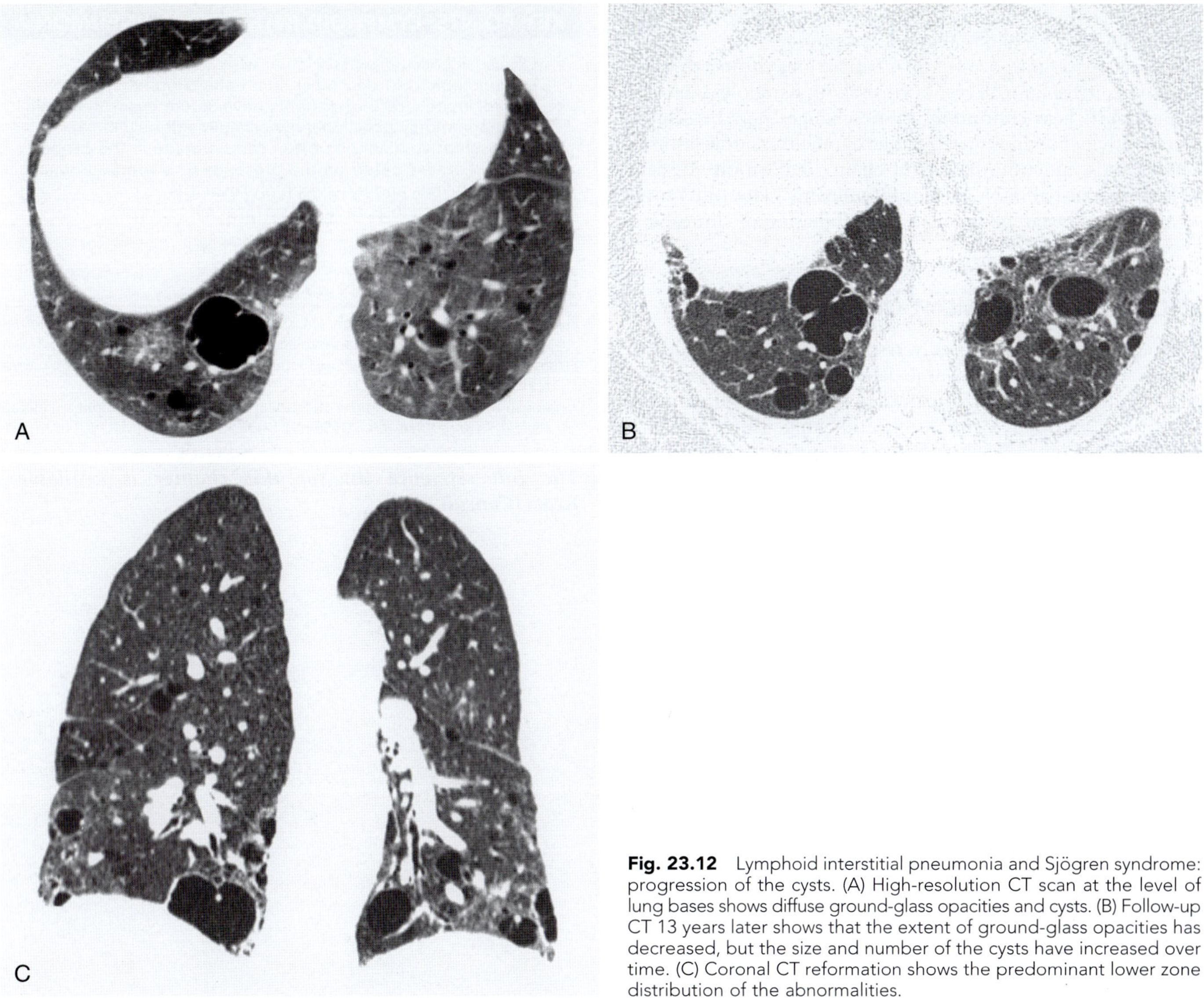

Fig. 23.12 Lymphoid interstitial pneumonia and Sjögren syndrome: progression of the cysts. (A) High-resolution CT scan at the level of lung bases shows diffuse ground-glass opacities and cysts. (B) Follow-up CT 13 years later shows that the extent of ground-glass opacities has decreased, but the size and number of the cysts have increased over time. (C) Coronal CT reformation shows the predominant lower zone distribution of the abnormalities.

LIP.[15] The findings on the initial CT scan consisted of ground-glass opacities (100%), thickening of interlobular septa (93%), centrilobular nodules (86%), cystic airspaces (71%), and airspace consolidation (29%). On follow-up CT nine patients improved, one showed no change, and four showed increased extent of disease. With the exception of cysts, the parenchymal opacities were reversible. On follow-up CT new cysts were seen in three patients; these developed mainly in areas with centrilobular nodules on initial CT. Honeycombing was seen on follow-up CT in four patients; in three patients it developed in areas of airspace consolidation, and in one patient it developed in an area with ground-glass opacity on initial CT.[15]

CLASSIC SIGNS OF LYMPHOID INTERSTITIAL PNEUMONIA

- Underlying immunologic disorder, most commonly Sjögren syndrome
- Serum dysproteinemia, most commonly polyclonal hypergammaglobulinemia
- Ground-glass opacities
- Thin-walled cysts
- Thickening of bronchovascular bundles
- Poorly defined centrilobular nodules

DIFFERENTIAL DIAGNOSIS

The main differential diagnosis of LIP histologically is lymphoma. This distinction usually requires immunohistochemical analysis to determine the presence of polyclonal lymphocytes.[1] High-resolution CT findings helpful in distinguishing LIP from lymphoma include the presence of cysts and the lack of pleural effusion. Honda and coworkers[16] compared the high-resolution CT findings of LIP with findings in patients who had malignant lymphoma. Cysts were more common in patients who had LIP (82%) than in patients who had malignant lymphoma (2%), whereas airspace consolidation and large nodules (11–30 mm in diameter) were more common in patients who had malignant lymphoma (66% and 41%, respectively) than in patients who had LIP (18% and

6%, respectively) ($P < .001$). Pleural effusions (25%) were seen only in patients who had malignant lymphoma.

Cystic airspaces may be seen on CT in various chronic diseases, including Langerhans cell histiocytosis, lymphangioleiomyomatosis, and LIP. Less commonly, cystic changes may be seen in hypersensitivity pneumonitis, catamenial pneumothorax, asthma, pneumocystis pneumonia, light-chain deposition disease, amyloidosis, and Birt-Hogg-Dubé syndrome. The differential diagnosis usually can be made by a combination of clinical and radiologic findings.[17,18]

SYNOPSIS OF TREATMENT OPTIONS

Most patients with LIP initially respond to corticosteroids or cytotoxic drugs or both.[7] In some patients the disease progresses despite treatment, however. The median survival is approximately 11 years.[7] Treatment with unilateral lung transplant has been described with excellent functional outcome and no evidence of recurrent LIP in the lung allograft after 4 years of follow-up.[7,14]

KEY POINTS: LYMPHOID INTERSTITIAL PNEUMONIA

- LIP usually occurs in association with an underlying immunologic disorder, most commonly Sjögren syndrome.
- Approximately 80% of patients have serum dysproteinemia, most commonly polyclonal hypergammaglobulinemia.
- A presumptive diagnosis often can be made in the proper clinical context based on the presence of bilateral ground-glass opacities and cysts on high-resolution CT.
- Definitive diagnosis requires surgical lung biopsy.

SUGGESTED READINGS

Hare SS, Souza CA, Bain G, Seely JM, Gomes MM, Quigley M. The radiological spectrum of pulmonary lymphoproliferative disease. *Br J Radiol.* 2012;85:848–864.

Swigris JJ, Berry GJ, Raffin TA, et al. Lymphoid interstitial pneumonia: a narrative review. *Chest.* 2002;122:2150–2164.

Tashtoush B, Okafor NC, Ramirez JF, Smolley L. Follicular bronchiolitis: a literature review. *J Clin Diagn Res.* 2015;9:OE1–OE5.

The full reference list for this chapter is available at ExpertConsult.com.

24 Non-Hodgkin Lymphoma

PATRICIA M. DE GROOT | CAROL C. WU | BRETT W. CARTER | KYUNG SOO LEE

Overview

Non-Hodgkin lymphoma (NHL) is a heterogeneous group of diseases that accounts for 90% of lymphoma diagnoses, with the other 10% being Hodgkin lymphoma (HL).[1,2] NHL arises during lymphocyte differentiation in either the humoral or cell-mediated immunity lineages of the immune system. Advances in molecular genetics and immunohistochemistry have increased the ability to differentiate distinct types of lymphoma, although not all of them are well understood.[3,4] The 2016 World Health Organization (WHO) classification of NHL contains numerous subtypes of both mature B-cell lymphomas (Table 24.1) and mature T-cell and natural killer (NK) cell neoplasms (Table 24.2).

ETIOLOGY, PREVALENCE, AND EPIDEMIOLOGY

NHL is a common malignancy, with 386,000 cases reported worldwide in 2012 and 199,700 deaths in that year, per GLOBOCAN statistics.[5,6] The incidence of NHL increased by 3% to 4% annually during the 1970s and 1980s, with relative stabilization in the mid-1990s.[7] An estimated 72,240 new lymphoma diagnoses (4.3% of new cancer cases) will be seen in 2017 in the United States.[8–10] The 5-year survival rate for NHL is 71% overall, and the 2014 prevalence of NHL in the United States was approximately 661,996 individuals.[9]

Geographic differences are seen in the incidence of NHL. Incidence is highest in North America, Western Europe, and Australia/New Zealand.[5] Annual incidence rates in the United States range from 19.9 to 21.4 per 100,000 people between 1994 and 2014.[9] Within the European Union, national NHL incidence is quite variable, with Finland and Italy having the highest rates and former Eastern bloc countries having the lowest numbers of new cases.[11]

Regional and socioeconomic factors also affect the distribution of lymphoma subtypes. Follicular lymphoma is most common in developed countries. The incidence of T-cell lymphoma and extranodal disease is greater in Asia. In Africa, Burkitt lymphoma is endemic, but overall incidence of NHL is low. Low-grade B-cell lymphomas are more common in high-income regions, whereas high-grade B-cell lymphoma is seen more commonly in low- and middle-income populations.[1,2,6,7]

B-cell lymphomas are the most frequent type of lymphoma, constituting 85% to 90% of NHL. Multiple subtypes exist; diffuse large B-cell lymphoma (DLBCL) is the most common, followed by follicular lymphoma. Together they represent 65% of NHL.[1] T/NK-cell lymphomas are much less common but equally varied. The principal subtypes of T-cell NHL are peripheral T-cell lymphoma, not otherwise specified; angioimmunoblastic T-cell lymphoma; and anaplastic large cell lymphoma.[2]

The most common risk factor for development of NHL is altered immune function, including autoimmune conditions, congenital immunodeficiency diseases, organ transplantation, and immunomodulatory infections, such as human immunodeficiency virus (HIV) and human T-cell leukemia virus type 1. Other infections, notably Epstein-Barr virus and hepatitis C virus, are implicated in lymphomagenesis.[1,2,6] Lymphoma is a disease of older people. Additional risk factors associated with development of B-cell lymphomas include medications, lifestyle factors, occupational exposures, and obesity.[1] Some known risk factors for T-cell lymphomas are tobacco smoking, celiac disease, chronic skin conditions such as psoriasis and eczema, and textile or electrical work.[1] Genetic factors also convey susceptibility.[1]

CLINICAL PRESENTATION

Non-Hodgkin lymphoma can affect any organ, and consequently symptoms at presentation may be varied and nonspecific. The most common finding is painless lymphadenopathy. B symptoms, such as night sweats, fever, pruritus, fatigue, and weight loss, may or may not be present.[1,8] More aggressive lymphomas may be more symptomatic.[2] In the thorax the most common sites of lymphoma involvement are the mediastinum, heart, lungs, pleura, and chest wall.[8,13] Symptoms specific to thoracic lymphomas can include cough, chest pain, dyspnea, congestive heart failure, and superior vena cava syndrome.[13,14]

Tissue sampling is required to make the diagnosis of NHL. Excisional biopsy is preferred, although core biopsy may be sufficient. Fine-needle aspiration and fluid cytology are not adequate for evaluation. Immunohistochemical studies and genetic analysis are recommended to accurately assign the lymphoma subtype and guide treatment planning.[1]

PATHOPHYSIOLOGY

B cell: All B lymphocytes originate in the bone marrow and travel to the spleen and lymph nodes, where they differentiate with the assistance of T cells into primary and secondary lymphoid follicles after encounter with an antigen. The secondary lymphoid follicle is characterized by germinal centers, which are the site of normal B-cell maturation. Within the germinal center, B cells proliferate rapidly and also undergo processes that require double-strand deoxyribonucleic acid (DNA) breaks: class-switch recombination, by which the immunoglobulin heavy chain may be converted from immunoglobulin (Ig)M to IgG, IgA, or IgE; and somatic hypermutation, which orchestrates mutations of the light-chain variable immunoglobulin, IgV, in response to specific antigens. These processes carry the potential for DNA damage.

Many B-cell lymphomas have been associated with chromosome translocations that activate protooncogenes. As an example, t(14;18)(q32:q21) translocation is a common mutation in

TABLE 24.1 2016 WHO CLASSIFICATION OF NON-HODGKIN LYMPHOMA B-CELL SUBTYPES[a]

MATURE B-CELL NEOPLASMS

- Chronic lymphocytic leukemia and small lymphocytic lymphoma
- Monoclonal B-cell lymphocytosis
- B-cell prolymphocytic leukemia
- Splenic marginal zone lymphoma
- Hairy cell leukemia
- Unclassifiable splenic B-cell lymphoma or leukemia[b]
- Splenic diffuse red pulp small B-cell lymphoma[b]
- Hairy cell leukemia variant
- Lymphoplasmacytic lymphoma
- Extranodal marginal zone lymphoma of mucosa-associated lymphoid tissue
- Nodal marginal zone lymphoma
- Pediatric nodal marginal zone lymphoma[b]
- Follicular lymphoma
- In situ follicular neoplasia
- Pediatric-type follicular lymphoma
- Large B-cell lymphoma with rearrangement of *IRF4*[b]
- Primary cutaneous follicle center lymphoma
- Mantle cell lymphoma
- In situ mantle cell neoplasia
- DLBCL, not otherwise specified
- T-cell–rich or histiocyte-rich large B-cell lymphoma
- Primary DLBCL of the CNS
- Leg-type primary cutaneous DLBCL
- EBV-positive DLBCL, not otherwise specified
- EBV-positive mucocutaneous ulcer[b]
- DLBCL associated with chronic inflammation
- Lymphomatoid granulomatosis
- Primary mediastinal (thymic) large B-cell lymphoma
- Intravascular large B-cell lymphoma
- ALK-positive large B-cell lymphoma
- Plasmablastic lymphoma
- Primary effusion lymphoma
- Human herpesvirus 8–positive DLBCL, not otherwise specified[b]
- Burkitt lymphoma
- Burkitt-like lymphoma with chromosome 11q aberrations[b]
- High-grade B-cell lymphoma with rearrangements of *BCL2* and *MYC* or of *BCL6* and *MYC*[b]
- High-grade B-cell lymphoma, not otherwise specified[b]
- Unclassifiable B-cell lymphoma with features that are intermediate between DLBCL and classic Hodgkin lymphoma

[a]Plasma cell neoplasms, Hodgkin lymphomas, posttransplant lymphoproliferative disorders, and tumors of histiocytic and antigen-presenting cells are not included in this panel.
[b]Provisional entities.
ALK, Anaplastic lymphoma kinase; *CNS*, central nervous system; *DLBCL*, diffuse large B-cell lymphoma; *EBV*, Epstein-Barr virus; *WHO*, World Health Organization.
Adapted from reference 1.

TABLE 24.2 2016 WHO CLASSIFICATION OF NON-HODGKIN LYMPHOMA T-CELL SUBTYPES[a]

MATURE T-CELL AND NATURAL KILLER (NK)-CELL NEOPLASMS

- T-cell prolymphocytic leukemia
- T-cell large granular lymphocytic leukemia
- Chronic lymphoproliferative disorder of NK cells[b]
- Aggressive NK-cell leukemia[b]
- EBV-positive T-cell lymphoproliferative diseases of childhood, including cutaneous chronic active EBV infection, hydroa vacciniforme-like lymphoma, severe mosquito-bite hypersensitivity, systemic chronic active EBV infection, and systemic EBV-positive T-cell lymphoma of childhood
- Adult T-cell leukemia or lymphoma
- Nasal-type extranodal NK–T-cell lymphoma
- Enteropathy-associated T-cell lymphoma
- Monomorphic epitheliotropic intestinal T-cell lymphoma
- Indolent T-cell lymphoproliferative disorder of the gastrointestinal tract[b]
- Hepatosplenic T-cell lymphoma
- Subcutaneous panniculitis-like T-cell lymphoma
- Mycosis fungoides
- Sézary syndrome
- Primary cutaneous CD30-positive T-cell lymphoproliferative disorders
- Lymphomatoid papulosis
- Primary cutaneous anaplastic large cell lymphoma
- Primary cutaneous γδ T-cell lymphoma
- Primary cutaneous CD8-positive aggressive epidermotropic cytotoxic T-cell lymphoma[b]
- Primary cutaneous acral CD8-positive T-cell lymphoma[b]
- Primary cutaneous CD4-positive small or medium T-cell lymphoproliferative disorder[b]
- Peripheral T-cell lymphoma, not otherwise specified
- Angioimmunoblastic T-cell lymphoma
- Follicular T-cell lymphoma[b]
- ALK-positive anaplastic large cell lymphoma
- ALK-negative anaplastic large cell lymphoma
- Breast implant–associated anaplastic large cell lymphoma[b]

[a]Plasma cell neoplasms, Hodgkin lymphomas, posttransplant lymphoproliferative disorders, and tumors of histiocytic and antigen-presenting cells are not included in this panel.
[b]Provisional entities.
ALK, Anaplastic lymphoma kinase; *DLBCL*, diffuse large B-cell lymphoma; *EBV*, Epstein-Barr virus; *NK*, natural killer; *WHO*, World Health Organization.
Adapted from reference 1.

follicular lymphoma and causes overexpression of the antiapoptotic protein BCL2, which blocks programmed cell death in the germinal center. The "double-hit" lymphomas have combined defects in the transcription factor genes *MYC* and *BCL2* or *BCL6*, and have particularly poor prognosis.[1,2,15]

Lymphomas can also originate in activated B cells once they leave the germinal centers. The prognosis for germinal center lymphomas is better than that of activated B cells, with a 5-year survival of 76% and 16%, respectively.[2]

T cell: Significantly less is understood of the pathophysiology of T-cell lymphomas, although they are thought to correlate with various stages of T-cell development. This is primarily because the diversity and rarity of the T-cell lymphoma subtypes hinder clinical and laboratory studies. Classification currently distinguishes between disease involving cells of innate immune system, such as NK cells and γδ T lymphocytes, and that affecting antigen-specific cells, including mature $CD4^+$ and $CD8^+$ αβ T cells and regulatory T cells.[1] Advances in immunohistochemical analysis now allow differentiation between the anaplastic lymphoma kinase (ALK)-positive and ALK-negative variants of anaplastic large cell lymphoma; one study showed that survival outcomes appear dependent on patient age and not the ALK status.[1,16]

IMAGING EVALUATION

Radiography: Radiography is no longer used as a tool for assessment of lymphomas. However, chest radiography is commonly used as a preliminary imaging modality for nonspecific thoracic symptoms and may therefore reveal the first indication of a mediastinal mass, lung consolidation, or pleural disease.

Computed tomography (CT): A CT examination is likely to be the initial study performed to assess abnormalities on chest radiography. This imaging modality is useful in identifying and characterizing the sites of disease in the thorax and developing a differential diagnosis.[8] It may prompt further evaluation with additional multiplanar imaging modalities, depending on the findings and the level of clinical suspicion. A contrast-enhanced CT study is preferred if not contraindicated by renal insufficiency or allergy profile of the patient.

Positron emission tomography (PET) and PET-CT: PET imaging with ^{18}F-fluorodeoxyglucose (FDG), particularly combined with CT, is now the imaging modality of choice for assessment of lymphoma.[1,8] PET-CT has a sensitivity of 94% and specificity of 100% in identifying nodal lymphoma as well as sensitivity of 88% and specificity of 100% for detecting extranodal disease.[17] It has been suggested to be as sensitive as bone marrow biopsy in ascertaining bone marrow involvement.[1] Different types of lymphoma can have different rates of FDG uptake: DLBCL and follicular and mantle cell lymphomas have avid uptake, whereas extranodal marginal zone lymphoma and T-cell lymphomas can have variable uptake (Table 24.3).[2,18]

TABLE 24.3 FDG AVIDITY OF NHL ACCORDING TO WHO CLASSIFICATION

Histology	% FDG Avid
Burkitt lymphoma	100
Mantle cell lymphoma	100
Anaplastic large T-cell lymphoma	100
Lymphoblastic lymphoma	100
Angioimmunoblastic T-cell lymphoma	100
Natural killer/T-cell lymphoma	100
Diffuse large B-cell lymphoma	97–100
Follicular lymphoma	91–100
Nodal marginal zone lymphoma	83–100
Small lymphocytic lymphoma	50–100
MALT marginal zone lymphoma	54–82

FDG, Fluorodeoxyglucose; *MALT*, mucosa-associated lymphoid tissue; *NHL*, non-Hodgkin lymphoma; *WHO*, World Health Organization.

Adapted from Weiler-Sagie M, Bushelev O, Epelbaum R, et al. (18) F-FDG avidity in lymphoma readdressed: a study of 766 patients. *J Nucl Med.* 2010;51:25–30. © by the Society of Nuclear Medicine and Molecular Imaging.

PET-CT is also useful in assessment of treatment response, and an end-of-therapy PET-CT examination is the standard of care.[1] The Deauville score has been developed to articulate a standard definition of remission (Table 24.4). The findings of complete remission include Deauville scores of 1, 2, and 3. Deauville scores of 4 and 5 indicate residual or recurrent disease.[1]

Magnetic resonance imaging (MRI): MRI has high temporal resolution leading to excellent soft tissue discrimination. Multiplanar imaging and the capability for dynamic cine sequences are also advantages. MRI before and after gadolinium contrast administration is the modality of choice in assessing primary cardiac lymphoma.[13] Thoracic MRI can also be helpful in assessing secondary cardiac or vascular involvement and chest wall invasion.[8] Both decreased gadolinium enhancement, compared with presentation, and decrease in T2 signal intensity indicate response to treatment. Diffusion-weighted imaging (DWI)-MRI may be useful in distinguishing active lymphoma, which has high restricted diffusion and low apparent diffusion coefficient mapping, unlike benign or treated lesions.[8]

IMAGING MANIFESTATIONS OF DISEASE

Mediastinum: Primary mediastinal large B-cell lymphoma (MLBCL), an uncommon type of NHL thought to arise from the thymic B cells, manifests predominantly in young adult women and on imaging appears as an anterior (prevascular) mediastinal mass of variable size (Fig. 24.1).[2] It originates from a medullary B-cell subpopulation in the thymus.[3] Local invasion is frequently present, and vascular involvement is common in this entity.[19] Primary MLBCL has been reported as a manifestation of acquired immune deficiency syndrome (AIDS)-related lymphoma (ARL), an AIDS-defining illness.[20] A mediastinal mass is also a typical manifestation of precursor T lymphoblastic lymphomas, usually in younger men.[1] The very rare mediastinal gray-zone lymphomas also manifest as a mediastinal mass in young patients; they have histologic features in between those of primary mediastinal LBCL and nodular sclerosing HL.[1,21] The mediastinum is also involved secondarily in the setting of systemic NHL, including DLBCL and follicular lymphoma, with lymphadenopathy as the most common feature.

CT imaging findings include bulky confluent soft tissue in the mediastinum that can measure up to several centimeters (Fig. 24.2; see Fig. 24.1). The anterior (prevascular) mediastinum is affected much more frequently than the middle (visceral) or posterior (paravertebral) mediastinal compartments. The mass may be homogeneous or contain necrosis or cystic elements. Mass effect on mediastinal structures may be present.[8] Superior vena cava syndrome is seen in up to 50% of patients with primary

TABLE 24.4 DEAUVILLE CRITERIA FOR RESPONSE ASSESSMENT ON FDG-PET

Deauville Score	FDG Uptake
1	No uptake
2	Uptake ≤ mediastinum
3	Uptake ≥ mediastinum < liver
4	Uptake moderately increased above liver
5	Markedly increased uptake > liver and/or new sites of disease

FDG, Fluorodeoxyglucose; *PET*, positron emission tomography.

Adapted from reference 1.

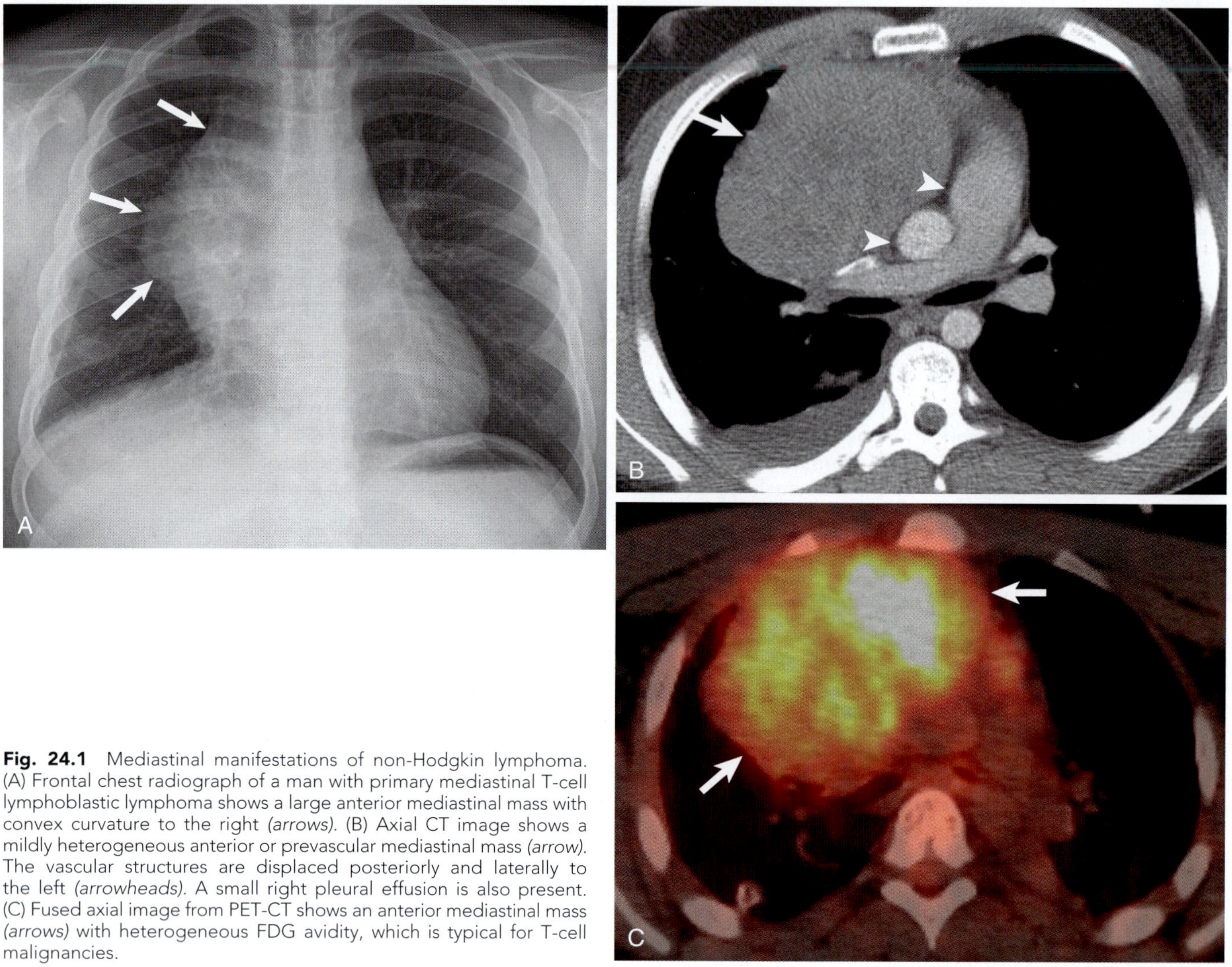

Fig. 24.1 Mediastinal manifestations of non-Hodgkin lymphoma. (A) Frontal chest radiograph of a man with primary mediastinal T-cell lymphoblastic lymphoma shows a large anterior mediastinal mass with convex curvature to the right *(arrows)*. (B) Axial CT image shows a mildly heterogeneous anterior or prevascular mediastinal mass *(arrow)*. The vascular structures are displaced posteriorly and laterally to the left *(arrowheads)*. A small right pleural effusion is also present. (C) Fused axial image from PET-CT shows an anterior mediastinal mass *(arrows)* with heterogeneous FDG avidity, which is typical for T-cell malignancies.

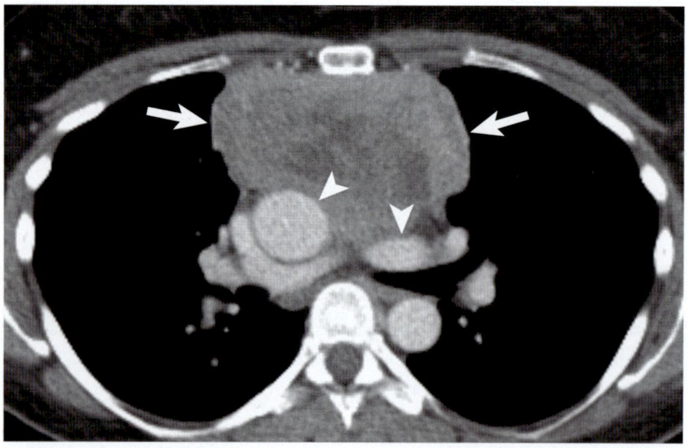

Fig. 24.2 Mediastinal manifestations of non-Hodgkin lymphoma (NHL). Axial CT image of a woman with primary mediastinal NHL demonstrates a heterogeneously enhancing anterior or prevascular mediastinal mass *(arrows)*. Note the posterior displacement of the mediastinal vascular structures *(arrowheads)*.

MLBCL.[19] Mediastinal lymphadenopathy is typically defined as lymph nodes measuring greater than 1 cm in short-axis diameter with prevascular, paratracheal, subcarinal, hilar, and posterior mediastinal stations as the most commonly affected sites (Fig. 24.3).[22]

On FDG–PET-CT mediastinal lymphoma demonstrates increased FDG uptake, consistent with metabolic activity indicative of active disease (see Figs. 24.1 and 24.3). PET-CT is also useful for detecting other sites of lymphoma involvement, including nodes and solid organs.[8] Residual soft tissue densities on CT may persist after therapy in the case of mediastinal or bulky abdominal disease; in the absence of FDG avidity, they are considered as nonviable treated malignancy.

On MRI mediastinal lymphoma is hypointense on T1-weighted images and hyperintense on T2-weighted images and demonstrates enhancement with gadolinium contrast administration. Posttreatment fibrosis does not enhance and is hypointense on all sequences.[8]

The differential diagnosis of primary mediastinal lymphoma includes secondary DLBCL with mediastinal involvement, Hodgkin lymphoma (see Fig. 24.3C), thymic neoplasms, germ

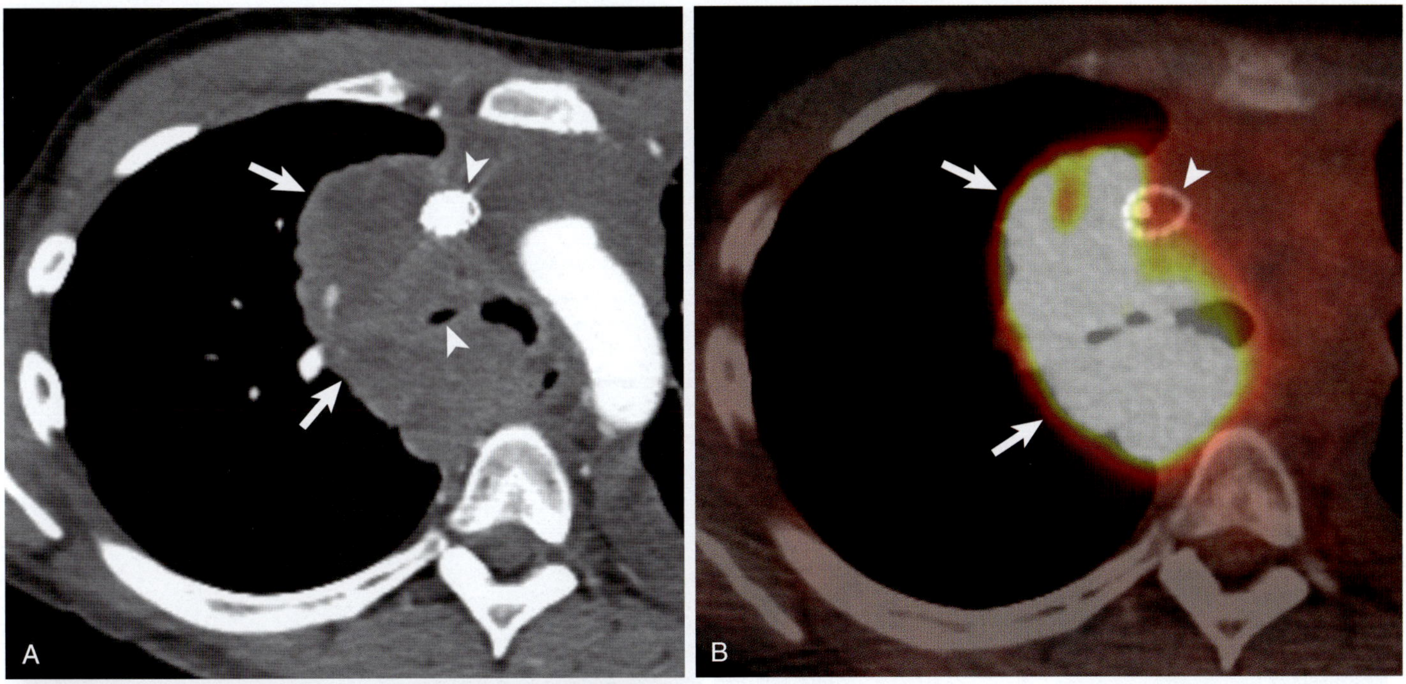

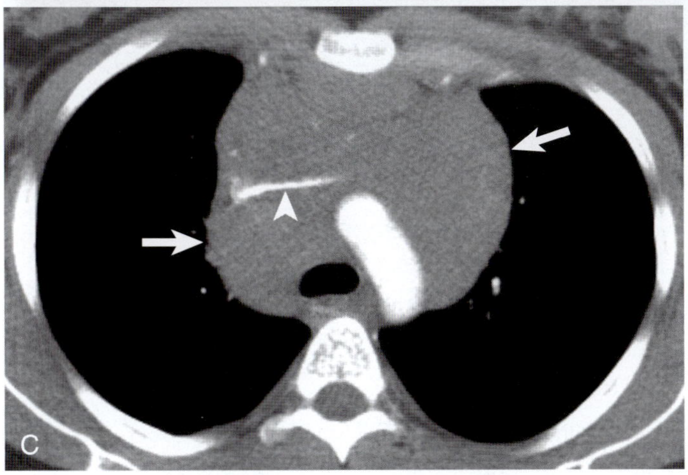

Fig. 24.3 Mediastinal manifestations of non-Hodgkin lymphoma. (A) Axial CT image of a man with secondary diffuse large B-cell lymphoma (DLBCL) of the mediastinum demonstrates conglomerate mediastinal soft tissue *(arrows)*. The superior vena cava is stented to prevent superior vena cava syndrome *(anterior arrowhead)*. The right main bronchus is compressed *(posterior arrowhead)*. (B) Axial fused PET-CT image shows marked FDG avidity associated with DLBCL. Note the difference from the FDG uptake of the T-cell neoplasm in Fig. 24.1C. (C) Axial CT image of a woman with classical Hodgkin lymphoma demonstrates infiltrative anterior (prevascular) and middle (visceral) mediastinal soft tissue mass *(arrows)* encasing the mediastinal vasculature and narrowing the left brachiocephalic vein *(arrowhead)*. This should be included in the differential diagnosis for mediastinal non-Hodgkin lymphoma.

cell tumors, and mediastinal nodal metastases from other primary malignancies.[3] Mediastinal mass and lymph nodes related to NHL, unlike thymic neoplasms or germ cell tumors, rarely contain internal calcification at presentation, although calcification can develop posttreatment.

Cardiac: Primary cardiac lymphoma is quite rare, less than 0.5% of extranodal lymphomas, but secondary involvement of the heart is seen in up to 25% of patients with widespread lymphoma.[13] Cardiac lymphoma typically involves the right heart chambers, both the right atrium and ventricle (Figs. 24.4 and 24.5). It is seen as one or more poorly enhancing masses of the myocardium that may extend along the epicardial surface and encase coronary vessels. The superior vena cava is affected in 25%. Pericardial thickening or nodularity and pericardial effusion may be present; a large pericardial effusion is suggestive of primary cardiac lymphoma in the absence of extensive extracardiac disease.[13] Pericardial effusion is also associated with T-cell lymphoblastic lymphoma of the mediastinum.[8] Most cardiac lymphomas are DLBCL, with high-grade disease found in immunocompromised patients.[13] Fibrin-associated large B-cell lymphoma is a rare variant of cardiac lymphoma seen with implanted prosthetic valves and grafts.[13]

On MRI cardiac lymphomas are typically hypointense on T1-weighted images and hyperintense on T2-weighted images. Variable enhancement is seen with contrast administration. Necrosis and hemorrhage are not common in cardiac lymphoma. Adherent thrombus may be present and is best identified on late gadolinium contrast sequences because of its failure to enhance.[13]

PET-CT can also detect cardiac lymphoma via increased FDG avidity of the lesion compared with physiologic cardiac uptake, which is generally concentrated in the left ventricular myocardium (see Figs. 24.4 and 24.5).[13]

The differential diagnosis of a cardiac mass includes metastatic malignancy, primary or secondary lymphoma, cardiac angiosarcoma, and benign cardiac neoplasms.[13]

Lungs: Primary pulmonary lymphoma is uncommon, representing 3.8% of extranodal lymphomas. Up to 80% of pulmonary lymphoma is NHL, primarily mucosa-associated lymphoid tissue (MALT) lymphoma. DLBCL is also seen in immunocompromised patients as a primary pulmonary lymphoma and may either

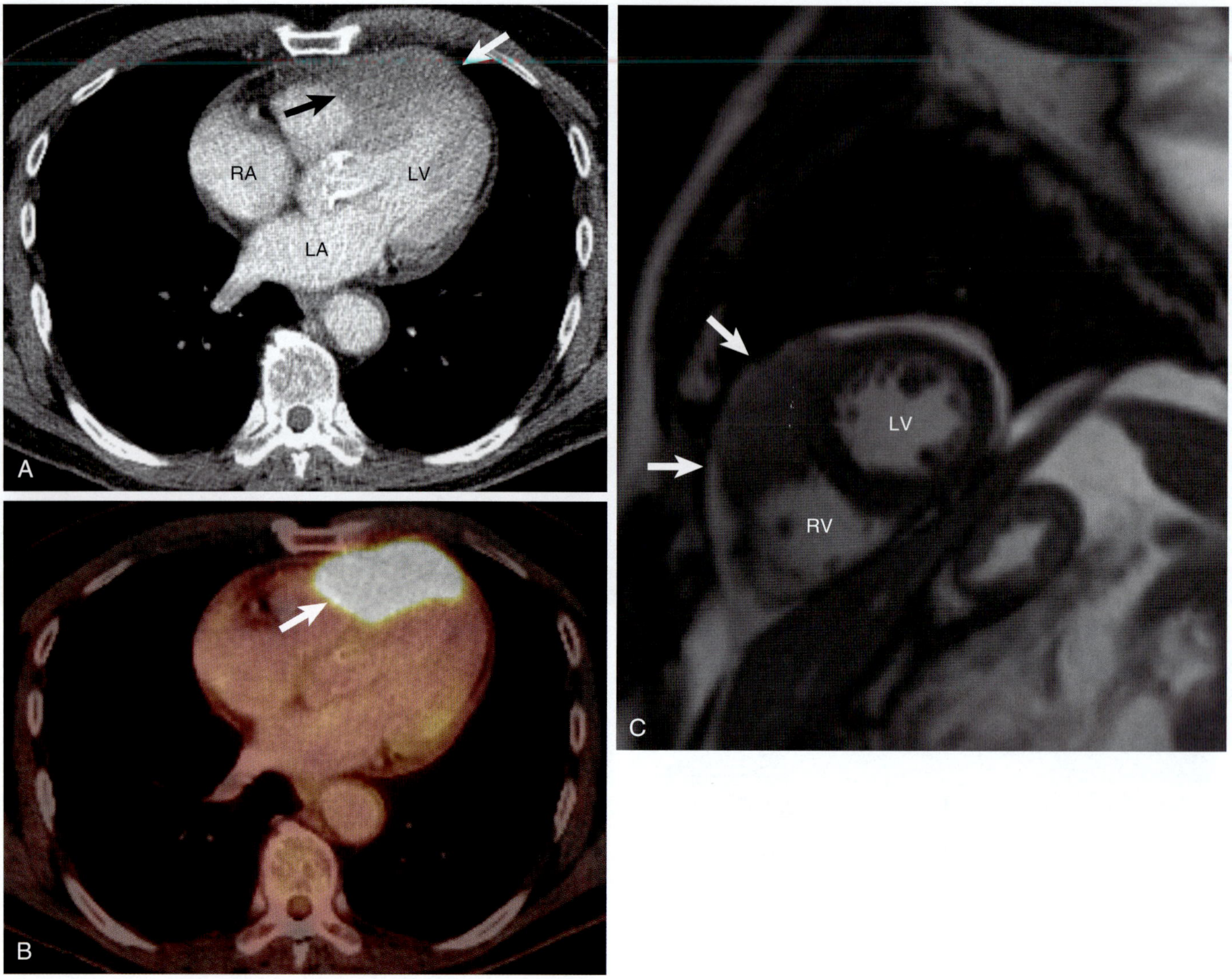

Fig. 24.4 Cardiac lymphoma. (A) Axial CT image of a man with primary large B-cell lymphoma of the heart, germinal center type, shows a soft tissue mass within the right ventricle *(arrows)* abutting the interventricular septum. (B) Axial fused PET-CT image shows intense FDG uptake, typical for diffuse large B-cell lymphoma *(arrow)*. (C) Sagittal MRI T1-weighted image shows the mass *(arrows)* involving the right ventricle and the right ventricular outflow tract. *LA*, Left atrium; *LV*, left ventricle; *RA*, right atrium; *RV*, right ventricle.

arise de novo or by aggressive transformation of MALT lymphoma.[8,19] The diagnostic criteria of primary pulmonary lymphoma require involvement of the lungs and/or airways by lymphoma without evidence of extrapulmonary disease for at least 3 months after diagnosis.[14] Pulmonary parenchymal involvement may manifest as single (Figs. 24.6 and 24.7) or multiple, unilateral or bilateral, nodules/masses, and/or consolidations (Fig. 24.8) with peribronchovascular distribution. Cavitation can be seen in primary DLBCL.[8] Nodule attenuation may be solid, subsolid, or ground-glass.[19] Airway involvement, hilar and mediastinal lymphadenopathy, and chest wall invasion may or may not be present.[23]

Secondary pulmonary lymphoma is more frequent, seen in 24% of NHL, usually from systemic DLBCL (Fig. 24.9).[8] It can occur via hematogenous spread or local invasion from lymph nodes.[14,19] Imaging findings of secondary pulmonary lymphoma involvement include nodules, masses, and mass-like consolidations (Fig. 24.10; see Fig. 24.9). A common pattern seen in NHL of the lung is peribronchial and/or septal thickening reflecting lymphangitic carcinomatosis. Air bronchograms and cavitation of nodules can be present. Pleural nodules and effusions can also be seen.[24] ARL constitutes a subset of B-cell lymphoma with pulmonary nodular manifestations in AIDS patients with CD4 counts less than 55 cells/μl.[8]

The differential diagnosis of primary or secondary pulmonary lymphoma includes primary lung malignancy, metastatic malignancy, infection, sarcoidosis, septic emboli, and the vasculitides.[8]

Tracheobronchial tree: Rare primary NHL of the tracheobronchial tree can occur, including MALT lymphoma. It tends to be indolent and limited with a good prognosis. Manifestations on imaging include mural or intraluminal nodules or airway wall infiltration.[8]

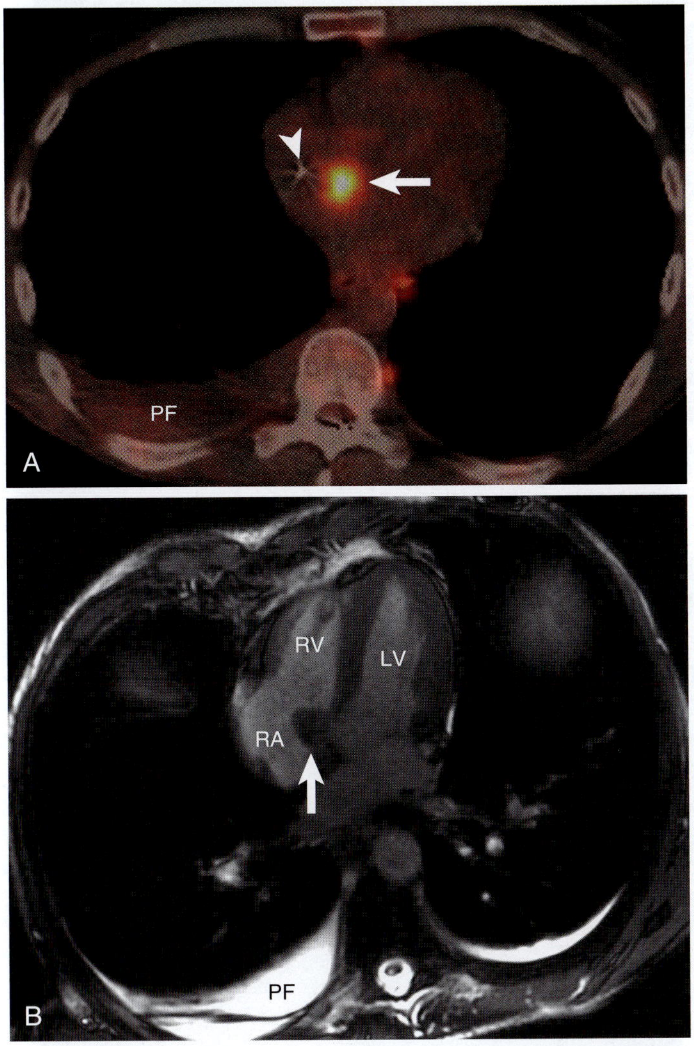

Fig. 24.5 Cardiac lymphoma. (A) Axial fused PET-CT image demonstrates an FDG-avid nodule within the heart *(arrow)* in this patient with double-hit diffuse large B-cell lymphoma. The tip of a central venous catheter is also noted *(arrowhead)*. (B) Axial T2-weighted MRI image demonstrates a hypointense 2-cm nodule *(arrow)* along the medial wall of the right atrium near the tricuspid annulus. *LV,* Left ventricle; *PF,* pleural fluid; *RA,* right atrium; *RV,* right ventricle.

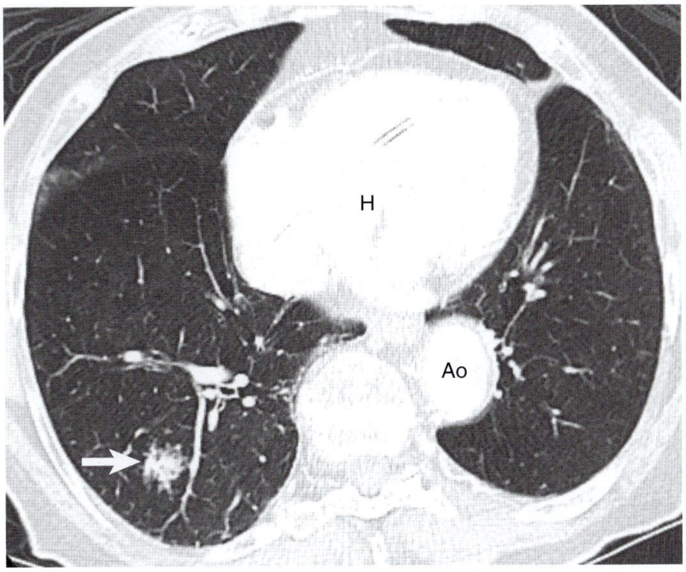

Fig. 24.6 Lung manifestations of primary non-Hodgkin lymphoma. Axial CT image in lung windows demonstrates an ill-defined subsolid right lower lobe nodule *(arrow)*, biopsy-proven to be follicular lymphoma of the lung. *Ao,* Aorta; *H,* heart.

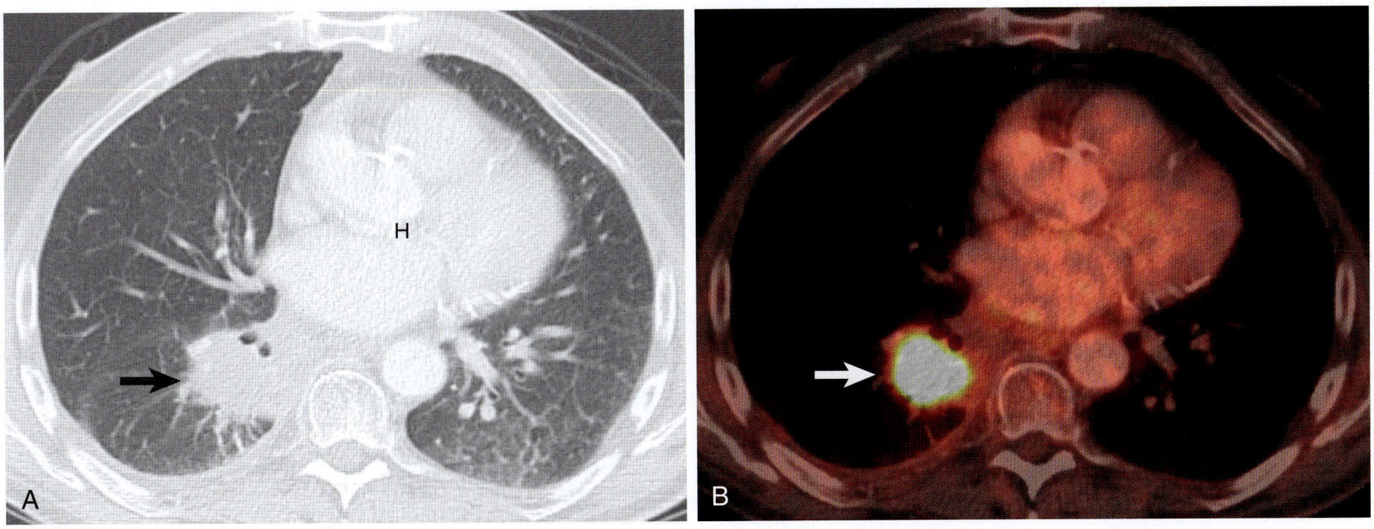

Fig. 24.7 Lung manifestations of primary non-Hodgkin lymphoma. (A) Axial CT image in lung windows demonstrates an ill-defined right lower lobe mass *(arrow)* in a man with primary anaplastic large cell lymphoma of the lung. (B) Axial fused PET-CT image shows intense FDG uptake *(arrow)* denoting the aggressive phenotype of the lymphoma. *H,* Heart.

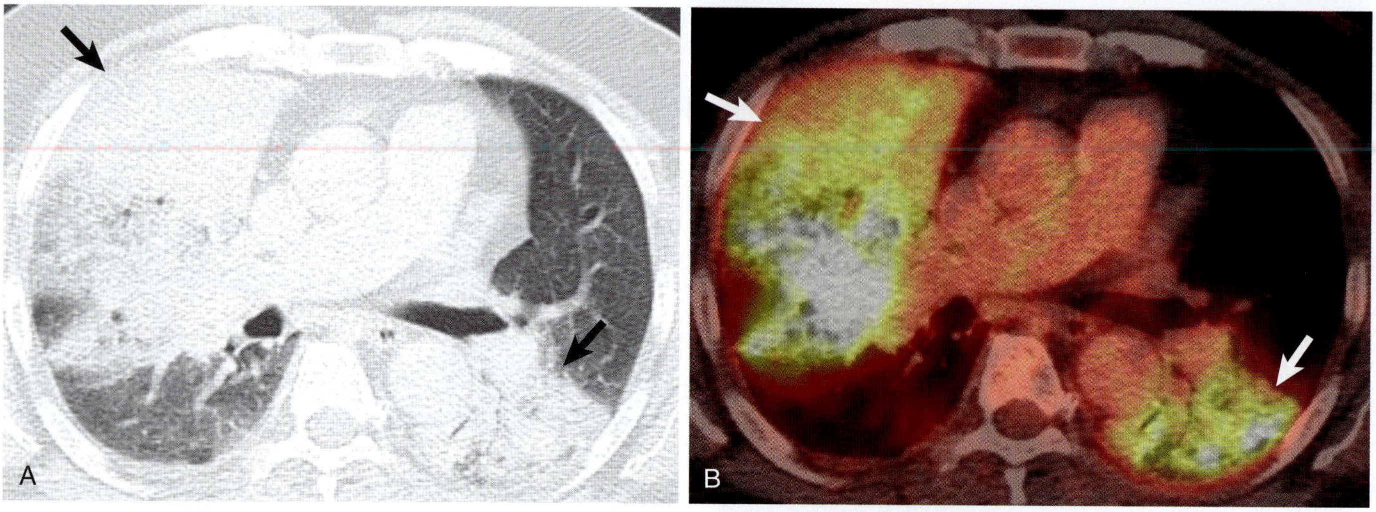

Fig. 24.8 Lung manifestations of primary non-Hodgkin lymphoma. (A) Axial CT image in lung windows shows solid and heterogeneous consolidations in both lungs *(arrows)*. Biopsy found extranodal marginal zone B-cell lymphoma of mucosa-associated lymphoid tissue of lung. (B) Axial fused PET-CT image shows heterogeneous fluorodeoxyglucose uptake in the lung consolidations *(arrows)*.

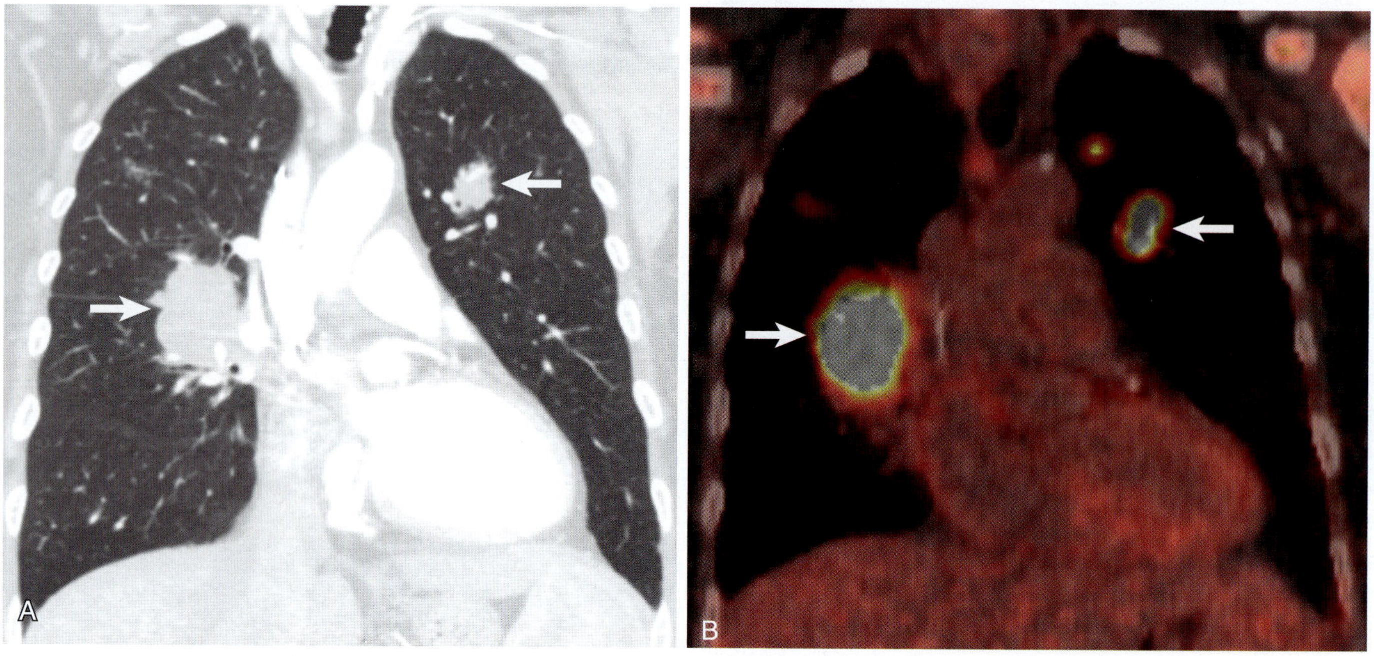

Fig. 24.9 Lung manifestations of secondary non-Hodgkin lymphoma. (A) Coronal CT image in lung windows demonstrates bilateral pulmonary masses with irregular margins *(arrows)*. Biopsy of the right lung mass found diffuse large B-cell lymphoma. (B) Coronal fused PET-CT image of the same patient shows marked FDG avidity in the bilateral lung masses *(arrows)*.

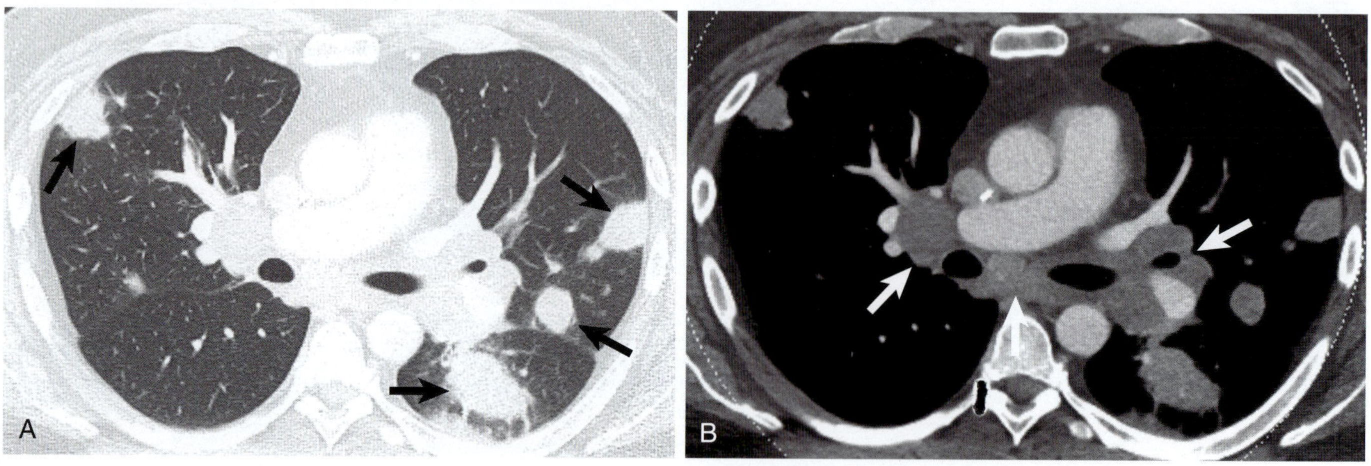

Fig. 24.10 Lung manifestations of secondary non-Hodgkin lymphoma. (A) Axial CT image in lung windows demonstrates multiple bilateral ill-defined nodules *(arrows)* in this man with disseminated mature T-cell/natural killer lymphoma, originally of the left nose and maxilla. (B) Axial contrast-enhanced CT image shows mediastinal and bilateral hilar lymphadenopathy *(arrows)*.

The differential diagnosis includes primary tracheobronchial neoplasms, such as adenoid cystic carcinoma, mucoepidermoid carcinoma, squamous cell carcinoma, and carcinoid tumor.

Pleura: Primary lymphoma of the pleura constitutes 7% of primary lymphomas. Most are B-cell lymphomas and are seen in cases of chronic pleural inflammation and HIV-infected patients. Secondary involvement of the pleura by DLBCL or follicular lymphoma is more common than primary disease, seen in up to 20% of patients. T-cell lymphoma can also have pleural manifestations. Findings on imaging include nodular pleural thickening with or without superimposed effusion (Figs. 24.11 to 24.13). It occurs more often in the left hemithorax.[8,19]

Primary effusion lymphoma manifests as an effusion without discrete nodularity and affects primarily the pleural space, although the pericardium and peritoneum may be affected. It is strongly associated with acquired infectious or posttransplant immunocompromise, human herpesvirus 8, and possibly Epstein-Barr virus and has a poor prognosis.[8,19]

The differential diagnosis for primary or secondary lymphoma of the pleural space includes metastatic carcinomas, particularly adenocarcinomas, and malignant pleural mesothelioma.

Chest wall: Lymphoma of the chest wall is most commonly secondary to direct invasion by an aggressive lymphoma of the mediastinum or osseous structures. It can also arise from axillary lymph nodes.[8] Primary NHL of the chest wall is extremely rare. Findings of chest wall invasion include elimination of fat planes, destruction of osseous structures, and incursion of soft tissue into the extrathoracic space. Disease involving the thoracic spine may encroach upon the spinal canal and thecal sac. MRI can identify invasion of the soft tissues in equivocal cases. It is the preferred modality for assessment of osseous involvement and potential spinal cord compression.[8]

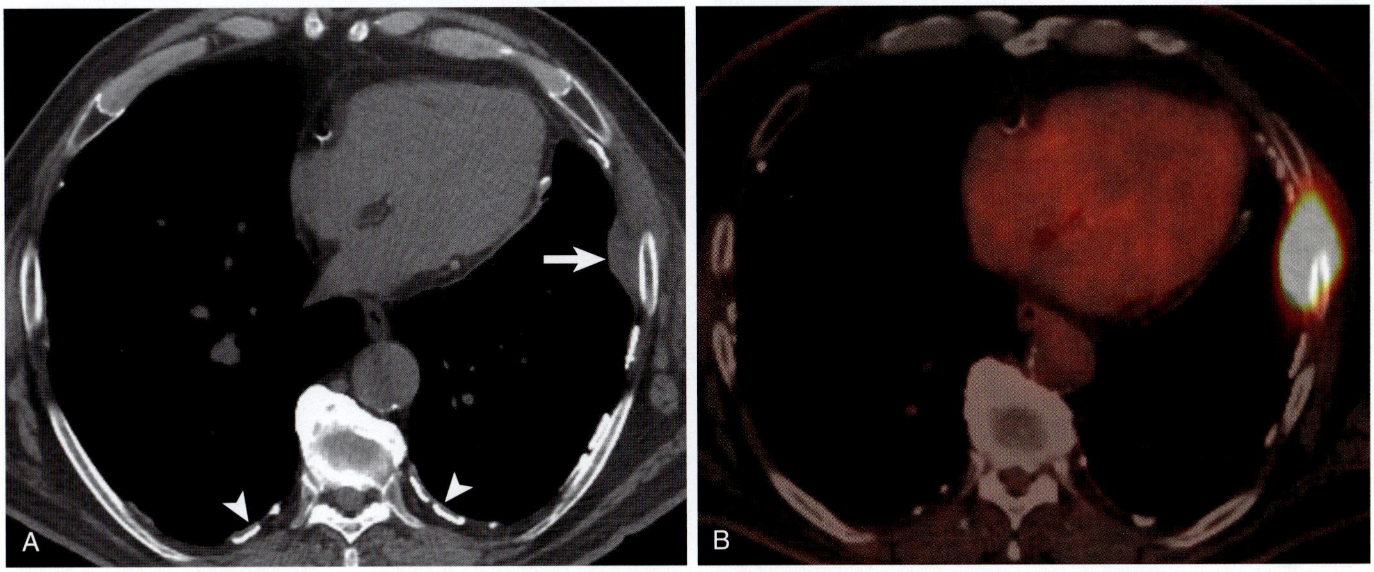

Fig. 24.11 Non-Hodgkin lymphoma of the pleura. (A) Axial noncontrast CT image shows a pleural nodule *(arrow)* in a man with large B-cell lymphoma. Note bilateral calcified pleural plaques *(arrowheads)* in keeping with asbestos-related pleural disease. (B) Axial fused PET-CT image demonstrates marked FDG uptake in the pleural nodule.

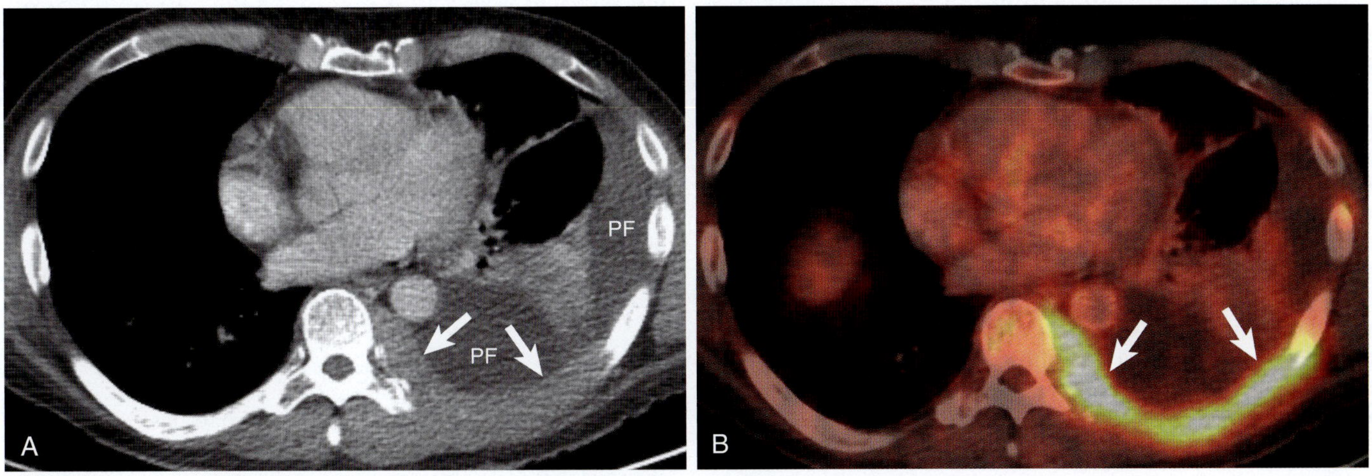

Fig. 24.12 Non-Hodgkin lymphoma of the pleura. (A) Axial contrast-enhanced CT image shows an enhancing posterior pleural rind *(arrows)* in the left hemithorax in this patient with marginal zone B-cell lymphoma. Note associated loculated pleural fluid *(PF)* and partial left lower lobe collapse. (B) Axial fused PET-CT image demonstrates FDG activity within the pleural rind *(arrows)*.

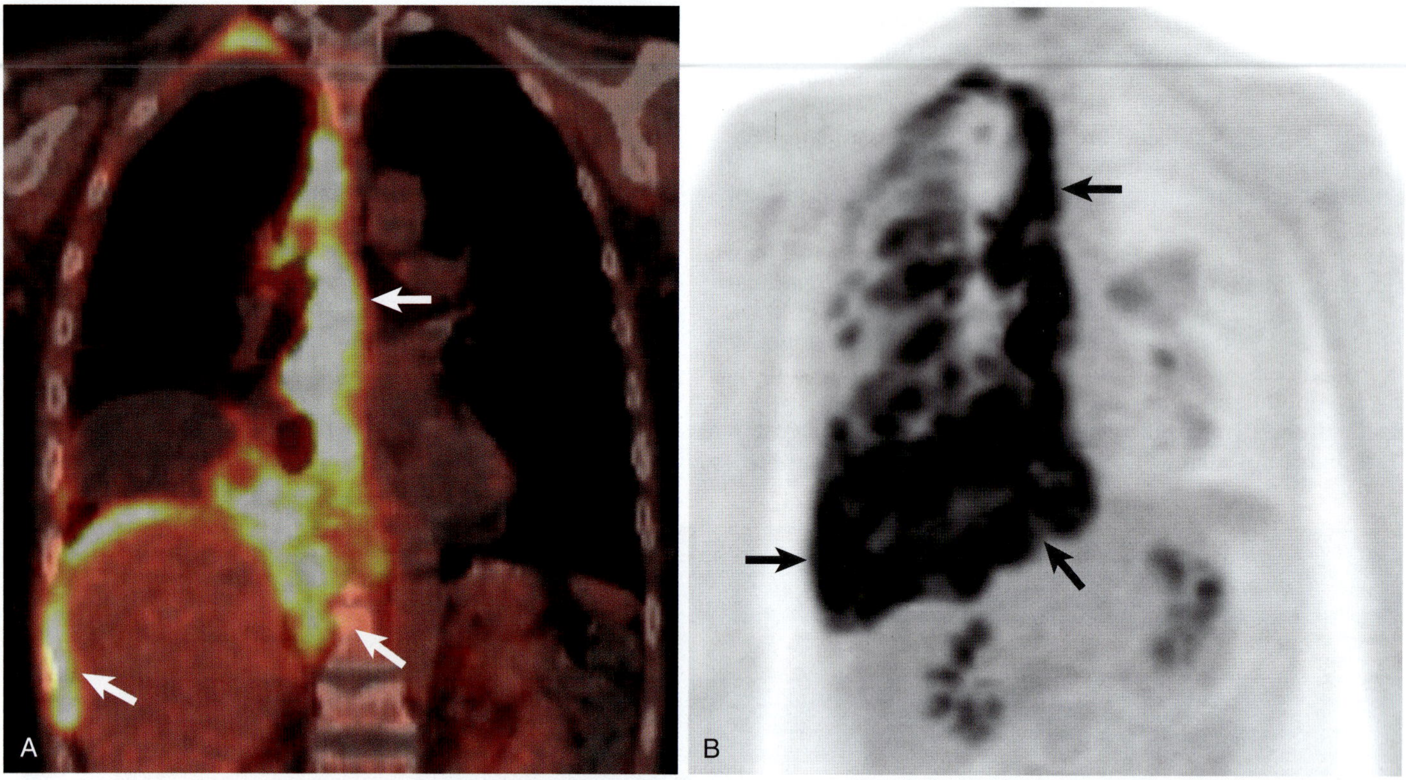

Fig. 24.13 Non-Hodgkin lymphoma of the pleura. (A) Coronal fused PET-CT image in a man with T-cell lymphoblastic lymphoma shows intense FDG activity within the diaphragmatic and mediastinal pleura *(arrows)*. (B) Maximum-intensity projection image from PET imaging shows the full extent of the circumferential pleural disease *(arrows)*. The differential diagnosis includes malignant pleural mesothelioma and metastatic adenocarcinoma.

The differential diagnosis of chest wall lymphoma includes primary malignancies of the chest wall, such as sarcomas, and fungal or tuberculous infections that can invade the chest wall.[8]

Breast: Lymphoma of the breast is infrequent, constituting only 1% to 2% of NHL and less than 0.5% of breast malignancies.[25] It is most prevalent in women, although there are a few case reports in men. The primary pathology is DLBCL, although other subtypes occur, including marginal zone lymphoma, small lymphocytic lymphoma, Burkitt lymphoma, and follicular lymphoma.[25] A variant of anaplastic large cell lymphoma is associated with breast implants (Figs. 24.14 to 24.16).[1]

Breast lymphoma typically manifests as a painless breast mass. Skin retraction, dimpling, and nipple discharge are rarely seen.[26] Imaging findings are not specific to distinguish lymphoma from other breast malignancies, and the diagnosis requires tissue sampling. Dedicated breast ultrasound typical shows a hypoechoic solid mass with indistinct or circumscribed margins. It demonstrates enhancement on cross-sectional imaging with intravenous contrast administration. CT and/or MRI are useful in cases of breast lymphoma for assessment of edema, lymphadenopathy, and involvement of other intrathoracic or extrathoracic sites.[27]

The differential diagnosis of breast lymphoma includes primary breast malignancies, metastatic malignancy, and infection.

STAGING

Staging of NHL requires a meticulous medical history; physical examination; laboratory assays, including measurement of lactate dehydrogenase in serum; and imaging studies.[1] PET-CT is used to stage FDG-avid lymphomas, whereas nonavid lymphomas are staged by CT.[28]

The staging system in current use for NHL is the Lugano classification, based on the older Ann Arbor system. It has been revised to distinguish limited stage I or II disease from more advanced stages III and IV. Stage I reflects a single node or regional nodal group. Stage II consists of two or more nodal groups on the same side of the diaphragm. An extranodal (E) designation may be used with either stage I or II to indicate extranodal involvement of disease. Stage III indicates disease on both sides of the diaphragm, and stage IV reflects noncontiguous extralymphatic involvement, such as presence of lung nodules or gastric mass.[28]

Risk stratification for NHL is usually based on the International Prognostic Index (IPI). Factors such as patient age (>60 years or ≤60 years), Eastern Cooperative Oncology Group (ECOG) performance status, elevated serum lactate dehydrogenase, stage, and number of extranodal sites of disease are used to predict prognosis. Some other variations of this system are also used.[1]

SYNOPSIS OF TREATMENT OPTIONS

B cell: The monoclonal antibody rituximab has revolutionized treatment of B-cell lymphomas. The addition of rituximab to existing chemotherapy regimens containing cyclophosphamide, doxorubicin, vincristine, and prednisone (R-CHOP) has significantly improved survival. It is the most common treatment regimen for DLBCL and follicular lymphoma. Bendamustine

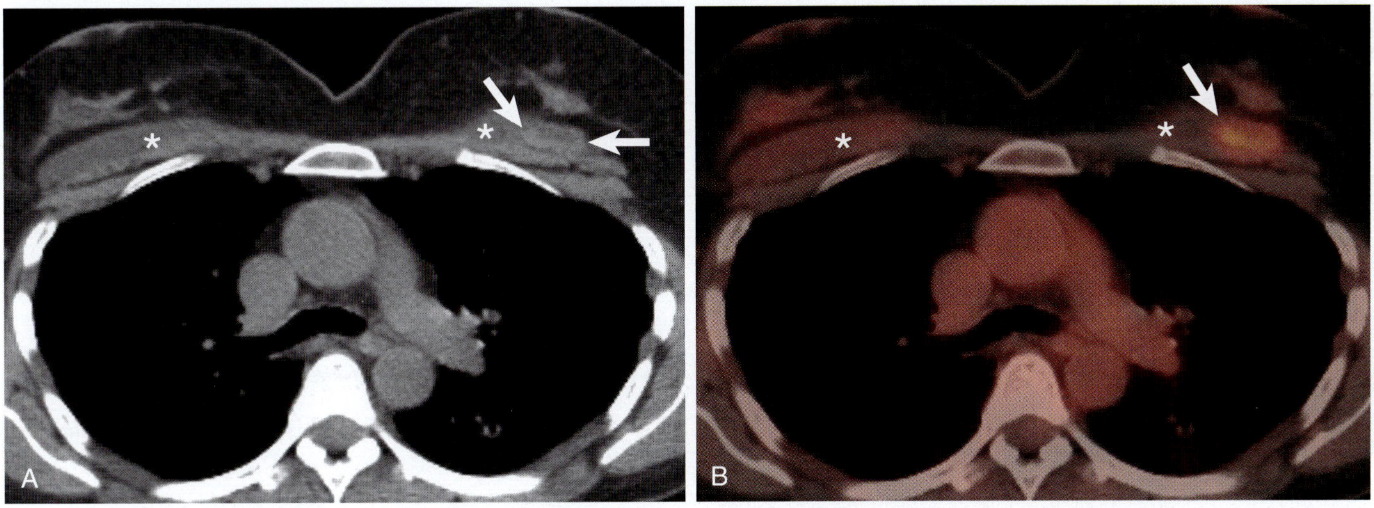

Fig. 24.14 Implant-associated non-Hodgkin lymphoma of the breast. (A) Axial CT image demonstrates a small oblong opacity *(arrows)* slightly hyperdense to muscle at the superior margin of the left breast prosthesis in this woman with anaplastic large cell lymphoma of the breast. (B) Axial fused PET-CT image shows mild FDG uptake within this nodule *(arrow)*. Breast prostheses *(asterisks)*.

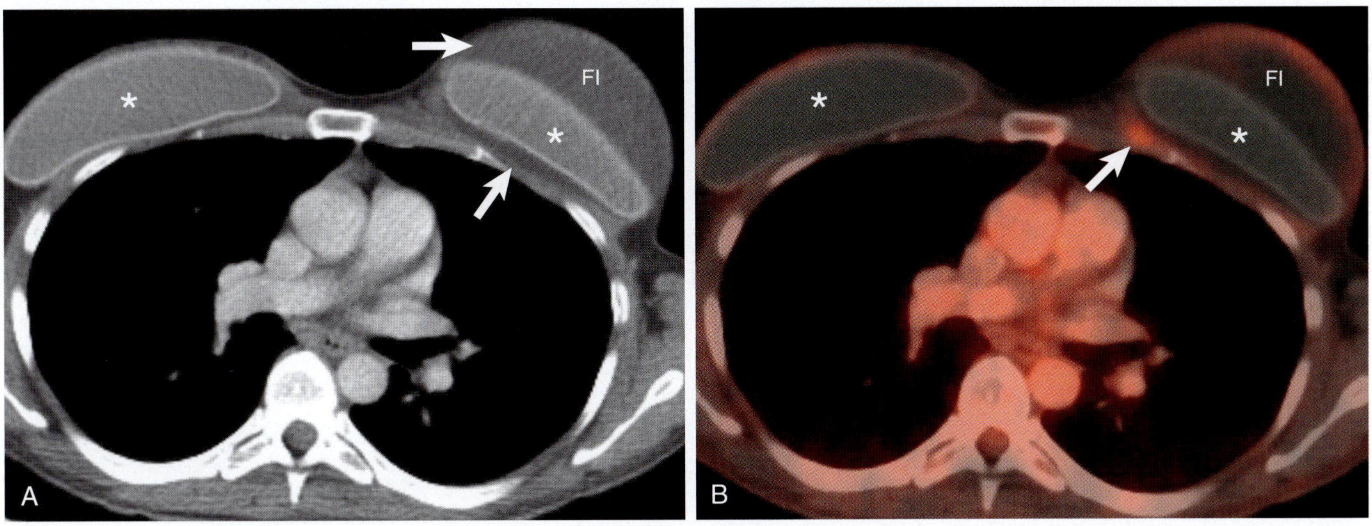

Fig. 24.15 Implant-associated non-Hodgkin lymphoma of the breast. (A) Axial contrast-enhanced CT image shows asymmetry of the breasts resulting from a pericapsular fluid collection *(Fl, arrows)* around the left breast implant in this 42-year-old woman. Fluid cytology was positive for anaplastic large cell lymphoma of the breast. (B) Axial fused PET-CT image shows only minimal focal FDG activity *(arrow)* at the posterior medial margin of the prosthesis. Breast prostheses *(asterisks)*.

plus rituximab and single-agent rituximab are also used in follicular lymphoma. Radiotherapy alone may be curative for localized DLBCL, but generally radiotherapy is used after chemotherapy. Traditionally, the indications for neoadjuvant radiation included bulky disease and osseous involvement. Patients with relapsed or incompletely responding disease may be candidates for potentially curative autologous stem cell transplantation if they respond to salvage chemotherapy.[1]

T cell: Because so much less is known about the pathophysiology and course of T-cell lymphomas, data are generally not adequate to inform treatment decisions, and therapy is based on expert consensus. Patients with peripheral T-cell lymphoma not otherwise specified have often been treated with CHOP. Autologous hematopoietic stem cell transplantation during remission can improve survival.[1]

KEY POINTS

- Non-Hodgkin lymphoma (NHL) is a heterogeneous group of hematologic malignancies with varied presentation. Primary or secondary thoracic involvement is common.
- PET-CT is the imaging modality of choice in the initial evaluation and staging of FDG-avid NHL and posttherapy assessment of response.
- Non–FDG-avid NHL is staged by CT.
- Thoracic MRI is useful for evaluation of mediastinal lymphomas, chest wall invasion, and spinal involvement. It is the preferred modality to evaluate cardiac lymphoma.
- The differential diagnosis for thoracic manifestations of NHL includes other primary malignancies, metastatic malignancies, infections, and, in some instances, vasculitides.

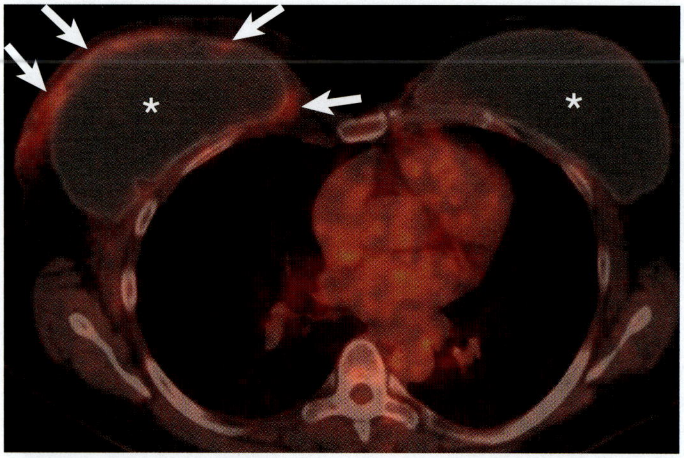

Fig. 24.16 Implant-associated non-Hodgkin lymphoma of the breast. Axial fused PET-CT image demonstrates mild circumferential FDG avidity around the right breast prosthesis *(asterisks)*. Histology revealed a CD30-positive anaplastic lymphoma kinase–negative anaplastic large cell lymphoma infiltrating the capsule of the implant.

SUGGESTED READINGS

Armitage JO, Gascoyne RD, Lunning MA, Cavalli F. Non-Hodgkin lymphoma. *Lancet*. 2017;390:298–310.

Barrington SF, Kluge R. FDG PET for therapy monitoring in Hodgkin and non-Hodgkin lymphomas. *Eur J Nucl Med Mol Imaging*. 2017;44(suppl 1):97–110.

Carter BW, Wu CC, Khorashadi L, et al. Multimodality imaging of cardiothoracic lymphoma. *Eur J Radiol*. 2014;83:1470–1482.

Cheson BD. Staging and response assessment in lymphomas: the new Lugano classification. *Chin Clin Oncol*. 2015;4:5.

Evens AM, Blum KA, eds. *Non-Hodgkin Lymphoma: Pathology, Imaging and Current Therapy. Cancer Treatment and Research*. Vol. 165. Switzerland, New York: Springer; 2015.

Kligerman SJ, Franks TJ, Galvin JR. Primary extranodal lymphoma of the thorax. *Radiol Clin North Am*. 2016;54:673–687.

The full reference list for this chapter is available at ExpertConsult.com.

25 Hodgkin Lymphoma

EMILY B. TSAI | CAROL C. WU | VICTORINE V. MUSE | KYUNG SOO LEE

Etiology, Prevalence, and Epidemiology

Hodgkin lymphoma (HL) is a neoplasm of B lymphocytes characterized by the presence of Reed-Sternberg cells. HL accounts for 10% of all cases of lymphoma and approximately 0.6% of all cancers diagnosed annually, with an annual incidence of 2 to 3 per 100,000 in Europe and the United States. Peak incidence occurs in two main age groups: young adults in the third decade and adults older than 50 years. It is slightly more common in men than in women, with a male to female ratio of 1.3:1 in the United States.[1,2] HL is less common in Asia. Risk factors for HL include Epstein-Barr virus infection, human immunodeficiency virus infection, and positive family history.

Intrathoracic involvement in HL is common and occurs most often in the form of lymph node enlargement. Approximately 85% of patients with HL have intrathoracic disease at initial presentation. Intrathoracic involvement usually is associated with evidence of HL elsewhere in the body. In one series of 1470 patients, only 44 (3%) had purely intrathoracic disease after appropriate clinical and pathologic staging.[3] Primary HL limited to the lung parenchyma is uncommon (<1%).[3,4]

Clinical Presentation

HL typically manifests as painless lymphadenopathy, involving the cervical and/or supraclavicular regions in 60% to 80% of patients, or as an incidental mediastinal mass on chest radiograph. Systemic B symptoms, defined as unexplained and persistent fever, night sweats, and weight loss, are present in less than 20% of patients with early-stage HL and up to 50% of patients with advanced disease. Pruritus is another characteristic systemic symptom seen in 10% to 15% of patients in the early course of the disease, which initially may be mild and localized but usually progresses and becomes generalized. Localized symptoms vary with organ involvement and include chest pain, cough or shortness of breath in patients with mediastinal involvement, or dry cough in patients with pulmonary involvement.[5,6]

Pathophysiology

HL is classified into two major types based on the immunophenotype of tumor cells: classic HL and nodular lymphocyte-predominant HL. Approximately 95% of cases of HL are classic HL, which is further classified histopathologically into four subtypes: nodular sclerosis (70%), mixed cellularity (10%–25%), lymphocyte-rich (5%), and lymphocyte-depleted (<1%–4%).

Of the classic HL, lymphocyte-rich and nodular sclerosis subtypes both have favorable prognosis. Nodular sclerosis HL usually occurs in young women, and most cases of HL in the mediastinum are of the nodular sclerosis subtype. The mixed-cellularity subtype tends to occur in middle-aged patients with systemic symptoms and extensive disease. The lymphocyte-depleted subtype has the worst prognosis because patients generally present with advanced-stage disease and systemic symptoms, and the bone marrow frequently is involved.[4] Nodular lymphocyte-predominant HL is usually diagnosed before age 35 years at an early stage with indolent course, although it is often associated with late or multiple relapses. There is also associated risk of development of secondary non-Hodgkin lymphoma, particular in those with splenic involvement.[7]

HL arises within a single lymphatic site and spreads contiguously to adjacent lymph nodes via lymphatic channels, typically spreading from the anterior mediastinal or paratracheal lymph nodes to involve, in decreasing order of frequency—hilar, subcarinal, internal mammary, pericardiophrenic, and posterior mediastinal nodes.[8–10] Eventual dissemination to distant sites and organs occurs hematogenously in advanced disease. As such, pulmonary involvement is rare without mediastinal and hilar lymph node involvement.[1a,11]

PATHOLOGY

Histologic diagnosis of HL is made by core-needle biopsy or excisional biopsy of an involved lymph node. Typical cases of classic HL may be diagnosed on routine light microscopy based upon the presence of Reed-Sternberg giant cells in association with appropriate stromal or cellular background. The Reed-Sternberg cell is a large, bilobed cell that has prominent eosinophilic nucleoli, perinucleolar clearing, thickened nuclear membrane, and abundant cytoplasm. Histologic subtypes are differentiated based on the composition of the background infiltrate and tumor cell morphology.

Confirmatory immunophenotyping is useful for distinguishing classic HL from nodular lymphocyte-predominant HL and other types of lymphoma. Classic HL tumor cells express CD15 (85%) and CD30 (nearly 100%) and lack global expression of pan–T antigens. CD20, a B-cell antigen, and BSAP/PAX5, a regulator of B-cell development, are variably expressed.[12] In nodular lymphocyte-predominant HL, cells are $CD20^+$ but $CD15^-$ and $CD30^-$.[7] Reed-Sternberg cells also may express the immune checkpoint inhibitor PD-L1, which suggests potential for therapy using PD-1/PD-L1 inhibitors.[13]

Bone marrow infiltration is seen in up to 15% of patients at diagnosis and typically occurs with advanced-stage disease. Bone marrow biopsy is no longer routinely recommended because it does not impact treatment decisions or patient outcomes, in part because of the universal use of chemotherapy and high sensitivity and specificity of positron emission tomography (PET)–computed tomography (CT) for the detection of bone marrow involvement.[14]

Manifestations of Disease

RADIOGRAPHY

HL involving the anterior mediastinum or paratracheal lymph nodes typically manifests radiographically as widening of the superior mediastinum by a lobulated mass (Fig. 25.1).

Three radiographic patterns of pulmonary parenchymal HL may occur. The most common is single or multiple pulmonary nodules, followed by lobar or segmental consolidation and reticular pattern with bronchovascular bundle and interlobular septal thickening (Figs. 25.2 and 25.3). Consolidation of lung parenchyma remote from the mediastinum is common. Reticular pattern with peribronchovascular and interlobular septal thickening can result from obstruction of lymphatic or venous drainage by enlarged hilar and mediastinal lymph nodes or from intrinsic tumor deposits within interstitial lymphatic pathways. Other findings include disseminated small nodules, cavitating masses, and endobronchial nodules.[8,15–17]

Up to 15% of patients who have HL present with bone involvement radiographically.[18] Osseous lesions can be lytic or blastic and are usually better seen on CT.

COMPUTED TOMOGRAPHY

Mediastinal Involvement

HL involves the anterior (prevascular) mediastinum or paratracheal regions in 90% to 100% of cases (see Fig. 25.1). In approximately

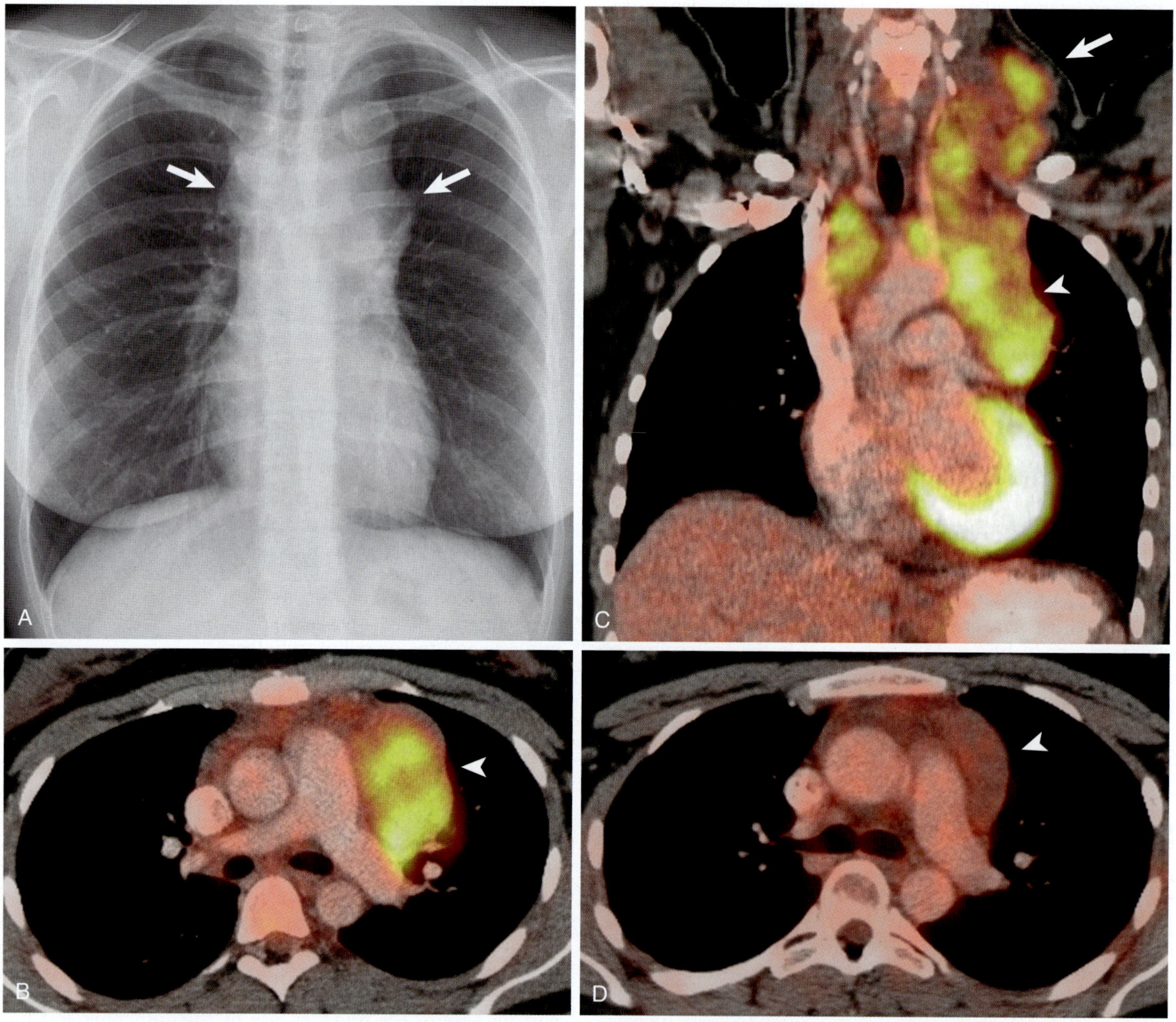

Fig. 25.1 Classic Hodgkin lymphoma with cervical and intrathoracic lymphadenopathy in a 21-year-old woman. (A) Chest radiograph shows widening of the upper mediastinum *(arrows)*. (B) and (C) Axial and coronal fused FDG–PET-CT show FDG-avid cervical *(arrow)* and prevascular *(arrowhead)* lymphadenopathy.

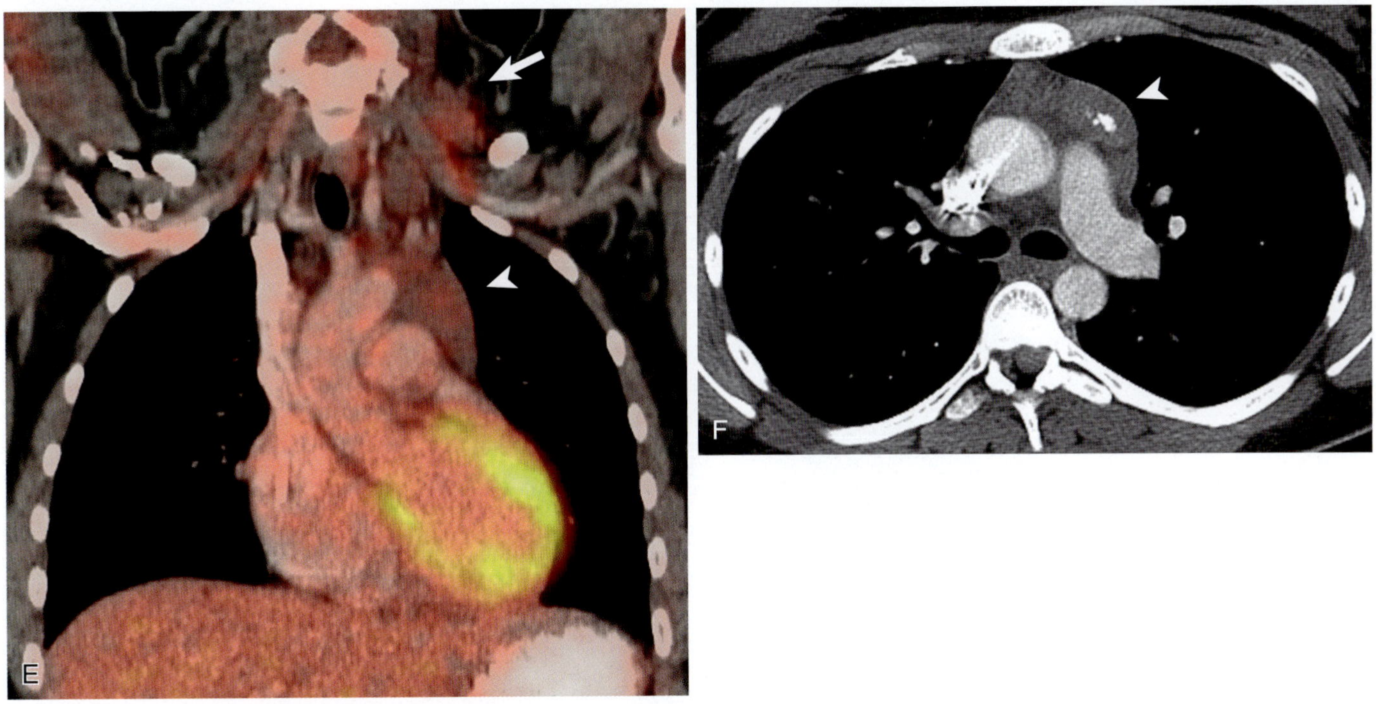

Fig. 25.1, cont'd (D) and (E) Axial and coronal fused FDG–PET-CT after treatment show decreased size and decreased FDG uptake of the cervical *(arrow)* and mediastinal *(arrowhead)* lymph nodes. (F) Subsequent posttreatment contrast-enhanced CT shows interval coarse calcification of the mediastinal lymph nodes *(arrowhead)*.

40% of cases the intrathoracic disease is confined to the anterior (prevascular) mediastinum. Enlarged lymph nodes most commonly have homogeneous soft tissue attenuation (see Fig. 25.1). In approximately 20% of cases, particularly in patients with large, coalescent masses, the involved lymph nodes or thymus may contain areas of low attenuation representing necrosis, hemorrhage, and cystic degeneration (Fig. 25.4).[19,20] Histologically, necrotic areas range from minute foci of fibrinoid necrosis to large areas of granular tissue destruction containing necrotic cells.[20] Necrosis is seen most commonly in the nodular sclerosis and mixed-cellularity cell subtypes of HL and is not seen in the lymphocyte-rich subtype. The necrotic or cystic appearance of mediastinal lymphadenopathy in patients with HL does not affect overall survival or length of remission.

HL also frequently involves the thymus and may result in diffuse thymic enlargement. Thymic involvement may be difficult to distinguish from anterior mediastinal lymph node involvement.

Dystrophic calcification may develop in involved lymph nodes after mediastinal radiation (Fig. 25.5; see also Fig. 25.1).[21,22] Although some investigators consider the complication to be unrelated to the degree of radiation,[23] others link it with relatively high doses.[22] The time interval between irradiation and the appearance of calcification ranges from 1 to 9 years.

HL may extend beyond affected lymph nodes into mediastinal interstitial tissue and invade the esophagus, superior vena cava, and pericardium (Fig. 25.6). Corresponding imaging manifestations, such as pericardial effusion, may be seen.[15,24] In contrast to lung cancer, HL rarely invades the phrenic nerve.[15,24] Involvement of the anterior mediastinal and internal mammary nodes (Figs. 25.7) may be associated with invasion of the sternum or the parasternal tissues (Fig. 25.8).[25,26]

Pleuropulmonary Disease

Lung parenchymal involvement occurs at initial presentation in 10% to 15% of patients with HL and eventually in 30% to 40% of cases and is almost always associated with hilar or mediastinal lymphadenopathy. Extension into the parenchyma may result in nodules or focal areas of consolidation.

The typical appearance of pulmonary Hodgkin lymphoma on CT consists of a single or multiple, irregularly marginated pulmonary nodules or masses (Fig. 25.9; see also Fig. 25.2). The size of the nodules ranges widely and may vary with time; individual foci may coalesce to form a large homogeneous nonsegmental mass (Fig. 25.10; see also Fig. 25.3), sometimes involving a whole lobe.[15,27] This type of parenchymal consolidation is not associated with lobar volume loss; its borders can be shaggy and ill defined, and an air bronchogram may be visible. Such masses can undergo necrosis and form a cavity that may have a thin or thick wall; in many cases masses are multiple.[28–30] Rarely, there is a generalized miliary or reticulonodular pattern.[29,31,32] Bronchial occlusion almost always is caused by tumor within the airway lumen or wall and can result in lobar or segmental atelectasis and obstructive pneumonitis.[33–36]

Pleural effusion is seen at presentation in approximately 10% of patients[8,9] and eventually develops in approximately 30%, most often in association with other intrathoracic manifestations of the disease (see Fig. 25.6).[15] The fluid can be serous, chylous, pseudochylous,[37] or rarely serosanguineous. The incidence of pneumothorax is increased in patients who have HL. Treatment with radiotherapy, lung involvement, radiation fibrosis, and infection seem to be risk factors.

Text continued on p. 421

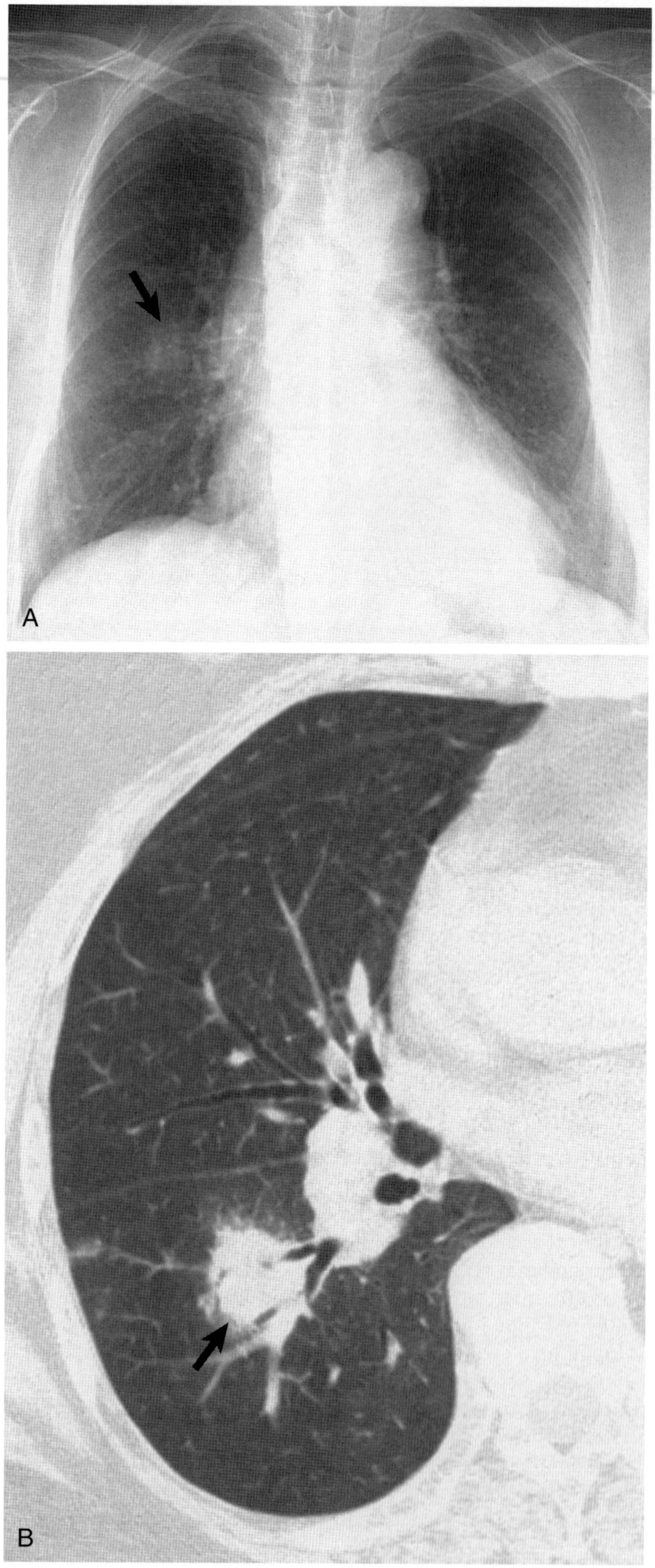

Fig. 25.2 Mixed-cellularity Hodgkin lymphoma with pulmonary involvement in a 70-year-old woman. (A) Chest radiograph shows poorly defined nodular lesion *(arrow)* in the right middle lung zone. (B) CT scan of right lung at the level of basal trunk shows a poorly defined nodule *(arrow)* containing air bronchograms.

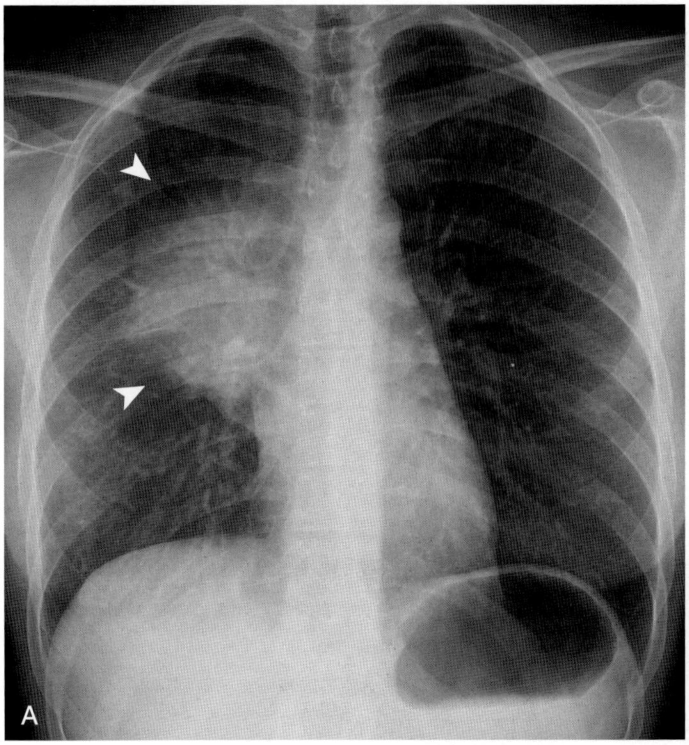

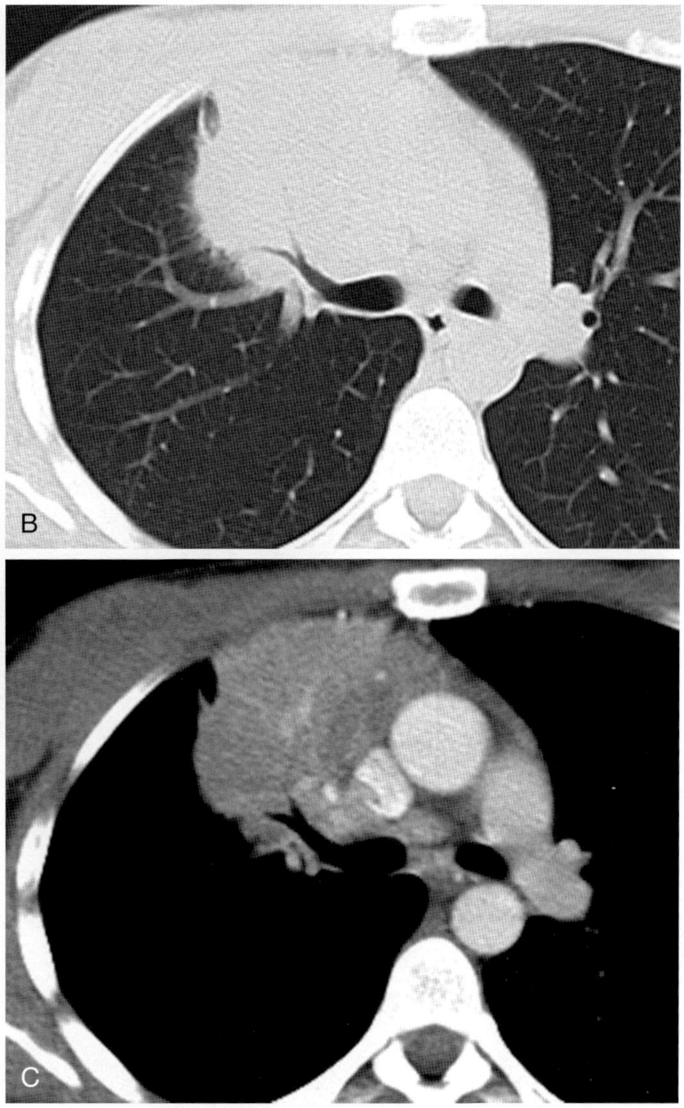

Fig. 25.3 Nodular sclerosis Hodgkin lymphoma with lung parenchymal involvement in a 38-year-old woman who presented with pruritus. (A) Chest radiograph shows a right upper lobe mass *(arrowheads)* with irregular borders that is contiguous with the mediastinum. (B) CT scan shows a right upper lobe mass with irregular borders and air bronchograms. (C) Contrast-enhanced CT scan shows that the right upper lobe lung mass is contiguous with anterior mediastinal soft tissue.

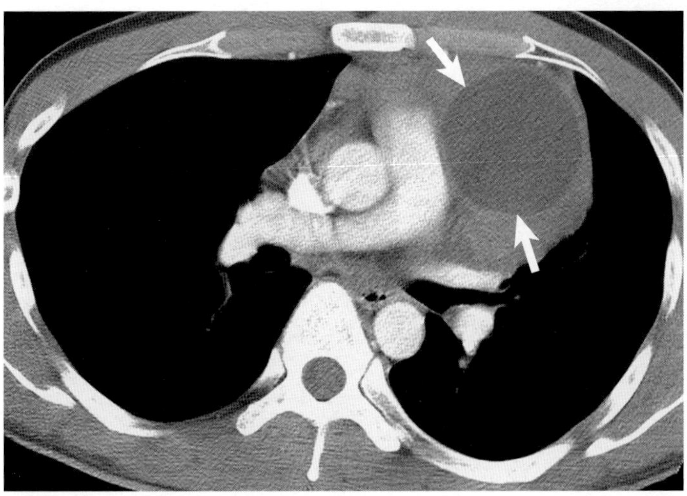

Fig. 25.4 Nodular sclerosis Hodgkin lymphoma with cystic area. Contrast-enhanced CT scan at level of the bronchus intermedius shows left anterior (prevascular) mediastinal mass containing a large round area of low attenuation *(arrows)*.

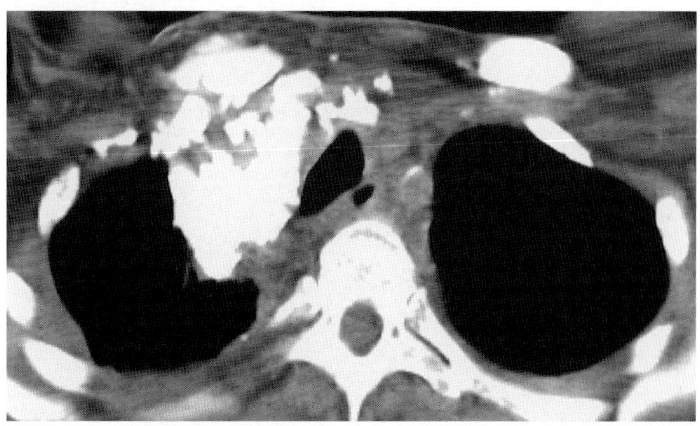

Fig. 25.5 Hodgkin lymphoma with dystrophic calcification after radiotherapy in a 47-year-old woman. CT scan shows extensive anterior mediastinal and right chest wall calcification.

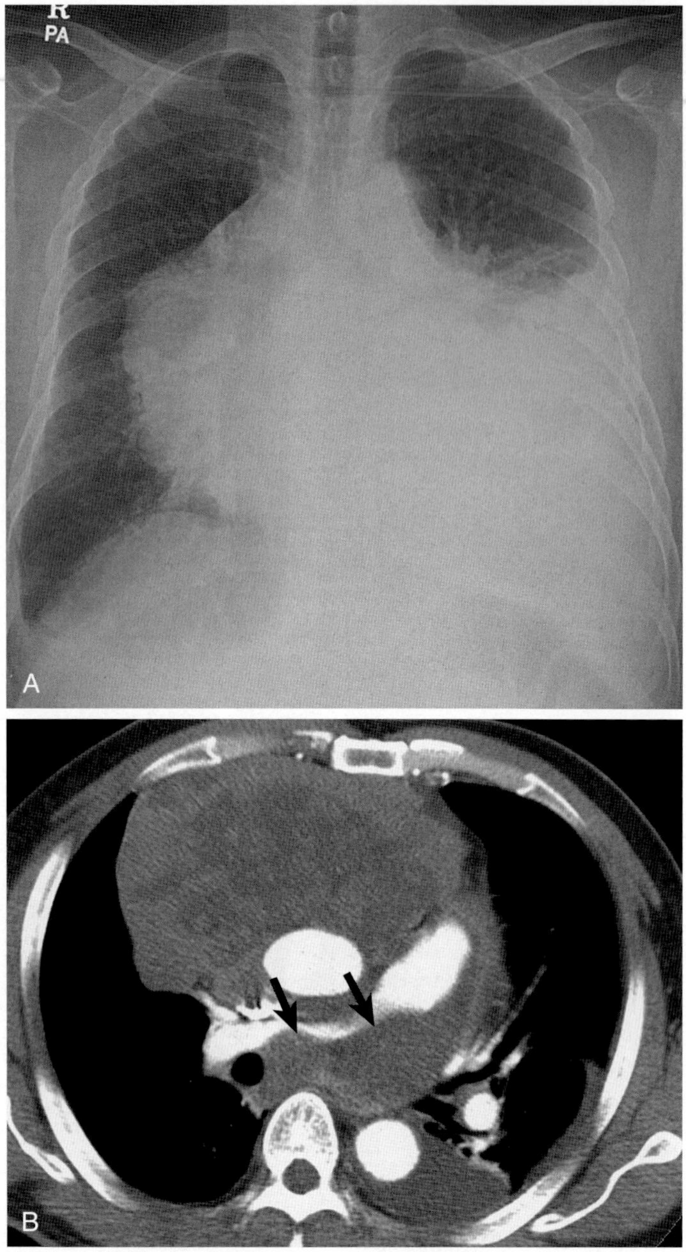

Fig. 25.6 Hodgkin lymphoma with intrapericardial extension. (A) Chest radiograph shows widened mediastinum with lobulated contour, obscuration of the right heart border, and left pleural effusion. (B) Contrast-enhanced CT scan shows large anterior (prevascular) mediastinal soft tissue mass with heterogeneous attenuation with intrapericardial involvement *(arrows)*. Note associated left pleural effusion.

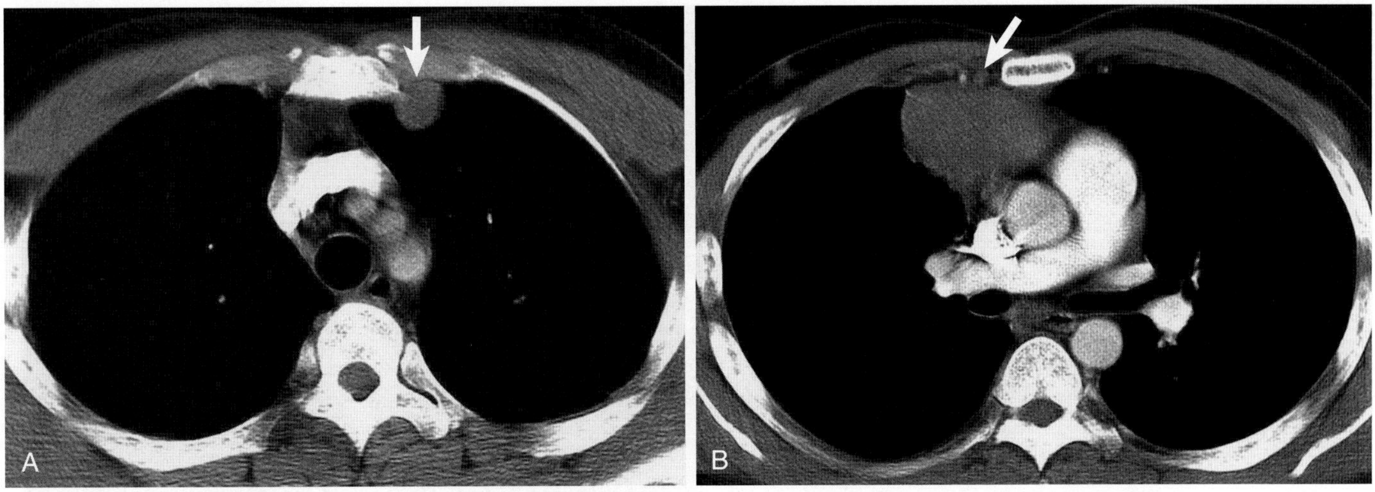

Fig. 25.7 Nodular sclerosis Hodgkin lymphoma in a 35-year-old man. (A) Contrast-enhanced CT scan at level of great vessels shows left internal mammary lymph node enlargement *(arrow)*. (B) CT scan at level of bronchus intermedius shows soft tissue mass in right anterior (prevascular) mediastinum. Also note slightly enlarged right internal mammary lymph node *(arrow)*.

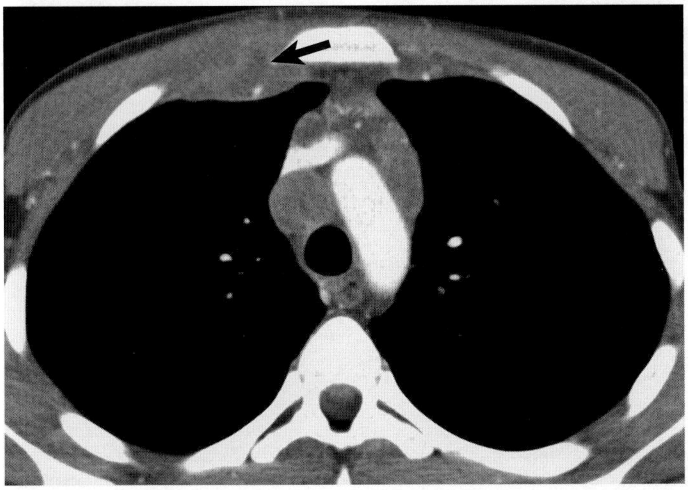

Fig. 25.8 Hodgkin lymphoma with chest wall extension in a 17-year-old boy. Contrast-enhanced CT scan shows enlarged anterior (prevascular) mediastinal and paratracheal lymph nodes and increased soft tissue in the region of the internal mammary lymph nodes with extension into the adjacent soft tissues and into the right parasternal region *(arrow)*.

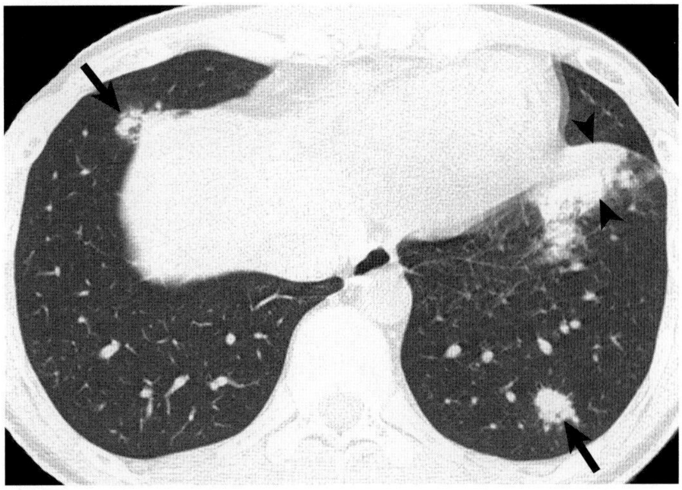

Fig. 25.9 Recurrent nodular sclerosis Hodgkin lymphoma with pulmonary involvement in a 23-year-old man. CT scan at the level of the right hemidiaphragm shows nodules *(arrows)* and airspace consolidation *(arrowheads)* in both lower lobes.

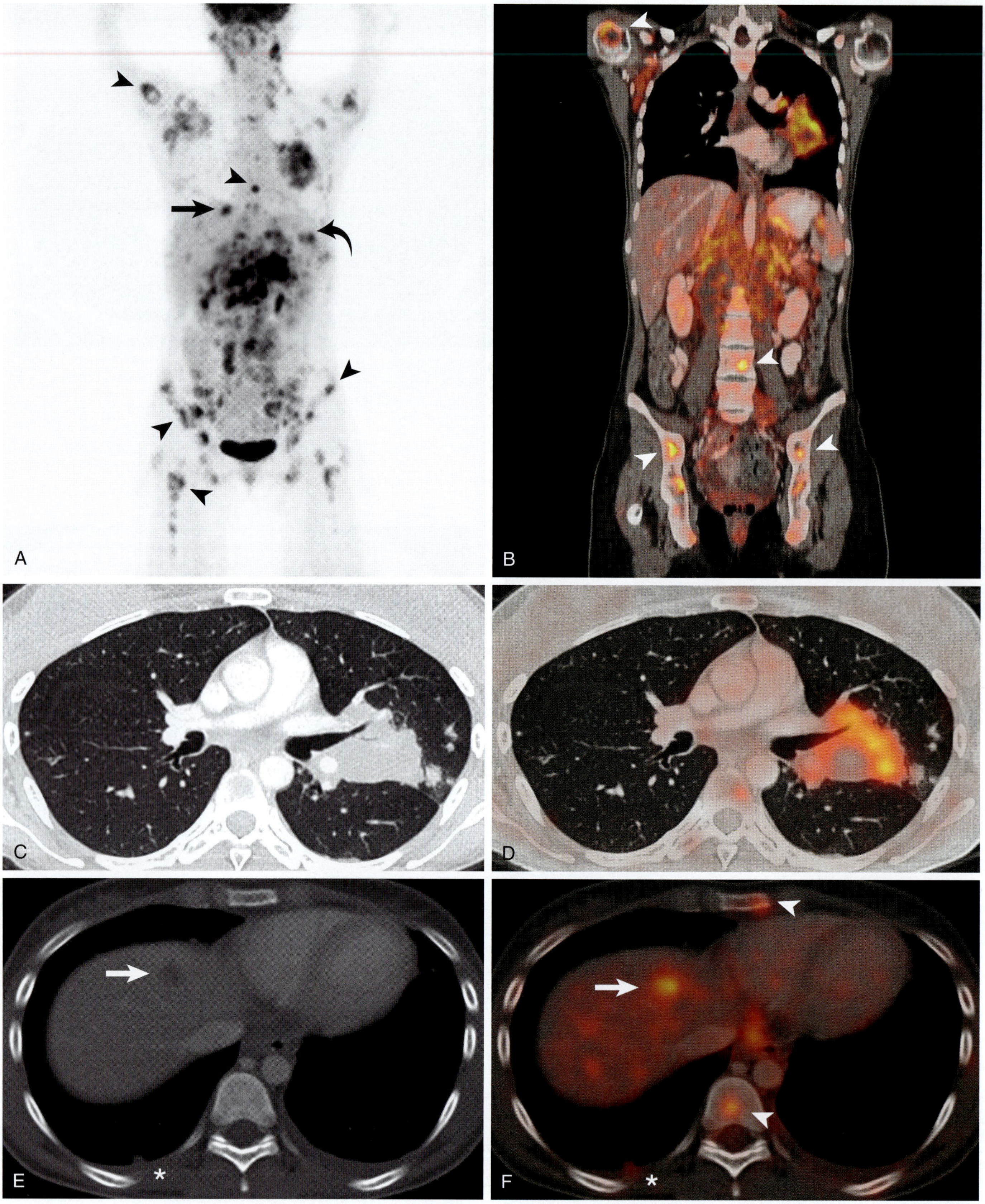

Fig. 25.10 Relapsed disease in a 38-year-old woman. (A) and (B) Coronal FDG-PET and fused FDG–PET-CT scans show widespread disease involving the cervical, thoracic, and abdominal lymph node stations; left lung; liver *(arrow)*; spleen *(curved arrow)*; and axial and appendicular osseous structures *(arrowheads)*. (C) and (D) Contrast-enhanced CT and fused FDG–PET-CT scans show an intensely FDG-avid left upper lobe mass. (E) and (F) Contrast-enhanced CT and fused FDG–PET-CT scans show an FDG-avid subpleural subcentimeter right lower lobe lung nodule *(asterisk)*, an intensely FDG-avid hepatic lesion *(arrow)* and radiographically occult, FDG-avid lesions in the sternum and visualized vertebral body *(arrowheads)*.

Although thoracic HL typically manifests with lymphadenopathy, a rare form of pulmonary Hodgkin lymphoma is restricted to the pulmonary parenchyma at presentation. Less than 100 cases of primary pulmonary HL have been reported in the English literature. It usually manifests as single or multiple nodules, which frequently cavitate. Occasionally, pulmonary Hodgkin lymphoma may manifest with an endobronchial mass in patients with a normal chest radiograph.[4,38]

Chest Wall and Extrathoracic Skeletal Involvement

The thoracic skeleton usually, but not invariably, is affected by direct extension of tumor from the mediastinum or lungs.[25,28,39] In such cases destruction of ribs, vertebrae, or the sternum typically results in focal lytic areas. By contrast, vertebral involvement other than by direct extension often is purely osteoblastic (ivory vertebra). Involvement of the extrathoracic skeleton (most commonly the spine or pelvis) usually results in mixed lytic and blastic lesions.[18]

POSITRON EMISSION TOMOGRAPHY

HD is almost always avid on fluorodeoxyglucose (FDG)-PET. FDG–PET-CT has improved the accuracy of pretreatment staging of HL and is now considered the standard of care. PET mostly upstages disease compared with CT alone (see Figs. 25.1 and 25.10).[40,41] Upstaging includes the detection of increased FDG uptake in normal-sized lymph nodes (usually <10 mm in diameter) and in extranodal sites, most commonly the liver, spleen, cortical bone, bone marrow, and skin (see Fig. 25.10). However, pulmonary involvement by Hodgkin lymphoma shows variable FDG uptake and may result in false-negative scans.[42]

More recently, use of interim PET-CT during treatment is under investigation to facilitate early identification of treatment failure and minimize treatment-related toxicities. PET-CT at the conclusion of treatment is considered the standard to confirm remission. Visual assessment of relative FDG uptake compared with the mediastinal background is recommended.[43,44] Residual or new metabolically active disease at the end of treatment represents treatment failure and requires further biopsy and treatment. In addition, a posttreatment baseline PET scan helps detect future relapse, which often occurs in the region of previous disease.[40]

After the completion of treatment and a negative posttreatment PET scan, the use of routine PET-CT for surveillance of HL is not recommended because of low positive predictive value, high false-positive rate, and lack of clear outcome benefit.[45]

DIFFERENTIAL DIAGNOSIS

The differential diagnosis of an anterior mediastinal mass includes HL, non-Hodgkin lymphoma, thymic neoplasms, substernal thyroid masses, germ cell tumors, and mycobacterial or fungal infection. Findings that favor Hodgkin lymphoma include lobulation and involvement of contiguous lymph node groups in the paratracheal and hilar regions.

The differential diagnosis of pulmonary HL includes infection, primary bronchogenic carcinoma, organizing pneumonia, granulomatosis with polyangiitis (Wegener granulomatosis), drug toxicity, and radiation pneumonitis.[27] Rarely, HL manifests with a generalized miliary or reticulonodular pattern,[31] which may be difficult or impossible to differentiate from lymphangitic spread of carcinoma or sarcoidosis.[29,32]

Staging

Staging is based on sites of involvement and clinical symptoms and is an important determinant of treatment and prognosis. For staging purposes, lymph nodes are divided into anatomic regions that can be encompassed by a single radiation field. The mediastinal region therefore encompasses thymus and prevascular, aortopulmonary, paratracheal, subcarinal, posterior mediastinal, and internal mammary lymph nodes. Right and left hilar lymph nodes are considered separate regions.

The Lugano staging classification,[46] published in 2014, is a modification of the Ann Arbor staging system:

- Stage I: Single lymph node region or single extralymphatic site (IE)
- Stage II: Two or more lymph node regions on the same side of the diaphragm or nodal stage I or II plus contiguous involvement of an extralymphatic site (IIE)
- Stage III: Lymph node regions on both sides of the diaphragm, which may include the spleen (IIIS) and/or limited contiguous extralymphatic organ or site (IIIE, IIIES)
- Stage IV: Disseminated noncontiguous extralymphatic involvement
- Additional subclassifications:
  - A or B: Absence (A) or presence (B) of systemic symptoms (fevers, night sweats, or unexplained weight loss)
  - E: Presence of limited extranodal extension from an adjacent nodal site that does not advance the stage
  - S: Presence of splenic involvement

In the Lugano classification, bulky disease is defined as a single nodal mass of 10 cm or a nodal mass greater than a third of the transthoracic diameter at any level of thoracic vertebrae as determined by CT. Additional scoring mechanisms have been designated to assess treatment response on PET-CT or CT only[44,46,47] and for patients treated with immunomodulatory therapy.[48]

Synopsis of Treatment Options

HL is curable in the majority of patients, even in cases of recurrence or relapse after initial treatment, because of more effective and less toxic combinations of radiotherapy and chemotherapy.[49] Patients with stage I and stage II disease are considered early stage and are further stratified into favorable and unfavorable prognosis disease based on clinical features, such as age, symptoms, number of sites of disease, and extent of mediastinal adenopathy. Patients with early-stage disease are treated with chemotherapy, typically ABVD (doxorubicin, bleomycin, vinblastine, dacarbazine), for two to six cycles depending on the extent of disease, with or without radiation therapy to the involved regions.[50]

Patients with stage III and stage IV disease and sometimes stage II disease with bulky nodal disease are considered to have advanced-stage disease and are treated with combination chemotherapy with or without consolidation radiation therapy. Patients with refractory or recurrent disease may undergo autologous hematopoietic stem cell transplantation. Treatment-related toxicities must be considered in deciding treatment regimens because of the high cure rates.

KEY POINTS: HODGKIN LYMPHOMA

- Hodgkin lymphoma (HL) is a neoplasm of B lymphocytes characterized by the presence of Reed-Sternberg cells.
- Peak ages of occurrence are 20 to 30 years and older than 50 years.
- The most common subtype is nodular sclerosis HL.
- Approximately 85% of patients with HL have intrathoracic disease at initial presentation, most commonly mediastinal lymph node enlargement.
- Pleuropulmonary involvement is present at diagnosis in 10%–15% of patients and eventually in 30%–40%.
- Purely intrathoracic disease is present in only 3% of cases and primary pulmonary disease in less than 1% of cases.
- FDG–PET-CT is the recommended imaging study for staging and may upstage disease in up to 25% of cases compared with CT alone.
- Imaging findings of lymph node involvement include:
  - Typically homogeneous soft tissue attenuation
  - May be necrotic or cystic-appearing in 20% of cases, most commonly in the nodular sclerosis and mixed-cellularity subtypes
  - Dystrophic calcification may develop after radiation therapy
- Imaging findings of pleuropulmonary involvement include:
  - Multiple pulmonary nodules, often with irregular margins
  - Less commonly, areas of consolidation or peribronchovascular and interlobular septal thickening
  - Pleural effusion at presentation in approximately 10% of patients and eventually in approximately 30%

SUGGESTED READINGS

Ansell SM. Hodgkin lymphoma: 2016 update on diagnosis, risk-stratification, and management. *Am J Hematol.* 2016;91(4):434–442.

Carter BW, Wu CC, Khorashadi L, Godoy MC, de Groot PM, Abbott GF, Lichtenberger JP 3rd. Multimodality imaging of cardiothoracic lymphoma. *Eur J Radiol.* 2014;83(8):1470–1482.

Cheson BD, Fisher RI, Barrington SF, Cavalli F, Schwartz LH, Zucca E, Lister TA. Recommendations for initial evaluation, staging, and response assessment of Hodgkin and non-Hodgkin lymphoma: the Lugano Classification. *J Clin Oncol.* 2014;32:3059–3067.

Gallamini A, Hutchings M, Ramadan S. Clinical presentation and staging of Hodgkin lymphoma. *Semin Hematol.* 2016;53(3):148–154.

The full reference list for this chapter is available at ExpertConsult.com.

26 Leukemia

GIRISH S. SHROFF | CAROL C. WU | CHITRA VISWANATHAN | MYLENE T. TRUONG

Etiology

Leukemias are a group of malignancies in which abnormal cells, usually abnormal white blood cells (leukocytes), are produced in the bone marrow. Leukemias may be classified as myeloid, also known as myelogenous or myeloblastic, or lymphoid, also known as lymphocytic or lymphoblastic, depending on the types of abnormal cells that are produced. In myeloid leukemias, myeloid stem cells, which normally develop into erythrocytes, platelets, and granulocytes or monocytes, are affected; in lymphoid leukemias, lymphoid stem cells, which normally develop into lymphocytes, are affected. Leukemias are classified as acute or chronic according to cellular maturity; immature, poorly differentiated cells (blast cells) predominate in acute leukemias, whereas chronic leukemias have more mature cells.[1] The four major leukemia types are acute myeloid leukemia (AML), chronic myeloid leukemia (CML), acute lymphoblastic leukemia (ALL), and chronic lymphocytic leukemia (CLL). Small lymphocytic lymphoma (SLL) is now grouped with CLL (CLL/SLL) because they are recognized as the same disease entity; differentiation is based on peripheral blood absolute lymphocyte count.[2,3] CML leads to the formation of the *BCR-ABL1* oncogene.[4] The World Health Organization (WHO) classification of leukemia has been recently revised to incorporate new clinical, morphologic, immunophenotypic, genetic, and prognostic data.[5]

Prevalence and Epidemiology

AML is much more common in adults than children and accounts for approximately 80% of acute leukemias in adults.[2] Median age at diagnosis is 67 years, and males are more commonly affected than females.[6] Among the four major leukemia types, AML has the worst prognosis, with a 5-year survival rate of approximately 20%.[2] CML is primarily a disease of adults and accounts for approximately 15% of leukemias in the adult population.[7] Median age at presentation is 44 to 55 years.[7] With the advent of tyrosine kinase inhibitor therapy, the annual mortality in CML has decreased to 1% to 2%, and consequently, its prevalence in the United States has increased.[4] ALL is the most common leukemia in young children, with a peak incidence between ages 2 and 5 years; ALL can also affect older adults age 65 years and older. CLL, the most frequent type of leukemia in the Western Hemisphere,[8] usually affects adults, most commonly older than 65 years.[3] The median survival of patients with CLL is 10 years, although life expectancy can range from about 2 to 3 years to 2 decades based on clinical stage; most patients have an indolent clinical course with prolonged survival.[3]

Risk factors for the development of leukemia include previous exposure to ionizing radiation or chemical agents, prior treatment with certain chemotherapeutic drugs, certain viral infections, chromosomal translocations, immunodeficiency disorders, chronic myeloproliferative disorders, and certain chromosomal disorders.[1]

Clinical Presentation

Clinical manifestations of leukemia are due to either suppression of normal marrow function or organ infiltration by leukemic cells.[1] Suppression of normal marrow function results in anemia, thrombocytopenia, and leukopenia, whereas organ infiltration can lead to lymphadenopathy, splenomegaly, hepatomegaly, and skeletal pain.[1]

Common presenting symptoms of AML are usually related to anemia, leukopenia, and thrombocytopenia and may include fatigue, infection, or bleeding.[6] Common presenting symptoms of ALL include lymphadenopathy, skeletal pain, bleeding, or fever. Patients with chronic leukemias are frequently asymptomatic at diagnosis. Between 20% and 50% of patients with CML are asymptomatic and are diagnosed by routine tests.[7,9] Common presenting symptoms include fatigue, bleeding, weight loss, abdominal fullness, and splenomegaly.[9] CLL patients often have lymphadenopathy that may involve the cervical, axillary, or inguinal regions.[10] The majority of patients with CLL have an indolent course, but some patients with aggressive disease can have frequent relapses.[3] Richter transformation occurs in patients with CLL and is a rare clinical entity associated with poor outcome defined by the development of diffuse large B-cell lymphoma or, much less frequently, classic Hodgkin lymphoma. The incidence rate of Richter transformation is 0.5% per year of observation.[11]

Clinical manifestations of leukemic pulmonary infiltration are nonspecific and include cough, dyspnea, and fever.[12] Diagnosis requires bronchoalveolar lavage or lung biopsy.[12]

Pathophysiology

All blood cells (red blood cells, platelets, and white blood cells) originate from hematopoietic stem cells. In the leukemias malignant transformation usually occurs at the pluripotent stem cell level.[1] As a result of abnormal proliferation, clonal expansion, and diminished apoptosis, normal blood elements are replaced with malignant leukemic cells.[1] Bone marrow failure—resulting from both marrow crowding by abnormal cells and inadequate production of normal marrow elements—and organ infiltration ensue.

Myeloid sarcoma, in the 2016 WHO classification, represents a unique presentation of any subtype of AML. It is defined as a tumor mass consisting of myeloid blasts, with or without maturation, occurring at an anatomic site other than the bone marrow.[13] It may present de novo, with concurrent AML, as extramedullary relapse of AML, or as progression of a prior myeloproliferative neoplasm.[5,13] It was formerly known as granulocytic sarcoma, chloroma, or myeloblastoma. The term *chloroma* is derived from the characteristic green color resulting from the high levels of the intracellular porphyrin-bearing enzyme myeloperoxidase. Bone (subperiosteal) and perineural involvement is common, whereas thoracic involvement is uncommon.[14]

Leukemic pulmonary infiltration is defined as extravascular collections of leukemic cells in regions of lung parenchyma not demonstrating other apparent causes for their presence (e.g., infection, hemorrhage, or venous congestion).[15] Leukemic pulmonary infiltration has been found at autopsy in a substantial percentage (>25%) of patients with leukemia.[15,16]

Other conditions of lung involvement seen in myeloid leukemias include leukostasis, leukemic cell lysis pneumopathy, and hyperleukocytic reaction. Pulmonary leukostasis is a condition that results from obstruction of pulmonary capillaries, arterioles, and small arteries by leukemic cells.[17] Leukostasis occurs most commonly in AML and less commonly in patients with CML in blast crisis.[17] Total white blood cell count is usually between 100,000 and 500,000/mm.[6,17] Leukemic cell lysis pneumopathy, a condition characterized by severe hypoxemia and diffuse pulmonary opacities that occurs within 48 hours after the initiation of chemotherapy in patients with high leukocyte counts,[17] can manifest as pulmonary hemorrhage, edema, and diffuse alveolar damage. Hyperleukocytic reaction is due to an increase in blast counts leading to intravascular accumulation of neoplastic cells, causing thrombi and alveolar hemorrhage.

Pulmonary alveolar proteinosis (PAP), a rare disorder with accumulation of excess surfactant within pulmonary alveoli resulting in cough and dyspnea, can be seen in association with hematologic malignancies. CML is the most commonly associated leukemia in reported cases of secondary PAP, although association with ALL and CLL have also been reported.[18]

In an autopsy review, pleural involvement was found in 15% of patients with leukemia.[16] In another review of autopsy findings in 495 patients with leukemia, pleural involvement was found to occur most commonly with ALL, occurring in 27% of patients with ALL.[19] Malignant pleural effusions can be seen at any time with acute leukemias but tend to occur in advanced disease in chronic leukemia.[20]

The pericardium, myocardium, and endocardium may be infiltrated by leukemia.[16,21,22] At autopsy, rates of cardiac involvement by leukemia range from 11% to 37%.[23–25] Leukemic cardiac involvement is frequently clinically silent.[25]

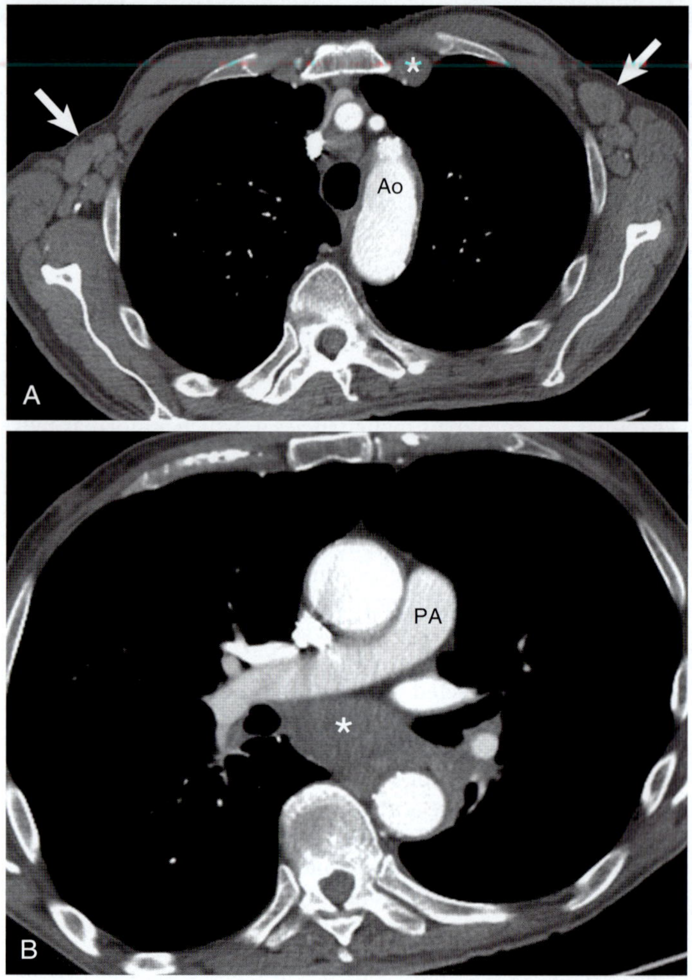

Fig. 26.1 Intrathoracic lymphadenopathy in chronic lymphocytic leukemia/small lymphocytic lymphoma in a 77-year-old man with longstanding loss of energy and weight loss. (A) CT image at the level of upper aortic arch (Ao) shows bilateral axillary *(arrows)* and left internal mammary lymphadenopathy *(asterisk)*. (B) CT image at the level of the pulmonary artery (PA) reveals subcarinal *(asterisk)* and left hilar lymphadenopathy.

Manifestations of the Disease

Intrathoracic imaging manifestations of leukemia include involvement of the mediastinum, lungs, pleura, heart, and axillae.[26]

MEDIASTINUM

Mediastinal lymphadenopathy is relatively common in patients with CLL and ALL, occurring in 25% of patients with CLL (Fig. 26.1) and 10% to 20% of patients with ALL.[26] Hilar lymphadenopathy is less common. Patients with ALL may present with a large symptomatic anterior mediastinal mass.[26] Mediastinal lymphadenopathy is less common in cases of AML or CML, occurring in 5% of these patients.[26]

Myeloid sarcoma may manifest as a focal mediastinal mass (Fig. 26.2), lymphadenopathy, or diffuse infiltration of mediastinal tissues.[14] Other less commonly affected sites include the hila, pleura, lungs, and pericardium.[14]

LUNG

In most cases pulmonary leukemic infiltration is not evident radiographically.[15,21] When evident it usually manifests as a bilateral reticular pattern with septal lines resembling interstitial edema or lymphangitic carcinomatosis. Nodules and focal homogeneous opacities may also be seen.[17,22]

On CT leukemic pulmonary infiltration usually manifests with smooth and/or nodular thickening of the interlobular septa and bronchovascular bundles as a result of the predilection of leukemic cells to infiltrate the pulmonary lymphatics.[22] Small nodules are also a common feature, although not usually the dominant finding.[17] Nodule distribution may be peribronchovascular, centrilobular, or random.[22] Areas of ground-glass attenuation and consolidation can also be seen, and the consolidation may be predominantly peribronchial in location (Fig. 26.3).[22]

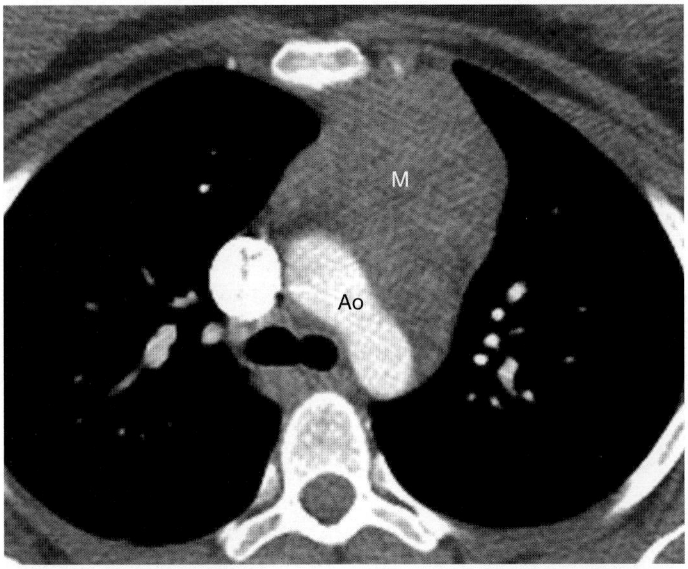

Fig. 26.2 Myeloid sarcoma in a 21-year-old woman with night sweats and slowly progressive fatigue and dyspnea on exertion. CT at the level of the aortic arch (Ao) shows an anterior mediastinal mass (M). Biopsy of the mass revealed myeloid sarcoma of the thymus, and the patient was diagnosed with acute lymphoblastic leukemia.

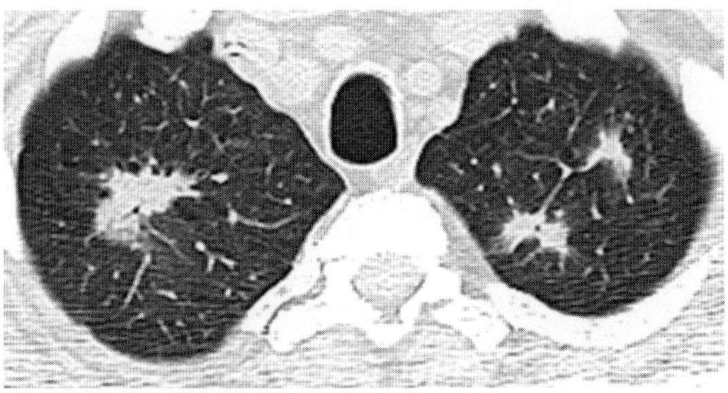

Fig. 26.3 Pulmonary leukemic infiltration in a 64-year-old man with relapsed acute lymphoblastic leukemia and disease progression despite multiple cycles of chemotherapy and stem cell transplant. CT demonstrates bilateral upper lobe peribronchiolar nodular opacities. Biopsy of the right upper lobe lesion confirmed leukemic infiltration. At autopsy, leukemic infiltrates were present in both lungs.

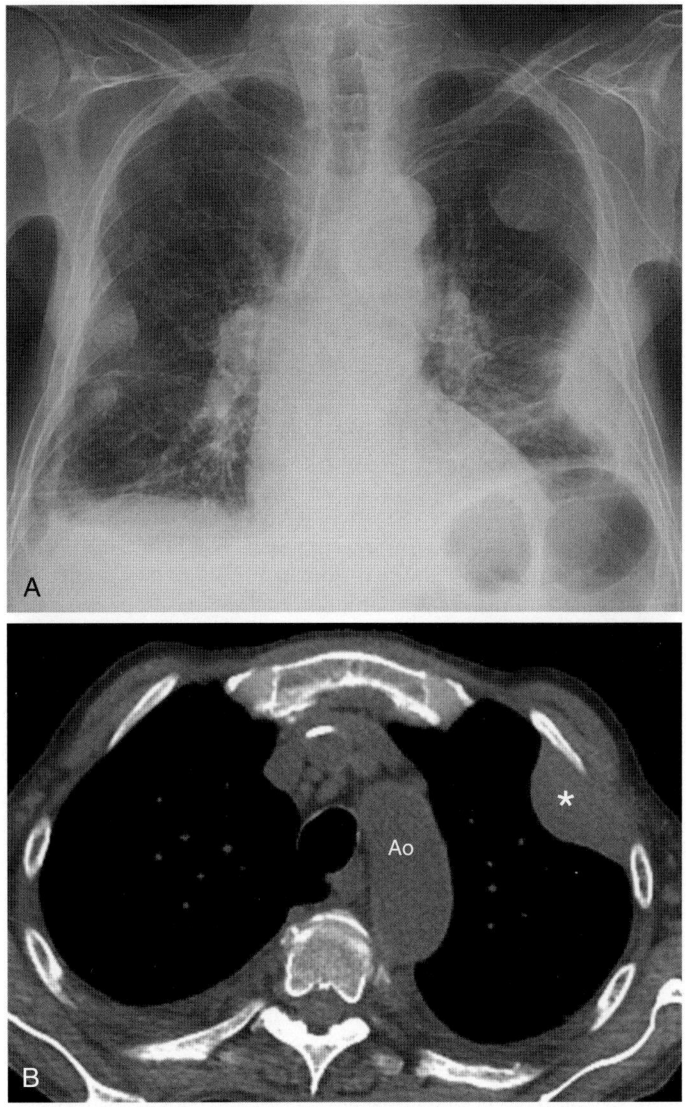

Fig. 26.4 Pleural leukemic involvement in a 73-year-old man with relapsed/refractory B-cell chronic lymphocytic leukemia. (A) Chest radiograph reveals bilateral peripheral lobular lesions manifesting the incomplete border sign, indicating a pleural or extrapleural process. Note small pleural effusions. (B) Noncontrast CT at the level of the aortic arch (Ao) shows a left upper pleural soft tissue mass *(asterisk)*. The other pleural lesions (not shown) were also soft tissue masses. Pleural biopsy revealed chronic lymphocytic leukemia/small lymphocytic lymphoma.

Pulmonary abnormalities on imaging are only rarely due to leukemic infiltration alone; coexisting abnormalities may include pneumonia, edema, hemorrhage, and drug-induced injury.

Imaging in patients with leukostasis may be normal or resemble interstitial or alveolar edema.[17,26] Leukemic cell lysis and hyperleukocytic reaction result in nonspecific bilateral consolidation.[17]

Imaging findings of secondary PAP are similar to findings in the idiopathic form of the disease, consisting of geographic ground-glass opacities with or without septal thickening.[27]

PLEURA

Pleural leukemic involvement can manifest on imaging as (1) pleural effusion, (2) pleural masses or pleural thickening, or (3) a combination of pleural effusion and pleural masses/pleural thickening (Fig. 26.4).[16,28]

Pleural effusions in leukemic patients are more commonly nonmalignant and a result of etiologies such as pneumonia, cardiac failure, or volume overload. In a review of 111 patients with acute leukemia ($n = 96$) and myelodysplastic syndrome/myeloproliferative neoplasm ($n = 15$) who underwent pleural procedures, infection (47%) was the most common cause of pleural effusion, followed by leukemic infiltration (36%) and volume overload (13%).[29]

HEART

Although a nonspecific finding, enlargement of the cardiac silhouette is the most common radiographic abnormality in patients with leukemic cardiac involvement.[21] Echocardiography or CT can help differentiate between cardiomegaly and pericardial effusion. Cardiomegaly in leukemia is much more likely to be secondary to anemia or heart failure than neoplastic involvement.[21] Similarly, a pericardial effusion in a patient with leukemia is more likely to be nonmalignant than malignant (Fig. 26.5). Nonmalignant pericardial effusions may be due to volume overload, heart failure, infection, drug reaction, or hypoalbuminemia.

AXILLAE

Axillary lymphadenopathy is most common in CLL, affecting 42% to 54% of CLL patients at diagnosis (see Fig. 26.1).[10]

ROLE OF POSITRON EMISSION TOMOGRAPHY–COMPUTED TOMOGRAPHY

Whole-body ^{18}F-FDG (fluorodeoxyglucose) positron emission tomography–computed tomography (PET-CT) is now a widely used imaging modality in the diagnosis and staging of malignant diseases, including the hematologic malignancies, particularly lymphoma. However, limited data has been reported on the utility of PET-CT in patients with leukemia. PET-CT is useful in staging patients suspected of having extramedullary involvement (i.e., involvement at a site other than bone marrow) or relapse of acute leukemia and in detecting Richter transformation in patients with CLL.

In patients with acute leukemia the sensitivity, specificity, and accuracy of PET-CT in diagnosing extramedullary involvement was 93%, 71%, and 80%, respectively.[30] PET-CT has high sensitivity for detecting early myeloid sarcoma in a patient with AML because lesions may show increased glycolytic activity (Fig. 26.6). PET-CT may increase specificity and help guide biopsy as well as provide a systemic overview of tumor burden and monitor treatment response.[31] Diffuse FDG uptake in extramedullary lesions may indicate leukemic involvement. An uncommon presentation of acute leukemia, extramedullary lesions may occur in up to 30% of patients with AML and has been increasingly reported in patients with ALL.[30] Identification of extramedullary involvement has a major impact on treatment. Associated with poor outcome, some extramedullary lesions cannot be effectively treated by standard chemotherapy alone and necessitate a more intensive chemotherapeutic regimen or allogeneic hematopoietic stem cell transplantation.

Similarly, PET-CT is also a useful diagnostic tool in patients with CLL and suspected Richter transformation. Patients with different CLL phases but similar maximum standard uptake values (SUVmax), the most common semiquantitative method of evaluation of lesions using PET, have similar outcomes. Nodal biopsy is the standard diagnostic procedure to determine CLL transformation. A cutoff SUVmax greater than or equal to 5 on PET/CT showed sensitivity, specificity, positive predictive value, and negative predictive value of 91%, 80%, 53%, and 97%, respectively, for detection of Richter's transformation.[32] PET-CT is useful to identify the sites most likely to be diagnostically informative. Therefore, in patients with suspected CLL transformation, biopsy of a lymph node with SUVmax greater than or equal to 5 is recommended.[33]

Differential Diagnosis

Leukemias and lymphomas can have similar manifestations, both clinically and radiologically. Intrathoracic lymphadenopathy can be seen with lymphoma, metastatic disease, or benign conditions such as sarcoidosis or infection. Diffuse thickening of interlobular septa and bronchovascular bundles can be secondary to lymphangitic spread of tumor (leukemia, lymphoma, or metastatic carcinoma) but can also be related to interstitial edema. A key distinguishing feature of tumor involvement is nodularity along the interlobular septa or bronchovascular bundles. Although sarcoidosis can also have nodular interstitial thickening, interlobular septal thickening is not usually a dominant feature. The differential diagnosis of pleural thickening and pleural masses includes metastatic disease, mesothelioma, fibrous tumor of the pleura, infection, or hematoma.

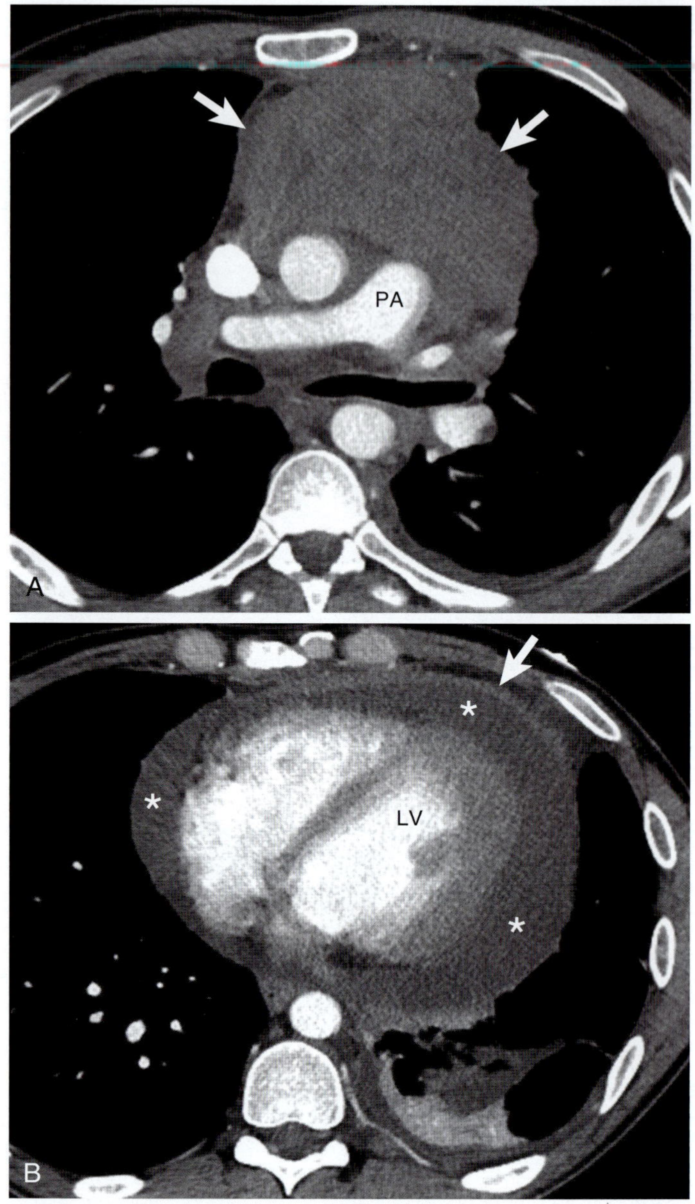

Fig. 26.5 Mediastinal and pericardial leukemic involvement in a 27-year-old man with T-cell acute lymphoblastic leukemia who presented with chest pain. (A) CT at the level of the pulmonary artery (PA) shows a large heterogeneous anterior mediastinal mass *(arrows)*. (B) CT at the level of the left ventricle (LV) shows a large pericardial effusion *(asterisks)* with pericardial thickening and enhancement *(arrow)*. Pericardiocentesis revealed numerous blasts, consistent with leukemic involvement.

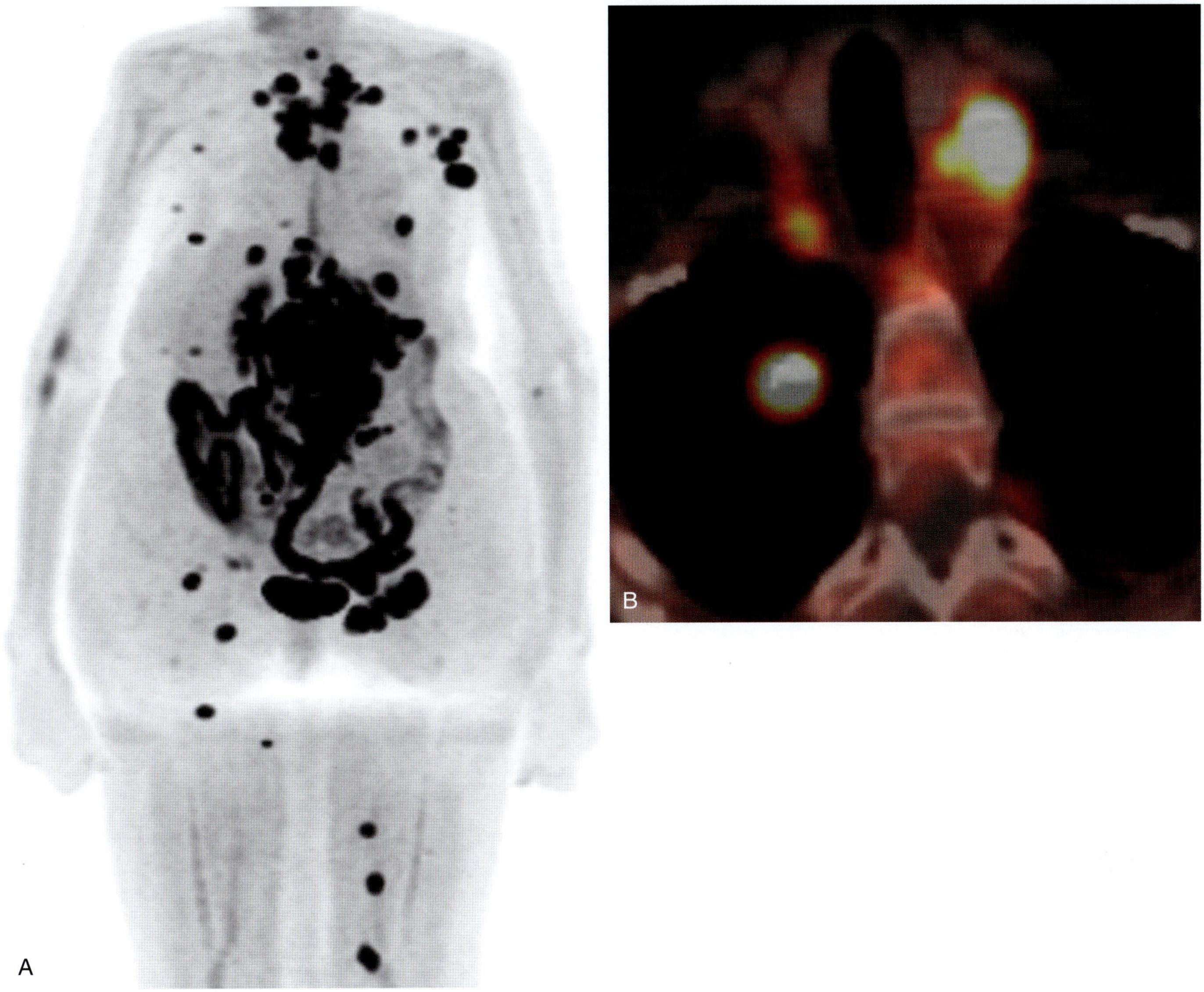

Fig. 26.6 Extramedullary acute myeloid leukemia and myeloid sarcoma in a 74-year-old woman with abdominal pain and fatigue. (A) Whole-body PET shows FDG-avid lesions in the lymph nodes of the neck, chest, abdomen, and pelvis, as well as multiple muscular and subcutaneous deposits. (B) Integrated axial PET-CT shows FDG-avid right upper lobe nodule and bilateral supraclavicular lymphadenopathy (maximum standard uptake value, 19.7, in the left supraclavicular lymph node). Biopsy of the left supraclavicular lymph node confirmed myeloid sarcoma. PET-CT is useful in staging patients suspected of having extramedullary involvement or relapse of acute leukemia and in identifying a biopsy target.

Synopsis of Treatment Options

Goals of therapy in leukemia are to eliminate leukemic cells and to allow normal hematopoiesis. Treatment is based on the specific subtype of leukemia. The different types of therapy used in the treatment of leukemia include chemotherapy, radiation therapy, biologic therapy, targeted therapy, and stem cell transplantation.

Conclusion

Leukemias are a varied group of malignancies classified as myeloid or lymphoid depending on the types of abnormal cells produced and acute or chronic based on cellular maturity. Intrathoracic imaging manifestations of leukemia include lymphadenopathy, pulmonary opacities, pleural and pericardial thickening, and/or effusion. These findings are nonspecific and can frequently be due to coexisting abnormalities, such as pneumonia, edema, hemorrhage, and drug-induced injury, instead of leukemic infiltration. Myeloid sarcomas are extramedullary masses of malignant myeloid blasts that can be found in the thorax in patients with AML. PET-CT is useful in staging patients suspected of having extramedullary involvement or relapse of acute leukemia and in detecting Richter transformation in patients with CLL. Awareness of the spectrum of intrathoracic manifestations of the leukemias is essential to aid radiologists in optimizing patient management.

KEY POINTS

- Leukemias may be classified as myeloid or lymphoid, depending on the types of abnormal cells produced.
- Leukemias are classified as acute or chronic according to cellular maturity; immature/blast cells predominate in acute leukemias, whereas chronic leukemias have more mature cells.
- Clinical manifestations are due to either suppression of normal marrow function resulting in anemia, thrombocytopenia, and leukopenia or organ infiltration by leukemic cells resulting in lymphadenopathy, hepatosplenomegaly, and skeletal pain.
- Intrathoracic imaging manifestations of leukemias include mediastinal mass or lymphadenopathy, pulmonary opacities, pleural and pericardial effusion/thickening.
- Myeloid sarcomas occur in patients with acute myeloid leukemia and are masses of malignant myeloid blasts found in an extramedullary location.
- Pulmonary abnormalities are only rarely due to leukemic infiltration alone; coexisting abnormalities may include pneumonia, edema, hemorrhage, and drug-induced injury.
- Pleural effusions in leukemic patients can be secondary to pneumonia, cardiac failure, volume overload, or leukemic infiltration.
- Pericardial effusions in leukemic patients are more commonly a result of volume overload, heart failure, infection, drugs, hypoalbuminemia, or autoimmune cause.
- PET-CT is useful in staging patients suspected of having extramedullary involvement or relapse of acute leukemia and in detecting Richter transformation in patients with chronic lymphocytic leukemia.

SUGGESTED READINGS

Averill LW, Acikgoz G, Miller RE, Kandula VV, Epelman M. Update on pediatric leukemia and lymphoma imaging. *Semin Ultrasound CT MR*. 2013;34:578–599.

Guillerman RP, Voss SD, Parker BR. Leukemia and lymphoma. *Radiol Clin North Am*. 2011;49:767–797.

Lee EY, Anthony MP, Leung AY, Loong F, Khong PL. Utility of FDG PET/CT in the assessment of myeloid sarcoma. *AJR Am J Roentgenol*. 2012;198:1175–1179.

Restrepo CS, Carrillo J, Rosado de Christenson M, Ojeda Leon P, Lucia Rivera A, Koss MN. Lymphoproliferative lung disorders: a radiologic-pathologic overview. Part II: neoplastic disorders. *Semin Ultrasound CT MR*. 2013;34:535–549.

Zhou WL, Wu HB, Wang LJ, Tian Y, Dong Y, Wang QS. Usefulness and pitfalls of F-18-FDG PET/CT for diagnosing extramedullary acute leukemia. *Eur J Radiol*. 2016;85:205–210.

The full reference list for this chapter is available at ExpertConsult.com.

27 Usual Interstitial Pneumonia/Idiopathic Pulmonary Fibrosis*

JONATHAN H. CHUNG | CHRISTOPHER M. WALKER

Etiology, Prevalence, and Epidemiology

Idiopathic pulmonary fibrosis (IPF) has been defined as "a specific form of chronic fibrosing interstitial pneumonia limited to the lung and associated with the histologic and/or CT appearance of usual interstitial pneumonia (UIP)."[1] IPF is the most common idiopathic interstitial lung disease.[2,3] Data from the late 1980s estimated a prevalence of 20 per 100,000 for men and 13 per 100,000 for women, and an incidence of 11 per 100,000 per year in men and 7 per 100,000 per year in women.[2] However, more recent data has shown that prevalence and incidence of IPF have increased, with a prevalence of 42.7 to 63 per 100,000 and an incidence of 16.3 to 17.4 per 100,000 per year, which may reflect the average increased life expectancy in that span of time.[4,5] Most patients with IPF are older than 50 years, and approximately 80% are older than 65 years.[3] Indeed, age older than 75 years has been shown to have an extremely high positive predictive value in IPF diagnosis.[6] IPF has been reported worldwide in rural and urban settings.[1] IPF is likely more common in Caucasians, although this has not been definitively proven.[7] IPF is more common in smokers; the odds ratio of IPF in smokers compared with lifelong nonsmokers in various studies ranges from 1.6 to 2.9.[1] Occasionally, clusters of IPF may occur in families. Although the prevalence of familial IPF is unknown, it has been estimated to account for 0.5% to 2.2% of patients with IPF.[8]

Clinical Presentation

Symptoms are nonspecific and include progressive dyspnea, nonproductive cough, weight loss, and fatigue.[1] Dyspnea is usually the main symptom and typically is present for more than 6 months before initial diagnosis.[1] Diagnosis is delayed by more than 1 year in up to half of patients. Finger clubbing occurs in 25% to 50% of patients. Auscultation typically reveals late inspiratory crackles (so-called Velcro rales). Cyanosis and signs of pulmonary hypertension and cor pulmonale are late manifestations.

The clinical course of IPF is typically one of relentless progressive increase in the extent of fibrosis and severity of clinical manifestations. The course of individual patients varies, however, and some patients remain stable for extended periods without treatment.[9] Acute deterioration with an abrupt and unexpected worsening of symptoms may occur secondary to infection, pulmonary embolism, pneumothorax, or heart failure. Often, no identifiable cause for the acute decline is identified, however, and these episodes are called "acute exacerbation" or "accelerated phase" of IPF.[10,11]

Acute exacerbations of IPF are defined as an acute, clinically significant respiratory deterioration characterized by new widespread alveolar abnormality and are considerably more common than previously recognized. In one retrospective study of 168 patients with IPF, 21% of patients died over a median period of 76 weeks, and 47% of these deaths followed an acute deterioration in the patient's clinical status.[12] In a second study of 147 patients with biopsy-proven IPF, the 1-year frequency of acute exacerbation was 8.5%, and the 2-year frequency was 9.6%.[13] As pointed out by the authors, however, the actual incidence of acute exacerbation could have been underestimated in their study because some of the patients were lost to follow-up and because the study included only patients with biopsy-proven IPF. In an autopsy series of 25 patients, 15 (60%) deaths in patients with IPF or nonspecific interstitial pneumonia (NSIP) associated with connective tissue disease were due to diffuse alveolar damage and consistent with acute exacerbation.[14] The reported mortality rates from acute exacerbation range from 20% to 86%.[15] Diagnostic criteria for acute exacerbation of IPF have recently been revised and include:[16]

1. Previous or concurrent diagnosis of IPF
2. Acute worsening or development of dyspnea typically of less than 1 month in duration
3. CT findings of bilateral ground-glass opacities and/or consolidation superimposed on a background pattern consistent with usual IPF
4. Deterioration not fully explained by cardiac failure or fluid overload

Pathophysiology

PATHOLOGY

It is currently believed that several components are involved in the pathogenesis of IPF, including repetitive lung injury, inflammation, exaggerated deposition of collagen and extracellular matrix, recruitment and proliferation of fibroblasts, inappropriate wound healing response, and excessive angiogenesis.[17] Epithelial injury and activation of fibroblast foci are currently considered the main early events that trigger a cascade of changes that eventually lead to extensive fibrosis.[18]

*The editors and the publisher would like to thank Drs. Nestor L. Müller and C. Isabela Silva Müller for contributing material on this topic to the prior edition of this work. It has served as the foundation for the current chapter.

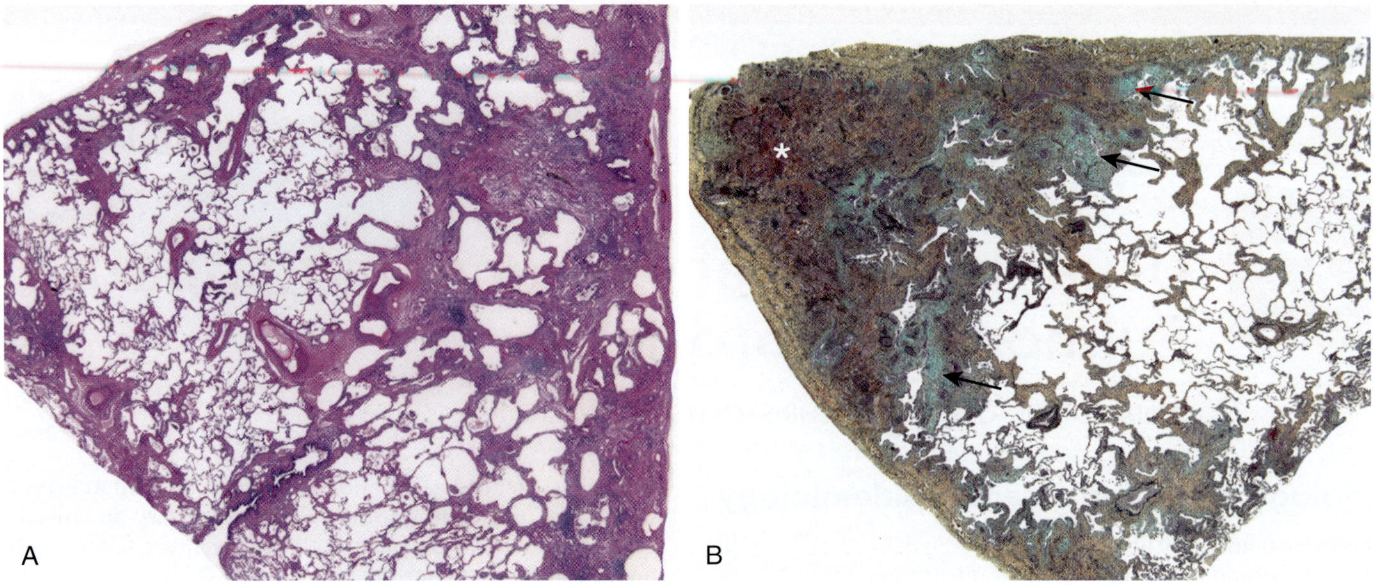

Fig. 27.1 Idiopathic pulmonary fibrosis: histologic findings. (A) Photomicrograph at low magnification shows characteristic heterogeneous appearance of usual interstitial pneumonia with areas of normal lung, foci of chronic inflammation and fibrosis, and honeycombing. The peripheral predominance of the fibrosis also is noted (hematoxylin-eosin stain). (B) Histologic specimen shows fibroblastic foci (blue areas, *arrows*) at interface between older subpleural fibrosis and muscle hyperplasia *(asterisk)* and normal and near-normal lung toward the center of the lobule (Movat pentachrome stain). *(Courtesy Dr. John English, Department of Pathology, Vancouver General Hospital, Vancouver, Canada.)*

IPF by definition is idiopathic UIP.[19] The key histologic features of UIP are temporal and geographic heterogeneity, presence of fibroblastic foci, and predilection for the periphery of the lobule and the subpleural regions (Fig. 27.1).[18,19] Additional features include smooth muscle hypertrophy, excessive collagen and extracellular matrix, destroyed alveolar architecture, traction bronchiectasis and bronchiolectasis, and honeycombing.[1,19] *Temporal heterogeneity* refers to the presence of active inflammation, scattered fibroblastic foci, and chronic scarring (i.e., findings ranging from relatively acute disease to established fibrosis). This is distinct from other interstitial pneumonias, such as NSIP, in which the changes seem to have occurred over a relatively narrow time span. *Geographic heterogeneity* refers to the presence of alternating areas of normal lung, interstitial inflammation, fibrosis, and honeycombing in different regions of the same tissue section and sometimes in a single lobule.[19] Fibroblast foci are aggregates of proliferating fibroblasts and myofibroblasts and represent microscopic zones of acute lung injury on a background of chronic scarring (see Fig. 27.1).[18] Fibroblastic foci are essentially areas of immature fibrosis that signify the active, advancing edge of lung remodeling.

Areas of honeycombing consist of cystic fibrotic airspaces, which frequently are lined by bronchiolar epithelium and filled with mucin.[19] Honeycombing usually represents markedly dilated transitional airways (respiratory bronchioles and alveolar ducts) and typically is associated with severe fibrosis and destruction of lung architecture. The honeycomb cysts usually range from 2 to 20 mm in diameter and are separated by a variable amount of fibrous tissue (Fig. 27.2). Although interstitial inflammation commonly is seen in UIP, it is typically mild and patchy.[18] Dystrophic calcification and osseous metaplasia occur occasionally.

In patients who undergo biopsy during an accelerated phase of their illness (acute exacerbation of IPF), the specimens show a prominent organizing pneumonia or diffuse alveolar damage pattern superimposed on the UIP pattern. Patients with organizing pneumonia have a better prognosis than patients with diffuse alveolar damage.[11,20]

Most patients with a histologic pattern of UIP have IPF, and by definition all patients with IPF have a histologic pattern of UIP. A histologic pattern of UIP is not diagnostic of IPF, however. A UIP pattern also may be seen in patients with connective tissue diseases, asbestosis, chronic hypersensitivity pneumonitis, certain drug-induced lung diseases, and familial IPF.[19] These conditions must be excluded before making a diagnosis of IPF.

LUNG FUNCTION

IPF results in restrictive lung function (decreased total lung capacity and vital capacity) and impaired gas transfer as assessed by the carbon monoxide diffusing capacity.[21,22] Most patients have normal or even increased expiratory flow rates when related to absolute lung volume. A few patients have evidence of airflow obstruction manifested by reduction in the maximal midexpiratory flow rate and forced expiratory volume in 1 second relative to the reduction in vital capacity, probably reflecting the effects of cigarette smoking.[23] Indices of airflow obstruction correlate closely with the presence of emphysema as determined by high-resolution CT.[24] Hypoxemia is common and is caused mainly by ventilation-perfusion inequality; however, in about 20% of cases, it can be attributed to a diffusion defect.[25]

Several studies have shown that the extent of abnormalities of high-resolution CT in patients with IPF correlates with severity of functional impairment.[26–28] Among the functional parameters, carbon monoxide diffusing capacity correlates best with extent of disease on CT.[26,27]

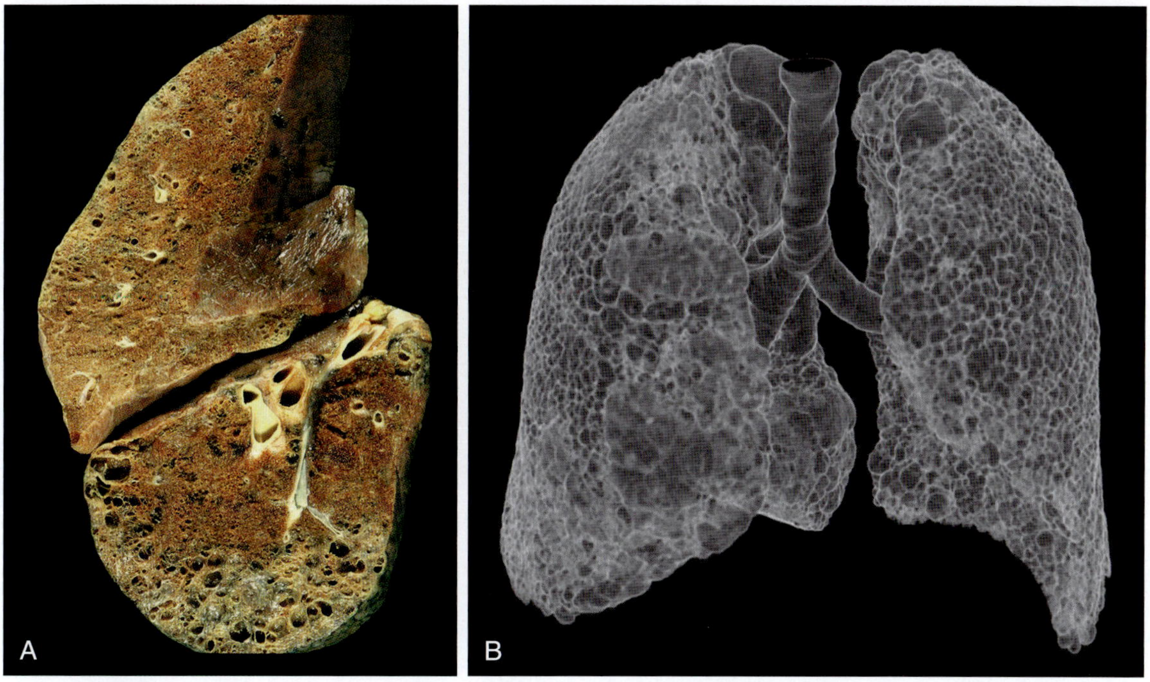

Fig. 27.2 Idiopathic pulmonary fibrosis. (A) Sagittal slice of the right middle and lower lobes shows honeycombing in the dorsal subpleural regions of the lower lobe and small foci of subpleural fibrosis in the remaining right lower lobe and middle lobe. (B) Coronal three-dimensional external volume-rendering (anterior view) image in another patient with end-stage usual interstitial pneumonia shows "cobblestone" appearance of the pleural surface as a result of extensive honeycombing.

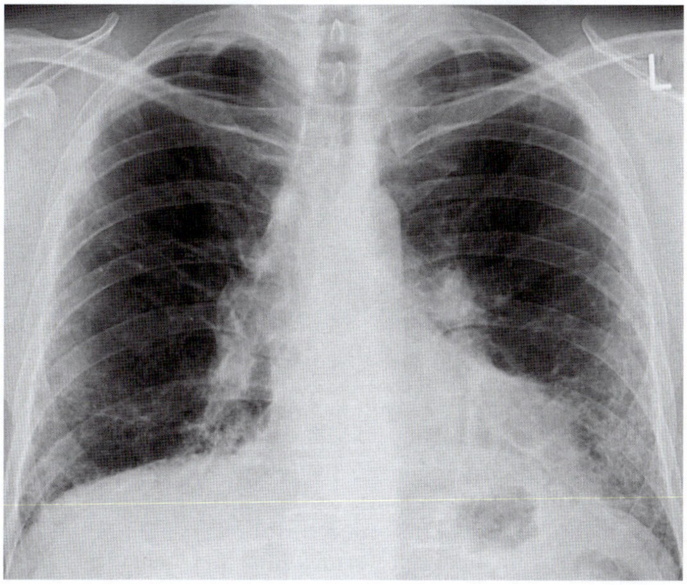

Fig. 27.3 Idiopathic pulmonary fibrosis: radiographic manifestations. Posteroanterior chest radiograph shows reticular pattern mainly in the peripheral regions and lower lung zones. Low lung volumes and enlargement of the central pulmonary arteries consistent with pulmonary arterial hypertension also are noted.

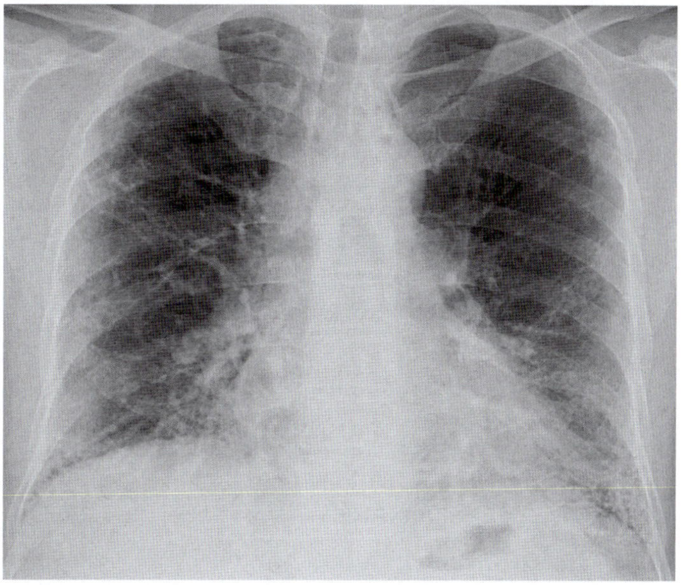

Fig. 27.4 Idiopathic pulmonary fibrosis: radiographic manifestations. Posteroanterior chest radiograph shows extensive bilateral reticular pattern worse in the lower lung zones.

Manifestations of the Disease

RADIOGRAPHY

The radiographic findings of UIP usually consist of symmetric, basal, small- to medium-sized irregular linear opacities resulting in a reticular pattern (Fig. 27.3). Although these opacities may be diffuse throughout both lungs, in 50% to 80% of cases they involve the lower lung zones predominantly or exclusively; in 60% a predominant peripheral distribution is apparent.[29,30] As the disease progresses the abnormalities become more diffuse and assume a coarser reticular or reticulonodular pattern associated with progressive loss of volume (Fig. 27.4). Advanced disease is characterized by the presence of honeycomb cysts measuring

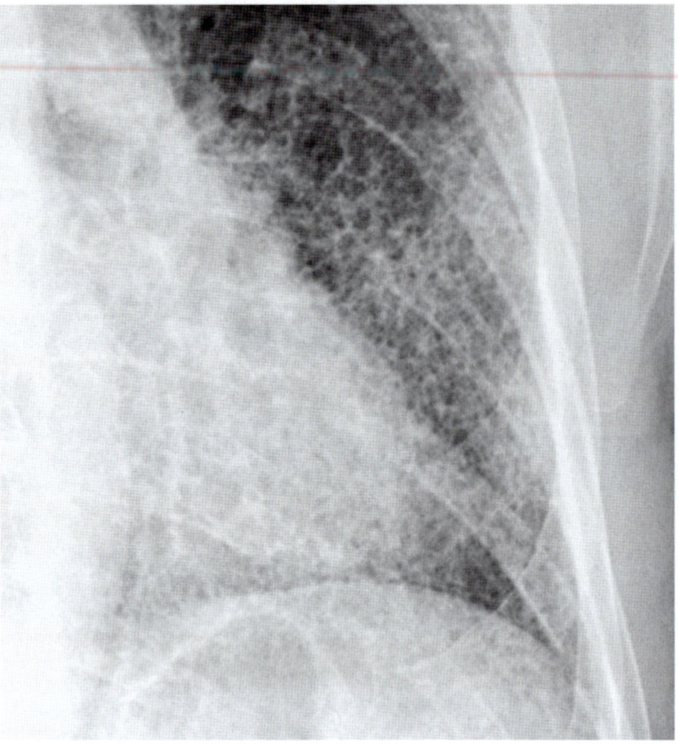

Fig. 27.5 Idiopathic pulmonary fibrosis (IPF): end-stage fibrosis. Magnified view of the left lower lobe from a posteroanterior chest radiograph shows coarse reticular pattern and cystic areas of honeycombing. The patient was a man with advanced IPF who underwent lung transplantation 1 year later.

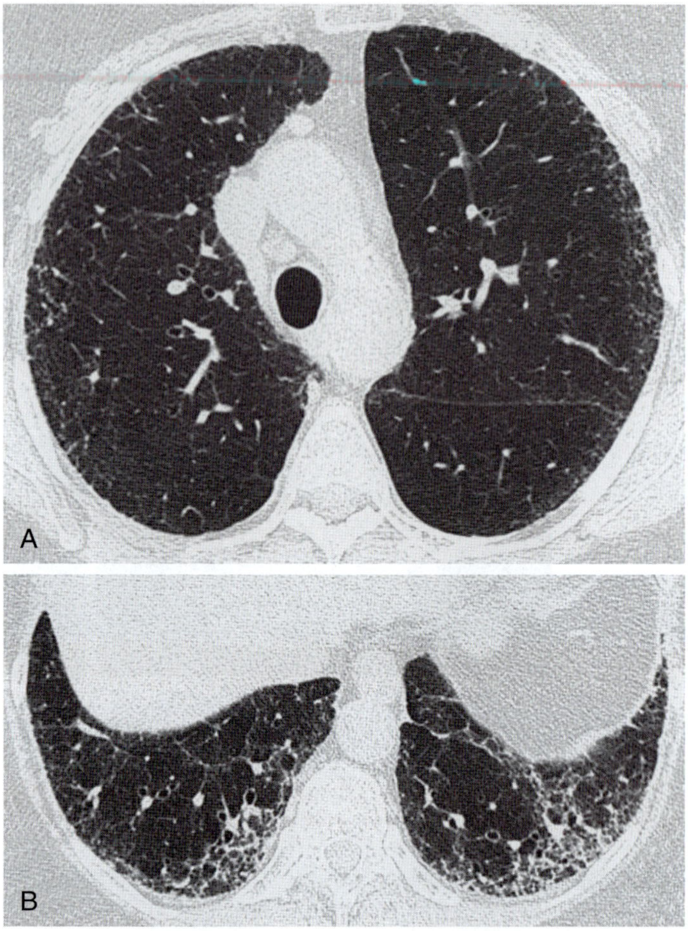

Fig. 27.6 Idiopathic pulmonary fibrosis: peripheral and basal reticulation. (A) High-resolution CT scan at the level of the upper lobes shows bilateral subpleural irregular intralobular linear opacities and irregular septal thickening resulting in a fine reticular pattern. (B) High-resolution CT scan at the level of the lung bases shows more severe subpleural reticulation and traction bronchiolectasis.

0.5 to 1 cm in diameter (Fig. 27.5). Evidence of pleural disease (effusion, pneumothorax, or diffuse thickening) is uncommon. Decreased lung volumes are radiographically evident at initial evaluation in 50% to 60% of cases.[31] The lung volumes decrease progressively over time. Most patients with IPF are smokers. In patients with associated emphysema the lung volumes may be normal or increased.

Virtually all patients with IPF have an abnormal chest radiograph at the time of presentation.[1] Basal reticular opacities are often evident on previous chest radiographs for several years before the development of symptoms.[1] A normal chest radiograph cannot be used, however, to exclude microscopic evidence of UIP.[1,32]

COMPUTED TOMOGRAPHY

UIP is characterized on high-resolution CT by the presence of patchy irregular intralobular lines resulting in a reticular pattern involving mainly the subpleural regions and the lower lung zones (Fig. 27.6).[33,34] The reticular pattern is associated with architectural distortion; dilation of bronchi and bronchioles (traction bronchiectasis and bronchiolectasis); and irregular pleural, vascular, and bronchial interfaces (Fig. 27.7).[35,36] The dilated bronchi and bronchioles in areas of fibrosis typically have a beaded appearance. Air-containing cysts lining up in rows or stacks in the subpleural lung measuring 2 to 20 mm in diameter (honeycombing) are seen in approximately 80% to 90% of patients (Figs. 27.8 and 27.9).[35] Honeycombing is the most specific sign of UIP on CT.

A predominantly subpleural distribution of the reticular pattern and honeycombing is evident on high-resolution CT in nearly all patients.[35,37,38] In approximately 80% of patients, the fibrosis is most severe in the lower lung zones; in about 15%, all zones are involved to a similar degree; and in 5%, mainly the upper lung zones are affected.[35,39] Although the reticulation and honeycombing in UIP tend to be most severe in the lower lung zones, in most patients the reticulation involves all lung zones. The geographic heterogeneity that is described on histologic specimens of UIP also is appreciated on high-resolution CT and refers to the presence of fibrosis (reticulation and honeycombing) alternating with areas of normal lung parenchyma (patchy distribution) (see Fig. 27.9).

Ground-glass opacities are present in most patients with UIP.[38,39] The ground-glass opacities in these patients are usually mild, however, and associated with evidence of fibrosis (Fig. 27.10). Ground-glass opacities away from areas of fibrosis are present in approximately 25% of patients and are typically less extensive than the reticulation.[35] Ground-glass opacities in UIP may reflect the presence of active inflammation or microscopic fibrosis (Fig. 27.11). Ground-glass opacities resulting from microscopic fibrosis usually are associated with reticulation, traction bronchiectasis, or bronchiolectasis (see Fig. 27.10).[40] Ground-glass opacities not associated with fibrosis correlate with interstitial inflammation.[36,41] On serial CT scans in patients with UIP, the

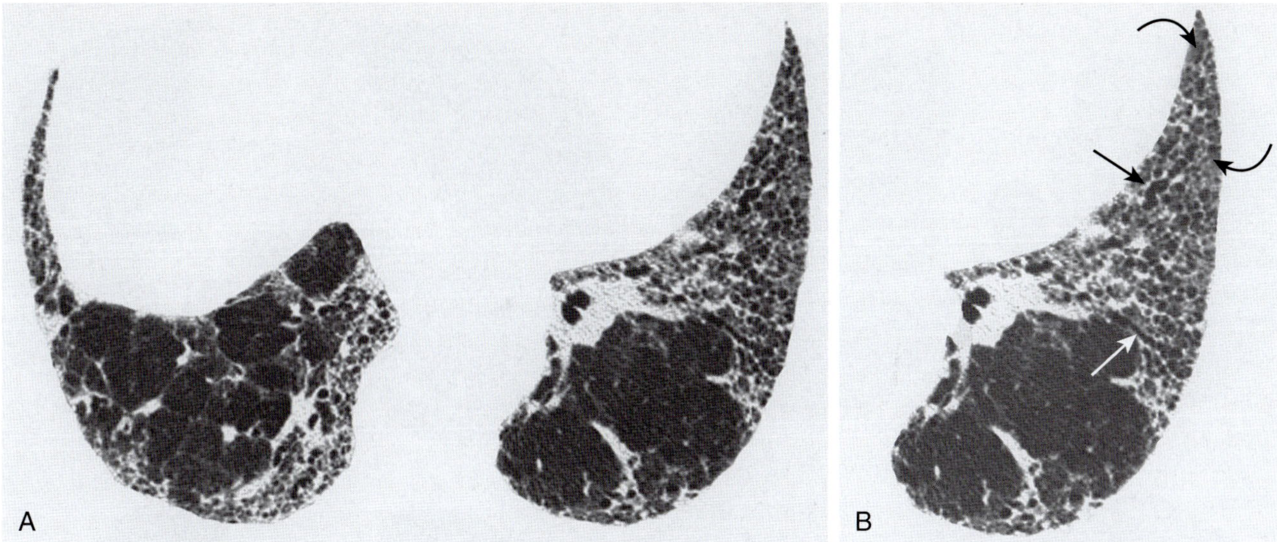

Fig. 27.7 Idiopathic pulmonary fibrosis with extensive reticulation, traction bronchiectasis, and traction bronchiolectasis. (A) High-resolution CT scan at the level of the lung bases shows reticular pattern in the peripheral regions of the lower lobes and diffusely in the middle lobe and lingula. (B) Magnified view of the left lower lung zone shows reticular pattern. Dilation and beading of bronchi (traction bronchiectasis) *(straight arrows)* also is noted. Dilated airways within approximately 0.5 to 1 cm from the pleura represent ectatic bronchioles (traction bronchiolectasis) *(curved arrows)*.

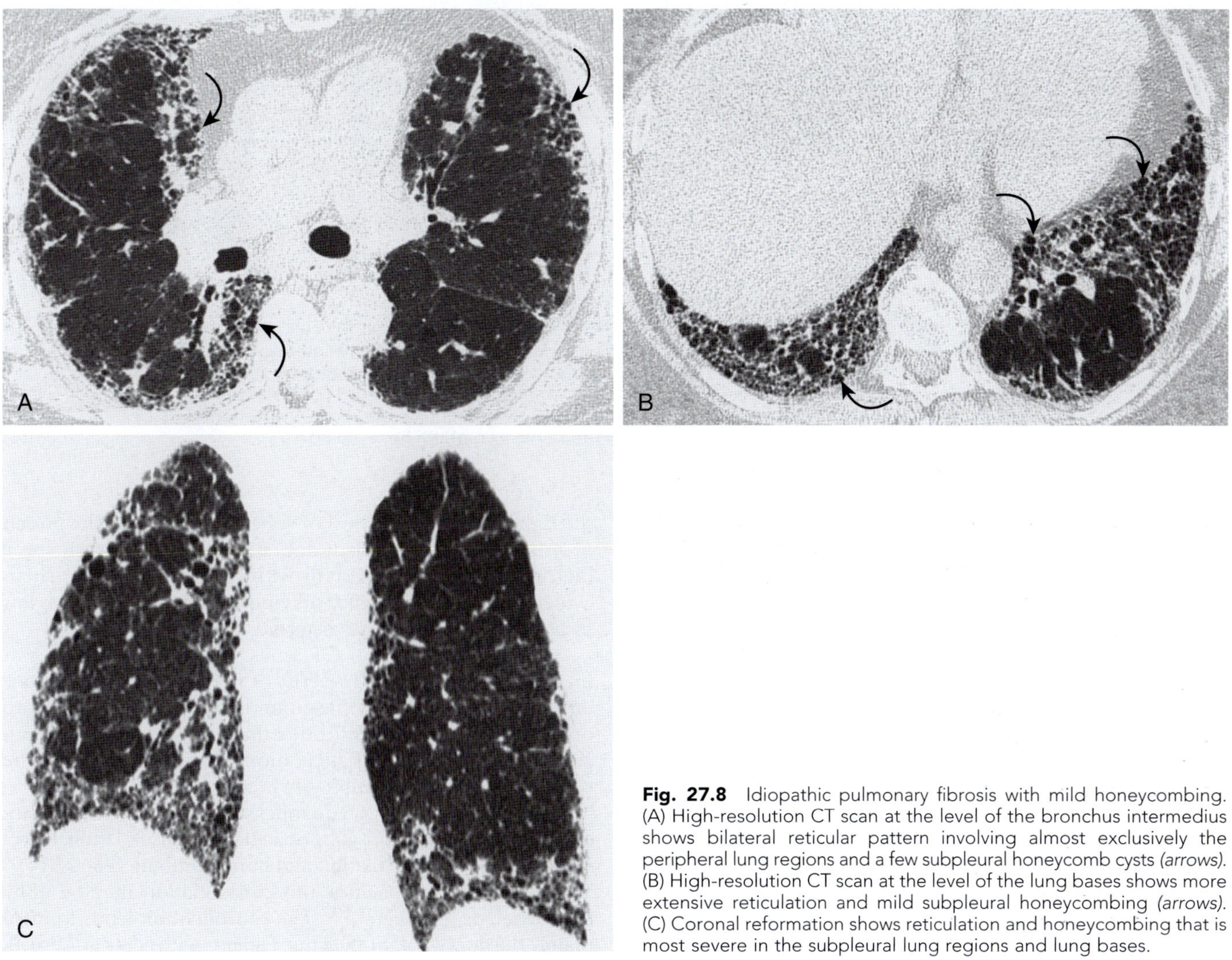

Fig. 27.8 Idiopathic pulmonary fibrosis with mild honeycombing. (A) High-resolution CT scan at the level of the bronchus intermedius shows bilateral reticular pattern involving almost exclusively the peripheral lung regions and a few subpleural honeycomb cysts *(arrows)*. (B) High-resolution CT scan at the level of the lung bases shows more extensive reticulation and mild subpleural honeycombing *(arrows)*. (C) Coronal reformation shows reticulation and honeycombing that is most severe in the subpleural lung regions and lung bases.

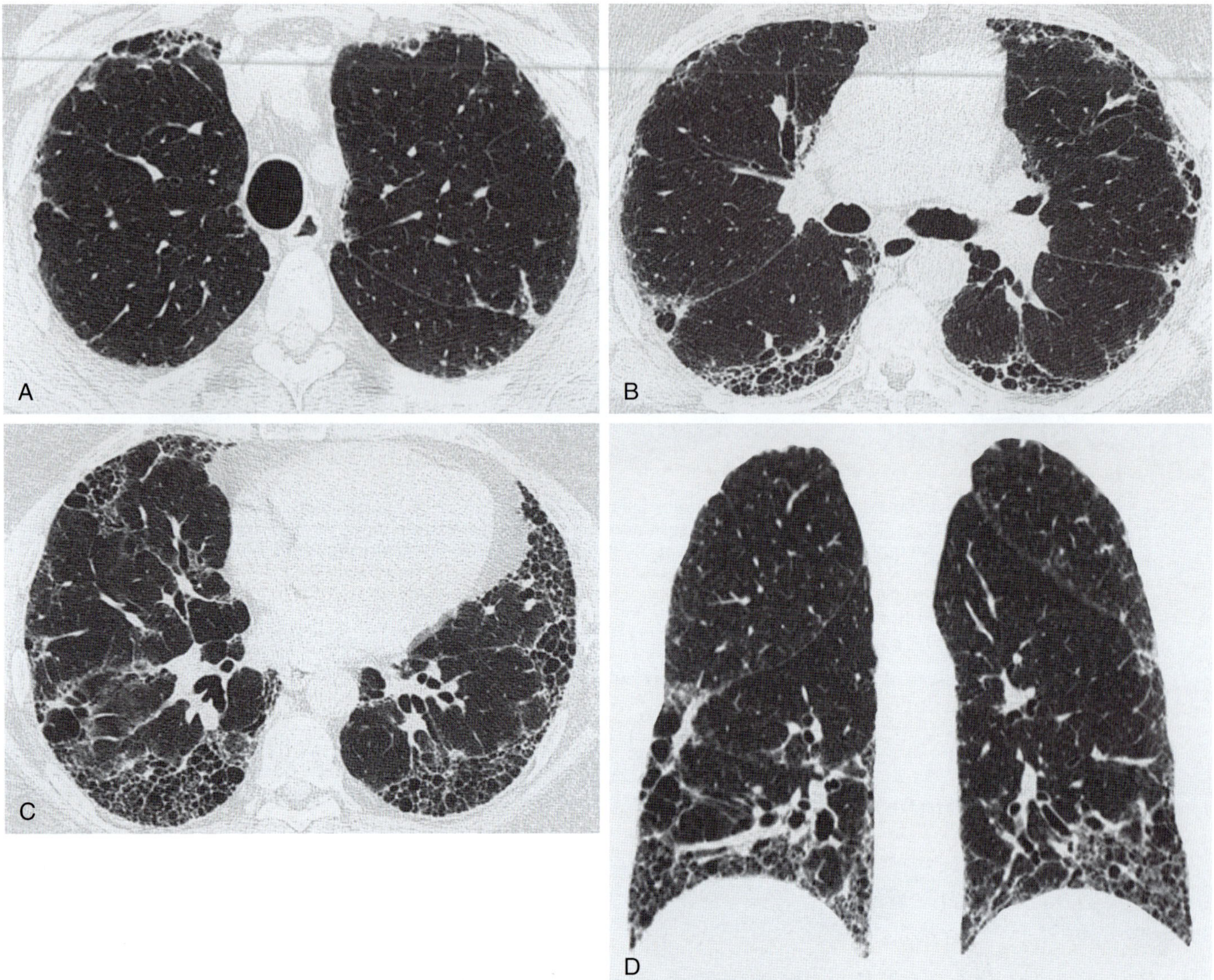

Fig. 27.9 Idiopathic pulmonary fibrosis with extensive honeycombing. (A) to (C) High-resolution CT scans at the level of the upper (A), middle (B), and lower (C) lung zones show extensive subpleural honeycombing mainly in the lower lobes (C). Note patchy distribution of the subpleural fibrosis alternating with areas of relatively normal lung parenchyma. (D) Coronal reformation image shows the peripheral distribution of the fibrosis in all lobes and the basal predominance of the honeycombing.

areas of ground-glass opacity may regress, but more commonly they progress to reticulation and honeycombing.[42,43]

Emphysema is evident on CT in approximately 30% of patients with UIP, with a few localized areas of decreased attenuation and vascularity (mosaic attenuation) in 4% to 43%, small areas of consolidation in 3%, and a few centrilobular nodules in 2% to 15%.[35,39,44] Not uncommonly, fine linear or small nodular foci of ossification are seen within areas of fibrosis as a result of diffuse or dendriform pulmonary ossification (Fig. 27.12).[45] Also, it is important to keep in mind that patients with IPF have an increased prevalence of pulmonary carcinoma, and careful inspection of the lungs for focal nodules or slowly growing lung lesions is mandatory.[46,47]

Mediastinal lymph node enlargement is evident on CT in approximately 70% of patients.[48,49] The enlargement is usually mild, with nodes measuring 10 to 15 mm in short-axis diameter and involving only one or two nodal stations (most commonly, the right lower paratracheal or subcarinal region). The presence of lymph node enlargement does not correlate with any specific high-resolution CT pattern or with extent of disease.[49] There is evidence that the prevalence of lymph node enlargement is lower in patients receiving corticosteroid therapy.[47]

Serial high-resolution CT scans typically show progressive increase in the extent and severity of fibrosis over several months or years (Fig. 27.13).[43,50] Some ground-glass opacities may improve or resolve with treatment, but others progress to reticulation and honeycombing.[42,43] Reticulation often progresses to honeycombing, and honeycomb cysts increase in size.[43,51]

The high-resolution CT manifestations of acute exacerbation of IPF consist of ground-glass opacities or consolidation, or both, superimposed on reticulation and honeycombing (Fig. 27.14).[20,52] The ground-glass opacities and consolidation may be diffuse, multifocal, or peripheral.[20,52] The consolidation tends to involve mainly the dorsal half of the lung. Patients with acute exacerbation and peripheral ground-glass opacities have a better prognosis than patients with multifocal or diffuse opacities.[20,52] The main differential diagnosis of acute exacerbation on high-resolution CT in patients with known IPF and acute clinical deterioration is pulmonary edema and opportunistic infection.

Several groups of investigators have assessed the diagnostic accuracy of high-resolution CT in the diagnosis of UIP/IPF. The overwhelming amount of data shows that CT is highly accurate when UIP is the confident first-choice diagnosis, although this can only be achieved in 50% to 70% of cases. The specificity of a confident UIP CT pattern is at least 95%, although sensitivity is lower in the range of 60% to 80%.[53–58]

Recently updated guidelines support use of four separate CT diagnostic patterns when considering an IPF diagnosis: typical UIP, probable UIP, indeterminate for UIP, and most consistent with non-IPF diagnosis.[58a] A confident high-resolution CT diagnosis of UIP requires clinical exclusion of known causes of UIP and the presence of all of the following four high-resolution CT criteria: (1) presence of a reticular pattern, (2) a predominantly peripheral and basal distribution, (3) presence of CT honeycombing, and (4) absence of atypical features (e.g., centrilobular nodules, peribronchovascular nodules, extensive consolidation, or extensive ground-glass opacities).[35,57] In these cases biopsy is obviated, given that approximately 95% of these patients will

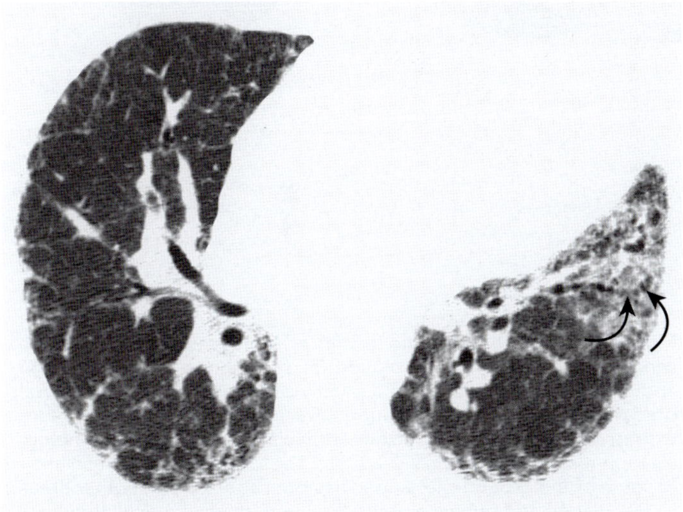

Fig. 27.10 Idiopathic pulmonary fibrosis with ground-glass opacities. High-resolution CT scan shows peripheral reticulation and patchy ground-glass opacities. Almost all areas of ground-glass opacity have superimposed reticulation or traction bronchiectasis *(arrows)*, suggesting that they probably represent microscopic fibrosis rather than inflammation.

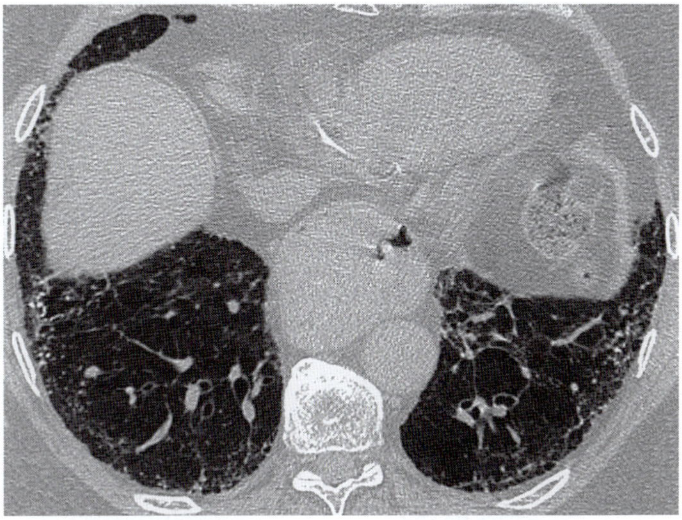

Fig. 27.12 Pulmonary ossification in idiopathic pulmonary fibrosis (IPF). High-resolution CT scan shows bilateral reticulation, honeycombing, and small foci of calcification characteristic of pulmonary ossification in IPF. A hiatal hernia is incidentally noted.

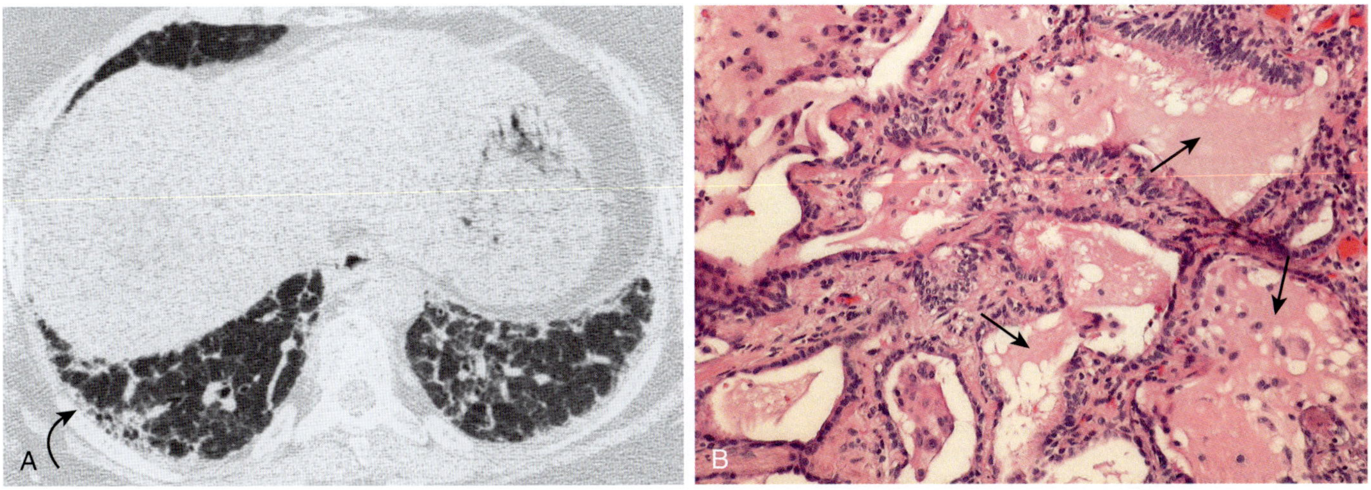

Fig. 27.11 Idiopathic pulmonary fibrosis: ground-glass opacities secondary to fibrosis. (A) High-resolution CT scan shows subpleural ground-glass opacities *(arrow)* and mild reticulation. (B) Photomicrograph of histopathologic specimen obtained from region showing ground-glass opacity on CT shows microscopic honeycombing with the airspaces filled by mucus and inflammatory cells *(arrows)*. *(From Souza CA, Müller NL, Flint J, et al: Idiopathic pulmonary fibrosis: spectrum of high-resolution CT findings. AJR Am J Roentgenol. 2005;185:1531–1539.)*

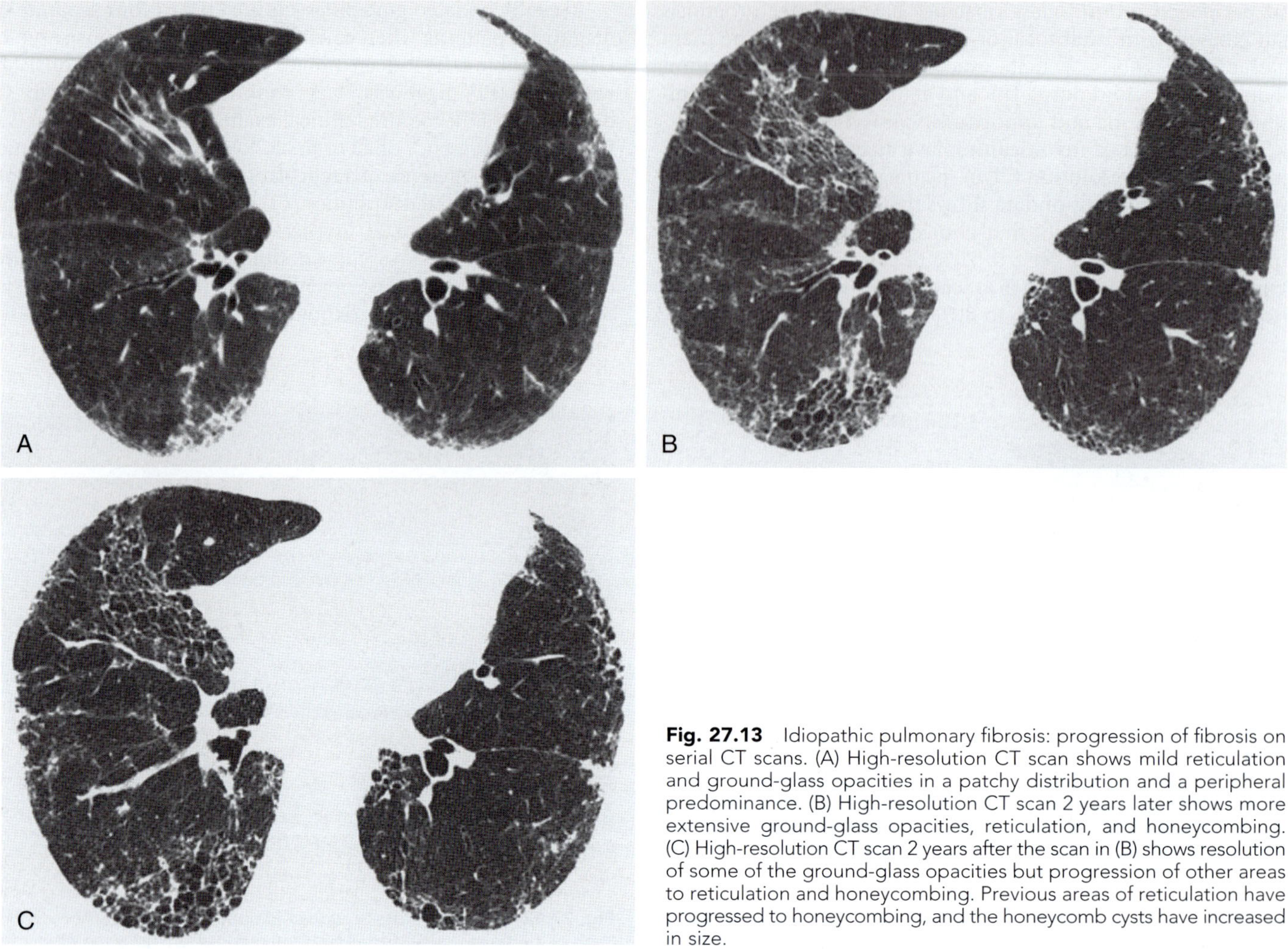

Fig. 27.13 Idiopathic pulmonary fibrosis: progression of fibrosis on serial CT scans. (A) High-resolution CT scan shows mild reticulation and ground-glass opacities in a patchy distribution and a peripheral predominance. (B) High-resolution CT scan 2 years later shows more extensive ground-glass opacities, reticulation, and honeycombing. (C) High-resolution CT scan 2 years after the scan in (B) shows resolution of some of the ground-glass opacities but progression of other areas to reticulation and honeycombing. Previous areas of reticulation have progressed to honeycombing, and the honeycomb cysts have increased in size.

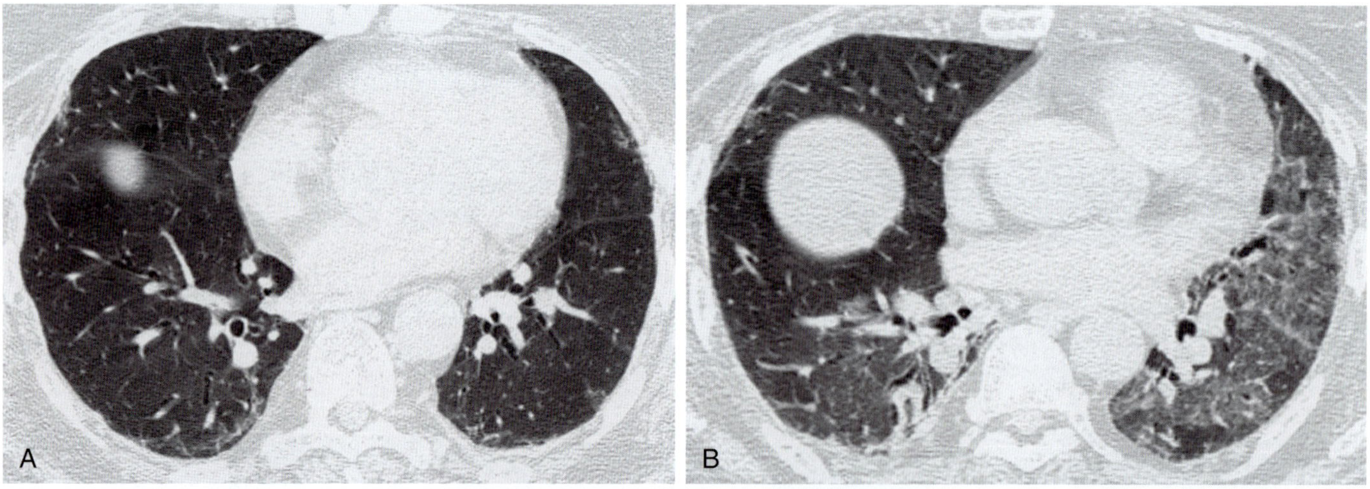

Fig. 27.14 Acute exacerbation of idiopathic pulmonary fibrosis. (A) High-resolution CT scan shows mild patchy subpleural reticulation. (B) High-resolution CT scan 7 months later, when the patient presented with acute respiratory failure, shows extensive bilateral ground-glass opacities superimposed on the reticulation. Surgical biopsy specimen showed diffuse alveolar damage superimposed on a background of interstitial fibrosis.

have UIP on pathology. If all criteria are met, except presence of CT honeycombing, the CT pattern is considered probable UIP, although 70% to 90% of these cases will also show UIP on pathology, especially in those older than 60 years and in current or former smokers.[35,59–61] The strongest predictors of IPF on high-resolution CT are lower lung honeycombing (odds ratio, 5.36) and upper lung reticulation (odds ratio, 6.28).[37] Although basal and peripheral honeycombing is a strong predictor of IPF, there is considerable interobserver agreement in the diagnosis of honeycombing.[35] Confident diagnosis of honeycombing requires the presence of clustered cystic subpleural airspaces measuring 2 mm to 1 cm in diameter that have well-defined thick walls that line up in rows or stack upon each other. They must be distinguished from traction bronchiolectasis, which may have a similar appearance but typically is located a few millimeters or more away from the pleura. The CT pattern, which is indeterminate for UIP, includes a variable or diffuse pattern of lung fibrosis or lung fibrosis with some mild features suggesting a non-UIP pattern such as scattered mosaic attenuation or expiratory air trapping. The CT features most consistent with a non-IPF diagnosis should be invoked if any one of the following findings are identified on CT: upper/middle or peribronchovascular distribution, extensive ground-glass opacity, consolidation, discrete cysts (not honeycombing), diffuse mosaic attenuation/air trapping, or profuse micronodules. However, even in these cases, UIP on pathology is not uncommon, occurring in 25% to 50% of cases depending on the patient population.[59,60,62]

CLASSIC HIGH-RESOLUTION COMPUTED TOMOGRAPHY SIGNS OF IDIOPATHIC PULMONARY FIBROSIS

- Subpleural and basal reticulation
- Subpleural and basal honeycombing
- Traction bronchiectasis and bronchiolectasis
- Irregular pleural, vascular, and bronchial interfaces
- Ground-glass opacities typically mild and associated with fibrosis
- Few or no centrilobular nodules
- Progressive increase of extent and severity of fibrosis
- Progressive decrease in lung volumes

Differential Diagnosis

Diagnosis in interstitial lung disease is unique in that it does not use pathology solely as the gold standard in diagnosis, and in recent years surgical lung biopsy is less often obtained for definitive diagnosis. The true gold standard for diagnosis is multidisciplinary discussion ideally involving clinicians, radiologists, and pathologists. Although the diagnosis of IPF is one of exclusion, careful attention to clinical, functional, and radiologic parameters allows accurate diagnosis in the absence of histologic confirmation in many patients. This is fortunate because surgical biopsy is an invasive procedure associated with potential complications.[63] The morbidity and mortality after surgical lung biopsy for interstitial lung disease are approximately 2.5% and 0.3%, respectively.[64] Several studies have shown that video-assisted thoracoscopic surgery biopsy is associated with less postoperative morbidity and mortality and with shorter hospital stays than limited thoracotomy.[65] The mortality after biopsy seems to be higher, however, in patients with IPF who present with atypical features and require lung biopsy for diagnosis.[63]

Surgical lung biopsy probably should be reserved for patients in whom the radiologic or clinical features of disease are atypical. Current guidelines support biopsy in patients with an indeterminate for UIP pattern and in patients whose CT suggests a non-IPF diagnosis. Conditions that commonly have similar parenchymal abnormalities as UIP/IPF are NSIP, chronic hypersensitivity pneumonitis, and asbestosis.[19] Reticular pattern and honeycombing also are commonly seen in chronic hypersensitivity pneumonitis. The distinction from UIP often can be made readily on high-resolution CT scan by the presence of centrilobular nodules, lobular areas of decreased attenuation and vascularity, and the relative sparing of the lung bases in patients with hypersensitivity pneumonitis.[44] Two studies have assessed the accuracy of high-resolution CT in distinguishing chronic hypersensitivity pneumonitis from UIP/IPF.[44,66] A confident high-resolution CT diagnosis was made in 62% of cases in one study and 53% of cases in the second study; this diagnosis was correct in 90% and 94% of cases.

Asbestosis usually can be distinguished readily from UIP/IPF by the presence of pleural plaques or diffuse pleural thickening. In one study the authors compared the high-resolution CT findings of 212 patients with IPF and 74 with asbestosis.[67] The CT findings were similar, except that overall the fibrosis in asbestosis was less extensive, was coarser, and was more likely to have a basal and subpleural distribution. None of the patients with IPF had pleural plaques, and only 4 (2%) had diffuse pleural thickening. Pleural plaques were seen in 58 (78%) patients with asbestosis, and diffuse pleural thickening was seen in 61 (82%). Of the 74 patients with asbestosis, 49 (66%) had pleural thickening and pleural plaques; 4 (5%) patients had no pleural disease.[67]

The interstitial lung disease that most commonly mimics UIP/IPF is NSIP, whether secondary or idiopathic (Table 27.1). One study showed that high-resolution CT had a sensitivity of 63% and specificity of 70% for UIP and a sensitivity of 70% and specificity of 63% for NSIP. The most helpful finding in distinguishing NSIP from IPF was the greater extent of ground-glass opacities (odds ratio, 1.04 for each 1% increase in the proportion of ground-glass opacities).[38] When all four independent observers agreed on the diagnosis (i.e., when the findings were characteristic of UIP or NSIP), the diagnostic accuracy was 96%; however, agreement of all four observers was present in only 45% of the cases.[38]

In a second study a confident CT diagnosis of IPF and NSIP was correct in 88% and 73%, respectively, of cases. The presence of honeycombing as a predominant feature had a specificity of 96%, sensitivity of 41%, and positive predictive value of 90% for IPF. This pattern was identified in only a single patient (by both readers) with fibrotic NSIP. Conversely, predominant ground-glass opacity or reticular opacity with minimal or no honeycombing was identified in 48 (96%) of 50 readings in patients with NSIP and in 26 (59%) of 44 readings in patients with UIP, giving a sensitivity of 96% and a specificity of 41% for the diagnosis of NSIP.[68]

A study using multivariate logistic regression analysis showed that the most useful finding for distinguishing IPF from NSIP was the extent of honeycombing.[39] The average extent of honeycombing was 4.4% of the parenchyma in IPF, 0.3% in cellular NSIP, and 0.6% in fibrotic NSIP.[39] These studies were limited by their retrospective design and reliance on pathology as the gold standard of diagnosis. In clinical practice only about 10%

TABLE 27.1 CLINICAL, HISTOLOGIC, AND HIGH-RESOLUTION COMPUTED TOMOGRAPHY FEATURES OF IDIOPATHIC PULMONARY FIBROSIS AND NONSPECIFIC INTERSTITIAL PNEUMONIA

	Idiopathic Pulmonary Fibrosis	Nonspecific Interstitial Pneumonia
CLINICAL FINDINGS		
Median age (yr)	50–70	40–50
Clinical symptoms	Progressive dry cough and dyspnea	Progressive dry cough and dyspnea
Response to corticosteroids	Poor	Good
Median survival	2–4 yr	6–14 yr for fibrotic NSIP; >15 yr for cellular NSIP
PATHOLOGIC FINDINGS		
Overall appearance	Heterogeneous	Homogeneous
Interstitial inflammation	Mild	Usually prominent
Interstitial fibrosis	Usually extensive; patchy	Mild to extensive; uniform
Fibroblastic foci	Prominent	Absent or scant
Honeycombing	Usually present	Uncommon
HIGH-RESOLUTION COMPUTED TOMOGRAPHY FINDINGS		
Reticulation	Typically most prominent feature; subpleural distribution	Variable; absent to extensive; often relative sparing of dorsal regions of lower lobes
Ground-glass opacity	Mild; usually associated with reticulation	Always present; typically most prominent feature
Traction bronchiectasis and bronchiolectasis	Common	Common
Honeycombing	Common; typically subpleural and basal	Uncommon at presentation; mild

NSIP, Nonspecific interstitial pneumonia.

to 15% of patients with suspected interstitial pulmonary fibrosis undergo surgical lung biopsy.[64,69] Therefore the presented data underestimates the accuracy of CT in distinguishing IPF from NSIP because many of the cases with high-confidence patterns would not have associated pathology. High-confidence UIP patterns on CT will almost always have UIP pathology if biopsy is pursued, and in the absence of a known cause for pulmonary fibrosis, the diagnosis will almost always be IPF.[57]

It has long been known that some degree of basilar interstitial abnormality is common in elderly patients. Unfortunately, postinfectious or postinflammatory scarring can mimic mild diffuse pulmonary fibrosis, although most cases of scarring can be differentiated from fibrosis by the more patchy and asymmetric distribution of scarring in contrast to the more symmetric and uniform distribution of true pulmonary fibrosis. Moreover, mild fibrosis at the lung bases may represent a normal part of the aging process. Copley and colleagues[70] found that in 60% of healthy patients older than 70 years of age, peripheral and basilar lung reticulation was evident on CT.[70] Other CT findings that have been described in the normal elderly population include segmental bronchial dilation and/or thickening, air-trapping, up to five pulmonary cysts, few thickened interlobular septa, subtle micronodules, and scattered ground-glass opacities.[71]

Synopsis of Treatment Options

Deterioration is gradual and inexorable in most patients, with increasing shortness of breath and eventually respiratory failure. The mean survival after the time of diagnosis ranges from 2 to 4 years (5-year survival range, 30% to 50%).[1]

Many attempts have been made to identify specific clinical, functional, laboratory, radiologic, and histologic features that predict disease progression and mortality. In one well-defined group of patients, survival was significantly worse in association with increased age at diagnosis, the presence of finger clubbing, absence of cigarette smoking, increased profusion of interstitial opacities, evidence of pulmonary hypertension on the chest radiograph, reduced lung volumes, and gas exchange abnormalities with exercise.[72] High-resolution CT findings associated with poor prognosis include extensive reticulation, extensive honeycombing, and the presence of reticulation as the predominant high-resolution CT pattern.[35]

Corticosteroid and standard immunosuppressive therapy has been shown ineffective in the setting of IPF and may in fact lead to increased patient morbidity and mortality.[73] Mitigation of factors that could potentially exacerbate patients' pulmonary fibrosis is essential. Obviously, smoking cessation is essential, as is adherence to routine demographically appropriate vaccinations. In recent years antifibrotic medications have become available (e.g., pirfenidone and nintedanib), which have been shown to slow the functional decline in IPF. Moreover, meta-analysis suggests possible improvement in survival, although this has not been definitively shown.[74] Unilateral lung transplantation should be considered for patients who show progressive deterioration despite optimal medical management and who meet the criteria for transplantation.[1]

KEY POINTS

- The diagnosis of idiopathic pulmonary fibrosis (IPF) is based on a high-resolution CT or histologic pattern of usual interstitial pneumonia (UIP) and clinical exclusion of other causes of UIP, such as asbestosis, chronic hypersensitivity pneumonitis, and connective tissue disease.
- In 50% to 70% of patients, a confident diagnosis of UIP/IPF can be made based on the high-resolution CT findings.
- A confident high-resolution CT diagnosis of UIP/IPF requires the presence of all of the following four high-resolution CT criteria: (1) presence of a reticular pattern, (2) a predominantly peripheral and basal distribution, (3) presence of CT honeycombing, and (4) absence of atypical features (e.g., centrilobular nodules, peribronchovascular nodules, extensive consolidation, or extensive ground-glass opacities).
- A probable UIP pattern on CT is identical to a high-confidence UIP pattern on CT, except for the absence of honeycombing. However, most of these patients will also have UIP on pathology and likely have IPF unless there is a known cause for pulmonary fibrosis.
- The indeterminate for UIP pattern on CT should be invoked in patients with variable or diffuse fibrosis or in patients with fibrosis but some features suggestive of a non-UIP diagnosis.
- The CT pattern most consistent with a non-IPF diagnosis should be invoked if any one of the following findings are identified on CT: upper/middle or peribronchovascular distribution, extensive ground-glass opacity, consolidation, discrete cysts (not honeycombing), diffuse mosaic attenuation/air-trapping, or profuse micronodules.

SUGGESTED READINGS

Chung JH, Lynch DA. The value of a multidisciplinary approach to the diagnosis of usual interstitial pneumonitis and idiopathic pulmonary fibrosis: radiology, pathology, and clinical correlation. *AJR Am J Roentgenol.* 2016;206(3):463–471.

Lynch DA, Sverzellati N, Travis WD, et al. Diagnostic criteria for idiopathic pulmonary fibrosis: a Fleischner Society White Paper. *Lancet Respir Med.* 2018;6:138–153.

Lynch DA, Travis WD, Müller NL, et al. Idiopathic interstitial pneumonias: CT features. *Radiology*. 2005;236:10–21.

Martin MD, Chung JH, Kanne JP. Idiopathic pulmonary fibrosis. *J Thorac Imaging.* 2016;31(3):127–139.

Raghu G, Rochwerg B, Zhang Y, et al; American Thoracic Society; European Respiratory society; Japanese Respiratory Society; Latin American Thoracic Association. An Official ATS/ERS/JRS/ALAT Clinical Practice Guideline: treatment of idiopathic pulmonary fibrosis. An update of the 2011 Clinical Practice Guideline. *Am J Respir Crit Care Med.* 2015;192(2):e3–e19.

The full reference list for this chapter is available at ExpertConsult.com.

28 Nonspecific Interstitial Pneumonia*

JONATHAN H. CHUNG | CHRISTOPHER M. WALKER

Etiology, Prevalence, and Epidemiology

Nonspecific interstitial pneumonia (NSIP) is a chronic interstitial lung disease characterized by homogeneous expansion of the alveolar walls by inflammation or fibrosis or both.[1,2] NSIP is the second most common chronic interstitial pneumonia, after usual interstitial pneumonia (UIP), accounting for 14% to 35% of cases.[2] NSIP may be idiopathic but more commonly occurs as a manifestation of connective tissue disease, hypersensitivity pneumonitis, drug-induced lung disease, and chronic interstitial lung disease complicating diffuse alveolar damage.[2]

The prognosis of NSIP is influenced by its predominant histologic component. Patients with a predominantly or exclusively inflammatory component (i.e., cellular NSIP) have an excellent prognosis with few reported deaths, whereas the reported median survival of patients with fibrotic NSIP ranges from approximately 6 to 14 years.[3] The prognosis of NSIP is considerably better than the prognosis of idiopathic pulmonary fibrosis (IPF), the clinical condition most commonly associated with UIP.

Clinical Presentation

The median age of onset of symptoms in NSIP is 40 to 50 years, which is more than 10 years younger than patients with IPF.[4] NSIP may occur in childhood and in the elderly, however, having been reported in patients 9 to 78 years old. The symptoms, similar to those of IPF, consist of progressive dyspnea and dry cough with a duration ranging from 6 months to 3 years before diagnosis.[3] Finger clubbing occurs in 10% to 35% of patients, which is less common than in patients with IPF. Auscultation reveals basal or widespread crackles.[4]

Pathophysiology

PATHOLOGY

The pathogenesis of NSIP is unknown. Because it is commonly seen in patients with connective tissue disease, especially systemic sclerosis, many investigators believe that NSIP is an autoimmune disease.[3] It also may be a subclinical form of other nonidiopathic interstitial lung diseases, such as hypersensitivity pneumonitis.[3]

NSIP is characterized histologically by homogeneous expansion of the alveolar walls by inflammation or fibrosis or both (Fig. 28.1).[1,2] The temporal and geographic homogeneity of NSIP, with the findings seeming to represent the same stage in the evolution of the disease, is distinct from the heterogeneity seen in UIP.[2] The histologic findings may range from inflammation (i.e., cellular NSIP) to predominant fibrosis (i.e., fibrotic NSIP). In cellular NSIP the alveolar septa are thickened by infiltrates of lymphocytes and plasma cells, whereas in fibrotic NSIP the thickening is mainly due to collagen accumulation.[2,4] The extent of interstitial fibrosis varies. The fibrosis may involve the alveolar septa, peribronchiolar interstitium, interlobular septa, and visceral pleura.[2] Areas of organizing pneumonia may be seen but are usually focal and mild.[2] Fibroblastic foci (i.e., aggregates of proliferating fibroblasts and myofibroblasts that give UIP the appearance of temporal heterogeneity) are absent or inconspicuous.[4]

The histologic differential diagnosis of NSIP includes hypersensitivity pneumonitis, lymphoid interstitial pneumonia, organizing pneumonia, and UIP.[2,4] In contrast to NSIP, the interstitial pneumonia in hypersensitivity pneumonitis has a bronchiolocentric distribution. Other helpful findings are the presence of chronic bronchiolitis and poorly formed granulomas, seen in 50% to 60% of patients with hypersensitivity pneumonitis.[2] Lymphoid interstitial pneumonia is similar to NSIP, except that it is typically associated with lymphoid hyperplasia in the form of peribronchiolar lymphoid aggregates.[2] Poorly sampled cases of cryptogenic organizing pneumonia may be misdiagnosed on biopsy as being NSIP.[2] A more difficult differential diagnosis is between NSIP and UIP because focal areas indistinguishable from NSIP commonly occur in what are otherwise typical cases of UIP.[5] Histologically, if one section has features diagnostic of UIP, and another section shows NSIP, the final diagnosis is UIP. Nonetheless, there is considerable interobserver variability even among expert histopathologists in the diagnosis of NSIP and in the distinction of fibrotic NSIP from UIP.[6,7]

LUNG FUNCTION

NSIP results in restrictive lung function (decreased total lung capacity and vital capacity) and impaired gas exchange as assessed by the carbon monoxide diffusing capacity.[4] The functional impairment varies but tends to be milder than in patients with IPF.[4]

Manifestations of the Disease

RADIOGRAPHY

The most common radiographic abnormalities are bilateral patchy or confluent hazy areas of increased opacity (ground-glass opacities) involving mainly the middle and lower lung zones (Fig. 28.2).[8,9] Other manifestations include a reticular pattern or a combination of reticular opacities, ground-glass opacities, and consolidation (Fig. 28.3).[1,9] In 15% of patients with NSIP and abnormal high-resolution computed tomography (CT) findings, the chest radiograph is normal.[9]

*The editors and the publisher would like to thank Drs. Nestor L. Müller and C. Isabela Silva Müller for contributing material on this topic to the prior edition of this work. It has served as the foundation for the current chapter.

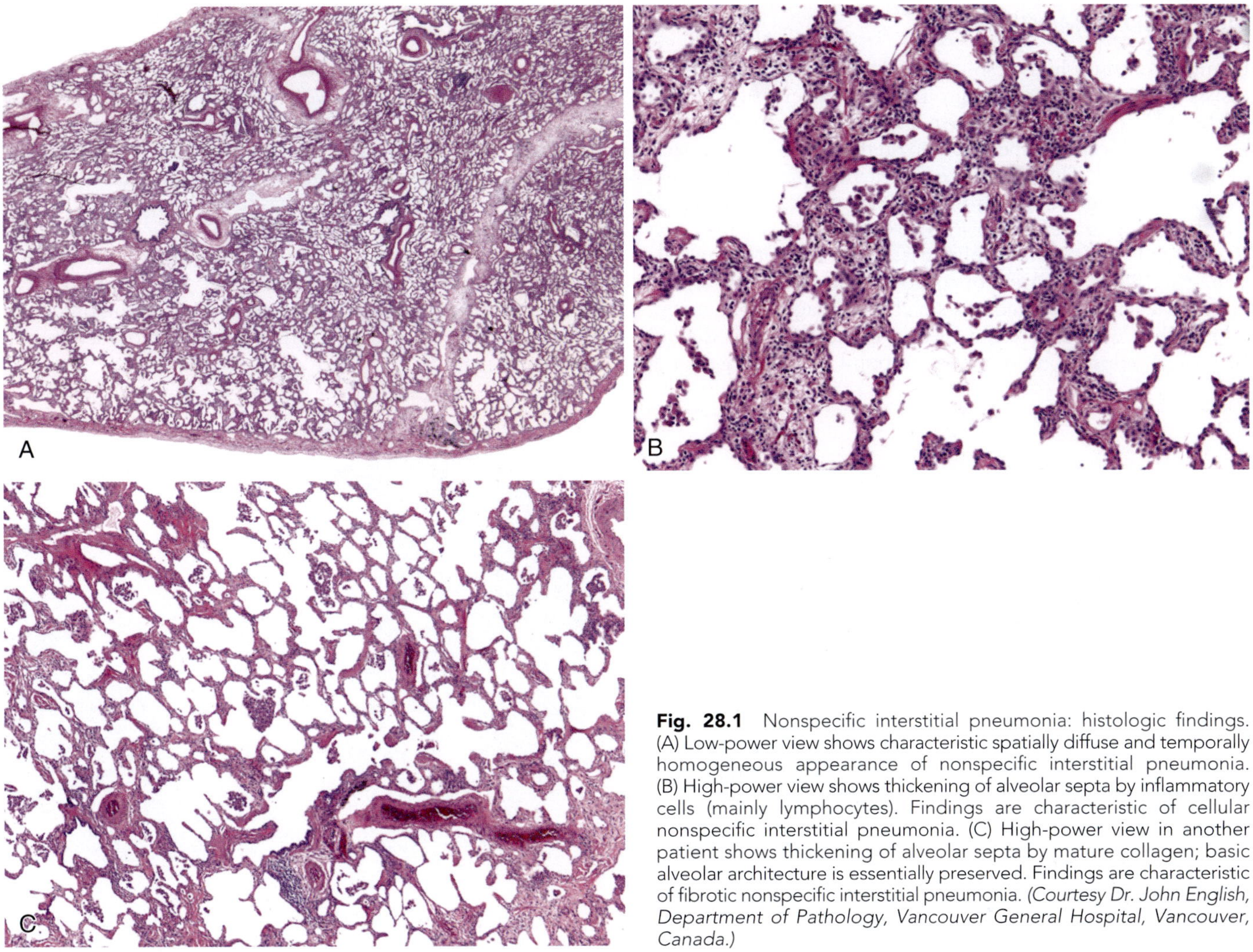

Fig. 28.1 Nonspecific interstitial pneumonia: histologic findings. (A) Low-power view shows characteristic spatially diffuse and temporally homogeneous appearance of nonspecific interstitial pneumonia. (B) High-power view shows thickening of alveolar septa by inflammatory cells (mainly lymphocytes). Findings are characteristic of cellular nonspecific interstitial pneumonia. (C) High-power view in another patient shows thickening of alveolar septa by mature collagen; basic alveolar architecture is essentially preserved. Findings are characteristic of fibrotic nonspecific interstitial pneumonia. *(Courtesy Dr. John English, Department of Pathology, Vancouver General Hospital, Vancouver, Canada.)*

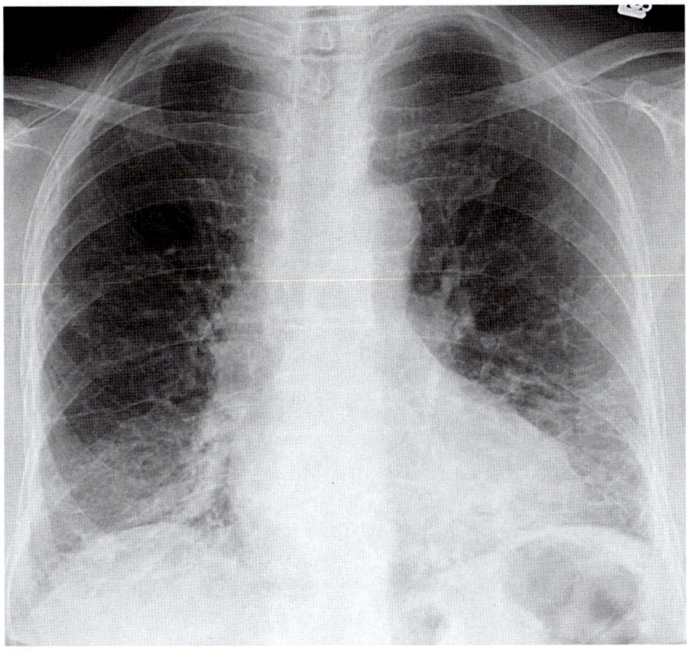

Fig. 28.2 Nonspecific interstitial pneumonia. Posteroanterior chest radiograph shows hazy increased opacity (ground-glass opacity) and irregular linear opacities in the middle and lower lung zones.

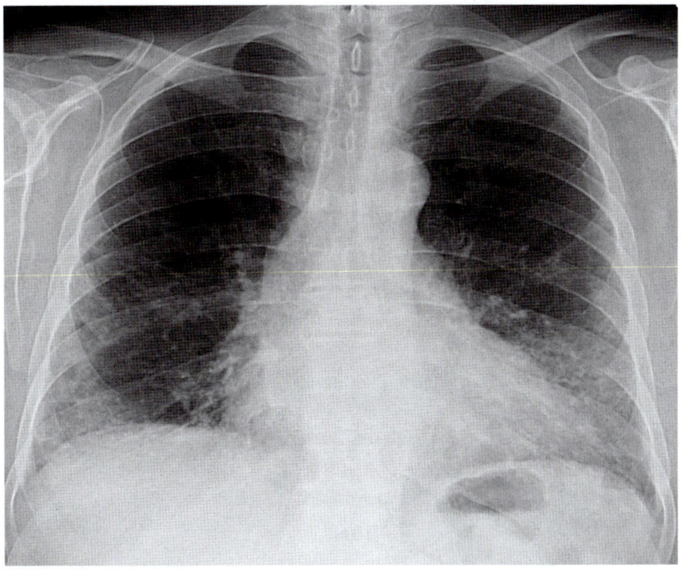

Fig. 28.3 Nonspecific interstitial pneumonia. Posteroanterior chest radiograph shows hazy increased opacity (ground-glass opacity) and reticulation mainly in lower lung zones.

COMPUTED TOMOGRAPHY

The most common high-resolution CT manifestation of NSIP consists of bilateral symmetric ground-glass opacities (Figs. 28.4 and 28.5).[10–12] Most patients have a fine reticular pattern and traction bronchiectasis superimposed on the ground-glass opacities (Fig. 28.6).[10–12] The prevalence of reticular opacities reported in various studies ranges from 50% to 100% of cases.[10–12] Honeycombing is seen in 10% to 30% of patients and, when present, tends to be mild, involving less than 10% of the parenchyma (Fig. 28.7).[10–13] Areas of consolidation and centrilobular nodules have been reported in a small percentage of patients in some studies[10,11] but were not seen in one other large study.[12] The areas of consolidation may correspond to focal organizing pneumonia and are seen most commonly in patients with collagen vascular disease. The abnormalities in NSIP may be diffuse but in 60% to 90% of cases involve mainly the lower lung zones and in 50% to 70% of patients involve predominantly the peripheral lung regions (Fig. 28.8).[10–14] A combination of predominant peripheral and peribronchovascular distribution is present in approximately 10% of patients.[13] Although the distribution of NSIP is frequently peripheral, it has been shown that in approximately 50% of patients with fibrotic NSIP the fibrosis tends to spare the lung immediately adjacent to the pleura at two or more levels in the dorsal regions of the lower lobes (Figs. 28.9 and 28.10).[13,14] This "relative subpleural sparing" is highly specific for fibrotic NSIP; conversely, UIP typically is most severe in the subpleural regions.[13]

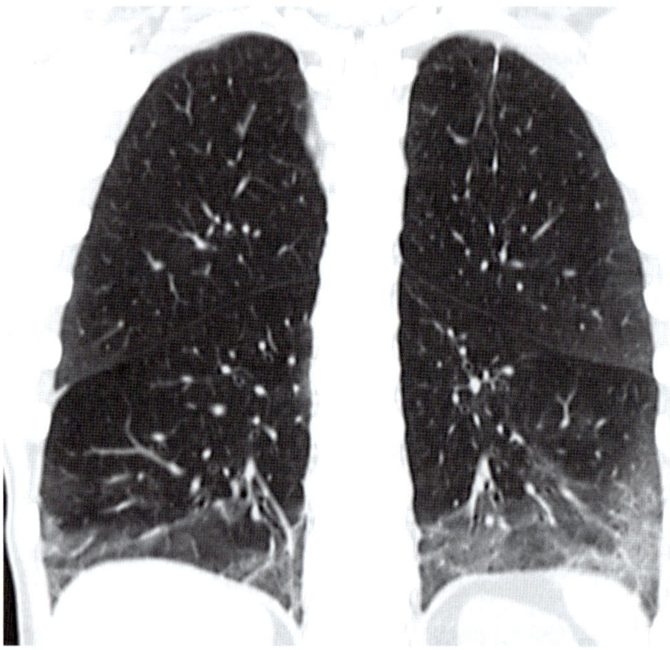

Fig. 28.4 Cellular nonspecific interstitial pneumonia (NSIP). Coronal image from chest CT shows extensive basilar ground-glass opacities without substantial traction bronchiectasis consistent with cellular NSIP.

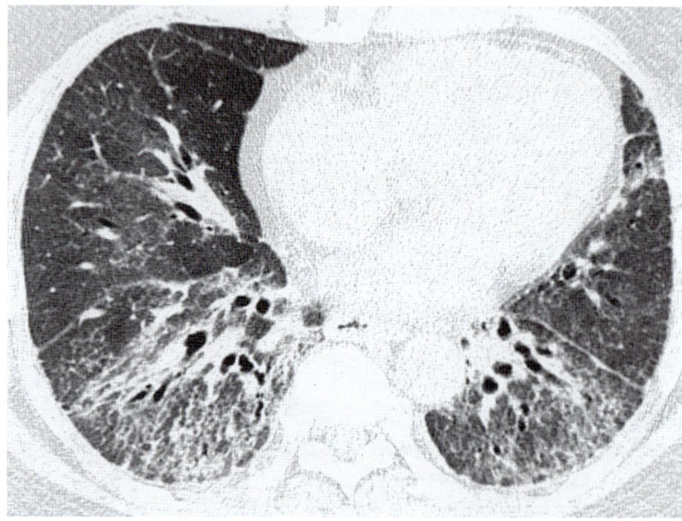

Fig. 28.6 Fibrotic nonspecific interstitial pneumonia. High-resolution CT scan shows extensive bilateral ground-glass opacities with associated traction bronchiectasis. Reticular pattern is present mainly in lower lobes and is associated with lower lobe volume loss with posterior displacement of major fissures owing to lower lobe fibrosis.

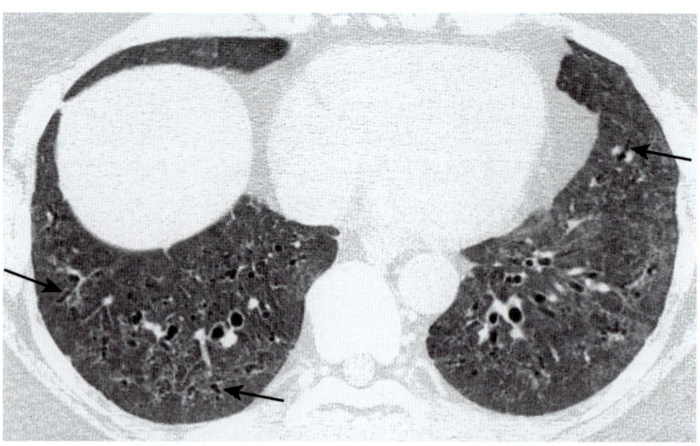

Fig. 28.5 Mixed cellular and fibrotic nonspecific interstitial pneumonia (NSIP). High-resolution CT shows diffuse bilateral ground-glass opacities. A few irregular linear opacities and mild traction bronchiectasis *(arrows)* also are present. The findings are consistent with mixed cellular and fibrotic NSIP.

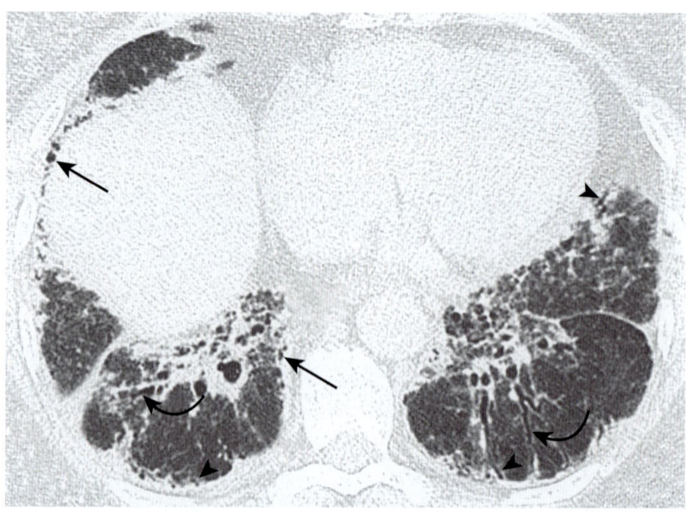

Fig. 28.7 Fibrotic nonspecific interstitial pneumonia. High-resolution CT scan shows bilateral ground-glass opacities, extensive reticulation, traction bronchiectasis *(curved arrows)*, traction bronchiolectasis *(arrowheads)*, and a few subpleural honeycomb cysts *(straight arrows)*.

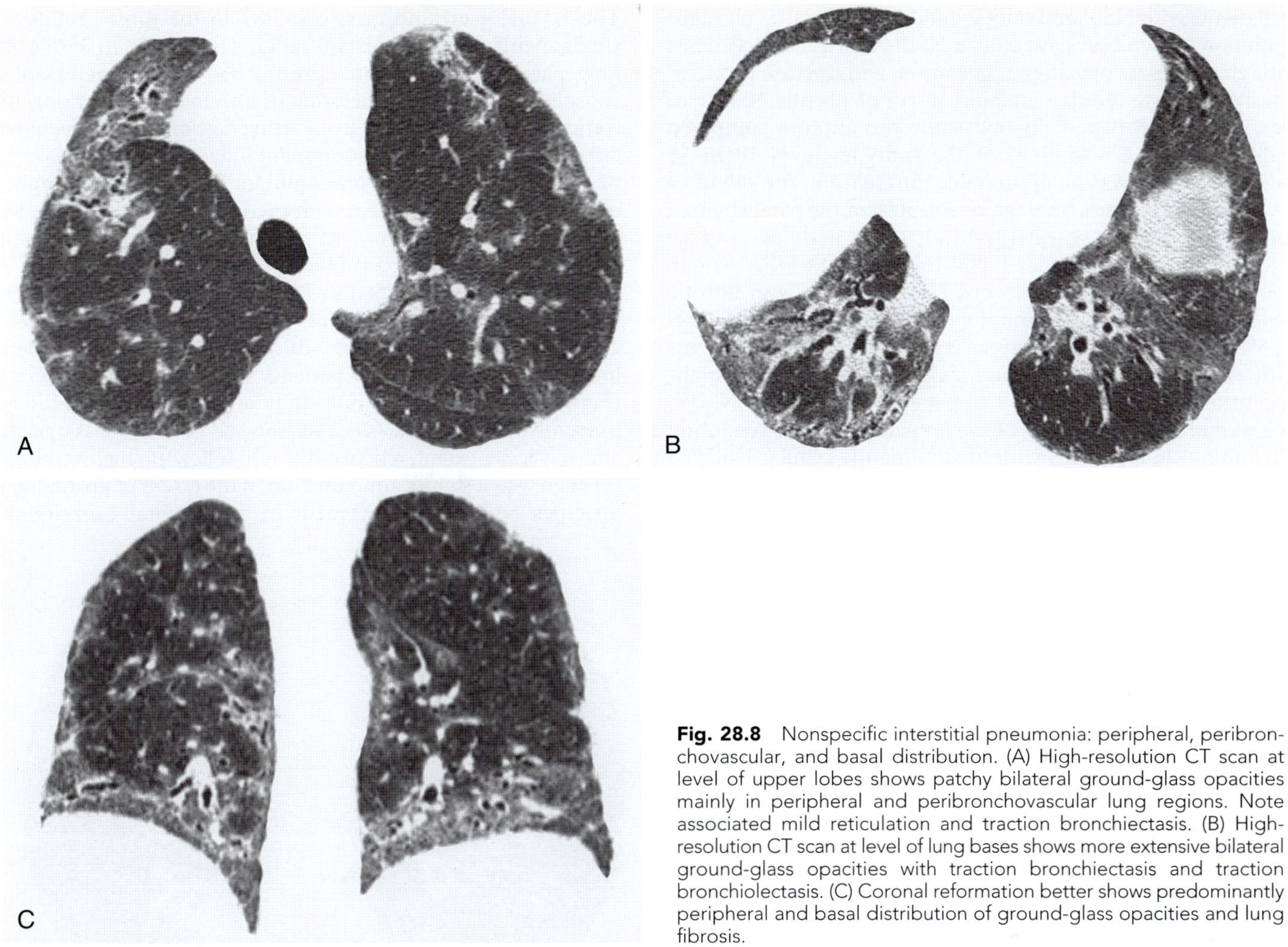

Fig. 28.8 Nonspecific interstitial pneumonia: peripheral, peribronchovascular, and basal distribution. (A) High-resolution CT scan at level of upper lobes shows patchy bilateral ground-glass opacities mainly in peripheral and peribronchovascular lung regions. Note associated mild reticulation and traction bronchiectasis. (B) High-resolution CT scan at level of lung bases shows more extensive bilateral ground-glass opacities with traction bronchiectasis and traction bronchiolectasis. (C) Coronal reformation better shows predominantly peripheral and basal distribution of ground-glass opacities and lung fibrosis.

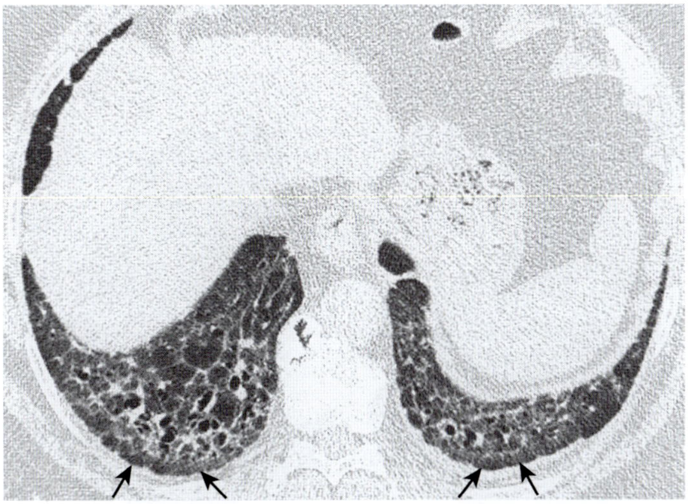

Fig. 28.9 Nonspecific interstitial pneumonia (NSIP): relative subpleural sparing. High-resolution CT scan shows extensive bilateral ground-glass opacities, traction bronchiectasis, and reticulation. The reticulation is less severe in the lung immediately adjacent to the pleura *(arrows)* than in the lung 1 cm away from the pleura (relative subpleural sparing), a characteristic finding seen in at least half of patients with NSIP.

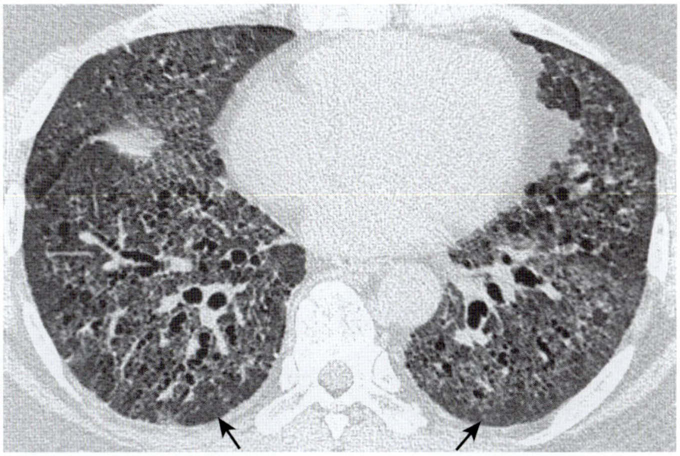

Fig. 28.10 Nonspecific interstitial pneumonia (NSIP): relative subpleural sparing. High-resolution CT scan shows extensive bilateral ground-glass opacities, traction bronchiectasis and bronchiolectasis, and reticulation. The reticulation is less severe in the lung immediately adjacent to the pleura *(arrows)* than in the lung 1 cm away from the pleura (relative subpleural sparing). This finding can be helpful in distinguishing NSIP from usual interstitial pneumonia.

Patients with NSIP and only ground-glass opacities on high-resolution CT typically have cellular NSIP (see Fig. 28.4). Patients with ground-glass opacities, reticulation, and traction bronchiectasis may have cellular (inflammatory) or fibrotic NSIP (see Figs. 28.5 to 28.10).[15,16] In one study the authors compared high-resolution CT findings of the subtypes of NSIP in 55 patients.[11] There was no appreciable difference in the extent of ground-glass opacities (average extent, 30% of the parenchyma), consolidation (average extent, 10%), small nodules (average extent, 9%), or interlobular septal thickening (average extent, 5%) between cellular and fibrotic NSIP. Patients with fibrotic NSIP had greater extent of intralobular lines (reticulation) (12% vs. 8%) and traction bronchiectasis (15% vs. 5%) than patients with cellular NSIP. Mild honeycombing was seen on high-resolution CT in 13 of 33 (39%) patients with fibrotic NSIP.[11] In a second study the investigators compared the high-resolution CT findings in 6 patients with predominantly cellular NSIP, 15 patients with equivalent extent of inflammation and fibrosis, and 15 patients with predominantly fibrosis on lung biopsy.[16] The extent of ground-glass opacities in the three groups was similar, with an average extent ranging from 25% to 35% of the lung parenchyma. All three groups had an average extent of consolidation of 10%. The extent of intralobular linear opacities (reticular pattern) ranged from an average of 13% of the parenchyma in patients with predominant inflammation to an average of 23% in patients with predominant fibrosis. Honeycombing was not seen in any patient with predominant inflammation or equivalent inflammation and fibrosis but was seen in patients with predominant fibrosis (average extent, 4%).[16]

Serial CT scans in patients with NSIP have shown that patients with predominant ground-glass opacities on the initial CT scan are more likely to improve with treatment and have a better long-term prognosis than patients with predominant fibrosis (Figs. 28.11 to 28.13). In one study of 13 patients with biopsy-proven NSIP, the initial CT scans showed ground-glass opacities and, to a lesser extent, reticulation.[17] On follow-up high-resolution CT there was a significant reduction in the extent of ground-glass opacities and an improvement in forced vital capacity that

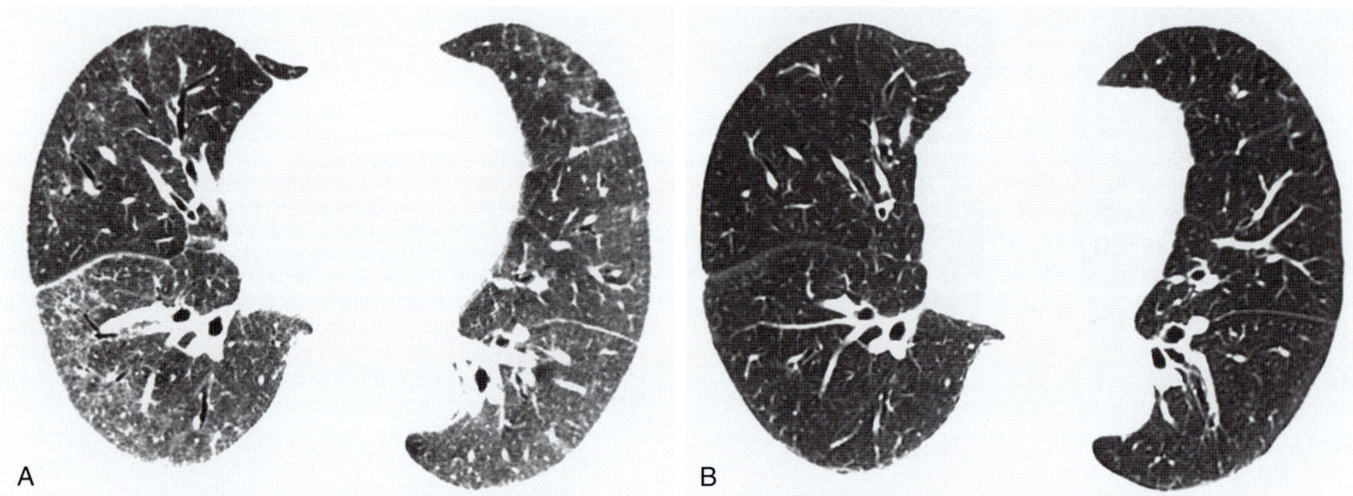

Fig. 28.11 Nonspecific interstitial pneumonia: improvement with treatment. (A) High-resolution CT scan shows patchy bilateral ground-glass opacities with reticulation. (B) Follow-up high-resolution CT scan 7 months later after treatment with corticosteroids shows resolution of ground-glass opacities.

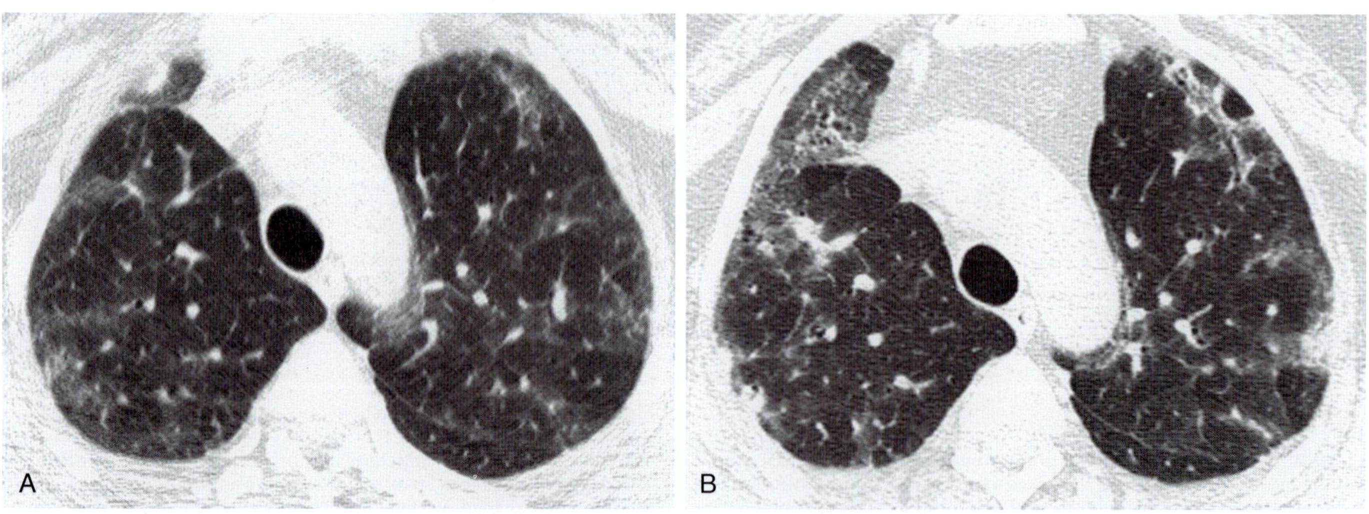

Fig. 28.12 Nonspecific interstitial pneumonia: mild progression over 5 years. (A) High-resolution CT scan shows patchy bilateral peripheral predominant ground-glass opacities. (B) Follow-up high-resolution CT scan 5 years later shows patchy ground-glass opacities, focal consolidation, and minimal fibrosis.

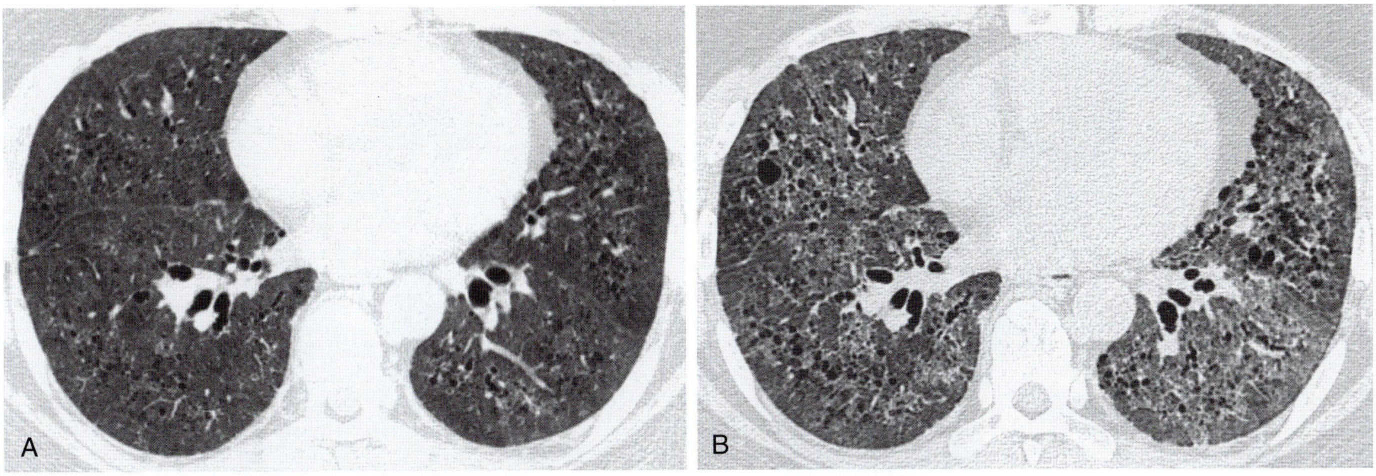

Fig. 28.13 Nonspecific interstitial pneumonia: progression of fibrosis over 2 years. (A) High-resolution CT scan shows extensive bilateral ground-glass opacities. Also noted are reticulation and traction bronchiectasis consistent with fibrosis. (B) High-resolution CT scan 2 years later shows progression of fibrosis with more extensive reticulation and traction bronchiectasis. Note relative subpleural sparing in dorsal regions.

correlated with the extent of reduction in ground-glass opacities on CT.[17] Similar results were described in a study of 14 patients with NSIP associated with polymyositis or dermatomyositis.[18] In a third study serial CT scans were performed in 38 patients with histologically proven NSIP, including 4 with cellular NSIP, 13 with mixed cellular and fibrotic NSIP, and 21 with fibrotic NSIP.[19] The predominant initial CT pattern was inflammatory (ground-glass opacities and consolidation) in 6 (16%) patients and fibrotic (reticulation and honeycombing) in 32 (84%) patients. The predominant pattern on initial high-resolution CT was significantly associated with change in extent of parenchymal abnormality on follow-up CT. At a mean follow-up of approximately 1 year, all of the patients with an inflammatory-predominant pattern on the initial CT scan improved, whereas of the 32 patients with a fibrosis-predominant pattern, 7 (22%) improved, 6 (19%) deteriorated, and 19 (59%) remained stable. There was no significant association between the histologic findings and the likelihood of improvement on follow-up CT.[19]

Mediastinal lymph node enlargement is evident on CT in approximately 80% of patients.[20,21] The nodal enlargement is usually mild, with lymph nodes measuring 10 to 15 mm in short-axis diameter and involving only one or two nodal stations (most commonly, the right lower paratracheal or subcarinal region). The prevalence of mediastinal lymph node enlargement in NSIP is similar to that in IPF.[20,21] No significant difference was found in the prevalence of lymph node enlargement in patients with predominant ground-glass opacity or predominant reticulation. There was a positive correlation, however, between the extent of disease in patients with NSIP and the likelihood of lymph node enlargement.[20,21]

Similar to patients with IPF, patients with NSIP may develop acute deterioration with an abrupt worsening of symptoms owing to infection, pulmonary embolism, pneumothorax, or heart failure. Occasionally, no identifiable cause for the acute decline is identified, however, and these episodes are called acute exacerbation or accelerated phase of NSIP.[22,23] The 1-year frequency of acute exacerbation has been estimated to be approximately 4% in patients with idiopathic NSIP and 3% in patients with NSIP associated with collagen vascular disease (rheumatoid arthritis and scleroderma).[24] The histologic findings consist of organizing pneumonia or, more commonly, diffuse alveolar damage superimposed on a background of NSIP.[22] The high-resolution CT findings consist of extensive ground-glass opacities and consolidation superimposed on reticulation (Fig. 28.14).[23]

Differential Diagnosis

Although the presence of extensive bilateral ground-glass opacities with superimposed fine reticulation in a patient with clinical findings consistent with chronic interstitial lung disease should suggest the possibility of NSIP, a confident diagnosis is seldom possible on high-resolution CT.[10,15] The high-resolution CT manifestations of NSIP can mimic those of cryptogenic organizing pneumonia, hypersensitivity pneumonitis, and IPF.[10] Cryptogenic organizing pneumonia usually can be distinguished by the predominance of consolidation, which typically involves mainly the peribronchial and subpleural lung regions.[25,26] Hypersensitivity pneumonitis typically manifests with bilateral ground-glass opacities, poorly defined centrilobular nodules, and lobular areas of air-trapping.[27] Occasionally, NSIP may be the predominant or only histologic pattern of hypersensitivity pneumonitis, however, and the high-resolution CT findings sometimes may be identical. Silva and associates[13] assessed the accuracy of high-resolution CT in distinguishing NSIP from chronic hypersensitivity pneumonitis and IPF in 66 patients. Two independent chest radiologists made a confident diagnosis in 70 (53%) of 132 readings. This diagnosis was correct in 66 (94%) of 70 readings. The high-resolution CT features that best differentiated NSIP were relative subpleural sparing, absence of lobular areas of decreased attenuation, and lack of honeycombing. The CT features that best differentiated chronic hypersensitivity pneumonitis were presence of lobular areas of decreased attenuation and vascularity and centrilobular nodules and absence of lower zonal predominance of abnormalities. The features that best differentiated IPF were basal predominance of honeycombing and absence of relative subpleural sparing and centrilobular nodules.[13]

The most important and often the most difficult differential diagnosis is between fibrotic NSIP and IPF (Table 28.1). One

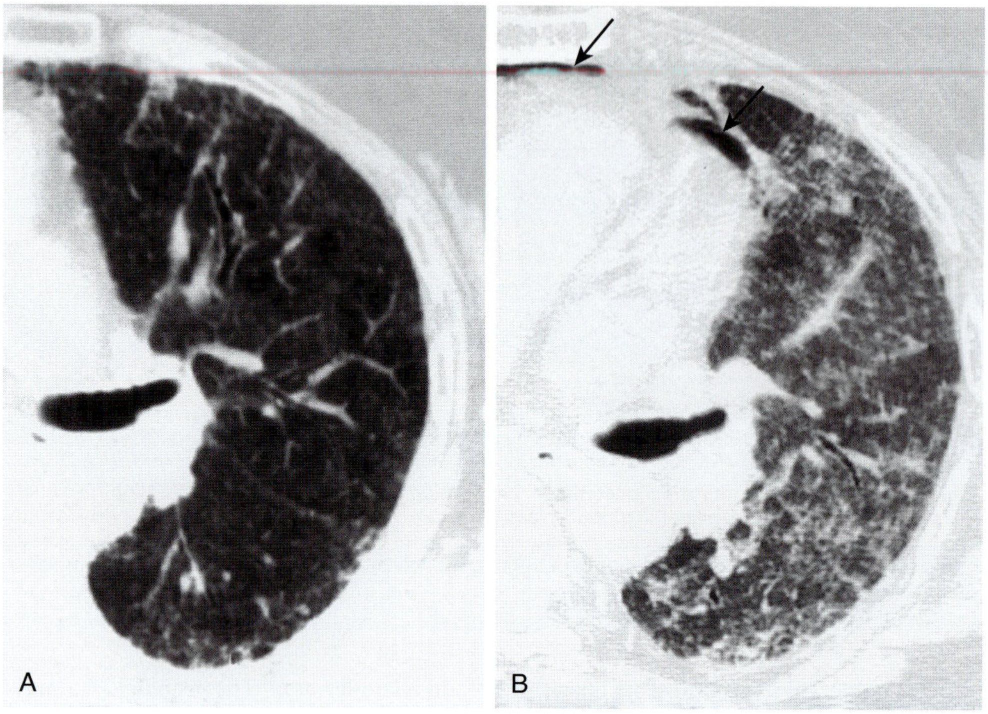

Fig. 28.14 Acute exacerbation of idiopathic nonspecific interstitial pneumonia (NSIP) in an 81-year-old woman. (A) High-resolution CT scan targeted to left lung at the level of the left main bronchus shows mild peripheral reticulation and patchy ground-glass opacities. (B) CT scan obtained at same level 6 months later, when the patient presented with acute deterioration, shows increased extent of ground-glass opacities and reticulation. A small pneumomediastinum *(arrows)* also is noted. The patient died 10 days later after the second CT scan. Autopsy showed diffuse alveolar damage and findings consistent with fibrotic NSIP. *(Courtesy Dr. Kiminori Fujimoto, Kurume University School of Medicine, Japan.)*

TABLE 28.1 CLINICAL, HISTOLOGIC, AND COMPUTED TOMOGRAPHY FEATURES OF USUAL INTERSTITIAL PNEUMONIA AND NONSPECIFIC INTERSTITIAL PNEUMONIA

	Usual Interstitial Pneumonia	Nonspecific Interstitial Pneumonia
CLINICAL FINDINGS		
Median age (yr)	50–70	40–50
Clinical symptoms	Progressive dry cough and dyspnea	Progressive dry cough and dyspnea
Response to corticosteroids	Poor	Good
Median survival	2–4 yr	6–14 yr for fibrotic NSIP 15 yr for cellular NSIP
PATHOLOGIC FINDINGS		
Overall appearance	Heterogeneous	Homogeneous
Interstitial inflammation	Mild	Usually prominent
Interstitial fibrosis	Usually extensive; patchy	Mild to extensive; uniform
Fibroblastic foci	Prominent	Absent or scant
Honeycombing	Usually present	Uncommon
HIGH-RESOLUTION COMPUTED TOMOGRAPHY FINDINGS		
Reticulation	Typically most prominent feature; subpleural	Variable; absent to extensive; often relative sparing of dorsal regions of lower lobes
Ground-glass opacity	Mild; usually associated with reticulation	Always present; typically most prominent feature
Traction bronchiectasis and bronchiolectasis	Common	Common
Honeycombing	Common; typically subpleural and basal	Uncommon at presentation; mild when present

NSIP, Nonspecific interstitial pneumonia.

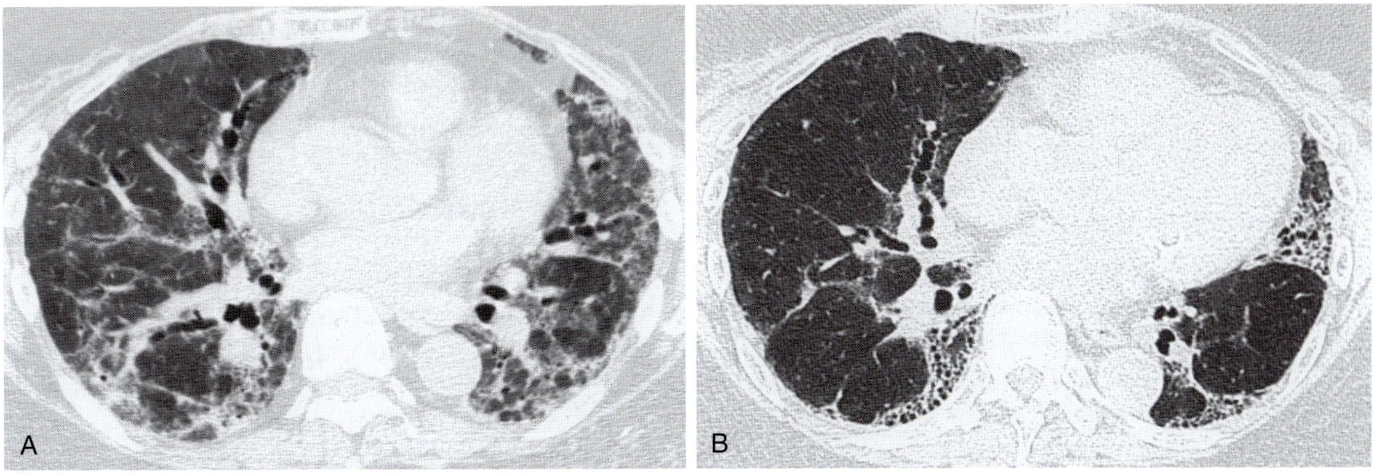

Fig. 28.15 Nonspecific interstitial pneumonia (NSIP): progression of findings that resemble idiopathic pulmonary fibrosis (IPF) over 4 years. (A) High-resolution CT scan at level of right middle lobe bronchus at presentation shows extensive ground-glass opacities, mild reticulation, and traction bronchiectasis. (B) Follow-up high-resolution CT scan at similar level 4 years later shows marked reduction in extent of ground-glass opacities, increase in reticulation and traction bronchiectasis, and development of a few subpleural honeycombing cysts. The follow-up CT findings resemble IPF. The patient was a 78-year-old man with biopsy-proven NSIP at the time of initial CT scan.

group of investigators compared the high-resolution CT findings of UIP and NSIP in 53 consecutive patients who had a clinical presentation consistent with IPF and who underwent lung biopsy.[12] The final diagnosis was IPF in 32 patients and NSIP in 21. High-resolution CT had a sensitivity of 63% and specificity of 70% for UIP and a sensitivity of 70% and specificity of 63% for NSIP. The most helpful finding in distinguishing NSIP from IPF was the greater extent of ground-glass opacities (odds ratio, 1.04 for each 1% increase in the proportion of ground-glass opacities).[12] When all four independent observers agreed on the diagnosis (i.e., when the findings were characteristic of UIP or NSIP), the diagnostic accuracy was 96%; however, agreement of all four observers was present in only 45% of the cases.[12]

In a second study 47 patients with biopsy-proven IPF (n = 22) or NSIP ($n = 25$) were independently reviewed by two chest radiologists.[28] A confident CT diagnosis of IPF and NSIP was correct in 88% and 73% of cases, respectively. The presence of honeycombing as a predominant feature had a specificity of 96%, sensitivity of 41%, and positive predictive value of 90% for IPF. This pattern was identified in only a single patient (by both readers) with fibrotic NSIP. Conversely, predominant ground-glass opacities, reticular opacities with minimal or no honeycombing, or both, were identified in 48 (96%) of 50 readings in patients with NSIP and in 26 (59%) of 44 readings in patients with UIP, giving a sensitivity of 96% and a specificity of 41% for the diagnosis of NSIP.[28]

A third group of investigators compared the high-resolution CT findings of various idiopathic interstitial pneumonias in 92 patients with a biopsy-proven diagnosis.[15] Two independent observers made the correct diagnosis in 79% of readings. Multivariate logistic regression analysis showed that the most useful finding for distinguishing IPF from NSIP was the extent of honeycombing. The average extent of honeycombing was 4.4% of the parenchyma in IPF, 0.3% in cellular NSIP, and 0.6% in fibrotic NSIP.[15]

In summary, these various studies show that in many patients high-resolution CT allows distinction of NSIP from IPF. Although the presence of predominantly peripheral and basal honeycombing in the appropriate clinical setting often allows a confident diagnosis of IPF on high-resolution CT, a confident diagnosis of NSIP usually requires surgical biopsy. Silva and colleagues[14] have shown that at long-term follow-up, approximately 30% of patients with an initial high-resolution CT pattern characteristic of NSIP progress to a pattern identical to IPF (Fig. 28.15).[14] In this study there were no CT features at presentation that distinguished NSIP that maintained its NSIP pattern at follow-up from NSIP that progressed to an IPF pattern.[14]

Even a histologic diagnosis of NSIP does not establish a final diagnosis. NSIP is a common reaction pattern to various drugs; is commonly associated with connective tissue diseases, particularly scleroderma; and can be a histologic manifestation of hypersensitivity pneumonitis.[2,4] These conditions need to be excluded by careful clinical assessment before making a diagnosis of idiopathic NSIP. In clinical practice, surgical biopsy is underused, being performed in less than 15% of patients with chronic interstitial lung disease.[29,30] Even if patients undergo lung biopsy, there is considerable disagreement among pathologists in the diagnosis of interstitial lung diseases, particularly NSIP.[6]

Synopsis of Treatment Options

Most patients with NSIP improve or stabilize after treatment with corticosteroids. Some patients may require the addition of immunosuppressive agents.[3]

KEY POINTS

- Nonspecific interstitial pneumonia (NSIP) is characterized histologically by homogeneous expansion of the alveolar walls by inflammation or fibrosis or both.
- Patients tend to be younger than patients with idiopathic pulmonary fibrosis (IPF) (median age, 40–50 years).
- Clinical and functional manifestations resemble those of IPF.
- NSIP has a better prognosis than IPF; prognosis is better in cellular NSIP than in fibrotic NSIP.
- Radiographic findings of NSIP consist of hazy increased opacities and reticulation mainly in the lower lung zones.
- High-resolution CT usually shows bilateral symmetric ground-glass opacities and superimposed fine reticulation and traction bronchiectasis.
- Lower lung zone predominance occurs in 60%–90% of cases.
- Peripheral predominance occurs in 50%–70% of cases.
- Relative sparing of the lung immediately adjacent to the pleura at two or more levels in the dorsal regions of the lower lobes occurs in approximately 50% of patients and is highly specific for the diagnosis.
- Patients with only ground-glass opacities have cellular NSIP.
- Patients with ground-glass opacities, reticulation, and traction bronchiectasis may have predominantly cellular (inflammatory) or fibrotic NSIP.
- Patients with predominantly ground-glass opacities on the initial CT scan are more likely to improve than patients with predominant reticulation.

SUGGESTED READINGS

Kligerman SJ, Groshong S, Brown KK, Lynch DA. Nonspecific interstitial pneumonia: radiologic, clinical, and pathologic considerations. *Radiographics*. 2009;29(1):73–87.

Lynch DA, Travis WD, Müller NL, et al. Idiopathic interstitial pneumonias: CT features. *Radiology*. 2005;236:10–21.

The full reference list for this chapter is available at ExpertConsult.com.

29 Cryptogenic Organizing Pneumonia/ Secondary Organizing Pneumonia*

JONATHAN H. CHUNG | CHRISTOPHER M. WALKER

Organizing pneumonia (OP) is a histologic pattern characterized by the presence of intraluminal granulation tissue polyps within alveolar ducts and surrounding alveoli associated with chronic inflammation of the surrounding lung parenchyma.[1,2] Because the granulation tissue polyps frequently also involve the bronchioles, the pattern was previously known as bronchiolitis obliterans organizing pneumonia (BOOP).[3] However, given the confusion of this entity with bronchiolitis obliterans (synonym: obliterative or constrictive bronchiolitis), this terminology has fallen out of favor.[1] OP may occur in association with several underlying conditions, including infections, connective tissue diseases, inflammatory bowel disease, inhalational injury, hypersensitivity pneumonitis, drug reaction, radiation therapy, and aspiration.[1,2,4] In some patients, no underlying cause is found, however, and the condition is termed *cryptogenic organizing pneumonia* (COP)[5] (Box 29.1).[3]

Etiology, Prevalence, and Epidemiology

COP accounts for 4% to 12% of cases of idiopathic interstitial pneumonias.[6] The exact incidence and prevalence of COP is not known as many cases are undiagnosed, and cases described in the literature are often based on presumptive diagnosis. Although COP and secondary OP are thought to occur at similar rates,[7] the cause for secondary OP is often difficult to identify or not exhaustively sought after. A population-based epidemiologic review of OP in Iceland estimated that the mean annual incidence of OP was 1.97 per 100,000 population, including 1.10 cases of COP and 0.87 cases of secondary OP per 100,000 population, respectively.[7] COP has an equal sex distribution and is approximately twice as common in nonsmokers than in smokers.[1] The average age of presentation is 50 to 60 years (range, 20–80 years).[8] Occasionally, COP may have seasonal recurrence. In one study the authors reported 12 patients with seasonal recurrence of COP for 3 to 11 years.[9] In all 12 patients symptoms recurred between late February and early May every year, tending to increase in severity each year. One case has been reported of recurrent COP starting 2 to 3 days before the menstrual period and resolving within 5 to 10 days.[10]

Clinical Presentation

Patients usually present with cough and progressive dyspnea of relatively short duration (median, <3 months).[1] The cough may be dry or productive of clear sputum. Other common manifestations include weight loss, chills, and intermittent fever. The clinical presentation mimics that of community-acquired pneumonia. Auscultation usually reveals localized or widespread crackles.[1] Finger clubbing is absent.

*The editors and the publisher would like to thank Drs. Nestor L. Müller and C. Isabela Silva Müller for contributing material on this topic to the prior edition of this work. It has served as the foundation for the current chapter.

Pathophysiology

PATHOLOGY

OP is characterized histologically by the presence of intraluminal plugs of granulation tissue within alveolar ducts and surrounding alveoli (Fig. 29.1), with or without concomitant granulation tissue polyps within the respiratory bronchioles (Fig. 29.2).[1,2] The distribution is typically patchy, and the connective tissue is of the same age. Mild associated interstitial inflammation is typically present with type II cell metaplasia and an increase in alveolar macrophages.[1] Even though the American Thoracic Society/European Respiratory Society consensus statement classifies COP as a form of idiopathic interstitial pneumonia, the abnormalities are mainly intraalveolar.[11]

LUNG FUNCTION

Pulmonary function tests usually show a mild to moderate restrictive ventilatory pattern with decrease in total lung capacity and vital capacity and impairment in gas exchange with decrease in carbon monoxide diffusing capacity.[1] The patients frequently are hypoxemic.

Manifestations of the Disease

RADIOGRAPHY

The most common radiographic manifestation of OP consists of bilateral symmetric or asymmetric areas of consolidation (Figs. 29.3 and 29.4).[12–14] The consolidation usually has a patchy distribution but may involve mainly the subpleural regions.[15] Occasionally, the areas of consolidation may be migratory, decreasing in size in one area and appearing in previously unaffected regions.[9] An unusual case of *levitating* consolidation has been described; the bilateral areas of consolidation migrated cephalad during a period of months and gradually disappeared after reaching the lung apices.[16]

The size of individual areas of consolidation ranges from about 1 cm to almost an entire lobe. Their margins are indistinct, and they may contain air bronchograms. The lung volume may appear preserved or decreased. Occasionally, the areas of consolidation may be round, resulting in multiple large nodular opacities or masses.[17] A pattern of small nodular, reticular, or

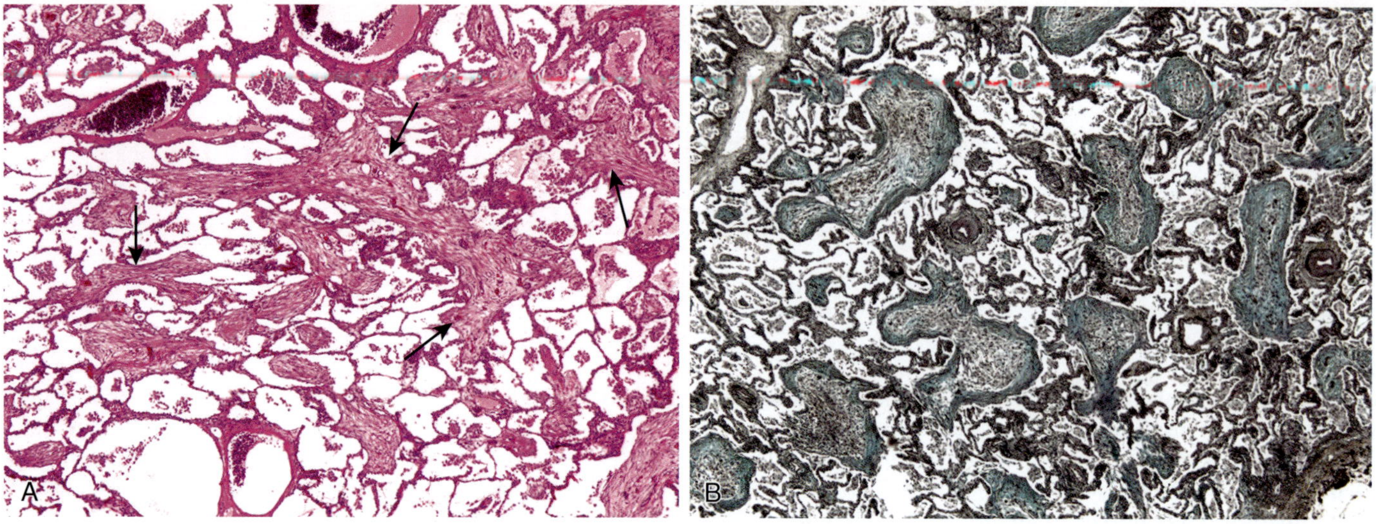

Fig. 29.1 Organizing pneumonia: classic histologic findings. (A) Photomicrograph at low magnification shows characteristic granulation tissue polyps *(arrows)* in the alveolar ducts and adjacent airspaces. Mild interstitial inflammation also is noted. (B) Movat pentachrome stain highlights the granulation tissue polyps in blue. *(Courtesy Dr. John English, Department of Pathology, Vancouver General Hospital, Vancouver, Canada.)*

BOX 29.1 CONDITIONS ASSOCIATED WITH ORGANIZING PNEUMONIA

- Idiopathic (cryptogenic organizing pneumonia)
- Connective tissue disease
- Drug reaction
- Infection (including bacteria, *Mycoplasma,* fungi, and *Pneumocystis*)
- Human immunodeficiency virus related
- Aspiration
- Hemorrhage
- Hypersensitivity pneumonitis
- Malignancy (solid tumor and hematologic)
- Posttransplantation (particularly stem cell transplantation)
- Postradiation
- Inhalational injury (toxic fume or smoke inhalation)
- Vasculitis syndromes (particularly granulomatosis with polyangiitis and eosinophilic granulomatosis with polyangiitis [Churg-Strauss syndrome])
- Inflammatory bowel disease
- Nonspecific reaction adjacent to other lesions (e.g., infarct, abscess, and neoplasm)
- Cocaine abuse
- Anthrax vaccination (rare)

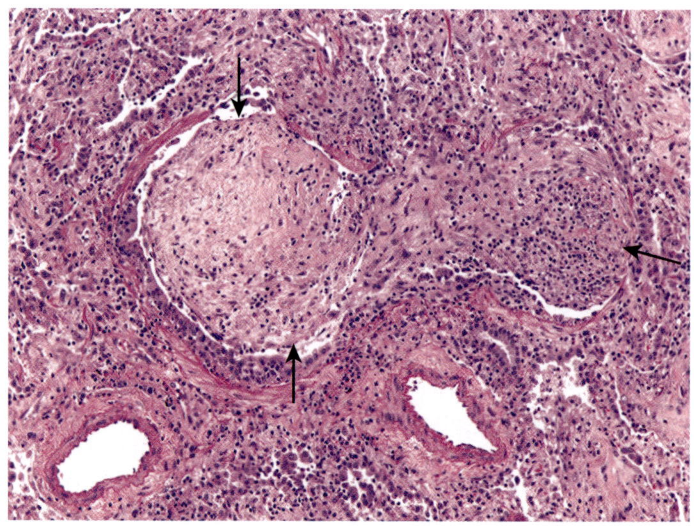

Fig. 29.2 Organizing pneumonia: histologic findings. High-power view shows granulation tissue polyp (Masson body) within bronchiolar lumen *(arrows)*. *(Courtesy Dr. John English, Department of Pathology, Vancouver General Hospital, Vancouver, Canada.)*

reticulonodular opacities may be seen in association with airspace opacities or occasionally as an isolated finding.[12,14] Small unilateral or bilateral pleural effusions are seen in about 20% of patients.[12,14]

COMPUTED TOMOGRAPHY

The characteristic high-resolution computed tomography (CT) manifestation of OP consists of patchy areas of consolidation.[18–20] The consolidation is usually bilateral and most commonly involves mainly the middle and lower lung zones.[20,21] In 60% to 80% of cases the consolidation has a predominantly peribronchial or subpleural distribution (Figs. 29.5 to 29.7).[20–22] The areas of consolidation may decrease in size in one area and appear in previously unaffected regions (Fig. 29.8).[9]

Another characteristic feature of OP is a perilobular pattern, seen in approximately 60% of patients (Fig. 29.9).[22] A perilobular pattern is defined as linear opacities that are of greater thickness and are less sharply defined than opacities encountered in thickened interlobular septa and that have an arcade-like or polygonal appearance.[19] The perilobular pattern frequently abuts the pleural surface and is surrounded by aerated lung parenchyma.[22] The perilobular pattern results from accumulation of organizing exudate in the perilobular alveoli, with or without interlobular septal thickening at histologic examination.[23] Less commonly, OP may result in crescentic or ring-shaped opacities surrounding areas of ground-glass opacification.[24] These have been referred to as the atoll sign[25] or as the reversed halo sign.[21] The reversed halo sign is seen in approximately 20% of patients with OP (Figs. 29.10 and 29.11).[21] Histopathologically, the central areas of ground-glass opacification were shown to correspond to alveolar septal inflammation, whereas the ring-shaped or crescentic periphery corresponds mainly to OP within alveolar ducts.[21] The atoll sign or reversed halo sign is not pathognomonic for OP and may be seen in pneumonias (classically mucormycosis and tuberculosis), granulomatosis with polyangiitis, pulmonary infarcts, and sarcoidosis; however, in the subacute to chronic setting, it is usually diagnostic of OP.[26]

Consolidation occurs in 90% to 95% of immunocompetent patients with OP[19,22] but is less common in immunocompromised patients, being seen in only 5 of 11 immunocompromised patients (45%) in one study.[19] Less common findings seen in OP include ground-glass opacities, small centrilobular nodules, and large

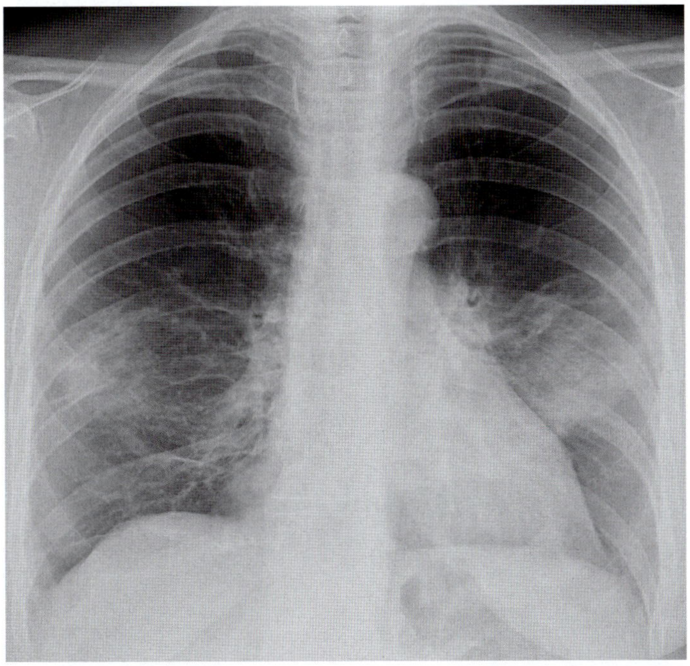

Fig. 29.3 Organizing pneumonia: radiographic findings. Posteroanterior chest radiograph shows patchy bilateral areas of consolidation and ground-glass opacities.

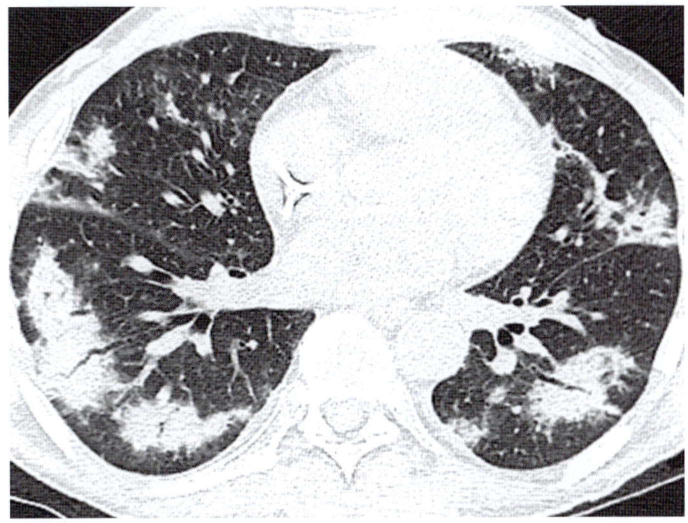

Fig. 29.5 Organizing pneumonia: round peripheral mass-like consolidation. CT scan shows bilateral round and oval peripheral and peribronchovascular areas of consolidation.

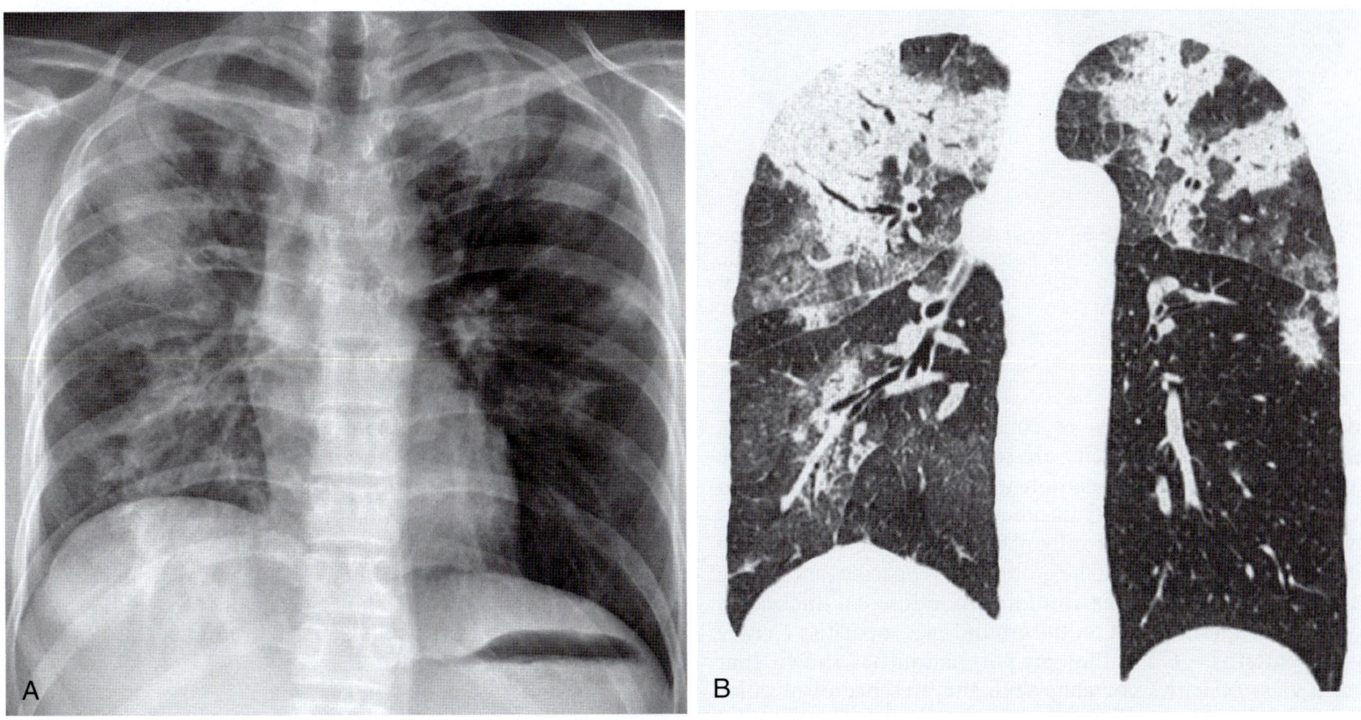

Fig. 29.4 Organizing pneumonia: radiographic and CT findings. (A) Posteroanterior chest radiograph shows bilateral multifocal and confluent consolidation involving mainly the upper lobes. (B) Coronal reformatted CT scan shows predominant peribronchial distribution of the consolidation. Bilateral ground-glass opacities also are noted.

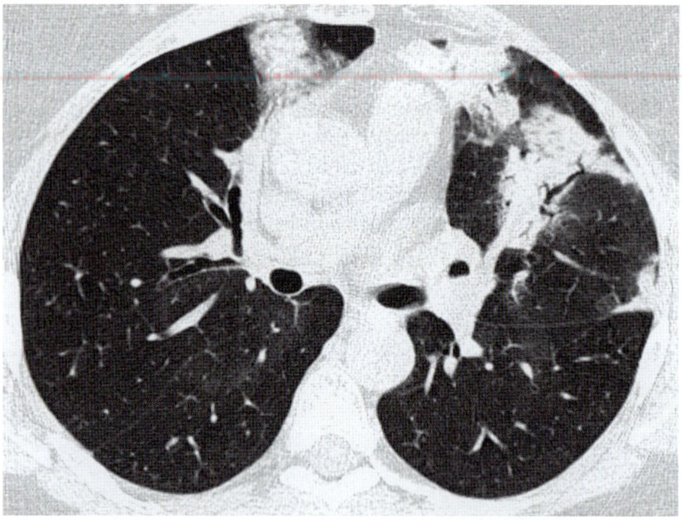

Fig. 29.6 Organizing pneumonia: high-resolution CT findings. High-resolution CT scan shows bilateral peripheral and peribronchial areas of consolidation in the upper lobes.

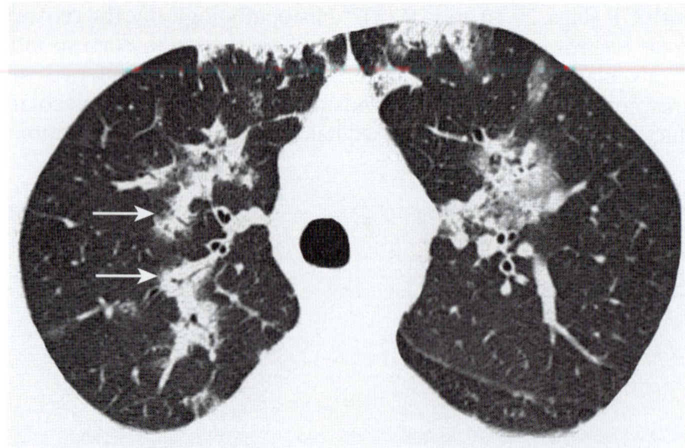

Fig. 29.7 Organizing pneumonia: high-resolution CT findings. High-resolution CT scan shows bilateral areas of consolidation in a peribronchial *(arrows)* and subpleural distribution.

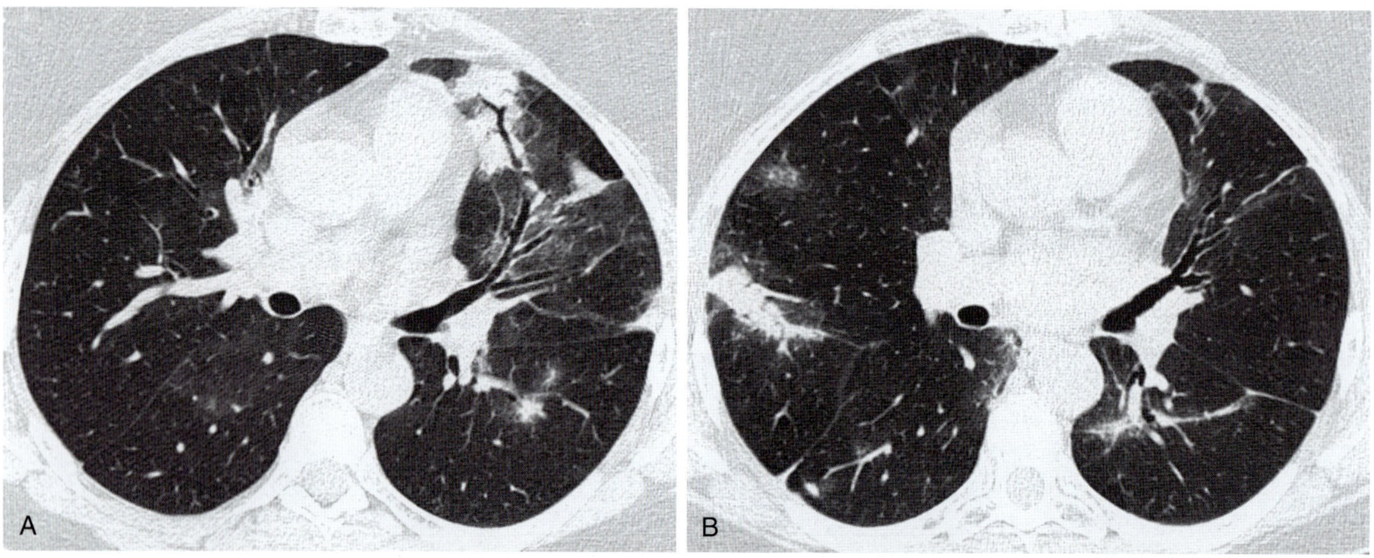

Fig. 29.8 Organizing pneumonia with migrating consolidation. (A) High-resolution CT scan shows peribronchial areas of consolidation in the left upper and lower lobes and patchy bilateral ground-glass opacities. (B) High-resolution CT scan 6 months later shows marked improvement in the areas of consolidation in the left lung but new foci of consolidation and ground-glass opacities in the right upper and both lower lobes.

nodules or mass-like areas of consolidation (see Fig. 29.5). Areas of ground-glass opacity are seen in approximately 60% of patients, usually in association with areas of consolidation (see Figs. 29.6 to 29.11).[19] Occasionally, ground-glass opacities may be the predominant or only manifestation of OP on high-resolution CT (Fig. 29.12).[19] The ground-glass opacities are usually bilateral and random in distribution. Smooth septal thickening may be seen superimposed on the ground-glass opacities ("crazy paving" pattern).[27] CT-pathologic correlation has shown that ground-glass opacities correlate with the presence of alveolar septal inflammation, but little granulation tissue, in the terminal airspaces.[28]

Nodular opacities measuring 1 to 10 mm are seen in 30% to 50% of patients, usually in association with areas of consolidation (Fig. 29.13).[19,20] CT-pathologic correlation has shown that the parenchymal nodules represent localized areas of OP, centered around abnormal bronchioles.[20] Occasionally, OP may manifest as large nodules or mass-like areas of consolidation.[17] In one study of 59 consecutive patients with COP, 12 (20%) had nodules and masses ranging from 8 mm to 5 cm in diameter as the primary manifestation of disease. The number of large nodules ranged from two to eight per patient. Of 60 lesions in the 12 patients, 53 (88%) had an irregular margin, and 27 (45%) had an air bronchogram.[17] Irregular linear opacities in a predominantly subpleural, peribronchial, or random distribution are seen in association with areas of consolidation in 5% to 25% of patients with COP.[18,19,22] This may be more common when secondary to stem cell transplantation; in one study, approximately half of

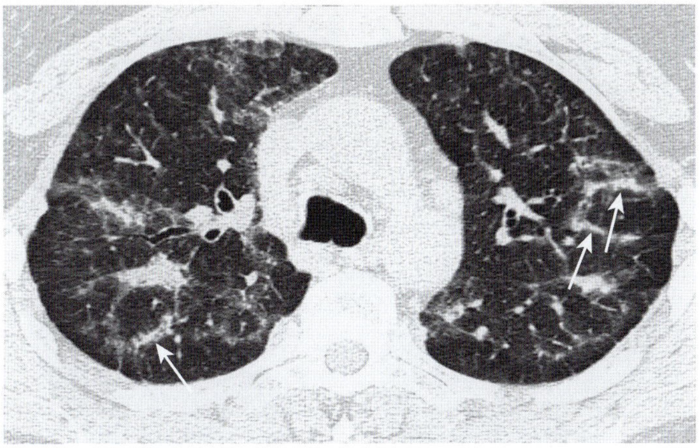

Fig. 29.9 Organizing pneumonia with perilobular opacities. High-resolution CT scan shows bilateral ground-glass opacities and polygonal linear opacities *(arrows)* marginating the secondary pulmonary lobules. These polygonal arcades reflect the presence of consolidation in the alveoli adjacent to the interlobular septa and are referred to as perilobular opacities or a perilobular pattern.

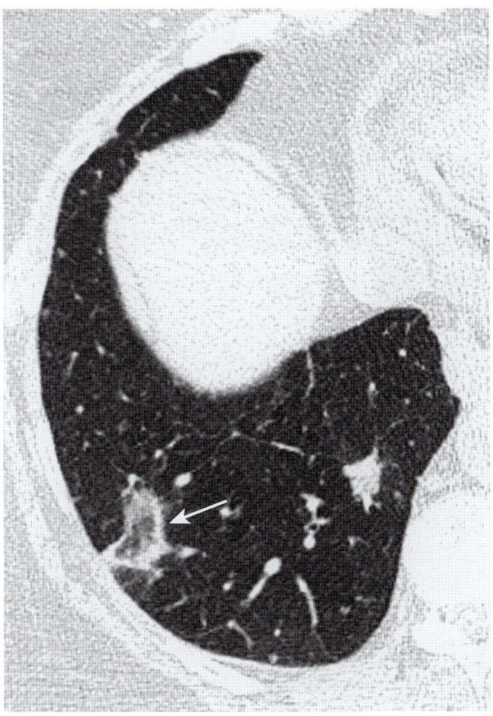

Fig. 29.10 Organizing pneumonia with reversed halo sign. View of the right lung from a high-resolution CT scan shows polyhedral opacity *(arrow)* surrounding area of ground-glass opacification (reversed halo sign). A small nodular area of consolidation in the medial right lower lobe also is noted.

cases of OP resulting from stem cell transplantation showed linear opacities on chest CT.[29] Occasionally, the reticular opacities may be the predominant finding.[30]

Bronchial wall thickening and dilation may be seen on high-resolution CT in patients who have extensive consolidation and usually is restricted to these areas.[19,20] The bronchial dilation is usually reversible; the bronchial diameter returns to normal after resolution of the parenchymal abnormalities. Slightly enlarged right paratracheal or subcarinal lymph nodes are seen in 20% to 40% of patients.[21,31] Small unilateral or bilateral pleural

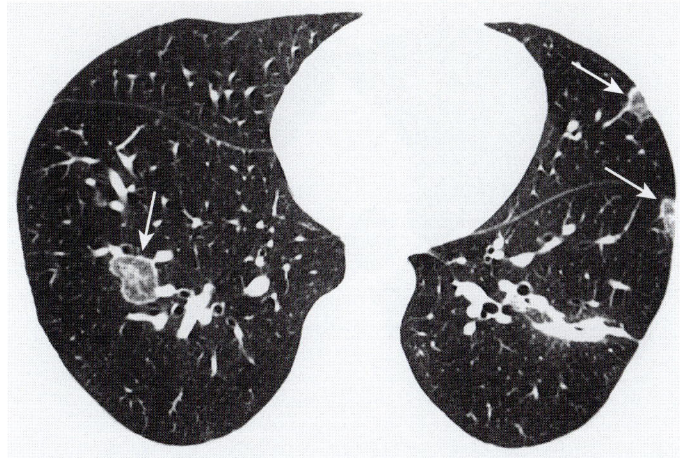

Fig. 29.11 Organizing pneumonia with reversed halo sign secondary to infection. High-resolution CT scan shows bilateral crescentic and ring-like consolidation *(arrows)* surrounding areas of ground-glass opacification (reversed halo sign). A bandlike area of consolidation in the left lower lobe also is noted.

effusions are evident on high-resolution CT in 10% to 30% of patients.[19–21]

IMAGING ALGORITHMS

The chest radiograph is usually the first and commonly the only imaging modality used in assessing patients with OP. High-resolution CT can be helpful in patients with a suspected diagnosis and nonspecific radiographic findings. It is superior to the radiograph in showing the characteristic and common peribronchial and subpleural distribution of OP and the presence of the perilobular pattern. OP is often fluorodeoxyglucose (FDG) avid on positron emission tomography (PET)-CT given its inflammatory nature (Fig. 29.14). Given the multifocality of OP and its often characteristic imaging findings, this is usually not a diagnostic issue; however, special care must be taken not to confuse cases of focal OP with lung cancer, given the similarity in imaging appearance with adenocarcinoma.

CLASSIC SIGNS

- Patchy areas of consolidation in 80%–90% of patients
- Usually bilateral
- Peribronchial or subpleural distribution in 60%–80%
- Perilobular pattern in 60%
- Crescentic or ring-shaped opacities surrounding areas of ground-glass opacification (reversed halo sign) in 20%
- Ground-glass opacity in 60% of patients, usually in association with consolidation
- Nodular opacities 1–10 mm in diameter in 30%–50% of patients

Differential Diagnosis

The differential diagnosis of COP includes OP secondary to underlying conditions, such as infection, connective tissue disease (particularly rheumatoid arthritis and polymyositis), inflammatory bowel disease, inhalational injury, hypersensitivity pneumonitis, drug reaction, radiation therapy, and aspiration. In the appropriate clinical context the presence of peribronchial or

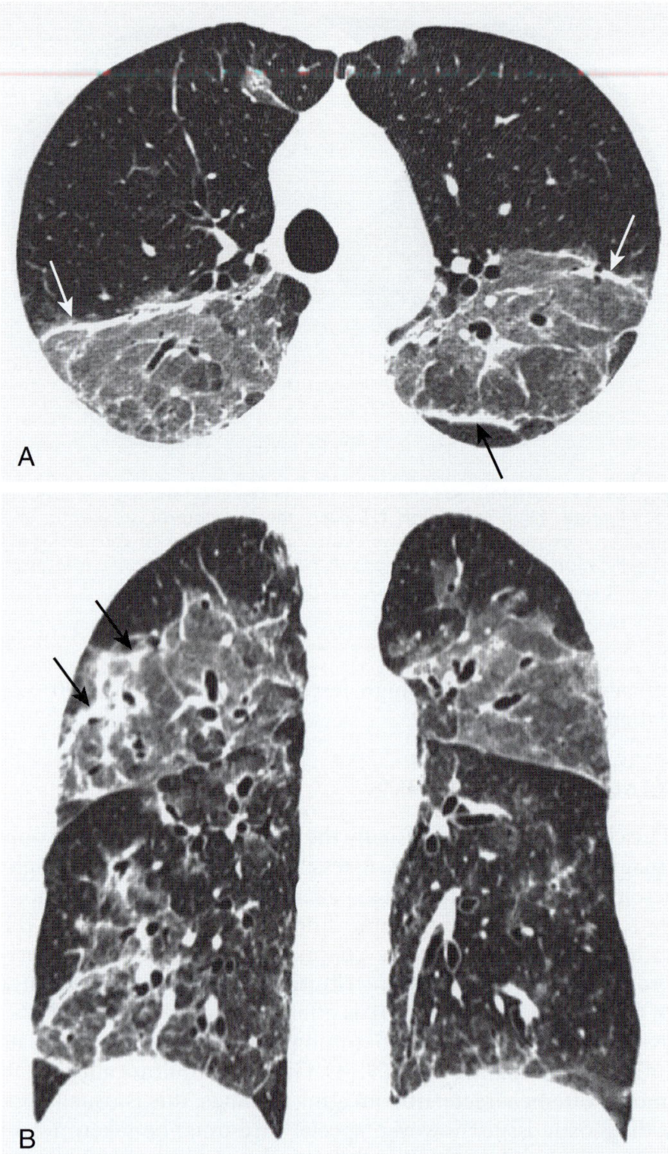

Fig. 29.12 Organizing pneumonia (OP): ground-glass opacity and reversed halo sign. (A) High-resolution CT scan in an immunocompromised woman with OP shows extensive bilateral ground-glass opacities, a few small nodular opacities, and bilateral crescentic and ring-like consolidation *(arrows)* surrounding areas of ground-glass opacification (reversed halo sign). (B) Coronal reformation shows the overall extent and distribution of the ground-glass opacities and the reversed halo sign (*arrows*).

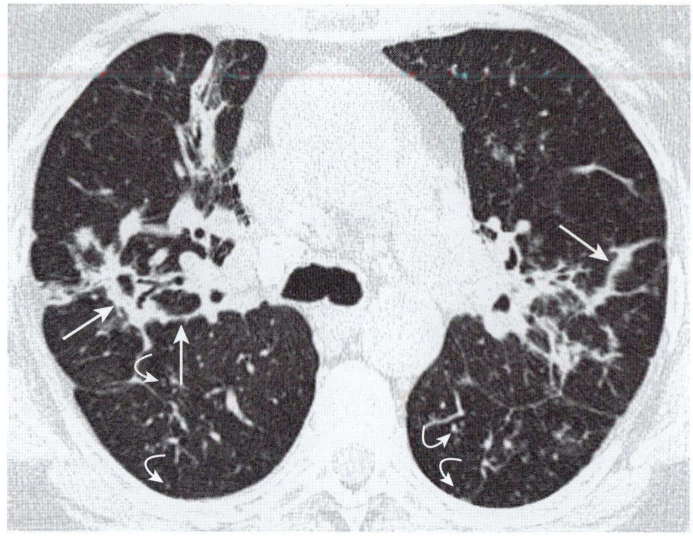

Fig. 29.13 Organizing pneumonia with small nodules. High-resolution CT scan shows perilobular pattern *(straight arrows)* and several small centrilobular nodules *(curved arrows)*. Patchy ground-glass opacities and a few irregular linear opacities also are noted.

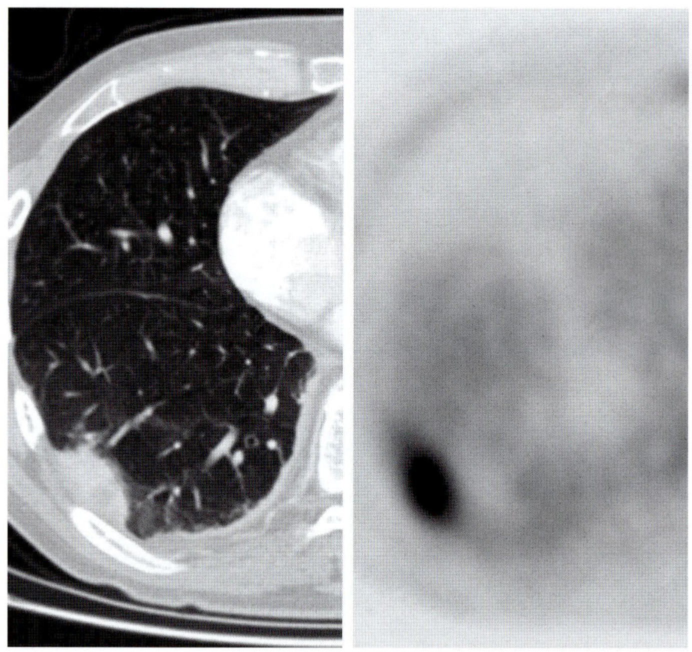

Fig. 29.14 Organizing pneumonia with FDG avidity. Composite image with axial contrast-enhanced CT scan *(left image)* and PET scan *(right image)* shows an FDG-avid right lower lobe subpleural mass initially thought to represent primary lung cancer.

subpleural consolidation that increases over several weeks despite antibiotics is highly suggestive of OP. The radiologic differential diagnosis in patients presenting with patchy bilateral consolidation includes bacterial, fungal, and viral pneumonia, adenocarcinoma, lymphoma, vasculitis, sarcoidosis, and chronic eosinophilic pneumonia (CEP). Most of these entities can be excluded by a combination of clinical findings, bronchoalveolar lavage, and transbronchial biopsy.

COP usually can be readily distinguished from other chronic interstitial and airspace lung diseases on high-resolution CT. One group of investigators reviewed the high-resolution CT findings in 129 patients who had various idiopathic interstitial pneumonias, including 24 with COP.[32] On average, based on the pattern and distribution of abnormalities on high-resolution CT, two independent observers made a correct first-choice diagnosis in 79% of 24 cases of COP, 71% of 35 cases of usual interstitial pneumonia, 63% of 23 cases of desquamative interstitial pneumonia, 65% of 20 cases of acute interstitial pneumonia, and 9% of 27 cases of nonspecific interstitial pneumonia.[32] The predominant subpleural distribution of COP resembles that of CEP.

In one study the authors compared the high-resolution CT findings in 38 patients with COP and 43 patients with CEP.[33]

Airspace consolidation was the most frequent high-resolution CT finding in COP (87%) and CEP (74%), and it had a predominantly peripheral distribution in 66% of patients with COP and 56% of patients with CEP. A peribronchial distribution of consolidation was seen more frequently in COP than in CEP (29% vs. 9%). There was no appreciable difference in the cephalocaudal distribution of the consolidation between COP and CEP. The most helpful distinguishing feature on CT was the presence of nodules, seen in 32% of patients with COP and only 5% of patients with CEP.[33] In clinical practice the differential diagnosis can be readily made based on clinical history and laboratory tests. Approximately 50% of patients with CEP have asthma, and most patients have peripheral eosinophilia.[34]

The differential diagnosis in patients who present with multiple large nodules and masses includes pulmonary metastases, lymphoma, granulomatosis with polyangiitis, and pulmonary infection, including septic emboli. Although in many cases a confident diagnosis of OP can be made based on the clinical findings and transbronchial biopsy, in some cases video-assisted thoracic surgery biopsy may be required for a definitive diagnosis.[11]

Synopsis of Treatment Options

In most patients the clinical and radiologic findings remit completely after treatment with oral corticosteroids or immunomodulators.[1] In a significant number of patients, however, the disease relapses when medical therapies are reduced or stopped.[1] Fifteen percent of patients with COP have progressive disease.[35,36] Patients with COP and reticular opacities on the chest radiograph or high-resolution CT are less likely to respond to treatment than patients without reticulation. In one study of seven patients with COP who had diffuse reticular opacities on the chest radiograph, three did not improve with steroid therapy, and two died of progressive pulmonary disease.[35] In a more recent study, none of the six patients who had reticular abnormality as the predominant pattern on initial CT showed complete resolution on follow-up imaging.[30] Occasionally, patients with OP may present with a fulminant course, leading to death or severe fibrosis.[37]

KEY POINTS

- Organizing pneumonia (OP) is a common histologic reaction pattern seen in association with or secondary to infections, connective tissue diseases, inflammatory bowel disease, inhalational injury, hypersensitivity pneumonitis, drug reaction, radiation therapy, and aspiration. These conditions must be excluded before making a diagnosis of cryptogenic organizing pneumonia.
- The clinical manifestations frequently mimic pneumonia and include cough, progressive dyspnea, and low-grade fever.
- In the proper clinical context, the presence of bilateral areas of consolidation that are increasing in extent over several weeks despite antibiotics suggests OP. In most patients a diagnosis of OP can be made based on a combination of clinical and radiologic findings and transbronchial biopsy.
- The characteristic high-resolution CT manifestation of OP consists of bilateral areas of consolidation in a peribronchial or subpleural distribution frequently associated with a perilobular pattern. In the subacute to chronic setting the atoll sign or reversed halo sign is quite specific for OP.

SUGGESTED READINGS

ATS/ERS Committee on Idiopathic Interstitial Pneumonias. An official American Thoracic Society/European Respiratory Society statement: update of the international multidisciplinary classification of the idiopathic interstitial pneumonias. *Am J Respir Crit Care Med*. 2013;188(6):733–748.

Kligerman SJ, Franks TJ, Galvin JR. From the radiologic pathology archives: organization and fibrosis as a response to lung injury in diffuse alveolar damage, organizing pneumonia, and acute fibrinous and organizing pneumonia. *Radiographics*. 2013;33(7):1951–1975.

Lynch DA, Travis WD, Müller NL, et al. Idiopathic interstitial pneumonias: CT features. *Radiology*. 2005;236:10–21.

The full reference list for this chapter is available at ExpertConsult.com.

30 Acute Interstitial Pneumonia*

JONATHAN H. CHUNG | CHRISTOPHER M. WALKER

Acute interstitial pneumonia (AIP) is a severe acute disease of unknown etiology that usually occurs in a previously healthy individual and produces histologic findings of diffuse alveolar damage.[1,2] The clinical, radiologic, and pathologic manifestations are identical to those of acute respiratory distress syndrome (ARDS); the only distinction is that no etiology is found. AIP is essentially idiopathic ARDS.[3]

Prevalence and Epidemiology

AIP is rare, has no sex predominance, and has no association with cigarette smoking. The average age at presentation is 50 to 60 years (range, 7–83 years).[1,4]

Clinical Presentation

A prodromal illness associated with symptoms suggestive of a viral upper respiratory tract infection is commonly present, with fever, chills, myalgias, and arthralgias.[1,4] This is followed by dry cough and rapidly progressive and severe dyspnea. Approximately two-thirds of patients have symptoms for less than 1 week, and one-third have symptoms for 60 days before diagnosis.[4]

Pathophysiology

PATHOLOGY

The histologic findings are those of diffuse alveolar damage (Fig. 30.1).[1–3] The acute, exudative phase shows edema, hyaline membranes, acute interstitial inflammation, and intraalveolar hemorrhage. The organizing (proliferative) phase shows loose organizing fibrosis and type II pneumocyte hyperplasia. Patients who survive more than 2 weeks may progress to the chronic phase with fibrosis that may be associated with extensive architectural remodeling resulting in honeycomb formation in severely fibrotic lung or, occasionally, development of cystic changes. There are no histologic features that distinguish diffuse alveolar damage in the setting of AIP from diffuse alveolar damage of known causes.

LUNG FUNCTION

The main functional abnormalities are restrictive ventilatory defect (decrease in total lung capacity and vital capacity) and impaired gas exchange leading to progressive hypoxemic respiratory failure.[4]

Manifestations of the Disease

RADIOGRAPHY

The radiographic manifestations are similar to those of ARDS and consist of bilateral airspace consolidation with air bronchograms (Figs. 30.2 and 30.3).[5,6] The consolidation is often initially patchy but tends to become rapidly confluent and diffuse, although it may have upper or lower lung zone predominance.[5,6] The lung volumes are usually decreased.

COMPUTED TOMOGRAPHY

The earliest manifestations of AIP on high-resolution CT consist mainly of patchy or diffuse bilateral ground-glass opacities (Figs. 30.4 and 30.5).[5,7–9] Most patients have smooth septal thickening and intralobular lines superimposed on the ground-glass opacity resulting in a "crazy paving" pattern (see Figs. 30.4 and 30.5).[8] Focal sparing of lung lobules frequently results in a geographic appearance (Fig. 30.6; see Figs. 30.4 and 30.5).[5,9,10] Consolidation is present in most patients (see Figs. 30.3 and 30.6). It may be patchy or confluent and tends to involve mainly the dependent lung. In 10% to 20% of cases the consolidation has a peripheral distribution.[5,8]

With progression of disease, the ground-glass opacities become diffuse, the areas of consolidation become more extensive, and architectural distortion and traction bronchiectasis become evident on thin-section CT (Fig. 30.7; see Fig. 30.6).[9,10] Honeycombing is seen in 10% to 26% of patients.[5,8] Other findings include small pleural effusions, seen in about 30% of patients, and mild mediastinal lymphadenopathy, present in 5% to 10%.[8]

CT-pathologic correlations have shown that areas of ground-glass opacity and consolidation without traction bronchiectasis occur in the exudative or early proliferative phase of AIP, whereas traction bronchiectasis is seen in the late proliferative and fibrotic phases of AIP.[10] Honeycombing correlates with the presence of dense interstitial fibrosis and restructuring of distal airspaces.[5,10] Patients who survive may have residual mild peripheral reticulation, traction bronchiectasis and bronchiolectasis, and honeycombing.[5]

IMAGING ALGORITHM

The chest radiograph is usually the first imaging modality used to assess patients who present with clinical findings of ARDS. CT is helpful mainly in the evaluation of patients with questionable or nonspecific radiographic findings and in the assessment of suspected complications.

*The editors and the publisher would like to thank Drs. Nestor L. Müller and C. Isabela Silva Müller for contributing material on this topic to the prior edition of this work. It has served as the foundation for the current chapter.

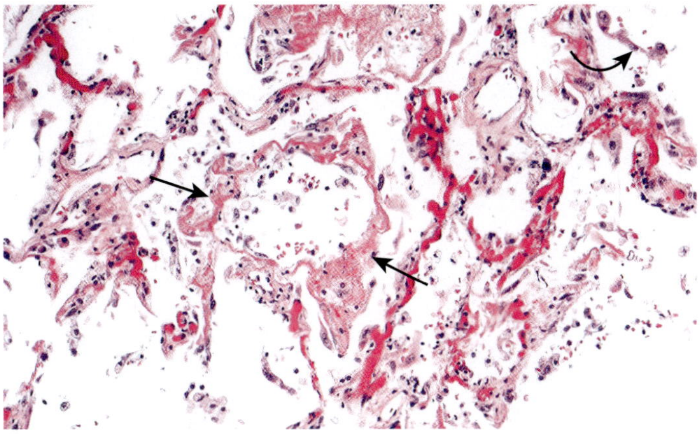

Fig. 30.1 Acute interstitial pneumonia: histologic findings. Micrograph shows hyaline membranes *(straight arrows)* and enlarged alveolar lining cells *(curved arrow)*, typical of diffuse alveolar damage (hematoxylin-eosin, 200×). *(Courtesy Dr. Andrew Churg, Department of Pathology, University of British Columbia, Vancouver, Canada.)*

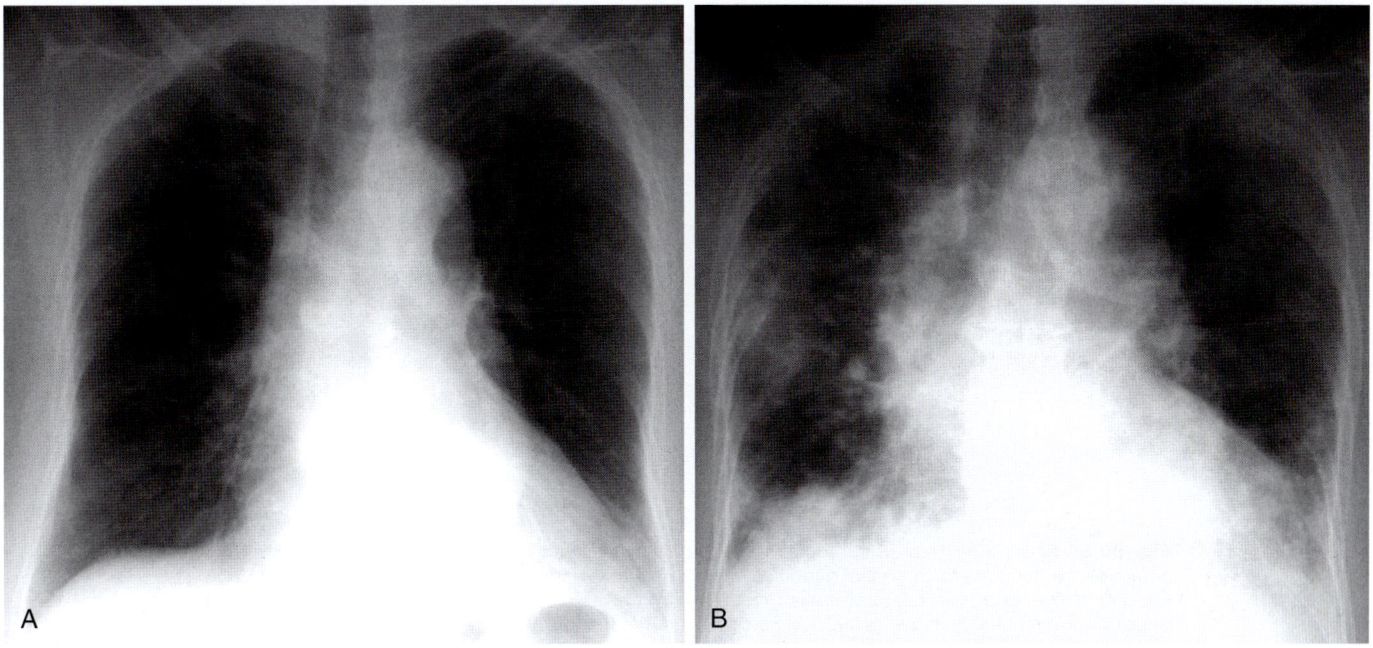

Fig. 30.2 Acute interstitial pneumonia: radiographic findings. (A) Chest radiograph is within normal limits except for the presence of mild scarring in the right upper lobe as a result of previous tuberculosis. (B) Chest radiograph 11 months later, when the patient developed acute shortness of breath, shows extensive bilateral consolidation. Surgical biopsy specimen revealed characteristic findings of diffuse alveolar damage. The diagnosis of acute interstitial pneumonia was made clinically after exclusion of known causes of acute respiratory distress syndrome.

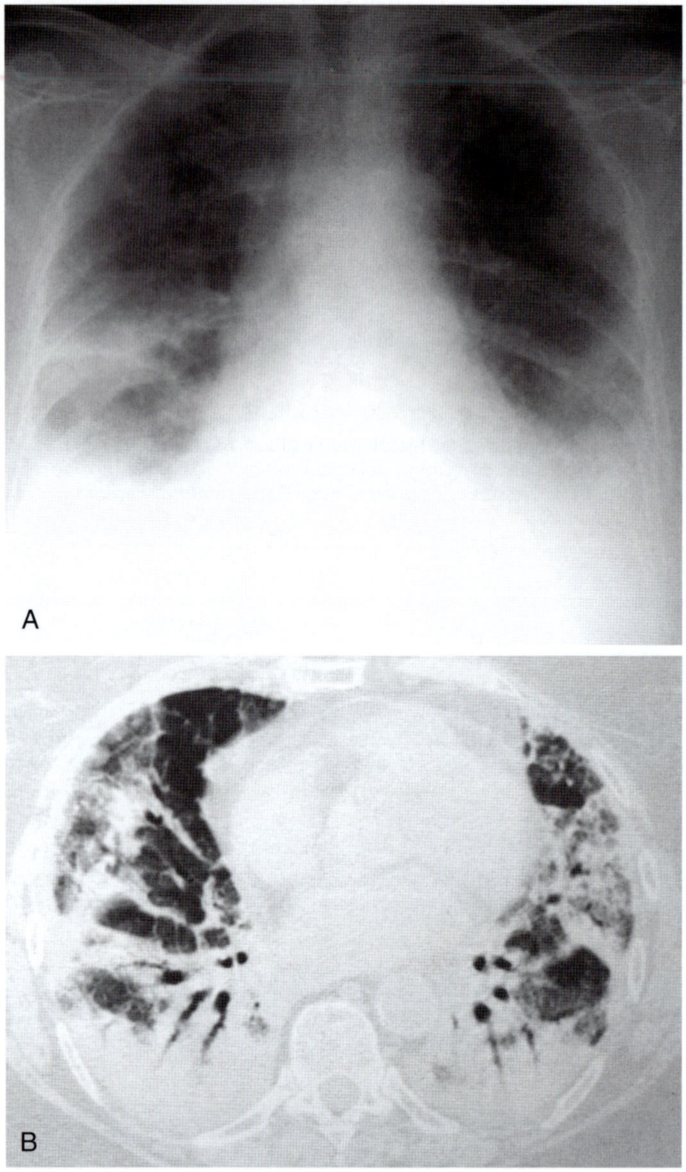

Fig. 30.3 Acute interstitial pneumonia: radiographic and CT findings. (A) Chest radiograph shows extensive bilateral areas of consolidation involving mainly the lower lung zones. (B) High-resolution CT scan shows extensive bilateral areas of consolidation with air bronchograms in a peripheral and dependent distribution. Focal ground-glass opacities are also noted.

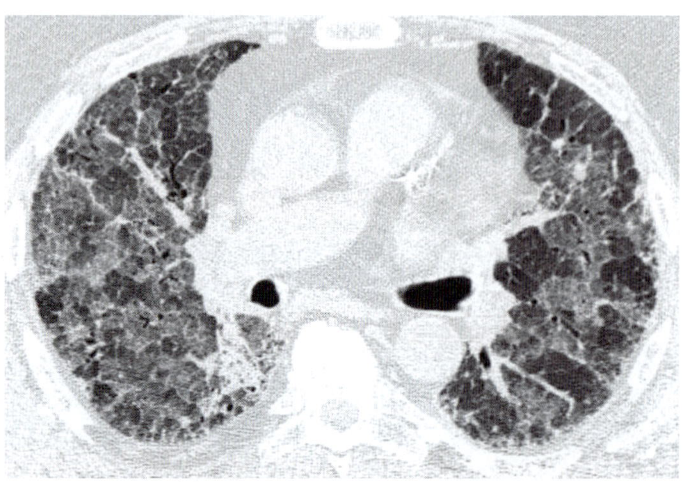

Fig. 30.4 Acute interstitial pneumonia: high-resolution CT findings. High-resolution CT scan shows extensive bilateral ground-glass opacities. Smooth septal thickening and intralobular lines are seen superimposed on the ground-glass opacities ("crazy paving" pattern) mainly in the right lung. Relative sparing of some of the secondary lobules results in a geographic appearance.

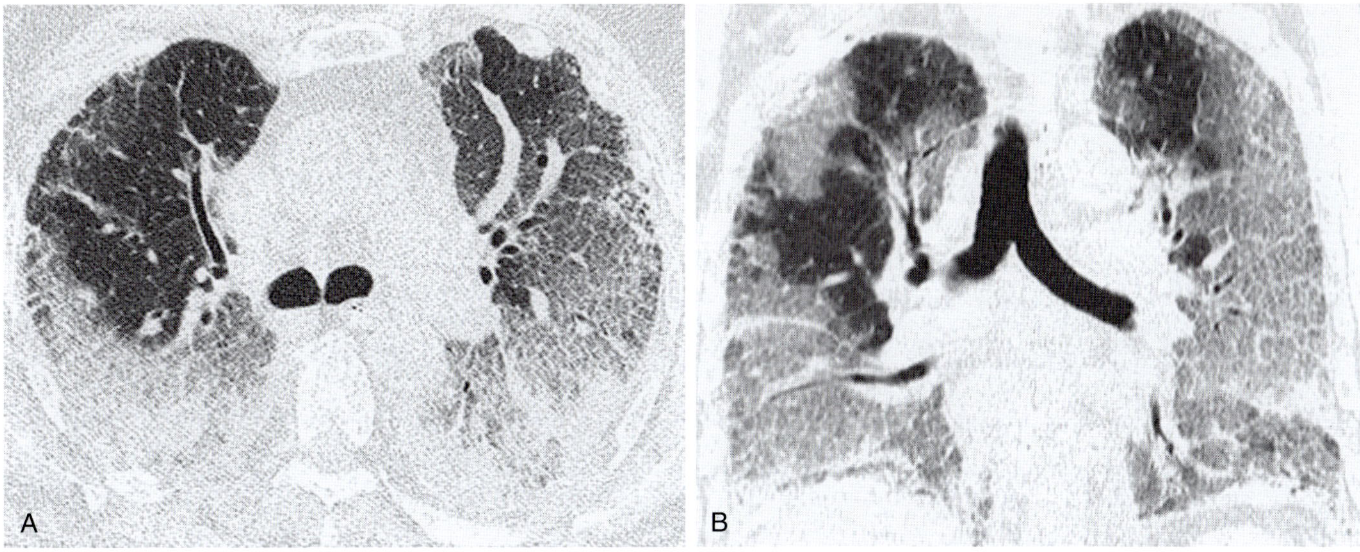

Fig. 30.5 Acute interstitial pneumonia: "crazy paving" pattern. (A) High-resolution CT scan shows bilateral ground-glass opacities with superimposed smooth linear opacities ("crazy paving" pattern) and dependent areas of consolidation. (B) Coronal reformation shows extensive bilateral ground-glass opacities and crazy paving pattern mainly in the left lung. Note relative sparing of some of the secondary lobules resulting in a geographic appearance.

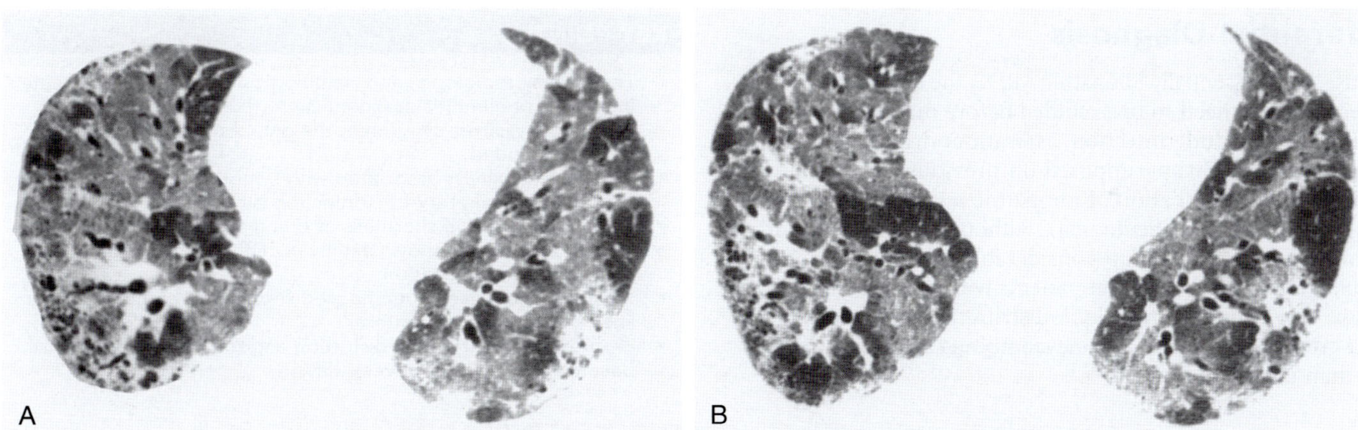

Fig. 30.6 Acute interstitial pneumonia: high-resolution CT findings. (A) and (B) High-resolution CT scans show extensive bilateral ground-glass opacities and small foci of consolidation. Mild traction bronchiectasis and bronchiolectasis are also noted. Relative sparing of some of the secondary lobules results in a geographic appearance.

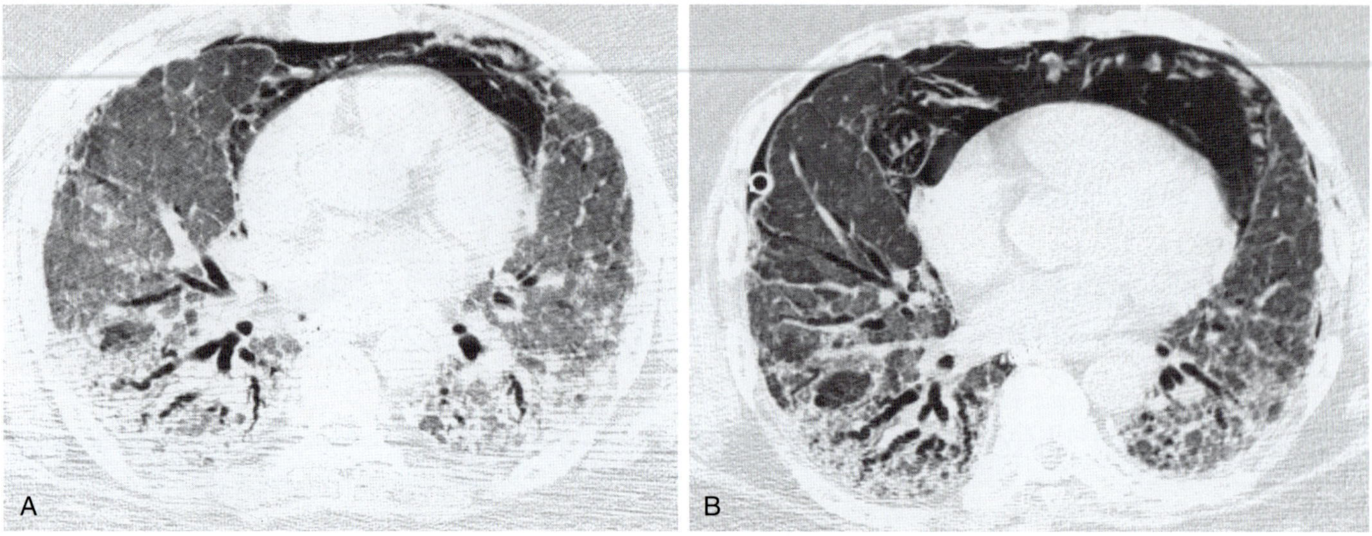

Fig. 30.7 Acute interstitial pneumonia: high-resolution CT findings on follow-up. (A) High-resolution CT scan performed a few days after hospital admission in newly diagnosed acute interstitial pneumonia shows extensive bilateral ground-glass opacities, dependent areas of consolidation, pneumomediastinum, and traction bronchiectasis and bronchiolectasis. (B) High-resolution CT scan 5 days later shows that the extent of dependent consolidation has decreased, but there is increased reticulation and traction bronchiectasis and bronchiolectasis. Extensive ground-glass opacities persist. Small bilateral pneumothoraces are present, and the pneumomediastinum has increased. A chest tube is in the right pleural space.

Differential Diagnosis

Because AIP is essentially idiopathic ARDS, the numerous possible causes of ARDS need to be excluded before making a diagnosis of AIP. These include infection, aspiration, drug-induced lung disease, and ARDS superimposed on previous interstitial lung disease (acute exacerbation of idiopathic pulmonary fibrosis or nonspecific interstitial pneumonia).[1] Although the high-resolution CT findings of AIP overlap considerably with the findings of ARDS, it has been shown that patients with AIP are more likely to have a symmetric lower lobe distribution of abnormalities and a greater prevalence of honeycombing (26% of patients vs. 8%) than patients with ARDS.[11]

Synopsis of Treatment Options

Patients usually require mechanical ventilation and are treated with corticosteroids. The prognosis is poor, with the mortality greater than 50% in most studies.[2–4] Patients with greater extent of ground-glass opacity or airspace consolidation without traction bronchiolectasis or bronchiectasis on high-resolution CT have been shown to have a better prognosis than patients with greater extent of either ground-glass opacity or airspace consolidation combined with traction bronchiolectasis or bronchiectasis.[12]

KEY POINTS

- The clinical, radiologic, and pathologic manifestations of acute interstitial pneumonia are identical to those of acute respiratory distress syndrome; the only distinction is that no etiology is found.
- A prodromal illness associated with symptoms suggestive of a viral upper respiratory tract infection is commonly present.
- Rapidly progressive shortness of breath occurs.
- Radiography or CT shows patchy or diffuse ground-glass opacities or consolidation.
- Most patients have superimposed septal lines and intralobular lines ("crazy paving" pattern).
- Progressive architectural distortion and traction bronchiectasis become evident after several days.

SUGGESTED READINGS

ATS/ERS Committee on Idiopathic Interstitial Pneumonias. An official American Thoracic Society/European Respiratory Society statement: update of the international multidisciplinary classification of the idiopathic interstitial pneumonias. *Am J Respir Crit Care Med.* 2013;188(6):733–748.

Sverzellati N, Lynch DA, Hansell DM, Johkoh T, King TE Jr, Travis WD. American Thoracic Society-European Respiratory Society Classification of the Idiopathic Interstitial Pneumonias: Advances in Knowledge since 2002. *Radiographics.* 2015;35(7):1849–1871.

The full reference list for this chapter is available at ExpertConsult.com.

31 Sarcoidosis*

JONATHAN H. CHUNG | CHRISTOPHER M. WALKER

Sarcoidosis is a systemic inflammatory disorder of unknown etiology that affects multiple organs and is characterized by the formation of noncaseating granulomas.[1] Intrathoracic lymph node and pulmonary parenchymal involvement occurs in more than 90% of cases. The granulomas have a characteristic distribution along the lymphatics in the pleura, interlobular septa, and bronchovascular bundles.[2] They may resolve spontaneously or with treatment or progress to fibrosis.

Etiology

The etiology is unknown. The presence of familial clustering and the racial variation in incidence suggest an important genetic contribution.[3] Clustering during certain times, in specific regions, and in close acquaintances of affected patients and variations in incidence with season indicate that environmental influences also have an important effect.[4,5] The nature of the immunologic disturbances suggests that sarcoidosis results from exposure of genetically susceptible individuals to specific environmental agents that trigger an exaggerated cellular immune response leading to granuloma formation.[6] Whether coincidental or linked via common susceptibility or exposure, sarcoidosis has been described in association with a variety of connective tissue disorders, including rheumatoid arthritis, ankylosing spondylitis, systemic lupus erythematosus, and progressive systemic sclerosis.[7]

Prevalence and Epidemiology

Sarcoidosis may occur at any age, but the disease is recognized most commonly in patients 20 to 40 years old and is slightly more common in women.[6] A second peak in incidence occurs in women older than 50 years.

There is considerable variation in the reported incidences and prevalences in different populations. Sarcoidosis is particularly common in African Americans, especially women. It is common in Scandinavian countries and Ireland and is seldom reported in South America and China.[4,8] The estimated lifetime incidence of sarcoidosis in the United States is 2.4% for African Americans and 0.85% for whites.[4] African Americans also have more severe lung disease than whites on presentation and a worse prognosis.[4] Sarcoidosis also is more prevalent in Irish living in London than in native Londoners and more prevalent in natives of Martinique living in France than in indigenous French.[4] Although the incidence in most nations of continental Europe is less than 1 per 100,000, the incidence in Scandinavian countries, such as Sweden (64 per 100,000) and Finland (11 per 100,000) is considerably higher.[4] Approximately 1 per 100,000 new cases of sarcoidosis are reported in Japan.[4] Overall mortality from sarcoidosis is 1% to 5%.[6]

Clinical Presentation

Approximately 30% to 50% of patients are asymptomatic, sarcoidosis being first suspected based on the presence of bilateral hilar lymphadenopathy on routine chest radiographs, and approximately 50% present with pulmonary symptoms. The most common pulmonary complaints are dyspnea, cough, and chest pain.[4,9] The mechanism for the development of chest pain is unclear.[9] Constitutional symptoms are common and include weight loss, fatigue, weakness, and malaise. Symptoms often develop insidiously and are frequently associated with evidence of multisystem involvement, most commonly the lungs, heart, skin, and eyes. In a study of 189 patients, 52% presented with pulmonary symptoms (26% with pulmonary symptoms alone), 13% with skin concerns, 6% with systemic symptoms, and 16% with other manifestations.[10] A characteristic acute manifestation is Löfgren syndrome, a triad of bilateral hilar lymphadenopathy, erythema nodosum, and polyarticular arthralgia, which is seen in 20% to 50% of patients with acute disease.[4] An acute onset of symptoms, usually with erythema nodosum, is particularly common in Scandinavian, Puerto Rican, and Irish women.

Five percent of patients with sarcoidosis develop pulmonary arterial hypertension.[11] The severity of pulmonary hypertension does not correlate well with the degree of pulmonary fibrosis and has been reported as an early primary manifestation of sarcoidosis, suggesting that other mechanisms may play a role. Such mechanisms include extrinsic compression of large pulmonary arteries or veins by enlarged lymph nodes, granulomatous vascular involvement, and pulmonary vasoconstriction by vasoactive factors.[11]

Myocardial involvement is evident at autopsy in approximately 25% of patients with sarcoidosis, but only approximately half of these patients have clinical evidence of myocardial involvement during their lifetime.[12] In the United States cardiac involvement accounts for 13% to 25% of deaths from sarcoidosis.[12] In Japan sarcoid heart disease is more common and responsible for 85% of deaths from sarcoidosis.[12] The most common cardiac manifestation of sarcoidosis is complete heart block. Other findings include atrial arrhythmias, congestive heart failure, ventricular aneurysm, rhythm disturbances, cor pulmonale caused by pulmonary hypertension, valvular regurgitation, or a combination of these processes.[12] Pericardial effusions occur in approximately 5% to 15% of patients with sarcoidosis, but they are usually small.[12]

Ocular involvement manifests in 25% to 60% of patients with systemic sarcoidosis.[13] The most common ocular manifestation is uveitis. More than 80% of uveitis cases manifest before or within 1 year after the onset of systemic disease. Ocular disease may progress to severe visual impairment or even blindness.[13]

Cutaneous involvement occurs in approximately 25% of patients and may be specific (granulomas present pathologically)

*The editors and the publisher would like to thank Drs. Nestor L. Müller and C. Isabela Silva Müller for contributing material on this topic to the prior edition of this work. It has served as the foundation for the current chapter.

or nonspecific.[14] The most frequent nonspecific abnormality is erythema nodosum.[15] This inflammatory reaction is a form of panniculitis that most commonly involves the shins and is characterized by the development of crops of transient, nonulcerating nodules that are generally tender, multiple, and bilateral. Erythema nodosum is the hallmark of acute sarcoidosis and is associated with a high rate of spontaneous resolution.[14] Lupus pernio ("purple lupus") is a chronic plaque-type, indurated, brown-to-purple lesion that progresses slowly and is usually located on the face, neck, shoulders, and digits and sometimes on the mucous membrane of the nose; it is often associated with involvement of the nasal bones.[14] Large plaques resembling psoriasis may develop over the trunk or extremities. Lupus pernio and plaques generally are associated with a chronic course and seldom, if ever, resolve completely.

Granulomas can be found in the liver and spleen at autopsy in approximately 75% of patients; however, palpable enlargement of these organs is seen in only 20%. Most such disease causes no symptoms. Occasionally, hepatic involvement may be associated with jaundice, chronic cholestasis, cirrhosis, and portal hypertension.[16]

Inflammatory arthralgia, which may be monarticular or polyarticular, occurs in 25% to 40% of patients with sarcoidosis.[6] The joints most commonly affected are the knees, ankles, elbows, and wrists. Symptoms are usually self-limited but occasionally recur.[17] True arthritis is uncommon.

Clinical or functional evidence of renal disease is uncommon despite the fact that granulomas are found in the kidneys in 5% to 20% of autopsied patients. Renal complications are usually secondary to the abnormal calcium metabolism in patients with sarcoidosis, which may result in hypercalcemia, hypercalciuria, and occasionally nephrocalcinosis, urolithiasis, or hypercalcemic renal failure.[18] Hypercalcemia occurs in about 2% to 10% of patients; hypercalciuria is about three times more frequent.[6] These abnormalities are due to dysregulated production of 1,25-$(OH)_2$-D_3 (calcitriol) by activated macrophages and granulomas.[6] Aside from the renal effects of hypercalcemia, metastatic calcification can occur in organs and tissues other than the kidney, including the eyes, lungs, and blood vessels.

Neurologic symptoms occur in 5% of patients with sarcoidosis.[19] The most common manifestations are cranial nerve palsies, headache, seizures, sensory and motor deficits, cerebellar symptoms, and neuropsychological deficits.[19] Cranial palsies are seen in 50% of patients with neurologic involvement. Although any cranial nerve can be affected, the facial nerve is the most commonly involved.[19] Psychiatric manifestations include delirium, psychosis, and personality change.

Pathophysiology

PATHOLOGY

Sarcoidosis is characterized by accumulation of large numbers of activated macrophages and T lymphocytes.[4] These cells release Th1-predominant cytokines, including interferon-γ, tumor necrosis factor-α, and various interleukins, and result in granuloma formation. The etiology of the initial stimulus and the reason why the granuloma formation is persistent are unknown.[4]

The histologic diagnosis of pulmonary sarcoidosis relies on three main findings: (1) the presence of tight, well-formed granulomas and a rim of lymphocytes and fibroblasts in the outer margin of granulomas; (2) perilymphatic interstitial distribution of granulomas; and (3) exclusion of an alternative cause.[6] The pathologic hallmark of sarcoidosis is the granuloma, composed of a central core of tightly clustered epithelioid histiocytes and occasional multinucleated giant cells surrounded by varying quantities of fibroblasts and collagen (Fig. 31.1).[2] Most granulomas are nonnecrotizing; however, some may show a small amount of central fibrinoid necrosis.[2] Fibroblasts are present at the periphery of more "mature" granulomas, and it seems that the fibrosis begins at this site.[20] In this circumstance concentric lamellae of collagen can be seen to separate the histologically "active" central portion of the granuloma from the adjacent tissue. With time the fibrosis proceeds inward until the entire granuloma is converted into a scar. This pattern of peripheral lamellar fibrosis is characteristic of healing sarcoidosis and is itself evidence in favor of the diagnosis.[20]

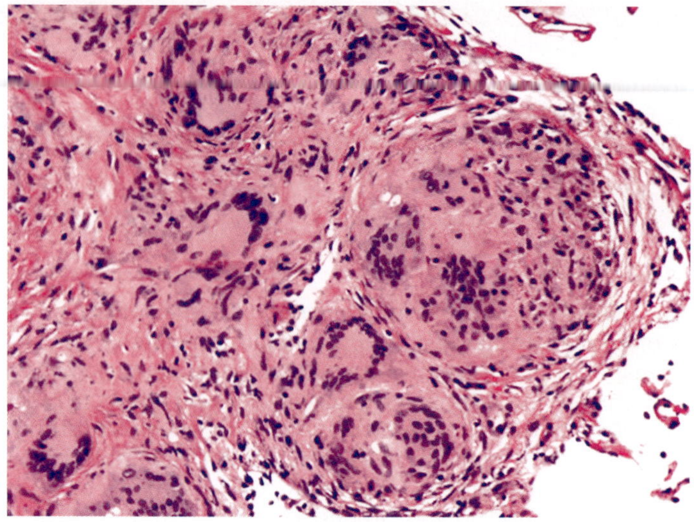

Fig. 31.1 Sarcoid granuloma. Histologic specimen shows characteristic well-formed sarcoid granulomas, central core of tightly clustered epithelioid histiocytes, and occasional multinucleated giant cells surrounded by varying quantities of fibroblasts and collagen. *(Courtesy Dr. Patrick O'Connor, Department of Pathology, Vancouver General Hospital, Vancouver, Canada.)*

The sarcoid granulomas have a characteristic perilymphatic distribution, pulmonary involvement being characteristically most prominent in the peribronchovascular, interlobular septal, and pleural interstitial tissue (Fig. 31.2).[2,21] In the early stages granulomas are discrete and histologically "active"; as the disease progresses, they often become confluent and undergo fibrosis, which results in more or less diffuse interstitial thickening.[20] The parenchymal interstitium also may be affected, although typically much less than in peribronchovascular, septal, and pleural locations. Possibly, because of the prominent peribronchovascular (Fig. 31.3) and septal location of the granulomatous inflammation, involvement of pulmonary arteries and veins is common.[20]

The gross appearance of pulmonary sarcoidosis depends on the stage and severity of disease. In the early, milder forms in which inflammation is most prominent in relation to peribronchovascular, interlobular, and pleural connective tissue, the appearance can resemble lymphangitic carcinomatosis. As disease progresses, involvement of the parenchymal interstitium becomes more evident, and entire lobules can be replaced by granulomas and fibrous tissue.[20] This process is usually most severe in the upper lobes, where it can take the form of more or less solid

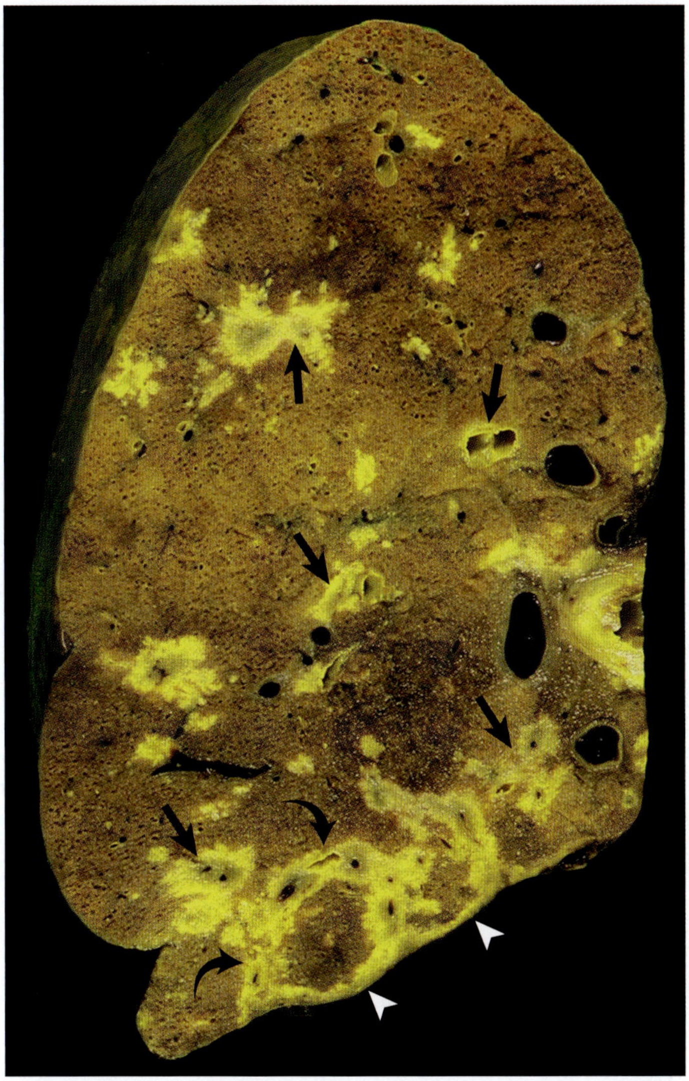

Fig. 31.2 Perilymphatic distribution of sarcoid granulomas. Surgical specimen from a lobectomy in a patient with sarcoidosis shows characteristic perilymphatic distribution of granulomas along bronchi and vessels *(straight arrows)*, interlobular septa *(curved arrows)*, and interlobar fissure *(arrowheads)*. *(Modified from Müller NL, Miller RR: Computed tomography of chronic diffuse infiltrative lung disease, part 2.* Am Rev Respir Dis. *1990;142:1440–1448.)*

areas of fibrous tissue associated with traction bronchiectasis.[20] The latter may be the site of aspergilloma formation.

Lymph node involvement is characterized by more or less diffuse replacement of the node by granulomas, often with a variable histologic appearance.[22] Initially, the granulomas are discrete and appear "active"; as in pulmonary disease, however, they tend to become confluent and undergo progressive fibrosis over time. In advanced disease this process can result in completely fibrotic nodes in which granulomas are difficult to recognize.

LUNG FUNCTION

Most patients with sarcoidosis and abnormal lung function have restrictive abnormalities; however, many have an obstructive deficit as well.[23] In a few patients the pattern is solely obstructive.[24] The frequency of airflow obstruction is greater in patients with

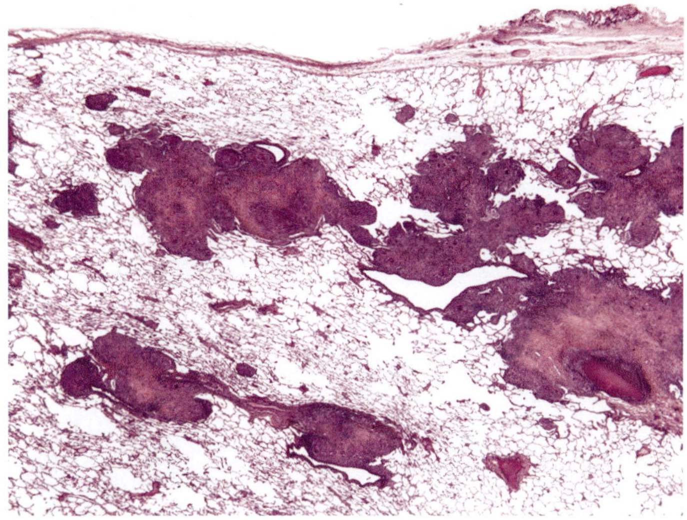

Fig. 31.3 Predominant peribronchial distribution of sarcoid granulomas. Histologic specimen shows well-formed confluent noncaseating granulomas adjacent to bronchioles. *(Courtesy Dr. John English, Department of Pathology, Vancouver General Hospital, Vancouver, Canada.)*

extensive fibrosis, older age, and smoking history.[25,26] Cigarette smoking seems to be the most important determinant of airflow obstruction in these patients,[27] although pulmonary fibrosis also plays an important role.[26] Restrictive lung function is manifested by a reduction in total lung capacity and vital capacity and obstructive lung function by reduction in the forced expiratory volume at 1 second–to–forced vital capacity ratio and by air-trapping (increase in the residual volume–to–total lung capacity ratio). Sarcoid patients also may have impairment in gas transfer as assessed by the carbon monoxide diffusing capacity and an increase in the alveolar-arterial oxygen gradient.

Manifestations of the Disease

RADIOGRAPHY

Radiographic abnormalities can be classified into five stages, as follows:[6,28]

Stage 0: No demonstrable abnormality

Stage I: Hilar and mediastinal lymph node enlargement without parenchymal abnormality (Fig. 31.4)

Stage II: Hilar and mediastinal lymph node enlargement plus parenchymal abnormality (Fig. 31.5)

Stage III: Parenchymal abnormality alone (Fig. 31.6)

Stage IV: Advanced fibrosis with evidence of reticulation, architectural distortion, hilar retraction, and occasionally honeycombing (Fig. 31.7)

In a multicentric case-control study of 736 patients with sarcoidosis, approximately 8% had stage 0, 40% had stage I, 37% had stage II, 10% had stage III, and 5% had stage IV disease.[28] The main utility of this staging system is in predicting outcome. Spontaneous remissions occur in 55% to 90% of patients with stage I disease, in 40% to 70% of patients with stage II, in 10% to 20% of patients with stage III disease, and in 0% of patients with stage IV sarcoidosis.[6]

The radiographic staging scheme applies only to the chest radiograph.[29] High-resolution computed tomography (CT) may show parenchymal abnormalities in patients with radiographic

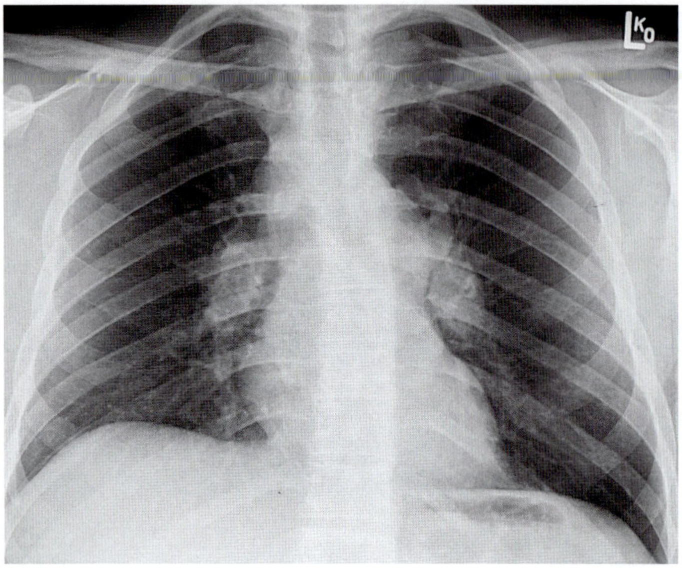

Fig. 31.4 Stage I sarcoidosis: radiographic findings. Posteroanterior chest radiograph in a man with sarcoidosis shows right paratracheal, aorticopulmonary window, and symmetric bilateral hilar lymph node enlargement.

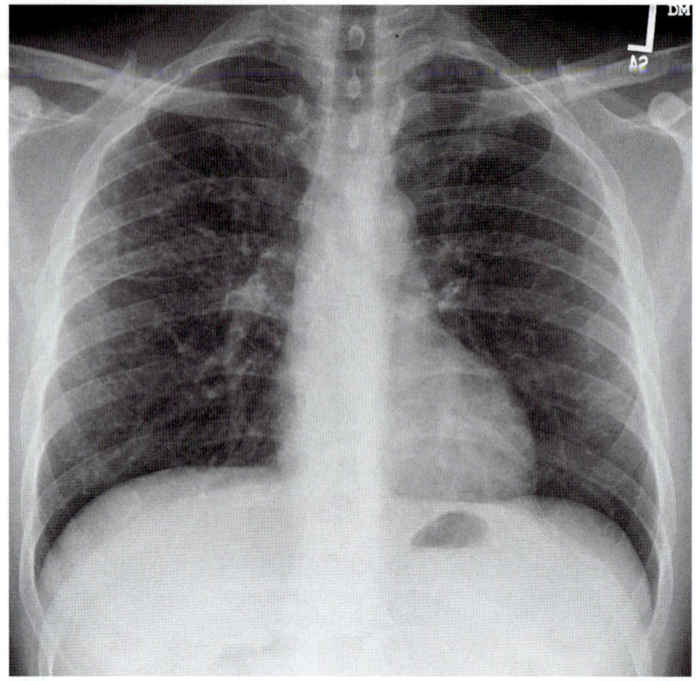

Fig. 31.6 Stage III sarcoidosis: radiographic findings. Posteroanterior chest radiograph in a man with sarcoidosis (same patient as Fig. 31.5A 4 years later) shows a reticulonodular pattern involving mainly the upper and middle lung zones. There is no evidence of hilar or mediastinal lymph node enlargement.

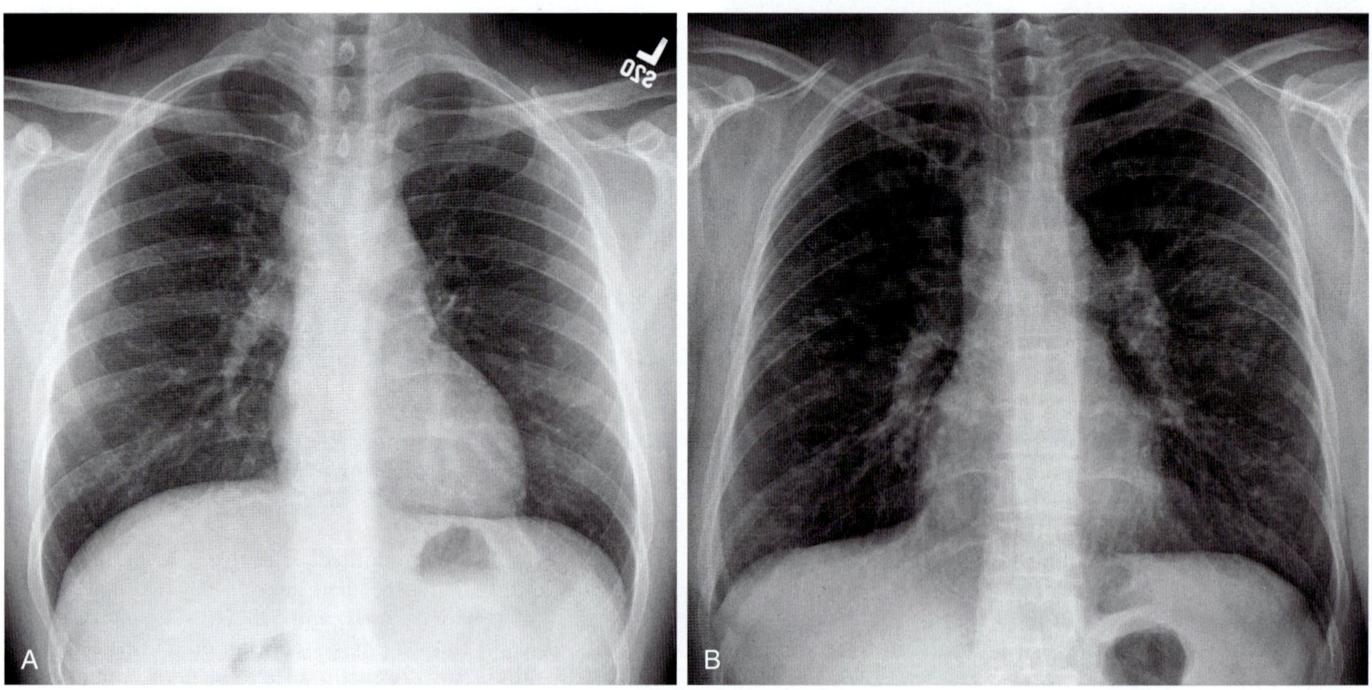

Fig. 31.5 Stage II sarcoidosis: radiographic findings. (A) Posteroanterior chest radiograph in a man with sarcoidosis shows right paratracheal, aorticopulmonary window, and symmetric bilateral hilar lymph node enlargement and small round and irregular opacities in the upper lung zones. Note medial deviation of the gastric bubble owing to splenomegaly. (B) Posteroanterior chest radiograph in a different patient with sarcoidosis shows more extensive parenchymal abnormalities characterized by small nodular opacities involving mainly the upper and middle lung zones. Symmetric bilateral hilar and right paratracheal lymphadenopathy also is noted.

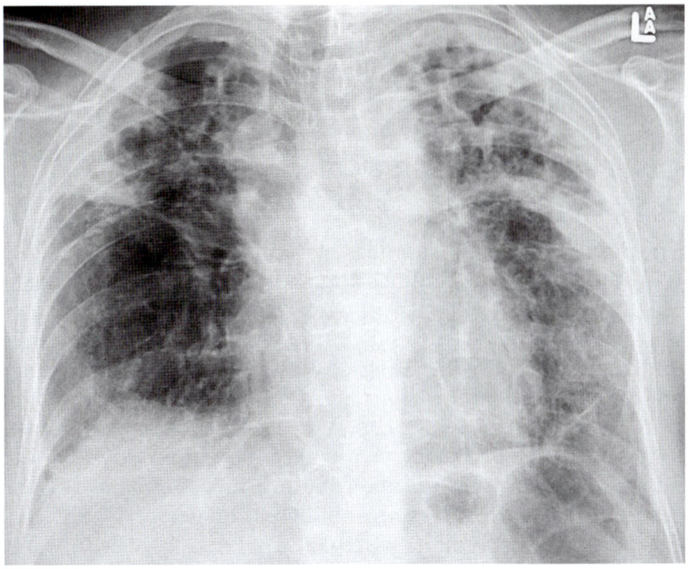

Fig. 31.7 Stage IV sarcoidosis: radiographic findings. Posteroanterior chest radiograph in a middle-aged woman with sarcoidosis shows a coarse reticulonodular pattern involving mainly the upper lobes. Note bilateral elevation of the hila and distortion of the lung architecture characteristic of fibrosis.

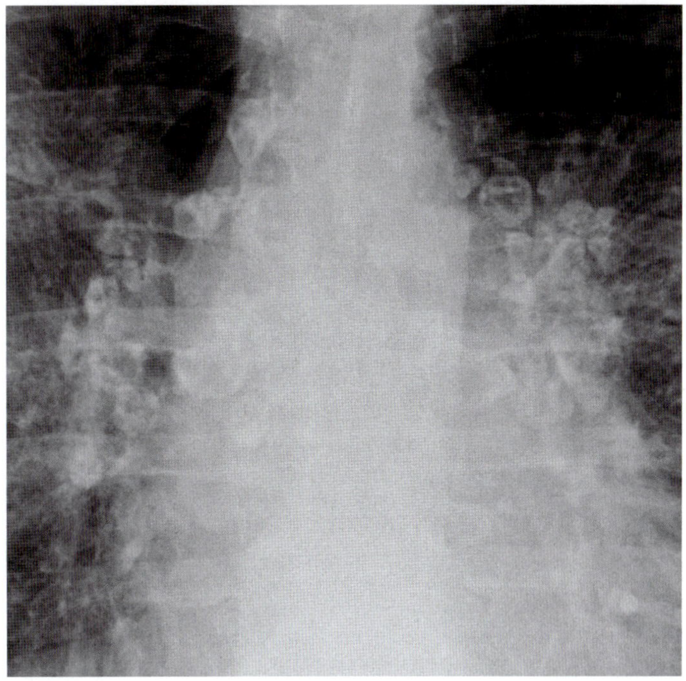

Fig. 31.8 Sarcoidosis: lymph node calcification. Magnified view of the middle and lower mediastinum from a posteroanterior chest radiograph shows extensive lymph node calcification. Most nodes show an eggshell pattern of calcification.

stage I disease; these abnormalities tend to be relatively mild and are unlikely to change the prognosis in these patients.[29]

Lymph Node Enlargement Without Pulmonary Abnormality

Lymph node enlargement without parenchymal disease is seen on the initial chest radiograph in approximately 40% of patients.[28] The combination of bilateral hilar and right paratracheal lymph node enlargement is a characteristic and common manifestation (see Fig. 31.4). Less common sites with lymphadenopathy evident on the radiograph include the aorticopulmonary window, subcarinal region, and anterior mediastinum. Hilar lymph node enlargement is usually bilateral and symmetric. Unilateral enlargement is uncommon, being reported in only 3% to 5% of proven cases.[30] Occasionally, hilar nodal enlargement is sufficient to compress adjacent bronchi and lead to atelectasis (most commonly involving the middle lobe).[31] Calcification of hilar lymph nodes is radiographically apparent in approximately 5% of patients initially and in more than 20% after 10 years of follow-up.[32] Eggshell calcification of hilar and mediastinal nodes may occur but is uncommon (Fig. 31.8).[31]

As with other interstitial diseases, the lungs can be involved by sarcoidosis in the absence of a demonstrable abnormality on the chest radiograph. The chest radiograph is normal (stage 0) in about 10% of patients who have biopsy-proven pulmonary sarcoidosis. Similarly, in a study of 21 consecutive patients with stage I disease who underwent surgical lung biopsy, typical sarcoid granulomas were present in the lung parenchyma in all; however, the extent of granulomatous inflammation was significantly less than that seen in lung biopsy specimens of patients who had radiographic evidence of diffuse lung involvement.[33] As might be expected, parenchymal abnormalities are seen more commonly on high-resolution CT scans than on radiography.[34]

Approximately 55% to 90% of patients who have stage I disease show complete radiographic resolution.[6] Occasionally, enlarged hilar and mediastinal nodes regress to normal size, only to undergo enlargement again at a later date. Node enlargement can persist unchanged for many years.

Diffuse Pulmonary Disease With or Without Lymph Node Enlargement

Parenchymal disease is seen on the chest radiograph at initial evaluation in approximately 55% of patients. This includes approximately 35% to 40% of patients with parenchymal disease associated with enlarged nodes (stage II), 10% with parenchymal disease not associated with enlarged nodes (stage III), and 5% with interstitial fibrosis (stage IV).[28]

The parenchymal abnormalities are typically bilateral and symmetric and involve mainly the upper lung zones in 50% to 80% of patients (see Figs. 31.5 and 31.6).[35,36] Occasionally, disease is asymmetric, unilateral, or diffuse (Fig. 31.9). The most frequent patterns are nodular and reticulonodular; less commonly, a reticular pattern, airspace consolidation, or, rarely, ground-glass opacities predominate.[29,37]

Nodular Pattern. A nodular pattern is present on chest radiographs in 30% to 60% of patients.[38,39] The nodules usually have irregular margins and involve mainly the middle and upper lung zones. They range from 1 to 10 mm in diameter, although most measure less than 3 mm (see Fig. 31.5).

Reticulonodular Pattern. A reticulonodular pattern is present in 25% to 50% of patients who have radiographically evident parenchymal abnormalities.[37,38] The pattern may result from a combination of nodules and thickening of the interlobular septa or a combination of nodules and intralobular linear opacities (see Fig. 31.9).

Parenchymal Consolidation. Parenchymal consolidation is present in 10% to 20% of patients who have sarcoidosis and

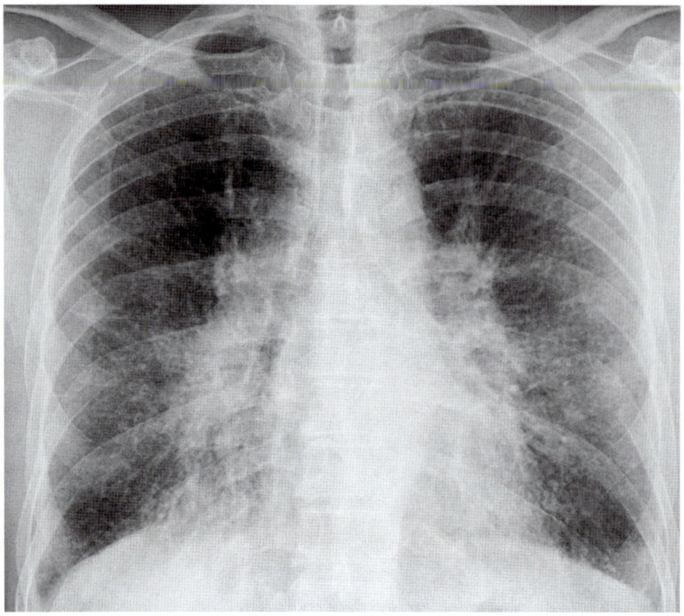

Fig. 31.9 Sarcoidosis: reticulonodular pattern. Posteroanterior chest radiograph shows diffuse reticulonodular pattern. Paratracheal, aorticopulmonary window, and symmetric bilateral hilar lymph node enlargement also is noted.

radiographically evident parenchymal disease.[34,40] The consolidation typically has a bilateral and symmetric distribution involving mainly the middle and upper lung zones (Fig. 31.10).

Fibrosis. Fibrosis is seen at presentation in approximately 5% of patients and eventually develops in 20% to 25% of patients.[28,41] The fibrosis in sarcoidosis typically involves mainly the perihilar regions of the middle and upper lung zones (Fig. 31.11).[42] It is usually associated with superior retraction of the hila, distortion of the bronchovascular bundles, bulla formation, traction bronchiectasis, and compensatory overinflation of the lower lobes.[42]

Cavitation and Mycetoma Formation. Cavitation is an uncommon manifestation of sarcoidosis and usually is seen in association with other parenchymal abnormalities. The cavities may resolve spontaneously or be complicated by superimposed infection or fungus ball formation (mycetoma).[43] Mycetomas develop in 1% to 3% of patients with sarcoidosis.[29,44] They typically occur in the upper lobes in patients with advanced (radiographic stage III or IV) sarcoidosis (Fig. 31.12).[29,44] The mycetomas are most often located in foci of bronchiectasis but also may be seen in bullae or cavities of uncertain origin.[45]

Pleural Disease. Pleural effusion has been documented in about 3% of patients.[31] Affected individuals typically have moderately advanced pulmonary sarcoidosis; nonnecrotizing granulomas are often identified on pleural biopsy. The effusion tends to clear in 4 to 8 weeks but may progress to chronic pleural thickening. Spontaneous pneumothorax has been estimated to occur in about 1% of patients.[46]

Cardiovascular Disease. Although abnormalities of the heart, pericardium, and pulmonary vasculature are commonly seen on histologic examination, they are usually of insufficient severity to cause radiographic manifestations. Radiographically evident enlargement of the cardiac silhouette may be the result of cardiomyopathy, valvular disease, pericardial effusion, or left ventricular aneurysm.[47] Pulmonary hypertension and cor pulmonale, caused by a combination of obliteration of the pulmonary vascular bed and hypoxic vasoconstriction, tend to occur in the late stage of the disease.

COMPUTED TOMOGRAPHY

Pulmonary Manifestations

The high-resolution CT findings of pulmonary sarcoidosis closely reflect the histologic findings and show a characteristic pattern of small nodules in a perilymphatic distribution.[21] The nodules are seen mainly adjacent to the bronchi and pulmonary arteries and veins and along the interlobular septa, interlobar fissures, and costal subpleural regions and result in nodular thickening of these structures (Figs. 31.13 and 31.14).[34,48,49] Sarcoid granulomas along the peribronchovascular interstitium extend to the peribronchiolar interstitium, resulting in prominence of the centrilobular core and centrilobular nodules (see Fig. 31.14). Although the distribution of sarcoidosis is typically perilymphatic, there is considerable variation in the extent to which it affects the various perilymphatic compartments. In some patients it is predominantly peribronchial or perivascular and in others predominantly subpleural; only occasionally does it involve mainly the interlobular septa. Although nodular septal thickening is commonly present, it is seldom extensive (Fig. 31.15), as this pattern is more commonly seen with lymphangitic carcinomatosis. Occasionally, the nodules may be small and result in a diffuse miliary pattern (Fig. 31.16) or involve predominantly or exclusively the subpleural lung regions. Conglomeration of subpleural granulomas in the costal regions may resemble pleural plaques (pseudoplaques) (Fig. 31.17).

Nodules are seen on high-resolution CT at initial evaluation in 90% to 100% of patients with parenchymal abnormalities secondary to sarcoidosis.[34,48] The nodules and the nodular thickening of the perilymphatic interstitium seen on high-resolution CT reflect confluence of microscopic granulomas.[21,50] The nodules may have smooth or irregular margins, are typically well defined, and most commonly measure 2 to 5 mm in diameter. Confluence of granulomas also may result in large nodules or masses measuring 1 to 4 cm in diameter, which are seen in 15% to 25% of patients (Fig. 31.18).[34,50] The large nodules predominate in the upper lobes and the peribronchovascular regions. The margins of these larger confluent nodules are typically poorly defined and demonstrate a combination of reticular and micronodular opacities, which has been labeled the galaxy sign.[51] Large nodules occasionally may cavitate.[35]

Extensive microscopic interstitial granulomas also may result in ground-glass opacities (Figs. 31.19 and 31.20) or areas of consolidation (see Fig. 31.10), usually superimposed on a background of interstitial nodules or fibrosis.[34,50] The areas of consolidation may be peribronchial or, less commonly, peripheral in distribution (see Fig. 31.10).[52] Air bronchograms can be seen in most cases.

Follow-up CT scans in patients with pulmonary sarcoidosis have shown that nodules, interlobular septal thickening, ground-glass opacities, and consolidation represent potentially reversible disease (Figs. 31.21 and 31.22).[53,54] Irregular lines and reticular opacities are usually irreversible but occasionally may improve or resolve.[54] Architectural distortion and honeycombing represent irreversible disease.[45,54] Except for showing such abnormalities, high-resolution CT is not helpful in predicting outcome because

Text continued on p. 472

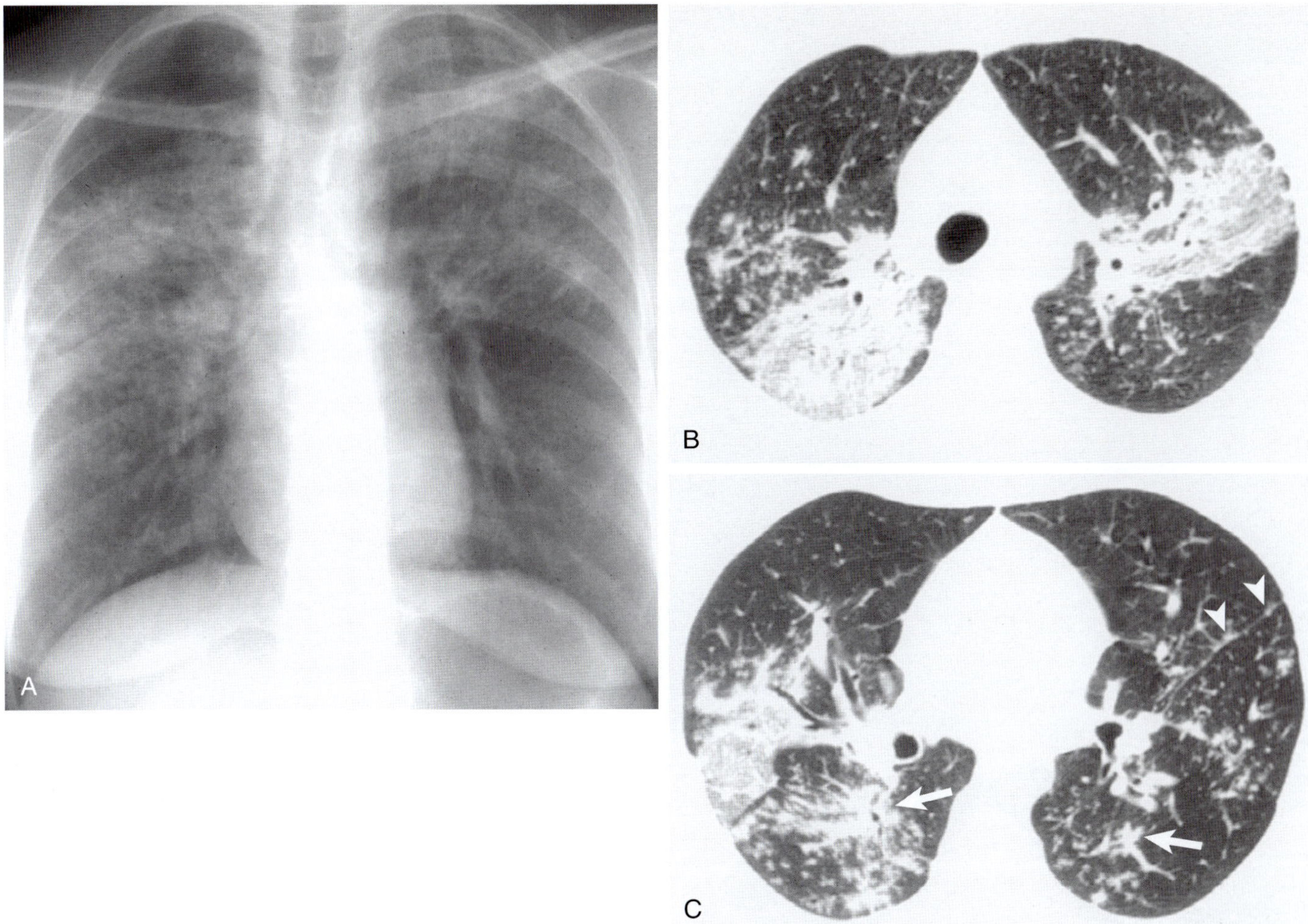

Fig. 31.10 Sarcoidosis: parenchymal consolidation. (A) Posteroanterior chest radiograph in a woman with stage II sarcoidosis shows bilateral areas of consolidation in the middle and upper lung zones. Air bronchograms can be seen. Poorly defined nodular opacities also are noted. (B) High-resolution CT scan at the level of the aortic arch shows bilateral areas of consolidation and ground-glass opacities. Note small nodules in a perilymphatic distribution. (C) High-resolution CT scan at the level of the middle lobe bronchus shows areas of consolidation in the right lung. Bilateral nodules mainly along the bronchi and vessels *(arrows)* and along the interlobar fissure *(arrowheads)* also are evident.

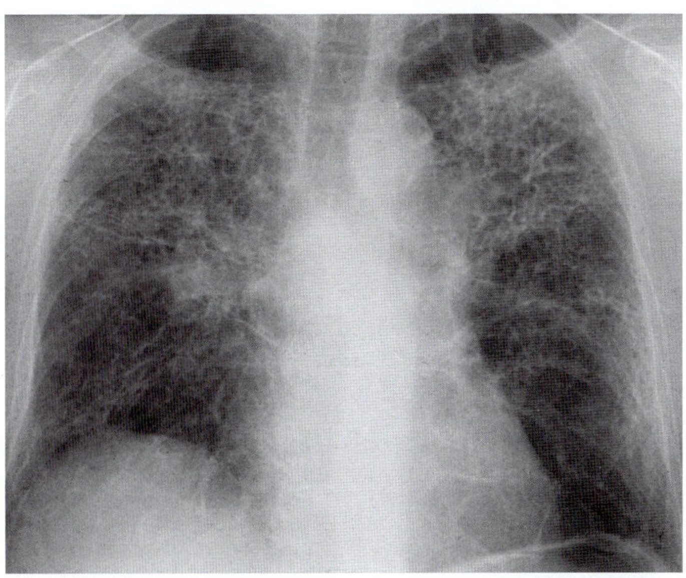

Fig. 31.11 Sarcoidosis: reticular pattern associated with fibrosis. Posteroanterior chest radiograph in woman with sarcoidosis shows a coarse reticular pattern involving mainly the perihilar regions of the middle and upper lung zones. *(From Müller NL, Fraser RS, Colman NC, et al:* Radiologic Diagnosis of Diseases of the Chest. *Philadelphia: Saunders; 2001.)*

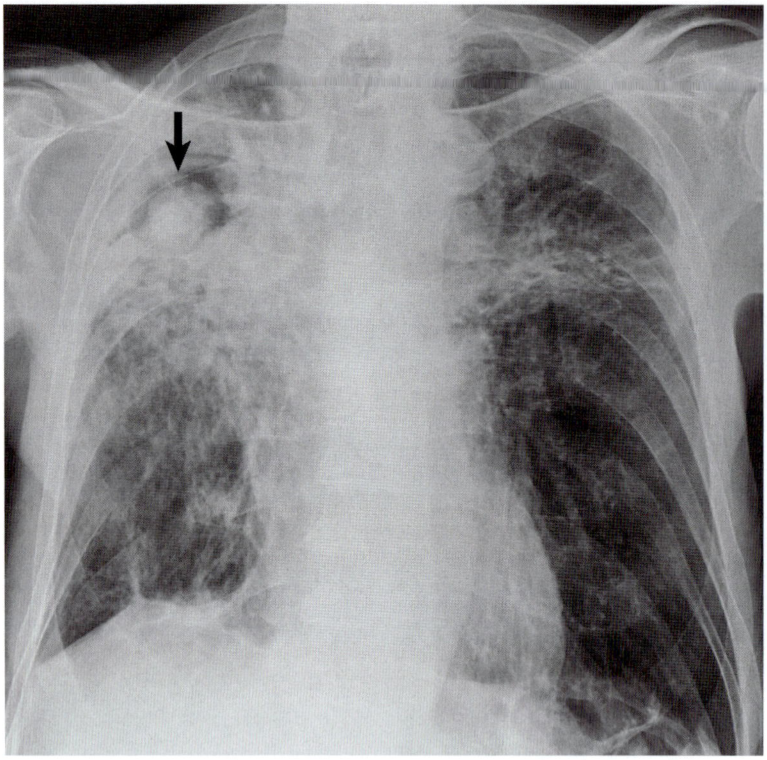

Fig. 31.12 Sarcoidosis: fungus ball formation. Posteroanterior chest radiograph shows a coarse reticulonodular pattern in the upper lobes associated with superior retraction of the hila (indicative of pulmonary fibrosis). A right upper lobe cavity is seen containing a fungus ball surrounded by a characteristic air crescent sign *(arrow)* in this patient with a history of hemoptysis.

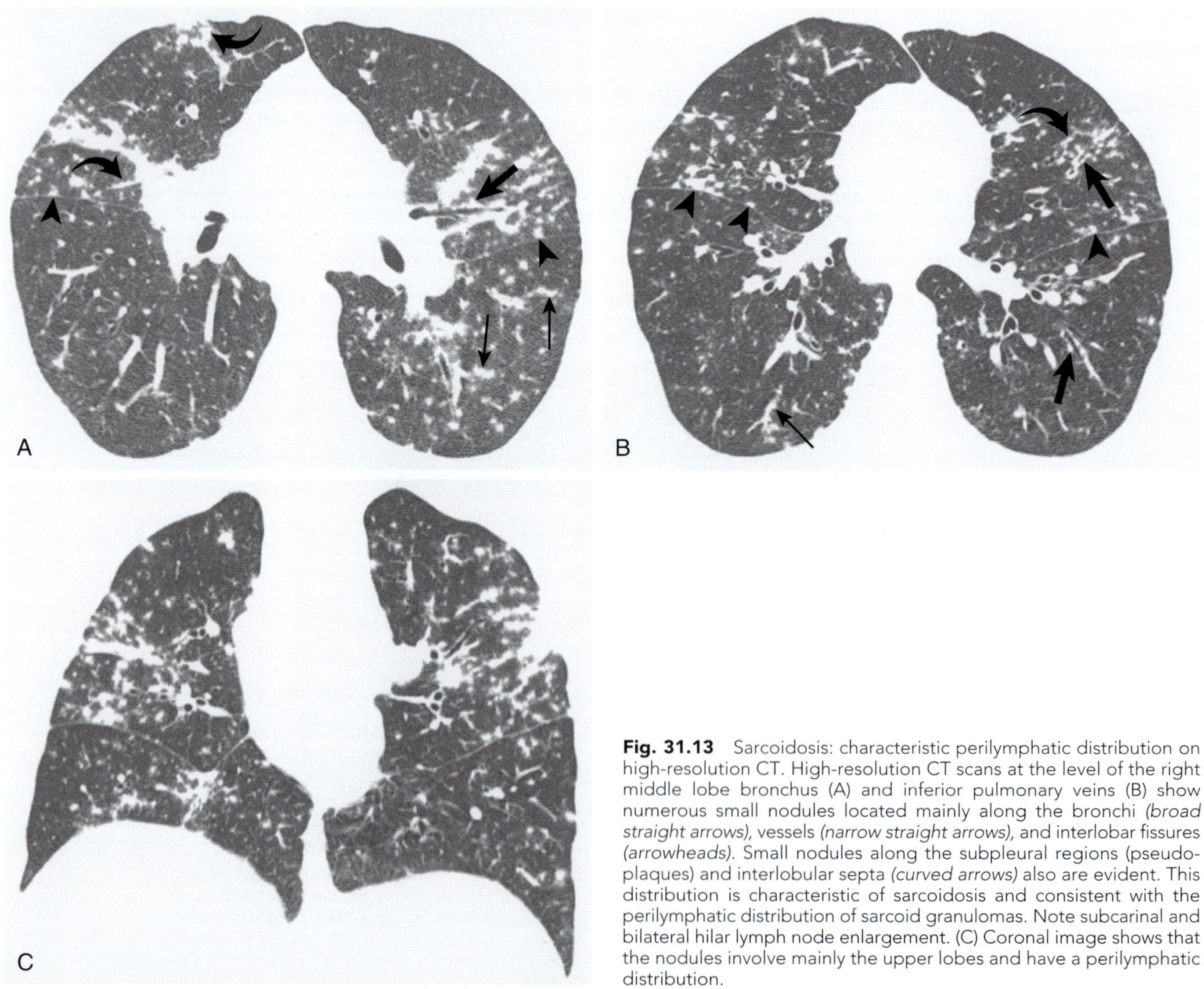

Fig. 31.13 Sarcoidosis: characteristic perilymphatic distribution on high-resolution CT. High-resolution CT scans at the level of the right middle lobe bronchus (A) and inferior pulmonary veins (B) show numerous small nodules located mainly along the bronchi *(broad straight arrows)*, vessels *(narrow straight arrows)*, and interlobar fissures *(arrowheads)*. Small nodules along the subpleural regions (pseudoplaques) and interlobular septa *(curved arrows)* also are evident. This distribution is characteristic of sarcoidosis and consistent with the perilymphatic distribution of sarcoid granulomas. Note subcarinal and bilateral hilar lymph node enlargement. (C) Coronal image shows that the nodules involve mainly the upper lobes and have a perilymphatic distribution.

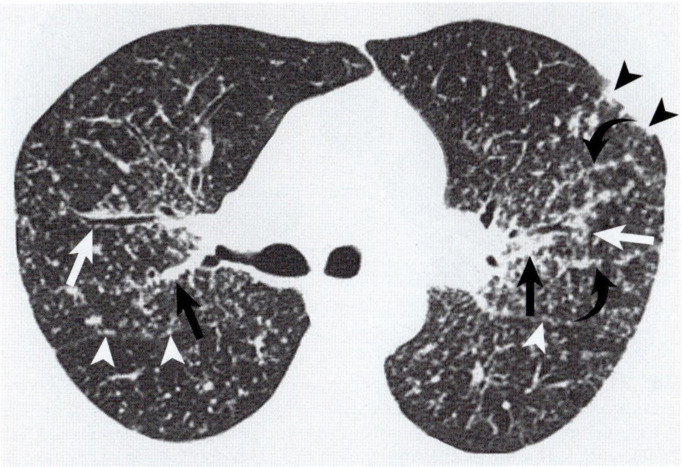

Fig. 31.14 Sarcoidosis: characteristic perilymphatic distribution on high-resolution CT. High-resolution CT scan shows nodular thickening of bronchi *(straight white arrows)*, vessels *(straight black arrows)*, interlobular septa *(curved arrows)*, and interlobar fissures *(white arrowheads)*. Conglomerate subpleural nodules resulting in pseudoplaques *(black arrowheads)* and prominence of the centrilobular core and centrilobular nodules secondary to involvement of the peribronchiolar interstitium also are noted.

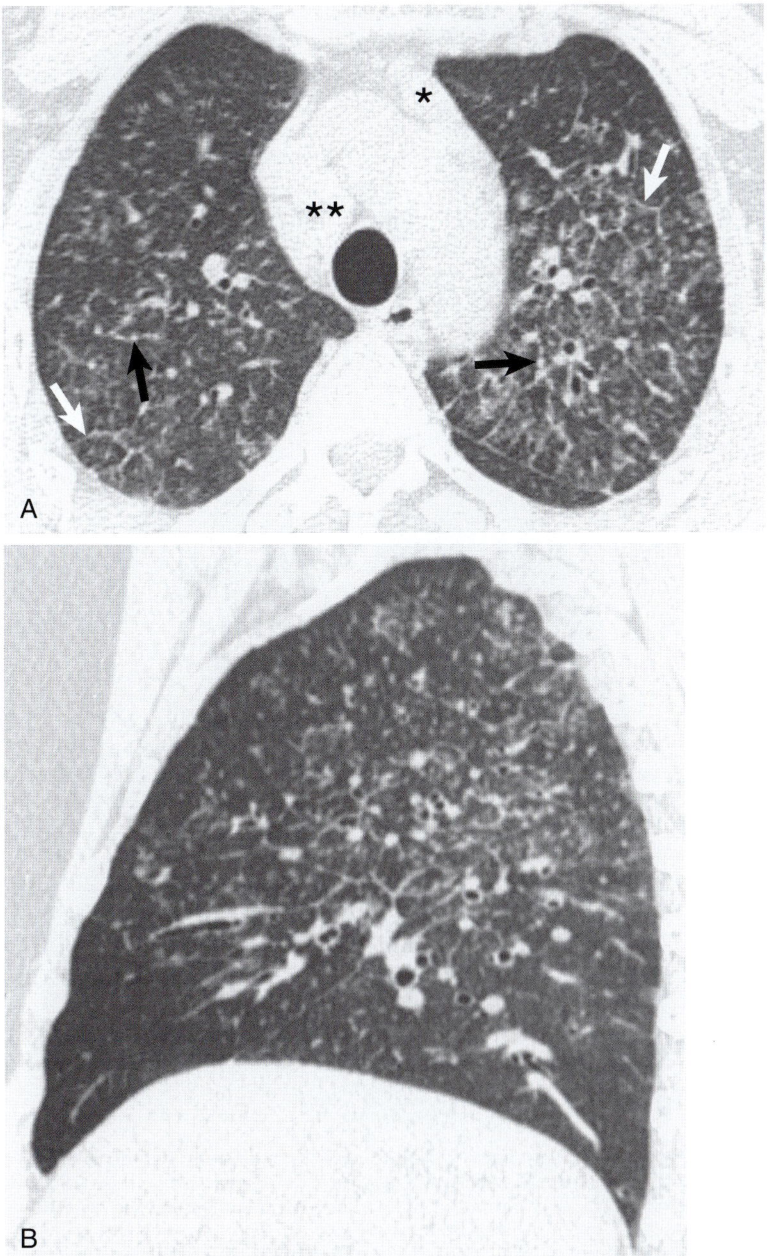

Fig. 31.15 Sarcoidosis: perilymphatic distribution on high-resolution CT. (A) High-resolution CT scan at the level of the aortic arch shows bilateral perilymphatic small nodules and extensive smooth *(white arrows)* and nodular *(black arrows)* interlobular septal thickening outlining the secondary lobule. Right paratracheal *(double asterisks)* and paraaortic *(single asterisk)* lymph node enlargement also is evident. The CT findings mimic the findings of lymphangitic carcinomatosis. (B) Sagittal reformation shows typical middle and upper lung zone distribution of perilymphatic nodules in sarcoidosis and extensive septal thickening.

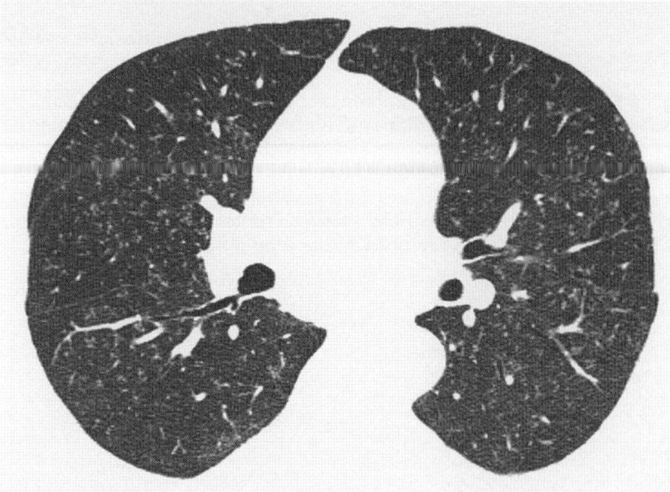

Fig. 31.16 Sarcoidosis: miliary pattern on high-resolution CT. High-resolution CT scan shows diffuse small nodules resulting in a miliary pattern. Subcarinal lymph node enlargement also is noted.

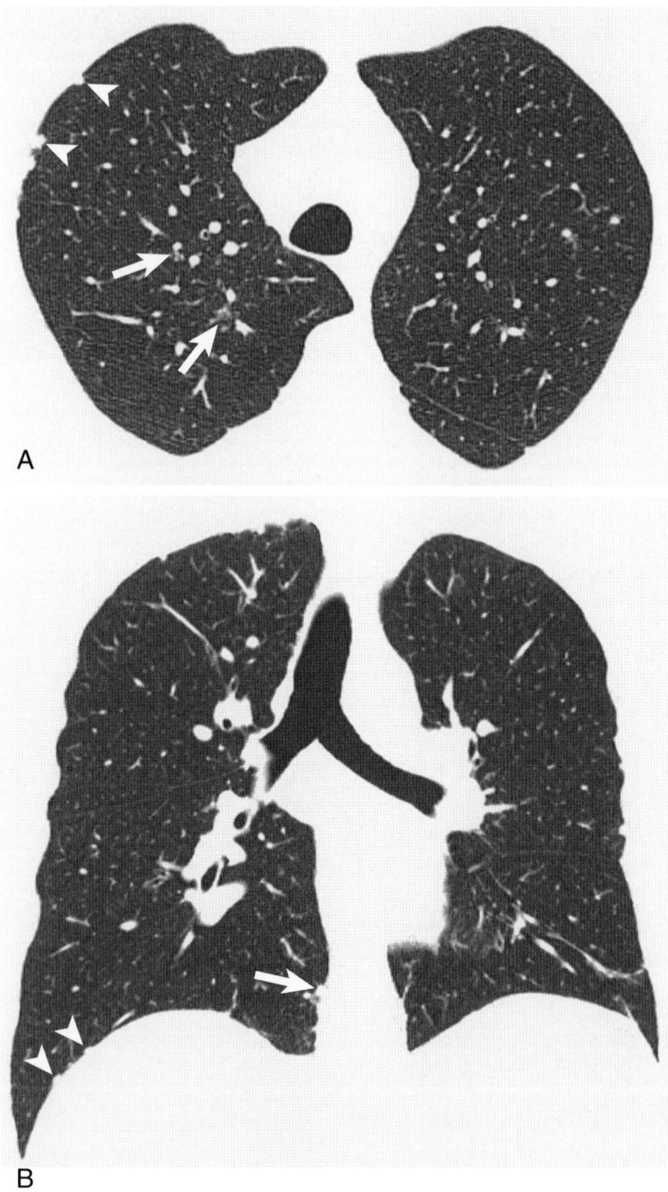

Fig. 31.17 Sarcoidosis: predominant subpleural distribution on high-resolution CT. (A) High-resolution CT scan shows a few nodules along the peribronchovascular interstitium *(arrows)* and subpleural nodules *(arrowheads)*. (B) Coronal reformation image shows better the distribution of subpleural nodules along the costal and paravertebral *(arrow)* regions and right hemidiaphragm *(arrowheads)*. In this patient the subpleural nodules of sarcoidosis resemble pleural plaques (pseudoplaques).

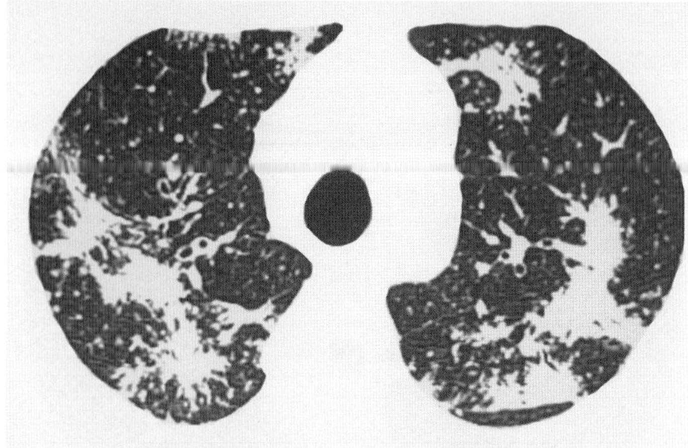

Fig. 31.18 Sarcoidosis: large nodules on high-resolution CT. High-resolution CT scan in a woman shows bilateral irregular nodular opacities in a perilymphatic and subpleural distribution with adjacent small nodules (galaxy sign). The large opacities result from the confluence of numerous small nodules (interstitial granulomas).

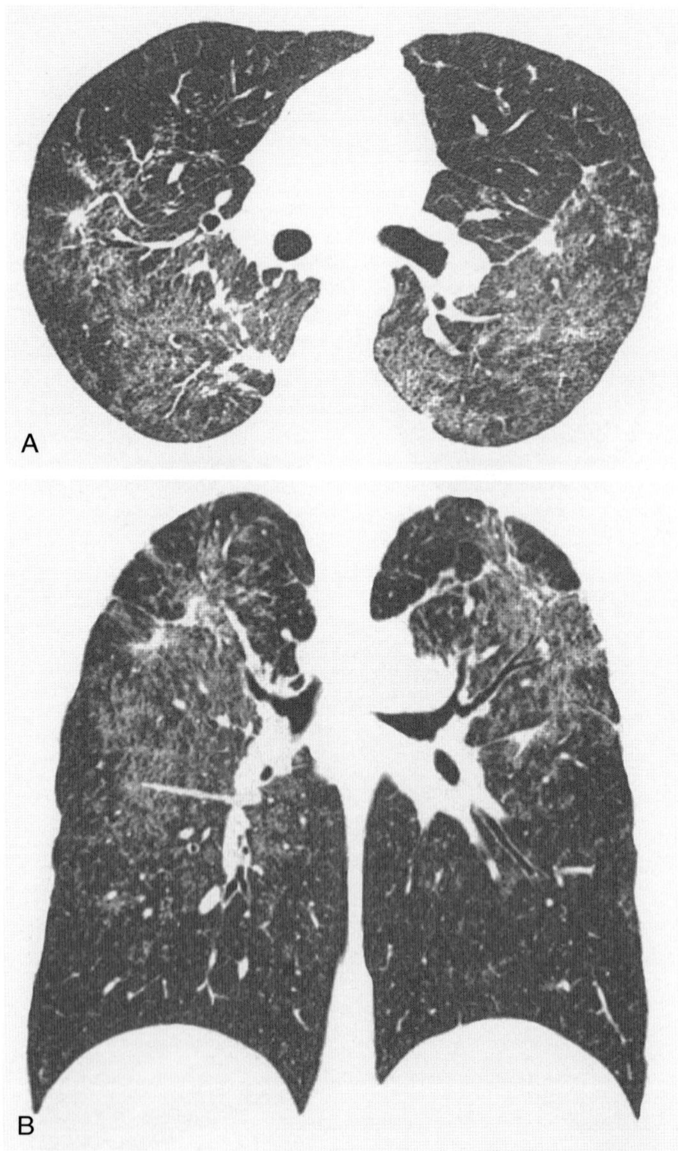

Fig. 31.19 Sarcoidosis: ground-glass opacities and fine nodularity on high-resolution CT. (A) High-resolution CT scan in a woman shows clusters of small nodules with areas of extensive confluence that give an appearance of ground-glass opacity on CT. (B) Coronal reformation shows upper and middle zonal predominance of abnormalities typical of sarcoidosis.

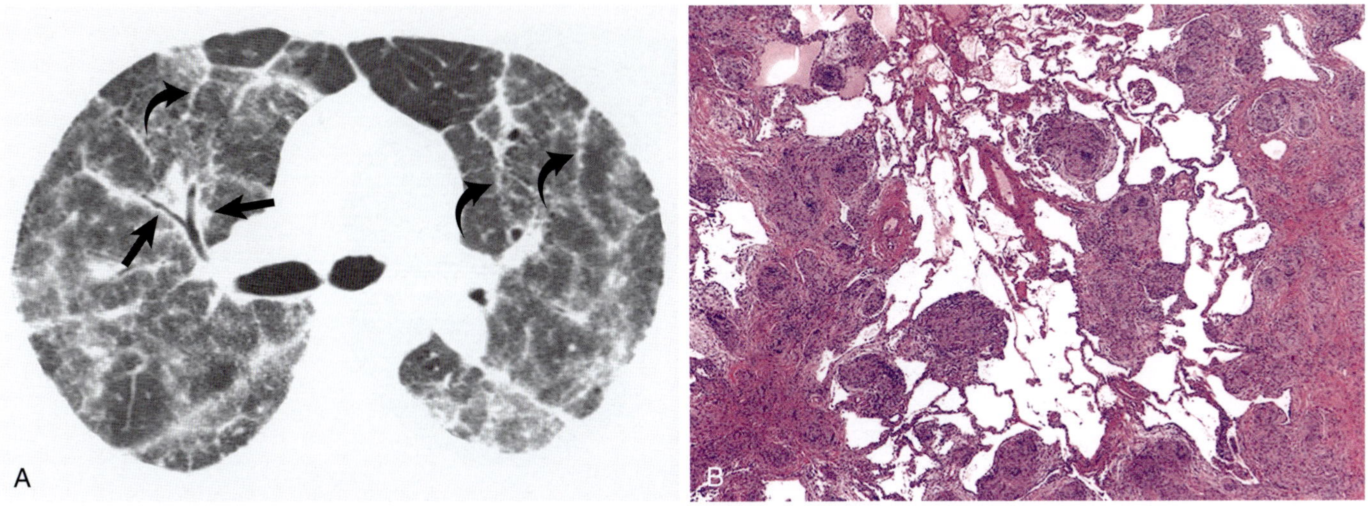

Fig. 31.20 Sarcoidosis: diffuse ground-glass opacities and fine nodularity on high-resolution CT. (A) High-resolution CT scan shows extensive bilateral ground-glass opacities and fine nodularity resulting in a granular appearance. Thickening of bronchi *(straight arrows)*, interlobular septa *(curved arrows)*, and interlobar fissures also are noted. (B) Histologic specimen from surgical biopsy shows septal and interstitial granulomas. The ground-glass opacities and fine granularity were due to the interstitial granulomas. There was no evidence of alveolitis.

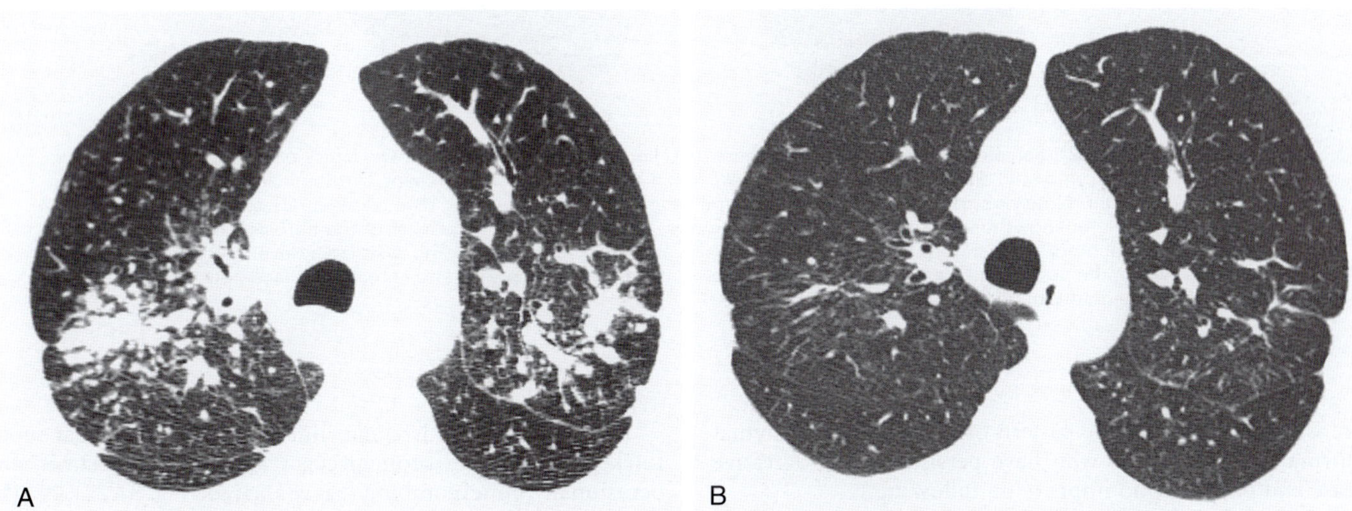

Fig. 31.21 Sarcoidosis: reversible findings. (A) Initial high-resolution CT scan shows nodules located mainly along the bronchi, vessels, and interlobar fissures. Small nodules along the subpleural costal regions and aorticopulmonary window lymph node enlargement also are evident. (B) Follow-up CT scan 10 years later shows marked improvement of abnormalities and aorticopulmonary window lymphadenopathy. Subtle peribronchovascular nodularity and bronchial and vascular distortion persist.

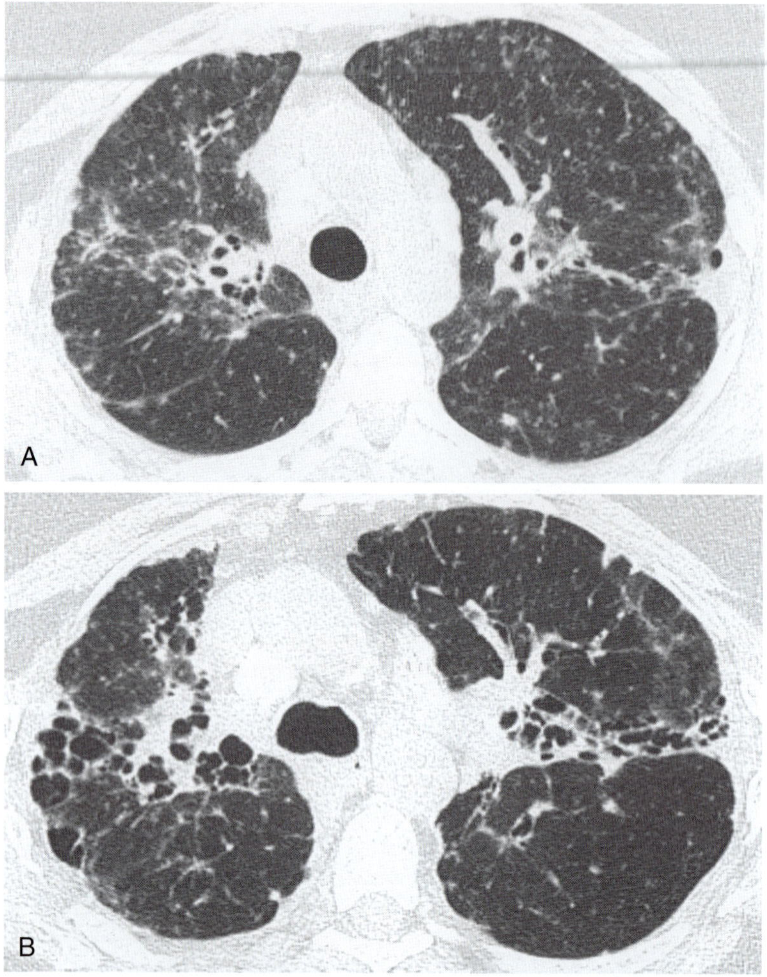

Fig. 31.22 Sarcoidosis: progression of disease. (A) High-resolution CT scan shows diffuse nodularity in a perilymphatic distribution. Minimal central bronchial distortion also is present, predominantly on the right. Note right paratracheal and paraaortic lymph node enlargement. (B) Follow-up CT scan 3 years later shows marked improvement of the diffuse nodularity but progression of the fibrosis. The central bronchial distortion has increased bilaterally, and subpleural honeycomb cysts have developed within the right lung. There is bilateral upper lobe volume loss with upward and anterior displacement of the interlobar fissures.

there is no difference in the pattern or extent of parenchymal abnormalities in patients who have persistent or progressive disease and patients who improve on follow-up.[45]

Regular and nodular bronchial wall thickening is common, but endoluminal abnormalities are seldom evident on CT even though mucosal thickening is frequently present at bronchoscopy.[55] Bronchial stenosis is uncommon. It may result from granulomatous inflammation of the bronchial wall, extrinsic compression by enlarged hilar lymph nodes, or bronchial distortion caused by pulmonary fibrosis.[29,56] Bronchial obstruction may result in distal atelectasis, most commonly the middle lobe. In a few patients focal areas of decreased attenuation and vascularity (i.e., mosaic attenuation) may be seen on inspiratory high-resolution CT in patients who have sarcoidosis. Air-trapping on expiratory high-resolution CT is relatively common, being seen in 90% of patients (Fig. 31.23).[26] The air-trapping may result from endoluminal or submucosal sarcoid granulomas or fibrotic obstruction of small airways.[26,57] The extent of air-trapping increases with extent of fibrosis.[26]

Fibrosis results in irregular linear opacities, irregular septal thickening, traction bronchiectasis and bronchiolectasis, and occasionally honeycombing (Fig. 31.24; see Fig. 31.22).[34,56] The fibrosis, similar to the nodules, involves mainly the peribronchovascular regions of the upper lobes and typically results in posterior displacement of the main and upper lobe bronchi, upward displacement of the hila, and compensatory overinflation of the lower lobes (Fig. 31.25).[34,42] Progressive fibrosis results in abnormal central conglomeration of perihilar bronchi and vessels associated with masses of fibrous tissue, typically most marked in the upper lobes. Subpleural honeycombing occurs in a small percentage of patients. Honeycombing usually is limited to patients who have severe fibrosis and central conglomeration of bronchi and involves mainly the middle and upper lung zones.[42,56] Rarely, the honeycombing may involve mainly the lower lung zones and mimic the appearance seen in idiopathic pulmonary fibrosis.[58] Fibrosis may result in large cystic spaces owing to traction bronchiectasis or bullae and development of intracavitary mycetomas (Fig. 31.26).[49,59]

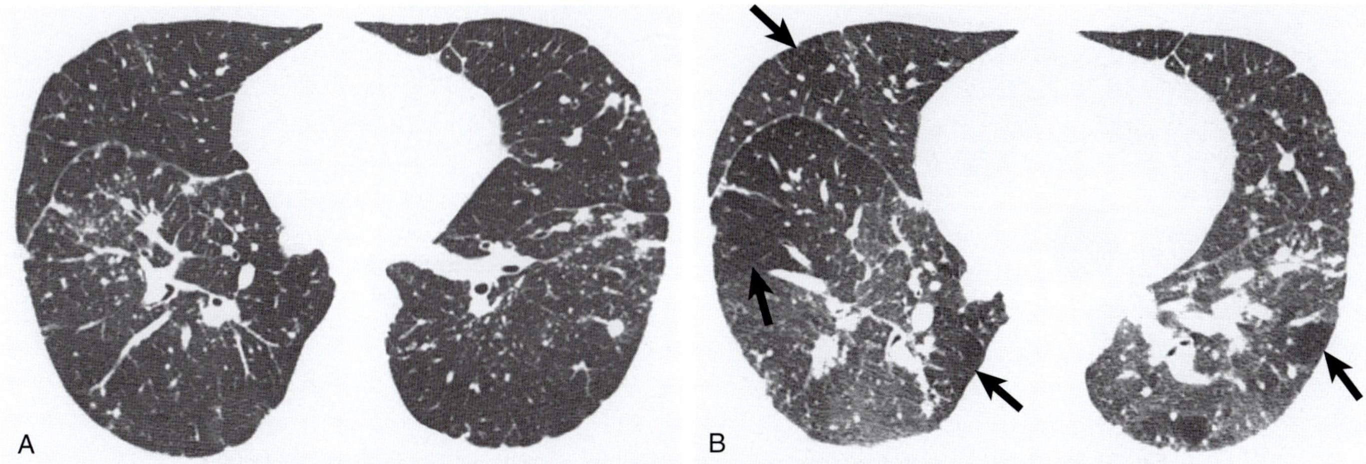

Fig. 31.23 Sarcoidosis: air-trapping on expiratory CT. (A) High-resolution CT scan in a man with sarcoidosis shows characteristic perilymphatic distribution of nodules along the interlobar fissures, subpleural regions, vessels, bronchi, and interlobular septa. (B) Expiratory image shows bilateral air-trapping *(arrows)*.

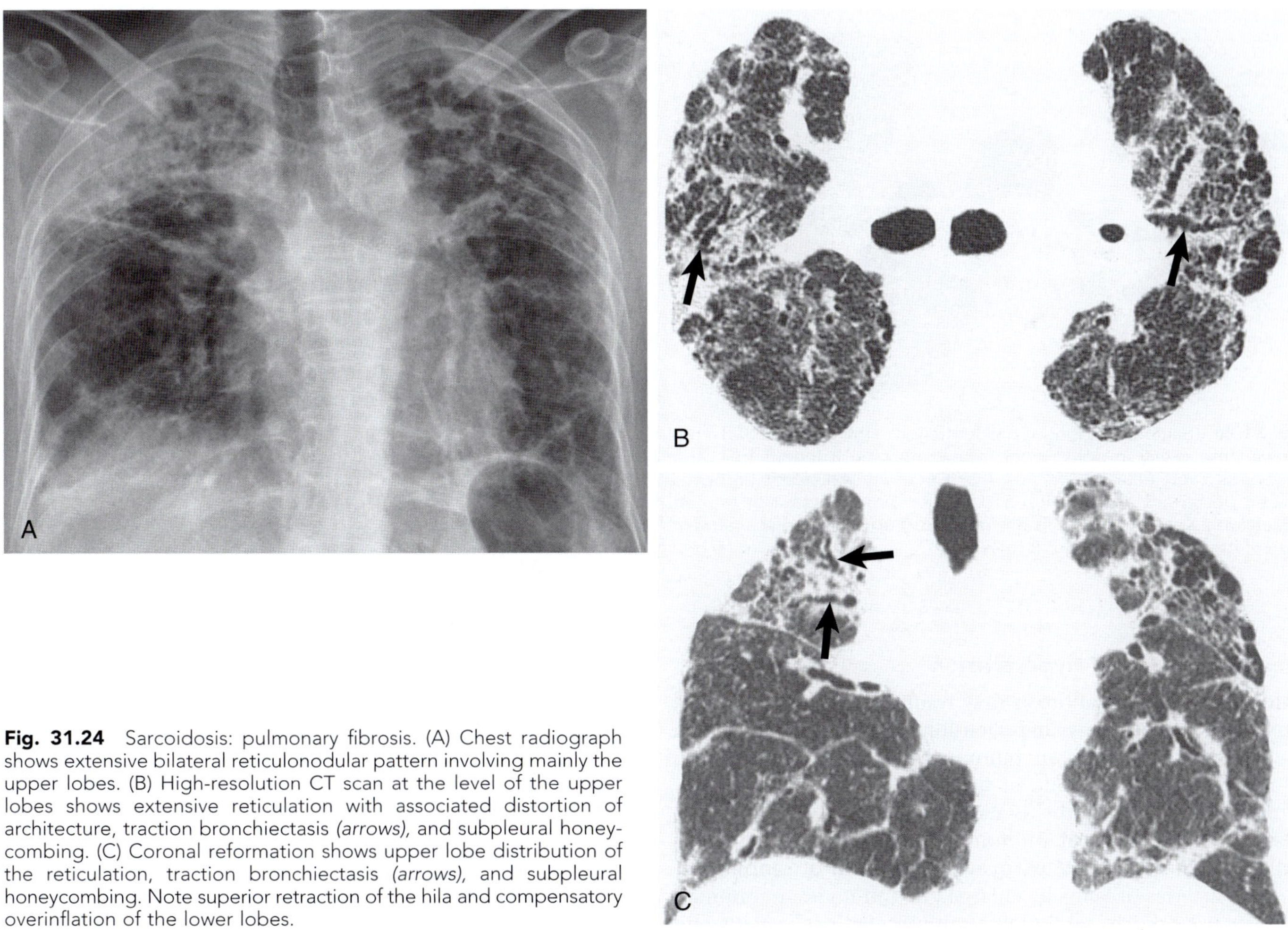

Fig. 31.24 Sarcoidosis: pulmonary fibrosis. (A) Chest radiograph shows extensive bilateral reticulonodular pattern involving mainly the upper lobes. (B) High-resolution CT scan at the level of the upper lobes shows extensive reticulation with associated distortion of architecture, traction bronchiectasis *(arrows)*, and subpleural honeycombing. (C) Coronal reformation shows upper lobe distribution of the reticulation, traction bronchiectasis *(arrows)*, and subpleural honeycombing. Note superior retraction of the hila and compensatory overinflation of the lower lobes.

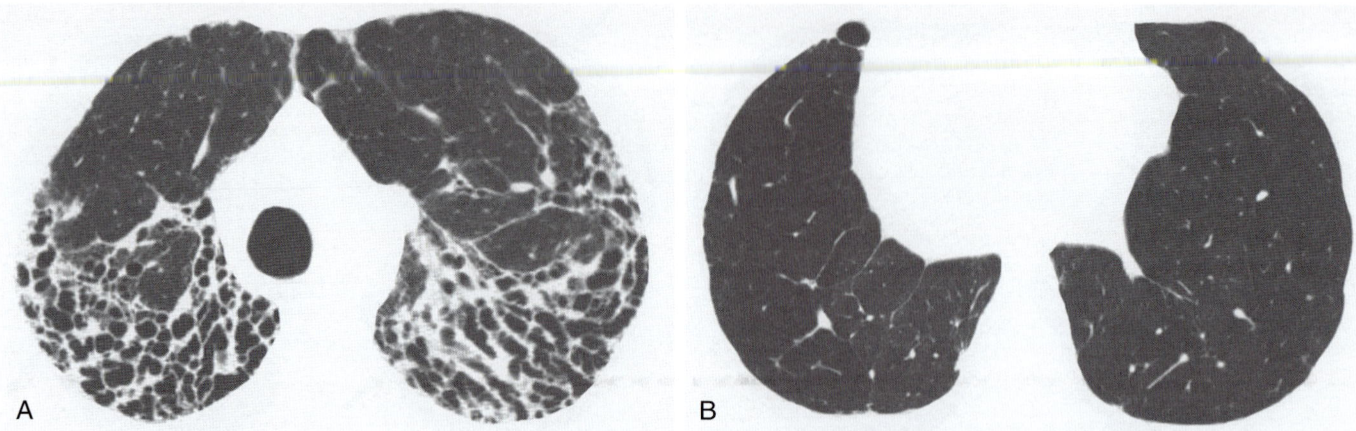

Fig. 31.25 Sarcoidosis: severe pulmonary fibrosis. (A) High-resolution CT scan at the level of the upper lobes shows architectural distortion, posterior displacement of the upper lobe bronchi, extensive traction bronchiectasis and bronchiolectasis, and a few subpleural cysts consistent with honeycombing. (B) High-resolution CT scan at the level of the lung bases shows compensatory hyperinflation.

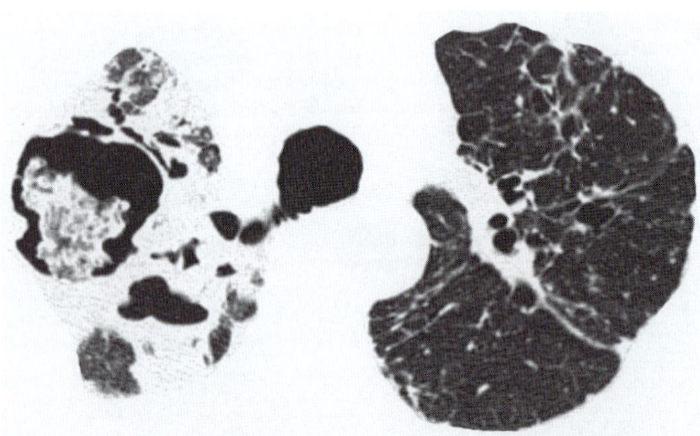

Fig. 31.26 Sarcoidosis: fungus ball formation. High-resolution CT scan shows large cavity in right upper lobe containing a fungus ball. The cavity was a very ectatic bronchus. A similar cavity-like ectatic bronchus is seen posteriorly. Reticulation and traction bronchiectasis in the left upper lobe also are noted. There is marked upward displacement of the ectatic bronchi owing to fibrosis.

Pulmonary Arterial Hypertension

Extensive pulmonary fibrosis may result in pulmonary arterial hypertension. Pulmonary hypertension is suspected on CT when the diameter of the main pulmonary artery is greater than 32 mm[60] or when the ratio of the diameters of the main pulmonary artery and of the ascending aorta is greater than 1.[61] Less common causes of pulmonary hypertension in patients with sarcoidosis include extrinsic compression of central pulmonary arteries or veins by enlarged lymph nodes, pulmonary venoocclusive disease, granulomatous vascular involvement, and pulmonary vasoconstriction by vasoactive factors.[11,56] Venoocclusive disease in these patients presumably results from obstruction of interlobular septal veins by intramural granulomas or perivascular fibrosis and is suspected on high-resolution CT by the presence of extensive septal thickening.[56]

Hilar and Mediastinal Nodes

Enlarged hilar and mediastinal nodes are seen on CT in approximately 90% of patients with sarcoidosis, a higher prevalence than is apparent on the chest radiograph.[62,63] CT also shows more extensive lymphadenopathy than is apparent on the radiograph.[63] The most commonly enlarged lymph nodes are the paratracheal and the hilar lymph nodes present in virtually all patients with enlarged nodes (Fig. 31.27). Lymphadenopathy also frequently is present in the aorticopulmonary window (90%), subcarinal (60%), anterior or prevascular mediastinal (50%), and posterior or paravertebral mediastinal (15%) lymph node groups.[63] Less commonly, lymph node enlargement may be seen in the axilla, internal mammary chain, and retrocrural region.[64]

Calcification of hilar and mediastinal lymph nodes is relatively common, being seen in 40% to 50% of patients with long-standing sarcoidosis.[54] The calcified nodes are most commonly bilateral, hilar, paratracheal, and subcarinal, and the pattern of calcification is most commonly focal but may be diffuse or eggshell.[65] The calcification of lymph nodes in sarcoidosis is initially focal and soft ("icing sugar" calcification) (Fig. 31.28) but over time becomes dense (Fig. 31.29).

Cardiac Sarcoidosis

CT plays a limited role in the assessment of cardiac abnormalities in patients with sarcoidosis. The most common finding is pericardial effusion, which occurs in 5% to 15% of patients.[12] Less common findings include cardiomegaly, signs of right ventricular strain, left heart failure, myocardial thinning at sites of involvement, and rarely ventricular aneurysm.[12,66]

Abdominal Manifestations

The most common abdominal manifestations of sarcoidosis are splenomegaly, hepatomegaly, lymphadenopathy, low-attenuation liver and splenic lesions, and punctate splenic and hepatic calcifications.[66,67] Splenic abnormalities occur in approximately 50% of patients, liver abnormalities in 15%, and lymphadenopathy in 40%.[67] There is no apparent correlation between the abdominal findings and stage of thoracic sarcoidosis. In approximately

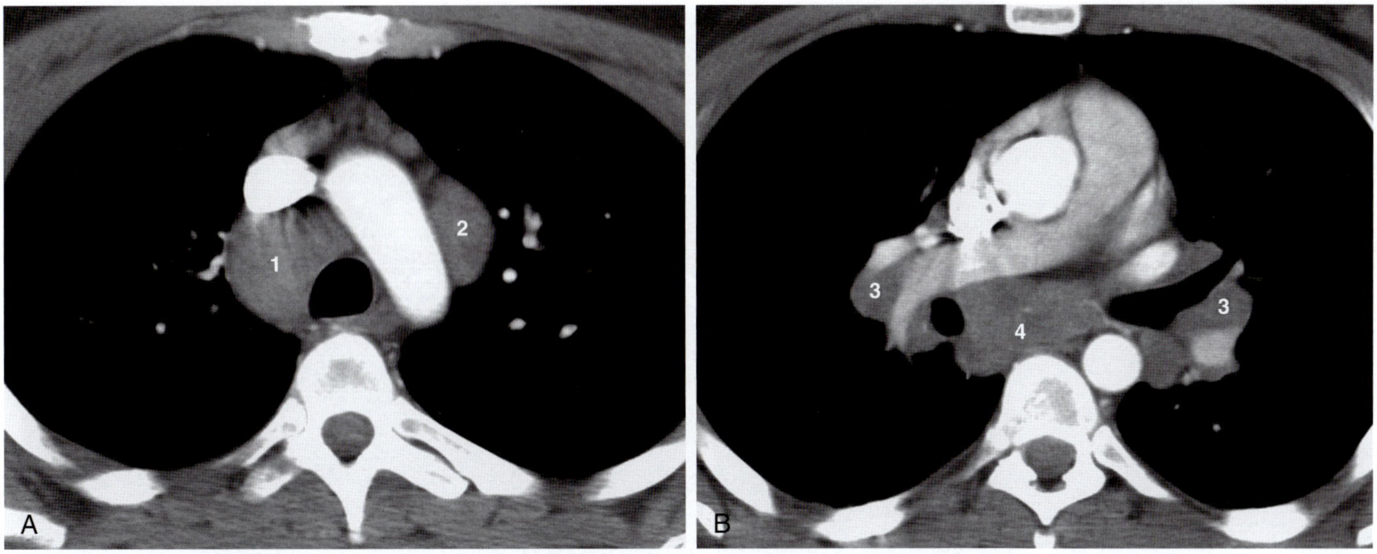

Fig. 31.27 Sarcoidosis: characteristic lymphadenopathy on CT. (A) Contrast-enhanced CT scan at the level of the aortic arch in a man with sarcoidosis shows enlarged paratracheal *(1)* and paraaortic *(2)* lymph nodes. (B) CT scan at the level of the bronchus intermedius shows enlarged bilateral hilar *(3)* and subcarinal *(4)* lymph nodes.

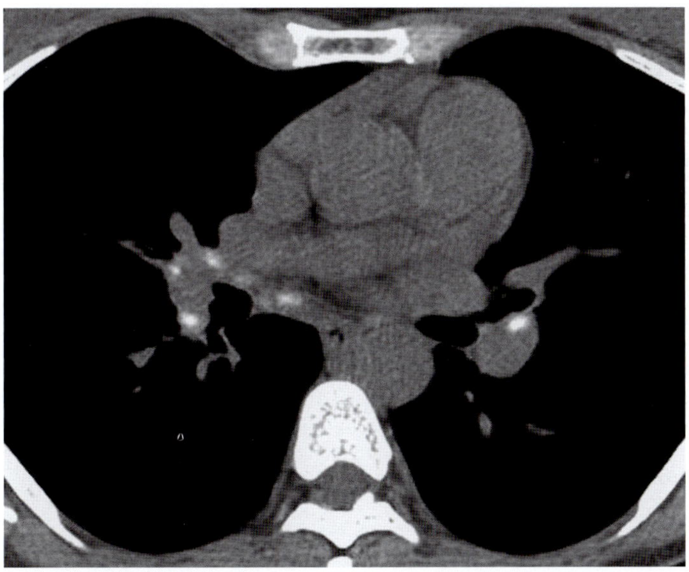

Fig. 31.28 Sarcoidosis: characteristic focal calcification of lymph nodes. CT scan in a woman with sarcoidosis shows soft ("icing sugar") calcification of bilateral hilar and subcarinal lymph nodes.

5% to 15% of patients, coalescing granulomas become apparent as hypoattenuating liver nodules.[66] Splenic nodules are larger and more common than hepatic lesions.[66] The abdominal lymphadenopathy typically involves several lymph nodes and is usually mild (1–2 cm diameter) but occasionally may be massive.[66,67]

MAGNETIC RESONANCE IMAGING

Magnetic resonance imaging (MRI) has a limited role in assessing pulmonary and nodal disease but is superior to CT in assessing cardiac and central nervous system (CNS) manifestations of sarcoidosis. Cardiac involvement may result in areas of increased signal intensity on T2-weighted MR images and hyperintensity on late gadolinium contrast-enhanced T1-weighted images.[66,68]

KEY POINTS: SARCOIDOSIS: HIGH-RESOLUTION COMPUTED TOMOGRAPHY FINDINGS

Characteristic high-resolution CT findings are as follows:

- Bilateral symmetric hilar and paratracheal lymphadenopathy
- Commonly enlarged subcarinal, aorticopulmonary window, and anterior or prevascular mediastinal nodes
- Well-defined, smooth or irregular nodules, measuring 2–5 mm, in a perilymphatic distribution
- Nodular thickening of bronchi, pulmonary vessels, interlobar fissures, costal pleura, and, to a lesser extent, interlobular septa
- Abnormalities usually most extensive in the middle and upper lung zones
- Fibrosis seen in 5% of patients at presentation and eventually in 20% of cases
- Fibrosis typically peribronchial and upper lung zone predominant with superior retraction of the hila
- Hilar and mediastinal nodes calcified in 40%–50% of patients with chronic sarcoidosis

MRI has a high sensitivity in detecting intracranial abnormalities resulting from neurosarcoidosis. The most characteristic manifestation is nodular or diffuse enhancing thickening of the leptomeninges mainly in the basal cisterns and hypothalamic regions after intravenous (IV) contrast administration.[19] Other findings include enhancement of the brain after administration of IV contrast and intracranial masses that are isointense on T1-weighted images and hyperintense on T2-weighted images.[19]

Gallium-67 Scintigraphy

Gallium-67 scintigraphy was used for many years as a marker of disease activity in sarcoidosis.[69] The use of gallium-67 for

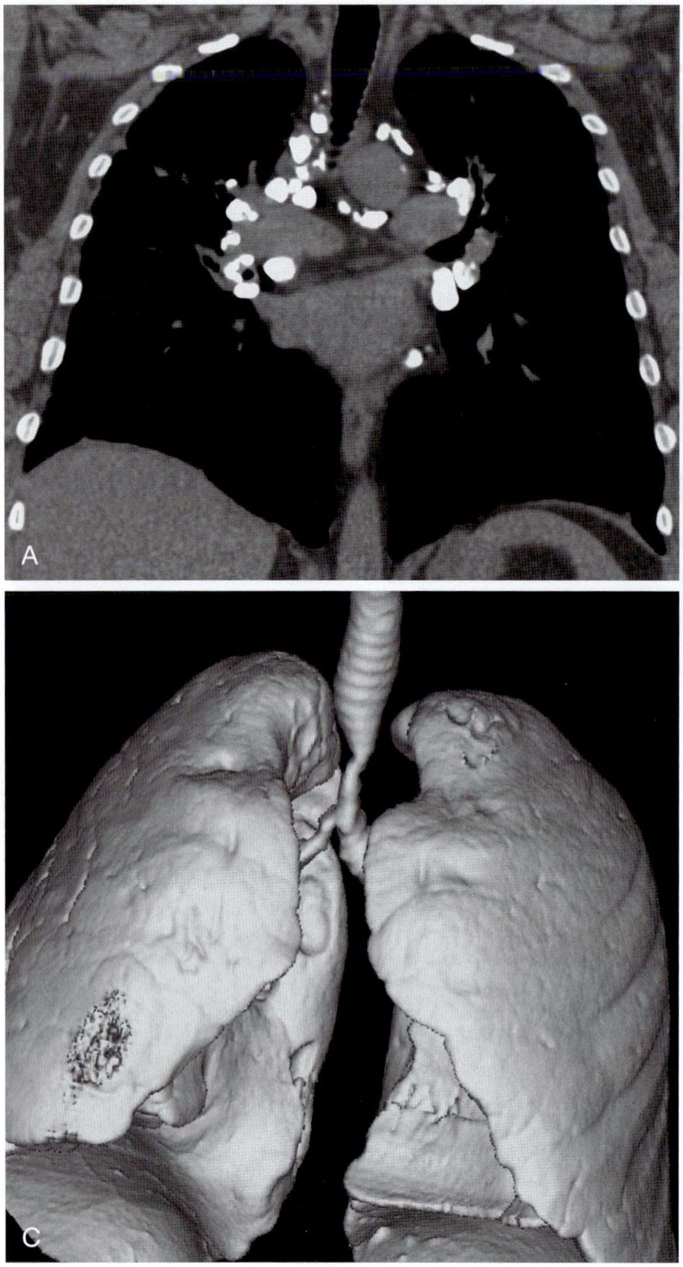

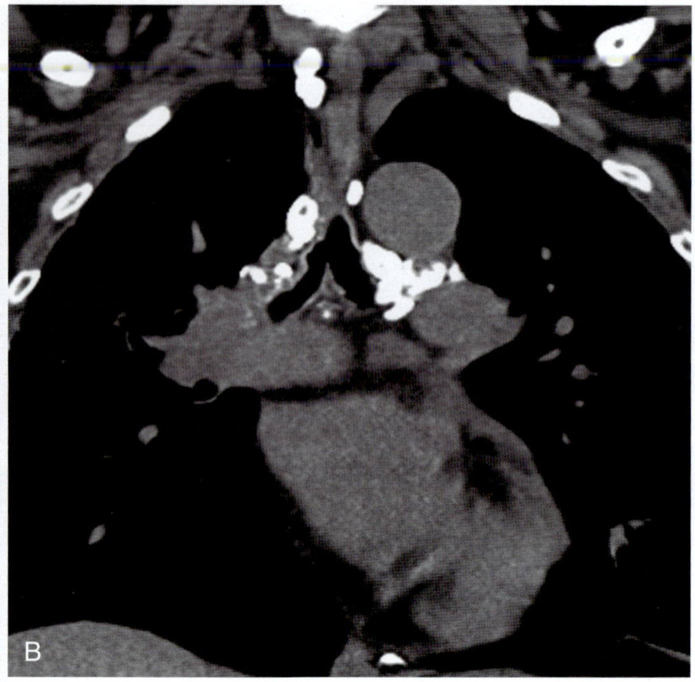

Fig. 31.29 Sarcoidosis: extensive nodal calcification on CT. (A) Coronal reformation CT scan in a patient with long-standing sarcoidosis shows numerous densely calcified mediastinal and bilateral hilar lymph nodes. (B) and (C) Coronal and volume-rendered CT images from a different patient show extensive densely calcified mediastinal lymph nodes resulting in narrowing of the distal trachea and proximal right main bronchus.

sarcoidosis diagnosis has essentially been replaced by thin section CT. Currently, it is not used in the setting of suspected sarcoidosis and is used mainly to diagnose difficult cases, such as when isolated extrathoracic disease seems to be present.[70] Gallium-67 scintigraphy can be used to detect cardiac sarcoidosis, although this has been supplanted by MRI and with fluorodeoxyglucose positron emission tomography–computed tomography (FDG–PET-CT).

POSITRON EMISSION TOMOGRAPHY

Increased uptake with FDG-PET has been shown in the lung and lymph nodes. FDG-PET is comparable to gallium-67 scintigraphy in detecting pulmonary sarcoidosis but is superior in assessing extrapulmonary involvement.[71] Uptake has been shown to decrease after high-dose steroid treatment.[72] FDG-PET accumulates in the myocardium of patients with cardiac sarcoidosis and has higher sensitivity for the detection of myocardial involvement than thallium-201 single-photon emission computed tomography and gallium-67 scintigraphy.[12] There is growing evidence that FDG-PET may have value in the detection of cardiac sarcoidosis, given its very good sensitivity for cardiac sarcoidosis, although lower specificity because of false positives from background FDG uptake in the normal myocardium is at times an issue.[12]

DIAGNOSTIC ALGORITHM

Approximately 75% of patients with sarcoidosis have characteristic radiographic manifestations consisting of bilateral hilar and paratracheal lymphadenopathy with or without concomitant parenchymal abnormalities.[28] In most of these asymptomatic patients, further imaging may be unnecessary but is frequently performed to help guide biopsy for diagnosis confirmation. In 15% to 20% of cases the radiologic findings are nonspecific or atypical, however, and high-resolution CT may be helpful. High-resolution CT can show parenchymal abnormalities in patients who have normal chest radiographs and in patients in whom only hilar adenopathy is apparent.[34] CT also has been shown to be superior to chest radiographs in showing early fibrosis and distortion of the lung parenchyma in patients who have sarcoidosis.[53]

The chest radiograph remains the first and foremost imaging modality used in the initial evaluation and follow-up of patients with sarcoidosis. The most common indications for CT in patients with suspected or proven sarcoidosis are (1) atypical clinical or chest radiographic findings; (2) detection of complications of the lung disease, such as bronchiectasis, aspergilloma, pulmonary fibrosis, or a superimposed infection or malignancy; and (3) a normal chest radiograph but high clinical suspicion of sarcoidosis.[6] High-resolution CT scans also may be helpful in selected patients with stage II or stage III sarcoidosis to discriminate between active inflammation and irreversible fibrosis.[29] Abdominal complications, such as hepatic and splenic involvement, also can be assessed using CT. MRI is superior to CT in the evaluation of cardiac and CNS involvement.

Differential Diagnosis

The presence of symmetric bilateral hilar lymph node enlargement, particularly in asymptomatic patients, is highly suggestive of sarcoidosis. In a study of 100 consecutive patients who had bilateral hilar lymphadenopathy, 74% had sarcoidosis.[73] Although malignancy (usually lymphoma) accounted for 11% of cases, all 11 patients with malignancy were symptomatic. All 47 patients who had no symptoms or only acute inflammatory features (e.g., uveitis, polyarthritis, or erythema nodosum) had sarcoidosis. Fifty of the 52 patients with normal physical examination had sarcoidosis. Anemia was present in only 1 of 74 sarcoid patients but was common in patients with malignancy. The authors concluded that the risk of malignancy was small in patients with bilateral hilar lymphadenopathy who had no prior history of malignancy, provided that physical examination and routine blood tests were normal.[73]

The radiographic findings of pulmonary involvement are often relatively nonspecific. In most of these patients a characteristic perilymphatic distribution of nodules is evident, however, on high-resolution CT. Conditions that may mimic the CT appearance of sarcoidosis include pulmonary lymphangitic carcinomatosis, immunoglobulin (Ig)G4-related lung disease, berylliosis, silicosis, and coal worker's pneumoconiosis. In sarcoidosis, IgG4-related lung disease and berylliosis, nodules tend to predominate in the peribronchovascular and subpleural regions; in lymphangitic carcinomatosis, nodules are most frequently septal and peribronchovascular; in silicosis and coal workers' pneumoconiosis, nodules usually appear centrilobular and subpleural in location on CT. When septal thickening is present in patients who have sarcoidosis, it is usually less extensive than that seen in patients who have lymphangitic carcinomatosis. Other findings that favor sarcoidosis are predominant involvement of the upper lobes, bilateral symmetric hilar lymphadenopathy, and lack of pleural effusion. In patients with symmetric bilateral hilar lymphadenopathy and characteristic parenchymal findings who have no history of occupational exposure, malignancy, or weight loss, a diagnosis of sarcoidosis can often be suggested based on the clinical and radiologic findings.

Synopsis of Treatment Options

Sarcoidosis has a tendency to wax and wane spontaneously or in response to therapy. Spontaneous remissions occur in nearly two-thirds of patients, but 10% to 30% of patients have a progressive course.[6] Most patients stabilize or improve with corticosteroid treatment, but relapse occurs in 75% of patients as the amount of drug is tapered or discontinued.[6] Use of immunomodulators is also a hallmark of therapy. Fatalities occur in 1% to 5% of patients owing to progressive respiratory insufficiency or CNS or myocardial involvement.[6] Clinical manifestations and causes of death vary in different geographic regions. In Japan approximately 75% of deaths ascribed to sarcoidosis are due to cardiac involvement, whereas in the United States most of the deaths are due to pulmonary complications.[6] Patients with end-stage pulmonary fibrosis may require lung transplantation. In some patients the disease may recur in the recipient lung. In one multicenter study that assessed the frequency and CT findings of recurrence of the primary disease after lung transplantation, recurrent sarcoidosis was found in 9 (35%) of 26 transplants.[74] The recurrent disease in these patients was mild.

KEY POINTS: SARCOIDOSIS

- Sarcoidosis is a systemic inflammatory disorder characterized by the presence of noncaseating granulomas.
- Intrathoracic lymph node and pulmonary parenchymal involvement occurs in more than 90% of cases.
- Prognosis correlates with radiographic stage at presentation.
- The main indications for CT are as follows:
  - Assessment of patients with a normal chest radiograph but high clinical suspicion of sarcoidosis
  - Assessment of patients with atypical clinical or chest radiographic findings
  - Detection of complications such as aspergilloma
  - Assessment of selected patients with stage II or stage III sarcoidosis to discriminate between active inflammation and irreversible fibrosis

SUGGESTED READINGS

Criado E, Sánchez M, Ramírez J, Arguis P, de Caralt TM, Perea RJ, Xaubet A. Pulmonary sarcoidosis: typical and atypical manifestations at high-resolution CT with pathologic correlation. *Radiographics*. 2010;30(6):1567–1586.

Hennebicque AS, Nunes H, Brillet PY, et al. CT findings in severe thoracic sarcoidosis. *Eur Radiol*. 2005;15:23–30.

Koyama T, Ueda H, Togashi K, et al. Radiologic manifestations of sarcoidosis in various organs. *Radiographics*. 2004;24:87–104.

Lynch JP 3rd. Computed tomographic scanning in sarcoidosis. *Semin Respir Crit Care Med*. 2003;24:393–418.

Prabhakar HB, Rabinowitz CB, Gibbons FK, O'Donnell WJ, Shepard JA, Aquino SL. Imaging features of sarcoidosis on MDCT, FDG PET, and PET/CT. *AJR Am J Roentgenol*. 2008;190(suppl 3):S1–S6.

The full reference list for this chapter is available at ExpertConsult.com.

32 Hypersensitivity Pneumonitis*

ANDREA L. MAGEE | CHRISTOPHER M. WALKER | JONATHAN H. CHUNG

Etiology

Hypersensitivity pneumonitis (HP), also known as extrinsic allergic alveolitis, is an immune-mediated inflammatory form of diffuse interstitial pulmonary disease caused by inhalation of various antigens that affect susceptible patients.[1–3] Occasionally, an HP reaction pattern may be seen in association with drug toxicity. Bacterial, mycobacterial, fungal, animal protein, and chemical compound causative antigens have been identified, with common examples listed in Table 32.1.[3]

HP occurs most commonly in middle-aged adults and is more common in nonsmokers when compared to demographically matched smokers, which is suspected to be due to the immunosuppressive effects of cigarette smoke on the intrapulmonary immune mediator cells that are implicated in HP.[4–7] Smokers who do develop HP are more likely to develop chronic disease, however, and have a worse prognosis than nonsmokers.[8] Certain occupations and hobbies that involve materials harboring the causative antigens have been described in the literature and should be queried during the collection of a detailed exposure history.[1,3,9–13]

The development of HP is influenced by the size, immunogenicity, duration of exposure, and number of inhaled organic particles and the immune response of the affected individual. Not all equal exposures lead to the development of HP. Farmer's lung (one of the most common types of HP), for instance, is estimated to occur in 9% to 12% of exposed farmers, and bird fancier's lung is estimated to occur in 15% of bird keepers.[14–16] It is not yet clear which variables determine the initial presentation and clinical course of the disease.[2] Regardless of the type of causative antigen or its environmental setting, only a small percentage of individuals with any given antigenic exposure develop HP.

The pathogenesis of HP is incompletely understood, but it is accepted that HP results from a non–immunoglobulin (Ig) E-mediated hypersensitivity reaction.[9] The antigens associated with the development of HP usually occur in aerosolized particles of less than 3 μm in diameter, which enables their deposition in the distal airspaces, resulting in type 3 (antigen-antibody complex) and type 4 (delayed cell-mediated) hypersensitivity reactions.[3,17–19] There is also evidence that alterations in neutrophil chemotaxis are involved in the pathophysiology of HP.[20,21]

Prevalence and Epidemiology

The prevalence and incidence of HP in the general population are difficult to evaluate, as disease manifestation is influenced by climatic, seasonal, and geographic conditions; differing diagnoses of the disease; methods to establish the diagnosis; intensity of exposure; smoking habits; and genetic risk factors.[22–27]

Clinical Presentation

Traditionally, HP has been described in terms of acute, subacute, and chronic manifestations.[28] Although this classification has merits, there is significant clinical overlap of these stages, and many patients present with findings not purely conforming to one category.[1,2,9,29]

An alternative classification scheme described in a 2011 publication by Lacasse and coworkers[30] sorted patients into clusters on the basis of clinical presentation, physical examination, laboratory results, chest radiograph findings, computed tomography (CT) findings, and bronchoalveolar lavage (BAL) results. This cluster system found that HP patients were most effectively grouped into two clusters. Cluster 1 patients had more recurrent systemic symptoms and fewer abnormal chest radiographs than those in cluster 2. Cluster 2 patients also had more severe restrictive lung disease patterns on pulmonary function testing and more pronounced fibrotic changes on CT. Although this classification scheme may best fit the HP patient population, the acute, subacute, and chronic subgroups persist in the literature and will be maintained throughout this chapter.

Acute HP manifests with abrupt onset of symptoms within 2 to 9 hours of antigenic exposure in a previously sensitized patient. Influenza-like symptoms often predominate, including chills, fever, myalgia, headache, and nausea. Respiratory symptoms range from mild cough to severe dyspnea and occasionally may progress to respiratory failure.[31] Symptoms gradually decrease within hours or days of exposure cessation but may recur after reexposure.

Subacute HP can be triggered by continuous exposure to antigen or repeated acute exposure. Symptoms may appear gradually over a period of several days to weeks. Patients usually present with milder symptoms compared with acute HP, often experiencing exertional dyspnea and cough with or without fever. Numerous exacerbations and remissions of subacute HP over an extended time may be seen in patients with subacute HP.

Chronic HP can develop as a progression from acute or subacute HP or may occur without any preceding HP history. Cough and exertional dyspnea are common initial manifestations, and fatigue and weight loss may be quite severe.[3,9] Bilateral crackles are commonly present on auscultation, and digital clubbing may occur. Chronic HP may progress either to emphysematous or fibrotic end-stage forms, which confer a worse prognosis (Figs. 32.1 and 32.2).[32–35] Pneumothorax, pneumomediastinum, and subcutaneous air are rare manifestations of HP.[33]

Diagnosis

Nonspecific clinical presentation and variable occurrence in exposed individuals require that physicians maintain a high index

*The editors and the publisher would like to thank Drs. Nestor L. Müller and C. Isabela Silva Müller for contributing material on this topic to the prior edition of this work. It has served as the foundation for the current chapter.

TABLE 32.1 MOST COMMON TYPES OF HYPERSENSITIVITY PNEUMONITIS AND COMMON INCITING AGENTS

Disease	Agent	Common Source
Farmer's lung	*Saccharopolyspora rectivirgula, Thermoactinomyces vulgaris, Absidia corymbifera*	Moldy hay, grain, silage
Humidifier lung	*T. vulgaris*	Contaminated forced-air systems; water reservoirs
Mushroom worker's lung	*Thermoactinomyces sacchari*	Moldy mushroom compost
Woodworker's lung, wood pulp worker's lung	*Alternaria tenuis*, wood dust	Oak, cedar, and mahogany dust; pine and spruce pulp
Japanese summer-type pneumonitis	*Trichosporum cutaneum (T. asahii)*	Contaminated old houses (tatami mats)
Hot tub lung	*Mycobacterium avium* complex	Hot tub water
Metal-working fluid–associated hypersensitivity pneumonitis	*Mycobacterium immunogenum*	Metal-working fluids
Bird fancier's lung, pigeon breeder's disease	Avian proteins	Avian droppings, feathers (parakeets, budgerigars, pigeons, chickens, turkeys)
Laboratory worker's lung	Proteins of rats, gerbils	Urine, serum, pelt proteins
Chemical worker's lung	Isocyanates; trimellitic anhydride	Polyurethane foams, spray paints, finishes, sealants, special glues

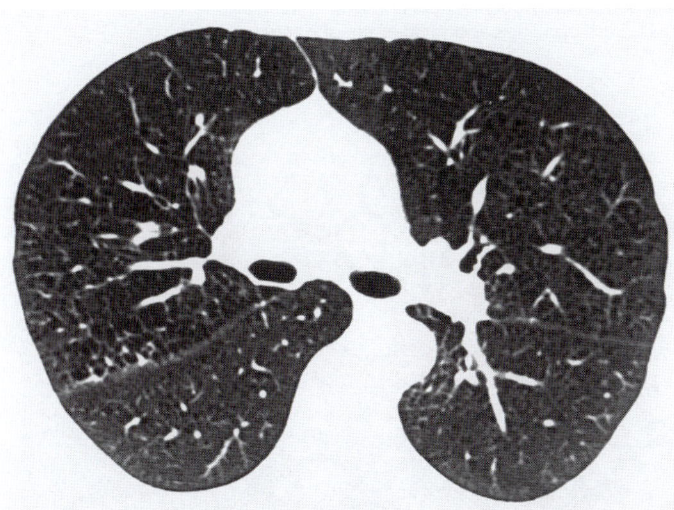

Fig. 32.1 Emphysema in hypersensitivity pneumonitis. High-resolution CT scan shows centrilobular emphysema. No other abnormalities are present. The patient was a lifelong nonsmoker. *(Courtesy Dr. Yvon Cormier, Hospital and University Laval, Ste. Foy, Quebec, Canada.)*

of suspicion and collect a meticulous history in making the diagnosis of HP. In up to 40% of histologically proven cases of HP, the offending agent is not identified.[23,34] In most cases, however, the diagnosis of HP can be made based on a combination of history of exposure to a possible allergen, clinical features, lung function tests, and consistent radiologic findings. The 2003 HP Study, a prospective multicenter study, identified factors that had significant predictive power in identifying active HP. These included known exposure to an offending antigen, onset of symptoms within 8 hours after exposure, the presence of precipitating antibodies, and the presence of inspiratory phase crackles on physical examination.[36]

LABORATORY FINDINGS

Laboratory testing in HP may include hematologic assessment, pulmonary function testing, testing for serum precipitins (precipitating antigens) to common causative antigens, specific inhalation challenge, BAL, and lung biopsy.

Hematologic evaluation in HP may reveal slight to moderate neutrophilic leukocytosis with lymphopenia, particularly during acute and subacute episodes. Nonspecific markers of inflammation, such as C-reactive protein and erythrocyte sedimentation rate, may be elevated.[1,37] Serum precipitating antibodies against the offending antigens may be present, and although these IgG antibodies are excellent markers of exposure to specific antigens in the environment, they are considered confirmatory evidence rather than pathognomonic for HP, and their absence does not exclude the diagnosis of HP. Numerous studies have documented the presence of serum precipitins in asymptomatic individuals with exposure to certain antigens, and conversely, the absence of serum precipitins in patients with HP has also been documented.[23,37,38]

BAL in active HP may show heightened overall cellularity, as well as an elevated proportion of lymphocytes.[1,20,21,37] Notably, during an acute exacerbation, the proportion of neutrophils may be higher than that of lymphocytes.[39,40] Specific inhalation challenge (SIC) tests involve nebulized antigenic exposure in a controlled clinical setting under medical supervision, with pulmonary function testing performed at multiple time points during the examination. SIC examinations are of questionable clinical utility in confirmation of HP diagnosis and may at best provide confirmatory evidence.[41–43]

LUNG FUNCTION

Functional abnormalities in HP include a reduction in the carbon monoxide diffusing capacity, predominantly restrictive lung function with a reduction of total lung capacity and forced vital capacity, and resting hypoxemia that usually worsens during exercise. Although restrictive lung function is the most commonly described long-term outcome in patients who have chronic HP, obstructive pattern findings are identified in some patients.[44–46]

Pathologic Findings

Classic histologic findings of HP have been described, regardless of the type of inciting antigen.[47–50] The histologic patterns of

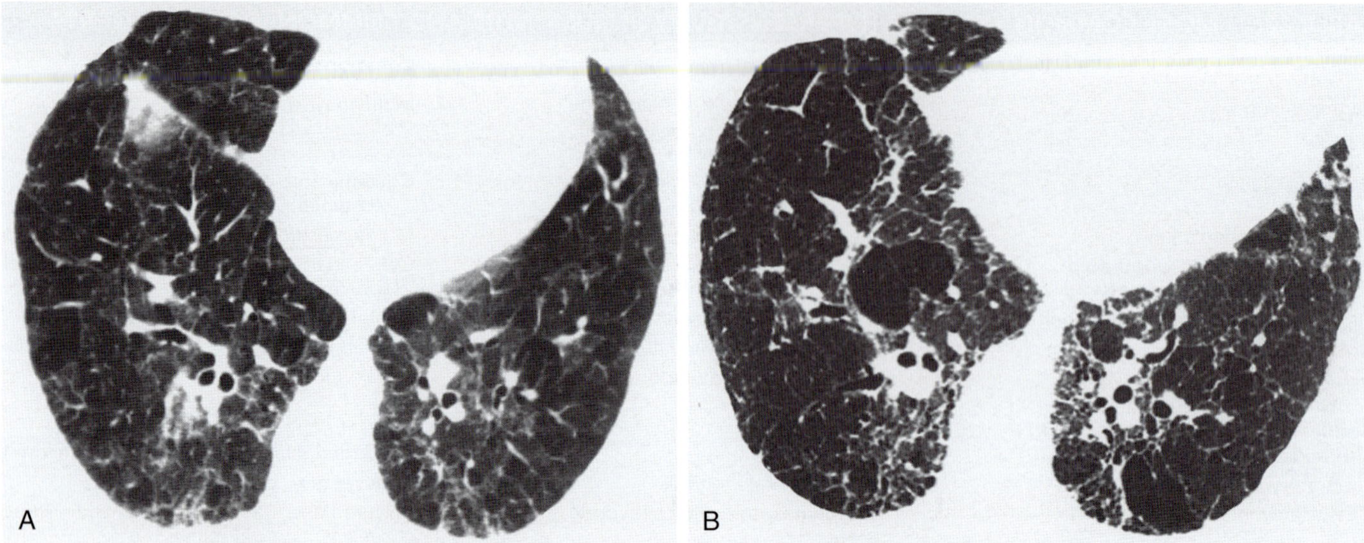

Fig. 32.2 Progression of fibrosis in a patient exposed to red cedar. (A) High-resolution CT scan through the lung bases shows patchy ground-glass opacities with minimal superimposed reticulation and lobular areas of decreased attenuation and vascularity. (B) CT scan 11 years later shows progression of reticulation and architectural distortion with development of traction bronchiectasis and bronchiolectasis and honeycombing resulting from fibrosis. Minimal ground-glass opacities and focal areas of decreased attenuation are present.

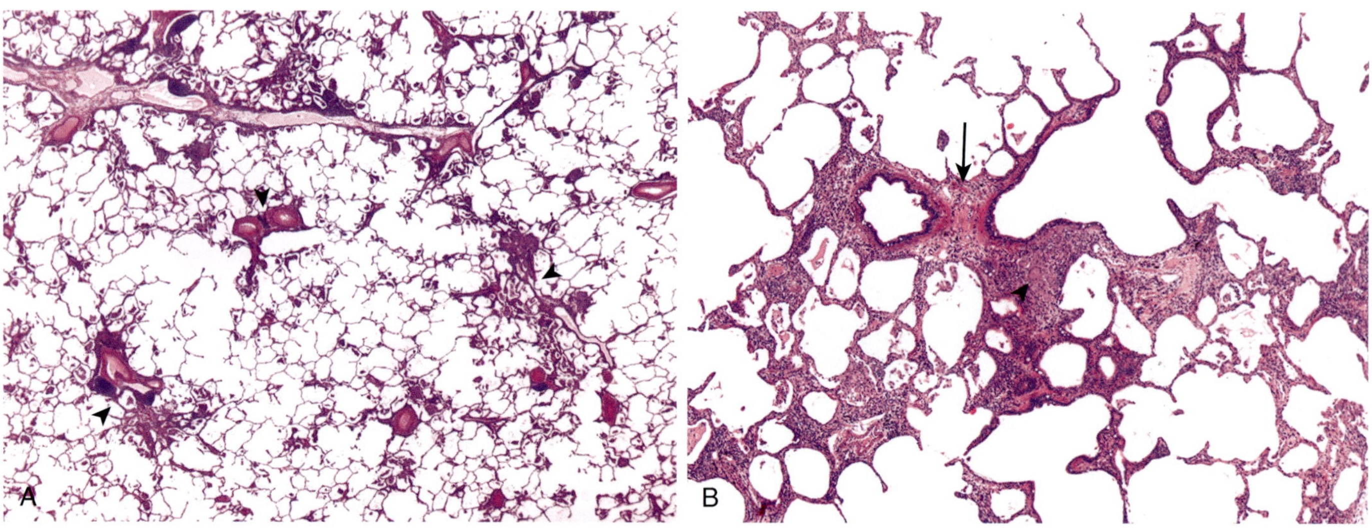

Fig. 32.3 Histologic findings of subacute hypersensitivity pneumonitis. (A) Photomicrograph of surgical lung biopsy specimen shows a moderate chronic lymphocytic inflammatory interstitial infiltrate in a predominantly peribronchiolar distribution *(arrowheads)*. (B) Higher-power view shows chronic lymphocytic inflammatory interstitial infiltrate in a peribronchiolar distribution, cellular bronchiolitis *(arrow)*, and a poorly formed granuloma *(arrowhead)*. These findings are characteristic of hypersensitivity pneumonitis and correlate with the poorly defined centrilobular nodules seen on high-resolution CT. *(Courtesy Dr. John English, Department of Pathology, Vancouver General Hospital, Vancouver, Canada.)*

HP vary with the stage of disease and may mimic the patterns of other interstitial lung diseases.[48,49,51]

Information about the lung biopsy findings of acute HP is limited, as biopsy is rarely performed. Histologic abnormalities described in these patients are nonspecific and include neutrophilic infiltration of the airspace and respiratory bronchioles combined with interstitial pneumonia, acute vasculitis, organizing pneumonia, and a pattern of diffuse alveolar damage.[1,3,29,50–52]

Subacute HP is characterized by a triad of cellular bronchiolitis; chronic bronchiolocentric cellular interstitial pneumonia composed predominantly of lymphocytes; and scattered, small, poorly formed noncaseating granulomas (Fig. 32.3).[47,53,54] Only approximately 60% of patients have all three findings at biopsy, however. In patients with only cellular interstitial pneumonia, the histologic features can be identical to the features of nonspecific interstitial pneumonia (NSIP). Other abnormalities that may be seen include areas of organizing pneumonia and constrictive bronchiolitis (or obliterative bronchiolitis) characterized by smooth muscle hypertrophy, peribronchiolar fibrosis, and partial airway obstruction.[47,54]

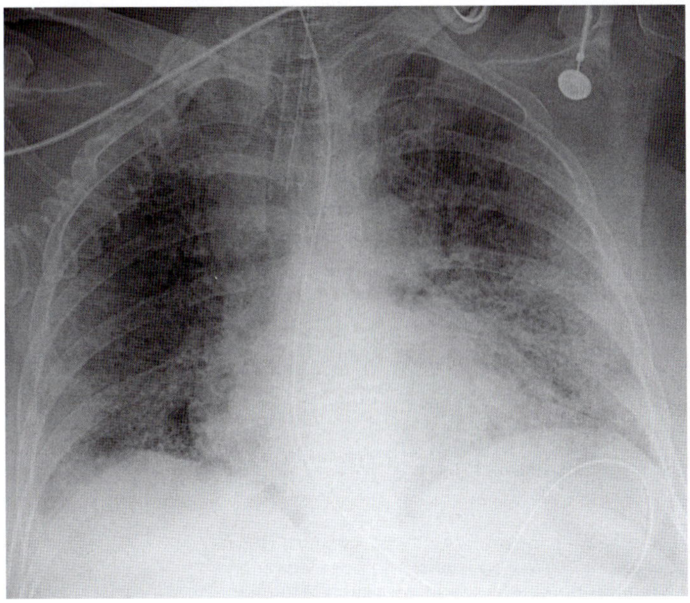

Fig. 32.4 Acute hypersensitivity pneumonitis on chest radiography. Anteroposterior chest radiograph shows extensive bilateral hazy areas of increased opacity (ground-glass opacities) and patchy areas of consolidation. The diagnosis of acute hypersensitivity pneumonitis (bird fancier's lung) was based on the clinical findings and history of exposure.

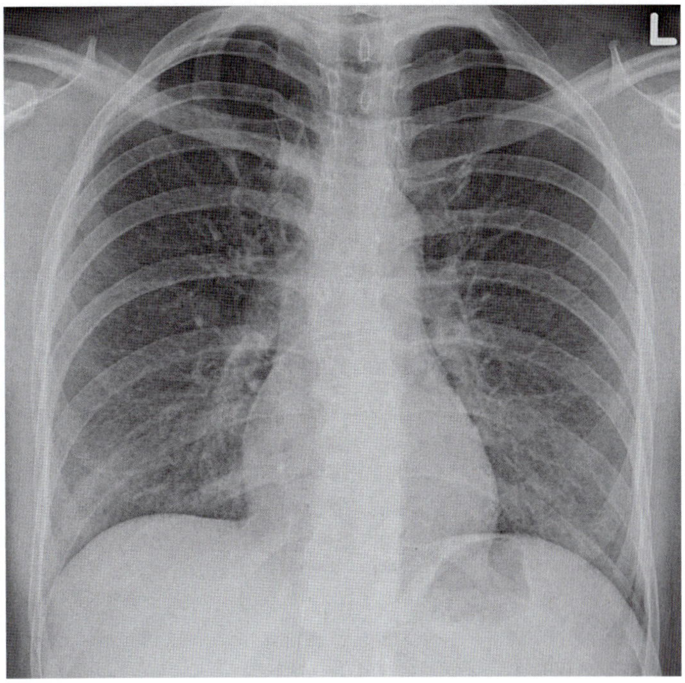

Fig. 32.5 Subacute hypersensitivity pneumonitis on chest radiography. Posteroanterior chest radiograph shows bilateral hazy areas of increased opacity (ground-glass opacities) involving mainly the lower lung zones. Incidental note is made of an accessory azygos fissure. The patient was a bird fancier with biopsy-proven hypersensitivity pneumonitis who presented with clinical findings of asthma.

Histologically, the chronic stage of HP often shows fibrosis superimposed upon findings of subacute HP. NSIP pattern and usual interstitial pneumonia pattern are histologic features of chronic HP and may be the predominant or the only histologic finding.[48,49,51,54,55]

Manifestations of the Disease

RADIOGRAPHY

HP may yield a radiograph with no significant abnormalities, and its only utility may be in excluding other differential considerations.[56] For instance, in a study of patients with bird breeder's lung and abnormal high-resolution CT, 7 (33%) of 21 patients with subacute HP and 1 (4%) of 24 patients with chronic HP had normal chest radiographs.[57] If abnormalities are present, acute HP most commonly manifests with middle or upper lung zone–predominant nodular or reticulonodular opacities (Fig. 32.4).[50,51]

The radiographic features of subacute HP include hazy areas of increased opacity (ground-glass opacities) (Fig. 32.5) and poorly defined nodular opacities (Fig. 32.6).[50,57–59] Although an upper lung zone predominance is commonly seen in other forms of HP, subacute HP has a more variable geographic pattern, and a diffuse or even lower lung zone predominance may be seen. Diffuse consolidation is rare in patients with subacute HP, and when present, superimposed infection should be considered (Fig. 32.7). Pneumomediastinum, pneumothorax, and subcutaneous air may be seen in some patients, presumably resulting from overdistention or disruption of alveoli with obliteration of the respiratory bronchioles (Fig. 32.8).[33]

The radiographic manifestations of chronic HP may include reticular opacities, honeycombing, and volume loss (Fig. 32.9).[50,60]

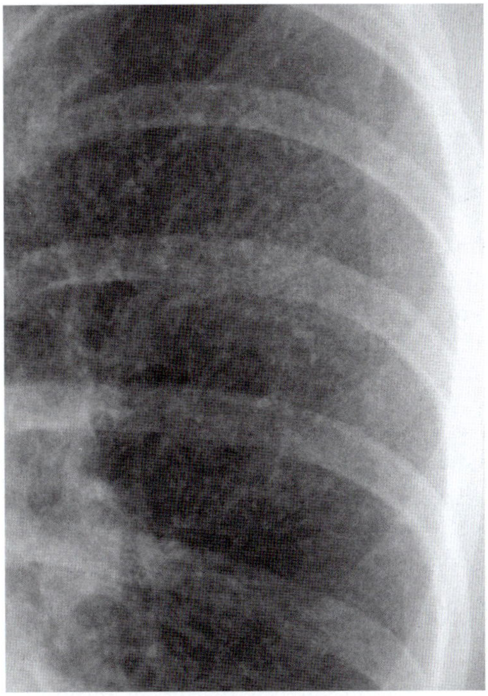

Fig. 32.6 Subacute hypersensitivity pneumonitis on chest radiography. Magnified view of left lung from a chest radiograph shows poorly defined small nodular opacities in a patient with pigeon breeder's lung. This appearance correlates with the poorly defined centrilobular nodules seen on high-resolution CT.

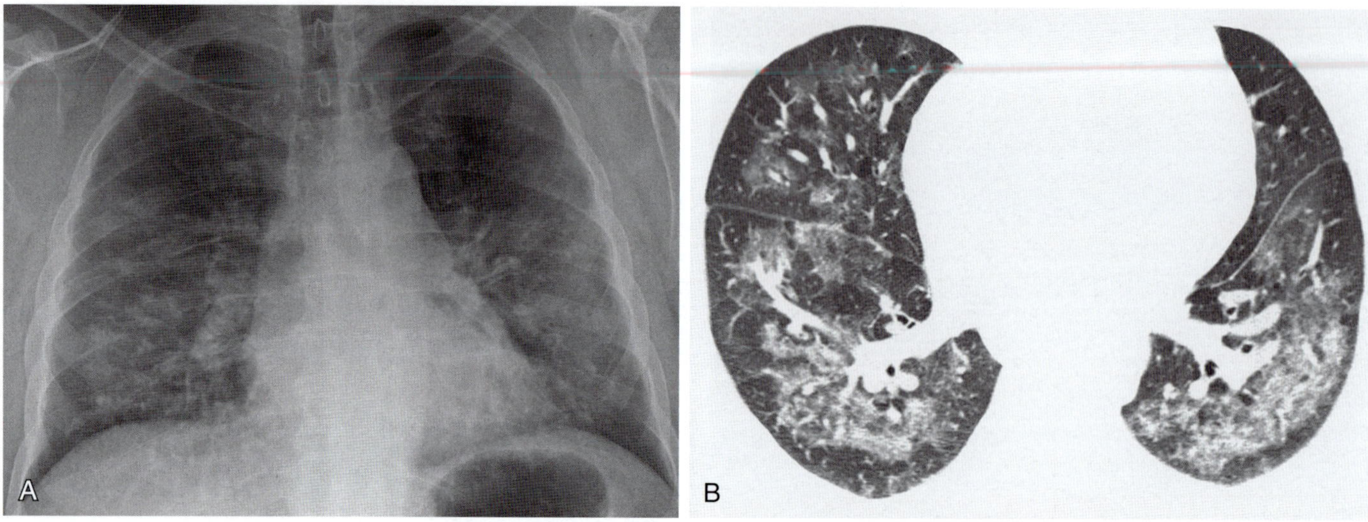

Fig. 32.7 Subacute hypersensitivity pneumonitis from isocyanate exposure. (A) Posteroanterior chest radiograph shows bilateral hazy areas of increased opacity (ground-glass opacities) and poorly defined nodular opacities in the middle and lower lung zones with relative peripheral sparing. (B) High-resolution CT at the level of the inferior pulmonary veins shows diffuse ground-glass opacities in a peribronchovascular distribution and minimal consolidation posteriorly secondary to organizing pneumonia.

The fibrosis may be diffuse and severe in all lung zones or have an upper or middle lung zone predominance.[59–61] Hilar and mediastinal lymph node enlargement may be seen and is a nonspecific finding (Fig. 32.10).[62]

COMPUTED TOMOGRAPHY

A multicenter study by Lacasse and coworkers[23] showed that the diagnosis of HP often can be made or rejected with confidence based on clinical history and high-resolution CT findings without the need for bronchoscopy or biopsy.[23] Transbronchial biopsy and surgical biopsy are generally considered for patients in whom bronchoalveolar lavage and high-resolution CT fail to yield a confident diagnosis.[63] High-resolution CT frequently shows characteristic findings in patients with normal or nonspecific chest radiographs (Fig. 32.11).[23,50,58,59,64]

Acute Phase

Because of the milder clinical manifestations and often rapid resolution of the symptoms, high-resolution CT is uncommonly performed in the assessment of patients with acute HP. CT in acute HP may be completely unremarkable. When abnormalities are present, the most common high-resolution CT findings consist of diffuse ground-glass opacities and consolidation.[50] Centrilobular nodules also may be seen. The diffuse airspace opacification seen in acute HP may be due to diffuse alveolar damage or acute organizing pneumonia.[54]

Subacute Phase

High-resolution CT in subacute HP may show poorly defined small centrilobular nodules (Fig. 32.12), symmetric patchy or diffuse bilateral ground-glass opacities, and lobular areas of decreased attenuation and vascularity on inspiratory images (mosaic attenuation) and air-trapping on expiratory images (Figs. 32.13 and 32.14).[a] Imaging abnormalities in subacute HP may show a diffuse distribution, an upper lung zone predominance, or may even show a middle and lower lung zone predominance with sparing of the bases.

Centrilobular nodules are seen in 40% to 76% of patients with subacute HP[57,59,65]; these nodules are often located several millimeters away from the pleural surfaces, interlobar fissures, and interlobular septa and are usually of ground-glass attenuation (see Figs. 32.12 and 32.13). Rarely, the nodules may appear well defined or have an apparent random distribution (Fig. 32.15). Histologically, the centrilobular nodules correspond to cellular bronchiolitis, noncaseating granulomas, and bronchiolocentric interstitial pneumonitis (see Figs. 32.3 and 32.15).

Ground-glass opacities are present in 82% of patients with subacute HP.[57,59,65] These ground-glass opacities reflect the presence of diffuse interstitial pneumonitis (Fig. 32.16).[54,58] The extent of ground-glass opacities has been shown to correlate with the severity of lung restriction and impairment in gas exchange.[65] Ground-glass opacities may be seen in conjunction with centrilobular nodules (see Figs. 32.8, 32.11, 32.13, and 32.14) or, less commonly, as an isolated finding (Fig. 32.17; see Fig. 32.16). Ground-glass opacities are also often present in conjunction with localized areas of decreased attenuation and vascularity, a finding that has been referred to as the "headcheese sign" (Fig. 32.18).[67] The headcheese sign is not specific for HP, however, and may be seen in any condition in which there is small airways disease and lung infiltration.

The areas of low attenuation in HP often have a striking lobular distribution and often correlate with regions of air-trapping on expiratory CT scans (see Fig. 32.18).[58,65,66] Such areas represent indirect signs of bronchiolar obstruction in HP and are presumably secondary to small airway obstruction by cellular bronchiolitis or, less commonly, constrictive bronchiolitis. The extent of lobular areas of decreased attenuation and vascularity correlates with an increase in residual volume and the residual volume–total lung capacity ratio.[65] Air-trapping on expiratory images may be the predominant or the only CT finding of

Text continued on p. 489

[a]References 23, 50, 54, 58, 59, 61, 65, 66.

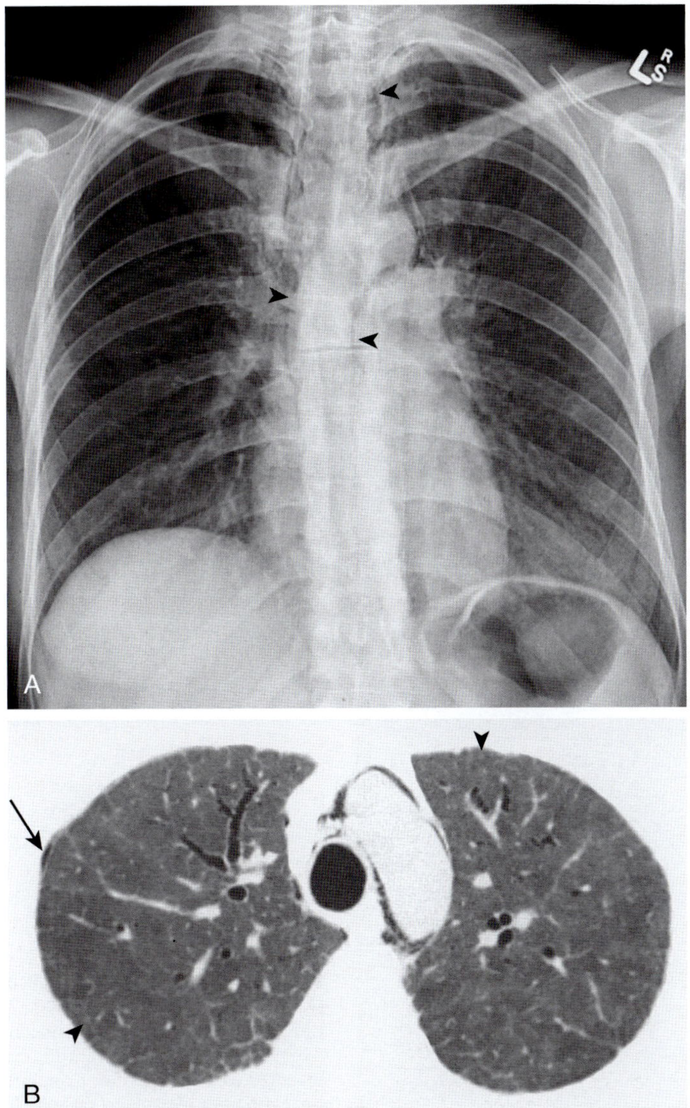

Fig. 32.8 Subacute hypersensitivity pneumonitis. (A) Posteroanterior chest radiograph shows bilateral hazy areas of increased opacity (ground-glass opacities) and pneumomediastinum *(arrowheads)*. (B) High-resolution CT at the level of the aortic arch shows diffuse ground-glass opacities and a few ill-defined centrilobular nodules *(arrowheads)* typical of hypersensitivity pneumonitis. Note small right pneumothorax *(arrow)* and pneumomediastinum. The patient had biopsy-proven hypersensitivity pneumonitis resulting from exposure to feathers in a bedcover (feather duvet), who presented with pneumomediastinum and right pneumothorax.

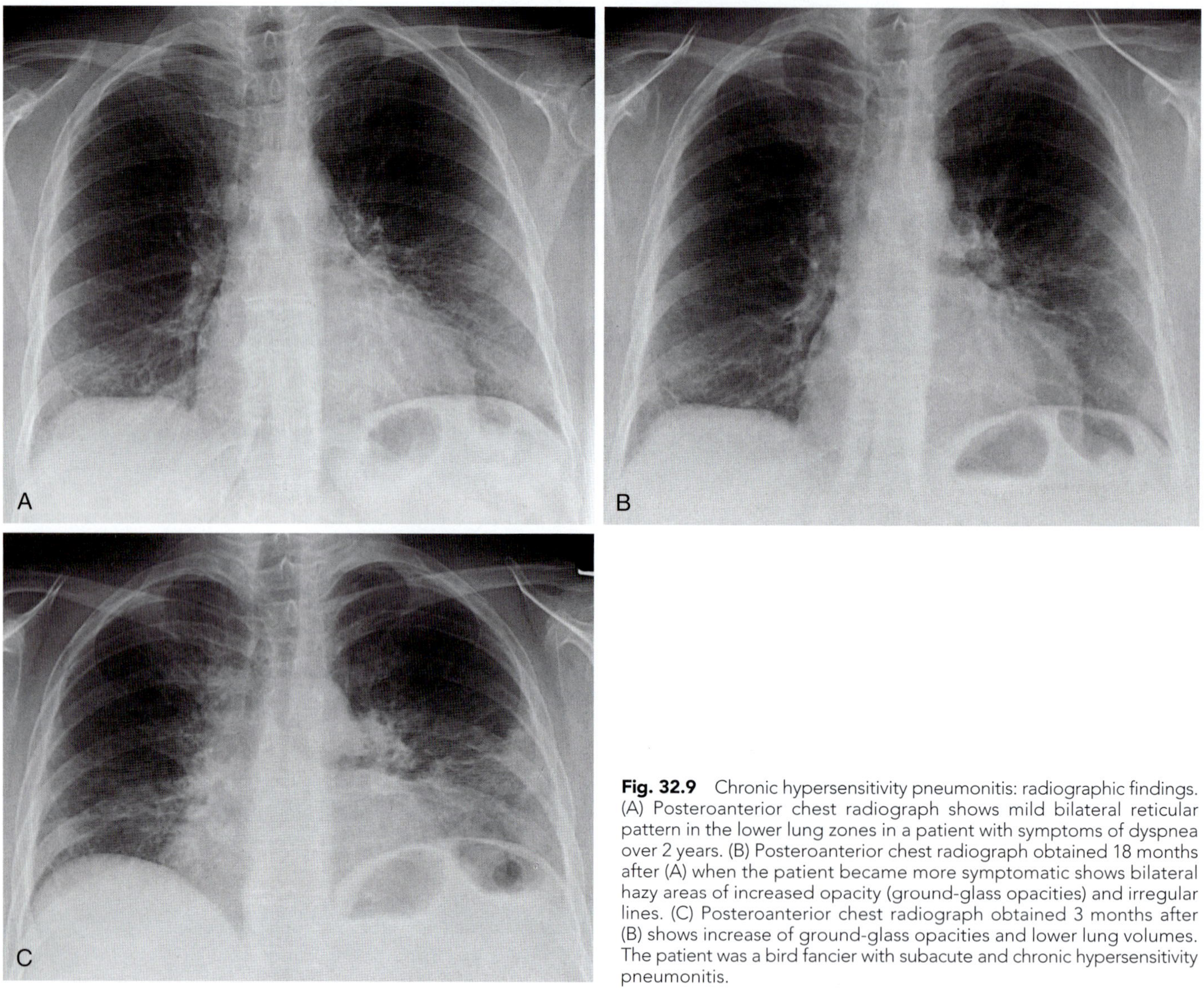

Fig. 32.9 Chronic hypersensitivity pneumonitis: radiographic findings. (A) Posteroanterior chest radiograph shows mild bilateral reticular pattern in the lower lung zones in a patient with symptoms of dyspnea over 2 years. (B) Posteroanterior chest radiograph obtained 18 months after (A) when the patient became more symptomatic shows bilateral hazy areas of increased opacity (ground-glass opacities) and irregular lines. (C) Posteroanterior chest radiograph obtained 3 months after (B) shows increase of ground-glass opacities and lower lung volumes. The patient was a bird fancier with subacute and chronic hypersensitivity pneumonitis.

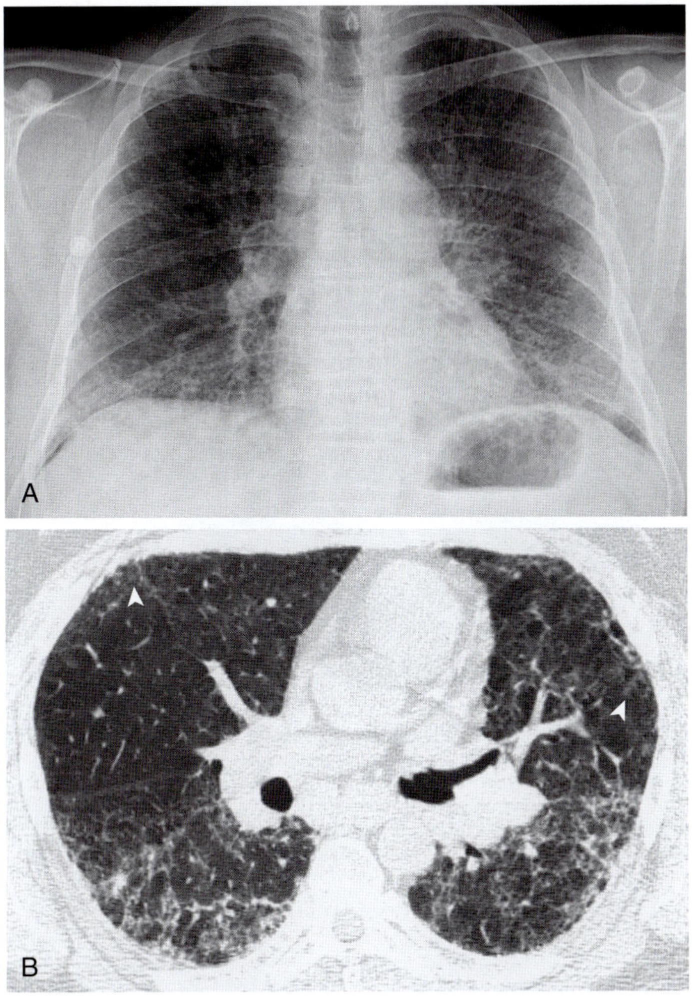

Fig. 32.10 Chronic hypersensitivity pneumonitis associated with lymph node enlargement in a patient exposed to feathers. (A) Posteroanterior chest radiograph shows extensive bilateral reticular pattern and mediastinal and bilateral hilar lymphadenopathy. (B) High-resolution CT scan at the level of the bronchus intermedius shows patchy ground-glass opacities and superimposed fine reticulation. A few ill-defined centrilobular nodules *(arrowheads)* and centrilobular emphysema are also present. Note subcarinal and bilateral hilar lymph node enlargement.

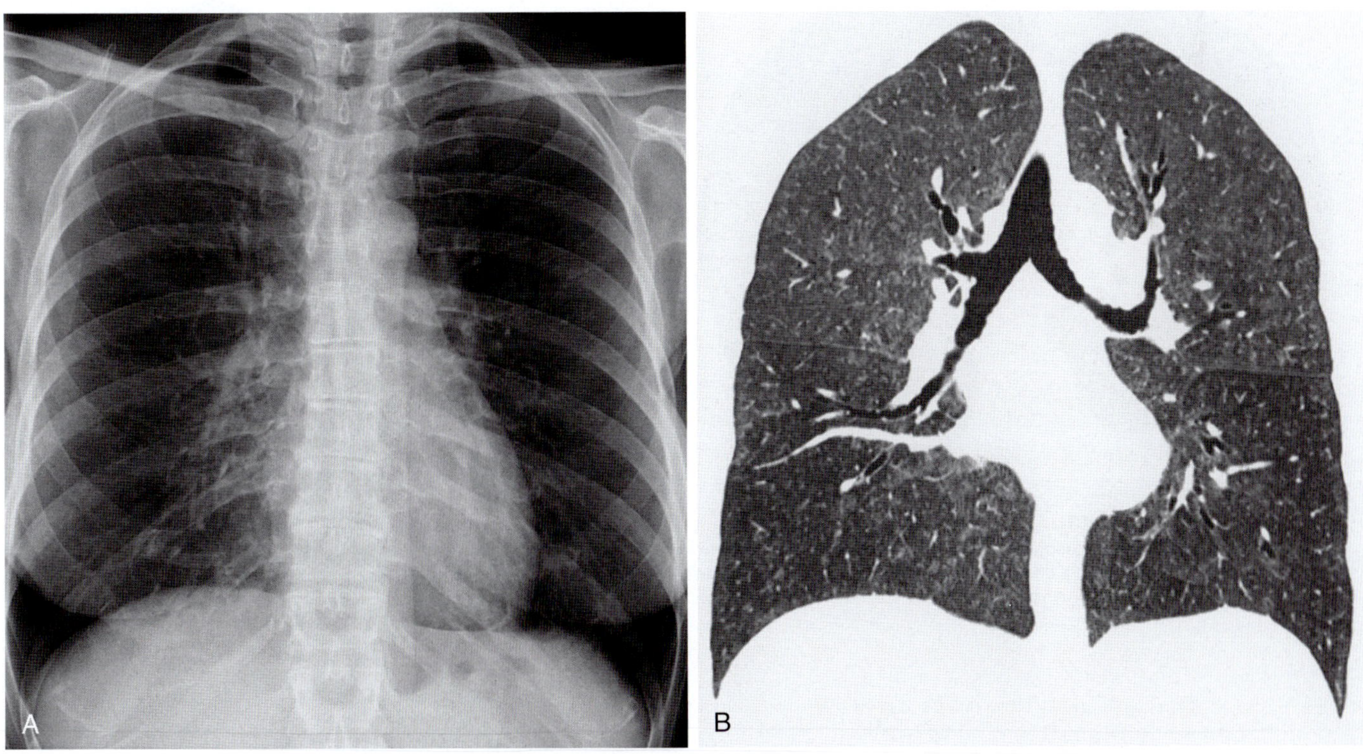

Fig. 32.11 Subacute hypersensitivity pneumonitis in patient with progressive dyspnea while working in a bird hospital. (A) Posteroanterior chest radiograph shows no definite abnormalities. (B) Coronal reformatted CT image obtained at the same day of the chest radiograph shows poorly defined centrilobular nodules and diffuse ground-glass opacities mainly in the upper and middle lung zones.

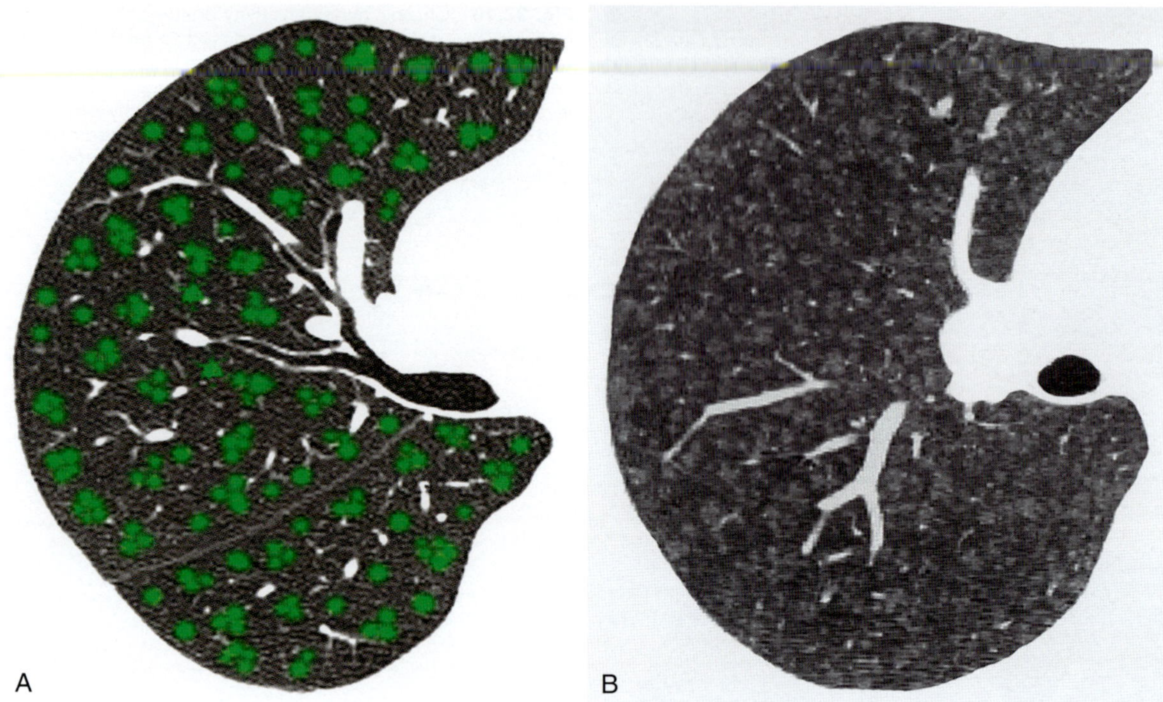

Fig. 32.12 Subacute hypersensitivity pneumonitis: schematic representation and CT appearance of centrilobular nodules. (A) Schematic representation shows typical distribution and appearance of nodular pattern of subacute hypersensitivity pneumonitis on high-resolution CT. The nodules are poorly defined and have ground-glass attenuation. The nodules usually measure 3–5 mm in diameter and typically appear as clusters. They are centered a few millimeters away from the pleural surfaces, interlobar fissures, and interlobular septa (centrilobular distribution). (B) High-resolution CT scan targeted to the right lung shows characteristic centrilobular nodules in a patient with bird breeder's lung.

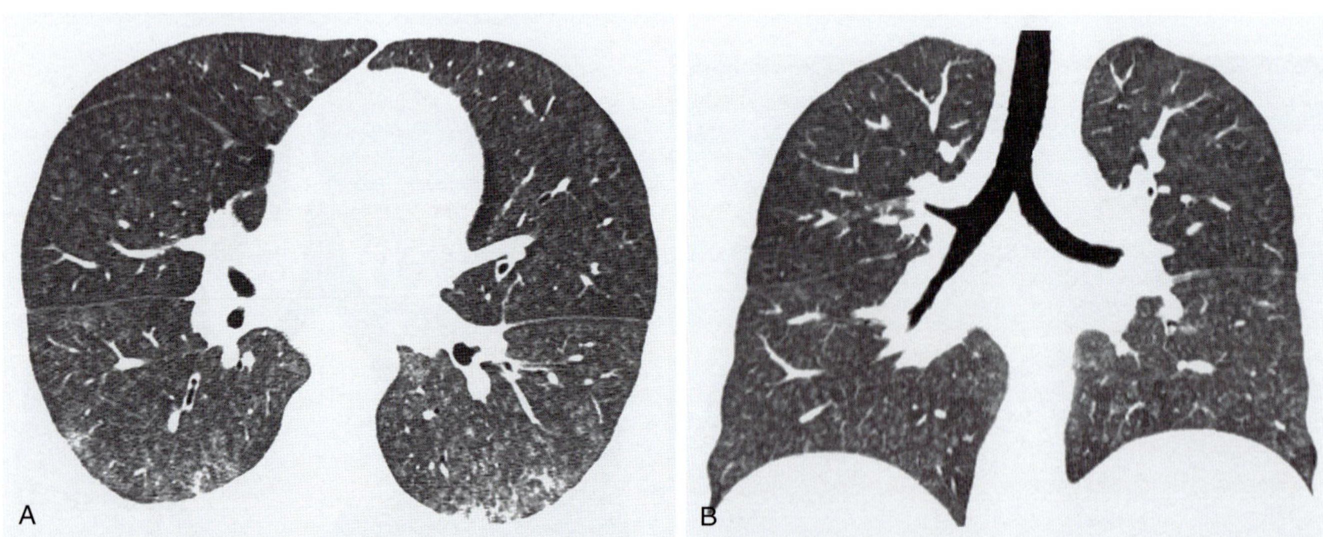

Fig. 32.13 Subacute hypersensitivity pneumonitis (bird fancier's lung): high-resolution CT findings. (A) High-resolution CT scan shows diffuse ground-glass opacities and bilateral poorly defined small nodules in a characteristic centrilobular distribution. (B) Coronal reformatted image shows diffuse distribution of abnormalities. A few subtle, localized areas of decreased attenuation and vascularity are seen in the lung bases.

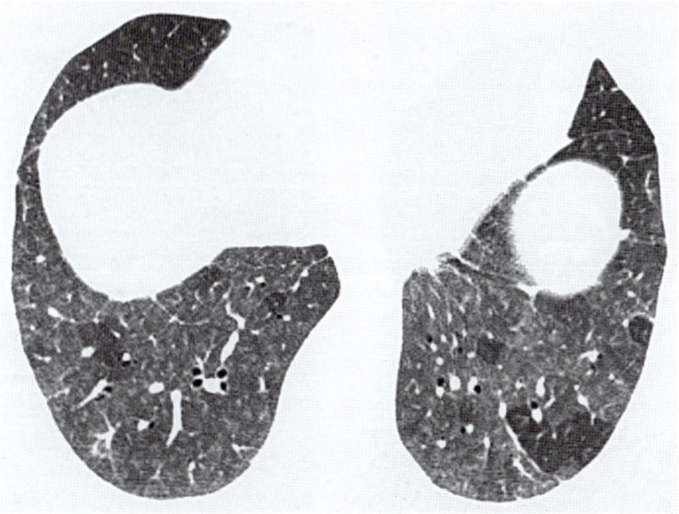

Fig. 32.14 Subacute hypersensitivity pneumonitis. High-resolution CT scan at the level of lung bases shows diffuse ground-glass opacities and poorly defined centrilobular nodules. Note lobular areas of decreased attenuation and vascularity reflecting cellular bronchiolitis or constrictive bronchiolitis associated with hypersensitivity pneumonitis.

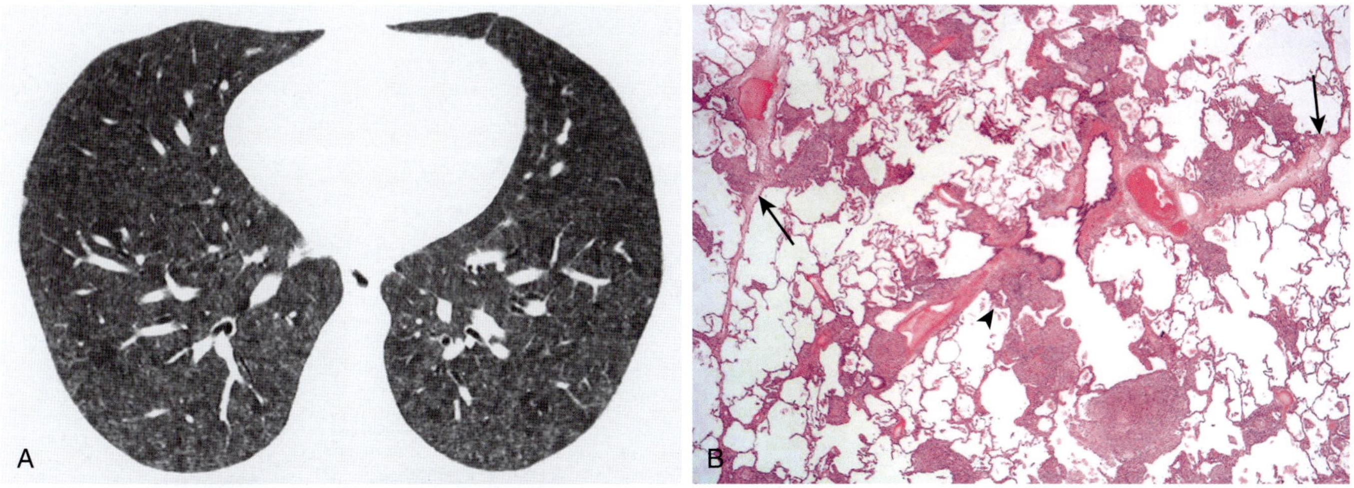

Fig. 32.15 Hot tub lung related to recurring exposure to *Mycobacterium avium* complex organisms contaminating hot tub water. (A) High-resolution CT scan shows diffuse ground-glass opacities and small nodules measuring approximately 1–2 mm. (B) Intermediate magnification of surgical lung biopsy specimen shows numerous prominent nonnecrotizing well-formed granulomas accompanied by a moderate chronic interstitial inflammatory infiltrate. Note the lack of definite predilection for anatomic distribution of the nonnecrotizing granulomas. They are seen along the interlobular septa *(arrows)* and bronchovascular bundles *(arrowhead)*, consistent with a random distribution. The nonnecrotizing granulomas correlate with the small nodules seen on CT, and the chronic interstitial inflammatory infiltrate correlates with the ground-glass opacities.

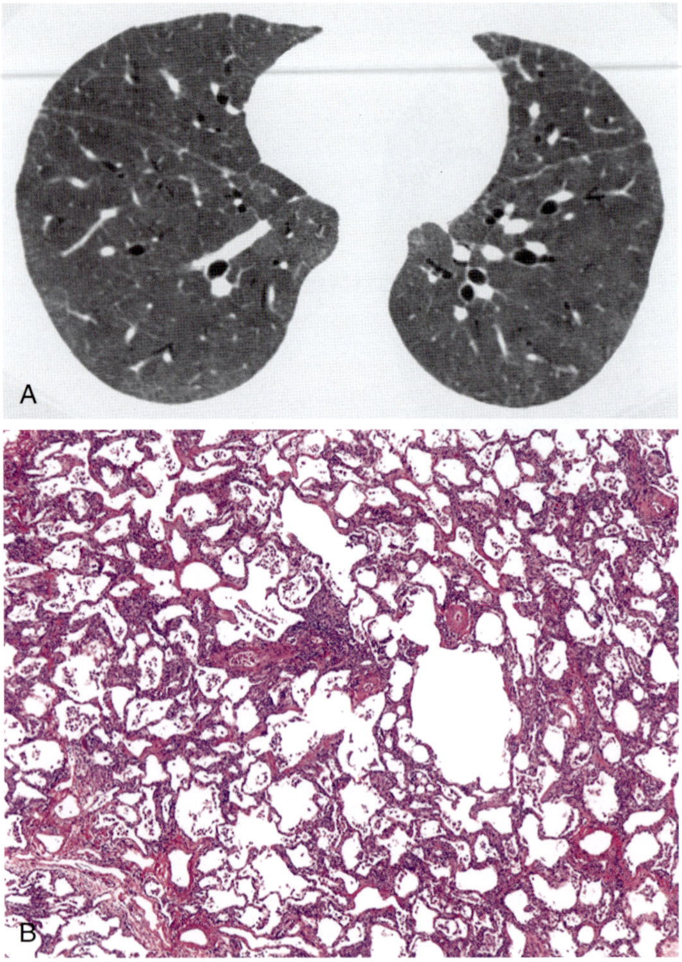

Fig. 32.16 Ground-glass opacity in subacute hypersensitivity pneumonitis: pathologic correlation. (A) High-resolution CT scan shows extensive ground-glass opacities. (B) Low-power view of surgical lung biopsy specimen shows moderate to diffuse chronic lymphocytic inflammatory interstitial infiltrate. This finding accounts for the ground-glass opacity seen on high-resolution CT. *(B, courtesy Dr. John English, Department of Pathology, Vancouver General Hospital, Vancouver, Canada.)*

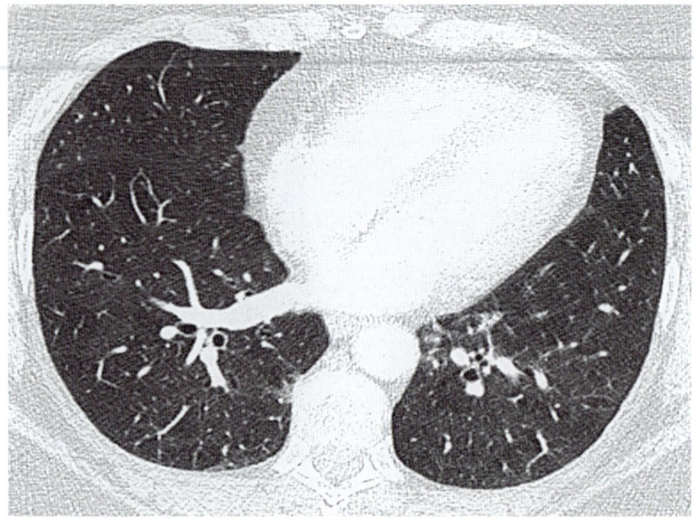

Fig. 32.17 Ground-glass opacity in subacute hypersensitivity pneumonitis in a bird breeder. High-resolution CT scan at the level of the right inferior pulmonary vein shows subtle abnormalities characterized by patchy lower lobe ground-glass opacities.

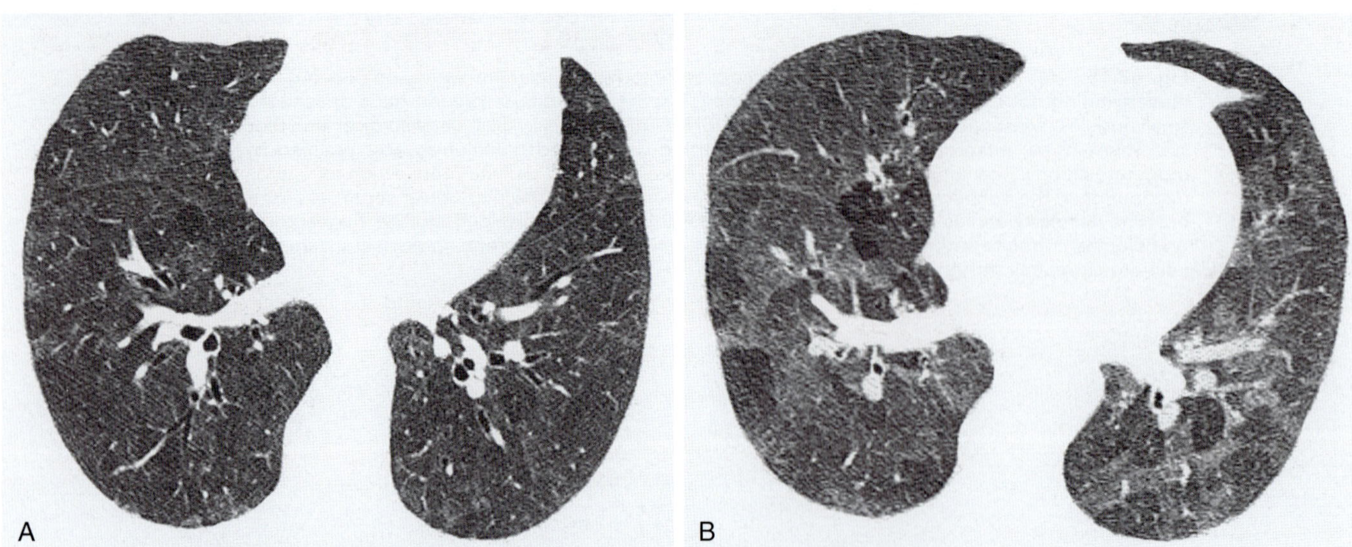

Fig. 32.18 Subacute hypersensitivity pneumonitis with the "headcheese sign." (A) High-resolution CT scan at the level of the right inferior pulmonary vein shows diffuse ground-glass opacity interposed with areas of normal lung and lobular areas of decreased attenuation and vascularity. The combination of ground-glass opacity, normal lung, and areas of decreased attenuation and vascularity gives the lung a geographic appearance called the headcheese sign. (B) Expiratory CT scan at the same level as (A) shows focal areas of air-trapping reflecting cellular bronchiolitis or, less commonly, constrictive bronchiolitis.

subacute HP (Fig. 32.19). Thus expiratory phase imaging should be incorporated into the chest CT protocol when there is clinical suspicion of HP. Focal areas of consolidation are seen occasionally and presumably reflect the presence of superimposed organizing pneumonia (see Fig. 32.7).

Thin-walled cysts in a random distribution are found in 13% of patients with subacute HP.[68] The cysts are typically few in number (1–15), range from 3 to 25 mm in maximal diameter, and are often geographically associated with ground-glass opacities.[68] These cysts are thought to arise in areas with bronchiolitis and bronchiolar obstruction.[69,70] Pneumomediastinum, pneumothorax, and subcutaneous air (air-leak syndrome) are rare (see Fig. 32.8).[33]

Chronic Phase

The high-resolution CT findings of chronic HP consist of findings of fibrosis with reticulation, architectural distortion, traction bronchiectasis and bronchiolectasis, and honeycombing (Fig. 32.20; see Fig. 32.10).[54,60,65,71,72] The fibrosis in chronic HP can be patchy, random, or peribronchovascular (Fig. 32.21) or have a predominantly subpleural distribution mimicking usual interstitial pneumonia (UIP) (Fig. 32.22).[60,65,72,73] The distribution of chronic HP findings in the cephalocaudal plane varies. CT may show middle lung zone predominance of fibrosis with sparing of the lung apices and bases (Fig. 32.23), upper lung zone predominance (see Fig. 32.21), lower lung zone predominance (Figs. 32.24 and 32.25), or no zonal predominance.[60,64,72]

Imaging is most helpful in diagnosing HP in cases with an upper lung zone predominance as this is atypical for UIP and NSIP. In most cases there are other contributory CT abnormalities (i.e., ground-glass opacities, lobular areas of decreased attenuation, and poorly defined centrilobular nodules) that usually aid in establishing the correct diagnosis (Fig. 32.26; see Fig. 32.20).[54,60,72] Ground-glass opacities are seen in most patients with chronic

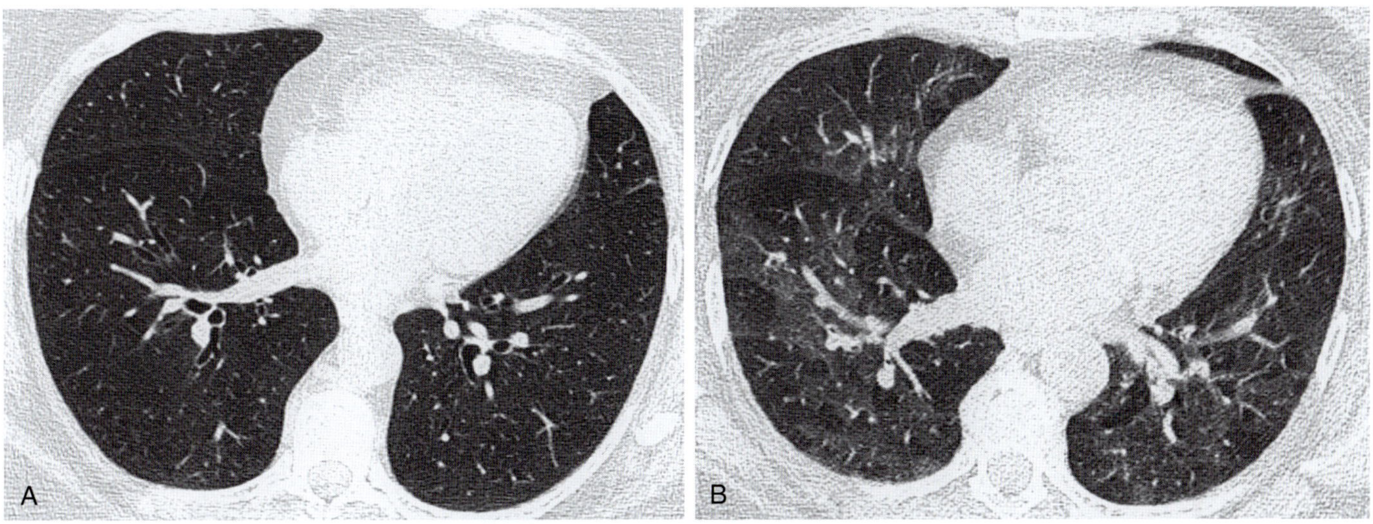

Fig. 32.19 Subacute hypersensitivity pneumonitis with normal inspiratory CT in a bird breeder with progressive shortness of breath and positive precipitins for avian antigen. (A) Inspiratory high-resolution CT scan at the level of the right inferior pulmonary vein is normal. (B) Expiratory CT scan at the same level as (A) shows patchy air-trapping.

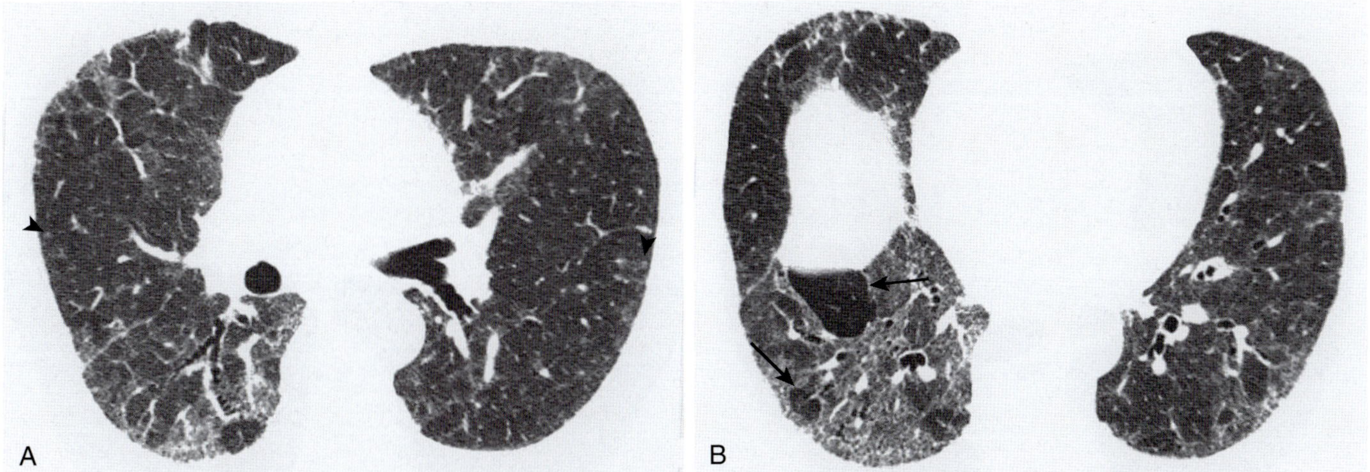

Fig. 32.20 Typical CT findings of biopsy-proven chronic hypersensitivity pneumonitis in a bird breeder. (A) and (B) High-resolution CT scans show mild reticulation with superimposed patchy ground-glass opacities and traction bronchiectasis and bronchiolectasis. A few poorly defined centrilobular nodules *(arrowheads)* and lobular areas of decreased attenuation and vascularity *(arrows)* are also present.

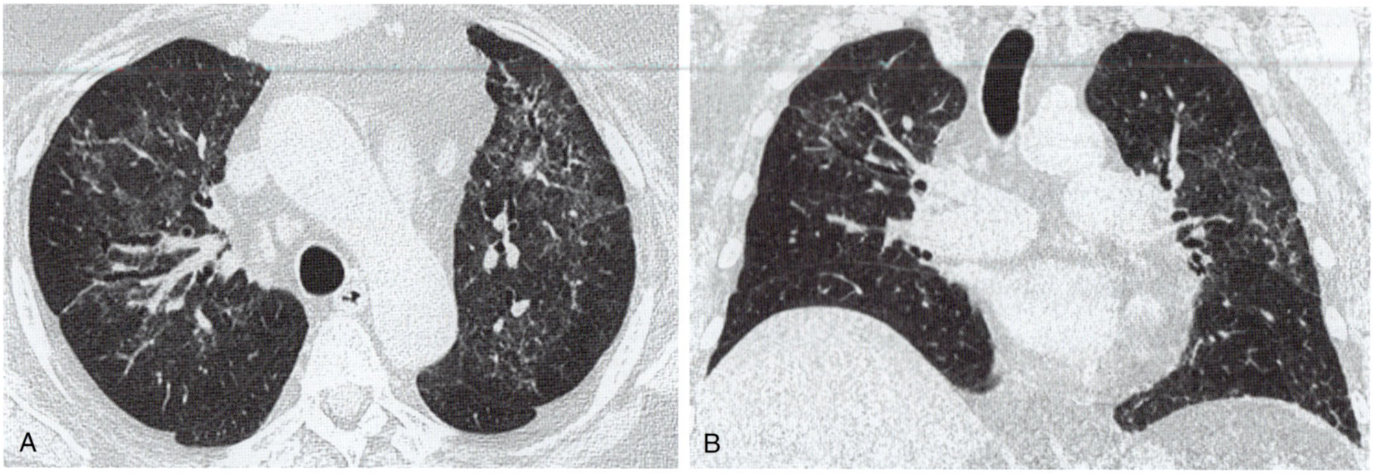

Fig. 32.21 Chronic hypersensitivity pneumonitis in a bird breeder. (A) High-resolution CT scan at the level of aortic arch shows mild ground-glass opacities with superimposed reticulation in a peribronchovascular/perihilar distribution. Note bilateral traction bronchiectasis indicating fibrosis. (B) Coronal reformatted image shows predominant upper zone distribution of the abnormalities.

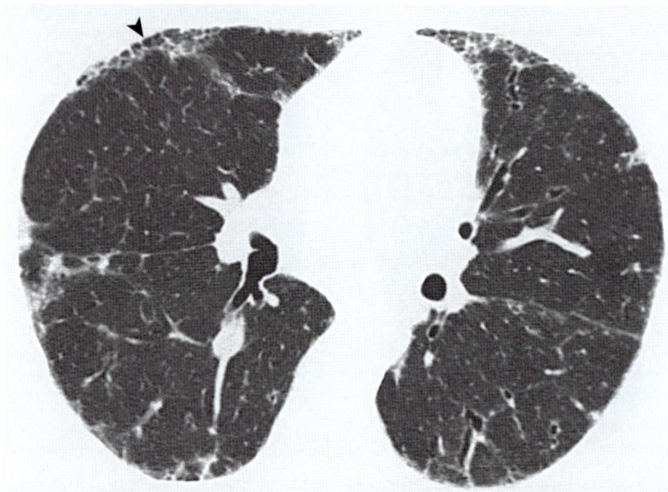

Fig. 32.22 Chronic hypersensitivity pneumonitis with usual interstitial pneumonia pattern secondary to inhalation of isocyanates. High-resolution CT scan shows mild peripheral reticulation and subpleural honeycombing *(arrowhead)*. Traction bronchiectasis and bronchiolectasis are also noted. No ground-glass opacities are present. These findings are similar to the findings seen in idiopathic pulmonary fibrosis.

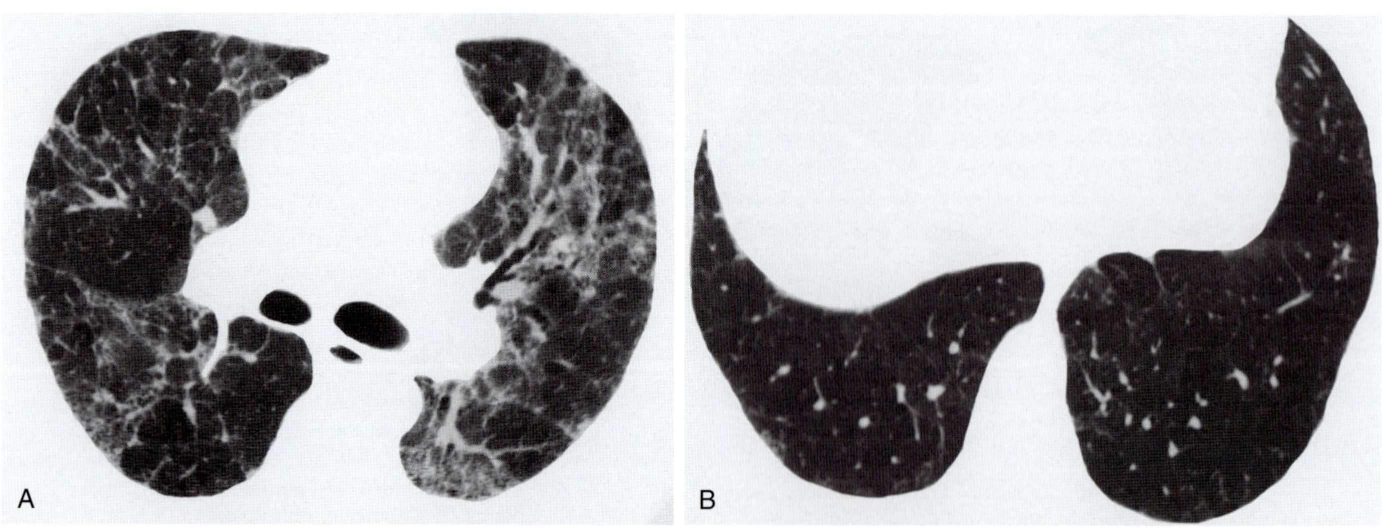

Fig. 32.23 Chronic hypersensitivity pneumonitis in a man exposed to red cedar. (A) High-resolution CT scan at the level of left main bronchus shows patchy ground-glass opacities, minimal reticulation, and lobular areas of decreased attenuation. (B) Note relative sparing at the lung bases, a characteristic finding of chronic hypersensitivity pneumonitis.

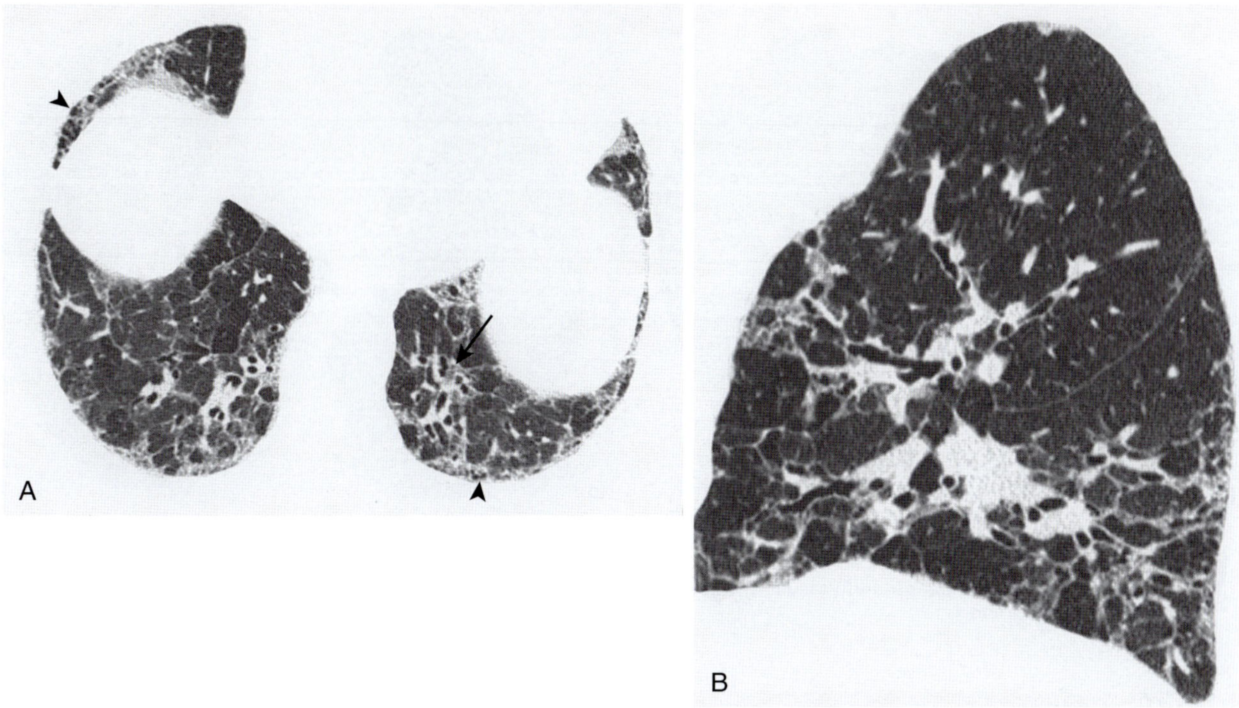

Fig. 32.24 Chronic hypersensitivity pneumonitis. (A) High-resolution CT scan at the level of the lung bases shows diffuse ground-glass opacities and patchy, peribronchovascular *(arrow)* and subpleural reticulation. Minimal subpleural honeycombing *(arrowheads)* and lobular areas of decreased attenuation are present. Note bilateral traction bronchiectasis suggesting fibrosis. (B) Sagittal reformatted image shows predominant lower zone distribution of the abnormalities. The presence of lobular areas of decreased attenuation, diffuse ground-glass opacities, and lack of subpleural predominance of fibrosis are typical for chronic hypersensitivity pneumonitis despite the lower zone predominance of abnormalities commonly seen in patients with usual interstitial pneumonia or nonspecific interstitial pneumonia.

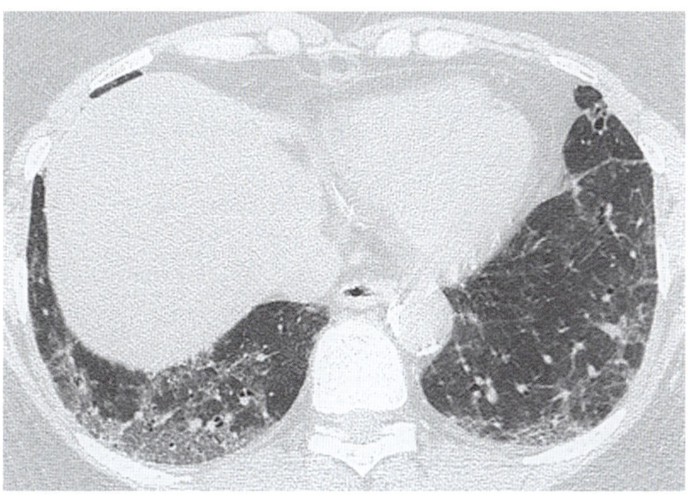

Fig. 32.25 Biopsy-proven chronic hypersensitivity pneumonitis with nonspecific interstitial pneumonia pattern. High-resolution CT scan through the lung bases shows subpleural ground-glass opacities with minimal superimposed reticulation, a pattern suggestive of nonspecific interstitial pneumonia.

HP but frequently involve less than 50% of the lung parenchyma and have a patchy distribution.[72] Lobular areas of decreased attenuation and vascularity are found in 80% of patients with chronic HP,[65,66,71,72] whereas poorly defined centrilobular nodules are identified in approximately 50%.[64,72] Cystic changes may be seen in up to 40% of chronic HP cases (Fig. 32.27).[72] Some extent of honeycombing occurs in 16% to 69% of patients with chronic HP (see Figs. 32.22 and 32.24).[57,60,64,72] In contrast to the honeycombing in patients with UIP, the honeycombing in patients with chronic HP seldom has a basal predominance.[72] Although emphysema is usually due to smoking, in farmer's lung, emphysema may be the predominant or only manifestation of chronic HP, even in nonsmokers (see Fig. 32.1). Lymph node enlargement is common, but usually only one or two nodes are enlarged, and their short-axis diameter is less than 15 mm (see Fig. 32.10).[62,74]

Acute Exacerbations

Acute exacerbations of HP often produce a precipitous deterioration in clinical status, and recognition of key imaging findings is essential if life-saving efforts are to be appropriately taken. The mechanism of acute exacerbations in HP remains under investigation. Acute exacerbations may represent a severe manifestation of the patient's underlying HP or may alternatively represent a pathophysiologically distinct process.[75] Several studies have demonstrated a relative increase in both fibrotic changes as well as ground-glass opacities on CT during an acute exacerbation of HP.[75,76] Histologic evaluation performed during an acute exacerbation as part of this same study revealed a relative increase in the proportion of neutrophils and decrease in the proportion of lymphocytes in BAL fluid.[76] Patients show very limited response to corticosteroid therapy and other attempts at symptomatic relief; patients often require mechanical ventilation and emergent lung transplantation.

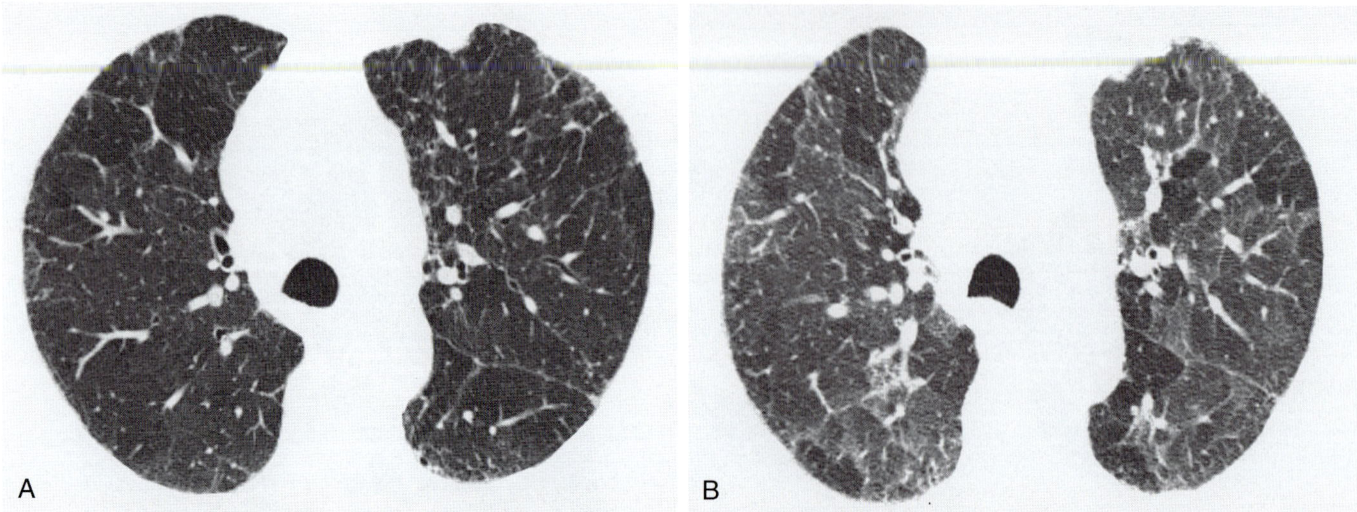

Fig. 32.26 Air trapping in chronic hypersensitivity pneumonitis. (A) High-resolution CT scan at the level of the upper lobes shows diffuse ground-glass opacities, minimal fibrosis, and focal areas of decreased attenuation and vascularity (mosaic attenuation). (B) Expiratory CT accentuates the areas of air-trapping.

CLASSIC SIGNS

ACUTE HYPERSENSITIVITY PNEUMONITIS

- Characterized by abrupt onset of symptoms within a few hours after heavy antigen exposure
- High-resolution CT rarely performed

SUBACUTE HYPERSENSITIVITY PNEUMONITIS

- Caused by intermittent or continuous exposure to low doses of antigen
- Radiographic findings
  - Hazy areas of increased opacity
  - Poorly defined nodular opacities
  - May be diffuse, but tend to involve mainly the upper lung zones
  - Pneumomediastinum and pneumothorax are rare
- High-resolution CT findings, more common:
  - Patchy or diffuse ground-glass opacities
  - Poorly defined centrilobular nodules
  - Lobular areas of decreased attenuation
  - Headcheese sign
  - Air-trapping
- High-resolution CT findings, less common:
  - Irregular nodules greater than 10 mm
  - Cysts, typically one to four in number, associated with ground-glass opacities in 13%
  - Consolidation as a result of organizing pneumonia
  - Pneumomediastinum, pneumothorax, and subcutaneous air are rare

CHRONIC HYPERSENSITIVITY PNEUMONITIS

- Results from very low level, persistent or recurrent exposure to antigen
- Characterized by the presence of fibrosis
- Radiographic findings
  - Reticular pattern
  - Volume loss
  - Honeycombing
  - Lymph node enlargement may be seen
- High-resolution CT findings
  - Patchy, peripheral, or peribronchovascular reticulation
  - Traction bronchiectasis and traction bronchiolectasis
  - Minimal honeycombing
  - Relative sparing of the lung bases
  - Superimposed findings of subacute disease are common
  - Emphysema in farmer's lung
  - Cysts in 40% of patients
  - Lymph node enlargement less than 15 mm in short-axis diameter may be seen

Differential Diagnosis

The CT appearance described above is not exclusively specific to HP. Each of the CT findings that characterize HP can also be seen in a variety of other conditions. For instance, the presence of poorly defined centrilobular nodules can be seen in various forms of bronchiolitis, including infectious bronchiolitis, diffuse panbronchiolitis,[77,78] and respiratory bronchiolitis-interstitial lung disease, as well as cholesterol granulomas and pulmonary capillary hemangiomatosis in the setting of pulmonary hypertension.[79] The main differential considerations for HP include respiratory bronchiolitis and atypical infections in the acute and subacute settings, as well as UIP and NSIP in the chronic setting. A positive smoking history and the presence of underlying emphysema favor etiologies such as respiratory bronchiolitis over HP. Diffuse ground-glass opacities in a characteristic pattern in a nonsmoking patient with an appropriate clinical history, implicating antigenic exposure, obviously favors HP.[23] Identical imaging findings in a patient with a diagnosis of acquired immunodeficiency syndrome, however, would favor *Pneumocystis jirovecii* pneumonia.[80] Similar findings in a patient with proven pulmonary hypertension may represent cholesterol granulomas or pulmonary capillary hemangiomatosis. Collection of a thorough clinical history, therefore, is paramount in making the correct diagnosis.

Distinction of chronic HP from idiopathic NSIP and UIP is important, given significant differences in management. Insidious chronic HP may mimic UIP or advanced fibrosis of any interstitial

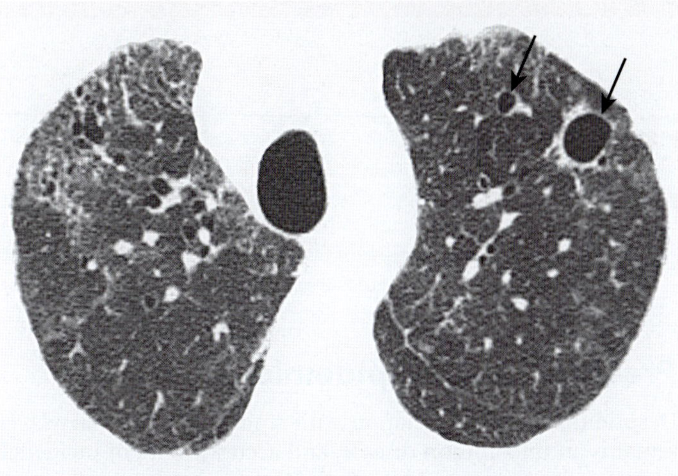

Fig. 32.27 Cysts in hypersensitivity pneumonitis. High-resolution CT scan at the level of the aortic arch shows patchy ground-glass opacities, minimal fibrosis, and a few poorly defined centrilobular nodules. Note thin-walled cysts *(arrows)*. The patient was a bird breeder (same patient shown in Fig. 32.20) with biopsy-proven subacute and chronic hypersensitivity pneumonitis.

lung disease. The CT features that best differentiate chronic HP from UIP and NSIP are the presence of lobular areas of decreased attenuation and vascularity and centrilobular nodules.[72] In some HP patients CT findings may be virtually indistinguishable from those of UIP (see Fig. 32.22) or NSIP (see Fig. 32.25). Silva and colleagues[72] found that the features that most reliably distinguish HP from UIP and NSIP are the presence of geographic regions of relative decreased attenuation, centrilobular and peribronchovascular distribution of nodularity, and a middle/upper lung zone predominance of CT abnormalities.[72] Because of the significant degree of overlap in clinical presentation and imaging findings between HP and other etiologies, most notably NSIP and UIP, a high degree of clinical suspicion is essential in making a correct diagnosis.

Synopsis of Treatment Options

The most effective treatment of HP consists of avoidance of the inciting antigen.[2,9] Systemic corticosteroids may alter or delay progression. In general, corticosteroids are reserved for patients with more severe symptoms or for patients who fail to respond to antigen avoidance. The prognosis is excellent with prompt recognition and initiation of treatment. Even after appropriate diagnosis and management, the course of the disease can be fatal. Single-lung transplantation has been performed in some patients with chronic HP.[34]

KEY POINTS

- Hypersensitivity pneumonitis (HP) occurs most commonly in adults; it is less common in smokers.
- HP is caused by inhalation of various antigens that affect susceptible patients; occasionally, it may be seen in association with drug toxicity.
- Three different types of presentation are described—acute, subacute, and chronic—with overlap between the stages being common.
- Histologic and radiologic findings are similar regardless of the type of inciting antigen and vary with the stage of disease; the findings may mimic those of other interstitial lung disease.
- Lymphocytosis in bronchoalveolar lavage, frequently greater than 50%, and the presence of serum precipitating antibodies against the offending antigens can support the diagnosis.
- The diagnosis of HP can be made based on a combination of history of exposure to a possible allergen, clinical features, lung function tests, and consistent radiologic findings.
- Avoidance of the inciting antigen is the most important factor in the management of HP.

SUGGESTED READINGS

Hirschmann JV, Pipavath SN, Godwin JD. Hypersensitivity pneumonitis: a historical, clinical, and radiologic review. *Radiographics*. 2009;29(7):1921–1938.

Lacasse Y, Cormier Y. Hypersensitivity pneumonitis. *Orphanet J Rare Dis*. 2006;1:25.

Matar LD, McAdams HP, Sporn TA. Hypersensitivity pneumonitis. *AJR Am J Roentgenol*. 2000;174:1061–1066.

Mohr LC. Hypersensitivity pneumonitis. *Curr Opin Pulm Med*. 2004;10:401–411.

Silva CIS, Müller NL, Churg A. Hypersensitivity pneumonitis: spectrum of high-resolution CT and pathologic findings. *AJR Am J Roentgenol*. 2007;188:334–344.

The full reference list for this chapter is available at ExpertConsult.com.

33 Pulmonary Langerhans Cell Histiocytosis*

STEPHEN B. HOBBS

Etiology

Langerhans cell histiocytosis (LCH) is an uncommon disease. Several synonyms, including histiocytosis X, eosinophilic granuloma, and Langerhans cell granulomatosis, have been used in the past, but the term *Langerhans cell histiocytosis* is now preferred. The previously used term *histiocytosis X* included several entities with similar morphologic but different clinical manifestations.[1] These entities included Letterer-Siwe disease, which is often fatal and occurs in children and infants with multiorgan involvement[2]; Hand-Schüller-Christian disease, which has a more indolent clinical course in children and adolescents and is characterized by lytic skull lesions, diabetes insipidus, and exophthalmos[2]; and eosinophilic granuloma, a disease of adults with lung and bone involvement.[2] The nomenclature of these various entities has been simplified, and LCH is now basically subdivided into single-organ or multiorgan involvement. Pulmonary involvement in LCH usually occurs in isolation but also is found in most adult cases with a multisystem disorder.[3]

Although viruses such as Epstein-Barr virus, papillomaviruses, and herpesviruses have been previously implicated as a cause of LCH, evidence from molecular biology studies has not substantiated the link.[4,5] However, the association of pulmonary LCH with cigarette smoking is strong, with supporting evidence from both clinical and pathologic studies. The exception is pulmonary LCH in children, which often occurs as part of a systemic disorder and is not associated with cigarette smoking.[6] Isolated pulmonary LCH in adults is almost exclusively encountered in smokers (>90%), with some studies reporting almost 100% of affected individuals being smokers.[7–10]

Supporting evidence for the association of LCH and smoking includes the fact that the earliest histopathologic finding in pulmonary LCH is a peribronchiolar interstitial infiltrate, a similar distribution to that seen in smoke-induced small airways disease.[11,12] In animal studies a Langerhans-like interstitial granulomatous reaction was seen to resolve when exposure to cigarette smoke was withdrawn.[13] Additionally, when compared with nonsmokers, smokers display an increased number of Langerhans cells in bronchoalveolar lavage fluid.[14] Despite these findings, the exact mechanism of the role of cigarette smoking in the pathogenesis of the condition is unclear.

A rare familial association has been reported, with an affected relative occurring in less than 1% of cases[15] in one large multicenter study showing only 1 of 274 adults (0.4%) as having familial LCH.[3] Further evidence for a genetic predisposition is provided by chromosomal instability in peripheral lymphocytes in LCH.[16]

*The editors and the publisher would like to thank Dr. Susan J. Copley for contributing material on this topic to the prior edition of this work. It has served as the foundation for the current chapter.

Prevalence and Epidemiology

Despite the strong association with smoking, pulmonary LCH remains an uncommon disease, and accurate data of incidence and prevalence are problematic.[17] With the widespread use of high-resolution CT today such surgical lung biopsy is performed much less frequently, and the diagnosis often is made based on a combination of clinical and imaging findings. In a study in which histopathologic confirmation was not obtained in all patients and diagnoses were made based on clinical and high-resolution CT appearances, pulmonary LCH was diagnosed in 6.6% of 1382 cases of diffuse interstitial lung disease.[18] Previously, pulmonary LCH was described as more common in men,[19] but more recently it has been described in women, and currently the sex incidence is thought to be approximately equal,[3,20] which may reflect the increasing number of female smokers.[7] It occurs more commonly in whites than in other ethnic groups,[21,22] and most individuals are in their 20s or 30s, with a mean age at onset of symptoms of 33 years and mean age at diagnosis of 35 years in a large multicenter study.[3]

Clinical Presentation

Patients usually present with cough and dyspnea. Other symptoms may include fever, malaise, and chest pain; however, in many patients the symptoms are mild and nonspecific.[12] Up to 25% of individuals may be asymptomatic with radiographically apparent disease.[23] Approximately 15% of patients may present initially with pneumothorax.[24] In one study of 102 patients with pulmonary LCH, 16% had pneumothorax and for those patients, the age at the time of initial diagnosis was significantly younger (median, 29 years) than in patients without pneumothorax (median, 41 years).[25] A significant proportion (60%) of patients may have recurrent pneumothorax.[25] Hemoptysis rarely may occur.[23] Bone lesions may cause chest wall pain and tenderness.[23] Physical examination frequently is normal, and finger clubbing is rare.[24]

In contrast to the pediatric form of the disease, multiple organ sites are less often affected but have been described, including pituitary, skin, eye, colon, heart, lymph nodes, and brain. In a large study multiple organ involvement occurred in only 28% of adult patients.[3] In all cases with single-organ and multiorgan involvement, the most common affected site was the lungs (58%).[3]

Pathophysiology

PATHOLOGY

Pulmonary LCH is characterized by histiocyte proliferation. Langerhans cells occur in the normal lung[9,12]; however, the histiocytic cells in LCH have distinguishing morphologic and immunohistochemical features, suggesting "activated" Langerhans cells (Figs. 33.1 and 33.2). Most studies have described clonal proliferation of histiocytes secondary to an abnormal inflammatory immunologic response.[5] Activated Langerhans cells are poorly susceptible to apoptosis, or programmed cell death, which may result in repeated stimulation of T cells.[26]

At a microscopic level, a cellular infiltrate is centered around the membranous bronchioles in the early stages of pulmonary LCH.[11,12] The interstitium becomes involved in more extensive disease, with varying proportions of Langerhans cells, eosinophils, lymphocytes, and fibroblasts, and a characteristic stellate appearance may occur as a result of central fibrosis. Although the stellate pattern is typical, a more symmetric nodular cellular infiltrate without central fibrosis, which may be related to an airway, also can be seen.[11] Occasionally, intraalveolar buds of granulation tissue may give an appearance similar to organizing pneumonia, although this appearance is relatively uncommon.[12] A "desquamative interstitial pneumonia–like reaction" is a frequent histopathologic accompaniment to LCH resulting from pigmented macrophages infiltrating the surrounding airspaces.[27] Respiratory bronchiolitis also may be seen, supporting the hypothesis that smoking-related interstitial lung disease is a spectrum with overlapping features.[27]

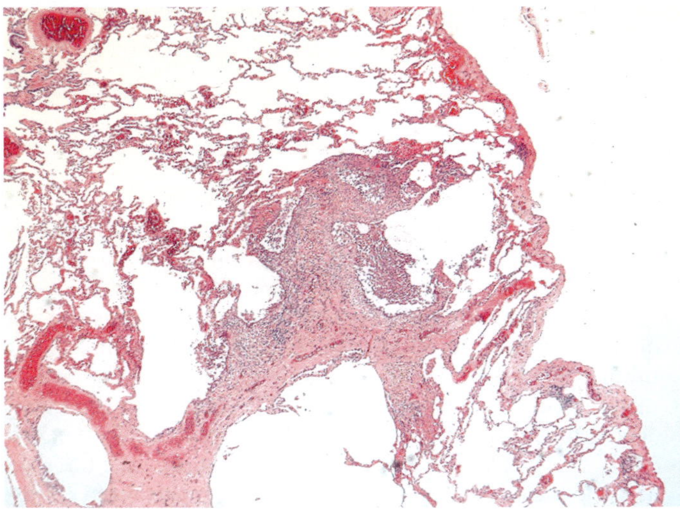

Fig. 33.1 Pulmonary Langerhans cell histiocytosis. Low-power view shows interstitial thickening, increased cellularity, and cystic spaces. *(Courtesy Dr. R. Dinas, Hammersmith Hospital.)*

The cystic spaces seen on macroscopic specimens (Fig. 33.3) and imaging seem to result from destruction of the bronchiolar wall and progressive enlargement of the airway lumen, with surrounding fibrous tissue.[28] It has been hypothesized that an increase in cyst size may occur as a result of a "ball-valve" effect secondary to partially obstructed bronchioles.[29] Concurrent emphysema is a frequent finding that is not surprising given the association with smoking. The lesions coalesce as the disease becomes more advanced, with increasing fibrosis, emphysema, and parenchymal destruction. In end-stage pulmonary LCH, the lung may be almost entirely replaced by fibrosis and cystic spaces. Pulmonary vascular involvement is a feature of late-stage LCH with luminal obliteration, intimal fibrosis, and medial hypertrophy. Progression of these features may result in pulmonary arterial hypertension, which may complicate end-stage pulmonary LCH.[30]

Several studies have correlated histopathologic features with high-resolution CT findings.[27,31,32] In early disease centrilobular nodules on CT correlate histopathologically with florid granuloma formation.[31] In contrast, cysts on high-resolution CT correlate with cavitary granulomas, cysts with fibrous walls, or a combination,[31] and an association between cysts and air-trapping has been reported.[32] The presence of ground-glass opacities on high-resolution CT correlates with respiratory bronchiolitis/desquamative interstitial pneumonia–like changes.[27] In advanced disease high-resolution CT may show large cysts and architectural distortion, with granulomas still seen on histopathologic specimens consistent with ongoing disease activity.[31]

LUNG FUNCTION

In early disease, despite the presence of radiologic abnormalities, many patients may have normal lung function; however, the most common pulmonary function abnormality is a reduction in diffusing capacity for carbon monoxide (DLCO).[24] The

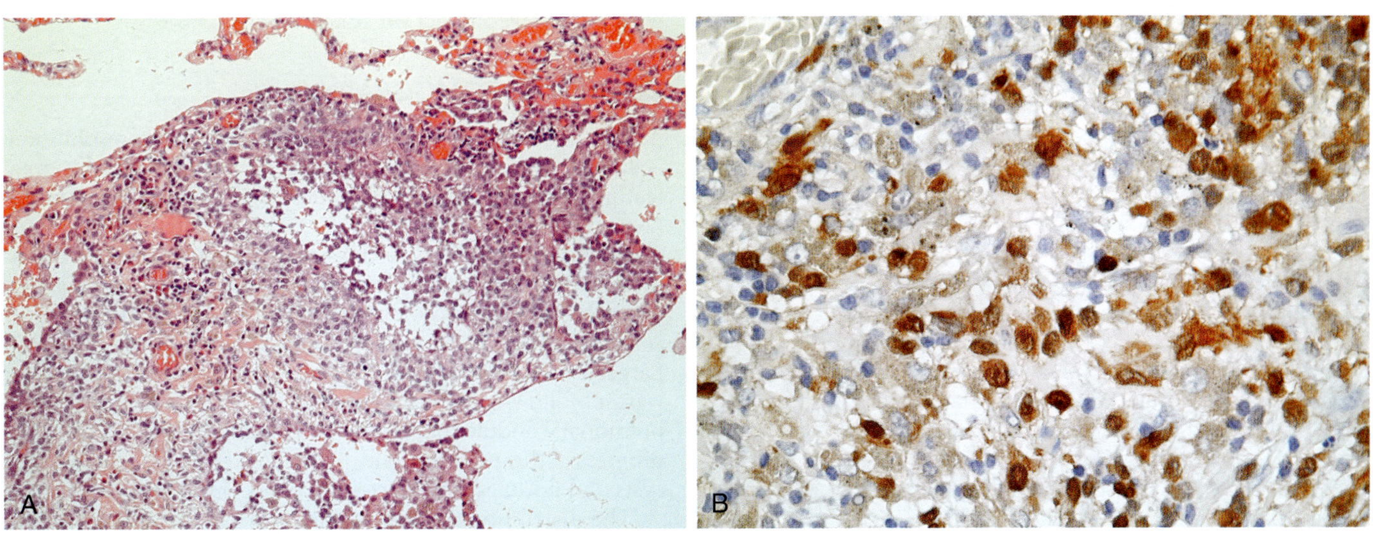

Fig. 33.2 Pulmonary Langerhans cell histiocytosis. High-power view (A) shows Langerhans cells, which stain positively for CD1a on immunohistochemistry (B). *(Courtesy Dr. R. Dinas, Hammersmith Hospital.)*

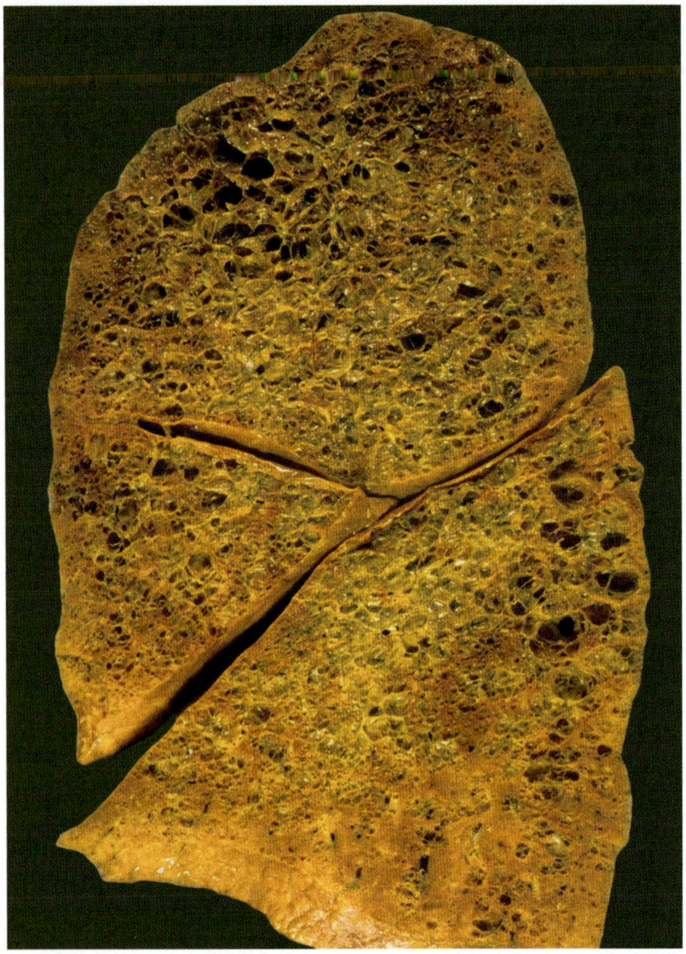

Fig. 33.3 Pulmonary Langerhans cell histiocytosis. Sagittal slice of the right lung shows numerous cystic spaces, most measuring about 0.5–1 cm in diameter. They are present in the central and peripheral regions and are more evident in the upper lobe and superior portions of the lower and middle lobes. Note relative sparing of the tip of the right middle lobe and the lung bases. *(Courtesy Dr. Roberta Miller.)*

reduction in DLCO is likely due to a combination of a pulmonary vasculopathy and parenchymal disease.[33] In advanced disease restrictive, obstructive, and mixed pulmonary function abnormalities have been described.[33] Obstruction may be due to bronchiolar narrowing secondary to peribronchiolar inflammation and fibrosis or coexisting emphysema. There is good correlation between the high-resolution CT appearances, including quantification of disease extent with objective measures, and functional parameters in pulmonary LCH.[34]

Manifestations of the Disease

RADIOGRAPHY

In early disease the radiograph may be normal, with abnormalities seen only on CT. The lung volumes are characteristically preserved or enlarged.[19,35] If disease is identifiable on radiography, the initial features are of a nodular or reticulonodular pattern with an upper and middle zone distribution that characteristically spares the costophrenic angles (Fig. 33.4).[19] Less commonly, significant involvement of the lower lobes occurs, but even in these cases the costophrenic angles are generally spared.[19] The distribution of nodules and curvilinear or reticular opacities is symmetric without central or peripheral predilection (Fig. 33.5).[19,36] As disease progresses a reticular pattern occurs from a composite of superimposed multiple cysts (Fig. 33.6).[37] Because of the evolving pattern from nodules to reticular abnormality/cysts, a combination of these features is frequently seen (see Fig. 33.5).[19]

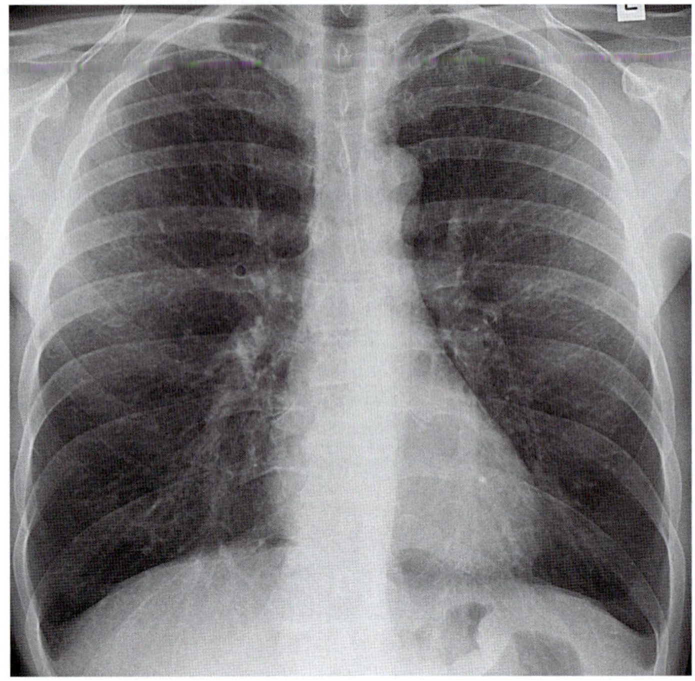

Fig. 33.4 Pulmonary Langerhans cell histiocytosis: early radiographic findings. Chest radiograph shows subtle nodularity in the upper zones.

As previously noted, pneumothorax is a common complicating radiographic feature.[25] Uncommon radiographic features include mediastinal lymphadenopathy,[38,39] consolidation,[38] pleural effusion,[40,41] and a solitary pulmonary nodule.[42] In advanced disease there may be large areas of destroyed lung with parenchymal distortion and hyperinflation, and distinguishing pulmonary LCH from advanced emphysema may be impossible (Fig. 33.7). Pulmonary arterial hypertension may result in enlargement of the pulmonary arteries in advanced disease and is associated with a negative impact on survival (Fig. 33.8).[43]

COMPUTED TOMOGRAPHY

As with other diffuse interstitial lung diseases, high-resolution CT is more sensitive than radiography.[44] The high-resolution CT features in early disease are multiple ill-defined micronodules (1–5 mm in diameter) with a bronchiolocentric (centrilobular) distribution (Fig. 33.9).[37] Nodules may be profuse and predominate in the upper and middle lung zones with typical sparing of the costophrenic angles and tips of the lingula and right middle lobe. A lower zone predominance is unusual but has been described.[45] Larger nodules (>1 cm in diameter) also can be seen and may warrant follow-up to evaluate for malignancy.[29,37] Rarely, a solitary pulmonary nodule may be the only manifestation. As the disease progresses the nodules tend to cavitate, and a combination of cysts and nodules is characteristic (Figs. 33.10 and 33.11).[29,37]

The distribution of cysts is the same as that of nodules, and the craniocaudal distribution of abnormalities may be convincingly shown on coronal and sagittal reformats.[46] The cysts initially

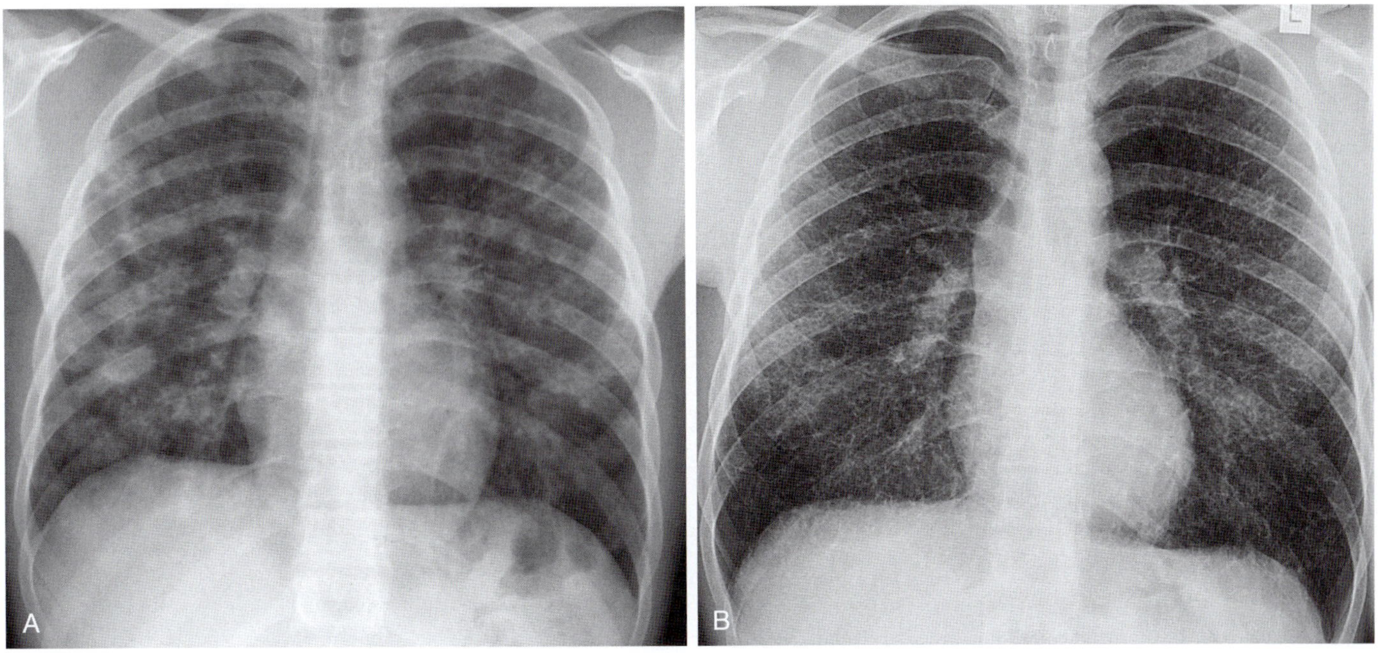

Fig. 33.5 Pulmonary Langerhans cell histiocytosis: progression of radiographic findings in a young man. (A) Chest radiograph shows confluent nodules with a middle and upper zone predominance. Ring shadows consistent with cysts also are seen. Note the characteristic sparing of the costophrenic angles. The corresponding high-resolution CT scan is shown in Fig. 33.12. (B) Chest radiograph 3 years later shows the typical progression to thin-walled cysts.

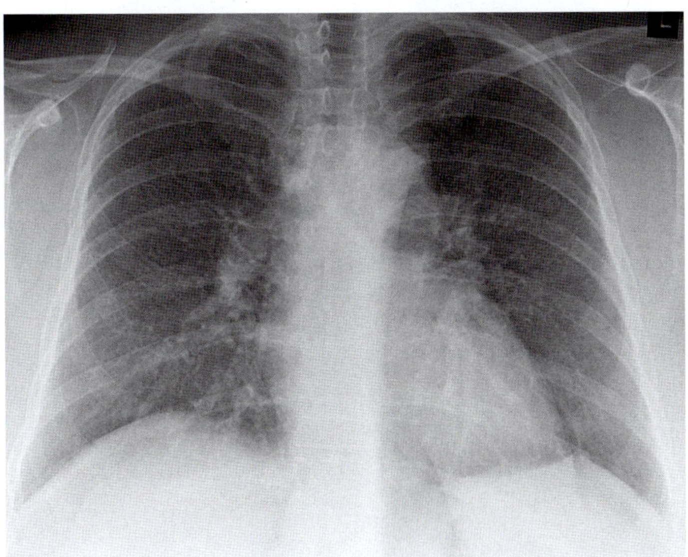

Fig. 33.6 Pulmonary Langerhans cell histiocytosis: reticular pattern. Chest radiograph shows subtle reticular pattern with a middle and upper zone predominance in histopathologically proven pulmonary Langerhans cell histiocytosis. The corresponding high-resolution CT scan is shown in Fig. 33.14.

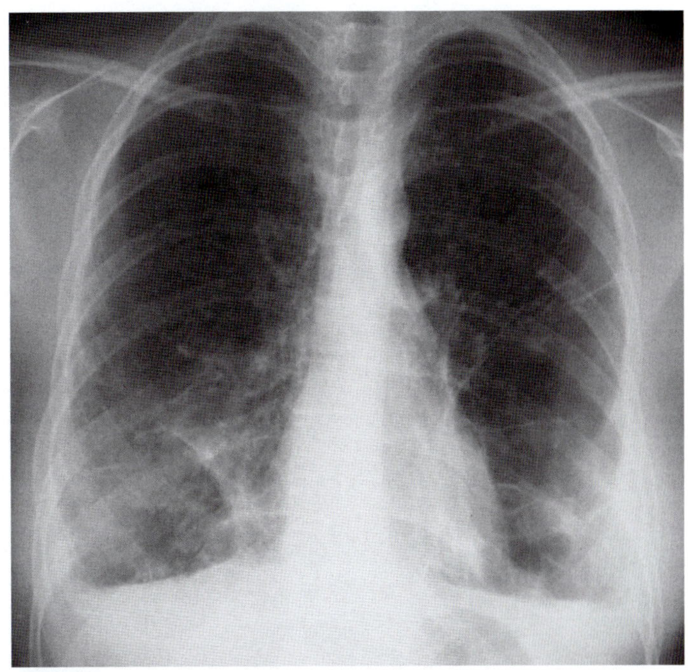

Fig. 33.7 Pulmonary Langerhans cell histiocytosis: "emphysema-appearance." Chest radiograph shows hyperinflation, large bullae, and areas of scarring. Lung biopsy specimen (see Figs. 33.1 and 33.2) showed pulmonary Langerhans cell histiocytosis.

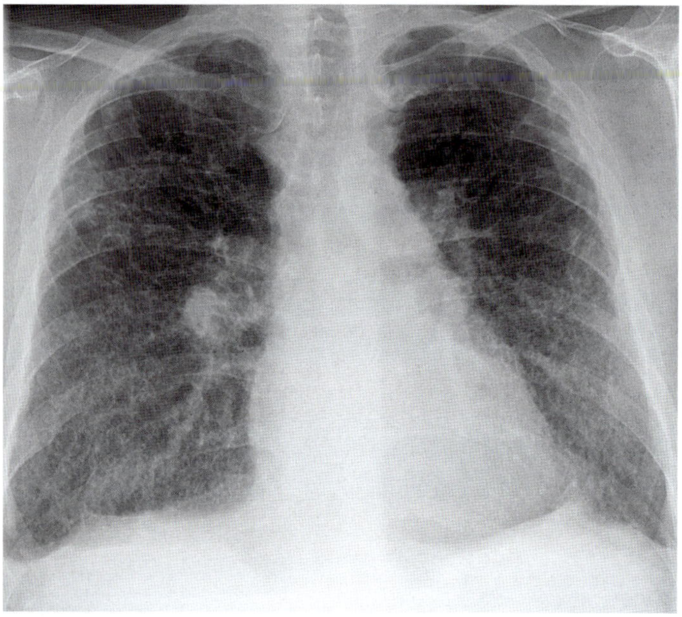

Fig. 33.8 Pulmonary Langerhans cell histiocytosis: end-stage. Chest radiograph shows widespread reticular pattern and pulmonary distortion. Note enlarged central pulmonary arteries in keeping with associated pulmonary hypertension.

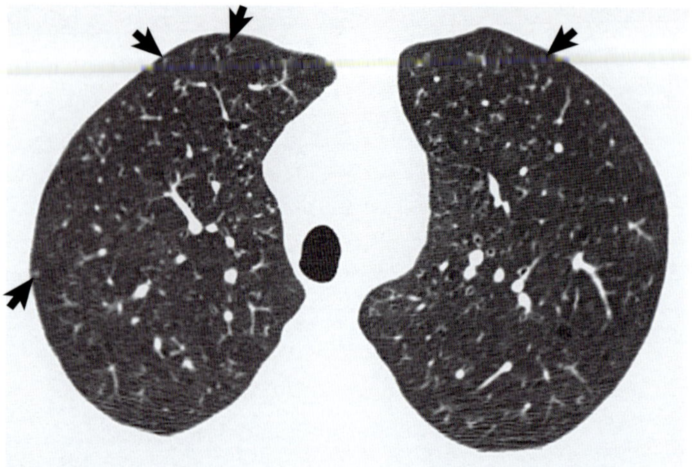

Fig. 33.9 Pulmonary Langerhans cell histiocytosis: micronodules on high-resolution CT. High-resolution CT scan shows subtle centrilobular nodules *(arrows)*, some of which are branching in a tree-in-bud pattern. Also evident is minimal emphysema.

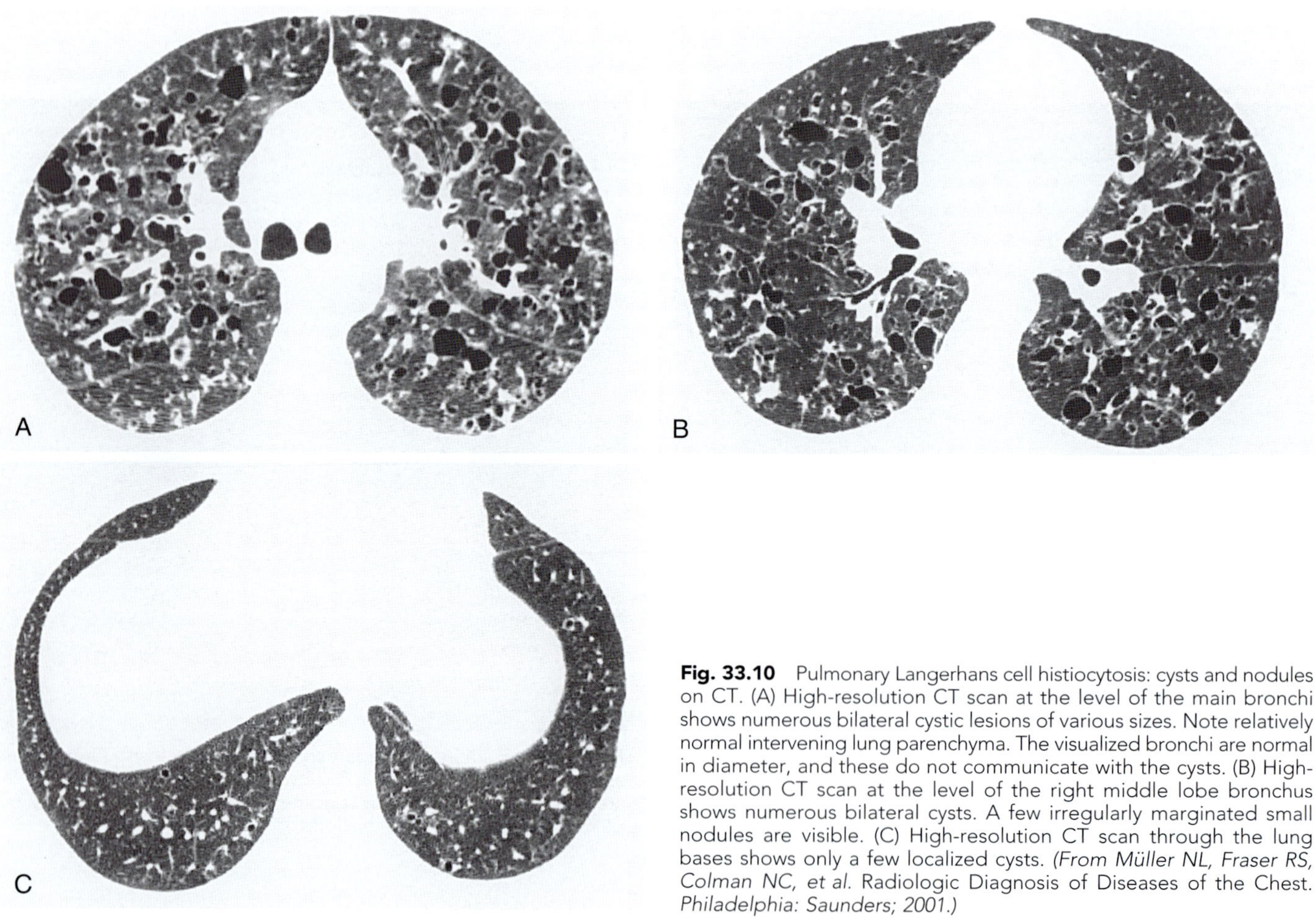

Fig. 33.10 Pulmonary Langerhans cell histiocytosis: cysts and nodules on CT. (A) High-resolution CT scan at the level of the main bronchi shows numerous bilateral cystic lesions of various sizes. Note relatively normal intervening lung parenchyma. The visualized bronchi are normal in diameter, and these do not communicate with the cysts. (B) High-resolution CT scan at the level of the right middle lobe bronchus shows numerous bilateral cysts. A few irregularly marginated small nodules are visible. (C) High-resolution CT scan through the lung bases shows only a few localized cysts. *(From Müller NL, Fraser RS, Colman NC, et al.* Radiologic Diagnosis of Diseases of the Chest. *Philadelphia: Saunders; 2001.)*

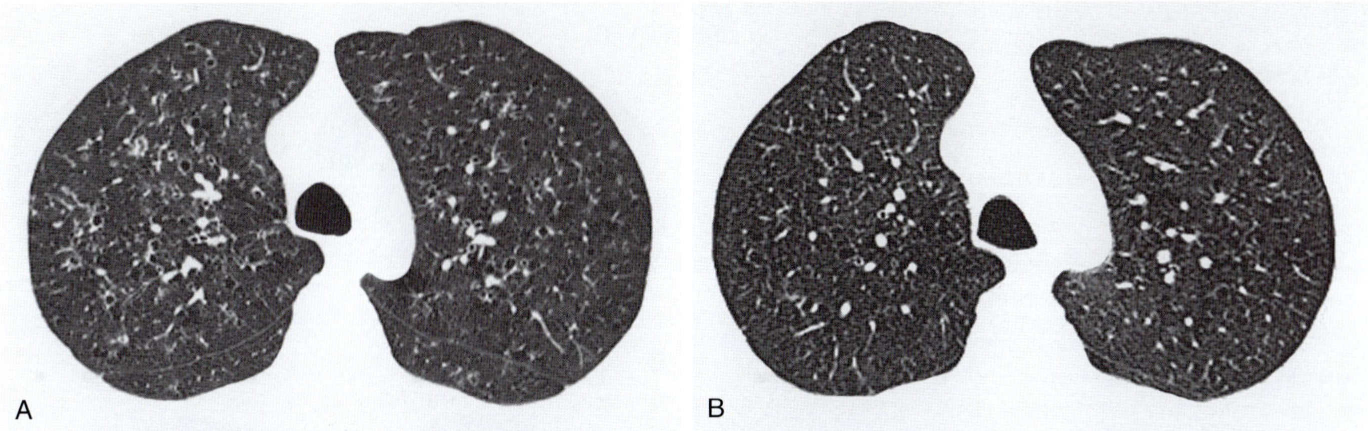

Fig. 33.11 Pulmonary Langerhans cell histiocytosis: progression of characteristic CT findings. (A) High-resolution CT scan shows the characteristic combination of micronodules and spherical cysts. (B) High-resolution CT scan 2 years later shows regression of the nodules and progression of the thin-walled cysts.

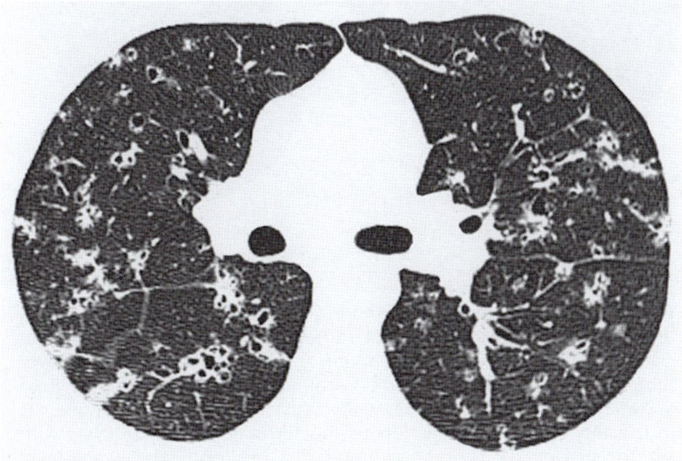

Fig. 33.12 Pulmonary Langerhans cell histiocytosis: characteristic thick-walled cysts. High-resolution CT scan of the same patient in Fig. 33.5 shows widespread thick-walled spherical cysts and a few irregular nodules.

may be thick walled and spherical with a diameter greater than 1 cm (Fig. 33.12; see Fig. 33.11) and then become thinner walled and more eccentric with coalescence in more advanced disease (Fig. 33.13; see Fig. 33.10).[37] Other features that have been described are centrilobular branching opacities (see Fig. 33.9), a reticular pattern (Fig. 33.14), and thickening of interlobular septa.[45] Large bullae may be seen,[29] resulting in difficulties in differentiation from extensive emphysema and end-stage pulmonary LCH. Ground-glass opacification also has been described but is not a common feature[37,45] (see Figs. 33.13 and 33.14) and is generally related to coexisting respiratory bronchiolitis, respiratory bronchiolitis–interstitial lung disease, and desquamative interstitial pneumonia. This is further histopathologic-radiologic evidence that there is a spectrum of smoking-related interstitial lung disease.[27]

The diagnostic accuracy of high-resolution CT is high,[47,48] and the combination of cysts and nodules with an appropriate distribution is relatively specific in the context of an adult cigarette smoker. This frequently obviates the need for open lung biopsy. Serial CT studies have shown that nodules may regress completely, indicating potentially reversible disease.[29] In contrast, older research suggested that cysts remain stable or enlarge on CT, suggesting irreversible damage.[29] However, more recent evidence does suggest that even thin-walled cysts contain active inflammatory cells on histopathology and as such can exhibit improvement on follow-up CT.[49]

POSITRON EMISSION TOMOGRAPHY

Recent studies have shown that positron emission tomographic (PET) scanning is a useful imaging modality to determine the extent of disease involvement in affected patients. Positive PET scans in pulmonary LCH usually occur in predominantly nodular lung disease, thick-walled cysts, bone, liver, and other extrapulmonary sites of involvement.[50,51]

ECHOCARDIOGRAPHY

Right heart failure and pulmonary arterial hypertension (PAH) are common in long-term disease patients and can be a significant cause of morbidity and mortality.[52] Echocardiography should be considered for all symptomatic patients to evaluate for pulmonary hypertension regardless of pulmonary artery disease on CT.[53] Referral for right heart catheterization should be obtained if echocardiography suggests PAH.[54]

IMAGING ALGORITHMS

Chest radiography is often the initial investigation and may be useful for follow-up or to show complicating pneumothorax. As in other diffuse interstitial lung diseases, high-resolution CT is more sensitive and specific and may provide information about disease reversibility, treatment response, and extrapulmonary disease sites.

Differential Diagnosis

The differential diagnosis based on clinical data includes emphysema and other diffuse interstitial lung diseases, especially ones related to smoking (e.g., respiratory bronchiolitis-interstitial lung disease and desquamative interstitial pneumonia). There is some overlap in appearance with other cystic lung diseases, however, and biopsy confirmation may be required in atypical cases.[45]

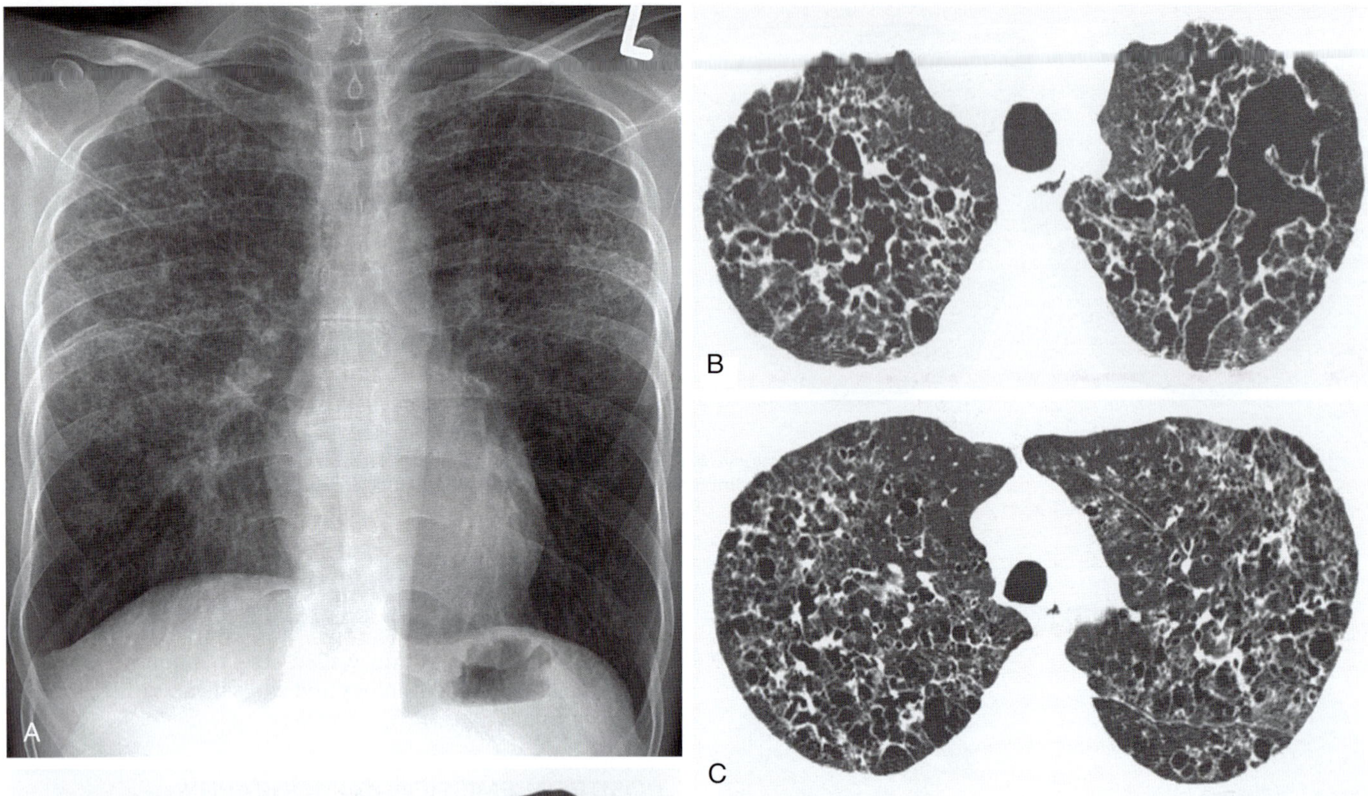

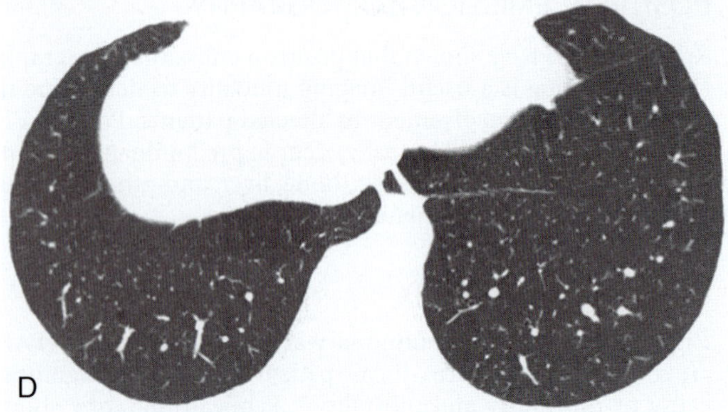

Fig. 33.13 Pulmonary Langerhans cell histiocytosis: nodules, cysts, and reticular pattern. (A) Chest radiograph shows diffuse reticular pattern in the upper and middle lung zones with sparing of the lower lung zones. (B) High-resolution CT scan at the level of the lung apices shows numerous bilateral thin-walled cysts. Conglomeration of cysts in the left upper lobe has led to the formation of large cysts with bizarre shapes. (C) High-resolution CT scan slightly above the level of the aortic arch shows numerous bilateral cysts, a few small nodules, and ground-glass opacities. (D) High-resolution CT scan at the level of the lung bases shows minimal abnormalities. The ground-glass opacities reflect the presence of respiratory bronchiolitis ("smoker's bronchiolitis").

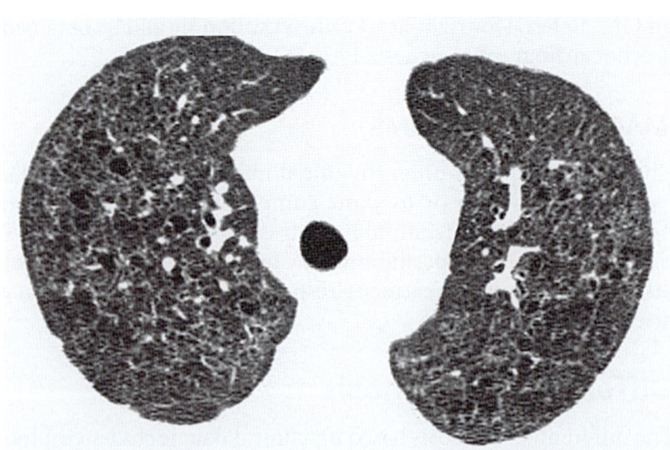

Fig. 33.14 Pulmonary Langerhans cell histiocytosis: cysts and reticular pattern. High-resolution CT scan of the same patient in Fig. 33.6 shows thin-walled cysts and a fine reticular pattern. Note associated ground-glass opacities reflecting the presence of smoking-related respiratory bronchiolitis.

The most frequent mimickers include lymphangioleiomyomatosis (LAM), lymphocytic interstitial pneumonia (LIP), and emphysema.[45] Distinguishing LAM and LIP from LCH is frequently possible by evaluating the distribution of cysts in the craniocaudal plane and the cyst shape. LCH cysts are upper lung predominant and bizarrely shaped; LAM cysts are more diffusely distributed and round; LIP cysts are lower lung predominant and frequently perivascular.

Synopsis of Treatment Options

MEDICAL

- Smoking cessation is critical, with many patients stabilizing or improving. Some patients may progress despite cessation.
- Medical treatment includes chemotherapeutic agents, such as vinblastine, cyclophosphamide, and busulfan, with or without corticosteroids.
- There is no consensus regarding optimal treatment; a formal clinical trial has been suggested.

SURGICAL

- Pneumothorax is a frequent complication and may require surgical pleurodesis.
- Patients with end-stage pulmonary LCH may develop pulmonary hypertension, and lung transplantation is a therapeutic option in this context, despite a disease recurrence rate of approximately 20%.
- Surgical options include single-lung transplant, double-lung transplant, and heart-lung transplant.

KEY POINTS

- Langerhans cell histiocytosis (LCH) may involve a single or multiple organs.
- Pulmonary LCH in an adult occurs almost exclusively in current or ex-smokers.
- Pulmonary disease is the most common form of single-organ disease.
- Radiographic appearances are nonspecific, most commonly consisting of a nodular or reticulonodular pattern.
- High-resolution CT usually progresses from ill-defined micronodules (1–5 mm in diameter) to a combination of cysts and nodules, with regression of nodules and increasing cysts (which may be bizarrely shaped) in more advanced disease.
- Pulmonary LCH has a characteristic upper and middle zone distribution with sparing of the costophrenic angles and tips of the lingula and right middle lobe.
- High-resolution CT findings often allow confident diagnosis; biopsy may be required in atypical cases.

SUGGESTED READINGS

Abbott GF, Rosado de Christenson ML, Franks TJ, et al. From the archives of the AFIP: pulmonary Langerhans' cell histiocytosis. *Radiographics*. 2004;24: 821–841.

Kim HJ, Lee KS, Johkoh T, et al. Pulmonary Langerhans cell histiocytosis in adults: high-resolution CT-pathology comparisons and evolutional changes at CT. *Eur Radiol*. 2011;21(7):1406–1415.

Seely JM, Salahudeen S, Cadaval-Goncalves AT, et al. Pulmonary Langerhans cell histiocytosis: a comparative study of computed tomography in children and adults. *J Thorac Imaging*. 2012;27(1):65–70.

Sundar KM, Gosselin MV, Chung HL, et al. Pulmonary Langerhans' cell histiocytosis: emerging concepts in pathobiology, radiology, and clinical evolution of disease. *Chest*. 2003;123:1673–1683.

Vassallo R, Ryu JH. Pulmonary Langerhans' cell histiocytosis. *Clin Chest Med*. 2004;25:561–571.

Vassallo R. Diffuse lung diseases in cigarette smokers. *Semin Respir Crit Care Med*. 2012;33(5):533–542.

The full reference list for this chapter is available at ExpertConsult.com.

34 Smoking-Related Interstitial Lung Disease*

STEPHEN B. HOBBS

Currently, the worldwide number of tobacco smokers is estimated at 1.1 billion people, with the World Health Organization estimating that tobacco use is responsible for approximately 6 million premature deaths each year.[1] In the United States 42 million adults are still smokers despite overall decreasing rates of smoking in the United States.[2] Despite a majority of the morbidity and mortality of smoking being related to lung cancer, coronary atherosclerosis, and chronic obstructive pulmonary disease, the smoking-related interstitial lung diseases are a commonly encountered and important clinical and radiologic entity.

The smoking-related interstitial lung diseases include a range of conditions, from those highly associated with smoking, such as respiratory bronchiolitis (RB), desquamative interstitial pneumonia (DIP), and pulmonary Langerhans cell histiocytosis (PLCH, see Chapter 33), to other conditions that are worsened or precipitated by smoking, such as acute eosinophilic pneumonia (AEP, see Chapter 37), pulmonary hemorrhage (see Chapter 2), and even pulmonary fibrosis.[3] This chapter focuses on the smoking-related interstitial pneumonias (RB, respiratory bronchiolitis–associated interstitial lung disease [RB-ILD], and DIP) and the smoking-related patterns of pulmonary fibrosis, including usual interstitial pneumonia (UIP), nonspecific interstitial pneumonia (NSIP), and combined pulmonary fibrosis and emphysema (CPFE).

Respiratory Bronchiolitis and Respiratory Bronchiolitis–Associated Interstitial Lung Disease

Etiology

RB is a common histopathologic finding in smokers,[4] which typically is not associated with symptoms or functional deficit. A few smokers develop symptoms and are classified as having RB-ILD. RB-ILD is a symptomatic clinical condition with radiologic and functional abnormalities that was first recognized in heavy cigarette smokers in the late 1980s.[5] Subsequent studies have confirmed a strong link with cigarette smokers, with very rare reports in nonsmokers,[6,7] although a link with inhalation of noxious substances in the workplace also has been suggested.[8]

Prevalence and Epidemiology

Despite the common habit of cigarette smoking in the general population and the frequency of RB in smokers approaching 100% in some studies,[9] the clinicopathologic entity of RB-ILD is comparatively rare, making accurate evaluation of prevalence difficult. RB-ILD was not yet a recognized disease in the earlier large milestone multicenter studies of interstitial lung disease that predated the 1990s.[10] In a study from a large tertiary referral center in the United Kingdom, the biopsy specimens in 168 cases over an 18-year period were retrospectively reviewed, and 13 (8%) of these showed a dominant pattern of RB-ILD.[8] The usual age at presentation is in the 30s and 40s, and men and women are almost equally affected, with a slight male preponderance.[5–8]

Clinical Presentation

Patients with RB-ILD are invariably middle-aged smokers and present with dyspnea that may be of insidious onset.[11] Cough also may be a feature and is sometimes severe. Less commonly, chest pain and, rarely, hemoptysis have been described. Bilateral end-inspiratory crackles, which may be predominantly basal, are common, but finger clubbing is very rare.[8]

Pathophysiology

PATHOLOGY

RB is characterized histologically by intraluminal and peribronchiolar airspace accumulation of pigmented macrophages (Fig. 34.1). These macrophages are called "smoker's macrophages" because they typically have granular brown cytoplasm. The pigmentation most likely represents the metabolites of cigarette smoke, given that the intensity of pigmentation correlates with pack-years of cigarettes smoked.[7] An ongoing inflammatory process is denoted by a mild peribronchiolar mononuclear inflammatory submucosal infiltrate, which may be associated with fibroblasts and collagen deposition, resulting in stellate fibrous scarring extending into surrounding alveolar walls.[5,6] Similar to macrophage pigmentation, peribronchiolar fibrosis also has been shown to correlate with the number of pack-years smoked.[7] Additional histopathologic findings include thickening of the peribronchiolar alveolar septa and alveolar ducts and histiocytes within the peribronchiolar fibrous tissue displaying anthracotic pigment, foci of goblet cell metaplasia, and metaplastic cuboidal epithelium in the airway epithelium.[6] Mild emphysema in the surrounding lung parenchyma is relatively common,[8] but honeycombing is not a recognized histopathologic feature and should raise the possibility of alternative diagnoses, with RB being an incidental finding.

Histopathologic findings in RB-ILD (Fig. 34.2) and DIP are similar, and differentiation between the two entities may be difficult. The distribution in RB-ILD is typically more patchy and bronchiolocentric, whereas DIP results in extensive uniform alveolar macrophage accumulation.[6] Currently, RB-ILD and DIP

*The editors and the publisher would like to thank Dr. Susan J. Copley for contributing material on this topic to the prior edition of this work. It has served as the foundation for the current chapter.

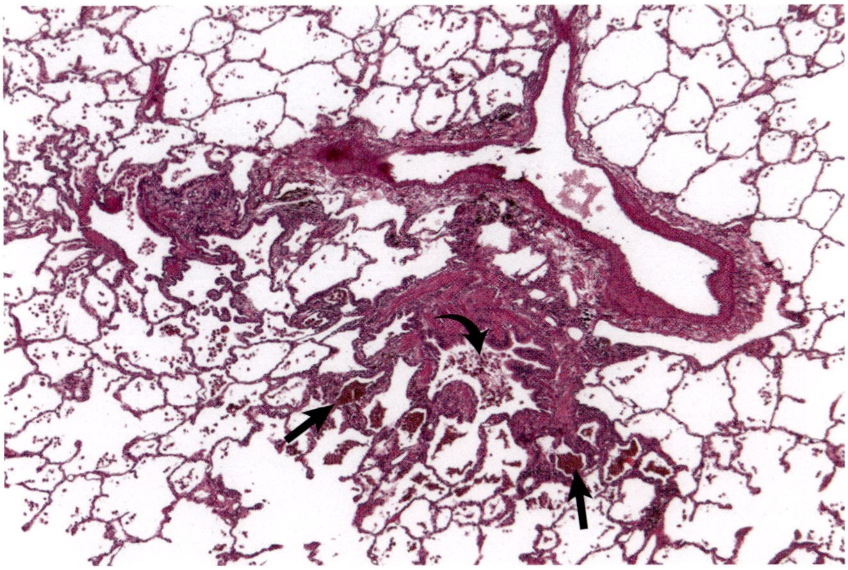

Fig. 34.1 Respiratory bronchiolitis: histologic findings. Histopathologic specimen shows respiratory bronchiole with increased intraluminal macrophages *(curved arrow)* and mural inflammation. Extension of the inflammation and macrophages *(straight arrows)* into the surrounding alveoli also is noted. *(Courtesy Dr. John English, Department of Pathology, Vancouver General Hospital, Vancouver, Canada.)*

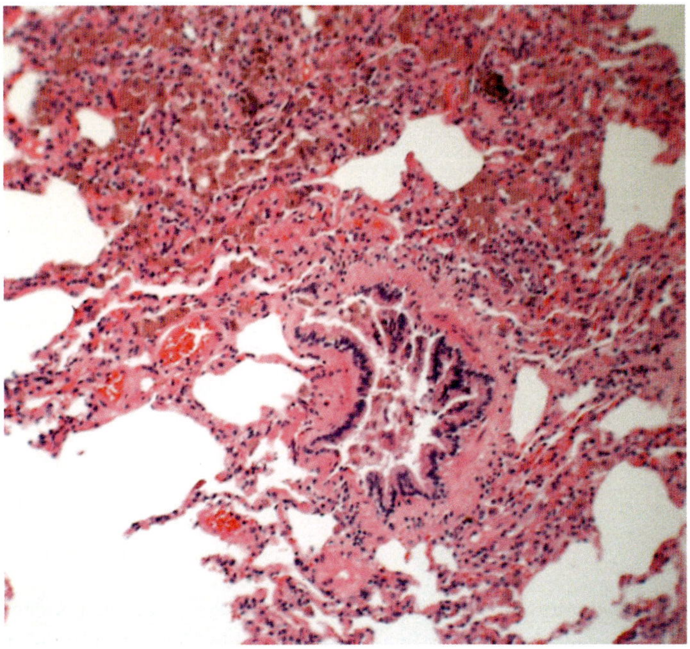

Fig. 34.2 Respiratory bronchiolitis–interstitial lung disease: histologic features. Histopathologic specimen shows extensive accumulation of pigmented macrophages in alveoli and bronchioles in a bronchiolocentric distribution. *(Courtesy Dr. S.R. Desai.)*

are considered to be a spectrum of smoking-related parenchymal disease that also may include PLCH.[6,12,13] Correlation with clinical and radiologic findings is vital in the diagnosis of RB-ILD, owing to the almost universal, usually incidental, histopathologic observation of RB in asymptomatic smokers.[8]

LUNG FUNCTION

Individuals with uncomplicated RB usually do not have lung function deficits. In contrast, the usual pulmonary function findings in RB-ILD are a mixed obstructive-restrictive defect. The carbon monoxide–diffusing capacity is often reduced, and the total lung capacity may be normal, reduced, or slightly increased.[5,6,8] In one study the most common functional deficit was a reduction in diffusing capacity.[14] There is an inverse correlation between the computed tomography (CT) extent of ground-glass opacity and arterial oxygen saturation.[15]

Manifestations of the Disease

RADIOGRAPHY

The radiographic features of biopsy-proven cases of RB-ILD have been described in numerous studies and are variable and nonspecific. A fine diffuse reticulonodular pattern with normal lung volumes has been described (Fig. 34.3).[6,8] In one study the main finding was the presence of ill-defined small nodules with lower zone predominance.[5] In another study the main abnormalities consisted of ground-glass opacities (Fig. 34.4) and airway wall thickening, with no cases showing a prominent reticulonodular pattern.[15] One-third of patients may have a normal radiograph, despite biopsy-proven disease.[5,6]

COMPUTED TOMOGRAPHY

Comparison of the high-resolution CT (HRCT) findings in 98 asymptomatic cigarette smokers with 175 nonsmoking controls showed ill-defined, upper zone–predominant parenchymal micronodules in 27% of smokers but not in control subjects.[16] Comparable differences were noted for areas of ground-glass opacity (20% of smokers and none of the control group). In a later study of heavy smokers with histopathologic correlation, parenchymal micronodules indicating the presence of RB (Fig. 34.5) and areas of ground-glass opacification, representing accumulations of inflammatory cells and a variable degree of fine interstitial fibrosis, were observed.[17] In another study investigating CT features in 57 smokers at baseline and follow-up

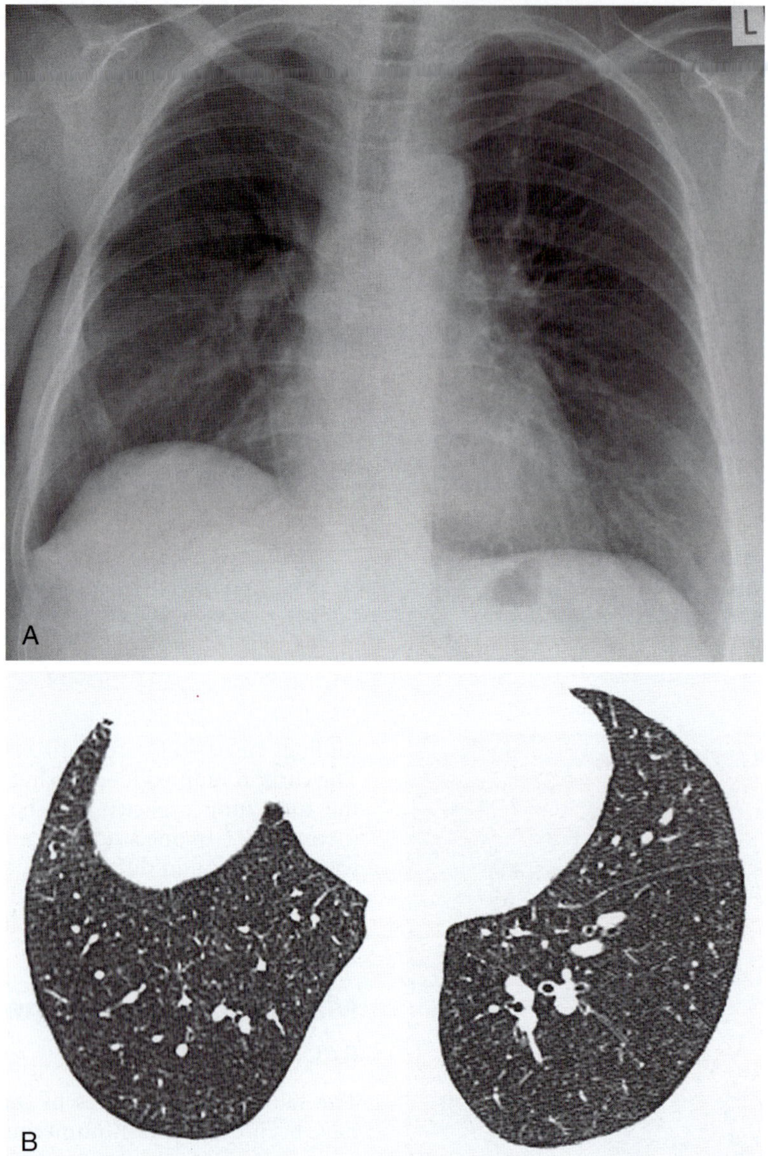

Fig. 34.3 Respiratory bronchiolitis–interstitial lung disease: radiologic findings. (A) Chest radiograph shows subtle reticulonodular pattern in the middle and lower zones. (B) The appearances are more apparent on a concurrent high-resolution CT scan, which shows ill-defined micronodules.

examinations, the percentages of patients with ground-glass opacity, emphysema, and ill-defined micronodules increased, respectively, from 28% to 42%, 26% to 40%, and 33% to 35% on follow-up.[18] Five patients displaying micronodules at baseline examination showed a replacement of this pattern by emphysema at follow-up.[18]

The HRCT findings of RB-ILD were initially described in five patients with biopsy-proven diagnosis.[19] Areas of ground-glass opacity (Fig. 34.6) were the most common finding. One patient had interlobular and intralobular thickening (Fig. 34.7). No patient had nodular opacities.[19] By contrast, a more recent study of 21 patients with pathologically proven RB-ILD documented centrilobular nodules in 71% of cases (see Fig. 34.7), areas of ground-glass opacity in 67%, and patchy areas of decreased attenuation (likely reflecting small airways disease) in 38%.[15] End-expiratory CT may emphasize the regional differences in lung density (Fig. 34.8). Most patients in the latter study showed wall thickening of proximal and distal airways, a similar appearance to that seen in chronic bronchitis. In another series of eight patients with RB-ILD, no single HRCT finding predominated.[12] Diffuse ground-glass opacification and centrilobular nodules were major features in about half of the patients, and emphysema was present in most patients.[12] Despite the fact that many patients are heavy smokers, the severity of the emphysema is usually mild or trivial, confined to the upper lobes, and with a centrilobular or paraseptal distribution. Some patients show thickening of interlobular septa, and features of established interstitial fibrosis are unusual but coexist in some patients with RB-ILD.[8,12] A mosaic attenuation pattern, representing constrictive bronchiolitis, is not usually a prominent feature, but when present, it is most obvious in the lower lobes. The combination of HRCT features of an infiltrative and small airways disease is similar to that seen in patients with subacute hypersensitivity pneumonitis (HP), and the distinction between these two conditions often rests on

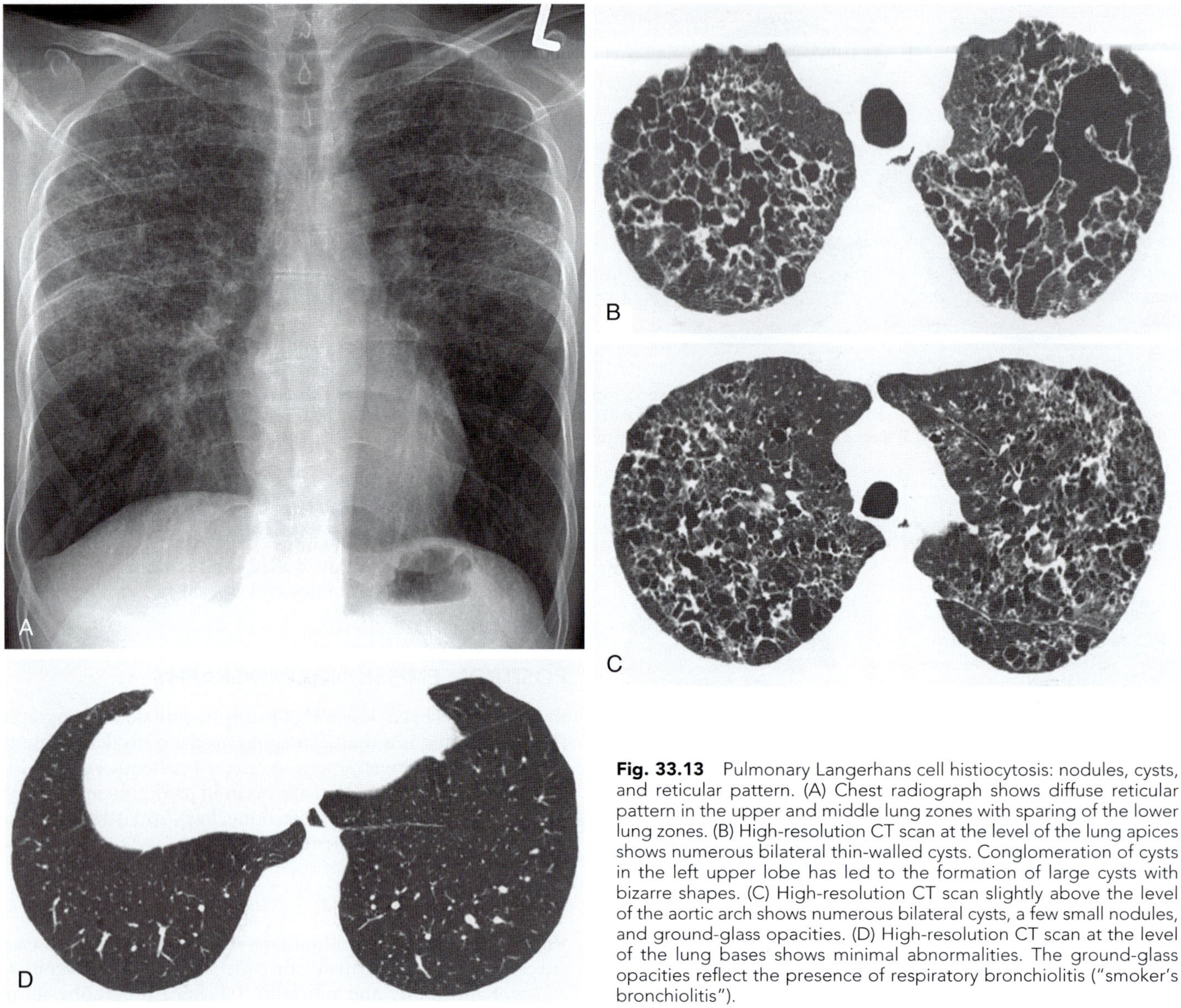

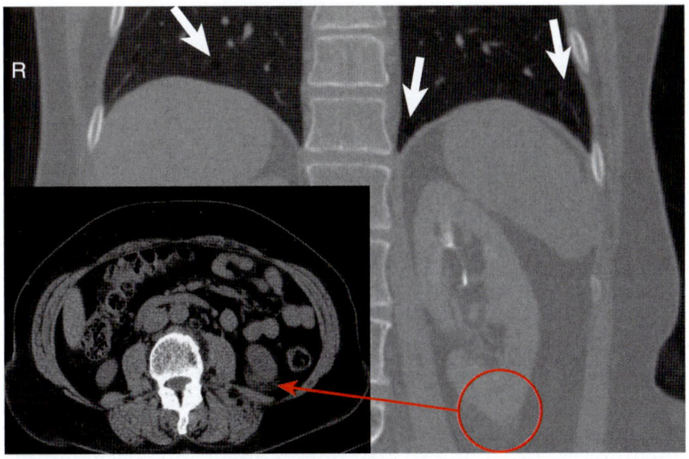

Fig. 35.12 Incidentally discovered lymphangioleiomyomatosis (LAM) in a 62-year-old woman who underwent abdominal CT for evaluating a left renal mass detected by ultrasound. Coronal reformatted CT of the upper abdomen shows a 4-cm mass *(red circle)* arising from the lower pole of the left kidney; the zoomed axial image, reformatted with a soft tissue window setting, better defines the fat and soft tissue–containing mass *(red arrow)*, consistent with an angiomyolipoma. Note small lung cysts in both lower lobes *(white arrows)*, suggesting LAM.

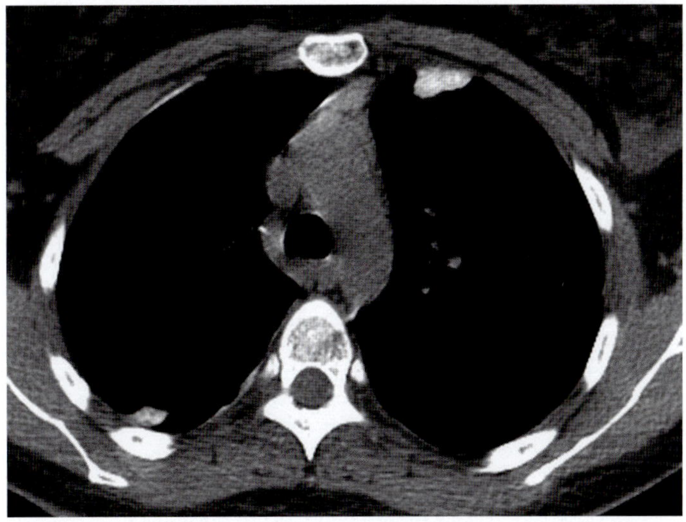

Fig. 35.13 Lymphangioleiomyomatosis with history of chemical pleurodesis in a 41-year-old woman. Axial CT image shows a calcified left pleural mass and high attenuation right pleural thickening located anteriorly and posteriorly secondary to the pleurodesis.

the aorta, renal and superior mesenteric arteries, and pelvic region.[46] They contain elements of water density, but their characteristics are nonspecific, and they are often similar in appearance to malignant abdominal and pelvic masses, such as lymphoma and ovarian cancer (see Fig. 35.3). Visualization of diurnal variation in lymphangioleiomyomas, on either sonography or CT, excludes a diagnosis of malignancy and avoids the need for biopsy.[102] Furthermore, the decreasing volume of the lymphangioleiomyomas during the fasting state represents another diagnostic clue.[46]

Sclerotic osseous lesions represent another extrapulmonary finding. They are often round in shape and range in size from 0.2 to 3.2 cm. They do not expand the bone or deform or extend beyond the cortex. They are more numerous in TSC-LAM than in S-LAM. It was shown, the presence of four or more sclerotic osseous lesions at whole-body CT differentiates patients with S-LAM from those with TSC-LAM or TSC, with high sensitivities and specificity.[103] Of importance, this observation suggests that any patient with LAM who is found to have multiple sclerotic bone lesions at CT should have a complete evaluation for TSC.

CT not only has a key diagnostic role but is also useful in assessing the severity of the disease and identifying complications. In general, the size of the cysts tends to be larger in more severe disease (see Figs. 35.8 and 35.10).[40,85,89] In a study by Müller and associates,[85] parenchymal involvement of less than 25% generally correlated with cysts measuring less than 0.5 to 1 cm, disease involving 25% to 80% of the lung correlated with cysts measuring 0.5 to 1 cm, and disease involving greater than 80% of the lung correlated with cysts measuring greater than 1 cm. The correlation between the extent of cysts on CT and the severity of symptoms seems to be unpredictable, however.[20,69] A subjective scoring method and quantitative thresholding technique provide measures of parenchymal disease extent that correlate directly with pulmonary function tests.[69,85,89,104,105] The prognostic value of CT will likely improve with the use of computer grading of the severity of disease based on texture patterns. It was shown that texture-based objective quantitative CT analysis correlated with subjective assessment, pulmonary functions, and progression of disease over time.[106]

Because of the high frequency of pleurodesis secondary to recurrent pneumothorax, an awareness of consequent CT findings is useful for the correct interpretation of pleural abnormalities in these patients.[107] Pleural abnormalities consist of pleural thickening, pleural effusion, loculated effusion, pneumothorax, focal or continuous plaque of high attenuation (probably caused by dystrophic calcification of the inflamed pleura after installation of talc or other sclerosing agents), and masses resulting from confluent fibrotic tissue or consistent with round atelectasis (Fig. 35.13).[107] An awareness of the posttransplantation imaging features also is mandatory for radiologists who work in lung transplantation centers. In addition to common transplant-related complications, morbidity is usually due to underlying disease.[13,108] LAM-related complications include native lung pneumothorax, chylothorax, chylous ascites, complications from renal AMLs, and recurrent LAM that might be evident only in lymph node sites.[108,109] A study of transplanted lungs with recurrent LAM has suggested metastatic spread of LAM cells to the graft from residual LAM tissue.[3]

IMAGING ALGORITHMS

The initial imaging modality used to evaluate patients with suspected LAM is the chest radiograph. If clinical data or chest radiography findings or both are supportive of LAM (young nonsmoking woman with unexplained pneumothoraces, chylous effusions, or obstructive functional impairment), a high-resolution CT study is indicated and may be supplemented, especially if TSC is suspected, with whole-body CT or MRI.

The presence of a characteristic CT scan in the absence of extrapulmonary findings is not diagnostic of LAM.[110] Therefore it is important to extend the chest CT scan down through the kidneys when evaluating patients with suspected LAM, and, conversely, it is important to carefully inspect the basal lung parenchyma for lung cysts on abdominal CT scans performed for renal AML evaluation (see Fig. 35.12).

There is less certainty as to whether patients with known TSC should be screened for pulmonary LAM.[28,88,93] The European Respiratory Society LAM task force recommends chest CT screening for females with TSC at the age of 18 years and, if negative, again at 30 to 40 years of age. If persistent respiratory symptoms develop, scanning should be performed as clinically appropriate.[88]

CLASSIC SIGNS

- The CT appearances of sporadic lymphangioleiomyomatosis (LAM) and tuberous sclerosis complex (TSC)-LAM are similar, consisting of scattered, bilateral, thin-walled cysts without a zonal predominance.
- Surrounding parenchyma is usually normal, but occasionally ground-glass opacities or interlobular septal thickening may be observed, usually representing foci of pulmonary hemorrhage.
- Spontaneous, often recurrent pneumothorax is the initial manifestation in half of patients.
- Angiomyolipoma is often associated with LAM.
- Chylous pleural effusion is more common in sporadic LAM and affects 14% of patients at presentation.
- Sclerotic osseous lesions, intramyocardial fat, and pulmonary nodules are more common with TSC-LAM.

Differential Diagnosis

The diagnosis of LAM may be delayed by 5 years after the onset of symptoms because it is often confused with more common lung disorders, such as asthma or chronic obstructive pulmonary disease.[111–113] The radiologist may be the first to suggest the diagnosis of LAM. On chest radiography the combination of a delicate reticular pattern and hyperexpansion of the lungs is typical of LAM, in contrast to the progressive loss of volume of most other fibrosing interstitial disorders. Such a combination may also occur in a few other conditions, including pulmonary Langerhans cell histiocytosis, sarcoidosis, and, rarely, hypersensitivity pneumonitis.

LAM can be confidently and correctly diagnosed in most cases on CT.[114,115] In some cases the distinction between LAM and centrilobular emphysema may present difficulties, particularly when centrilobular emphysema takes on a "cyst-like" morphology.[111] In LAM cysts are variably demarcated by a thin wall that ranges from invisible[44,47] to nearly 2-mm thick in most cases; as a rule, cyst walls are exquisitely thin. Vessels are seen at the periphery of the cysts and generally are not displaced (see Fig. 35.9), as is often the case in centrilobular and bullous emphysema. LAM cysts do not contain a "dot-like" centrilobular core structure.[111,116] Indeed, identification of residual core lobular structures in the center of "cysts," typical of emphysema, may be helpful in differentiating these conditions.

Other cystic lung diseases occasionally may be confused with LAM, particularly pulmonary Langerhans cell histiocytosis. In pulmonary Langerhans cell histiocytosis, cavitating nodules are present, particularly in the early stages of the disease, and the resulting cysts are more irregular with thicker walls and tend to occur predominantly in the upper and middle lung zones, sparing the costophrenic sulci. Nevertheless, advanced pulmonary Langerhans cell histiocytosis, when the distribution characteristics are less obvious, may be difficult to distinguish from severe LAM. Even neoplastic lesions, such as multiple mesenchymal cystic hamartomas, benign metastasizing leiomyoma, and metastases from primary squamous cell carcinoma, occasionally can be confused with LAM, although these cystic lesions generally have thicker walls, are associated with solid nodules, and tend to be less numerous.[111,112]

Birt-Hogg-Dubé syndrome (BHDS) is an autosomal-dominant inherited genodermatosis stemming from a defect in the folliculin gene that has to be differentiated from LAM.[117] The two diseases have similar radiologic manifestations, including pulmonary cysts, pneumothorax, and renal tumors. In contrast to LAM cysts, the cysts in BHD are less numerous, larger in size, oval in shape, and tend to predominantly involve the lower lung zones, particularly the paracardial regions. Furthermore, patients with BHDS often report family history of pneumothorax.[117]

Usually, the clinical history and other parenchymal features rule out more easily the possibility of lymphoid interstitial pneumonia, usual interstitial pneumonia, and *Pneumocystis jirovecii* pneumonia.

KEY POINTS: DIFFERENTIAL DIAGNOSIS

- The absence of residual core lobular structures and the presence of vessels at the periphery of thin walls suggest lymphangioleiomyomatosis (LAM) instead of centrilobular emphysema.
- Cavitating nodules and cysts sparing the costophrenic sulci occur in Langerhans cell histiocytosis, not in LAM.
- LAM cysts are more numerous and smaller than those associated with Birt-Hogg-Dubé syndrome.

DIAGNOSTIC CRITERIA

- Diagnosis of tuberous sclerosis complex (TSC) should be made according to established criteria.[53] It is usually made clinically by recognition of the somatic features; imaging plays a pivotal role in detection of associated pulmonary or extrapulmonary pathology.
- It is important to consider sporadic LAM or TSC-LAM in a young or middle-aged woman who presents with pneumothorax, dyspnea, or obstructive lung disease.
- Biopsy confirmation of LAM is not required when the CT appearance is characteristic in a patient with known TSC or when pulmonary cysts are associated with other typical manifestations (i.e., angiomyolipoma [AML]), lymphangioleiomyoma, chylous pleural effusion, or chylous ascites).[41,118]
- Vascular endothelial growth factor (VEGF)-D testing is recommended to establish the diagnosis of LAM before proceeding to lung biopsy in patients whose CT scan shows abnormalities characteristic of LAM but who have no other confirmatory clinical or extrapulmonary radiologic features of LAM.[118]
- Elevated VEGF-D level has a sufficient positive predictive value for use as a diagnostic test for LAM. When used in combination with the European Respiratory Society diagnostic criteria, 80% of patients could avoid lung biopsy for diagnosis.[17,88]
- The gold standard for the diagnosis of LAM is thoracoscopic lung biopsy. In patients unable to undergo a thoracoscopic lung biopsy, the diagnosis can be made on the basis of a transbronchial biopsy, especially in conjunction with immunohistochemical staining with HMB45.[88]
- All patients with LAM should undergo a careful clinical examination for stigmata of TSC. The diagnosis of TSC is often difficult because an increasing number of patients with mild disease are being identified in adulthood, including some with LAM as the initial manifestation.
- All patients with LAM or suspected LAM should have an abdominal and pelvis CT at diagnosis or during workup to identify AML and other abdominal lesions. Brain imaging is recommended for all patients with TSC and in women with sporadic LAM before treatment with progesterone. Patients with TSC should undergo annual brain MRI studies until 21 years of age and then every 2–3 years to diagnose and monitor giant cell tumors.[84]

SUGGESTED READINGS

Abbott GF, Rosado de Christenson ML, Frazier AA, et al. From the archives of the AFIP: lymphangioleiomyomatosis: radiologic-pathologic correlation. *Radiographics*. 2005;25:803–828.

Avila N, Dwyer AJ, Moss J. Imaging features of lymphangioleiomyomatosis: diagnostic pitfalls. *AJR Am J Roentgenol*. 2011;196:982–986.

Gupta N, Meraj R, Tanase D. Accuracy of chest high-resolution computed tomography in diagnosing diffuse cystic lung diseases. *Eur Respir J*. 2015;46:1196–1199.

Hancock E, Osborne J. Lymphangioleiomyomatosis: a review of the literature. *Respir Med*. 2002;96:1–6.

Johnson SR. Lymphangioleiomyomatosis. *Eur Respir J*. 2006;27:1056–1065.

Johnson SR, Cordier JF, Lazor R, et al. European Respiratory Society guidelines for the diagnosis and management of lymphangioleiomyomatosis. *Eur Respir J*. 2010;35:14–26.

McCormack FX. Lymphangioleiomyomatosis. *Medgenmed*. 2006;8:15.

McCormack FX, Gupta N, Finlay GR, et al. Official American Thoracic Society/Japanese Respiratory Society Clinical Practice Guidelines: lymphangioleiomyomatosis diagnosis and management. *Am J Respir Crit Care Med*. 2016;194:748–761.

Pacheco-Rodriguez G, Kristof AS, Stevens LA, et al. Filley Lecture. Genetics and gene expression in lymphangioleiomyomatosis. *Chest*. 2002;121:56–60.

Pallisa E, Sanz P, Roman A, et al. Lymphangioleiomyomatosis: pulmonary and abdominal findings with pathologic correlation. *Radiographics*. 2002;22:S185–S198.

Roach ES, Sparagana SP. Diagnosis of tuberous sclerosis complex. *J Child Neurol*. 2004;19:643–649.

Tobino K, Hirai T, Johkoh T, et al. Differentiation between Birt-Hogg-Dubé syndrome and lymphangioleiomyomatosis: quantitative analysis of pulmonary cysts on computed tomography of the chest in 66 females. *Eur J Radiol*. 2012;81:1340–1346.

The full reference list for this chapter is available at ExpertConsult.com.

36 Idiopathic Pleuroparenchymal Fibroelastosis

ROBERT M. DEWITT | STEPHEN K. FRANKEL

Amitani and colleagues[1] first described a unique pattern of upper lobe–predominant, idiopathic pulmonary fibrosis (IPF) in 13 patients in the Japanese literature in 1992. The currently preferred term in the English-language literature, *idiopathic pleuroparenchymal fibroelastosis* (iPPFE), was coined by Frankel and colleagues[2] in 2004 in a case series of five patients presenting with unique clinical and radiographic findings distinct from any of the previously characterized idiopathic interstitial pneumonias (IIPs).[2] Since that time, a number of cases of pleuroparenchymal fibroelastosis (PPFE) have been identified in patients with compelling etiologic correlates commonly associated with the development of interstitial lung disease (ILD), including familial interstitial pneumonitis[3]; recurrent lower respiratory tract lung infections[4]; lung, bone marrow, and hematopoietic cell transplantation[5]; chemotherapeutic medications (drug-induced PPFE)[6]; occupational exposure to aluminosilicate dust[7] or asbestosis[8]; and systemic autoimmune diseases, such as rheumatoid arthritis and scleroderma. As with the other IPs/ILDs, PPFE is described as idiopathic when no associated causative etiology can be identified. iPPFE was recently recognized as a distinct entity in the American Thoracic Society/European Respiratory Society 2013 update on the IIPs and was categorized as one of the two rare IIPs, along with lymphoid IP.[9]

Prevalence and Epidemiology

As of January 2017, approximately 120 cases have been reported overall in the published literature.[10] To date, iPPFE appears to have no gender preference and no association with cigarette smoking. The average age at presentation is highly variable, ranging from 13 to 87 years with a median of approximately 53 years.[11]

Clinical Presentation

Patients most often present with insidious onset of dyspnea, exercise intolerance, and nonproductive cough, similar to other patients with fibrosing ILD. Additional symptoms include chest discomfort (pain, tightness, inability to take a satisfying breath), pneumothorax, and constitutional symptoms, such as fatigue, malaise, and weight loss. Patients have been described as having a slender stature with associated "flattened thoracic cage" or "platythorax," potentially signifying a decrease in the anterior-posterior dimension of the thorax.[12]

Pathology

Although there are no well-defined consensus criteria regarding the histopathologic diagnosis of PPFE, in a 2013 review von der Thüsen[13] proposed a working definition of iPPFE with "definite" and "consistent with" histologic criteria. "Definite" criteria of iPPFE include (1) upper zone fibrosis of the visceral pleura; (2) prominent, homogeneous, subpleural intraalveolar fibrosis with alveolar septal elastosis; (3) sparing of the parenchyma distant from the pleura; (4) at most, mild, patchy lymphoplasmocytic infiltrates; and (5) at most, small numbers of fibroblastic foci. Criteria that are "consistent with" iPPFE also have intraalveolar fibrosis as just described; however, (1) this may not be associated with significant pleural fibrosis, (2) may not be predominantly subpleural, or (3) may not occur in an upper lobe biopsy. Additional criteria for iPPFE were proposed by Rosenbaum and colleagues[14] in 2015, which included (1) fibrous IP with 80% fibroelastic changes in nonatelectatic lung; (2) subpleural and/or centrilobular distribution; (3) overall inflammation absent to mild; (4) no specific lobe predilection, typically multilobar; and (5) rare or no granulomas. A recent quantitative assessment of elastic fibers (EF) demonstrated twice the number of EF in iPPFE compared with IPF.[15] That said, it is important to note that the two conditions are not mutually exclusive and often appear to coexist.[4,16] Although an experienced pathologist may be able to recognize the characteristic features of PPFE on standard eosin and hematoxylin stains, incorporating the routine use of EF-specific agents, such as orcein or Verhoeff–van Gieson stains, could greatly facilitate identifying PPFE histologically (Fig. 36.1).

Physiology

The main physiologic abnormality is a restrictive ventilatory impairment similar to other fibrosing ILDs. Often there is a disproportionate reduction in forced vital capacity relative to the reduction seen in the diffusion capacity of carbon monoxide compared with the degree of impairment seen in these parameters in patients with other ILDs, such as IPF. Additionally, disproportionate upper lobe fibrotic collapse with compensatory hyperinflation of the lower lobes may increase the ratio of residual volume to total lung capacity distinguishing PPFE from IPF.[12]

Imaging

Radiographs in early iPPFE may demonstrate bilateral apical pleural irregularity or be normal as subtle visceral pleural nodularity, and intraalveolar fibrosis may be radiographically occult (Fig. 36.2). Indeed, patients often present with physiologic impairment and symptoms that are more pronounced than what would be expected based upon the radiographic findings alone. Later-stage disease classically demonstrates increased severity in the apical pleural thickening, with upper lobe–predominant reticulonodular opacities and retracted, elevated hila. Lateral radiographs may illustrate anterior-posterior dimensional narrowing. Recurrent pneumothorax may occur in PPFE.[12,17]

Early in the disease course, high-resolution computed tomography demonstrates apical-predominant subpleural nodular and reticular opacities that may coalesce into areas of dense consolidation with associated traction bronchiectasis, architectural distortion, and intraalveolar fibrosis (Fig. 36.3). As with chest radiography, the upper lobe volume loss may be associated with superior hilar retraction. As the disease progresses, multilobar pleuroparenchymal thickening can be seen, and the apical disease may evolve to include upper lobe bullae or cysts. Again, additional ILD patterns may coexist with PPFE, most commonly usual interstitial pneumonia (UIP) and nonspecific interstitial pneumonia (NSIP) patterns of lung fibrosis.[4,16]

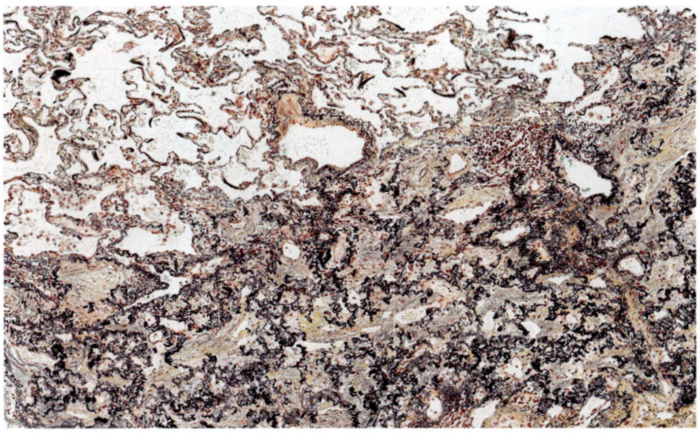

Fig. 36.1 Pleuroparenchymal fibroelastosis: histologic findings. Micrograph shows pentachrome (Movat)-stained sections photographed at 4x objective magnification showing fibroelastotic changes in the subpleural parenchyma of the lower right portion of the image, contrasted against the preserved normal architecture of the lung in the upper left corner. Yellow corresponds to the mature collagen of fibrotic lung, whereas the black highlights the increased number and fragmentation of the elastin fibers embedded within the fibrosis. *(Courtesy Dr. Steve Groshong, Department of Pathology, National Jewish Health, Denver, Colorado.)*

Differential Diagnosis

Differential diagnosis includes those entities that manifest with apical or upper lobe–predominant disease, as well as those entities that manifest with a combination of parenchymal and pleural abnormalities. As such, competing diagnostic considerations may include apical capping, tuberculosis, sarcoidosis, silicosis, hypersensitivity pneumonitis, radiation-induced lung injury/fibrosis, asbestos-related lung disease and connective tissue disease–associated lung diseases, such as rheumatoid arthritis and ankylosing spondylitis.

Treatment and Management

Prognosis is highly variable with clinically significant disease progression occurring in 60% of patients and death attributable to the disease occurring in 40%.[4,10] A worse prognosis appears to exist in patients with PPFE plus a concomitant UIP pattern,[17] as well as those with familial forms of the disease. Patients are often treated empirically with corticosteroids and/or immunosuppressive/cytotoxic agents, although efficacy has not been confirmed. In one case report pirfenidone treatment appeared to sustain pulmonary function.[18] In patients with a combination of iPPFE and IPF, the antifibrotic agents pirfenidone and nintedanib have been used to treat the IPF, but the secondary effects on the PPFE are as of yet unknown/unreported. Lung transplant has been successfully performed in advanced cases.[19]

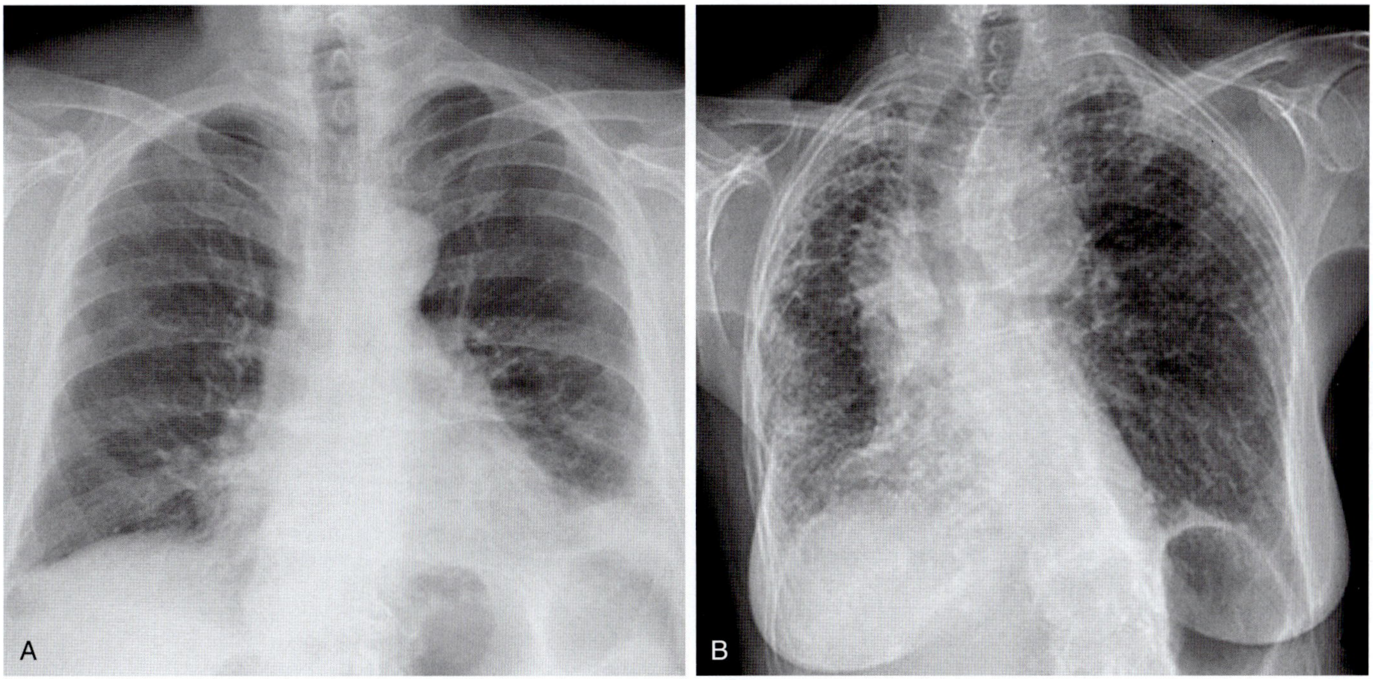

Fig. 36.2 Idiopathic pleuroparenchymal fibroelastosis: radiographic findings. (A) Chest radiograph shows no lung fibrosis. There is a small left pleural effusion. (B) Chest radiograph 4 years later demonstrates apical predominant pleural thickening with diffuse, course reticular markings, retracted and elevated hila, and right greater-than-left lung volume loss with compensatory rightward tracheal deviation.

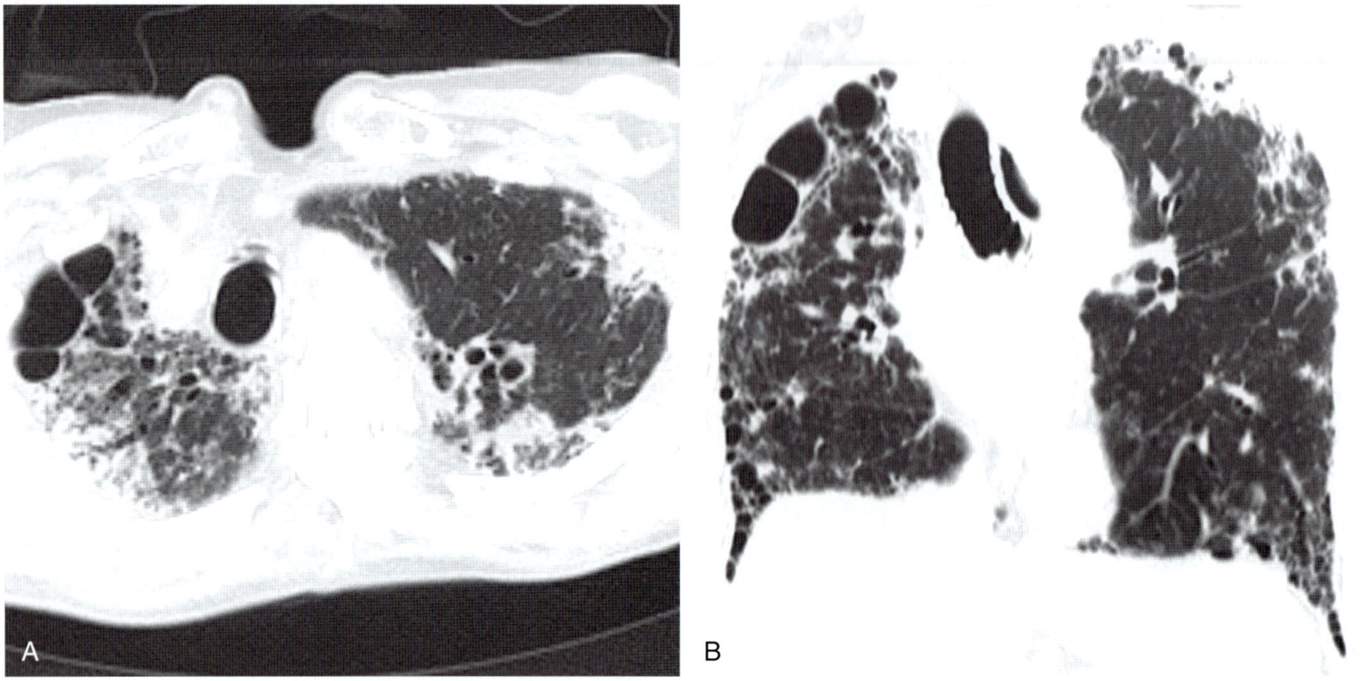

Fig. 36.3 Idiopathic pleuroparenchymal fibroelastosis: high-resolution CT findings. Axial (A) and coronal (B) high-resolution CT scan shows apical predominant subpleural thickening, dense subpleural consolidation and volume loss with right apical bullae. Basilar honeycombing is consistent with patient's concomitant usual interstitial pneumonia.

Beyond directed pharmacologic therapy, many experts emphasize the importance of a comprehensive approach to disease management, including pulmonary rehabilitation, oxygen therapy, achieving and maintaining ideal body weight through proper nutrition and exercise, and vaccinations per Advisory Committee on Immunization Practices guidelines. Additionally, screening for and treatment of commonly seen comorbid conditions, such as gastric esophageal reflux disease, pulmonary hypertension, bronchiectasis, osteoporosis, UIP/NSIP, depression, and anxiety, is also recommended. Longitudinal care with a team of experts in the care of ILD patients may often be beneficial given the rarity of the disease.

KEY POINTS

- Idiopathic pleuroparenchymal fibroelastosis (iPPFE) requires a multidisciplinary approach for accurate diagnosis.
- iPPFE is likely to increase in prevalence as more specialists become aware of this distinct entity.
- Although classically upper lobe predominant, at time of diagnosis, PPFE often evolves with disease progression to be a multilobar process.
- iPPFE may coexist with other histopathologic lesions, such as usual interstitial pneumonia and nonspecific interstitial pneumonia.
- Further study is necessary to establish optimal idiopathic PPFE management and treatment guidelines.

SUGGESTED READINGS

ATS/ERS Committee on Idiopathic Interstitial Pneumonias. An official American Thoracic Society/European Respiratory Society statement: update of the international multidisciplinary classification of the idiopathic interstitial pneumonias. *Am J Respir Crit Care Med*. 2013;188(6):733–748.

Reddy TL, Tominaga M, Hansell DM, et al. Pleuroparenchymal fibroelastosis: a spectrum of histopathological and imaging phenotypes. *Eur Respir J*. 2012;40(2):377–385.

The full reference list for this chapter is available at ExpertConsult.com.

37 Eosinophilic Lung Diseases*

MELISSA PRICE | CAROL C. WU | MATTHEW D. GILMAN

Eosinophilic diseases of the lung include a heterogeneous group of pulmonary disorders that characteristically feature peripheral or tissue eosinophilia.[1] Patients with these illnesses have a variable clinical presentation and may be asymptomatic or may exhibit organ dysfunction or clinical symptoms of severe respiratory illness.[1,2] Histologically, eosinophilic lung diseases demonstrate infiltration of eosinophils in the pulmonary interstitium and alveolar spaces with preservation of the lung architecture. As a result, these illnesses respond dramatically to corticosteroid treatment and typically heal without significant lung parenchymal damage.[3]

The diseases are classified as idiopathic or secondary to a known primary disease process or well-defined cause.[2] Established causes of eosinophilic lung disease include primary airways diseases, such as allergic bronchopulmonary aspergillosis (see Chapter 57), drug reaction (see Chapter 65), and toxin exposure and parasitic infections (see Chapter 14).[3] The idiopathic eosinophilic diseases of the lung are simple pulmonary eosinophilia (Löffler syndrome), acute and chronic eosinophilic pneumonia, and the systemic conditions such as hypereosinophilic syndrome and eosinophilic granulomatosis with polyangiitis (formerly known as Churg-Strauss, which is discussed in Chapter 46).[2]

The diagnosis of eosinophilic lung disease can be made in the presence of one of the following criteria: (1) peripheral eosinophilia (>1000/mm^3) in conjunction with pulmonary parenchymal opacities on chest radiography, (2) tissue eosinophilia on surgical or transbronchial lung biopsy, or (3) eosinophilia in bronchoalveolar lavage (BAL) fluid (differential cell count > 25).[1,3]

Simple Pulmonary Eosinophilia

Etiology, Prevalence, and Epidemiology

Simple pulmonary eosinophilia (SPE) was originally identified and described in 1932 by Löffler. Patients with SPE typically have fleeting pulmonary opacities on chest radiography in the presence of blood eosinophilia. Approximately one-third of cases of SPE are idiopathic. The majority of cases occur secondary to drug toxicity or parasitic infection.[4,5] The incidence of SPE in oncologic patients undergoing follow-up CT imaging has been reported to be 0.95%. These individuals typically lack respiratory symptoms and have subsolid nodules on chest CT.[6]

*The editors and the publisher would like to thank Dr. Takeshi Johkoh for contributing material on this topic to the prior edition of this work. It has served as the foundation for the current chapter.

Clinical Presentation

Individuals may be asymptomatic or may experience minimal respiratory symptoms, fever, or malaise. Symptoms and radiologic findings are self-limited and resolve spontaneously within 30 days with or without treatment.[7]

Pathophysiology

Data is limited on the pathophysiology of this disease entity, but there is an association with alveolar infiltration with eosinophils and giant cells.[5]

Manifestations of the Disease

RADIOGRAPHY

The characteristic radiographic findings are nonsegmental opacities, which are frequently ill-defined and peripheral in distribution.[1,7] The opacities may be unilateral or bilateral and are characteristically transient or migratory[8,9] (Fig. 37.1).

COMPUTED TOMOGRAPHY

Ground-glass opacities and consolidation, the most common CT findings, either showed a random distribution or upper and middle lung zone predominance (Fig. 37.2; see Fig. 37.1). Pulmonary parenchymal nodules were reported to be present in 42% of cases.[10] The CT features and distribution of opacities present in SPE and chronic eosinophilic pneumonia are similar; the important distinguishing feature is that the imaging findings in SPE will spontaneously fluctuate over a period of days as opposed to chronic eosinophilic pneumonia (CEP), where the consolidations and ground-glass opacities will persist for weeks to months and be accompanied by more significant respiratory symptoms.[11] In individuals with SPE found at oncologic surveillance or routine screening, pulmonary nodules (either solitary or multiple) with a ground-glass halo are the most common CT finding.[6,9,12]

Differential Diagnosis

The presence of consolidation on chest radiography can be seen in the setting of pneumonia, alveolar pulmonary edema, or diffuse alveolar damage. The absence of or minimal pulmonary symptoms associated with SPE, along with peripheral blood eosinophilia, strongly suggests the diagnosis. It is important to exclude known associations with pulmonary eosinophilia, the most common of which are parasitic infection and drug toxicity.

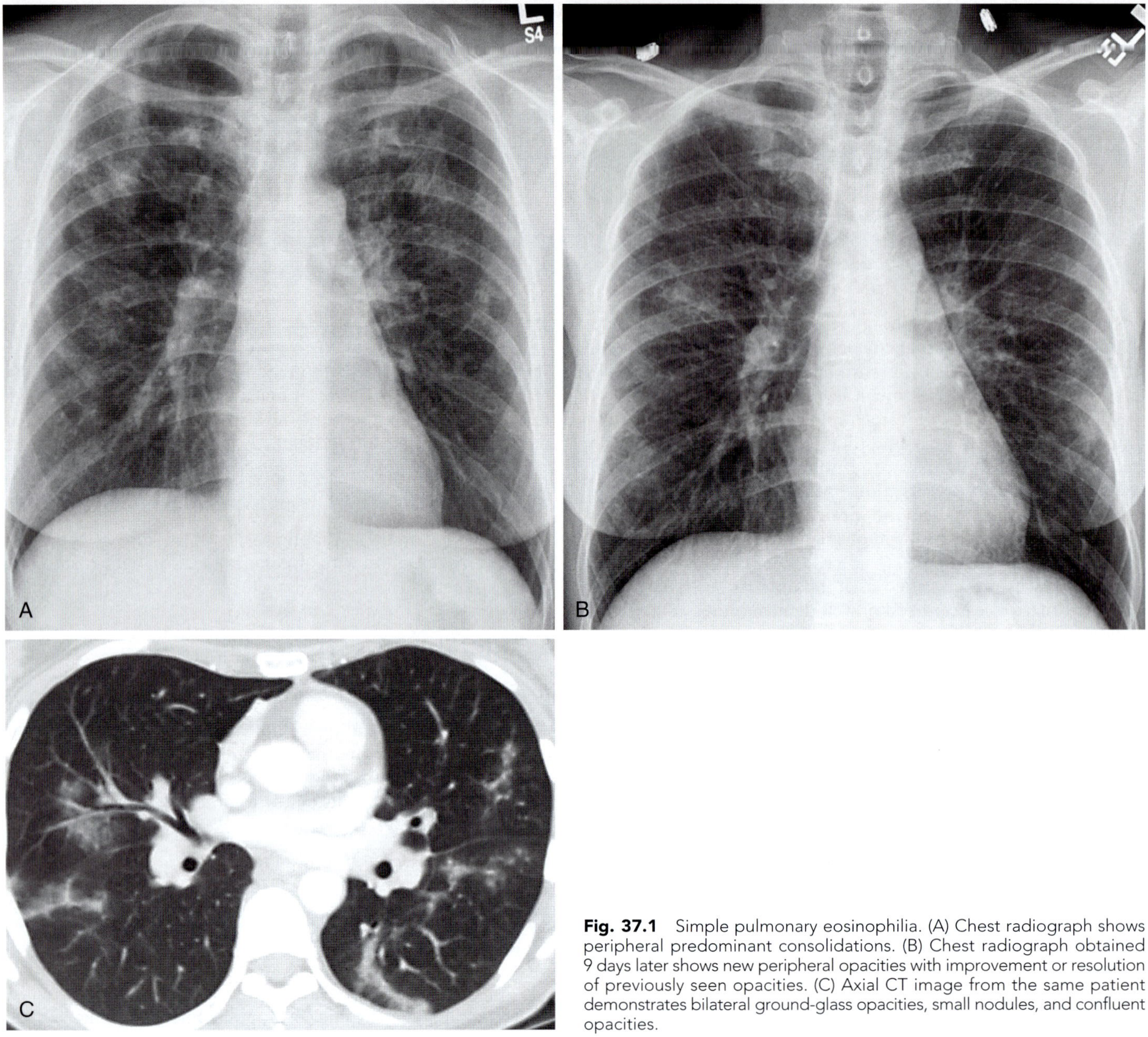

Fig. 37.1 Simple pulmonary eosinophilia. (A) Chest radiograph shows peripheral predominant consolidations. (B) Chest radiograph obtained 9 days later shows new peripheral opacities with improvement or resolution of previously seen opacities. (C) Axial CT image from the same patient demonstrates bilateral ground-glass opacities, small nodules, and confluent opacities.

Synopsis of Treatment Options

No treatment is required because SPE is asymptomatic and self-limited.

KEY POINTS: SIMPLE PULMONARY EOSINOPHILIA

- Approximately one-third of cases are idiopathic; infectious etiologies and drug toxicity are more common and should be excluded.
- Clinical course is mild and self-limited, with symptoms resolving spontaneously within a month.
- Radiography shows nonsegmental, peripheral opacities that are transient and/or migratory.
- Subsolid nodules, ground-glass opacities, and consolidation may be seen on CT.

Chronic Eosinophilic Pneumonia

Etiology, Prevalence, and Epidemiology

Idiopathic chronic eosinophilic pneumonia (ICEP) is a respiratory illness characterized by alveolar eosinophilia, typically greater than 25% at BAL and/or blood eosinophilia of at least 6%.[1,13] Although blood eosinophilia is present in most patients, up to 12% of patients with ICEP do not have peripheral eosinophilia.[13] The disease is more common among women[14] and tends to occur around the fifth decade.[1,14,15] There is an association of ICEP with asthma,[13,16–18] which has been reported to occur in up to 53% of patients with ICEP.[15] Unlike in eosinophilic granulomatosis with polyangiitis and hypereosinophilic syndrome (HES),

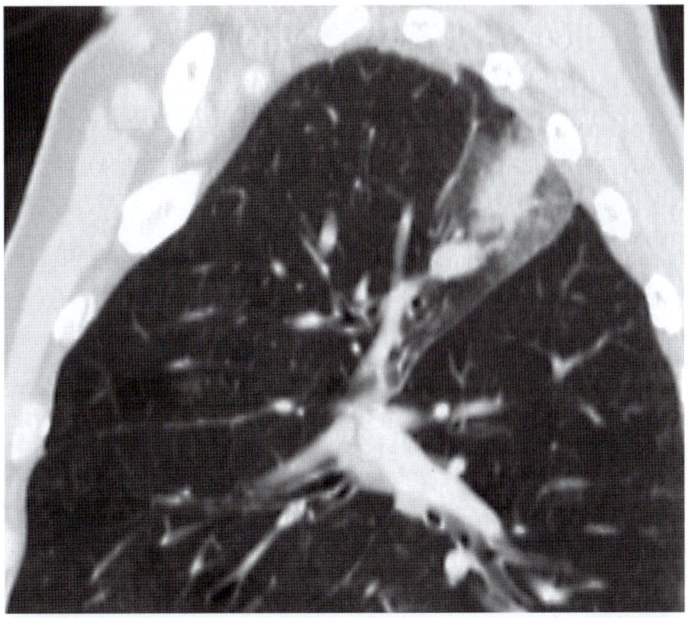

Fig. 37.2 Simple pulmonary eosinophilia. Sagittal CT image shows nodular subpleural consolidation in the posterior segment of the right upper lobe with adjacent ground-glass opacity in this man with peripheral eosinophilia. The consolidation nearly resolved at follow-up CT imaging 4 weeks later.

extrathoracic symptoms and organ dysfunction are not present in ICEP.[16]

Clinical Presentation

Systemic symptoms associated with ICEP, such as fever, weight loss, and night sweats in addition to dyspnea and cough,[14] are typically present for 1 month on average before clinical presentation.[18] The mean time to diagnosis is 7.7 months,[13] reflecting the confounding factors that make the diagnosis of ICEP challenging. Other features seen in a minority of patients include anorexia, chills, and hemoptysis.[13]

Pathophysiology

At histology there is an alveolar infiltration of eosinophils and to a lesser extent macrophages, lymphocytes, and plasma cells,[14] and in approximately half of patients, there will be foci of interstitial fibrosis.[13] In more rare cases, eosinophilic microabscesses and regions of intraalveolar necrosis will also be present.[13]

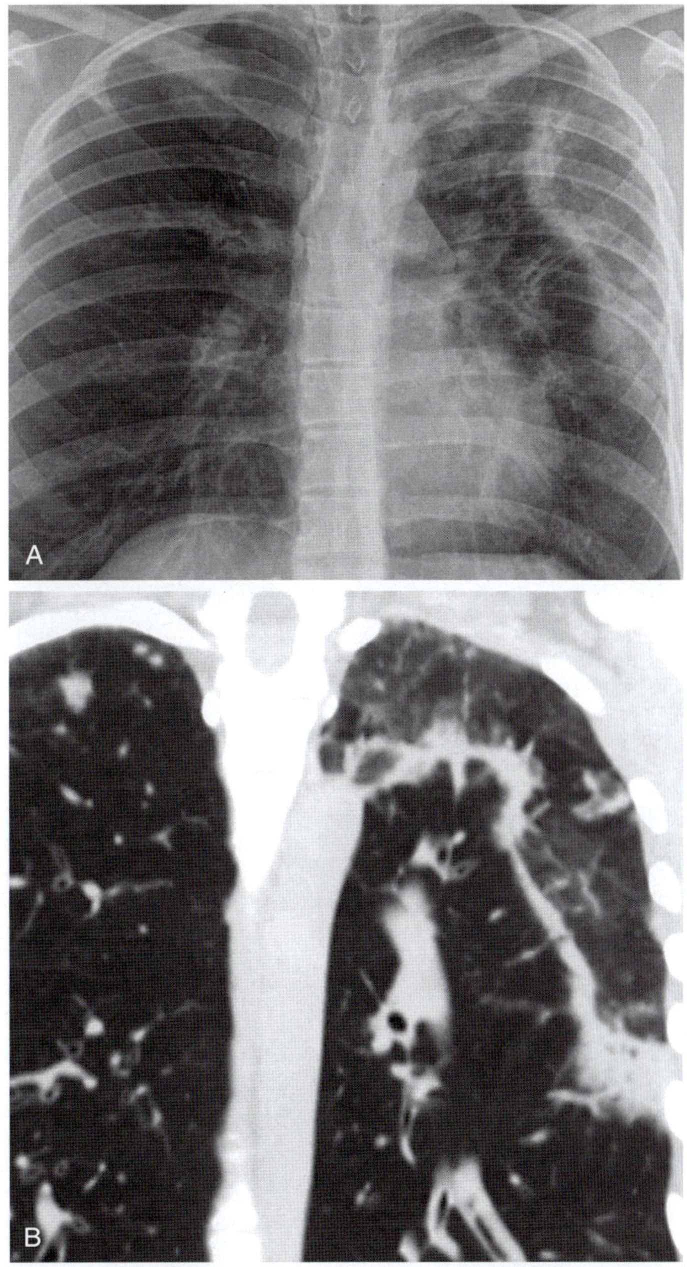

Fig. 37.3 Chronic eosinophilic pneumonia. (A) Chest radiograph in a woman with a 7-month history of cough shows bilateral upper lobe opacities, greater on the left. (B) Coronal CT image reveals ground-glass opacity in the apical left upper lobe with surrounding peripheral consolidation. The patient had a bronchoalveolar lavage eosinophilia of 71% at bronchoscopy.

Manifestations of the Disease

RADIOGRAPHY

The characteristic radiographic finding in ICEP is peripheral airspace opacities.[1,14] In their 1969 article that first described the disease, Carrington and colleagues[14] identified the unique presence of three features in ICEP: progressive peripheral dense consolidations, prompt resolution with corticosteroid treatment, and recurrence in the same unique locations upon relapse. The dense peripheral consolidation in ICEP has been described as the "photographic negative" of pulmonary edema.[14,19] There is typically no lobar or segmental distribution to the opacities, which can be unilateral or bilateral and show ill-defined margins. An apical or axillary location is common (Fig. 37.3), and opacities may be mistaken for loculated pleural fluid.[19]

COMPUTED TOMOGRAPHY

Subpleural and upper lung zone–predominant consolidation and areas of ground-glass opacity are present in the vast majority of patients (Figs. 37.4 and 37.5).[10] In some patients mediastinal lymphadenopathy will be evident on CT (Fig. 37.6).[10,11] Unlike in acute eosinophilic pneumonia, pleural effusions are rare.[10]

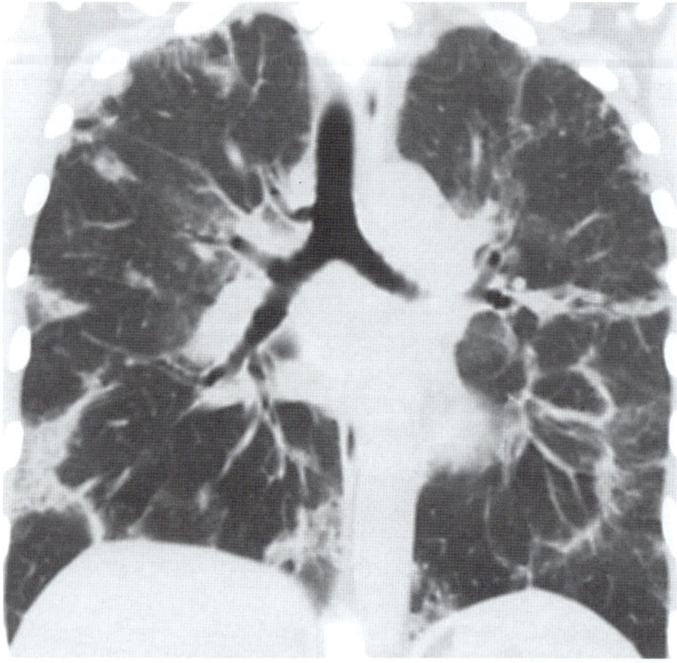

Fig. 37.4 Chronic eosinophilic pneumonia. Coronal CT image shows patchy bilateral consolidation and ground-glass opacities without craniocaudad zonal predominance.

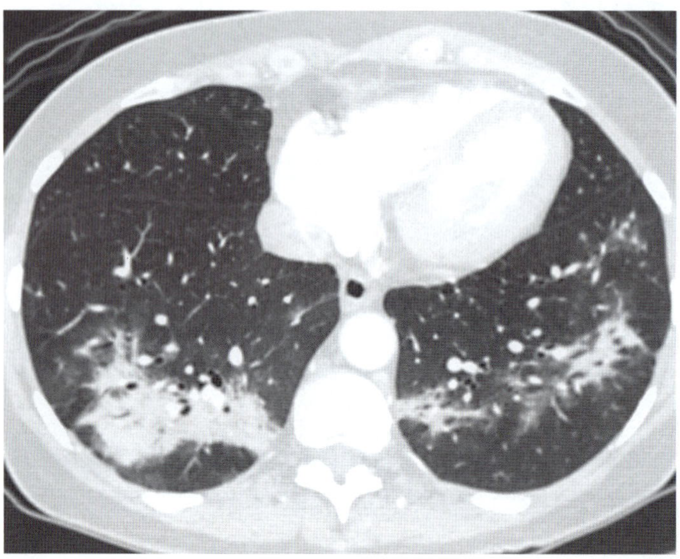

Fig. 37.5 Chronic eosinophilic pneumonia. Axial CT image demonstrates lower lobe consolidations, an atypical distribution for chronic eosinophilic pneumonia as the disease is generally upper lung zone predominant.

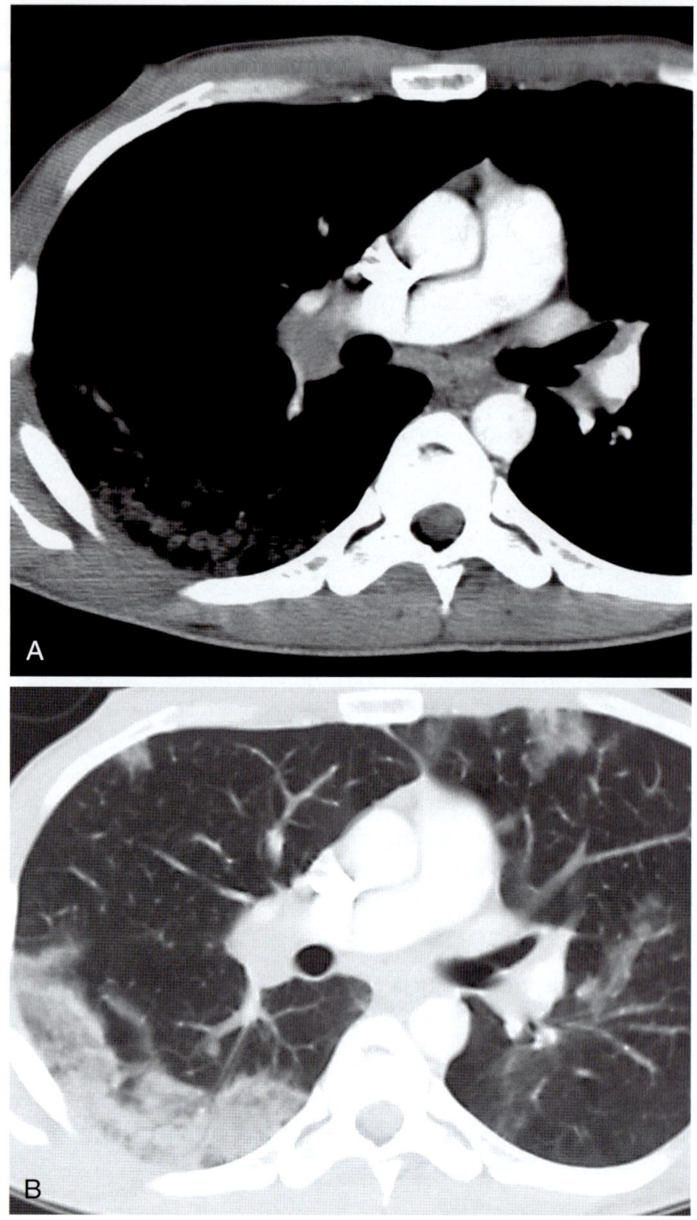

Fig. 37.6 Chronic eosinophilic pneumonia. (A) Axial CT image with soft tissue window shows right hilar and subcarinal lymphadenopathy in this man with a history of asthma and recurrent sinusitis who presented with 3 months of productive cough and a 10-lb weight loss. (B) Axial CT image shows bilateral peripheral ground-glass and confluent opacities. The patient's bronchoalveolar lavage eosinophilia was 65%.

Less common CT findings include nodules, bronchiectasis, and interlobular septal thickening.[10] In patients who have had at least 2 months of symptoms at the time of CT imaging, band-like opacities and lobar atelectasis can be seen.[20]

Differential Diagnosis

The primary differential consideration in patients who have ICEP is an infectious pneumonia, given the airspace opacities and febrile respiratory illness that characterize the disease. Other diagnoses that may be considered include organizing pneumonia, drug toxicity, and sarcoidosis.[1] The upper lobe–predominant opacities, constitutional symptoms, and rare hemoptysis may raise concern for tuberculosis.[14,19] SPE may appear identical to ICEP on imaging; however, patients with SPE will have transient opacities that fluctuate over a period of days, a relative paucity of constitutional symptoms, and spontaneous resolution.[8,11] The presence of blood and alveolar eosinophilia, dramatic clinical and radiographic response to steroids, and peripheral airspace opacities favor the diagnosis of ICEP.

Synopsis of Treatment Options

ICEP is extremely steroid sensitive, and opacities seen on imaging improve or resolve rapidly on initiation of corticosteroid therapy.[8,11,14,19] After discontinuation or tapering of steroid therapy, there is a tendency for symptoms to recur and opacities to reappear, often in the same location and configuration as seen initially.[14]

KEY POINTS: CHRONIC EOSINOPHILIC PNEUMONIA

- Idiopathic chronic eosinophilic pneumonia features filling of the alveoli with a mixed inflammatory infiltrate, primarily of eosinophils.
- Peripheral eosinophilia is typically present, but absence of elevated blood eosinophils does not exclude the diagnosis.
- Systemic symptoms include fever, nonproductive cough, weight loss, and dyspnea. In contrast to acute eosinophilic pneumonia, hypoxemic respiratory failure is uncommon.
- As many as 50% of patients have a history of asthma or atopy.
- The characteristic pattern is peripheral opacities favoring the upper lobes: "photographic negative" of pulmonary edema.
- Response to corticosteroids is rapid, although recurrence is frequent with steroid withdrawal.

Acute Eosinophilic Pneumonia

Etiology, Prevalence, and Epidemiology

Acute eosinophilic pneumonia (AEP) is an idiopathic respiratory illness associated with cigarette smoking—in particular, new-onset cigarette smoking.[21–24] There was a relatively high incidence of AEP among military personnel who had been stationed in Iraq or nearby during Operation Iraqi Freedom, and 78% of these individuals reported recent-onset cigarette smoking. The illness has also been linked with toxin inhalation[25,26] and various medications.[27,28] Unlike CEP, there is no association of AEP with asthma; however, allergic rhinitis has been found in 38% of patients with AEP in one series.[18]

Clinical Presentation

AEP is a febrile respiratory illness in which patients present with acute dyspnea and hypoxemic respiratory failure.[1,29] The average age of presentation of AEP is early adulthood,[30] and it occurs more frequently among males.[18,30] Fever, dyspnea, cough, and pleuritic chest pain are the most common clinical symptoms.[1,30]

Pathophysiology

AEP affects the lung diffusely, with histology demonstrating diffuse alveolar damage and eosinophilic infiltration of the lung interstitium and alveoli. Acute interstitial pneumonia (i.e., idiopathic acute respiratory distress syndrome) also demonstrates a diffuse alveolar damage pattern at histology but lacks the tissue eosinophilia.[31] AEP is diagnosed when there are greater than 25% eosinophils in BAL fluid and diffuse pulmonary opacities are present on chest radiograph in the absence of an infectious source.[29,32] Peripheral eosinophil levels are often normal at the time of diagnosis but may become elevated several days after treatment.[18,29,33]

Manifestations of the Disease

RADIOGRAPHY

The radiographic findings are variable but may include both bilateral reticular and diffuse or patchy confluent opacities. Alternatively, either the reticular pattern or confluent opacity pattern may only be visible (Figs. 37.7 and 37.8).[30,34] Small bilateral

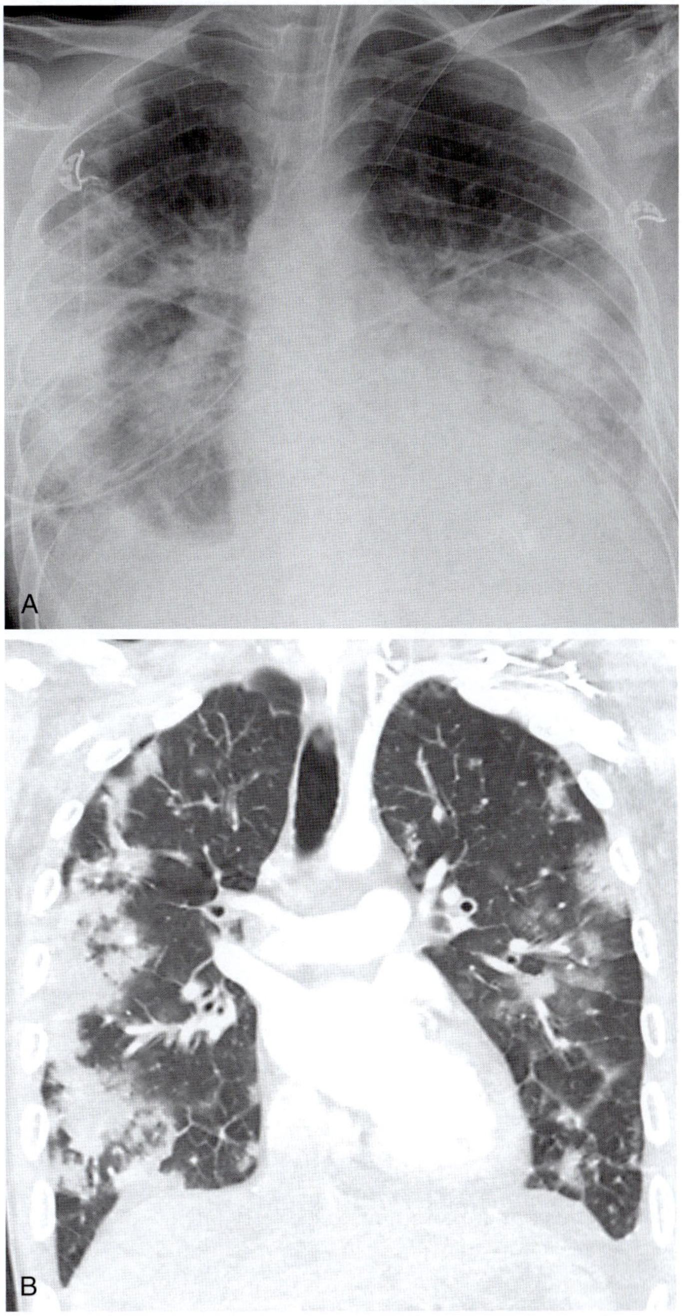

Fig. 37.7 Acute eosinophilic pneumonia. (A) Portable chest radiograph in a young man with acute eosinophilic pneumonia shows bilateral confluent and patchy opacities involving the lung periphery. The patient had a history of asthma and developed hypoxemic respiratory failure over a period of days, which required mechanical ventilation. (B) Coronal CT image shows bilateral consolidations with surrounding ground-glass opacities and diffuse bronchial wall thickening.

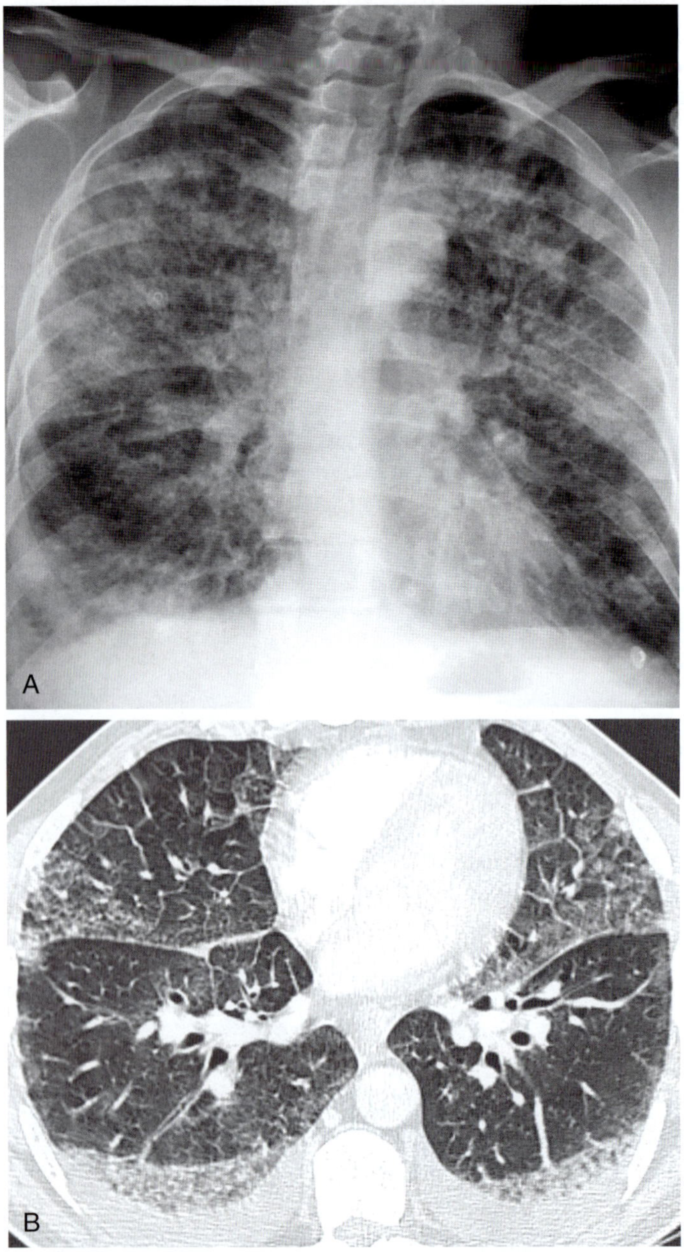

Fig. 37.8 Acute eosinophilic pneumonia. (A) Portable chest radiograph in a 41-year-old male firefighter who presented with acute respiratory failure shows bilateral reticular and confluent opacities. (B) Axial CT image shows peripheral ground-glass opacities and interlobular septal thickening producing the "crazy paving" pattern as well as small bilateral pleural effusions, which are commonly present in acute eosinophilic pneumonia.

pleural effusions are common. The disease often appears similar to pulmonary edema.[34]

COMPUTED TOMOGRAPHY

On CT a patient with AEP shows smooth interlobular septal thickening, diffuse ground-glass opacities, consolidation, and bilateral pleural effusions (Fig. 37.9; see also Figs. 37.7 and 37.8).[10,35,36] There is typically no zonal predominance in the cephalocaudad plane for these findings.[10,35] Pulmonary nodules

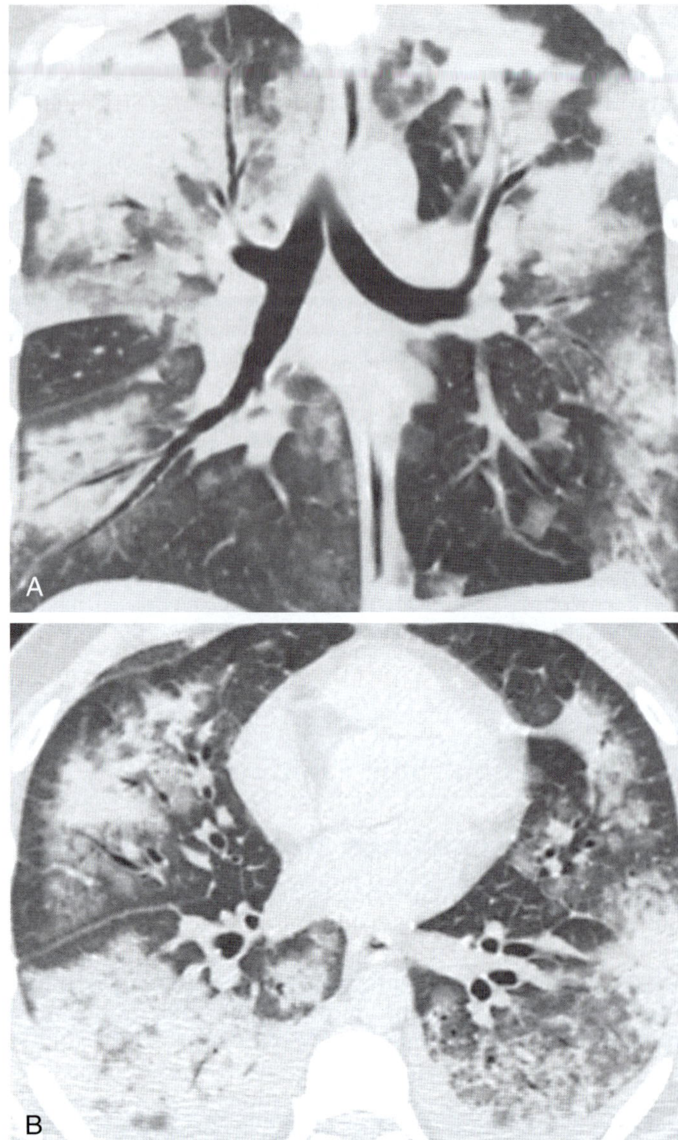

Fig. 37.9 Acute eosinophilic pneumonia. (A) and (B) Coronal and axial CT images of a 38-year-old man who presented with one week of fever, night sweats, fatigue, and shortness of breath, show multifocal, bilateral consolidations and ground-glass opacities with small bilateral pleural effusions.

occur in some of the patients.[10] Thickening of the peribronchovascular interstitium is also frequently observed.[35,36] The diffuse ground-glass opacities in conjunction with interlobular septal thickening can produce the nonspecific "crazy paving" pattern in patients with AEP (see Fig. 37.8).[35] Cardiac enlargement, in contrast to cardiogenic pulmonary edema, is not associated with the illness. Intrathoracic lymphadenopathy may be present but is not common.[10]

Differential Diagnosis

Pulmonary edema, multifocal pneumonia, pulmonary hemorrhage, and acute interstitial pneumonia are differential considerations. Suspecting the diagnosis of AEP can be particularly challenging in the absence of bronchoscopy and BAL because at initial presentation blood eosinophils are usually normal. The presence of BAL eosinophilia in conjunction with the clinical and radiologic findings should raise suspicion for the illness. In all cases it is important to exclude an underlying infection and drug toxicity.[1]

Synopsis of Treatment Options

Many patients will require mechanical ventilation at some time during their illness.[30] AEP resolves rapidly with steroids or spontaneously, which is a distinguishing feature from CEP.[18,30] After recovery from AEP, patients do not relapse,[30,37] and there is typically no residual fibrosis after recovery.[34]

KEY POINTS: ACUTE EOSINOPHILIC PNEUMONIA

- Rapidly progressive hypoxic respiratory failure with fever and dyspnea in the absence of infectious source are characteristic features of acute eosinophilic pneumonia.
- Bronchoalveolar lavage eosinophilia should be present for diagnosis: differential cell count of >25% eosinophils.
- Absence of blood eosinophilia does not exclude the diagnosis and is common.
- Infection and drug toxicity should be excluded.
- Tends to occur in young adults with a slight male predominance.
- Associated with recent-onset cigarette smoking.
- Response to corticosteroid therapy is rapid, but patients may recover spontaneously.
- Imaging findings often closely resemble pulmonary edema.

Hypereosinophilic Syndrome

Etiology, Prevalence, and Epidemiology

Hypereosinophilic syndrome (HES) is a rare condition characterized by marked peripheral eosinophilia with organ infiltration and resultant dysfunction.[7,38] The diagnostic criteria of HES based on the 2010 revision by Simon and colleagues[39] include (1) an elevation of the absolute eosinophil count (AEC) greater than $1500/mm^3$ on at least two occasions or evidence of prominent tissue eosinophilia with associated symptoms and marked blood eosinophilia and (2) exclusion of secondary causes of eosinophilia, such as parasitic or viral infections, allergic disease, drug-induced or chemical-induced eosinophilia, hypoadrenalism, and neoplasms. Subcategories of HES include a myeloproliferative form that includes myeloproliferative-HES (M-HES) and chronic eosinophilic leukemia, lymphocytic form (L-HES), and other HES variants.[39,40] The mean age at diagnosis is 52.5 years,[41] and the disease is more common in men.[41,42] Cardiac dysfunction in HES has the highest associated mortality.

Pathophysiology

Patients with M-HES have mutations of hematopoietic stem cells and expansion of the eosinophil population. In L-HES, activated T lymphocytes generate increased amounts of at least one eosinophil hematopoietin (interleukin [IL]-3 and/or IL-5), resulting in polyclonal blood hypereosinophilia. Patients with HES may also develop cutaneous, cardiac, and neurologic involvement and dysfunction resulting from eosinophil infiltration.[43] Cardiac involvement, present in 40% to 60% of patients, can result in complete heart block, eosinophilic myocarditis, ventricular thrombus formation, and cardiomyopathy.[40,43–45] In advanced stages of disease the eosinophilic-induced cardiac damage features fibrosis and mitral and tricuspid valvular regurgitation leading to a restrictive cardiomyopathy.[38] Eosinophilic infiltration of the lung is difficult to distinguish from other eosinophilic pneumonias.

Clinical Presentation

The initial presentation of HES can vary greatly. Some of the reported presenting symptoms include fever, recurrent abdominal pain, pruritic rash, and weight loss.[46] Patients with M-HES can present with hepatosplenomegaly, anemia, and thrombocytopenia typical of myeloproliferative diseases. The disease involves the lung in 40% of cases, with symptoms of cough, bronchospasm, and dyspnea.[43] In cases with cardiac involvement, patients experience congestive heart failure.[42]

Manifestations of the Disease

RADIOGRAPHY

Cardiac enlargement and findings related to pulmonary edema are among the more common radiographic findings.[42] Pleural effusions may also be present. In many cases the chest radiograph of patients with HES will be normal.[46,47] Focal or diffuse opacities can also be seen.[40]

COMPUTED TOMOGRAPHY

Patients with HES may have pulmonary nodules, which when present often have a surrounding ground-glass halo.[47] Other CT findings include interlobular septal and bronchial wall thickening and patchy or diffuse opacities (Fig. 37.10). Unlike ICEP, there is no zonal predominance of opacities in the craniocaudad plane.[10] Pulmonary embolism and intrathoracic lymphadenopathy with mildly enlarged mediastinal or hilar lymph nodes have also been reported.[48]

Synopsis of Treatment Options

HES is typically treated with corticosteroids and hydroxyurea. Survival has improved since the disease was first described; however, the prognosis remains poorer than other eosinophilic lung diseases.[44] Imatinib, a tyrosine kinase inhibitor, is used in M-HES.[40]

KEY POINTS: HYPEREOSINOPHILIC SYNDROME

- Rare disease featuring marked peripheral eosinophilia.
- Clinical presentation is variable, and pulmonary involvement is seen in approximately half of cases.
- CT findings include pulmonary nodules with ground-glass halos, interlobular septal thickening, and consolidation and ground-glass opacities.
- Greatest morbidity and mortality is associated with cardiac involvement.

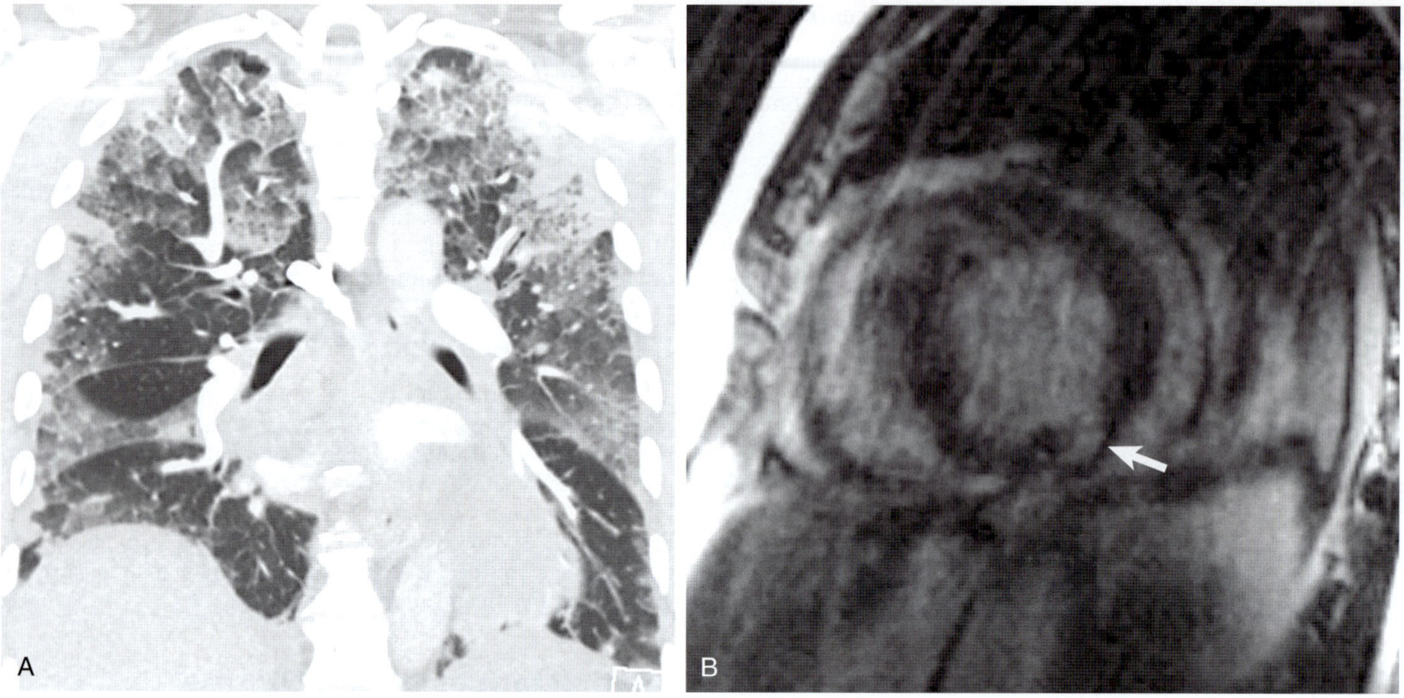

Fig. 37.10 Hypereosinophilic syndrome. (A) Coronal CT image of a 70-year-old man demonstrates upper lobe and peripheral predominant ground-glass opacities and interlobular septal thickening. The patient was admitted with dyspnea and cough and found to have myocarditis and cardiogenic shock. He had marked peripheral eosinophilia, and bronchoalveolar lavage showed 44% eosinophils. (B) Postcontrast short-axis cardiac MRI shows late gadolinium enhancement in the basal inferolateral wall *(arrow)* of the left ventricle.

SUGGESTED READINGS

Bernheim A, McLoud T. A review of clinical and imaging findings in eosinophilic lung diseases. *AJR Am J Roentgenol.* 2017;208(5):1002–1010.

Cottin V. Eosinophilic lung diseases. *Clin Chest Med.* 2016;37(3):535–556.

Curtis C, Ogbogu P. Hypereosinophilic syndrome. *Clin Rev Allergy Immunol.* 2016;50(2):240–251.

Price M, Gilman MD, Carter BW, Sabloff BS, Truong MT, Wu CC. Imaging of eosinophilic lung diseases. *Radiol Clin North Am.* 2016;54(6):1151–1164.

Rose DM, Hrncir DE. Primary eosinophilic lung diseases. *Allergy Asthma Proc.* 2013;34(1):19–25.

The full reference list for this chapter is available at ExpertConsult.com.

38 Metabolic and Storage Lung Diseases*

CHRISTOPHER M. WALKER | JONATHAN H. CHUNG

Metabolic and storage lung diseases are a broad group of diseases and syndromes characterized by underlying biochemical or metabolic dysfunctions. Accurate diagnosis is difficult because these diseases are often indolent, are rarely encountered in clinical practice, and because their manifestations are often vague and nonspecific. These groups of disorders may affect the lung solely or as part of a systemic disorder.

Metabolic Pulmonary Diseases

Pulmonary Alveolar Proteinosis

ETIOLOGY

Pulmonary alveolar proteinosis (alveolar lipoproteinosis) is a rare disease characterized by the accumulation of protein- and lipid-rich material resembling surfactant within the parenchymal airspaces.[1] Three distinct subtypes of the disease are recognized: autoimmune or acquired, secondary, and genetic. More than 90% of cases are acquired and likely of autoimmune etiology related to a mutation in the surfactant gene or the presence of an antibody to granulocyte-macrophage colony-stimulating factor. These mutations and antibodies result in the defective clearance of surfactant by alveolar macrophages, as well as impaired function of lung neutrophils.[1–3] Less commonly, pulmonary alveolar proteinosis is secondary, occurring in association with conditions that result in functional impairment or reduced numbers of alveolar macrophages, as may occur in inorganic dust inhalation, particularly acute silicosis; immunodeficiency syndromes, such as acquired immunodeficiency syndrome or immunoglobulin deficiency; and hematologic malignant neoplasms, such as acute myelogenous leukemia.[1,4] Rarely, it may be congenital and rapidly fatal.[2]

PREVALENCE AND EPIDEMIOLOGY

The prevalence of pulmonary alveolar proteinosis has been estimated to be approximately 4 per million persons.[2] Pulmonary alveolar proteinosis occurs predominantly in patients between the ages of 20 and 50 years and has a male-to-female preponderance of about 2.5 : 1.[1] About 70% of patients are smokers.

CLINICAL PRESENTATION

Patients may be asymptomatic in up to a third of all cases.[3] The most frequent symptom is shortness of breath on exertion that is usually slowly progressive. Cough, usually nonproductive, is also common. A low-grade fever develops or is evident at initial evaluation in some patients and should suggest concomitant infection. Clubbing of the fingers has been identified in about a third of patients.[5]

PATHOPHYSIOLOGY

On histologic examination the alveoli can be seen to be filled with finely granular, lipoproteinaceous material that stains eosinophilic with hematoxylin and eosin and purple with periodic acid–Schiff (Fig. 38.1). The alveolar architecture is usually preserved, but septal thickening may be due to edema, dilated lymphatics, or lymphocytic infiltration.[5] Ultrastructural examination by transmission electron microscopy shows the intraalveolar material to consist of amorphous granular debris containing numerous relatively discrete osmiophilic granules or lamellar bodies. These structures represent phospholipids and are identical to inclusions found in normal type II pneumocytes.[5]

Pulmonary function test results may be normal or show a restrictive ventilatory defect with reduction in vital capacity and total lung capacity and a disproportionately severe decrease in the carbon monoxide diffusing capacity (DLCO).[4] Extensive disease may result in hypoxemia and increased alveolar-arterial pressure gradient (PAO_2-PaO_2), which increases further with exercise.[5]

MANIFESTATIONS OF THE DISEASE

Radiography

The characteristic radiographic pattern of pulmonary alveolar proteinosis consists of bilateral, symmetric patchy areas of consolidation that have a vaguely nodular appearance.[1,5] In up to 50% of cases, the consolidation is perihilar (bat wing or butterfly distribution; Fig. 38.2); in the remaining cases, it is random or has a predominantly peripheral or basal distribution (Fig. 38.3). In up to 84% of cases, there is regional sparing, most commonly the lung apices, costophrenic sulci, or lung periphery.[2] Characteristically, patients may have extensive consolidation and relatively mild respiratory symptoms ("clinicoradiologic discrepancy").[5] In patients who have less severe disease, the appearance may be one of ground-glass opacities.[6] Frequently, the parenchymal involvement is asymmetric or rarely unilateral.[2,7] In some patients a linear interstitial pattern can be seen superimposed on consolidation or ground-glass opacities.

High-Resolution Computed Tomography

High-resolution computed tomography (HRCT) is superior to chest radiography in assessment of the pattern and distribution of abnormalities and may show lesions even when radiography is normal.[7,8] The predominant abnormality typically consists of bilateral ground-glass opacities, although consolidation may also be present, particularly in the dorsal lung regions.[8,9] The

*The editors and the publisher would like to thank Drs. Nestor L. Müller and C. Isabela Silva Müller for contributing material on this topic to the prior edition of this work. It has served as the foundation for the current chapter.

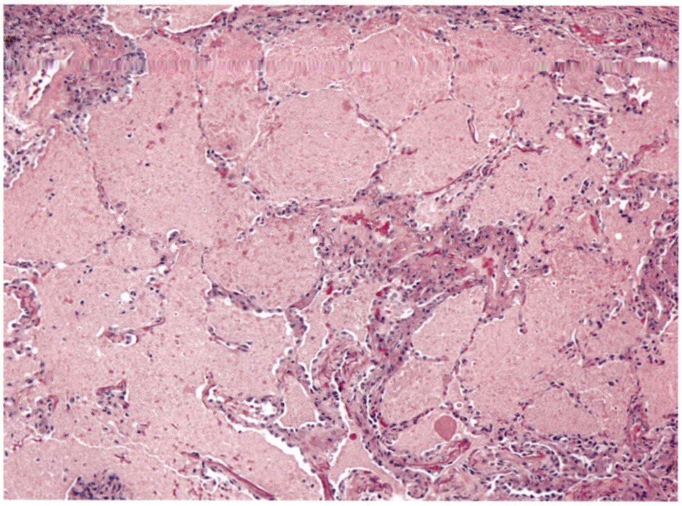

Fig. 38.1 Pulmonary alveolar proteinosis. Histologic specimen shows filling of the alveolar airspaces with a granular eosinophilic proteinaceous material. *(Courtesy Dr. John English, Department of Pathology, Vancouver General Hospital, Vancouver, Canada.)*

ground-glass opacities tend to involve all lung zones to a similar extent but can have a predominant lower zone distribution. In about 75% of cases in one series, a fine linear pattern forming polygonal shapes, measuring 3 to 10 mm in diameter, can be seen superimposed on the ground-glass opacities ("crazy paving" pattern; see Figs. 38.2 and 38.3).[2,9,10] The pattern reflects the presence of interstitial edema or the accumulation of lipoproteinaceous material in the airspaces adjacent to the interlobular septa.[10,11] There is typically sharp demarcation between normal and abnormal parenchyma. Pleural effusions and lymphadenopathy are always absent and should raise suspicion for an alternative diagnosis, secondary pulmonary alveolar proteinosis, or the possibility of coexistent infection.[2] The radiologic manifestations of secondary pulmonary alveolar proteinosis are often similar to those of the more common idiopathic form (Fig. 38.4). However, some subtypes, such as silicoproteinosis, may manifest with dependent consolidation, often containing foci of calcification, as well as diffuse solid centrilobular nodules and patchy ground-glass opacities. Affected patients also have calcified mediastinal and hilar lymph nodes, and the "crazy paving" pattern is usually absent.[12,13]

In reviewing the radiographic and CT images in a patient with known pulmonary alveolar proteinosis, it is important also to look for complications. The main complication is infection, including community-acquired pneumonia and infection caused by unusual organisms such as *Nocardia, Aspergillus,* and *Pneumocystis.*[1] The increased susceptibility to pulmonary infection may be due to impaired macrophage and neutrophil function, as well as the presence of intraalveolar lipoproteinaceous fluid that may facilitate the growth of microorganisms.[1] The prevalence of opportunistic infections has decreased considerably since the use of bronchoalveolar lavage (BAL) for the treatment of these patients.[1]

Interstitial fibrosis occasionally develops in patients with pulmonary alveolar proteinosis manifesting as airway irregularity and fissural displacement (Fig. 38.5).[2,14,15] Other rare complications include the development of emphysematous bullae and pneumothorax.[1] Pulmonary alveolar proteinosis has been shown to demonstrate increased fluorodeoxyglucose uptake, which is thought to be related to glucose use by the inflammatory components.[16]

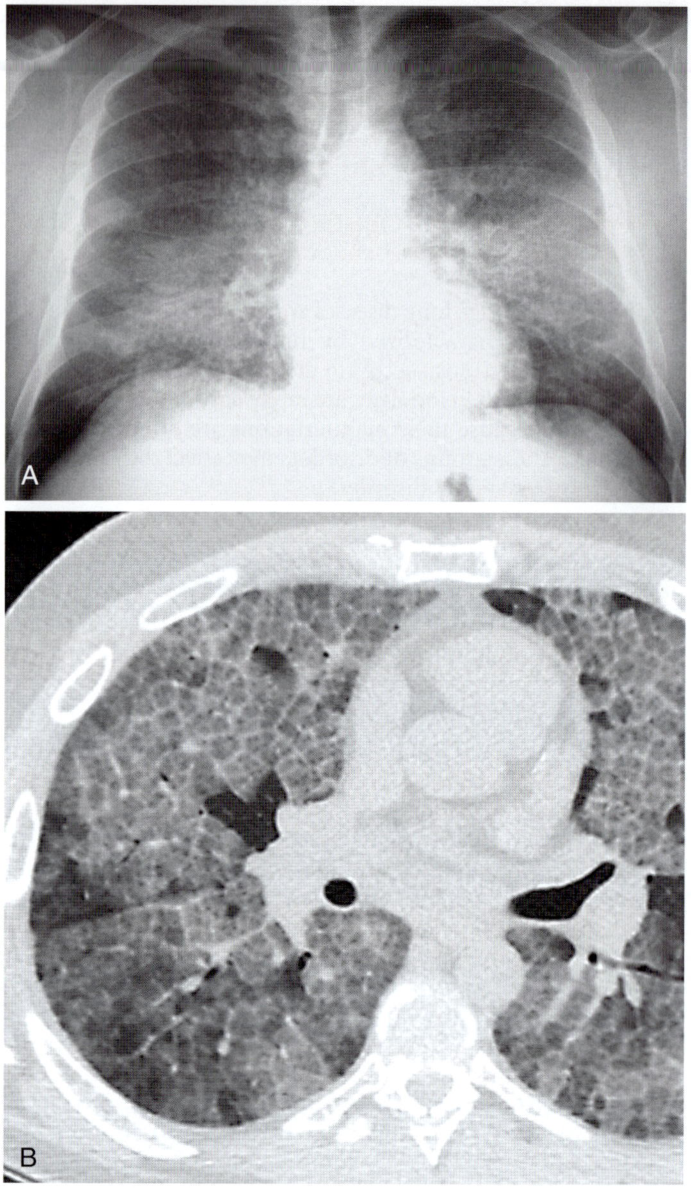

Fig. 38.2 Pulmonary alveolar proteinosis: imaging findings. (A) Posteroanterior chest radiograph shows airspace consolidation and ground-glass opacities mainly in the perihilar regions (butterfly pattern) with sparing of the peripheral regions. Note vaguely nodular appearance. (B) High-resolution CT demonstrates extensive bilateral ground-glass opacities and a superimposed fine linear pattern forming polygonal arcades ("crazy paving" pattern). Note sharp demarcation of normal lung from abnormal lung.

DIFFERENTIAL DIAGNOSIS

The findings on the chest radiograph mimic those of pneumonia, pulmonary edema, and hemorrhage, but unlike those other conditions, a patient with pulmonary alveolar proteinosis is much less symptomatic than the radiographic appearance would suggest. The diagnosis of pulmonary alveolar proteinosis can often be suggested by the characteristic manifestations on HRCT. However, although it is characteristic of pulmonary alveolar proteinosis,

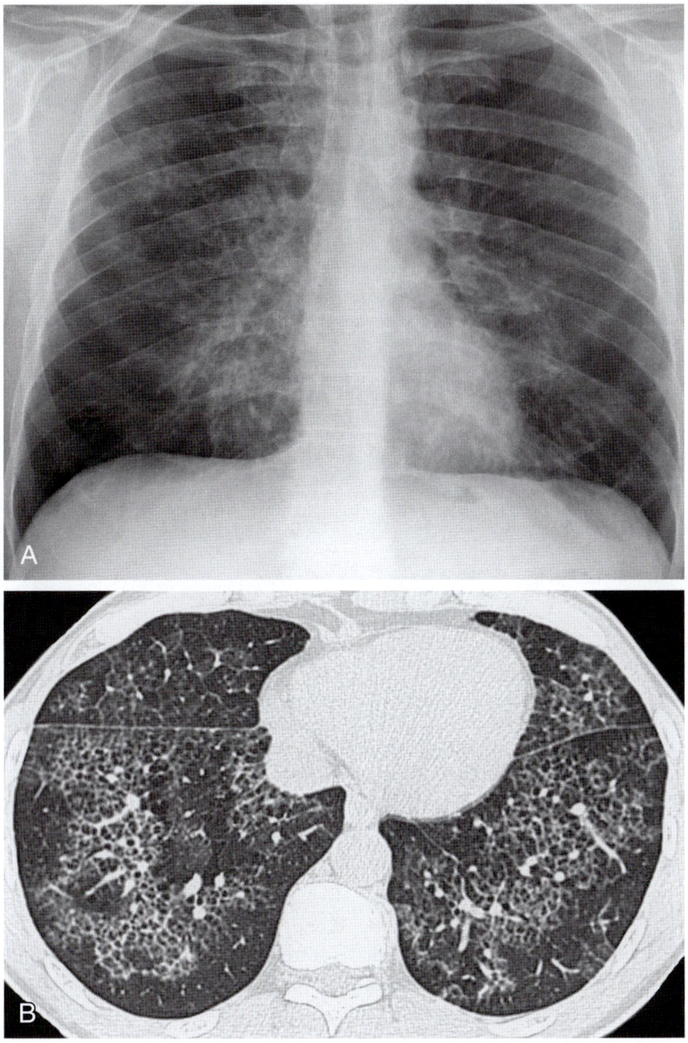

Fig. 38.3 Pulmonary alveolar proteinosis: imaging findings. (A) Posteroanterior chest radiograph shows asymmetric hazy areas of increased opacity (ground-glass opacities) and faint reticulonodular pattern in the right middle and bilateral lower lung zones. (B) High-resolution CT shows bilateral ground-glass opacities and superimposed fine linear pattern forming polygonal arcades ("crazy paving" pattern). Note the sharp demarcation between normal and abnormal parenchyma, a feature that usually reflects lobular boundaries. Also note the presence of mild emphysema.

the "crazy paving" pattern can also be seen in a variety of other conditions, including primary lung or metastatic adenocarcinoma, lipoid pneumonia, pulmonary hemorrhage or edema, and infections, including bacterial or *Pneumocystis* pneumonia.[17] The diagnosis of pulmonary alveolar proteinosis can usually be confirmed by examination of BAL.[5] Characteristic features of pulmonary alveolar proteinosis include milky BAL fluid; relatively few inflammatory cells, including alveolar macrophages; large acellular eosinophilic bodies in a diffuse background of granular basophilic material; periodic acid–Schiff staining of the proteinaceous material; elevated levels of surfactant proteins; and characteristic ultrastructural features with abundant lamellar bodies and cellular debris. The main constituent of the BAL fluid in pulmonary alveolar proteinosis is phospholipid, mainly lecithin, the main component of surfactant.[5] If it is deemed necessary to confirm the diagnosis by tissue examination, transbronchial biopsy is likely to be sufficient.

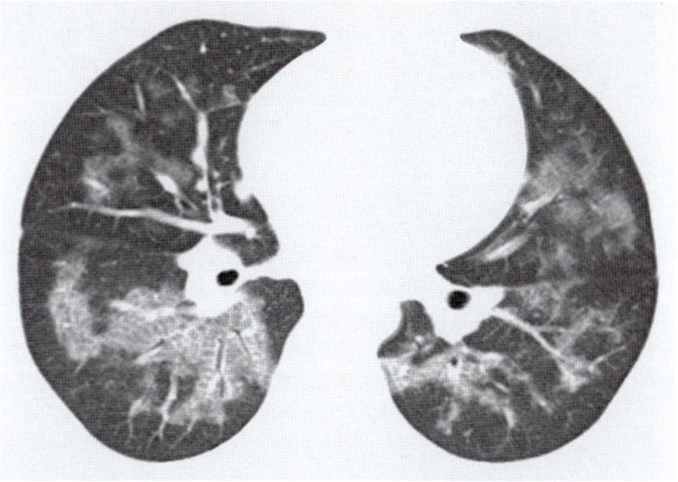

Fig. 38.4 Secondary pulmonary alveolar proteinosis in an 11-year-old girl undergoing immunosuppressive therapy for aplastic anemia. High-resolution CT shows bilateral ground-glass opacities with sparing of the peripheral lung. Mild superimposed linear opacities ("crazy paving" pattern) are present in the lower lobes.

SYNOPSIS OF TREATMENT OPTIONS

Treatment of acquired pulmonary alveolar proteinosis is with unilateral or bilateral whole-lung lavage. Some patients require only one or two procedures, whereas a few require that lavage be repeated semiannually or annually. The overall prognosis for alveolar proteinosis treated by whole-lung lavage is excellent. Corticosteroids should not be used as empirical treatment of alveolar proteinosis because of its potential to exacerbate opportunistic infections.[1] Spontaneous resolution without treatment may occur in up to 25% of patients.[5] On occasion, patients may not respond to BAL and may require lung transplantation or experimental therapy with granulocyte-macrophage colony-stimulating factor or rituximab.[3] As might be expected in view of the pathogenesis, recurrence of the condition has been documented after lung transplantation.[18]

Therapy for secondary pulmonary alveolar proteinosis is aimed at treatment of the underlying condition. For example, in patients with pulmonary alveolar proteinosis secondary to hematologic malignant disease, the pulmonary findings improve or resolve after successful chemotherapy or bone marrow transplantation.[4]

KEY POINTS: PULMONARY ALVEOLAR PROTEINOSIS

- It is a rare disease, usually of autoimmune etiology.
- Lipoproteinaceous material (surfactant) fills the airspaces.
- Imaging findings:
  - Ground-glass opacities or consolidation.
  - Perihilar, peripheral, or random distribution.
  - High-resolution CT usually shows a characteristic pattern of smooth interlobular septal thickening and intralobular lines superimposed on ground-glass opacities ("crazy paving" pattern).
  - Abnormal lung is sharply demarcated from normal lung.
  - Pleural effusion or lymphadenopathy is rare and should suggest an alternative diagnosis—secondary pulmonary alveolar proteinosis or coexistent infection.
- Bronchoalveolar lavage is usually diagnostic.

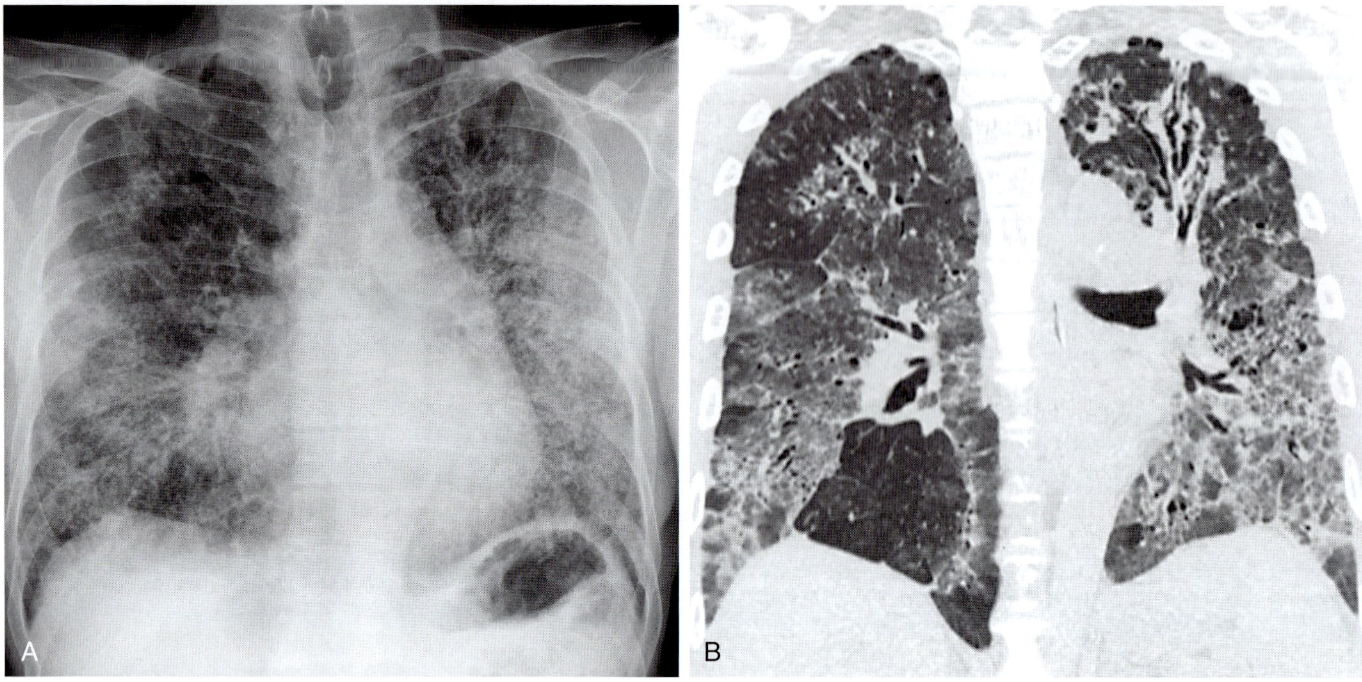

Fig. 38.5 Pulmonary alveolar proteinosis with fibrosis. (A) Posteroanterior chest radiograph shows patchy bilateral opacities with reticulation. (B) Coronal CT shows asymmetric ground-glass opacities with interlobular septal thickening and intralobular lines ("crazy paving" pattern). Note traction bronchiectasis and traction bronchiolectasis, as well as bilateral major fissure distortion indicating a component of lung fibrosis. As is typically seen, there are several areas of lung that are relatively spared, best visualized in the right lower lobe.

Amyloidosis

ETIOLOGY

Amyloidosis is a generic term for a heterogeneous group of disorders characterized by accumulation of various insoluble fibrillar proteins (amyloid).[19,20] The abnormal proteins are deposited in the extracellular space and cause disease by compression of the adjacent cells and tissues. Amyloidosis can be hereditary or acquired, localized, or systemic.

PREVALENCE AND EPIDEMIOLOGY

Amyloidosis is rare. It affects the respiratory tract in about 50% of cases.[21] Amyloid may involve the trachea, bronchi, mediastinum, pleura, heart, or, more commonly, the lung parenchyma.[22]

CLINICAL PRESENTATION

Tracheobronchial amyloidosis typically manifests after the fifth decade with dyspnea, cough, and occasionally hemoptysis.[19] Less commonly, it causes symptoms that simulate asthma. Discrete tracheal and endobronchial nodules are usually asymptomatic but occasionally may result in airway obstruction with distal atelectasis or bronchiectasis. Symptoms and signs in such cases depend on the volume of lung affected and whether infection is present. The presence of amyloid in other sites is rare.[23]

The nodular parenchymal form of amyloidosis usually is asymptomatic and is discovered incidentally on the chest radiograph.[24] The majority of patients have no evidence of extrathoracic disease (either amyloidosis or otherwise).

Diffuse interstitial amyloidosis frequently results in progressive dyspnea and respiratory insufficiency.[24] Diffuse involvement is most often seen as part of multisystem disease (primary amyloidosis), in which amyloid type L is typically present and may be associated with multiple myeloma.[25]

PATHOPHYSIOLOGY

Amyloidosis is a disorder of protein folding rather than of amino-acid sequence, and amyloid deposits consist mainly of protein fibrils.[19] Amyloid is not a single substance but consists of several proteins, each of which resembles the others morphologically but is distinctive biochemically.[26] The most important proteins associated with respiratory tract disease are amyloid L and amyloid A. Amyloid L is derived from immunoglobulin light chains and is therefore usually associated with abnormal plasma cell function, either as part of a systemic disease, such as multiple myeloma or macroglobulinemia, or, more commonly, localized to the lungs without evidence of systemic disease. Amyloid A is derived from a serum acute-phase reactant synthesized in the liver that can be formed in several chronic inflammatory diseases, including connective tissue disease, particularly rheumatoid arthritis; chronic infection, particularly tuberculosis; bronchiectasis; and certain neoplasms, such as Hodgkin disease.[19] The majority of cases of respiratory tract amyloidosis are amyloid type L; the main exceptions are in patients with chronic inflammatory disease or a family history of amyloidosis.[19] On histologic examination, amyloidosis is characterized by the presence of amorphous, eosinophilic, extracellular material that shows a characteristic apple-green birefringence when it is

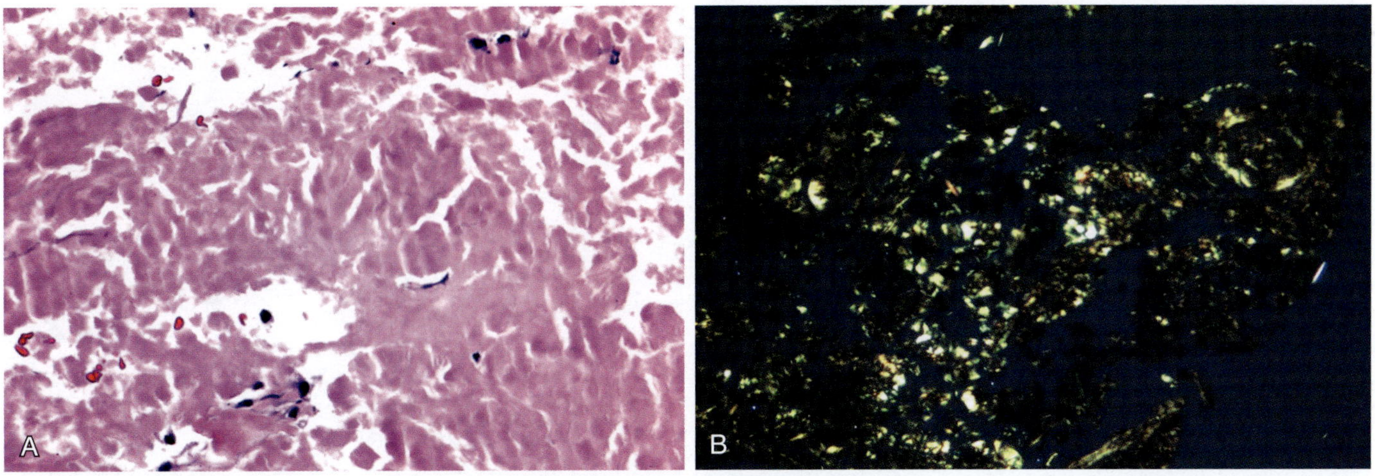

Fig. 38.6 Amyloidosis. (A) Histologic specimen shows extracellular amorphous eosinophilic material. (B) Specimen stained with Congo red and examined with polarizing microscopy shows characteristic apple-green birefringence.

stained with Congo red and examined by polarizing microscopy (Fig. 38.6).[20]

There are three major forms of amyloidosis in the lower respiratory tract: tracheobronchial, nodular parenchymal, and diffuse parenchymal (alveolar septal, interstitial).[27] Although these forms can occur in combination, in many cases the amyloid is deposited predominantly at one site. In addition to airway and pulmonary parenchymal disease, amyloidosis can also affect the hilar and mediastinal lymph nodes, pulmonary arteries, pleura, heart, and diaphragm.[27]

Airway involvement occurs most commonly in the trachea and proximal bronchi. Although overlap does occur, it is usually manifested in one of two ways: a localized nodule or, more commonly, multiple discrete or confluent intramural plaques that distort the airway wall and cause stenosis of its lumen.[27] On histologic examination the amyloid is situated in the subepithelial interstitial tissue and often surrounds tracheobronchial gland ducts and acini.[27]

The parenchymal nodules of localized pulmonary amyloid can be solitary or multiple and are usually fairly well defined. Amyloid is often identifiable in the alveolar interstitium at the periphery of the nodule; however, in the central region the normal parenchymal architecture is generally obscured by a more or less solid mass of amyloid that typically contains fairly numerous multinucleated giant cells and variable numbers of lymphocytes and plasma cells.[27] Calcification and ossification are relatively common. The nodular parenchymal form of amyloidosis is usually of amyloid type L and localized to the lung. It is the most common respiratory form of amyloidosis. In one series of 48 patients with localized respiratory tract amyloidosis, 34 had parenchymal deposits, of which 28 cases were nodular and 6 were diffuse alveolar septal.[24]

Diffuse interstitial (alveolar septal) amyloidosis involves the parenchymal interstitium and the media of small blood vessels. The amyloid deposition is typically adjacent to endothelial and epithelial basement membranes and can appear in a uniform and more or less linear pattern or as multiple small nodules.[27]

Lung Function

Pulmonary function tests may show evidence of restriction and impaired gas transfer in patients who have diffuse alveolar septal amyloidosis and air-trapping and fixed upper airway obstruction in those who have proximal tracheobronchial involvement.[27]

MANIFESTATIONS OF THE DISEASE

Radiography

In the majority of patients with tracheobronchial amyloidosis, the chest radiograph is normal. When present, the findings include focal or diffuse thickening of the airway wall with associated narrowing of the airway lumen (Fig. 38.7).[25] The findings are often difficult to see on the radiograph.

Nodular primary parenchymal amyloidosis manifests as solitary or, less commonly, multiple nodules usually ranging from 0.5 to 15 cm in diameter.[25] The nodules occur most commonly in the lower lobes and are usually peripheral. Disease may progress slowly during a period of several years, with a slight increase in size of the nodules and the development of additional nodules.

Diffuse interstitial (alveolar septal) amyloidosis results in a reticular, nodular, or reticulonodular pattern that may be diffuse or involve mainly the lower lobes.[25]

Pleural effusions may occur in amyloidosis but are usually due to heart failure caused by cardiac involvement.[21] Pleural amyloid deposits are rare.

Computed Tomography

The CT manifestations of tracheobronchial amyloidosis consist of thickening of the airway wall, narrowing of the lumen, and, in some cases, foci of calcification (Fig. 38.8; see Fig. 38.7).[28,29] The airway wall thickening may be focal or diffuse and nodular, plaque-like, or circumferential; it is generally confined to the trachea but can extend to the main, lobar, and segmental bronchi.[25,29] Bronchial involvement is frequently associated with distal atelectasis, bronchiectasis, or air-trapping.[21]

Nodular primary parenchymal amyloidosis manifests as solitary or, less commonly, multiple nodules usually ranging from 0.5 to 5 cm in diameter (Fig. 38.9).[30] On occasion, nodular parenchymal amyloidosis may result in a large mass (Fig. 38.10). Calcification is seldom evident on radiographs but is seen in 20% to 50% of nodules on CT.[30,31] The nodules tend to be more common in the periphery of the lower lobes but may be seen anywhere in the parenchyma (see Fig. 38.9). Rarely, nodules will

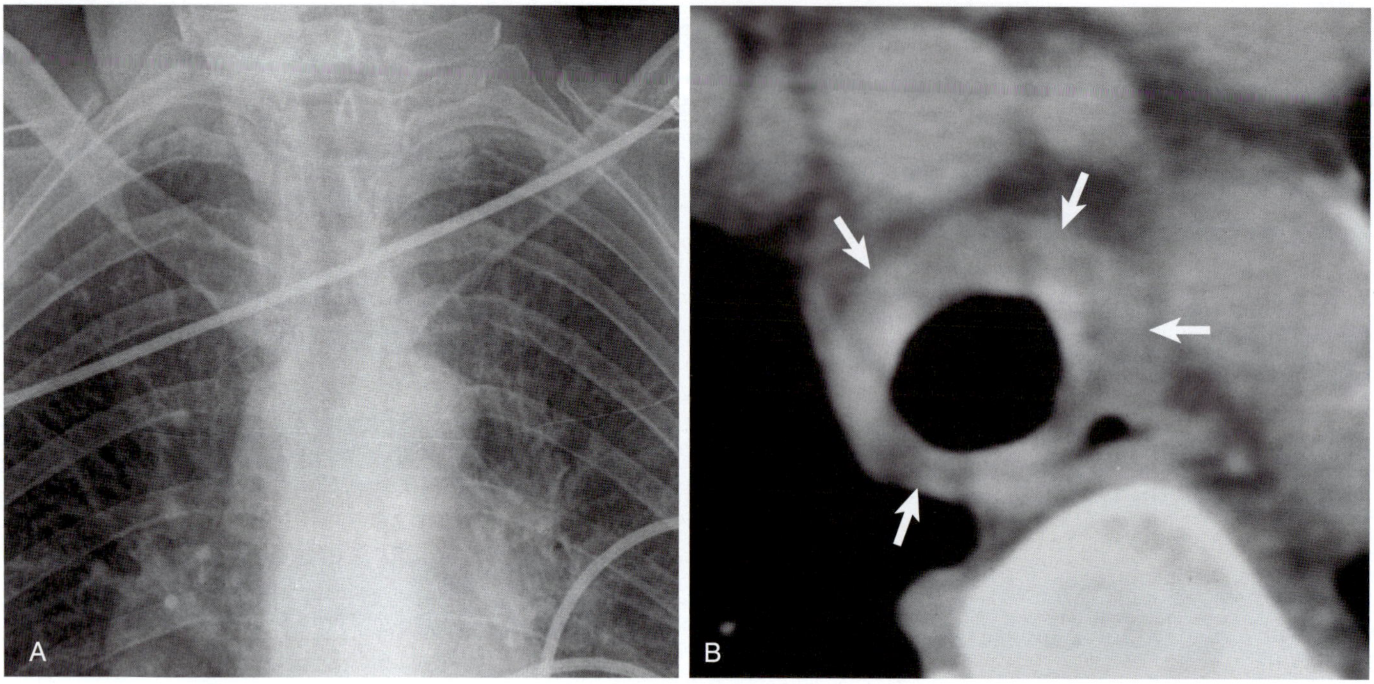

Fig. 38.7 Diffuse tracheal amyloidosis. (A) Magnified view from a chest radiograph shows narrowing of the mid trachea. (B) Axial CT from a different patient immediately above the level of the aortic arch shows marked circumferential thickening of the trachea *(arrows)*. On CT and at bronchoscopy, the entire trachea was abnormal. *(B from Müller NL, Fraser RS, Colman NC, Paré PD.* Radiologic Diagnosis of Diseases of the Chest. *Philadelphia: WB Saunders; 2001.)*

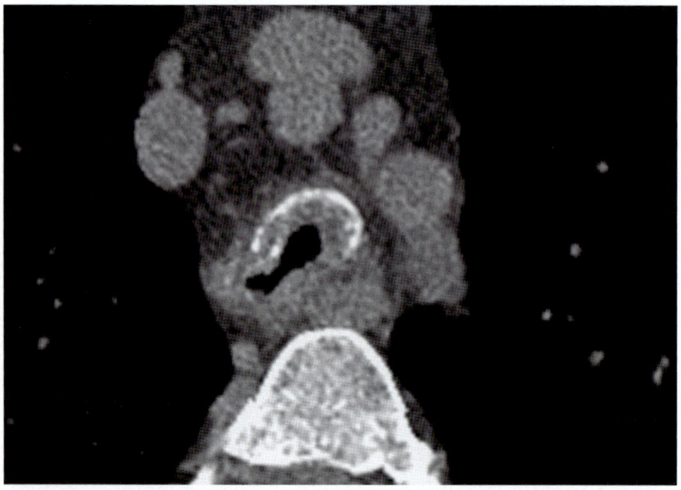

Fig. 38.8 Diffuse tracheobronchial amyloidosis. Magnified view of the trachea shows circumferential thickening and foci of calcification.

cavitate.[22] Cysts may occasionally be present adjacent to the nodules. Cysts and nodular amyloid deposits have been described most commonly in patients with Sjögren syndrome, with or without associated lymphoid interstitial pneumonia (Fig. 38.11).[32]

The HRCT findings of diffuse interstitial amyloidosis consist mainly of reticular opacities and interlobular septal thickening.[21,30] Multiple subpleural micronodules can often be seen in association with the reticular opacities. Less common HRCT findings include ground-glass opacities, consolidation, traction bronchiectasis, and honeycombing.[30] Punctate calcification may be seen in some of the nodules and areas of consolidation.

Mediastinal and hilar lymphadenopathy is rare in localized disease but occurs in approximately 75% of patients with amyloid L-type systemic amyloidosis (Fig. 38.12). It is seen most commonly with diffuse interstitial amyloidosis.[25]

DIFFERENTIAL DIAGNOSIS

The radiologic and CT findings are relatively nonspecific. The differential diagnosis of tracheal wall thickening includes relapsing polychondritis, tracheobronchopathia osteochondroplastica (TBO), granulomatosis with polyangiitis (formerly Wegener granulomatosis), inflammatory bowel disease, and adenoid cystic carcinoma. Unlike amyloidosis, both relapsing polychondritis and TBO typically spare the noncartilaginous posterior membrane.[33] The main differential diagnosis of the parenchymal nodular form of amyloidosis is granulomatous infection or primary or metastatic tumors. The differential diagnosis of the diffuse interstitial form includes a large number of interstitial and airspace lung diseases, such as nonspecific interstitial pneumonia, usual interstitial pneumonia, and primary lung and metastatic adenocarcinoma. The diagnosis of amyloidosis usually requires histologic confirmation by needle, bronchial, transbronchial, or surgical biopsy. The diagnosis is based on demonstration of amyloid by Congo red staining, which produces characteristic apple-green birefringence under crossed polarized light.[27]

SYNOPSIS OF TREATMENT OPTIONS

The treatment of symptomatic tracheobronchial amyloidosis may involve intermittent bronchoscopic resection, surgical resection, or laser ablation.[19] Repeated bronchoscopic intervention is considered preferable to surgical resection, but recurrence is

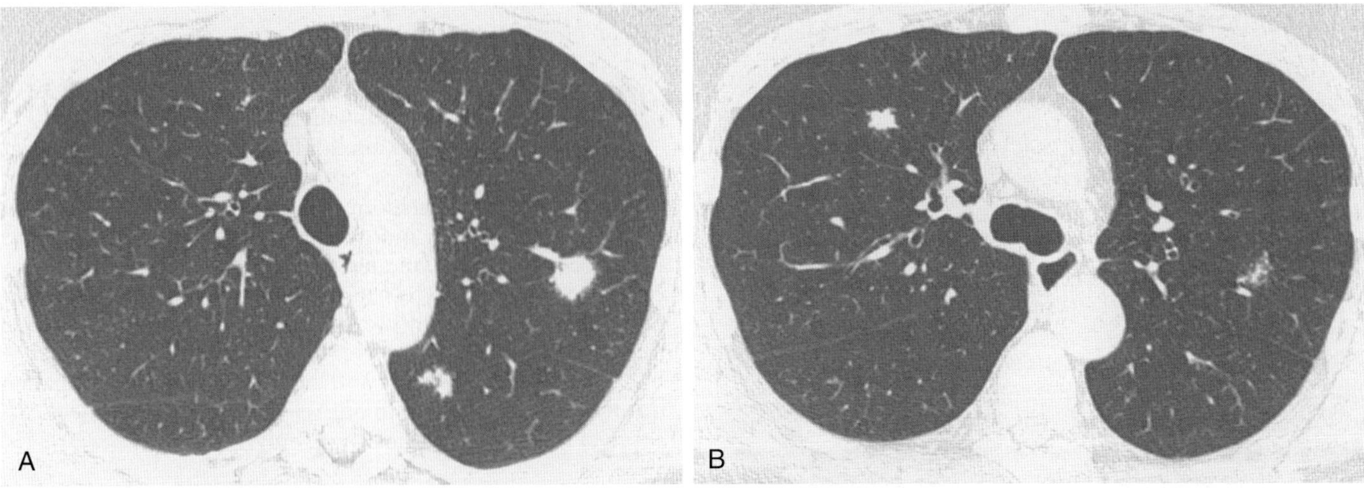

Fig. 38.9 Nodular parenchymal amyloidosis proven at surgical resection. High-resolution CT images at the level of the aortic arch (A) and tracheal carina (B) show bilateral nodules with spiculated margins.

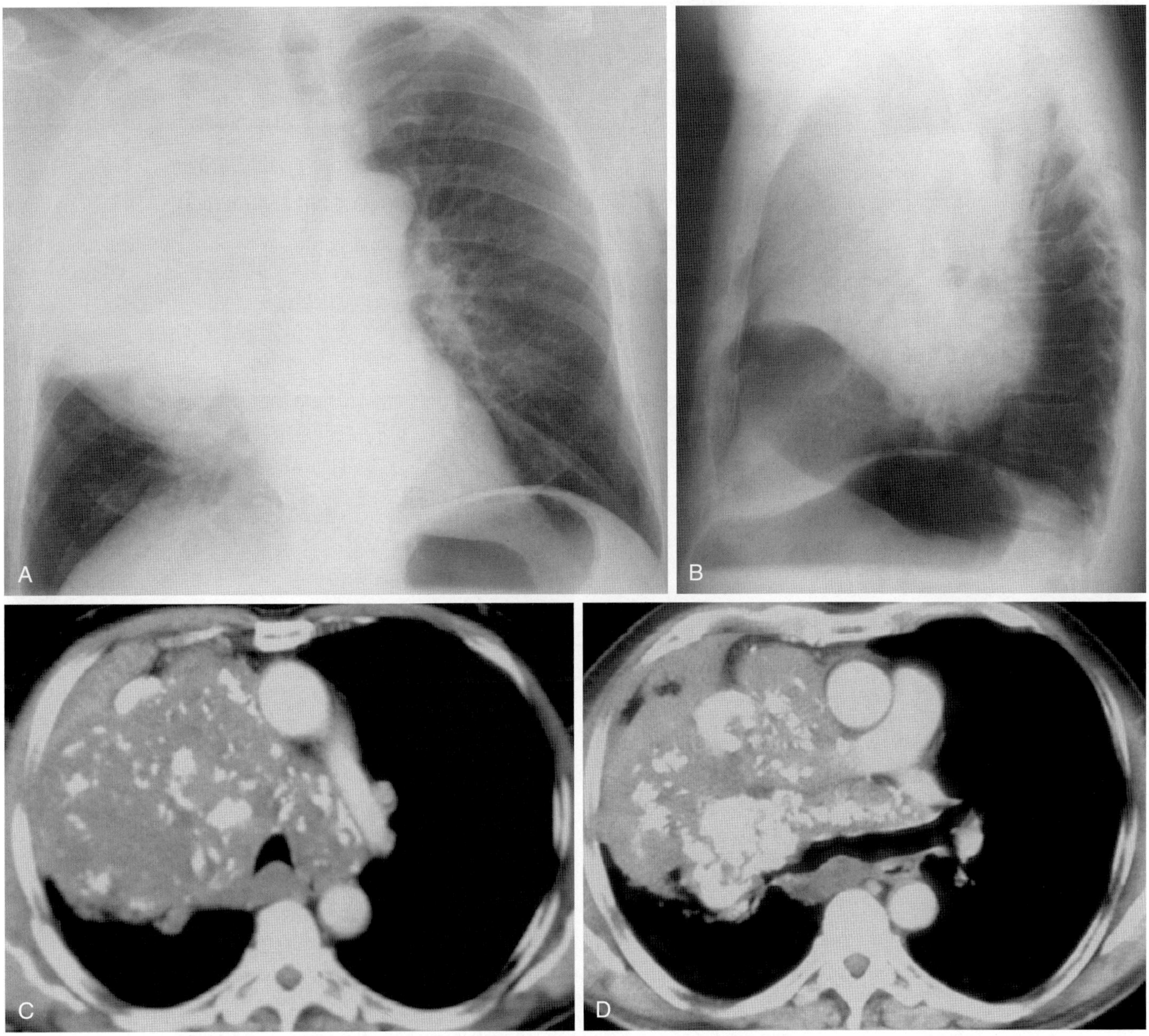

Fig. 38.10 Nodular parenchymal amyloidosis. Posteroanterior (A) and lateral (B) chest radiographs show a homogeneous mass occupying most of the right hemithorax. CT at the level of the lower trachea (C) and left main bronchi (D) show a large right upper and middle lobe mass with numerous coarse foci of calcification. The mass extends into the mediastinum, is associated with calcified mediastinal lymph nodes, and compresses the trachea and right bronchi.

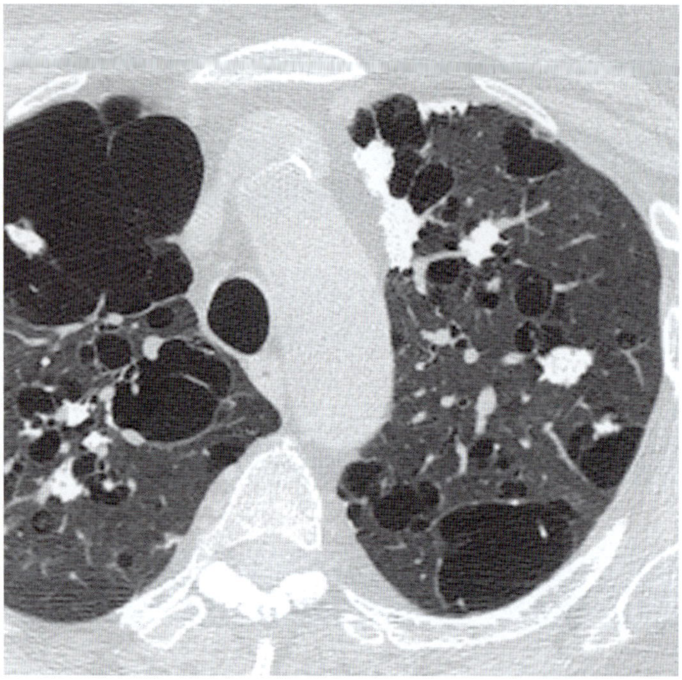

Fig. 38.11 Nodular parenchymal amyloidosis with lymphoid interstitial pneumonia in a patient with Sjögren syndrome. Axial CT shows calcified nodules and cysts throughout both lungs. Pulmonary cysts associated with amyloidosis are most commonly seen in patients with Sjögren syndrome and may be secondary to coexistent lymphoid interstitial pneumonia or amyloidosis itself.

common.[19] Stenting may have a role in the treatment of airway narrowing and complications thereof.

Nodular parenchymal amyloidosis is usually asymptomatic and remains stationary or progresses slowly. It usually has a good prognosis and seldom requires treatment. By contrast, diffuse interstitial amyloidosis frequently progresses. Treatment includes oral melphalan and prednisolone or peripheral stem cell transplantation.[19] The natural history and prognosis of disease in patients who have diffuse interstitial pulmonary involvement may be determined by the presence of amyloid elsewhere in the body, particularly the heart and kidneys; however, many patients die of respiratory failure. In one series of 35 patients, the median survival time after diagnosis was only 16 months.[25]

Pulmonary Alveolar Microlithiasis

ETIOLOGY

Pulmonary alveolar microlithiasis is a rare disease characterized by innumerable tiny calculi (microliths) within alveolar airspaces.[34] Although it can occur at any age, most reported cases have been in patients between the ages of 20 and 50 years.[35] The disorder is autosomal recessive and is caused by a mutation in the *SLC34A2* gene.[36]

PREVALENCE AND EPIDEMIOLOGY

Alveolar microlithiasis is rare. A total of 500 to 800 cases had been published in the literature before 2016.[36,37] Approximately

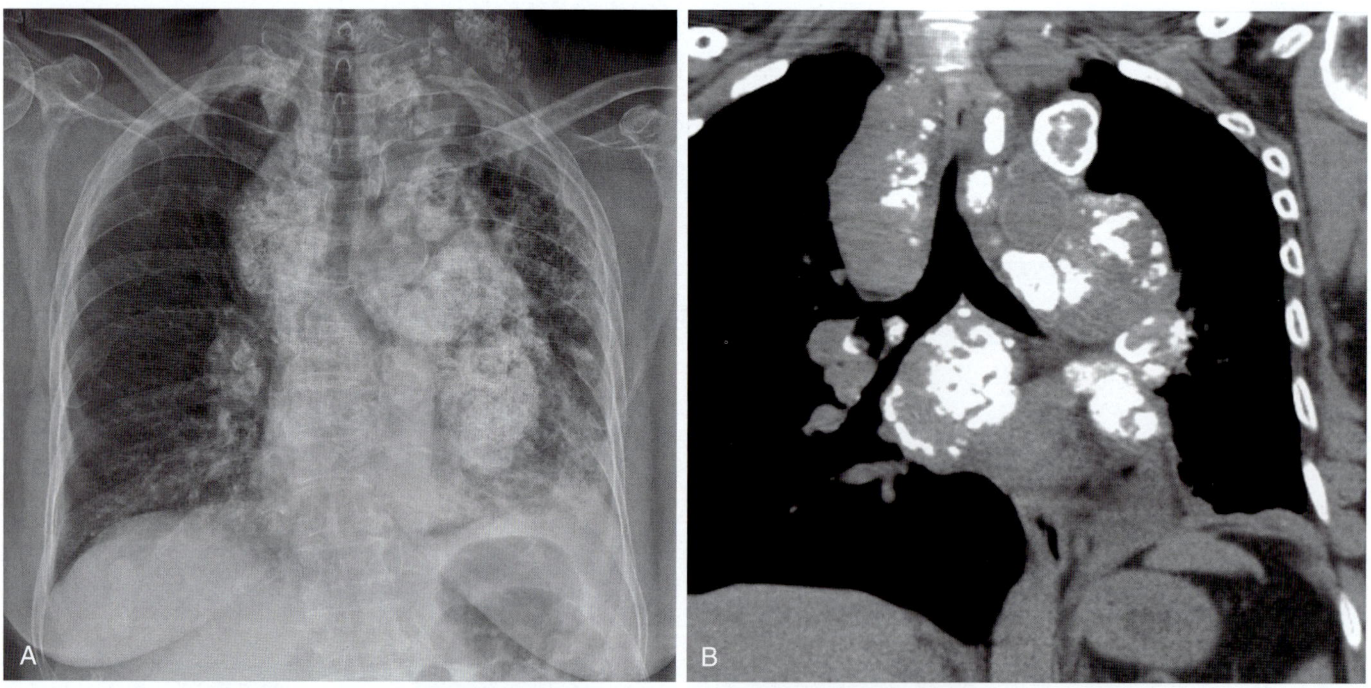

Fig. 38.12 Calcified lymph nodes with lung fibrosis from systemic (light-chain) AL amyloidosis associated with monoclonal gammopathy of undetermined significance. (A) Posteroanterior chest radiograph shows enlarged mediastinal and left neck calcified lymph nodes. Note left lung volume loss with fibrosis secondary to long-standing left pulmonary artery and left main bronchus compression. (B) Coronal noncontrast CT shows massive partially calcified mediastinal and hilar lymphadenopathy, which causes occlusion of the distal left main bronchus.

KEY POINTS: AMYLOIDOSIS

- Abnormal protein is deposited in extracellular tissues.
- Amyloidosis is a disorder of protein folding rather than of amino-acid sequence.
- The three main manifestations are tracheobronchial, parenchymal nodular, and diffuse interstitial.
- Tracheobronchial amyloidosis
  - Clinical symptoms: dyspnea and cough; focal or diffuse thickening of the trachea or central bronchi that involves the posterior membrane
  - Foci of calcification common
  - Atelectasis and obstructive pneumonitis
- Nodular parenchymal amyloidosis
  - Usually asymptomatic
  - Single or multiple nodules or masses
  - Mainly lower lobe and peripheral location
  - Foci of calcification common
- Diffuse interstitial amyloidosis
  - Clinical symptoms: progressive shortness of breath, dry cough
  - Reticular pattern
  - Ground-glass opacities on high-resolution CT (HRCT)
  - Interlobular septal thickening on HRCT
  - May be associated with lymphadenopathy and cardiac involvement

43% of cases came from Europe and 41% from Asia; the remaining cases were from the United States and other countries. The disease does not have any preference for specific races, and the incidence is similar in both sexes.[35] However, it has been described in premature twins.[35] Family history for the disease is found in one-third of the patients and is often associated with consanguineous marriage.[34,36,37]

CLINICAL PRESENTATION

There is typically dissociation between the radiologic findings, which can be striking and extensive, and the clinical manifestations, which are usually mild. More than 50% of patients are asymptomatic when the disease is first discovered, the diagnosis being made on the basis of the typical pattern seen on a chest radiograph.[37] The most common symptom is dyspnea on exertion; cough develops occasionally. The disease can remain stable for many years or progress slowly. As the disease progresses, respiratory insufficiency may develop in association with cyanosis, clubbing of the fingers, and evidence of pulmonary hypertension.[38]

PATHOPHYSIOLOGY

The pathogenesis of microlithiasis is related to a defective phosphate transporter that is important for type II pneumocytes, which results in the formation of calcium phosphate microliths in the alveolar spaces.[36] On histologic examination, microliths consist of calcareous concentric lamellae placed around a central nucleus. The microliths may fill the pulmonary alveolar airspaces. The microliths are most numerous in the lower lung zones. They range in size from about 250 to 750 μm in diameter and are round, oval, or irregular in shape.[39] Chemical analysis and energy-dispersive x-ray microanalysis have shown them to be composed mainly of calcium phosphate.[40,41] In early disease the alveolar walls are normal; eventually, interstitial fibrosis develops, sometimes associated with multinucleated giant cell formation.[40]

MANIFESTATIONS OF THE DISEASE

Radiography

The characteristic radiographic pattern is one of a fine sand–like micronodulation ("sandstorm lung") that may be diffuse but tends to be most severe in the middle and lower lung zones.[34,42] Regardless of the effect of superimposition or summation of shadows, individual deposits are usually identifiable as sharply defined nodules measuring less than 1 mm in diameter. On occasion, there is a reticular pattern or septal lines superimposed on the characteristic sandstorm appearance (Fig. 38.13). Other findings may include bullae in the lung apices, a zone of increased lucency between the lung parenchyma and the ribs (known as a black pleural line), and pleural calcification (Fig. 38.14).[42,43]

Computed Tomography

HRCT manifestations consist of calcific nodules measuring 1 mm or less in diameter, sometimes confluent, and distributed predominantly along the cardiac borders and dorsal portions of the lower lung zones (see Fig. 38.13).[42,44] The higher attenuation in the dorsal portion of the lungs persists when scans are obtained with the patient in the prone position. Other common findings on HRCT include ground-glass opacities, interlobular septal thickening (often with apparent extensive calcification), subpleural interstitial thickening, and paraseptal emphysema (see Fig. 38.14).[42,44] HRCT-pathologic correlation has shown that the apparent calcification of interlobular septa on CT is due to accumulation of microliths in the periphery of the secondary lobules rather than interstitial disease.[11] Correlation of HRCT with radiographic findings has shown that the black pleural line on the radiograph can be caused by subpleural cysts along the costal and mediastinal pleura (see Fig. 38.14) or by a layer of extrapleural fat.[44,45]

Nuclear Medicine

Technetium-99m methylene diphosphonate (^{99m}Tc-MDP) bone scintigraphy usually shows diffuse uptake of radiotracer in both lungs.[46]

DIFFERENTIAL DIAGNOSIS

The differential diagnosis of microlithiasis includes miliary tuberculosis, sarcoidosis, talcosis caused by intravenous drug use, amyloidosis, idiopathic pulmonary ossification, and metastatic pulmonary calcification. The diagnosis can generally be made with confidence on the basis of the classic radiographic pattern of sand-like nodules in a predominantly middle and lower lung zone distribution and the striking radiologic-clinical disparity in severity of disease. Values from chemical analysis of blood are invariably within the normal range. Microliths can be identified in sputum, BAL fluid, and transbronchial biopsy specimens.[41]

SYNOPSIS OF TREATMENT OPTIONS

Treatment is palliative and includes the use of diphosphonate, steroids, and therapeutic BAL, although the effectiveness of these therapies is debatable.[35,36] On occasion, patients progress to respiratory failure and may require lung transplantation.[47] Once the diagnosis has been established, the patient's family should be screened for the disorder because of its autosomal-recessive inheritance.

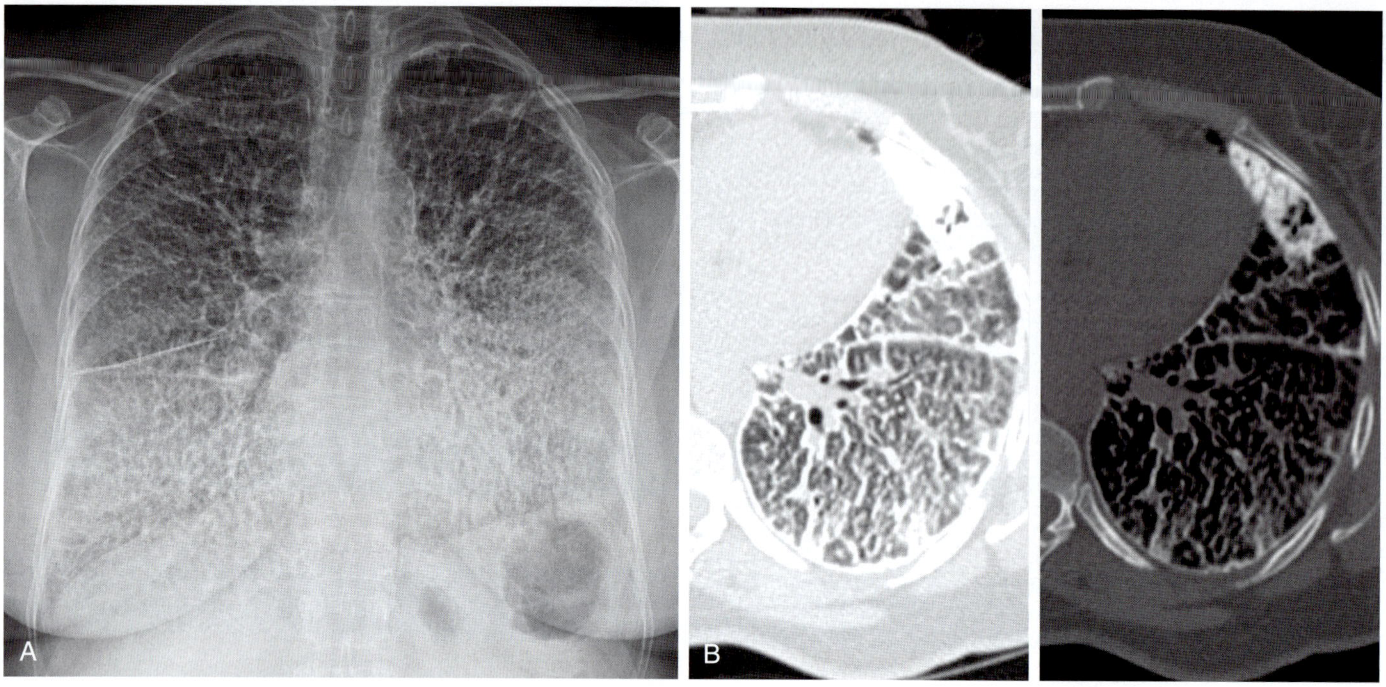

Fig. 38.13 Alveolar microlithiasis. (A) Posteroanterior chest radiograph shows bilateral high-attenuation nodularity with septal lines and thickening of the subpleural interstitium with a middle and lower lung zone predominance. (B) Composite image with axial CT in lung window *(left image)* and axial CT in bone window *(right image)* shows extensive high-attenuation deposits involving the periphery of the secondary pulmonary lobules. Note confluent calcification in the lingula adjacent to the heart border. *(Courtesy Dr. Christian Cox, Mayo Clinic, Rochester, MN.)*

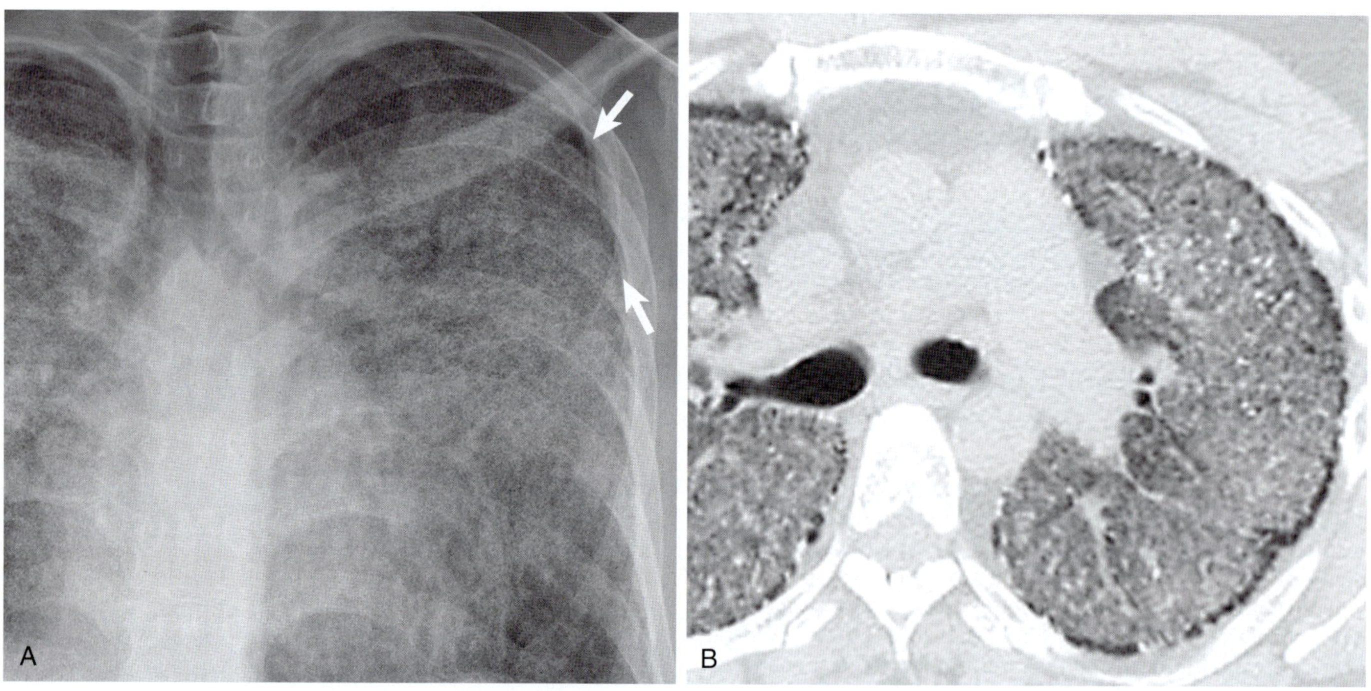

Fig. 38.14 Alveolar microlithiasis. (A) View of the left lung from a posteroanterior chest radiograph shows numerous small calcific opacities, resulting in a sandstorm appearance. Note zone of increased lucency *(arrows)* between the ribs and the peripheral lung (black pleural line). (B) Axial CT shows diffuse bilateral ground-glass opacities with scattered small calcific nodules. Note subpleural cysts along the periphery of the lung, which give rise to the black pleural line on chest radiography. *(Courtesy Dr. Christian Cox, Mayo Clinic, Rochester, MN.)*

KEY POINTS: PULMONARY ALVEOLAR MICROLITHIASIS

- Idiopathic accumulation of innumerable tiny calculi (microliths) within alveolar airspaces is seen.
- It is often asymptomatic and may result in progressive shortness of breath.
- Innumerable sand-like nodules (<1 mm in diameter) are apparent on the radiograph and CT.
- Predominance of distribution is in the middle and lower lung zones.
- Calcified septal lines and ground-glass opacities are commonly seen on high-resolution CT.

Metastatic Pulmonary Calcification

ETIOLOGY, PREVALENCE, AND EPIDEMIOLOGY

Metastatic calcification typically occurs in patients who have hypercalcemia, usually associated with chronic renal failure and less often with an intraosseous malignant neoplasm such as multiple myeloma; it has also been reported after kidney and liver transplantation, primary hyperparathyroidism, hypervitaminosis D, and excess exogenous administration of calcium and vitamin D (milk-alkali syndrome).[48,49] The abnormality is especially common in patients undergoing maintenance hemodialysis.[48] For example, in one investigation of 23 such patients, 14 (61%) had pulmonary uptake on ^{99m}Tc-diphosphonate scanning.[50] Rarely, metastatic pulmonary calcification may occur in patients with no apparent biochemical abnormality.[51]

CLINICAL PRESENTATION

Clinical manifestations of metastatic calcification are typically absent. However, pulmonary function abnormalities may be seen, including restrictive lung function with a decrease in vital capacity and impairment in gas exchange with a decrease in DLCO.[48] Rarely, patients may develop progressive shortness of breath and respiratory failure.[48]

PATHOPHYSIOLOGY

Ectopic metastatic calcification is influenced by serum calcium and phosphate concentration, alkaline phosphatase activity, and local pH.[48] It occurs when there is a release of excess calcium salts from bone and their transport through the circulation. Metastatic pulmonary calcification has a predilection for the apical and subapical lung zones, a feature attributable to regional differences in pulmonary ventilation and perfusion.[49] Because the ventilation-perfusion ratio is higher at the apex than at the base of the lung, the local milieu at the apex has a higher partial pressure of oxygen, a lower partial pressure of carbon dioxide, and a higher pH (approximately 7.50 vs. 7.39 at the base).[48] This relative alkalinity favors the precipitation of calcium salts in the apical region.

On pathologic examination, deposits of calcium phosphate are seen in a more or less linear fashion in alveolar septa and the walls of small pulmonary vessels and bronchi.[52] Interstitial fibrosis may or may not be present. Airspaces are typically unaffected.

Metastatic calcification occurs in normal lung tissue and is therefore distinct from dystrophic calcification, which occurs in tissue that is degenerating or dead. Dystrophic calcification is by far more common and in the lung is associated most often with foci of previous granulomatous inflammation.

MANIFESTATIONS OF THE DISEASE

Radiography

In the majority of patients with metastatic calcification, the chest radiograph is normal.[49] When present, the findings consist of numerous 3- to 10-mm diameter fluffy, poorly defined nodular opacities mimicking airspace nodules or patchy parenchymal opacification (Fig. 38.15).[49] The nodules tend to involve mainly the upper lobes. Calcification of the nodules is seldom evident on the radiograph.

Computed Tomography

The HRCT manifestations of metastatic calcification typically consist of fluffy, poorly defined nodular opacities measuring 3 to 10 mm in diameter (see Fig. 38.15).[49,53] The nodules are centrilobular in distribution and tend to be most numerous in the upper lung zones.[54] Occasionally, the nodules may coalesce and become mass-like opacities (Fig. 38.16). Less commonly, the nodules may be diffuse or occasionally involve mainly the lower lung zones; although usually fluffy, the nodules may be well defined. In one series of seven patients with metastatic calcification, calcification of the nodules was evident on CT in four cases and calcification of vessels in the chest wall in six cases (see Fig. 38.15).[49] The nodule calcification may be stippled, diffuse, or occasionally ring-like.[49,55] Calcified vessels are typically seen between the pectoralis major and minor. Other findings that may be present include extensive ground-glass opacities, patchy consolidation, and, less commonly, calcification of pulmonary arteries and the left atrial wall.[49,55]

Magnetic Resonance Imaging

Metastatic calcification lesions may manifest with high T1 signal intensity relative to skeletal muscle.[56]

Nuclear Medicine

The calcific nature of the opacities can be confirmed by scanning with bone-imaging agents such as ^{99m}Tc-diphosphonate.[57,58]

DIFFERENTIAL DIAGNOSIS

The differential diagnosis of metastatic pulmonary calcification includes pneumonia, respiratory bronchiolitis, hypersensitivity pneumonitis, cholesterol granulomas, sarcoidosis, silicosis, talcosis, amyloidosis, and idiopathic pulmonary ossification. The diagnosis of metastatic calcification can usually be based on a clinical history of chronic renal failure, lack of significant respiratory symptoms, characteristic appearance of fluffy and poorly defined 3- to 10-mm-diameter upper lobe nodules on HRCT, and demonstration of calcification on CT or ^{99m}Tc-MDP scintigraphy. In assessing for the presence of metastatic calcification, it is important to perform the CT with thin sections (1 mm or less) to minimize volume averaging and to reformat the images by a standard algorithm to minimize artifacts caused by the reconstruction algorithm.

SYNOPSIS OF TREATMENT OPTIONS

Treatment is aimed at the primary disease, usually chronic renal failure, and normalization of calcium, phosphate, and parathyroid hormone levels. Metastatic pulmonary calcification may occasionally resolve without treatment.[51]

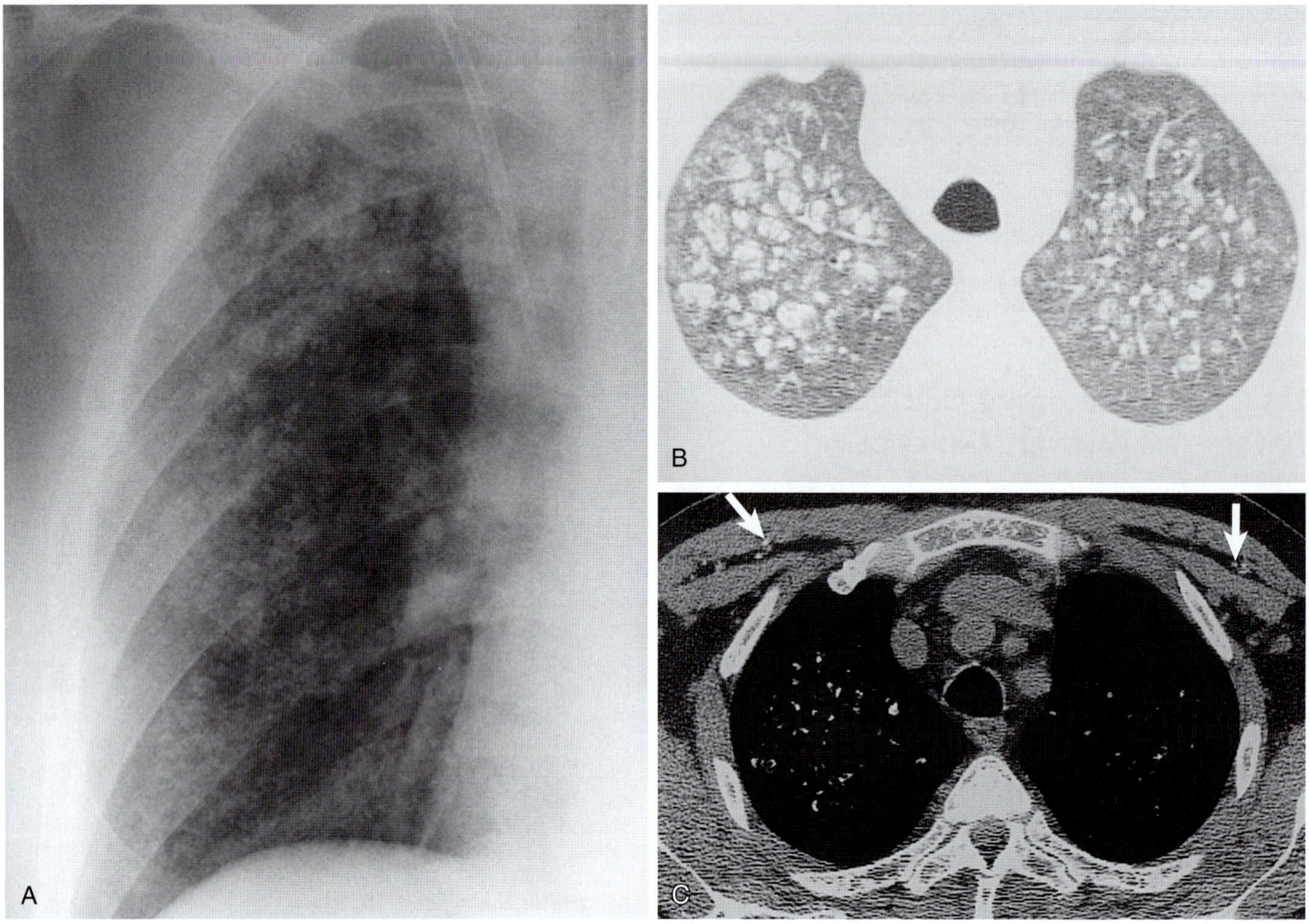

Fig. 38.15 Metastatic pulmonary calcification in chronic renal failure. (A) Close-up view of the right lung from a posteroanterior chest radiograph shows poorly defined nodular opacities involving mainly the upper lobe. Similar findings were present in the left lung. A hemodialysis catheter is in place. (B) High-resolution CT through the lung apices shows nodular areas of increased attenuation. (C) Soft tissue windows show calcification within the opacities. Vascular calcification in the chest wall also is evident *(arrows). (From Müller NL, Fraser RS, Colman NC, Paré PD.* Radiologic Diagnosis of Diseases of the Chest. *Philadelphia: WB Saunders; 2001.)*

KEY POINTS: METASTATIC PULMONARY CALCIFICATION

- It occurs most commonly in patients with chronic renal failure.
- It is usually asymptomatic.
- Radiographic findings consist of poorly defined nodular opacities or consolidation.
- Predominance of distribution is in the upper lobes.
- Fluffy 3- to 10-mm diameter centrilobular nodules are seen on high-resolution CT.
- Calcification of nodules is seen on CT in about 60% of cases.
- Calcification of chest wall arteries is frequently seen on CT.
- Uptake in the lung is demonstrated on bone scintigraphy.

Lipid Storage Diseases

Gaucher Disease

ETIOLOGY, PREVALENCE, AND EPIDEMIOLOGY

Gaucher disease is an autosomal-recessive abnormality characterized by mutations in the glucocerebrosidase gene, leading to decreased enzyme activity.[59] This deficiency results in an accumulation of glucocerebroside predominantly in the reticuloendothelial cells (Gaucher cells) of the liver, spleen, lymph nodes, and bones and in the brain in the infantile form of the disease. The majority of patients are female, and more than 95% are Ashkenazi Jews.

Symptomatic lung involvement in Gaucher disease is rare, being restricted to patients with other severe manifestations. In one review of 411 patients, only 8 (5%) had prominent pulmonary signs or symptoms; these included 4 adults and 4 children.[60]

CLINICAL PRESENTATION

Clinical symptoms and signs include dyspnea, tachypnea, cyanosis, and finger clubbing.[60]

PATHOPHYSIOLOGY

On histologic examination, Gaucher cells may be found in the perilymphatic interstitium, alveolar septa, alveolar airspaces, or alveolar capillary lumina.[61]

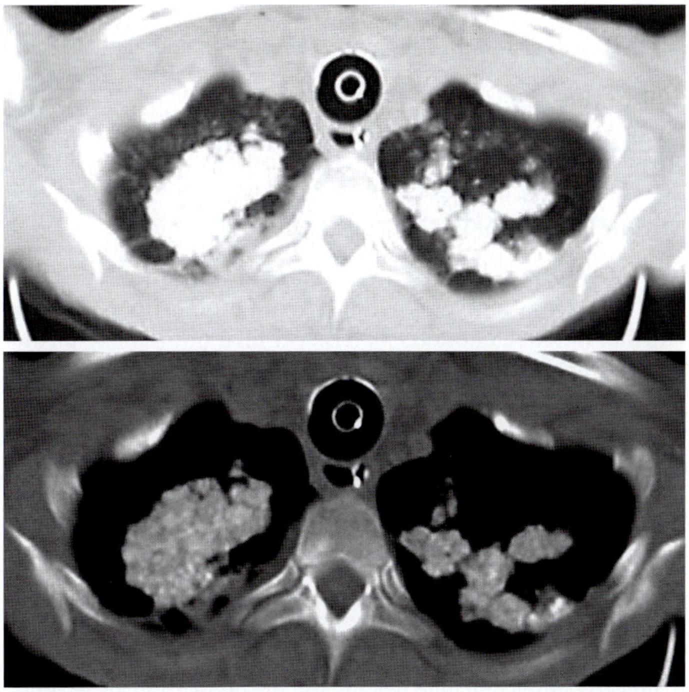

Fig. 38.16 Metastatic pulmonary calcification. Composite image with axial CT in lung window *(top image)* and bone window *(bottom image)* shows upper lobe mass-like opacities containing dense calcification. Note ill-defined centrilobular ground-glass nodules adjacent to the masses. *(Courtesy Dr. Christian Cox, Mayo Clinic, Rochester, MN.)*

MANIFESTATIONS OF THE DISEASE

Radiography

Radiologic manifestations consist of a reticulonodular or miliary pattern affecting both lungs diffusely.[60] Lytic lesions are occasionally seen in the ribs.

Computed Tomography

CT findings include interlobular septal thickening, intralobular linear opacities, and extensive ground-glass opacities; the abnormalities may be diffuse or involve mainly the lower lung zones.[60,62] Other abnormalities that may be seen include signs of pulmonary arterial hypertension, rib lesions, extramedullary hematopoiesis, and hepatosplenomegaly.[60,63]

TREATMENT OPTIONS

Treatment is with enzyme replacement therapy. This often results in decreased hepatosplenomegaly, improved hematologic parameters, and improvement in the dyspnea.[60] However, the pulmonary abnormalities do not resolve, and the pulmonary hypertension may progress.[60]

KEY POINTS: GAUCHER DISEASE

- Glucocerebroside accumulates in reticuloendothelial cells.
- It affects mainly the liver, spleen, lymph nodes, and bones.
- Symptomatic pulmonary involvement occurs in 5% of cases.
- Chest radiograph: reticulonodular pattern mainly in lower lung zones.
- High-resolution CT: interlobular septal thickening, intralobular linear opacities, and extensive ground-glass opacities.
- Hepatomegaly and splenomegaly may be seen.

Niemann-Pick Disease

ETIOLOGY, PREVALENCE, AND EPIDEMIOLOGY

Niemann-Pick disease is caused by an autosomal-recessive inherited defect in the production of sphingomyelinase, a deficiency that results in the deposition of sphingomyelin in the liver, spleen, lungs, bone marrow, and brain. Three subtypes that depend on the age at onset, genetic defect, and the predominant organs affected have been described. Many patients die in infancy or childhood; however, some survive into adulthood, occasionally exhibiting the first manifestations of the disease at that time.

CLINICAL PRESENTATION

Pulmonary involvement can be asymptomatic or (rarely) severe enough to cause respiratory failure.[64]

PATHOPHYSIOLOGY

The histologic findings consist of diffuse endogenous lipoid pneumonia, aggregates of large multivacuolated "foam" cells, and mild fibrosis.[65]

MANIFESTATIONS OF THE DISEASE

Radiography

The radiographic manifestations consist of a reticular or reticulonodular pattern involving mainly the lower lung zones.[66]

Computed Tomography

HRCT demonstrates patchy bilateral ground-glass opacities, smooth thickening of the interlobular septa, and commonly smooth intralobular lines (Fig. 38.17).[66–68] The various patterns may occur separate from each other or be admixed, resulting in a pattern known as "crazy paving."[67] The abnormalities may be diffuse but tend to involve mainly the lower lung zones.[67] Hepatomegaly, splenomegaly, and peripheral lymph node enlargement are common.

Although HRCT provides excellent depiction of the extent of parenchymal abnormalities, there is poor correlation between the extent of abnormalities on CT and the functional impairment in patients with Niemann-Pick disease. Thus patients with severe interstitial lung disease on CT may have normal gas transfer, whereas patients with moderate to severe gas transfer defect may have mild interstitial disease.[67]

KEY POINTS: NIEMANN-PICK DISEASE

- Accumulation of sphingomyelin characterizes the disease.
- It affects mainly the liver, spleen, lung, bone marrow, and brain.
- Pulmonary involvement is often asymptomatic.
- Chest radiograph: reticular pattern involving mainly the lower lung zones.
- High-resolution CT: bilateral ground-glass opacities, smooth thickening of the interlobular septa, and smooth intralobular lines.
- Hepatomegaly and splenomegaly are common.

Hermansky-Pudlak Syndrome

ETIOLOGY, PREVALENCE, AND EPIDEMIOLOGY

Hermansky-Pudlak syndrome is an autosomal-recessive disease characterized by tyrosinase-positive oculocutaneous albinism,

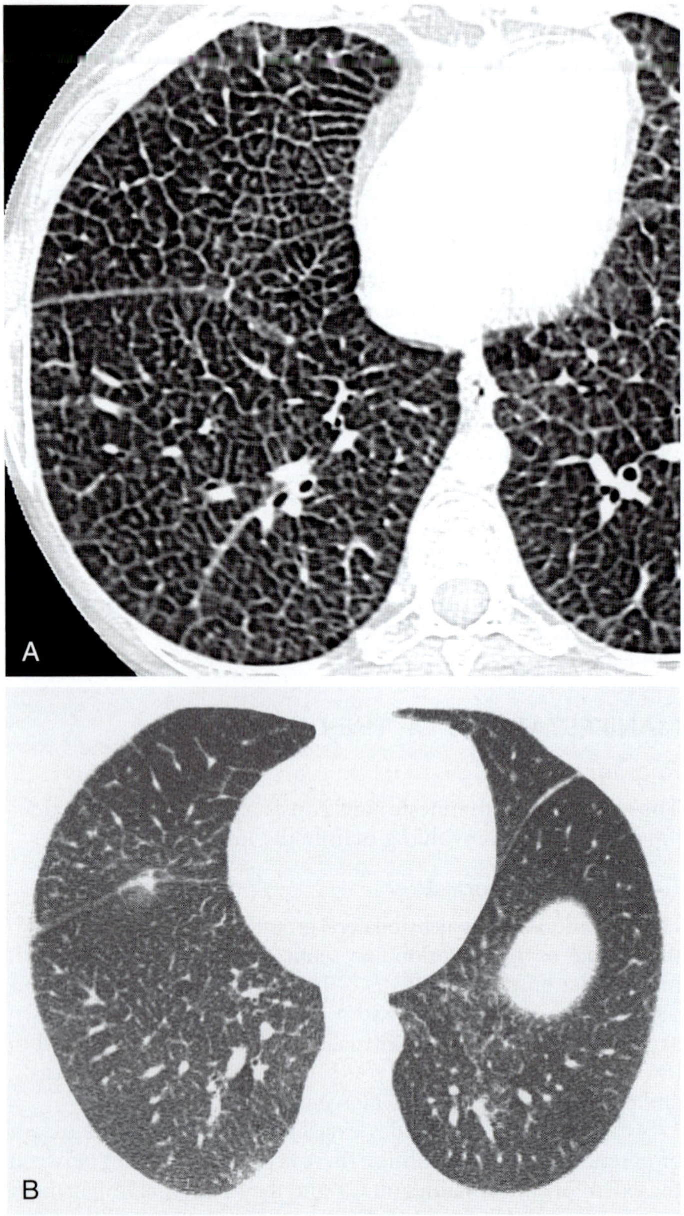

Fig. 38.17 Niemann-Pick disease. (A) Axial CT shows diffuse interlobular septal thickening with mild ground-glass opacities. (B) Axial CT from a different patient shows mild thickening of the interlobular septa and patchy ground-glass opacities. *(Image A courtesy Tomás Franquet, MD, PhD.)*

a defect in platelet function, and the accumulation of ceroid pigment in macrophages throughout the body.[69] It has been documented most often in persons from Puerto Rico and southern Holland.[70]

CLINICAL PRESENTATION

Patients experience progressive dyspnea and are susceptible to infection and to a bleeding tendency.

PATHOPHYSIOLOGY

The histologic findings consist of variably severe parenchymal fibrosis associated with ceroid-laden macrophages.[71] Ceroid, a complex chromolipid, appears histologically as a brown pigment that is periodic acid–Schiff positive, diastase resistant, and acid fast.

Lung Function

Pulmonary function studies reveal a restrictive pattern. Hypoxemia at rest is characteristic.

MANIFESTATIONS OF THE DISEASE

Radiography

The most common radiographic manifestation is a bilateral reticular or reticulonodular pattern, perihilar fibrosis, and pleural thickening (Fig. 38.18).[72]

Computed Tomography

HRCT is more sensitive than chest radiography in assessing the presence and the extent of pulmonary disease in patients with Hermansky-Pudlak syndrome.[73] The main HRCT findings consist of interlobular septal thickening, ground-glass opacities, and peribronchovascular thickening.[72,73] HRCT findings in the more advanced stages of disease include moderate to severe reticulation, traction bronchiectasis, honeycombing, and peribronchovascular thickening (see Fig. 38.18).[73] The abnormalities tend to involve mainly the subpleural lung regions and the middle and lower zones.

SYNOPSIS OF TREATMENT OPTIONS

The only treatment for pulmonary fibrosis in these patients is lung transplantation.[74]

KEY POINTS: HERMANSKY-PUDLAK SYNDROME

- Oculocutaneous albinism, a defect in platelet function, and the accumulation of ceroid pigment in macrophages characterize the disease.
- Patients have dyspnea, susceptibility to infection, and bleeding tendency.
- Chest radiograph: bilateral reticulation, perihilar fibrosis, and pleural thickening.
- High-resolution CT: septal thickening, ground-glass opacities, and peribronchovascular thickening; extensive reticulation and honeycombing may develop.

Erdheim-Chester Disease

ETIOLOGY, PREVALENCE, AND EPIDEMIOLOGY

Erdheim-Chester disease is a multisystemic disorder classified as a non–Langerhans cell histiocytosis characterized by the deposition of lipid-laden macrophages in a variety of tissues, particularly bones, that results in symmetric osteosclerosis. Pulmonary involvement has been reported in 14% to 23% of patients, and extraskeletal involvement affects about half of all patients.[75,76]

CLINICAL PRESENTATION

The most common clinical manifestation is bone pain, usually in the lower limbs. Other relatively common findings are exophthalmos and diabetes insipidus. Respiratory manifestations include dyspnea and cough. Progression to respiratory failure and death has been seen in a number of patients.

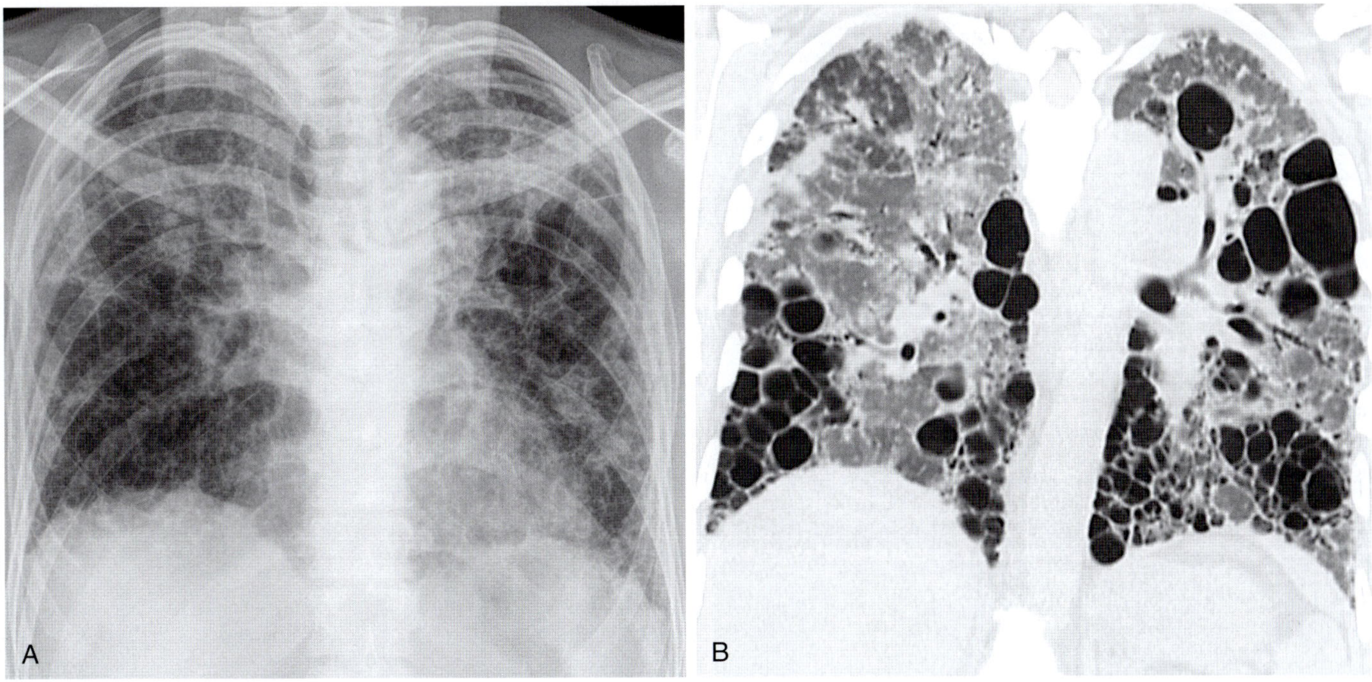

Fig. 38.18 Hermansky-Pudlak syndrome. (A) Posteroanterior chest radiograph shows low lung volume with diffuse reticular opacities and architectural distortion most severe in the middle and lower lung zones. (B) Coronal CT shows diffuse ground-glass opacities, reticulation, and severe honeycombing greatest in the periphery and lung bases.

PATHOPHYSIOLOGY

Lung biopsy specimens show an infiltrate of foamy histiocytes, lymphocytes, and scattered giant cells with associated fibrosis in a perilymphatic distribution. The infiltrate involves visceral pleura, interlobular septa, and bronchovascular bundles.[77]

MANIFESTATIONS OF THE DISEASE

Radiography

The characteristic radiographic feature of Erdheim-Chester disease is osteosclerosis of the metadiaphysis of the long bones (Fig. 38.19).[78] The intrathoracic manifestations include bilateral reticular opacities, interlobular septal thickening, and pleural effusions.[79,80]

Computed Tomography

HRCT demonstrates ground-glass opacities, interlobular septal thickening, reticular opacities, and centrilobular nodules.[80] The parenchymal abnormalities may be diffuse but tend to involve mainly the upper lung zones.[77] Other common findings include pleural effusions or thickening, pericardial effusion or thickening, and perirenal and aortic soft issue encasement (Fig. 38.20).[80]

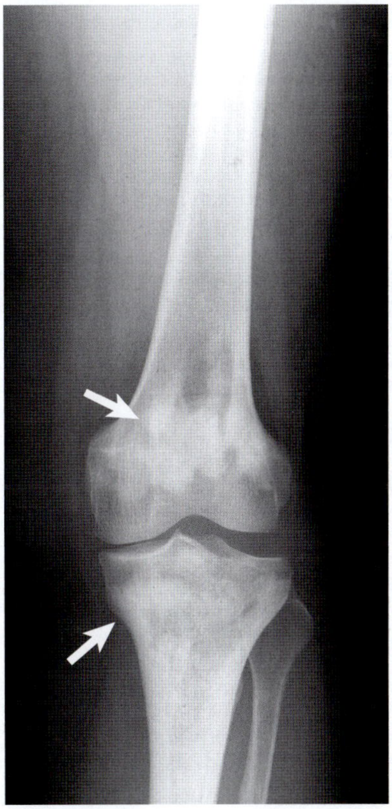

Fig. 38.19 Erdheim-Chester disease. Anteroposterior knee radiograph shows osteosclerosis *(arrows)* involving the distal femoral metaphysis and proximal tibial metadiaphysis. The contralateral knee showed similar findings. *(Reproduced with permission from Walker CM, et al. Tumorlike conditions of the pleura.* Radiographics. *2012;32:971-985.)*

Plasma Cell and Lymphocyte Deposition Disorders

Immunoglobulin G4 (IgG4)-Related Disease

ETIOLOGY AND PATHOPHYSIOLOGY

Immunoglobulin G4 (IgG4)-related disease is a diverse group of immune-mediated conditions of unknown etiology characterized

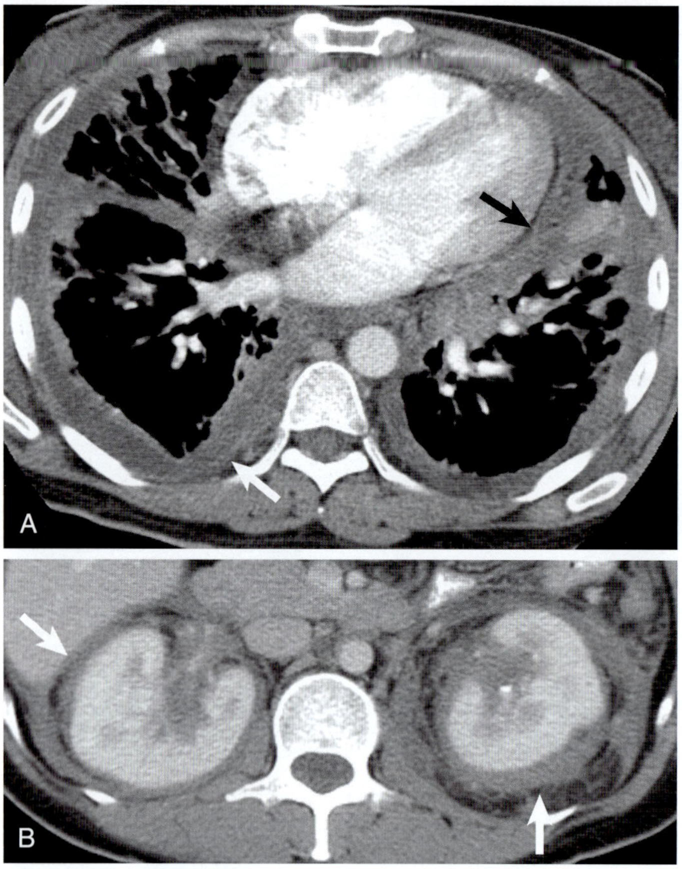

Fig. 38.20 Erdheim-Chester disease. (A) Axial contrast-enhanced CT shows circumferential pleural *(white arrow)* and pericardial *(black arrow)* thickening. The pleural thickening extends into the major fissures. Note interlobular septal thickening in the middle and left lower lobes. (B) Axial CT through the upper abdomen shows circumferential soft tissue thickening *(arrows)* surrounding both kidneys, a finding characteristic of Erdheim-Chester disease. *(Reproduced with permission from Walker CM, et al. Tumorlike conditions of the pleura.* Radiographics. *2012;32:971-985.)*

KEY POINTS: ERDHEIM-CHESTER DISEASE

- Symmetric osteosclerosis and deposition of lipid-laden macrophages in a variety of tissues, particularly bones, characterize the disease.
- The most common symptom is bone pain, usually in the lower limbs.
- Respiratory manifestations include dyspnea and cough.
- Chest radiograph: bilateral reticular opacities, interlobular septal thickening, and pleural effusions.
- High-resolution CT: ground-glass opacities, pleural thickening/effusions, interlobular septal thickening, reticular opacities, and centrilobular nodules.
- Perirenal and/or periaortic soft tissue thickening may occur with pulmonary findings and is helpful in suggesting this diagnosis.

by infiltration of organ systems by IgG4-positive plasma cells and lymphocytes, which leads to fibrosis and tumefactive lesions. About 70% of all patients will have an elevated serum IgG4 level. This disease may affect nearly every organ system, but the pancreas is most commonly involved.[81] IgG4-related disease has findings consistent with both an autoimmune and an allergic disorder.

Three major diagnostic criteria have been proposed: (1) diffuse or localized swelling in one or more organs, (2) elevated serum IgG4 level greater than 135 mg/dL, and (3) histology showing lymphoplasmacytic infiltration and storiform fibrosis and organ

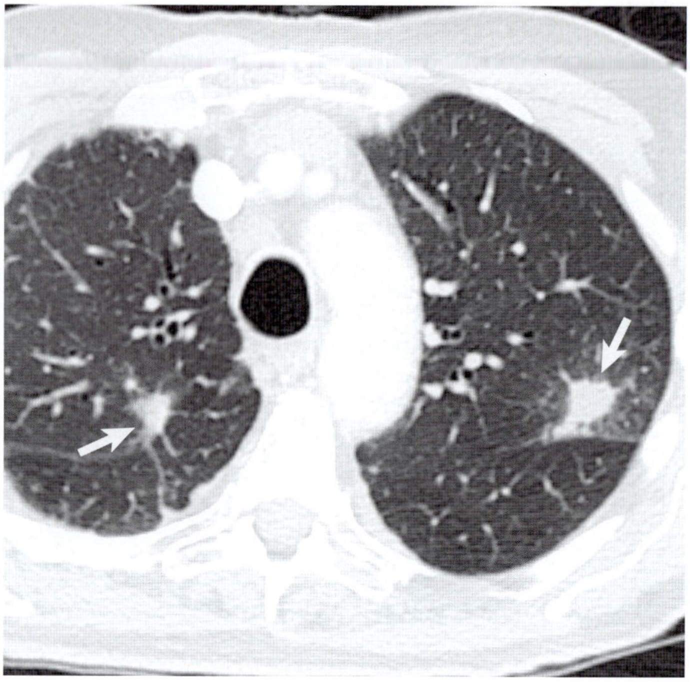

Fig. 38.21 Immunoglobulin G4 (IgG4)-related disease, nodular form. Axial CT shows two spiculated lung nodules *(arrows)* shown to represent IgG4-related disease on biopsy. Note surrounding ground-glass opacities adjacent to the left upper lobe nodule.

infiltration by IgG4-positive plasma cells. The diagnosis of IgG4-related disease is considered definitive if all three criteria are met, probable if criteria 1 and 3 are met, and possible if criteria 1 and 2 are met.[82]

CLINICAL PRESENTATION

Patients with involvement of the lung may be asymptomatic or may present with cough, dyspnea, hemoptysis, chest pain, or respiratory failure.

MANIFESTATIONS OF THE DISEASE

Four major types of IgG4-related pulmonary involvement have been described: (1) nodular or mass-like lesions (Fig. 38.21), (2) round ground-glass nodules, (3) alveolar interstitial disease manifesting with diffuse ground-glass opacities and honeycombing, and (4) bronchovascular disease (Fig. 38.22) manifesting with mediastinal and hilar lymphadenopathy and interlobular septal thickening that often mimics the appearance of sarcoidosis. Patients may also develop visceral or parietal pleural thickening and nodularity.[81] Treatment is with corticosteroids, and response is excellent in most patients.[81]

KEY POINTS: IMMUNOGLOBULIN G4–RELATED DISEASE

- Diverse group of immune-mediated conditions of unknown etiology characterized by infiltration of organ systems by immunoglobulin G4–positive plasma cells and lymphocytes
- Four major intrathoracic manifestations:
  - Nodular or mass-like lesions
  - Round ground-glass nodules
  - Alveolar interstitial disease that can mimic nonspecific interstitial pneumonia
  - Bronchovascular disease that can mimic sarcoidosis

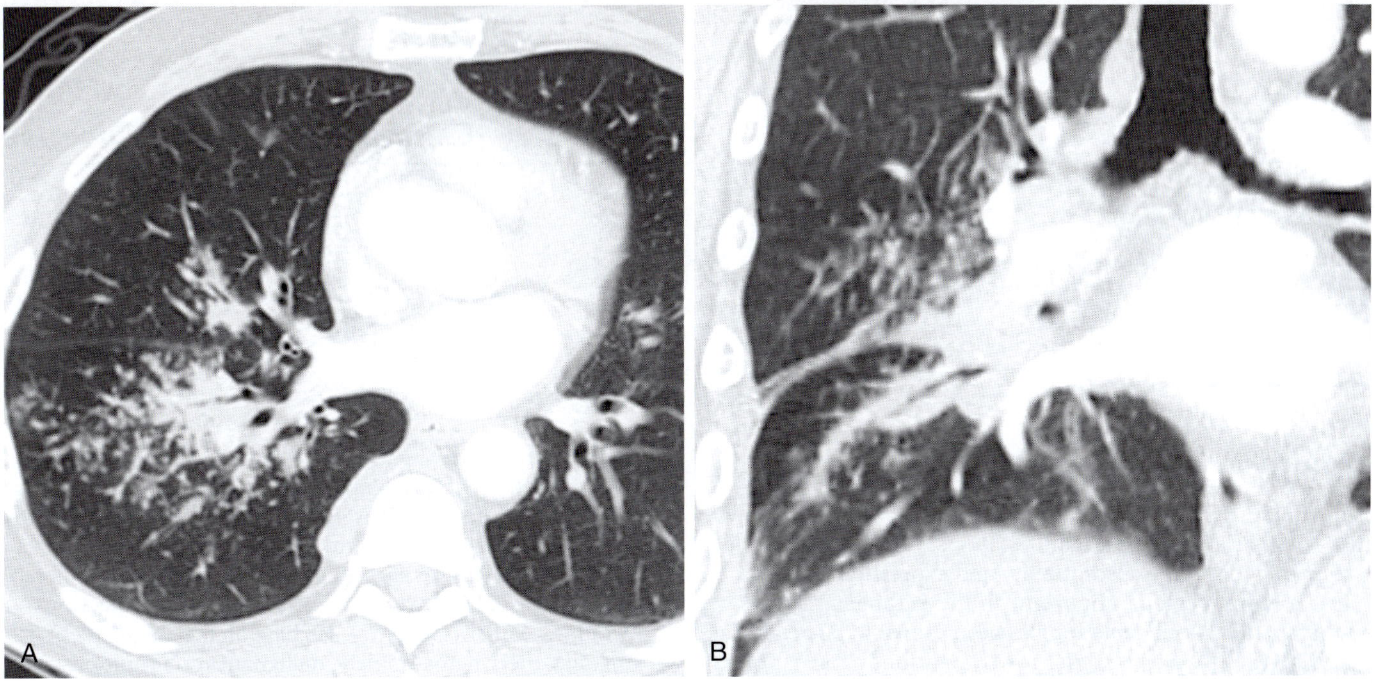

Fig. 38.22 Immunoglobulin G4–related disease, bronchovascular form. Axial (A) and coronal (B) CT shows asymmetric right lung peribronchovascular thickening with nodularity typical of a perilymphatic distribution of nodules. This appearance may mimic that seen with sarcoidosis, and there is often associated mediastinal and hilar lymphadenopathy (not present in this case).

SUGGESTED READINGS

Czeyda-Pommersheim F, et al. Amyloidosis: modern cross-sectional imaging. *Radiographics*. 2015;35:1381–1392.

Frazier AA, et al. From the archives of the AFIP: pulmonary alveolar proteinosis. *Radiographics*. 2008;28:883–899, quiz 915.

Ngo AV, et al. Tumors and tumorlike conditions of the large airways. *AJR Am J Roentgenol*. 2013;201:301–313.

Renapurkar RD, Kanne JP. Metabolic and storage lung diseases: spectrum of imaging appearances. *Insights Imaging*. 2013;Sep 27. Available at: https://www.ncbi.nlm.nih.gov/pubmed/24078438. [Epub ahead of print].

Walker CM, et al. Tumorlike conditions of the pleura. *Radiographics*. 2012;32:971–985.

The full reference list for this chapter is available at ExpertConsult.com.

39 Rheumatoid Arthritis*

STEPHEN B. HOBBS

Etiology

Rheumatoid arthritis (RA) is an autoimmune disorder of unknown cause with variable clinical manifestations. Genetic factors play a major role in disease susceptibility and expression.[1]

The B lymphocyte is important in the pathogenesis of RA, and therapeutic B-cell depletion has been shown to be beneficial in active RA.[2] The exact trigger for autoantibody formation is unknown, but in animal models, both B cells and non–B-cell antigen-presenting cells are required for the development of autoimmunity.[3] Most connective tissue diseases (CTDs) have known human leukocyte antigen (HLA) associations, and the link with the *HLA-DRB1* gene is best understood.[1] In RA, $CD4^+$ T cells have a role in the development of pulmonary parenchymal disease inasmuch as the interstitial pneumonias seen in patients with RA are characterized by increased $CD4^+$ cells (T-helper/inducer cells) when compared with those with idiopathic interstitial pneumonia.[4]

Prevalence and Epidemiology

RA is estimated to affect 1% of the adult population worldwide, but there are some marked demographic differences.[5] RA has a higher incidence in North American Indians (5.3%) and is two to three times more common in women,[1] but some manifestations of RA, such as pleural effusions, necrobiotic nodules, and pulmonary fibrosis, are more frequent in men. Patients with RA have a shortened life expectancy by 5 to 10 years.[6]

Cigarette smoking has a synergistic effect on the pulmonary manifestations of RA, and smoking is the most consistent independent (and preventable) predictor of interstitial lung disease (ILD) in RA.[7] The exact pathogenic role of cigarette smoke remains unclear, but the gradient of risk associated with the development of pulmonary involvement in RA increases with exposure to cigarette smoke.[7] Smokers frequently have several abnormalities on high-resolution computed tomography (HRCT), and it can be difficult to tease out the contribution of pulmonary involvement in RA versus smoking-related disease.

A positive rheumatoid factor (RF) early in the course of the disease is a prognostic marker for premature mortality. The relative risk of dying has been estimated to be six times higher in seropositive patients.[8]

More than a third of patients with RA die of infections; in half of such cases this is not recognized before death. The most common sites of infection are the respiratory and urinary tracts.[9] A national study of RA patients in Finland demonstrated that the life span of subjects with RA was shortened by up to 20%,[10] and the excess deaths were usually due to cardiovascular causes, infections, and amyloidosis. Patients with RA also have an increased risk of death from lung cancer, hematopoietic malignancies, chronic obstructive pulmonary disease, and renal failure.[11–13] Disease-modifying drugs are associated with malignancy, and there are several case reports of methotrexate-induced lymphoma.[14,15]

Individuals with rheumatoid arthritis–associated interstitial lung disease (RA-ILD) are often asymptomatic. Among patients with joint symptoms for less than 2 years (early rheumatoid disease), 58% had evidence of interstitial lung disease, but only 14% of those patients were clinically symptomatic.[16] In an autopsy study of long-standing RA in 81 patients, only 35% had evidence of RA-ILD, but the cause of death was respiratory failure related to that ILD in 9%.[17] Patients with a definite or probable usual interstitial pneumonia (UIP) pattern of lung fibrosis of RA-ILD have a shorter survival than those with nonspecific interstitial pneumonia (NSIP) pattern.[18] However, regardless of HRCT pattern, a lower forced vital capacity or decline in forced vital capacity is independently associated with risk of death.[19]

Clinical Presentation

RA is manifested insidiously as arthralgia, joint swelling, and stiffness.[6] Pleural effusions and pleuritis are the most common pulmonary manifestations of RA. Approximately 20% of patients have symptomatic pleural disease, with the majority having "mild pleurisy."[20] Pleural effusions are more frequent in middle-aged men with RA and typically occur during episodes of active arthritis.[21] In RA pleural effusions can resolve over a period of weeks to months, but they may persist for years. Although RF may be present in the exudative effusion, it is a nonspecific finding that can also be present in effusions caused by systemic lupus erythematosus, tuberculosis, and malignancy. The most frequent respiratory symptoms in RA are exertional dyspnea or cough; airway disease may be manifested as wheezing but can be asymptomatic.

Pathophysiology

PATHOLOGY

More than 20 pathologic processes have been described in the lung parenchyma of RA patients, and they can occur synchronously,

*The editors and the publisher would like to thank Drs. Maureen Quigley and David M. Hansell for contributing material on this topic to the prior edition of this work. It has served as the foundation for the current chapter.

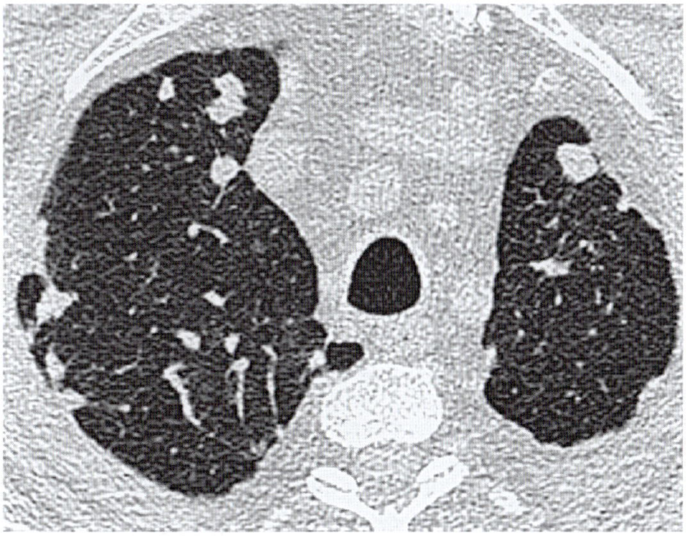

Fig. 39.1 Necrobiotic nodules. High-resolution CT shows bilateral nodules and pleural effusions. This man with rheumatoid arthritis had multiple histologically proven necrobiotic nodules and died from massive hemoptysis when one of the nodules eroded an adjacent bronchial vessel.

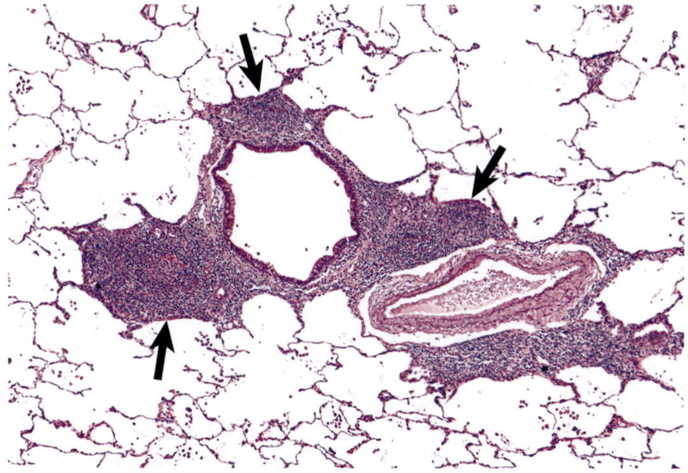

Fig. 39.2 Follicular bronchiolitis. A histologic specimen demonstrates hyperplastic lymphoid follicles *(arrows)* along the bronchovascular bundle. The appearance is characteristic of hyperplasia of bronchus-associated lymphoid tissue. *(Courtesy Dr. John English, Department of Pathology, Vancouver General Hospital, Vancouver, Canada.)*

with up to six different pathologic patterns reported in the same lung biopsy specimen (personal communication with T.V. Colby). Separating subclinical disease from symptomatic disease is an important clinical distinction because pulmonary complications are a common cause of death in patients with RA.[17,22]

No large series have correlated the histopathologic and HRCT appearances in patients with CTDs, and in general, some extrapolation is needed from series that characterize the appearances of the individual idiopathic ILDs. Pulmonary involvement may precede the articular manifestations of disease.[23]

In a study of surgical lung biopsy results in patients with various CTDs, the majority of those with RA had a histologic diagnosis of NSIP, and the rest had follicular bronchiolitis, UIP, or organizing pneumonia.[23] There is a selection bias in patients who come to surgical biopsy, and UIP is likely underrepresented because patients with a confident HRCT diagnosis of UIP are not generally referred for biopsy. This perhaps explains why UIP is usually thought to be the predominant radiologic pattern in RA,[24] whereas biopsy studies generally favor NSIP.

Although pulmonary rheumatoid (necrobiotic) nodules are frequently mentioned in the literature, they appear to be relatively rare in clinical practice, and in one autopsy study of nearly 1000 patients, no examples were documented.[25,26] However, HRCT studies have reported pulmonary nodules in up to 28% of cases,[27] but because these nodules do not have a pathologic correlate, the exact nature of the nodules is not known. Pulmonary rheumatoid nodules can vary in size from 0.5 to 7 cm and are pathologically identical to subcutaneous rheumatoid nodules (Fig. 39.1). Rheumatoid nodules contain a necrotic center surrounded by palisaded histiocytes and leukocytes. The occurrence of pulmonary rheumatoid nodules can antedate the arthritis, and although nodules are generally asymptomatic, they can cavitate and result in catastrophic hemoptysis or pneumothorax. Pulmonary nodules are usually found in patients with subcutaneous nodules and positive RF,[28] and they can occasionally regress and disappear spontaneously. Because patients with RA are frequently immunosuppressed, cavitating nodules can become infected. Caplan syndrome represents an association of pulmonary nodules and pneumoconiosis in patients with RA[29]; it was initially described in coal miners, but similar syndromes have been reported in foundry workers, roof tile makers, and individuals exposed to various mineral dusts.[29]

Follicular bronchiolitis is characterized by lymphoid hyperplasia of bronchus-associated lymphoid tissue, with the follicles distributed along the bronchioles (Fig. 39.2). In one series the majority of patients with biopsy-proven follicular bronchiolitis had RA,[30] and it is important to remember there is considerable overlap between lymphocytic interstitial pneumonia (LIP) and follicular bronchiolitis. The two conditions are distinguished pathologically by expansion of the interstitium in LIP versus the degree to which mononuclear cells are concentrated around the airways in follicular bronchiolitis.[31]

There have been a few reports of a triad of recurrent alveolar hemorrhage, crescentic immune complex–mediated glomerulonephritis, and RA. These patients have nail bed hemorrhage and necrotizing vasculitis.[30] In an attempt to characterize the vasculopathy seen in some patients with RA, a survey of rheumatologists revealed that most practitioners see fewer than five patients with RA vasculitis annually.[32] Pulmonary vascular involvement is infrequently recognized either clinically or pathologically.

Pulmonary amyloid deposition in patients with RA is rare, but there are isolated case reports, including a patient with diffuse septal pulmonary amyloidosis.[33] Amyloidosis, follicular bronchiolitis, and smoking-related ILD are all potentially responsible for the small pulmonary nodules that are so frequently seen on HRCT.

LUNG FUNCTION

Patients with RA frequently have abnormal pulmonary function test (PFT) findings as a result of the various pathologic processes. There are several studies that describe a range of PFT abnormalities, but these studies often contain cigarette smokers. A study of PFT abnormalities in lifelong nonsmokers who had significant

RA (defined by treatment of the disease with an antirheumatic drug) but no clinical evidence of ILD found that more than a quarter of this cohort had abnormal PFT results but no pulmonary symptoms, and these abnormalities were both restrictive and obstructive.[34] The mixture of an obstructive or restrictive picture is not surprising in view of the range of pulmonary diseases encountered in RA. There is good correlation between evidence of air-trapping on HRCT and functional indices of early airway obstruction in patients with RA.[35] Subtle changes in PFT values can alert the clinician to occult disease, and when the patient has mild pulmonary hypertension, diffusing lung capacity for carbon monoxide (DLCO) can be reduced in the presence of normal HRCT findings.[36] Lung function tests may have an important role in monitoring disease progression; however, joint disease can limit a patient's ability to exercise, and therefore altered exercise tolerance cannot always be used as an indicator of clinical deterioration, and the debility caused by RA itself may limit patients' ability to perform lung function testing.

Manifestations of the Disease

In most patients with RA the onset of disease is insidious, but in a fifth of patients the joint involvement has a more acute onset. Joint symptoms include pain, swelling, and stiffness, with the number of involved joints increasing over a period of weeks to months. Approximately 10% of patients have a fulminant onset, and a few start with episodic symptoms, which then progress to persistent disease. The arthropathy in RA typically involves the small joints of the hands and feet and then progresses to large joints in a symmetric distribution. There is abnormal proliferation of the synovium of joints and resultant pannus. In chronic disease deformities of the hands can be very severe. The cervical spine is often involved in patients with RA, and subluxation or impaction of C1 on C2 is a frequent complication.

The wide range of extraarticular manifestations in RA is summarized in Table 39.1.

RADIOGRAPHY

The radiographic manifestations of pulmonary disease in RA patients can be broadly divided into pleural and parenchymal involvement. Pleural disease reflects the "polyserositis," and thus pericardial effusions are a frequent accompaniment. Pleural effusions tend to be asymptomatic[37] and small to moderate in size.[38] Radiographic evidence of a pleural effusion has been reported in 1% of all RA cases.[39] The effusions are generally unilateral but can be bilateral,[40] and on chest radiography, 20% of patients with RA demonstrate pleural thickening (Fig. 39.3).[39] Long-standing effusions may become loculated, simulating empyema despite sterility. Rheumatoid pleural involvement can result in thickening of both parietal and visceral pleura, resulting in pleural fibrosis and trapped lung. Core biopsy of this thickening typically shows nonspecific inflammatory changes rather than rheumatoid granulomas or malignancy.

A readily recognizable but rare form of lung involvement on chest radiography is the presence of cavitating necrobiotic nodules (Fig. 39.4). The plethora of ILDs encountered in patients with RA are generally nonspecific; furthermore, some of these diseases may not be readily detected by chest radiography (e.g., follicular bronchiolitis). The relative insensitivity of chest radiography is especially evident in patients with constrictive bronchiolitis; even in individuals with functionally severe airflow limitation, the chest radiograph may be normal.

The classic radiologic pattern of pulmonary fibrosis in RA is a reticular or reticulonodular pattern (Fig. 39.5). There may be evidence of honeycombing, and the disease is usually symmetric and basal in distribution. Diffuse reticulonodular fibrosis is seen in 5% of all RA patients, and pulmonary fibrosis is more frequently found in those with subcutaneous nodules, antinuclear antibodies, and RF titers.[39]

Patchy consolidation may represent organizing pneumonia or infection. Organizing pneumonia typically shows changing, bilateral peripheral consolidation on chest radiography[41]; however, infection, drug-induced lung disease, and malignancy are differential diagnoses.

In a prospective study of patients with early RA (preceding chest symptoms), chest radiographs showed ILD in 6% of patients, whereas HRCT showed ILD in 33% of patients.[16] Chest radiography has been reported to have a sensitivity of 23% for "fibrosing alveolitis" in RA, which implies that chest radiography is not good at detecting fibrotic lung disease in patients with RA.[42]

COMPUTED TOMOGRAPHY

HRCT is particularly helpful in the context of RA-ILD because it often shows more than one pulmonary disease, which may not be evident on chest radiography. Diagnostic precision in RA-ILD is challenging as a result of (1) the wide range of potential simultaneous pathologies, (2) the possibility of a concurrent CTD, and (3) the need to determine the significance of limited pulmonary disease. Further possible diagnostic confounders include the presence of smoking or drug-related disease and immunosuppression-related infection. Because the reported lifelong prevalence of significant lung disease has not been higher than 20% in any series of RA patients, it seems that HRCT may be detecting truly subclinical pulmonary disease.[43] RA patients with pulmonary symptoms have bronchiectasis, pulmonary nodules, and areas of ground-glass opacity and honeycombing

TABLE 39.1 OVERVIEW OF THE NONPULMONARY EXTRAARTICULAR MANIFESTATIONS OF RHEUMATOID ARTHRITIS

Dermatologic	Palmar erythema, subcutaneous rheumatoid nodules, vasculitis
Ocular	Keratoconjunctivitis sicca, episcleritis, scleritis, choroiditis
Cardiac	Pericarditis, myocarditis, coronary vasculitis, valvular nodules
Neuromuscular	Entrapment neuropathy, peripheral neuropathy, mononeuritis multiplex
Hematologic	Felty syndrome (rheumatoid arthritis, splenomegaly, and leukopenia), large granular lymphocyte syndrome, lymphomas
General	Fever, lymphadenopathy, weight loss, fatigue
Other	Amyloidosis, secondary Sjögren syndrome

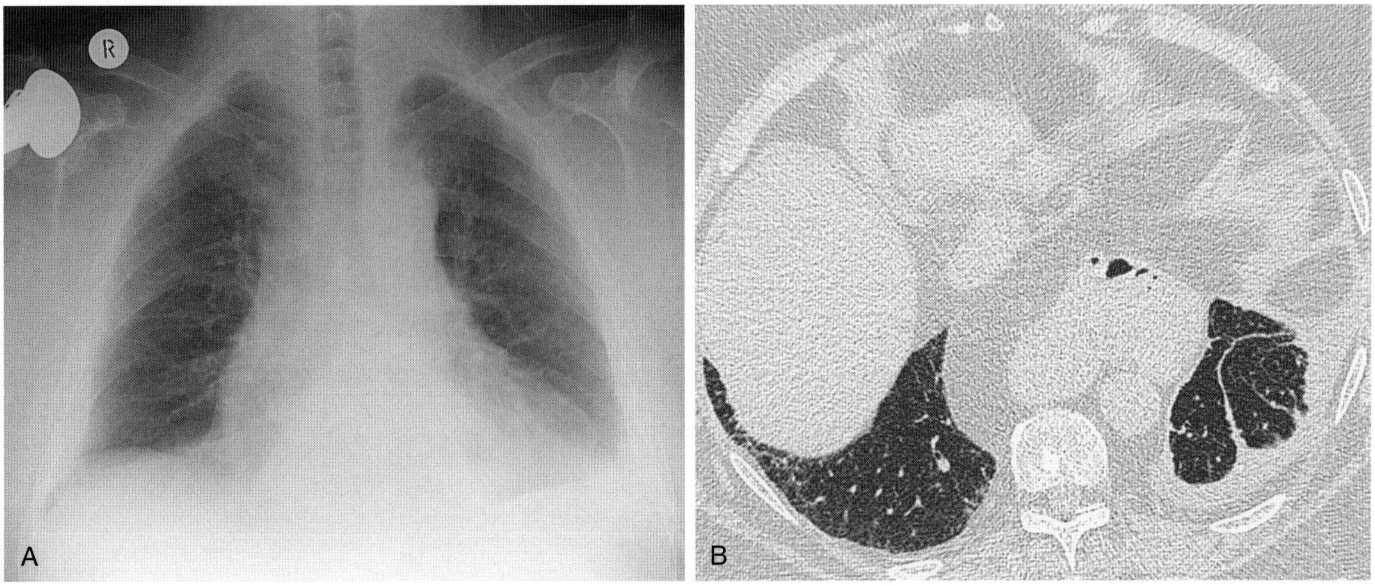

Fig. 39.3 Pleural involvement in rheumatoid arthritis. (A) A chest radiograph shows bilateral pleural thickening. Also note the right shoulder hemiarthroplasty performed for rheumatoid involvement of the shoulder joint. (B) CT shows pleural thickening more pronounced on the left. Parenchymal bands are seen secondary to previous exudative effusions. Incidental note is made of a hiatal hernia.

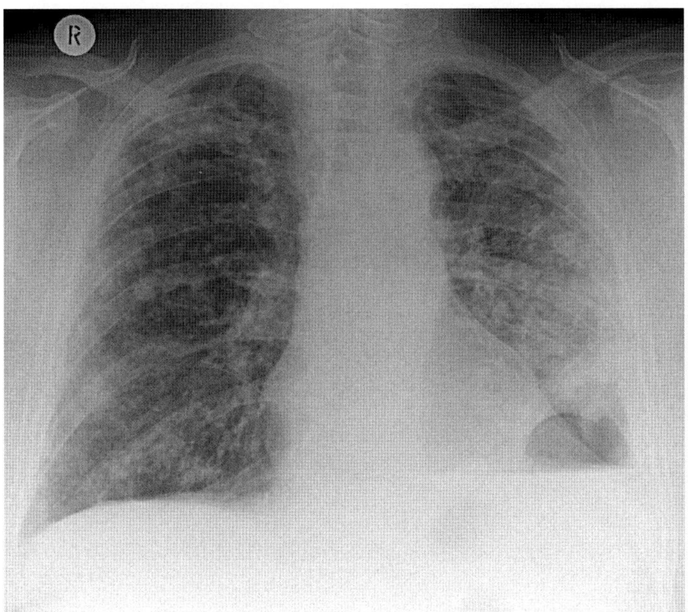

Fig. 39.4 Necrobiotic nodules. A chest radiograph shows bilateral, poorly defined nodules and pleural thickening in rheumatoid arthritis. Also noted is an air-fluid level at the left base, which was due to hemo-pneumothorax secondary to rupture of a subpleural necrobiotic nodule. This is the chest radiograph of the same patient shown in Fig. 39.1.

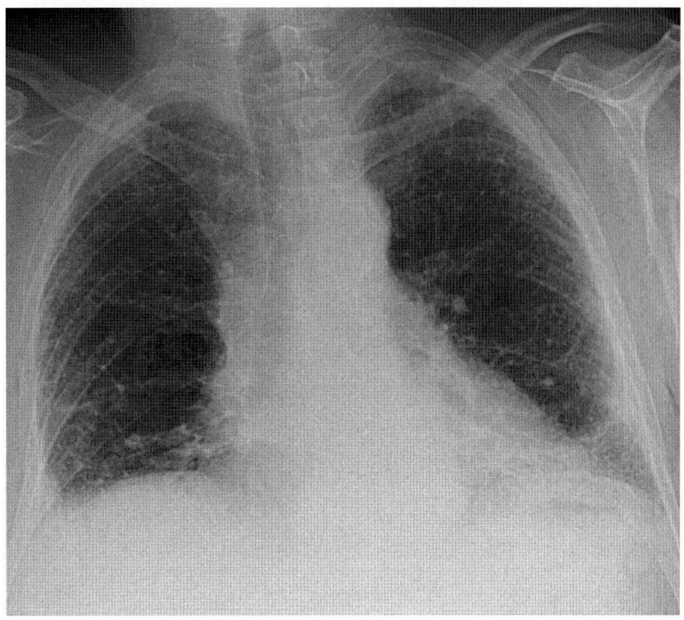

Fig. 39.5 Interstitial lung disease in rheumatoid arthritis. A chest radiograph shows a peripheral reticulonodular pattern. Surgical lung biopsy revealed end-stage lung fibrosis.

on HRCT.[44] These same findings, with the exception of honeycombing, are seen to a lesser degree in RA patients without respiratory symptoms.[44] See Table 39.2 for a summary of HRCT findings and patterns in connective tissue disease, including RA.

The most common fibrotic lung diseases in RA are UIP and NSIP (Figs. 39.6 and 39.7). Many studies of RA were undertaken before the recognition of NSIP, and these early series combine UIP and NSIP as "fibrosing alveolitis." In a study that attempted to characterize the HRCT patterns seen in RA, four major morphologic patterns were identified: UIP (37%), NSIP (30%), constrictive bronchiolitis (17%), and organizing pneumonia (8%). In patients who underwent biopsy, the CT findings correlated with the pathologic findings in the majority of cases.[24] Organizing pneumonia is usually seen in the middle or lower zones, frequently in a peribronchovascular or peripheral distribution.[45] Organizing pneumonia can have several morphologic manifestations: focal areas of consolidation (Fig. 39.8), a perilobular pattern, bands of consolidation, airspace opacities, and nodules.

TABLE 39.2 CORRELATION BETWEEN PATHOLOGIC PROCESSES DESCRIBED IN CONNECTIVE TISSUE DISEASE AND THEIR MORPHOLOGIC APPEARANCE ON HIGH RESOLUTION COMPUTED TOMOGRAPHY

Pathologic Diagnosis	High-Resolution Computed Tomography Appearance
Nonspecific interstitial pneumonia (fibrotic subtype)	Predominantly ground-glass opacity with underlying distortion and fine reticulation, which may or may not be subpleural and basal
Usual interstitial pneumonia	Reticulation with honeycombing in a peripheral and basal distribution. The disease tends to creep anteriorly and subpleurally in the upper lobes
Organizing pneumonia	Consolidation that is most commonly peripheral or peribronchovascular; often around the perimeter of the secondary pulmonary lobules (perilobular distribution)
Respiratory bronchiolitis–associated interstitial lung disease	Indistinct centrilobular nodules and patchy ground-glass opacities; minor lobular air trapping
Desquamative interstitial pneumonia	Usually random distribution of extensive ground-glass opacity; sometimes small cysts
Diffuse alveolar damage	Widespread ground-glass opacity and consolidation
Lymphoid interstitial pneumonia	Ground-glass opacity and/or nodules; cysts in approximately 50% of cases
Follicular bronchiolitis	Small centrilobular/peribronchial nodules and ground-glass opacity
Constrictive bronchiolitis	Mosaic attenuation, attenuated pulmonary vessels in areas of decreased lung density, and abnormalities of the large airways (bronchial dilation and/or wall thickening)
Lymphoproliferative disease	Consolidation, masses, nodules, or ground-glass opacity; thickened interlobular septa may be seen
Amyloid	Variable appearances; bronchovascular structures may be infiltrated. Reticulonodular/linear pattern in the lungs. Large nodules may calcify.

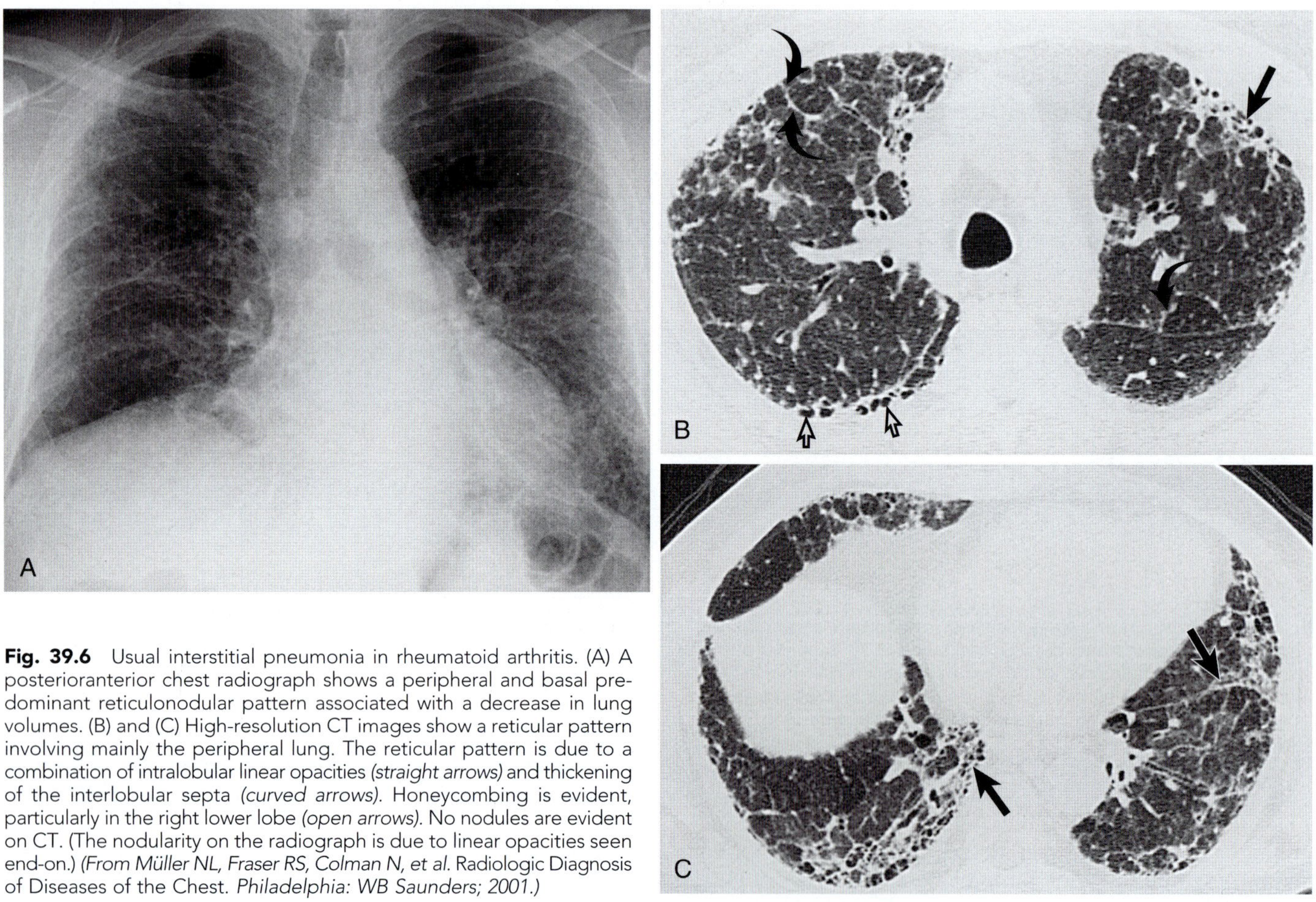

Fig. 39.6 Usual interstitial pneumonia in rheumatoid arthritis. (A) A posterioranterior chest radiograph shows a peripheral and basal predominant reticulonodular pattern associated with a decrease in lung volumes. (B) and (C) High-resolution CT images show a reticular pattern involving mainly the peripheral lung. The reticular pattern is due to a combination of intralobular linear opacities *(straight arrows)* and thickening of the interlobular septa *(curved arrows)*. Honeycombing is evident, particularly in the right lower lobe *(open arrows)*. No nodules are evident on CT. (The nodularity on the radiograph is due to linear opacities seen end-on.) *(From Müller NL, Fraser RS, Colman N, et al.* Radiologic Diagnosis of Diseases of the Chest. *Philadelphia: WB Saunders; 2001.)*

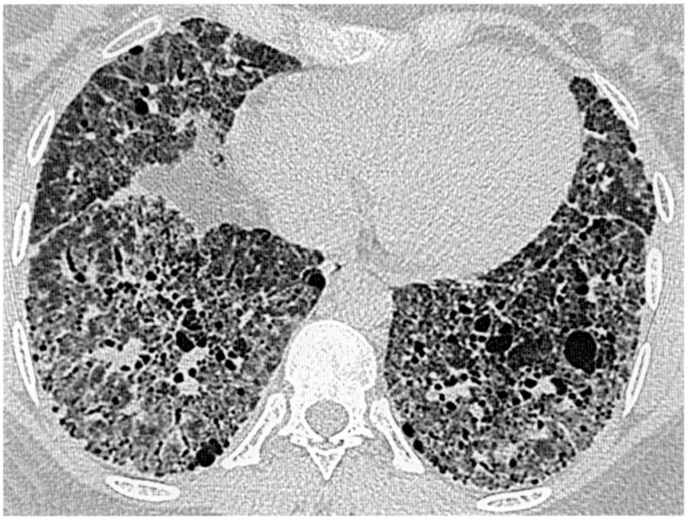

Fig. 39.7 Nonspecific interstitial pneumonia in rheumatoid arthritis. High-resolution CT shows extensive ground-glass opacities and reticulation reflecting severe fibrosis.

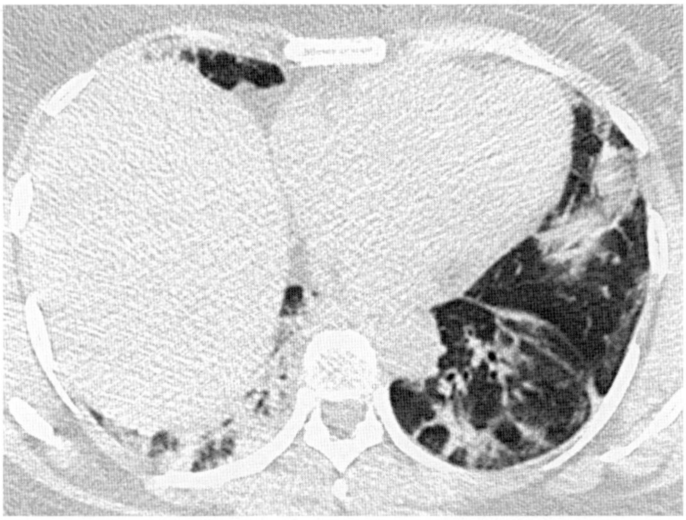

Fig. 39.8 Organizing pneumonia in rheumatoid arthritis. A high-resolution CT image shows patchy peripheral and perilobular consolidation, typical of organizing pneumonia.

There is a strong association between RA and airway disease, with bronchiectasis and constrictive bronchiolitis frequently coexisting. On HRCT bronchiectasis has been reported in 15% of asymptomatic RA patients who were lifelong nonsmokers (Fig. 39.9).[22] However, there is a spectrum of estimates of the prevalence of bronchiectasis in RA, and a long list of contributing factors for the development of bronchiectasis has been proposed, including secondary Sjögren syndrome, α_1-antitrypsin deficiency, and particular HLA subtypes, with some authors speculating that bronchiectasis is a risk factor for the development of RA.[46]

Constrictive bronchiolitis, which is associated with RA, is probably subclinical in many patients with RA.[44,47] Although early reports of constrictive bronchiolitis in RA were characterized by a rapidly progressive course that was often fatal,[48] more recently it has become clear that there is considerable heterogeneity in severity and progression, with a number of patients deteriorating slowly. The characteristic HRCT findings of constrictive bronchiolitis consist of areas of decreased attenuation and vascularity (see Fig. 39.9), with redistribution of blood flow to more normal lung resulting in areas of relatively increased lung attenuation and vascularity (i.e., mosaic attenuation).[49] The relationship of large airways disease to small airways disease, in terms of natural history and which develops first, has not been fully addressed.[50]

Pulmonary vasculopathy in RA affects the smaller vessels and is difficult to diagnose based on imaging. In one study 20% of patients with RA had mild pulmonary arterial hypertension without evidence of other pulmonary or cardiac disease.[36] Pulmonary hypertension may also develop in patients with RA secondary to ILD or cardiac disease, and in total, almost a third of unselected hospitalized RA patients had pulmonary hypertension as judged by echocardiography. In patients younger than 50 years, there is a strong correlation between the diameter of the pulmonary trunk on CT and mean pulmonary artery pressure. If the diameter of the pulmonary trunk is greater than that of the adjacent (nonaneurysmal) ascending aorta, there is a high probability of pulmonary arterial hypertension, and this is a useful CT sign that should be sought.[51]

In a study of histopathologic and CT findings in follicular bronchiolitis, the cardinal features were centrilobular nodules measuring 1 to 12 mm in diameter, some of which were peribronchovascular, and patchy areas of ground-glass opacity (Fig. 39.10).[31] The ground-glass opacities were generally bilateral and diffuse in distribution. Mild bronchial dilation with wall thickening is seen in some cases of follicular bronchiolitis. As previously discussed, follicular bronchiolitis forms a continuum with LIP. The HRCT appearances of LIP are usually characterized by the presence of ground-glass opacities, poorly defined centrilobular nodules, interlobular septal thickening, and cysts (Fig. 39.11).[45] However, the majority of LIP case reports are associated with Sjögren syndrome rather than RA.

Amyloidosis, although common in pathologic series, can be difficult to identify on HRCT because the appearances are nonspecific. Amorphous or irregular calcifications are occasionally identifiable within large amyloid deposits, which often have odd shapes, but definitive diagnosis usually requires biopsy confirmation.[52]

A personal or family history of RA is associated with an increased risk for Hodgkin lymphoma,[53] and this risk is substantially increased in patients with severe RA.[54] An increased risk for hematologic malignancies has been shown in patients with RA,[55] and lymphoproliferative disease should be considered in the differential diagnosis for any RA patient with nonresolving consolidation on HRCT.

A large assortment of disease-modifying antirheumatic drugs are used to treat CTDs. These drugs can produce a broad spectrum of systemic side effects, and the pulmonary consequences of these drugs are of particular relevance. It may be difficult to separate the contribution of the CTD itself from that of the drug in causing the pulmonary disease. Many of these disease-modifying drugs are used for their immunosuppressive effects, which increases the risk for opportunistic infections with organisms such as *Pneumocystis jirovecii, Aspergillus, Cryptococcus,* and *Nocardia,*[56,57] and, more controversially, increases the risk for lymphoproliferative disease.[58] See Chapter 65 for a broader discussion of drug-induced lung injury.

Methotrexate is often the disease-modifying drug of choice in the treatment of RA, and its most serious complication is pneumonitis. The mean estimated prevalence of "methotrexate

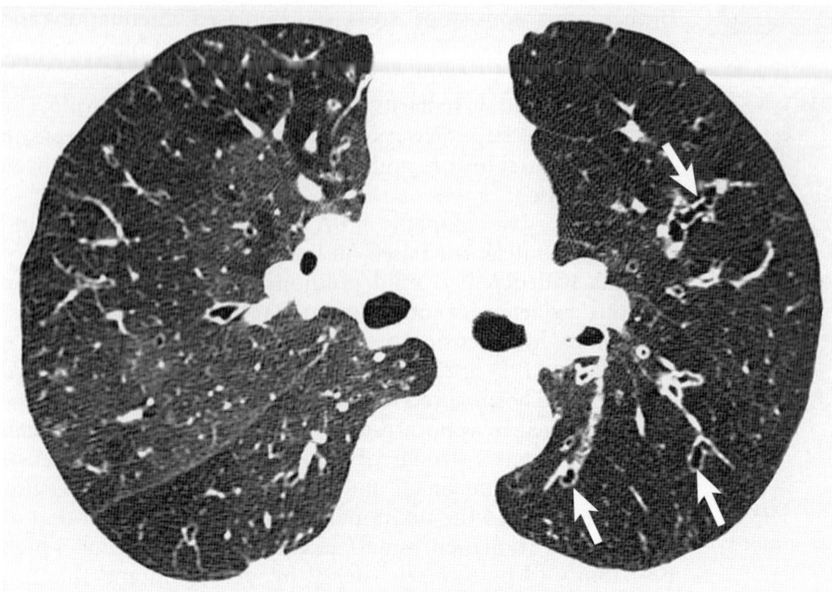

Fig. 39.9 Constrictive bronchiolitis and bronchiectasis in rheumatoid arthritis. High-resolution CT shows mosaic attenuation with areas of decreased attenuation and vascularity, bronchiectasis *(arrows)*, and bronchial wall thickening.

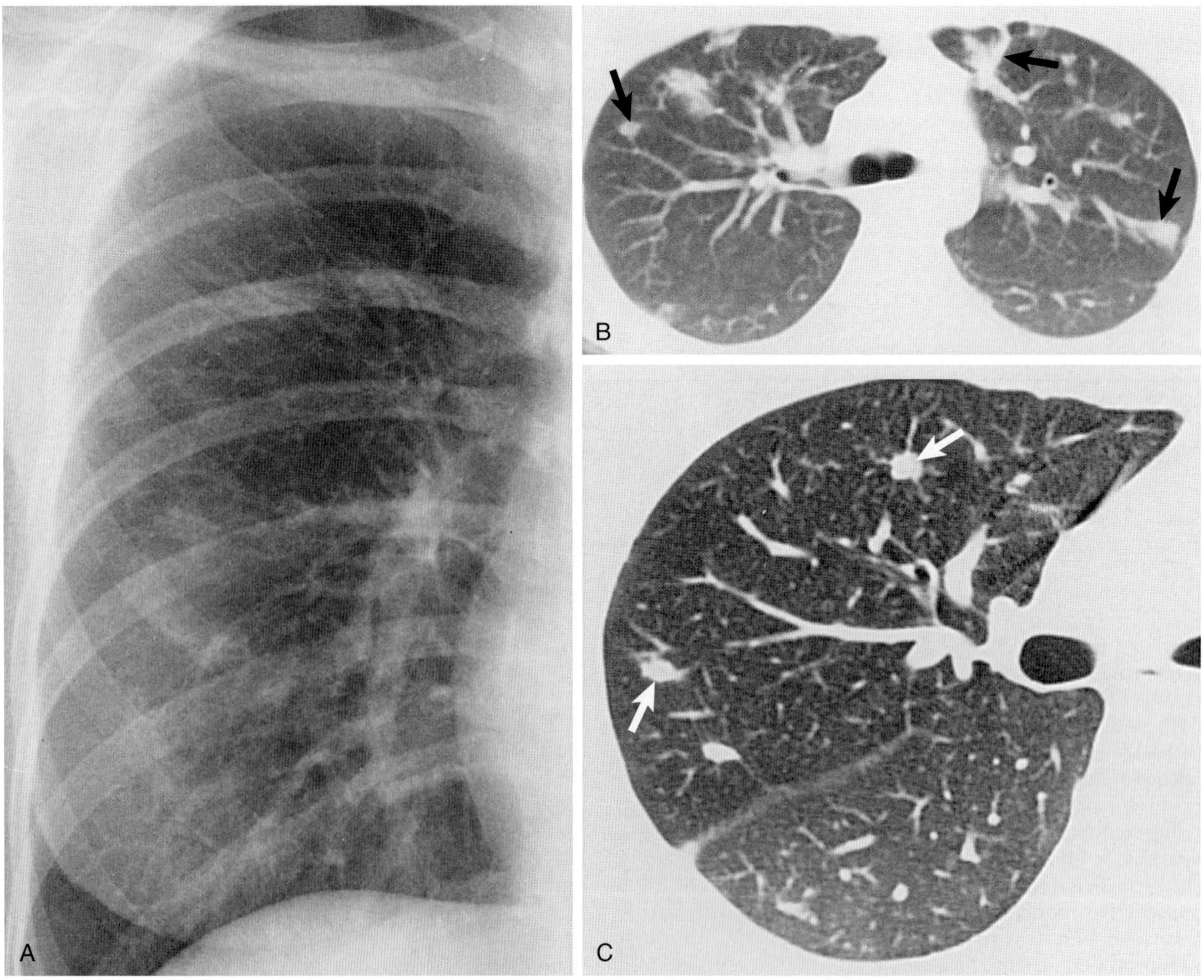

Fig. 39.10 Follicular bronchiolitis in rheumatoid arthritis. (A) A view of the right lung from a posterior-anterior chest radiograph shows ill-defined nodular opacities. A similar pattern was present in the left lung. (B) Axial CT shows focal nodular areas of consolidation *(arrows)* in both lungs, located in a predominantly peribronchovascular distribution. (C) A high-resolution CT image targeted to the right lung shows sharply defined peribronchovascular nodular opacities *(arrows)* in the right upper lobe. *(From Müller NL, Fraser RS, Colman N, et al.* Radiologic Diagnosis of Diseases of the Chest. *Philadelphia: WB Saunders; 2001.)*

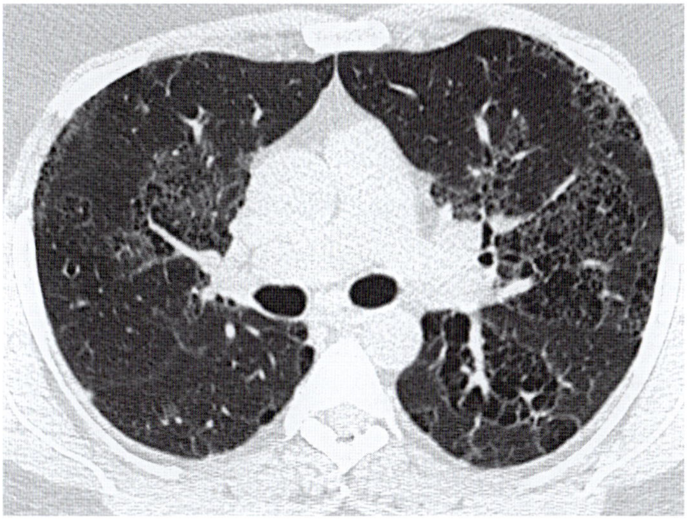

Fig. 39.11 Lymphoid interstitial pneumonia in rheumatoid arthritis. High-resolution CT shows ground-glass opacities and "soap bubble" cystic destruction, in keeping with lymphoid interstitial pneumonia.

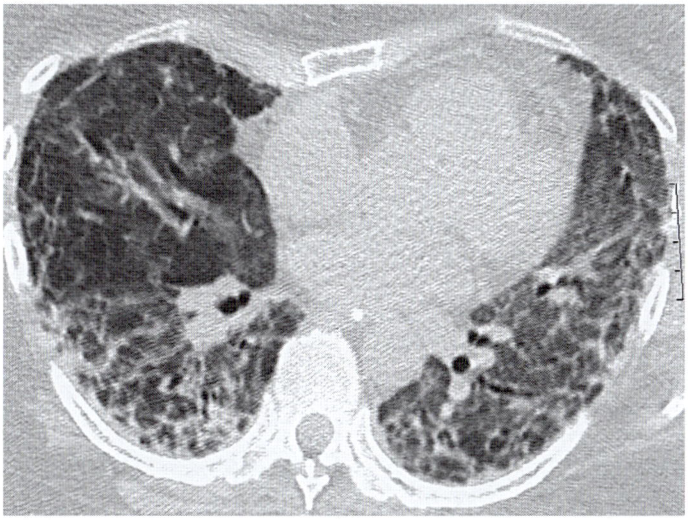

Fig. 39.12 Gold-induced diffuse alveolar damage in rheumatoid arthritis. High-resolution CT demonstrates widespread ground-glass opacities and patchy consolidation, in keeping with diffuse alveolar damage. This woman had established rheumatoid arthritis when she went into fulminant respiratory failure after commencing gold treatment.

lung" is 3.3%,[59] with a fatality rate of 22%.[58] Methotrexate-induced pneumonitis can develop weeks to years after commencing therapy, and the mechanism of injury is idiosyncratic; of interest, the pneumonitis does not always recur when the patient is rechallenged with the drug.[58]

Gold salts are used to treat RA, and pulmonary toxicity has been reported in 1% of patients (Fig. 39.12).[60] Gold treatment may elicit a hypersensitivity response, diffuse alveolar damage, pulmonary fibrosis, organizing pneumonia, and constrictive bronchiolitis. It has been suggested that the pulmonary effects of gold treatment can be differentiated from those produced by RA.[61] However, there is considerable overlap between the two, and HRCT alone cannot distinguish between them.

Penicillamine is used to treat RA, and it is associated with constrictive bronchiolitis, but debate exists whether this is a true association or whether the constrictive bronchiolitis is related to RA alone.[62]

ULTRASONOGRAPHY

Doppler echocardiography is a noninvasive method for diagnosing pulmonary hypertension.[36] Thoracic ultrasonography may be useful for assessing pleural effusions and localizing the optimal site for thoracentesis.

IMAGING ALGORITHMS

The chest radiograph is a useful first-line investigation for symptomatic thoracic disease in RA because it may reveal a pleural effusion or evidence of ILD. A normal chest radiograph does not exclude diffuse interstitial or airway disease, and HRCT may be helpful. Echocardiography should be performed to investigate for pulmonary hypertension, and even in the presence of normal HRCT findings, a decreased DLCO may alert the clinician to the presence of a subtle pulmonary vasculopathy.

Differential Diagnosis

FROM CLINICAL DATA

Both rheumatologic and nonrheumatologic diseases are included in the differential diagnosis for RA, and there is considerable clinical overlap between CTDs. A diagnosis other than RA should be considered in patients with asymmetric arthritis, a migrating pattern of joint disease, predominantly large-joint arthritis, distal interphalangeal involvement, rash, thoracic or lumbar vertebral pain, renal disease, RF-negative status, hypocomplementemia, or the lack of development of erosions on joint radiographs.

FROM SUPPORTIVE DIAGNOSTIC TECHNIQUES

Rheumatoid factor refers to a series of antibodies that recognize the Fc portion of an immunoglobulin G molecule as their antigen. These antibodies probably developed as a mechanism to remove immune complexes from the circulation, and therefore many conditions characterized by chronic inflammation are associated with RF positivity, most notably systemic lupus erythematosus and mixed cryoglobulinemia. Of patients with RA, positive RF occurs in approximately 70% to 80%. Patients with ILD have been reported to have increased serum and lavage RF titers. The extent and severity of lung fibrosis in RA have been shown to relate to the RF titer, but the exact pathogenic role of RF in the lung remains obscure.

More recently, antibodies to citrullinated peptides and proteins have been evaluated with a similar sensitivity to identifying cases of RA but with much higher specificity (95%–98%). The high degree of specificity is greatest in patients with anti–cyclic citrullinated peptide (CCP) antibodies (ACPA) at least three times the upper limit of normal.[63]

Synopsis of Treatment Options

- Analgesics—for instance, nonsteroidal antiinflammatory drugs
- Corticosteroids
- Disease-modifying antirheumatic drugs—for instance, gold, azathioprine, D-penicillamine, methotrexate
- Immunomodulation—for instance, B-cell depletion
- Angiogenesis inhibitors
- Gene therapy
- Antiinflammatory cytokines—for instance, anti–tumor necrosis factor

KEY POINTS

- Rheumatoid arthritis affects 1% of the worldwide population.
- Rheumatoid arthritis is two to three times more common in women, but pleural effusions, interstitial fibrosis, and necrobiotic nodules are more frequent in men.
- Pleural disease, including effusions and pleural thickening, is the most common thoracic manifestation but is frequently asymptomatic.
- "Pleuritis" is the most common pulmonary symptom seen in rheumatoid arthritis (RA).
- Parenchymal lung disease is frequent in RA patients and a common cause of death in affected patients but may be subclinical as well.
- In a few patients (10%) pulmonary symptoms predate the arthropathy.
- There is a wide spectrum of pulmonary diseases in RA, and they are not mutually exclusive. Approximately a third of patients have fibrotic lung disease.
- Rheumatoid factor positivity is associated with more severe pulmonary disease, extraarticular manifestations, and increased mortality.
- Smoking cigarettes has a synergistic effect with RA, and patients who smoke appear to have more severe pulmonary and articular disease.
- Interstitial lung disease is slightly more commonly usual interstitial pneumonia than nonspecific interstitial pneumonia; occasionally, organizing pneumonia is seen.
- Other common findings include bronchiectasis, constrictive bronchiolitis, follicular bronchiolitis, vasculitis, and pulmonary arterial hypertension.
- Necrobiotic pulmonary nodules are rare, and a solitary nodule in an RA patient is more likely to be lung cancer than necrobiotic.

SUGGESTED READINGS

Chansakul T, et al. Intra-thoracic rheumatoid arthritis: imaging spectrum of typical findings and treatment related complications. *Eur J Radiol.* 2015;84(10):1981–1991.

Tanaka N, Kim JS, Newell JD, et al. Rheumatoid arthritis–related lung diseases: CT findings. *Radiology*. 2004;232:81–91.

The full reference list for this chapter is available at ExpertConsult.com.

40 Systemic Sclerosis (Scleroderma)*

BRENT P. LITTLE

Etiology

Systemic sclerosis (scleroderma) has three cardinal features: excessive collagen production, vascular damage, and inflammation/autoimmunity. The pathogenesis of systemic sclerosis is obscure, but there are several contributing factors, including genetic, environmental, and autoimmune influences. Familial aggregation for systemic sclerosis, although infrequent (1.2%–1.5% of families), has been established and lays a firmer foundation for genetic studies of its etiopathogenesis.[1]

Systemic sclerosis is considered to be an autoimmune process, possibly resulting from deleterious effects of cytokines on extracellular matrix proteins and tissue healing.[2] Some studies have also implicated cellular microchimerism in its pathogenesis. Microchimerism results from persistence of fetal cells in the maternal circulation from previous pregnancies. The demonstration of fetal $CD3^+$ T cells in the maternal circulation and fetal cells in affected tissues suggests that microchimerism may, in some patients, initiate a graft-versus-host–like response that results in systemic sclerosis.[3]

Prevalence and Epidemiology

Systemic sclerosis is uncommon, with an annual incidence of 20 per million population per year and an estimated prevalence of 500 cases per million population.[4] The incidence of systemic sclerosis increases with age, and it most frequently affects women in their childbearing years. There is no overall racial predilection.[5] Systemic sclerosis is associated with significant mortality,[6–8] and approximately a third of patients die within 10 years of diagnosis. Variables that best predict reduced survival include older age (>64 years), reduced renal function, anemia, reduced gas diffusing capacity for carbon monoxide (DLCO), reduced total serum protein level, and decreased pulmonary reserve (forced vital capacity).[9] Individuals with anticentromere antibody (ACA) have a better prognosis than those with anti–topoisomerase I (Scl-70) antibody.[10] The poorer prognosis of those with anti–Scl-70 probably relates to the fact that fibrotic lung disease is more likely to develop in these patients and to be manifested as diffuse systemic sclerosis.

Clinical Presentation

Only 1% of patients initially have respiratory symptoms,[11] usually shortness of breath on exertion, but in established disease, dyspnea is the most common pulmonary symptom in systemic sclerosis and occurs in about 60% of patients.[11] Approximately 16% of patients with systemic sclerosis have pleuritic chest pain at some time in their disease. Unlike patients with rheumatoid arthritis or systemic lupus erythematosus, clinically significant pleural effusion rarely develops in patients with systemic sclerosis.[12] Nevertheless, pleural fibrosis and adhesions are frequently identified at autopsy.[13]

Approximately 41% of patients with systemic sclerosis have pulmonary hypertension,[14] and dyspnea on exertion is usually the first symptom of pulmonary hypertension. The risk for pulmonary hypertension in patients with systemic sclerosis increases with the age at disease onset[15]; gas diffusing capacity may be significantly decreased for many years before the diagnosis of pulmonary hypertension is made (perhaps indicating subclinical disease).[16]

Cardiac symptoms reflect a wide range of possible involvement: right-left ventricular dysfunction (fatigue), pulmonary hypertension (dyspnea), congestive heart failure (edema), pericarditis/angina (chest pain), autonomic dysfunction (palpitations), and rhythm disturbances and conduction defects (dizziness, syncope, sudden death).[17]

Gastrointestinal symptoms, particularly swallowing difficulties, are common. The severity of esophageal motor involvement in systemic sclerosis has been shown to correlate with the severity of pulmonary manifestations of the disease (quantified by decreased DLCO) and evidence of interstitial lung disease on high-resolution computed tomography (HRCT).[18] This may be due to the fact that there is a relationship between gastroesophageal reflux and interstitial lung disease, but an alternative explanation is that they both reflect the severity of the systemic vasculopathy.[18] Systemic sclerosis is accompanied by joint pain in 15% of patients and by inflammatory myopathy in 10% of patients. Muscle weakness, cutaneous pruritus, and Raynaud phenomenon are common.[13] Renal failure can be manifested as hypertensive/normotensive renal failure or as an abrupt onset of a renal emergency.[19]

Scleroderma can be localized to the skin or be systemic. Systemic disease is further divided into limited cutaneous and diffuse cutaneous types. *Limited cutaneous systemic sclerosis* encompasses the now outdated term "CREST variant" (*c*alcinosis, *R*aynaud disease, *e*sophageal dysmotility, *s*clerodactyly, and *t*elangiectasia). Limited cutaneous systemic sclerosis is defined by skin thickening in areas distal to the elbows and knees, with or without facial scleroderma. By contrast, *diffuse cutaneous systemic sclerosis* is defined by the presence of skin thickening proximal as well as distal to the elbows and knees, with or without facial or truncal disease.[20] Although lung involvement occurs more frequently in the diffuse form of systemic sclerosis, it is evident in approximately a third of patients with limited cutaneous disease.[21]

*The editors and the publisher would like to thank Drs. Maureen Quigley and David M. Hansell for contributing material on this topic to the prior edition of this work. It has served as the foundation for the current chapter.

Pathophysiology

PATHOLOGY

Scleroderma is characterized by fibrosis and vascular obliteration of the skin, gastrointestinal tract, lungs, heart, and kidneys. The lungs are the second most common site of visceral involvement, and pulmonary disease is a major cause of death in patients with systemic sclerosis.[22]

The two main pulmonary manifestations are interstitial fibrosis and pulmonary hypertension; the latter reflects a primary vasculopathy, but it may be secondary to cardiac or pulmonary disease. A postmortem study has reported that three quarters of patients with systemic sclerosis had interstitial fibrosis.[13] Pulmonary fibrosis has been estimated to ultimately develop in 80% of patients with systemic sclerosis and pulmonary arterial hypertension in 50% of cases.[23] Patients with systemic sclerosis generally fall into one of two categories: those in whom fibrotic lung disease develops and who have anti–Scl-70 antibodies (and in whom pulmonary hypertension may develop secondary to their heart or lung disease) and those who have solely pulmonary hypertension and positive serology for ACA.[24] Of interest, ACA and anti–Scl-70 antibodies are almost always mutually exclusive, being simultaneously present in less than 0.5% of patients with systemic sclerosis. Patients with diffuse cutaneous systemic sclerosis and anti–Scl-70 antibody are at especially high risk for fibrotic lung disease.[25]

The most frequent histologic subtype of pulmonary fibrosis is nonspecific interstitial pneumonia (NSIP). A review of lung biopsy specimens taken from patients with systemic sclerosis found that more than 75% of this cohort had NSIP on histologic review.[26] The high frequency of NSIP in this study can probably be extrapolated to a wider population of patients with systemic sclerosis who have not undergone lung biopsy.[27] The prevalence of usual interstitial pneumonia (UIP) in the systemic sclerosis population has been estimated to be less than 10%.[26,27] There are case reports of diffuse alveolar damage in systemic sclerosis, but it is rare.[28] A few cases of diffuse alveolar hemorrhage have also been reported; in most instances the diffuse alveolar hemorrhage occurs in the setting of preexisting fibrotic lung disease.[29,30]

Cardiac involvement is virtually always present to some degree in the form of patchy myocardial fibrosis, sometimes causing ventricular diastolic dysfunction.[17] Ventricular systolic dysfunction is also seen in patients with concomitant coronary or hypertensive heart disease. Patients with systemic sclerosis are prone to the development of conduction defects and autonomic cardiac neuropathy.[17]

In a postmortem series, the esophagus was involved in 75% of patients with systemic sclerosis,[13] and at autopsy most organs show evidence of patchy fibrosis or atrophy, or both.

LUNG FUNCTION

In systemic sclerosis, a diffusing capacity (DLCO) of 50% or less of predicted and reduced spirometric reserve predict reduced survival.[9] Diminished diffusing capacity is the earliest detectable pulmonary function abnormality in patients with systemic sclerosis, and it correlates with clinical symptoms of dyspnea and the presence of pulmonary fibrosis.[31] The diffusing capacity can be reduced because of pulmonary fibrosis or vasculopathy. Reduced diffusing capacity is the best predictor of the extent of fibrotic lung disease in systemic sclerosis.[32]

Manifestations of the Disease

The hallmark of systemic sclerosis is thickened skin. In diffuse scleroderma with facial involvement, a cardinal sign is exaggerated radial furrowing around the lips (tobacco pouch sign). Skin thickening starts with the fingers and hands in virtually all cases; progression of the skin tightening and thickening is variable. Calcinosis is seen over the periarticular surfaces of the hands, elbows, and knees. Telangiectases occur on the hands, face, lips and gastrointestinal mucosal surfaces. The cutaneous macules are a harmless cosmetic problem, but those in the gastrointestinal tract can bleed and lead to iron deficiency anemia.[19] Patients with systemic sclerosis commonly have Raynaud phenomenon (reversible vasomotor instability precipitated by cold or emotion). It is usually manifested as changes in color of the extremities (pallor to cyanosis and eventually erythema).

RADIOGRAPHY

The most frequent abnormality on chest radiography is a widespread, symmetric basal reticulonodular pattern (Fig. 40.1).[33] Depending on the severity of the pulmonary fibrosis, honeycombing, reduced lung volumes, and traction bronchiectasis can be appreciated on the chest radiograph. However, as with all interstitial lung disease, chest radiography lacks the sensitivity of HRCT for the detection of limited parenchymal disease.[27,34] A dilated air-filled esophagus can be identified in many patients (see Fig. 40.1).[35] Because there is no anatomic obstruction, a fluid level is not usually a feature on erect chest radiographs.

COMPUTED TOMOGRAPHY

The majority of patients with fibrosing lung disease and systemic sclerosis have a histologic pattern of NSIP rather than UIP (Fig. 40.2; see Fig. 40.1). Evidence for this comes from both histopathologic and radiologic studies.[26]

The typical HRCT appearances of NSIP consist of predominantly ground-glass opacities involving mainly the lower lung zones and often mainly the subpleural regions, reticulation, architectural distortion (traction bronchiectasis and volume loss), and occasional limited honeycombing.[36–38] Although ground-glass opacities may initially be the predominant or only abnormality, over time, progressive reticulation, traction bronchiectasis, traction bronchiolectasis, and, less commonly, areas of honeycombing tend to develop (see Fig. 40.2). In many patients traction bronchiectasis is a predominant abnormality. In patients with symptomatic pulmonary involvement in systemic sclerosis, pulmonary fibrosis and ground-glass opacity are common findings, with honeycombing seen more frequently in the limited than the diffuse cutaneous form of systemic sclerosis subtypes.[39] The extent of involvement at HRCT correlates with patient prognosis in systemic sclerosis; in an important study, patients with less than 20% involvement of the lungs had an average 10-year survival of 67%, whereas a group with greater than 20% involvement had an average survival of 43%.[40]

Lymphadenopathy is frequent in patients with systemic sclerosis and interstitial lung disease, and the degree of lymph node enlargement is related to the extent, but not the type, of interstitial disease.[41]

In patients with isolated pulmonary arterial hypertension (and limited scleroderma), evidence of raised pulmonary artery

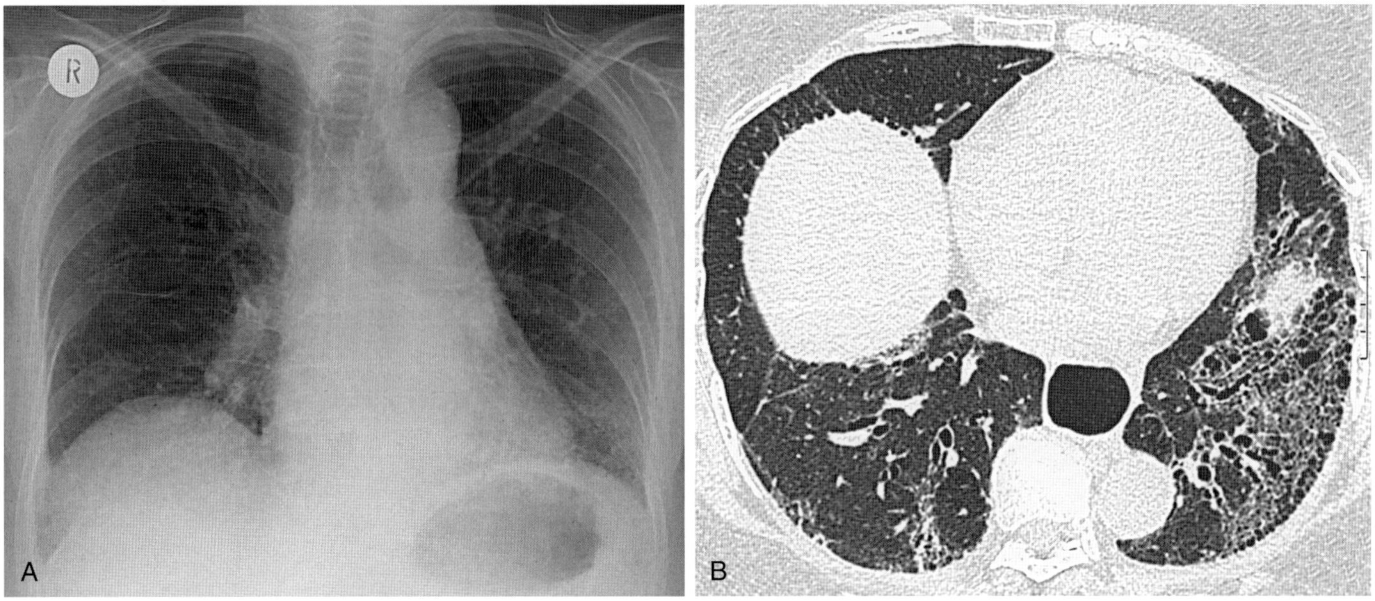

Fig. 40.1 (A) Systemic sclerosis: radiographic and high-resolution computed tomography (HRCT) findings. Posteroanterior chest radiograph shows left greater than right lower lung zone reticular pattern with decreased lung volumes. Note an air-filled tubular structure in the left paratracheal region caused by a dilated esophagus. (B) HRCT shows ground-glass opacities, extensive reticulation, and traction bronchiectasis and bronchiolectasis in the left lower lobe. Mild fibrosis is seen in the right lower and middle lobes and lingula, along with minimal bilateral subpleural honeycombing. The parenchymal findings were confirmed to be nonspecific interstitial pneumonia. Note the dilated air-filled esophagus.

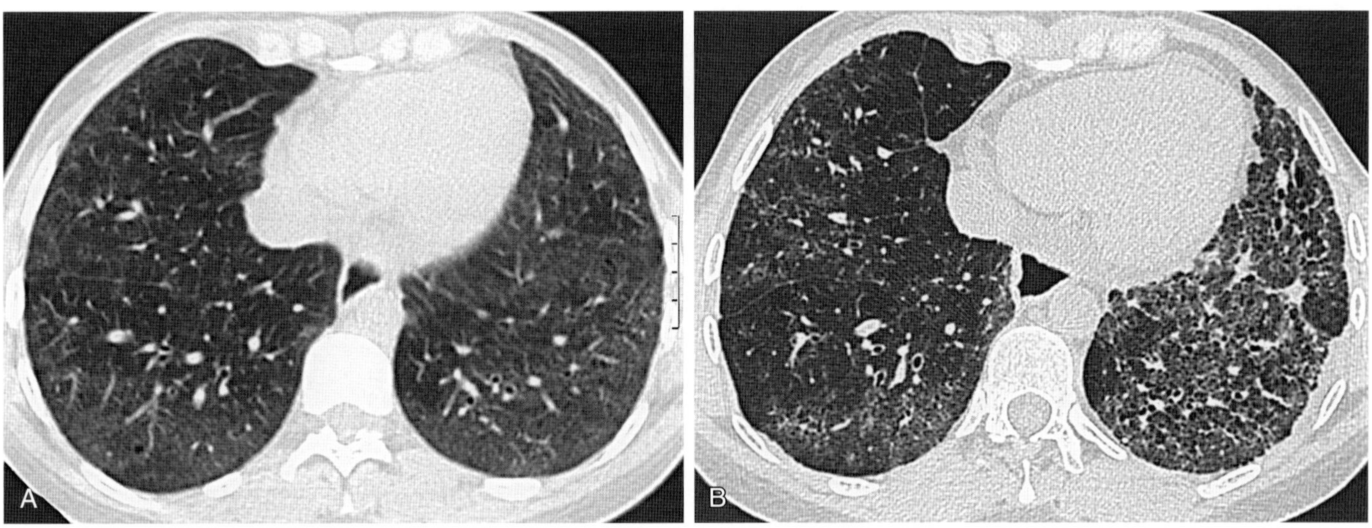

Fig. 40.2 (A) Nonspecific interstitial pneumonia in systemic sclerosis. High-resolution computed tomography (HRCT) shows diffuse bilateral ground-glass opacities. Note the minimal bilateral peripheral reticulation and dilated esophagus. (B) HRCT approximately 10 years later shows extensive reticulation and traction bronchiectasis superimposed on the ground-glass opacities, consistent with progressive fibrosis.

pressure may be a diameter of the main pulmonary artery greater than 3.2 cm, or a diameter larger than that of the adjacent ascending aorta (Fig. 40.3)[42]; however, a nondilated pulmonary artery does not necessarily exclude pulmonary hypertension.

A number of studies have shown an increased risk for lung cancer (usually adenocarcinoma) in patients with systemic sclerosis, including nonsmokers,[43–45] and this is relevant in the evaluation of incidental pulmonary nodules.

There are a few isolated case reports of diffuse alveolar damage[28] and diffuse alveolar hemorrhage[29,30] in patients with systemic sclerosis, and both diseases have similar and nonspecific appearances on HRCT (widespread consolidation and/or ground-glass opacities).

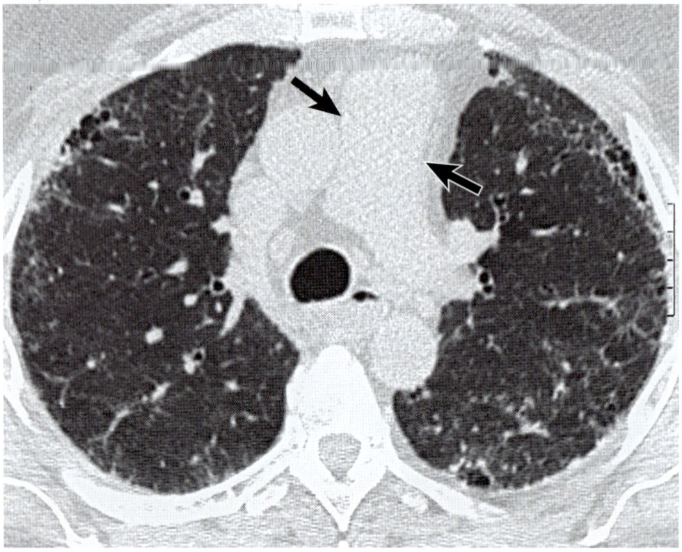

Fig. 40.3 Pulmonary hypertension confirmed by right heart catheterization with fibrotic lung disease in systemic sclerosis. CT shows bilateral ground-glass opacities and peripheral predominant reticulation and minimal honeycombing, consistent with interstitial fibrosis. The diameter of the pulmonary artery *(arrows)* is greater than that of the adjacent ascending aorta, indicating pulmonary hypertension.

KEY POINTS: MANIFESTATIONS OF SYSTEMIC SCLEROSIS ON HIGH-RESOLUTION COMPUTED TOMOGRAPHY

- Pulmonary fibrosis: fibrotic nonspecific interstitial pneumonia is the most common pattern
- Ground-glass opacities with extensive traction bronchiectasis
- Fine reticular pattern or limited honeycombing (subpleural and basal)
- Dilated esophagus
- Dilated main pulmonary artery
- Mediastinal and hilar lymphadenopathy
- Consolidation possible as a result of infection, aspiration, organizing pneumonia, diffuse alveolar damage, or occasionally diffuse pulmonary hemorrhage

CLASSIC SIGNS

The Diagnostic and Therapeutic Criteria Committee of the American Rheumatism Association proposed preliminary criteria for systemic sclerosis in 1980. Proximal scleroderma was the single major criterion and had a sensitivity of 91% and a specificity of 99%. Sclerodactyly, digital pitting scars of the fingertips or loss of substance of the distal finger pad and basal pulmonary fibrosis were further minor criteria in the absence of proximal scleroderma.[46] Updated criteria were published in 2013 by the American College of Rheumatology and the European League Against Rheumatism. Similar to the prior criteria, skin thickening of the fingers extending proximal to the metacarpophalangeal joints is sufficient for a diagnosis of scleroderma. However, several additional criteria were added to increase sensitivity for early or mild scleroderma cases, including nail fold capillary abnormalities, and presence of autoantibodies (anti–Scl-70, anticentromere, and anti–ribonucleic acid polymerase III).[47]

Differential Diagnosis

The differential diagnosis of systemic sclerosis includes connective tissue diseases, such as rheumatoid arthritis, mixed connective tissue disease, and overlap syndromes with other connective tissue diseases. The serologic autoantibody profile is important in all autoimmune diseases. ACA is associated with limited cutaneous involvement in systemic sclerosis.[1] It is relatively specific for scleroderma and in one study had a sensitivity of 32%.[48] This antibody is rarely found in healthy patients, and its presence in "normal" sera may predict the future development of systemic sclerosis.[1] ACAs are associated with isolated pulmonary hypertension secondary to a proliferative vasculopathy,[49] and anti–Scl-70 antibodies are associated with the severity and presence of pulmonary fibrosis.[3]

The antinucleolar system is also a heterogeneous group of antibodies that are not routinely screened for, but anti–PM-Scl antibodies are found in 50% of patients with overlap of scleroderma and dermatomyositis.[50] They are less frequently seen in patients with "pure" systemic sclerosis (3%–8% of patients)[4]; their presence can predict limited cutaneous involvement.[5]

Granulocytosis on bronchoalveolar lavage has been shown to predict progression of fibrotic lung disease with deterioration of lung function, which is most sensitively monitored by measurements of DLCO.[25]

Treatment

Immunosuppressive or immunomodulatory agents are often used as systemic disease-modifying therapies. Cyclophosphamide and mycophenolate mofetil have shown modest benefit in systemic disease; cyclophosphamide treatment led to a slower progression of measures of fibrosis at HRCT than did patients treated with placebo in the landmark Scleroderma Lung Study.[51,52] Organ-based therapies targeted to specific symptoms include proton-pump inhibitors and H1-blockers for gastroesophageal reflux, vasodilators and calcium channel blockers for digital ulcers, and angiotensin-converting enzyme inhibitors for renal and cardiovascular disease. Additional therapies under consideration include stem cell transplantation and monoclonal antibodies.[53]

KEY POINTS

- Lung involvement occurs in a majority of patients with scleroderma.
- Patients with systemic sclerosis and pulmonary involvement have one of two patterns: (1) fibrotic lung disease with or without secondary pulmonary arterial hypertension or (2) "primary" pulmonary arterial hypertension without fibrotic lung disease. The patient's autoantibody profile determines whether pattern 1 or 2 is more likely.
- Fibrotic lung disease is seen in approximately 80% of patients and usually manifests with a nonspecific interstitial pneumonia pattern; a usual interstitial pneumonia pattern is uncommon.
- Patients with systemic sclerosis have an increased incidence of lung cancer.

SUGGESTED READINGS

Ahuja J, Arora D, Kanne JP, et al. Imaging of pulmonary manifestations of connective tissue diseases. *Radiol Clin North Am.* 2016;54(6):1015–1031.

Arroliga AC, Podell DN, Matthay RA. Pulmonary manifestations of scleroderma. *J Thorac Imaging.* 1992;7:30–45.

Bolster MB, Silver RM. Lung disease in systemic sclerosis (scleroderma). *Baillieres Clin Rheumatol.* 1993;7:79–97.

Goldin JG, Lynch DA, Strollo DC, et al. High-resolution CT scan findings in patients with symptomatic scleroderma-related interstitial lung disease. *Chest.* 2008;134(2):358–367.

The full reference list for this chapter is available at ExpertConsult.com.

41 Systemic Lupus Erythematosus*

BRENT P. LITTLE

Etiology

The pathogenesis of systemic lupus erythematosus (SLE) involves genetic and environmental factors, hormonal influences, and cell-mediated responses. In SLE, B lymphocytes lose self-tolerance and inappropriately produce autoantibodies. Serologic positivity for antinuclear antibodies (ANAs) is found in nearly all patients,[1] but anti–deoxyribonucleic acid (DNA) antibodies, although less frequent than ANAs, are far more specific for SLE. A high titer of anti–double-stranded DNA (dsDNA) is considered the best marker of disease activity in SLE.[2]

Genetic evidence for a hereditary tendency comes from the concordance rate in monozygotic twins (≈25% vs. 2% in dizygotic pairs).[3] The search for lupus susceptibility genes has uncovered considerable genetic variance, and human leukocyte antigen associations vary according to ethnicity.[4]

Apoptosis (the process of cell death precipitated by various insults) is thought to be crucial to the development of SLE. The autoimmunity of SLE is suspected to be triggered by exposure to both Epstein-Barr virus and cytomegalovirus.[5,6] Sex hormones may have a role in developing or modulating SLE because the disease primarily affects women of childbearing age and is exacerbated by estrogen in lupus-prone mice.[7]

Prevalence and Epidemiology

The prevalence of SLE ranges from 17 to 48 per 100,000 population.[8] Most patients are female (female-to-male ratio, 8 : 1) and between the ages of 15 and 45 years.[9] During childhood and after menopause the female-to-male ratio is closer to 2 : 1. Survival statistics have improved in patients with SLE, and in a large cohort of European patients, 92% were found to have survived for 10 years after onset of the disease.[10] The highest mortality is in patients with infections, renal disease, non-Hodgkin lymphoma, and lung cancer. Mortality risk is greatest with female gender, younger age, disease duration of less than 1 year, and African-American ethnicity. Overall, the most frequent causes of mortality in SLE are active disease, thrombotic complications, and infections.[2]

Clinical Presentation

The most frequent symptoms of SLE are arthritis, malar rash, photosensitivity, and neurologic involvement.[2] In the first 5 years after a diagnosis of SLE, the most common cause of death is infection, but after this period thrombotic disease becomes the most frequent cause of mortality.[2] The diagnosis of SLE is often elusive, and it may take up to 2 years from the first manifestations of the disease to make a firm diagnosis of SLE.[2]

Recurrent pleuritic chest pain due to serositis is the most common thoracic symptom in patients with SLE.[11,12] Pulmonary embolism is another common cause of pleuritic chest pain, particularly in those who have antiphospholipid syndrome (see later). Finally, pericarditis and/or pericardial effusion may result in chest pain.

Lower respiratory tract infections can be caused by either common or opportunistic pathogens because patients are frequently immunosuppressed. Patients with lupus can have fulminant respiratory failure; important causes include opportunistic infections, drugs, impaired renal or cardiac function, diffuse alveolar hemorrhage, or lupus pneumonitis.[13]

In autopsy studies chronic pulmonary disease is common in SLE, with some form of pleural or parenchymal disease found in up to 98% of patients; however, chronic pulmonary involvement may be mild and asymptomatic in many patients.[11,14] "Shrinking lung" syndrome—low lung volumes possibly caused by a combination of diaphragmatic weakness and chest wall restriction—can cause progressive chronic dyspnea that can occasionally be fatal.[15]

Antiphospholipid syndrome is common in SLE patients, characterized by vascular thrombosis or obstetric complications (or both), thrombocytopenia, and the presence of certain antibodies, such as anticardiolipin and lupus anticoagulant.[16]

Pulmonary hypertension affects up to 8% of patients with SLE, with half of cases classified as primary and half as secondary pulmonary hypertension in one cohort.[17] Patients with SLE are at increased risk for atherosclerosis, and SLE is an independent risk factor for stroke and myocardial infarction. Women 18 to 44 years of age with SLE are twice as likely as those without lupus to have a myocardial infarction or stroke, and heart failure is nearly four times as likely to develop.[18]

Renal disease affects about a third of patients with SLE and remains one of the most dangerous life-threatening complications.[19] Gastrointestinal involvement commonly results in nonspecific abdominal pain and dyspepsia.[20] Hepatosplenomegaly can fluctuate with disease activity, and although mesenteric vasculitis is very rare, it can be life threatening.[19]

Arthralgia and myalgia occur in most patients with SLE; the classic "Jaccoud arthropathy" affects the hands of up to half of patients with SLE and is characterized by reducible, nonerosive joint deformities with preservation of hand function. Skin involvement in SLE is very common and includes the classic malar rash, discoid rash, and generalized photosensitivity. Sun sensitivity, mouth ulcers, and dry mouth can occur.

Hematologic features include normocytic normochromic anemia, thrombocytopenia, and leukopenia.[21]

Manifestations of neuropsychiatric lupus can include headache, seizures, and psychiatric diagnoses, including depression, psychosis, and neuropathy.

*The editors and the publisher would like to thank Drs. Maureen Quigley and David M. Hansell for contributing material on this topic to the prior edition of this work. It has served as the foundation for the current chapter.

Pathophysiology

PATHOLOGY

Other than infection, "lupus pneumonitis" has been described as the most common acute lung disease in lupus patients. However, the incidence of lupus pneumonitis has likely been overestimated and may be lower than 4% overall; although the condition is characterized by diffuse alveolar damage, many cases of pneumonia and aspiration were found to have been mistaken clinically for lupus pneumonitis in a large autopsy series.[22] When it occurs, lupus pneumonitis has a high mortality of almost 50%.[11] The frequency of acute lupus pneumonitis in hospitalized patients with lupus is up to 6%,[13,23] and the outcome of patients with diffuse alveolar damage is either healing and fibrinolysis or parenchymal scarring; chronic fibrotic lung disease occurs in a subset of patients.[24]

In a description of surgical lung biopsy specimens from two patients with SLE, one demonstrated usual interstitial pneumonia and the other follicular bronchiolitis with a minor component of cellular nonspecific interstitial pneumonia.[25] The proportion of patients with SLE who have primarily fibrotic lung disease has been estimated to be less than 10%.[26] Organizing pneumonia is not a common pulmonary manifestation of SLE.[27–29]

Diffuse alveolar hemorrhage is rare in SLE but has a high mortality rate.[13] Diffuse alveolar hemorrhage in SLE is pathogenetically similar to lupus renal microangiopathy. There are isolated case reports of lymphoid interstitial pneumonia in SLE, usually in the presence of an overlap with Sjögren syndrome.[30,31]

The myopathy of SLE can affect the diaphragm and result in a raised diaphragm and basal atelectasis, the so-called shrinking lung syndrome.[32] There has been much debate concerning the pathogenesis of this phenomenon,[15] and the cause remains controversial. In one study the majority of patients with "shrinking lung" syndrome had normal neuromuscular diaphragmatic function.[33]

There is an association between SLE and certain neoplasms, particularly hematologic malignancies and non-Hodgkin lymphoma and possibly lung and hepatobiliary cancer.[34]

LUNG FUNCTION

A range of pulmonary function abnormalities occur in patients with SLE, and as a generalization, abnormal pulmonary function test results are reported in approximately two-thirds of patients with SLE.[35,36]

Manifestations of the Disease

RADIOGRAPHY

The most common radiographic abnormalities in SLE are the presence of bilateral pleural effusions or pleural thickening (Fig. 41.1) and enlargement of the cardiopericardial silhouette because of pericardial effusion or cardiomegaly. The most common pulmonary finding is consolidation secondary to infection.[12] Other acute manifestations of SLE include pulmonary embolism; acute lupus pneumonitis, which occurs in less than 4% of SLE patients; and pulmonary hemorrhage, which occurs in less than 2% of patients.[12]

In acute lupus pneumonitis the chest radiograph often shows unilateral or bilateral hazy pulmonary opacities or consolidation, predominantly in the lower zones (Fig. 41.2).[13] Bacterial pneumonia can have an identical appearance.[12] The manifestations of pulmonary hemorrhage usually consist of bilateral ground-glass opacities or consolidation that may be patchy or diffuse (Fig. 41.3).

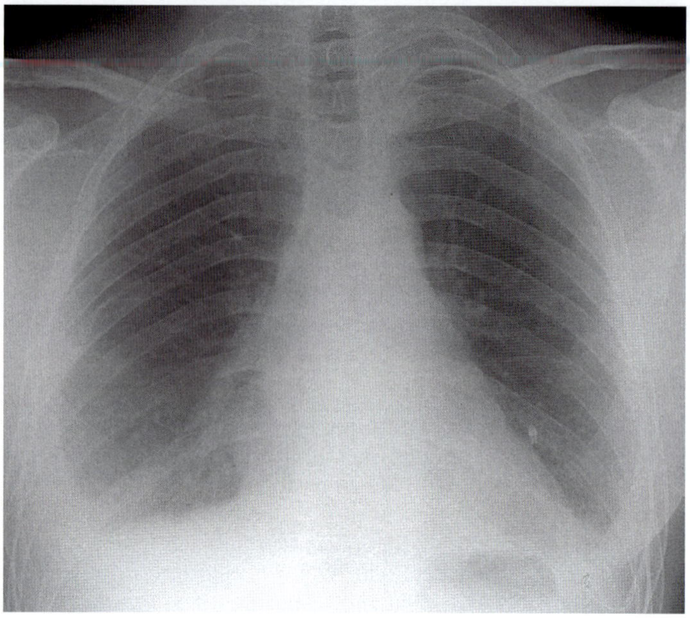

Fig. 41.1 Bilateral pleural effusions in systemic lupus erythematosus. A chest radiograph shows bilateral small pleural effusions (a left-sided pleural catheter is present).

In "shrinking lung" syndrome the chest radiograph and computed tomography (CT) characteristically show elevated hemidiaphragms, adjacent atelectasis, and occasionally, small pleural effusions (Fig. 41.4).[15]

The radiographic manifestations of interstitial disease are usually mild and consist mainly of a reticular pattern in a predominantly basal distribution (Fig. 41.5).

COMPUTED TOMOGRAPHY

There are few high-resolution computed tomography (HRCT) studies of SLE. In a prospective series of 34 consecutive patients with SLE, 70% were found to have HRCT abnormalities.[37] The most frequent CT findings were interstitial lung disease in a third of patients, bronchiectasis in 21%, axillary and mediastinal lymphadenopathy in 18%, and pleuropericardial abnormalities in 15%. The proportion of patients with SLE and interstitial lung disease on HRCT was higher than expected from previous studies, which, based mainly on clinical and radiographic findings, estimated that interstitial fibrosis developed in 3% to 8% of patients with SLE.[12] The bronchiectasis seen in patients with SLE is usually mild and may be due to repeated infections or reflect an occult overlap disease.[38]

Another CT study that focused on lung involvement in patients with SLE excluded all those with pulmonary symptoms or an abnormal chest radiograph.[39] More than a third of patients had abnormalities on HRCT. Bronchial dilation was seen in 18% of subjects, and 13% had pleural irregularities. A third of patients had interlobular septal thickening and intralobular linear opacities, and 22% had architectural distortion. These abnormalities were located mainly in the subpleural and basal lung regions and were interpreted as representing fibrosis (Fig. 41.6).

The proportion of patients with interstitial lung disease is more frequent in SLE patients with respiratory symptoms, up to 60% in

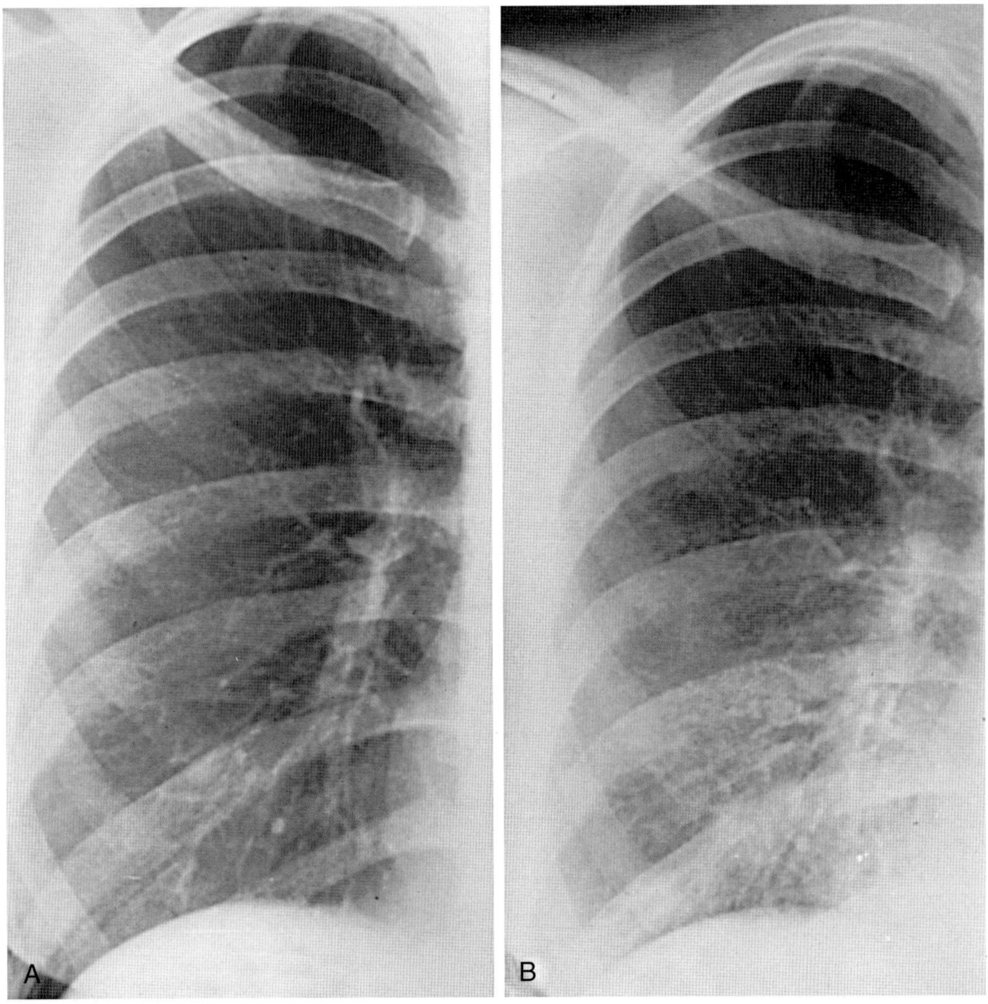

Fig. 41.2 Acute lupus pneumonitis. A detailed view of the right lung from a posteroanterior radiograph (A) is normal. Two days later, after the onset of dyspnea and cough in this patient who had systemic lupus erythematosus (B), the right lung shows increased opacity and poorly defined lung markings in the middle and lower portions of the chest, representing acute noncardiogenic pulmonary edema. Similar features were identified in the left lung. *(From Müller NL, Fraser RS, Colman N, et al.* Radiologic Diagnosis of Diseases of the Chest. *Philadelphia: WB Saunders; 2001.)*

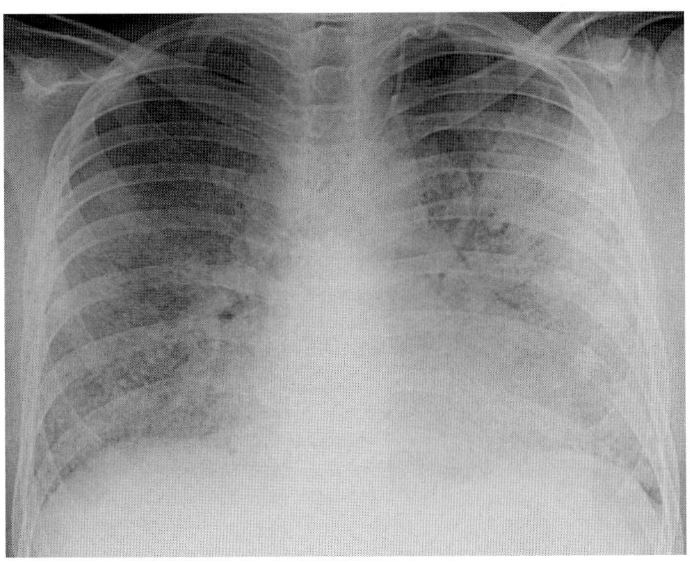

Fig. 41.3 Diffuse pulmonary hemorrhage in a patient with hemoptysis and systemic lupus erythematosus. A chest radiograph shows diffuse left greater than right lung consolidation.

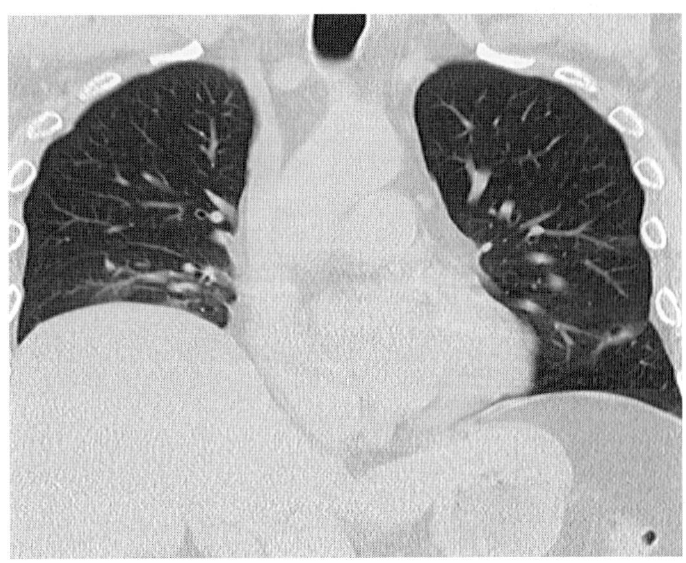

Fig. 41.4 "Shrinking lung" syndrome in systemic lupus erythematosus. A coronal CT image shows elevated hemidiaphragms and adjacent atelectasis. The syndrome refers to the presence of persistently low lung volumes in SLE not explained by parenchymal fibrosis or visible pleural disease.

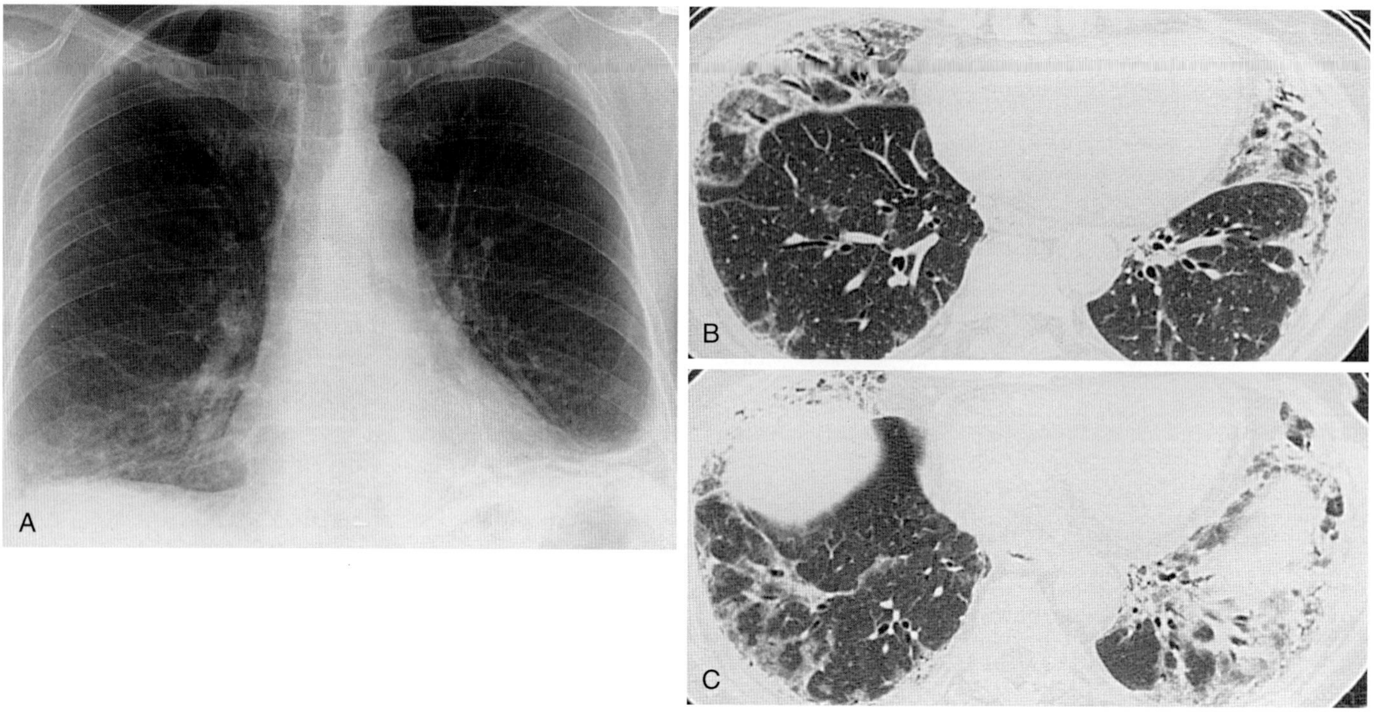

Fig. 41.5 Pulmonary fibrosis in systemic lupus erythematosus. A posteroanterior chest radiograph (A) shows irregular linear opacities in the lower lung zones. High-resolution CT images (B) and (C) show ground-glass opacity, irregular linear opacities, architectural distortion, and traction bronchiectasis indicative of fibrosis. *(From Müller NL, Fraser RS, Colman N, et al.* Radiologic Diagnosis of Diseases of the Chest. *Philadelphia: WB Saunders; 2001.)*

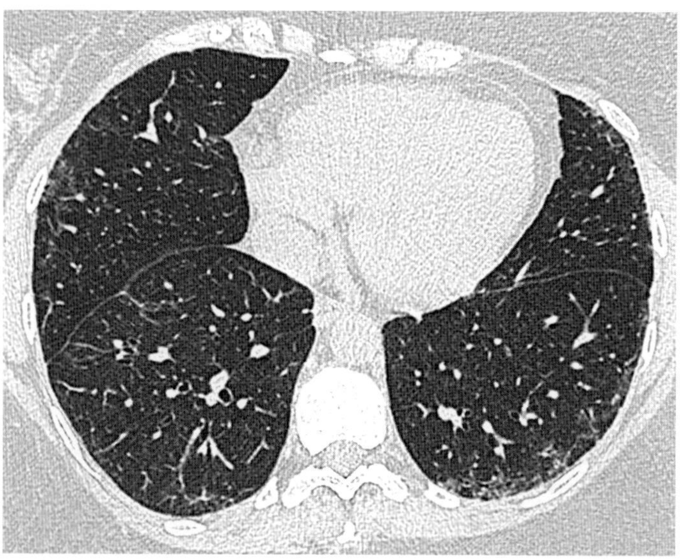

Fig. 41.6 Fibrosis in systemic lupus erythematosus. High-resolution CT in a patient with SLE shows a subpleural, basilar predominant reticular pattern that is suggestive of a fibrotic nonspecific interstitial pneumonia or early usual interstitial pneumonia (UIP) (i.e., probable UIP pattern by Fleischner society criteria).

some studies.[38] Frank honeycombing was not described in the two largest CT studies,[37,39] which may have been due to the fact that both series focused on SLE patients without known lung disease.

The CT appearances of diffuse alveolar hemorrhage are nonspecific and consist of widespread ground-glass opacity and airspace consolidation (Fig. 41.7). The CT features of diffuse alveolar hemorrhage may be indistinguishable from those of pneumonia or diffuse alveolar damage (Fig. 41.8). In acute lupus pneumonitis, extensive ground-glass opacities or confluent consolidation and air bronchograms are evident on HRCT,[40] and the consolidation is often accompanied by pleural effusions[41]; effusions are rarely associated with uncomplicated diffuse alveolar hemorrhage.

More than 50% of patients with SLE have antiphospholipid syndrome and are prone to the development of pulmonary embolism (Fig. 41.9). Most of these patients have deep vein thrombosis, although rarely, pulmonary artery or vein thrombosis may occur.[42,43]

KEY POINTS: COMMON RADIOLOGIC FEATURES OF SYSTEMIC LUPUS ERYTHEMATOSUS

- Pleural effusions or pleural thickening (usually bilateral)
- Pericardial effusion or cardiac enlargement
- Areas of ground-glass opacity and/or consolidation (infection, diffuse alveolar damage, or hemorrhage)
- Low lung volumes with elevated hemidiaphragms ("shrinking lung" syndrome)
- Interstitial fibrosis in a subpleural and basal distribution with only occasional honeycombing on high-resolution CT
- Deep vein thrombosis and pulmonary thromboembolism in the presence of anticardiolipin antibodies and antiphospholipid syndrome
- Enlarged pulmonary trunk secondary to pulmonary hypertension

NUCLEAR MEDICINE

Patients with suspected pulmonary embolism may be evaluated with ventilation-perfusion scintigraphy.

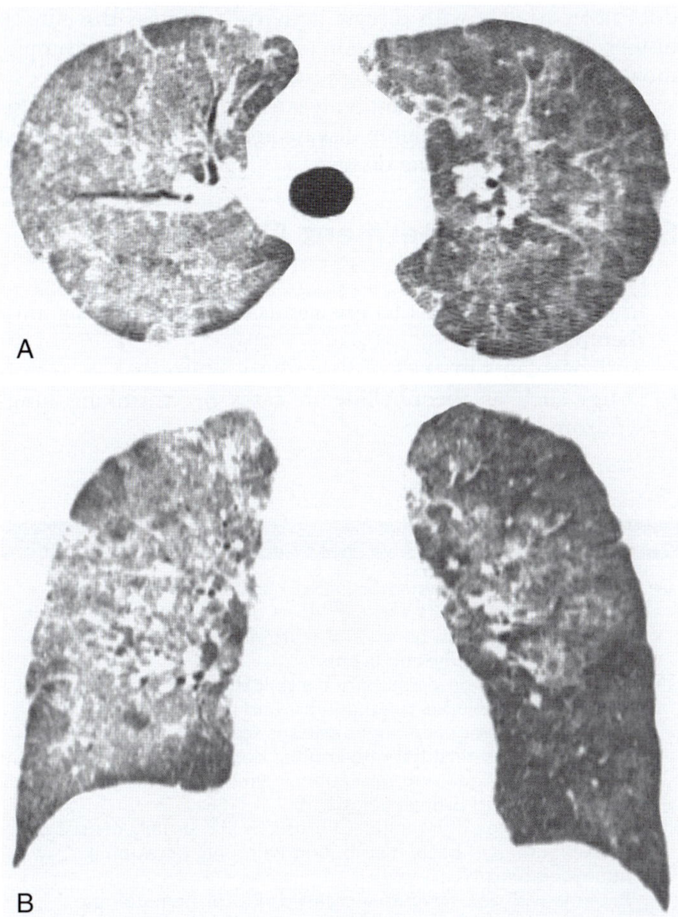

Fig. 41.7 Diffuse pulmonary hemorrhage in systemic lupus erythematosus. (A) Axial CT at the level of the upper lobes shows bilateral ground-glass opacity, patchy consolidation, mild septal thickening, and poorly defined nodular opacities, more severe on the right. (B) A coronal reformatted image demonstrates the overall extent and asymmetric distribution of the findings.

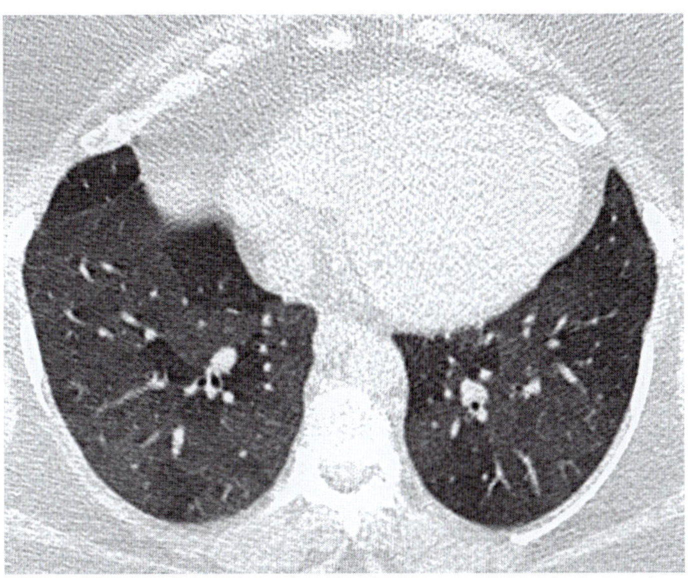

Fig. 41.8 Acute lupus pneumonitis with acute respiratory compromise. High-resolution CT shows widespread ground-glass opacity. Subtle fibrosis eventually developed in the same distribution as the ground-glass opacity.

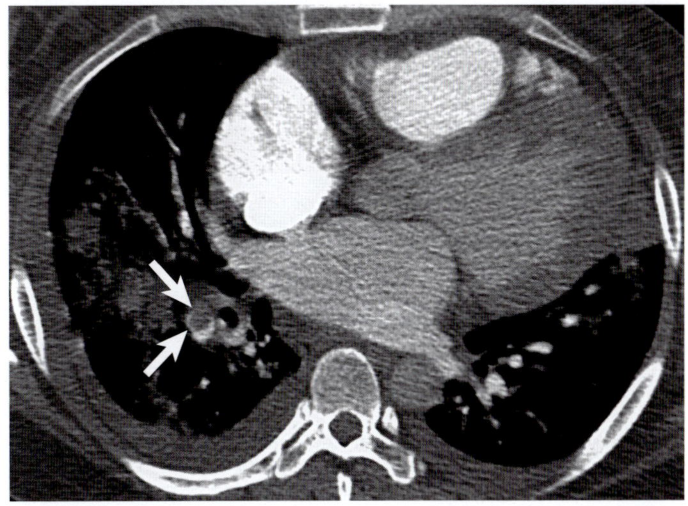

Fig. 41.9 Acute pulmonary embolism in systemic lupus erythematosus with antiphospholipid syndrome. Contrast-enhanced CT demonstrates a filling defect in the right lower lobe pulmonary artery *(arrows)*. Consolidation is secondary to pulmonary hemorrhage. Small bilateral pleural effusions and cardiomegaly are present.

IMAGING ALGORITHMS

A patient with SLE and respiratory symptoms may have a chest radiograph that refines the potentially wide differential diagnosis —for example, showing a pleural effusion or signs of a lower respiratory tract infection—and these findings may not require further imaging. Suspected pulmonary embolism should be investigated by pulmonary CT angiography or ventilation-perfusion scintigraphy. HRCT is the test of choice for the investigation of known or suspected interstitial lung disease.

CLASSIC SIGNS

The American College of Rheumatology diagnostic criteria for systemic lupus erythematosus (SLE) were radically altered in 1982, with more recent minor amendments; satisfaction of any 4 of 11 criteria yields a diagnosis of SLE (Box 41.1). More recently, the Systemic Lupus International Collaborating Clinics (SLICC) group published refinements to the diagnostic criteria; satisfaction of 4 of the revised criteria, including at least 1 immunologic criterion, *or* presence of a biopsy-proven nephritis in the setting of antinuclear antibody or anti–double-stranded deoxyribonucleic acid antibodies is sufficient to establish a diagnosis of SLE.[44]

Differential Diagnosis

FROM CLINICAL DATA

In patients with multiorgan disease, both rheumatic and nonrheumatic illnesses can mimic SLE. The diagnostic criteria and autoantibody profile refine the differential diagnosis but are not definitive. The nonrheumatic processes that mimic SLE are systemic infections and include human immunodeficiency virus infection, mononucleosis, viral polyarthropathy, and poststreptococcal glomerulonephritis.

Lupus can resemble other rheumatic diseases, including rheumatoid arthritis, scleroderma, and mixed connective tissue disease. SLE can also be induced by drugs, most frequently procainamide and hydralazine. Drug-induced lupus typically

BOX 41.1 1982 REVISED CRITERIA FOR THE CLASSIFICATION OF SYSTEMIC LUPUS ERYTHEMATOSUS WITH THE 2005 AMERICAN COLLEGE OF RHEUMATOLOGY RECOMMENDED AMENDMENTS

1. Malar rash: fixed erythema, flat or raised, over the malar eminences; tending to spare the nasolabial folds
2. Discoid rash: erythematous raised patches with scaling and follicular plugging
3. Photosensitivity rash: unusual reactivity to sunlight with rash
4. Oral ulcers: oral or nasopharyngeal ulceration, usually painless
5. Arthritis: nonerosive arthritis involving two or more peripheral joints and characterized by tenderness, swelling, or effusion
6. Serositis: pleuritis or pericarditis
7. Renal disorder: persistent proteinuria or cellular casts—may be red cell, hemoglobin, granular, tubular, or mixed
8. Neurologic disorder seizures or psychosis in the absence of causative drugs
9. Hematologic disorder hemolytic anemia: with reticulosis, leukopenia, lymphopenia, or thrombocytopenia
10. Immunologic disorder anti-DNA antibody to native DNA in abnormal titer or anti-Sm: presence of antibody to Sm nuclear antigen or positive finding of antiphospholipid antibodies based on (1) an abnormal serum level of immunoglobulin (Ig)G or IgM anticardiolipin antibodies, (2) a positive test result for lupus anticoagulant, or (3) false-positive serologic test for syphilis for at least 6 months and confirmed by *Treponema pallidum* immobilization or the fluorescent treponemal antibody absorption test
11. Antinuclear antibodies (ANA): elevated titers of ANA in the absence of drugs known to induce lupus

From Tan EM, Cohen AS, Fries JF, Masi AT, McShane DJ, Rothfeld NF, et al. The 1982 revised criteria for the classification of systemic lupus erythematosus. *Arthritis Rheum*. 1982;25:1271–1277.

starts after prolonged drug administration, and the symptoms usually disappear a few weeks after cessation of administration of the drug. Symptoms of drug-induced lupus include muscle and joint pain, flu-like symptoms, and serositis (patients are frequently ANA positive).

FROM SUPPORTIVE DIAGNOSTIC TECHNIQUES

More than 98% of patients with SLE have elevated ANA. Testing for ANA is especially sensitive for SLE but has low specificity; that is, most individuals with a positive ANA do not have SLE, but most with SLE have a positive ANA. In SLE the ANA titer does not correlate with disease activity,[45] whereas the clinical history, erythrocyte sedimentation rate, anti-dsDNA, and complement levels provide some prognostic information.[46]

A high titer of anti-Sm antibody is a criterion for the diagnosis of SLE, and although highly disease specific, it is encountered in other connective tissue disease.[47]

Synopsis of Treatment Options

- Corticosteroids
- Immunomodulatory therapy agents/disease-modifying antirheumatic drugs
- Anticoagulants in cases of thrombotic episodes
- Drugs such as theophylline in cases of "shrinking lung" syndrome

KEY POINTS

- Systemic lupus erythematosus (SLE) has a wide variety of clinical manifestations and can affect almost any organ system.
- Mortality in SLE can be due to acute disease exacerbations, infections, or thrombotic events.
- The most common pulmonary complications of SLE are infection, acute lupus pneumonitis, and pulmonary embolism. Occasional pulmonary manifestations include interstitial fibrosis (usual interstitial pneumonia, nonspecific interstitial pneumonia), organizing pneumonia, lymphoid interstitial pneumonia, and bronchiectasis.
- The CT findings of interstitial fibrosis in SLE usually consist of a subpleural and basal distribution with only occasional honeycombing.
- Patients with SLE have an increased risk for hematologic malignancies, lymphoma, and lung cancer.
- Many patients without respiratory symptoms have abnormalities on imaging or on physiologic testing, but the majority of these patients have a subclinical course of lung disease.

SUGGESTED READINGS

Manson JJ, Rahman A. Systemic lupus erythematosus. *Orphanet J Rare Dis.* 2006;1:6.

Wiedemann HP, Matthay RA. Pulmonary manifestations of systemic lupus erythematosus. *J Thorac Imaging*. 1992;7:1–18.

The full reference list for this chapter is available at ExpertConsult.com.

42 Polymyositis/Dermatomyositis*

STEPHEN B. HOBBS

Etiology

Immune-mediated muscle inflammation and vascular damage are the hallmarks of polymyositis (PM) and dermatomyositis (DM). In PM the immune system is primed to act against muscle antigens, whereas in DM there is complement-mediated damage to both endomysial vessels and the microvasculature of the dermis. The trigger for the autoimmune malfunction in PM/DM is unknown. As with other connective tissue diseases, B-cell and T-cell autoregulation is disrupted. Viruses have a possible etiologic role, but direct evidence is lacking. However, a seasonal pattern of development of the disorders provides some epidemiologic evidence for an infectious agent having a causative role in PM and DM. In patients with anti–Jo-1 antibodies, weakness is more likely to develop in April, and those with a different autoantibody (anti–signal recognition particle) are more likely to have an onset of weakness in November.[1] Animal models have been used to provide supportive evidence for virally induced myositis,[2] and many different infectious agents have been proposed, including coxsackievirus, parvovirus, enterovirus, human T-lymphotropic virus, and human immunodeficiency virus.[3]

Prevalence and Epidemiology

PM/DM has an incidence of approximately 5 to 10 cases per million per year,[4] and in DM there are two population age peaks: children and young to middle-aged adults.[5] PM affects women more frequently than men (2 : 1 ratio) and has a higher incidence in African Americans than in whites.[6,7] In PM/DM pulmonary disease can overshadow the primary muscle disorder, and patients with PM/DM and interstitial lung disease (ILD) have higher mortality than those with isolated ILD.[8] Estimates of PM/DM-related death rates vary between 10% and 27%,[9–11] and these deaths are usually the consequence of cancer or pulmonary complications. Predictors of poor outcome include old age at onset, male gender, dysphagia, long-standing symptoms before diagnosis or therapy, pulmonary and cardiac involvement, and the presence of anti–Jo-1 antibodies.[9] The majority of survivors have a chronic continuous or polycyclic disease course (80%).[9]

Clinical Presentation

PM and DM are usually considered part of the same disease spectrum, and the main clinical difference is thought to be the prominent lilac "heliotrope" facial rash seen in DM. Nevertheless, DM and PM are pathogenetically distinct. DM is a humorally mediated microangiopathy, whereas PM is a cell-mediated immune response to muscle fibers. However, PM and DM are usually grouped together in many clinical studies, and for the purposes of this discussion they will be frequently considered a single entity.

The onset of PM/DM may be acute or insidious. Acute infection can precede or perhaps incite symptoms; children with juvenile DM frequently have symptoms of systemic illness 3 months before the onset of disease.[12] DM (but not PM) is seen in the pediatric population, and symptoms are similar in children and adults, although childhood onset is more likely to be acute and florid.

The clinical hallmark of PM is proximal muscle weakness with muscle tenderness and myalgia. Patients may also have dyspnea, dysphagia, aspiration pneumonia, fever, weight loss, secondary Sjögren syndrome, Raynaud phenomenon, polyarthritis, and cardiac myopathy. The frequency of ILD is not definitively known in PM/DM patients; however, depending on inclusion criteria and follow-up length, upwards of 75% of patients will have some evidence of ILD.[13] With the use of chest radiography alone, the incidence of ILD in patients with PM/DM has been estimated to be much lower at 9% to 10%, but this likely reflects the lesser sensitivity of radiography than high-resolution CT (HRCT).[14,15] The association between polyarthritis and ILD in PM/DM is well known,[14,16] and the pulmonary manifestations of PM/DM are thought to precede symptoms of the inflammatory myopathy in almost a third of cases.[17] There are various modes of pulmonary involvement, ranging from fulminant and acute (diffuse alveolar damage, pneumonia) to chronic progressive symptoms (fibrotic lung disease, pulmonary hypertension, respiratory muscle weakening). Pulmonary involvement may be asymptomatic.

Patients with established PM/DM are at risk for infection. They are frequently immunosuppressed, and both opportunistic and nonopportunistic infections develop.[18] In one study a majority of PM/DM patients (89%) exhibited an opportunistic infection at some time after the onset of their PM/DM. A variety of organisms were responsible for these infections, but more than half were due to fungi.[10]

Pulmonary hypertension can develop in patients with PM/DM, and in concert with the myositis, which affects the respiratory muscles, the result may be markedly abnormal physiologic parameters even with relatively normal imaging results. The pulmonary hypertension seen in those with PM/DM is usually secondary to ILD, although primary pulmonary vascular disease has been described.[19]

Weakness of the respiratory muscles may lead to respiratory failure; nevertheless, mild respiratory failure has a good prognosis[20] and mechanical ventilation is rarely required for respiratory muscle weakness alone.[14]

Weakness of the laryngeal musculature may cause dysphonia, and esophageal involvement is usually manifested as dysphagia. Esophageal disease is estimated to be present in up to half of patients with inflammatory arthropathy, and the esophageal myopathy can be proximal as a result of striated muscle

*The editors and the publisher would like to thank Drs. Maureen Quigley and David M. Hansell for contributing material on this topic to the prior edition of this work. It has served as the foundation for the current chapter.

involvement or distal as a result of smooth muscle involvement, particularly in overlap connective tissue disease.[21]

Fulminant myositis can precipitate acute renal failure as a consequence of severe rhabdomyolysis and myoglobinuria.

Cutaneous eruptions, which occur in DM, tend to be dusky and erythematous. Periorbital edema with a heliotrope (purplish appearance) hue is pathognomonic for DM. The skin lesions frequently fade completely but may be followed by brownish pigmentation, atrophy, scarring, or vitiligo. Subcutaneous calcification may occur, particularly in childhood DM. This is similar in distribution to that encountered in systemic sclerosis but tends to be more extensive (calcinosis universalis), particularly in untreated or undertreated disease. Polyarthralgia, accompanied at times by joint effusions, joint swelling, and other evidence of nondeforming arthritis, occurs in about 30% of patients but tends to be mild.[22]

Although symptomatic cardiac involvement is not common in PM/DM,[21] it is of prognostic importance.[9,23] Cardiac involvement is recognized as the third leading cause of death in this condition, after sepsis and malignancy.[24] Various cardiac manifestations have been described in the literature, including conduction abnormalities, myocarditis, cardiomyopathy, coronary artery atherosclerosis, valvular disease, and pericardial abnormalities.[25]

There is an association with malignancy and the inflammatory myopathies, but the association is strongest with adult-onset DM.[26] Even though the link was refuted in an analysis of 102 patients with adult-onset DM,[27] more recent evidence from population-based cohort studies has confirmed an association between malignancy and DM and PM.[28] These studies show an even stronger association between PM and malignancy, with recent data confirming that the association of DM and PM with malignancy is not purely due to various biases.[28] The majority of these malignancies are adenocarcinomas, with the strongest correlation with ovarian carcinoma. Other associations include cervical, lung, pancreas, bladder, and gastric adenocarcinomas. Of interest, the peak incidence of cancer diagnosis occurs within the first year of diagnosis of the myopathy. In some patients the diagnosis of cancer occurs during relapse of previously dormant myositis.[29,30]

The classification of PM/DM is potentially confusing. Amyopathic DM is DM without muscle weakness, and although pulmonary fibrosis is uncommon in these patients, isolated case reports do appear.[31] Antisynthetase syndrome occurs in a subgroup of inflammatory myopathy patients who have antisynthetase antibodies; anti–Jo-1 antibody is one of these antisynthetase antibodies. These patients have features similar to those of PM and DM, but they are more likely to have significant ILD. Antisynthetase syndrome is also associated with "mechanic's hands," a condition in which the skin of the patient's fingers is thickened and cracked with accompanying polyarthritis and Raynaud phenomenon.[22]

Pathophysiology

PATHOLOGY

The most common parenchymal lung diseases associated with PM/DM are nonspecific interstitial pneumonia (NSIP), organizing pneumonia (OP), diffuse alveolar damage (DAD), usual interstitial pneumonia (UIP), and alveolar hemorrhage (secondary to capillaritis).[32] In a review of surgical lung biopsy specimens from patients with PM/DM, the predominant histologic process was NSIP.[33] In another series by Douglas and coworkers,[17] 70 patients with PM/DM and ILD were examined. In this group 22 patients underwent surgical lung biopsy, and the majority in this series had NSIP histologically (81%). The remaining patients had DAD, OP, and UIP.

PM/DM patients can progress through the pathologic sequence of DAD, then OP, and finally fibrotic NSIP. The first step is acute epithelial injury, and then organization occurs with the production of intraalveolar buds of granulation tissue (OP).[34] On serial evaluation this patchy consolidation, which is presumed to be OP, may be partially reversible; alternatively, it may progress to reticular abnormality.[35] OP and NSIP are frequently found together on lung biopsy specimens.

Acute ILD in patients with PM/DM may have a rapidly progressive course, and in a study of 81 patients with inflammatory myopathy, 5 had acute ILD and all 5 had died within 6 months of disease onset.[20] These 5 patients had histologically proven DAD, and in all cases the muscle involvement was typical of DM but was classified as mild. Acute ILD in PM/DM has high mortality, and all the patients were seronegative for antisynthetase antibodies. Seronegativity for antisynthetase antibodies is considered a poor prognostic indicator in DAD associated with PM/DM.[20]

Active and healed vasculitis has been demonstrated pathologically in PM/DM.[8] Unlike rheumatoid arthritis and systemic lupus erythematosus, pleural disease is not commonly described, but fibrinous pleuritis has been recorded at autopsy (12%). Pleural effusions were also present in a quarter of cases and were presumed to be secondary to heart failure or malignancy.[8]

LUNG FUNCTION

Lung function testing is useful for the early diagnosis of pulmonary involvement in PM/DM. The earliest abnormality detected is usually a decrease in the diffusing capacity for carbon monoxide (DLCO). A restrictive pattern subsequently develops if pulmonary fibrosis occurs. An important parameter is KCO, defined as the ratio of the rate of DLCO to the accessible alveolar volume (VA). KCO values less than 70% of predicted in a nonsmoker can be helpful in suggesting an occult vasculopathy.[36] In patients with PM, half have a 50% reduction in respiratory muscle strength, and hypercapnia is likely to occur when respiratory muscle strength is less than 30% of normal.[37] The hallmark of respiratory muscle weakness is a reduction in maximum inspiratory and expiratory pressure.[20]

Manifestations of the Disease

Primary thoracic manifestations of PM/DM include one or more of the following ILDs: NSIP, OP, UIP, and DAD. Vascular manifestations include vasculitis, capillaritis/hemorrhage, and pulmonary hypertension. Secondary manifestations include respiratory failure, atelectasis, pneumonia, aspiration, drug-related disorders, heart failure, and various neoplasms.

RADIOGRAPHY

Evidence of ILD, especially OP, may precede the frank myositis and skin lesions.[38,39] In PM/DM chest radiographs commonly demonstrate bilateral irregular linear opacities (reticulation) at the lung bases and occasionally consolidation.[17] In most series of PM/DM the proportion of patients with evidence of ILD on

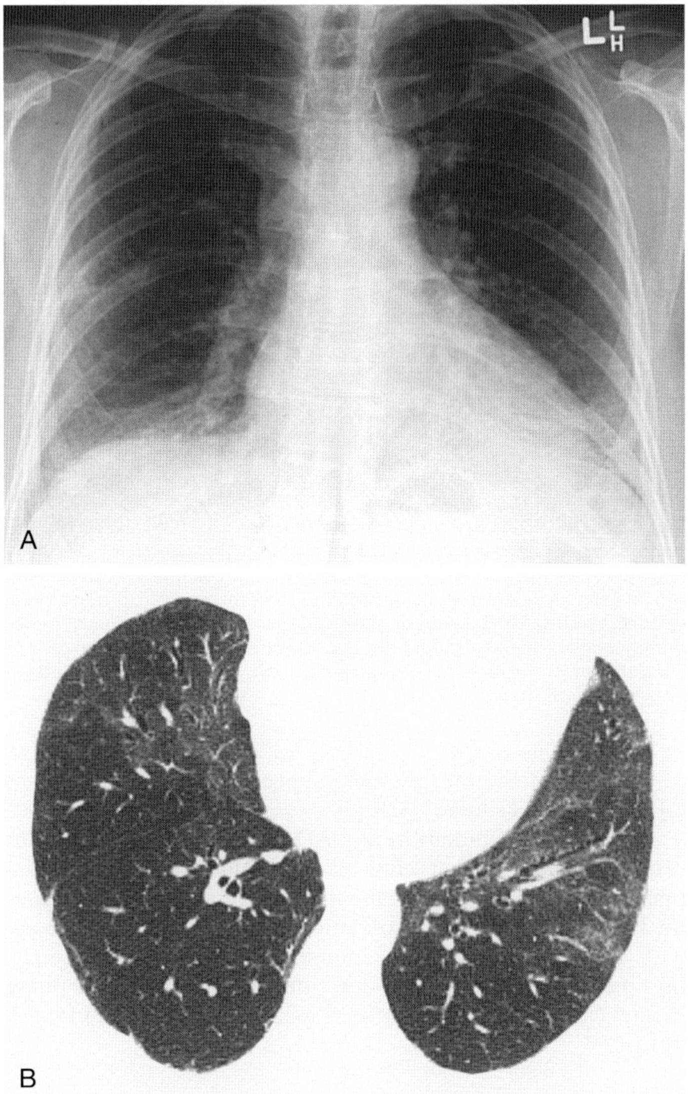

Fig. 42.1 Nonspecific interstitial pneumonia in polymyositis. (A) A chest radiograph shows low lung volumes, hazy increased opacity (ground-glass opacities) in the lower lung zones, and mild basal reticulation. (B) High-resolution CT through the lower lungs shows extensive bilateral ground-glass opacities and minimal reticulation without honeycombing.

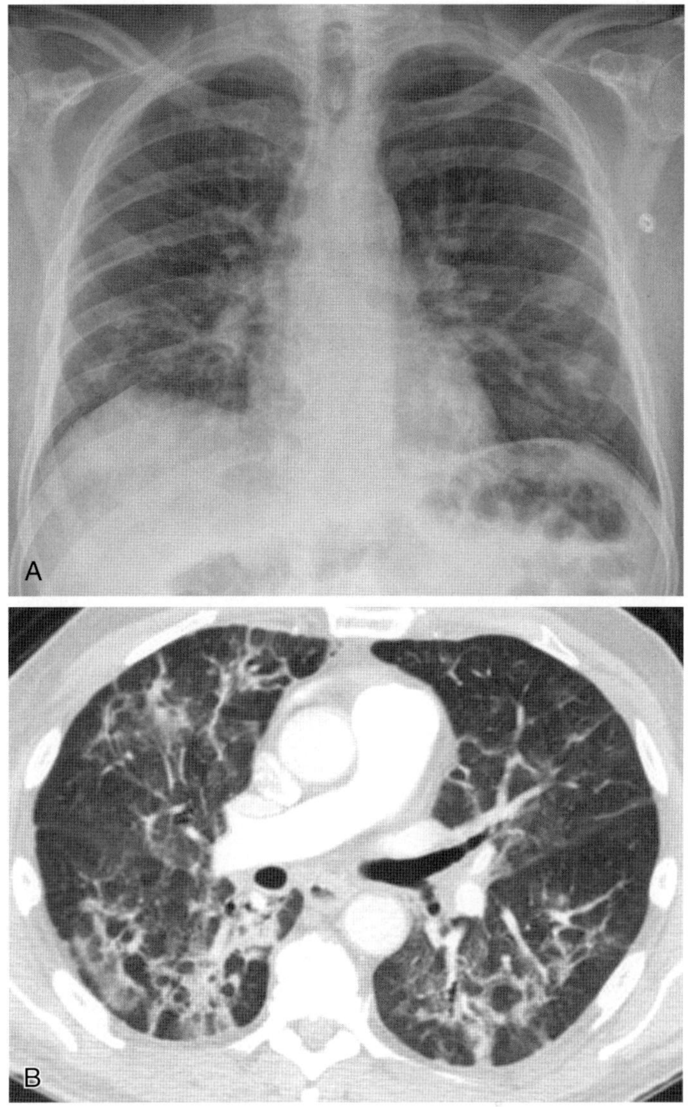

Fig. 42.2 Organizing pneumonia in polymyositis. (A) A chest radiograph shows bilateral areas of consolidation involving mainly the lower lung zones. (B) Axial CT demonstrates bilateral consolidation in a bronchovascular and perilobular distribution.

chest radiography is approximately 10%.[14,15] In one of the largest studies of PM/DM-ILD,[17] abnormalities on chest radiography included irregular linear opacities (95%), consolidation (25%), honeycombing (4%), and pleural effusions (4%). These findings most commonly reflect the presence of NSIP, OP, or DAD.

The most common ILD in patients with PM/DM is NSIP. The main radiographic manifestations of NSIP consist of a reticular pattern and hazy increased opacity (ground-glass opacities) in the lower lung zones (Fig. 42.1). The most frequent manifestations of OP consist of bilateral areas of consolidation that may be patchy, mainly peribronchial or subpleural, and that may involve any lung zone (Fig. 42.2). Patients with PM often have findings of both NSIP and OP radiologically and histologically (Fig. 42.3). DAD is characterized by a sudden onset and rapid progression from ground-glass opacities to extensive bilateral consolidation. The main differential diagnosis of areas of consolidation is aspiration or pneumonia. Pleural disease is relatively uncommon in PM/DM. The majority of pleural effusions seen in these patients are related to heart failure, infection, or malignancy.

COMPUTED TOMOGRAPHY

Abnormalities seen on HRCT in PM/DM include linear opacities (63%), consolidation (53%–100%), ground-glass opacities (43%), and rarely, honeycombing.[17,40] These abnormalities most commonly reflect the presence of NSIP, OP, or DAD. The manifestations of NSIP typically consist of ground-glass opacities with or without superimposed intralobular linear opacities; these findings result in a reticular pattern that is situated mainly in the lower lung zones (Fig. 42.4). The reticulation may be absent (cellular NSIP) or minimal (see Fig. 42.1), but with progression of fibrosis, it can gradually become the predominant finding (fibrotic NSIP). In patients with fibrosis the reticular pattern is typically associated

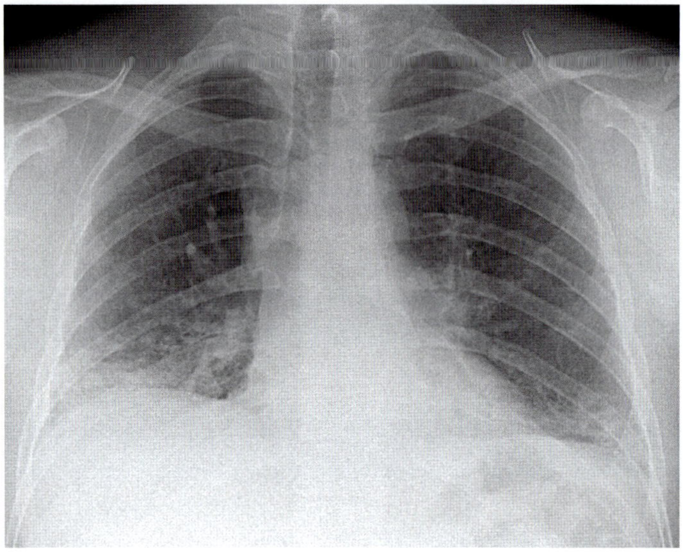

Fig. 42.3 Mixed nonspecific interstitial pneumonia and organizing pneumonia in polymyositis. A chest radiograph shows basal reticulation with volume loss. Also noted are focal areas of consolidation in the right lung base.

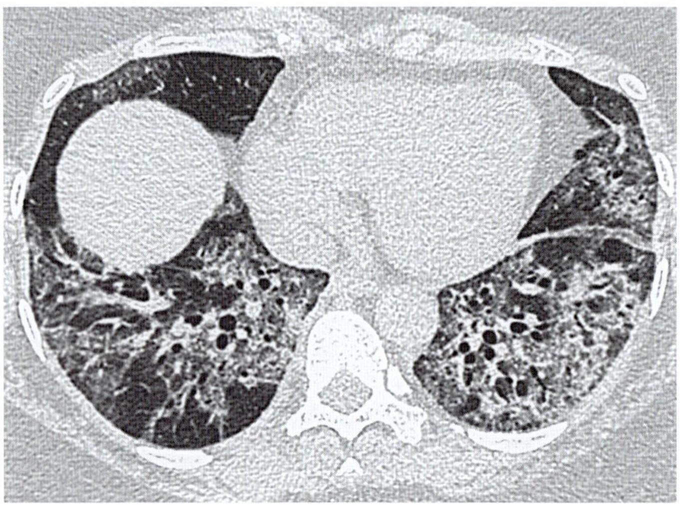

Fig. 42.4 Nonspecific interstitial pneumonia in polymyositis. High-resolution CT shows bilateral ground-glass opacities and mild reticulation.

with architectural distortion, traction bronchiectasis, and traction bronchiolectasis. As mentioned previously, patients with inflammatory myopathies may have CT and histologic features of NSIP and OP simultaneously (Fig. 42.5).

The consolidation in PM/DM is usually presumed to be due to areas of OP, with ground-glass opacities representing either DAD or fine intralobular fibrosis. However, lower respiratory tract infection is an important differential diagnosis in patients with PM/DM.[10] The consolidation on HRCT in patients with OP can be patchy and random but often has a predominantly subpleural (see Fig. 42.2),[40,41] perilobular, or peribronchovascular distribution (see Fig. 42.5).[42] Linear opacities or parenchymal bands are nonspecific and may reflect previous OP or interlobular/intralobular fibrosis. In one study the patchy consolidation, parenchymal bands, and irregular bronchovascular thickening had improved or disappeared in virtually all patients with PM/DM, and although this study lacked pathologic correlation, the

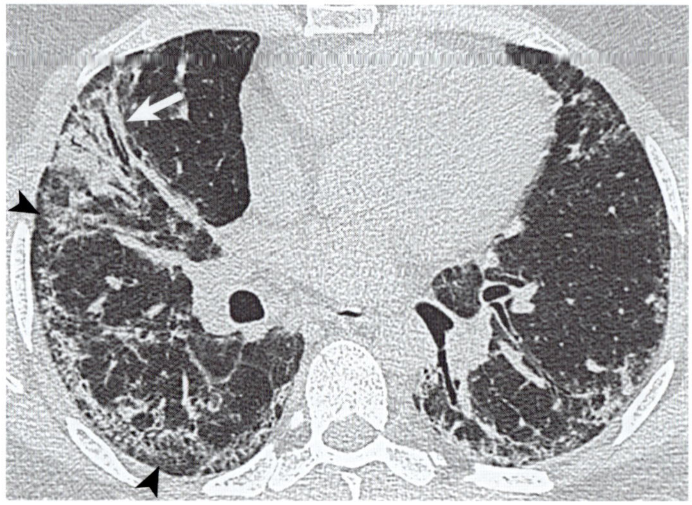

Fig. 42.5 Mixed nonspecific interstitial pneumonia (NSIP) and organizing pneumonia in a patient with myositis and anti–Jo-1 antibody positivity (antisynthetase syndrome). High-resolution CT shows bilateral peripheral reticulation and peribronchial consolidation *(arrow)*. Mild ground-glass opacity and relative subpleural sparing *(arrowheads)* of the lung immediately adjacent to the pleura are also evident. These appearances are consistent with mixed organizing pneumonia and NSIP (confirmed on surgical lung biopsy).

reversibility of the morphologic appearance was suggestive of OP or possibly cellular NSIP.

The acute manifestation of DAD in PM/DM is a fulminant respiratory failure that clinically resembles acute interstitial pneumonia. The findings in the majority of acute PM/DM cases on HRCT are patchy consolidation and ground-glass opacity with or without features of interstitial fibrosis.[43–45] These CT findings are similar to those described in the accelerated phase (acute exacerbation) of patients with idiopathic pulmonary fibrosis.[46]

MAGNETIC RESONANCE IMAGING

Gadolinium-enhanced cardiac magnetic resonance imaging (MRI) has been used for the investigation of myocarditis associated with PM; the typical enhancing pattern for myositis is patchy uptake of gadolinium not following a vascular distribution.[47] Additionally, MRI can characterize inhomogeneous inflammation in muscle of PM/DM patients and may be used to guide muscle biopsies.[48,49]

IMAGING ALGORITHMS

Chest radiography is performed routinely in patients with PM/DM, usually to exclude occult disease or lower respiratory tract infection, to which these patients are prone. However, the limited sensitivity of chest radiography for mild interstitial lung disease should prompt consideration for HRCT imaging if there is clinical or radiographic suspicion of thoracic involvement.

Differential Diagnosis

FROM CLINICAL DATA

There are numerous inflammatory myopathies, including drug-induced myopathy, virus-induced myopathy, Cushing syndrome, hypothyroidism, hyperthyroidism, systemic lupus erythematosus, sarcoidosis, and fibromyalgia. DM can be difficult to distinguish from subacute cutaneous lupus erythematosus, but muscle lesions have different distributions, and cutaneous lupus seldom has the accompanying features of DM.[21]

FROM SUPPORTIVE DIAGNOSTIC TECHNIQUES

Disease assessment in PM/DM is conventionally based on clinical evaluation, muscle biopsy, serum enzyme levels, such as creatine kinase, and electromyography.

Antisynthetase antibodies are highly antigen and disease specific. They include multiple different aminoacyl–transfer RNA synthetases—most prominently, anti–Jo-1, anti–PL-7, anti–PL-12, anti-EJ, and anti-OJ. These antibodies target the synthetases for histidine, threonine, alanine, glycine, and isoleucine, respectively. Of these, anti–Jo-1 antibodies are present in 30% of patients with inflammatory myositis,[50] and figures of 20% to 30% sensitivity are quoted for anti–Jo-1 in PM.[51] The presence of anti–Jo-1 antibodies correlates strongly with the presence of fibrotic lung disease in PM, and the normal incidence of pulmonary fibrosis in PM/DM rises from 10% to 60% to 70% in patients who are antibody positive.[52] Patients with antisynthetase antibodies and PM/DM are considered to be a subgroup of those with inflammatory arthropathies and are said to have "antisynthetase syndrome." Patients with this syndrome have a higher prevalence of ILD than do those who are antibody negative and have an inflammatory myositis. More recently, anti-MDA5 (melanoma differentiation-associated gene 5) antibody has been linked with amyopathic myositis and rapidly progressive ILD, severe skin lesions, and overall poor prognosis.[53]

Muscle biopsy is crucial in securing the diagnosis of PM and in excluding other rare muscle diseases. In PM muscle biopsy shows muscle fibers in varying stages of inflammation, necrosis, and regeneration. Findings include predominantly endomysial inflammatory infiltrates that are enriched with T-suppressor/cytotoxic (CD8) cells.[54] The finding of endomysial lymphoid inflammation is one of the major diagnostic criteria for PM. By contrast, DM infiltrates are concentrated in a perivascular distribution, and more B lymphocytes and T-helper (CD4) lymphocytes are present than in PM.

Bronchoalveolar lavage provides information about lung involvement. Early in the disease, findings compatible with lymphocytic alveolitis with high counts of $CD8^+$ T cells have been reported.[51] The presence of eosinophils and neutrophils is less common and indicates fibrosis with adverse prognostic significance. Similarly, in those with antisynthetase syndrome, disappearance of the lymphocytosis in bronchoalveolar lavage fluid indicates progression to fibrosis.[22]

Synopsis of Treatment Options

- Corticosteroids as the mainstay of treatment
- Analgesics—for instance, nonsteroidal antiinflammatory drugs
- Immunoglobulins—for instance, Gamimune
- Disease-modifying antirheumatic drugs—for instance, azathioprine

KEY POINTS

- The diagnosis of polymyositis/dermatomyositis (PM/DM) is usually made by following established diagnostic criteria.
- As with other connective tissue diseases, PM/DM has a plethora of clinical manifestations and pathologic entities.
- Pulmonary manifestations may precede symptoms of the inflammatory myopathy.
- The most common diffuse lung diseases in PM/DM are nonspecific interstitial pneumonia (NSIP), organizing pneumonia, and diffuse alveolar damage.
- Consolidation may be due to infection, organizing pneumonia, or diffuse alveolar damage. The consolidation in organizing pneumonia tends to be bilateral and to be mainly peribronchial or subpleural (or both).
- Diffuse ground-glass opacity may represent NSIP, diffuse alveolar damage, or occasionally, diffuse alveolar hemorrhage or opportunistic infection.
- Fibrotic lung disease usually has an NSIP pattern—that is, lower lung zone–predominant ground-glass opacities with superimposed reticulation.
- Patients who have antisynthetase antibodies are more likely to have interstitial lung disease. Patients without antisynthetase antibodies in whom acute interstitial pneumonitis develops have an unfavorable prognosis.
- Both PM and DM are associated with an increased risk for malignancy, and screening for malignancy may be considered in adult-onset DM, but guidelines for this do not yet exist.

SUGGESTED READINGS

Ahuja J, et al. Imaging of pulmonary manifestations of connective tissue diseases. *Radiol Clin North Am*. 2016;54(6):1015–1031.

Dalakas MC, Hohlfeld R. Polymyositis and dermatomyositis. *Lancet*. 2003;362:971.

Kolasinski SL, et al. Current perspectives on imaging for systemic lupus erythematosus, systemic sclerosis, and dermatomyositis/polymyositis. *Rheum Dis Clin North Am*. 2016;42(4):711–732.

Mandel DE, et al. Idiopathic inflammatory myopathies: a review of the classification and impact of pathogenesis. *Int J Mol Sci*. 2017;18(5).

The full reference list for this chapter is available at ExpertConsult.com.

43 Sjögren Syndrome*

STEPHEN B. HOBBS

Etiology

Sjögren's syndrome, or "sicca syndrome," is a disorder of the immune system that is largely defined by its two most common symptoms—dry eyes and a dry mouth; these symptoms frequently accompany other autoimmune disorders. Distinction is usually made between Sjögren's syndrome that occurs in the absence of an accompanying connective tissue disease (primary Sjögren's syndrome) and Sjögren's syndrome accompanied by another connective tissue disease (secondary Sjögren's syndrome) such as systemic lupus erythematosus, rheumatoid arthritis (RA), scleroderma, systemic sclerosis, cryoglobulinemia, and polyarteritis nodosa. Both primary and secondary types occur with similar frequency, and virtually all organs may be involved.

The etiology of the disease is not fully understood, but it is speculated that environmental factors trigger the human leukocyte antigen (HLA)-DR–dependent immune system, which affects the exocrine glandular vascular endothelium. Infiltration of the exocrine glands by lymphocytes leads to apoptosis and glandular dysfunction.[1] There is evidence that certain HLA class II antigens are increased in these patients; in Caucasian individuals, Sjögren syndrome is associated with HLA-DR3 and certain HLA-DQ alleles.[2] Possible triggering environmental factors include viruses, such as Epstein-Barr, human T-lymphotropic virus-1, human herpesvirus 6, human immunodeficiency virus, hepatitis C, and cytomegalovirus. Damage or cell death caused by viral infection or other causes may provide triggering antigens to Toll-like receptors on dendritic or epithelial cells.[1]

Prevalence and Epidemiology

Sjögren syndrome can develop at any age, but 59 years of age is the average at diagnosis (range, 43–75 years).[3] There are two age peaks for primary disease—the first in the third decade and the second after menopause.[4] The worldwide prevalence of Sjögren syndrome is 14.4 per 100,000 population, and the condition is nine times more frequent in women than in men.[5]

Clinical Presentation

Keratoconjunctivitis, the characteristic ophthalmologic feature of Sjögren syndrome, is caused by a lack of tear film secondary to destruction of the lacrimal gland. Patients complain of dry eyes, irritation, or photophobia. Careful assessment of patients with dry eyes is important; in particular, the integrity of the corneal surface needs to be evaluated.

Dryness of the mouth makes swallowing and talking difficult. Sudden swelling of a salivary gland suggests infection, whereas a more insidious onset of salivary gland enlargement can signal lymphomatous transformation.[1]

Exocrine glandular involvement is typically the first manifestation of Sjögren syndrome, with a subsequent slow deterioration in salivary and lacrimal function.[6] In a cohort of patients with primary disease, musculoskeletal (60%), urogenital (40%), hematologic (24%), cutaneous (20%), pulmonary (11%), gastrointestinal (7%), neurologic (8%), and renal (3%) manifestations were noted. Symptoms of myalgia and arthralgia are frequent, whereas arthritis is rare.[7] There are few descriptions of the type of arthritis found in these patients, but it tends to be similar to RA.[1] Urogenital symptoms are secondary to vulval dryness and pruritus, which leads to dyspareunia.[8] Many patients with primary Sjögren syndrome have a normocytic, normochromic anemia, and leukopenia,[8] as well as an increased risk for hematologic malignancies (leukemia, myeloma, Hodgkin and non-Hodgkin lymphoma).[9] Given that the syndrome is characterized by a lymphocytic infiltrate, it can be anticipated that a spectrum of lymphoproliferative disorders may develop in patients with Sjögren syndrome, including lymphocytic (lymphoid) interstitial pneumonia (LIP), follicular bronchiolitis, nodular lymphoid hyperplasia, and mucosa-associated lymphatic tissue (MALT) lymphoma, in addition to frank lymphoma. Amyloid deposition in conjunction with LIP has also been described.[10]

The incidence of cutaneous vasculitis has been estimated at 9%, and it is usually manifested as purpura, urticarial lesions, and maculopapules.[4] Raynaud phenomenon has been reported in 30% of patients,[11] and in patients with primary Sjögren syndrome and Raynaud phenomenon, the density of nail fold capillaries is significantly reduced.[12]

Patients with primary Sjögren syndrome have an increased risk for additional autoimmune diseases,[13] particularly RA, scleroderma, and primary biliary cirrhosis.[14] Clinical or biochemical evidence of liver disease, or both, is found in up to 10% of patients,[15] and the incidence of Sjögren syndrome in patients with chronic liver disease suggests a link between hepatitis C virus and Sjögren syndrome.[16]

Pathophysiology

PATHOLOGY

In one of the few computed tomography (CT)-pathology correlative studies of primary Sjögren syndrome, the major histologic patterns of lung disease found on biopsy were nonspecific interstitial pneumonia (NSIP) (61%), bronchiolitis, type not specified (12%), malignant lymphoma (12%), amyloidosis (6%), atelectatic fibrosis (6%), and honeycomb fibrosis, histologic subtype not specified (3%).[17] The CT appearance of an NSIP pattern had a high positive predictive value for the presence of NSIP on biopsy.[17] The relative scarcity of usual interstitial pneumonia (UIP) in this study may be a result of the small size

*The editors and the publisher would like to thank Drs. Maureen Quigley and David M. Hansell for contributing material on this topic to the prior edition of this work. It has served as the foundation for the current chapter.

of the series and also because those with typical UIP on high-resolution CT (HRCT) may not have undergone surgical lung biopsy. Conversely, in a smaller series of lung biopsy specimens ($n = 9$),[18] two-thirds of the patients had histologic UIP, and a third had NSIP.

Malignant lymphoma (see Chapter 24) is the major cause of morbidity and mortality in patients with primary Sjögren syndrome, and these patients have a 44-fold increased risk for the development of non-Hodgkin lymphoma.[19]

LIP is a diffuse interstitial proliferation of mature small lymphocytes and plasma cells,[20] and it commonly occurs in patients with Sjögren syndrome, autoimmune thyroid disease, acquired immune deficiency syndrome, and Castleman disease (see Chapter 23).[21] Other diffuse interstitial lung diseases encountered in connective tissue diseases, such as diffuse alveolar damage[22] and diffuse pulmonary hemorrhage, are not commonly associated with Sjögren syndrome.

LUNG FUNCTION

It is difficult to obtain a clear picture of the pattern of abnormal pulmonary function in primary Sjögren syndrome from the literature,[23] and some studies report both restrictive and obstructive abnormalities. However, a 10-year follow-up of pulmonary function in patients with primary Sjögren syndrome found that most patients do not have progressive lung disease.[24]

Manifestations of the Disease

The most frequently observed clinical manifestations of primary Sjögren syndrome are dry mouth, dry eyes, and parotid swelling. The main extraglandular manifestations are arthralgia and myalgia. The range of extraglandular pathology can significantly delay diagnosis in this condition, but in patients with known connective tissue disease, it is important to be alert to symptoms of "sicca syndrome."

KEY POINTS: THORACIC MANIFESTATIONS OF SJÖGREN SYNDROME

Parenchymal disease: common
- Nonspecific interstitial pneumonia
- Usual interstitial pneumonia
- Lymphocytic interstitial pneumonia
- Organizing pneumonia
- Lymphoma
- Amyloid deposits

Airway disease: common
- Follicular bronchiolitis
- Bronchiectasis

Vascular disease: uncommon
- Pulmonary hypertension

Pleural disease: uncommon
- Pleural effusion
- Pleural thickening

RADIOGRAPHY

One in 10 patients with primary Sjögren syndrome has pulmonary involvement evident on the chest radiograph.[25] The most common pulmonary manifestations (NSIP, UIP, or LIP) give rise to a reticular or reticulonodular pattern and ground-glass opacities usually involving mainly the lower lung zones (Fig. 43.1). Patients with pure LIP have a reticulonodular pattern on chest radiography, with or without ground-glass opacities and patchy areas of consolidation.[26] The prevalence of chest radiographic abnormalities varies between studies, and in one series, all patients with primary Sjögren syndrome had bilateral consolidation, reticulonodular opacities, or multiple cysts.[17] The majority of these abnormalities occurred in the lower zones. Pleural disease is rare in primary Sjögren syndrome.

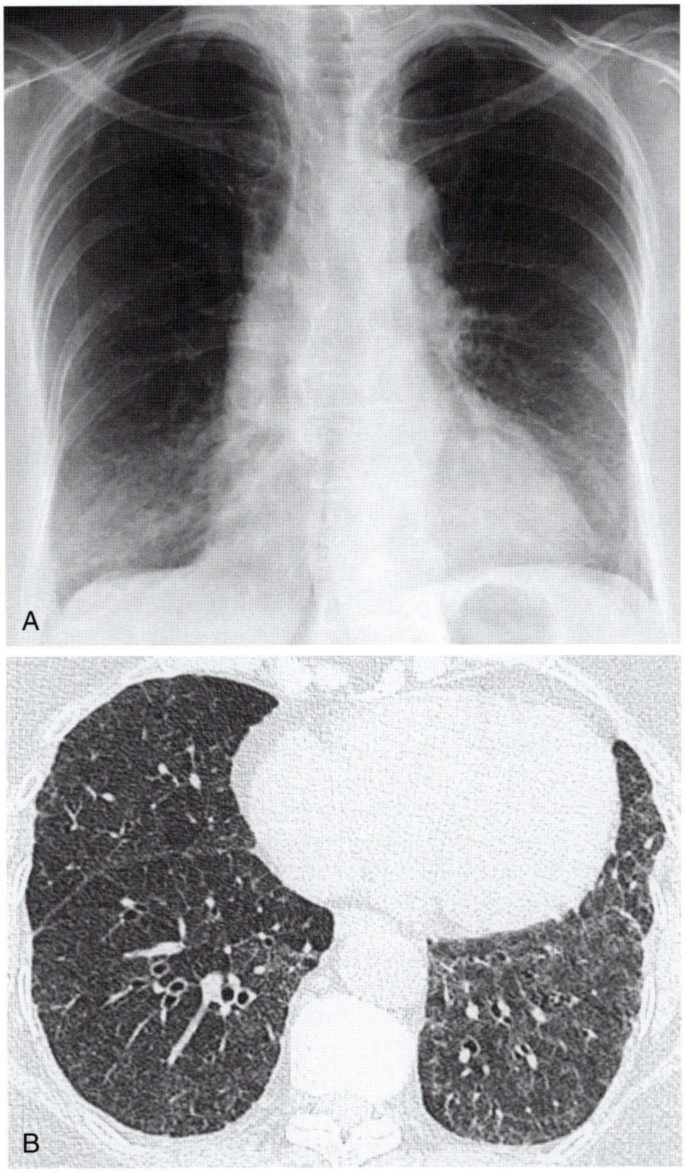

Fig. 43.1 Nonspecific interstitial pneumonia in Sjögren syndrome. (A) Chest radiograph shows hazy increased opacity (ground-glass opacities) in the middle and lower lung zones and a mild reticular pattern at the lung bases. (B) High-resolution CT demonstrates extensive bilateral ground-glass opacities and minimal reticulation.

Patients with Sjögren syndrome and supervening lymphoma are likely to have abnormal mediastinal and hilar contours on chest radiography, but a normal chest radiograph does not preclude nodal disease. In patients with the rarer primary lymphomas of lung parenchyma or MALT lymphoma, a chest radiograph may show patchy ground-glass opacity and sometimes indolent or, indeed, static areas of consolidation on serial radiographs.

COMPUTED TOMOGRAPHY

Few studies have concentrated exclusively on Sjögren syndrome of the lung, and because its prevalence is approximately equal to that of RA, it can be presumed that Sjögren syndrome either tends to not be associated with lung involvement or runs a subclinical course. The prevalence of HRCT "abnormalities" in those who fulfill the diagnostic criteria is between 34% and 65%,[27,28] but the majority of patients recruited to these studies had no respiratory symptoms.

Koyama and colleagues[29] studied 60 patients with abnormal HRCT findings who fulfilled the diagnostic criteria for primary Sjögren syndrome. The most common CT findings were areas of ground-glass opacity (92%), subpleural small nodules (78%), nonseptal linear opacity (75%), interlobular septal thickening (55%), bronchiectasis (38%), cysts (30%), and airspace consolidation (25%). The nodules and septal thickening, although nonspecific, would be consistent with LIP or follicular bronchiolitis (Fig. 43.2). The cysts are also consistent with LIP, and the consolidation could represent lower respiratory tract infection, lymphoproliferative disease, or organizing pneumonia.

Another study that attempted to characterize the appearances of primary Sjögren syndrome on HRCT[27] recruited nonsmokers, and most of the CT abnormalities were found in those with respiratory symptoms. Similar to the previous study, the most frequent findings on HRCT were ground-glass opacities, linear opacities (reticulation), and airspace consolidation. The histologic correlate for the ground-glass opacities (frequently seen in the various HRCT studies of Sjögren syndrome) is uncertain; NSIP, LIP, infection, and organizing pneumonia are all possible explanations for the ground-glass opacity.[17] The proportion of patients with honeycombing on HRCT varies between 8% and 25%.[27,28] In Sjögren syndrome there is an increased prevalence of micronodules and interlobular septal thickening,[28] but the pathologic correlate for these lesions is unknown.

A CT-pathologic correlation in primary Sjögren syndrome found that the NSIP pattern on HRCT had a high positive predictive value (94%) for the presence of NSIP in the pathologic specimen; however, cases without an NSIP pattern correlated poorly with the histologic diagnosis.[17] In this study there were no cases of biopsy-proven LIP despite three patients having cysts on CT; in these three patients, amyloidosis and malignant lymphoma were diagnosed histologically. The HRCT manifestations of NSIP consist of predominantly ground-glass opacities commonly with superimposed reticulation, traction bronchiectasis, and bronchiolectasis and typically involving mainly the lower lung zones (see Fig. 43.1). More extensive reticulation, with or without associated honeycombing, may result from NSIP or UIP (Fig. 43.3).

The HRCT appearance of LIP is characterized by the presence of ground-glass opacities, poorly defined centrilobular nodules, and interlobular septal thickening (Fig. 43.4.)[30] Patients with LIP frequently have cysts and perivascular cysts that may actually be the most distinctive finding or even the sole finding (see Chapter 23). This can lead to a misdiagnosis of lymphangioleiomyomatosis (LAM) in some cases, but the cysts in LIP usually are predominant in the lower lungs around bronchi and vessels in contrast to the more diffuse distribution of LAM-related cysts (see Chapter 35).

A spectrum of lymphoproliferative pathology may be encountered in patients with primary Sjögren syndrome (Fig. 43.5). The cardinal feature of nonpulmonary lymphoma on chest radiography or CT is mediastinal or hilar lymphadenopathy, with the anterior mediastinal and paratracheal nodes being the most frequently involved groups.[31,32] Primary pulmonary Hodgkin lymphoma is rare, and the frequency of lymphomas primarily arising in the lung is less than 1% of all lymphomas.[33] Primary lymphoma is usually manifested as localized areas of consolidation, and air bronchograms are commonly present. Lymphangitic infiltration is the second most frequent radiologic finding in primary lymphoma.[33] Patients with pulmonary MALT lymphoma typically do not have mediastinal lymphadenopathy, and MALT lymphomas

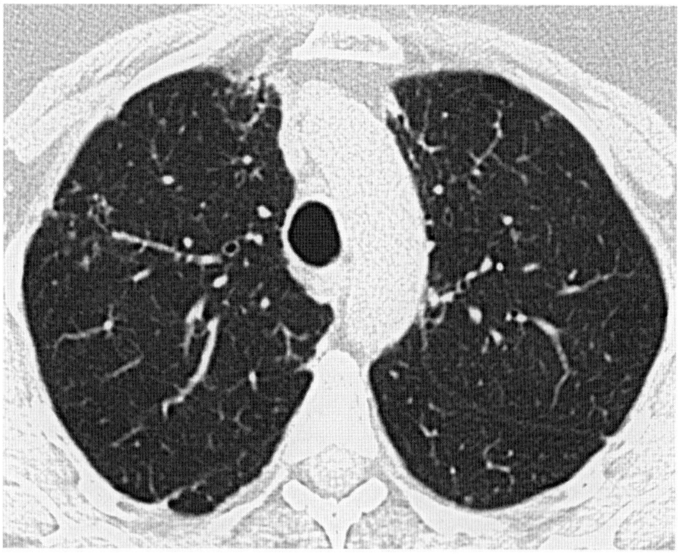

Fig. 43.2 Nonspecific parenchymal findings frequently seen in primary Sjögren syndrome. High-resolution CT shows nonspecific findings, including small peribronchial and subpleural nodules and mild bronchial dilation. These abnormalities are likely to represent follicular bronchiolitis. Cystic changes are also evident in the anterior left upper lobe.

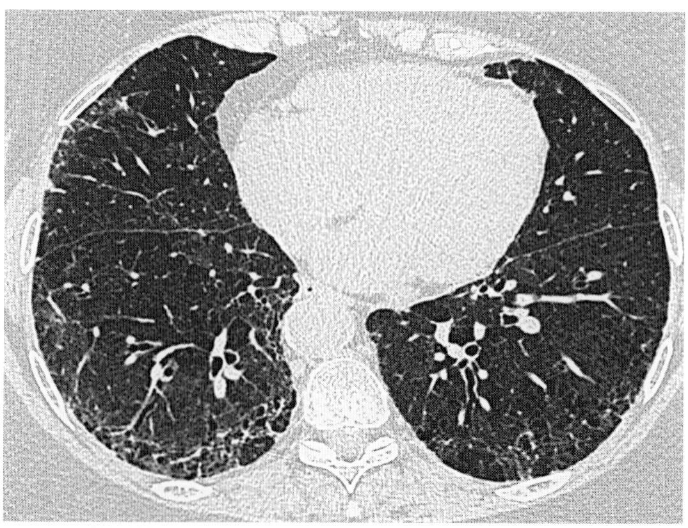

Fig. 43.3 Fibrotic lung disease in Sjögren syndrome likely representing nonspecific interstitial pneumonia. High-resolution CT shows a subpleural and basal reticular pattern with areas of subpleural sparing.

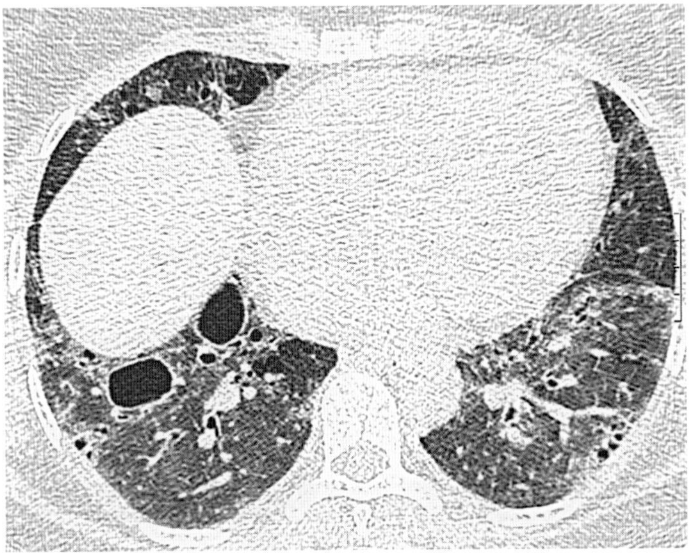

Fig. 43.4 Lymphoid interstitial pneumonia in Sjögren syndrome. High-resolution CT shows cystic airspaces, ground-glass opacities, and small nodules.

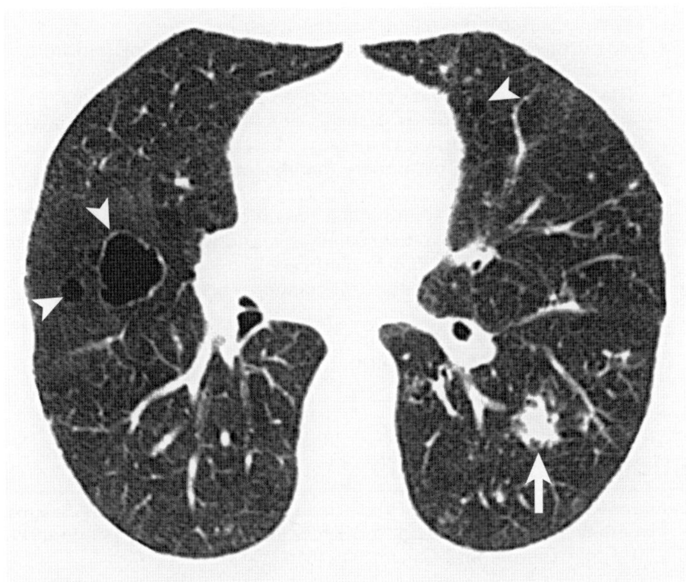

Fig. 43.5 Lymphoid interstitial pneumonia (LIP) and B-cell lymphoma in Sjögren syndrome. High-resolution CT shows diffuse ground-glass opacities, bilateral cysts *(arrowheads)*, and an irregular nodule in the left lower lobe *(arrow)*. The patient was a middle-aged woman with LIP proven by surgical biopsy and with B-cell lymphoma proven by bone marrow biopsy.

are generally indolent lesions with single or multiple areas of consolidation or ground-glass opacity, adjacent interlobular septal thickening, and prominent air bronchograms.[34,35] However, prominent adenopathy in the chest is not necessarily indicative of lymphoma because benign lymphadenopathy, thymic lymphoid hyperplasia, and multilocular thymic cysts can also occur in the setting of Sjögren syndrome. Systemic lymphoplasmacytic inflammation can result in lymph node enlargement throughout the chest, including the mediastinum, and thymic lymph node hyperplasia can manifest as nodules and increased attenuation in the anterior mediastinal fat as well.[36] Multilocular thymic cysts

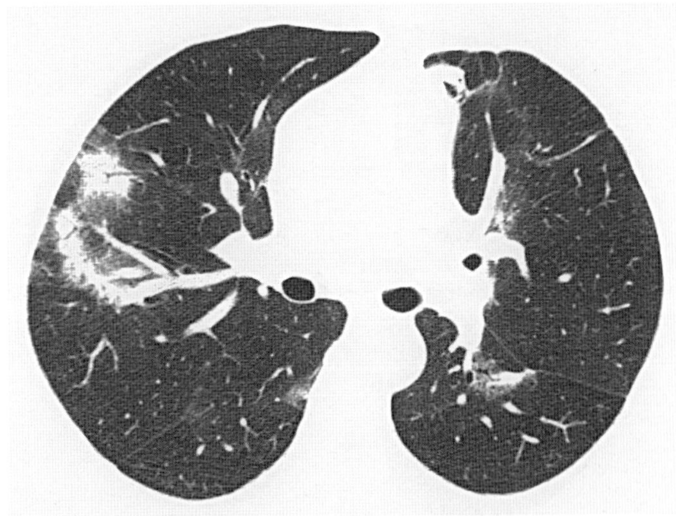

Fig. 43.6 Organizing pneumonia in Sjögren syndrome. High-resolution CT shows bilateral areas of consolidation in a predominantly peribronchial distribution surrounded by a halo of ground-glass opacity. Also noted is a perilobular distribution in the right upper lobe.

can manifest as thin-walled, anterior mediastinal cysts in Sjögren syndrome, likely as the result of chronic noninfectious inflammation. Occasionally, they may demonstrate internal heterogeneity or increased attenuation suggesting internal hemorrhage or proteinaceous fluid.[37–39] A significant solid component or irregular wall thickening of these multilocular cysts should raise the possibility of a malignancy (see Chapter 77).

Case reports of organizing pneumonia and follicular bronchiolitis have been associated with primary Sjögren syndrome.[40] The HRCT manifestations of organizing pneumonia (see Chapter 29) typically consist of bilateral areas of consolidation that frequently have a predominantly peribronchial, perilobular, or subpleural distribution (Fig. 43.6). The cardinal HRCT features of follicular bronchiolitis are centrilobular nodules measuring 1 to 12 mm in diameter, variably associated with peribronchial nodules and patchy areas of ground-glass opacity.[41] Follicular bronchiolitis is, however, infrequently described in Sjögren syndrome, and it is difficult to know whether this is because few biopsy studies of Sjögren syndrome have been conducted or whether it reflects the true prevalence of follicular bronchiolitis in these patients.

A study that focused on patients who had primary Sjögren syndrome and respiratory symptoms found that large or small airways disease, or both, affected more than half the patients in this cohort.[42] Bronchiectasis has been described in HRCT studies in 4% to 38% of patients with primary Sjögren syndrome,[27,28,43] and it has been postulated that the bronchiectasis occurs because lymphocytic invasion of the tracheobronchial mucous glands results in atelectasis and recurrent infection (Fig. 43.7). A single case of middle lobe syndrome has been attributed to lymphocytic bronchiolitis in a patient with primary Sjögren syndrome.[44] Patients with primary Sjögren syndrome frequently have bronchial hyperresponsiveness and increased epithelial airway damage compared with healthy control persons.[45] There are a few descriptions of air-trapping on HRCT in Sjögren syndrome, and in one study the extent of air-trapping did not correlate with pulmonary function test results, and the authors suggested that this may be due to a subclinical bronchiolar inflammatory process that preceded the functional changes.[46]

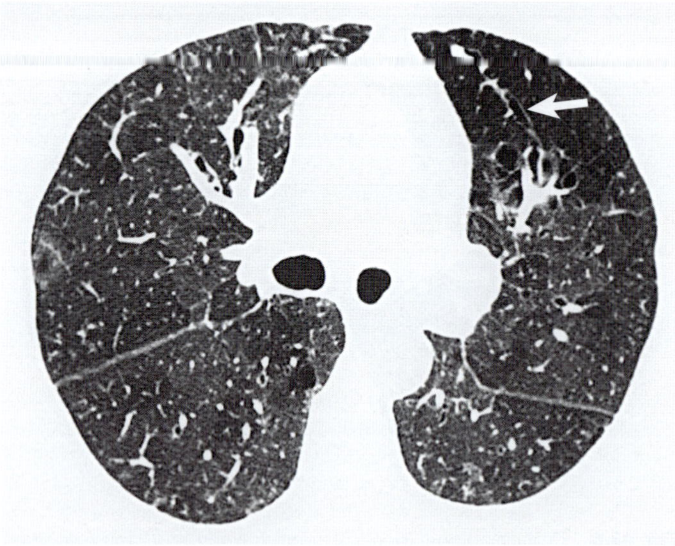

Fig. 43.7 Bronchiectasis in Sjögren syndrome. High-resolution CT shows left upper lobe bronchiectasis *(arrow)* and focal areas of decreased attenuation and vascularity, consistent with constrictive bronchiolitis. Also evident is minimal bilateral ground-glass opacities.

Primary pulmonary hypertension has been recognized in a few isolated case reports,[47] and it may be a rare association of Sjögren syndrome. Antiphospholipid syndrome occurs in a small subgroup of patients and could be a cofactor for the development of pulmonary hypertension. However, the incidence of lupus anticoagulant is estimated to be only 11% in those with primary Sjögren syndrome, and this value is far lower than in systemic lupus erythematosus.[48]

ULTRASONOGRAPHY

Echocardiography in Sjögren syndrome shows a higher-than-expected rate of pericarditis and diastolic dysfunction, although overt clinical cardiac involvement is rare.[49]

IMAGING ALGORITHMS

Because the frequency of clinically significant interstitial lung disease is not high, patients tend to be imaged only if they have respiratory symptoms. A chest radiograph may be initially performed in a symptomatic patient to exclude gross parenchymal or neoplastic disease, but because of the relative insensitivity of the chest radiograph, HRCT is the investigation of choice to exclude interstitial or airway disease.

Differential Diagnosis

The imaging differential diagnosis varies widely, depending on the pattern of pulmonary parenchymal disease, airways disease, vascular disease, and pleural disease. Each pattern would result in a tailored differential. For example, if the primary pulmonary parenchymal pattern consisted of an NSIP-type chronic fibrosing interstitial pneumonia, the differential may include other connective tissue diseases, chronic hypersensitivity pneumonitis, or drug toxicity.

KEY POINTS

- Sjögren syndrome can be primary or secondary; primary Sjögren syndrome has its own set of diagnostic criteria, and secondary Sjögren syndrome is associated with other connective tissue diseases.
- Sjögren syndrome is relatively common, especially in the older female population, but symptomatic lung disease is infrequent.
- The most common clinical manifestations are dry mouth, dry eyes, and parotid swelling.
- No curative agent exists. Treatment is essentially for symptom palliation and prevention of complications.
- The majority of patients with Sjögren syndrome will have abnormal HRCT findings, but this does not necessarily equate with clinically important disease.
- The most common pulmonary manifestations include interstitial fibrosis (most commonly, nonspecific interstitial pneumonia and usual interstitial pneumonia), lymphocytic interstitial pneumonia, bronchiectasis, and lymphoma.
- The most common HRCT findings are ground-glass opacities, intralobular linear opacities (reticulation), cystic airspaces, and mild bronchiectasis.
- There is an increased risk for malignant lymphoma in patients with primary Sjögren syndrome.

SUGGESTED READINGS

Egashira R, et al. CT findings of thoracic manifestations of primary Sjögren syndrome: radiologic-pathologic correlation. *Radiographics*. 2013;33:1933–1949.
Fox RI. Sjögren's syndrome. *Lancet*. 2005;366:321–331.

The full reference list for this chapter is available at ExpertConsult.com.

44 Mixed Connective Tissue Disease*

BRENT P. LITTLE

Etiology

Mixed connective tissue disease (MCTD) is a disease with certain features of polymyositis, scleroderma, and systemic lupus erythematosus. Much of the evidence that MCTD is a distinct clinical entity stems from the identification of antiribonucleoprotein (anti-RNP) antibody, disease-specific human leukocyte antigen (HLA) profiles, suggestive clinical features, and because in the vast majority of patients, MCTD does not evolve into other connective tissue disease–related entities.[1]

The etiology of MCTD is unknown, but the presence of antibodies to RNPs implies that the immune system has become sensitized to ribonucleic acid synthesis or metabolism. Infectious agents have been investigated as a potential trigger for MCTD. Retroviral sequences have been found in a high proportion of MCTD patients,[2] and most studies have revealed a strong association with MCTD and HLA-DR4.[3]

Prevalence and Epidemiology

The incidence of MCTD is not known but is estimated to be higher than that of polymyositis, lower than that of systemic lupus erythematosus, and similar to that of systemic sclerosis.[4] The majority of patients are women, with an average age at diagnosis of 37 years (range, 4–80 years).[4] Pediatric-onset MCTD carries less mortality than adult-onset MCTD,[5] probably because pulmonary hypertension is less frequent in the younger group. The prognosis for patients with MCTD is highly variable, but a severe, progressive disease course is unusual.[6] In five series of MCTD (total of 194 patients), mortality was generally low (mean, 13%; range, 4%–35%); nevertheless, the fact that MCTD affects young women indicates a greater risk for premature death.[6] Pulmonary hypertension is the most serious complication of MCTD, with severe infection secondary to immunosuppression being the other frequent cause of death.[6,7]

Clinical Presentation

Most patients with MCTD have one or more of the following: Raynaud phenomenon, arthralgia, arthritis, swollen hands, sclerodactyly, or acrosclerosis (i.e., stiffness and atrophy of the skin of hands and feet), and two-thirds suffer from frank myositis.[7,8] Esophageal dysmotility and reflux are reportedly frequent in MCTD, and generalized lymphadenopathy has been observed in 50% of patients.[8] The most common cardiac abnormality is pericarditis; less common cardiac manifestations include myocarditis and complete heart block.[4] The most frequent clinical manifestations of pulmonary involvement are dyspnea, pleuritic chest pain, and bibasilar rales.[4] Secondary Sjögren syndrome is relatively common.[9] Cutaneous manifestations include photosensitivity, livedo reticularis (a net-like vascular skin discoloration in the trunk or extremities), and calcinosis.

When Sharp and colleagues[10] first described MCTD, it was considered a benign condition requiring little treatment. It is now realized that serious renal[11] and pulmonary involvement does occur; interstitial lung disease occurs in 21% to 66% of patients.[12]

Pleural effusion is one of the most common clinical manifestations of MCTD, but it is usually small and resolves spontaneously. In a retrospective review of the chest radiographs of 81 patients with MCTD, 6% had small pleural effusions, and even fewer had pleural thickening. Although a prospective study of patients with "MCTD" reported "pleuritis" in 35%,[13] this study was undertaken before modern diagnostic criteria had been published.[14] The incidence of pleuritis and effusions is likely to fall in the middle of this range because chest radiography may underestimate disease (compared with computed tomography [CT]) and, conversely, modern diagnostic criteria for MCTD are more rigorous.

MCTD is associated with pulmonary hypertension, commonly manifested insidiously as progressive dyspnea on exertion.[15] A surveillance study of a drug (bosentan) used to treat pulmonary hypertension found that connective tissue disease–related pulmonary hypertension and idiopathic pulmonary hypertension were each responsible for approximately a third of cases treated with this drug. In this cohort the majority of patients with connective tissue disease–associated pulmonary hypertension had systemic sclerosis (75%), and the next largest group consisted of patients with MCTD (9%).[16] Although having a lower incidence in MCTD than in systemic sclerosis, pulmonary hypertension should be considered as a possible cause of dyspnea in both diseases.

Pathophysiology

PATHOLOGY

In patients with pulmonary hypertension in MCTD, plexiform lesions in small- and medium-sized arteries can occur, similar to primary pulmonary hypertension.[17–20] In other connective tissue diseases, pulmonary vasculopathies are often associated with diffuse alveolar hemorrhage, but reports of diffuse alveolar hemorrhage in patients with MCTD are rare.[15] Pulmonary thromboembolism may occur,[21,22] possibly secondary to coexisting antiphospholipid syndrome.

Pulmonary hemorrhage, diffuse alveolar damage, organizing pneumonia, nonspecific interstitial pneumonia, usual interstitial

*The editors and the publisher would like to thank Drs. Maureen Quigley and David M. Hansell for contributing material on this topic to the prior edition of this work. It has served as the foundation for the current chapter.

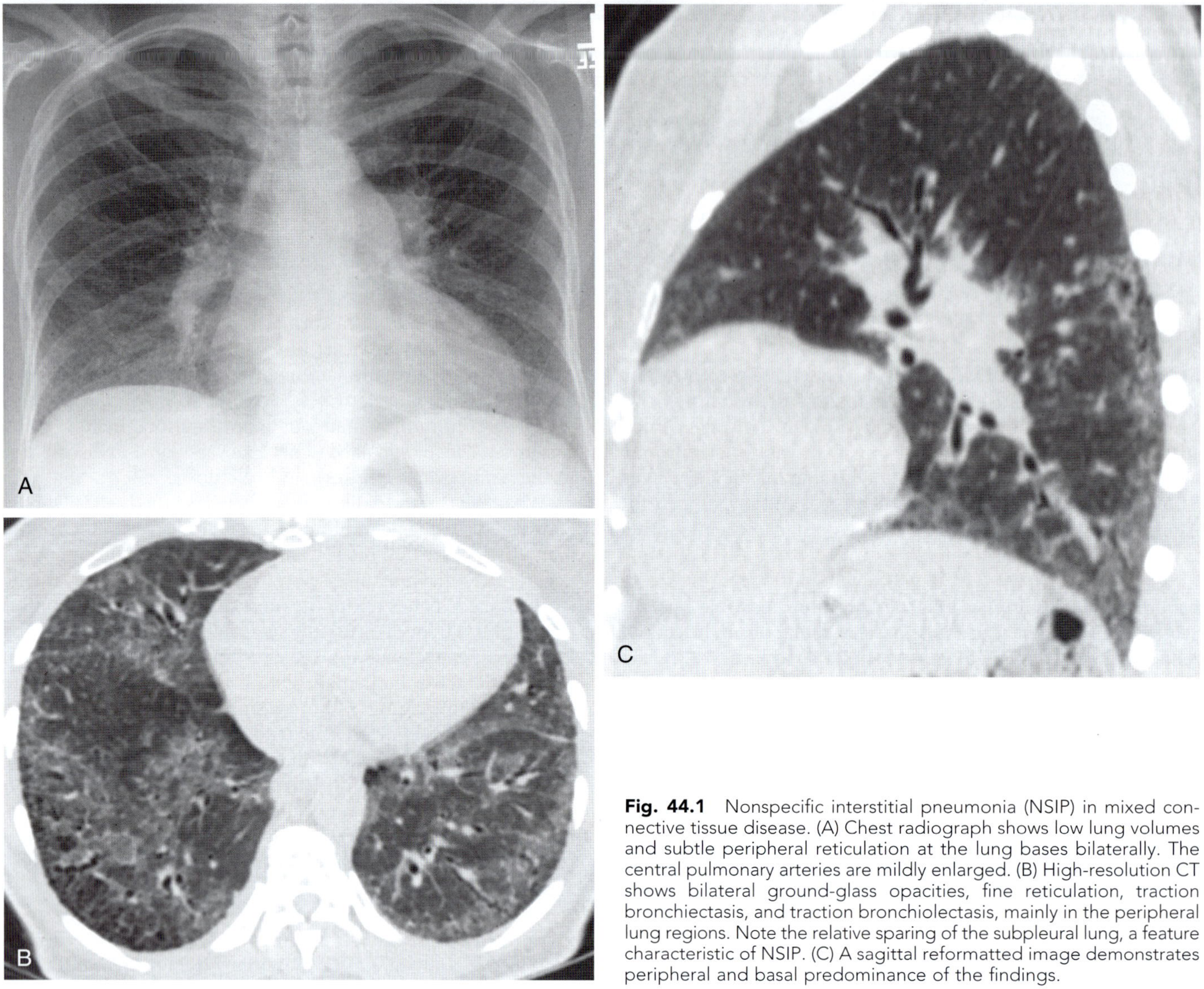

Fig. 44.1 Nonspecific interstitial pneumonia (NSIP) in mixed connective tissue disease. (A) Chest radiograph shows low lung volumes and subtle peripheral reticulation at the lung bases bilaterally. The central pulmonary arteries are mildly enlarged. (B) High-resolution CT shows bilateral ground-glass opacities, fine reticulation, traction bronchiectasis, and traction bronchiolectasis, mainly in the peripheral lung regions. Note the relative sparing of the subpleural lung, a feature characteristic of NSIP. (C) A sagittal reformatted image demonstrates peripheral and basal predominance of the findings.

pneumonia (UIP), and airway disease may be seen in MCTD. These findings are consistent with the clinical manifestations of MCTD, which commonly have features of systemic sclerosis, systemic lupus erythematosus, or polymyositis/dermatomyositis.

LUNG FUNCTION

Pulmonary disease has been reported in 73% of patients with MCTD on the basis of pulmonary function tests, chest radiography, or both.[13] The most common abnormality in pulmonary function testing is decreased lung diffusing capacity for carbon monoxide (DLCO)[13]; nearly half of patients in a small series had a decreased DLCO.[23] In this study the value of DLCO correlated with the duration of the disease, but the cause of the impaired diffusing capacity was not explored. Some of this group may have had a proliferative vasculopathy associated with MCTD, but other possibilities include fibrotic lung disease and emphysema. Patients with MCTD have been reported as having functional small airway obstruction, but there is no high-resolution CT (HRCT) or pathologic confirmation of this finding.[13,23] However, large airway disease has been described in a single HRCT study that reported bronchiectasis in a few individuals.[24]

Manifestations of the Disease

RADIOGRAPHY

The true burden of lung disease in MCTD is unclear. On chest radiography interstitial lung disease has been reported to affect between 21% and 85% of patients.[13,25] The typical radiographic abnormality is a reticular or reticulonodular pattern in the lower zones (Fig. 44.1).[13] Pleural effusions or thickening is seen on less than 10% of chest radiographs. Because these patients are often immunosuppressed, it is important to rule out infection in the face of nonspecific pulmonary abnormalities. Chest radiographs are less sensitive than HRCT for the detection of interstitial lung disease,[26] and an apparently normal radiograph does not rule out interstitial lung disease.

COMPUTED TOMOGRAPHY

Nonspecific interstitial pneumonia (NSIP) is the most frequent pattern of interstitial lung disease in MCTD; UIP and lymphocytic interstitial pneumonia are less commonly observed patterns.[12] One study of MCTD reviewed 41 HRCT scans with lung abnormalities in patients with MCTD.[24] Most patients had an NSIP pattern of disease, with micronodules, ground-glass opacities, and intralobular lines (reticulation), predominantly in the lower zones (see Fig. 44.1). Nearly 50% of scans showed evidence of fibrosis, including intralobular lines, architectural distortion, and traction bronchiectasis.[24] A small proportion of patients had airspace consolidation, honeycombing, cysts, and bronchiectasis resembling a UIP pattern of fibrosis (Fig. 44.2). Therefore the HRCT manifestations of MCTD include findings seen in patients with systemic sclerosis, systemic lupus erythematosus, and polymyositis/dermatomyositis.

In a second large CT study of pulmonary involvement in MCTD, 144 sequential patients were scanned at diagnosis, and 67% were said to have "active interstitial lung disease" diagnosed on the basis of ground-glass opacity on HRCT and an abnormal clearance time for technetium 99m–labeled diethylenetriamine-pentaacetic acid (DTPA).[27] In more than two-thirds of patients with active disease at baseline, HRCT findings had reverted to normal at the 6-month follow-up scan. The majority of DTPA scans also normalized at 6 months. The authors suggested that ground-glass opacity may be reversible with early treatment; however, a proportion of patients progressed despite early treatment. The pathologic process that the ground-glass opacities represented is unknown, but a cellular infiltrate or, less likely, hemorrhage would be an explanation for this reversible disease.

Pulmonary arterial hypertension may manifest as pulmonary arterial enlargement on chest radiography or CT[28]; accompanying small pericardial effusion or small poorly defined centrilobular nodules are uncommon.[29] Pulmonary arterial hypertension may be associated with interstitial lung disease or may be the only intrathoracic manifestation of MCTD (Fig. 44.3).

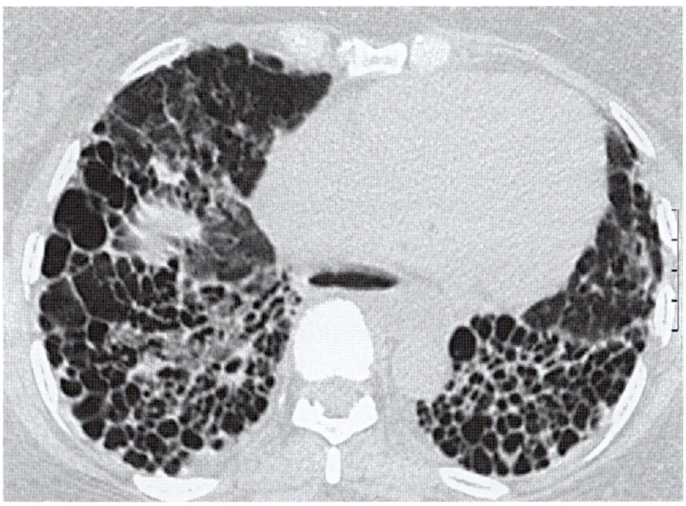

Fig. 44.2 Honeycombing and usual interstitial pneumonia pattern of lung fibrosis in mixed connective tissue disease. High-resolution CT shows marked honeycombing and a dilated esophagus with a peripheral and lower lung zone predominance.

KEY POINTS: FINDINGS OF MIXED CONNECTIVE TISSUE DISEASE ON HIGH-RESOLUTION COMPUTED TOMOGRAPHY

- Small pleural effusions and pleural thickening
- Ground-glass opacities representing either fine fibrosis or reversible disease, usually in a nonspecific interstitial pneumonia pattern
- Reticulation, traction bronchiectasis and bronchiolectasis, and occasional honeycombing; lower lung zone predominance
- Micronodules, presumably reflecting lymphoid hyperplasia
- Occasional bronchiectasis
- Pulmonary arterial enlargement as a result of pulmonary hypertension

IMAGING ALGORITHMS

Although MCTD is estimated to have the same incidence as systemic sclerosis, the frequency of clinically significant lung disease is far less. In symptomatic patients a chest radiograph may show pleural involvement, but suspected interstitial lung disease should be investigated with HRCT. Echocardiography, in conjunction with the clinical history and assessment of DLCO, can assist in identifying pulmonary hypertension.

Differential Diagnosis

FROM CLINICAL DATA

The differential diagnosis includes primary pulmonary hypertension, systemic sclerosis, systemic lupus erythematosus, polymyositis/

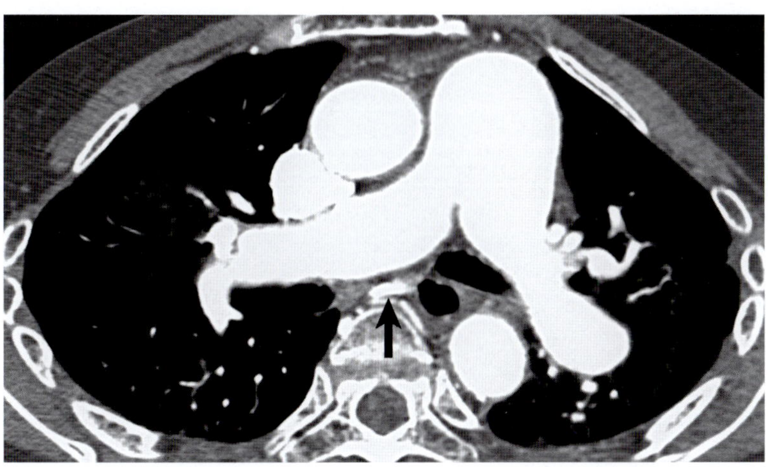

Fig. 44.3 Pulmonary hypertension in mixed connective tissue disease. Contrast-enhanced CT shows marked dilation of the main, right, and left pulmonary arteries. Also note the enlarged bronchial arteries *(arrow)*.

CLASSIC SIGNS

Four sets of criteria have been published for the diagnosis of MCTD.[10,30–32] The criteria of Alarcon-Segovia and Cardiel have the highest sensitivity when tested on patients with well-defined connective tissue disease (100% specificity and 99.6% sensitivity).[30] They are the simplest of the published criteria, and the key component is the presence of anti-RNP antibodies at a hemagglutination titer of 1:1600 or greater. At least three of the following five clinical criteria must also be present: (1) edema of the hands, (2) synovitis, (3) myositis, (4) Raynaud phenomenon, and (5) acrosclerosis.[30] Returning to the Sharp et al[10] original description of MCTD, some of these patients did not have anti-RNP antibodies, and because these antibodies are described in other connective tissue diseases, there is debate about the weight that is put on the serologic profile in MCTD.[1]

dermatomyositis, rheumatoid arthritis, and Raynaud phenomenon. MCTD is associated with specific autoantibodies, including anti-RNP antibodies, but these can also be seen in other connective tissue diseases. A rheumatologic diagnosis is made by applying the specific diagnostic criteria, but patients may "evolve" into other connective tissue diseases.

FROM SUPPORTIVE DIAGNOSTIC TECHNIQUES

The serologic presence of anti–U1-RNP antibodies is the essential diagnostic criterion for MCTD, but the specificity of the antibody has not been fully defined. Frandsen and coworkers[33] studied 151 patients with high-titer U1-RNP, and MCTD was diagnosed in 26% of these patients; 7% had systemic lupus erythematosus, and 3% had systemic sclerosis. There were 84 patients with possible undifferentiated connective tissue disease, but over a mean follow-up of 7 years, MCTD developed in a further 58, systemic sclerosis in 4, and systemic lupus erythematosus in 2. In 64% of those with high-titer anti–U1-RNP antibodies, MCTD subsequently developed.[33]

Synopsis of Treatment Options

- Analgesics, for instance, nonsteroidal antiinflammatory drugs
- Corticosteroids
- Disease-modifying antirheumatic drugs, for instance, cyclophosphamide, methotrexate
- Calcium channel blocking agents to control Raynaud phenomenon
- Endothelin receptor blockade with bosentan for pulmonary hypertension

KEY POINTS

- Mixed connective tissue disease (MCTD) has defined clinical/serologic diagnostic criteria.
- The literature on pulmonary involvement in MCTD is sparse, which may reflect the difficulty in studying a group undergoing metamorphosis or may reflect a true paucity of lung disease.
- Pulmonary hypertension and severe infections are the most serious pulmonary manifestations of MCTD.
- A large proportion of patients with early MCTD appear to have steroid-responsive and "reversible" interstitial lung disease

SUGGESTED READINGS

Henry TS, Little BP, Veeraraghavan S, et al. The spectrum of interstitial lung disease in connective tissue disease. *J Thorac Imaging*. 2016;31:65–77.

Prakash UB. Lungs in mixed connective tissue disease. *J Thorac Imaging*. 1992;7:55–61.

Prakash UB. Respiratory complications in mixed connective tissue disease. *Clin Chest Med*. 1998;19:733–746.

The full reference list for this chapter is available at ExpertConsult.com.

45 Interstitial Pneumonia With Autoimmune Features

MICHAEL A. KADOCH | JUSTIN M. OLDHAM

Interstitial pneumonia with autoimmune features (IPAF) refers to the clinical entity of interstitial lung disease (ILD) in patients with features of autoimmunity but without overt connective tissue disease (CTD). IPAF was introduced in 2015 by an international consensus panel in an attempt to standardize the nomenclature and diagnostic criteria for this entity, which represents an intermediary on the spectrum between the idiopathic interstitial pneumonias (IIPs) and CTD-associated ILD. The high-resolution computed tomography (HRCT) pattern is a critical component of IPAF criteria, and the prognostic significance of individual patterns and pattern features were recently described. As such, IPAF remains an area of active multidisciplinary investigation, and knowledge of this clinical entity is essential for a comprehensive understanding of ILD.

Background

ILD often arises in the context of an established CTD, such as rheumatoid arthritis, systemic lupus erythematosus, polymyositis, dermatomyositis, Sjögren syndrome, scleroderma, and mixed connective tissue disease. Nonspecific interstitial pneumonia (NSIP) is the most commonly encountered ILD pattern on HRCT in those with CTD, with the exception of rheumatoid arthritis, where a usual interstitial pneumonia (UIP) pattern is more commonly observed. Current international guidelines for the diagnosis of the IIPs recommend excluding CTD,[1] which is typically performed by assessing for extrathoracic manifestations, autoantibody testing, and multidisciplinary discussion.

It is not uncommon, however, for ILD to be the first, or only, manifestation of autoimmunity. Many patients with ILD exhibit features of CTD but do not satisfy rheumatologic criteria for a specific CTD diagnosis. These patients have been previously described in the pulmonary medicine and radiology literature by various names, including: lung-dominant CTD,[2] undifferentiated CTD-associated ILD,[3] and autoimmune-featured ILD.[4] The diagnostic criteria used to define these entities were overlapping but varied. Despite the associated features of autoimmunity, few of these patients will go on to develop overt CTD.

The need for a standardized nomenclature and diagnostic criteria for this patient population led to the formation of the European Respiratory Society (ERS)/American Thoracic Society (ATS) Task Force on Undifferentiated Forms of Connective Tissue Disease–Associated Interstitial Lung Disease. In 2015 this group produced an official ERS/ATS research statement proposing criteria for patients with IPAF.[5] Patients with IPAF can be thought of as intermediary on the spectrum between the IIPs and those with overt CTD-associated ILD.

Diagnostic Criteria

The diagnosis of IPAF requires[1]: the presence of ILD by HRCT or surgical lung biopsy,[2] exclusion of an alternate etiology for the ILD,[3] failure to meet criteria for a defined CTD, *and*[4] at least one feature from at least two of these domains: clinical, serologic, and morphologic (Table 45.1).[5]

The clinical domain comprises features that are strongly associated with CTD. These include distal digital fissuring ("mechanic's hands"), digital tip ulceration, inflammatory arthritis or polyarticular morning stiffness lasting more than 60 minutes, palmar telangiectasia, Raynaud phenomenon, unexplained digital edema, and unexplained fixed rash on the digital extensor surfaces (Gottron sign). The serologic domain includes autoantibodies with strong CTD association and requires moderately elevated titers for less specific autoantibodies, such as the antinuclear antibody (ANA) and rheumatoid factor (RF).

The morphologic domain includes three subdomains: radiologic, pathologic, and multicompartment. The radiologic subdomain is focused on HRCT features that are commonly associated with CTD, including NSIP (Fig. 45.1), organizing pneumonia (OP) (Fig. 45.2), NSIP with OP overlap (Fig. 45.3), and lymphocytic interstitial pneumonia (LIP). UIP is not included in the IPAF criteria because it lacks specificity. The pathologic subdomain similarly includes NSIP, OP, NSIP with OP overlap, and LIP. Interstitial lymphoid aggregates with germinal centers and diffuse lymphoplasmacytic infiltration are also included because they are strongly associated with CTD.[6] UIP is again not included because it lacks specificity for CTD.

Extraparenchymal thoracic manifestations are commonly encountered in the setting of CTD, leading to the inclusion of a multicompartment subdomain. The multicompartment subdomain includes unexplained pleural or pericardial effusion or thickening, intrinsic airways disease (airflow obstruction, bronchiolitis, or non–traction bronchiectasis), and pulmonary vasculopathy.

Clinical Features

Application of IPAF criteria has resulted in the description of highly heterogeneous IPAF cohorts around the world. The largest North American cohort of 144 patients was predominantly white, had a mean age of 63 years, had a slight female predominance, and had a history of smoking in over half.[7] Most patients (51%) met IPAF criteria through a combination of serologic and morphologic domains, and only 26% met all three domains. The most common clinical feature was Raynaud phenomenon (28%), and the most common serologic feature was ANA seropositivity

TABLE 45.1 DIAGNOSTIC CRITERIA FOR INTERSTITIAL PNEUMONIA WITH AUTOIMMUNE FEATURES

CLINICAL DOMAIN	"Mechanic's hands," distal digital tip ulceration, inflammatory arthritis, polyarticular morning joint stiffness, palmar telangiectasia, Raynaud phenomenon, unexplained digital edema, Gottron sign	
SEROLOGIC DOMAIN	ANA ≥ 1:320, RF ≥ 2× upper limit of normal, anti-CCP, anti-dsDNA, anti-Ro (SS-A), anti-La (SS-B), anti-ribonucleoprotein, anti-Smith, antitopoisomerase (Scl-70), anti-tRNA synthetase, anti–PM-Scl, anti-MDA5	
MORPHOLOGIC DOMAIN	**HRCT**	NSIP, OP, NSIP with OP overlap, LIP
	Histopathology	NSIP, OP, NSIP with OP overlap, LIP, interstitial lymphoid aggregates with germinal centers, diffuse lymphoplasmacytic infiltration
	Multicompartment Involvement	Unexplained pleural effusion/thickening, unexplained pericardial effusion/thickening, unexplained intrinsic airways disease, unexplained pulmonary vasculopathy

The diagnosis of IPAF requires: (1) the presence of an interstitial pneumonia on HRCT or biopsy, (2) exclusion of alternative etiologies, (3) exclusion of a defined CTD, *and* (4) at least one feature from at least two of these domains: clinical, serologic, and morphologic.

ANA, Antinuclear antibodies; *CCP*, cyclic citrullinated peptide; *CTD*, connective tissue disease; *dsDNA*, double-stranded deoxyribonucleic acid; *HRCT*, high-resolution computed tomography; *IPAF*, interstitial pneumonia with autoimmune features; *LIP*, lymphocytic interstitial pneumonia; *MDA5*, melanoma differentiation-associated gene 5; *NSIP*, nonspecific interstitial pneumonia; *OP*, organizing pneumonia; *PM-Scl*, polymyositis-scleroderma; *RF*, rheumatoid factor; *SS-A*, Sjögren syndrome A antibody; *SS-B*, Sjögren syndrome B antibody; *tRNA*, transfer ribonucleic acid.

Reproduced with permission from the © ERS 2015. *Eur Respir J*. 2015;46:976-987. DOI: 10.1183/13993003.00150-2015.

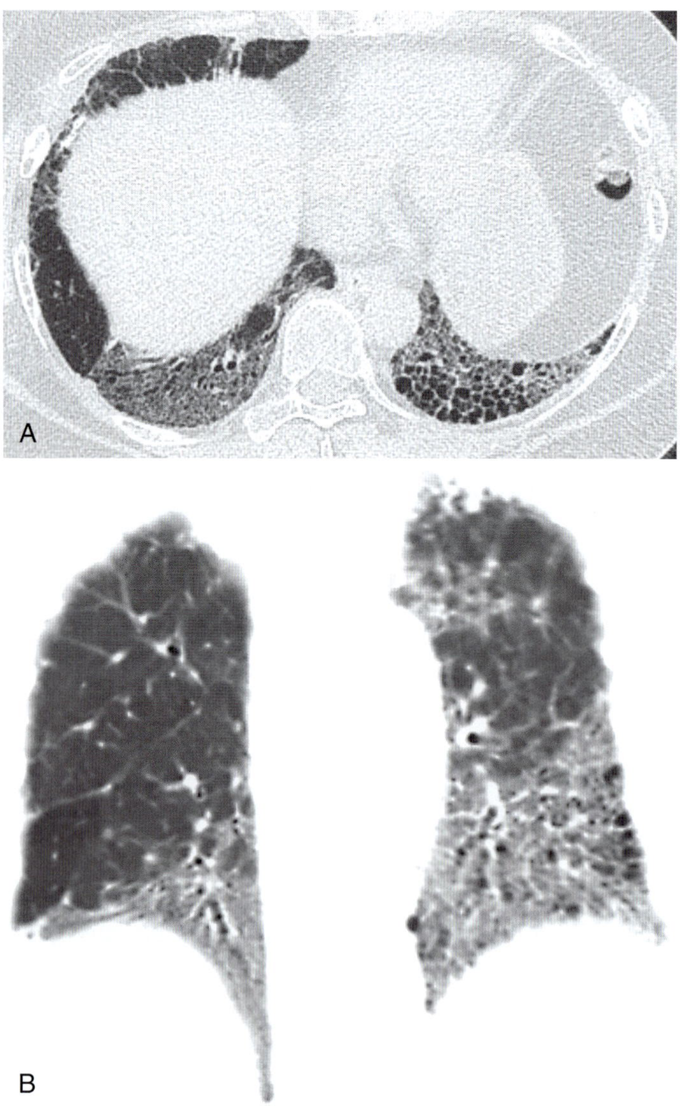

Fig. 45.1 A 60-year-old woman with interstitial pneumonia with autoimmune features and a fibrotic nonspecific interstitial pneumonia (NSIP) pattern. Supine axial (A) and coronal (B) high-resolution computed tomography images demonstrate basilar predominant peribronchovascular ground-glass opacities and traction bronchiectasis with some superimposed honeycombing. Findings are most compatible with a fibrotic NSIP pattern.

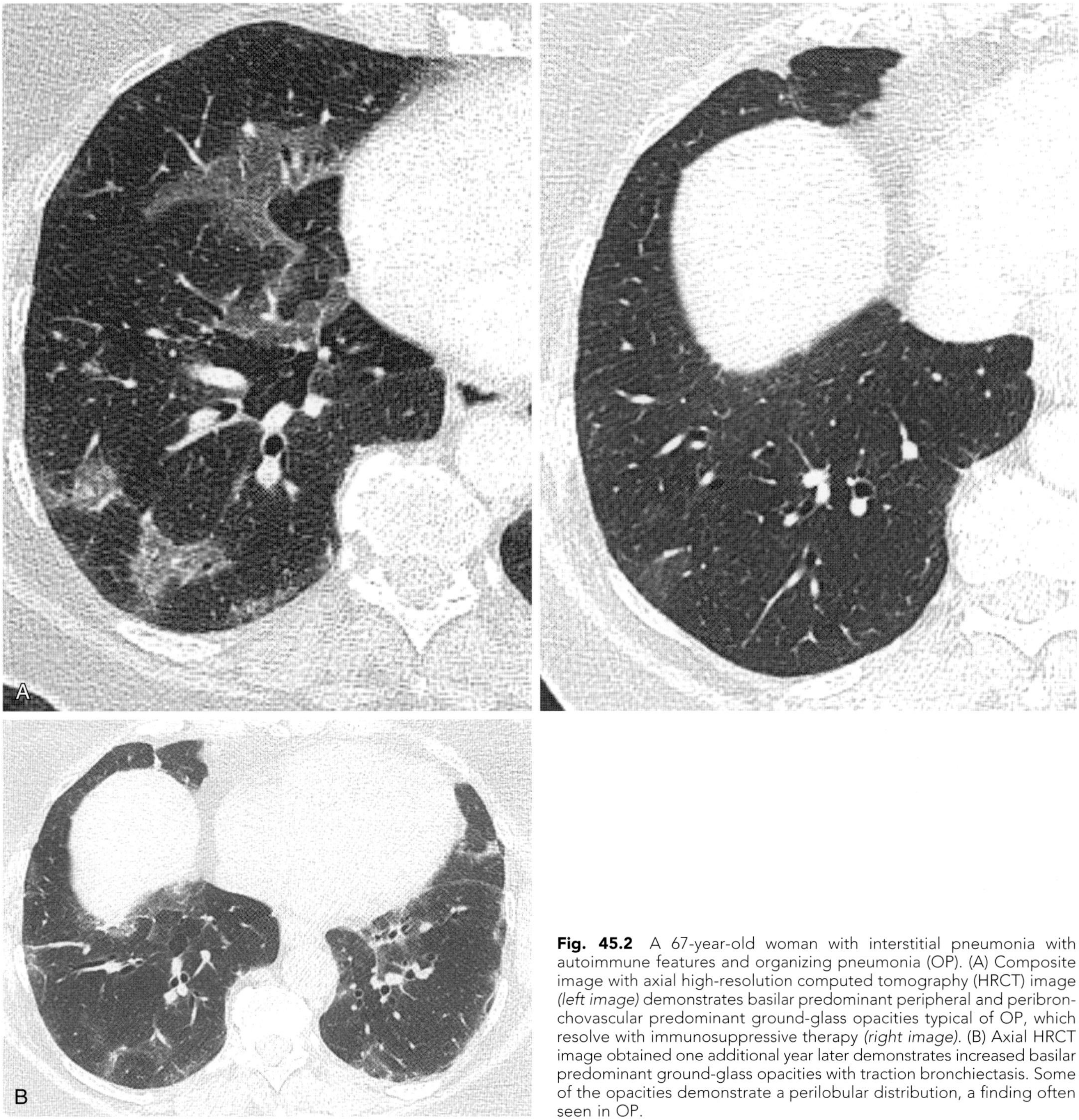

Fig. 45.2 A 67-year-old woman with interstitial pneumonia with autoimmune features and organizing pneumonia (OP). (A) Composite image with axial high-resolution computed tomography (HRCT) image *(left image)* demonstrates basilar predominant peripheral and peribronchovascular predominant ground-glass opacities typical of OP, which resolve with immunosuppressive therapy *(right image)*. (B) Axial HRCT image obtained one additional year later demonstrates increased basilar predominant ground-glass opacities with traction bronchiectasis. Some of the opacities demonstrate a perilobular distribution, a finding often seen in OP.

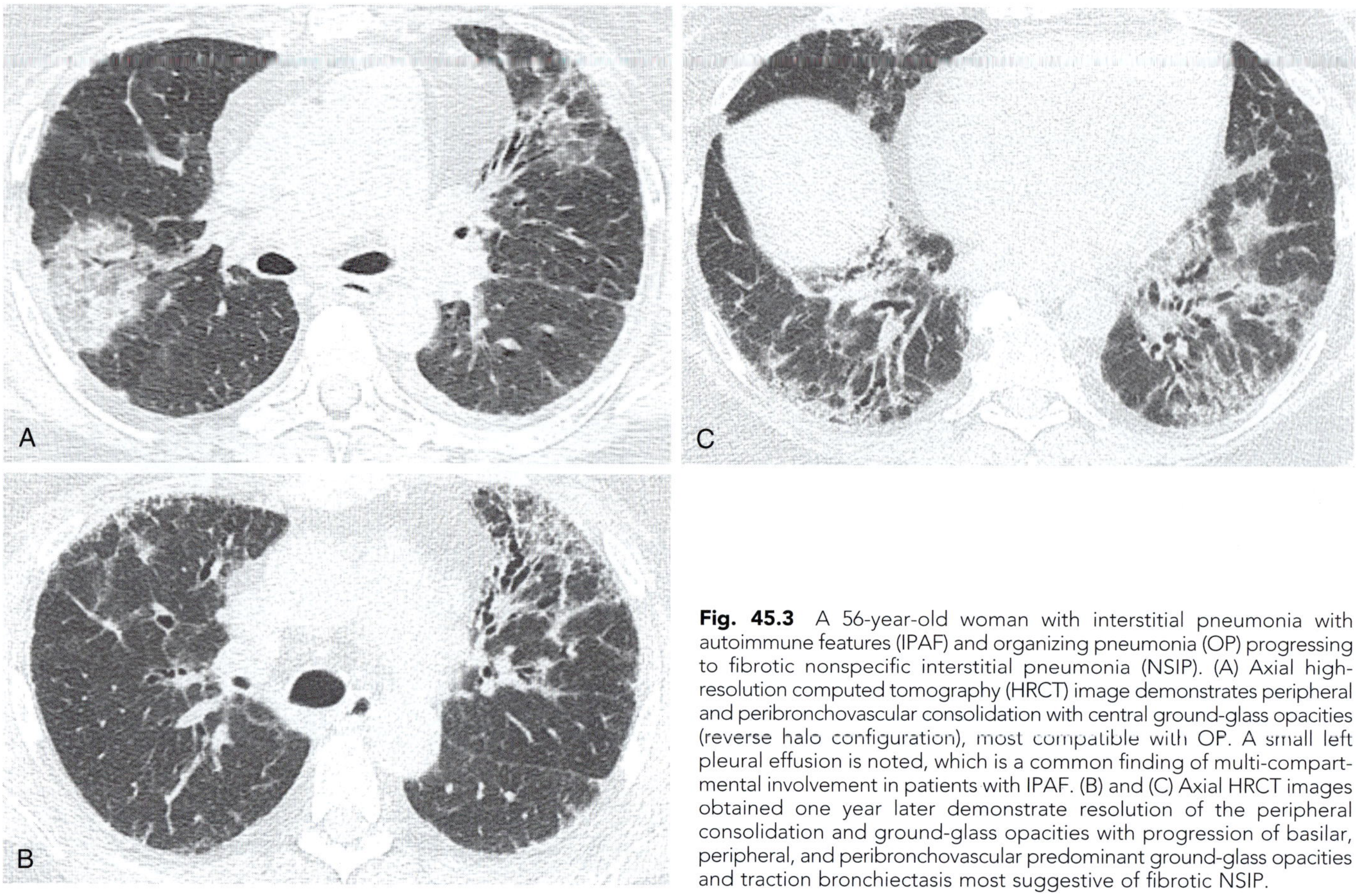

Fig. 45.3 A 56-year-old woman with interstitial pneumonia with autoimmune features (IPAF) and organizing pneumonia (OP) progressing to fibrotic nonspecific interstitial pneumonia (NSIP). (A) Axial high-resolution computed tomography (HRCT) image demonstrates peripheral and peribronchovascular consolidation with central ground-glass opacities (reverse halo configuration), most compatible with OP. A small left pleural effusion is noted, which is a common finding of multi-compartmental involvement in patients with IPAF. (B) and (C) Axial HRCT images obtained one year later demonstrate resolution of the peripheral consolidation and ground-glass opacities with progression of basilar, peripheral, and peribronchovascular predominant ground-glass opacities and traction bronchiectasis most suggestive of fibrotic NSIP.

(76%), which is similar to findings reported in a smaller North American cohort[8] and the European cohorts.[9,10] There is discrepancy among the various IPAF cohorts with regard to the predominant pattern of ILD (UIP vs. NSIP) on either HRCT or biopsy.

Imaging Features

The radiographic patterns of IPAF have not been described but likely resemble those seen with the different CT patterns. The CT patterns of IPAF and their prognostic significance were recently described for the largest North American cohort.[11] A definite UIP pattern was most commonly encountered (51%) (Fig. 45.4). Fewer patients had a probable UIP pattern (14%) and findings most consistent with a non-IPF diagnosis (35%). On the basis of the imaging pattern alone, UIP was most common (51%), followed by NSIP (27%), hypersensitivity pneumonitis (HP) (8%), NSIP with OP (7%), and OP (4%) (Table 45.2). These findings are discrepant with previous cohorts that found NSIP to be more common than UIP in IPAF patients.[8,10] Of particular interest is the presence of an HP pattern in nearly one-tenth of IPAF patients (Fig. 45.5), suggesting a possible relationship between autoimmunity and HP.[12]

Three CT findings were recently described that may be more prevalent in a UIP pattern associated with CTDs when compared with a UIP pattern associated with idiopathic pulmonary fibrosis (IPF).[13] The "anterior upper lobe sign" represents anterior upper lobe–predominant lung fibrosis with relative sparing of the remainder of the upper lobes, which is associated with concomitant lower lobe fibrosis. The "exuberant honeycombing sign" represents extensive honeycombing comprising greater than 70% of the fibrotic portions of lung (see Fig. 45.4). Finally, the "straight edge sign" represents isolation of fibrosis in the lung bases, with a sharp demarcation in the craniocaudal plane and without general extension along the lateral lung margins on coronal images.

TABLE 45.2 CT PATTERNS IN A COHORT OF 136 PATIENTS WITH INTERSTITIAL PNEUMONIA WITH AUTOIMMUNE FEATURES

CT Pattern	Number (%) of Patients
Usual interstitial pneumonia	70 (51)
Nonspecific interstitial pneumonia	37 (27)
Hypersensitivity pneumonitis	11 (8)
Nonspecific interstitial pneumonia with overlapping organizing pneumonia	9 (7)
Organizing pneumonia	5 (4)
Other	4 (3)

CT, Computed tomography; *IPAF*, interstitial pneumonia with autoimmune features.

136 patients with diagnostic-quality chest CT scans were available for review among a cohort of 144 total IPAF patients.

Adapted from Chung JH, Montner SM, Adegunsoye A, et al. CT findings, radiologic-pathologic correlation, and imaging predictors of survival for patients with interstitial pneumonia with autoimmune features. *AJR Am J Roentgenol*. 2017;208:1229-1236.

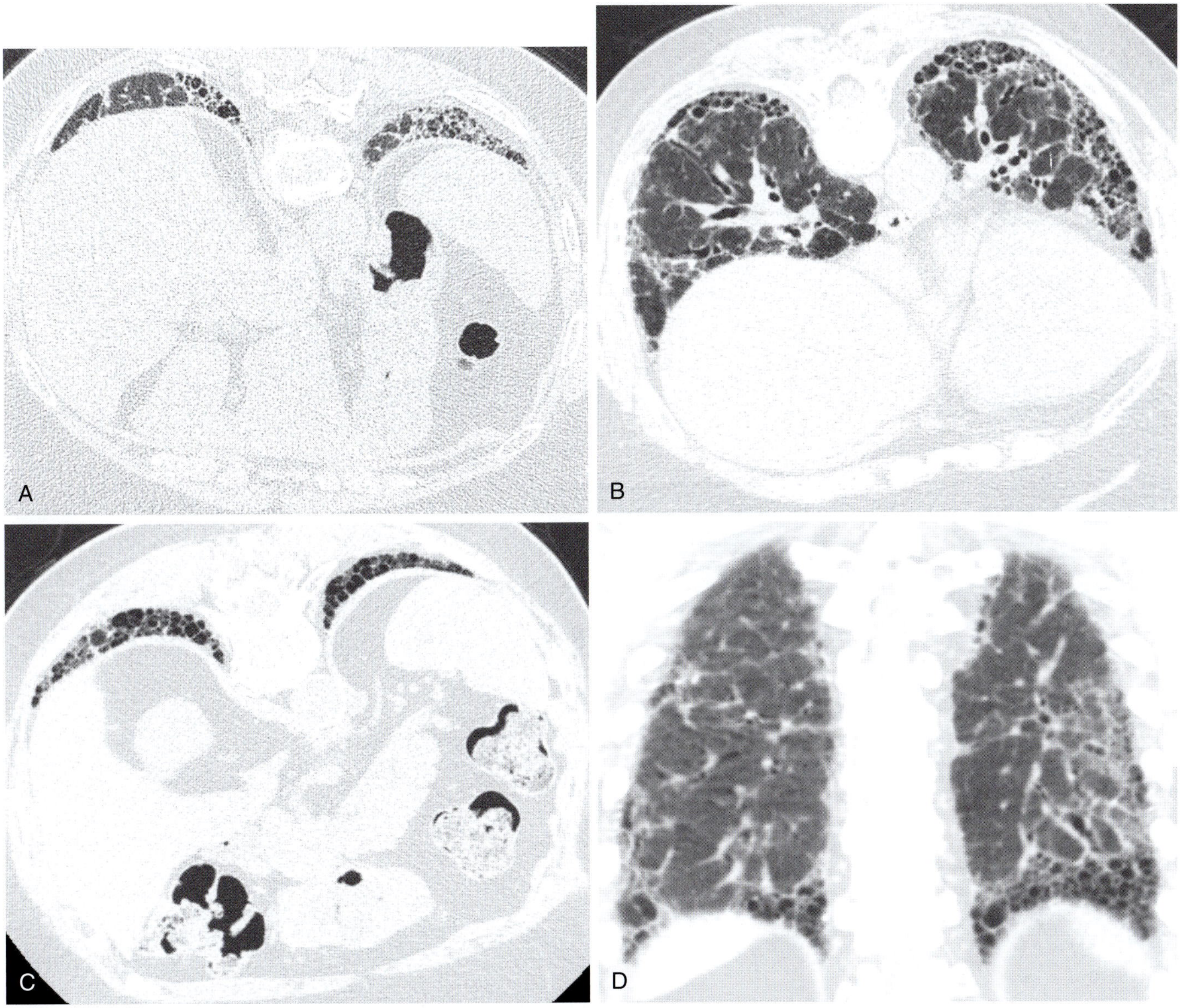

Fig. 45.4 A 73-year-old woman with interstitial pneumonia with autoimmune features and a progressive usual interstitial pneumonia pattern (UIP). (A) Prone axial high-resolution computed tomography (HRCT) image demonstrates basilar predominant subpleural reticular opacities and early honeycombing. (B to D) Prone axial and coronal HRCT images obtained three years later demonstrate progression of basilar predominant traction bronchiectasis and honeycombing, which is most pronounced at the costophrenic angles. Findings are compatible with a definite UIP pattern. This is typical of the "exuberant honeycombing sign" (i.e., the majority of fibrosis is composed solely of honeycombing), which has been described as more often associated with connective tissue disease–associated interstitial lung disease.

Most patients in the largest North American cohort had a basilar (89%) and peripheral-predominant (74%) disease distribution. Approximately 60% of patients had honeycombing, which was one of two independent predictors of mortality. Nearly all patients (96%) had traction bronchiectasis. Ground-glass opacity was present in 28% of patients and was the most common finding on CT scans, with a pattern most consistent with a non-IPF diagnosis. Mosaic attenuation without CT evidence of emphysema was present in 35% of patients, and air-trapping was present in 10% of patients. Multicompartment involvement was common, with pleural effusion or thickening present in 13% of patients and pericardial effusion or thickening present in 2% of patients. Pulmonary artery enlargement (≥3.3 cm), suggestive of possible pulmonary hypertension, was present in 27% of patients and was the only other independent predictor of mortality. Percentage of reticulation and mosaic attenuation corrected for emphysema were not predictive of mortality.

Outcomes and Treatment

In the largest North American cohort, IPAF patients demonstrated significantly worse survival than a CTD-associated ILD cohort

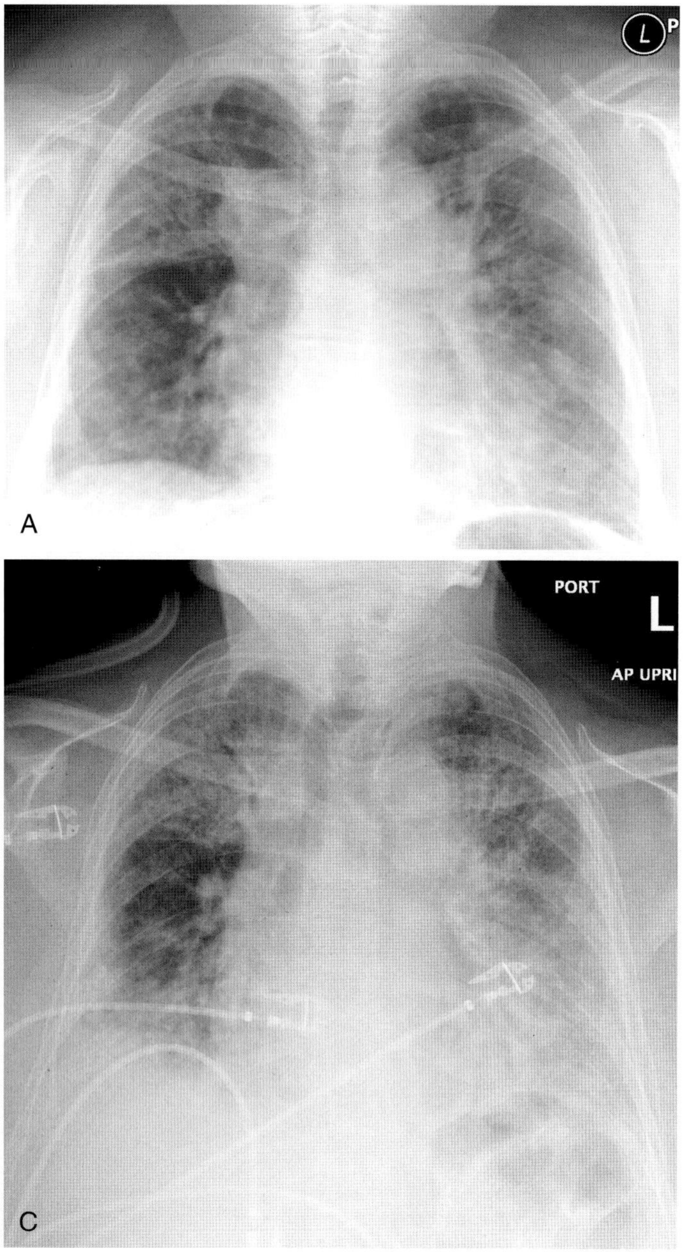

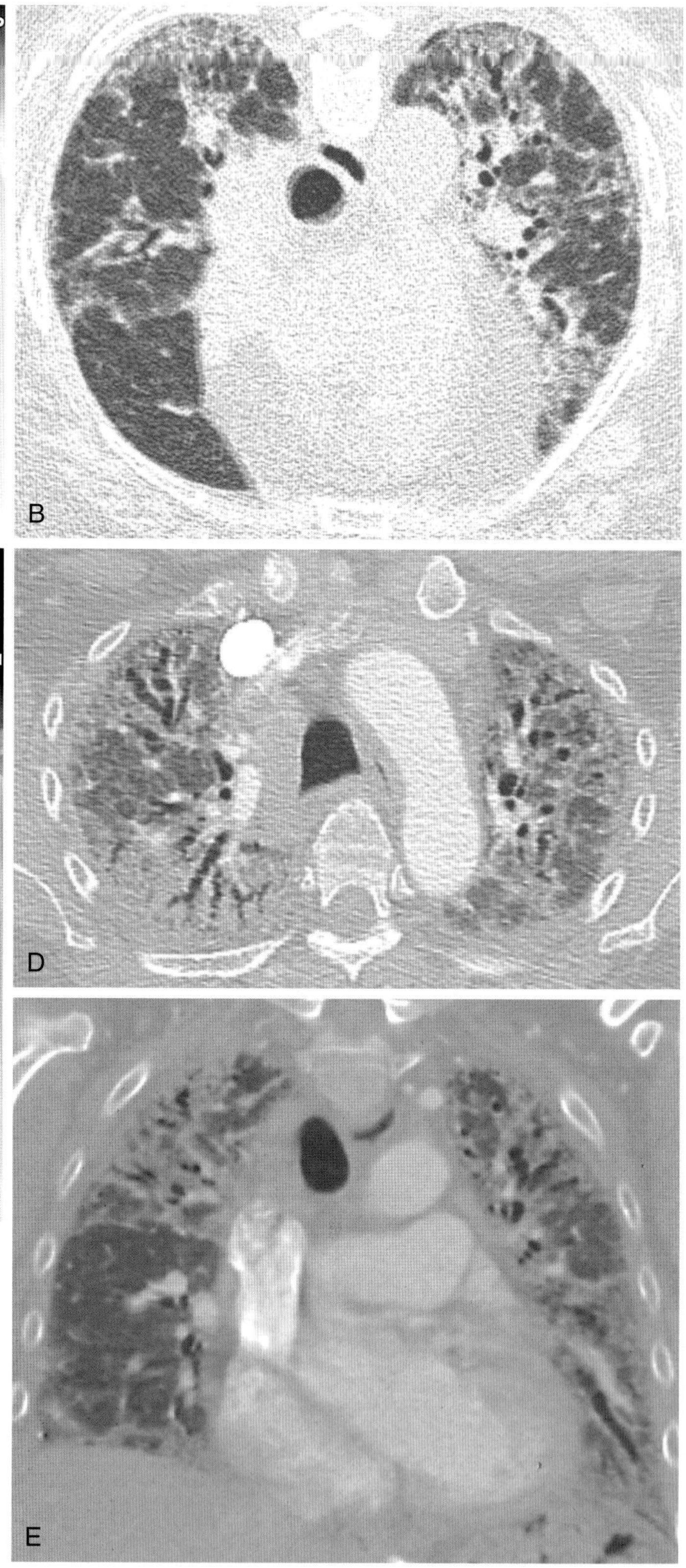

Fig. 45.5 A 62-year-old woman with interstitial pneumonia with autoimmune features and a hypersensitivity pneumonitis (HP) pattern. Frontal chest radiograph (A) and prone axial high-resolution CT image (B) demonstrate traction bronchiectasis and peribronchovascular ground-glass opacities with a middle to upper lung zone predominance. Frontal chest radiograph (C) along with axial (D) and coronal (E) CT images obtained 2 years later demonstrate progression of upper lung zone–predominant traction bronchiectasis and peribronchovascular ground-glass opacities. Findings are most compatible with a progressive chronic HP pattern.

KEY POINTS: INTERSTITIAL PNEUMONIA WITH AUTOIMMUNE FEATURES

- Interstitial pneumonia with autoimmune features (IPAF) criteria are intended to identify patients with ILD and features of autoimmunity who fail to meet overt connective tissue disease (CTD) criteria.
- Previous terms used to describe this entity include lung-dominant CTD, undifferentiated CTD-associated interstitial lung disease (ILD), and autoimmune-featured ILD.
- Diagnosis requires ILD; exclusion of alternative etiologies, including overt CTD; and additional features from defined clinical, serologic, and morphologic domains.
- The most common clinical feature is Raynaud phenomenon.
- The most common serologic feature is antinuclear antibody seropositivity.
- There is discrepancy among the IPAF cohorts with regard to the predominant pattern of ILD (usual interstitial pneumonia [UIP] vs. nonspecific interstitial pneumonia) on high-resolution computed tomography or biopsy.
- A UIP pattern, along with presence of honeycombing, pulmonary artery enlargement, and a history of cigarette smoking are reported independent predictors of mortality.
- Multicompartment involvement is common and is associated with worse survival, as this may lead to the inclusion of UIP patients with concurrent airways disease and/or pulmonary vasculopathy.
- The optimal treatment strategy for patients meeting IPAF criteria has yet to be defined.
- Outcomes are variable and highly dependent on the center under study and methods used in applying IPAF criteria.

and only marginally better survival than an IPF cohort.[7] IPAF patients without UIP had similar survival to CTD-associated ILD patients, whereas those with UIP had similar survival to IPF patients (see Fig. 45.4). Patients who satisfied morphologic subdomain criteria for HRCT had improved survival, whereas those with multicompartment involvement had worse survival. The IPAF cohorts with NSIP predominance[8,10] demonstrated more variable outcomes. A history of cigarette smoking was shown to be an independent predictor of mortality in one cohort.[10]

The optimal treatment strategy for patients meeting IPAF criteria has yet to be defined. Immunosuppression with systemic corticosteroids or steroid-sparing agents, such as mycophenolate mofetil or azathioprine, is commonly pursued but with little data to support this approach. Two recent investigations suggested that immunosuppression was associated with stability in pulmonary function over time.[8,14] The role of antifibrotic therapy in appropriately selected IPAF patients is currently under investigation.

SUGGESTED READINGS

Chung JH, Montner SM, Adegunsoye A, Lee C, Oldham JM, Husain AN, et al. CT findings, radiologic-pathologic correlation, and imaging predictors of survival for patients with interstitial pneumonia with autoimmune features. *AJR Am J Roentgenol*. 2017;208(6):1229–1236.

Fischer A, Antoniou KM, Brown KK, Cadranel J, Corte TJ, du Bois RM, et al. An official European Respiratory Society/American Thoracic Society research statement: interstitial pneumonia with autoimmune features. *Eur Respir J*. 2015;46(4):976–987.

The full reference list for this chapter is available at ExpertConsult.com.

46 Antineutrophil Cytoplasmic Antibody–Associated Vasculitis*

STEPHANE L. DESOUCHES | CHRISTOPHER M. WALKER | JONATHAN H. CHUNG

Etiology, Prevalence, and Epidemiology

Pulmonary vasculitis is traditionally characterized by size of vessel involvement as defined by the Chapel Hill nomenclature.[1] Within the small-vessel vasculitides, antineutrophil cytoplasmic antibody (ANCA)-associated vasculitis represents a diverse group of entities, and although the inciting stimulus has not been fully elucidated, an immune-mediated response is implicated.

Although rare, with an overall incidence of 20 to 100 cases per million and a prevalence of 150 to 450 cases per million,[2] pulmonary vasculitis remains one of the most challenging diagnoses and management concerns in the care of critically ill patients.[3] This in part is due to the nonspecific disease manifestations and diagnosis through a combination of clinical and imaging criteria.[2,4]

Because of the tremendous overlap in clinical and laboratory manifestations among the systemic vasculitides and an absence of validated criteria for diagnosis, determining the exact vasculitis affecting the patient and initiation of the appropriate treatment can be difficult. A recent multinational observational study, endorsed by the American College of Rheumatology and the European League Against Rheumatism, the Diagnostic and Classification Criteria for Vasculitis study (DCVAS) was started, seeking to develop and validate diagnostic and classification criteria for the primary vasculitides.[5]

Three entities are traditionally grouped within the small-vessel vasculitis class, specifically, antineutrophil cytoplasmic antibody (ANCA)-associated vasculitis: granulomatosis with polyangiitis (GPA, formerly Wegener granulomatosis), eosinophilic granulomatosis with polyangiitis (eGPA, formerly Churg-Strauss syndrome), and microscopic polyangiitis (MPA). Antineutrophil cytoplasmic antibodies activate neutrophils and monocytes that express the ANCA antigens myeloperoxidase (MPO) and proteinase 3 (PR3) on their surfaces. Cytoplasmic-pattern ANCA (c-ANCA) targets the MPO antigen, whereas perinuclear-pattern ANCA (p-ANCA) targets PR3.[6]

Although each of these entities is associated with a positive ANCA, GPA is associated with c-ANCA reactivity, eGPA is usually associated with perinuclear p-ANCA activity, and MPA can have c-ANCA or p-ANCA positivity. GPA has an annual incidence of approximately 30 cases per million,[7] whereas eGPA is the least common ANCA-associated vasculitis, with an annual incidence of approximately 2.4 cases per million.[8] MPA has an annual incidence similar to GPA, with 10 to 30 cases per million, and represents the most common cause of pulmonary-renal syndrome.[2]

*The editors and the publisher would like to thank Drs. Nestor L. Müller and C. Isabela Silva Müller for contributing material on this topic to the prior edition of this work. It has served as the foundation for the current chapter.

Granulomatosis With Polyangiitis (Formerly Wegener Granulomatosis)

Clinical Presentation

Formerly referred to as Wegener granulomatosis,[9] GPA may manifest as a systemic disease or involve primarily or exclusively the respiratory tract.[10] This limited GPA is not a distinct process but instead exists along a continuum and often precedes systemic disease.[2]

Most patients present with upper and lower respiratory symptoms, including epistaxis, sinusitis, cough, hemoptysis, dyspnea, and pleuritic chest pain.[11] Systemic symptoms include fever, malaise, weight loss, and fatigue; with joint involvement taking the form of arthralgia or arthritis. Fifty percent to 80% of patients have glomerulonephritis.[11]

Pathophysiology

Characteristic histopathologic findings consist of granulomatous inflammation with vasculitis and parenchymal necrosis.[12] A mixed cellular infiltrate of neutrophils, lymphocytes, plasma cells, histiocytes, and eosinophils tends to be aggregated in small microabscess-like clusters. As these clusters become necrotic, they enlarge, coalesce, and result in a characteristic appearance of geographic necrosis (Figs. 46.1 and 46.2). Inflammation is typically parenchymal, although mucosal or submucosal granulomatous inflammation of the airways is also common.[13] On occasion, patients may present with or develop capillaritis, which results in focal or diffuse hemorrhage that remains an important cause of morbidity and mortality in patients with GPA.[6]

Manifestations of the Disease

RADIOGRAPHY AND COMPUTED TOMOGRAPHY

The most common radiographic abnormality consists of lung nodules or masses, seen in up to 90% of patients with GPA

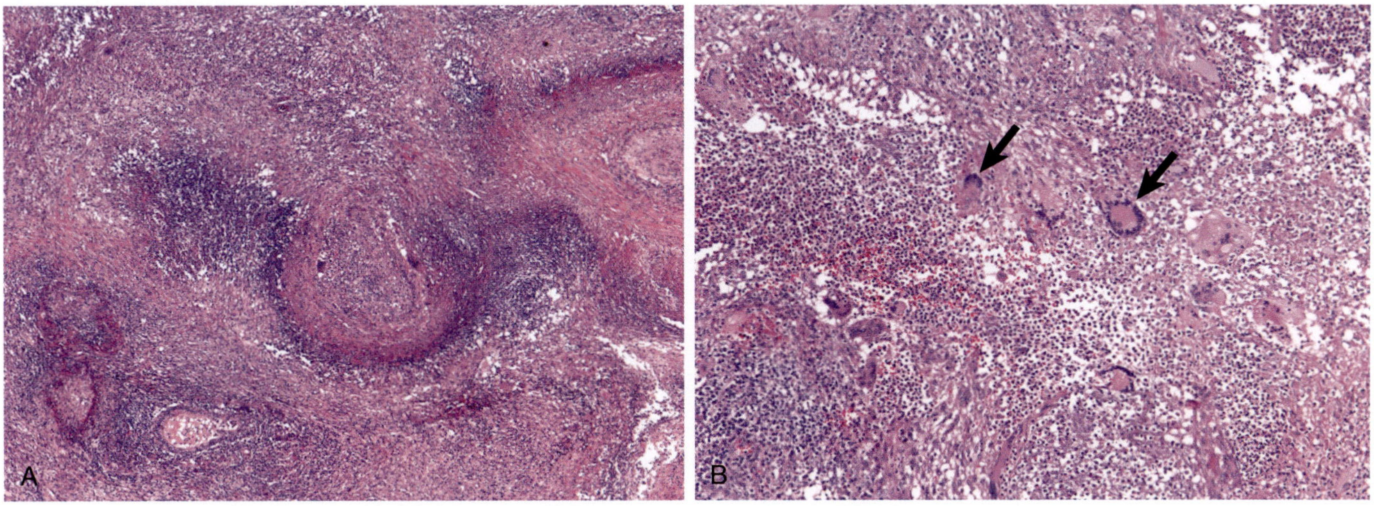

Fig. 46.1 Granulomatosis with polyangiitis: geographic necrosis. (A) Histologic specimen demonstrates areas of basophilic necrosis with irregular border, resulting in a geographic appearance. The necrotic regions are surrounded by a mixed inflammatory infiltrate. (B) High-power view demonstrates granulomatous inflammation and multinucleated giant cells *(arrows)*. *(Courtesy Dr. John English, Department of Pathology, Vancouver General Hospital, Canada.)*

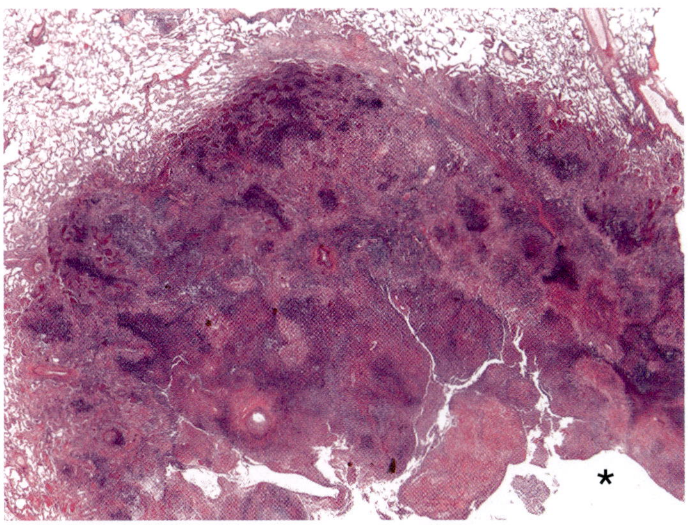

Fig. 46.2 Granulomatosis with polyangiitis: necrosis and cavitation. Histologic specimen shows nodule with necrosis and cavitation *(asterisk)*. *(Courtesy Dr. John English, Department of Pathology, Vancouver General Hospital, Canada.)*

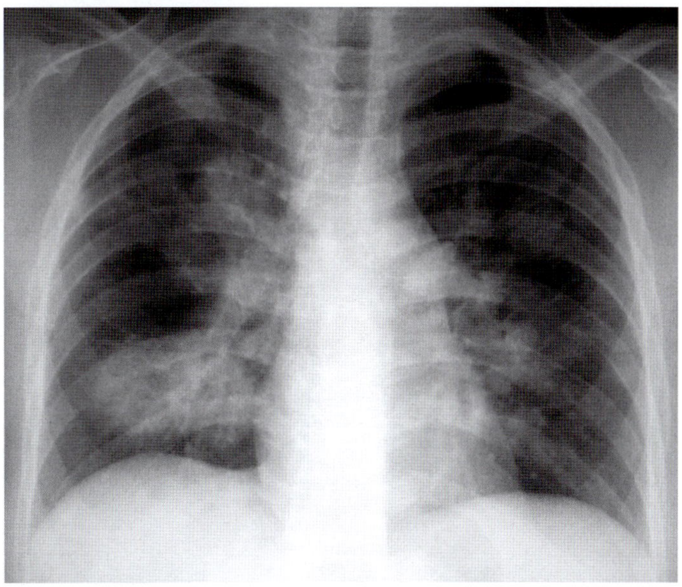

Fig. 46.3 Granulomatosis with polyangiitis: bilateral nodules and masses. Chest radiograph demonstrates bilateral nodules, masses, and focal areas of consolidation in a central distribution.

(Fig. 46.3).[13,14] The nodules and masses can range from a few millimeters to greater than 10 cm in diameter. The nodules tend to be bilateral and show no apicobasal gradient.[13,14] An increase in size and number of nodules is associated with disease progression. Computed tomography (CT) often will show nodules that are not apparent on radiography and is more sensitive for the presence of cavitation, which is evident on CT scan in most nodules larger than 2 cm in diameter (Fig. 46.4).[2] When cavitation occurs, masses tend to be thick walled and have an irregular, shaggy inner lining (Fig. 46.5).[13,14] In up to 15% of cases, one or more of the nodules or masses are surrounded by a rim of ground-glass opacity representing the CT halo sign (Fig. 46.6).[14] Less commonly, areas of ground-glass opacity can be surrounded by consolidation in the so-called reversed halo sign, which likely represents an organizing pneumonia-like reaction (Fig. 46.7).

Areas of airspace consolidation, or less commonly ground-glass opacities, are seen in approximately 25% to 50% of patients (Figs. 46.8 to 46.10).[13] Foci of cavitation may occasionally be seen within the areas of consolidation.[15] Diffuse consolidation or ground-glass opacities usually reflects the presence of pulmonary hemorrhage and can be seen in up to 10% of patients (see Fig. 46.9).[2]

Other less common parenchymal abnormalities include centrilobular nodules, tree-in-bud opacities, septal lines, and foci of calcification within the nodules, masses, or areas of consolidation.[13,14,16]

Tracheal and bronchial involvement is usually inferred on radiography by secondary signs of airway obstruction, such as

Text continued on p. 598

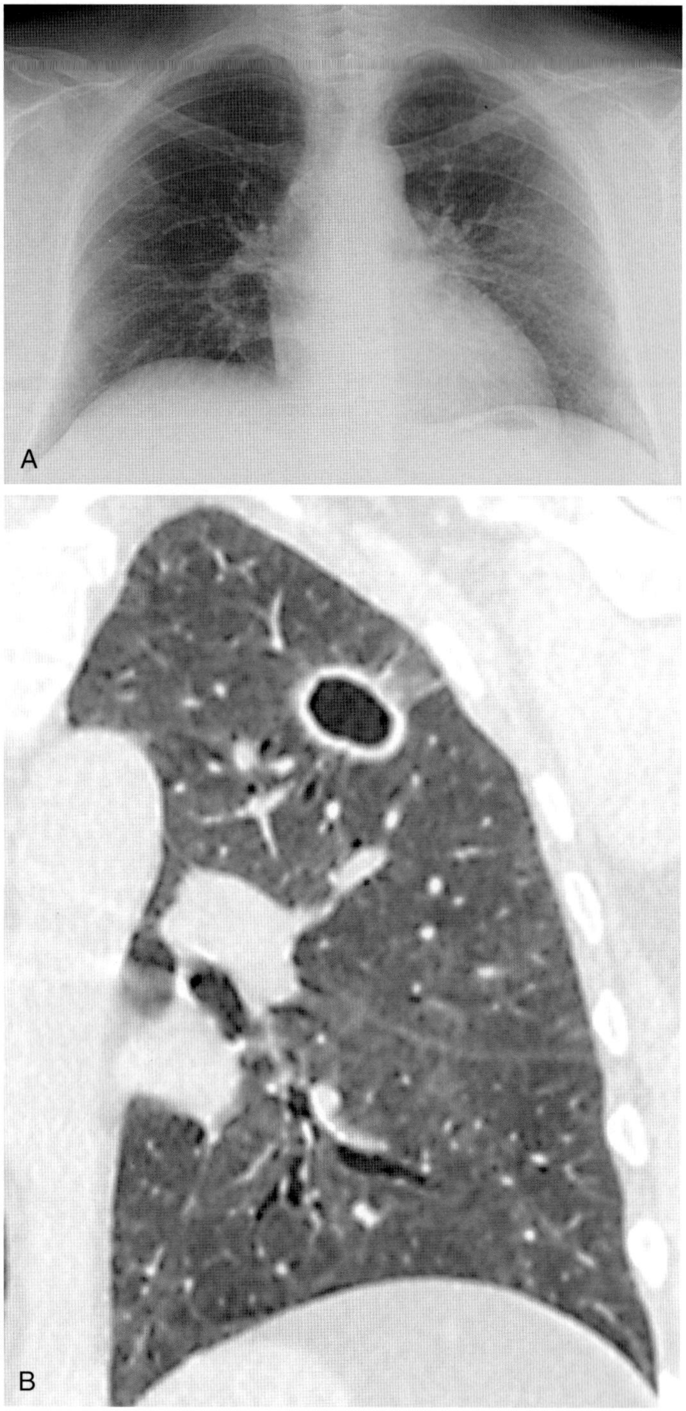

Fig. 46.4 Granulomatosis with polyangiitis: cavitary nodules. (A) Chest radiograph shows bilateral thin-walled cavitary nodules. (B) Coned-down coronal reformatted CT image demonstrates thin-walled left upper lobe cavitary nodule, with mild surrounding ground-glass opacities suggestive of hemorrhage.

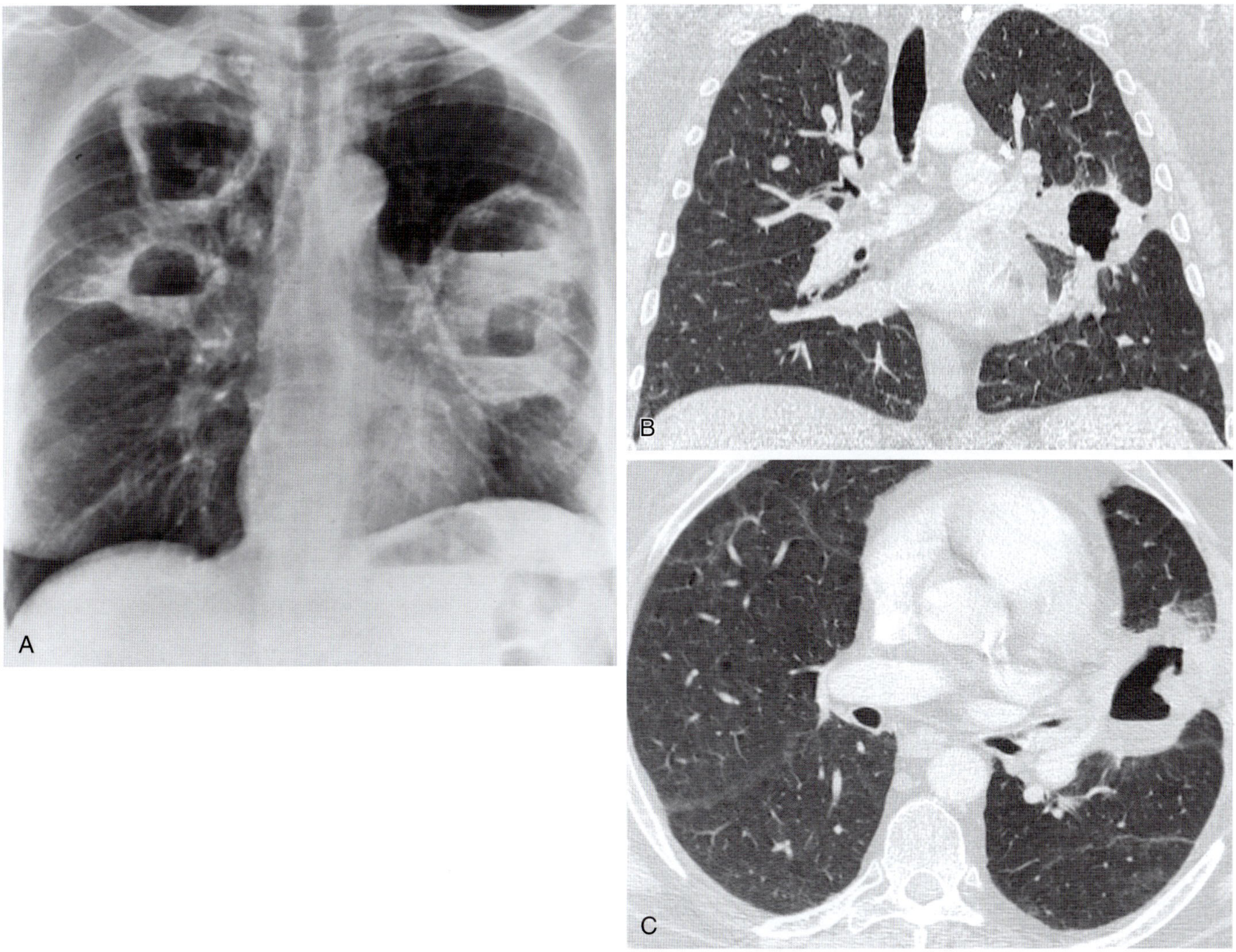

Fig. 46.5 Granulomatosis with polyangiitis: cavitating nodules and masses. (A) Posteroanterior chest radiograph shows multiple large thick-walled cavities with air-fluid levels. The left upper lung zone is oligemic, suggesting the possibility of compromise of the left upper lobe bronchus and resulting hypoxic vasoconstriction. (B) Coronal reformatted CT image from a different patient shows a thick-walled cavitary mass in the left upper lobe perihilar region. (C) CT image from the same patient as (B) shows an air-fluid level within the cavitary mass. *(Fig. 46.5A from Müller NL, Fraser RS, Colman NC, Paré PD.* Radiologic Diagnosis of Diseases of the Chest. *Philadelphia: WB Saunders; 2001.)*

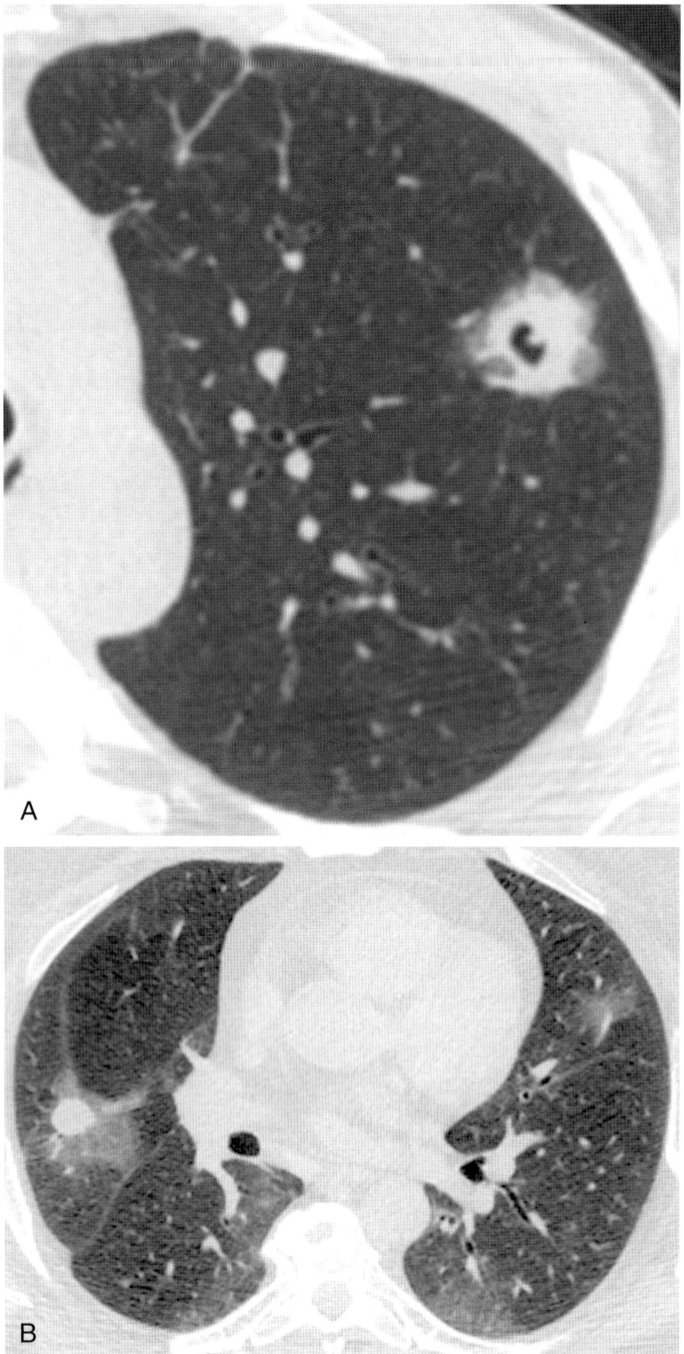

Fig. 46.6 Granulomatosis with polyangiitis: CT halo sign. (A) CT image shows peripheral cavitary nodule in the left upper lobe surrounded by a halo of ground-glass opacity. (B) CT image at the level of the minor fissure shows a noncavitary right upper lobe nodule with surrounding halo of ground-glass opacity. Foci of left upper and bilateral lower lobe ground-glass opacities likely represent pulmonary hemorrhage.

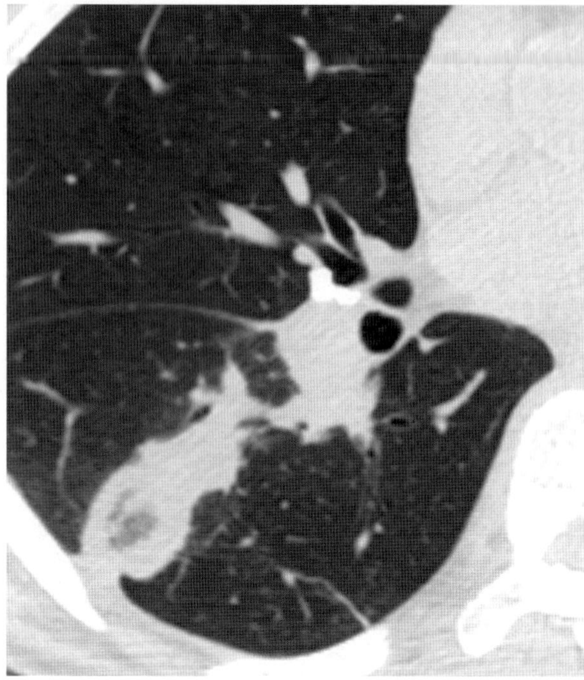

Fig. 46.7 Granulomatosis with polyangiitis: reversed halo sign. CT image shows ground-glass opacity with rim of surrounding consolidation. Histopathologic analysis of these types of nodules usually show central hemorrhage and a rim of organizing pneumonia reaction pattern.

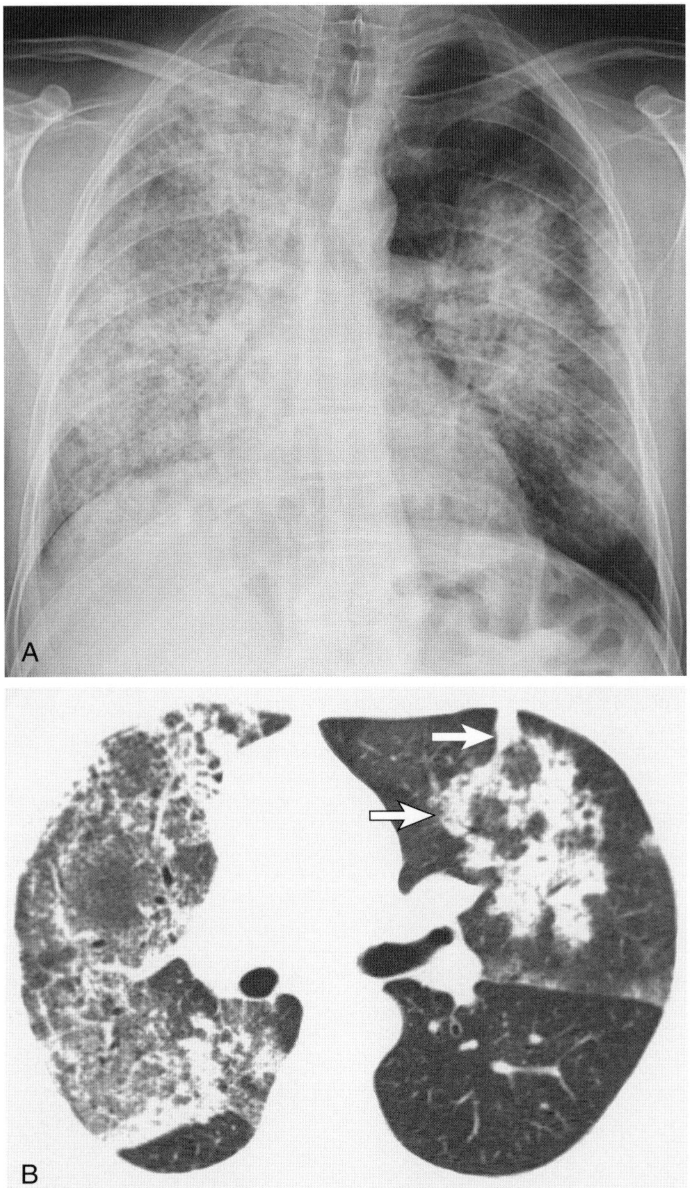

Fig. 46.8 Granulomatosis with polyangiitis: ground-glass opacities and consolidation. Chest radiograph (A) and CT image (B) show asymmetric bilateral ground-glass opacities and areas of consolidation. On CT the consolidation in the left upper lobe has a perilobular distribution of consolidation *(arrows)* that surrounds ground-glass opacities, a finding consistent with organizing pneumonia secondary to pulmonary hemorrhage.

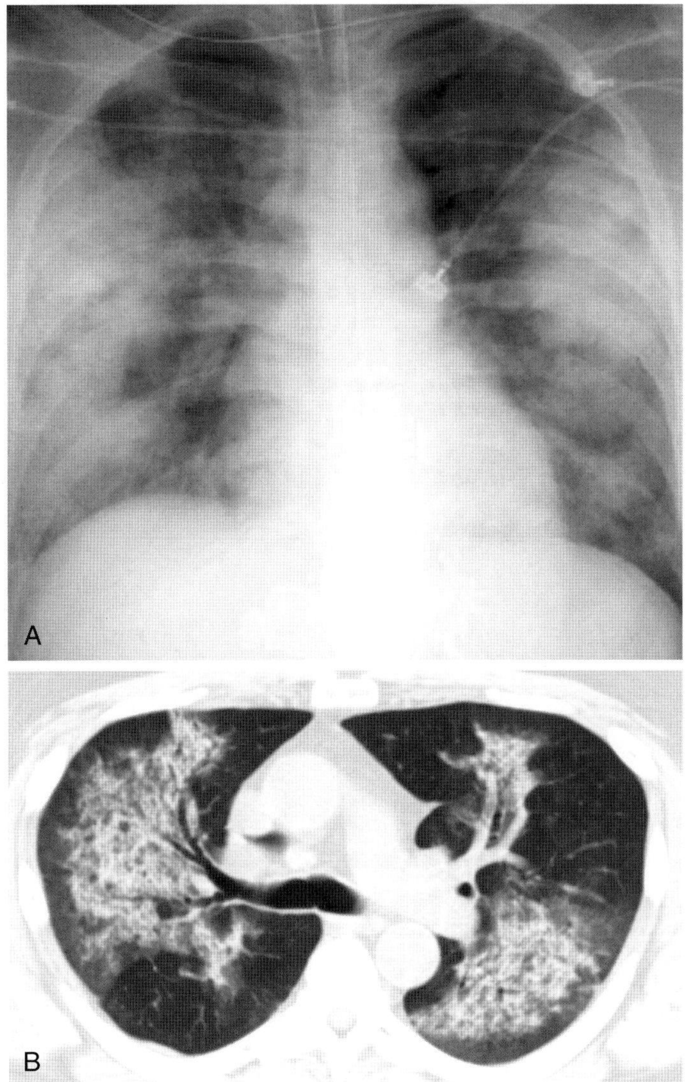

Fig. 46.9 Granulomatosis with polyangiitis: pulmonary hemorrhage. (A) Chest radiograph shows perihilar predominant consolidation that spares the lung apices and bases. (B) Axial CT image shows perihilar predominant consolidation and ground-glass opacities that spare the lung periphery, which is typical of pulmonary hemorrhage. *(From Lichtenberger JP 3rd, Digumarthy SR, Abbott GF, et al. Diffuse pulmonary hemorrhage: clues to the diagnosis.* Curr Probl Diagn Radiol. *2014;43:128–139.)*

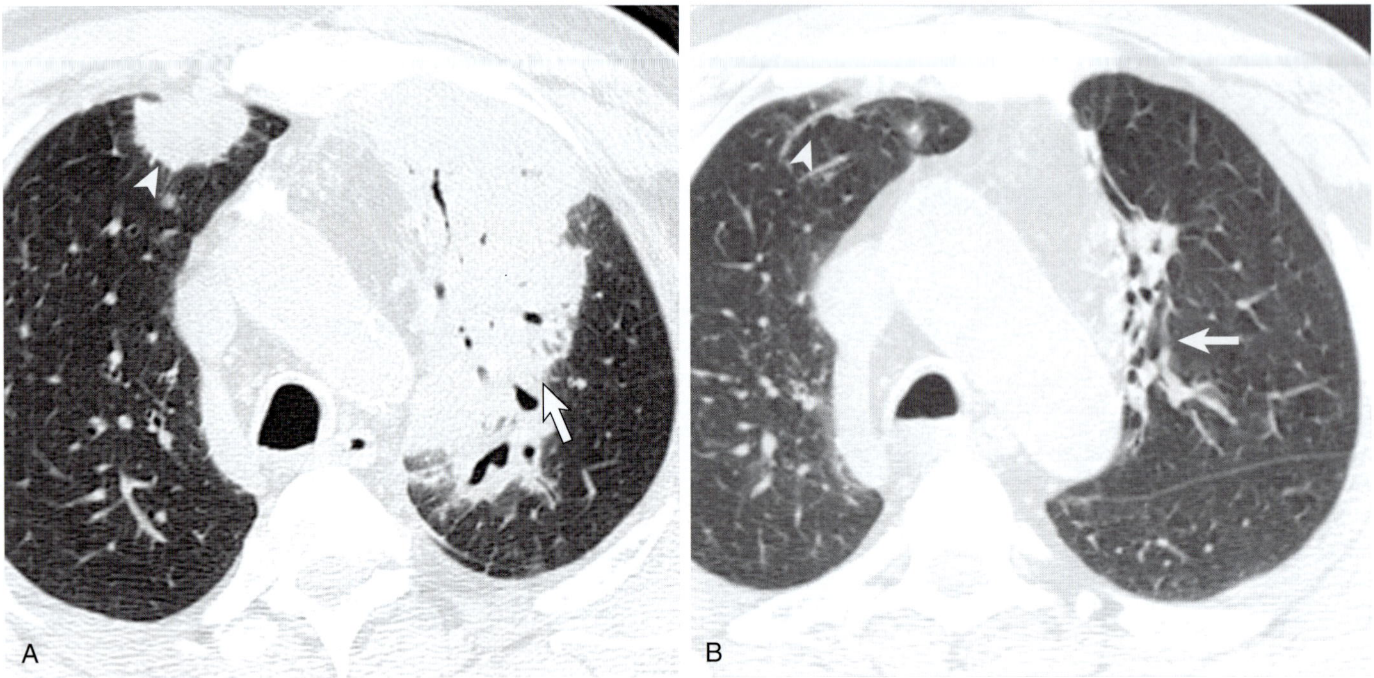

Fig. 46.10 Granulomatosis with polyangiitis: mass and consolidation before and after treatment. (A) CT image shows a right upper lobe mass *(arrowhead)* and left upper lobe consolidation *(arrow)* containing air bronchograms. (B) Repeat CT image 9 months after initiation of treatment demonstrates considerable improvement of the right upper lobe mass *(arrowhead)* and left upper lobe consolidation *(arrow)* with residual scarring. *(From Martinez F, Chung J, Digumarthy S, et al. Common and uncommon manifestations of Wegener granulomatosis at chest CT: radiologic-pathologic correlation.* Radiographics. *2012;32:51–69.)*

atelectasis or air-trapping.[15] When focal airway stenosis is visualized, it most commonly affects the subglottic trachea (Fig. 46.11). With CT central bronchial wall thickening is seen in 50% to 60% of patients and tracheal wall thickening in 15% (Fig. 46.12).[13,14] Multiplanar reconstructions are essential for optimal imaging assessment of the presence and severity of airway stenosis (see Fig. 46.12).[16]

Pleural effusions occur in 15% to 20% of patients and pleural thickening in 10%.[13,14] Mediastinal lymph node enlargement is seen on CT in approximately 20% of cases and hilar lymph node enlargement in 3%.[13]

Approximately 50% of nodules and masses will resolve completely with disease treatment, and another 40% will decrease in size.[2] However, intralobular linear opacities and areas of bronchiectasis tend to remain stable.[17] This reinforces the theory that ground-glass opacities, consolidation, cavitated nodules, and masses represent active inflammatory lesions, whereas intralobular linear opacities and areas of bronchiectasis more often represent chronic fibrosis. Rarely, hemosiderin can accumulate in the alveoli from repeated hemorrhage, resulting in diffuse centrilobular nodules (Fig. 46.13).

Interstitial fibrosis with a pattern resembling idiopathic nonspecific interstitial pneumonia or idiopathic pulmonary fibrosis may occasionally be the first manifestation of GPA.[18] Uncommonly, GPA will involve the aorta and great vessels, the heart, the cardiac valves, or the pulmonary arteries.

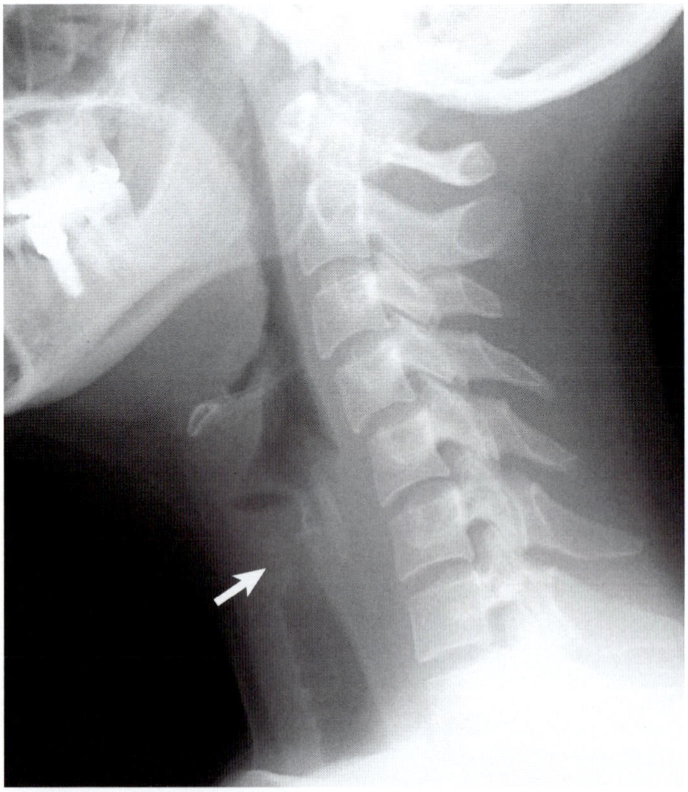

Fig. 46.11 Granulomatosis with polyangiitis: subglottic stenosis. Lateral view of the neck shows focal wall thickening of the subglottic trachea *(arrow)* with associated stenosis.

NUCLEAR IMAGING

Evaluation of multisystem involvement and monitoring treatment response and maintenance can be facilitated with nuclear imaging.

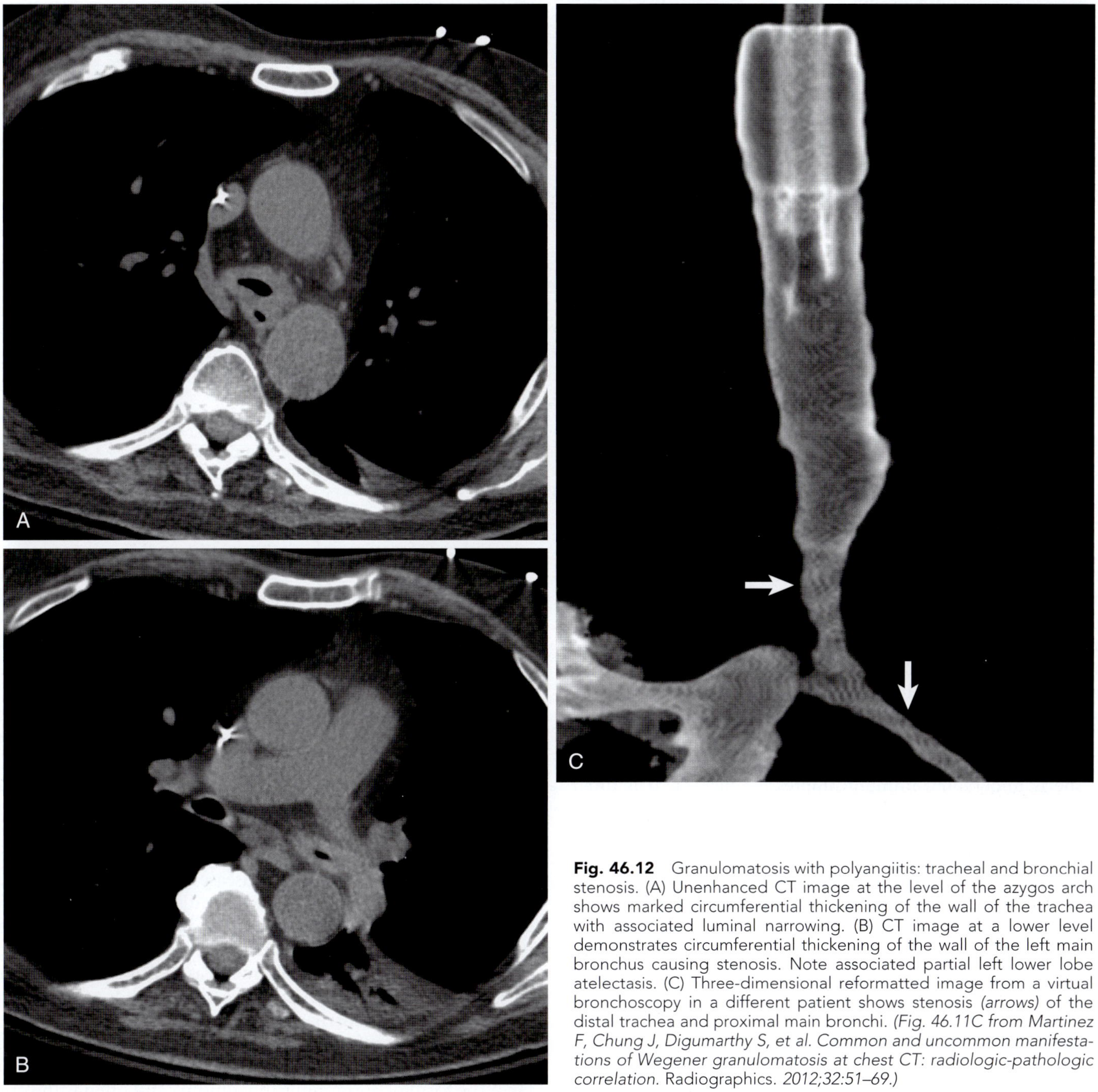

Fig. 46.12 Granulomatosis with polyangiitis: tracheal and bronchial stenosis. (A) Unenhanced CT image at the level of the azygos arch shows marked circumferential thickening of the wall of the trachea with associated luminal narrowing. (B) CT image at a lower level demonstrates circumferential thickening of the wall of the left main bronchus causing stenosis. Note associated partial left lower lobe atelectasis. (C) Three-dimensional reformatted image from a virtual bronchoscopy in a different patient shows stenosis *(arrows)* of the distal trachea and proximal main bronchi. *(Fig. 46.11C from Martinez F, Chung J, Digumarthy S, et al. Common and uncommon manifestations of Wegener granulomatosis at chest CT: radiologic-pathologic correlation.* Radiographics. *2012;32:51–69.)*

Imaging with gallium-67 has been shown to be helpful as a negative scan virtually excludes active disease. Unfortunately, specificity is lower in these scans as inflammation from other sources, including bacterial or viral infection, can result in a false-positive interpretation.[19]

Imaging of GPA with fluorodeoxyglucose (FDG) PET with CT improves upper respiratory tract lesion detection.[7] Increased uptake on FDG-PET can help localize active lesions for biopsy during initial workup, and maximum standardized uptake value correlates with disease activity, allowing use for treatment response and maintenance.[7]

Differential Diagnosis

The radiologic manifestations of GPA, although multiple and variable, consist mainly of bilateral subpleural or peribronchovascular nodules or masses with and without cavitation. The main differential diagnoses for this pattern include infections (septic embolism, fungal infection, multiple lung abscesses) and neoplasms (hematogenous metastases, lymphoma). Septic emboli and multiple lung abscesses usually favor the lower lobes and seldom measure more than 3 cm in diameter. There is also commonly a clinical history suggestive of infection, such as fever.

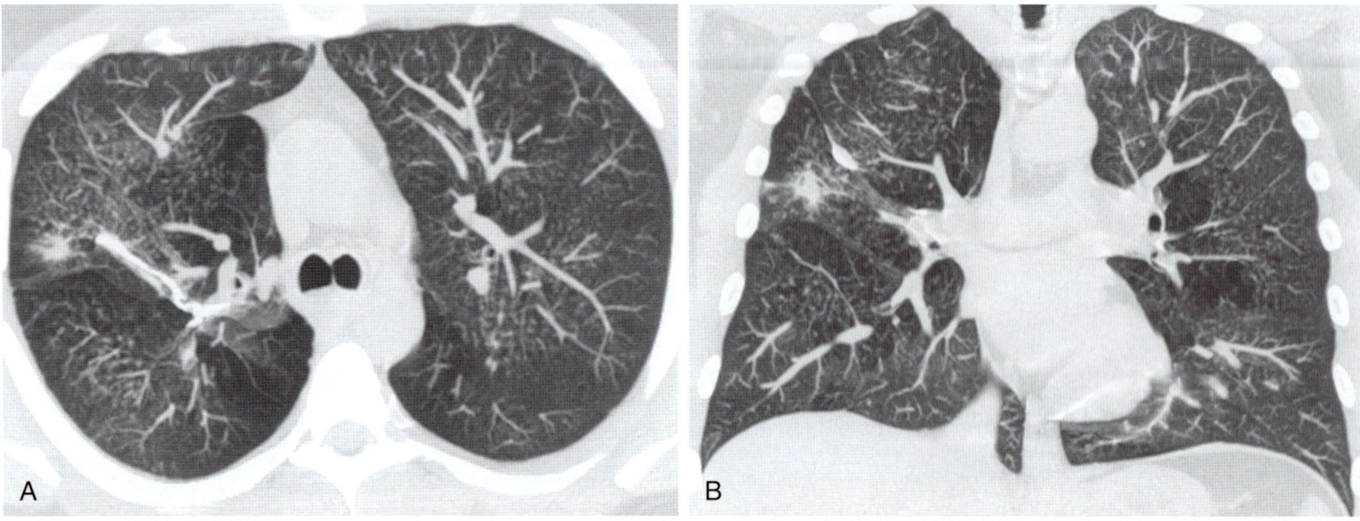

Fig. 46.13 Granulomatosis with polyangiitis (GPA): hemosiderosis. Axial (A) and coronal (B) maximum-intensity projection images show diffuse bilateral centrilobular nodules. A spiculated right upper lobe nodule is also noted relating to patient's known GPA. Surgical biopsy showed the centrilobular nodules represented hemosiderin secondary to repeated alveolar hemorrhage.

Hematogenous metastases and lymphoma may be multiple and range in size from a few millimeters to greater than 10 cm in diameter but also usually show a lower lobe predominance and rarely if ever cavitate. The distinction of GPA from these other conditions can usually be made clinically by the presence of upper respiratory symptoms, including sinusitis and epistaxis, laboratory findings indicative of glomerulonephritis, and the presence of serum c-ANCA.

A particular issue arises when new nodules or masses are detected in a person who has known GPA, especially when he or she is undergoing immunosuppressive therapy. It is often difficult to differentiate opportunistic infections (e.g., fungal organisms or *Nocardia*) or a new malignancy from simply a worsening of GPA. In these patients bronchoscopy and occasionally biopsy is needed to exclude infection or malignancy before initiating higher doses of immunomodulatory therapy.

Eosinophilic Granulomatosis With Polyangiitis (Formerly Churg-Strauss Syndrome)

Clinical Presentation

Formerly referred to as Churg-Strauss syndrome, eGPA nearly always manifests with the classic clinical triad of asthma, hypereosinophilia, and vasculitis.[2] This entity exists as three distinct clinical phases; there is prodromal stage of adult-onset asthma, usually lasting years, generally requiring corticosteroid therapy and often preceded by allergic rhinitis. This is usually followed by a second phase with marked peripheral blood eosinophilia and eosinophilic tissue infiltrates. The third stage consists of an often life-threatening vasculitic phase that can manifest with acute respiratory distress syndrome and pulmonary hemorrhage.[20,21] The disease can, but does not always, progress through each stage in turn. Cardiac involvement, seen in 13% to 47% of cases, may result in angina, myocardial infarction, myocarditis, left-sided heart failure, and pericarditis.[22] The majority of patients respond to treatment with corticosteroids and immunomodulators, with about 25% experiencing relapses of disease. Among those patients who relapse, most will respond to repeat treatment. Mortality among treated patients who relapse approaches 3%.[23]

Pathophysiology

Although the exact pathophysiology of eGPA is not clear, its association with asthma and atopy, as well as eosinophilia, suggests an autoimmune or allergic process.[20] Markers of eosinophil activation parallel disease activity and seem to predict relapses; it is also known that direct tissue injury is caused by eosinophils and neutrophil degranulation products.[22] ANCAs are present in about 40% to 75% of patients with eGPA, and both the frequency and levels seem to correlate with disease activity.[22,24] The presence or absence of ANCA usually allows a distinction between two subtypes of eGPA. ANCA positivity is associated with a higher prevalence of renal (rapidly progressive glomerulonephritis), nervous system, and skin involvement, as well as alveolar hemorrhage. Alternatively, ANCA-negative disease tends to have more cardiac and nonhemorrhagic pulmonary involvement.

The characteristic feature of the early phase of eGPA is extravascular tissue infiltration by eosinophils.[25] In the lung this takes the form of eosinophilic pneumonia and often is the only abnormality seen on surgical biopsy.[25] In the vasculitic phase eosinophilic tissue infiltration is almost always present, but findings of vasculitis are also seen (Fig. 46.14). These are characterized by an eosinophil-rich necrotizing vasculitis involving primarily small arteries, arterioles, venules, and veins and necrotizing granulomas centered on necrotic eosinophils.[25] On histologic examination, the only specific finding of healed vasculitis is thrombosed small vessels.[25]

Manifestations of the Disease

RADIOGRAPHY

Radiography typically shows bilateral nonsegmental airspace opacities without an apicobasal gradient (Fig. 46.15).[2,20] The areas

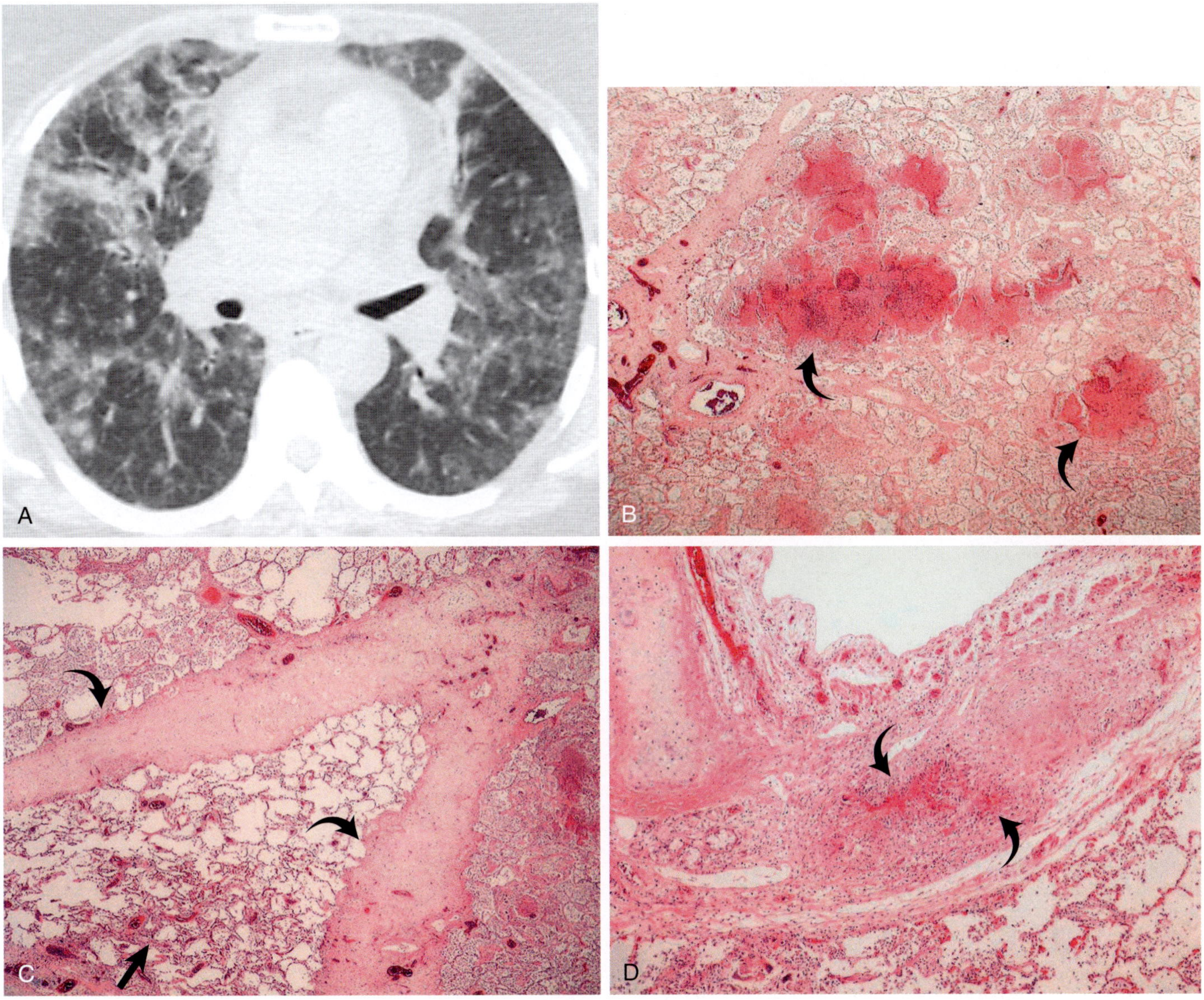

Fig. 46.14 Eosinophilic granulomatosis with polyangiitis: CT and histologic findings. (A) CT image shows predominantly peripheral ground-glass opacities bilaterally. Small areas of consolidation are noted in both upper lobes. Also noted are thickening of the interlobular septa best visualized in the anterior right upper lobe. (B) Photomicrograph of histopathologic specimen shows eosinophilic pneumonia pattern with large number of partially necrotic eosinophils *(arrows)*. (C) Photomicrograph from a different patient shows edematous and fibrotic interlobular septa *(curved arrows)*. A focus of very early eosinophilic pneumonia is present between the interlobular septa *(straight arrow)*. Such small foci could result in poorly defined centrilobular ground-glass nodules. A focus of well-developed eosinophilic pneumonia with eosinophil necrosis is present to the right of the thickened septum. (D) Photomicrograph shows necrotizing focus *(arrows)* in the wall of a large bronchus. *(From Silva CI, Müller NL, Fujimoto K, et al. Churg-Strauss syndrome: high-resolution CT and pathologic findings.* J Thorac Imaging. *2005;20:74–80.)*

of consolidation may have a peripheral distribution, overlapping with findings of chronic eosinophilic pneumonia (Fig. 46.16), or may be transient and migratory and be indistinguishable from simple pulmonary eosinophilia (Löffler syndrome).[26,27] In contrast to GPA, even when these airspace opacities become confluent, cavitation is rare.[26,27] Cardiac involvement may result in cardiomegaly from myocarditis or ischemic cardiomyopathy and pericardial effusion. Unilateral or bilateral pleural effusions are seen on the chest radiograph in approximately 10% of patients.[22]

COMPUTED TOMOGRAPHY

Seen in up to 90% of patients, bilateral areas of ground-glass opacities or consolidation are the most common abnormalities on CT.[20,26,27] These usually have a symmetric distribution and often a peripheral predominance similar to chronic eosinophilic pneumonia (see Fig. 46.16).[26,27] Another relatively common finding on CT is the presence of interlobular septal thickening, seen in approximately 50% of patients (see Fig. 46.14), which may reflect the presence of interstitial pulmonary edema secondary to cardiac involvement or eosinophilic infiltration of the

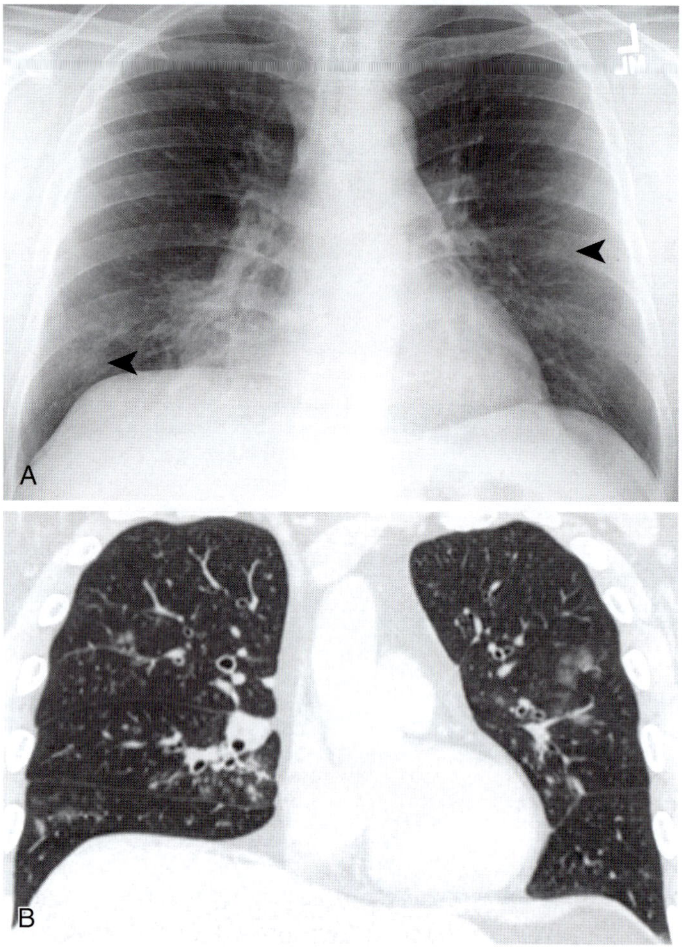

Fig. 46.15 Eosinophilic granulomatosis with polyangiitis (eGPA): patchy distribution and tree-in-bud opacities. (A) Chest radiograph shows subtle patchy bilateral airspace opacities *(arrowheads)*. (B) Coronal reformatted CT image demonstrates patchy bilateral ground-glass opacities with tree-in-bud opacities in the right middle lobe. Many of the airway-associated findings of eGPA (e.g., bronchial wall thickening, endoluminal mucous plugging, tree-in-bud opacities) are in part explained by asthma, which is present in nearly all affected patients.

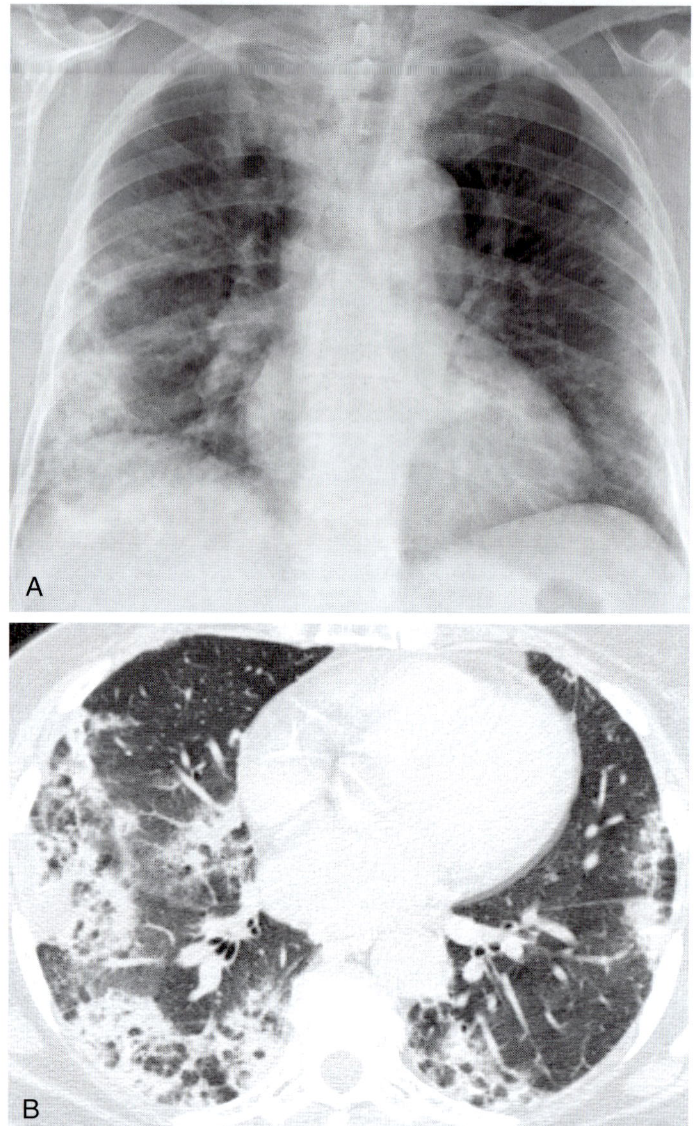

Fig. 46.16 Eosinophilic granulomatosis with polyangiitis: chronic eosinophilic pneumonia pattern. (A) Chest radiograph shows patchy bilateral areas of consolidation in a predominantly subpleural distribution. (B) CT image shows bilateral peripheral, subpleural areas of consolidation.

septa.[27,28] Less common findings, partially explained by coexistent asthma, include small centrilobular nodules, bronchial wall thickening, bronchial dilation, and tree-in-bud opacities.[21] Unilateral or bilateral pleural effusions are seen on CT in 10% to 50%[22] and may be caused by left-sided heart failure resulting from cardiomyopathy or by eosinophilic pleuritis.[22,27] Mediastinal lymphadenopathy can be observed but is uncommon.[21]

Differential Diagnosis

In clinical practice the diagnosis of eGPA is made through a combination of imaging findings, chronicity, and clinical presentation. The imaging findings of transient, patchy nonsegmental ground-glass opacities or consolidation without predilection for any lung zone, seen in a patient with a history of asthma, should raise suspicion for eGPA, although simple pulmonary eosinophilia and chronic eosinophilic pneumonia could manifest similarly. By imaging alone, the differential diagnosis would also include allergic bronchopulmonary aspergillosis, simple pulmonary eosinophilia, chronic eosinophilic pneumonia, organizing pneumonia, bacterial pneumonia, fungal pneumonia, and viral pneumonia.

The diagnosis of eGPA—as distinct from simple pulmonary eosinophilia or chronic eosinophilic lung disease in patients with asthma—is based on systemic manifestations, including rash, peripheral neuropathy, and presence of serum p-ANCA.[23]

Pneumonia as a cause of bilateral opacities in patients with asthma, as in other patients, needs to be excluded on the basis of clinical findings and appropriate cultures or serologic tests. The main considerations are infections that may result in symmetric bilateral ground-glass opacities or consolidation. These include mainly bacterial, mycoplasmal, or viral bronchopneumonia and opportunistic infections, such as those caused by *Pneumocystis jirovecii* and cytomegalovirus, which can be seen in asthmatic patients being treated with corticosteroids.

Microscopic Polyangiitis

Clinical Presentation

MPA often has a subacute prodromal phase, including fever, chills, weight loss, arthralgias, and myalgias lasting weeks to months before onset of the more characteristic acute vasculitic symptoms.[3] The vasculitis manifestations are usually renal and, less commonly, pulmonary. Rapidly progressive glomerulonephritis occurs in more than 90% of patients and diffuse pulmonary hemorrhage in 10% to 30%.[2] Other relatively common manifestations include skin lesions, peripheral neuritis, and gastrointestinal hemorrhage.[29]

Involvement of the sinuses, upper airway, or the eyes is uncommon in MPA and more often seen in patients with GPA. Although clinical symptoms of MPA and polyarteritis nodosa (PAN) may overlap, involvement of the pulmonary arteries suggests MPA as this is very rare in PAN.[30]

Pathophysiology

Like the other ANCA-associated vasculitides, the pathogenesis of MPA is unknown. Serum ANCAs are present in the majority of patients, including p-ANCAs directed against MPO in 50% to 75% of cases (as seen in eGPA) and c-ANCAs directed against PR3 in 10% to 15% (as seen in GPA).[31] The available data suggest that ANCAs are a pathogenic factor in the development of small-vessel vasculitis.[32] However, because not all patients with MPA have serum ANCA positivity and the antibody can be found in association with other diseases, other factors are probably involved.

The most common manifestation is renal disease with rapidly progressive glomerulonephritis. The main pulmonary histologic findings are neutrophilic capillaritis and alveolar hemorrhage.[33] Alveolar hemorrhage and capillaritis represent a histologic reaction pattern rather than a specific disease entity.[34] This pattern may be seen in a variety of diseases, including MPA, GPA, connective tissue diseases (particularly systemic lupus erythematosus), antiphospholipid syndrome, and drug hypersensitivity.[34]

Manifestations of the Disease

RADIOGRAPHY

The radiographic features consist of patchy or diffuse bilateral airspace opacities and consolidation representing alveolar hemorrhage (Fig. 46.17).[3] These airspace opacities and consolidations

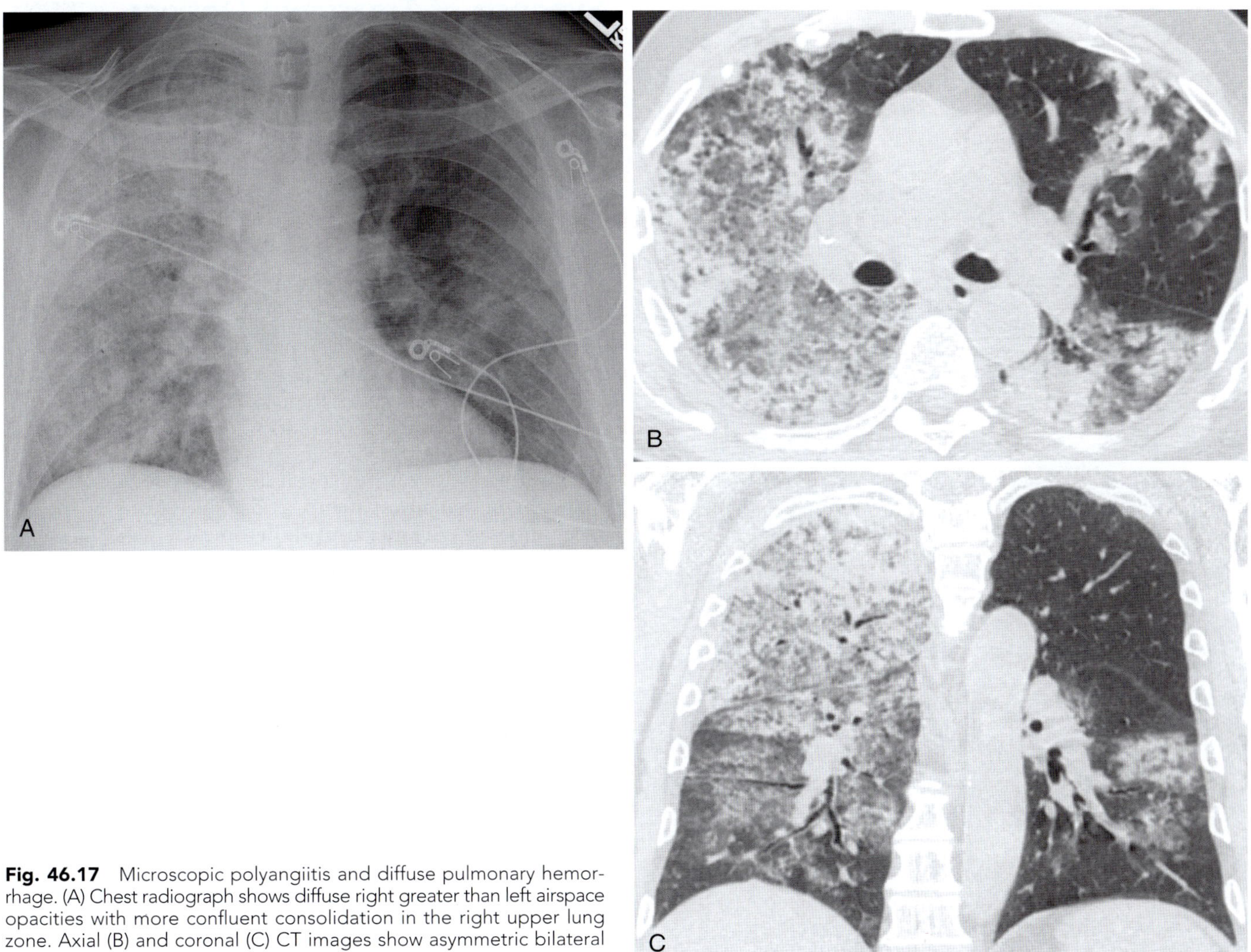

Fig. 46.17 Microscopic polyangiitis and diffuse pulmonary hemorrhage. (A) Chest radiograph shows diffuse right greater than left airspace opacities with more confluent consolidation in the right upper lung zone. Axial (B) and coronal (C) CT images show asymmetric bilateral ground-glass opacities and consolidation.

are usually widespread but may be more prominent in the perihilar areas and in the middle and lower lung zones.[35–37]

COMPUTED TOMOGRAPHY

Imaging findings on CT usually consist of bilateral ground-glass opacities and consolidation that may be patchy or diffuse (see Fig. 46.17).[30] The ground-glass opacity corresponds to alveolar hemorrhage from capillaritis and interstitial chronic inflammation in the alveolar septa. Repeated hemorrhage in patients with MPA can lead to interstitial fibrosis, which portends a worse prognosis. Appropriate treatment can result in complete resolution of symptoms and imaging findings (Fig. 46.18).

Differential Diagnosis

The diagnosis of MPA should be suspected in patients with rapidly progressive glomerulonephritis and presence of p-ANCA who present with clinical and radiologic findings consistent with diffuse pulmonary hemorrhage.

Lung biopsy shows nonspecific findings, including diffuse alveolar hemorrhage and capillaritis. Similar findings may be seen in GPA, systemic lupus erythematosus, and drug hypersensitivity. Furthermore, lung biopsy is not recommended in patients with immune-mediated alveolar hemorrhage when a specific diagnosis can be established by biopsy of other tissues and by serum ANCA assays.[38]

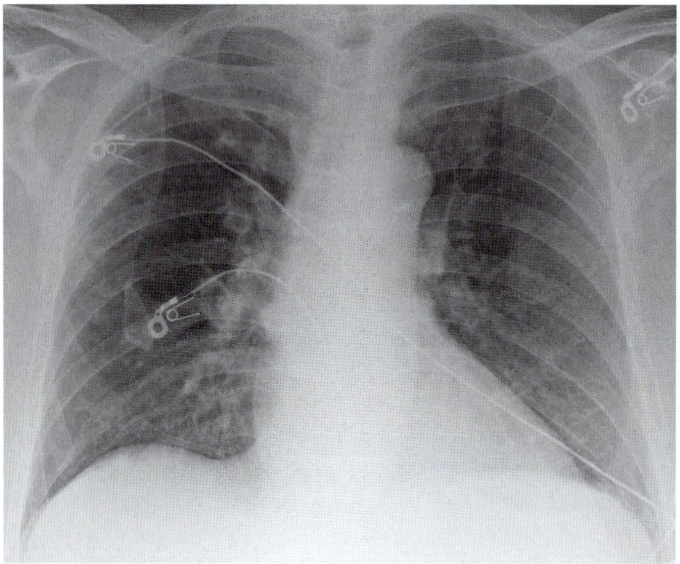

Fig. 46.18 Microscopic polyangiitis: resolution after treatment. Chest radiograph from same patient as in Fig. 46.17 obtained 2 months after onset of treatment shows complete resolution of pulmonary opacities.

MPA is the most common cause of the pulmonary-renal syndrome. The main differential diagnosis clinically is with other conditions that may cause pulmonary and renal manifestations, particularly Goodpasture syndrome, GPA, and systemic lupus erythematosus. Goodpasture syndrome is usually diagnosed by demonstration of circulating or tissue-bound anti–glomerular basement membrane antibodies. MPA is distinguished from GPA by the lack of granulomatous inflammation and from systemic lupus erythematosus and other small-vessel vasculitides by the lack of immune deposits on surgical lung biopsy.

IMAGING ALGORITHM

Chest radiography is the main imaging modality used in the initial assessment and follow-up of patients with ANCA-associated vasculitis. Unless certain findings are seen on chest radiography to suggest a specific diagnosis, such as cavitary nodules in GPA, further evaluation is often warranted using chest CT. If there is high clinical suspicion for vasculitis, high-resolution CT is recommended, allowing evaluation for findings of air-trapping, bronchiectasis, or other signs of airway involvement. Even with high-resolution CT, imaging findings can be indeterminate, and close correlation with clinical history and laboratory results is important to arrive at a specific diagnosis.

Synopsis of Treatment Options

Treatment of ANCA-associated vasculitis has significantly improved even over the past decade. Immunosuppression with cyclophosphamide has been a mainstay of treatment since 1971, although high toxicity, including marrow suppression and hemorrhagic cystitis, has limited its use.[39]

Current treatment strategies revolve around a short course of cyclophosphamide induction with chronic suppression either with corticosteroids or other immunomodulators, such as methotrexate or azathioprine.[39]

The advent of monoclonal therapies, such as rituximab, have greatly improved the long-term prognosis of patients with ANCA-associated vasculitis with prolonged remission and reduced recurrence of disease. Side effects of these newer medications are also considerably better than older treatment options.[39]

An additional treatment option for induction of remission is intravenous immunoglobulin, which is highly effective in the acute setting. This treatment is usually reserved for life-threatening illness or in pediatric patients as the side effects of the other medications would be particularly detrimental to the still developing body.[40]

As with all immunomodulation therapies, patients are at increased risk for opportunistic infections and must be closely monitored for this complication. Before immunosuppressive therapy, almost all patients died within 6 months of diagnosis. Currently, the estimated median survival after diagnosis is in excess of 20 years; most deaths are due to either the disease or complications of therapy.

KEY POINTS

- Chest radiography is the main imaging modality used in the initial assessment and follow-up of patients with antineutrophil cytoplasmic antibody (ANCA)-associated vasculitis.
- CT is indicated in patients with suspected granulomatosis with polyangiitis (GPA) for optimal assessment of the extent of parenchymal abnormalities and detection of mild disease that may not be apparent on the radiograph. In the setting of suspected eosinophilic (e)GPA or microscopic polyangiitis (MPA) with classic radiographic findings, CT seldom adds additional information.
- Serum cytoplasmic (c)-ANCA are present in 90% to 95% of cases of systemic GPA and in 60% of cases of organ-limited GPA. Approximately 70% of patients with eGPA have serum perinuclear-pattern (p)-ANCA. The majority of patients with MPA have p-ANCA) reactivity, although a minority may be c-ANCA positive.
- Most patients with GPA present with upper and lower respiratory symptoms, including epistaxis, sinusitis, cough, hemoptysis, dyspnea, and pleuritic chest pain.
- The most common radiologic findings in GPA are lung nodules or masses, seen in up to 90% of patients. Cavitation occurs eventually in about 50% of cases.
- The most common clinical manifestations of eGPA are asthma, allergic rhinitis, neuropathy, and peripheral eosinophilia, which occur in most patients.
- Almost exclusively, eGPA occurs in patients with asthma.
- The most common radiographic findings in eGPA consist of transient or migratory opacities, or consolidation in a peripheral distribution, resembling those of simple pulmonary eosinophilia (Löffler syndrome) and chronic eosinophilic pneumonia, respectively.
- MPA is the most common cause of the pulmonary-renal syndrome, a syndrome characterized by the coexistence of pulmonary hemorrhage and glomerulonephritis.
- The radiologic findings in MPA are those of diffuse pulmonary hemorrhage and range from patchy bilateral ground-glass opacities to confluent consolidation that may spare the lung periphery or extreme lung apices and bases.

SUGGESTED READINGS

Brown KK. Pulmonary vasculitis. *Proc Am Thorac Soc.* 2006;3:48–57.

Castaner E, Alguersuari A, Gallardo X, et al. When to suspect pulmonary vasculitis: radiologic and clinical clues. *Radiographics.* 2010;30:33–53.

Chung MP, Yi CA, Lee HY, et al. Imaging of pulmonary vasculitis. *Radiology.* 2010;255:322–341.

Thickett DR, Richter AG, Nathani N, et al. Pulmonary manifestations of anti-neutrophil cytoplasmic antibody (ANCA)-positive vasculitis. *Rheumatology.* 2006;45:261–268.

The full reference list for this chapter is available at ExpertConsult.com.

47 Goodpasture Syndrome (Anti–Basement Membrane Antibody Disease)*

JONATHAN H. CHUNG | CHRISTOPHER M. WALKER

Etiology, Prevalence, and Epidemiology

Goodpasture syndrome, also known as anti–basement membrane antibody disease, is an autoimmune disorder characterized by repeated episodes of pulmonary hemorrhage, usually associated with glomerulonephritis and the presence of anti–glomerular basement membrane (anti-GBM) antibodies. Goodpasture syndrome is rare, with an incidence of approximately one patient per million population per year.[1] It has a bimodal distribution with respect to age, with peaks at 20 to 30 and 60 to 70 years of age and a male-to-female ratio of approximately 3 : 2.[2,3]

Clinical Presentation

The most common presenting symptom is hemoptysis, which occurs in about 80% to 95% of patients.[3,4] The hemoptysis may range from mild to copious and life threatening. In more than 50% of patients, it precedes glomerulonephritis.[3] On occasion, the hemoptysis may occur late in the course of the disease or be absent altogether. Other presenting symptoms include dyspnea, fatigue, weakness, pallor, cough, and, occasionally, frank hematuria.[3] Although results of the initial urinalysis may be normal, proteinuria, hematuria, and cellular and granular casts almost invariably develop at some stage.[5] More than 90% of patients have anti-GBM antibodies, and approximately 80% have crescentic glomerulonephritis on renal biopsy.[3] More than 90% of patients have iron deficiency anemia resulting from blood loss from pulmonary hemorrhage.[3]

Pathophysiology

Goodpasture syndrome is an autoimmune disorder characterized by the presence of autoantibodies against the glomerular and alveolar basement membranes.[3] It has been suggested that environmental factors, such as smoking, previous hydrocarbon exposure, and infection, may play a role in triggering Goodpasture syndrome.[2] In the kidney complement activation and inflammatory cell enzymes are responsible for glomerular damage. The precise pathogenesis of the pulmonary hemorrhage is unknown.

The main histologic findings of Goodpasture syndrome consist of pulmonary alveolar capillaritis, which results in diffuse pulmonary hemorrhage, and a segmental necrotizing glomerulonephritis, which progresses to a crescentic nephritis.[1] The capillaritis is identical to that of granulomatosis with polyangiitis (formerly Wegener granulomatosis) and microscopic polyangiitis and appears as a neutrophil infiltrate intimately associated with alveolar septa with or without fibrin thrombi and necrosis. Other histologic changes depend on the duration and severity of the disease at the time of examination but usually include hemosiderin-laden macrophages in alveolar airspaces and interstitial tissue and mild to moderate interstitial fibrosis.[5] Immunofluorescence studies show characteristic linear staining most readily recognized in the glomerulus but also frequently evident in the alveolar capillary walls.[1,6] Immunoglobulin (Ig)G is the usual antibody detected, although IgA and IgM are occasionally present as well.[5]

Manifestations of the Disease

RADIOGRAPHY

In the early stages of the disease, the radiographic pattern is one of patchy hazy areas of increased opacity (ground-glass opacities) scattered fairly evenly throughout the lungs (Fig. 47.1). With more severe hemorrhage, the pattern may progress to focal or confluent areas of consolidation often associated with air bronchograms (Fig. 47.2). The opacities usually are widespread but may be more prominent in the perihilar areas and in the middle and lower lung zones.[7] The apices and costophrenic angles are often spared. Although parenchymal involvement usually is bilateral, it is commonly asymmetric and occasionally may be unilateral.[7,8] The chest radiograph may be normal in patients with diffuse pulmonary hemorrhage. In one review of 39 episodes of diffuse pulmonary hemorrhage in 23 patients, the radiograph was normal in 7 (18%) episodes.[8] Serial radiographs show that within 2 to 3 days, the areas of consolidation are gradually replaced by a reticular or reticulonodular pattern, the distribution of which is identical to that of the airspace disease (Fig. 47.3).[7,9] This reticular pattern diminishes gradually during the next several days, and the appearance of the chest radiograph usually returns to normal about 10 to 12 days after the original episode.[9] With repeated episodes of hemorrhage, increasing amounts of hemosiderin are deposited within the interstitial tissue and are associated with progressive fibrosis. In most cases the chest radiograph shows only partial clearing after each hemorrhagic episode, revealing persistence of a fine reticulonodular pattern indicative of the irreversible interstitial disease.[9] Once these changes have developed, new episodes of pulmonary hemorrhage usually result in the typical pattern of airspace consolidation superimposed on the diffuse interstitial disease.

*The editors and the publisher would like to thank Drs. Nestor L. Müller and C. Isabela Silva Müller for contributing material on this topic to the prior edition of this work. It has served as the foundation for the current chapter.

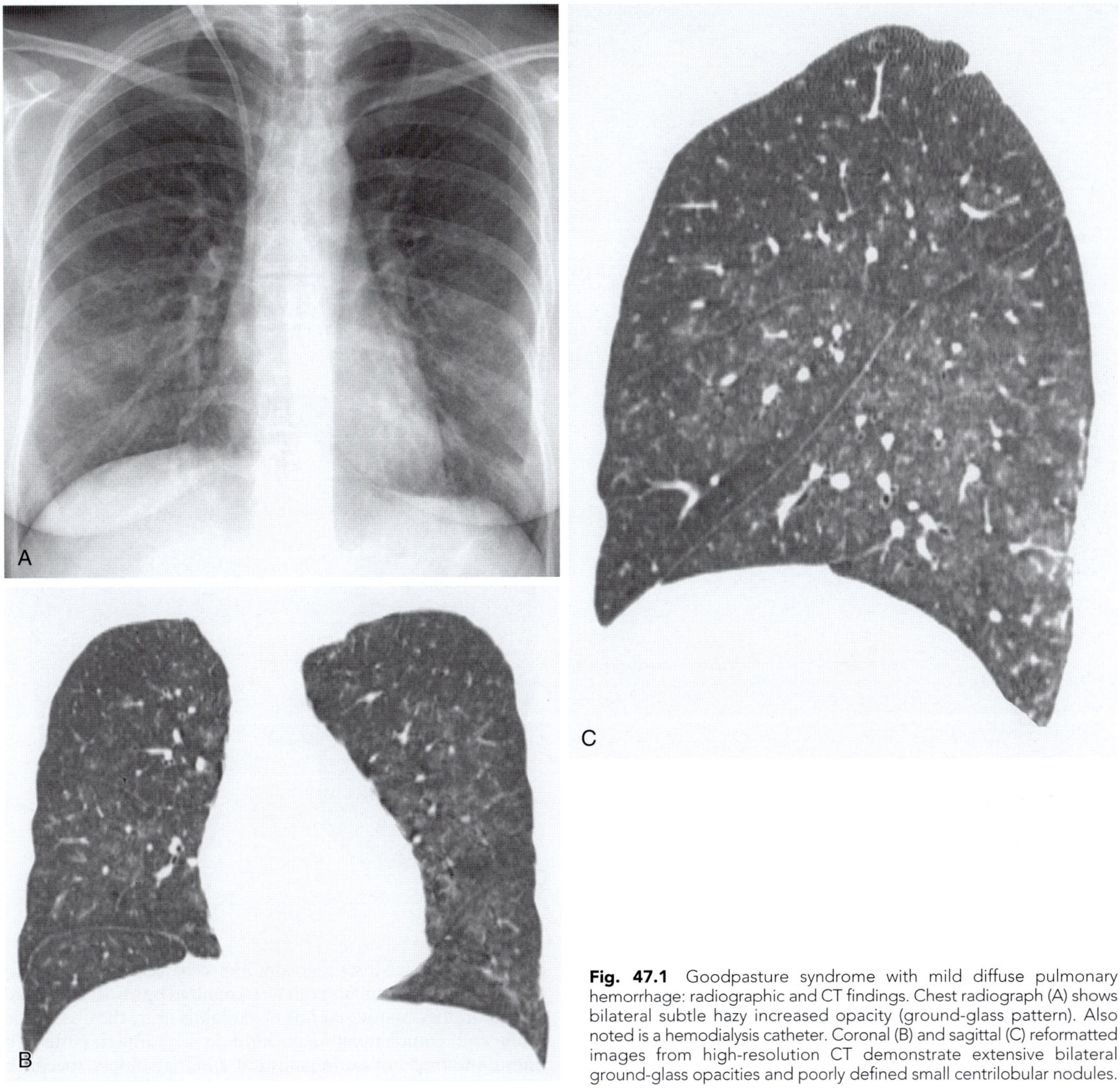

Fig. 47.1 Goodpasture syndrome with mild diffuse pulmonary hemorrhage: radiographic and CT findings. Chest radiograph (A) shows bilateral subtle hazy increased opacity (ground-glass pattern). Also noted is a hemodialysis catheter. Coronal (B) and sagittal (C) reformatted images from high-resolution CT demonstrate extensive bilateral ground-glass opacities and poorly defined small centrilobular nodules.

COMPUTED TOMOGRAPHY

The computed tomography (CT) manifestations of acute pulmonary hemorrhage consist of bilateral ground-glass opacities and, less commonly, areas of consolidation (see Figs. 47.1 and 47.2).[7,10] The ground-glass opacities may have a patchy distribution or be diffuse. CT scans performed 2 to 3 days after the acute episode show decrease in the ground-glass opacities and consolidation and presence of small, poorly defined centrilobular nodules and, less commonly, interlobular septal thickening.[10] These findings are presumably secondary to the lymphatic resorption of the blood and gradually resolve during the next 1 to 2 weeks. Pulmonary fibrosis and interstitial hemosiderin deposition may develop in those with recurrent hemorrhage and typically manifests as reticulation, traction bronchiectasis, and architectural distortion (Fig. 47.4). Frank honeycombing may develop and signals more severe fibrosis.

IMAGING ALGORITHM

The chest radiograph is usually the initial imaging modality used in the evaluation of patients with diffuse pulmonary hemorrhage and Goodpasture syndrome. In the proper clinical setting, when the radiograph demonstrates bilateral ground-glass opacities or consolidation, no further imaging is required. In some patients with diffuse pulmonary hemorrhage, the radiograph may be normal or show only questionable abnormalities. Thin-section

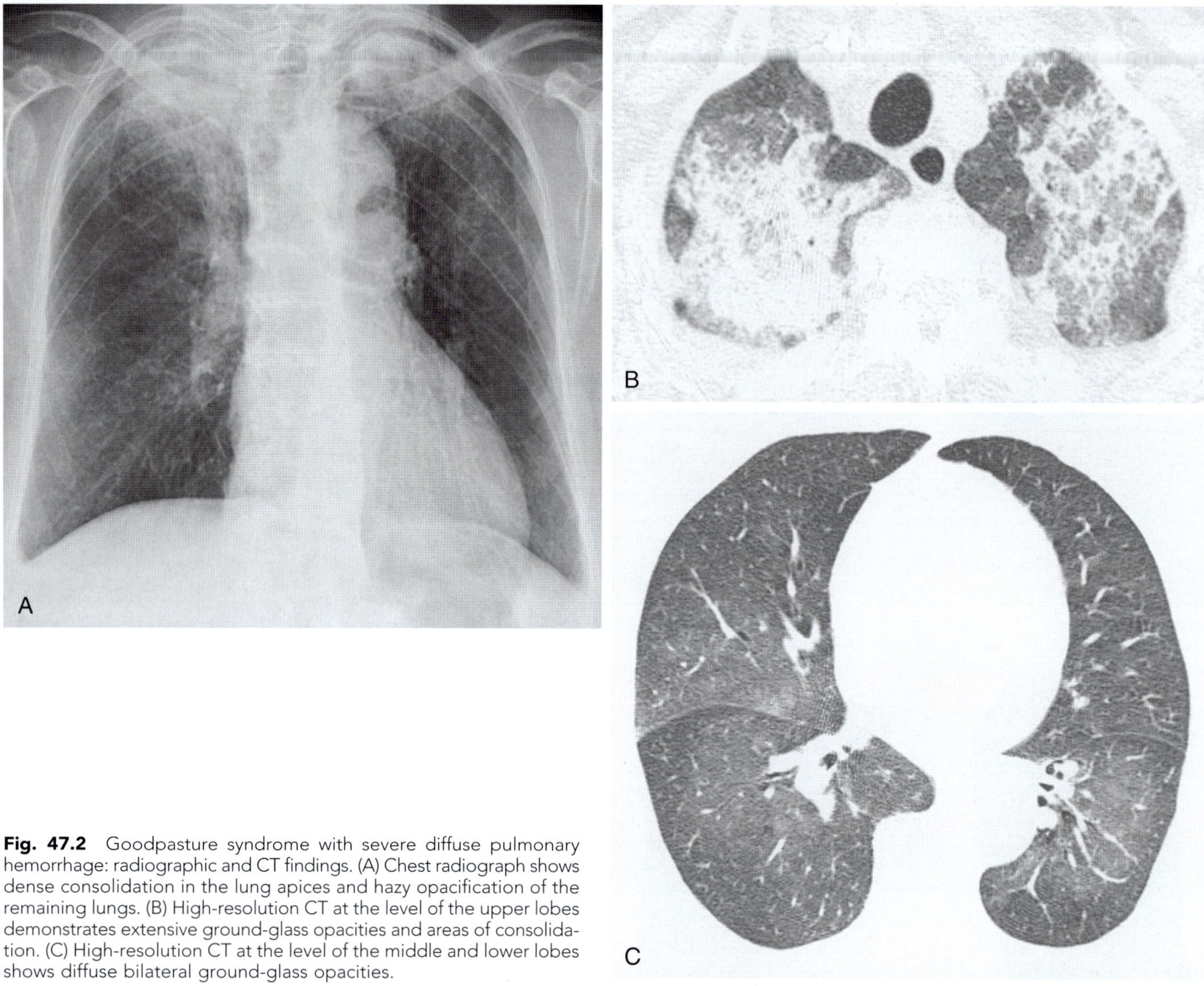

Fig. 47.2 Goodpasture syndrome with severe diffuse pulmonary hemorrhage: radiographic and CT findings. (A) Chest radiograph shows dense consolidation in the lung apices and hazy opacification of the remaining lungs. (B) High-resolution CT at the level of the upper lobes demonstrates extensive ground-glass opacities and areas of consolidation. (C) High-resolution CT at the level of the middle and lower lobes shows diffuse bilateral ground-glass opacities.

CT is indicated in patients with clinically suspected diffuse pulmonary hemorrhage and questionable or nonspecific radiographic findings. Thin-section CT is also indicated in patients with hemoptysis in whom the clinical presentation is not characteristic of Goodpasture syndrome. In these cases thin-section CT is helpful to rule out other causes of hemoptysis, such as bronchiectasis and bronchogenic carcinoma.[11]

Differential Diagnosis

Approximately 20% of patients with glomerulonephritis and pulmonary hemorrhage have Goodpasture syndrome, 50% have some form of systemic vasculitis, and most of the remainder have diffuse alveolar hemorrhage in association with other forms of glomerulonephritis.[12] The diagnosis of Goodpasture syndrome should be suspected when an adult patient has hemoptysis and bilateral airspace consolidation on the chest radiograph, particularly when manifestations of renal disease are also present. Confirmation can be obtained by demonstration of circulating or tissue-bound anti-GBM antibodies by enzyme-linked immunosorbent assay or immunofluorescent examination.[13] If the diagnosis remains uncertain, it can be confirmed by demonstration of autoantibodies on kidney biopsy. Most other conditions characterized by hemoptysis and renal dysfunction can be recognized by associated clinical and laboratory manifestations of vasculitis or by the observation of Ig and complement deposition in a granular pattern on immunofluorescent examination of a kidney biopsy specimen.[5] Because renal involvement in Goodpasture syndrome may not be apparent initially, the diagnosis must be considered in any patient who has radiologic and clinical findings consistent with diffuse alveolar hemorrhage and no evidence of kidney disease.[5] The differential diagnosis in this situation is large and includes various connective tissue diseases (especially systemic lupus erythematosus), systemic vasculitis (e.g., granulomatosis with polyangiitis), aspirated blood after vascular disruption, and occasionally certain metastatic neoplasms, such as choriocarcinoma.[14,15]

Synopsis of Treatment Options

The treatment of Goodpasture syndrome is aimed at removal of circulating autoantibodies, which is accomplished by plasmapheresis and stopping the production of anti-GBM antibodies with use of immunosuppressive medications, typically corticosteroids and cyclophosphamide.[3]

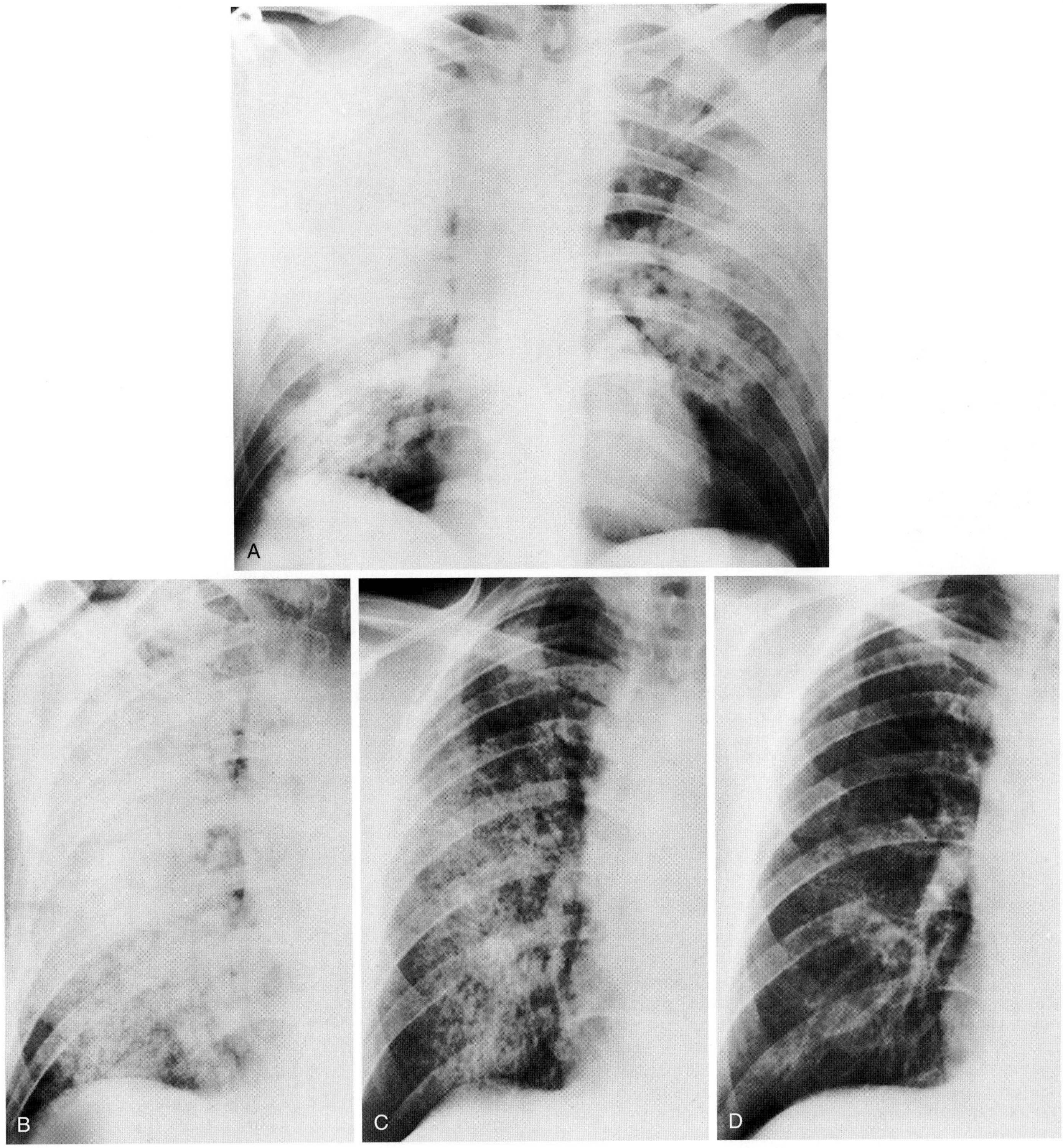

Fig. 47.3 Goodpasture syndrome: changes on sequential radiographs after massive pulmonary hemorrhage. Posteroanterior radiograph (A) shows extensive consolidation of both lungs. A well-defined air bronchogram is visualized. Three days later (B), the pattern was somewhat more granular, and 10 days after the initial episode (C), the pattern had become distinctly reticular. Six days later (D), only a fine reticular pattern remains in an anatomic distribution identical to the original involvement. *(From Müller NL, Fraser RS, Colman NC, Paré PD.* Radiologic Diagnosis of Diseases of the Chest. *Philadelphia: WB Saunders; 2001.)*

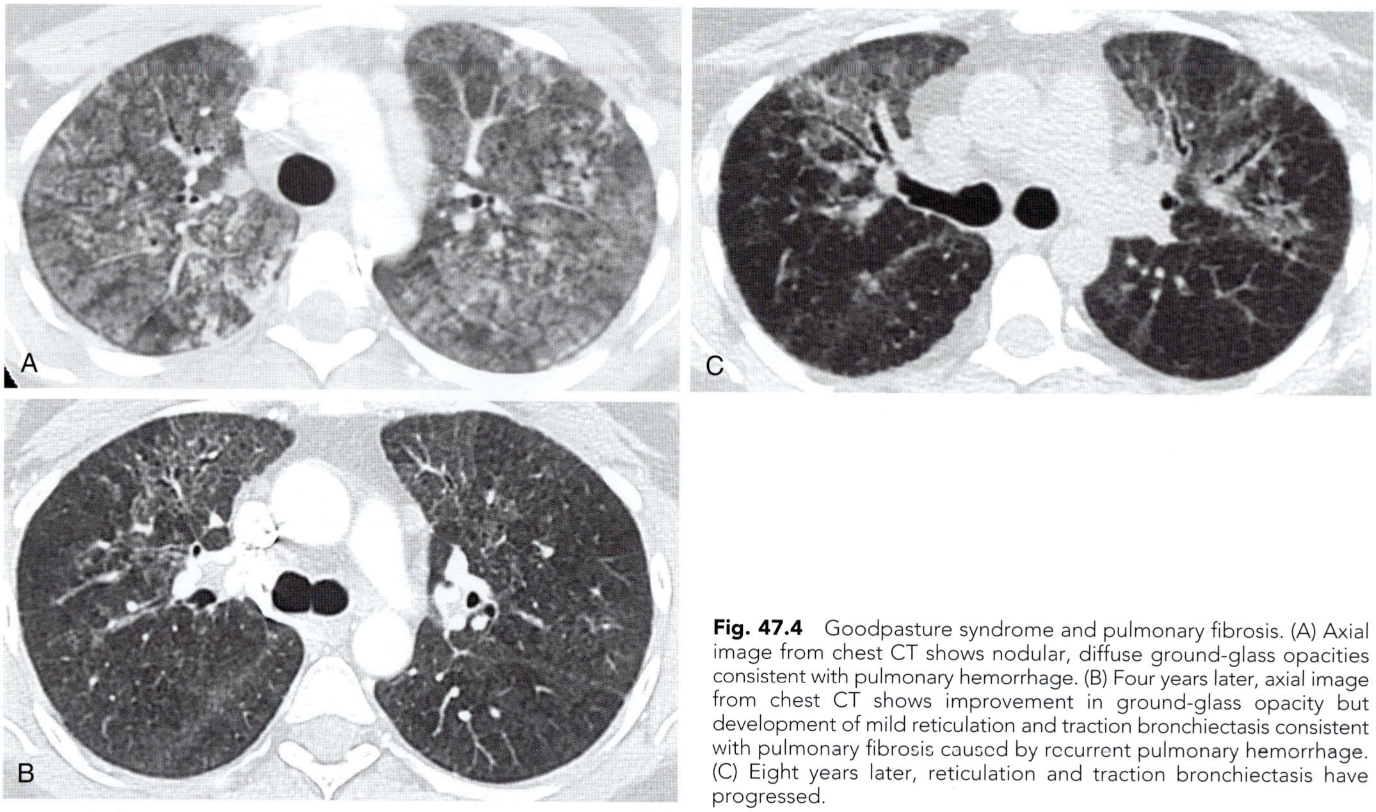

Fig. 47.4 Goodpasture syndrome and pulmonary fibrosis. (A) Axial image from chest CT shows nodular, diffuse ground-glass opacities consistent with pulmonary hemorrhage. (B) Four years later, axial image from chest CT shows improvement in ground-glass opacity but development of mild reticulation and traction bronchiectasis consistent with pulmonary fibrosis caused by recurrent pulmonary hemorrhage. (C) Eight years later, reticulation and traction bronchiectasis have progressed.

KEY POINTS

- Goodpasture syndrome has a bimodal age distribution with peaks at 20–30 and 60–70 years of age.
- It is more common in men than in women (3:2).
- It is characterized by repeated episodes of pulmonary hemorrhage and presence of serum anti–glomerular basement membrane antibodies.
- The presenting symptom is hemoptysis in 80%–95% of patients.
- Respiratory symptoms often precede renal manifestations.
- The radiologic findings are those of diffuse pulmonary hemorrhage and range from patchy bilateral ground-glass opacities to confluent consolidation.
- CT is indicated in patients with hemoptysis in whom the clinical presentation is not characteristic of Goodpasture syndrome. In these cases CT is helpful to rule out other causes of hemoptysis, such as bronchiectasis and bronchogenic carcinoma.

With treatment the 5-year survival ranges from 63% to 94%, depending on the initial renal function.[16] In one study approximately 20% of patients had normal recovery, 39% were receiving maintenance hemodialysis, 12% received transplants and were doing well, 5% were awaiting transplants, and 24% died.[3] The prognosis is closely associated with the degree of initial renal impairment. Predictors of poor prognosis include initial creatinine levels greater than 5 mg/dL, crescent formation in more than 50% of glomeruli, and oligoanuria (i.e., <100 mL of urine produced per day).[3] On occasion, Goodpasture syndrome may recur years later in patients whose disease remits spontaneously or as a result of therapy.[17]

SUGGESTED READINGS

Chung MP, Yi CA, Lee HY, Han J, Lee KS. Imaging of pulmonary vasculitis. *Radiology*. 2010;255:322–341.

Peto P, Salama AD. Update on antiglomerular basement membrane disease. *Curr Opin Rheumatol*. 2011;23:32–37.

Sanders JS, Rutgers A, Stegeman CA, Kallenberg CG. Pulmonary: renal syndrome with a focus on anti-GBM disease. *Semin Respir Crit Care Med*. 2011;32:328–334.

The full reference list for this chapter is available at ExpertConsult.com.

48 Behçet Disease*

JONATHAN H. CHUNG | CHRISTOPHER M. WALKER

Etiology, Prevalence, and Epidemiology

Behçet disease is an uncommon systemic disorder of unknown etiology characterized by vasculitis and the triad of recurrent ulcers of the oral and genital mucosa with relapsing uveitis.[1] Vascular complications develop in 20% to 40% of patients with Behçet disease and include subcutaneous thrombophlebitis, deep venous thrombosis, and pulmonary and systemic arterial aneurysms and occlusions.[1,2] The reported frequency of pulmonary complications is highly variable, ranging from less than 1% to 18% of patients.[1] The main pulmonary manifestations are pulmonary artery aneurysm, embolism, hemorrhage, and infarction. Although relatively infrequent, pulmonary complications are one of the most common direct causes of death in patients with Behçet disease.[1]

Behçet disease affects men much more commonly than women (ratio of 10:1), and the mean age at presentation is 30 years (range, 10–59 years).[1] Although it has a worldwide distribution, most cases cluster along the ancient Silk Road, which extends from the Middle East to East Asia. The highest prevalence rate is in Turkey (4 cases per 1000 population).[3] The prevalence in other Asian countries ranges from 2 to 30 cases per 100,000.[4] The prevalence in Europe and the United States is less than 1 case per 100,000 population. Of interest, there is heterogeneity in the clinical presentation of Behçet disease in nonendemic areas, suggesting that environmental factors may play a role in patient phenotype.[5]

Clinical Presentation

The diagnosis of Behçet disease is based on the presence of recurrent oral ulcerations along with two of the following criteria: recurrent genital ulcerations; eye lesions, including uveitis and retinal vasculitis; skin lesions (folliculitis, erythema nodosum); and positive result of skin pathergy test (pustule formation 24–48 hours after skin prick).[6] The symptoms typically wax and wane. Pulmonary manifestations may be the initial manifestation of the disease or, more commonly, develop several years after the diagnosis (mean, 5.5 years after diagnosis; range, 6 months to 26 years).[1] Nearly all patients with pulmonary artery aneurysms have hemoptysis.[1] Other symptoms include chest pain, dyspnea, and cough. The pulmonary symptoms may be secondary to formation of pulmonary artery aneurysms, arterial and venous thrombosis, pulmonary infarction, hemorrhage, recurrent pneumonia, or pleurisy. Hemoptysis may be massive and is a common cause of death. Behçet disease may also result in thrombosis of the superior vena cava and other mediastinal veins.

*The editors and the publisher would like to thank Drs. Nestor L. Müller and C. Isabela Silva Müller for contributing material on this topic to the prior edition of this work. It has served as the foundation for the current chapter.

Pathophysiology

The pathogenesis of Behçet disease is unknown. The greater incidence in certain ethnic groups, the strong association with human leukocyte antigen (HLA)-B51 in many ethnic groups, the genetic association with mutations of factor V Leiden, and reports of familial clustering of disease unrelated to HLA-B51 imply that a genetic influence is important.[4,7,8]

The histologic features of Behçet disease consist of systemic vasculitis and perivascular inflammatory infiltrates.[9] The vasculitis can involve large, medium, and small vessels of both the arterial and venous circulation. There is a tendency to thrombus formation and for the thrombi to show evidence of inflammation. The earliest pulmonary vascular abnormalities histologically consist of transmural vascular inflammation by lymphocytes, plasma cells, and polymorphonuclear leukocytes.[10] The inflammatory process can extend into adjacent airways and cause bronchial or pulmonary artery erosion and hemoptysis. With progression of disease, there is thinning of the muscular and elastic layers, resulting in aneurysm formation. The aneurysms are in fact pseudoaneurysms that arise as complications of vasculitis and transmural necrosis.[6,11] In the majority of patients the aneurysms are multiple, bilateral, saccular, and partially or completely thrombosed; the pulmonary arteries distal to the pseudoaneurysms also are thrombosed.[1,11] Other findings include organized thrombi and parenchymal infarcts, which can be related to local vasculitis and thrombosis or to thromboembolism secondary to systemic thrombophlebitis.[12] Approximately 80% of patients with pulmonary artery aneurysms have concomitant extrapulmonary venous thrombi or thrombophlebitis.

Manifestations of the Disease

RADIOGRAPHY

The radiologic manifestations are usually those of pulmonary artery aneurysms and thrombosis of the pulmonary arteries and systemic veins. Pulmonary artery aneurysms manifest radiographically as round perihilar opacities or as rapidly developing unilateral hilar enlargement (Fig. 48.1).[13] The aneurysms may be single or more commonly multiple and unilateral or bilateral; they usually measure 1 to 3 cm in diameter.[14,15] When they are associated with an acute episode of hemoptysis, they appear poorly marginated; otherwise, they have a distinct outline. Thrombotic occlusion of the pulmonary vasculature most commonly involves the right interlobar artery and less often the lobar and segmental arteries.[16] It may result in localized areas of consolidation resulting from infarction, areas of oligemia, and areas of atelectasis. Unilateral or bilateral pleural effusions may be seen in association with infarction. Pulmonary hemorrhage caused by vasculitis or pulmonary artery rupture occasionally

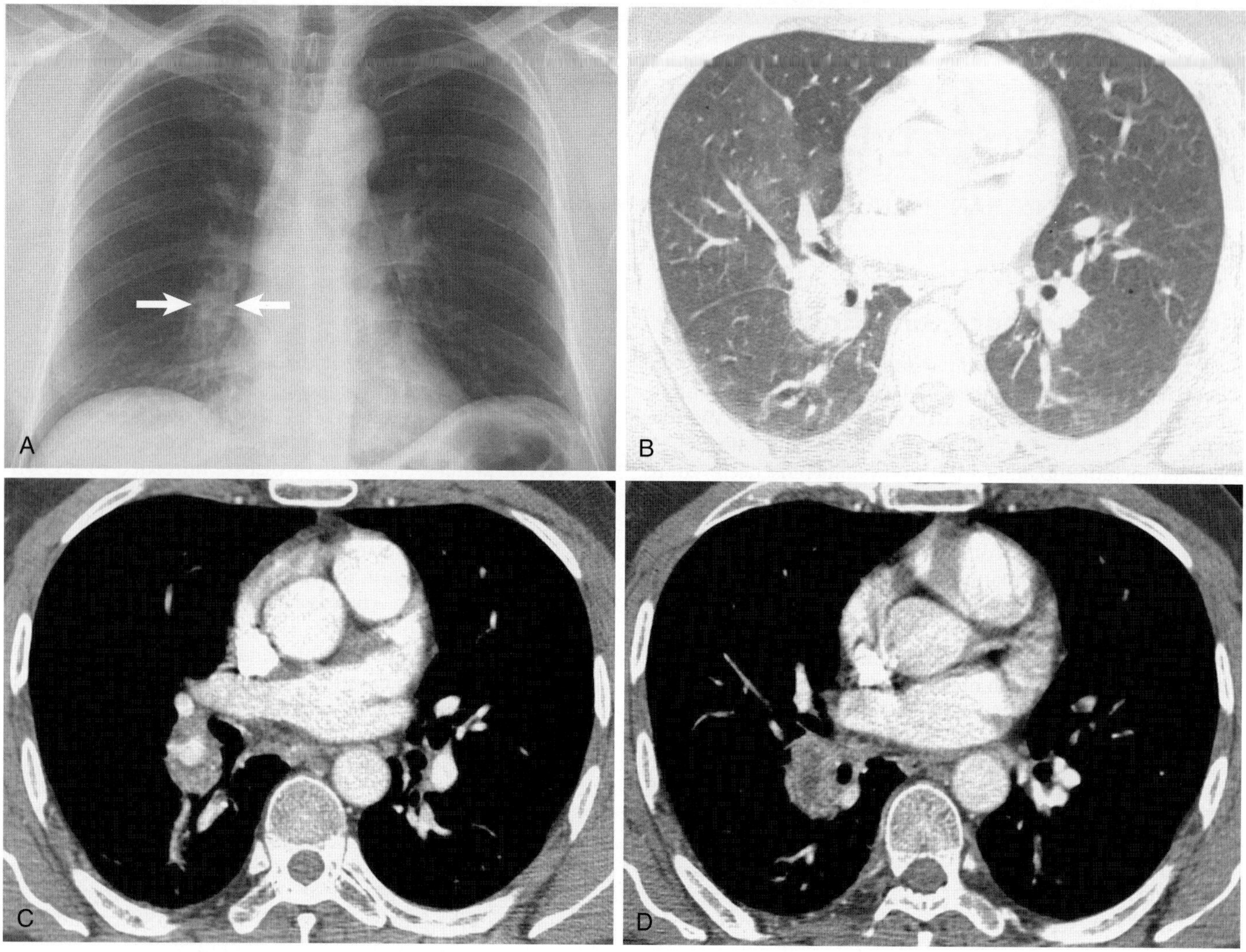

Fig. 48.1 Behçet disease. (A) Chest radiograph reveals increased size of the right interlobar and lower lobe pulmonary arteries *(arrows)*. (B) CT image shows increased diameter of the right interlobar and lower lobe pulmonary arteries and asymmetric bilateral ground-glass opacities consistent with pulmonary hemorrhage. (C) Contrast-enhanced CT image shows partially thrombosed aneurysm of the right interlobar pulmonary artery. (D) CT image at a slightly lower level demonstrates thrombosis of the right lower lobe pulmonary artery.

results in focal, multifocal, or diffuse airspace consolidation.[14] Thrombosis of the superior vena cava is relatively common and may be manifested on the chest radiograph as mediastinal widening resulting from associated collateral circulation and mediastinal edema (Fig. 48.2).[15] Mediastinal widening may also be due to aortic aneurysm formation.

COMPUTED TOMOGRAPHY

The presence, size, and location of the pulmonary aneurysms are best assessed on contrast-enhanced computed tomography (CT).[14,15] Aneurysms are seen as saccular or fusiform dilatations that show homogeneous filling by contrast material simultaneously with the pulmonary artery (see Fig. 48.1). The aneurysms are often multiple and range from 1 to 7 cm in diameter. The wall of the involved pulmonary artery is often thickened and enhances after intravenous administration of contrast material.[15] The aneurysms most commonly involve the right interlobar artery, followed in decreasing order by lobar and segmental arteries. Partial or complete thrombosis of the aneurysm may occur and result in localized areas of consolidation resulting from infarction, areas of decreased attenuation and vascularity, and atelectasis. Pulmonary hemorrhage from vasculitis or pulmonary artery rupture can result in focal, multifocal, or diffuse ground-glass opacities or consolidation (see Fig. 48.1). Other pulmonary manifestations include recurrent pneumonia and organizing pneumonia.[1,2] Organizing pneumonia is a nonspecific pathologic response to lung injury characterized by organizing granulation tissue in the airspaces, alveolar ducts, and bronchioles. It is seen with increased prevalence in a variety of conditions, including collagen vascular diseases, hematologic disorders, and Behçet disease. It may occur in patients with or without evidence of pulmonary artery aneurysm or vasculitis. The CT findings typically consist of bilateral areas of consolidation involving mainly the peribronchial and peripheral lung regions.

Thrombosis of major veins, including the superior vena cava, is a common finding in patients with or without pulmonary artery aneurysms (see Fig. 48.2). Thrombosis of the brachiocephalic and subclavian veins may accompany superior vena caval occlusion.[17] Thrombosis of the superior vena cava is well demonstrated on contrast-enhanced CT. It may result in partial or complete obstruction of the superior vena cava, collateral circulation, and mediastinal

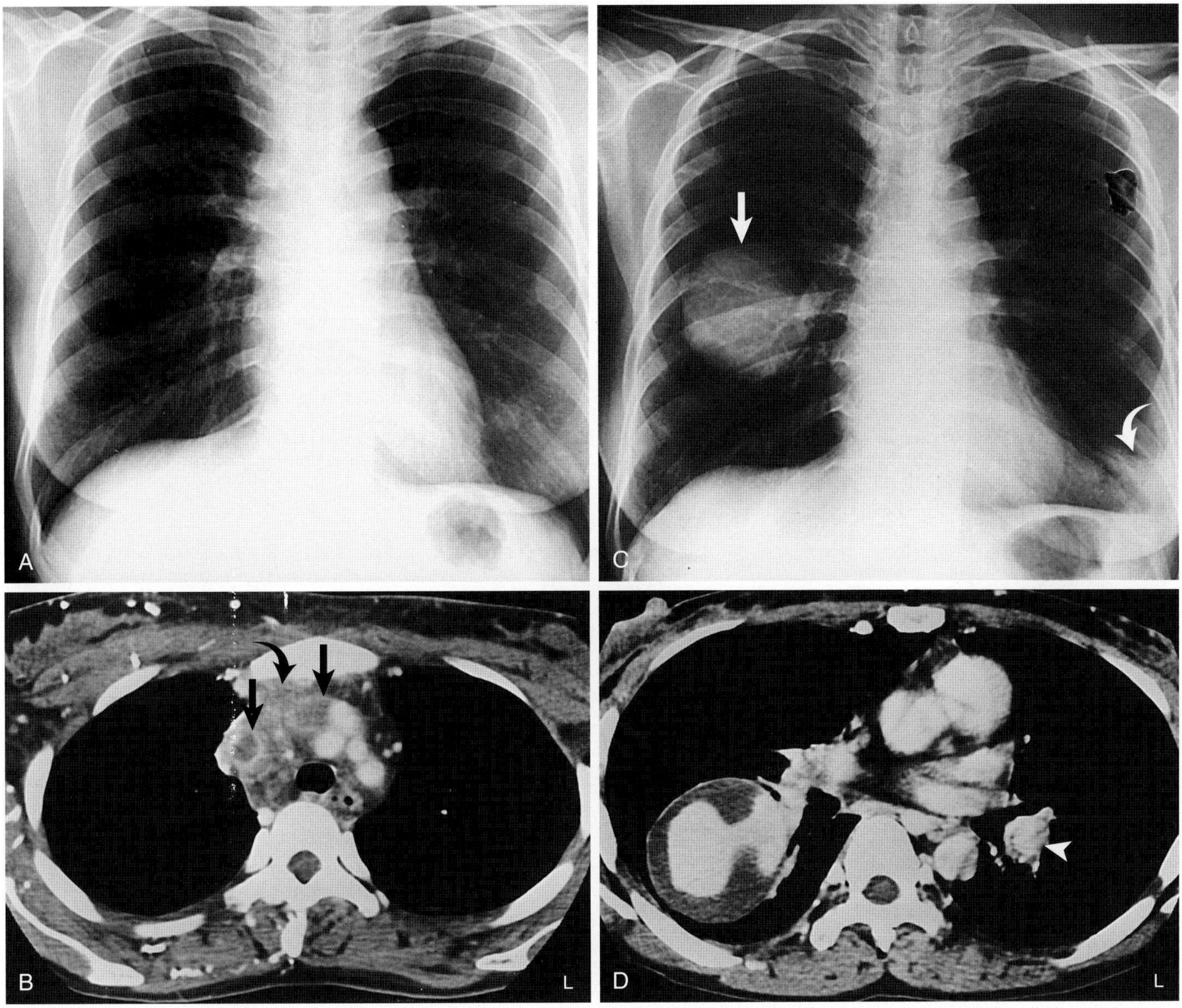

Fig. 48.2 Behçet disease with thrombosis of the superior vena cava and pulmonary artery aneurysm. (A) Posteroanterior chest radiograph in a woman with Behçet disease shows widening of the right upper mediastinum. (B) Contrast-enhanced CT scan shows thrombosis of the right and left brachiocephalic veins *(straight arrows)* and increased attenuation of the mediastinal fat *(curved arrow)*, a finding that is suggestive of edema. Collateral veins are visible in the mediastinum and chest wall. (C) Posteroanterior chest radiograph obtained 6 months later shows a round, well-defined mass in the right lower lobe *(straight arrow)* and localized consolidation in the left lower lobe *(curved arrow)*. The upper mediastinum appears normal. (D) Contrast-enhanced CT scan obtained at the same time as the posteroanterior chest radiograph (C) shows a large aneurysm of a branch of the right pulmonary artery with enhancement of the patent lumen and a circumferential thrombus. Note a dilated left interlobar pulmonary artery *(arrowhead)*. *(From Ahn JM, Im JG, Ryoo JW, et al. Thoracic manifestations of Behçet syndrome: radiographic and CT findings in nine patients.* Radiology. *1995;194:199–203. Case courtesy Dr. Jung-Gi Im, Department of Radiology, Seoul National University Hospital, Seoul, South Korea.)*

edema. Less common findings of Behçet disease include pseudoaneurysms of the thoracic aorta and subclavian and coronary arteries, mediastinitis (including fibrosing mediastinitis) (Fig. 48.3), and pleural effusion.[4,18,19] Unilateral or bilateral pleural effusions may result from thrombosis of the superior vena cava, pulmonary infarction, or vasculitis of the pleura.[4,14]

MAGNETIC RESONANCE IMAGING

The presence, size, and location of the pulmonary aneurysms and superior vena caval thrombosis can be well assessed on magnetic resonance (MR) angiography (Fig. 48.4).[2,20] Magnetic resonance imaging (MRI), however, is considered to be less sensitive than contrast-enhanced CT in demonstrating small pulmonary artery aneurysms.

IMAGING ALGORITHM

The diagnosis of pulmonary artery aneurysm can be suspected on a radiograph in the presence of sudden hilar enlargement or the appearance of polylobular and round opacities. Contrast-enhanced CT is the imaging modality of choice in the evaluation of patients

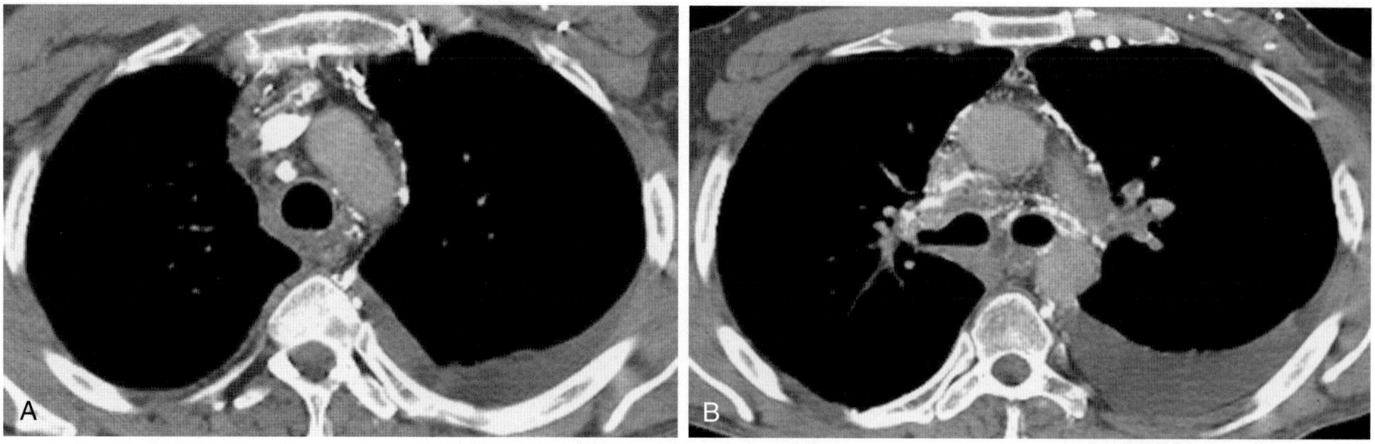

Fig. 48.3 Behçet disease with fibrosing mediastinitis. Contrast-enhanced CT images at the level of the aortic arch (A) and aortopulmonary window (B) demonstrate complete occlusion of the superior vena cava and increased soft tissue density in the adjacent soft tissues consistent with fibrosing mediastinitis. Note associated extensive venous collateral circulation and left pleural effusion. *(Courtesy Dr. Jeffrey P. Kanne, Madison, WI.)*

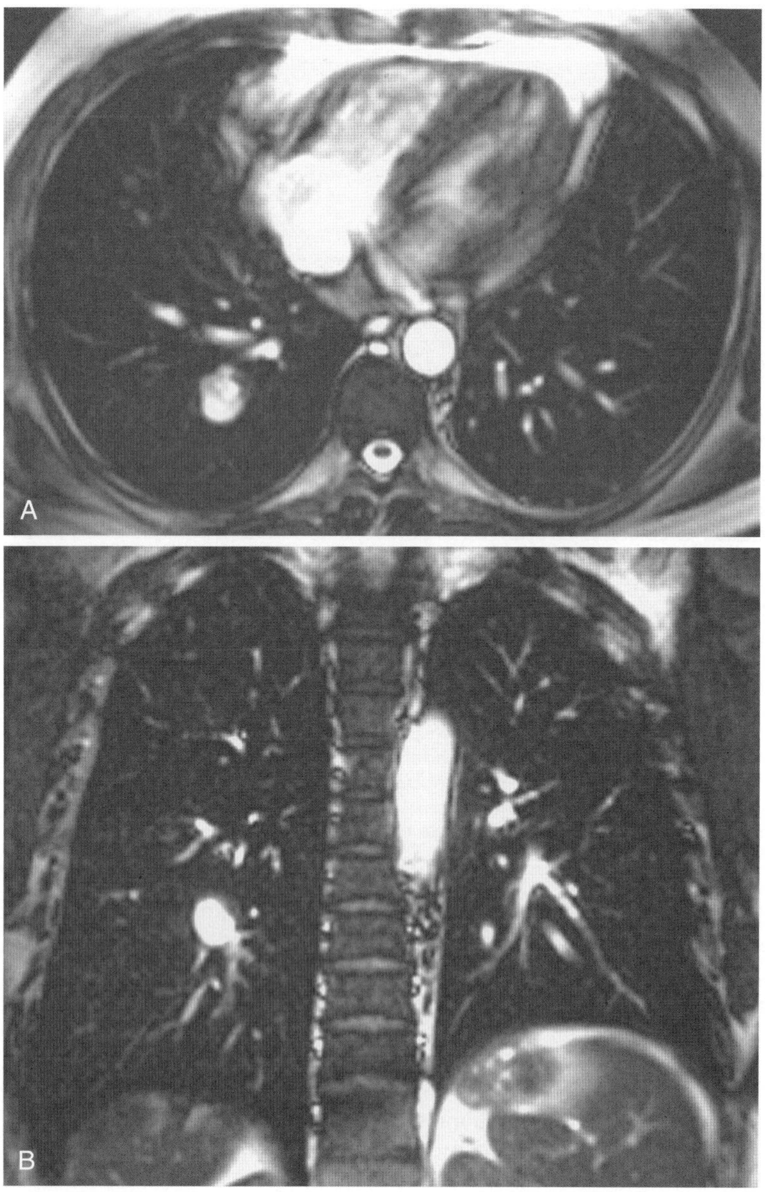

Fig. 48.4 Behçet disease: magnetic resonance (MR) findings. (A) Cross-sectional MR image shows a right lower lobe pulmonary artery aneurysm. (B) Coronal MR angiogram better demonstrates the location of the aneurysm. *(Courtesy Dr. Erkan Yilmaz, Turkey.)*

with Behçet disease and suspected pulmonary artery aneurysms.[4] It is also the imaging modality of choice for the assessment of suspected aortic aneurysms and thrombosis of the superior vena cava. These findings can also be seen on MRI.

The presence, size, and location of aortic and pulmonary artery aneurysms and superior vena caval thrombosis can also be well seen at angiography. Angiography, however, may be inadequate if aneurysms or vessels are completely thrombosed. Furthermore, aortography, venography, and pulmonary angiography carry a risk of aneurysm formation at the arterial puncture site and venous thrombosis after contrast material injection and therefore are not recommended in patients with Behçet disease.[2]

Differential Diagnosis

Pulmonary artery aneurysms and pseudoaneurysms are uncommon. The differential diagnosis includes Behçet disease, Hughes-Stovin syndrome, infection (mycotic pseudoaneurysm), and previous trauma (often iatrogenic, such as malpositioned pulmonary arterial catheter).[21] Hughes-Stovin syndrome is characterized by recurrent thrombophlebitis, pulmonary artery aneurysm formation, and rupture.

The diagnosis of Behçet disease as the cause of pulmonary artery aneurysm is usually straightforward on the basis of the characteristic history of associated recurrent oral and genital ulcerations and uveitis.

Synopsis of Treatment Options

Pulmonary artery aneurysm formation is associated with a very poor prognosis; it is one of the leading causes of death in Behçet disease. The mean survival after the onset of hemoptysis and pulmonary artery aneurysm is approximately 1 year.[4] The most common treatment consists of corticosteroids, cyclophosphamide, and other immunosuppressive medications.[4] Patients with pulmonary artery aneurysms and mild to moderate hemoptysis may respond to medical treatment. Life-threatening massive hemoptysis, however, necessitates intervention. The treatment of choice is selective transcatheter embolization of the aneurysms. The technique of embolization varies from one center to another; some interventional radiologists use coils, and others favor acrylic glue.[11] The main limitations to embolization are the presence of superior or inferior vena caval occlusion and the potential complication of severe bleeding.[4] Surgery is seldom indicated. Surgical treatment consists mostly of major anatomic resection rather than preservation of lung tissue. Surgery is associated with a high risk of complications and an approximately 25% incidence of recurrent anastomotic aneurysms. The cumulative 1-year and 5-year survival rates of patients with Behçet disease and pulmonary artery aneurysms are 57% and 39%, respectively.[1] Aortic aneurysms associated with Behçet disease can often be successfully treated with stent grafts.[22]

KEY POINTS

- Behçet disease occurs mainly in the Middle East and East Asia. Young adults are most commonly affected; it is much more common in men.
- Recurrent oral and genital ulcers, uveitis, and skin lesions characterize Behçet disease.
- Vascular complications, most commonly thrombophlebitis, deep venous thrombosis, and pulmonary and systemic arterial aneurysms and occlusions, occur in 20%–40% of patients.
- Pulmonary manifestations occur in 1%–18% of patients.
- The main pulmonary abnormality is the formation of pulmonary artery aneurysms. The aneurysms are usually multiple and most commonly bilateral.
- The main symptoms are hemoptysis, chest pain, and cough.
- Common radiologic findings:
  - Hilar mass or perihilar nodule on chest radiography
  - Pulmonary artery aneurysm on contrast-enhanced CT and MR images
  - Aneurysm and partial or complete thrombosis of distal vessels
  - Pulmonary artery wall is often thickened and enhances after intravenous contrast administration
  - Thrombosis of the superior vena cava and aortic aneurysm

SUGGESTED READINGS

Guillaume B, Vendrell A, Stefanovic X, Thony F, Ferretti GR. Acquired pulmonary artery pseudoaneurysms: a pictorial review. *Br J Radiol.* 2017;90:20160783.

Hiller N, Lieberman S, Chajek-Shaul T, et al. Thoracic manifestations of Behçet disease at CT. *Radiographics.* 2004;24:801–808.

Leccese P, Yazici Y, Olivieri I. Behçet's syndrome in nonendemic regions. *Curr Opin Rheumatol.* 2017;29:12–16.

Seyahi E, Yazici H. Behçet's syndrome: pulmonary vascular disease. *Curr Opin Rheumatol.* 2015;27:18–23.

Uzun O, Akpolat T, Erkan L. Pulmonary vasculitis in Behçet disease: a cumulative analysis. *Chest.* 2005;127:2243–2253.

The full reference list for this chapter is available at ExpertConsult.com.

49 Takayasu Arteritis*

CHRISTOPHER M. WALKER | JONATHAN H. CHUNG

Etiology, Prevalence, and Epidemiology

Takayasu arteritis, also known as pulseless disease or Martorell syndrome, is an idiopathic chronic granulomatous arteritis affecting medium and large arteries with a predilection for the aorta and its main branches.[1] It is seen most commonly in Japan, Southeast Asia, India, Mexico, and Brazil.[1,2] Although it occurs most commonly in girls and women from eastern Asia, it has been recognized worldwide in both sexes.[1] The incidence in North America is very low, estimated to be 2.6 cases per million population per year.[1] The female-to-male ratio is about 10:1 in Japan but is likely lower in non-Asians (approximately 3:1 in South Africa).[3,4] The patients are usually between 10 and 40 years of age at the time of initial diagnosis.[1]

In a national survey in Japan from 1998 to 2000, Takayasu arteritis was shown to involve the aortic arch in 59% of cases, descending aorta in 45%, ascending aorta in 30%, left subclavian artery in 60%, left common carotid artery in 40%, brachiocephalic artery in 19%, and pulmonary arteries in 15%.[3] It involved the abdominal aorta in 28% of cases and the renal arteries in 13%. Approximately 28% had concomitant thoracic and abdominal aortic lesions. Abdominal aorta and renal artery involvement is considerably more common in other south Asian countries.[3] Coronary arterial involvement is not uncommon and may be seen in 10% to 30% of all patients at conventional angiography and up to 53% at coronary computed tomography (CT) angiography.[5]

Clinical Presentation

Constitutional symptoms of fever, myalgias, arthralgias, and weight loss are typically present for months to years before the more specific features of the disease become evident. These are usually related to vascular stenosis, the most common being diminished or absent pulses in as many as 96% of patients, typically in association with limb claudication and blood pressure discrepancies.[1,6] Clinical examination reveals vascular bruits in 80% to 94% of patients, often multiple and affecting mainly the carotid, subclavian, and abdominal arteries.[1,7] Other common findings are hypertension in 33% to 83% of patients, usually reflecting renal artery stenosis, which is seen in 28% to 75% of patients; aortic regurgitation caused by dilatation of the ascending aorta and separation of the valve leaflets; and left-sided heart failure associated with hypertension, aortic regurgitation, and dilated cardiomyopathy.[1,7]

Evidence of pulmonary involvement almost always occurs in patients who have systemic findings; rarely, it is the first manifestation of disease.[8] Many patients are asymptomatic despite the presence of clinical signs or radiologic findings of pulmonary disease. Chest pain and hemoptysis occur occasionally.[8]

Various classification schemes have been proposed. The best known is the one by Numano's group, which divided the disease into six types[2,9]:

- Type I involves only the branches of the aortic arch.
- Type IIa involves the aorta only at its ascending portion or at the aortic arch. The branches of the aortic arch may be involved as well. The rest of the aorta is not affected.
- Type IIb affects the descending thoracic aorta with or without involvement of the ascending aorta or the aortic arch with its branches. The abdominal aorta is not involved.
- Type III is concomitant involvement of the descending thoracic aorta, the abdominal aorta, or the renal arteries. The ascending aorta and the aortic arch and its branches are not involved.
- Type IV involves only the abdominal aorta or the renal arteries.
- Type V is a generalized type, with combined features of the other types.

In this classification scheme, involvement of the coronary and pulmonary arteries is indicated as C^+ or P^+, respectively.[9,10]

Pathophysiology

The pathogenesis of Takayasu arteritis is unclear, and familial onset indicates a genetic contribution beyond ethnicity.[11] The disease has been shown to be associated with different human leukocyte antigen (HLA) alleles in different populations and may coexist with autoimmune disorders, including systemic lupus erythematosus, rheumatoid arthritis, and sarcoidosis.[12,13] Although the HLA association suggests the possibility of an autoimmune process, no specific autoantigens have been identified.[1] Takayasu arteritis has also been associated with infections caused by *Mycobacterium tuberculosis* and streptococcal species.[14]

The main histologic finding consists of patchy panarteritis involving the large elastic vessels of the systemic and pulmonary circulations. On microscopic examination the vasculitis may be divided into an acute inflammatory phase and a healed fibrotic phase.[1] The acute phase is characterized by vasculitis of the vasa vasorum in the adventitia; infiltration of the media by lymphocytes; and thickening of the intima by mucopolysaccharides, smooth muscle cells, and fibroblasts.[1] The inflammation tends to be most marked in the adventitia, with infiltration of B and T lymphocytes.[15] In the chronic phase there is fibrosis with destruction of elastic tissue and narrowing of the arterial lumen in a patchy distribution, often affecting multiple areas. Marked inflammation and more acute progression may cause degeneration of smooth muscle cells with loss of elastic fibers and subsequent aneurysm formation or rupture of the involved arteries.[11,16]

*The editors and the publisher would like to thank Drs. Nestor L. Müller and C. Isabela Silva Müller for contributing material on this topic to the prior edition of this work. It has served as the foundation for the current chapter.

Manifestations of the Disease

RADIOGRAPHY

The most common radiographic abnormalities consist of a wavy or scalloped contour of the descending thoracic aorta and dilated of the aortic arch. Aneurysms of the ascending and descending thoracic aorta are seen less frequently.[17]

COMPUTED TOMOGRAPHY

Multidetector CT angiography with or without electrocardiography gating has a high sensitivity and specificity in the diagnosis of Takayasu arteritis.[18] It depicts the presence and extent of luminal stenosis or aneurysm formation and provides information about vessel wall thickness and inflammation and presence of mural calcification.[19] Precontrast CT often shows high attenuation wall thickening relative to the aortic lumen.[10] Postcontrast imaging in early-stage Takayasu arteritis shows aortic wall thickening with the "double-ring" sign. This sign consists of a poorly enhanced internal ring (swollen intima) and an enhancing outer ring (inflamed media and adventitia).[14] In patients with active inflammation, delayed-phase CT obtained 20 to 40 minutes after intravenous injection shows circumferential enhancement of the vessel wall.[20] Aortic (Fig. 49.1) or branch vessel stenosis (Fig. 49.2) is the most common luminal change and occurs in up to 90% of patients. Vascular occlusion (Fig. 49.3) and aneurysm formation (Fig. 49.4) are less common disease manifestations, with the latter being associated with fatal rupture or aortic dissection (Fig. 49.5).[10] Aortic wall calcification is usually transmural (see Fig. 49.5), occurs in up to 27% of patients, and is typically seen in chronic Takayasu arteritis. Pulmonary artery involvement occurs in 15% to 63% of patients (Fig. 49.6).[3,10]

The most common abnormalities consist of stenosis or occlusion of segmental or subsegmental branches, usually in an upper lobe. These abnormalities are associated with localized areas of low attenuation and decreased vascularity on high-resolution CT and perfusion defects on technetium-99m–macroaggregated

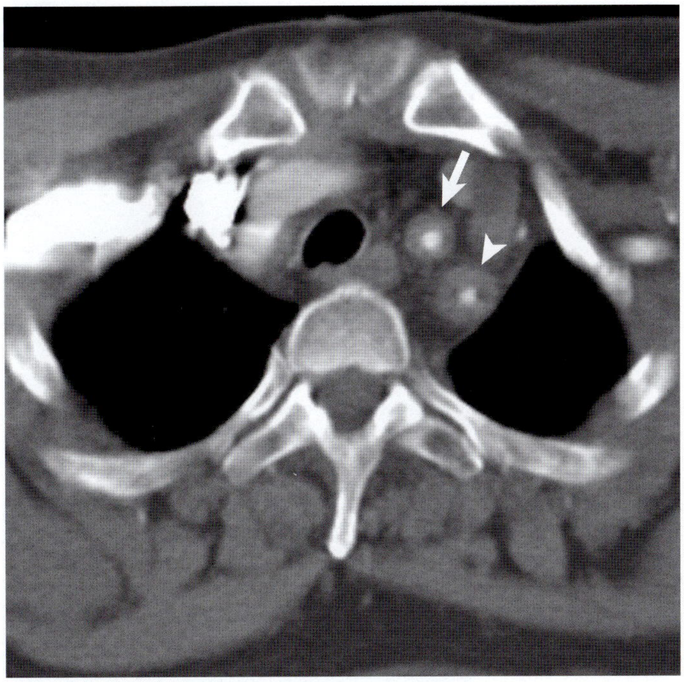

Fig. 49.2 Takayasu arteritis with wall thickening. Axial contrast-enhanced CT shows marked concentric wall thickening with resultant stenosis of the left common carotid *(arrow)* and left subclavian *(arrowhead)* arteries.

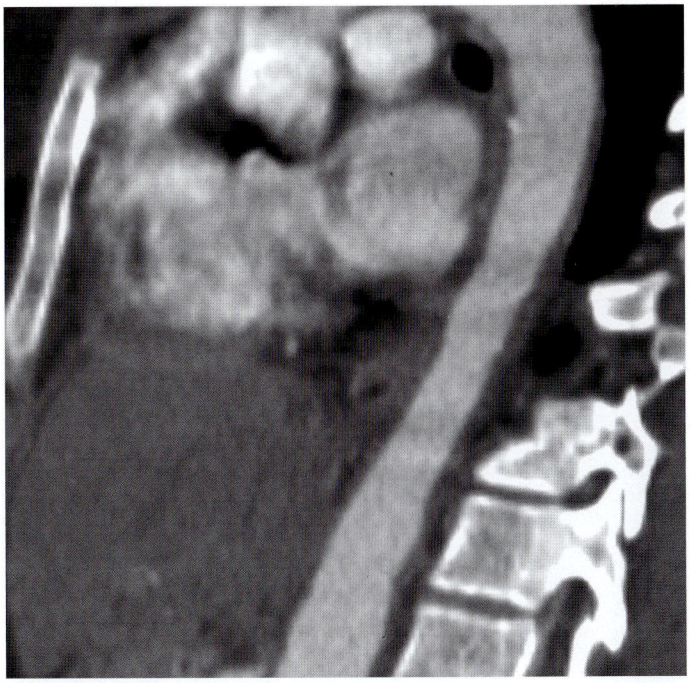

Fig. 49.1 Takayasu arteritis with stenosis. Oblique sagittal contrast-enhanced CT shows a smooth tapered stenosis of the middle descending thoracic aorta.

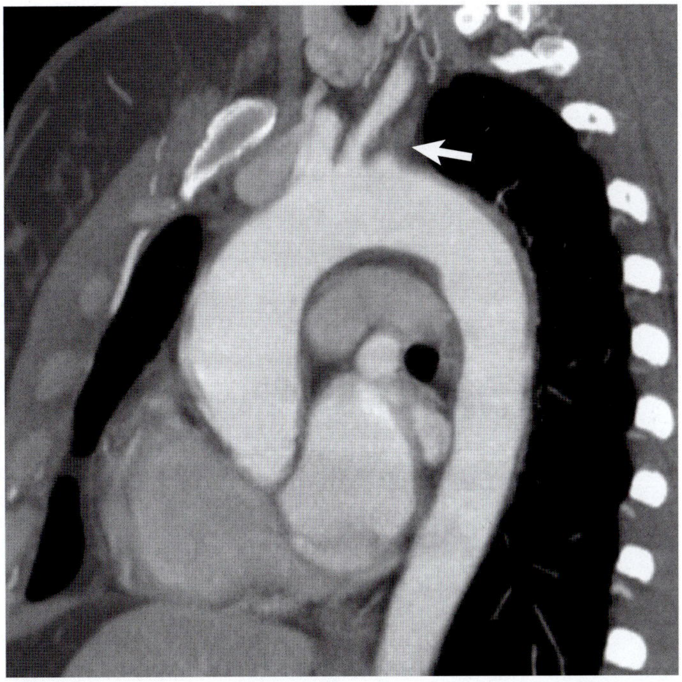

Fig. 49.3 Takayasu arteritis causing vascular occlusion. Oblique sagittal contrast-enhanced CT shows occlusion of the left subclavian artery *(arrow)* and mild wall thickening with stenosis of the left common carotid artery.

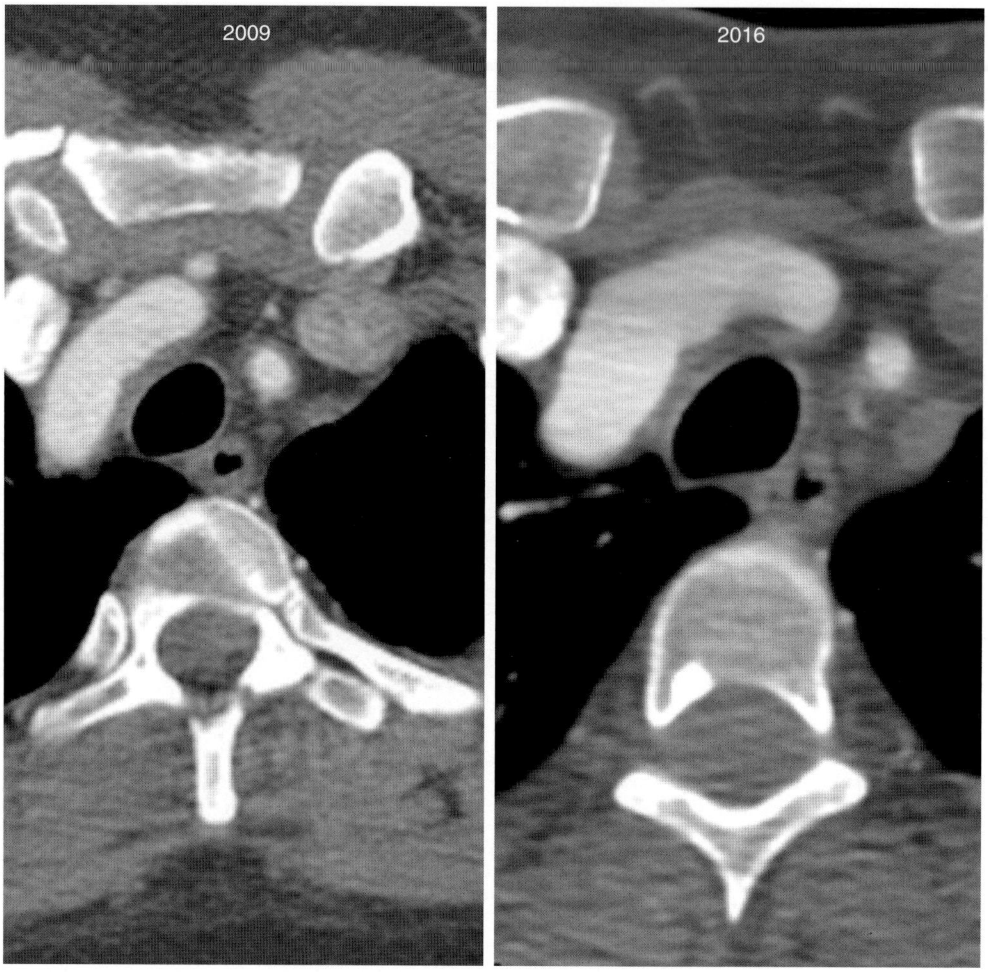

Fig. 49.4 Takayasu arteritis causing aneurysm formation. Composite image with axial contrast-enhanced CT in 2009 *(left image)* and 2016 *(right image)* shows progressive aneurysmal enlargement of the brachiocephalic artery.

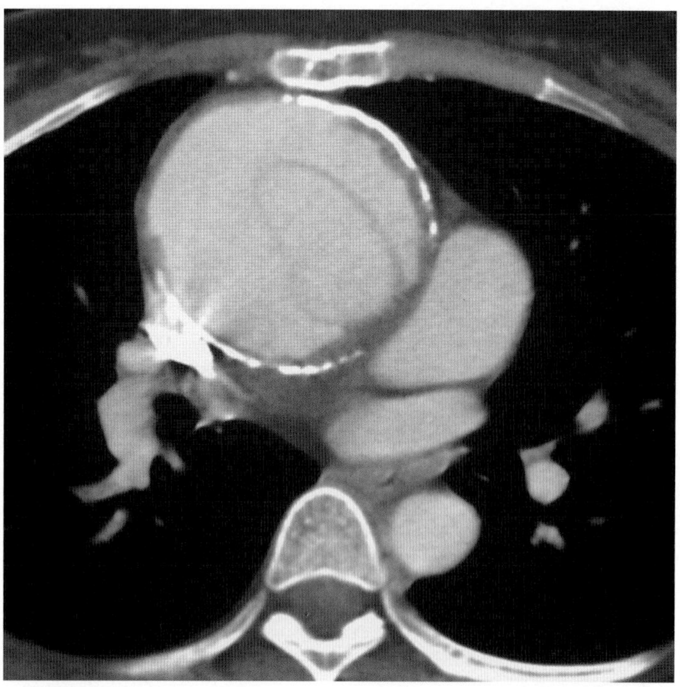

Fig. 49.5 Takayasu arteritis with aortic aneurysm and dissection. Contrast-enhanced CT demonstrates aneurysm of the ascending aorta, extensive calcification of the aortic wall, and intimomedial flap indicating aortic dissection.

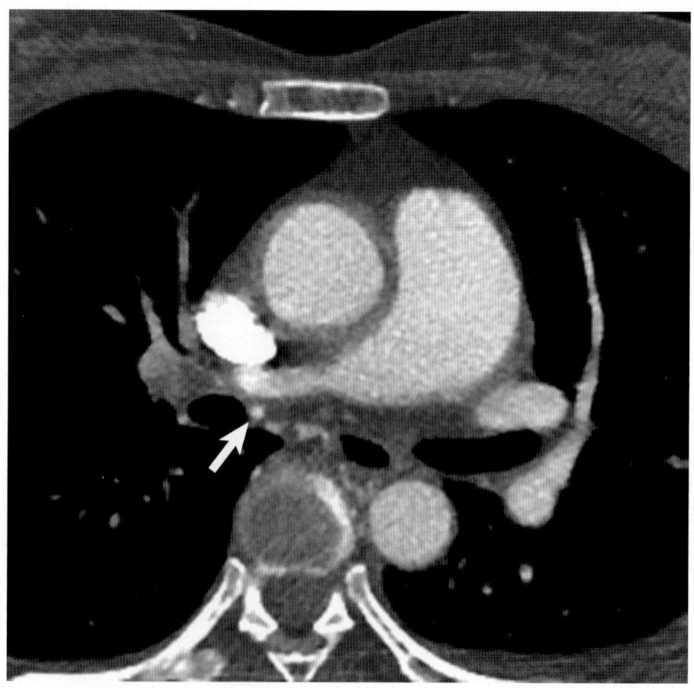

Fig. 49.6 Takayasu arteritis with pulmonary artery involvement. Axial contrast-enhanced CT shows smooth, tapered narrowing of the right pulmonary artery and its branches with enlargement of bronchial artery collaterals *(arrow)*. *(Reproduced with permission from Walker CM, Rosado-de-Christenson ML, Martínez-Jiménez S, et al. Bronchial arteries: anatomy, function, hypertrophy, and anomalies.* Radiographics. *2015;35:32–49.)*

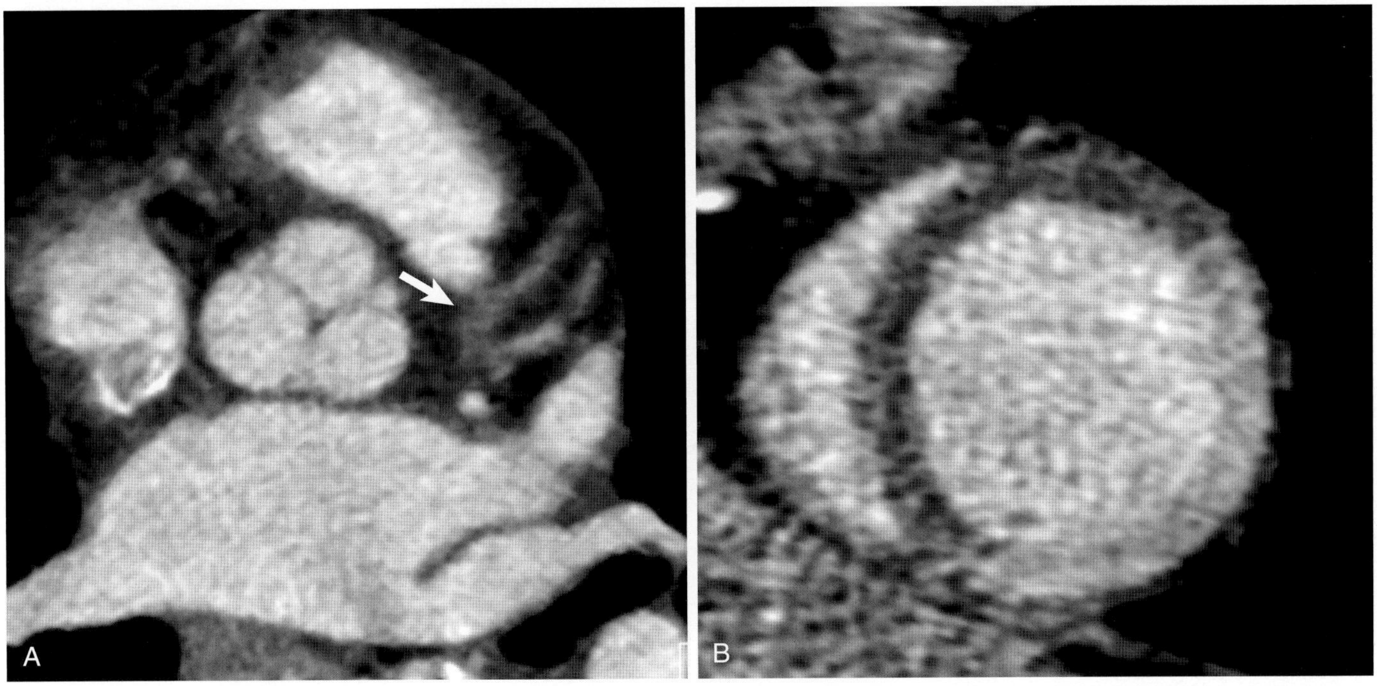

Fig. 49.7 Takayasu arteritis with coronary artery occlusion. (A) Axial contrast-enhanced CT shows occlusion *(arrow)* of the left anterior descending coronary artery. (B) Cardiac short-axis CT shows hypoenhancement of the anterior and septal walls of the left ventricle corresponding to the left anterior descending coronary artery territory. The lateral and inferior walls enhance normally.

albumin perfusion scintigraphy.[21] The main limitations of CT are radiation dose and need for iodinated contrast material. Coronary artery involvement is common, affecting greater than 50% of all patients. Common manifestations include ostial and nonostial coronary artery stenoses and occlusions (Fig. 49.7) and, less commonly, aneurysm formation.[5]

MAGNETIC RESONANCE IMAGING

Magnetic resonance imaging (MRI) is the imaging modality of choice for the assessment of patients with suspected or proven Takayasu arteritis.[16,18] It avoids radiation exposure, which is an important consideration in these young patients, and the risks of iodinated contrast load. Manifestations of Takayasu arteritis on MRI include concentric wall thickening of the aorta and other involved vessels (Fig. 49.8), signal alterations within and surrounding inflamed vessels, intraluminal thrombi, multifocal stenoses, vascular dilation, and aneurysm formation.[22,23] Approximately 90% to 95% of patients with clinical and laboratory evidence of disease activity have a segment of vessel wall edema demonstrated by MRI.[24] MRI has also been shown to demonstrate edema in patients in apparent clinical remission but who subsequently develop arterial stenosis.[7]

The recommended techniques for MRI in patients with Takayasu arteritis include T2-weighted fat-suppressed multiplanar sequences to detect vessel wall edema; T1-weighted fast spoiled gradient-echo or fast spin-echo double-inversion–recovery multiplanar sequences before and after the intravenous administration of the contrast agent, to detect vessel wall thickening and enhancement by the contrast material; and MR angiography (MRA) to evaluate luminal narrowing and dilatations.[2] MRA techniques include noncontrast three-dimensional steady-state free-precession images and three-dimensional angiography with contrast material.[2,25]

Limitations of MRI include low sensitivity in the detection of abnormalities in small branches of the aorta; overestimation of moderate stenosis; and no information about plaque content, which limits its value in distinguishing vasculitic and atherosclerotic disease.[26] In a double-blind study of 30 consecutive patients with use of fast low-angle–shot sequences to acquire gadolinium-enhanced three-dimensional MRA sequences, the sensitivity and specificity of MR compared with those of conventional angiography were 100%.[27] MRA accurately depicted 323 (98%) of 330 arteries, but 7 (2%) stenotic arteries were overestimated as occluded.[27]

ANGIOGRAPHY

Previously, angiography, particularly digital subtraction angiography, was the procedure of choice for the diagnostic evaluation of Takayasu arteritis.[22] The angiographic features of Takayasu arteritis typically consist of long, smooth, tapered stenoses ranging from mild to severe; occlusions; and collateral circulation. Angiography, however, does not depict the vessel wall and cannot distinguish stenoses caused by acute mural inflammation from stenoses caused by chronic transmural fibrosis.[22] Furthermore, it is invasive and associated with substantial radiation dose, and it can be difficult to perform in patients with long-segment stenoses or extensive arterial calcification. Therefore angiography has been replaced by MRI or contrast-enhanced CT in the initial evaluation of patients with Takayasu arteritis.

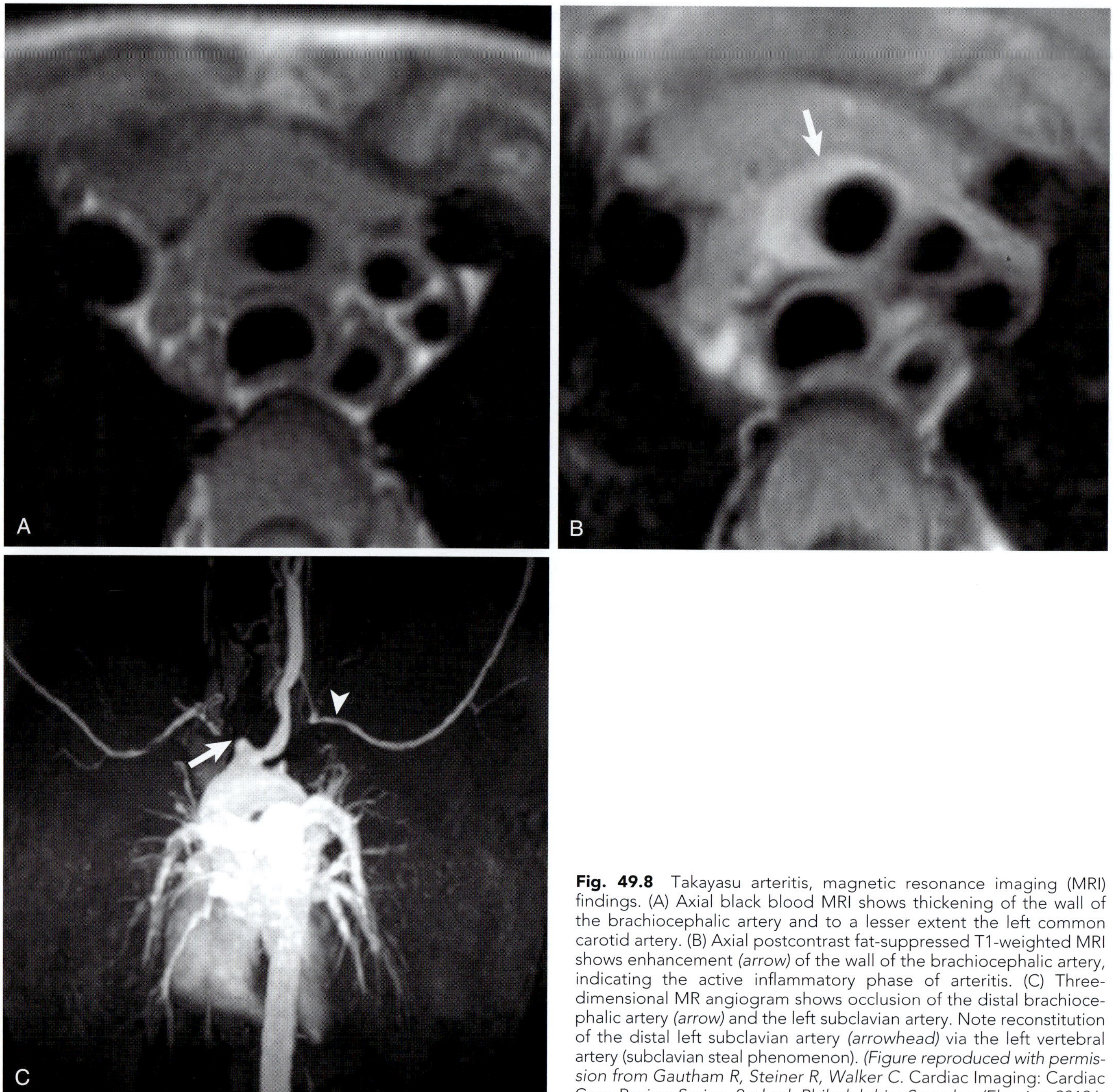

Fig. 49.8 Takayasu arteritis, magnetic resonance imaging (MRI) findings. (A) Axial black blood MRI shows thickening of the wall of the brachiocephalic artery and to a lesser extent the left common carotid artery. (B) Axial postcontrast fat-suppressed T1-weighted MRI shows enhancement *(arrow)* of the wall of the brachiocephalic artery, indicating the active inflammatory phase of arteritis. (C) Three-dimensional MR angiogram shows occlusion of the distal brachiocephalic artery *(arrow)* and the left subclavian artery. Note reconstitution of the distal left subclavian artery *(arrowhead)* via the left vertebral artery (subclavian steal phenomenon). *(Figure reproduced with permission from Gautham R, Steiner R, Walker C.* Cardiac Imaging: Cardiac Case Review Series. *2nd ed. Philadelphia: Saunders/Elsevier; 2013.)*

POSITRON EMISSION TOMOGRAPHY

Several studies have shown high uptake of ^{18}F-fluorodeoxyglucose (FDG) on positron emission tomography (PET) imaging in patients with Takayasu arteritis and other forms of aortitis, reflecting the presence of active inflammation (Fig. 49.9).[28,29] It has been suggested that FDG-PET imaging may be comparable to MRI in the diagnosis of aortitis but that FDG-PET imaging may identify more vascular regions involved in the inflammatory process and therefore may be more reliable in monitoring disease activity during immunosuppressive therapy.[28,30] However, a recent meta-analysis of eight studies comprising 170 vasculitis patients and 230 control patients identified a pooled sensitivity of 75.9% and pooled specificity of 93.0% for detection of large-vessel vasculitis among untreated patients with elevated inflammatory markers, suggesting that a negative FDG-PET study does not exclude a diagnosis of large-vessel vasculitis.[29]

Synopsis of Treatment Options

Medical treatment is aimed at control of active inflammation and prevention of further vascular damage. The main treatment is with high-dose corticosteroids, to which approximately 50% of patients respond. Patients with corticosteroid resistance or relapsing disease require treatment with cytotoxic or biological agents, including methotrexate and anti–tumor necrosis factor (TNF) therapy.[1,11] Treatment of symptomatic stenoses or occlusions includes percutaneous angioplasty, stenting, and surgical revascularization.[31]

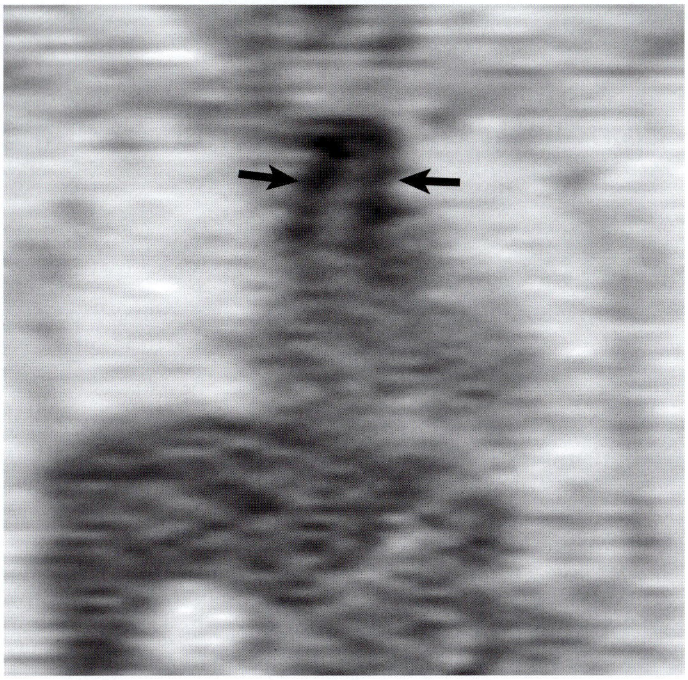

Fig. 49.9 Takayasu arteritis, positron emission tomography (PET) findings. Coronal fluorodeoxyglucose (FDG)-PET shows increased FDG uptake *(arrows)* along the ascending aortic wall, indicating the active inflammatory phase of Takayasu arteritis. *(Figure reproduced with permission from Gautham R, Steiner R, Walker C.* Cardiac Imaging: Cardiac Case Review Series. *2nd ed. Philadelphia: Saunders/Elsevier; 2013.)*

KEY POINTS

- Takayasu arteritis is an idiopathic chronic arteritis affecting predominantly the aorta and its main branches.
- It occurs most commonly in Japan, Southeast Asia, India, Mexico, and Brazil and usually affects patients between 10 and 40 years of age.
- The female-to-male ratio ranges from 10:1 in Japan to 3:1 in South Africa.
- The most common clinical presentation is diminished or absent pulses evident in 84%–96% of patients.
- Cross-sectional imaging manifestations include:
  - Concentric wall thickening of the aorta and other involved vessels
  - Vessel wall edema during active inflammation
  - Multifocal stenoses
  - Aneurysm formation

SUGGESTED READINGS

Gotway MB, Araoz PA, Macedo TA, et al. Imaging findings in Takayasu's arteritis. *AJR Am J Roentgenol.* 2005;184:1945–1950.

Serra R, et al. Updates in pathophysiology, diagnosis and management of Takayasu arteritis. *Ann Vasc Surg.* 2016;35:210–225.

Steeds RP, Mohiaddin R. Takayasu arteritis: role of cardiovascular magnetic imaging. *Int J Cardiol.* 2006;109:1–6.

Zhu FP, et al. Takayasu arteritis: imaging spectrum at multidetector CT angiography. *Br J Radiol.* 2012;85:e1282–e1292.

The full reference list for this chapter is available at ExpertConsult.com.

50 Acute Pulmonary Embolism*

CAROL C. WU | MATTHEW D. GILMAN

Etiology

Pulmonary embolism (PE) refers to blood clot(s) within the pulmonary arterial system, usually caused by migration of deep vein thrombosis (DVT) from the lower extremities. Rarely, emboli are from other sources, such as the iliac veins, renal veins, inferior vena cava, right heart chambers, or upper extremity veins. More recently, there are speculations of PE developing de novo.[1] Risk factors for PE are the same as those for DVT, including immobilization, trauma, surgery, active malignancy, prior history of venous thromboembolism (VTE), pregnancy, use of oral contraceptives, indwelling catheters, and hereditary hypercoagulable states, such as deficiency of protein C or S.

Prevalence and Epidemiology

The reported incidence for PE ranges from 29 to 78 per 100,000 person-years. The incidence rates increase with age.[2] An increase in the incidence rate from 2001 to 2009 has been observed, thought to reflect, at least in part, increased use of multidetector computed tomography (MDCT) and improved image resolution.[2] In a recent study, 54% of all PE in oncologic patients and 19% of all PE in non-oncologic patients are diagnosed incidentally on CT performed for purposes other than to look for PE, such as for cancer restaging or evaluation of pleural effusions or pneumonia.[3] The recurrence rate of PE is 15 to 29 per 100,000 person-years.[2]

PE is the third most common cause of cardiovascular death after myocardial ischemia and stroke,[4] with an untreated mortality of 30%.[5] The mortality rate is lower with treatment, although it is estimated that in one-quarter of patients experiencing PE, the initial clinical presentation is sudden death. Predictors of poor survival after PE include syncope and systemic hypotension.[2]

Clinical Presentation

The clinical manifestations of acute PE depend on several factors that individually or in combination influence the effect of vascular occlusion on the lung parenchyma: the presence or absence of associated cardiopulmonary disease; the size, number, and location of emboli; the presence of multiple embolic episodes and the time interval between them; and the rate of thrombus organization and lysis, whether spontaneously or with therapy.[6] The most common symptoms are dyspnea, tachypnea, and pleuritic chest pain. A sudden onset of these symptoms in the absence of underlying respiratory disease is highly suggestive of acute PE. On the contrary, the clinical diagnosis of acute PE is difficult in patients with chronic respiratory diseases, and this situation is exemplified by patients with chronic obstructive pulmonary disease (COPD), in whom acute PE may mimic COPD exacerbation.

The clinical probability assessment, an important component of strategies for optimal diagnosis of acute PE based on noninvasive tests, is therefore much more helpful in patients devoid of underlying cardiopulmonary disease[7] than in patients with COPD.[8] Various clinical probability assessment scores have been validated—the Wells score,[9] the Geneva score (recently revised),[7,10] and the Pisa score.[11] The use of a combination of clinical probability scores and serum D-dimer test, which has a very high negative predictive value for VTE, has been shown to be effective in reducing the use and improving the positive yield of computed tomography pulmonary angiography (CTPA)[12,12a] and is recommended by the American College of Physicians' Best Practice Advice in the evaluation of patients with suspected acute PE.[13] Both the American College of Radiology Appropriateness Criteria[14] and American Thoracic Society and American College of Chest Physicians Choosing Wisely campaign[15] stated that CTPA should not be performed in patients with a low clinical probability and negative result of a highly sensitive D-dimer assay.

Pathology

The potential consequences of acute PE are hemorrhage or, less commonly, infarction within the lung parenchyma; acute pulmonary hypertension; and right ventricular dysfunction. The last is sometimes responsible for left ventricular failure because of impairment of left ventricular preload and decreased coronary arterial perfusion.

In most cases PEs are degraded through the effects of fibrinolysis. Less commonly, they may break down into small fragments that embolize to the peripheral arterial branches. Delayed recanalization can also be seen with creation of multiple small vascular channels within the endoluminal clot.

The effect of thromboemboli in individual patients is influenced by the degree of obstruction of the pulmonary circulation, the presence and extent of underlying lung abnormalities, and the status of the patient's fibrinolytic system.

Manifestations of the Disease

RADIOGRAPHY

The chest radiograph has an important role in excluding other diagnoses that can mimic the clinical picture of acute PE, such

*The editors and the publisher would like to thank Drs. Martine Remy-Jardin and Jacques Remy for contributing material on this topic to the prior edition of this work. It has served as the foundation for the current chapter.

as a pneumothorax or pneumonia. The chest radiograph, however, is both insensitive and nonspecific in the diagnosis of acute PE.

The radiographic manifestations of acute PE include a spectrum of abnormalities ranging from a normal chest radiograph to a series of focal changes reflecting the pleural or parenchymal consequences of acute pulmonary vascular obstruction.

Radiographic Features Observed in the Absence of Infarction or Hemorrhage

Peripheral oligemia caused by obstruction of the pulmonary artery or vasoconstriction of distal hypoxic lung result in peripheral hyperlucency, referred to as the Westermark sign (Fig. 50.1).

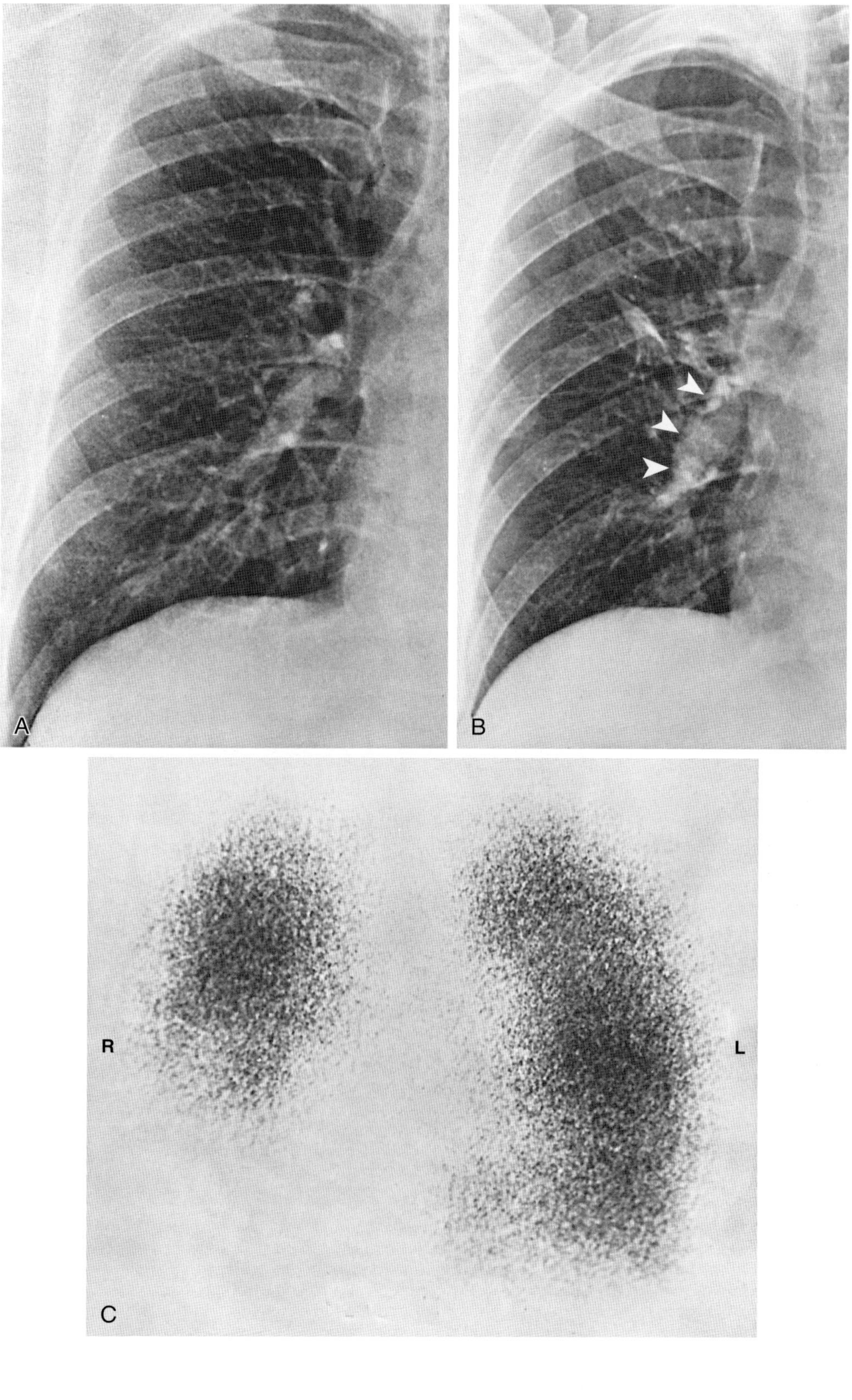

Fig. 50.1 Fleischner sign and Westermark sign in acute pulmonary embolism. On admission to the hospital, posteroanterior radiograph (A) revealed no significant abnormalities. Several days after abdominal surgery, the patient experienced abrupt onset of right-sided chest pain and dyspnea. A radiograph at this time (B) showed an obvious increase in diameter and a change in configuration of the right interlobar artery (Fleischner sign; *arrowheads*); also the distal end of this artery appeared knuckled and the vessels peripheral to it diminutive. The right lower zone showed increased radiolucency, indicating diminished perfusion (Westermark sign). Scintigraphy (C) revealed absence of perfusion of the lower half of the right lung. *(From Müller NL, Fraser RS, Colman NC, Paré PD.* Radiologic Diagnosis of Diseases of the Chest. *Philadelphia: WB Saunders; 2001.)*

Dilatation of a major pulmonary artery (Fleischner sign; see Fig. 50.1) is identified more easily in the right hilum and can be seen in conjunction with a truncated appearance of the enlarged vessel, reflecting the arterial amputation. These findings are seen only in patients with massive acute PE.

Radiographic Features Suggestive of Infarction or Hemorrhage

Pulmonary consolidation in acute PE is usually due to parenchymal hemorrhage and edema. On occasion, it may be the result of pulmonary infarction. Infarction is suggested by the finding of a homogeneous wedge-shaped consolidation in the periphery of the lung, with a rounded, convex apex toward the hilum, referred to as the Hampton hump (Fig. 50.2). Cavitation can occur but is rare. The pattern of resolution of infarction has been described as the "melting ice cube" sign, where the opacity retains its typical shape as it resolves. This feature helps differentiate this entity from pneumonia.

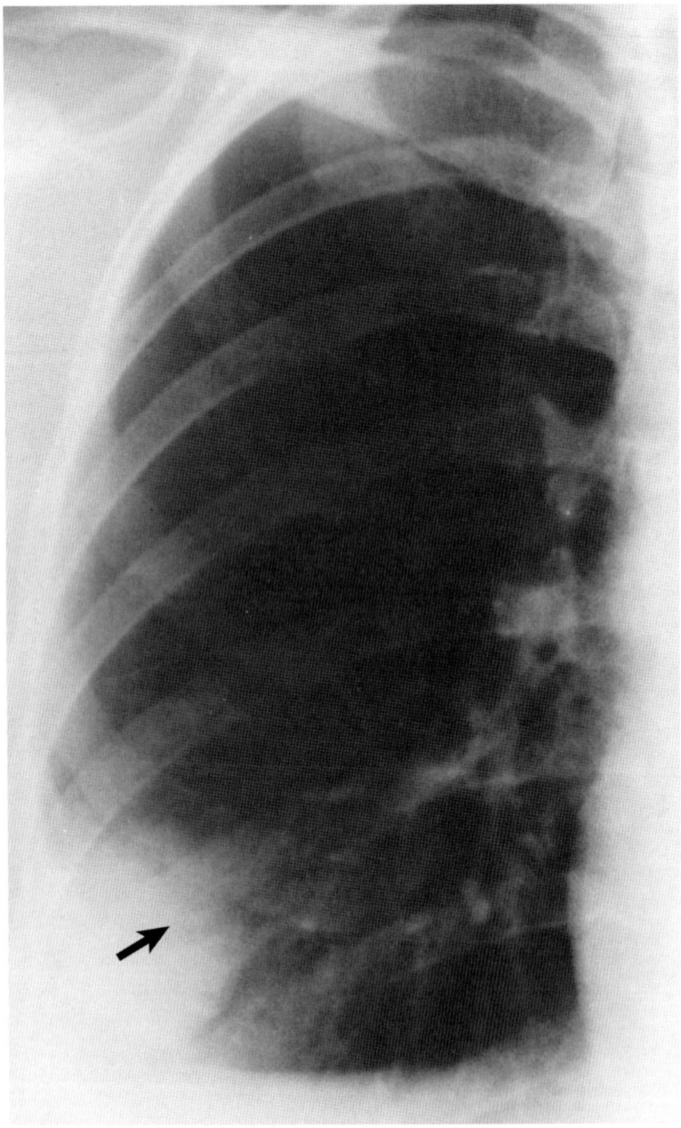

Fig. 50.2 The Hampton hump in acute pulmonary embolism. View of the right lung on posteroanterior radiograph reveals a homogeneous opacity in the right costophrenic angle with a convex contour *(arrow)* toward the hilum. This constitutes the typical feature of the Hampton hump and is highly suggestive of a pulmonary infarct. *(From Müller NL, Fraser RS, Colman NC, Paré PD.* Radiologic Diagnosis of Diseases of the Chest. *Philadelphia: WB Saunders; 2001.)*

Additional Findings

Pleural effusion can be seen, either as an isolated abnormality or, more commonly, in patients who have infarction or hemorrhage. Acute PE may also be responsible for radiographic features suggestive of right-sided cardiac dysfunction, such as dilatation of the azygos vein and superior vena cava, reflecting systemic venous hypertension. Radiographic findings of pulmonary arterial hypertension are rarely observed.

COMPUTED TOMOGRAPHY

With the advent of MDCT technologies resulting in short image acquisition time and improved image quality, CT pulmonary angiography (CTPA), with high sensitivity and specificity, has become the imaging modality of choice in the evaluation of suspected PE.[14]

Computed Tomography Findings

The CT criteria for acute PE are partial or complete filling defects within a contrast-opacified pulmonary artery (Fig. 50.3). A partial filling defect is defined as an intravascular central or marginal area of low attenuation surrounded by a variable amount of contrast material (Fig. 50.4; see also Fig. 50.3). A variant has been described as the "railway track" sign when the endoluminal clot is surrounded by a rim of contrast material on both sides. A complete filling defect is defined by an intraluminal area of low attenuation that occupies the entire cross-section of the

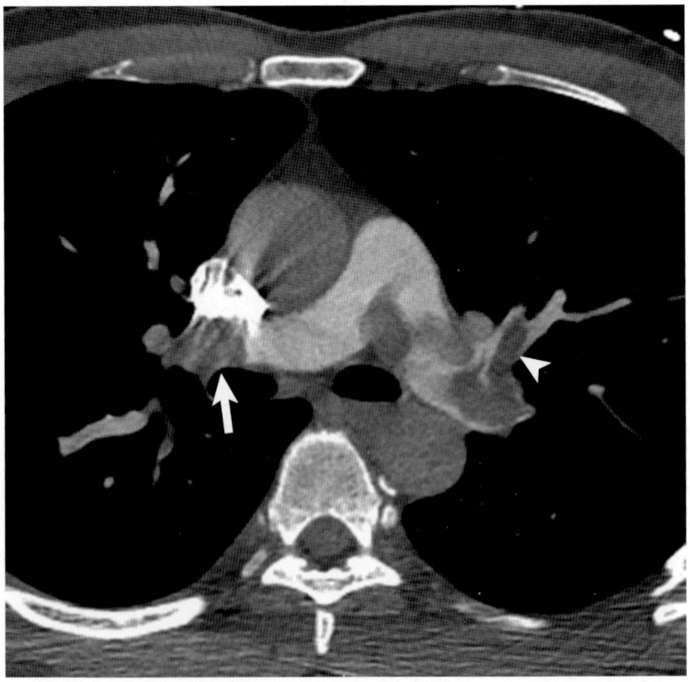

Fig. 50.3 CT features of acute pulmonary embolism. Contrast-enhanced CT scan shows endoluminal filling defects in the right interlobar pulmonary artery *(arrow)* and left-sided pulmonary arteries. The arrow points to a complete filling defect. The arrowhead points to partial filling defects extending into the anterior segmental artery of the left upper lobe and left lower lobe pulmonary arteries.

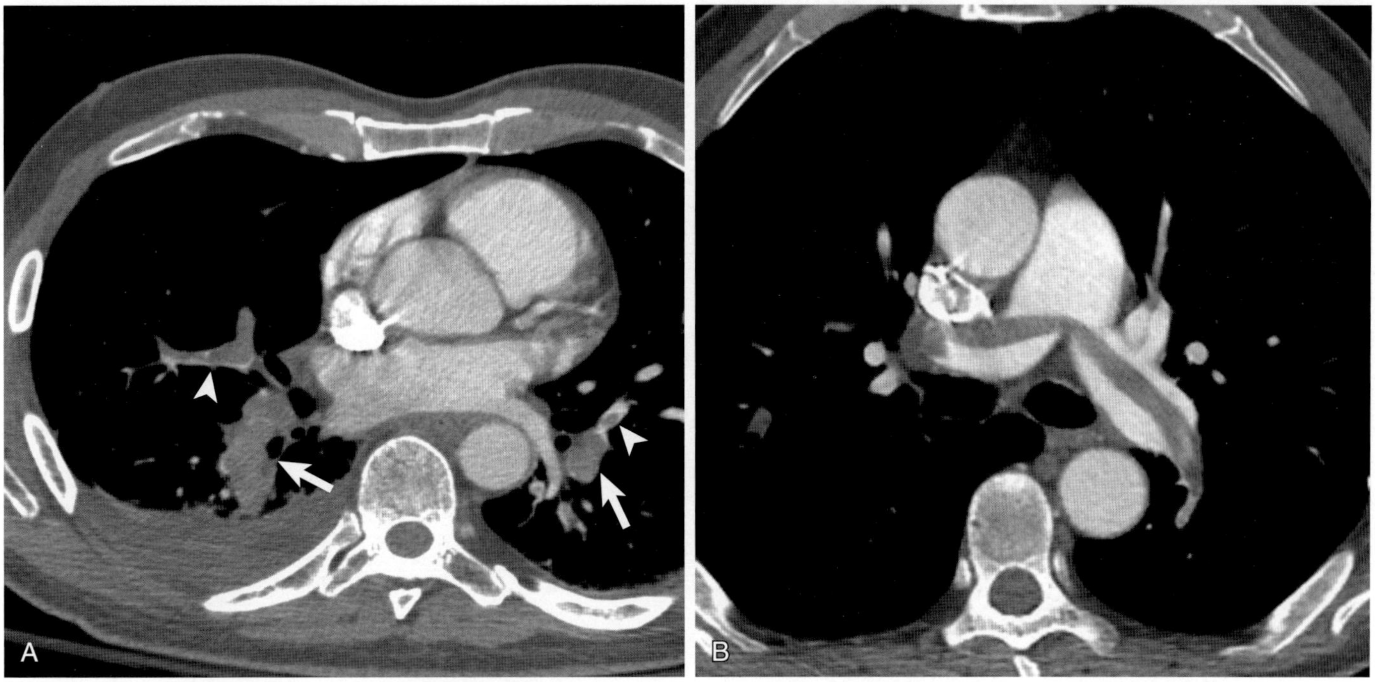

Fig. 50.4 Acute pulmonary embolism with partial and complete filling defects. (A) Contrast-enhanced CT image shows partial filling defects *(arrowheads)* in the right middle lobe and lingular pulmonary arteries. Complete filling defects *(arrows)* are noted in bilateral lower lobe pulmonary arteries. (B) CT image in another patient demonstrates saddle embolus bridging the pulmonary arteries.

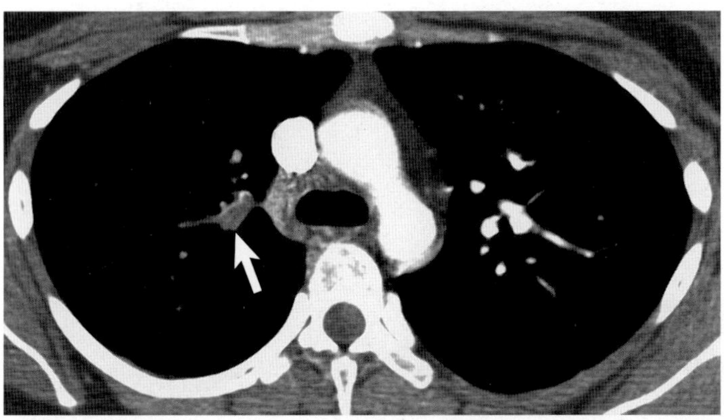

Fig. 50.5 Acute pulmonary embolism (PE) with complete filling defect. Contrast-enhanced CT image shows complete obstruction of the right upper lobe vessels *(arrow)* caused by acute PE.

vessel (Fig. 50.5; see also Fig. 50.3). The involved pulmonary artery branch may dilate in the setting of acute PE, particularly if the embolus is occlusive. On noncontrast CT hyperattenuation within the central pulmonary arteries should raise suspicion for PE. This is referred to as the hyperdense lumen sign, which has poor sensitivity but high specificity (Fig. 50.6).[16]

Indirect findings of PE include peripheral areas of consolidation or ground-glass opacities resulting from pulmonary hemorrhage or infarction and pleural effusions (Fig. 50.7). The reverse halo sign, where an area of ground-glass opacity is surrounded by a rim of consolidation, has been described for pulmonary infarction.[17] The reverse halo sign, when observed in the subpleural lung, should prompt consideration or search for PE. Areas of decreased attenuation and vascularity in affected portions of lungs may occur but are uncommon in acute PE (Fig. 50.8).

In the absence of endovascular defects to suggest acute PE, analysis of lung, pleural, and mediastinal compartments can often help identify an alternative explanation for the patient's symptoms.

Assessment of Pulmonary Embolism Severity. The prognosis and optimal therapy for patients with PE are strongly influenced by the presence or absence of hemodynamic events. Recent management guidelines classify patients as those with massive PE, submassive PE, and nonmassive PE. Massive PE, defined by signs of hemodynamic instability, such as shock and/or a systolic blood pressure less than 90 mm Hg, is an indication for thrombolysis.[18] Submassive PE refers to acute PE without systemic hypotension but with right ventricular dysfunction on CT or echocardiogram and/or signs of myocardial necrosis. These patients have a guarded prognosis and are usually not suitable for outpatient treatment, which is increasingly used in patients with nonmassive PE.[18,19] As most PE is now diagnosed on CTPA, attention has been directed to the use of morphologic criteria on CT scans to investigate the severity of acute PE, relying on the recognition of signs indicating right-sided heart failure,[20,21] quantification of the obstruction of the pulmonary arterial bed,[22–26] and evaluation of lung perfusion. The right ventricle to left ventricle–diameter ratio of greater than or equal to 1, measured on axial images (Fig. 50.9), has been shown to have the best predictive value of poor clinical outcome and death.[27,28] Ventricular diameters are measured as the maximum distance from the interventricular septum to the endocardial border perpendicular to the long axis of the ventricular chamber. Each axial ventricular diameter is measured on the axial image, where it is largest.[28] Other CT findings of right heart strain, such as bowing of the interventricular septum and reflux of intravenous contrast into the inferior vena cava or hepatic veins, are less reliable (Fig. 50.10).[27]

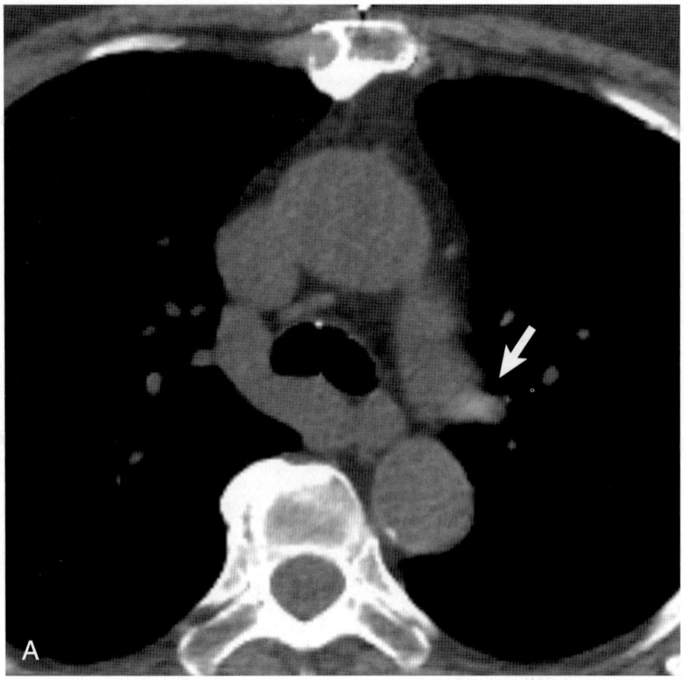

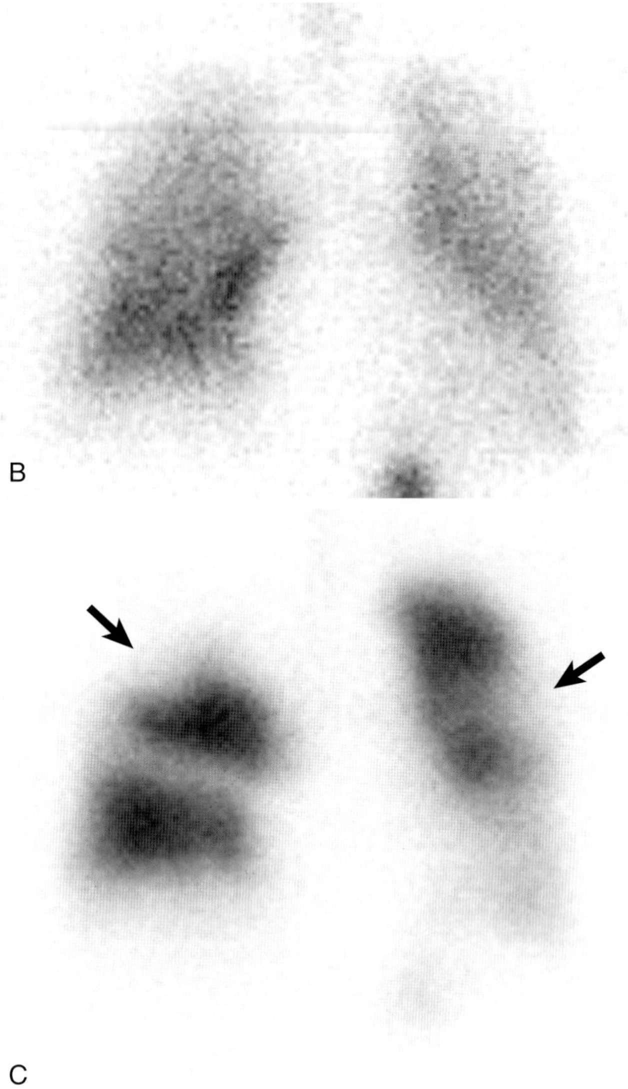

Fig. 50.6 Acute pulmonary embolism (PE) on noncontrast CT. (A) Noncontrast CT image shows hyperdensity *(arrow)* within the left upper lobe anterior segmental pulmonary artery. Subsequent ventilation (B) and perfusion (C) scintigraphy revealed large mismatched segmental perfusion defects *(arrows)* in the right upper lobe apical segment and left upper lobe anterior segment consistent with high probability of PE.

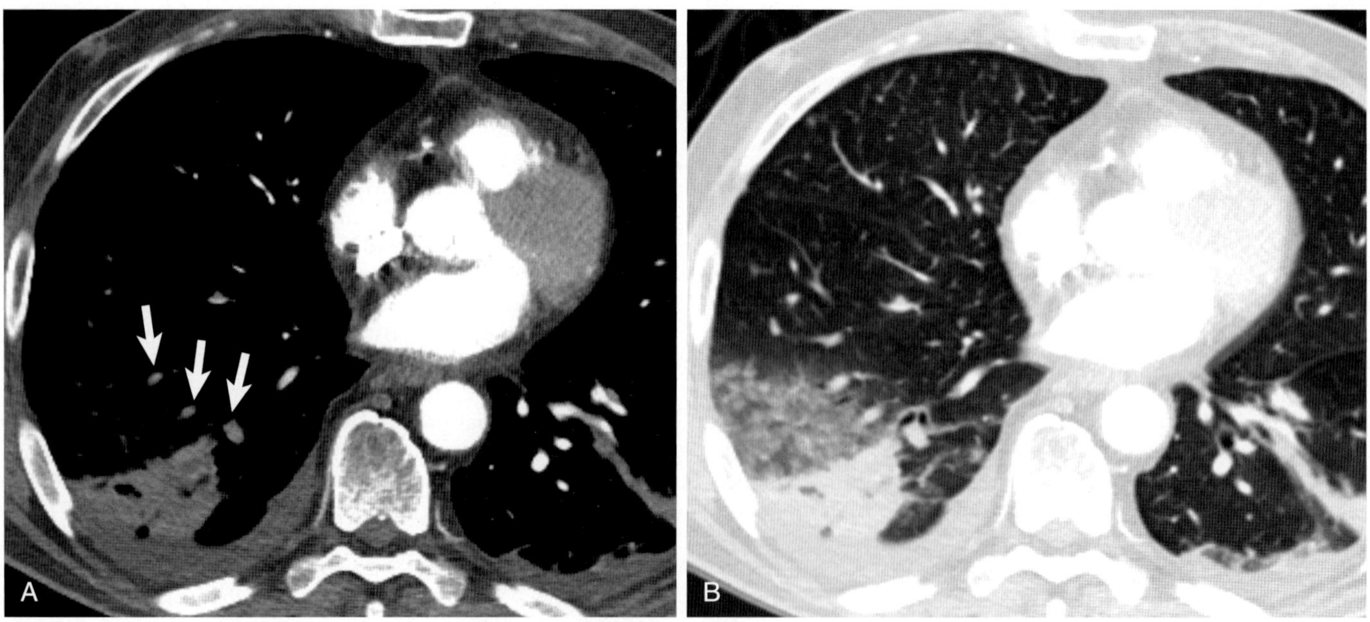

Fig. 50.7 Pulmonary infarcts in acute pulmonary embolism. Contrast-enhanced CT scan in soft tissue window (A) shows filling defects consistent with pulmonary emboli *(arrows)* in multiple right lower lobe pulmonary artery branches. Corresponding lung window image (B) shows right lower lobe wedge-shaped subpleural consolidation and ground-glass opacity most consistent with pulmonary infarct and hemorrhage. A small right pleural effusion is evident.

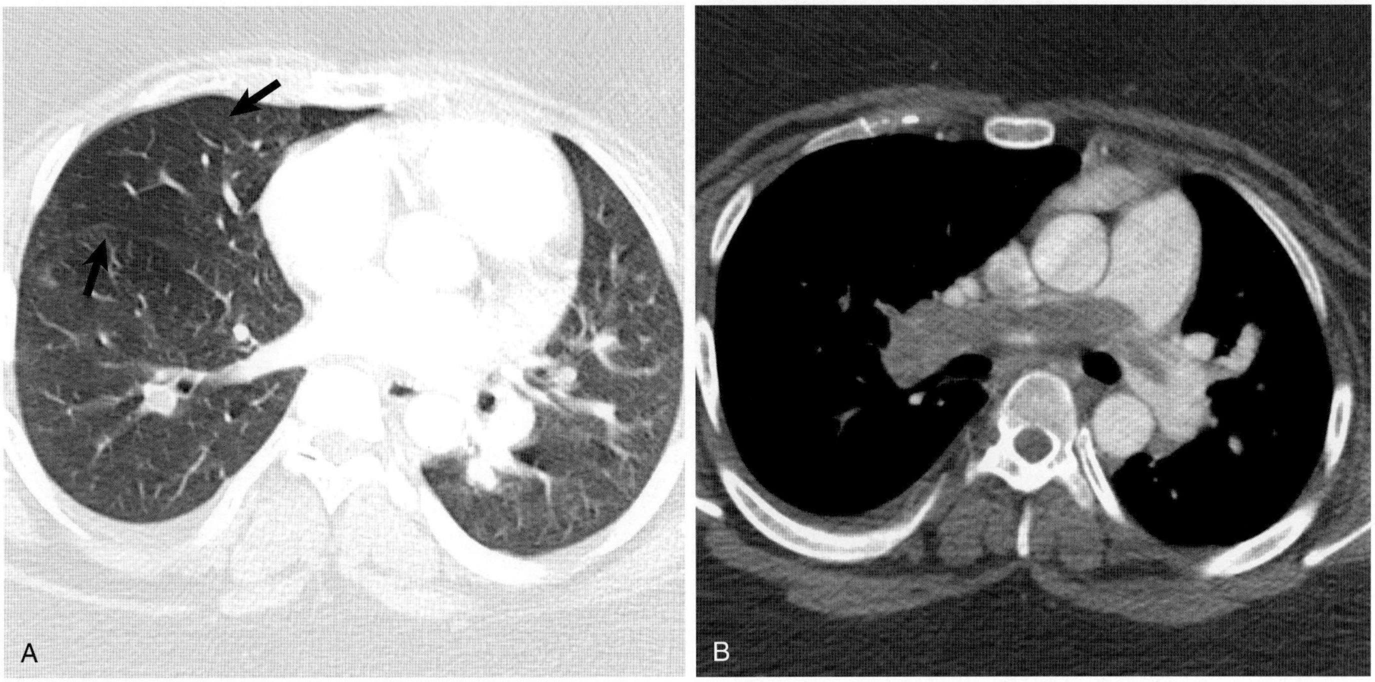

Fig. 50.8 Decreased attenuation in acute pulmonary embolism. (A) CT scan shows decreased vascularity and attenuation *(arrows)* of the right middle and lower lobes. (B) Contrast-enhanced CT scan shows a large saddle embolus with a larger amount of thrombus extending into the right pulmonary artery and its branches.

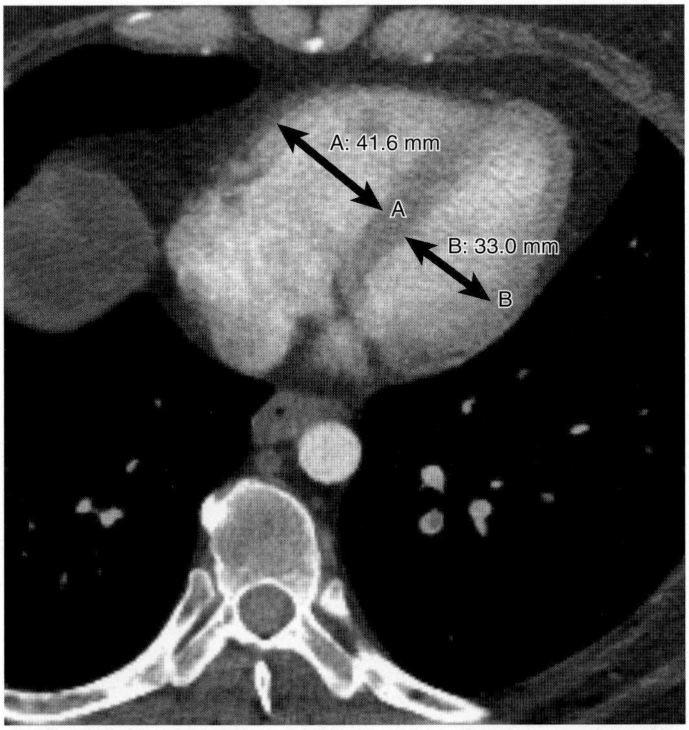

Fig. 50.9 Measurement of right ventricular (RV) to left ventricular (LV)–diameter ratio. Ventricular diameters are measured as the maximum distance from the interventricular septum to the endocardial border perpendicular to the long axis of the ventricular chamber. Each axial ventricular diameter is measured on the axial image where it is largest. RV to LV–diameter ratio ≥1 has been shown to correlate with pulmonary embolism–related mortality.

Scoring systems such as the Quanadli index[23] have been developed to quantify clot burden but are not in common clinical use as they are cumbersome. The most proximal level of pulmonary artery involvement should, however, be reported as this finding does have treatment implications. For patients with subsegmental PE (Fig. 50.11) and no proximal DVT in the legs, who have a low risk for recurrent VTE, clinical surveillance is recommended over anticoagulation.[18] In selected patients with acute central PE, catheter-assisted or surgical embolus removal is an option.[18,29,30]

Dual-energy CT, with datasets acquired at different tube voltage levels, allows creation of perfusion maps similar to scintigraphy. Wedge-shaped pulmonary parenchymal perfusion defects distal to PE can be visualized (Fig. 50.12). These perfusion maps improve the detection of peripheral PE,[31] and the extent of perfusion defects has been correlated with adverse clinical outcome.[32,33]

Standard Multidetector Computed Tomography Protocols. Technologic advances in MDCT have allowed high-quality CTPA to be performed routinely and reliably. Remy-Jardin and colleagues[34] observed that an accurate interpretation down to the subsegmental arteries was more often possible not only in otherwise healthy patients (65% vs. 10%) but also in patients with underlying respiratory disease (47% vs. 15.5%). The improvement in image quality is particularly important for the management of dyspneic patients, such as those with COPD (see Fig. 50.11) and those in the intensive care unit (Fig. 50.13). High-pitch, low tube-voltage image acquisitions and iterative reconstruction are now used to lower the dose of radiation and contrast agent.[35–37] To ensure optimal contrast opacification of the pulmonary arteries, a test bolus or bolus tracking with the region of interest placed in the pulmonary trunk or main pulmonary artery should be used. Careful instruction should be given to patients to ensure

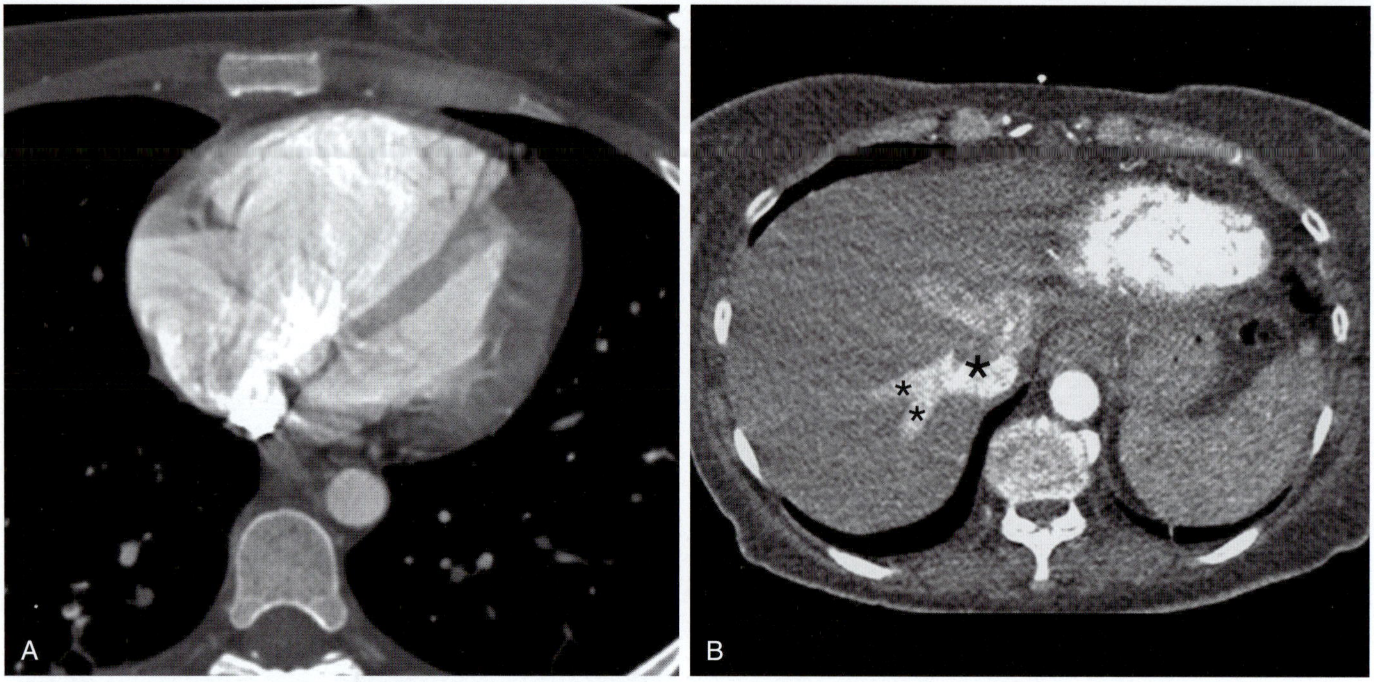

Fig. 50.10 Assessment of pulmonary embolism severity: CT features of right heart dysfunction/failure. (A) Contrast-enhanced CT image obtained at the level of the ventricular cavities shows leftward shift of the interventricular septum resulting from right ventricular dilatation. Note the enlarged right atrium and reflux of contrast within the coronary sinus. The RV to LV–diameter ratio is clearly >1 in this case. (B) CT image obtained at a slightly more caudal level demonstrates reflux of contrast into the inferior vena cava *(large star)* and hepatic veins *(small stars)*.

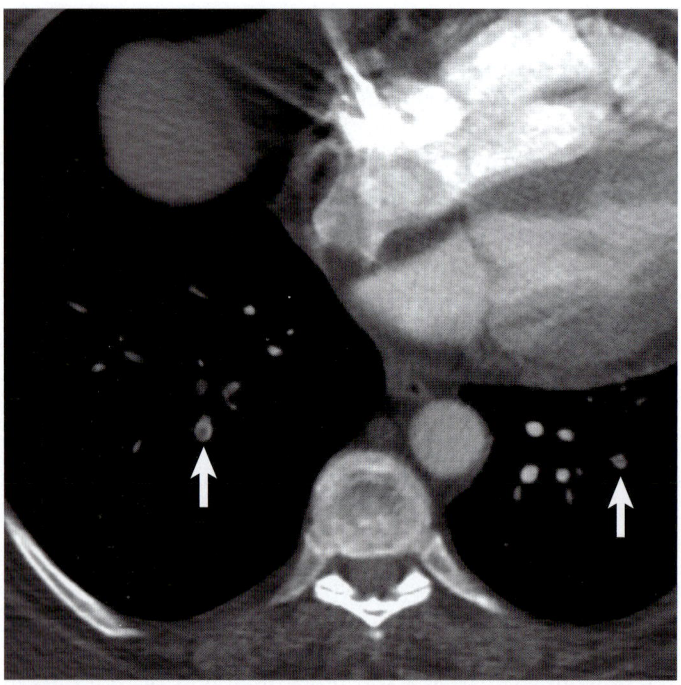

Fig. 50.11 Pulmonary embolism in a dyspneic patient with chronic obstructive pulmonary disease. Contrast-enhanced CT image obtained at the level of the lower lobes shows subsegmental filling defects *(arrows)* in both lower lobes.

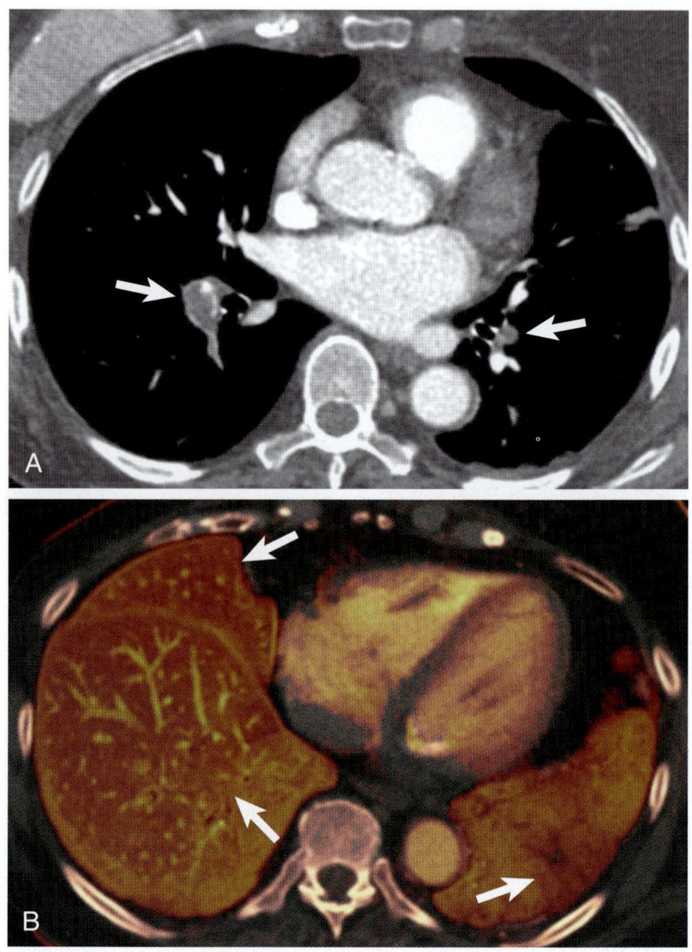

Fig. 50.12 Acute pulmonary embolism on dual-energy multidetector CT. (A) Axial CT image shows occlusive filling defects *(arrows)* at the origin of the right middle and lower lobar pulmonary arteries and left lower lobe lateral basal segmental pulmonary artery. (B) Perfusion map demonstrates perfusion deficits as darker colors *(arrows)* in areas of the lung supplied by the affected pulmonary artery branches.

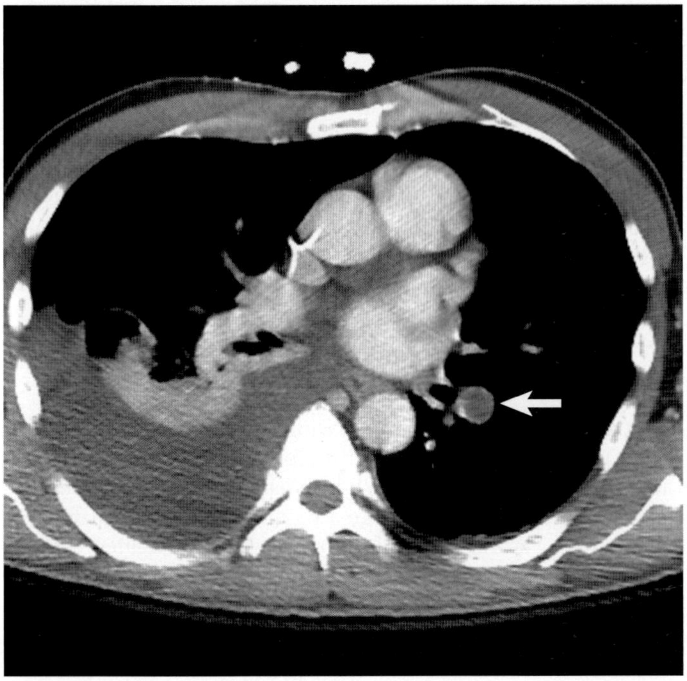

Fig. 50.13 Pulmonary embolism in a patient referred from the intensive care unit. Contrast-enhanced CT image shows endoluminal clot *(arrow)*.

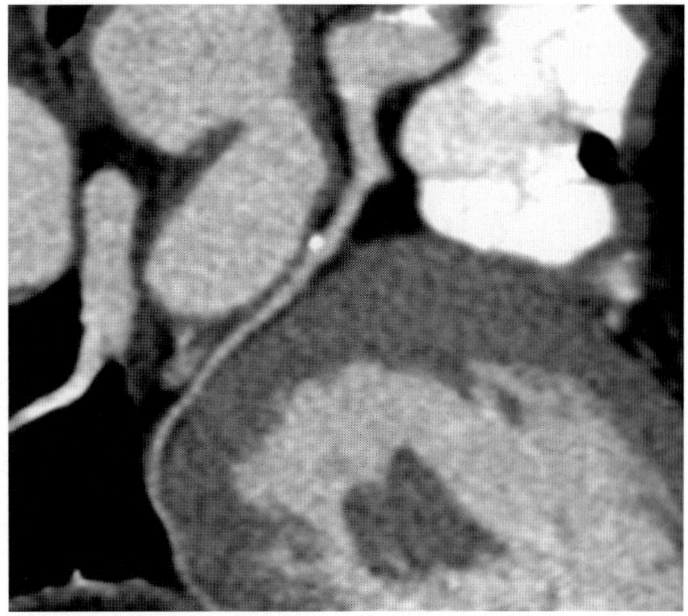

Fig. 50.14 Acute chest pain investigated with electrocardiography (ECG)-gated 64-slice multidetector CT angiography. Curved planar reformatted image of the left circumflex coronary artery was reconstructed from an ECG-gated CT examination of the entire chest. Note the excellent image quality, enabling demonstration of the patency of the vessel lumen despite calcified plaque.

adequate breath-holding and to avoid the Valsalva maneuver, which can cause interruption of contrast bolus because of influx of unopacified blood from the inferior vena cava resulting in dense contrast in the superior vena cava and aorta but less opacified blood in the pulmonary arteries.[38] Performance of CTPA in middle inspiratory or expiratory phase, instead of at maximal inspiration, can help reduce the incidence of transient interruption of contrast. Patients can be instructed to avoid deep inspiration or expiration and simply hold their breath.[39] Alternatively, patients can take a breath in, a breath out, and then suspend breathing.[40]

To obtain optimal contrast opacification of the pulmonary arteries, high-contrast injection rates of 3 to 4 mL/s are often used. However, in patients with poor peripheral venous access, low flow rates of 2.0 or 2.5 mL/s can be used with diagnostic results in most patients.[41] The total volume of contrast administered should be tailored to the patient's body habitus and renal function.[38] Objectively, density of greater than or equal to 200 Hounsfield units in the pulmonary trunk is considered diagnostic for the evaluation of PE.[41,42]

Triple-rule-out protocols with electrocardiography-gating are performed at some institutions for patients with acute chest pain to simultaneously evaluate for PE, acute coronary syndrome, and acute aortic syndrome (Fig. 50.14).[43,44]

Gadolinium-based contrast agents have been used as an alternative to iodinated contrast agents for patients with relative or absolute contraindications to iodinated contrast agents in whom contrast-enhanced CT of the chest was the examination of choice. With use of a 16–detector-row system, 92% (55 of 60) of gadolinium-enhanced CT angiographic examinations yielded good to excellent vascular enhancement and enabled radiologists to provide clinicians with diagnostic information, including successful detection of acute PE (Fig. 50.15).[45]

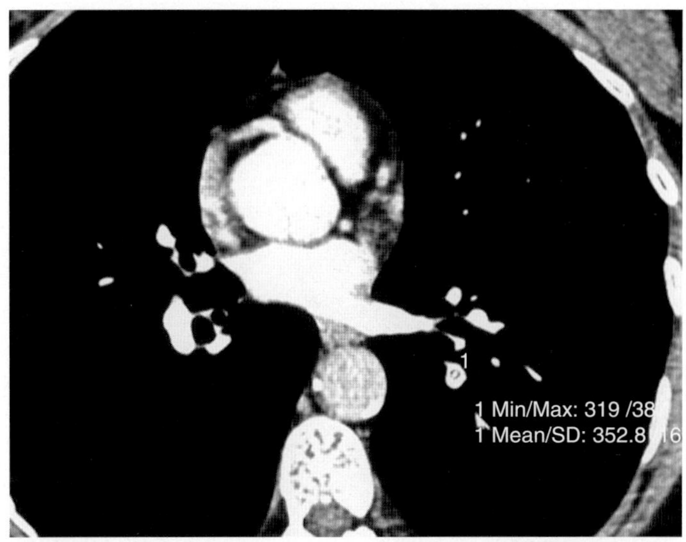

Fig. 50.15 Computed tomography (CT) pulmonary angiography obtained after administration of gadolinium in a patient thought to have acute pulmonary embolism (PE) with a history of severe allergic reaction to iodinated contrast media. Axial CT scan obtained at the level of the lower lobes illustrates the excellent degree of arterial enhancement within the pulmonary arteries, measured at 352 Hounsfield units in the posterobasal segmental artery of the left lower lobe. Findings were negative for acute PE.

Clinical Validity of a Negative Computed Tomography Pulmonary Angiography

In a meta-analysis of 15 studies that used contrast-enhanced chest CT to rule out the diagnosis of acute PE in a total of 3500 patients with a minimum of 3-month follow-up, Quiroz and colleagues[46] concluded that the clinical validity of using a CT scan to rule out PE is similar to that reported for conventional pulmonary angiography—namely, 1% to 2.8% for CT (including single-slice CT, MDCT, and electron-beam CT) versus 1.1% to 2.9% for conventional pulmonary angiography. The majority of studies that were included in this meta-analysis used conventional single-slice CT, which may have missed the diagnosis of peripheral PE. The low incidence of venous thromboembolic events during follow-up across all these studies suggests that even if peripheral pulmonary emboli were missed and subsequently not treated on the basis of a normal CT scan, the patient outcome was not adversely affected. According to the guidelines of the British Thoracic Society, no further examination or treatment is needed for patients with a high-quality normal CT angiogram performed on a multidetector scanner.[47] A recent study has also shown that the incidence of PE is only 2.5% on ventilation and perfusion (VQ) imaging performed after suboptimal CTPAs, likely because of the ability of most suboptimal CTPAs to exclude central PE.[48]

MAGNETIC RESONANCE IMAGING

Magnetic resonance imaging (MRI) also allows direct and noninvasive demonstration of acute PE. It has the advantage of not requiring radiation. It can be used in patients with severe allergic reactions to iodinated contrast. Its diagnostic accuracy has been shown to be very high for MR angiography,[49] MR perfusion,[50] real-time MRI,[51] and combined protocols (Fig. 50.16).

However, MRI suffers from several disadvantages in the diagnostic workup of PE. First, and despite remarkable results in the detection of acute PE with contrast-enhanced MR angiography, the overall image quality is inferior to that achievable on CT angiography because of a lower spatial resolution, motion artifacts, and overlapping pulmonary veins. Second, MRI is suboptimal for the evaluation of pulmonary parenchyma and hence limited in ability to provide differential diagnosis of acute PE. Third, the availability of MRI units is lower than that of CT scanners, especially in the context of emergency departments. Last, an MRI scanner is generally a hostile environment for patients who are clinically unstable, particularly if they need life-support equipment, which frequently is incompatible with a highly magnetized field.

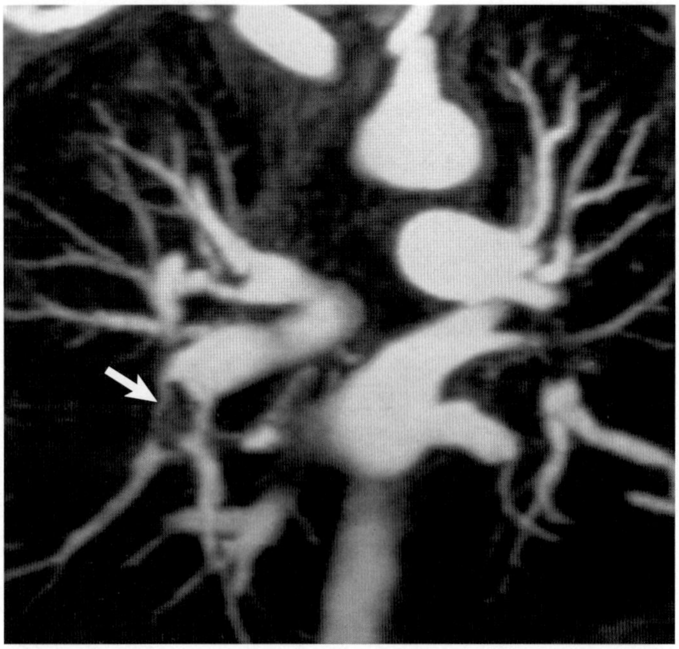

Fig. 50.16 MRI of acute pulmonary thromboembolism. Coronal MRI shows filling defect *(arrow)* in the right interlobar pulmonary artery. *(Case courtesy Dr. Jaime Fdez-Cuadrado, Hospital La Paz, Madrid, Spain. From* Müller NL, Fraser RS, Colman NC, Paré PD. Radiologic Diagnosis of Diseases of the Chest. *Philadelphia: WB Saunders; 2001.)*

ULTRASONOGRAPHY

Apart from the detection of DVT with venous duplex sonography, which is beyond the scope of this chapter, thoracic ultrasonography for diagnosis of acute PE is usually limited to the bedside management of massive acute PE. An original approach was reported by Mathis and colleagues,[52] who investigated the use of thoracic ultrasonography to diagnose peripheral PE on the basis of the identification of triangular or rounded subpleural parenchymal lesions. In the absence of CTPA, they found that thoracic ultrasonography could be a suitable tool to demonstrate PE at the bedside and in the emergency setting. Transthoracic echocardiography, used to detect evidence of right heart strain, such as dilated right ventricle, abnormal septal motion and tricuspid regurgitation, has been shown to have low sensitivity but relatively high specificity and is used at the bedside in critical care settings in patients who are not able to receive a CTPA.[53]

NUCLEAR MEDICINE

Before the advent of CTPA, VQ scintigraphy was widely used in the evaluation of patients thought to have acute PE. Its use has decreased considerably with the increased availability and improved diagnostic accuracy of MDCT. The diagnosis of acute PE on scintigraphy is based on the identification of VQ mismatch —that is, the presence of ventilation in the absence of perfusion distal to the obstructing emboli (Fig. 50.17; see Fig. 50.6). The findings are classified into five categories—normal, near-normal, low probability, intermediate probability, and high probability— on the basis of the probability of embolism, known as the PIOPED I criteria (Prospective Investigative Study of Acute Pulmonary Embolism Diagnosis I).

Because the original PIOPED I criteria led to a large proportion of nondiagnostic scans, several amendments have been made, enabling a decrease in the number of intermediate interpretations and a more accurate assessment of angiographically proven cases of acute PE.[54,55] The modified PIOPED II criteria classify findings as "PE present" (high probability), "PE absent" (very low probability or normal), or "nondiagnostic" (intermediate or low probability). These changes allow VQ scans to be more definitive in a majority of patients.[56] Another way of improving the diagnostic accuracy of scintigraphy is to eliminate the ventilation scan, focusing on the perfusion scan.[57,58] When the chest radiograph is normal, this approach can reduce both cost and radiation dose.[59] VQ scan is the preferred imaging modality for evaluation of suspected PE in pregnancy for patients with normal chest radiograph and in the absence of leg symptoms. VQ scan allows lower radiation dose to the maternal breast and lung tissue compared with CTPA, and the radiation dose to the fetus is thought to be low for both imaging modalities.[60]

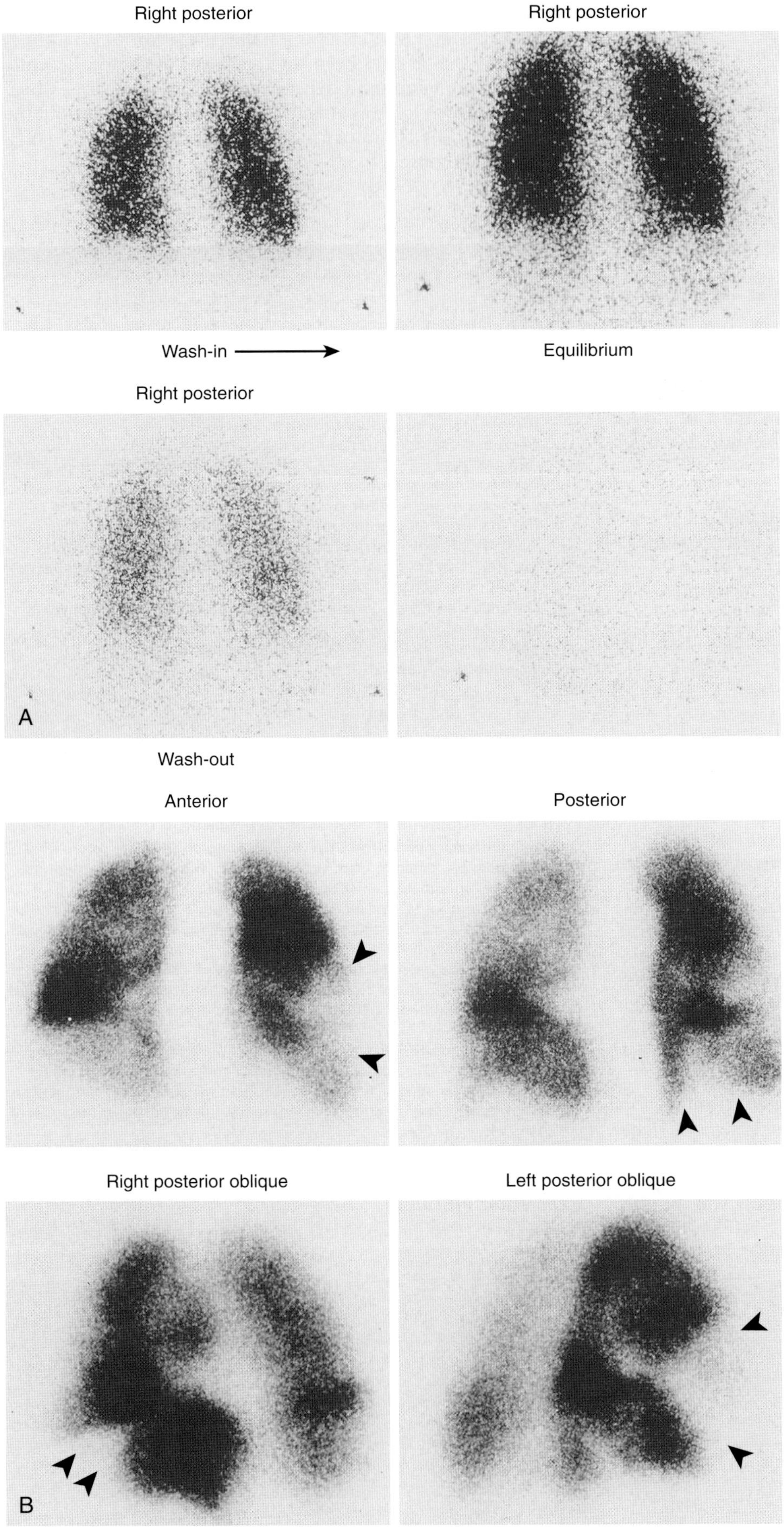

Fig. 50.17 Ventilation-perfusion scintigraphy in acute pulmonary embolism. (A) Xenon-133 posterior inhalation lung scan shows normal ventilation during the wash-in, equilibrium, and wash-out phases. (B) Corresponding Technetium-99m labeled macroaggregated albumin perfusion lung scans in anterior, posterior, and right and left posterior oblique projections identify multiple large segmental filling defects throughout both lungs *(arrowheads)*. These findings, in concert with the ventilation study, are virtually diagnostic (high probability) of pulmonary thromboembolism. *(From Müller NL, Fraser RS, Colman NC, Paré PD.* Radiologic Diagnosis of Diseases of the Chest. *Philadelphia: WB Saunders; 2001.)*

Differential Diagnosis

PITFALLS IN THE INTERPRETATION OF ENDOLUMINAL FILLING DEFECTS ON COMPUTED TOMOGRAPHY PULMONARY ANGIOGRAPHY

- Technically related pitfalls
  - Cardiac and respiratory motion artifacts
  - Suboptimal opacification of pulmonary arteries
  - Partial volume averaging
- Anatomically related pitfalls
  - Juxtahilar lymph nodes
  - Misidentification of a pulmonary vein as a pulmonary artery
  - Mucus-filled bronchi
- Patient-related pitfalls
  - Unilateral increase in pulmonary vascular resistance: large pleural effusion; extensive consolidation, hyperinflation, hypoxic vasoconstriction, conditions with elevated venous pressure
  - Left-to-right shunt
  - Right-to-left shunt (patent foramen ovale)
  - Right-sided heart failure and pulmonary hypertension
- Nonthrombotic emboli
  - Tumoral: pulmonary artery sarcoma, right heart myxoma, tumor emboli
  - Foreign body: bullet, catheter fragment, cement used for orthopedic procedures or vertebroplasty
- In situ thrombosis
  - Pulmonary hypertension
  - Postsurgical (lobectomy, pneumonectomy)
  - Pulmonary artery stenosis
  - Chronic atelectasis

Synopsis of Treatment Options

Treatment of acute PE is dependent on mortality risks. Patients with massive PE, with an estimated 30-day PE-related mortality rate of greater than 15%, should be treated with systemic thrombolysis in the absence of contraindications. Surgical and catheter-directed pulmonary embolectomy or catheter-directed thrombolysis can be considered in patients with massive PE who failed to respond to thrombolytic therapy during the first hour or in whom thrombolytic therapy is contraindicated.

Hemodynamically stable patients are further stratified for close monitoring versus outpatient treatment using signs of right heart dysfunction on CT or echocardiogram; laboratory biomarkers, such as brain-type natriuretic peptides and troponin levels; and clinical criteria, such as the Hestia decision rule or the Pulmonary Embolism Severity Index (PESI). Low-molecular-weight heparin (LMWH) and parallel initiation of vitamin K antagonists (VKAs) has been the treatment of choice. Recently introduced nonvitamin K–dependent oral anticoagulants, which have been shown to be as effective as LMWH/VKAs without the need for frequent laboratory monitoring and preceding LMWH, are increasingly used.[61]

KEY POINTS

- With the advent of multidetector CT technologies resulting in short image-acquisition time and improved image quality, CT pulmonary angiography (CTPA), with high sensitivity and specificity, has become the imaging modality of choice in the evaluation of suspected pulmonary embolism (PE).
- The use of clinical decision rule and serum D-dimer level in the evaluation of patients with suspected PE can help decrease use and improve positive yield of CTPA.
- CTPA allows direct visualization of PE as endoluminal filling defects within pulmonary artery branches.
- CT signs of right heart dysfunction are an important factor in the management of hemodynamically stable patients with acute PE. Right ventricular to left ventricular–diameter ratio greater than or equal to 1 on axial CT images has been shown to be a predictor of poor outcome.
- Diagnosis of PE on ventilation-perfusion (VQ) scintigraphy scanning relies on the presence of mismatched VQ defects. The VQ scan is the test of choice in pregnant women suspected of having PE.

SUGGESTED READINGS

Albrecht MH, Bickford MW, Nance JW Jr, Zhang L, De Cecco CN, Wichmann JL, Vogl TJ, Schoepf UJ. State-of-the-art pulmonary CT angiography for acute pulmonary embolism. *AJR Am J Roentgenol.* 2017;208(3):495–504.

Konstantinides SV, Barco S, Lankeit M, Meyer G. Management of pulmonary embolism: an update. *J Am Coll Cardiol.* 2016;67(8):976–990.

Metter D, Tulchinsky M, Freeman LM. Current status of ventilation-perfusion scintigraphy for suspected pulmonary embolism. *AJR Am J Roentgenol.* 2017;208(3):489–494.

Meyer M, Haubenreisser H, Sudarski S, Doesch C, Ong MM, Borggrefe M, Schoenberg SO, Henzler T. Where do we stand? Functional imaging in acute and chronic pulmonary embolism with state-of-the-art CT. *Eur J Radiol.* 2015;84(12):2432–2437.

Ruggiero A, Screaton NJ. Imaging of acute and chronic thromboembolic disease: state of the art. *Clin Radiol.* 2017;72(5):375–388.

van der Hulle T, Dronkers CE, Klok FA, Huisman MV. Recent developments in the diagnosis and treatment of pulmonary embolism. *J Intern Med.* 2016;279(1):16–29.

The full reference list for this chapter is available at ExpertConsult.com.

51 Chronic Pulmonary Thromboembolism*

BRENT P. LITTLE

Etiology

Chronic pulmonary thromboembolism is an uncommon entity resulting from an incomplete resolution of thrombi, leading to complex restructuring processes within pulmonary arteries. Extensive clinical experience from the literature suggests that failure of thromboembolic resolution after a single embolic event or after recurrent thromboembolic events represents the predisposing condition in most patients with the disease. Although the clinical signs and symptoms are nonspecific, a confident diagnosis can usually be made on computed tomography angiography (CTA).

Prevalence and Epidemiology

It has been estimated that in the United States approximately 600,000 episodes of pulmonary embolism occur each year. Although the natural history of adequately treated acute pulmonary embolism is not well characterized, data based predominantly on clinical follow-up suggest that thromboembolic resolution occurs in the overwhelming majority of patients who experience an acute embolic event (Fig. 51.1). Evolution toward chronic thromboembolic disease has been estimated to range between 2% and 18% of patients when serial perfusion scans have been performed,[1–3] and it has been reported in 13% of patients with CT follow-up (Fig. 51.2).[4] The basis for this alternative natural history has not been clearly established. Despite extensive investigation the only identifiable thrombotic predisposition has been the presence of lupus anticoagulant in approximately 10% of patients. Less than 1% of patients have had deficiencies of antithrombin III, protein C, or protein S. In a subset of patients, long-standing increase in pulmonary artery pressure resulting from the chronic obstruction of the pulmonary arterial bed leads to chronic thromboembolic pulmonary hypertension, and can be complicated by cor pulmonale and right-sided heart failure. At this stage there is a poor prognosis of the disease with a 5-year survival rate of only 30%.

Clinical Presentation

The spectrum of symptoms associated with chronic pulmonary thromboembolism depends on the percentage of the pulmonary arterial bed chronically obstructed and the development of pulmonary hypertension. In the absence of pulmonary hypertension the symptoms are nonspecific, including progressive dyspnea and exercise intolerance. A diagnostic delay, particularly in the absence of an acute history of venous thromboembolism, is common. The mean time from onset of symptoms to diagnosis usually exceeds 3 years.

The symptomatic history has been well described.[5] After a documented venous thromboembolic event, symptomatic recovery occurs, although often not to a level equivalent to that before the acute event. In patients without a documented acute thromboembolic event, several data confirm the often subtle clinical manifestations of a venous thromboembolic event and the frequency with which misdiagnosis occurs.[6] After a period of clinical stability that may range from months to years, increasing exertional dyspnea, hypoxemia, and right ventricular dysfunction ultimately ensue.

Chronic thromboembolic pulmonary hypertension (CTEPH) can develop in up to 3.8% of patients after an acute episode and in up to 10% of patients with recurrent pulmonary embolism. CTEPH is classified as group IV pulmonary hypertension according to the Fifth World Symposium of Pulmonary Hypertension (Nice, France, 2013). The diagnosis can be made in the setting of elevated pulmonary artery pressure (mean pressure ≥25 mm Hg, with wedge pressure ≤15 mm Hg), with evidence of chronic emboli as assessed by a ventilation-perfusion (VQ) scan or cross-sectional imaging, such as CT or magnetic resonance imaging (MRI).[7]

Pathophysiology

ANATOMY

Fresh thrombus may fragment and disperse into smaller pulmonary arteries, but within a few days, thrombotic emboli undergo organization and become firmly adherent to the vessel wall. In 4 to 6 weeks they are converted into fibrous tissue, often with recanalization. Some emboli may disappear, and it is presumed that they are destroyed by plasmin. Thin fibrous bands stretching across the lumen of major pulmonary arteries are sometimes the only evidence of previous thromboembolism. More often, the lumen of smaller arteries is divided into multiple channels by the usual process of recanalization.[8] A mixed pattern of vascular stenosis, intraluminal webs, and abnormal tapering of vessel diameter can be seen.[9] As a consequence of the presence of pulmonary hypertension, a secondary, small-vessel arteriopathy, also described as plexogenic arteriopathy, may develop.[10]

PATHOLOGY

Early resolution of pulmonary vascular obstruction occurs by two mechanisms: mechanical changes in thrombus location and endogenous thrombolysis. After these early events, organization and recanalization further alleviate the degree of pulmonary vascular obstruction.[11] However, significant organized residual disease may persist, and therefore abnormal pulmonary hemodynamics at rest or with exercise may be present in patients whose perfusion scans (i.e., the most frequent means of follow-up) return to normal.[12]

---

*The editors and the publisher would like to thank Drs. Martine Remy-Jardin and Jacques Remy for contributing material on this topic to the prior edition of this work. It has served as the foundation for the current chapter.

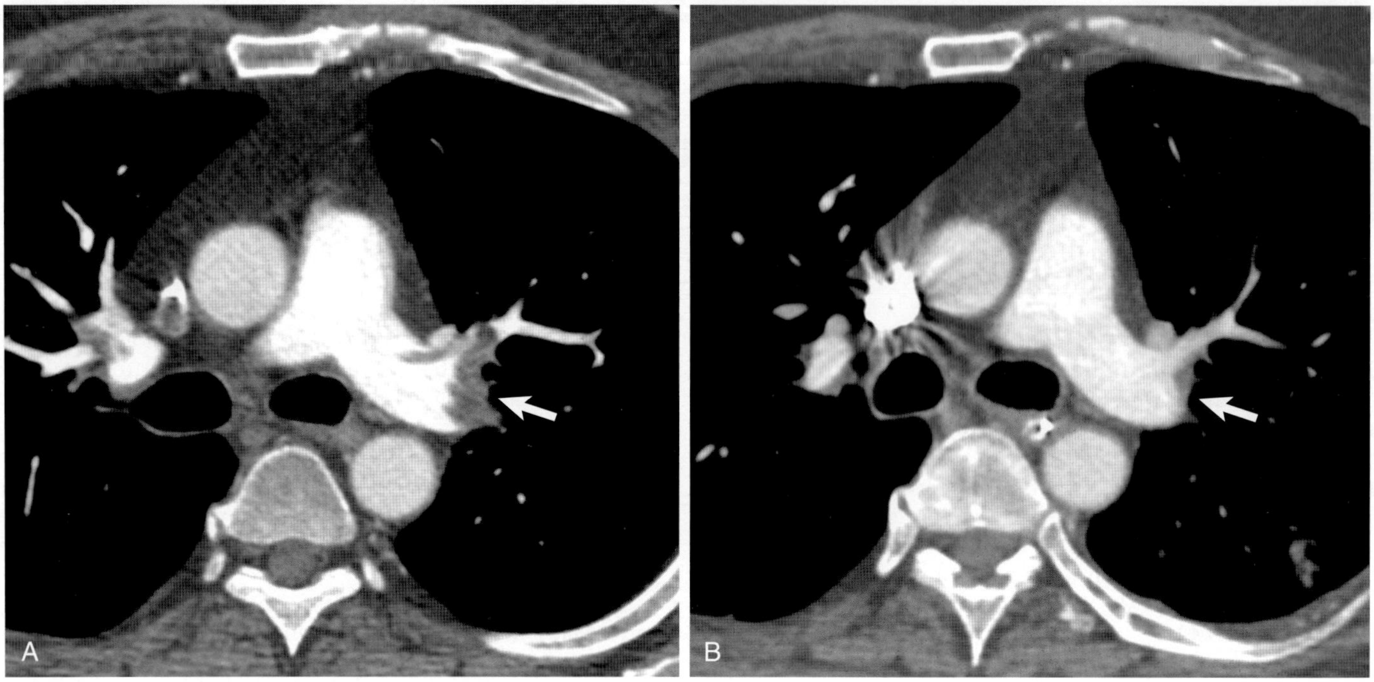

Fig. 51.1 Natural history of acute pulmonary embolism: complete resolution. (A) Axial CT scan shows acute pulmonary emboli in the left main and left upper lobe anterior segmental pulmonary arteries *(arrow)*. Additional right upper lobe pulmonary artery embolism is also noted. (B) Axial CT scan obtained 2 months later, after adequate anticoagulant treatment, shows complete resolution of the endoluminal clot *(arrow)*.

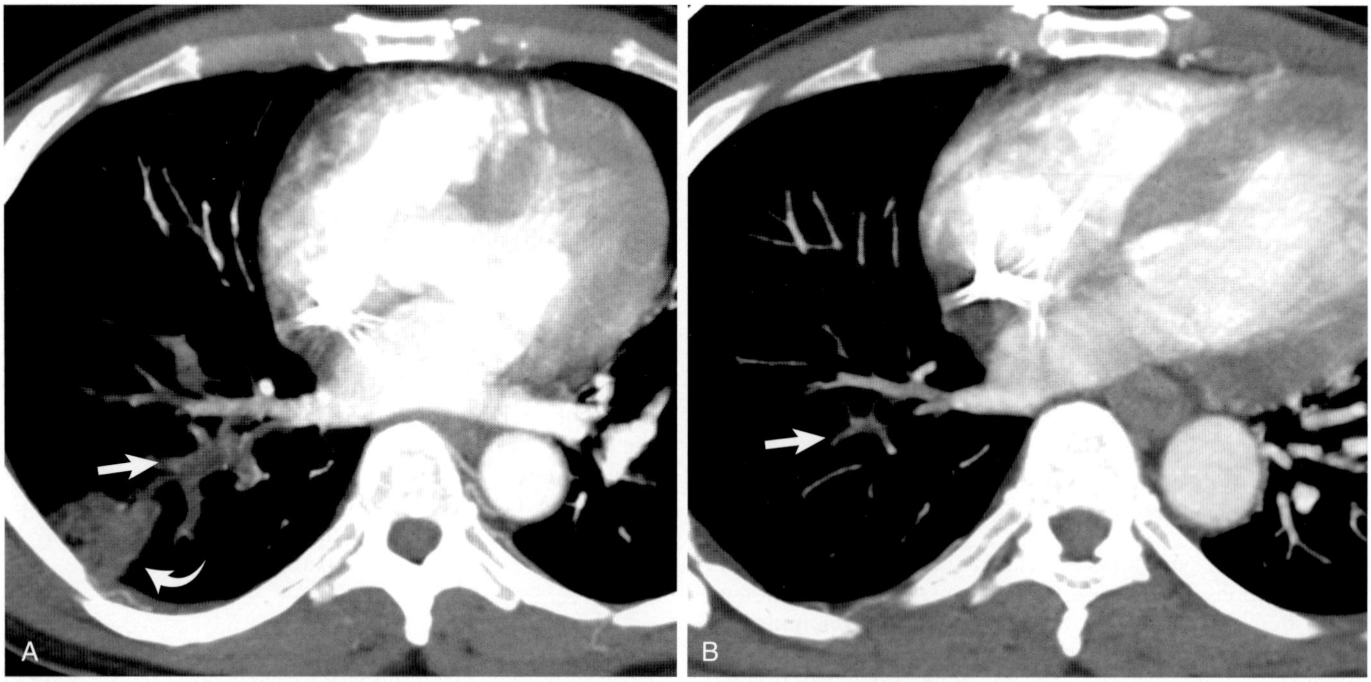

Fig. 51.2 Natural history of acute pulmonary embolism: evolution to chronic pulmonary embolism. (A) Axial CT scan shows acute right lower lobe pulmonary emboli *(straight arrow)*, with a pulmonary infarct *(curved arrow)*. (B) CT image obtained 1 year later, after adequate anticoagulation, shows chronic emboli in the same distribution, with a marked decrease in diameter of the right lower lobe pulmonary arteries *(arrow)*.

Chronic pulmonary thromboembolism may show a silent clinical period lasting months or years, followed by clinical deterioration that parallels the loss of right ventricular functional capacity. This decline may be due to recurrent thromboembolism, in situ pulmonary artery thrombosis, and a hypertensive pulmonary arteriopathy similar to that encountered in patients with pulmonary hypertension from other causes.[13,14]

LUNG FUNCTION

The results of spirometry, often performed as part of the evaluation of the patient's dyspnea, are usually within normal limits.[15] Approximately 20% of patients show mild to moderate restriction, to a large extent caused by parenchymal scarring related to prior infarcts. A reduction in single-breath diffusing capacity for carbon monoxide (DLCO) can be observed, ranging from mild to severe; a normal value does not exclude the diagnosis.

Manifestations of the Disease

RADIOGRAPHY

Chest radiography may be normal or may demonstrate findings of pulmonary hypertension. Asymmetry in size of the central pulmonary arteries can be seen in conjunction with areas of relative hypoperfusion and hyperperfusion. The asymmetry of the central pulmonary arteries may be so dramatic that it may suggest pulmonary artery agenesis, whereas areas of increased perfusion may suggest consolidation with pneumonia or interstitial lung disease. Chest radiography may also reveal parenchymal or pleural scars, consistent with prior infarcts, and enlargement of the right ventricle in the advanced forms of the disease.

COMPUTED TOMOGRAPHY

Cardiovascular Signs of Chronic Pulmonary Thromboembolism

Vascular Signs. The CT features of chronic pulmonary thromboembolism are similar to those described with conventional angiography (Box 51.1). Chronic emboli are usually identified on the basis of at least two of the following features: emboli eccentric and contiguous with the vessel wall, recanalization within an area of arterial hypoattenuation, arterial stenosis or web, reduction of more than 50% of the overall arterial diameter, or complete occlusion of a stenosed artery (Figs. 51.3 to 51.7). A recanalized thrombus perpendicular to the artery wall generates webs or bands and focal stenoses with mild poststenotic dilatation

BOX 51.1 VASCULAR COMPUTED TOMOGRAPHIC FEATURES SUGGESTIVE OF CHRONIC THROMBOEMBOLISM

- Organized embolic material
  - Partial or complete filling defects
  - Emboli eccentric and contiguous with the vessel wall
  - Irregular contours of the intimal surface
- Retracted embolic material
  - Complete filling defects at the level of stenosed pulmonary arteries
  - Abrupt cutoffs and narrowing
- Recanalized embolic material
  - Webs, bands, or stenoses with poststenotic dilatation
- Calcified embolic material
  - Calcifications within filling defects

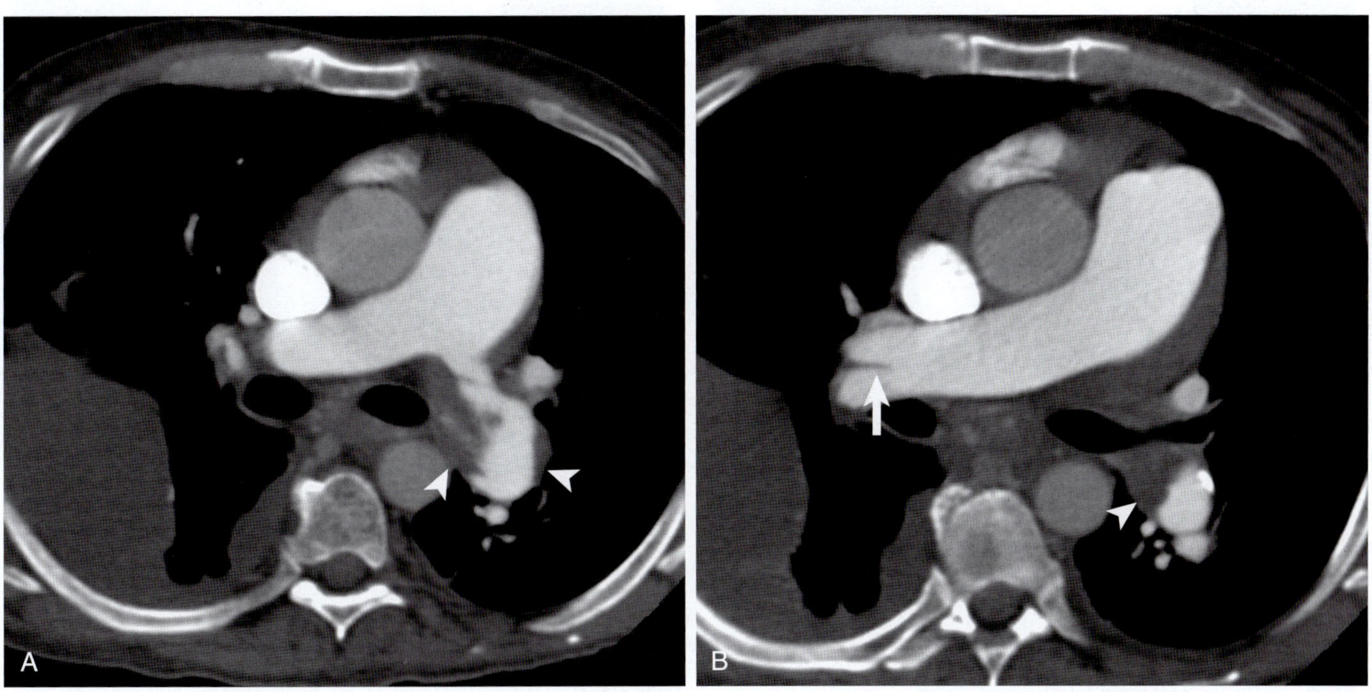

Fig. 51.3 CT angiographic signs of chronic thromboembolic disease: chronic mural clot. (A) and (B) Axial CT scans show mural defects involving the outer wall of the left main and left interlobar pulmonary arteries *(arrowheads)*. Note linear web in the distal right pulmonary artery *(arrow)*. A dilated pulmonary trunk indicates pulmonary hypertension.

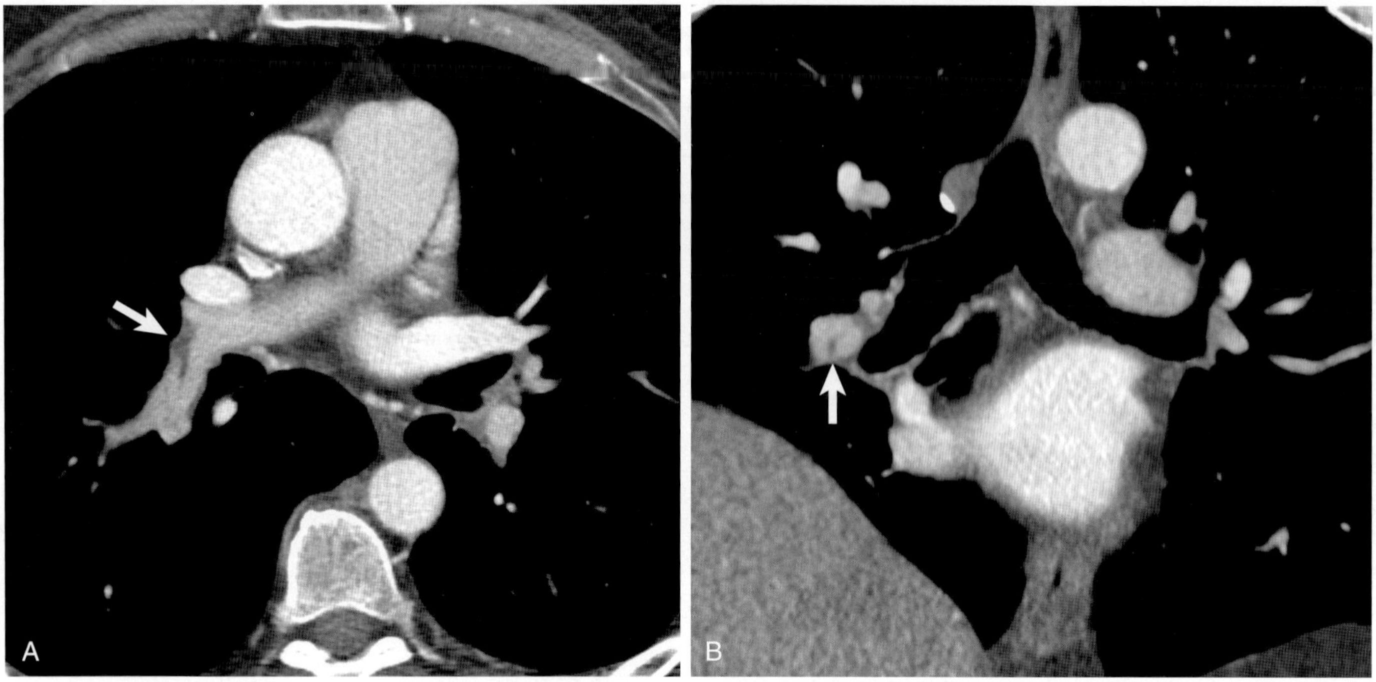

Fig. 51.4 CT angiographic signs of chronic thromboembolic disease: eccentric filling defect and incomplete recanalization resulting in an intraluminal web. (A) Axial CT scan shows an eccentric filling defect *(arrow)* within the right interlobar pulmonary artery. (B) Coronal CT image shows a linear web *(arrow)* in a right lower lobe pulmonary artery.

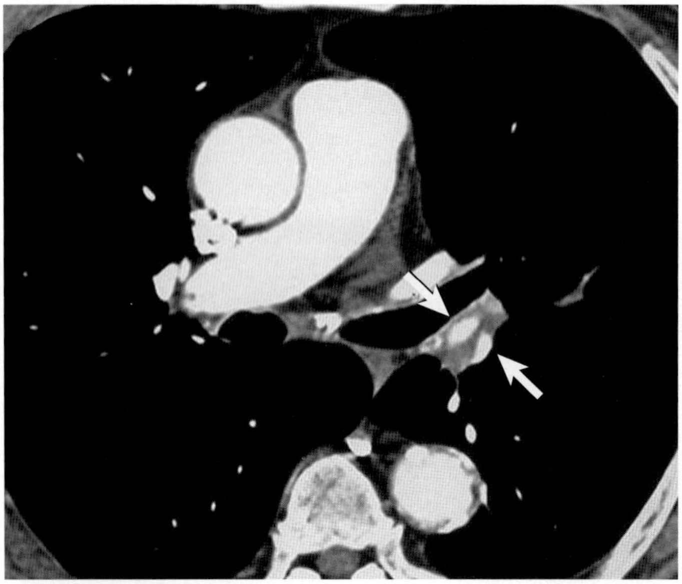

Fig. 51.5 CT angiographic signs of chronic thromboembolic disease: recanalized embolic material. Axial CT scan obtained at the level of the left upper lobe bronchus shows two circulating channels *(arrows)* within the left interlobar pulmonary artery, consistent with incomplete recanalization.

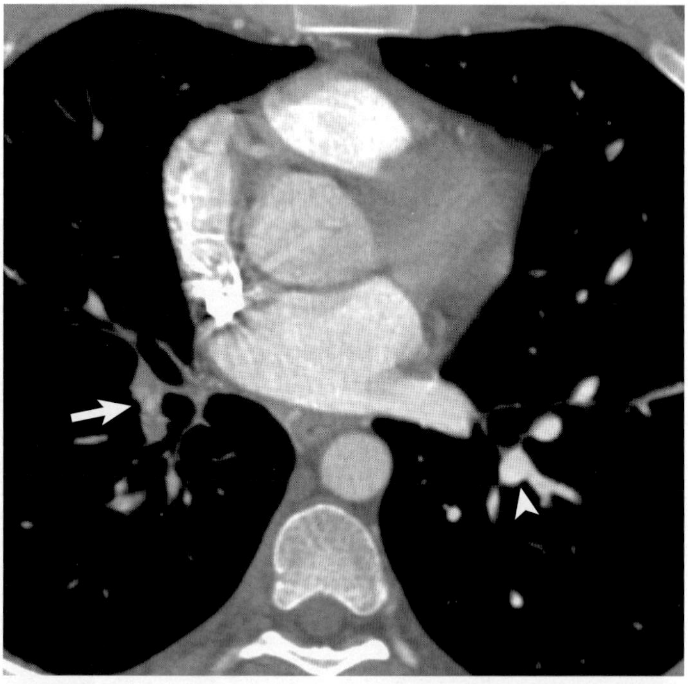

Fig. 51.6 CT angiographic signs of chronic thromboembolic disease: retraction of chronically obstructed pulmonary arteries. Axial CT scan obtained at the level of the lower lobes shows complete obstruction and retraction of the right lower lobe pulmonary artery *(arrow)* compared with the normally perfused left lower lobe pulmonary artery *(arrowhead)*.

(Fig. 51.8). Parallel to the arterial lumen, the incomplete recanalization thickens the artery wall, sometimes resulting in an irregular contour of the intimal surface. Calcifications within chronic thrombi are seen in a small number of patients.

Most cases of chronic pulmonary thromboembolism have multiple and bilateral arterial abnormalities.

Because partial or complete filling defects of normal-sized pulmonary arteries can be seen in acute and chronic pulmonary embolism, these features alone should not lead to the assessment of chronic pulmonary embolism. A study has pointed out that the mean attenuation value of chronic clots is higher than that of acute filling defects, possibly because of enhancement of organizing thrombi.[16] The additional presence of dilated bronchial arteries (Fig. 51.9) is a strong argument in favor of chronic or

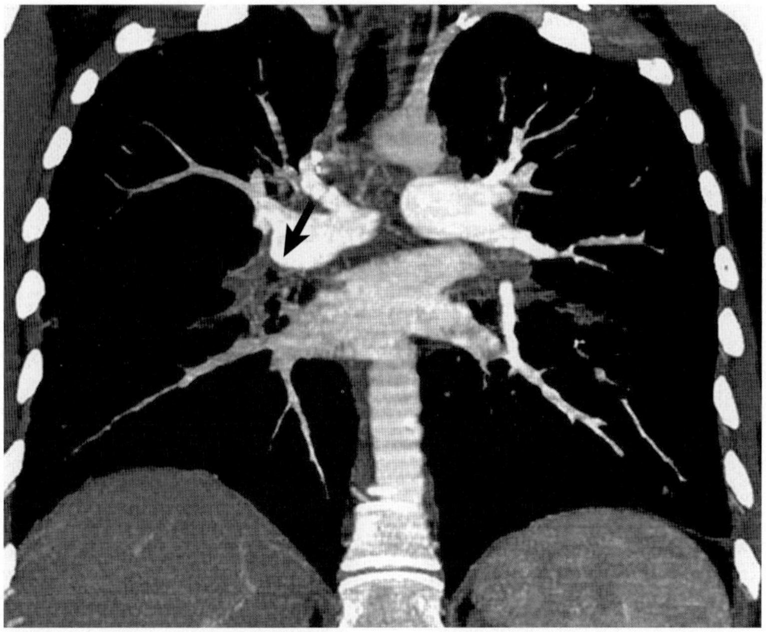

Fig. 51.7 CT angiographic signs of chronic thromboembolic disease: complete arterial occlusion. Coronal maximum-intensity projection image shows abrupt cutoff of the right interlobar pulmonary artery *(arrow)*.

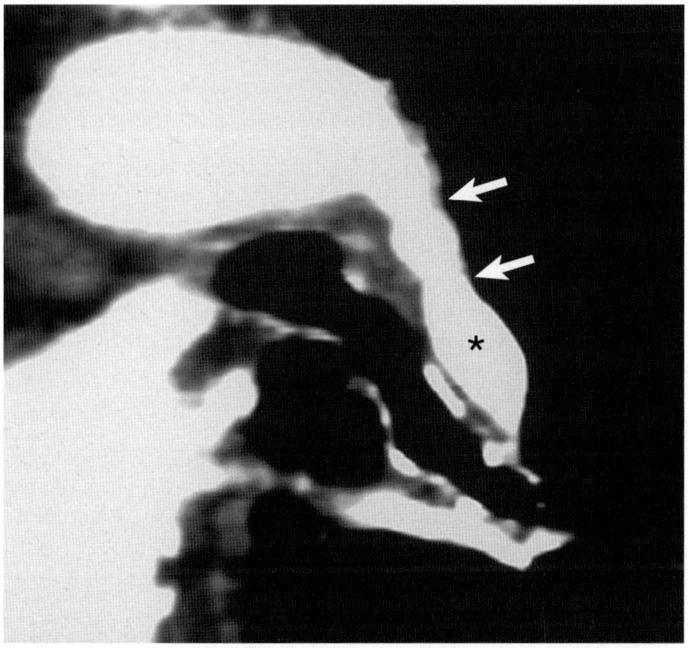

Fig. 51.8 CT angiographic signs of chronic thromboembolic disease: incomplete recanalization leading to focal stenoses. Multiplanar reformatted image of the left interlobar pulmonary artery shows two focal stenoses *(arrows)* with poststenotic dilatation *(star)*.

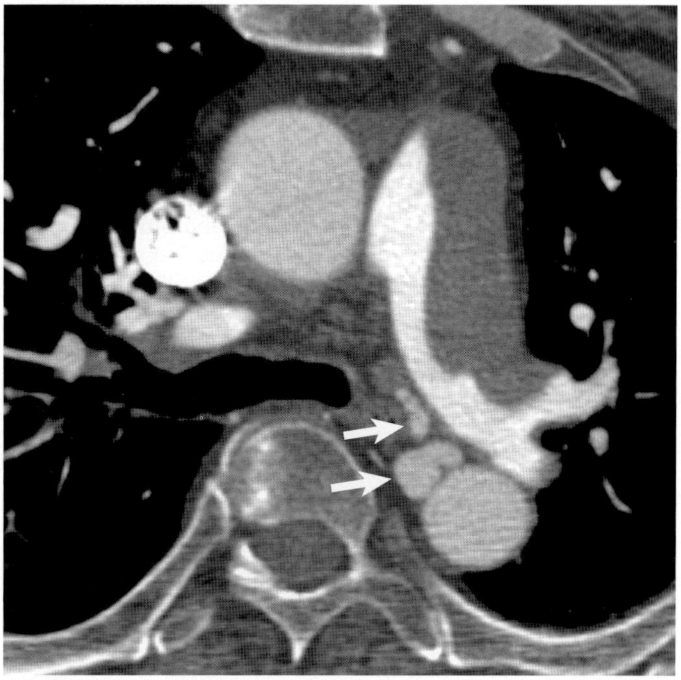

Fig. 51.9 Systemic collateral supply in a patient with chronic pulmonary thromboembolism. Axial CT scan shows a large eccentric filling defect in the pulmonary trunk and left pulmonary arteries. Dilated bronchial arteries *(arrows)* represent collateral circulation to the left lung. *(Reproduced with permission from Walker CM, Rosado-de-Christenson ML, Martínez-Jiménez S, et al. Bronchial arteries: anatomy, function, hypertrophy, and anomalies.* Radiographics. *2015;35:32–49.)*

recurrent pulmonary embolism instead of acute pulmonary embolism (50% vs. 7%).[17]

Pulmonary Hypertension. Pulmonary hypertension can be suspected on the basis of the dilatation of the main pulmonary artery (upper limit of normal, 2.8–3.2 cm). Its diameter can be compared with that of the ascending aorta and is suggestive of pulmonary hypertension when the ratio of the pulmonary artery diameter to the ascending aorta diameter is equal to or greater than 1. The diameters of the right and left pulmonary arteries are also increased (upper limit of normal, 1.6 cm).

Arterial dilatation and subsequent changes in lung attenuation on CT scans are unevenly distributed, an important criterion for differential diagnosis between chronic thromboembolic pulmonary hypertension and pulmonary hypertension of other causes. The marked variation in the diameter of segmental vessels reported by Bergin and colleagues[18] probably reflects the irregular distribution of emboli and subsequent sequelae within the lungs.

Systemic Collateral Supply. CTA allows assessment of the systemic collateral supply frequently seen in patients with chronic pulmonary thromboembolism.[19] Bronchial dilation in patients with chronic pulmonary thromboembolism resembles that seen in chronic bronchial disease. The CT findings of bronchial artery hypervascularization consist of abnormal dilatation of the proximal portions of bronchial arteries (i.e., a diameter >1.5 mm) and arterial tortuosity. In chronic pulmonary thromboembolism, the bronchial circulation is considerably increased because of the development of systemic to pulmonary arterial anastomoses. These anastomoses occur beyond the level of arterial obstruction and help maintain pulmonary blood flow (see Fig. 51.9).

Systemic perfusion of the peripheral pulmonary arterial bed accounts for areas of ground-glass opacity in patients with chronic pulmonary thromboembolic disease.[20] It is likely that subpleural septal lines sometimes identified in these patients reflect the presence of dilated bronchial arteries or other collaterals within interlobular septa. Development of bronchial hypervascularization is also responsible for recurrent or massive hemoptysis.[21] In this specific context, CTA of the bronchial arteries may help identify their ostia before a therapeutic embolization procedure.

Nonbronchial systemic arteries may also be involved in the collateral systemic supply in chronic thromboembolic disease. Their detection on CTA can help distinguish chronic thromboembolic from primary pulmonary hypertension.[22] This systemic to pulmonary collateral shunt has been estimated to represent approximately 30% of the systemic blood flow by studies using a contrast medium dilution method[23] and MRI.[24]

Cardiac Signs. Over time, right ventricular function deteriorates, even in the absence of recurrent embolism, presumably because of the development of hypertensive vascular abnormalities in the unobstructed pulmonary artery bed. The main signs suggestive of right ventricular dysfunction include right ventricular enlargement, reflux of contrast into dilated hepatic veins and the inferior vena cava, and straightening or leftward bowing of the interventricular septum (Fig. 51.10).[25]

Parenchymal Signs of Chronic Pulmonary Thromboembolism

Mosaic Attenuation. Mosaic attenuation can be recognized on CT scans as sharply demarcated regions of variable attenuation in the lung parenchyma that predominantly conform to the boundaries of secondary pulmonary lobules, without evidence of destruction or displacement of pulmonary vessels and with obvious disparity in the size of pulmonary vessels compared with areas of decreased attenuation (Fig. 51.11).[26,27] As demonstrated by Sherrick and colleagues,[27] the mosaic pattern of lung attenuation is more frequently seen in patients with pulmonary hypertension caused by cardiac or pulmonary disease.

Prior studies have shown that the areas of low attenuation within the lung parenchyma are due to hypoperfusion,[28] which explains the concurrent presence of fewer and smaller vessels within these areas. Regions of increased attenuation are due to the redistribution of blood flow in the patent arterial bed, which is subsequently dilated. A potential limitation in the sensitivity of CT scans for depicting areas of hypoperfusion may be collateral blood flow established from the bronchial circulation, which can be abundant in chronic thromboembolism.

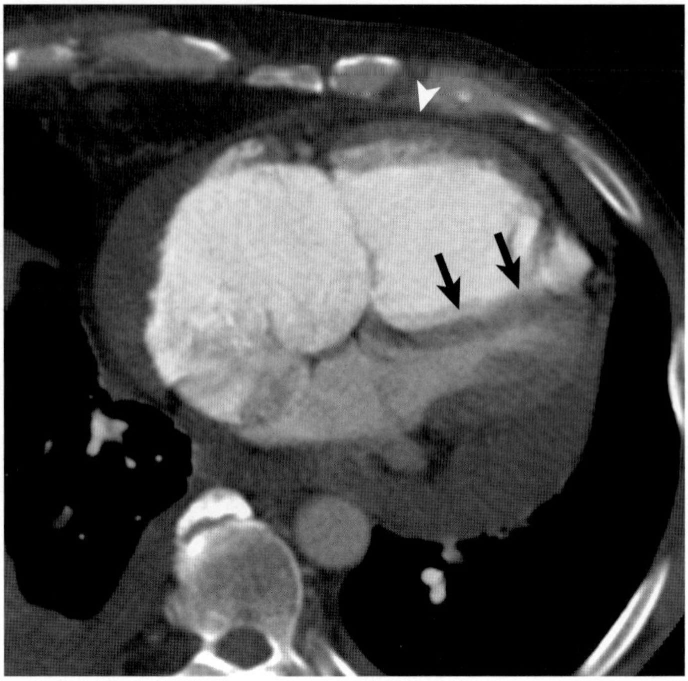

Fig. 51.10 CT features of right ventricular dysfunction in chronic pulmonary thromboembolic disease. Axial CT scan obtained at the level of the ventricles shows right ventricular enlargement and leftward displacement of the interventricular septum *(arrows)*. Note the abnormal thickening of the right ventricular myocardium *(arrowhead)*, suggestive of longstanding pulmonary hypertension.

Parenchymal Scarring. A common but nonspecific finding is the presence of wedge-shaped peripheral parenchymal areas of high attenuation with their tips pointing to the perihilar area, which are often multiple and favor the lower lung zones.[29] These areas do not enhance after administration of contrast material and likely represent fibrosis from pulmonary infarctions. They have been reported to occur in 10% to 15% of the thromboembolic events.

Miscellaneous Signs

In patients with chronic thromboembolic pulmonary hypertension, enlarged hilar lymph nodes can be seen, which is related to vascular transformation of the lymph node sinuses. An accurate knowledge of the position of hilar lymph nodes in relation to the major pulmonary arteries is essential to differentiate hilar lymphadenopathy from mural thrombi.[30]

The presence of bronchial dilatation in patients without clinical and functional evidence of chronic obstructive lung disease raises the hypothesis that chronic pulmonary thromboembolism may directly affect airways. In a study of 33 patients with chronic pulmonary thromboembolic disease, Remy-Jardin and colleagues[31] reported cylindric bronchial dilatation in 64% of patients (Fig. 51.12). The dilatation was observed at the level of segmental and subsegmental bronchi and was associated with severely stenosed arterial branches.

MAGNETIC RESONANCE IMAGING

The implementation of high-performance gradient systems decisively improved the quality of contrast-enhanced MR angiography. Hemodynamic parameters of the right ventricle

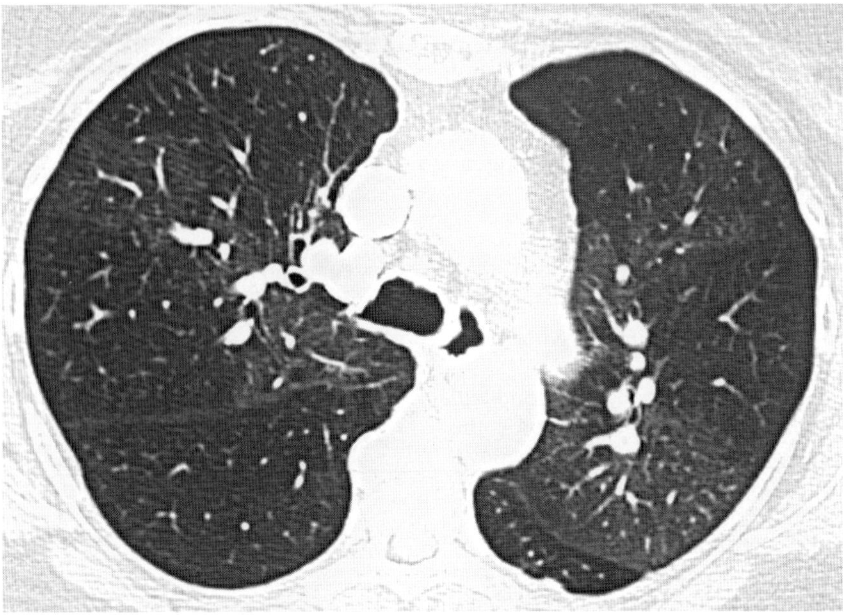

Fig. 51.11 Mosaic attenuation. Axial CT image obtained at the level of the carina shows enlarged vessels within areas of increased attenuation. Decreased vessel diameters and lower attenuation are found in the remaining portions of both lungs.

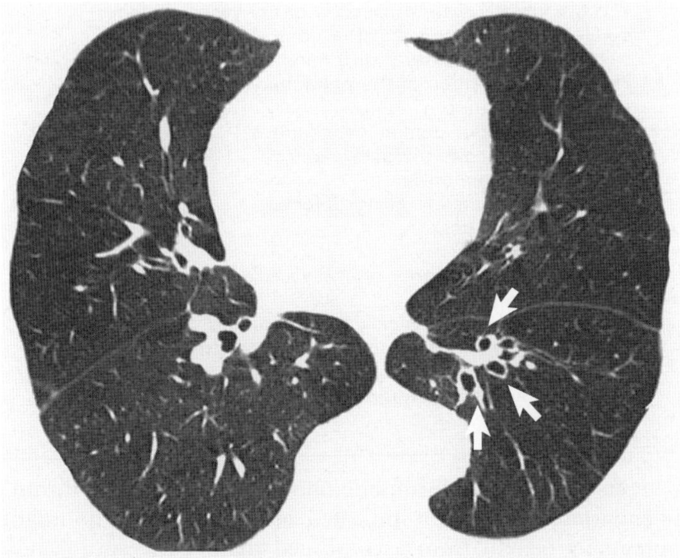

Fig. 51.12 Bronchial dilatation in chronic pulmonary thromboembolism. Axial CT image at the level of the right inferior pulmonary vein shows marked reduction in size of all pulmonary arterial branches in the left lower lobe consistent with chronic pulmonary thromboembolism. Note mild dilatation of the accompanying bronchi *(arrows).*

and blood flow velocities in the pulmonary arteries can also be assessed with MRI. This combination makes it a promising complementary tool to CT in the preoperative workup of chronic thromboembolic pulmonary hypertension.[32]

ULTRASONOGRAPHY

Transthoracic echocardiography is the initial method of choice for the diagnosis of pulmonary hypertension. Depending on the stage of the disease when echocardiography is performed, it may demonstrate variable degrees of right atrial and right ventricular enlargement, abnormal right ventricular systolic function, tricuspid regurgitation, leftward displacement of the interventricular septum, decreased left ventricular size, and abnormal left ventricular systolic and diastolic function.[33] Contrast echocardiography may also demonstrate a patent foramen ovale.

NUCLEAR MEDICINE

VQ scintigraphy remains an important modality for the evaluation of chronic thromboembolic disease. Compared with conventional catheter pulmonary angiography, VQ has a sensitivity, specificity, and accuracy of up to 100%, 93.7%, and 96.5%, respectively.[34] In chronic thromboembolic disease, at least one or, more commonly, several segmental or larger mismatched perfusion defects are present on scintigraphy.[35] The perfusion defects in chronic thromboembolic disease are often qualitatively different from those encountered in acute disease. Rather than demonstrating a complete absence of perfusion, the scan often is characterized by areas of diminished activity that are the consequence of different resistances and therefore different relative flows within the branches of the pulmonary vascular bed. VQ scan abnormalities often understate, in certain cases to a remarkable degree, the actual extent of vascular obstruction.

IMAGING ALGORITHMS

Diagnosis and Treatment of Chronic Thromboembolic Pulmonary Hypertension

Modalities of Diagnosis. VQ scintigraphy has a high sensitivity and specificity for detection of chronic thromboembolic disease and is still used as a first-line imaging modality at some institutions.[36,37] However, CTA has become a popular technique in the evaluation of suspected CTEPH and also has very high accuracy.[20,29,38] CTA has the advantage of depicting the location and morphology of emboli, which is important for treatment planning. CTA also accurately depicts peripheral emboli and completely occlusive clots. Reformatted images are mandatory for the detection of mild arterial stenoses and small concentric thrombi that are adherent to the arterial wall or located tangentially at the bottom or the roof of a vessel.

Selection of Surgical Candidates

The goals of pulmonary endarterectomy are to decrease the extent of pulmonary vascular obstruction, leading to a reduction in pulmonary artery pressure and therefore improved cardiac function.

After assessment of hemodynamic dysfunction, the second and most absolute criterion for potential surgical intervention is the accessibility of thrombi.[39] Present surgical techniques allow removal of chronic thrombi for which the proximal location extends to the main, lobar, and segmental arteries. Those that begin more distally are not accessible to endarterectomy, which explains why this determination is critical. Several studies have demonstrated that the surgical accessibility of chronic clots is accurately depicted by CTA, which can detect residual thromboembolic material incorporated concentrically in vessel walls.[20,29,38,40]

Differential Diagnosis

The differential diagnosis of vascular features of chronic pulmonary thromboembolism is listed in Box 51.2.

Synopsis of Treatment Options

Treatments for CTEPH include surgical therapy with thromboendarterectomy, balloon angioplasty of the pulmonary arteries, and medical therapy. Although thromboendarterectomy is the only potentially curative approach, patients with a peripheral distribution of emboli and extensive arterial remodeling may not benefit from surgery or angioplasty. Medical therapy consists of any of a variety of drugs that have effects on endothelial function, such as sildenafil, bosentan, epoprostenol, and the newer riociguat.[41]

At experienced centers, the performance of pulmonary thromboendarterectomy in patients with CTEPH can restore normal or nearly normal pulmonary hemodynamics, even in the presence of severe pulmonary hypertension or right-sided heart failure. The risk of recurrence is low because patients generally have preoperative placement of an inferior vena cava filter and are treated indefinitely with oral anticoagulants once surgery has been performed.[42] At centers with experience in performing thromboendarterectomy, a mortality rate of less than 5% has been quoted, which is a remarkable achievement when one considers the severity of cardiopulmonary disease and the hemodynamic fragility of these patients.

The major cause of death, other than reperfusion pulmonary edema, after pulmonary thromboendarterectomy is persistent postoperative pulmonary hypertension and right ventricular failure in patients for whom pulmonary thromboendarterectomy failed to result in a substantial improvement in pulmonary hemodynamics. This latter group includes patients whose disease involves a substantial component of distal, surgically inaccessible embolic obstruction and patients who have developed severe secondary pulmonary hypertensive changes in their distal pulmonary bed. The ability to identify the central and peripheral component of the disease could help identify that cohort of patients with chronic thromboembolic disease in whom thromboendarterectomy is not indicated, as well as those who might potentially benefit from a combined therapeutic approach—thromboendarterectomy to manage the central component of the disease followed by aggressive medical intervention to manage the distal component.[12] In patients with established distal arteriopathy deemed unsuitable for surgical intervention, medical treatment of pulmonary hypertension may offer an option by which to delay the progression of the disease.[43,44]

BOX 51.2 DIFFERENTIAL DIAGNOSIS OF VASCULAR FEATURES OF CHRONIC THROMBOEMBOLIC DISEASE

- Congenital pulmonary artery stenosis
  - Usually diagnosed in children (vs. diagnosis of chronic thromboembolic disease in adults)
  - Isolated proximal arterial stenoses versus proximal arterial stenosis associated with mural thrombi and mural and luminal calcifications without poststenotic dilatation in chronic thromboembolic disease
- Fibrosing mediastinitis
  - Partially calcified soft tissue causing narrowing of adjacent pulmonary arteries
  - Presence of mediastinal lymphadenopathy
  - Clinical context with history of histoplasmosis, tuberculosis, and other endemic granulomatous diseases. Sarcoidosis can occasionally cause a similar appearance.
- Takayasu arteritis
  - High-attenuation wall thickening
  - Delayed enhancement after contrast administration (after 1 or 2 minutes)
  - Smooth tapering of the pulmonary artery without intraluminal thrombus
  - Systemic arteritis (involvement of the aortic and supraaortic branch vessel walls)
- Neurofibromatosis
  - Severe intimal fibrosis
  - Responsible for multiple bilateral filling defects on CT scans
  - Specific clinical context
- Pulmonary artery sarcoma
  - Isolated proximal filling defects, sometimes bilateral
  - Mass usually extends outside of the vessel lumen
  - Delayed enhancement after contrast material administration (after 2 or 3 minutes)
- Proximal interruption of the pulmonary artery
  - Abrupt tapering of the pulmonary artery without endoluminal or periluminal changes
  - Occurs opposite the aortic arch
- Acute thromboembolism
  - Partial or complete filling defects
  - Smooth margins
  - Vessel expansion
  - Absence of any other typical vascular features of chronic thromboembolism
- Anatomically and technically related pitfalls
  - Partial volume effect on obliquely oriented vessels misinterpreted as abrupt narrowing
  - Hilar lymph nodes misinterpreted as mural thrombi

KEY POINTS

- The diagnosis of chronic pulmonary thromboembolism should be considered in all patients who have unexplained dyspnea.
- CT is helpful in determining whether there is surgically treatable disease by demonstrating chronic pulmonary thromboembolism in the main, lobar, and segmental arteries.
- Newer medications now allow treatment of chronic pulmonary thromboembolism involving the pulmonary arteries beyond the segmental level.

SUGGESTED READINGS

Fedullo PF, Auger WR, Kerr KM, Rubin LJ. Chronic thromboembolic pulmonary hypertension. *N Engl J Med*. 2001;345:1465–1472.

Jamieson SW, Kapelanski DP, Sakakibara N, et al. Pulmonary endarterectomy: experience and lessons learned in 1,500 cases. *Ann Thorac Surg*. 2003;76(5):1457–1462, discussion 1462–1464.

Renapurkar RD, Shrikanthan S, Heresi GA, et al. Imaging in chronic thromboembolic pulmonary hypertension. *J Thorac Imaging*. 2017;32(2):71–88.

Rich S, McLaughlin VV. Chronic thromboembolic pulmonary hypertension. *Clin Chest Med*. 2001;22:561–581.

The full reference list for this chapter is available at ExpertConsult.com.

52 Nonthrombotic Pulmonary Embolism*

CHRISTOPHER M. WALKER | JONATHAN H. CHUNG

Fat Embolism

Etiology, Prevalence, and Epidemiology

The term *fat embolism* refers to the presence of globules of free fat within the pulmonary vasculature. Fat embolism is common among trauma patients, especially those with long bone or pelvic fractures.[1] In the context of trauma, fat embolism is also common after extensive injury to subcutaneous fat, such as occurs in severe beatings or liposuction.[1] Fat embolism must be differentiated from fat embolism syndrome, which is defined by the presence of clinical signs and symptoms resulting from fat emboli.[1] The clinical manifestations of fat embolism syndrome consist of the triad of hypoxia (95%), confusion (60%), and petechial rash (33%). Unfortunately, the classic triad is rarely present, and the clinical manifestations of fat embolism syndrome range from an indolent course to fulminant respiratory failure.[2] The incidence of clinically significant disease in patients who have simple tibial or femoral fractures is generally believed to be about 1% to 3%.[3] In individuals who have more severe trauma, the incidence of clinically evident embolism is probably in the range of 10% to 20%.[3,4] Less common causes of fat embolism include severe beatings (embolism of subcutaneous fat), orthopedic procedures (e.g., intramedullary prosthesis insertion, arthroplasty), liposuction, severe pancreatitis, sickle cell disease, hematopoietic stem cell (bone marrow) transplantation and harvesting, and venous hyperalimentation.[1,2,5]

Clinical Presentation

The symptoms of fat embolism syndrome usually appear gradually; dyspnea, neurologic symptoms, fever, and petechial rash typically develop 12 to 36 hours after injury.[3,6] The delay in the development of clinical symptoms is presumably due to the time required for hydrolysis of neutral fat to toxic free fatty acids.[6] Cough, hemoptysis, and pleuritic chest pain occur occasionally. Signs include pyrexia, tachypnea, and tachycardia. Acute cor pulmonale with cardiac failure, cyanosis, and circulatory shock may occur.

Symptoms of systemic fat embolism are seen in up to 85% of patients who have pulmonary disease.[3] The symptoms are mainly related to the central nervous system and include confusion, restlessness, stupor, delirium, seizures, and coma. A petechial rash often develops 2 to 3 days after embolization, particularly along the anterior axillary folds and in the conjunctiva and retina.

Pathophysiology

Two pathogenetic mechanisms have been implicated in the development of pulmonary abnormalities after fat embolism.[7] The first is mechanical vascular obstruction, predominantly by fat globules themselves and possibly enhanced in some cases by platelet or red blood cell aggregates. A second potential mechanism involves conversion of neutral triglycerides, the form in which fat appears to be transported to the lungs, into free fatty acids by endothelial lipases. On histologic examination, the presence of fat within pulmonary arterioles and capillaries can be suspected on hematoxylin and eosin–stained sections when there are round to oval spaces, 20 to 40 μm in diameter, apparently compressing red blood cells to one side. Definitive histologic diagnosis requires the use of fat-soluble dyes on unfixed (frozen) tissue or other special techniques.[7]

Manifestations of the Disease

RADIOGRAPHY

The radiographic findings may be subtle and consist of bilateral hazy areas of increased opacity (ground-glass opacities) or patchy consolidation (Fig. 52.1). In more severe cases, widespread consolidation resembles the radiographic appearance of acute respiratory distress syndrome from any cause.[8] In one review of 22 patients with fat embolism syndrome, 2 had normal chest radiographs throughout hospitalization, and 20 developed pulmonary abnormalities.[9] In all cases the radiographic findings consisted of bilateral areas of consolidation consistent with diffuse pulmonary edema. The time to appearance of evident radiographic lung injury was within 24 hours of initial trauma in 50% of cases, between 24 and 48 hours in 20%, and more than 48 hours in 30%. Of the patients with abnormal radiographs, 10 of 20 (50%) had complete resolution of the edema pattern within 1 week of development of opacities and 30% within 1 to 4 weeks; 20% died without resolution of the radiographic findings.[9] Pleural effusions are typically absent.

COMPUTED TOMOGRAPHY

The computed tomography (CT) findings of fat embolism syndrome include bilateral patchy or diffuse ground-glass opacities, patchy or confluent areas of consolidation, and poorly defined centrilobular nodules measuring less than 10 mm in diameter (Fig. 52.2; see also Fig. 52.1).[10–13] CT may demonstrate parenchymal abnormalities in patients with normal chest radiographs. In an investigation of 9 patients with fat embolism syndrome who had normal radiographs, all were found to have abnormalities on high-resolution CT; 7 had ground-glass opacities, and 2 had small nodular opacities.[14] A CT review of 18 patients with fat embolism syndrome demonstrated consolidation with a dependent distribution (see Fig. 52.2) and

*The editors and the publisher would like to thank Drs. Nestor L. Müller and C. Isabela Silva Müller for contributing material on this topic to the prior edition of this work. It has served as the foundation for the current chapter.

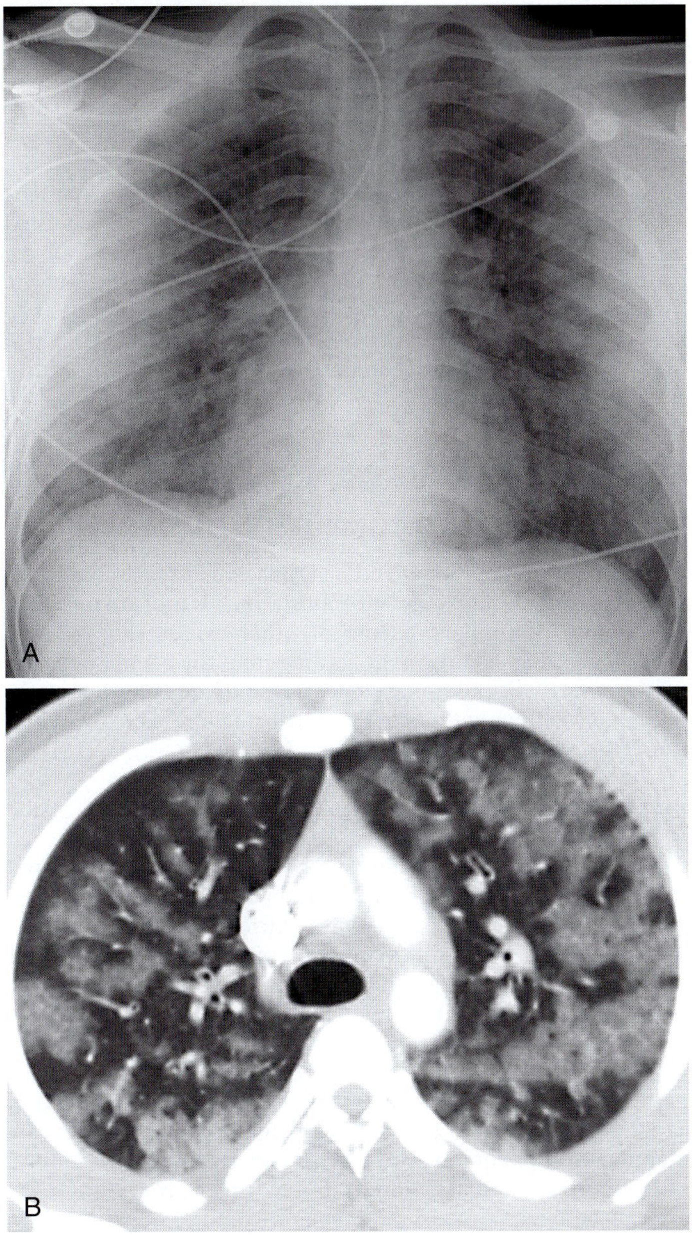

Fig. 52.1 Mild fat embolism after motor vehicle accident: radiographic and CT findings. (A) Anteroposterior chest radiograph 2 days after motor vehicle collision shows peripheral predominant consolidation. (B) Axial CT demonstrates patchy bilateral ground-glass opacities with well-defined lobular sparing.

patchy or peripheral predominant ground-glass opacities in the majority of patients. There was often lobular sparing with sharp margination between areas of involved and noninvolved lung that is thought to be secondary to variations in perfusion at time of embolization (see Fig. 52.1).[12] Less common manifestations included lobular ground-glass opacities or consolidation, smooth septal thickening, bronchial wall thickening, and a crazy paving pattern.[13] The degree and extent of consolidation and ground-glass opacities correlate well with disease severity.[12] Centrilobular and subpleural nodules are usually seen in association with ground-glass opacities but may be the predominant or only abnormality evident on high-resolution CT in patients with fat embolism.[14,15] The nodular opacities tend to be located in the centrilobular regions, along the interlobular septa, and along the interlobar fissures. Tree-in-bud

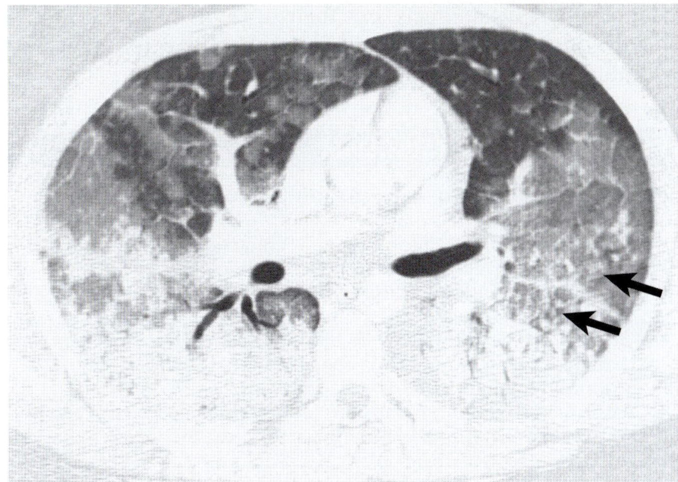

Fig. 52.2 Fat embolism after hip arthroplasty: CT findings. Axial CT demonstrates extensive bilateral consolidation, ground-glass opacities, lobular sparing, and a few poorly defined centrilobular nodules *(arrows)*. The consolidation and ground-glass opacities have a dependent distribution.

opacities are uncommon but have been reported. Intraarterial fat is usually not seen, but the pulmonary trunk is often dilated (size >29 mm). Rarely, there are reports of patients developing pulmonary fibrosis months after fat embolization.[12]

Differential Diagnosis

The time lapse between trauma and radiographic signs of fat embolism is usually 12 to 36 hours.[3,6,16] This delay differentiates fat embolism from traumatic lung contusion, in which the radiographic opacity invariably appears immediately after injury. In addition, although the lung contusion usually clears rapidly (in about 24 hours), resolution of fat embolism generally takes 7 to 10 days and occasionally as long as 4 weeks. Further differentiation lies in the extent of lung involvement; contusion seldom affects both lungs diffusely and symmetrically.

Several tests have been evaluated to identify fat embolism, but none of these is specific for the diagnosis.[6] Thrombocytopenia is frequently present and may be associated with disseminated intravascular coagulation (DIC). Hypocalcemia may develop because of the affinity of calcium ions for free fatty acids released by the hydrolysis of embolized fat.[17] Lipiduria is relatively common, and hematuria and proteinuria are seen occasionally.[3]

The diagnosis can be difficult to make, partly because of the relative nonspecificity of signs and symptoms and partly because clinical abnormalities may be related more directly to the cause of the emboli (e.g., trauma-associated shock). Some investigators have advocated the use of bronchoalveolar lavage and analysis of harvested macrophages for the presence of fat.[18] However, patients who do not have fat embolism syndrome may also have lipid-laden macrophages in their bronchoalveolar lavage fluid, and the definitive diagnostic threshold is unclear; some investigators propose a value as low as 5% and others a value as high as 30%.[18]

Synopsis of Treatment Options

There is no specific treatment available for fat embolism syndrome.[19] The mainstay of treatment is therefore supportive. Prophylactic corticosteroids (methylprednisolone) and heparin may have beneficial effects, but their utility is controversial.[2,19] The outcome in patients who receive supportive care is generally favorable; the mortality is less than 10%.[13]

KEY POINTS: FAT EMBOLISM

- Common causes are severe trauma and long bone and pelvic fractures.
- Typical symptoms include dyspnea, confusion, and petechial rash, which develop 12 to 36 hours after injury.
- Radiographic findings consist of bilateral ground-glass opacities or consolidation.
- CT findings include patchy or diffuse ground-glass opacities, patchy or confluent areas of consolidation, lobular sparing, and poorly defined centrilobular nodules.
- As distinct from lung contusion, radiographic findings of fat embolism are not present immediately after the injury.

Amniotic Fluid Embolism

Etiology, Prevalence, and Epidemiology

Amniotic fluid embolism is a rare but severe complication of pregnancy. In a population-based cohort of 3 million hospital deliveries in Canada between 1991 and 2002, the total rate of amniotic fluid embolism was 14.8 per 100,000 multiple-birth deliveries and 6.0 per 100,000 singleton deliveries.[20] Of the 180 cases of amniotic fluid embolism in women with singleton deliveries during the study period, 24 (13%) were fatal. Medical induction of labor nearly doubled the overall cases of amniotic fluid embolism, and the association was stronger for fatal cases. Maternal age of 35 years or older, cesarean or instrumented vaginal delivery, polyhydramnios, cervical laceration or uterine rupture, placenta previa or abruption, eclampsia, and fetal distress were also associated with an increased risk.[20]

Clinical Presentation

The majority of patients are in the 35th to 42nd week of pregnancy at the time of embolization. The clinical manifestations are typically abrupt, with sudden onset of cardiovascular collapse, cyanosis, and hemorrhage or DIC.[21] In less severe cases the initial manifestation is progressive dyspnea.[22] Although these abnormalities begin during spontaneous labor in most patients, they occur after delivery in about 30% (10% spontaneous and 20% after cesarean section).[23] The majority of patients experience seizures.

Pathophysiology

It is likely that little if any amniotic fluid enters the maternal circulation during normal labor and that significant embolism occurs only when there is disruption of the uterine wall in association with rupture of the placental membranes.[24] Such disruption can occur at several sites, the most common probably being the endocervix or lower uterine segment. Traumatic tears in the small veins in these regions can occur during normal labor but are of no significance if they are covered by fetal membranes; however, if such veins have separated from the fetal membranes, uterine contractions can "pump" amniotic fluid into the maternal venous circulation.[7] Amniotic fluid can also enter the maternal circulation at the placental site, usually in cases of uterine rupture, placenta previa, or cesarean section when the incision involves the site.[7]

The pathophysiologic consequences of intravascular amniotic fluid are complex and probably related to several processes. These include pulmonary vascular obstruction by amniotic fluid particulates, such as meconium; left ventricular dysfunction, possibly as a result of ischemia secondary to pulmonary hypertension and right ventricular dysfunction; pulmonary edema, related to the left ventricular dysfunction just described or to damage to the vascular endothelium by some constituent of amniotic fluid; and an immunologic reaction pathogenetically similar to anaphylaxis.[22] The main histologic abnormality is the presence of squames, mucin, and bile derived from meconium within small pulmonary vessels.[7]

Manifestations of the Disease

RADIOGRAPHY AND COMPUTED TOMOGRAPHY

The principal radiographic finding is bilateral airspace consolidation with or without pleural effusions, which is indistinguishable from acute pulmonary edema of other causes (Fig. 52.3).[25] Whether cardiac enlargement accompanies the edema depends on the severity of pulmonary hypertension and consequent cor pulmonale with or without left ventricular failure. The consolidation may persist or resolve within a few days.[25]

Differential Diagnosis

The diagnosis of amniotic fluid embolism is based on the rapid development of a complex constellation of findings with sudden cardiovascular collapse: acute left ventricular failure with pulmonary edema, DIC, and neurologic impairment. Because the predominant radiographic manifestation is widespread airspace consolidation, the main differential diagnoses are massive pulmonary hemorrhage and aspiration of liquid gastric contents. The diagnosis of amniotic fluid embolism should be considered, particularly in patients with risk factors such as medical induction of labor and placenta previa or abruption; it is supported by identification of squames, mucin, or hair fragments in samples of pulmonary capillary blood aspirated through a pulmonary arterial catheter.[26]

Synopsis of Treatment Options

There are no specific pharmacologic or other therapies that prevent or treat the amniotic fluid embolism syndrome.[27] The treatment is therefore supportive and involves aggressive management of multiple types of shock simultaneously.[27] The mortality rate of clinically recognized cases remains high at 19% in a recent study and up to 61% in older cohort studies; 25% to 50% of patients die within the first hour of the disease and most of the rest within 12 hours.[23,28] Serious neurologic sequelae are common in survivors.[23]

Tumor Embolism

Etiology, Prevalence, and Epidemiology

Hematogenous pulmonary metastases are derived from tumor fragments lodged within pulmonary vessels. In most cases these

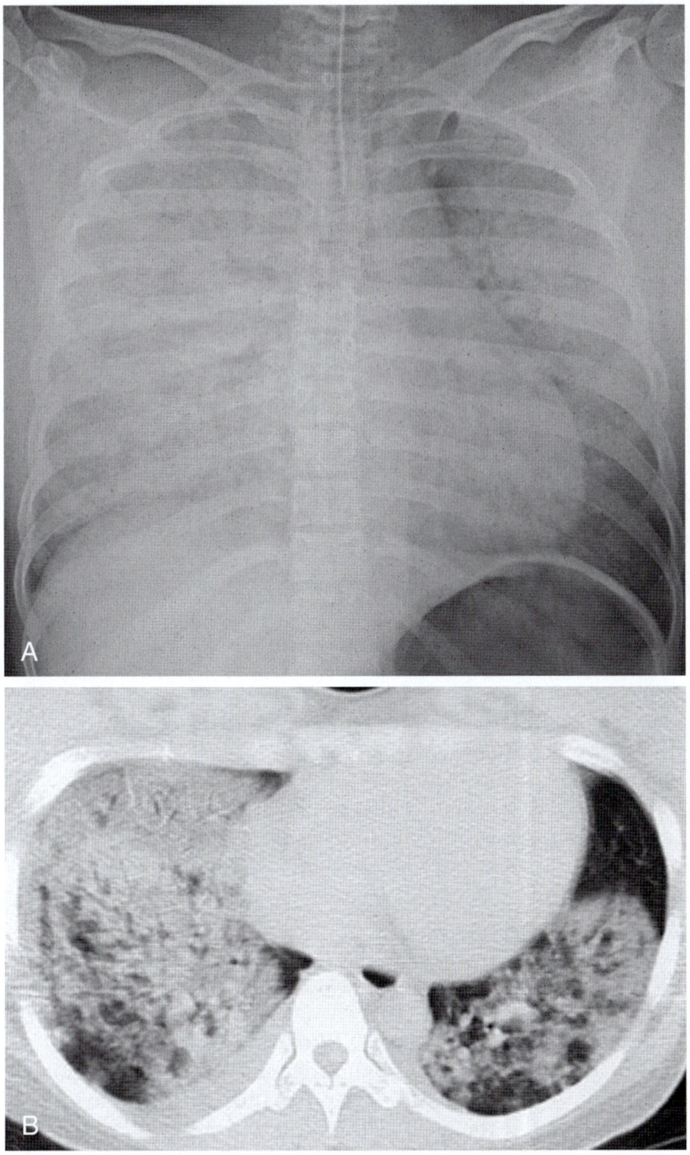

Fig. 52.3 Amniotic fluid embolism. (A) Anteroposterior chest radiograph shows diffuse bilateral consolidation with endotracheal intubation. (B) Axial CT shows bilateral consolidation with ground-glass opacities as well as small pleural effusions. *(From Bach AG, Restrepo CS, et al. Imaging of nonthrombotic pulmonary embolism: biological materials, nonbiological materials, and foreign bodies.* Eur J Radiol. *2013;82:e120–e41.)*

KEY POINTS: AMNIOTIC FLUID EMBOLISM

- Amniotic fluid embolism occurs in 14.8 per 100,000 multiple-birth deliveries and 6.0 per 100,000 singleton deliveries and carries a substantial mortality rate.
- Main risk factors are multiple-birth deliveries, medical induction of labor, cervical laceration, uterine rupture, placenta previa or abruption, and eclampsia.
- Clinical presentation: dyspnea, cyanosis, sudden onset of cardiovascular collapse, hemorrhage, or disseminated intravascular coagulopathy. Symptoms usually begin during labor and before giving birth.
- Radiologic manifestation: bilateral airspace consolidation that resembles pulmonary edema.

tumor fragments are small and therefore do not result in clinically or radiologically apparent vascular obstruction. However, when tumor emboli are of sufficient size or number, the clinical, pathologic, and radiographic manifestations can be identical to those of pulmonary thromboembolism. The manifestations can include pulmonary infarction, acute cor pulmonale and sudden death, and a slowly progressive syndrome of dyspnea and pulmonary hypertension.[29] Tumor embolism is seen most commonly in metastatic renal cell carcinoma, hepatocellular carcinoma, carcinoma of the breast, carcinoma of the stomach, and carcinoma of the prostate.[29,30] Tumor embolism may be more frequent after interventions that increase the fragmentation of the tumor mass, such as surgery, radiation therapy, or chemotherapy.[31]

Manifestations of the Disease

RADIOGRAPHY

Intravascular tumor emboli are seldom recognized on the chest radiograph.

COMPUTED TOMOGRAPHY AND NUCLEAR MEDICINE

Tumor emboli may be seen as filling defects in the central pulmonary arteries (Fig. 52.4), as nodular or beaded thickening of the peripheral pulmonary arteries, or as nodular and branching centrilobular opacities (tree-in-bud pattern) representing enlarged centrilobular arteries (Fig. 52.5).[30,32,33] In contrast to thromboembolic disease, tumor macroembolism is resistant to fibrinolytics and anticoagulation therapy.[31] Occasionally, tumor microembolism and lymphangitic carcinomatosis may manifest on nuclear medicine perfusion scintigraphy with contour mapping of the pulmonary segments, whereby numerous small perfusion defects outline the bronchopulmonary segments (see Fig. 52.5).[34]

KEY POINTS: INTRAVASCULAR TUMOR EMBOLISM

- Common primaries: renal cell carcinoma; hepatocellular carcinoma; carcinomas of the breast, stomach, and prostate
- Seldom evident on the chest radiograph
- Findings on CT:
  - Intravascular filling defects
  - Nodular or beaded thickening of the peripheral pulmonary arteries
  - Nodular and branching centrilobular opacities (tree-in-bud pattern)

Air Embolism

Etiology, Prevalence, and Epidemiology

Air emboli may have their origin in either the greater or the lesser circulation. In venous air embolism the air enters the systemic venous circulation and passes to the right side of the heart and then to the lungs; clinical and functional manifestations are therefore related to obstruction of the pulmonary circulation and affect predominantly the lungs. In systemic (arterial) air embolism air typically enters the pulmonary venous circulation and passes to the left side of the heart and then to the systemic

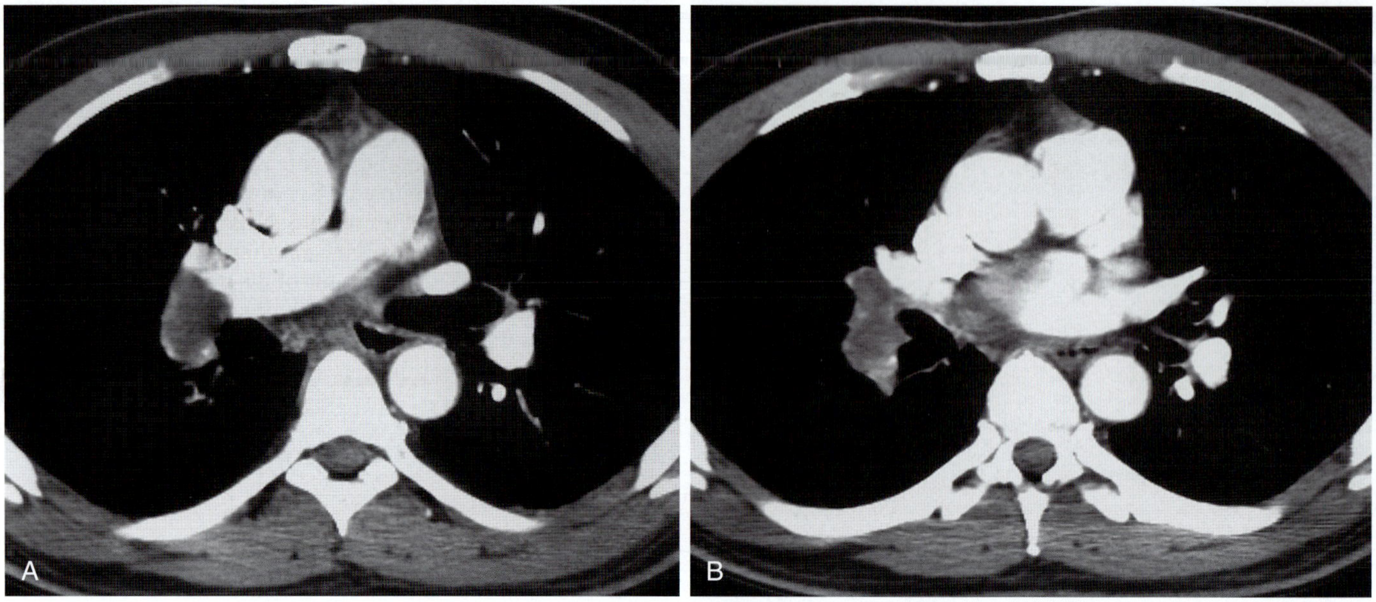

Fig. 52.4 Intravascular metastases from renal cell carcinoma. Contrast-enhanced CT images at the level of the right interlobar (A) and lower lobe (B) pulmonary arteries demonstrate large intraluminal filling defects. The appearance is indistinguishable from pulmonary thromboembolism.

arteries; the effects are therefore manifested mainly in the heart, the spinal cord, and the brain. Venous air embolism is a frequent iatrogenic complication, occurring most commonly with surgery, insertion and maintenance of intravenous (IV) devices, diagnostic or therapeutic air injection (e.g., arthrography), and barotrauma caused by positive-pressure ventilation.[7,35] Venous air embolism has been reported to occur in more than half of all cesarean sections.[36] Small quantities of air can be found in the central veins in up to 23% of patients during contrast material administration for CT.[37] Noniatrogenic air embolism sometimes occurs in scuba divers as a result of gas bubble formation in the blood, which is due to rapid reduction in the ambient pressure during a diver's ascent.[38]

Systemic air embolism occurs when the wall of a vessel exposed to air is disrupted and the pressure of the air exceeds the pressure in the vessel. The most common cause is probably penetrating thoracic trauma, either iatrogenic or accidental.[7] Other causes include open-heart surgery (residual air in pulmonary veins released into the circulation after cross-clamping is terminated), transthoracic needle biopsy, and thoracentesis.[7] Embolism can also occur in several situations in which the thorax is intact. One of the most common is scuba diving, in which the pathogenesis may be related to poor ventilation of a bulla or cyst because of partial or complete obstruction of its feeding airway.[39] Identical barotrauma of ascent can occur in airplane passengers.[40] In both these situations, tissue disruption is related to the increase in air pressure in an enclosed space as a result of a decrease in ambient pressure. Systemic air embolization can also occur in a variety of situations in which there is underlying lung disease, such as severe asthma, and during assisted positive-pressure ventilation.[41]

Clinical Presentation

The majority of patients with pulmonary air embolism are asymptomatic. Clinical symptoms include dyspnea and lightheadedness; chest pain occurs occasionally.[7] Physical findings include tachycardia, tachypnea, and systemic hypotension. Signs of pulmonary edema may also be evident. Migration of air into systemic vessels supplying the brain or heart may result in convulsions, coma, or chest pain.

Pathophysiology

The effects of embolized air in the pulmonary circulation depend on its quantity and rate of entry. Rapid injection of a large amount of air may result in the formation of an air block in the outflow tract of the right ventricle that prevents pulmonary arterial blood flow.[7] Smaller amounts, infused slowly, appear to exert an effect at the level of the distal pulmonary arteries and arterioles.[7] Some of this effect is probably related to vascular obstruction by air bubbles themselves; however, reflex vasoconstriction and the formation of fibrin emboli as blood and air are whipped together in the right-sided heart chambers may also be important. The overall effect of these processes is a transient increase in pulmonary vascular resistance and arterial pressure.[42] Both clinical and experimental observations indicate that pulmonary edema complicates some cases of pulmonary air embolism, probably as a result of increased microvascular permeability.[43]

Another cause of pulmonary air embolism is related to the air that reaches the pulmonary vasculature as part of the decompression syndrome. When a diver spends a prolonged period breathing gas at greater than atmospheric pressure, excess air dissolves in the blood and tissue fluids. With too rapid an ascent and return of partial pressures to lower values, air comes out of solution and forms small bubbles that can be carried in the systemic veins to the right side of the heart and pulmonary vasculature. Oxygen coming out of solution can be disposed of easily by metabolic consumption, but the inert nitrogen is much slower to be cleared. The bubbles cause lung microvascular damage and noncardiac pulmonary edema.[7] This form of pulmonary decompression sickness, which has been called the chokes, is a

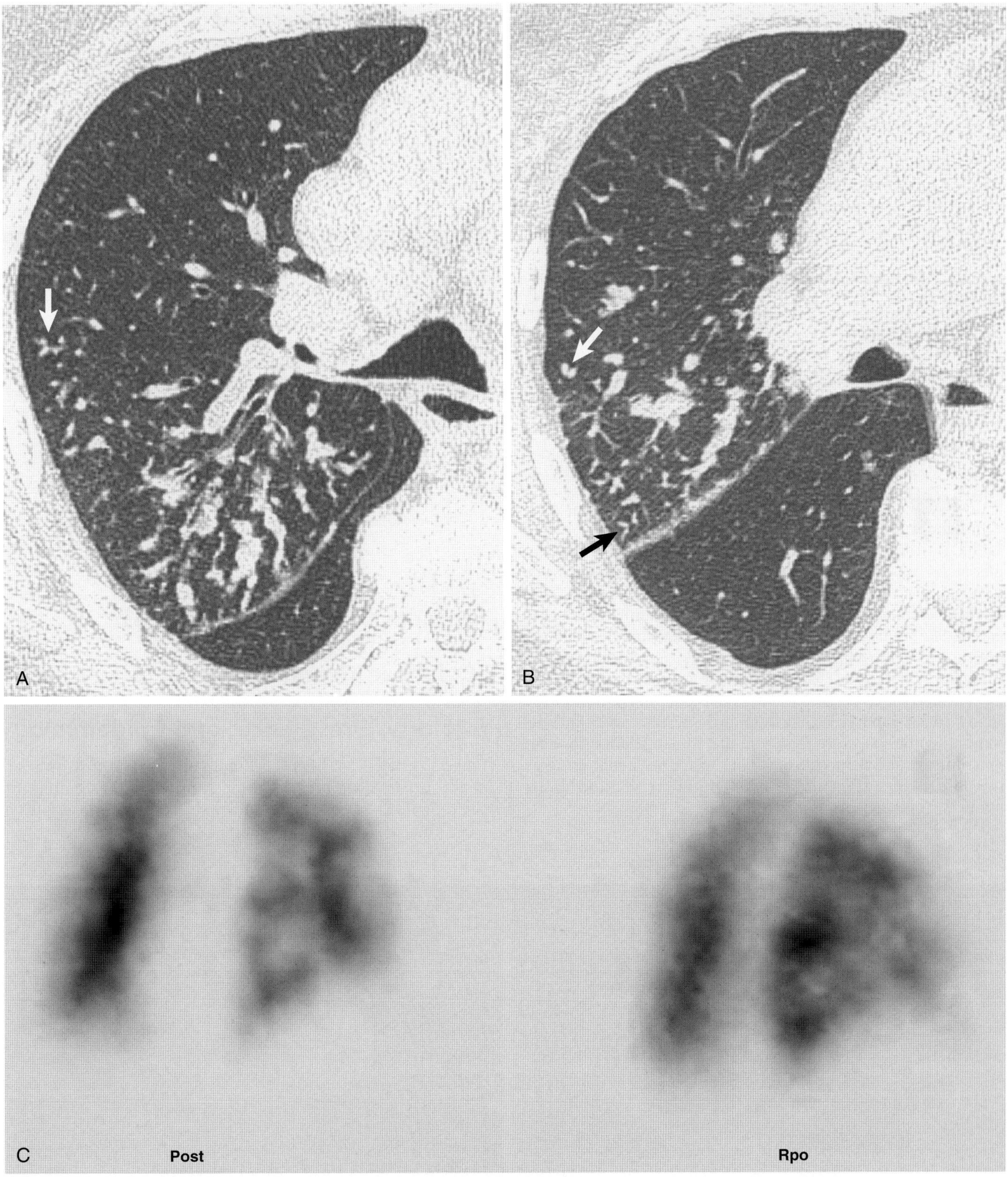

Fig. 52.5 Intravascular metastases from renal cell carcinoma. Views of the right lung at the level of the tracheal carina (A) and bronchus intermedius (B) demonstrate nodular thickening of the pulmonary vessels and centrilobular nodular and branching opacities (tree-in-bud pattern; *arrows*). (C) Perfusion scintigraphy from a different patient with tumor microembolism and lymphangitic carcinomatosis shows contour mapping where small perfusion defects outline the bronchopulmonary segments. *Rpo*, Right posterior oblique. *(Fig. 52.5C courtesy Daniel Applebaum, MD, University of Chicago, Chicago, IL.)*

relatively uncommon form of decompression illness that is sometimes fatal.[44]

Manifestations of the Disease

RADIOGRAPHY

The principal sign of air embolism is the presence of gas in cardiac chambers or pulmonary or systemic vessels.[35] In pulmonary air embolism the gas is present in the right-sided heart chambers and central pulmonary arteries; in systemic air embolism it can be identified in the left-sided heart chambers, aorta, or more peripheral branches of the systemic arterial tree, such as the neck, shoulder girdles, or upper part of the abdomen. Other manifestations of pulmonary air embolism include pulmonary edema, focal oligemia, enlarged central pulmonary arteries, and atelectasis.[35] The radiographic findings associated with air embolism in a study of 31 scuba divers included pneumomediastinum ($n = 8$), subcutaneous air ($n = 3$), pneumopericardium ($n = 2$), and pneumothorax and pneumoperitoneum ($n = 1$ each).[45]

COMPUTED TOMOGRAPHY

Pulmonary air embolism is seen particularly well on CT (Fig. 52.6). In a study of 100 patients who received IV contrast material that was injected by hand and followed by a drip infusion, asymptomatic venous air embolism was documented in 23.[37] The most common site was the pulmonary trunk. In another series of 677 patients who underwent contrast-enhanced CT, air emboli were detected in 79 (12%).[46] They were located in the pulmonary trunk in 54 (8%), the superior vena cava in 12 (1.8%), the right ventricle in 10 (1.5%), the subclavian or brachiocephalic vein in 6 (0.9%), and the right atrium in 5 (0.7%).[46] Seven patients (1%) had emboli at more than one site. Systemic air embolism is uncommon and is most commonly seen after penetrating or iatrogenic trauma. It manifests as air within the left-sided heart chambers, aorta, or systemic arteries (Fig. 52.7).

Synopsis of Treatment Options

Treatment is largely supportive. Therapeutic interventions include mechanical measures, such as positioning and measures aimed at reducing bubble size, including placement in the left lateral decubitus position to prevent right ventricular outflow tract obstruction.[31,47] Hyperbaric oxygen therapy is often helpful, particularly if it is started within 6 hours after venous or systemic air embolism.[48]

KEY POINTS: AIR EMBOLISM

- Venous air embolism
  - Pathogenesis: air typically enters systemic veins and affects mainly the lungs
  - Common causes: surgery, intravenous (IV) devices
  - Symptoms: dyspnea, chest pain
  - Radiographic findings: air in pulmonary vessels; occasionally pulmonary edema
  - CT findings: small amount of venous air commonly seen during IV administration of contrast material
- Systemic air embolism
  - Pathogenesis: air typically enters pulmonary veins and affects mainly the brain and heart
  - Common causes: penetrating thoracic trauma, scuba diving
  - Symptoms: chest pain, seizures, coma
  - Radiographic and CT findings: air in systemic vessels

Embolism of Talc, Starch, and Cellulose (Intravenous Talcosis, Talc Granulomatosis, Cellulose Granulomatosis)

Etiology, Prevalence, and Epidemiology

Emboli of talc, starch, and cellulose are seen almost invariably in chronic IV drug users.[49] In most instances the complication occurs with medications intended solely for oral use; pills are

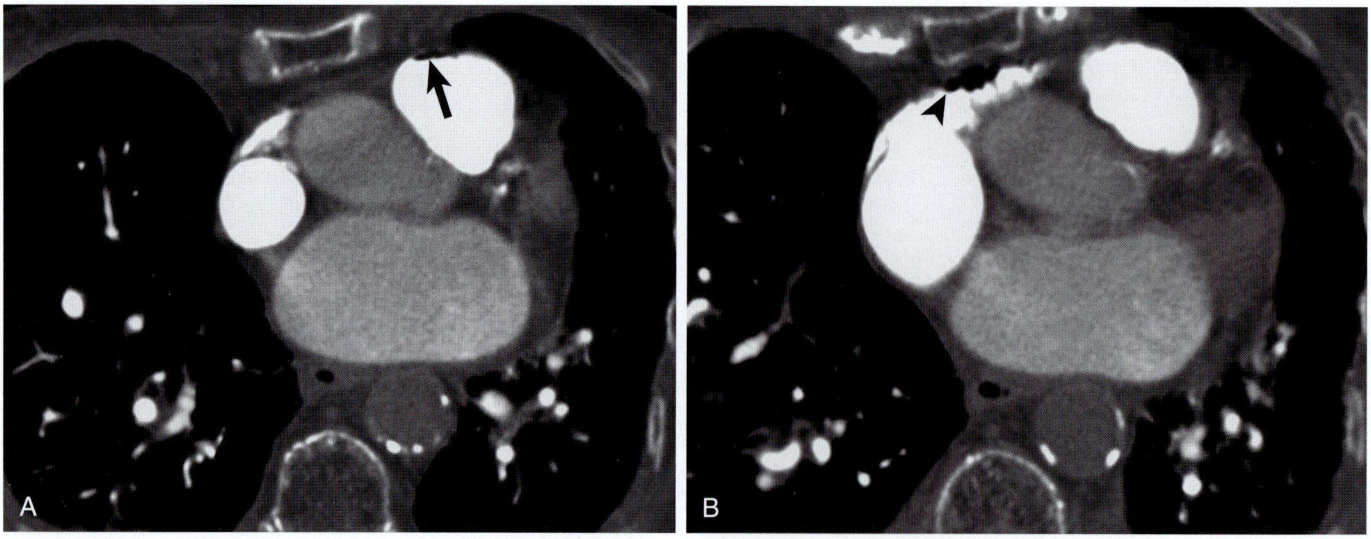

Fig. 52.6 Intravenous air embolism after administration of contrast material. Contrast-enhanced CT images at the level of the pulmonary trunk (A) and right ventricular outflow tract (B) demonstrate small amount of air in the pulmonary trunk (*arrow* in A) and right atrium (*arrowhead* in B).

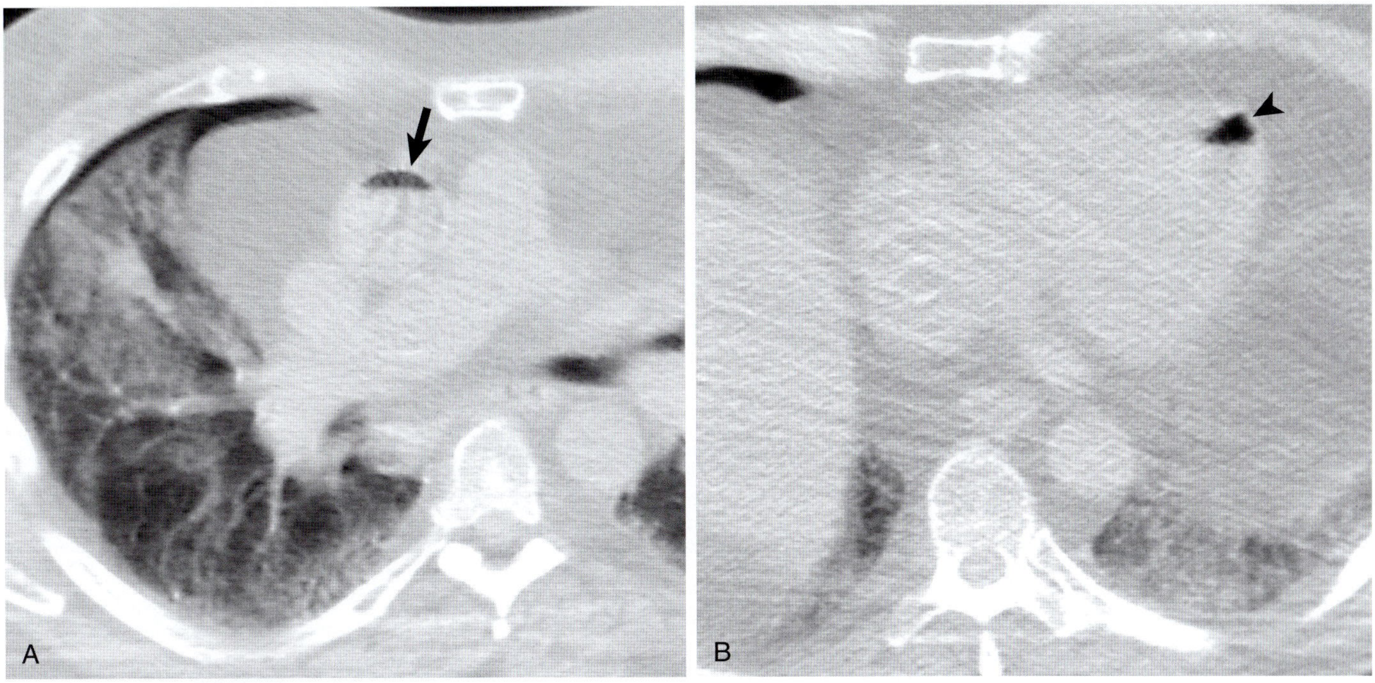

Fig. 52.7 Systemic air embolism following right lung biopsy. Axial CT images at the level of the right pulmonary artery (A) and lung bases (B) shows air within the ascending aorta *(arrow)* and left ventricular apex *(arrowhead)*. Note right pneumothorax, right middle lobe nodule, and peripheral reticulation with architectural distortion compatible with interstitial lung disease.

crushed in a spoon or bottle top, water is added, and the mixture is drawn into a syringe and injected. Oral medications misused in this way include amphetamines and closely related drugs, such as methylphenidate hydrochloride (Ritalin), methadone hydrochloride, hydromorphone hydrochloride (Dilaudid), propoxyphene (Darvon), and pentazocine (Talwin).[7] All these medications have in common the addition of an insoluble filler to bind the medicinal particles together and to act as a lubricant to prevent the tablets from sticking to punches and dies during manufacture. The commonly used fillers are talc, cornstarch, and microcrystalline cellulose.

Clinical Presentation

Most addicts are asymptomatic; granulomas are found incidentally at autopsy in those who die of other causes. Typically, symptoms develop only in heavy users and consist of slowly progressive dyspnea and, occasionally, persistent cough. Cor pulmonale may be evident as a result of extensive disease. As in silicosis, disease may progress, and disability may increase after cessation of exposure.[49] Organized thrombi and scars are visible on the forearms of nearly all addicts who inject drugs intravenously. Glistening particles can be seen in the fundi and may be the earliest clue to the drug use.[49]

Pathophysiology

When injected intravenously, the insoluble fillers contained in tablets meant for oral use become trapped within pulmonary arterioles and capillaries and cause vascular occlusion. In time the foreign particles migrate through the vessel wall and come to lie in the adjacent perivascular and parenchymal interstitial tissue, where they result in a foreign-body giant-cell reaction and fibrosis.[7] Chronic pulmonary hypertension typically develops at this stage if the quantity of foreign material is sufficient.

On pathologic examination the lungs initially show variable numbers of more or less discrete parenchymal nodules measuring up to 1 mm in diameter. On histologic examination the small nodules consist of loosely formed granulomas containing large multinucleated giant cells.[7] In long-standing disease, the nodules tend to become confluent, especially in the upper lobes, and produce large areas of consolidation resembling the progressive massive fibrosis seen in the pneumoconioses. Sections of the large foci of upper lobe consolidation seen in long-standing disease show sheets of multinucleated giant cells, usually not organized in discrete granulomas; a variable degree of fibrosis is also present. Talc is recognized as irregular, plate-like crystals that are strongly birefringent (Fig. 52.8).[50] Panacinar emphysema, sometimes with bulla formation, is often evident.[51] The pathogenesis of the emphysema is unclear.

Manifestations of the Disease

RADIOGRAPHY

The earliest radiologic manifestation of IV talcosis is the presence of widespread nodules ranging from barely visible to about 1 mm in diameter (Fig. 52.9). They are distinct and "pinpoint" in character, similar to alveolar microlithiasis. In the early stages the nodules are usually distributed diffusely and uniformly throughout the lungs.[52] In more advanced disease the upper lobe nodules may coalesce to form an almost homogeneous opacity that resembles end-stage sarcoidosis or the progressive massive fibrosis of silicosis or coal workers' pneumoconiosis, except for the frequent presence of an air bronchogram (Fig. 52.10).[49] In the late stages of the disease, increasing disability

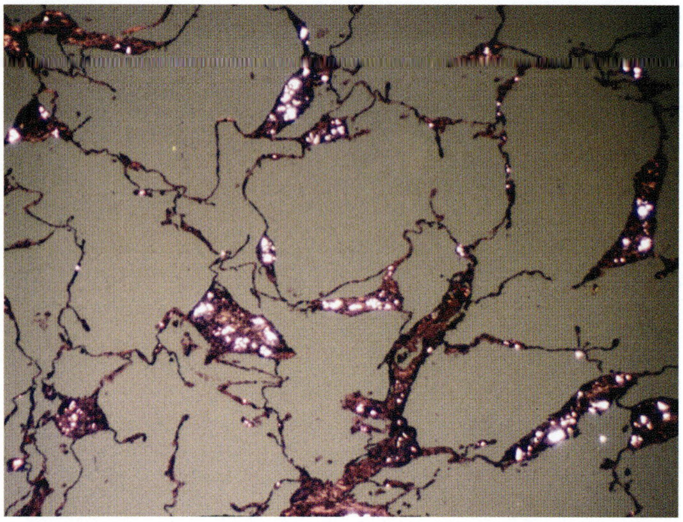

Fig. 52.8 Intravenous (IV) talcosis: histologic findings. Lung biopsy specimen from a patient with IV talcosis demonstrates irregular birefringent crystals characteristic of talc.

and deteriorating function are associated with radiographic evidence of emphysema and bullae.[49] In patients who inject crushed Ritalin tablets, the appearance mimics that of α1-antitrypsin deficiency with basilar-predominant emphysema.[53]

COMPUTED TOMOGRAPHY

The earliest high-resolution CT findings consist of widespread nodules ranging from barely visible to about 1 mm in diameter, a fine granular pattern, or ground-glass opacities (Fig. 52.11).[52,54] The nodules of cellulose granulomatosis have been referred to as a vascular tree-in-bud pattern with nodules distributed diffusely throughout the lungs, differentiating them from the more common tree-in-bud opacities seen with infectious bronchiolitis or aspiration. The nodules are more easily characterized with the help of maximum-intensity projection images. An ancillary clue usually seen with this diagnosis is enlargement of the central pulmonary arteries, indicating coexistent pulmonary hypertension (Fig. 52.12). Over time, the nodules coalesce, resulting in dense foci of consolidation or masses with associated volume loss, superior retraction of the hila, and overinflation of the remaining lung, characteristic of progressive massive fibrosis. These conglomerate areas of fibrosis typically contain foci of high attenuation consistent with talc deposition (see Fig. 52.10).[52,55] On occasion, IV talcosis may result in more extensive fibrosis and honeycombing and resemble end-stage sarcoidosis (Fig. 52.13).

The radiographic and CT findings of IV abuse of methylphenidate (crushed Ritalin tablets) differ somewhat from those of other types of IV drug abuse. The main abnormality closely mimics α1-antitrypsin deficiency and characteristically consists of bilateral, symmetric emphysema involving mainly the lower lung zones without bulla formation (Fig. 52.14).[52,53]

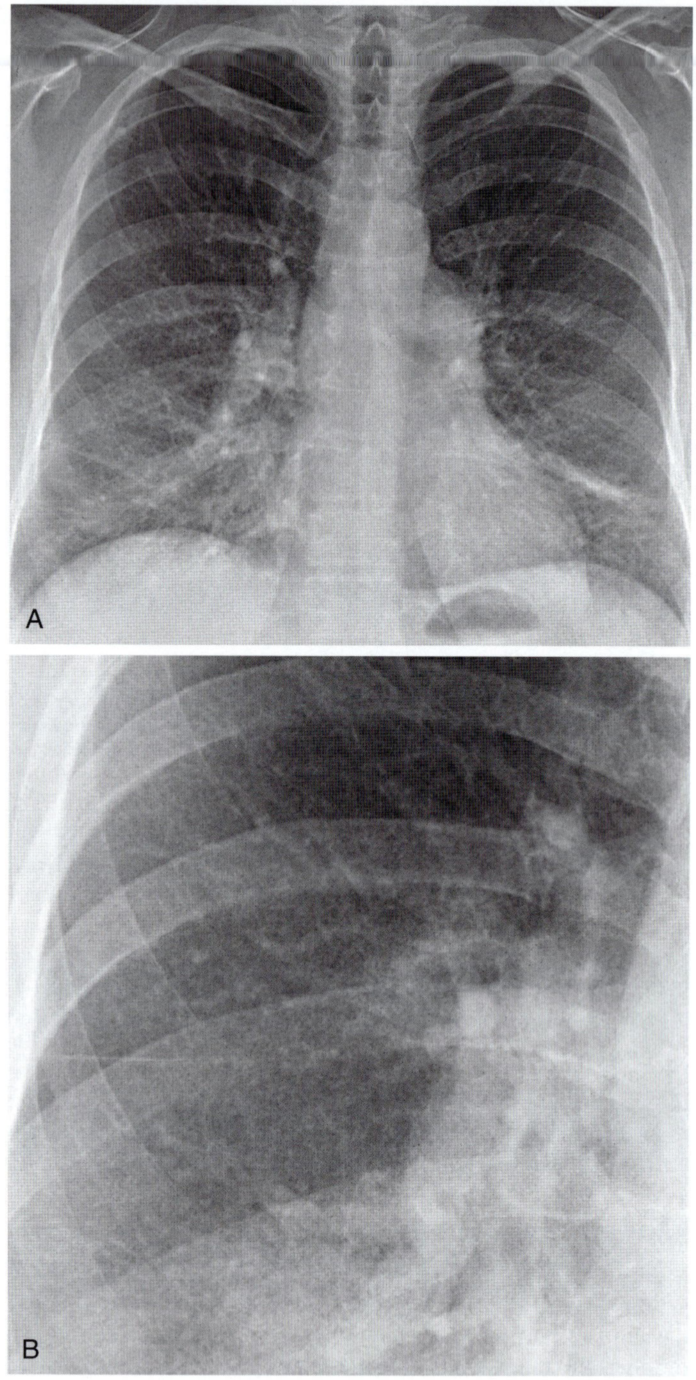

Fig. 52.9 Intravenous (IV) talcosis in an IV drug user: diffuse pinpoint nodular pattern on the chest radiograph. (A) Chest radiograph shows diffuse nodular pattern. The nodules measure 1 mm or less in diameter. Also noted is enlargement of the pulmonary trunk indicating pulmonary hypertension. (B) Magnified view of the right middle lung zone better demonstrates the fine nodular pattern.

Liquid Acrylates and Acrylic Cement

Etiology, Prevalence, and Epidemiology

Liquid acrylate glues, most commonly isobutyl-2-cyanoacrylate and *n*-butyl-2-cyanoacrylate, are frequently used in embolization therapy for vascular malformations and in endoscopic sclerotherapy for gastric variceal bleeding. Acrylic cement (polymethyl methacrylate) is used in vertebroplasty. Asymptomatic pulmonary embolism associated with these procedures is probably more frequent than is generally appreciated, occurring in 4% to 23% of cases[31]; however, symptomatic embolization is uncommon.[56,57]

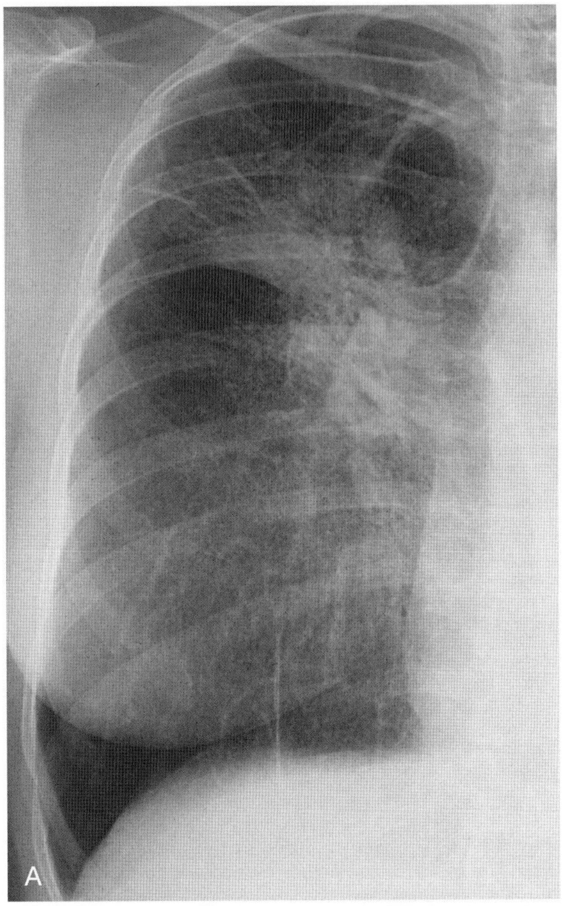

Fig. 52.10 Intravenous (IV) talcosis with conglomerate massive fibrosis in an IV drug user. (A) View of the right lung from a chest radiograph shows conglomerate mass in the perihilar region of the right upper lobe with associated superior retraction of the hilum. Also noted are numerous well-defined 1- to 2-mm-diameter nodules. (B) Composite image with high-resolution CT of the right upper lobe in lung window *(left image)* and soft tissue window *(right image)* shows numerous small nodules, diffuse ground-glass opacities, and a conglomerate mass with foci of high attenuation consistent with talc deposition. Note associated architectural distortion and anterior tenting of the right major fissure, indicating a component of fibrosis.

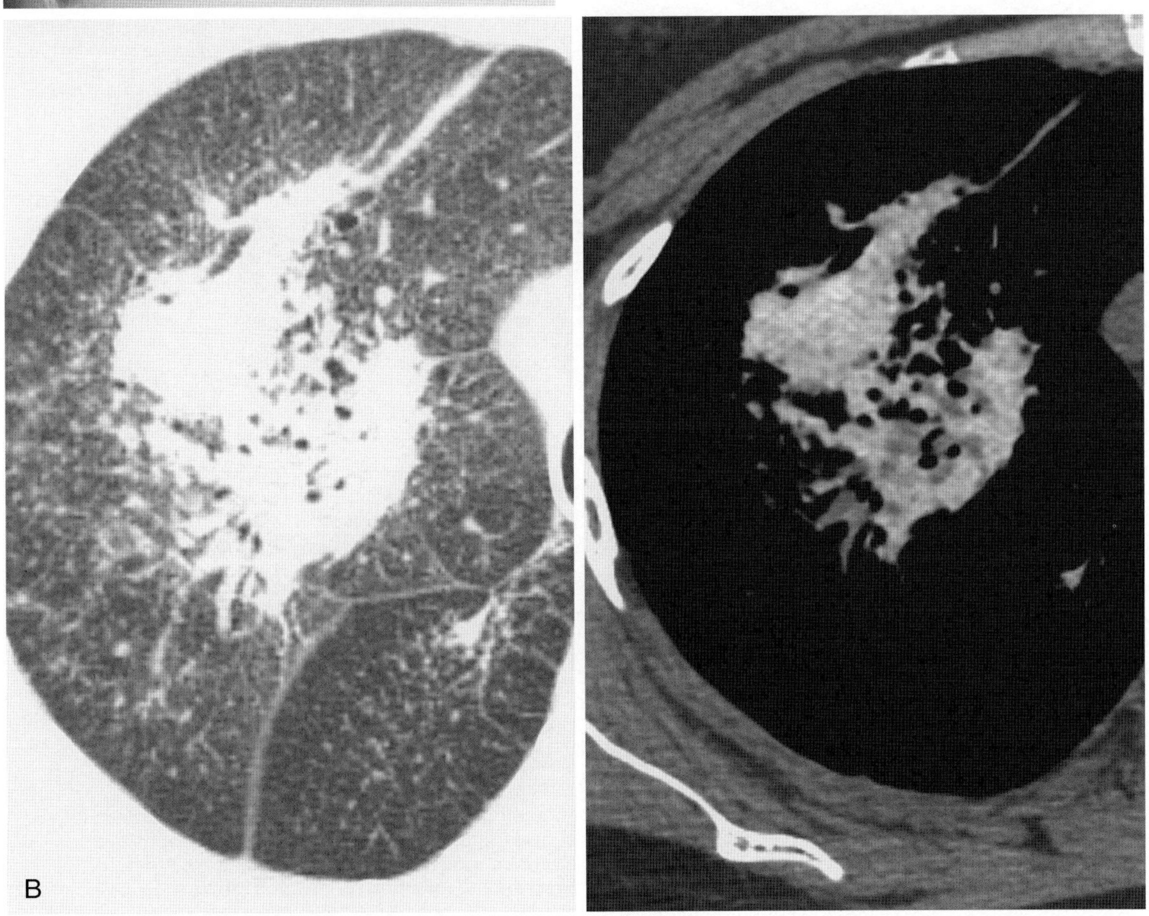

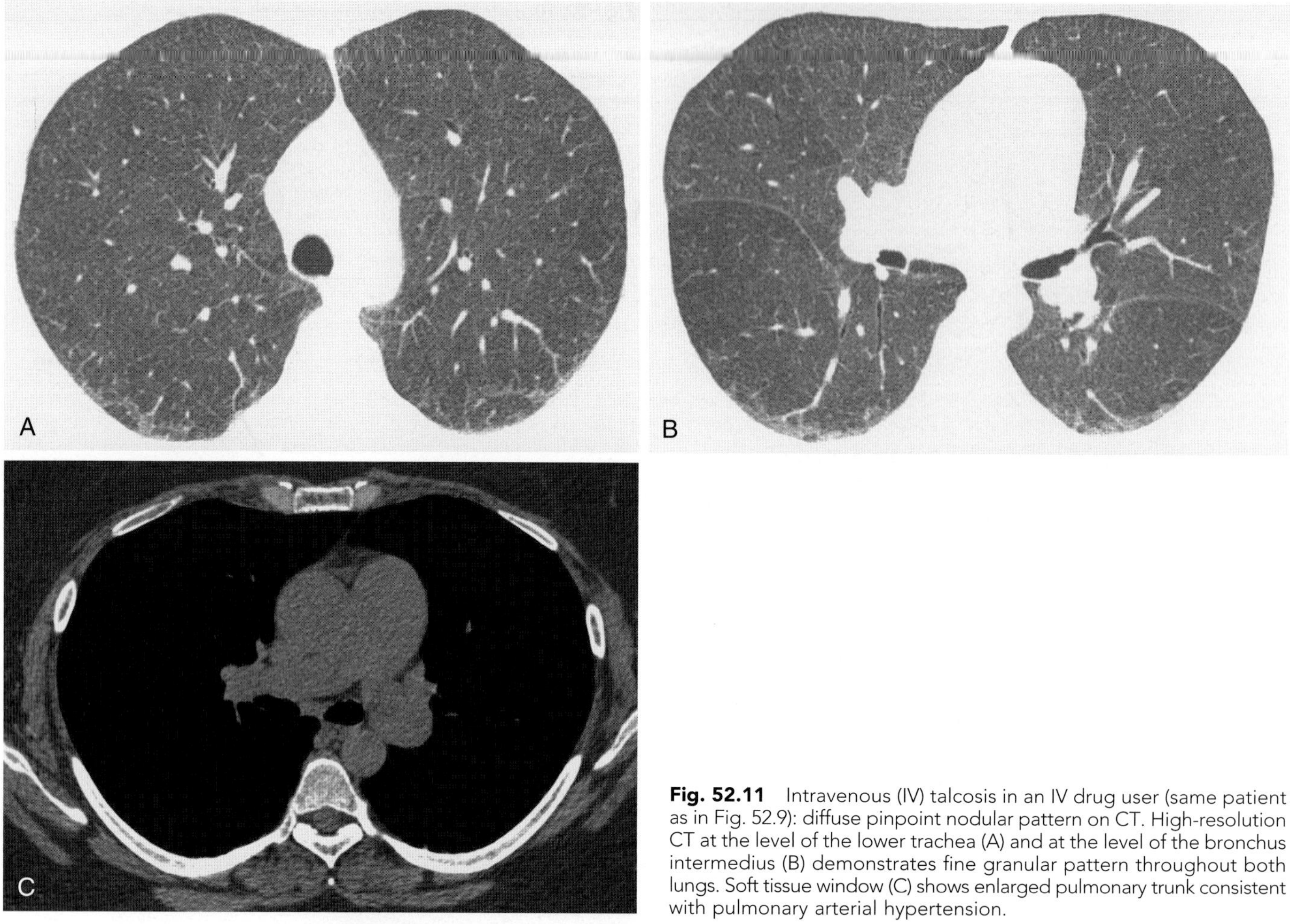

Fig. 52.11 Intravenous (IV) talcosis in an IV drug user (same patient as in Fig. 52.9): diffuse pinpoint nodular pattern on CT. High-resolution CT at the level of the lower trachea (A) and at the level of the bronchus intermedius (B) demonstrates fine granular pattern throughout both lungs. Soft tissue window (C) shows enlarged pulmonary trunk consistent with pulmonary arterial hypertension.

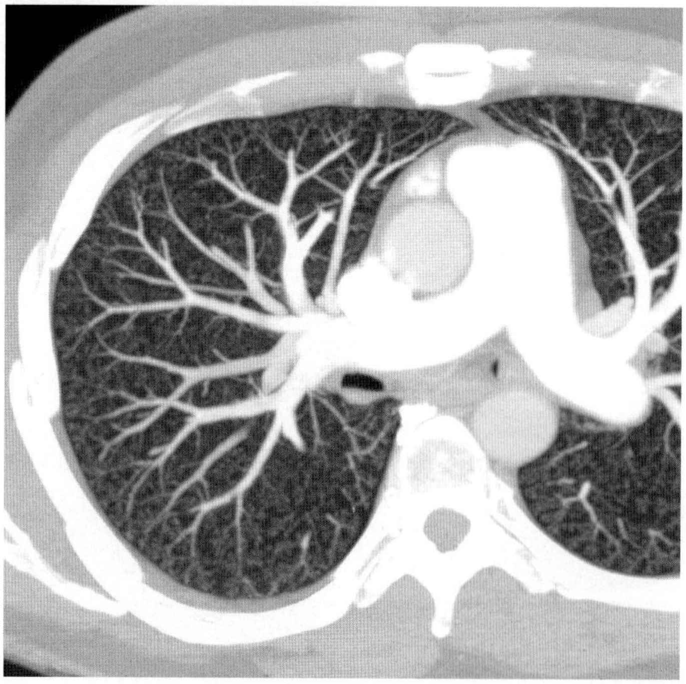

Fig. 52.12 Cellulose granulomatosis from intravenous (IV) injection of crushed morphine tablets. Axial maximum-intensity projection image demonstrates diffuse and uniform tree-in-bud opacities throughout both lungs. Enlarged central pulmonary arteries suggest pulmonary hypertension. A diffuse tree-in-bud pattern may be seen with diffuse panbronchiolitis or after IV injection of crushed oral medications such as opioids or amphetamines.

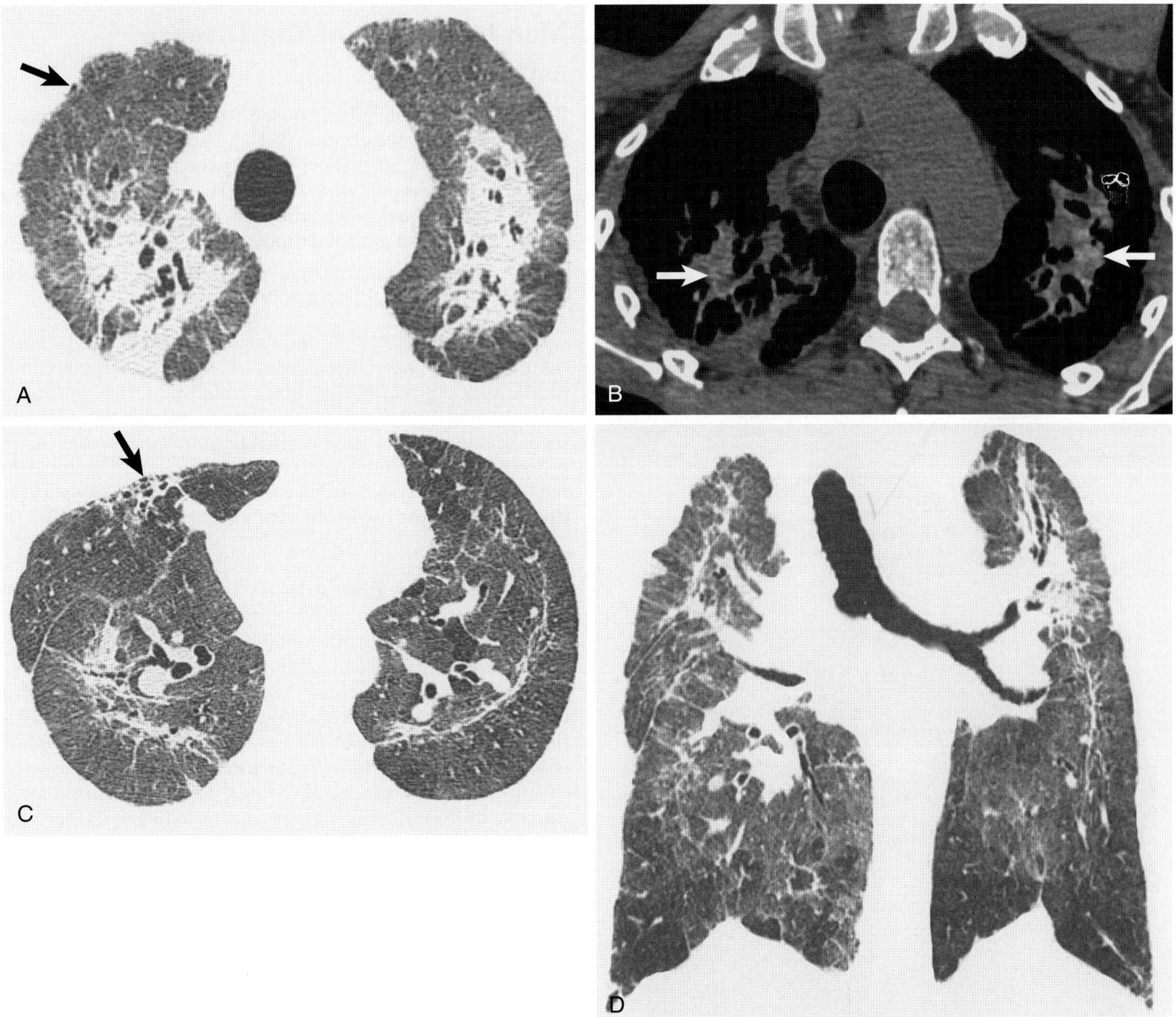

Fig. 52.13 Intravenous talcosis with extensive fibrosis after intravenous drug use. (A) High-resolution CT at the level of the aortic arch shows conglomerate fibrosis with air bronchograms, architectural distortion, subpleural cyst *(arrow)* consistent with early honeycombing, and mild emphysema. Also evident are diffuse ground-glass opacities. (B) CT in soft tissue windows shows foci of increased attenuation *(arrows)* within the conglomerate fibrosis consistent with talc deposition. (C) CT at the level of lower lung zones shows diffuse ground-glass opacities, peribronchial fibrosis with traction bronchiectasis in the right lower and middle lobes, and subpleural honeycombing *(arrow)*. (D) Coronal CT demonstrates predominantly upper lobe distribution of the fibrosis with upward retraction of the hila, overinflation of the lung bases, and tenting of the hemidiaphragms. The predominantly peribronchial and upper lobe distribution of fibrosis resembles end-stage sarcoidosis or an occupational lung disorder such as silicosis.

KEY POINTS: INTRAVENOUS TALCOSIS AND CELLULOSE GRANULOMATOSIS

- Intravenous (IV) talcosis is seen almost exclusively in chronic IV drug users.
- The complication usually occurs with medications intended solely for oral use.
- Most patients are asymptomatic. Symptoms include progressive dyspnea and cough.
- Radiographic findings:
  - Widespread nodules ranging from barely visible to 1 mm in diameter
  - Upper lobe conglomerate masses
  - Lower lobe panlobular emphysema in methylphenidate (Ritalin) users
- CT findings:
  - Widespread nodules ranging from barely visible to 1 mm in diameter and may include a diffuse vascular tree-in-bud pattern
  - Diffuse ground-glass opacities
  - Upper lobe conglomerate masses containing areas of high attenuation
  - Lower lobe panacinar emphysema in methylphenidate (Ritalin) users

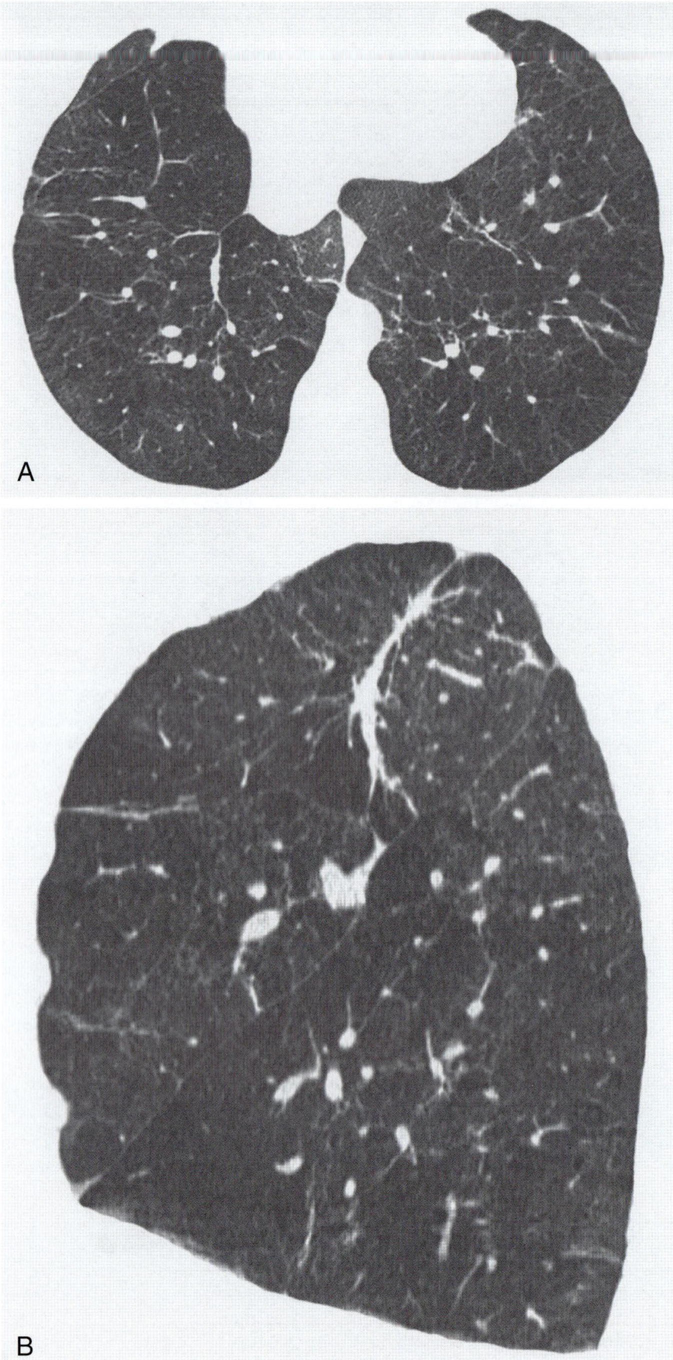

Fig. 52.14 Ritalin lung with panacinar emphysema after intravenous use of crushed methylphenidate tablets (Ritalin). (A) High-resolution CT at the level of the lower lobes demonstrates extensive areas of decreased attenuation and focal areas of scarring. (B) Sagittal reformatted CT of the right lung demonstrates increased lung volumes, focal areas of scarring, and predominantly lower lung zone distribution of the areas of low attenuation. This CT appearance closely mimics α1-antitrypsin deficiency.

Clinical Presentation

Most patients are asymptomatic. Patients may complain of pleuritic chest pain with or without associated cough and bloody sputum. Severe manifestations can include hypotension and arrhythmia.[56]

Manifestations of the Disease

RADIOGRAPHY

Because the acrylate glue is mixed with radiopaque substances to allow accurate localization during embolization therapy, the chest radiograph may show tubular or nodular high-density opacities along the pulmonary vessels (Fig. 52.15).[58] Other findings in patients with extensive embolism include subsegmental or segmental areas of consolidation.[57]

COMPUTED TOMOGRAPHY

CT scans show tubular or nodular radiopaque material within the pulmonary vessels (see Fig. 52.15).[58] The material is often most easily appreciated on bone windows. Other findings in patients with extensive cyanoacrylate pulmonary embolism include subsegmental, predominantly subpleural wedge-shaped areas of consolidation consistent with infarction.[57] On occasion, the filling defects may be large enough to manifest with perfusion defects on nuclear medicine scintigraphy (see Fig. 52.15).

Iodized Oil Embolism

In the past, pulmonary oil embolism was usually a complication of lymphangiography with ethiodized poppy seed oil (Ethiodol). More recently, it has been described as a complication of iodinated oil embolism that occurs after transcatheter oil chemoembolization for the treatment of hepatocellular carcinoma.[59] Lipiodol is also mixed with *n*-butyl cyanoacrylate in endoscopic sclerotherapy for gastric variceal bleeding.[60] Lipiodol is mixed for the purpose of fluoroscopic monitoring and dilution of the cyanoacrylate to delay hardening.

Clinical Presentation

Few patients develop symptoms after lymphangiography.[61] Patients with iodinated oil embolism after transcatheter oil chemoembolization are more likely to develop respiratory symptoms, including cough, hemoptysis, and dyspnea.[59] In a review of 336 patients with hepatocellular carcinoma who underwent transcatheter oil chemoembolization through the hepatic artery, 14 patients received more than 20 mL of iodized oil. Respiratory symptoms of cough, hemoptysis, and dyspnea developed in 6 of these 14 patients 2 to 5 days after therapy.[59]

Manifestations of the Disease

RADIOGRAPHY

The radiographic findings usually consist of a fine reticular pattern, which may persist for 1 to 2 weeks.[61] In addition, small peripheral vessels may be so filled with contrast material that they have an arborizing pattern similar to that seen on pulmonary arteriography.[62] In patients with extensive embolism the radiograph may demonstrate diffuse ground-glass opacities and consolidation.[59] Embolization of Lipiodol mixed with cyanoacrylate in endoscopic sclerotherapy for gastric variceal bleeding may result in multiple radiopaque emboli within the central pulmonary arteries without evidence of pulmonary parenchymal abnormality.[60]

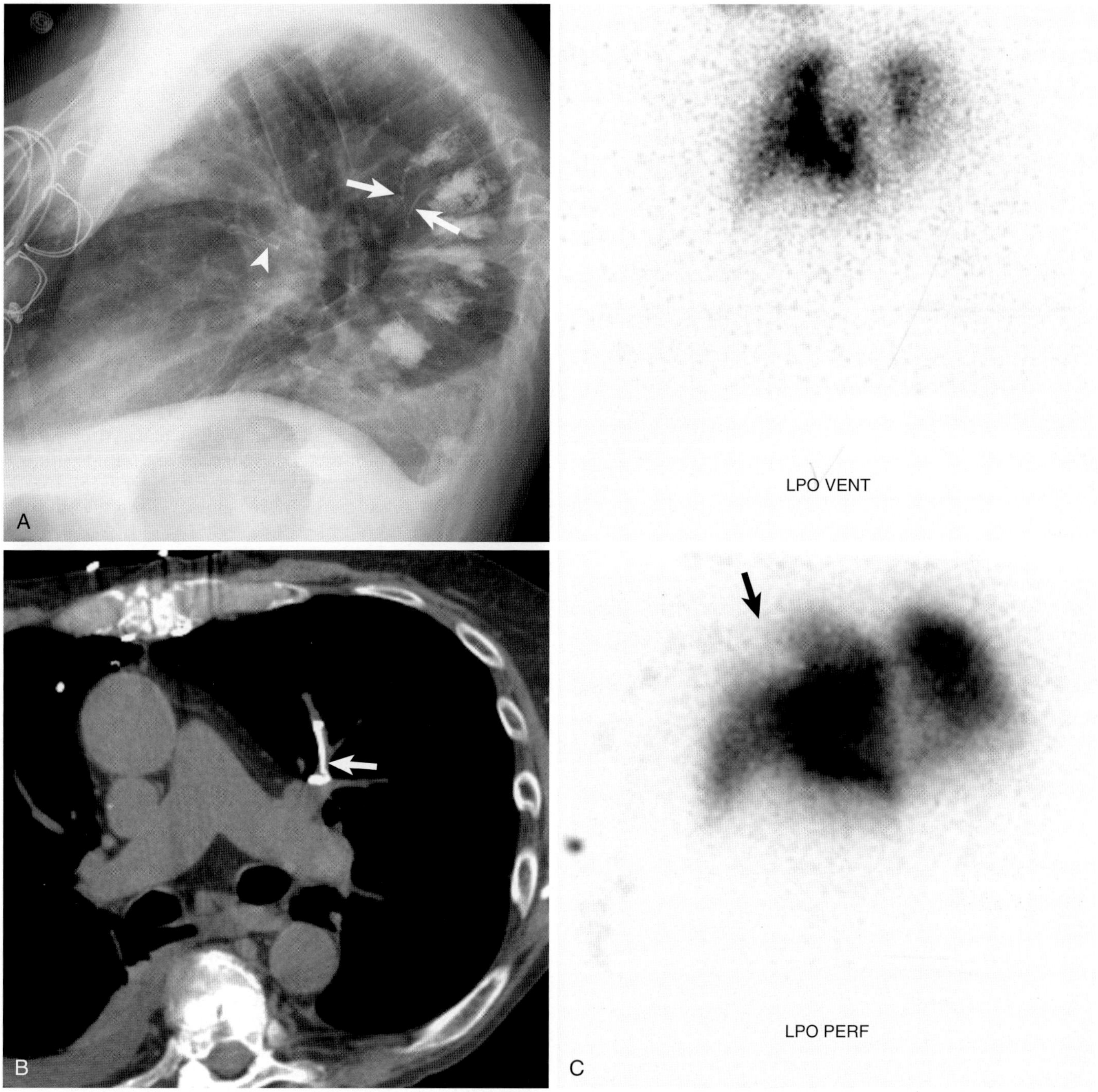

Fig. 52.15 Methylmethacrylate embolization following vertebroplasty. (A) Lateral chest radiograph shows multilevel thoracic spine vertebroplasty with methylmethacrylate entering paravertebral veins *(arrows)* with resultant embolization to the lungs *(arrowhead)*. (B) Oblique axial noncontrast CT shows a high-attenuation filling defect *(arrow)* in the anterior segmental pulmonary artery of the left upper lobe. (C) Ventilation perfusion scintigraphy shows a large wedge-shaped mismatched perfusion defect *(arrow)* in the anterior left upper lobe corresponding to the embolized methylmethacrylate. *LPO*, Left posterior oblique; *Perf*, perfusion; *Vent*, ventilation.

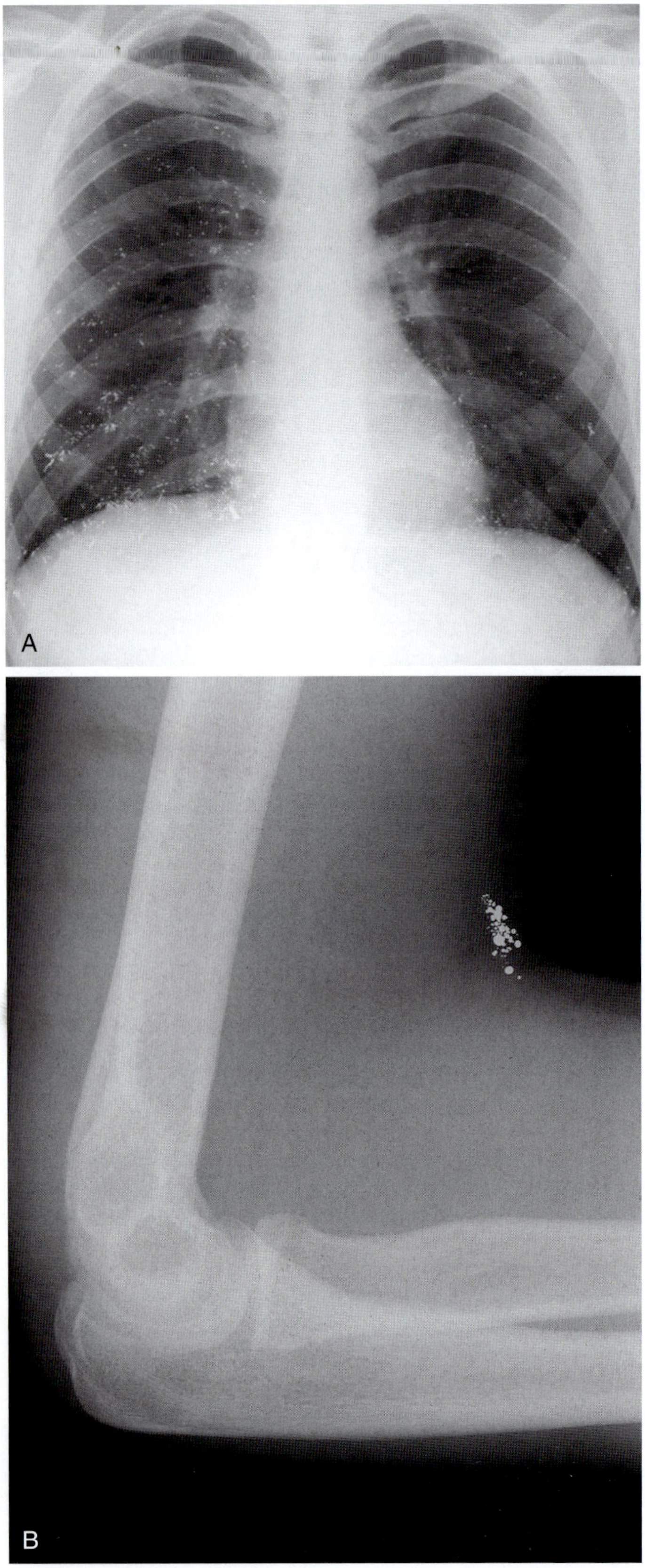

Fig. 52.16 Mercury injection with suicide attempt. (A) Posteroanterior chest radiograph shows diffuse high-attenuation mercury spherules, many with a branching configuration throughout both lungs. (B) Lateral radiograph of the elbow confirms that the mercury was injected intravenously rather than aspirated, given the presence of mercury in the antecubital fossa. *(Fig. 52.16A reproduced with permission from Peterson N, Harvey-Smith W, Rohrmann CA. Radiographic aspects of metallic mercury embolism.* AJR Am J Roentgenol. *1980;135:1079-1081; Fig. 52.16B courtesy C. Rohrmann, Seattle, WA.)*

Other Materials

Mercury

The iatrogenic, suicidal, or accidental injection of mercury is generally well tolerated, but patients may have some symptoms of pulmonary obstruction or systemic toxicity. After injection, the high-attenuation mercury spherules are found within the lungs, heart, and other parts of the body (Fig. 52.16). The spherules disappear gradually, remaining within the lungs for a prolonged period of time.[63]

Bullets and Shrapnel

Uncommonly, these agents enter the extrathoracic systemic veins or the right side of the heart, are carried to the lungs, and then lodge within pulmonary arteries.[64] Such foreign bodies can remain in the right ventricle or within the pulmonary vasculature for prolonged periods without untoward effects. In one case a bullet was present in the right ventricle 59 years after a bullet wound to the left side of the neck.[65] In another report the authors described the case of an 11-year-old girl who was struck in the suboccipital region with a "soft-nosed" bullet fired at close range. Several months later the patient was found to have asymptomatic pulmonary emboli.[66]

Radiopaque Foreign Bodies

A variety of devices, such as wire loops and balloons filled with contrast medium, have been used therapeutically in both the pulmonary and systemic circulations to obliterate arteriovenous malformations or to control intractable hemorrhage. Escape of such material into the systemic veins can result in opacities of metallic density within the lungs.[67] Other devices, such as catheter fragments or inferior vena cava filters, may embolize to both the lungs and right-sided cardiac chambers (Fig. 52.17).

Plastic Intravenous Catheters

These devices, either whole or in fragments, usually embolize to the lungs when they are cut by the sharp bevel of the needle housing them. On occasion, they are detached from their connector or fracture spontaneously.[68]

Silicone

Silicone fluid (polydimethylsiloxane) embolism has been reported in some patients in whom the substance has been injected subcutaneously for breast augmentation.[69] Radiographs have shown a combination of interstitial and airspace disease, which

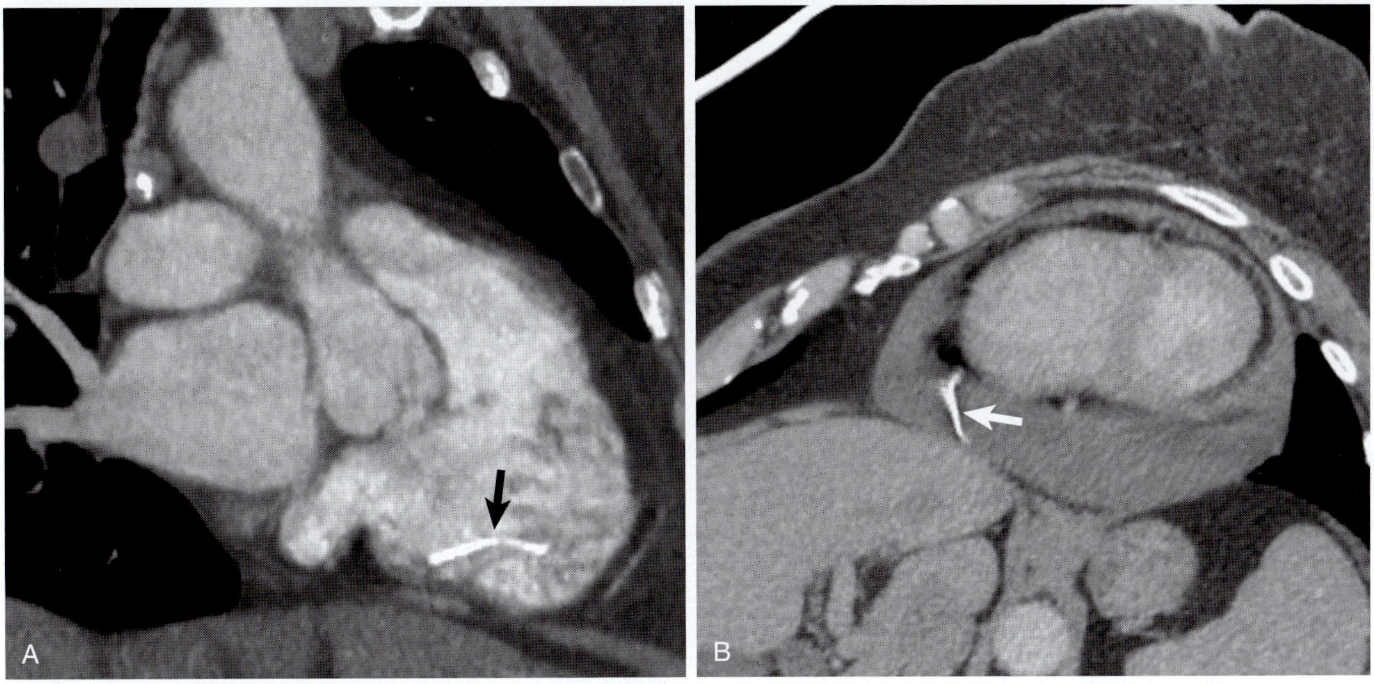

Fig. 52.17 Inferior vena cava (IVC) filter embolization with subsequent hemopericardium. (A) Oblique coronal contrast CT shows an embolized IVC filter fragment within the right ventricle. (B) Follow-up oblique axial CT shows perforation of the right ventricular myocardium with the filter fragment *(arrow)* now residing within the pericardial cavity with resultant large hemopericardium.

in severe cases progresses to a pattern of acute respiratory distress syndrome.

SUGGESTED READINGS

Bach AG, et al. Imaging of nonthrombotic pulmonary embolism: biological materials, nonbiological materials, and foreign bodies. *Eur J Radiol*. 2013;82: e120–e141.

Han D, Lee KS, Franquet T, et al. Thrombotic and nonthrombotic pulmonary arterial embolism: spectrum of imaging findings. *Radiographics*. 2003;23:1521–1539.

Talbot M, Schemitsch EH. Fat embolism syndrome: history, definition, epidemiology. *Injury*. 2006;37:S3–S7.

The full reference list for this chapter is available at ExpertConsult.com.

53 Pulmonary Arterial Hypertension*

VEDANT GUPTA | STEPHEN B. HOBBS

Pulmonary arterial hypertension (PAH) is defined as a mean pulmonary arterial pressure of greater than 25 mm Hg at rest or 30 mm Hg with exercise, with an elevated pulmonary vascular resistance (PVR) greater than 3 Wood units. Although pulmonary pressures may be elevated in many conditions, PAH fundamentally requires changes in the pulmonary vasculature. Mean pressures of 26 to 40 mm Hg are considered mild; 41 to 55 mm Hg, moderate; and greater than 55 mm Hg, severe.

Although the inciting factor may be from any number of conditions, PAH is due to progressive increase of PVR, leading to increased right ventricle (RV) pressure load. As PAH progresses, the RV is unable to compensate, leading initially to exertional symptoms (usually dyspnea) but eventually to florid right heart failure, cardiogenic shock, and death.

The diagnosis of PAH continues to be a challenge, predominantly because of nonspecific initial symptoms. Although pathologic findings are definitive for the diagnosis, routine biopsies are not performed, and therefore noninvasive imaging is essential for diagnosis. Largely, this is achieved via echocardiography, but this is not ordered unless clinical suspicion of PAH is high. Other imaging modalities are essential in increasing or decreasing the index of suspicion. Once PAH is suspected, imaging is also essential for identifying the underlying etiology and comorbid conditions. However, evaluation of the degree of pulmonary pressure elevation, changes in PVR, and any contribution of left-sided heart disease is best done by hemodynamic catheterization (right heart catheterization), especially if considering PAH-specific therapy.

Etiology and Classification

PAH can be usefully classified according to the predominant site of pathologic insult, into precapillary and postcapillary causes (Box 53.1). Precapillary causes include small-vessel vasculopathy affecting the arterioles, thrombotic or embolic disease, proximal vascular obstruction by tumor or vasculitis, congenital heart disease (CHD), and pleuroparenchymal disease. Postcapillary causes of pulmonary hypertension include causes of chronically raised pulmonary venous pressure, such as left ventricular failure, valvular heart disease, atrial myxoma, mediastinal fibrosis, and, rarely, congenital venous stenosis, as well as predominantly postcapillary vasculopathies, such as pulmonary venoocclusive disease, and pulmonary capillary hemangiomatosis (PCH).

A more clinically based classification of pulmonary hypertension has been developed and refined, aiming to individualize different categories sharing similarities in pathophysiologic mechanisms, clinical presentation, and therapeutic options. These two classifications inevitably bear many similarities. The World Health Organization meeting in 1973 was the first to endorse standardized nomenclature.[1] Since then, the clinical classification has been reclassified multiple times. The most recent classification system was devised in 2009 in Dana Point, California, and was essentially maintained, with some minor adjustments, at the Fifth World Symposium on Pulmonary Hypertension in Nice, France (Box 53.2).[2,3] The last three iterations have largely been minor reclassifications to try to better align the pathophysiology of PAH in different conditions.

Group 1 PAH is a varied group of underlying conditions that result in increased pulmonary vascular tone from intrinsic issues in the pulmonary vasomotor tone or a secondary increase in PVR from an increase in pulmonary vascular flow. Group 2 is pulmonary hypertension related to left-sided heart disease, whereas pulmonary hypertension associated with pulmonary parenchymal disease and/or hypoxemia is group 3. Chronic thrombotic or embolic diseases comprise group 4, and group 5 is a heterogeneous group with multifactorial or unclear mechanisms (see Box 53.2).

Some important developments in the understanding of group 1 PAH over the years include recognition of specific genetic mutations associated with PAH, as well as drug- and toxin-mediated PAH. Familial PAH is an autosomal-dominant condition with incomplete penetrance, caused in 50% of cases by mutations in the bone morphogenetic protein receptor type II, and it is clinically and radiologically indistinguishable from idiopathic PAH.[4] The most recognized drugs associated with PAH are the anorexigenic drugs, namely, aminorex fumarate, fenfluramine, and dexfenfluramine. Cocaine, amphetamine, and chemotherapeutic agents have also been implicated.

Group 1 PAH may also develop from a sustained congenital left-to-right shunt. This includes both high-pressure shunts, such as truncus arteriosus, ventricular septal defects, and patent ductus arteriosus (PDA), and low-pressure high-flow shunts, such as atrial septal defects and partial anomalous pulmonary venous return. Other conditions, such as chronic renal failure, portopulmonary hypertension, and thyrotoxicosis, which increase pulmonary blood flow, can also result in pulmonary hypertension.

Initially, the presence of a shunt exposes the pulmonary circulation to high flow, preventing it from adapting normally to extrauterine life. Ongoing high flow during extended periods results in a progressive pulmonary vasculopathy with associated in situ thrombosis. The position and size of the cardiac defect and the magnitude of the shunt govern the time taken for these changes to occur. Left uncorrected, rising pulmonary arterial pressures lead to bidirectional and then reversed flow across the shunt (Eisenmenger syndrome). Even after apparently effective corrective surgery, patients may go on to develop significant pulmonary hypertension.

Pulmonary hypertension occurs in a wide variety of collagen vascular diseases and confers a worse prognosis. Incidences vary among the diseases but can be as high as 12% in patients with the limited form of scleroderma.[5] Pulmonary hypertension is

*The editors and publisher would like to thank Drs. Nicholas J. Screaton and Deepa Gopalan for contributing material on this topic to the prior edition of this work. It has served as the foundation for the current chapter.

BOX 53.1 CAUSES OF PULMONARY HYPERTENSION

PRECAPILLARY HYPERTENSION

Small-vessel disease
- Idiopathic pulmonary arterial hypertension
- Portopulmonary hypertension
- Anorexigen abuse
- Connective tissue associated
- Human immunodeficiency virus infection

Pulmonary arterial obstruction and stenosis
- Chronic thromboembolic disease
- Nonthrombotic emboli (metastatic neoplasm, parasites, talc)
- Sickle cell disease

Increased blood flow
- Congenital heart disease or shunts

Pleuropulmonary disease
- Chronic obstructive pulmonary disease
- Interstitial lung disease
- Bronchiectasis, cystic fibrosis

Chest wall deformities

Alveolar hypoventilation
- Neuromuscular disease
- Obesity
- Obstructive sleep apnea

POSTCAPILLARY HYPERTENSION

Pulmonary venoocclusive disease
Pulmonary capillary hemangiomatosis
Left-sided heart failure
- Mitral valve disease
- Myxoma

Mediastinal fibrosis
Congenital venous stenosis
Anomalous pulmonary venous connections

BOX 53.2 CLINICAL CLASSIFICATION OF PULMONARY HYPERTENSION (NICE, 2013)

Group 1. Pulmonary arterial hypertension
- 1.1. Idiopathic
- 1.2. Heritable
- 1.3. Drug and toxin induced
- 1.4. Associated with
  - 1.4.1. Collagen vascular disease
  - 1.4.2. Human immunodeficiency virus infection
  - 1.4.3. Portal hypertension
  - 1.4.4. Congenital heart disease
  - 1.4.5. Schistosomiasis
  - 1.4.6. Chronic hemolytic anemia
- 1.5. Pulmonary venoocclusive disease or pulmonary capillary hemangiomatosis
- 1.6. Persistent pulmonary hypertension of the newborn

Group 2. Pulmonary hypertension with left-sided heart disease
- 2.1. Systolic dysfunction
- 2.2. Diastolic dysfunction
- 2.3. Left-sided valvular heart disease
- 2.4. Congenital/acquired left ventricular inflow or outflow obstruction or congenital cardiomyopathy

Group 3. Pulmonary hypertension associated with lung disease or hypoxemia
- 3.1. Chronic obstructive pulmonary disease
- 3.2. Interstitial lung disease
- 3.3. Other pulmonary diseases with mixed restrictive and obstructive pattern
- 3.4. Sleep-disordered breathing
- 3.5. Alveolar hypoventilation disorders
- 3.6. Chronic exposure to high altitude
- 3.7. Developmental abnormalities

Group 4. Pulmonary hypertension resulting from chronic thrombotic or embolic disease

Group 5. Pulmonary hypertension with unclear, multifactorial mechanisms
- 5.1. Hematologic disorders: myeloproliferative disorders, splenectomy
- 5.2. Systemic disorders: sarcoidosis, Langerhans cell histiocytosis, lymphangioleiomyomatosis, neurofibromatosis, vasculitis
- 5.3. Metabolic disorders: glycogen storage disease, Gaucher disease, thyroid disorders
- 5.4. Others: compression of pulmonary vessels, fibrosing mediastinitis, chronic renal failure on dialysis, segmental pulmonary hypertension

the cause of up to 50% of disease-related deaths in patients with limited scleroderma. Isolated pulmonary hypertension is less common in diffuse scleroderma; when it is present, it is often seen in patients with the nucleolar antibody anti-U3 ribonucleoprotein.[6] In mixed connective tissue disease (CTD), one long-term follow-up study found that pulmonary hypertension was the most common cause of death, occurring in 38% of patients.[7] Although elevated PA pressures can be seen with any CTD, it is less frequently seen in systemic lupus erythematosus, rheumatoid arthritis (RA), and polymyositis. In RA, pulmonary hypertension is more frequently a late manifestation of rheumatoid interstitial lung disease than of vasculopathic changes. Systemic lupus erythematosus can be complicated by a hypercoagulable state; therefore chronic thromboembolic pulmonary hypertension (CTEPH) should always be considered an alternative cause of pulmonary hypertension in these patients.

Pulmonary hypertension is thought to affect 0.1% of the human immunodeficiency virus (HIV)-infected population annually, representing a relative risk of 500, compared with an HIV-negative individual.[8,9] Pulmonary thromboembolic disease represents another cause of pulmonary hypertension in patients with chronic HIV infection, being present in 3% of patients with pulmonary hypertension and HIV infection or acquired immune deficiency syndrome.[10,11]

Pulmonary venoocclusive disease (PVOD) and PCH are considered together because they share several common features, particularly in relation to their management. Although an arterial component is usually present, both diseases predominantly affect the venules immediately downstream from the capillary bed. The venous occlusion in PCH is due to an abnormal uncontrolled proliferation of capillaries that infiltrate the interstitium, the vessels, and, less commonly, the airways. In both PVOD and PCH, venous occlusion results in increased transcapillary hydrostatic pressure, with consequent focal areas of edema and hemorrhage. There is limited epidemiologic data available on both diseases. PVOD is rare, with an incidence of 0.1 to 0.3 per million, although up to 5% to 10% of idiopathic PAH patients have been found on pathology to have PVOD.[12–17] PCH is rarer still. Unlike idiopathic PAH, one-third of PVOD cases occur in children, with equal sex distribution; there is a (2:1) male predominance in adult patients.[18]

The etiology of both diseases is unknown and may be multifactorial. Cytotoxic drugs, including bleomycin,[19] herbal "bush" tea,[20] bone marrow transplantation, and thoracic radiotherapy have all been implicated in PVOD, although the majority of cases are currently considered idiopathic. Clinically, the triad of severe PAH, radiographic evidence of pulmonary edema, and normal pulmonary artery occlusion pressure is considered to be diagnostic of PVOD. In conjunction, these findings can obviate the need for tissue diagnosis. However, many patients with PVOD do not have this triad. As these diseases are often difficult to distinguish from idiopathic pulmonary hypertension and from interstitial lung disease, radiologic investigations, particularly computed tomography (CT), have an important role to play in diagnosis.

Many chronic lung conditions can lead to pulmonary hypertension through an increase in PVR. This is partly due to destruction of the vascular bed and partly due to vascular remodeling in response to chronic alveolar hypoxia. Although the resulting pulmonary hypertension is often mild and associated with a preserved cardiac output, its presence worsens prognosis. Approximately 90% of patients with severe chronic obstructive pulmonary disease will have pulmonary hypertension.[21]

In CTEPH thrombi from untreated or recurrent acute emboli organize and become incorporated into the wall of the pulmonary arteries. Thrombi in smaller vessels often recanalize, forming a trabecular mesh. This process, which may occur in repeated cycles, leaves endothelialized residua that obstruct or narrow pulmonary arteries, resulting in progressive pulmonary hypertension, hypoxemia, and right-sided heart failure.[22,23] The true prevalence of CTEPH is unknown as many cases may remain undiagnosed. CTEPH may complicate up to 3.8% of cases of acute pulmonary embolism[24] and carries a poor prognosis if it is left untreated.[25]

The importance of aggressively identifying etiology cannot be understated. In particular, PAH-specific vasodilator therapy has been indicated in group 1 (excluding PVOD and PCH). Vasodilator therapy has been studied inconsistently in group 3 (PAH associated with parenchymal lung disease) or group 4 (CTEPH), although it is likely still efficacious. Postcapillary causes of PAH (PVOD, PCH, and group 2 PAH) do not typically benefit from pulmonary vasodilator therapy. Furthermore, the approach to transplantation is varied based on the underlying etiology (single-lung vs. double-lung transplantation vs. multiorgan transplantation).

Epidemiology

Given the challenges in recognition and diagnosis, the true incidence and prevalence have been difficult to capture. There are no large international registries, and national registries have some variance. In addition, most of the registry data has been limited to group 1 PAH, and the epidemiology of other PAH groups is still not entirely clear. However, group 1 PAH still remains a relatively rare disease with an annual incidence of 1.1 to 3.6 per million population and a prevalence of 6.6 to 52 per million population.[26–31] There is a female preponderance (anywhere from 60%–80%) that has been fairly consistent over time.[32] Although early registries suggested this to be a disease of the young, the median age of more recent registries seems to range from 50 to 65 years of age.

Idiopathic PAH in these registries represents anywhere from 39% to 60% of all group 1 PAH patients, with anywhere from 11% to 43% being PAH associated with CHD and 15% to 30% PAH associated with CTD.[32] Familial or heritable PAH is an increasingly recognized etiology for group 1 PAH; however, idiopathic cases outnumber familial cases of pulmonary hypertension by more than 10:1.

Pathophysiology

At birth the pulmonary arterial circulation is histologically similar to the systemic circulation. However, as the newborn adapts to extrauterine life, the pulmonary arterial circulation rapidly develops into a high-flow low-pressure system. Increase in vascular compliance allows the pulmonary circulation to accommodate systemic cardiac outputs with little rise in pulmonary arterial pressure.

Pulmonary arteries more than 1 mm in diameter have walls that consist of numerous parallel elastic laminae. These "elastic" arteries act predominantly as conductance vessels and contribute little to resistance. As the vessel diameter narrows to between 1 mm and 100 μm, the elastic component is replaced by smooth muscle. The precapillary "muscular" arteries contribute significantly to PVR and are, in health, the site of the greatest pressure drop within the circulation. In general, the muscular arteries or resistance vessels are also the site most affected in disease, as occurs in idiopathic PAH.

PAH, regardless of cause, results in dilation of the large elastic pulmonary arteries and may result in pulmonary arterial atherosclerosis. Other common findings include intimal fibrosis of elastic and large muscular arteries and thickening of the media of small muscular arteries. In addition to muscle hypertrophy-hyperplasia, several abnormalities are often present in small- to medium-sized muscular arteries that together characterize plexogenic pulmonary arteriopathy. These abnormalities include cellular intimal proliferation and fibrosis, plexiform lesions, fibrinoid "necrosis," and vasculitis (Fig. 53.1). Plexiform lesions are seen in small supernumerary arteries a short distance beyond their origin from the parent vessel. The lesion consists of a localized focus of vascular dilation associated with an intraluminal plexus of slit-like vascular channels (see Fig. 53.1). This plexogenic arteriopathy is the hallmark of idiopathic PAH and PAH associated with congenital systemic-pulmonary shunts (most commonly CHD). The histologic findings of pulmonary hypertension resulting from chronic thromboembolism include thrombi in various stages of organization in the large and small pulmonary arteries. The most common findings in small pulmonary vessels are medial hypertrophy and intimal fibrosis, which may be eccentric, concentric, or in a colander pattern consistent with recanalized thrombus (Fig. 53.2). Venoocclusive disease is characterized by stenosis or obliteration of the lumina of small pulmonary veins and venules by intimal fibrous tissue (Fig. 53.3). Other common findings are engorged venules, dilated lymphatics, and septal thickening (see Fig. 53.3). Histologic evidence of PAH is usually present, but changes of plexogenic arteriopathy are absent. The main histologic abnormality in PCH consists of patchy interstitial proliferation of thin-walled blood vessels the size of capillaries. The vessels appear to invade the walls of pulmonary veins and to a lesser extent the pulmonary arteries. The venular infiltration is often accompanied by intimal fibrosis, which may lead to stenosis.

Clinical Presentation and Outcomes

Pulmonary hypertension is often difficult to diagnose because it manifests insidiously with nonspecific clinical findings. Patients initially complain of exertional breathlessness, representing right-sided cardiac insufficiency in the face of an increased workload. As disease progresses, exercise tolerance steadily deteriorates, and exertional syncope or chest pain may develop. Once the right ventricle fails to sustain an appropriate cardiac output at rest, patients develop ongoing symptoms of overt right-sided heart failure, including fatigue, loss of appetite, ascites, and pedal edema. Hence, not uncommonly, pulmonary hypertension can be

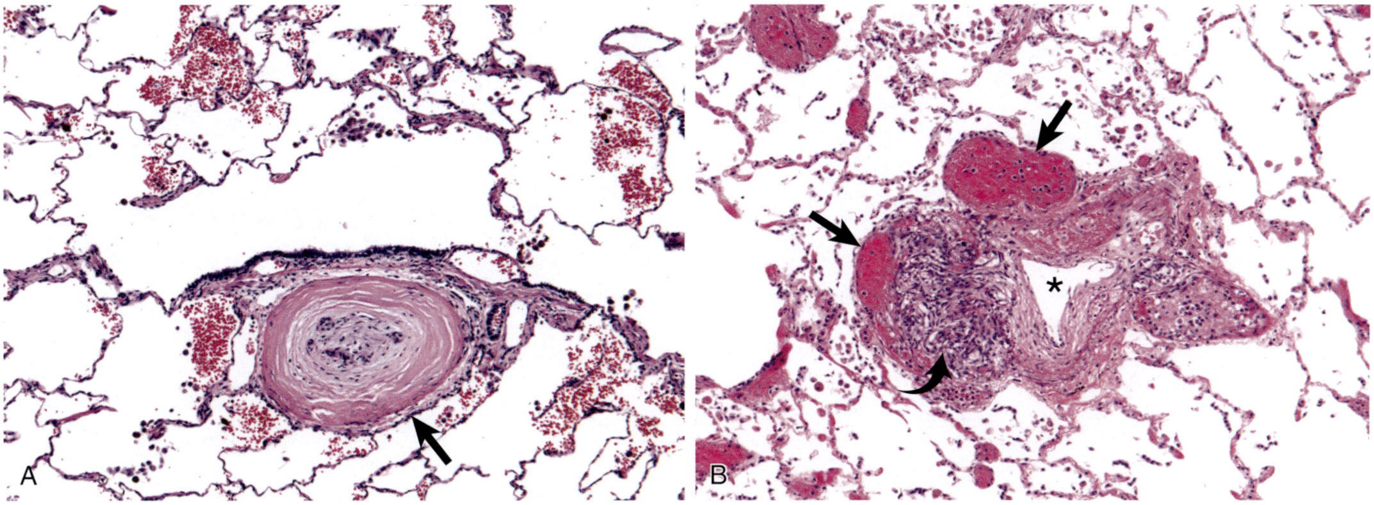

Fig. 53.1 Histologic findings of pulmonary arterial hypertension (PAH). (A) Histologic specimen (hematoxylin-eosin stain, original magnification ×100) in patient with PAH shows concentric laminar fibrosis. The normal pulmonary artery *(arrow)* is replaced by a concentrically arranged intimal proliferation of myofibroblasts and collagen with occlusion of the lumen and atrophy of the arterial media. (B) Histologic specimen (hematoxylin-eosin stain, original magnification ×100) shows plexiform and dilation lesions. The plexiform lesion *(curved arrow)* consists of an aneurysmal segment of pulmonary artery *(asterisk)* that is typically filled with a knot-like proliferation of endothelium-like cells. Its appearance has been likened to that of a renal glomerulus. The degree of cellularity may vary, and thrombi can sometimes be seen. Dilation lesions *(straight arrows)* are identified in their characteristic position around the plexiform lesion and probably represent postobstructive or bypass microaneurysms. *(Courtesy Dr. John English, Department of Pathology, Vancouver General Hospital, Vancouver, Canada.)*

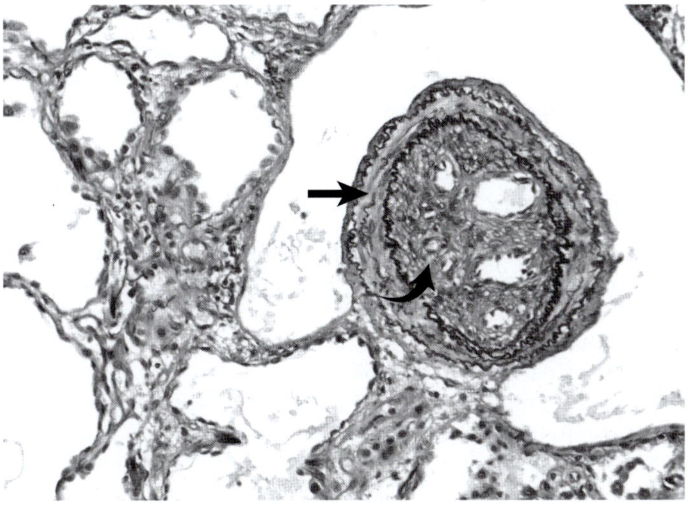

Fig. 53.2 Recanalized thrombus in pulmonary arterial hypertension. Histologic specimen (elastic stain, original magnification ×200) shows pulmonary artery with recanalized thrombus ("colander lesion"). The arterial lumen *(curved arrow)* is occupied by a fibroproliferative lesion that represents an old organized thrombus. The sharply punched-out spaces are recanalized lumina that give the lesion its name and also allow pathologists to distinguish it from a plexiform lesion. The arterial tunica media *(straight arrow)* is marginally hypertrophic. *(Courtesy Dr. John English, Department of Pathology, Vancouver General Hospital, Vancouver, Canada.)*

misdiagnosed as asthma, hyperventilation syndrome, or lack of fitness. The delay in diagnosis compounded by the fact that the pulmonary circulation has an extensive reserve means that by the time the diagnosis is made, much of the circulation has already been compromised.

Prognosis in PAH is still poor long term but has improved over time. National Institutes of Health registry data published in 1991 estimated median survival of 2.8 years for idiopathic PAH, with 1-year, 3-year, and 5-year survival rates of 68%, 48%, and 34%, respectively.[33] More recent data from the REVEAL Registry (Registry to Evaluate Early and Long-Term PAH Disease Management) shows 1-year, 3-year, and 5-year survival rates of 85%, 68%, and 57%, respectively.[34] Prognosis does vary based on etiology, with PAH associated with CHD or drugs and toxins having a better long-term prognosis and PAH associated with portopulmonary hypertension and CTD having a worse long-term prognosis, compared with idiopathic PAH, heritable PAH, or PAH associated with HIV (all with similar prognosis). The prognosis in severe portopulmonary hypertension (coexisting portal hypertension and PAH) is poor, with median survival of 6 months and 5-year survival of 10% in one series,[35] compared with a 5-year survival of 50% for patients with hepatopulmonary syndrome (hypoxemia caused by pulmonary vasodilation and shunting in the setting of liver disease).[36] There are also risk stratification tools proposed by guideline committees that include clinical features (progression of symptoms, syncope), functional parameters (New York Heart Association classification, 6-minute walk distance), and hemodynamic parameters and imaging findings. Specifically, RA area greater than 26 cm^2 and presence of pericardial effusion are considered a high risk for early mortality (1-year mortality >10%).[37]

Synopsis of Treatment Options

Originally, treatment for PAH was limited to anticoagulation, calcium channel blockers,[38,39] oxygen, and diuretics for symptomatic relief. This is still often the guideline-directed medical

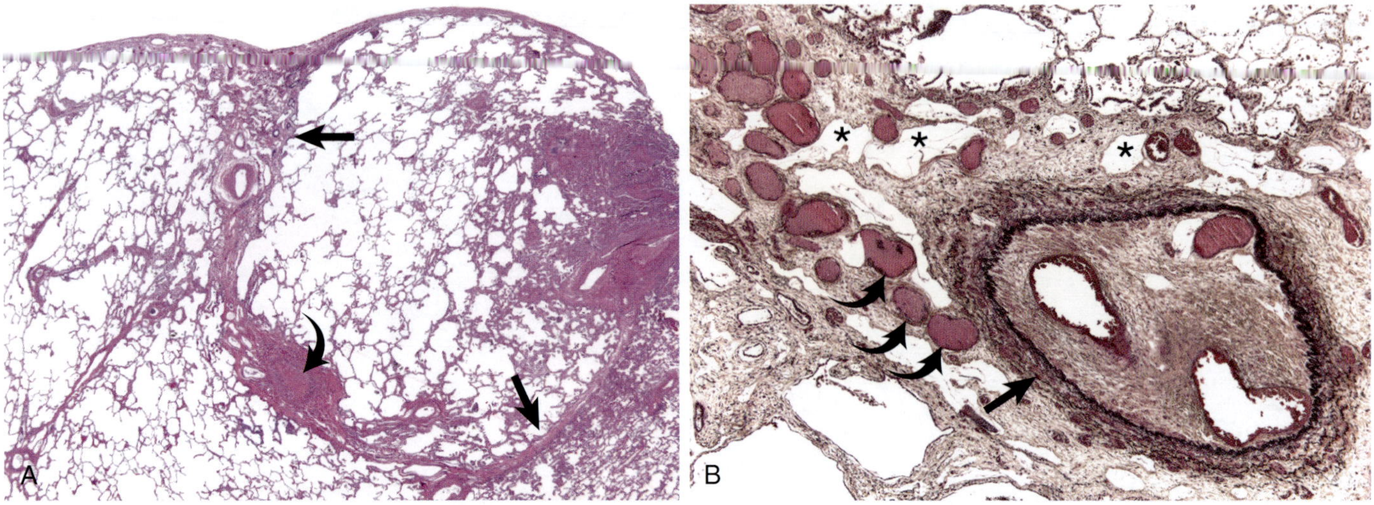

Fig. 53.3 Venoocclusive disease. (A) Low-power photomicrograph (hematoxylin-eosin stain, original magnification ×12.5) demonstrates thickening of the interlobular septa *(straight arrows)*. Within the thickened septum is a vein that is totally occluded by an old, organized thrombus *(curved arrow)*. (B) Medium-power photomicrograph (Movat pentachrome stain) shows an interlobular septal vein *(straight arrow)* that contains an old organized thrombus with several recanalization lumina. Surrounding the vein is a leash of dilated and congested venules *(curved arrows)* and dilated lymphatic channels *(asterisks)*. Some of the pulmonary parenchyma adjacent to the vein is fibrotic. *(Courtesy Dr. John English, Department of Pathology, Vancouver General Hospital, Vancouver, Canada.)*

therapy for patients who show pulmonary vasoreactivity on testing during right heart catheterization. However, targeted therapies have revolutionized the management of patients for many causes. Targeted therapies modify disease by reversal of the vascular remodeling process, inhibiting platelet aggregation, and causing vasodilatation. The first of these, intravenous epoprostenol, has proven benefits in exercise tolerance, hemodynamics, and survival.[40,41] Subsequent modifications to improve the stability of the compound have allowed improvement in ease of administration; however, it still remains a continuous infusion with all of the associated risks. Other prostanoids, such as treprostinil (intravenous, subcutaneous, inhaled, and oral formulations) and inhaled iloprost, have subsequently been developed and also appear to be effective in improving functional capacity and survival.[42–44] Other classes of vasodilators, such as dual endothelin receptor antagonists, selective endothelin receptor antagonists, phosphodiesterase inhibitors, and cyclic guanosine monophosphate antagonists have also been shown to be efficacious in improving functional capacity.[45,46] These are generally administered orally and are therefore easier to take with fewer logistical issues than continuous infusions. As such, targeted therapy is now more accessible to a wider proportion of patients with pulmonary hypertension, reinforcing the need to make an early diagnosis. Also, combination therapy has been shown to be synergistic and is often used.[47–61]

Apart from lung transplantation, long-term oxygen therapy is the only measure that has been shown to significantly improve survival in patients with PAH associated with parenchymal lung disease (group 3 PAH).[62,63] In the diagnostic workup of patients being considered for lung transplantation, particularly in the setting of emphysema, CT permits detection of small primary lung cancers that are not radiographically apparent and can thus significantly influence management. When unilateral lung transplantation is being considered, perfusion scintigraphy is widely used to select the side with the most compromised function.

The treatment of CTEPH is discussed in detail in Chapter 51.

Manifestations of the Disease

Given the significant crossover in imaging findings of PAH among different subtypes, the remainder of the chapter is organized by specific imaging modalities. As many of the comorbid or inciting disease states, such as acute and chronic pulmonary thromboembolism, intrinsic lung pathologies, and so forth, are discussed separately; specific diagnostic or prognostic findings will be emphasized here.

RADIOGRAPHY

Chest radiography is usually the initial imaging study in patients with suspected pulmonary hypertension. It is useful to assess heart size, pattern of cardiac chamber dilatation, and enlargement of proximal pulmonary arteries, as well as to detect any underlying pulmonary parenchymal disorder.

The radiographic features of pulmonary hypertension consist of central pulmonary arterial dilatation down to the segmental level, with attenuation of peripheral pulmonary blood vessels, giving rise to "peripheral pruning" (Fig. 53.4). Hilar artery enlargement is assessed by measuring the diameter of the interlobar arteries. The upper limit for the transverse diameter of the right interlobar artery measured from its lateral aspect to the bronchus intermedius is 15 mm in women and 16 mm in men.[64] The transverse diameter of the left interlobar artery is difficult to appreciate on the posteroanterior view. On a lateral view the upper limit measured from the circular lucency of the left upper lobe bronchus to the posterior margin of the vessel is 18 mm.[65]

Calcification within the pulmonary arteries may be seen in pulmonary hypertension associated with intracardiac shunts and usually results from prolonged and severe pulmonary hypertension that has resulted in calcific atherosclerosis.[66] Pulmonary artery calcification is usually associated with high PVR and irreversible vascular disease.[66]

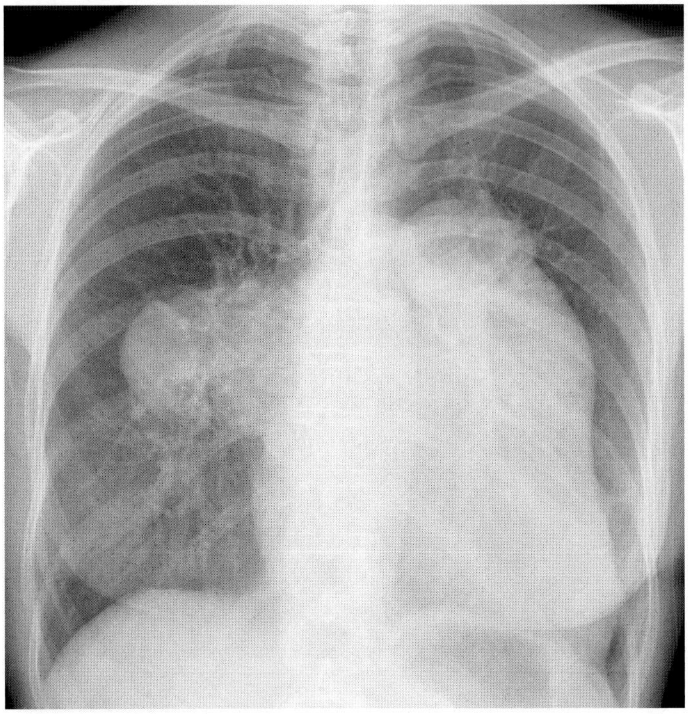

Fig. 53.4 Idiopathic pulmonary arterial hypertension. Posteroanterior chest radiograph demonstrates gross enlargement of the proximal pulmonary arteries with tapering of the peripheral vasculature (peripheral pruning) and cardiomegaly resulting from dilated right-sided heart chambers.

Heart size as assessed by cardiothoracic ratio may be normal or enlarged in pulmonary hypertension. Enlargement of the right ventricle causes reduction of the retrosternal clear space on the lateral radiograph. Right atrial dilatation is seen as a widening of the right border of the heart on the frontal projection. Enlargement of the right atrial appendage causes an increase in the retrosternal opacity above the expected location of the right ventricle on the lateral projection.

There is no correlation between the extent of the radiographic abnormalities and the degree of pulmonary hypertension.[67] The accuracy of the chest radiograph in detecting pulmonary hypertension is unknown.

The chest radiograph is useful in defining coexistent conditions, such as pulmonary venous congestion, chest wall and vertebral deformities, emphysema, interstitial lung fibrosis, and other parenchymal and pleural abnormalities. In 90% of patients with idiopathic PAH, the chest radiograph is abnormal at the time of diagnosis.[68] The typical features include enlarged proximal pulmonary arteries with peripheral pruning, cardiomegaly with right-sided chamber enlargement, and pulmonary oligemia (Fig. 53.5). The lungs are otherwise normal, enabling differentiation from pulmonary hypertension secondary to parenchymal lung disease.

Congenital Systemic-Pulmonary Shunts (Congenital Heart Disease)

The radiographic features of pulmonary hypertension caused by chronic shunt physiology include the familiar complex of a dilated pulmonary trunk and central pulmonary arteries.[69] Increased flow results initially in prominence of peripheral pulmonary vessels in proportion to the proximal vessels. On radiographic examination, pulmonary plethora is characterized by vessels being identifiable within 2 cm of the pleural surface. Vasculopathy and the development of pulmonary hypertension may be difficult to identify on the chest radiograph. Peripheral oligemia with rapid tapering of the peripheral vessels and disparity between the proximal and distal calibers is a late manifestation often indicating shunt reversal and Eisenmenger syndrome.

The right ventricle and atrium typically enlarge in proportion to the degree of volume overload. Paradoxically, increased PVR and the development of pulmonary hypertension may lead to reduction in size of the cardiac silhouette.[69]

Atrioseptal defects are characterized by cardiomegaly with enlargement of the right atrium and ventricle (Fig. 53.6); ventriculoseptal defects, by right ventricular hypertrophy and dilatation of the atria and eventually the left ventricle; and PDA, by enlargement of the left atrium, left ventricle, and aortic arch. In addition, there may be calcification of the ductus diverticulum.[70]

Pulmonary Venoocclusive Disease and Pulmonary Capillary Hemangiomatosis

The specific diagnosis of PVOD is suggested radiographically when features of PAH are accompanied by evidence of diffuse pulmonary interstitial edema and a normal-sized left atrium.[71,72] Back-pressure from the obstructed venular side of the pulmonary circulation results in dilatation of the right-sided heart chambers and central pulmonary arteries, pleural effusions, and signs of pulmonary interstitial edema. The central pulmonary veins and the left atrium are not enlarged, in contrast to patients with mitral stenosis, cor triatriatum, or left atrial myxoma. Mediastinal lymphadenopathy caused by vascular congestion may be present.

In PCH the chest radiograph shows the typical features of pulmonary hypertension. In addition, a reticulonodular or fine nodular pattern may be present, which can suggest an interstitial process.

Left-Sided Heart Disease

Left-sided cardiac diseases, such as myocardial dysfunction, mitral valve disease (Fig. 53.7), and left atrial myxoma, are characterized by pulmonary venous hypertension, interstitial edema, and pleural effusions. Normally, in the erect position the hydrostatic pressure gradient causes higher flow and therefore greater vessel caliber in the dependent lung regions. Pulmonary venous hypertension results in loss or reversal of this normal-caliber gradient, with narrowing of lower lobe and distention of upper lobe vessels. This so-called cephalization, upper zone vascular distention or recruitment, is present in 95% of patients with critical mitral stenosis[73] and 33% to 76% of patients with mild left ventricular dysfunction admitted to coronary care.[65,74] Upper zone vascular distention is the earliest radiographic feature of pulmonary venous hypertension.

The development of pulmonary interstitial edema is characterized by thickening of the interlobular septa (Kerley B lines) and loss of the sharp margins of vessels and bronchi (perihilar haze and peribronchial cuffing). Finally, frank pulmonary edema results in airspace filling.

The presence of left atrial enlargement can help distinguish left-sided cardiac lesions from PVOD. Hemosiderosis caused by long-standing pulmonary venous hypertension produces fine reticular opacities on chest radiographs. Small (1–3 mm) calcified ossific nodules are the hallmark of mitral stenosis but are now rarely seen. In rare cases a left atrial myxoma is manifested as a heavily calcified mass.

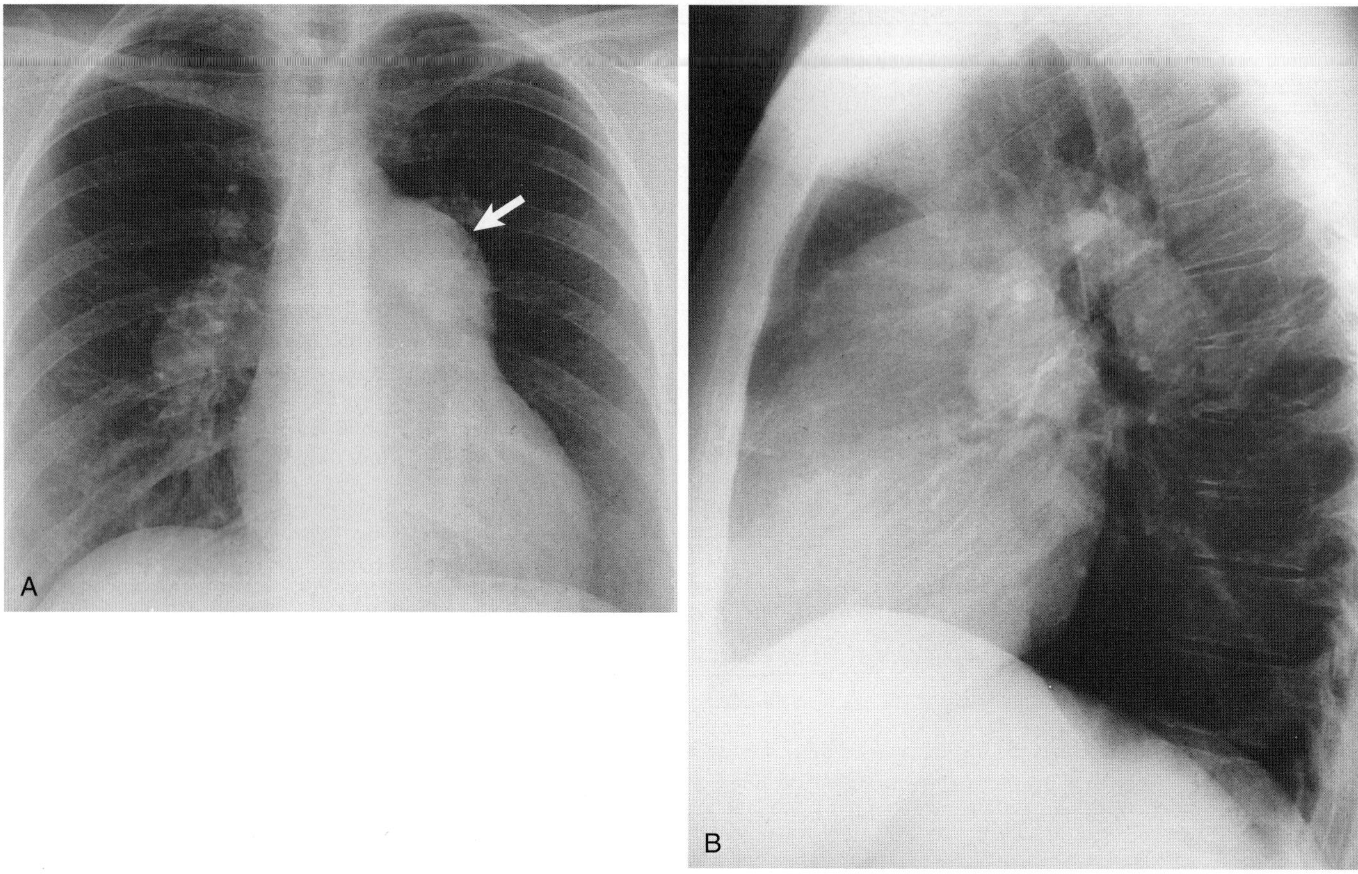

Fig. 53.5 Pulmonary arterial hypertension (PAH) in a woman with idiopathic PAH. Posteroanterior (A) and lateral (B) chest radiographs show enlargement of the central pulmonary arteries with rapid tapering of the vessels. On the posteroanterior view, marked enlargement of the main pulmonary artery results in a focal convexity *(arrow)* immediately below the level of the aortic arch. On the lateral view, right ventricular enlargement and dilation of the pulmonary outflow tract result in filling of the lower retrosternal clear space. *(From Müller NL, Fraser RS, Colman NC, Paré PD.* Radiologic Diagnosis of Diseases of the Chest. *Philadelphia: WB Saunders; 2001.)*

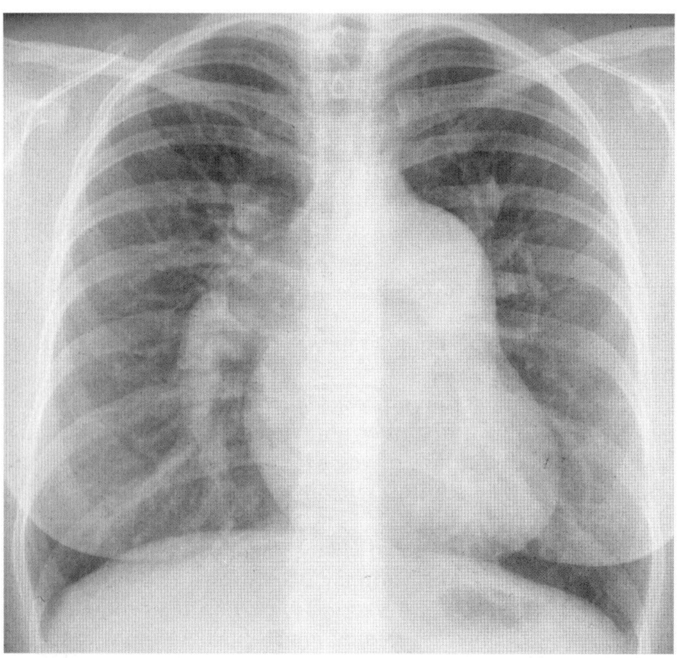

Fig. 53.6 Pulmonary hypertension caused by atrial septal defect. Chest radiograph shows cardiomegaly and enlarged central pulmonary arteries.

Chronic Thromboembolic Pulmonary Hypertension

Chest radiography in CTEPH reveals the familiar complex of cardiomegaly and right-sided chamber dilatation. The central pulmonary arteries may be asymmetrically enlarged with abrupt cutoff. The peripheral pulmonary vessels are disorganized with regional areas of hypoperfusion and hyperperfusion. Pleural thickening or effusions and peripheral scarring from previous infarction and atelectasis may be present.[75] Please see Chapter 51 for a more complete discussion of CTEPH.

COMPUTED TOMOGRAPHY

CT is an important tool for the assessment of patients with suspected pulmonary hypertension. The combination of CT pulmonary angiography and high-resolution CT allows a comprehensive assessment of the pulmonary vasculature and lung parenchyma, an assessment of the pattern of cardiac chamber dilatation and the severity of tricuspid regurgitation, and a limited evaluation of right-sided heart function.[76]

Dilation of central pulmonary arteries is a cardinal sign of pulmonary hypertension on CT and magnetic resonance imaging (MRI) (Fig. 53.8). On CT the diameter of the main pulmonary artery is most frequently measured at the level of its bifurcation at a right angle to its long axis and just lateral to the ascending

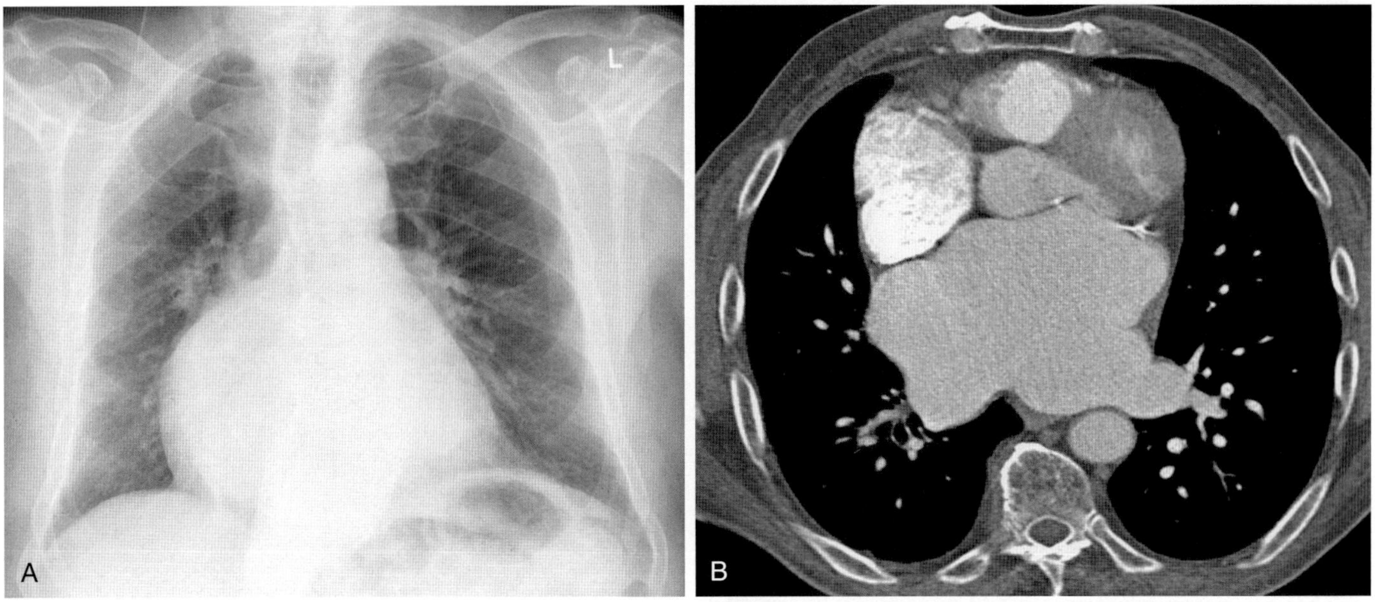

Fig. 53.7 Mitral stenosis and regurgitation. (A) Chest radiograph in a patient with mitral stenosis and regurgitation with classic features of left atrial enlargement, including a double right border of the heart, splaying of the carina, and straightening of the left heart border resulting from enlargement of left atrial appendage. (B) CT image at the level of mitral valve confirms massively enlarged left atrium with calcified mitral valve leaflets, features typical of mitral stenosis and regurgitation.

aorta. The most frequently cited study evaluating absolute pulmonary artery size suggests that a main pulmonary artery of 29 mm or larger on CT is suggestive of pulmonary hypertension with a sensitivity of 69% to 87% and a specificity of 89% to 100%.[77] However, more recent studies have called use of absolute pulmonary artery size into question. A study from 2013 suggested that using a cutoff of greater than or equal to 29.5 mm resulted in only a specificity of 79.4%, and the authors suggested using a cutoff of greater than or equal to 32 mm, which results in a specificity of 90.2%.[78] A study from 2016 demonstrated an even lower specificity of 62% when using the same cutoff, and the authors suggested that such evaluation of absolute pulmonary artery diameter may not be adequate for clinical use.[79] It is our current clinical practice to suggest the possibility of PAH when the main pulmonary artery diameter is greater than or equal to 32.5 mm, while recognizing that a significant number of these patients will be considered falsely positive after evaluation by echocardiography. Of interest, despite these issues with pulmonary artery size, there is some evidence that changes in size over time in an individual patient may have significant prognostic value, with one study demonstrating increasing mortality (hazard ratio, 1.33) for every 1-mm increase in pulmonary artery size over time.[80]

An alternative simple method is to assess the relative diameters of pulmonary artery and thoracic aorta at the same anatomic level. When pulmonary artery diameter exceeds that of the thoracic aorta, pulmonary hypertension is likely with a specificity of 92% and a positive predictive value of 93%. However, given the propensity for the aorta to dilate, particularly in the elderly, the pulmonary artery to aorta ratio has a relatively low negative predictive value and sensitivity of 44% and 70%, respectively.[81]

Within the lungs, the diameter of the pulmonary artery should be approximately equal to that of its neighboring bronchus in normal subjects. In patients with pulmonary hypertension or increased blood flow or volume, significant dilatation of these small vessels relative to adjacent bronchi may be present.[82] There may be concomitant attenuation of peripheral pulmonary vascular markings (pruning). In a study by Tan and colleagues,[83] a main pulmonary artery diameter of 29 mm or more, accompanied by a segmental artery to bronchus ratio of greater than 1 in three of four pulmonary lobes, had a 100% specificity for pulmonary hypertension in patients with intrinsic lung disease.

Cardiac morphology should not be overlooked in evaluating thoracic CT. Dilatation of the right-sided heart chambers and hypertrophy of the right ventricle can be readily appreciated. Although echocardiography and MRI enable assessment of true long and short cardiac axes, measurements have been validated on CT transverse images. The upper limits for the transverse diameter of the right atrium and right ventricle are 35 mm and 45 mm, respectively.[84] The enlarged right ventricle may encroach on the left ventricular cavity, resulting in abnormal systolic and diastolic function of the left ventricle. Enlargement of the central pulmonary veins at the level of the left atrium is usually subjective. Early opacification of the inferior vena cava or hepatic veins on first-pass contrast-enhanced CT almost invariably indicates tricuspid regurgitation (see Fig. 53.8).[85] CT is also reasonably good for detecting intracardiac shunts and anomalous pulmonary venous drainage.

Pericardial thickening or effusion is a frequent finding in patients with severe pulmonary hypertension.[86] Rarely, thrombus may be present in the right atrium or ventricle. Ancillary findings indicating right-sided heart failure are the presence of ascites, features of hepatic congestion and cirrhosis, and peripheral edema.

Idiopathic PAH shows a dilated main pulmonary artery on CT with abrupt tapering of tortuous peripheral pulmonary vessels. As with other forms of pulmonary hypertension, there is right-sided cardiac chamber enlargement that may or may not be associated with tricuspid regurgitation. In a study by Baque-Juston

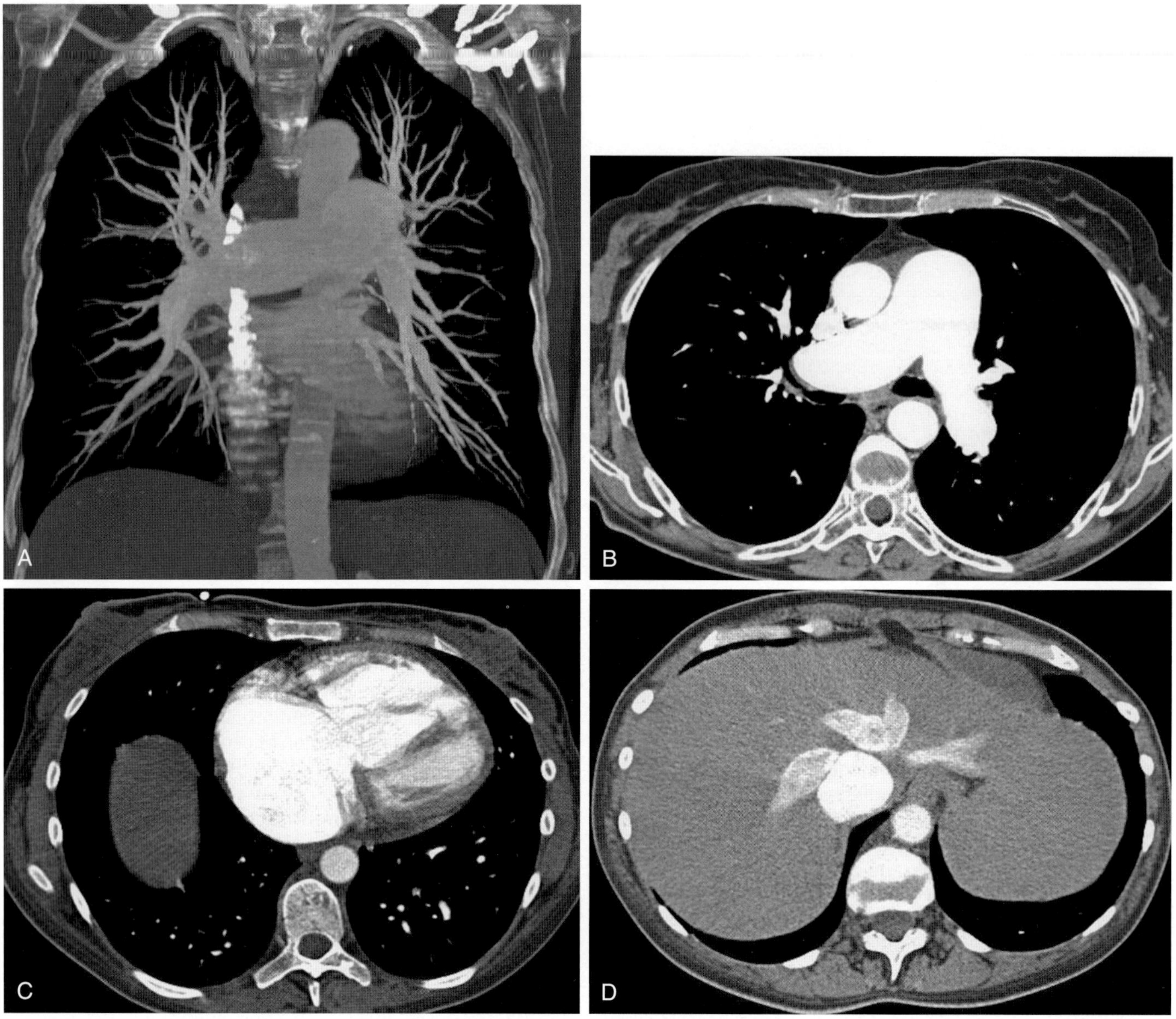

Fig. 53.8 Idiopathic pulmonary arterial hypertension. (A) Coronal maximum-intensity projection image from a CT scan demonstrates enlarged central pulmonary arteries. (B) Contrast-enhanced CT image at the level of the right pulmonary artery demonstrates dilatation of the main pulmonary artery, which is larger than the adjacent ascending aorta. (C) CT image at the level of the tricuspid valve shows enlargement of the right atrium and ventricle with leftward bowing of the interventricular septum. (D) CT image at the level of the liver shows reflux of contrast medium into the inferior vena cava and hepatic veins, indicating tricuspid regurgitation.

and colleagues,[86] moderate pericardial thickening of more than 2 mm or effusion was seen in 53% of a subgroup of patients with severe pulmonary hypertension. The presence of a pericardial effusion is a poor prognostic sign. In general, the lungs are normal; however, cholesterol granulomas are seen in cases of severe pulmonary hypertension and are manifested on CT as small, poorly defined, low-attenuating centrilobular nodules mimicking the appearance of infection, respiratory bronchiolitis, hypersensitivity pneumonitis, or aspiration.[87] Regional variations in parenchymal perfusion can cause a mosaic pattern of lung attenuation.[88]

In situ thrombosis caused by reduced flow in the proximal vessels is often identified on CT in severe idiopathic PAH. It is typically central and nonocclusive, permitting its differentiation from chronic organized emboli in CTEPH, which is usually occlusive and predominates in the lower lobes.[89]

Congenital Systemic-Pulmonary Shunts (Congenital Heart Disease)

Although CT is not the primary imaging modality in patients with known cardiac shunts, it is a front-line investigation in patients with suspected pulmonary hypertension, and therefore careful evaluation for features suggestive of a shunt is essential, with the caveat that CT has limited use in functional evaluation of shunts (Fig. 53.9). Linear calcification and in situ nonocclusive thrombus may be evident in the central pulmonary arteries at

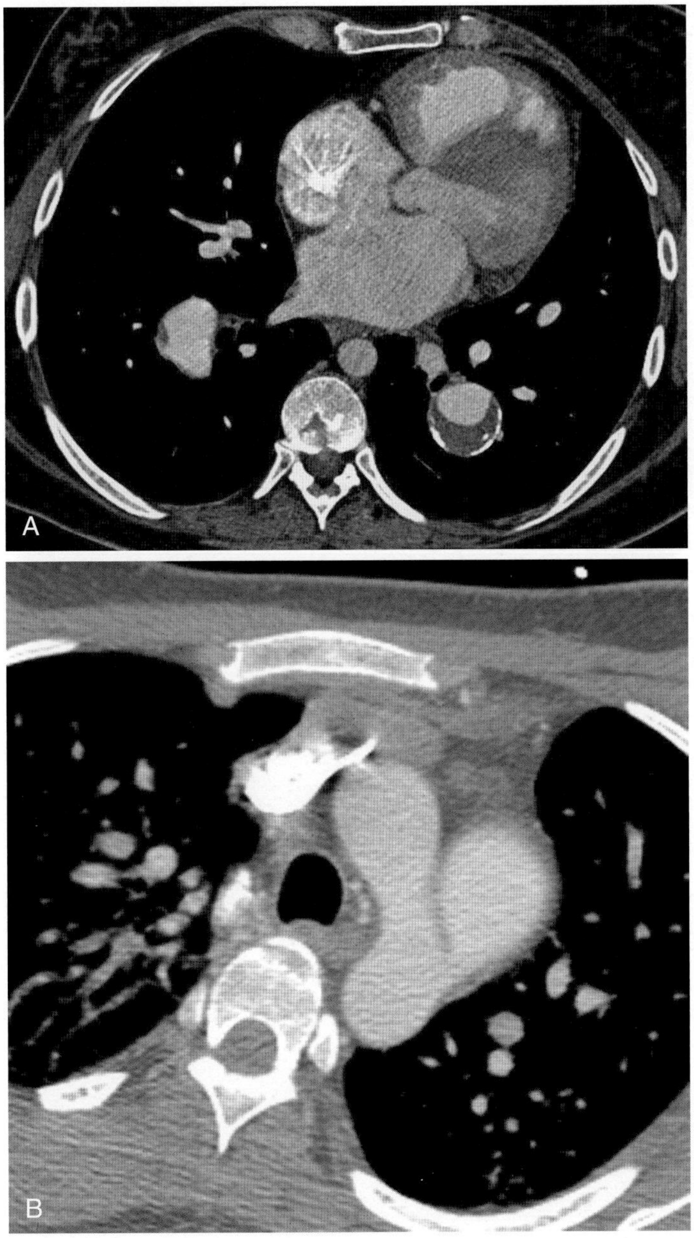

Fig. 53.9 Pulmonary hypertension caused by congenital shunt detected on CT pulmonary angiogram performed as a part of routine workup for pulmonary hypertension. (A) CT angiogram depicts a large atrial septal defect with in situ thrombus in the left lower lobe pulmonary artery. Peripheral calcification is seen around the thrombus. (B) CT angiogram shows a communication between the left pulmonary artery and the aortic isthmus characteristic of a patent ductus arteriosus. *(Fig. 53.9B reproduced with permission from Abbara S, Walker CM. Patent ductus arteriosus. In: Abbara S.* Diagnostic Imaging: Cardiovascular. *2nd ed. Philadelphia: Amirsys; 2013.)*

CT. In case of a PDA, mural calcification or aneurysmal dilatation of the ductus may be identified. A significant challenge in assessing shunts is the limited functional data CT provides.

Pulmonary Venoocclusive Disease and Pulmonary Capillary Hemangiomatosis

PVOD causes interstitial edema and fibrosis resulting from venular obstruction. On CT this is manifested by widespread smooth, interlobular septal thickening, which is both more frequent and extensive than in patients with idiopathic pulmonary hypertension

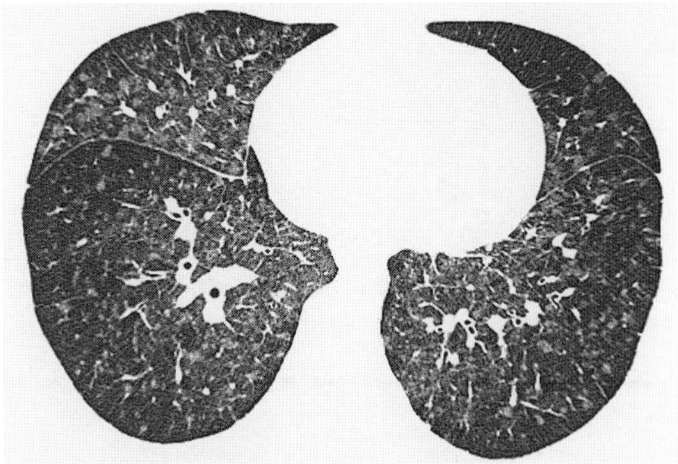

Fig. 53.10 Pulmonary venoocclusive disease. High-resolution CT image in a patient with pulmonary hypertension associated with significant venous involvement shows widespread ground-glass opacities with centrilobular nodules and smooth interlobular septal thickening in histologically proven pulmonary venoocclusive disease.

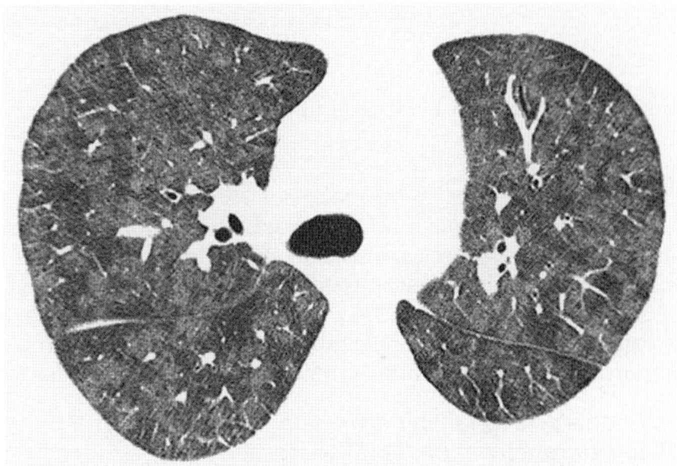

Fig. 53.11 Pulmonary capillary hemangiomatosis (PCH). High-resolution CT image in a patient with pulmonary hypertension associated with significant capillary involvement shows heterogeneous parenchymal attenuation with patchy ground-glass opacity in PCH.

(Fig. 53.10). Other common CT findings include central and gravity-dependent ground-glass opacity, multiple small centrilobular nodules, and areas of consolidation associated with normal-caliber or small central pulmonary veins (see Fig. 53.10).[90,91] Ground-glass opacities are more frequent in PVOD than in other causes of pulmonary hypertension.[88,92] The pathologic correlate of ground-glass opacity in PVOD is uncertain but may result from alveolar septal thickening with associated hyperplasia of lining epithelium and is believed to represent varying regions of underperfusion and interstitial edema.[93] Hilar and mediastinal lymphadenopathy is significantly more frequent in PVOD than in other causes of idiopathic pulmonary hypertension.[94] Small pericardial effusions can also be present.

The high-resolution CT findings of PCH consist of peribronchial cuffing, patchy areas of ground-glass opacity (Fig. 53.11), and poorly defined centrilobular ground-glass nodules caused by capillary proliferation.[95] Smooth interlobular septal thickening may be present as well. There may therefore be overlap between the imaging and hemodynamic findings in PVOD and PCH,

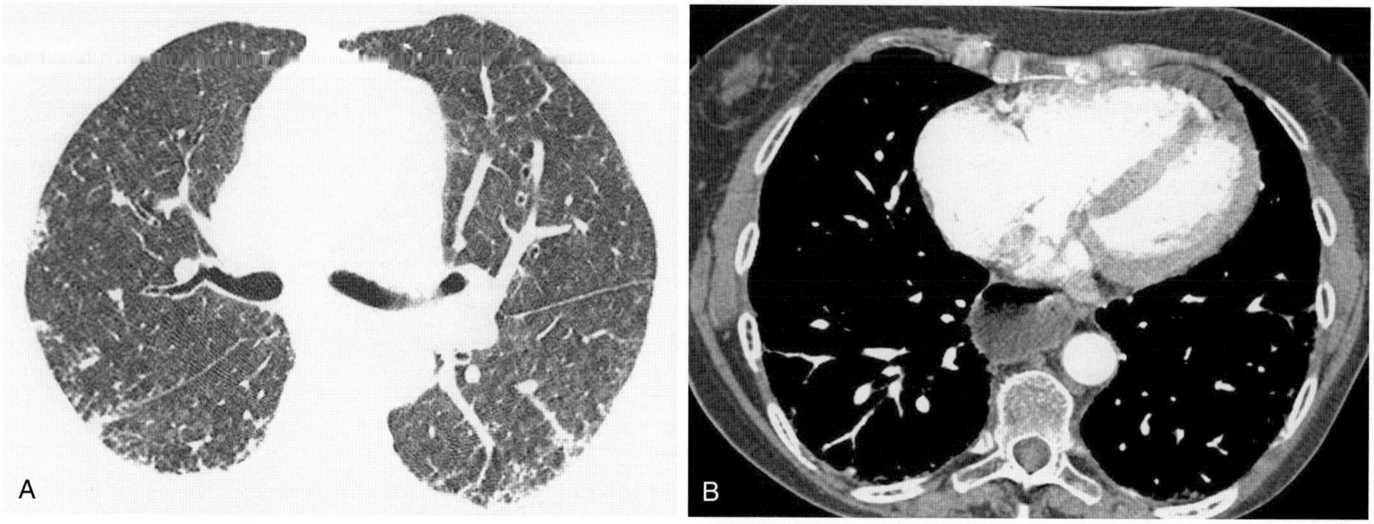

Fig. 53.12 Pulmonary hypertension in systemic sclerosis and CREST (calcinosis, *R*aynaud disease, *e*sophageal dysmotility, *s*clerodactyly, and *t*elangiectasia) syndrome. (A) CT image at the level of the main bronchi shows mild peripheral reticulation in keeping with interstitial fibrosis in addition to subtle heterogeneity of lung attenuation consistent with a pulmonary vasculopathy. (B) CT image at the level of the tricuspid valve shows right-sided cardiac chamber enlargement, a small pericardial effusion, and a dilated fluid-filled esophagus in keeping with esophageal dysmotility.

but these differ from those seen in other causes of pulmonary hypertension.

Left-Sided Heart Disease

CT often complements echocardiography by demonstrating an intracardiac soft tissue mass with additional evidence of extracardiac extension when it is present, interstitial edema, vascular congestion, pleural effusions, and enlargement of central vessels resulting from secondary PAH.[96] Cardiac chamber enlargement and valvular abnormalities can be identified sometimes as well (see Fig. 53.7).

Pulmonary Arterial Hypertension Associated With Pleuroparenchymal Lung Disease

Radiographic and CT findings consist of a combination of the features of the underlying pleuroparenchymal disorder and signs of pulmonary hypertension, with dilated right-sided heart chambers and proximal pulmonary vasculature (Fig. 53.12). In patients with interstitial fibrosis, the severity of pulmonary hypertension in affected individuals correlates with the degree of central pulmonary artery dilatation and the extent of parenchymal disease.[97] In CTD, when there is a combination of interstitial fibrosis and pulmonary vasculopathy, the severity of pulmonary hypertension may be disproportionate to the severity of parenchymal lung disease.[98]

Chronic Thromboembolic Pulmonary Hypertension

CT is often used to visualize central- and segmental-vessel thromboembolism.[23,99] It has greater sensitivity and accuracy for depicting central CTEPH than either pulmonary angiography or MRI does,[100] and it is more specific than scintigraphy.[101] Ventilation-perfusion (VQ) scintigraphy has a high sensitivity and specificity for detection of chronic thromboembolic disease and is still used as a first-line imaging modality at some institutions.[102,103] However, CTA has become a more popular technique in the evaluation of suspected CTEPH and also has very high accuracy. CT features in CTEPH consist of eccentric flattened mural thrombi that may be occlusive or have areas of recanalization.[104] Chronically occluded vessels are often smaller than expected. Calcifications can be observed in approximately 10% of patients.[105] The wall-adherent organized thrombotic material is much more easily visualized on CT than at angiography. Please see Chapter 51 for a more complete discussion of CTEPH.

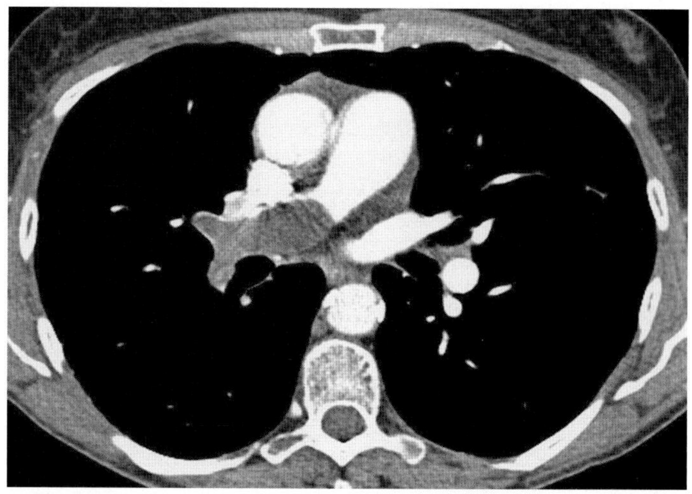

Fig. 53.13 Pulmonary artery sarcoma. Contrast-enhanced CT image shows a large intravascular filling defect in the right pulmonary artery extending into the proximal lobar vessels. This is occlusive and unilateral, features suggestive of tumor.

Primary Pulmonary Artery Sarcoma

Sarcoma is an uncommon cause of an intraluminal arterial filling defect. These intravascular tumors are manifested as unilateral, lobulated, heterogeneously enhancing masses at CT. They may demonstrate vascular distention and local extravascular spread. Unlike acute and chronic pulmonary embolism, pulmonary artery sarcoma demonstrates enhancement. Pulmonary artery sarcoma is lobulated and forms acute angles with the vessel wall (Fig. 53.13), whereas chronic pulmonary embolism forms obtuse angles.[106]

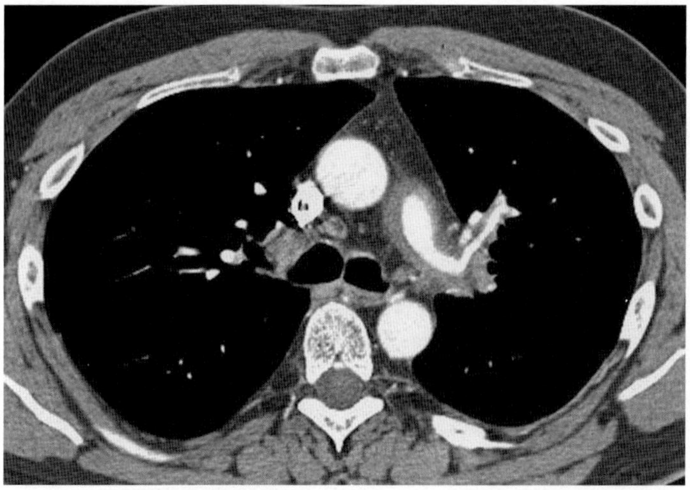

Fig. 53.14 Takayasu arteritis. Contrast-enhanced CT image demonstrates diffuse thickening of the wall of the left and upper lobe pulmonary arteries in a patient with biopsy-proven Takayasu arteritis. The aorta and supraaortic vessels were normal.

Vasculitis

Takayasu arteritis is a large-vessel arteritis that affects the proximal pulmonary vasculature (Fig. 53.14). Aortic and systemic artery involvement usually overshadows any pulmonary manifestations, although isolated pulmonary artery involvement with consequent pulmonary hypertension has been described. Multiple pulmonary stenoses resulting from focal thickening of vessel wall can be mistaken for CTEPH, but the vessel contour is smooth, and there may be delayed contrast enhancement on CT and MRI resulting from the inflammatory nature of the disease.[107]

Fibrosing Mediastinitis

Fibrosing mediastinitis can result in pulmonary hypertension and may be difficult to distinguish from unilateral chronic thromboembolism. Pulmonary vascular occlusion is produced by fibrous encasement of the pulmonary arteries or veins in a nonuniform pattern. There may be constriction of individual pulmonary veins with asymmetric mediastinal widening and calcifications accompanied by a hilar mass and ipsilateral Kerley B lines and peripheral wedge-shaped consolidation resulting from venous infarction.[108] Pulmonary angiography reveals unilateral or asymmetric narrowing of central pulmonary arteries and distal arterial cutoffs when mediastinal fibrosis affects the arterial side of the pulmonary circulation. With involvement of pulmonary veins, the venous-phase angiograms show nonuniform pulmonary vein obstruction, stenosis, or focal dilatation near the left atrium. Contrast-enhanced CT elegantly demonstrates the degree of vascular compromise while also demonstrating the extent of mediastinal involvement.

Nonthrombotic Emboli

Please see Chapters 14 and 52 for a complete discussion on nonthrombotic pulmonary emboli, including pulmonary tumor emboli, parasitic emboli, pulmonary talcosis, fat emboli, and foreign-body emboli.

In sickle cell disease, recurrent episodes of acute chest syndrome, with capillary obstruction and accompanying in situ thrombosis,[109] may lead to chronic changes. Approximately half of patients show evidence of interstitial disease, probably reflecting scarring from small pulmonary infarcts. Ultimately, if there is sufficient and permanent occlusion of the microvascular bed, cor pulmonale develops, with dilatation of the central pulmonary arteries and evidence of right ventricular hypertrophy.[110]

MAGNETIC RESONANCE IMAGING

MRI techniques enable noninvasive morphologic and functional assessment. MRI permits evaluation of cardiac chamber dimensions, ventricular muscle mass, and wall motion. Contrast-enhanced MR angiography (MRA) depicts the pulmonary vasculature, and morphologic images show good correlation with those of angiography. However, the additional functional data provided by velocity-encoded cine phase-contrast MRI also permit accurate and precise assessment of pulmonary and systemic blood flow and shunt quantification.

It is important to note that the main role in MRI is to help identify the functional impact of PAH on the right heart, assess prognosis in PAH as well as aid in identification of etiology. However, it lacks necessary sensitivity to rule out PAH. In general, MRI studies of patients with pulmonary hypertension show the characteristic anatomic changes of right ventricular hypertrophy, reversal of septal curvature, and dilatation of pulmonary arteries. Another observation is abnormal intravascular signal corresponding to slow pulmonary arterial blood flow on gated spin-echo MRI in 92% of cases of PAH, notably with a direct relationship to elevated PVR.[111]

As in CT, a basic linear correlation has been demonstrated between pulmonary arterial pressure and the ratio of pulmonary artery to aortic size.[112] Additionally, because the pulmonary artery plays an important role in converting the pulsatile right ventricular flow into nearly steady flow at the capillary level, evaluation of pulmonary artery distensibility or stiffness has been a subject of investigation. Multiple studies dating to 1989 have found that increased stiffness (or decreased distensibility) of the pulmonary artery between diastole and systole corresponds with increased RV workload and increased energy transmission from the RV to the small pulmonary vessels, leading to increased vascular damage.[113–120] More recent data suggests that reductions in pulmonary artery elasticity occur before overt pressure elevations occur, and such an evaluation could be useful for early detection of PAH.[121] Similar data has been achieved in multiphase CTA as well.[122]

Gradient-echo and balanced steady-state free precession cine MRI permits assessment of right and left ventricular function and is the gold standard for biventricular structure and function. Specifically, the assessment of right-sided heart structure and function is largely performed via cardiac MRI. Direct measurement of right and left ventricular stroke volume, ejection fraction, cardiac output, and shunt fractions is a sensitive, noninvasive method of detecting hemodynamic changes in patients with pulmonary hypertension.[123] In pulmonary hypertension the ventricular geometry is disturbed, and therefore accurate volume estimations are difficult to obtain from single-plane acquisitions. With volumetric MRI, ventricular volumes can be measured independently of any geometric assumption, in contradistinction to echocardiography.[124]

In addition, MRI is the gold standard examination for the evaluation of CHD, given the ability to not only assess anatomy but also physiology. Velocity-encoded cine phase-contrast MRI allows direct calculation of pulmonic and systemic flow, allowing reliable shunt fractions. It is particularly useful for the evaluation of supracristal ventricular septal defect, atrioventricular septal defect, and partial anomalous pulmonary venous drainage, in which echocardiography and conventional angiography have

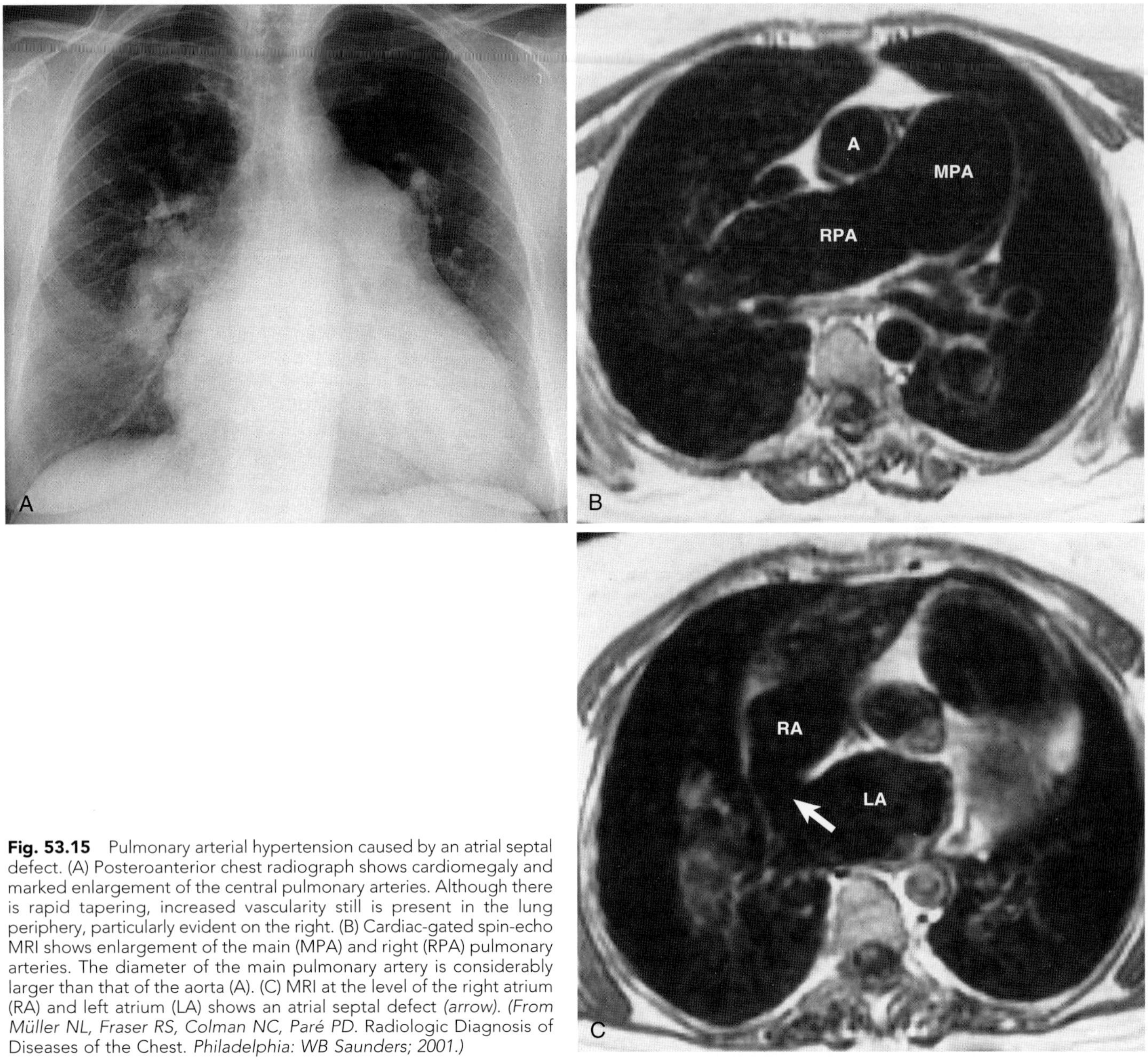

Fig. 53.15 Pulmonary arterial hypertension caused by an atrial septal defect. (A) Posteroanterior chest radiograph shows cardiomegaly and marked enlargement of the central pulmonary arteries. Although there is rapid tapering, increased vascularity still is present in the lung periphery, particularly evident on the right. (B) Cardiac-gated spin-echo MRI shows enlargement of the main (MPA) and right (RPA) pulmonary arteries. The diameter of the main pulmonary artery is considerably larger than that of the aorta (A). (C) MRI at the level of the right atrium (RA) and left atrium (LA) shows an atrial septal defect *(arrow). (From Müller NL, Fraser RS, Colman NC, Paré PD.* Radiologic Diagnosis of Diseases of the Chest. *Philadelphia: WB Saunders; 2001.)*

limited use (Fig. 53.15). The combination of fast MR perfusion imaging and high-spatial-resolution MRA with parallel acquisition techniques also enables the differentiation of idiopathic PAH from CTEPH with high accuracy.[125]

On MRI, in addition to the generic features such as right ventricular hypertrophy and dilatation, idiopathic PAH demonstrates symmetrically enlarged central pulmonary arteries, diffuse pattern of abruptly tapering and pruned subsegmental vessels, filamentous or "corkscrew" peripheral arteries, and occasionally subpleural collateral vessels, similar to the findings on angiography. MRI permits monitoring of cardiac function in response to therapy in patients with idiopathic pulmonary hypertension without the use of ionizing radiation. A study by Bergin and colleagues[126] demonstrated that MRA had accuracy identical to that of radionuclide scanning (92%) in distinguishing patients with CTEPH from those with idiopathic PAH.

ECHOCARDIOGRAPHY

Doppler echocardiography is the most common and readily available noninvasive method for assessing cardiac anatomy and function. Because echocardiography permits assessment of right-sided heart function and the estimation of pulmonary artery pressure, it forms part of both the initial diagnostic workup and the follow-up of patients with clinically suspected pulmonary hypertension.

Tricuspid regurgitation is detected in more than 90% of patients with severe pulmonary hypertension. The velocity of the regurgitant jet across the tricuspid valve as assessed by Doppler echocardiography can be used to estimate peak pulmonary artery pressure, although its accuracy is imperfect. A tricuspid regurgitant velocity of 3.0 m/s on echocardiography corresponds to pulmonary pressure greater than 30 mm Hg. Although in general these estimates correlate well with invasive measurements of right ventricular pressures, an individual estimate may be inaccurate. In particular, echocardiography has only limited ability to differentiate between mild pulmonary hypertension and normal pulmonary hemodynamics.[127]

Right ventricular myocardial hypertrophy, paradoxical septal motion, abnormal systolic intervals, and abnormal pulmonary valve motion may become apparent as disease progresses. Transesophageal echocardiography may be used to detect intracardiac shunts, particularly small patent foramen ovale and sinus venosus atrioseptal defects, which are notoriously difficult to diagnose on transthoracic echocardiography. Transesophageal echocardiography is also valuable for the assessment of valvular structures and other structural lesions, such as left atrial myxomas.

NUCLEAR MEDICINE

The main role of VQ lung scintigraphy is to differentiate chronic thromboembolic disease from other causes of pulmonary hypertension as it is often nonspecifically abnormal in the setting of nonthromboembolic disease (Fig. 53.16). In thromboembolic

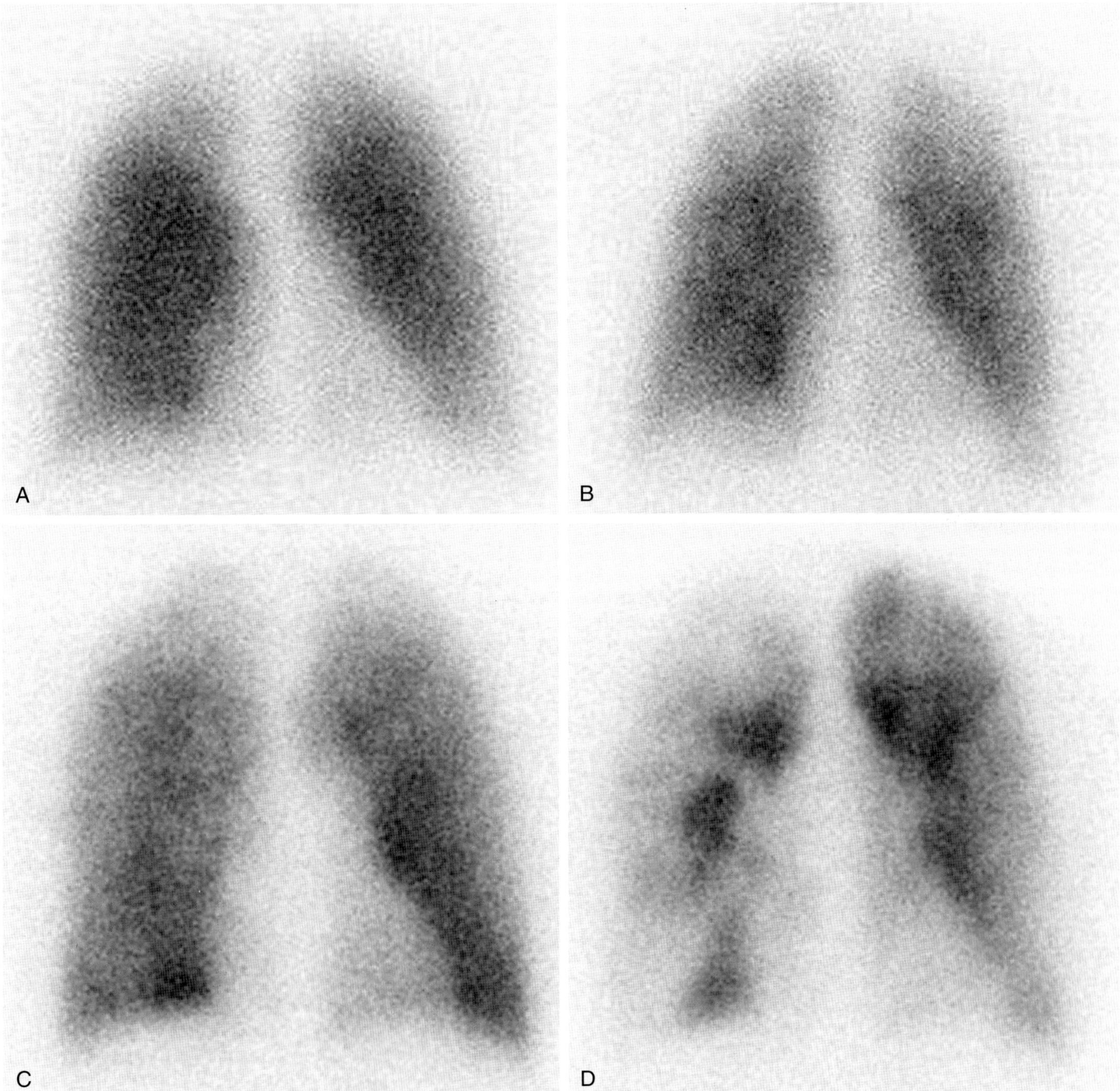

Fig. 53.16 Comparison of idiopathic pulmonary arterial hypertension (PAH) and chronic thromboembolic disease: ventilation and perfusion lung scintigraphy in two different patients. (A) and (B) In a patient with idiopathic PAH, anterior views show normal ventilation (A) with heterogeneous, mottled perfusion pattern (B). (C) and (D) In a patient with chronic thromboembolic disease, anterior views show normal ventilation (C) and multiple segmental perfusion defects (D).

disease there is segmental reduction in perfusion with maintenance of normal ventilation, leading to mismatch of perfusion and ventilation in the affected bronchopulmonary segment. VQ scintigraphy has a sensitivity of 90% to 100% and a specificity of 94% to 100% for distinguishing between idiopathic pulmonary hypertension and CTEPH, a higher sensitivity than CT angiography.[128,129]

Mismatched segmental perfusion defects may be seen with other processes that result in obstruction of the central pulmonary arteries, such as mediastinal lymphadenopathy, fibrosing mediastinitis, large-vessel arteritis, pulmonary vascular or bronchogenic tumors, and pulmonary venoocclusive disease. Whereas segmental or lobar perfusion defects are typical in CTEPH, the perfusion scan in idiopathic PAH is either normal or has low probability for pulmonary embolism with patchy subsegmental areas of reduced perfusion or "mottling" (see Fig. 53.16).[130] However, there are issues about the potential fallibility of the perfusion lung scan in making the differential diagnosis and the decisions regarding anticoagulant therapy.

In some patients with advanced primary pulmonary hypertension, there is scintigraphic evidence of reversed mismatching (i.e., pulmonary perfusion of areas of lung showing little or no ventilation). CT studies have demonstrated that such areas show normal or engorged pulmonary vasculature, with areas of increased parenchymal attenuation that are shown to have ventilatory defects at scintigraphy.[95]

The role of perfusion scintigraphy in other conditions is less clear. On perfusion scintigraphy in the presence of right-to-left shunt, activity in the thyroid or kidneys can be seen and used to calculate shunt fraction. VQ scintigraphy in parenchymal lung disease may demonstrate matched ventilation and perfusion defects. When unilateral lung transplantation is being considered, perfusion scintigraphy can be used to select the side with the most compromised function.

Pulmonary Venoocclusive Disease

In PVOD perfusion scans commonly reveal patchy distribution of tracer material without clear segmental or subsegmental defects; ventilation scans are normal. This VQ mismatch may lead to a misdiagnosis of CTEPH. Unilateral absence of perfusion can be due to severe asymmetric involvement of the major pulmonary veins.

ANGIOGRAPHY

Right-sided heart catheterization is often performed independently but may be performed at the same time as pulmonary angiography. A flotation catheter is passed from the vena cava through to a lobar pulmonary artery. It permits evaluation of pulmonary hemodynamics and cardiac function and assessment of dynamic response to pharmacologic stimuli. Measurement of oxygen saturations in the vena cava, the right chambers of the heart, and the pulmonary artery may identify previously unsuspected left-to-right shunting. In addition, an acute vasodilator challenge can be performed during right-sided heart catheterization to identify patients likely to respond to specific therapy.[131]

Pulmonary angiography is the gold standard technique for defining the pulmonary vascular anatomy, but modern CT and MRI techniques are now commonplace as noninvasive alternatives. With careful monitoring and modification of standard angiographic procedures, pulmonary angiography can be performed safely even in patients with severe pulmonary hypertension. The procedure has a 1.5% incidence of serious complications, with a mortality rate of 0.5%.[132] It has excellent temporal resolution, with resultant decrease in motion artifact and venous contamination compared with CT and MRI. Pulmonary angiography can also be used in the setting of CTEPH, in which it may help confirm disease location and surgical accessibility in cases where CTA is equivocal. Although pulmonary angiography is now seldom performed in PVOD, it typically shows enlarged central pulmonary arteries and right ventricle, with a prolonged parenchymal enhancement phase resulting in delayed filling of normal-sized or small pulmonary veins and a normal or small left atrium.[133] Pulmonary venography shows focal venous obstructions, a finding highly suggestive of the diagnosis of PVOD.

IMAGING ALGORITHM

Pulmonary hypertension presents with nonspecific symptoms and signs. Imaging plays a pivotal role, not only in confirming the presence of pulmonary hypertension but also in elucidating an underlying cause. Although there exists a range of available imaging modalities, consideration should be given to factors such as ionizing radiation exposure and the invasive nature of some examinations with their attendant risks. The diagnostic strategy should be tailored to suit an individual institution, depending on local expertise, ease of access, and cost.

All patients presenting with suspected pulmonary hypertension will have chest radiography. If it shows the now familiar complex of proximal pulmonary artery enlargement and cardiomegaly, further investigation with echocardiography is warranted. In the context of a normal radiograph but high clinical suspicion, echocardiography provides a simple and noninvasive method to rule pulmonary hypertension in or out. Echocardiography not only can confirm pulmonary hypertension but also can provide a clue as to the underlying mechanism. No further investigation is required if the echocardiogram is completely normal.

If a cardiac cause of pulmonary hypertension is identified on echocardiography or the patient is seen to have an unexpected shunt, patients should proceed to MRI for definitive evaluation. This might be sufficient if patients need conservative or medical management only. However, when surgery is considered, right-sided heart catheterization is useful for further disease definition.

Where there is no definitive cardiac cause on echocardiography, a combination of CT pulmonary angiography and/or high-resolution CT provides a diagnosis in the majority of patients. Any further testing will depend on the result of CT.

Not infrequently, unexpected intracardiac shunts can be seen on CT angiography. These cases will need further assessment with right-sided heart catheterization and MRI. Parenchymal lung disease is readily detected on CT and should be correlated with lung function test results. Pulmonary venoocclusive disease may be confused with pulmonary edema or interstitial fibrosis. Idiopathic pulmonary hypertension is a diagnosis of exclusion.

When the CT findings are equivocal, VQ scintigraphy may be useful to exclude distal thromboembolic disease. Many centers use VQ scintigraphy as a frontline examination before CT. Undoubtedly, it is a useful screening test valuable for the exclusion of CTEPH. However, in other conditions, the findings are too nonspecific to be reliable. In the absence of a normal or high-probability VQ scan, the diagnostic conundrum continues, and the pathway may have to revert to CT or MRI.

KEY POINTS: PULMONARY HYPERTENSION

- Causes of pulmonary hypertension can be divided into precapillary and postcapillary etiologies. The alternative World Health Organization classification scheme includes pulmonary arterial hypertension (PAH) (group 1), pulmonary hypertension related to left heart disease (group 2), pulmonary hypertension related to pulmonary parenchymal disease (group 3), chronic thromboembolic pulmonary hypertension (group 4), and multifactorial or unclear disease (group 5).
- Prognosis in patients with idiopathic PAH has improved with newer targeted medical therapies.
- Echocardiography permits estimation of pulmonary artery pressure and is useful as a screening tool and in follow-up.
- Echocardiography and MRI are the imaging modalities of choice for detection of cardiac abnormalities.
- Right-sided cardiac chamber size, function, and hemodynamics are key predictors of prognosis, with cardiac MRI being the gold standard for assessment.
- Radiographs are frequently abnormal in cases of pulmonary hypertension, but a negative chest radiograph does not exclude disease.
- CT evaluation of the pulmonary arteries and/or lung parenchyma can provide important insights into the etiology of the pulmonary hypertension.
- CT features of pulmonary venoocclusive disease and pulmonary capillary hemangiomatosis include smooth interlobular septal thickening, ground-glass opacities, centrilobular nodules, pleural effusion, and mediastinal lymphadenopathy. Differentiation of these from precapillary vasculopathy is important as vasodilator therapy can lead to fatal pulmonary edema.
- The main role of ventilation-perfusion lung scintigraphy is to differentiate chronic thromboembolic disease from other causes of pulmonary hypertension.

SUGGESTED READINGS

Ascha M, et al. A review of imaging modalities in pulmonary hypertension. *Ann Thorac Med.* 2017;12(2):61–73.

Francois CJ, Schiebler ML. Imaging of pulmonary hypertension. *Radiol Clin North Am.* 2016;54(6):1133–1149.

Ruggiero A, Screaton NJ. Imaging of acute and chronic thromboembolic disease: state of the art. *Clin Radiol.* 2017;72(5):375–388.

The full reference list for this chapter is available at ExpertConsult.com.

54 Hydrostatic Pulmonary Edema*

CHRISTOPHER M. WALKER | JONATHAN H. CHUNG

Etiology

Pulmonary edema is defined as an abnormal accumulation of fluid in the extravascular compartments (interstitial and airspace) of the lung. Traditionally, pulmonary edema has been divided into hydrostatic edema and permeability edema based on the presumed mechanism. Hydrostatic edema is caused by an elevation in pulmonary capillary pressure, and permeability edema is caused by disruption of the capillary endothelium, resulting in protein leakage into the surrounding tissue. This distinction into two categories is problematic. First, severe elevation in pulmonary capillary pressure in left ventricular failure may result in endothelial cell damage, resulting in a mixture of hydrostatic and permeability edema. Second, permeability edema is now known to occur in conditions that do not cause diffuse alveolar damage, such as hantavirus pulmonary syndrome and interleukin therapy. Permeability edema in these settings behaves very differently from permeability edema in patients with diffuse alveolar damage (acute respiratory distress syndrome [ARDS]). For these reasons, a modern definition of pulmonary edema should incorporate four main categories based on pathophysiology: hydrostatic edema, permeability edema with diffuse alveolar damage (DAD), permeability edema without DAD, and mixed edema caused by both hydrostatic and permeability edema.[1]

The most common cause of hydrostatic pulmonary edema is a rise in pulmonary venous pressure secondary to disease of the left side of the heart. Increased pressure within the left atrium is transmitted to the pulmonary veins as a result of back pressure, most often from a failing left ventricle or obstruction to left atrial outflow. Rarely, venous hypertension is caused by stenosis of the pulmonary veins themselves, such as occurs in congenital or acquired venoocclusive disease or fibrosing mediastinitis.[2] Other common causes of hydrostatic pulmonary edema are renal disease, hypervolemia, and liver failure. Both acute and chronic renal disease, with or without uremia, can be associated with acute pulmonary edema. A major contributing cause in these cases is left ventricular failure; however, it is likely that decreased protein osmotic pressure, hypervolemia, and increased capillary permeability also have roles.[3] Administration of large volumes of intravenous fluids has been shown to cause pulmonary edema in patients who do not have underlying heart disease.[4] Fluid overload is an important cause of hydrostatic edema in the postoperative period, in the elderly, and in patients with borderline cardiac or renal failure. Pulmonary edema occurs with increased frequency in patients who have cirrhosis or acute hepatic failure or have undergone liver transplantation.[5] It is likely that the edema in these patients is due to a combination of increased capillary pressure, increased endothelial permeability, and decreased plasma osmotic pressure.[2] Finally, hydrostatic pulmonary edema is also a well-described but uncommon complication of head trauma, seizures, and raised intracranial pressure.

COMMON CAUSES OF HYDROSTATIC PULMONARY EDEMA

- Cardiogenic
  - Left ventricular failure
  - Mitral valve disease
  - Left atrial myxoma
- Obstruction of the pulmonary veins
  - Primary (idiopathic) venoocclusive disease
  - Fibrosing mediastinitis
- Neurogenic
  - Head trauma
  - Seizures
  - Increased intracranial pressure
- Decreased capillary osmotic pressure
  - Renal disease
  - Fluid overload
  - Cirrhosis

Clinical Presentation

The main clinical manifestations of acute hydrostatic pulmonary edema are dyspnea, tachypnea, and orthopnea.[2,6] Clinical findings include peripheral and central cyanosis, tachycardia, pallor, peripheral edema, and elevated jugular venous pressure. In the most severe cases the patient may expectorate frothy, blood-tinged fluid.

In patients in whom pulmonary edema develops insidiously, the symptoms may be mild, and dyspnea may occur only during exertion. Other suggestive symptoms in these patients include a history of orthopnea and paroxysmal nocturnal dyspnea. Some patients with chronic left-sided heart failure may have minimal symptoms even in the presence of extensive pulmonary edema evident on the chest radiograph.[2,6] Laboratory testing, including B-type natriuretic peptide (BNP) and N-terminal fragment (NT-proBNP), are elevated in situations causing increased myocardial stress or in patients with renal failure. A normal laboratory value can be used to essentially rule out heart failure in patients presenting to the emergency department with dyspnea.[7]

Pathophysiology

Under normal steady-state conditions, there is continual flow of fluid and protein from the pulmonary microvasculature to the interstitium; these substances are then returned to the bloodstream

*The editors and publisher would like to thank Drs. Nestor L. Müller and C. Isabela Silva Müller for contributing material on this topic to the prior edition of this work. It has served as the foundation for the current chapter.

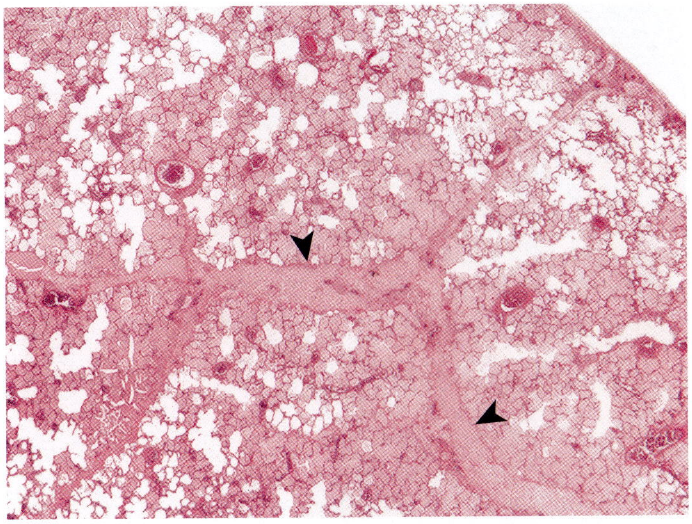

Fig. 54.1 Pathologic findings of pulmonary edema. Histologic specimen shows thickening of the interlobular septa *(arrowheads)* and partial filling of the airspaces by fluid. *(Courtesy Dr. John English, Department of Pathology, Vancouver General Hospital, Vancouver, Canada.)*

by the lymphatics. The volume of water and protein movement is dependent on the balance of pressure across the pulmonary microvasculature and on the permeability of the microvascular membrane. The factors that govern the formation and removal of extravascular water within the lungs are described by the fluid transport equation originally proposed by Starling.[8]

An increase in microvascular hydrostatic pressure or a decrease in protein osmotic pressure in the microvascular lumen will result in the transudation of fluid from the microvessels into interstitial tissue (hydrostatic pulmonary edema). Sufficient accumulation of fluid in this compartment constitutes interstitial edema; when the storage capacity of the interstitial space is exceeded and epithelial cell damage occurs, edema floods into the alveolar airspaces (Fig. 54.1).[9] The pulmonary interstitium itself can be divided into two compartments: an alveolar septal (parenchymal) compartment and a peribronchovascular and interlobular septal (axial) compartment. Although the alveolar septal compartment constitutes a large percentage of the total interstitial space, its relatively low compliance means that fluid tends to accumulate to a much lesser extent within it than in the peribronchovascular and interlobular septal connective tissue.[10]

The pathogenesis of acute pulmonary edema secondary to head trauma, seizures, and raised intracranial pressure is poorly understood but likely is secondary to both hydrostatic and permeability mechanisms. Most studies suggest that the main mechanism is increased microvascular pressure (hydrostatic pulmonary edema).[11,12] Experimental studies have shown transient, massive sympathetic discharge from the central nervous system, which results in generalized vasoconstriction, shift of blood volume into the pulmonary vascular compartment, and elevation of pulmonary microvascular pressure.[13] It has also been shown that the sympathetic activity increases pulmonary vasomotor tone, causing constriction of pulmonary veins and a subsequent increase in pulmonary capillary hydrostatic pressure.[12] There is also evidence that a direct negative inotropic effect on the heart contributes to the pathogenesis of the edema.[14,15] Finally, elevated hydrostatic pressure may cause endothelial injury resulting in secondary permeability edema manifesting with high protein–content edema fluid.[1]

Manifestations of the Disease

RADIOGRAPHY

Hydrostatic edema results in two principal radiologic patterns related to whether the fluid remains localized in the interstitial space or whether it also occupies the airspaces.

Predominantly Interstitial Edema

Transudation of fluid into the interstitial spaces of the lung inevitably constitutes the first stage of pulmonary edema because the capillaries are situated in this compartment. Although this transudation of fluid constitutes the first stage of fluid accumulation in the lungs, classic teaching and radiology dogma state that the initial radiographic sign in interstitial pulmonary edema is pulmonary venous hypertension. This sign manifests with redistribution of blood flow from the lower to the upper lung zones (Fig. 54.2), with the upper lobe arteries becoming larger than the accompanying bronchus (Fig. 54.3).[16,17] This redistribution is termed by many authors as cephalization of the vasculature. Unfortunately, this sign is often not present in interstitial pulmonary edema or is difficult to accurately determine on radiography.[1,18,19] Furthermore, redistribution of blood flow can be assessed reliably only on radiographs performed at maximal inspiration in the erect position. In a study of 86 patients with acute myocardial infarction, pulmonary vascular redistribution (cephalization) was present in only 1 patient with an elevated wedge pressure.[19] Pistolesi and colleagues[20] determined that redistribution of pulmonary blood flow (cephalization) does not correlate with wedge pressure but likely reflects chronic structural vascular changes and occurs in patients with chronically elevated venous pressures, such as those with chronic and recurrent heart failure or in patients with long-standing mitral stenosis (see Fig. 54.2).

Therefore the first reliable radiographic evidence of interstitial pulmonary edema is fluid accumulating within the perivascular interstitial tissue and interlobular septa. As a result of this localization, edema fluid produces a characteristic radiographic pattern of loss of definition of segmental and subsegmental pulmonary vessels (i.e., vascular indistinctness) and thickening of the interlobular septa (Kerley A and B lines; Fig. 54.4).[21] Unfortunately, vascular indistinctness relies on subjective assessment and can be caused by many factors other than interstitial edema, including motion, differences in equipment, lung volume, and patient rotation. A more objective finding, and often the most reliable radiographic sign of early interstitial edema, is subpleural interstitial edema. This sign manifests with thickening of the interlobar fissures (thick fissures) caused by fluid accumulation in the interstitium beneath the visceral pleura (see Fig. 54.4).[1] Thick fissures are usually visible earlier than Kerley B lines because there are two layers of visceral pleural that contribute to the thickening, and the fissures are larger and longer than interlobular septa. It is important to note that a thick fissure does not represent pleural effusion within the fissure but rather thickening of the subpleural interstitium.[1]

In circumstances in which edema fluid accumulates in the parenchymal interstitial tissue before the development of overt airspace edema, the accumulation is usually invisible or only faintly discernible radiographically as a "haze," which tends to

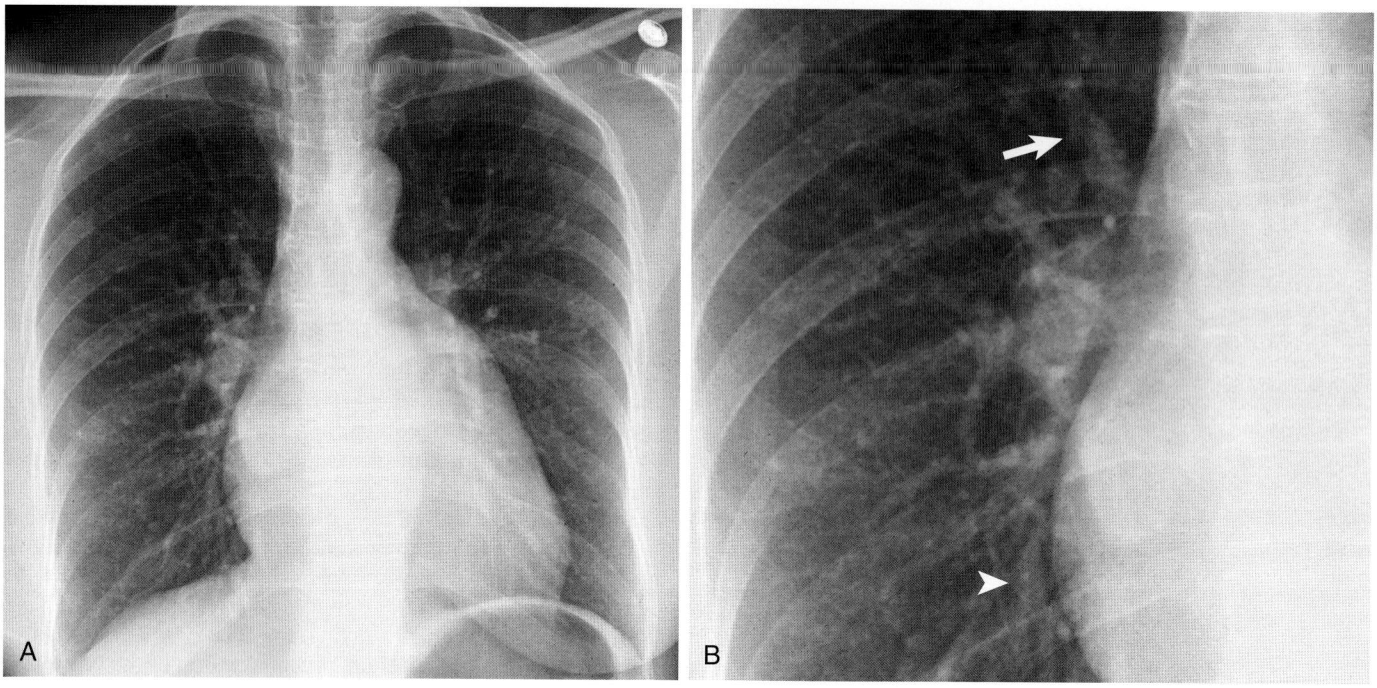

Fig. 54.2 Redistribution of blood flow to upper lung zones caused by pulmonary venous hypertension in a woman with mitral stenosis and mitral regurgitation. (A) Posteroanterior radiograph shows unusually prominent vascular markings in the upper lung zones and sparse markings in the lower lung zones. Note left atrial appendage and left atrial dilation indicating mitral stenosis and regurgitation. (B) Detail radiograph of the right lower lung zone shows discrepancy in size of the upper lung zone pulmonary arteries *(arrow)* relative to lower lung zone pulmonary arteries *(arrowhead)*. Pulmonary venous hypertension (cephalization) is most commonly noted with long-standing heart failure or mitral stenosis and is often not present or discernible in acute interstitial edema.

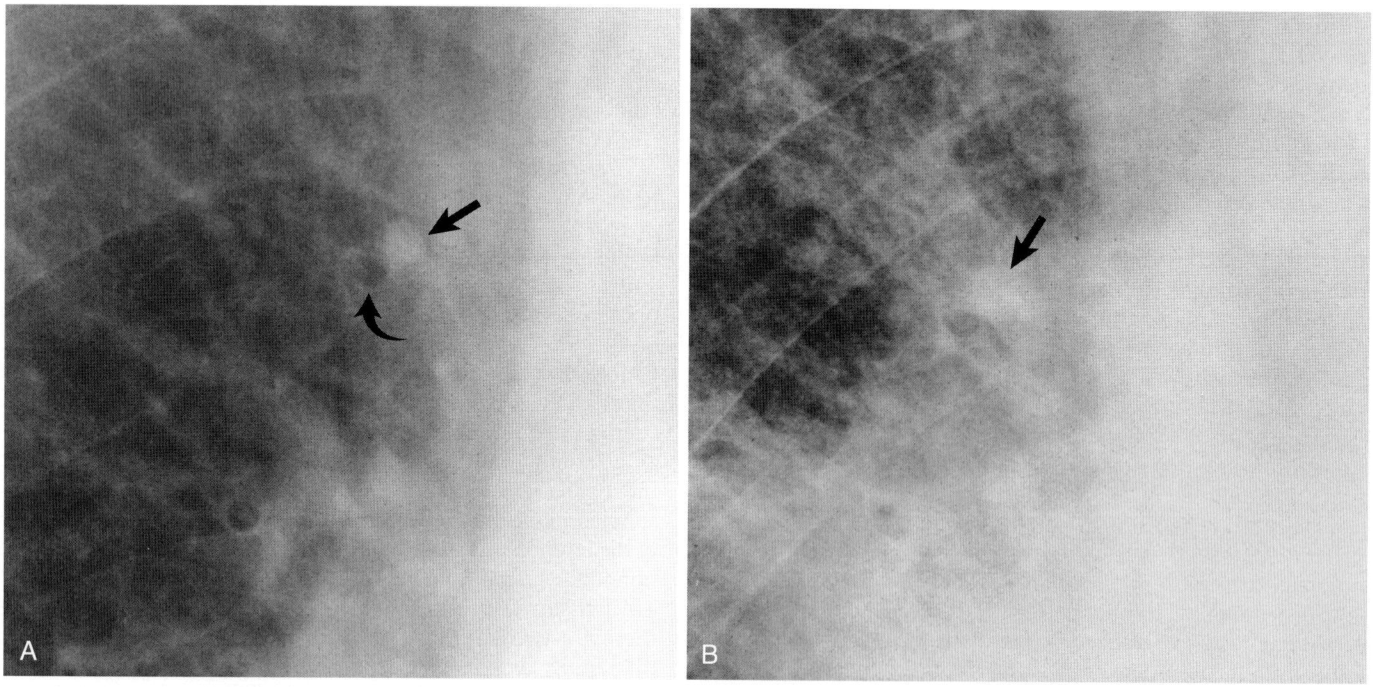

Fig. 54.3 Increased upper lung zone ratio of pulmonary artery to bronchus diameter in hydrostatic pulmonary edema. (A) View of the right upper lung zone from anteroposterior radiograph shows a normal ratio of pulmonary artery to bronchus diameter. The external diameter of the pulmonary artery *(straight arrow)* is similar to that of the external diameter of its accompanying bronchus *(curved arrow)*. (B) Erect anteroposterior radiograph 3 years later after acute myocardial infarction and development of pulmonary edema shows increased diameter of the pulmonary artery *(arrow)*. Perihilar haze with vascular indistinctness is also evident. *(From Müller NL, Fraser RS, Colman NC, Paré PD.* Radiologic Diagnosis of Diseases of the Chest. *Philadelphia: WB Saunders; 2001.)*

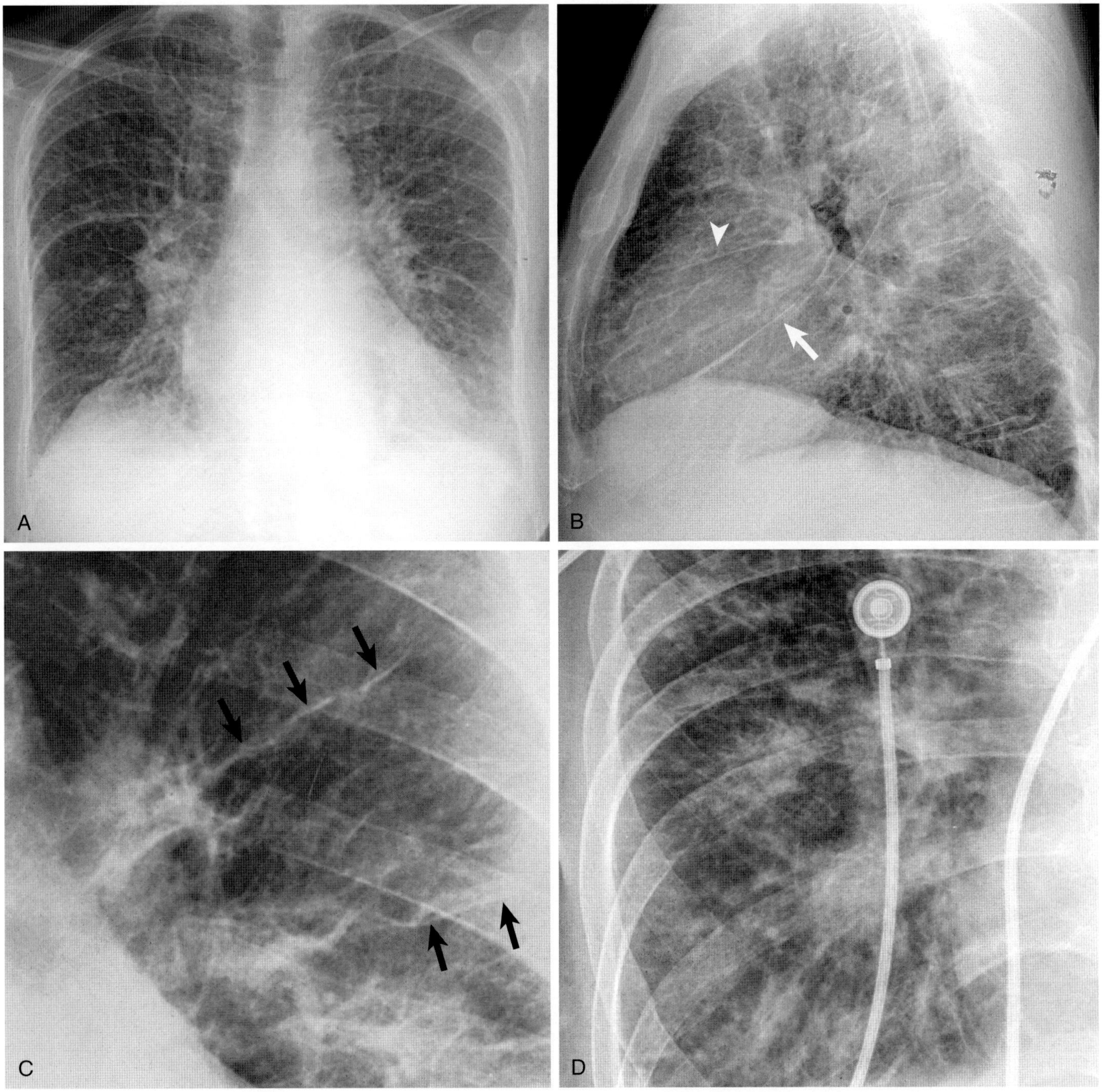

Fig. 54.4 Interstitial pulmonary edema from left-sided heart failure. Posteroanterior (A) and lateral (B) radiographs show multiple linear opacities throughout both lungs. These lines consist of a combination of long septal lines (Kerley A lines), predominantly in the middle lung zones (*arrows* in C), and shorter peripheral septal lines (Kerley B lines best seen in D). In lateral projection (B), the interlobar fissures are thick (*arrow* and *arrowhead*) as a result of subpleural interstitial edema. *(Fig. 54.4A from Gutschow SE, Walker CM. Acute thoracic conditions in the ICU. In: Shepherd J.* Thoracic Imaging Requisites, *3rd ed. Philadelphia: Elsevier; 2018; Fig. 54.4C from Müller NL, Fraser RS, Colman NC, Paré PD.* Radiologic Diagnosis of Diseases of the Chest. *Philadelphia: WB Saunders; 2001.)*

be predominantly lower zonal or perihilar in distribution. Although the severity of radiographic abnormalities correlates somewhat with pulmonary wedge pressure, there is often a phase lag between the elevation in wedge pressure and radiographic signs of pulmonary edema, possibly because of the time required for transudation of fluid into the extravascular space.[22,23] The heart is generally enlarged; however, like pulmonary vascular redistribution, the heart size may be normal when the cause of the edema is recent myocardial infarction, coronary insufficiency, or restrictive cardiomyopathy.[24]

Evidence for interstitial pulmonary edema is also provided by an increase in the thickness of the walls of bronchi seen

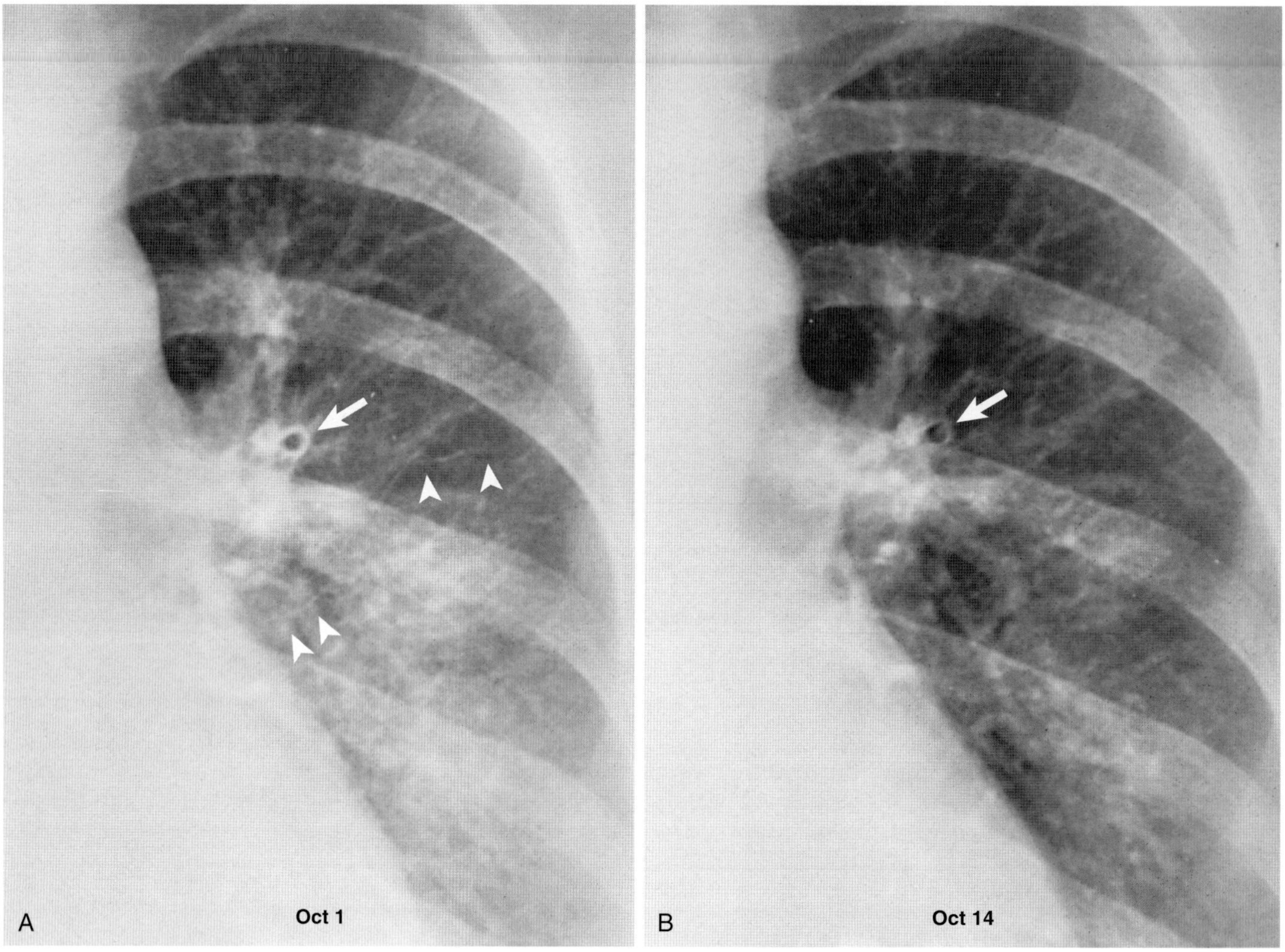

Fig. 54.5 Peribronchial cuffing in pulmonary edema from renal failure. (A) Detailed view of the upper half of the left lung from posteroanterior radiograph shows distended upper lobe vessels, perihilar haze, septal A lines *(arrowheads)*, and thickened bronchial wall viewed end-on *(arrow)*. (B) A few weeks later, after diuretic therapy, signs of pulmonary edema had resolved. Note decreased thickness of the bronchial wall *(arrow)*. *(From Müller NL, Fraser RS, Colman NC, Paré PD.* Radiologic Diagnosis of Diseases of the Chest. *Philadelphia: WB Saunders; 2001.)*

end-on in the perihilar zones.[21] In the absence of chronic airway disease, such as bronchitis or asthma, these structures measure less than 1 mm in thickness. When fluid accumulates in the interstitial tissue surrounding them, their shadow thickens and loses its sharp definition (Fig. 54.5). After adequate treatment of edema, all these radiologic signs may disappear within a matter of hours to as long as a few days.

The vascular pedicle is the width of the superior mediastinum measured from the right lateral border of the superior vena cava, at the point where it crosses the right main bronchus, to the left lateral margin of the left subclavian artery, where it arises from the aortic arch. A change in the width of the vascular pedicle is a useful indicator of a patient's intravascular volume status but only when comparison radiographs performed with similar positioning and depth of inspiration are available.[1] In the majority of normal patients, the vascular pedicle measures between 38 and 58 mm wide. Because of its wide normal range, a change in the vascular pedicle as opposed to absolute size, obtained in similar radiographic positions, is a more useful determinant of volume status. With fluid overload, the vascular pedicle widens (Fig. 54.6), whereas in patients with left-sided heart failure, the vascular pedicle is widened in only 50% of patients. Patients with permeability edema generally do not have a widened vascular pedicle.

Airspace Edema

Airspace pulmonary edema tends to develop with epithelial damage after the transmural pressure becomes greater than 25 mm Hg.[21] Although interstitial edema usually precedes airspace edema, the chest radiograph may show evidence of both simultaneously. The characteristic radiographic abnormality is the presence of patchy or confluent bilateral areas of consolidation that tend to be symmetric and to involve mainly the perihilar regions and the lower lung zones (Fig. 54.7).[25] Air bronchograms are uncommon. In the majority of cases the shadows are confluent and create irregular, poorly defined patchy opacities scattered randomly throughout the lungs; in the medial third of the lungs particularly, coalescence of areas of consolidation is common (Fig. 54.8). In less than 10% of cases, airspace hydrostatic pulmonary edema has a central, nongravitational distribution with sparing of the

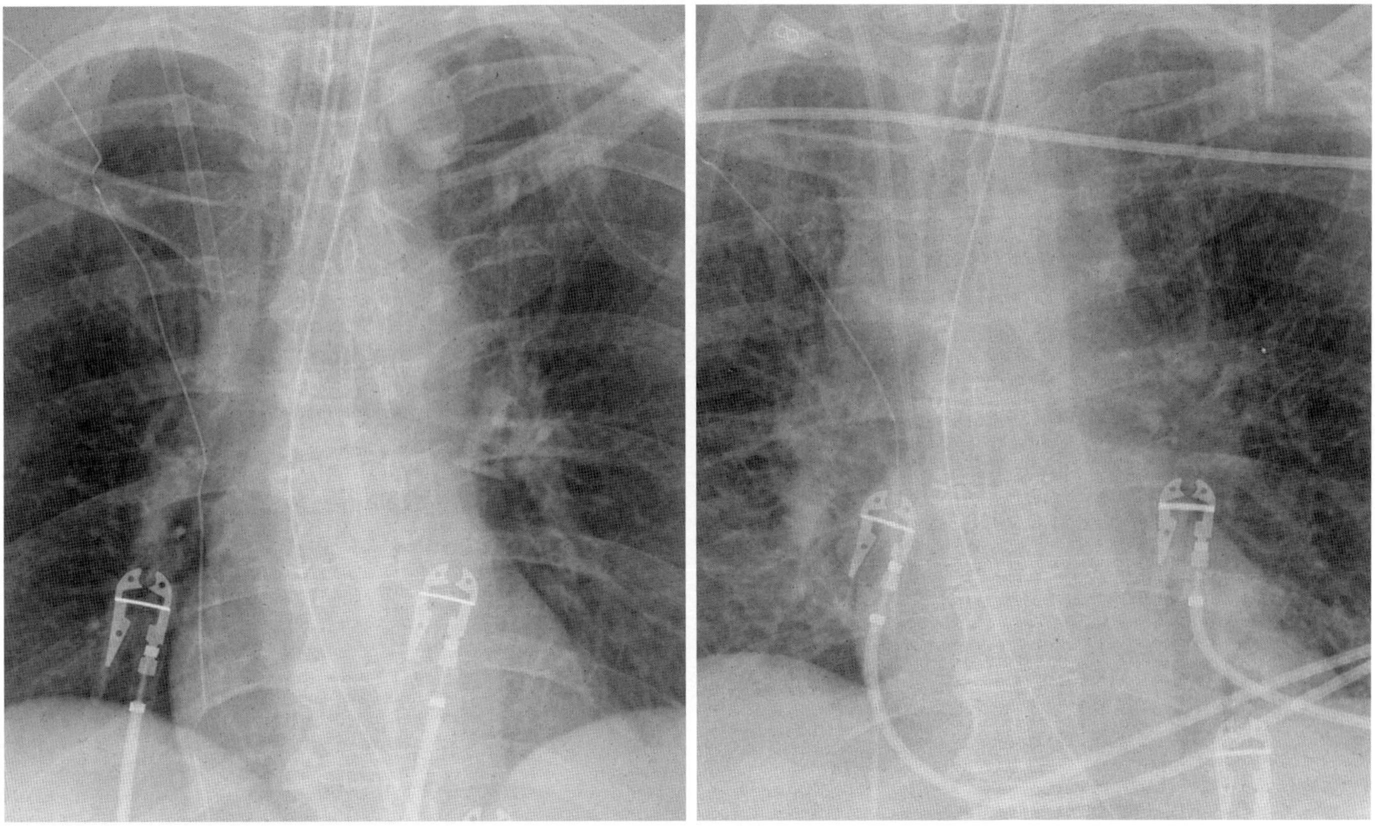

Fig. 54.6 Fluid overload pulmonary edema. Composite image with frontal radiograph before *(left image)* and after *(right image)* the administration of 12 L of intravenous fluids shows widening of the vascular pedicle, enlargement of the azygos vein, and diffuse interstitial pulmonary edema. *(From Gutschow SE, Walker CM. Acute thoracic conditions in the ICU. In: Shepherd J.* Thoracic Imaging Requisites, *3rd ed. Philadelphia: Elsevier; 2018.)*

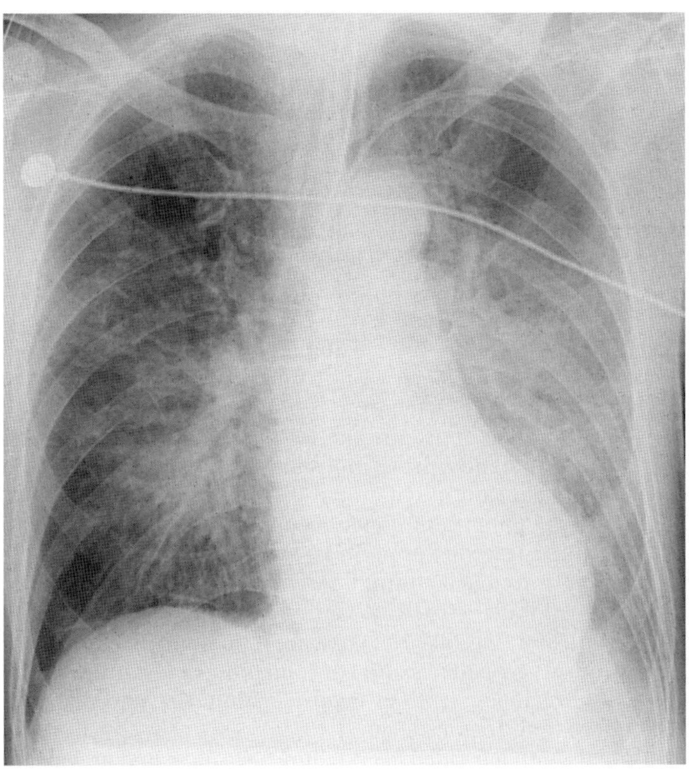

Fig. 54.7 Interstitial and airspace pulmonary edema in left-sided heart failure. Anteroposterior radiograph demonstrates enlarged and poorly defined pulmonary vessels, perihilar haze in the right lung, and perihilar haze and consolidation in the left lung. Also noted are an endotracheal tube and left subclavian central venous catheter.

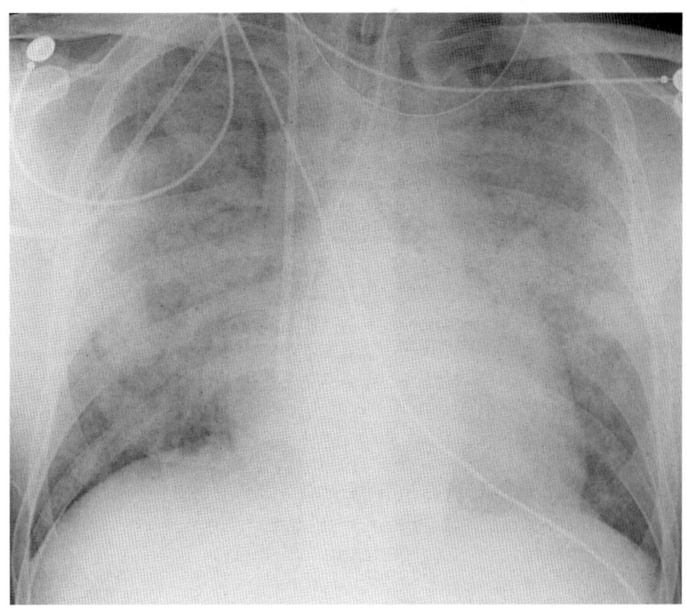

Fig. 54.8 Airspace pulmonary edema from left-sided heart failure. Anteroposterior radiograph demonstrates extensive bilateral consolidation with slight central predominance. Also noted are a right internal jugular central venous catheter and nasogastric tube.

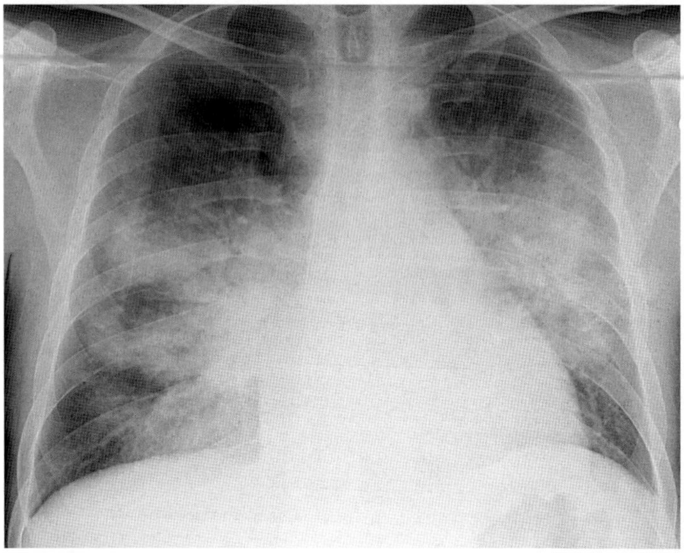

Fig. 54.9 Bat wing pattern of pulmonary edema. Posteroanterior radiograph shows consolidation in the perihilar portions of both lungs, creating a bat wing or butterfly appearance; the periphery of both lungs is relatively unaffected. The consolidation is fairly homogeneous and is associated with well-defined bilateral air bronchograms. Also noted is a left peripherally inserted central catheter with the tip at the superior cavoatrial junction.

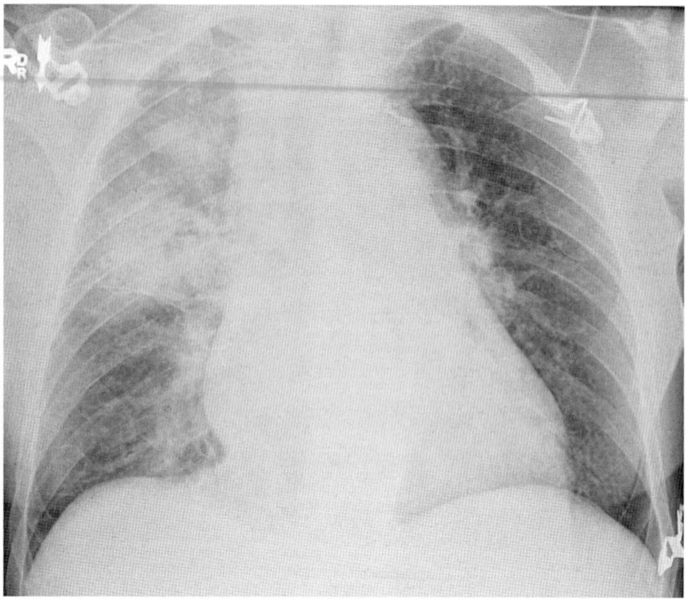

Fig. 54.10 Right upper lobe pulmonary edema caused by acute mitral regurgitation. Anteroposterior radiograph shows prominent and ill-defined pulmonary vascular markings and septal lines consistent with interstitial pulmonary edema. Also noted is extensive right upper lobe consolidation. Although the upper lobe consolidation is most suggestive of pneumonia, it was proved to be due to airspace pulmonary edema secondary to acute mitral regurgitation after myocardial infarction.

peripheral lung, a pattern known as bat wing or butterfly edema (Fig. 54.9).[21] Bat wing edema tends to occur with rapidly developing severe cardiac failure as seen in acute mitral insufficiency (associated with papillary muscle rupture or massive myocardial infarct) or renal failure.[21]

Edema secondary to cardiac disease is generally bilateral and fairly symmetric. On occasion, it is predominantly unilateral or occupies zones of one or both lungs out of keeping with the "expected" distribution of disease arising from a central influence. Unilateral pulmonary edema can occur in a wide variety of conditions in which the pathogenetic mechanism exists either on the same side as the edema (ipsilateral edema) or on the opposite side (contralateral edema). The most common causes of asymmetric hydrostatic pulmonary edema are a patient preferring to lie on one side or morphologic changes in the lung parenchyma in chronic obstructive pulmonary disease. Extensive emphysema or marked destruction and fibrosis as seen in end-stage tuberculosis or sarcoidosis will result in pulmonary edema in the regions that are less affected by these disease processes. Mitral regurgitation, particularly in the setting of acute myocardial infarction, tends to result in edema involving mainly the right upper lobe because the reflux stream is directed toward the right superior pulmonary vein (Fig. 54.10).[21,26] Such asymmetric distribution occurs in 9% of adults and 22% of children with grade 3 or 4 mitral regurgitation.[27,28]

Like hydrostatic interstitial pulmonary edema, airspace edema usually clears fairly rapidly in response to adequate treatment of the underlying condition. Resolution appears to be radiographically complete in less than 3 days in most cases.

Chest radiography plays an important role in the initial evaluation of patients with hydrostatic pulmonary edema. However, there may be as much as a 12-hour delay between the onset of symptoms and the development of significant radiographic abnormalities when the onset of pulmonary edema is abrupt.[27] Additionally, there may be a therapeutic lag with the pulmonary venous pressures returning to normal with resolution of patient symptoms but with persistent edema on chest radiography.[19]

COMPUTED TOMOGRAPHY

Although a diagnosis of hydrostatic pulmonary edema is usually based on clinical information and findings on conventional chest radiography, it is important to recognize its appearance on computed tomography (CT), both because it can mimic other diseases and because it is seen occasionally in patients not suspected clinically to have edema.

The most common findings of interstitial pulmonary edema on high-resolution CT consist of septal thickening and ground-glass opacities (Fig. 54.11).[29,30] Some patients may have almost exclusively septal thickening or ground-glass opacities.[29,30] The interlobular septal thickening is smooth and uniform, except for a focal nodular appearance resulting from prominent septal veins or intraparenchymal lymph nodes.[30] The edema tends to have a perihilar and gravitational distribution, but this is not always present. Other common findings include increased vascular caliber, thickening of the perihilar peribronchovascular interstitium (peribronchial cuffing), interlobar fissures, prominence of the centrilobular structures caused by interstitial edema, and pleural effusion (Fig. 54.12).[30] Airspace pulmonary edema results in ground-glass opacities and consolidation that, similar to the interstitial changes, tend to involve mainly the perihilar and dependent lung regions (Fig. 54.13).

Patients with left-sided heart failure have increased prevalence of enlarged mediastinal lymph nodes and hazy opacification of the mediastinal fat (Fig. 54.14). The abnormalities resolve after

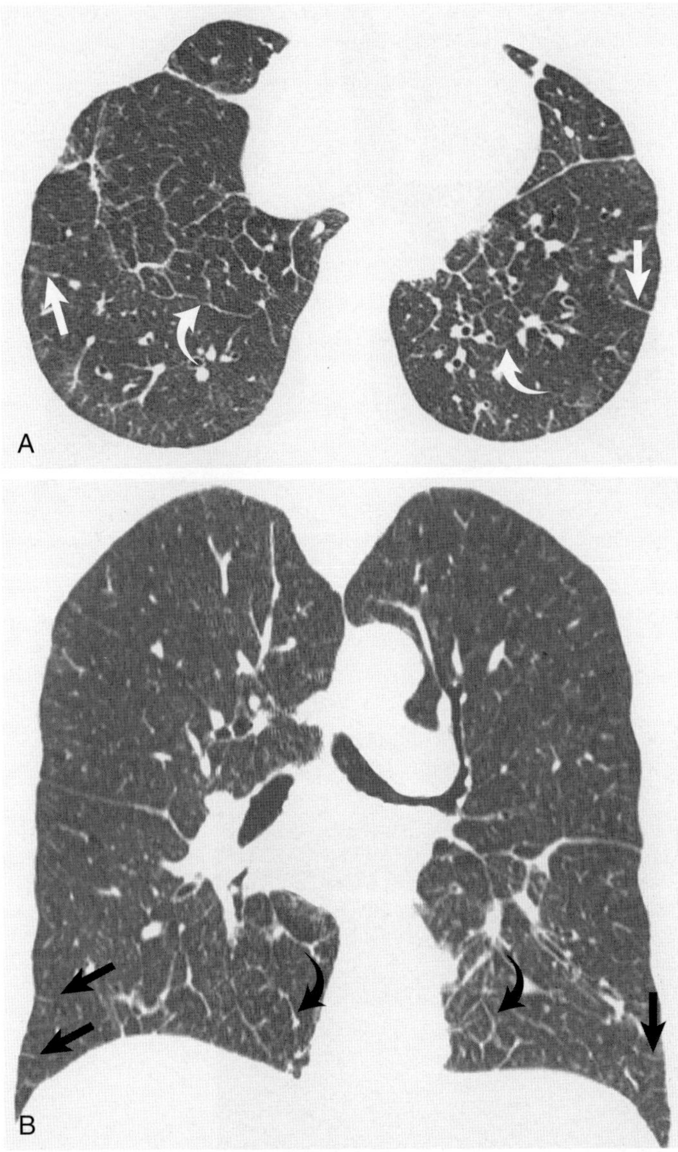

Fig. 54.11 Interstitial pulmonary edema in left-sided heart failure: CT findings. (A) CT at the level of the lower lung zones shows smooth interlobular septal thickening perpendicular to the pleura *(straight arrows)* and more centrally as polygonal arcades *(curved arrows).* (B) Coronal reformatted CT demonstrates septal pattern mainly in the lower lung zones. The thickened interlobular septa are seen as smooth lines perpendicular to the pleura *(straight arrows)* and as polygonal arcades *(curved arrows).* The thickened interlobular septa are the CT equivalent of Kerley B lines seen on radiography.

successful treatment of the heart failure. In a review of 46 patients who had major and minor clinical signs of congestive heart failure and had undergone chest CT during their symptomatic period, enlarged mediastinal lymph nodes and hazy mediastinal fat were seen in 55% and 33% of cases, respectively.[31] A recent retrospective study involving 215 patients with congestive heart failure who underwent CT showed enlarged mediastinal lymph nodes in 68%. Of importance, lymph node enlargement usually involved more than one nodal station and generally spared the hilar lymph node stations.[32] It is also common for intraparenchymal lymph nodes to enlarge during episodes of pulmonary edema. These lymph nodes manifest as triangular- or rectangular-shaped nodules located along fissures and interlobular septa. Lymphadenopathy in patients with left-sided heart failure therefore does not necessarily indicate an infectious process or malignant neoplasm.

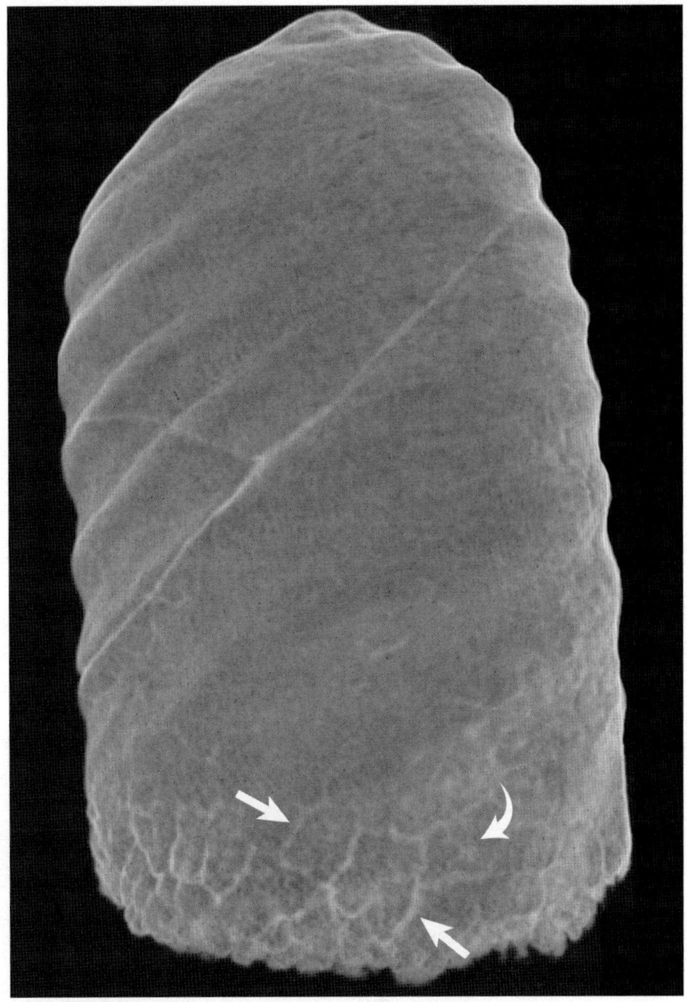

Fig. 54.12 Interstitial pulmonary edema in left-sided heart failure: septal lines and prominent centrilobular structures on volume-rendering CT. Volume-rendered CT image of the right lung shows thickening of the interlobular septa *(straight arrows)* and prominence of the centrilobular structures *(curved arrow)* resulting from interstitial edema. Note that the edema involves almost exclusively the dependent regions of the lower lobe.

ECHOCARDIOGRAPHY

Bedside transthoracic echocardiography allows assessment of myocardial and valvular function and can play an important role in the assessment of patients with hydrostatic pulmonary edema.[6,33] In one study of 49 critically ill patients with unexplained pulmonary edema or hypotension, transthoracic echocardiography results were in agreement with data generated from a pulmonary artery catheter in 86% of cases.[34] It has been suggested that transthoracic echocardiography should be the first approach to assessment of left ventricular and valvular function in patients in whom the clinical, laboratory, and radiologic findings fail to establish the cause of pulmonary edema.[6]

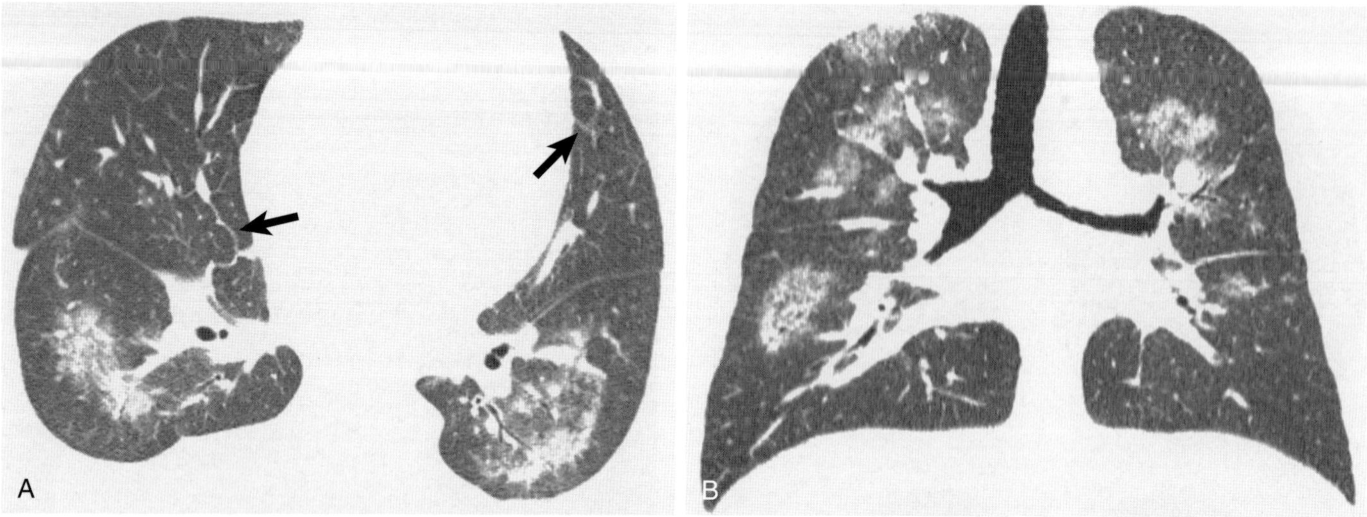

Fig. 54.13 Perihilar distribution of airspace pulmonary edema (bat wing edema) in left-sided heart failure. (A) High-resolution CT shows consolidation and ground-glass opacities in the lower lobes. Note mild interlobular septal thickening *(arrows)* and small pleural effusions. (B) Coronal reformatted CT demonstrates predominantly perihilar (bat wing) distribution of the consolidation and ground-glass opacities.

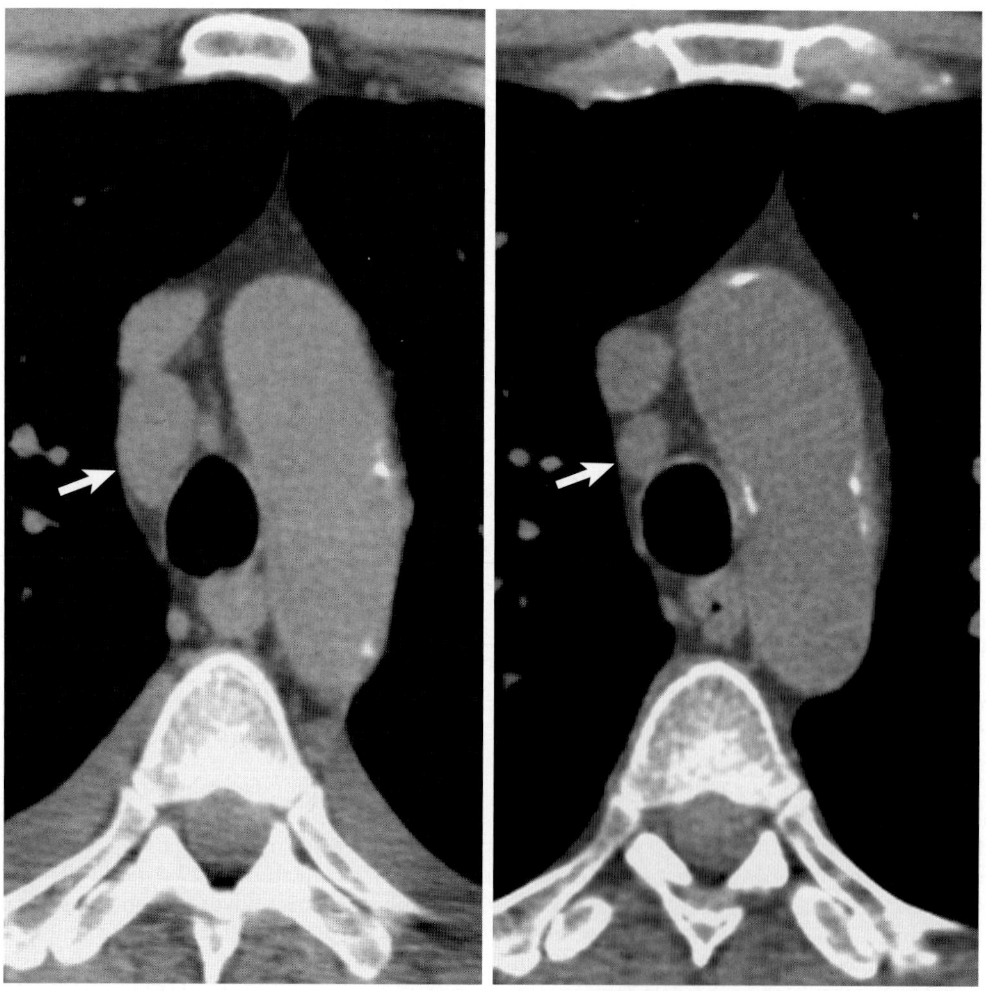

Fig. 54.14 Enlarged mediastinal lymph node in patient with pulmonary edema. Composite image with CT at time of pulmonary edema *(left image)* and 2 months later after resolution of pulmonary edema *(right image)* shows resolution of small pleural effusions and decreased size of a right paratracheal station lymph node *(arrows)*.

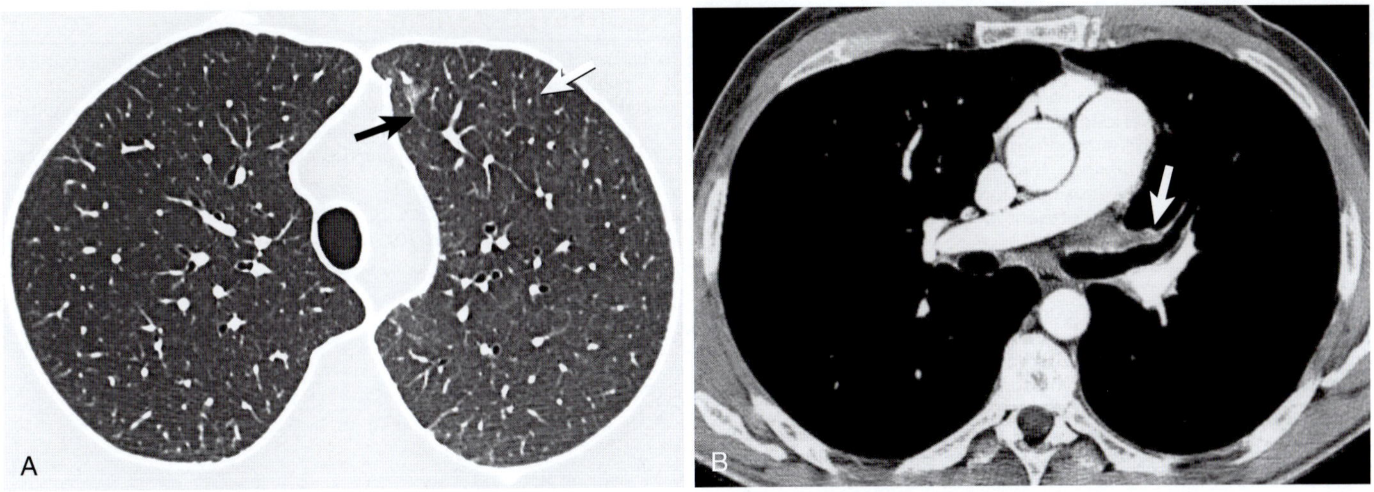

Fig. 54.15 Unilateral pulmonary edema caused by venous obstruction after radiofrequency ablation. (A) High-resolution CT image at the level of the upper lobes demonstrates thickening of the interlobular septa *(arrows)* and diffuse ground-glass opacities in the left upper lobe. (B) Contrast-enhanced CT at the level of the left upper lobe bronchus shows lack of enhancement of the left superior pulmonary vein *(arrow)* consistent with complete obstruction.

CLASSIC SIGNS

- Thickening of interlobar fissures
- Loss of definition of subsegmental and segmental vessels (vascular indistinctness)
- Septal (Kerley) lines
- Perihilar or diffuse consolidation
- Air bronchograms uncommon
- Small pleural effusions commonly evident on radiograph
- Cardiomegaly common

Differential Diagnosis

The differential diagnosis of hydrostatic pulmonary edema includes pneumonia, exacerbation of chronic obstructive pulmonary disease or asthma, pulmonary hemorrhage, and upper airway obstruction.[2] Making the diagnosis can be difficult. It has been estimated that the clinical diagnosis of acute heart failure is incorrect in more than 50% of cases, with frequent overdiagnosis and underdiagnosis.[35,36]

On radiologic examination the most common difficulty is the differentiation of hydrostatic from permeability pulmonary edema with or without diffuse alveolar damage. Findings most suggestive of hydrostatic pulmonary edema include cardiomegaly, predominantly perihilar distribution of the edema, thick fissures, and presence of septal lines and pleural effusion.[37,38] Radiographic features most suggestive of permeability edema include inhomogeneous or predominantly peripheral distribution of the edema, presence of air bronchograms, and lack of septal lines and pleural effusion.[37,38] A combination of findings permits correct identification of hydrostatic pulmonary edema in 80% to 90% of patients and correct identification of permeability edema in 60% to 90% of cases.[37,38] However, patients with ARDS frequently have superimposed hydrostatic edema, and it is often difficult or impossible to determine to what extent the parenchymal abnormalities are due to permeability edema or hydrostatic edema. In these patients measurement of the pulmonary arterial wedge pressure with a pulmonary artery catheter is often required.

The most common causes of hydrostatic pulmonary edema are left-sided heart failure (cardiogenic pulmonary edema), acute and chronic renal disease, and fluid overload. Less commonly, unilateral or bilateral pulmonary edema may be the result of pulmonary venous obstruction. Abnormalities of the pulmonary veins that may result in pulmonary edema include congenital pulmonary vein stenosis, pulmonary venoocclusive disease, stenosis that follows surgery or radiofrequency ablation, fibrosing mediastinitis, and pulmonary vein compression or invasion by tumor. Pulmonary venoocclusive disease is a rare idiopathic condition that results in progressive occlusion of the pulmonary veins, chronic interstitial edema, and severe pulmonary hypertension. The clinical, radiographic, and CT findings are mainly those of pulmonary hypertension (see Chapter 53). However, unlike those with idiopathic and chronic thromboembolic pulmonary arterial hypertension, patients with pulmonary venoocclusive disease typically also have findings of interstitial edema, particularly thickening of the interlobular septa.[39] Radiofrequency ablation is commonly used for the elimination of focal arrhythmogenic triggers arising within pulmonary veins in patients with atrial fibrillation. Radiofrequency energy delivery outside the pulmonary vein ostia in these patients may result in vein stenosis or occlusion and pulmonary edema distal to the obstructed vein (Fig. 54.15).[40] The pulmonary vein stenosis and obstruction and the edema can be well demonstrated on CT[40] and on contrast-enhanced MR angiography.[41]

Synopsis of Treatment Options

In patients with acute hydrostatic pulmonary edema, in the absence of contraindications, empirical treatment is often started with diuretic therapy.[6] Other fairly standard medical therapy options include supplemental oxygen provided by a face mask, vasodilators, and inotropics. In patients with acute cardiogenic pulmonary edema, noninvasive support ventilation with continuous positive airway pressure or bilevel noninvasive pressure support ventilation has been shown to reduce intubation rate and mortality.[42]

KEY POINTS

- Common causes of hydrostatic pulmonary edema include left ventricular failure, mitral valve disease, renal failure, liver disease, and fluid overload.
- Characteristic findings include thick fissures, ill-defined pulmonary vascular markings, thickened interlobular septa (Kerley B lines), pleural effusions, and cardiomegaly.
- Cardiomegaly may not be present in patients with acute pulmonary edema.
- Classic bat wing distribution of edema is seen in less than 10% of patients.
- There may be a lag of 12 hours or more between the onset of symptoms and the development of radiologically visible abnormalities. Additionally, there may be up to a 3-day lag in clearing of edema after symptom resolution.
- Radiographic findings are of limited value in differentiating hydrostatic from permeability edema. The most helpful signs in diagnosing hydrostatic edema are presence of septal lines and pleural effusion, lack of air bronchograms, and predominantly central distribution of edema.

SUGGESTED READINGS

Gluecker T, Capasso P, Schnyder P, et al. Clinical and radiologic features of pulmonary edema. *Radiographics*. 1999;19:1507–1531.

Ketai LH, Godwin JD. A new view of pulmonary edema and acute respiratory distress syndrome. *J Thorac Imaging*. 1998;13:147–471.

Ware LB, Matthay MA. Clinical practice. Acute pulmonary edema. *N Engl J Med*. 2005;353:2788–2796.

The full reference list for this chapter is available at ExpertConsult.com.

55 Permeability Pulmonary Edema*

STEPHEN B. HOBBS

Etiology

Pulmonary edema is defined as an excess of fluid in the extravascular compartment of the lung and is classified into four categories based on pathophysiology: hydrostatic edema, permeability edema with diffuse alveolar damage, permeability edema without diffuse alveolar damage, and mixed edema resulting from hydrostatic and permeability edema. Permeability pulmonary edema is almost always a manifestation of capillary endothelial injury or alveolar epithelial damage with resultant loss of fluid and protein into the airspaces or interstitium. Less commonly, permeability edema may occur in the absence of diffuse alveolar damage, such as in patients with the hantavirus pulmonary syndrome or after interleukin therapy.[1] Patients who have permeability edema were originally classified clinically into two groups: those with acute lung injury and those with acute respiratory distress syndrome (ARDS).[2–4] However, this definition, which was recommended by the American-European Consensus Conference in 1994, was refined in 2011, with the new outline being referred to as the *Berlin definition*.[5] That updated definition removes the term *acute lung injury* and includes four clinical criteria for a diagnosis of ARDS. Those criteria focus on (1) timing (acute onset within 1 week of clinical insult or onset of respiratory symptoms), (2) chest imaging (bilateral opacities representing an airspace process on chest radiography or computed tomography [CT]), (3) origin of edema (respiratory failure not fully explained by cardiac failure or fluid overload), (4) oxygenation (now based on PaO_2/FiO_2 [partial pressure of oxygen in arterial blood/forced inspiratory oxygen] ratio while on 5 cm of continuous positive airway pressure [CPAP]). The three categories of oxygenation are mild (PaO_2/FiO_2 of 201–300), moderate (PaO_2/FiO_2 of 101–200), and severe (PaO_2/FiO_2 of ≤100).

The majority of patients who are at increased risk for the development of ARDS can be classified into two categories: pulmonary (or direct injury) and extrapulmonary (or indirect injury). The main causes of direct lung injury are pneumonia and aspiration; the main causes of indirect lung injury are sepsis, major trauma, and multiple transfusions. A large cohort study reported that the most common risk factor is severe sepsis with a suspected pulmonary source, followed by severe sepsis with a suspected extrapulmonary source.[6] In some series, sepsis (pulmonary or extrapulmonary), pneumonia, aspiration of gastric contents, and major trauma account for more than 85% of causes of ARDS.[7] Other more rare causes include burns, drug overdose, near drowning, postperfusion injury after cardiopulmonary bypass, pancreatitis, fat embolism, and high-altitude pulmonary edema.

Prevalence and Epidemiology

An accurate estimate of the incidence of ARDS has been hampered by the lack of a uniform definition and the heterogeneity of the causes and clinical manifestations. An early estimate by the National Institutes of Health (NIH) suggested that the annual incidence in the United States was 75 per 100,000 population,[2] and a more recent study from 2005 demonstrated an incidence of 86 per 100,000.[6] It is currently estimated that there are approximately 190,000 case annually in the United States, resulting in 75,000 deaths.[6]

Clinical Presentation

Patients with permeability edema typically present with acute onset of shortness of breath (generally <72 hours after initial onset or inciting event), bilateral parenchymal opacities on imaging, and refractory hypoxemia and no significant evidence of left-sided heart failure.

ARDS is often associated with other organ failure.[8–10] Patients who die early (within the first 72 hours of ARDS onset [26%–44%]) usually die of the presenting injury or illness that resulted in ARDS. Patients whose deaths occur late (>72 hours after ARDS onset [56%–74%]) most often die of complications (i.e., new organ failures) that arose during the course of ARDS.[10,11] Although the mortality rate for patients with ARDS has declined from 50% to 70% in the 1980s to 35% to 46% in 2014, the distribution of causes of death has not changed.[3,11,12] Sepsis with multiorgan failure is the most common cause of death (30%–50%), whereas respiratory failure results in a smaller percentage of deaths (13%–19%).[11] The increased survival during the past 2 decades is due largely to advances in supportive care, such as dialysis, and a decrease in extrapulmonary organ failure.[13] Nevertheless, survival for those patients who have sepsis syndrome has not changed appreciably.[11]

PREDICTIVE CLINICAL RISK FACTORS

Results of multivariate regression analyses have shown an association of death due to ARDS with increasing age (>70 years),[8] underlying liver cirrhosis,[9] high McCabe score for prognosis of the underlying disease, high Acute Physiology and Chronic Health Evaluation II (APACHE II) score for general severity,[10] and high Sequential Organ Failure Assessment (SOFA) score for associated multiorgan failure.[10] Pulmonary factors independently associated with mortality are direct lung injury as the cause of ARDS and the extent of oxygenation impairment on day 3 after the onset of

*The editors and publisher would like thank Dr. Kazyua Ichikado for contributing material on this topic to the prior edition of this work. It has served as the foundation for the current chapter.

ARDS.[10,11] Semiquantitative evaluation of fibroproliferative changes by high-resolution CT scan in patients with a clinically early stage of ARDS is also an independent predictor of survival and shows a significant inverse association with the number of ventilator-free days (i.e., days without mechanical ventilation).[14]

Pathophysiology

The histologic features of ARDS are characterized by diffuse alveolar damage and represent a time-dependent, stereotypic response to acute lung injury.[14,15] The changes can be viewed as evolving from epithelial and endothelial necrosis to alveolar collapse and eventually to fibroblast proliferation and fibrosis. Permeability edema is prominent in the early stages and heralds the onset of rapidly progressive fibroblast proliferation, which predominates in the late phase of disease. The microscopic appearance varies according to both the time interval between injury and biopsy and the extent and localization of the injury. Diffuse alveolar damage has traditionally been divided into three sequential and overlapping phases: the acute exudative phase of edema and hemorrhage, the subacute proliferative phase of organization and repair, and the fibrotic phase of collagen deposition and end-stage fibrosis. The last two phases are designated the fibroproliferative phase. It is of clinical importance that the histologic features of diffuse alveolar damage correlate with the duration of injury more than with its initiating cause.

The acute exudative phase predominates within the first 7 days of injury and is characterized by edema, intraalveolar hemorrhage, and hyaline membrane formation (Fig. 55.1). The histologic changes

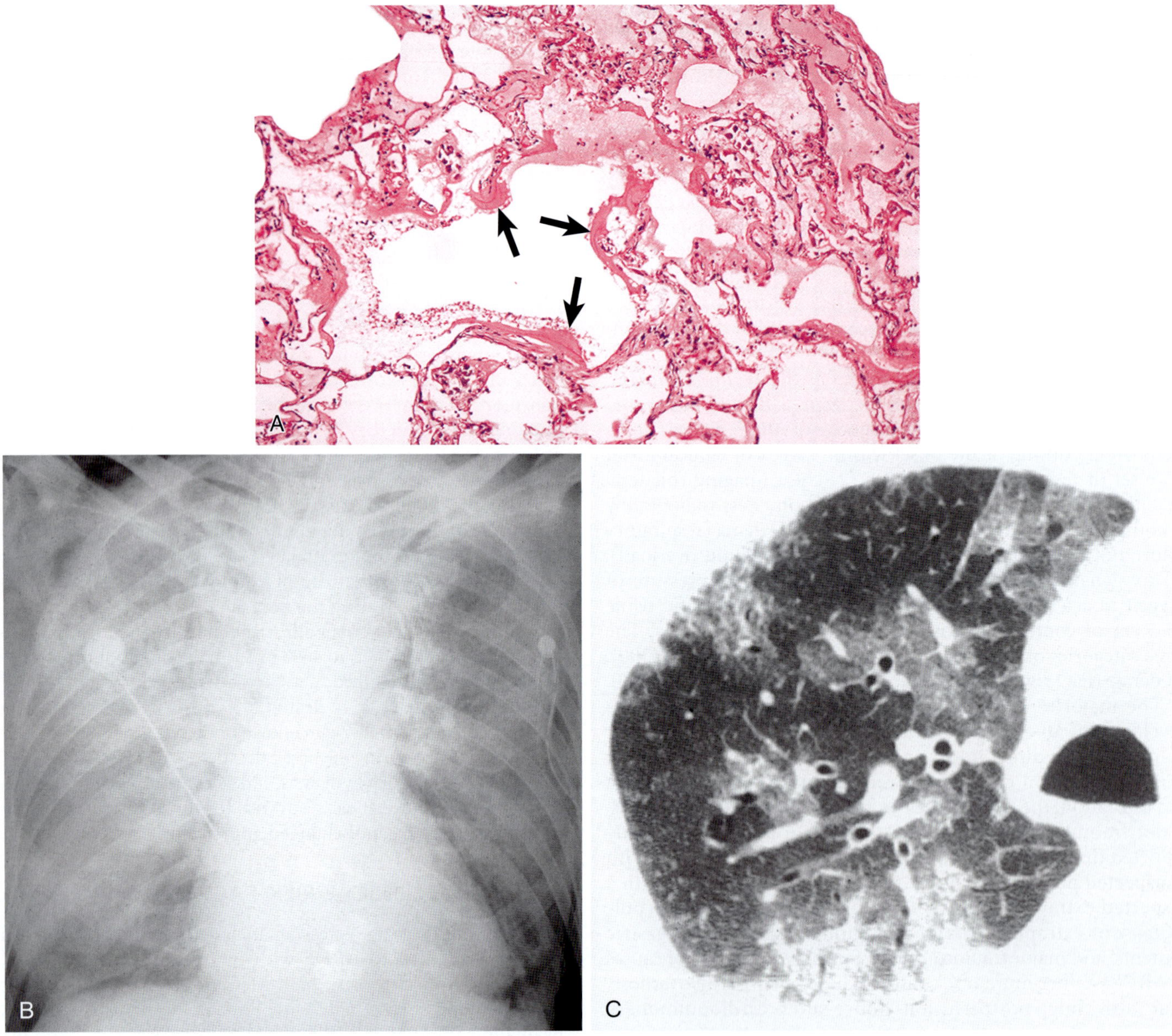

Fig. 55.1 Acute exudative phase of diffuse alveolar damage caused by sepsis. (A) Pathologic specimen shows characteristic intraalveolar hyaline membranes *(arrows)* and exudates. (B) Chest radiograph shows extensive bilateral ground-glass opacities and consolidation. (C) High-resolution CT scan at the level of the right upper lobe shows patchy ground-glass opacities demarcated by secondary lobules and associated with dependent consolidation.

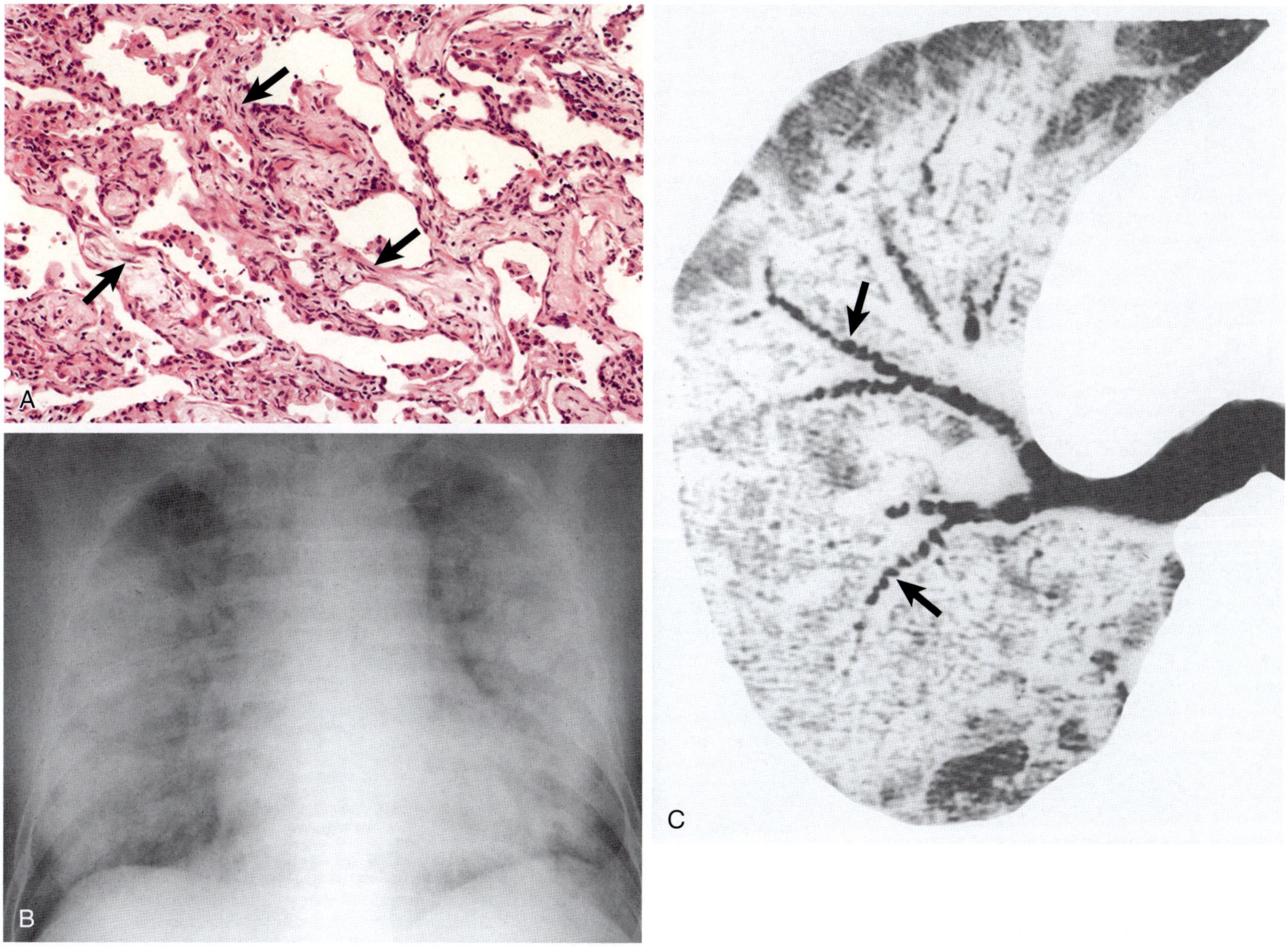

Fig. 55.2 Subacute proliferative phase of diffuse alveolar damage caused by viral pneumonia (3–7 days after the onset of lung injury). (A) Pathologic specimen shows diffuse fibroblastic proliferation *(arrows)* within the interstitium associated with organized hyaline membranes. (B) Chest radiograph demonstrates bilateral ground-glass opacities, consolidation, and low lung volumes. (C) High-resolution CT scan at the level of the right upper lobe bronchus shows extensive ground-glass opacities with associated reticulation and traction bronchiectasis *(arrows)*.

in the early exudative phase consist of capillary congestion, alveolar edema, and intraalveolar hemorrhage. Hyaline membranes, the histologic hallmark of this stage of the lesion, develop later and are most numerous 3 to 7 days after injury. Fibrin thrombi may be seen in the alveolar capillaries and pulmonary arterioles.

In the subacute proliferative phase of diffuse alveolar damage, fibroblast proliferation, mainly within the interstitium but also within airspaces, becomes prominent (Fig. 55.2). The proliferation of alveolar type 2 pneumocytes, which is seen as early as 3 days after injury and is a reparative phenomenon, occurs in the early proliferative phase and persists throughout this phase. Within the interstitium, fibroblasts and myofibroblasts proliferate and subsequently migrate into fibrinous intraalveolar exudate and convert the exudate to cellular granulation tissue. With the proliferation of fibroblasts (subacute proliferative phase), there is remodeling of the parenchyma, resulting in dilatation of the bronchi (traction bronchiectasis) and bronchioles (traction bronchiolectasis). Subsequently, typically 2 weeks or more after the injury, there is progressive fibrosis with collagen deposition (chronic fibrotic phase; Fig. 55.3). Microcystic airspaces 1 mm or larger in diameter (microscopic honeycombing) and traction bronchiectasis and bronchiolectasis are most pronounced in the late fibrotic phase. Cyst-like spaces in end-stage ARDS may also result from chronic interstitial emphysema.

Manifestations of the Disease

RADIOGRAPHY

In the initial phase of ARDS, the parenchymal abnormalities may be mild and the chest radiograph normal. In some cases the lung volumes may be decreased because of shallow breathing and tachypnea. Characteristic radiographic findings of the exudative phase of ARDS consist of extensive bilateral ground-glass opacities and consolidation (Fig. 55.4; see also Fig. 55.1). Their distribution may be patchy or diffuse and symmetric or asymmetric, and they may involve all lung zones to a similar extent or mainly the upper or lower lung zones. The bronchi

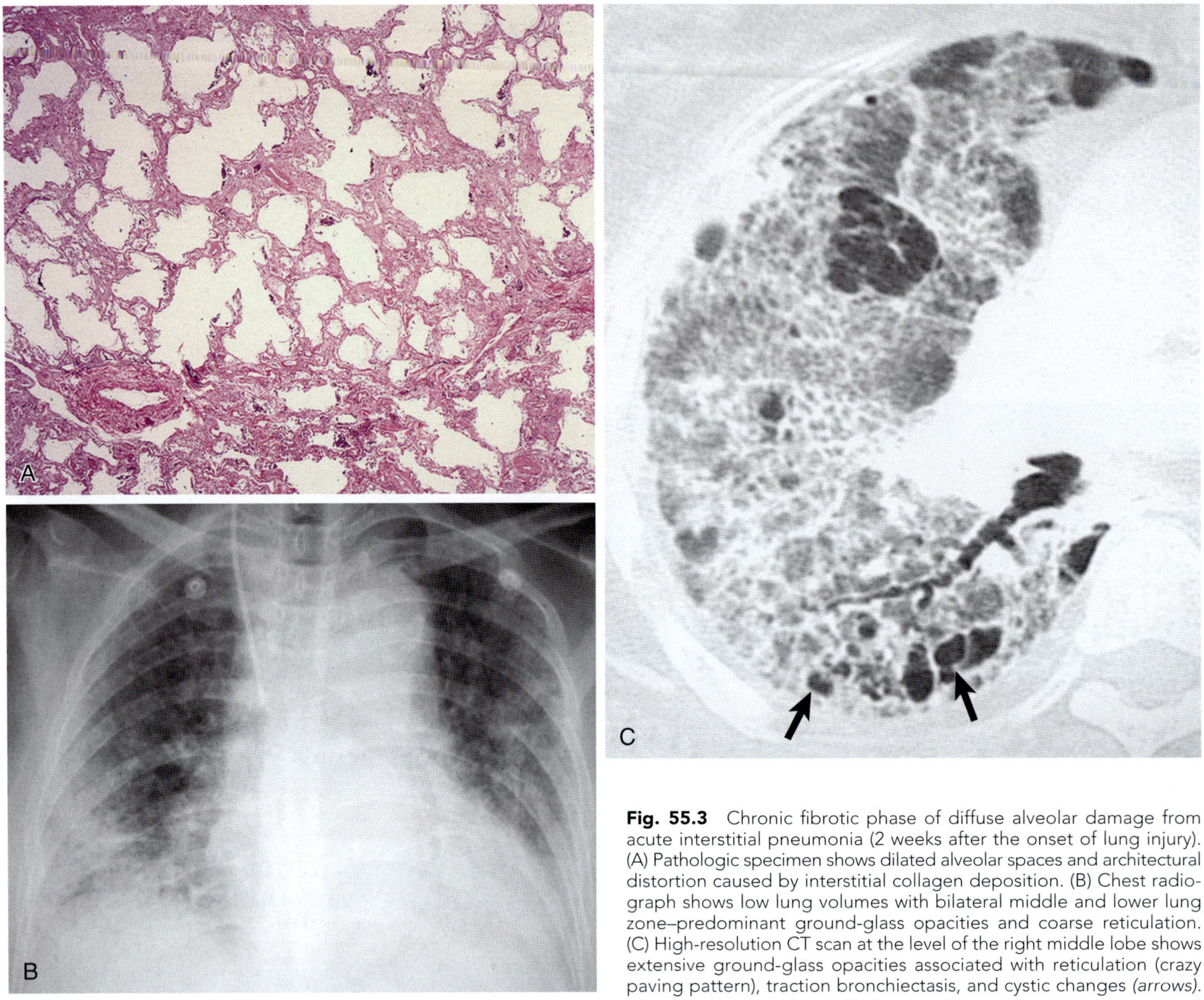

Fig. 55.3 Chronic fibrotic phase of diffuse alveolar damage from acute interstitial pneumonia (2 weeks after the onset of lung injury). (A) Pathologic specimen shows dilated alveolar spaces and architectural distortion caused by interstitial collagen deposition. (B) Chest radiograph shows low lung volumes with bilateral middle and lower lung zone–predominant ground-glass opacities and coarse reticulation. (C) High-resolution CT scan at the level of the right middle lobe shows extensive ground-glass opacities associated with reticulation (crazy paving pattern), traction bronchiectasis, and cystic changes *(arrows)*.

typically remain patent, resulting in air bronchograms (see Fig. 55.4). With progression to the fibroproliferative phase, a coarse reticular pattern is seen superimposed on the ground-glass opacities, and there is progressive volume loss (see Figs. 55.2 and 55.3). The radiographic findings are markedly influenced by the positive end-expiratory pressure ventilation that is routinely used in patients with extensive permeability edema.[16–18]

COMPUTED TOMOGRAPHY

Similar to the radiograph, the CT findings may be normal in the early phase of ARDS, but an abnormality is usually detected within 12 hours. The CT findings have been shown to correlate well with the pathologic phases of diffuse alveolar damage.[19–21] In the exudative and early proliferative phase of diffuse alveolar damage, CT typically shows extensive bilateral ground-glass opacities with or without associated consolidation (Fig. 55.5; see also Fig. 55.1). Interlobular septal thickening is frequently superimposed on the ground-glass opacities, resulting in a pattern known as crazy paving (Fig. 55.6). This interlobular septal thickening corresponds histologically to edematous thickening in the exudative phase and to alveolar collapse adjacent to interlobular septa and subsequent organization in the proliferative or fibrotic phase of diffuse alveolar damage. In the early stages the consolidation, when present, tends to have a patchy distribution. Later in the exudative phase, the consolidation becomes more homogeneous and gravity dependent (see Fig. 55.6). In the late proliferative and fibrotic phase, the CT findings also include traction bronchiectasis and bronchiolectasis associated with loss of lung volume (as demonstrated by displacement or distortion of interlobar fissures, bronchi, or vessels; see Figs. 55.2 and 55.3). In the fibrotic phase, coarse reticular opacities and small cystic spaces caused pathologically by marked restructuring of distal airspaces and interstitial dense fibrosis are also seen (Fig. 55.7; see also Fig. 55.3). In some patients the distribution of residual fibrosis after resolution of the airspace disease will be anterior lung predominant (Fig. 55.8).

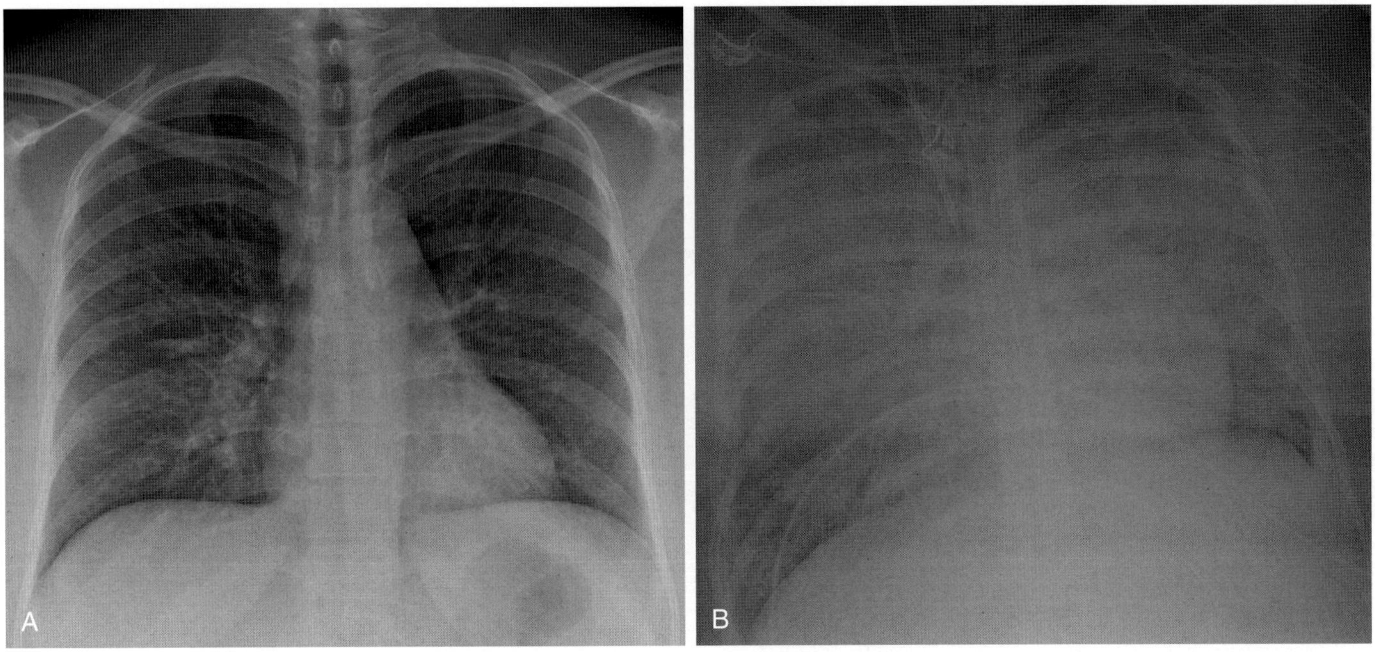

Fig. 55.4 Acute respiratory distress syndrome: radiographic findings. (A) Admission radiograph showing mild bronchial wall thickening and diffuse interstitial opacities. (B) Thirty-six hours later, both lungs show extensive consolidation with air bronchograms.

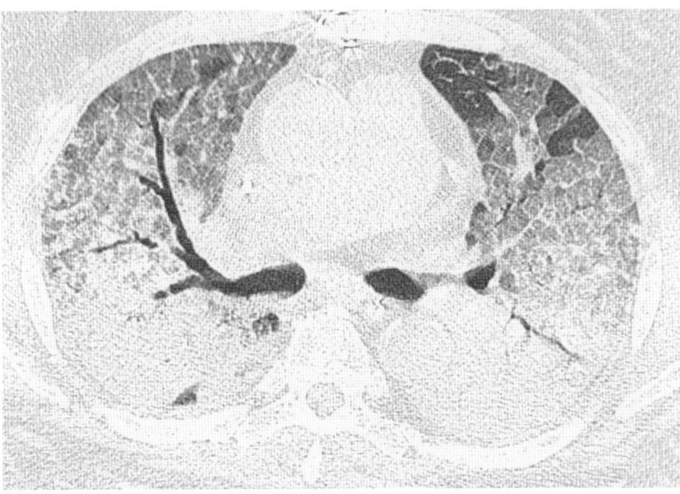

Fig. 55.5 Diffuse alveolar damage caused by amiodarone. Axial CT demonstrates extensive bilateral ground-glass opacities and dependent areas of consolidation. Note focal lobular areas of sparing and smooth lines superimposed on the ground-glass opacities, resulting in a crazy paving pattern. The patient presented with progressive shortness of breath and developed respiratory failure.

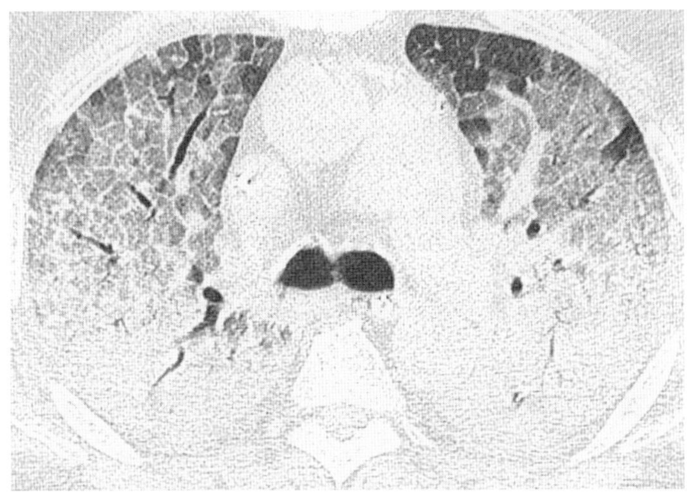

Fig. 55.6 Acute respiratory distress syndrome with crazy paving pattern on CT. High-resolution CT image shows extensive ground-glass opacities with superimposed smooth septal thickening (crazy paving pattern). Also noted are bilateral areas of consolidation with air bronchograms in the dependent lung regions.

MONITORING OF DISEASE PROGRESSION OR REGRESSION

The chest radiograph plays an important role in the diagnosis of ARDS, in monitoring of disease progression, and in assessment of clinically suspected complications.[18,19] Chest radiographs are particularly helpful in detecting and monitoring pneumothorax (Fig. 55.9).[22,23]

The radiographic findings in patients with ARDS are influenced by a number of factors, including stage of diffuse alveolar damage, positive end-expiratory pressure, inspiratory volume, and timing of x-ray exposure. A high positive end-expiratory pressure may result in increased lucency and apparent improvement of ARDS. Therefore the radiographs must be interpreted with awareness of the ventilator settings. With regression of disease, the radiographic findings begin to improve and may resolve completely. However, in some cases there may be residual coarse reticular opacities and cysts.[17,18]

PREDICTION OF ETIOLOGY (DIRECT PULMONARY VS. EXTRAPULMONARY INJURY)

The differentiation between pulmonary or direct and extrapulmonary or indirect injury may be supported by findings on

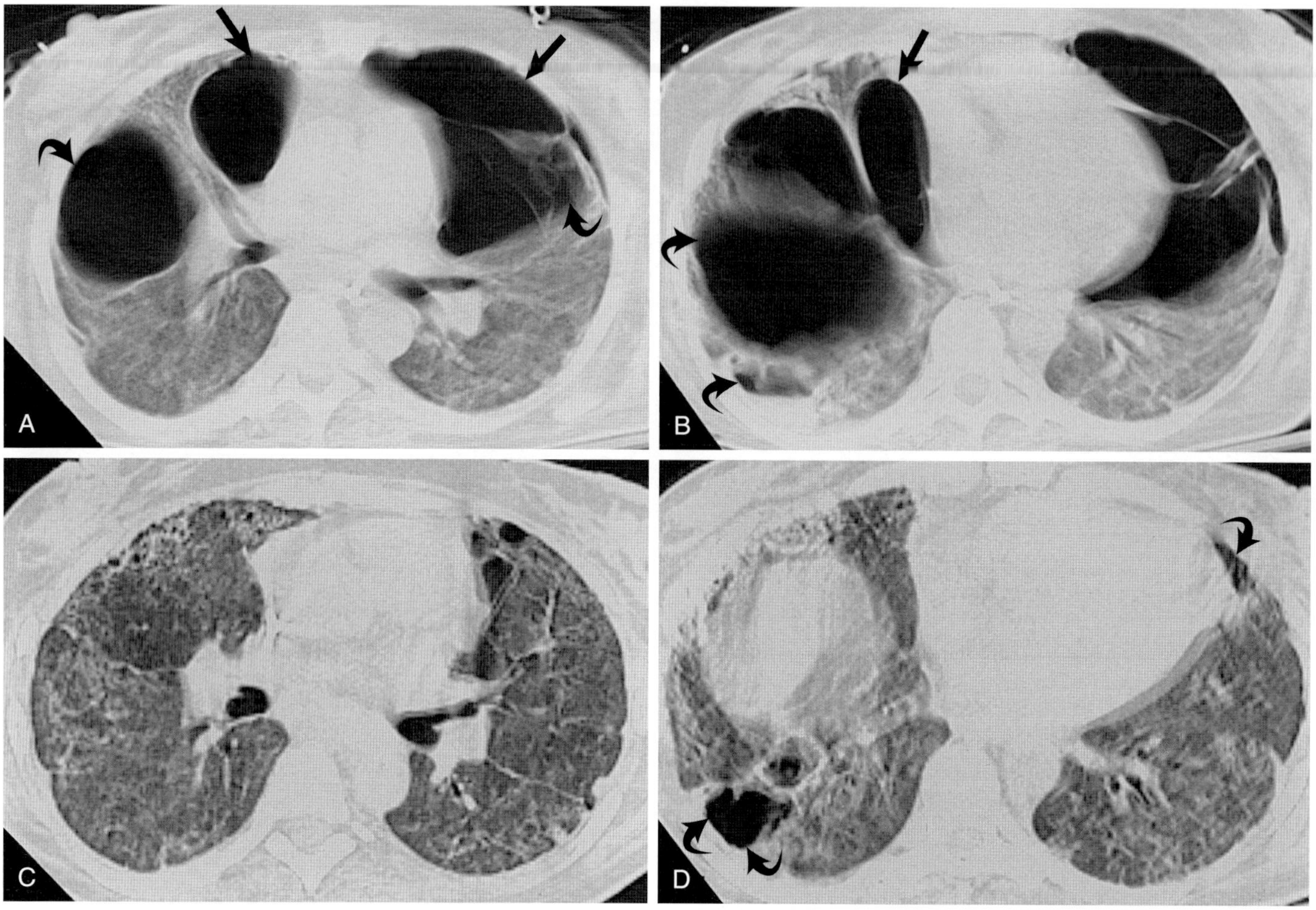

Fig. 55.7 Cystic changes in acute respiratory distress syndrome (ARDS) in a woman who developed sepsis and ARDS after cesarean section. High-resolution CT scans 1 week later (A and B) show bilateral loculated pneumothoraces *(straight arrows)* and cystic changes *(curved arrows)* in both lungs. High-resolution CT scans 1 month later (C and D) show bilateral areas of ground-glass opacity, irregular linear opacities, and residual cystic changes (D, *curved arrows*). *(Case courtesy Dr. Maura Brown, Vancouver, Canada; from Müller NL, Fraser RS, Colman NC, Paré PD.* Radiologic Diagnosis of Diseases of the Chest. *Philadelphia: WB Saunders; 2001.)*

computed tomography,[24] respiratory mechanics, and response to positive end-expiratory pressure.[25] Goodman and colleagues[26] reported that patients with ARDS secondary to direct lung injury tend to have an asymmetric distribution of the ground-glass opacities and consolidation on CT (Fig. 55.10), whereas patients with ARDS secondary to indirect injury tend to have bilateral symmetric distribution of findings (Fig. 55.11). Desai and colleagues[27] reported that there was considerable overlap in the findings between ARDS resulting from direct lung injury and ARDS resulting from extrathoracic causes. However, ARDS resulting from extrathoracic causes was more likely to be associated with extensive dependent consolidation, whereas ARDS resulting from direct lung injury was more likely to have more extensive nondependent consolidation and cysts.[27] Therefore bilateral symmetric distribution of findings characterized by dependent areas of dense consolidation merging with nondependent ground-glass opacity and apparently normally aerated lung is most frequently seen in patients with ARDS secondary to indirect lung injury.

PREDICTION OF PATHOLOGIC STAGES AND PROGNOSIS

As mentioned previously, the high-resolution CT findings correlate with the pathologic stage of diffuse alveolar damage.[19–21] Traction bronchiolectasis or bronchiectasis within areas of increased attenuation (ground-glass opacity, consolidation) on high-resolution CT usually indicates progression from the exudative to the fibroproliferative and fibrotic phases of diffuse alveolar damage. During these phases, the lung parenchyma undergoes extensive remodeling with some degree of pulmonary fibrosis. The extent of coarse reticular pattern associated with CT signs of lung fibrosis, including architectural distortion and traction bronchiectasis, correlates with the length of time that patients receive pressure-controlled inverse-ratio ventilation.[28]

Extensive CT abnormalities indicative of fibroproliferative changes were independently predictive of poor prognosis in patients with early ARDS.[29] Such findings were also associated with requirements for longer duration of ventilator assistance. The accurate determination of disease stage by means of CT

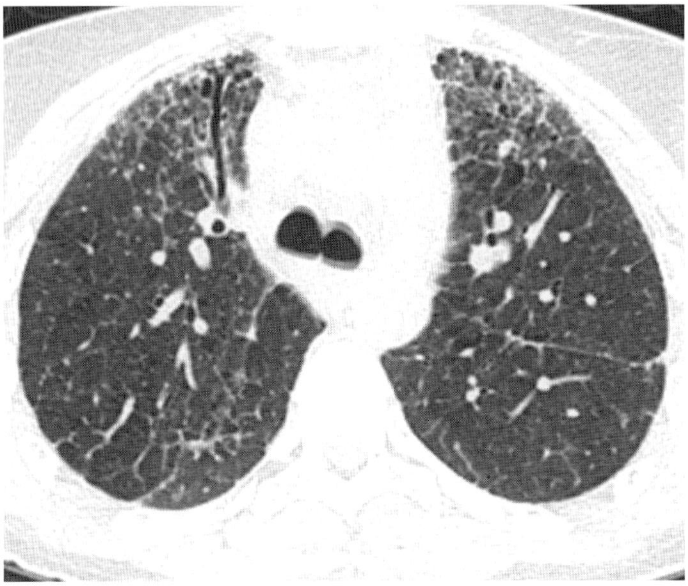

Fig. 55.8 Fibrotic stage of acute respiratory distress syndrome after severe influenza virus H1N1 infection. High-resolution CT scan demonstrates bilateral anterior lung reticulation, architectural distortion, and traction bronchiectasis.

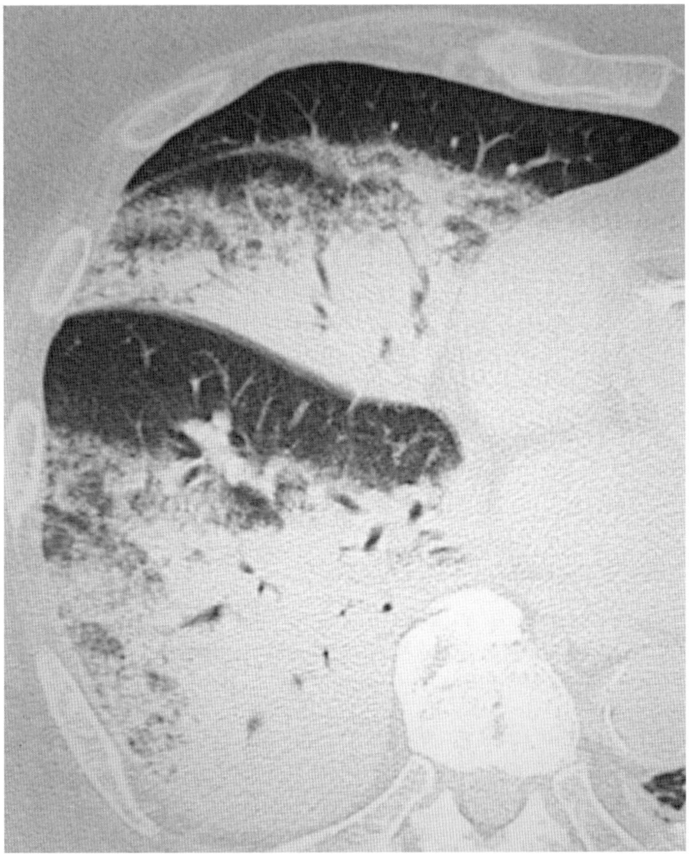

Fig. 55.10 Acute respiratory distress syndrome caused by *Streptococcus pneumoniae* pneumonia. High-resolution CT scan at the level of the right middle lobe demonstrates dependent consolidation in the middle and lower lobes. The left lung was normal.

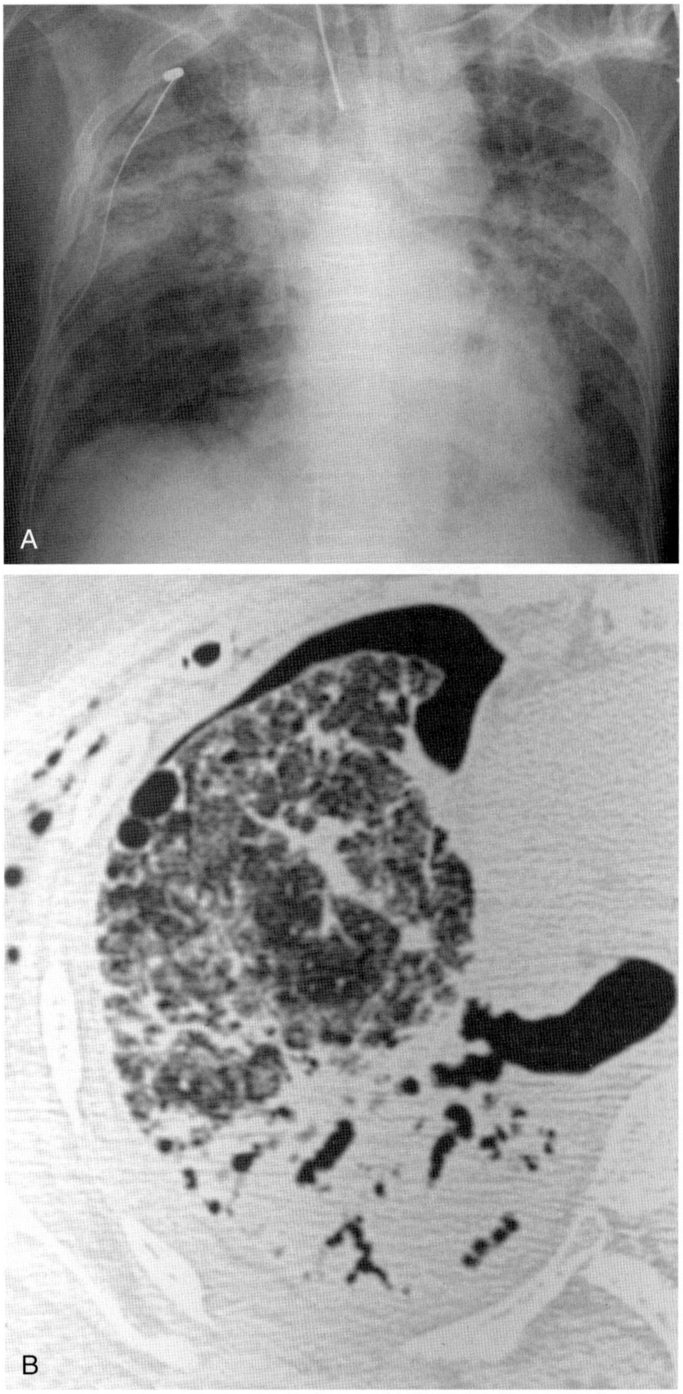

Fig. 55.9 Barotrauma (pneumothorax) in acute respiratory distress syndrome after prolonged ventilator assistance. (A) Chest radiograph shows right pneumothorax associated with bilateral coarse reticulation and volume loss. A right chest tube is in place. (B) High-resolution CT scan at the level of the right upper lobe demonstrates a small anterior right pneumothorax. Also noted are anterior ground-glass opacities, dependent consolidation, and findings of the fibrotic stage of diffuse alveolar damage with coarse reticulation, traction bronchiectasis, and cystic changes.

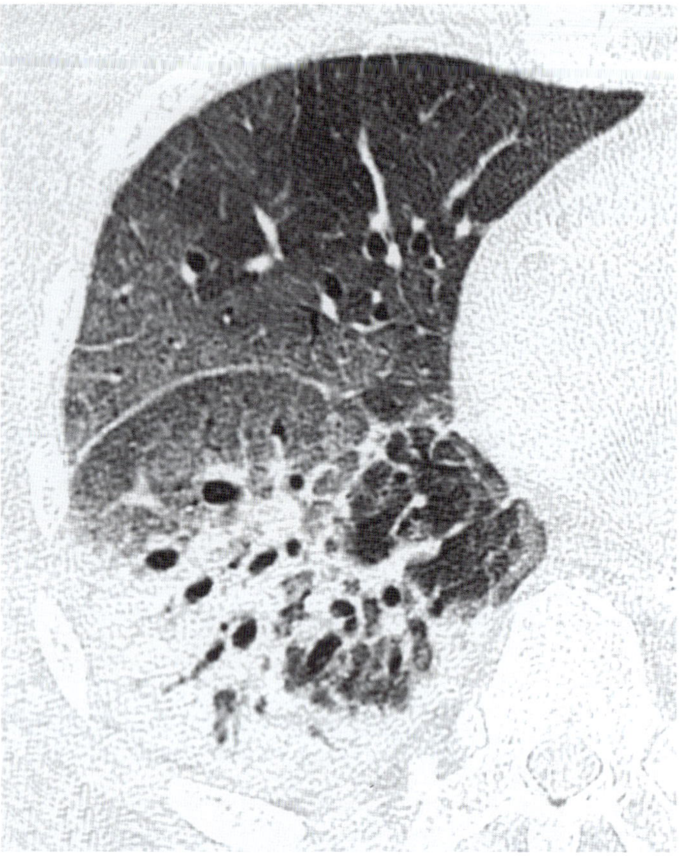

Fig. 55.11 Acute respiratory distress syndrome caused by sepsis. High-resolution CT scan at the level of the right middle lobe shows dependent consolidation and nondependent ground-glass opacity. The left lung showed similar findings.

assessment may be informative regarding the potential for ventilator-induced lung injury and the response to treatment in patients with ARDS.

DETECTION OF COMPLICATIONS

Computed tomography is superior to radiography in the detection of complications. It has been reported that up to 40% of cases of pneumothorax and 80% of cases of pneumomediastinum seen on the CT scan may not be apparent on the radiograph.[30] Pleural effusions and lung abscesses are also detected more frequently on CT than on radiographs.[31] The onset of barotrauma (pneumothorax, pneumomediastinum, and subcutaneous air) is more likely to occur late in the course of disease and is related to worsening lung compliance and increased fibroproliferative change over time (see Fig. 55.9).[29,32]

Differential Diagnosis

In the majority of patients the diagnosis of ARDS can be readily made on the basis of a combination of clinical, radiologic, and laboratory findings. In patients with no apparent risk factors for ARDS who present with acute dyspnea and diffuse parenchymal abnormalities, the differential diagnosis includes other causes of acute airspace disease, such as hydrostatic pulmonary edema, diffuse alveolar hemorrhage, drug reaction, and pneumonia. The differential diagnosis requires careful clinical history and appropriate laboratory tests, including serology.[33] Depending on the clinical findings, further investigation may include bronchoscopy with bronchoalveolar lavage. Transbronchial and surgical lung biopsy may be required in selected cases.[34,35]

Several diffuse parenchymal lung diseases may manifest acutely and mimic the clinical, physiologic, and radiographic criteria for ARDS. These include acute interstitial pneumonia (see Chapter 30), acute eosinophilic pneumonia (see Chapter 37), organizing pneumonia (see Chapter 29), diffuse alveolar hemorrhage (see Chapter 2), and acute hypersensitivity pneumonitis (see Chapter 32).[33] Acute interstitial pneumonia is essentially idiopathic ARDS. The patients have clinical, imaging, and histologic findings identical to those of patients with ARDS, but no etiology is identified. Compared with patients with ARDS, patients with acute interstitial pneumonia are more likely to have a predominantly lower lung zone and bilateral symmetric distribution of parenchymal abnormalities.[33]

Radiographic features most suggestive of permeability edema include patchy or predominantly peripheral distribution of the edema, presence of air bronchograms, and lack of septal lines and pleural effusion.[36–38] Findings most suggestive of hydrostatic pulmonary edema include cardiomegaly, blood flow redistribution (upper lobe vessel size > lower lobe vessel size), predominantly perihilar distribution of the edema, thick fissures, and presence of septal lines and pleural effusion.[36–38] A combination of findings permits correct identification of hydrostatic pulmonary edema in 80% to 90% of patients and correct identification of permeability edema in 60% to 90%.[36–38] However, patients with ARDS frequently have superimposed hydrostatic edema, and it is often difficult or impossible to determine to what extent the parenchymal abnormalities are due to permeability edema or hydrostatic edema. In these patients, measurement of the pulmonary arterial wedge pressure with a Swan-Ganz catheter is often required.

Synopsis of Treatment Options

Several large well-controlled trials of ARDS therapies have been completed through the NIH-sponsored ARDS Clinical Trials Network. Currently, there is no specific therapy for ARDS, but treatment of the underlying condition, if known, is critical. Other therapies are supportive, and the mechanical ventilation strategy used has proven most important to overall mortality. Other supportive therapies focus on complication minimalization and include deep venous thrombosis prophylaxis, stress ulcer prophylaxis, and early mobilization.

VENTILATOR MANAGEMENT

The cornerstone of supportive therapy is mechanical ventilation, but ARDS is characterized by stiff, low-compliance lungs with impaired gas exchange. Correspondingly, there is strong evidence to support the use of volume- and pressure-limited lung-protective ventilation in adult patients with ARDS.[39] Because there is often marked heterogeneity of distribution of disease, positive-pressure ventilation must focus on recruitment and ventilation of diseased units and avoidance of injury to healthy units. Mechanical ventilatory support of ARDS has therefore shifted during the past decade to providing smaller (and thus less injurious) tidal volumes.

The oxygenation in patients with ARDS is improved when they are maneuvered into the prone position or are ventilated with positive end-expiratory pressure. Prone positioning causes

KEY POINTS

- Permeability edema is usually clinically manifested by acute respiratory distress syndrome (ARDS).
- Diagnostic criteria of ARDS relate to
  - Timing (acute onset within 1 week of clinical insult)
  - Chest imaging (airspace process on chest radiography or CT)
  - Origin of edema (limited contribution of cardiac failure or fluid overload)
  - Oxygenation (PaO_2/FiO_2 [partial pressure of oxygen in arterial blood/forced inspiratory oxygen] ratio while on 5 cm of continuous positive airway pressure)
- Etiology
  - Direct lung injury: pneumonia, aspiration of gastric contents
  - Extrapulmonary injury: sepsis, major trauma, and multiple transfusions
- Chest radiography findings include bilateral ground-glass opacities or consolidation in the exudative phase, which may progress to a superimposed coarse reticular pattern with volume loss in the fibroproliferative and fibrotic phases.
- The CT findings mirror the chest radiographic abnormalities, with extensive bilateral ground-glass opacities and predominantly dependent consolidation. Traction bronchiectasis and bronchiolectasis with architectural distortion are seen in the fibroproliferative and fibrotic stages.
- The radiologic findings of ARDS are relatively nonspecific. The main radiologic differential diagnosis includes severe pneumonia, hydrostatic pulmonary edema, and diffuse alveolar hemorrhage.
- Extrathoracic causes of ARDS are more likely to be associated with extensive dependent consolidation. ARDS caused by direct lung injury is more likely to have more extensive nondependent consolidation and cysts.

recruitment of poorly aerated or nonaerated areas of dorsal lung. A study has shown that the alveolar recruitment response to positive end-expiratory pressure is nonuniform; the most recruitment occurs in the nondependent and more cephalic lung.[32]

PHARMACOLOGIC INTERVENTION

No specific pharmacologic therapy has proved effective for ARDS.

Corticosteroids

Numerous trials of short-course, high-dose corticosteroids in humans at risk for, or in the early phase of, ARDS have failed to demonstrate benefit.[3] The ARDS Network has reported that methylprednisolone therapy may be harmful when it is initiated more than 2 weeks (chronic phase) after the onset of ARDS.[40]

SUGGESTED READINGS

ARDS Definition Task Force, Ranieri VM, Rubenfeld GD, Thompson BT, Ferguson ND, Caldwell E, et al. Acute respiratory distress syndrome: the Berlin definition. *JAMA*. 2012;307:2526–2533.

Bernard GR. Acute respiratory distress syndrome. A historical perspective. *Am J Respir Crit Care Med*. 2005;172:798–806.

Desai SR. Acute respiratory distress syndrome: imaging of the injured lung. *Clin Radiol*. 2002;57:8–17.

Goodman LR, Fumagalli R, Tagliabue P, et al. Adult respiratory distress syndrome due to pulmonary and extrapulmonary causes: CT, clinical, and functional correlations. *Radiology*. 1999;213(2):545–552.

Milne EN, Pistolesi M, Miniati M, et al. The radiologic distinction of cardiogenic and noncardiogenic edema. *AJR Am J Roentgenol*. 1985;144(5):879–894.

The full reference list for this chapter is available at ExpertConsult.com.

56 Tracheal Diseases*

BRENT P. LITTLE

The wide variety of tracheal diseases includes both benign and malignant conditions that may manifest as tracheal masses, focal or diffuse tracheal thickening, or tracheal calcification. Tracheal tumors, inflammatory conditions involving the trachea, infections, and posttraumatic or iatrogenic injuries are among the variety of tracheal pathologies that can be characterized at imaging. Structural abnormalities of the trachea include acquired or congenital tracheal stenosis, tracheomalacia, and tracheomegaly.

Although a subset of tracheal diseases may be first suspected at chest radiography, computed tomography (CT) is requisite for characterizing the extent and morphology of tracheal pathology. Volumetric acquisitions with multiplanar and three-dimensional (3D) reformats can accurately depict tracheal abnormalities, and the use of inspiratory and expiratory imaging is typically used to assess for tracheomalacia and potential air-trapping within the lungs.

Tracheal Neoplasms

Etiology

A majority of primary tracheal neoplasms in adults are malignant.[1,2] The most common cell type is squamous cell carcinoma, which is associated with cigarette smoking.[1,2] The second most common cell type is adenoid cystic carcinoma, which is not smoking related.[1,2] The most common benign tracheal neoplasm is squamous cell papilloma, which may be solitary or multiple.[1,2] Solitary papillomas have an association with cigarette smoking, whereas multiple papillomas (also referred to as *papillomatosis*) are linked to infection by the human papillomavirus.[1,2] A variety of other benign and malignant neoplasms may also arise in the trachea (Box 56.1).

Prevalence and Epidemiology

Primary tracheal neoplasms are rare. It has been estimated that a primary tracheal tumor is roughly 180 times less common than a primary lung cancer.[3] In a retrospective chart review of all cases of primary tracheal malignancy seen at the MD Anderson Cancer Center between 1945 and 2005, the authors identified 74 patients with primary tracheal cancers.[4] Among these, 34 (46%) were squamous cell carcinomas, 19 (26%) were adenoid cystic carcinomas, and 21 (28%) were of other histologic types. Squamous cell carcinoma and squamous cell papilloma have a male predominance and are associated with cigarette smoking, whereas adenoid cystic carcinoma has no sex predilection and is not related to smoking.[1,2]

Clinical Presentation

Primary tracheal neoplasms are often clinically silent until the tracheal lumen is narrowed by approximately 75%.[5] At the time of clinical presentation, symptoms include dyspnea, cough, hemoptysis, wheezing, and stridor.[1,5] Of interest, up to one-third of adult patients with primary tracheal neoplasms are initially misdiagnosed with "adult-onset" asthma. Thus this diagnosis should always raise the suspicion for a tracheal neoplasm.

The average age at presentation of squamous cell carcinoma is between 50 and 60 years.[1] In contrast, patients with adenoid cystic carcinoma typically present approximately 1 decade earlier. However, adenoid cystic carcinoma may occur over a broad spectrum of ages, ranging from the third to the ninth decade.[1] The average age at presentation for squamous cell papilloma is approximately 50 years, whereas diffuse papillomatosis most commonly presents in childhood.[1]

Pathophysiology

ANATOMY

Tracheal neoplasms are usually characterized by an endoluminal tracheal mass, which may have smooth, irregular, or lobulated margins.[1,2] Although some overlap exists between benign and malignant lesions, benign lesions are typically less than 2 cm in diameter, with well-defined smooth borders and without evidence of contiguous tracheal thickening or mediastinal invasion. In contrast, malignant lesions usually vary in size between 2 and 4 cm in diameter, with a flat or polypoid shape and irregular or lobulated borders. Contiguous tracheal wall thickening and mediastinal invasion are frequently observed.

Manifestations of the Disease

RADIOGRAPHY

On careful scrutiny, an intraluminal tracheal mass is often visible on chest radiographs of patients with tracheal neoplasms (Fig. 56.1). However, these lesions are frequently initially overlooked. Extraluminal involvement is not usually detectable by

*The editors and publisher would like to thank Drs. Nestor L. Müller, C. Isabela Silva Müller, Maryellen Sun, Phillip M. Boiselle, and Karen S. Lee for contributing material on this topic to the prior edition of this work. It has served as the foundation for the current chapter.

BOX 56.1 MALIGNANT AND BENIGN TRACHEAL NEOPLASMS

MALIGNANT TRACHEAL NEOPLASMS

Epithelial

- Squamous cell carcinoma
- Adenoid cystic carcinoma
- Carcinoid
- Mucoepidermoid carcinoma
- Adenocarcinoma
- Small cell carcinoma
- Large cell carcinoma
- Acinic cell carcinoma
- Malignant salivary gland–type mixed tumors
- Carcinomas with pleomorphic, sarcomatoid, or sarcomatous elements

Mesenchymal

- Fibrosarcoma
- Rhabdomyosarcoma
- Angiosarcoma
- Kaposi sarcoma
- Liposarcoma
- Osteosarcoma
- Leiomyosarcoma
- Chondrosarcoma
- Paraganglioma
- Spindle cell sarcoma
- Lymphoma
- Malignant fibrous histiocytoma

BENIGN TRACHEAL NEOPLASMS

Epithelial

- Squamous cell papilloma
- Papillomatosis
- Pleomorphic adenoma
- Glandular papilloma
- Adenomas of salivary gland type
- Mucous gland adenoma
- Monomorphic adenoma
- Oncocytoma

Mesenchymal

- Hamartoma
- Neurofibroma
- Chondroma
- Fibroma
- Hemangioma
- Granular cell tumor
- Schwannoma
- Fibrous histiocytoma
- Pseudosarcoma
- Hemangioendothelioma
- Leiomyoma
- Chondroblastoma
- Lipoma
- Glomus tumor

radiographs unless it is sufficiently extensive to distort the normal mediastinal contours.

Computed Tomography

Multidetector CT has a high sensitivity (97%) for detection of tracheal neoplasms and is typically used for characterization of morphology and the extent of involvement of the trachea and adjacent structures.[6] On CT a tracheal mass typically appears as a polypoid or sessile intraluminal mass of soft tissue attenuation (Fig. 56.2; see also Fig. 56.1). Necrosis and ulceration may be observed, especially in squamous cell carcinomas. CT scans frequently suggest whether a lesion is malignant or benign (see Figs. 56.1 and 56.2). Although CT usually cannot distinguish between neoplastic cell types, detection of fat within a lesion on CT is nearly pathognomonic for a hamartoma or lipoma (Fig. 56.3), and identification of calcification within a lesion is highly suggestive of a chondroid tumor (chondroma, chondrosarcoma).

CT also provides an assessment of submucosal spread and local extratracheal invasion (see Fig. 56.2). Regional lymph node metastases and complications such as tracheoesophageal fistula may also be detected by CT. However, CT does not reliably detect microscopic mediastinal invasion or neural invasion.[7]

Eccentric or circumferential tracheal wall thickening is less common than an intraluminal mass as a manifestation of malignant tracheal neoplasms.[1,2] This feature is not associated with benign tracheal neoplasms. CT readily detects the presence of circumferential tracheal wall thickening and luminal narrowing. It readily distinguishes an intrinsic tracheal abnormality from extrinsic compression. Multiplanar and 3D reconstructions complement axial images by enhancing the accuracy of assessment of craniocaudad extent of disease and extratracheal extension (Fig. 56.4).

Magnetic Resonance Imaging

Magnetic resonance imaging (MRI) is useful for tissue characterization and assessment of mediastinal invasion.[8] Although most tracheal neoplasms have intermediate signal intensity on T1-weighted images and high signal intensity on T2-weighted images, MRI may show characteristic signal patterns in cases of leiomyomas, fibromas, hamartomas, and lipomas.[8]

Imaging Algorithms

Chest radiographs are typically the first-line imaging test for a patient presenting with central airway symptoms. However, a high level of suspicion is required, as lesions are often overlooked at routine imaging.

CT is the imaging modality of choice for the detection and staging of tracheal neoplasms. MRI plays a secondary role complementary to CT in selected cases in which additional information is deemed necessary with regard to tissue characterization or when CT is indeterminate for mediastinal invasion. MRI is more sensitive than CT for detecting mediastinal invasion or submucosal growth of tumor.[8]

Fluorodeoxyglucose–positron emission tomography (FDG-PET)–CT can be helpful in the diagnosis and staging of tracheal malignancies. Tracheal malignancies are almost universally FDG avid, and PET is highly sensitive for the detection of nodal metastases.[9] PET-CT is more sensitive for the detection of tracheal tumors than CT alone and may be helpful in characterizing the full extent of tumors with submucosal spread, such as adenoid cystic carcinoma. In addition, PET-CT can be used to detect tumor recurrence after treatment.[9]

Differential Diagnosis

FROM CLINICAL DATA

Primary tracheal neoplasms are frequently misdiagnosed clinically as adult-onset asthma. Thus this diagnosis should prompt careful assessment of the trachea on chest radiographs. The clinical symptoms of central airway obstruction also overlap with other tracheal disorders, including tracheal stenosis and tracheomalacia. Thus it is not possible to establish a diagnosis of a tracheal tumor on clinical grounds alone.

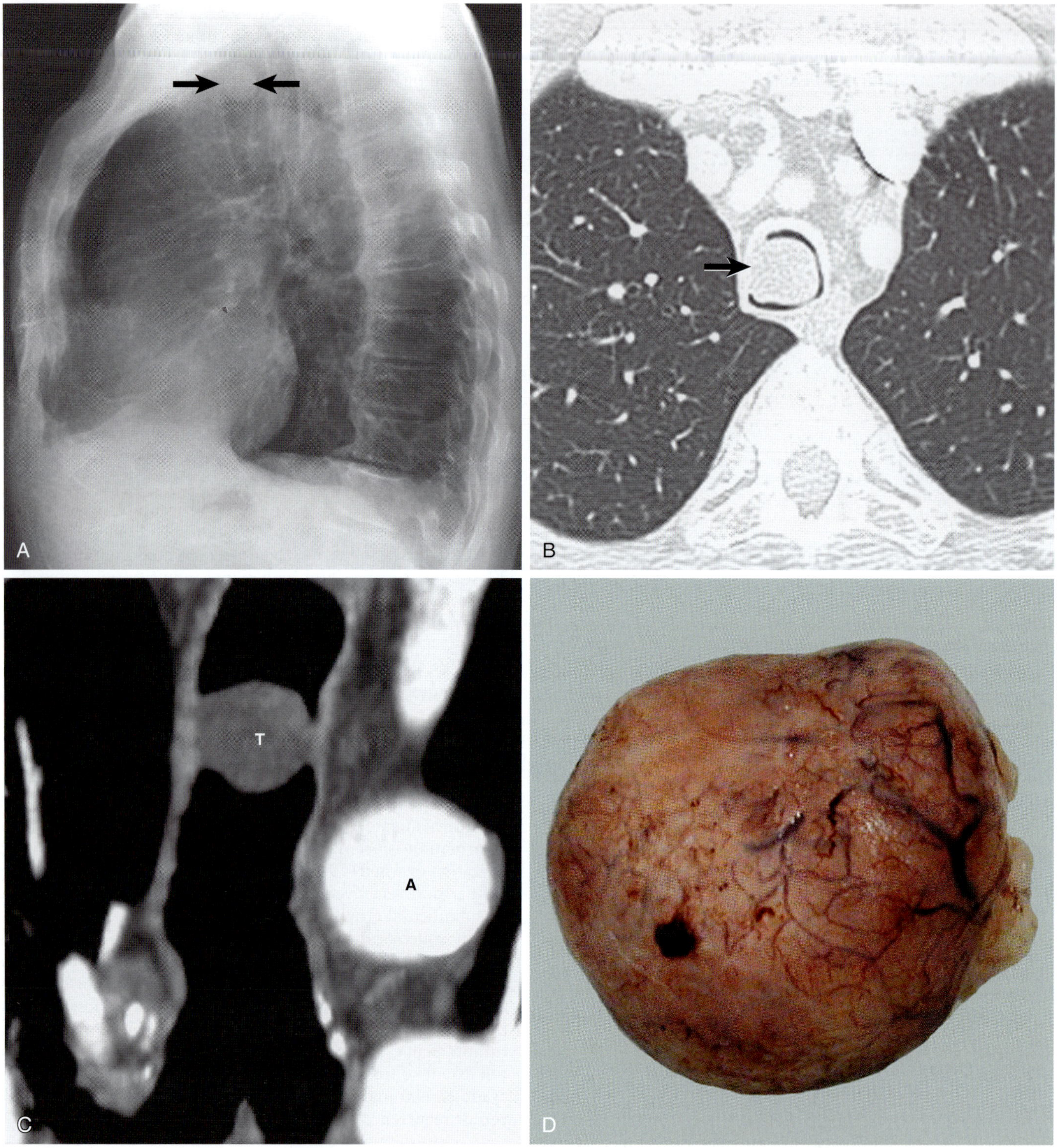

Fig. 56.1 Benign tracheal neoplasm, neurofibroma. (A) Lateral chest radiograph demonstrates a smoothly marginated round mass within the tracheal lumen *(arrows)*. (B) Axial CT image shows near complete occlusion of the tracheal lumen *(arrow)*. (C) Coronal reformatted image demonstrates a round contour, a diameter less than 2 cm, smooth margins, and lack of extratracheal extension, all suggestive of a benign lesion. *A*, Aortic arch; *T*, tumor. (D) Gross pathology specimen shows round mass with smooth margins.

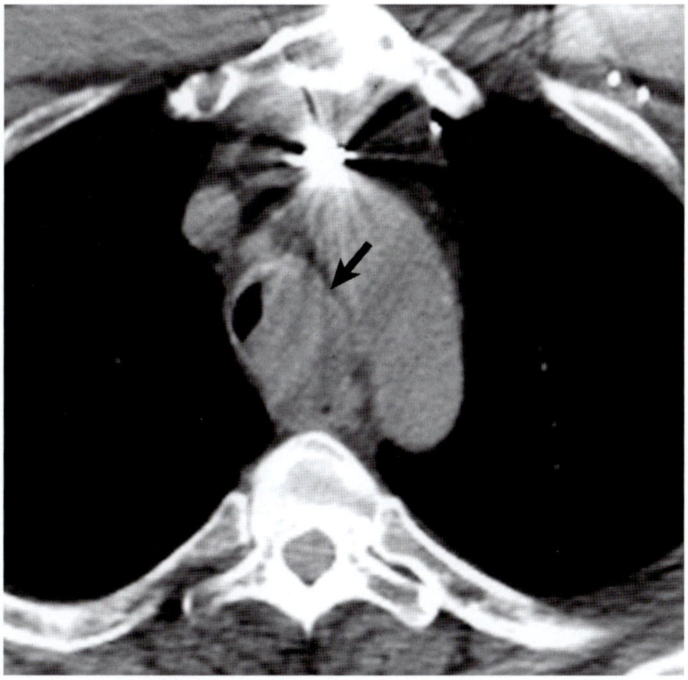

Fig. 56.2 Malignant tracheal neoplasm, metastatic renal cell carcinoma. Axial CT image demonstrates a lobulated intraluminal mass with invasion of the airway wall *(arrow)*. *(Figure reproduced with permission from Walker CM, Bueno J. Airway metastases. In: Rosado-de-Christenson ML, Carter BW, eds.* Specialty Imaging: Thoracic Neoplasms. *1st ed. Philadelphia: Amirsys-Elsevier; 2015.)*

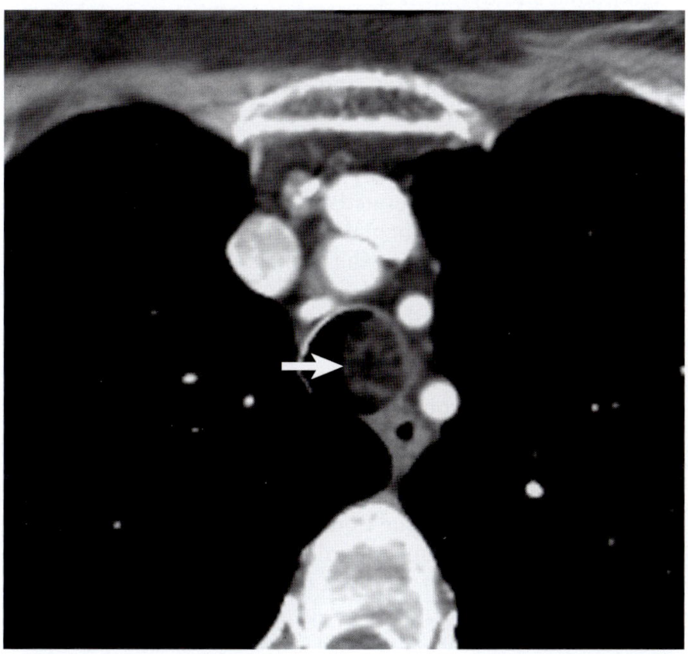

Fig. 56.3 Tracheal hamartoma. Axial CT image demonstrates a tracheal mass *(arrow)* arising from left lateral wall containing macroscopic foci of fat.

FROM SUPPORTIVE DIAGNOSTIC TECHNIQUES

When a discrete tracheal mass is identified on imaging studies, the diagnosis of a primary tracheal neoplasm can usually be made with a high degree of confidence. Cross-sectional imaging, including CT and MRI, readily differentiate a primary tracheal neoplasm from invasion by an extratracheal malignant neoplasm, such as

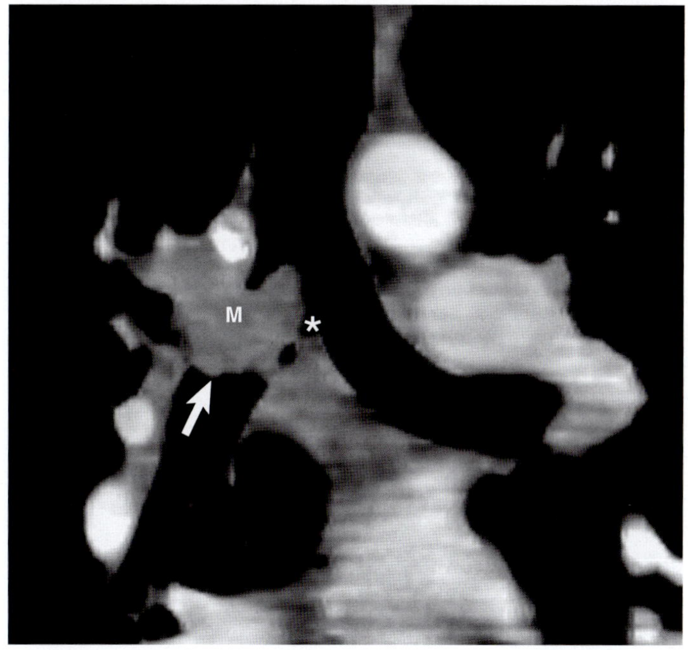

Fig. 56.4 Multiplanar reconstruction for assessment of extent of adenoid cystic carcinoma. Coronal reformatted image demonstrates a mass *(M)* arising at the level of the carina *(asterisk)*, with extension into the right main bronchus *(arrow)* and paratracheal soft tissues.

thyroid carcinoma. In addition, CT and MRI can often distinguish benign and malignant lesions and may rarely provide a specific diagnosis. Although a discrete tracheal mass usually represents a primary tracheal neoplasm, the differential diagnosis also includes metastatic disease from an extrathoracic primary neoplasm, including breast cancer, colorectal carcinoma, renal carcinoma, melanoma, and lung cancer.[10] A variety of nonneoplastic lesions, including granulation polyps, amyloidosis, and retained secretions, may also mimic a tracheal neoplasm on imaging studies. Secretions can sometimes be differentiated from a fixed tracheal lesion by identification of small foci of air within secretions; strands of additional secretions within the airway may also be identified. Alternatively, a repeat CT in a prone position after coughing can document a change in position or clearing of secretions.

In contrast, when a tracheal neoplasm manifests as eccentric or circumferential tracheal wall thickening rather than as a discrete mass, the differential diagnosis includes tracheal stenosis from a variety of nonmalignant entities, including iatrogenic (postintubation stenosis), infectious (tuberculosis), and inflammatory causes (e.g., granulomatosis with polyangiitis, relapsing polychondritis).

In general, the presence of marked irregularity of tracheal wall thickening and the presence of extratracheal extension favor a primary tracheal neoplasm, but biopsy is usually necessary to establish the diagnosis.

TYPES OF TRACHEAL NEOPLASMS

Squamous Cell Carcinoma

Squamous cell carcinomas are often large (4 cm) at the time of initial diagnosis, and their endoluminal component may be either exophytic or ulcerative.[1] These lesions are often sessile and frequently result in asymmetric narrowing of the tracheal lumen.[1] Regional lymph node metastases and local mediastinal invasion are relatively common. Extension from the trachea into the main

KEY POINTS: TRACHEAL NEOPLASMS

- Tracheal neoplasms are usually malignant and most commonly manifest as an intraluminal tracheal mass and less commonly as eccentric or circumferential tracheal wall thickening.
- The most common cell types are squamous cell carcinoma and adenoid cystic carcinoma.
- Features suggestive of malignancy include size larger than 2 cm, irregular margins, contiguous tracheal wall thickening, and extratracheal extension.
- Tracheal neoplasms are often overlooked on chest radiographs but can usually be identified retrospectively on careful inspection of the trachea.
- CT is the imaging modality of choice; multiplanar and 3D reconstructions enhance assessment of craniocaudal extent of disease and extratracheal involvement.

bronchus and development of a tracheoesophageal fistula are observed in 25% and 15% of cases, respectively.[1]

Adenoid Cystic Carcinoma

Adenoid cystic carcinoma is the most common variety of tracheobronchial gland neoplasm, accounting for about 75% to 80% of cases. It usually arises from the trachea or the main bronchi and only occasionally from more distal bronchi or lung periphery. The mean age at diagnosis is 45 to 50 years.[11,12] Cigarette smoking does not seem to be an etiologic factor.[13] The most common clinical manifestations are cough, hoarseness, hemoptysis, dyspnea, wheeze, and recurrent pneumonitis.[14,15] The symptoms of dyspnea and wheeze frequently lead to a misdiagnosis of asthma.[14,15]

Adenoid cystic carcinomas grossly appear as polypoid or broad-based and infiltrative intraluminal tracheal masses. At diagnosis, the lesions are usually less than 2 cm, and their surface may be either smooth or ulcerated.[1,16] These neoplasms are nonencapsulated and characteristically spread along perineural surfaces or perineural lymphatics.[1] At the time of diagnosis, the lesion has often already infiltrated long segments of the tracheal submucosa.[1] The extent of microscopic invasion is typically greater than that estimated by imaging assessment and direct visualization at surgery.[16]

CT is superior to radiography in identifying the tumors and is particularly helpful in assessing the presence of extraluminal extent and mediastinal invasion.[15,17] The most common finding on CT consists of a lobulated, polypoid endoluminal mass with associated focal thickening of the airway wall (Fig. 56.5).[15,18] Less commonly, adenoid cystic carcinoma may be associated with extensive thickening of the tracheal or bronchial wall (Fig. 56.6).[19] Adenoid cystic carcinoma has a tendency to infiltrate beneath the mucosa; its longitudinal extent may be underestimated on CT.[14] Optimal assessment requires thin sections (preferably 1 mm or less) and multiplanar or 3D reformations.[6,15,20]

KEY POINTS: ADENOID CYSTIC CARCINOMA

- Adenoid cystic carcinoma is the most common tracheobronchial gland neoplasm and the second most common primary malignant tumor of the trachea (after squamous cell carcinoma).
- Most tumors arise in the trachea or main bronchi.
- Imaging findings include the following:
  - Polypoid endoluminal mass
  - Circumferential tracheal wall thickening

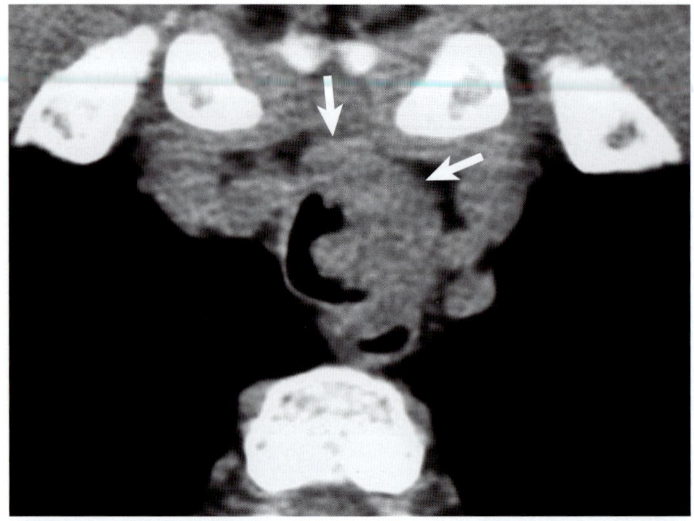

Fig. 56.5 Adenoid cystic carcinoma of the trachea. Axial CT scan shows a lobulated polypoid endotracheal tumor with extensive involvement of the tracheal wall and extension into the adjacent mediastinum *(arrows)*.

Mucoepidermoid Carcinoma

Mucoepidermoid carcinoma (MEC) is the second most common form of tracheobronchial gland neoplasm but accounts for less than 0.2% of pulmonary carcinomas.[21] Patients vary in age from 3 months to 78 years, but almost half are younger than 30 years.[22,23] Symptoms are related predominantly to growth in the airway wall and lumen and include cough, hemoptysis, recurrent pneumonia, and dyspnea.[22,24]

MECs are composed of cells that show glandular (typically mucus production) and "epidermoid" features and are classified histopathologically into low- and high-grade neoplasms. They usually are located in segmental bronchi and, less commonly, arise within the lobar or main bronchi or trachea.[14] Most grow within the airway lumen and produce a polypoid mass with an intact or occasionally ulcerated surface epithelium; peripheral extension within the bronchial lumen may occur.[22] Low-grade tumors often are confined to the bronchial wall; by contrast, the high-grade form commonly extends into the peribronchial interstitium or adjacent lung parenchyma with propensity for lymph node metastases.

Radiographic findings are related to tumor location and size and may consist of a solitary nodule or mass, lobar or segmental consolidation or atelectasis, or a central mass with associated obstructive pneumonitis or atelectasis (Fig. 56.7).[22]

The CT manifestations of MECs usually consist of a smoothly oval or lobulated soft tissue nodule or mass measuring at least 1 cm in diameter.[19,22] Punctate calcification within the tumor is seen on CT scan in 25% to 50% of cases.[22] High-grade MECs typically show high FDG uptake, whereas low-grade tumors show low uptake that may be similar to a mediastinal blood pool.[25,26] The tumors are homogeneous and show slight enhancement after the administration of contrast medium (Fig. 56.8). The direction of the longest diameter of the oval or lobulated tumor in the lobar or segmental bronchus is typically parallel to that of the branching pattern in the corresponding airways containing the tumor. Associated CT findings include distal bronchial dilation with mucoid impaction, postobstructive pneumonia, atelectasis, and air-trapping.[22]

Occasionally, the tumors may involve the trachea rather than the bronchi and appear as a polypoid intraluminal nodule on

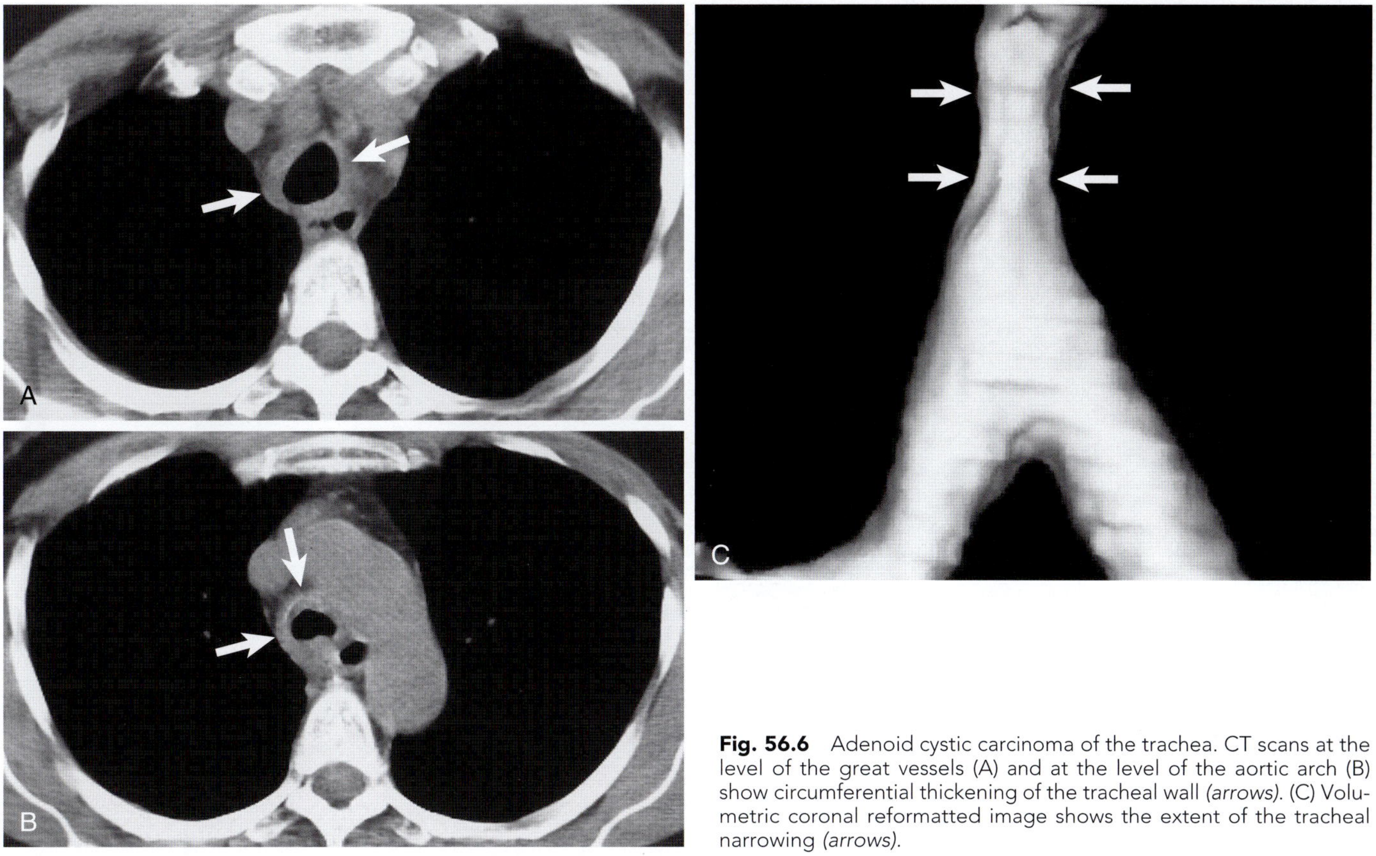

Fig. 56.6 Adenoid cystic carcinoma of the trachea. CT scans at the level of the great vessels (A) and at the level of the aortic arch (B) show circumferential thickening of the tracheal wall *(arrows)*. (C) Volumetric coronal reformatted image shows the extent of the tracheal narrowing *(arrows)*.

radiograph and CT scan (Fig. 56.9).[22] CT is superior to radiographs in the assessment of intraluminal tumor and the extent of involvement of the bronchial or tracheal wall and mediastinum. Metastatic disease, including hilar or mediastinal lymphadenopathy, pleural nodularity, osseous lesions, and liver lesions, is uncommon except in high-grade MECs.[22]

KEY POINTS: MUCOEPIDERMOID CARCINOMA

- Mucoepidermoid carcinoma (MEC) accounts for less than 0.2% of pulmonary carcinomas.
- MEC most commonly involves segmental bronchi.
- Imaging findings include the following:
  - 1- to 4-cm nodule or mass
  - Distal obstructive pneumonitis, atelectasis, or air-trapping
  - Close association with bronchus usually evident on CT

Tracheal Papilloma

A solitary papilloma typically appears as a small, sessile or pedunculated growth arising from the tracheal wall.[1] Larger lesions may demonstrate a cauliflower-like appearance.[1,16] A range of squamous dysplasia, as well as in situ or invasive carcinoma, may also be identified within squamous cell papillomas.[16]

Synopsis of Treatment Options

MEDICAL

Medical therapy does not play a primary role in the treatment of tracheal tumors. Antibiotic therapy may be administered to treat postobstructive pneumonia or bronchitis.

SURGICAL

Surgery is the treatment of choice, with resection of the involved portion of the trachea and reconstruction of the remaining uninvolved portions of the trachea.[27] Accurate preoperative identification of the precise level and length of resection is critically important.[27]

Surgical treatment is usually curative for benign tracheal neoplasms. Complete excision of a solitary papilloma is recommended to exclude an invasive malignant neoplasm and to prevent recurrence.[16]

Treatment of malignant tracheal neoplasms is usually by segmental resection and reconstruction performed in a single stage and adjuvant preoperative and postoperative irradiation.[28] For patients in whom squamous cell or adenoid cystic carcinoma is unresectable, palliative methods that yield good success rates are available, including laser photoresection, external beam irradiation, and brachytherapy.[28,29]

MECs have a 5-year survival after surgery of approximately 80% in patients with low-grade malignancy at histology and 30% in patients with carcinomas with high-grade malignancy.[24] It is recommended that MECs be treated by radical surgery with lymph node sampling and dissection.[24]

Tracheal Stenosis

Etiology

Tracheal stenosis refers to narrowing of the tracheal lumen. A variety of iatrogenic, inflammatory, infectious, and neoplastic processes may result in focal or diffuse tracheal narrowing. This

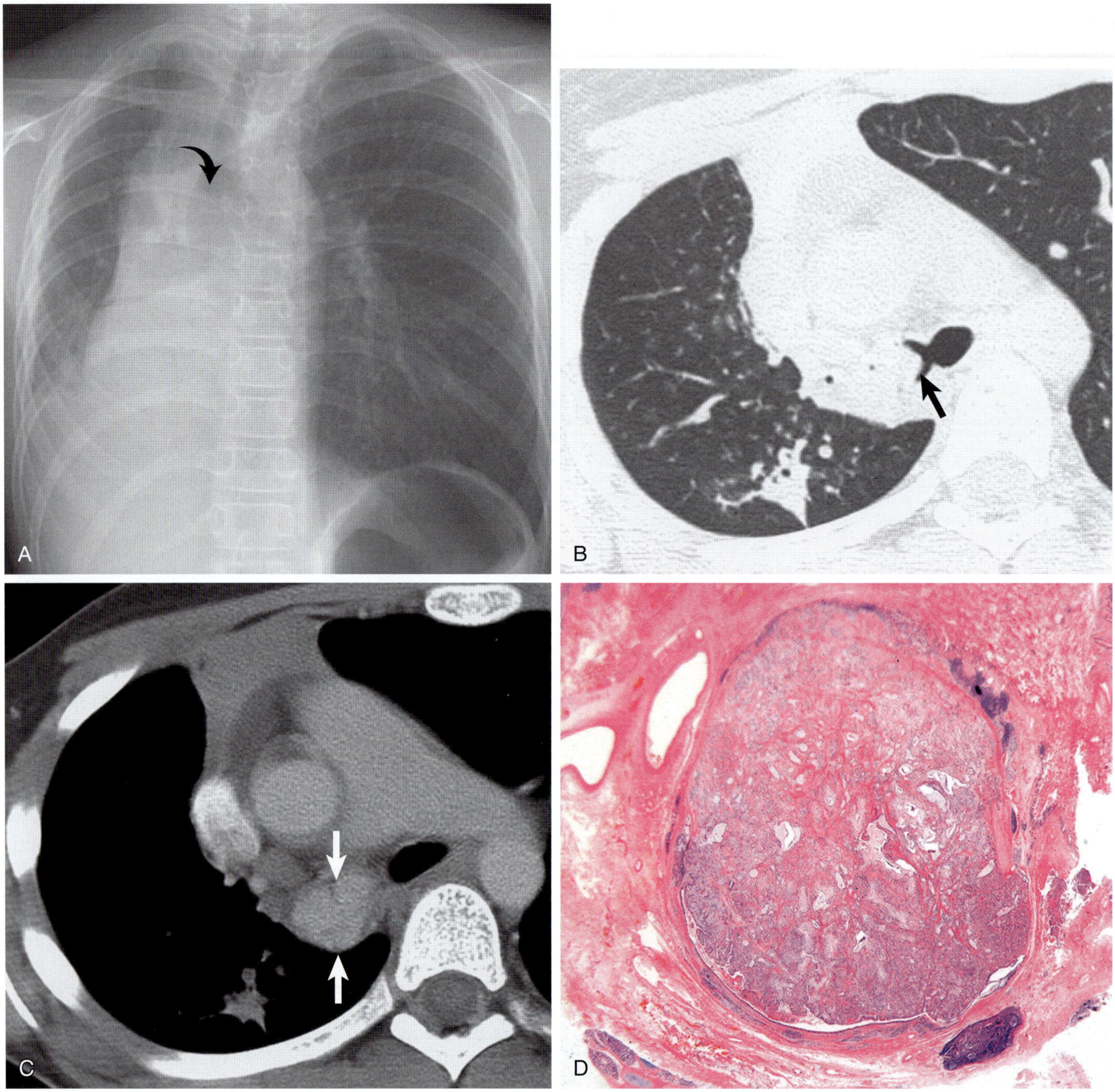

Fig. 56.7 Mucoepidermoid carcinoma (MEC) originating in the right main bronchus. (A) Chest radiograph shows a poorly defined soft tissue mass in the right main bronchus *(arrow)* and marked volume loss of the right lung with ipsilateral shift of the mediastinum and elevation of the right hemidiaphragm. (B) CT scan shows an endobronchial tumor *(arrow)* with almost complete obstruction of the right main bronchus and associated volume loss of the right lung. (C) CT scan at soft tissue windows shows a large endobronchial tumor *(arrows)*. (D) Low-power view of the surgical specimen after pneumonectomy shows an endobronchial MEC. *(Courtesy Dr. Joungho Han, Department of Pathology, Samsung Medical Center, Sungkyunkwan University School of Medicine, Seoul, South Korea.)*

section focuses on postintubation tracheal stenosis, which is by far the most common cause of acquired tracheal stenosis.[30–32]

Postintubation stenosis occurs secondary to injury of the trachea from the high pressure of an endotracheal tube balloon against the wall of the trachea.[30,33] This initially results in mucosal necrosis, followed by scarring and stenosis.[30,33]

Prevalence and Epidemiology

The true prevalence of postintubation tracheal stenosis is unknown. Although it was initially reported in up to 20% of cases after endotracheal intubation, its prevalence has decreased substantially to an estimated 1% with the introduction of low-pressure cuff endotracheal tubes.[31,33] The prevalence of tracheal

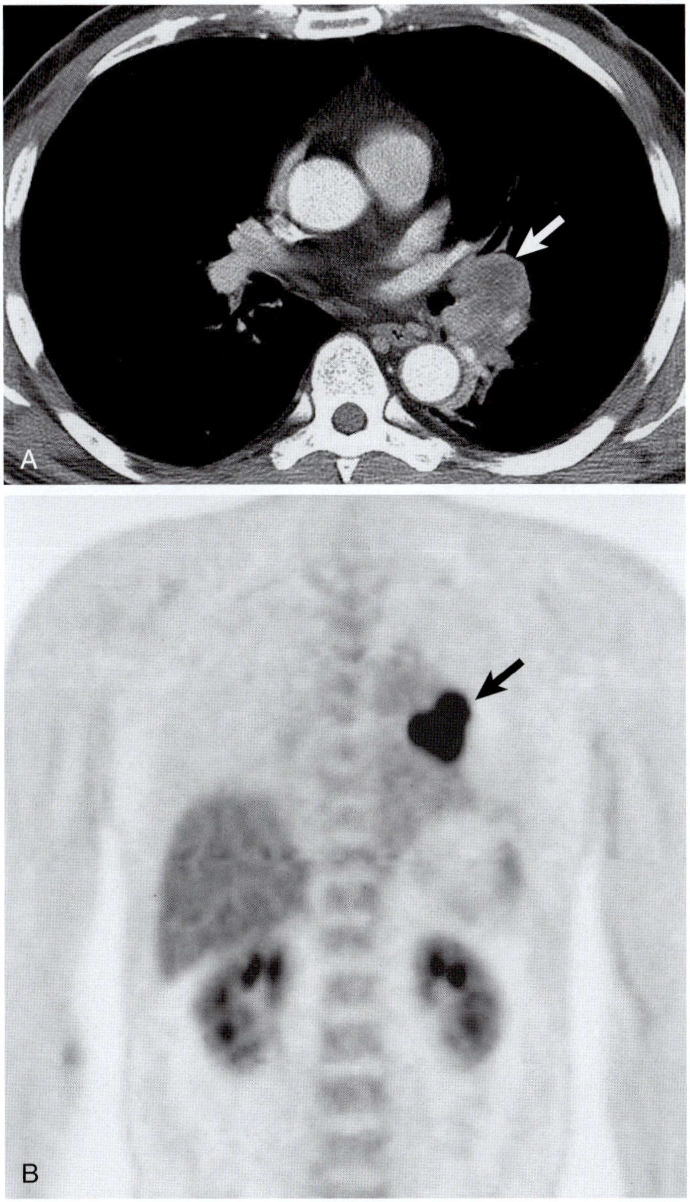

Fig. 56.8 Mucoepidermoid carcinoma (MEC) originating in the lingular bronchus. (A) CT scan shows a large tumor *(arrow)* originating from the lingular bronchus and extending into adjacent hilum and lung parenchyma. Also evident is associated volume loss of the left lung. (B) Positron emission tomography image shows marked fluorodeoxyglucose uptake typical of high-grade MEC *(arrow)*. *(Courtesy Dr. Kyung Soo Lee, Samsung Medical Center, Seoul, South Korea.)*

stenosis has been estimated at approximately 30% after long-standing tracheostomy tube placement.[34]

Risk factors include difficult or prolonged intubation, infection, mechanical irritation, steroid administration, and use of positive-pressure ventilation.[33]

Clinical Presentation

Affected patients typically present with dyspnea on exertion, stridor, and wheezing.[33] Symptoms of upper airway obstruction are often delayed several weeks after extubation. Patients with mild stenoses may initially be asymptomatic. However, such patients may eventually develop symptoms when tracheal luminal

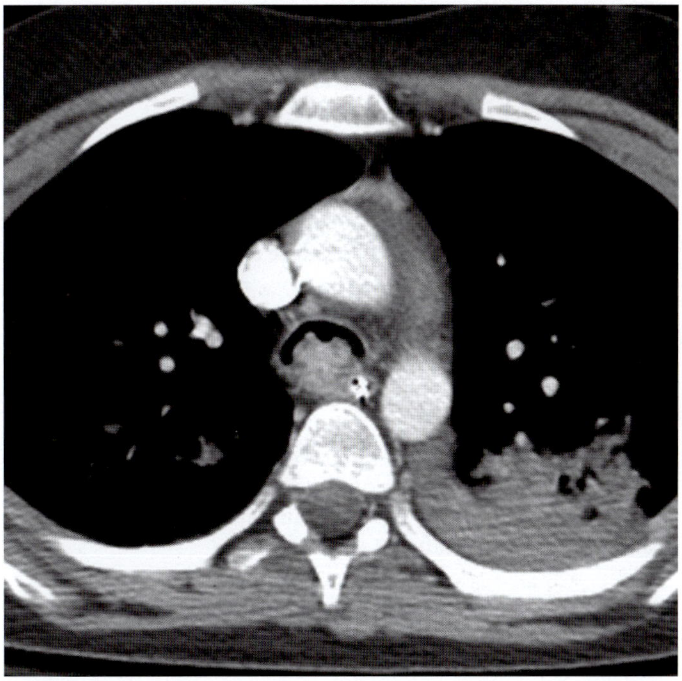

Fig. 56.9 Mucoepidermoid carcinoma of the trachea. CT scan shows a heterogeneously enhancing tumor along the posterior tracheal membrane. Note left lower lobe consolidation and small left pleural effusion from aspiration pneumonia. *(Figure reproduced with permission from Walker CM. Mucoepidermoid carcinoma. In: Rosado-de-Christenson ML, Carter BW, eds.* Specialty Imaging: Thoracic Neoplasms. *1st ed. Philadelphia: Amirsys-Elsevier; 2015.)*

narrowing is worsened by airway edema and secretions from a coexistent respiratory infection.[35]

Pathophysiology

ANATOMY

Postintubation stenosis is characterized by eccentric or concentric tracheal wall thickening and associated luminal narrowing. The craniocaudal length usually ranges from 1.5 to 2.5 cm.[30,32] In patients who have undergone tracheostomy tube placement, the stenosis occurs most commonly at the stoma site and less commonly at the site where the tip of the tube has impinged on the tracheal mucosa.[30,33,36] In patients who have undergone endotracheal intubation, stenosis occurs most commonly in the subglottic region at the level of the endotracheal tube balloon.[32]

PATHOLOGY

Acutely, ischemic necrosis is due to compromise of the blood supply to the tracheal mucosa.[30] This is followed by a superficial tracheitis with shallow ulcerations. The exposed cartilaginous rings subsequently soften and become fragmented. This is followed by fibrosis and granulation tissue formation, resulting in concentric or eccentric wall thickening with associated luminal narrowing.

LUNG FUNCTION

Flow-volume loops may show characteristic changes of airway obstruction.[35] Such changes typically precede abnormalities in spirometric volumes.[35]

Manifestations of the Disease

FOCAL TRACHEAL NARROWING

General

The most common imaging finding in postintubation stenosis is a focal area of tracheal luminal narrowing measuring approximately 2 cm in craniocaudal length.[30,32,33] The focal nature and circumferential narrowing may produce a characteristic hourglass configuration.

Less commonly, one may observe a thin membrane projecting into the tracheal lumen or a long segment of eccentric soft tissue thickening.[30,33]

Radiography

Postintubation stenoses are often overlooked on conventional radiographs, in part because of a proximal location.[33] On careful scrutiny of radiographs, however, airway narrowing is usually visible in cases of significant stenosis.

Computed Tomography

CT is the imaging modality of choice to detect and characterize tracheal stenosis. On axial images, CT demonstrates eccentric or concentric soft tissue thickening with associated luminal narrowing (Fig. 56.10).[32] Multiplanar reconstruction and 3D external rendering of images help detect focal stenoses and aid in assessment of craniocaudal length, which is often underestimated on axial images (Fig. 56.11, see Fig. 56.10).[30]

Less commonly, tracheal stenosis may manifest as a thin membrane of granulation tissue projecting into the tracheal lumen.[30,33] This finding may be difficult to detect on axial CT images, but thin-section and reformatted images may aid in its visibility.

Because long-standing tracheal stenoses may be complicated by coexistent tracheomalacia resulting from weakness and fragmentation of the tracheal cartilage, the addition of a dynamic expiratory CT sequence can help detect excessive airway collapsibility.

Magnetic Resonance Imaging

Similar to CT, MRI demonstrates eccentric or concentric soft tissue thickening internal to the tracheal cartilage. Multiplanar images along the axis of the trachea accurately depict the craniocaudal extent of stenosis.

Imaging Algorithms

Chest radiographs are usually the initial imaging obtained for the assessment of patients with central airway symptoms and suspected tracheal stenosis. However, a normal chest radiograph does not exclude this diagnosis. CT with multiplanar and 3D renderings is the study of choice for detection and characterization of tracheal stenosis. MRI may be considered an alternative to CT in younger patients in whom radiation exposure may be a concern.

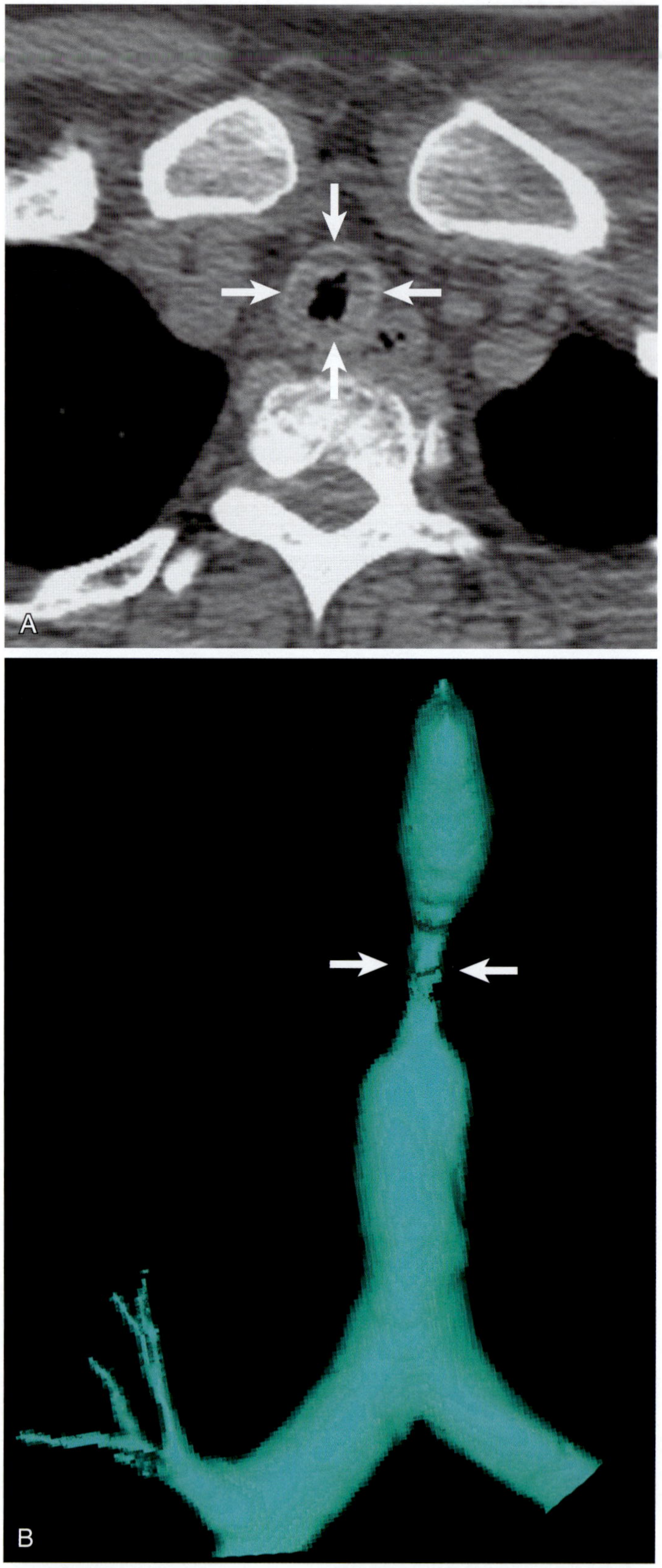

Fig. 56.10 Postintubation stenosis. (A) Axial CT image of the proximal trachea demonstrates circumferential wall thickening *(arrows)* and luminal narrowing caused by postintubation stenosis. (B) Three-dimensional (3D) external rendering of the trachea demonstrates hourglass-shaped focal stenosis *(arrows)*. Craniocaudad extent of stenosis was more accurately assessed on the 3D image than on the contiguous axial CT images.

Differential Diagnosis

FROM CLINICAL DATA

Although the symptoms of postintubation stenosis overlap with those of other causes of central airway obstruction, the diagnosis should be suspected when a patient with a recent history of

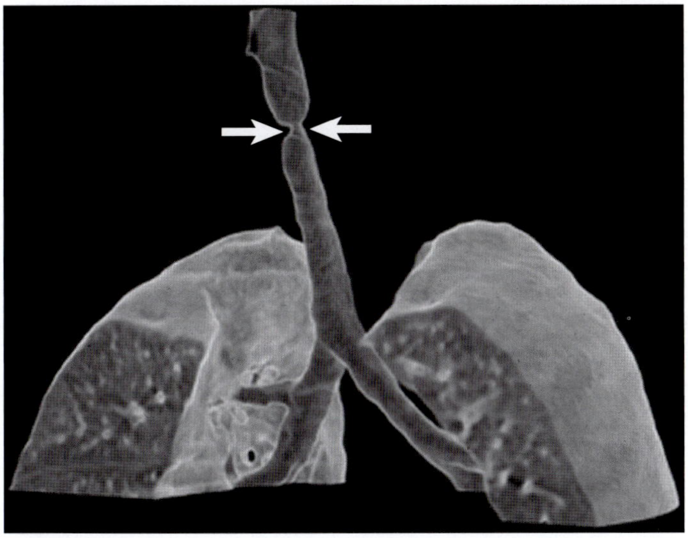

Fig. 56.11 Postintubation stenosis. Three-dimensional external rendering of the trachea demonstrates focal high-grade subglottic stenosis *(arrows)*. The stenosis was nearly overlooked on axial CT images (not shown).

intubation or tracheostomy tube placement presents with upper airway symptoms.

FROM SUPPORTIVE DIAGNOSTIC TECHNIQUES

The diagnosis may be suggested by the detection of focal airway narrowing on chest radiographs or CT scans. A characteristic hourglass narrowing at the typical location of the endotracheal tube cuff is highly suggestive of this diagnosis in a patient with a prior history of tracheostomy or endotracheal intubation. Biopsy may be required in equivocal cases to exclude underlying neoplasms.

Synopsis of Treatment Options

A variety of interventional bronchoscopic (balloon dilation, laser therapy, stent placement) and surgical (resection and end-to-end anastomosis) techniques may be used to treat symptomatic tracheal stenoses.[35] Specific treatment decisions depend on patient factors, characteristics of the stenosis, and local expertise.

KEY POINTS: TRACHEAL STENOSIS

- Tracheal stenosis is the most common complication of endotracheal intubation and tracheostomy tube placement, although the prevalence has decreased substantially since the introduction of low-pressure cuffs.
- Postintubation stenosis most commonly manifests as a focal, hourglass-shaped tracheal stenosis.
- CT with multiplanar and three-dimensional reconstructions is the imaging modality of choice.
- A variety of bronchoscopic and surgical interventions may be used to treat this condition.

Tracheomalacia

Etiology

Tracheomalacia is a condition characterized by increased compliance and excessive collapsibility of the trachea caused by weakness of the airway walls or supporting cartilage and may be congenital or acquired.[37,38] Primary or congenital tracheomalacia is associated with congenital weakness of the airway wall, which may arise in the setting of abnormal cartilaginous matrix, inadequate maturity of cartilage (e.g., premature infants), or congenital tracheoesophageal fistula.[37] Secondary or acquired tracheomalacia has been associated with a variety of conditions, including chronic obstructive pulmonary disease (COPD), prior intubation, prior surgery (e.g., lung resection or transplantation), radiation therapy, long-standing extrinsic compression (e.g., thyroid goiter or vascular ring), and chronic inflammation (e.g., relapsing polychondritis).[37] Acquired tracheomalacia may also be idiopathic in some cases.

Prevalence and Epidemiology

The true prevalence of tracheomalacia is unknown because this functional disorder usually escapes detection on routine chest radiographs and routine CT scans.[38] The congenital form is most commonly observed in premature infants[37] and is often associated with cardiovascular abnormalities, bronchopulmonary dysplasia, and gastroesophageal reflux. The acquired form of tracheomalacia has been reported in 5% to 23% of bronchoscopic studies performed in patients with respiratory symptoms.[38]

Clinical Presentation

The congenital form typically manifests in the first weeks to months of life with symptoms of expiratory stridor, cough, and difficulty feeding.[37] Patients with the acquired form may present at any age, but the prevalence of this condition increases with advancing age.[37] When tracheomalacia occurs secondary to prior intubation, symptoms may arise several weeks to several years after intubation.

The most common symptoms in patients with acquired tracheomalacia are intractable cough, dyspnea, wheezing, and recurrent respiratory infections.[37]

Pathophysiology

ANATOMY

The trachea is often normal in appearance on routine end-inspiratory imaging studies, but it may also show preferential widening of the coronal (lunate) or sagittal (saber-sheath) dimension in some cases. At autopsy in patients with acquired tracheomalacia, the pars membranacea is often dilated and flaccid.[37]

PATHOLOGY

Tracheomalacia is characterized pathologically by weakening of the cartilage or posterior membranous wall, with degeneration and atrophy of the longitudinal elastic fibers.[37]

LUNG FUNCTION

Pulmonary function test results may be suggestive of tracheomalacia, but they are not diagnostic.[37] Spirometry usually shows obstruction proportional to the severity of tracheomalacia. The characteristic pattern is a decreased forced expiratory volume in 1 second (FEV1) and a low peak flow rate with a rapid decrease in flow.[37]

Manifestations of the Disease

GENERAL

The hallmark of tracheomalacia is excessive expiratory collapse. Although once defined as more than 50% reduction in cross-sectional luminal area of the trachea during expiration, many now suggest using a threshold of 70% collapse[39] because healthy subjects have been shown to demonstrate degrees of collapse that overlap with this value.[40]

RADIOGRAPHY

Because it escapes detection on routine end-inspiratory imaging studies, tracheomalacia is not detectable on routine chest radiographs. Fluoroscopy may be rarely used to diagnose this condition.

COMPUTED TOMOGRAPHY

Paired inspiratory-expiratory CT imaging is the method of choice for diagnosis of this condition (Fig. 56.12). Dynamic expiratory imaging (during a forced exhalation) is more sensitive than end-expiratory imaging for detection of this condition.[38,41,42] Cine CT imaging during a coughing maneuver is highly sensitive for detection of tracheomalacia but requires multiple acquisitions to image the entirety of the trachea.[43]

A "lunate" configuration of the trachea, in which the coronal tracheal diameter is larger than the sagittal diameter, is uncommon but highly specific for tracheomalacia.[44] The detection of a lunate configuration on inspiratory CT should always prompt consideration of tracheomalacia, which can be confirmed at expiratory CT.[39]

Although precise cross-sectional area measurements are recommended for diagnosis of mild to moderate tracheomalacia, the presence of complete expiratory collapse is diagnostic of severe tracheomalacia. At expiratory imaging, a crescentic, frown-like configuration of the tracheal lumen with less than 6 mm of distance between the anterior and posterior walls is highly suggestive of tracheomalacia (Fig. 56.13).[45] Recognition of this characteristic appearance may aid in the detection of tracheomalacia on routine CT scans in which patients inadvertently breathe during the CT acquisition.

MAGNETIC RESONANCE IMAGING

Dynamic MRI during breathing maneuvers or coughing may be used to diagnose tracheomalacia.[46]

IMAGING ALGORITHMS

Fluoroscopy is highly operator dependent and has been supplanted by cross-sectional imaging with CT or MRI. Paired inspiratory–dynamic expiratory CT is the imaging method of choice and provides simultaneous information about airway anatomy and compliance. Because MRI lacks ionizing radiation, it may be considered an alternative imaging modality for younger patients and those undergoing serial follow-up examinations.

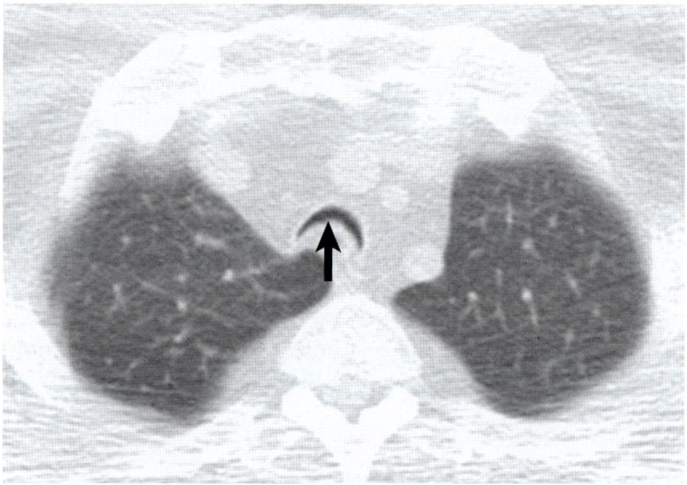

Fig. 56.13 Tracheomalacia with frown sign. Dynamic expiratory CT image demonstrates frown-like crescentic configuration of the tracheal lumen *(arrow)*, highly suggestive of tracheomalacia.

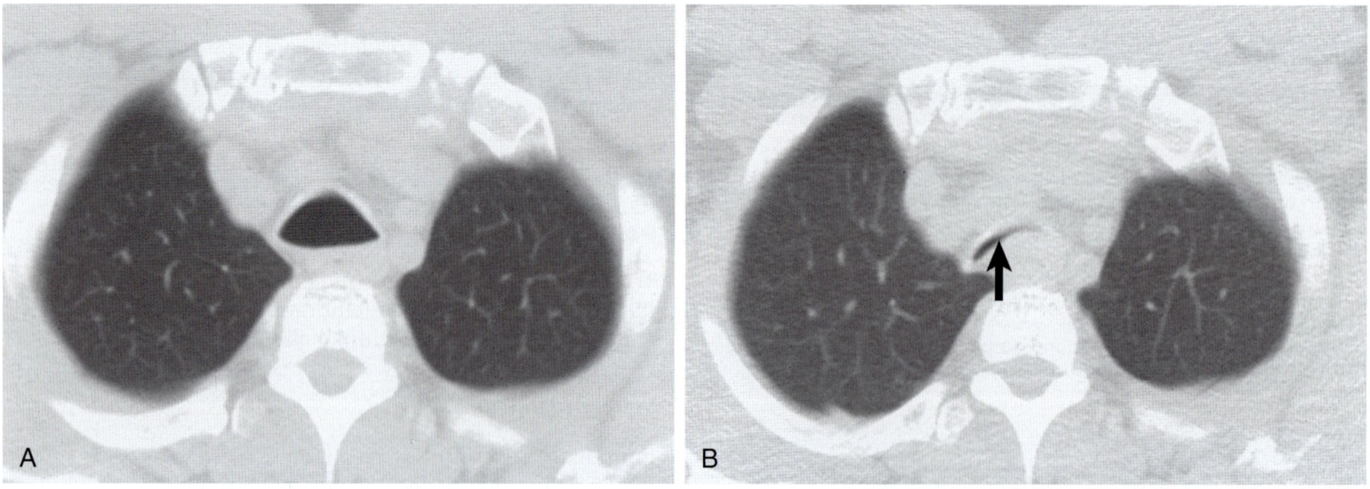

Fig. 56.12 Tracheomalacia. (A) Axial CT image at end inspiration demonstrates patency of the tracheal lumen. Note relative widening of the coronal dimension with respect to the sagittal dimension ("lunate" shape), which is suggestive of underlying tracheomalacia. (B) Axial CT image during dynamic expiration demonstrates near-complete collapse of the tracheal lumen *(arrow)*, consistent with severe tracheomalacia.

Differential Diagnosis

FROM CLINICAL DATA

There are no clinical features that allow one to distinguish tracheomalacia from other respiratory conditions such as emphysema, chronic bronchitis, and asthma.[37] Moreover, these conditions often coexist with tracheomalacia. The diagnosis requires a high index of suspicion among patients at risk for this condition.

FROM SUPPORTIVE DIAGNOSTIC TECHNIQUES

A definitive diagnosis can be made by identifying excessive expiratory tracheal lumen collapse by paired inspiratory–dynamic expiratory CT, dynamic MRI, fluoroscopy, or bronchoscopy.

Tracheomalacia should be distinguished from the entity known as "excessive dynamic airway collapse" (EDAC). Although tracheomalacia is due to abnormal cartilage and results in collapse of the anterior and posterior walls of the trachea, EDAC is thought to be a result of peripheral airway obstruction (as in asthma or COPD) and results in collapse of primarily the posterior membranous trachea.[47]

Synopsis of Treatment Options

MEDICAL

Treatment of patients with mild to moderate symptoms is conservative. Continuous nasal positive airway pressure helps with nocturnal symptoms.[37] Antibiotics are used to treat respiratory infections.

SURGICAL

Severely symptomatic patients may benefit from surgical intervention with tracheoplasty.[37,48,49] This surgical technique involves remodeling of the tracheal lumen and an increase in its rigidity by placement of a graft along the posterior wall. It is best suited to patients with excessive expiratory motion of the posterior wall of the trachea. Stents are a potential option for severely symptomatic patients who are not surgical candidates, but long-term use of stents is limited by a relatively high complication rate.[37]

KEY POINTS: TRACHEOMALACIA

- Tracheomalacia refers to excessive expiratory collapsibility of the trachea.
- It may be congenital or acquired.
- It is widely considered an underdiagnosed condition.
- Paired inspiratory–dynamic expiratory CT imaging is the best imaging method of diagnosis.
- The frown sign and lunate configuration of the trachea are highly suggestive of this condition.
- Treatment is usually conservative, but severely symptomatic patients may benefit from surgery.

Relapsing Polychondritis

Etiology

Relapsing polychondritis is a multisystem disorder characterized by recurrent inflammation of the cartilaginous structures of the external ear, nose, peripheral joints, larynx, trachea, and bronchi.[50,51] Its etiology is unknown, but it is likely to be immune mediated.[50] Recent research suggests a genetic susceptibility, an overlap with other disorders associated with immunologic abnormalities, and the potential for multiple inciting events, including chemical insults.[51]

Prevalence and Epidemiology

Relapsing polychondritis is very rare, with an estimated prevalence of 4.5 to 9 per million individuals.[52,53] It is most prevalent among white individuals. Most studies report that men and women are equally affected,[51] but a female predominance has also been reported.[50] Airway involvement is present in up to 50% of patients and is a major cause of morbidity and mortality.[50,51,54] Women are more likely than men to experience serious airway problems.[51]

Clinical Presentation

The average age at onset is the fifth and sixth decades, but the disease may rarely occur in childhood.[51] The diagnosis is established when any three of the following clinical features are present: bilateral auricular chondritis, nonerosive seronegative inflammatory arthritis, nasal chondritis, ocular inflammation, respiratory tract chondritis, or audiovestibular damage.[55] Alternative diagnostic criteria include one or more of these clinical findings with positive histologic confirmation or chondritis at two or more separate anatomic locations with response to steroids or dapsone.[56]

The clinical manifestations and course of disease are highly variable. For this reason, there is often a substantial delay in diagnosis of approximately 3 years.[50] Auricular involvement is the most common clinical feature.[51] A saddle-nose deformity, which results from collapse of the cartilaginous nasal septum but preservation of the bony nasal septum, is highly characteristic of this condition.

Patients with laryngotracheobronchial involvement may present with a variety of symptoms, including hoarseness, aphonia, wheezing, inspiratory stridor, nonproductive cough, dyspnea, and recurrent infections.[51] Notably, airway involvement may be asymptomatic in the early stages. Airway involvement may uncommonly occur as an isolated manifestation of relapsing polychondritis, without other perceptible features of this condition.[57]

Pathophysiology

ANATOMY

The airway may be involved focally or diffusely. The larynx and upper trachea are most commonly affected, but the disease may also involve the airways more distally to the level of the subsegmental bronchi.[51]

Glottic, subglottic, laryngeal, or tracheobronchial inflammation may result in luminal encroachment. Loss of structural cartilaginous support resulting from cartilaginous inflammation and destruction may result in excessive compliance and dynamic expiratory collapsibility (tracheomalacia). In the late stages of the disease, there is fibrosis-induced luminal contraction of the airway, with severe luminal narrowing.

PATHOLOGY

The tracheal mucosa may be edematous. The tracheal cartilaginous rings may demonstrate abnormalities varying from mild inflammation to total resorption by granulation tissue.[51]

There is no biopsy finding that is pathognomonic for relapsing polychondritis, but specimens of inflamed cartilage may show characteristic features.[50] Histologic features of the cartilage include loss of basophilic staining of the matrix and perichondral inflammation.[51] Eventually, the cartilage is destroyed and replaced by fibrous tissue.

LUNG FUNCTION

The effects of this condition on major airways can be fixed or variable. Variable obstruction is due to increased expiratory compliance and flaccidity, resulting in tracheomalacia. In late stages the airway obstruction is fixed because of cicatricial narrowing of the airway. The degree of airflow obstruction, as measured by FEV1, may be severe and does not improve after inhalation of bronchodilators.[51]

Pulmonary function tests, especially flow-volume loops, are helpful for discerning the nature (fixed or dynamic) of airway obstruction and its location (intrathoracic or extrathoracic).[50] Pulmonary function tests have also been reported to be useful for monitoring of disease status over time.[50]

Manifestations of the Disease

RADIOGRAPHY

Calcification of the tracheal wall or airway narrowing is occasionally visible on chest radiographs, but it is better visualized at CT.

COMPUTED TOMOGRAPHY

Increased attenuation of the tracheal wall is the most common imaging manifestation of relapsing polychondritis and may range from subtle to frankly calcified (Fig. 56.14).[58–61] Increased wall thickness is also common and may be calcified or noncalcified (Fig. 56.15; see also Fig. 56.14). Both of these features characteristically spare the posterior membranous wall of the trachea unless the inflammation is severe, at which point it may secondarily involve the posterior wall.[59–62] CT readily identifies wall thickening, but it is unable to distinguish fibrosis from inflammation. Tracheal luminal narrowing is a common manifestation of airway involvement, ranging in prevalence from 33% to 89%.[58–61] It may be diffuse or focal in distribution and is often accompanied by bronchial narrowing (Fig. 56.16). Compared with axial CT images, multiplanar and 3D external renderings of the trachea improve the detection of subtle airway stenoses and enhance the accuracy of determining the craniocaudad extent of disease (see Fig. 56.16).[63] Paired inspiratory–dynamic expiratory CT is highly sensitive for the detection of tracheomalacia in patients with known or suspected relapsing polychondritis (Fig. 56.17).[64–66] Early in the course of disease, this finding may precede detectable morphologic abnormalities; thus dynamic expiratory CT should be routinely performed in the assessment of symptomatic patients with known or suspected relapsing polychondritis.[66]

MAGNETIC RESONANCE IMAGING

Increased wall thickness may be observed at MRI, but calcification is better visualized with CT. A potential advantage of MRI is its ability to distinguish fibrosis from inflammation.[67] Dynamic MRI is a potential CT alternative for the evaluation of tracheomalacia.[68]

IMAGING ALGORITHMS

Chest radiographs play a minor role in patients with relapsing polychondritis and are most useful for the assessment of

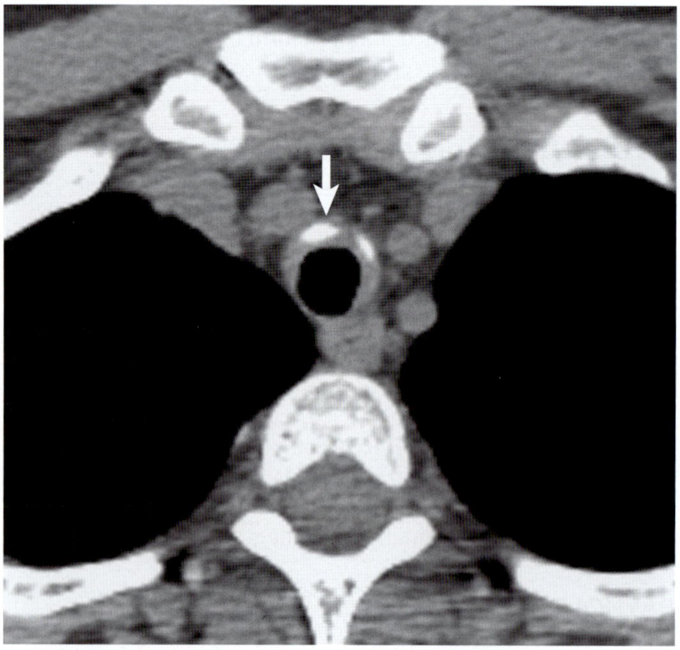

Fig. 56.14 Tracheal wall thickening and calcification resulting from relapsing polychondritis. Axial CT image at the thoracic inlet demonstrates marked tracheal wall thickening with calcification *(arrow)*. Note the characteristic sparing of the posterior noncartilaginous wall.

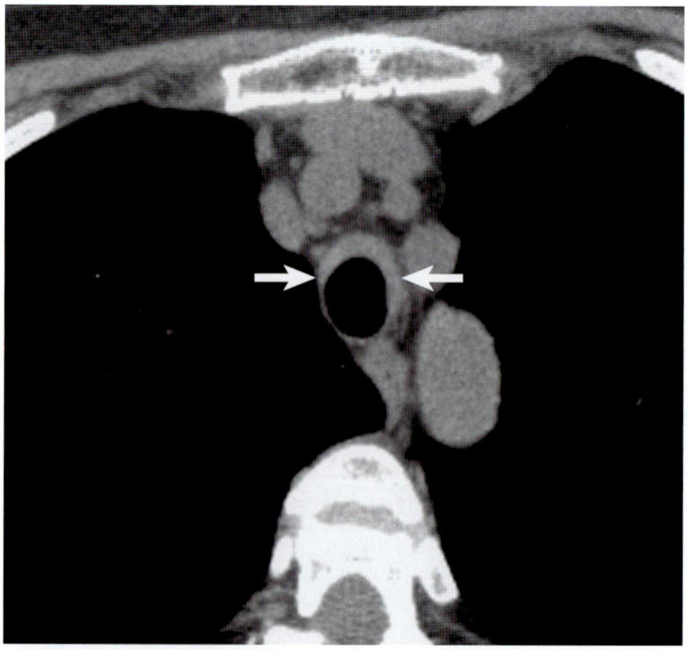

Fig. 56.15 Tracheal wall thickening without calcification in relapsing polychondritis. Axial CT image at the top of the aortic arch demonstrates marked tracheal wall thickening *(arrows)* without calcification.

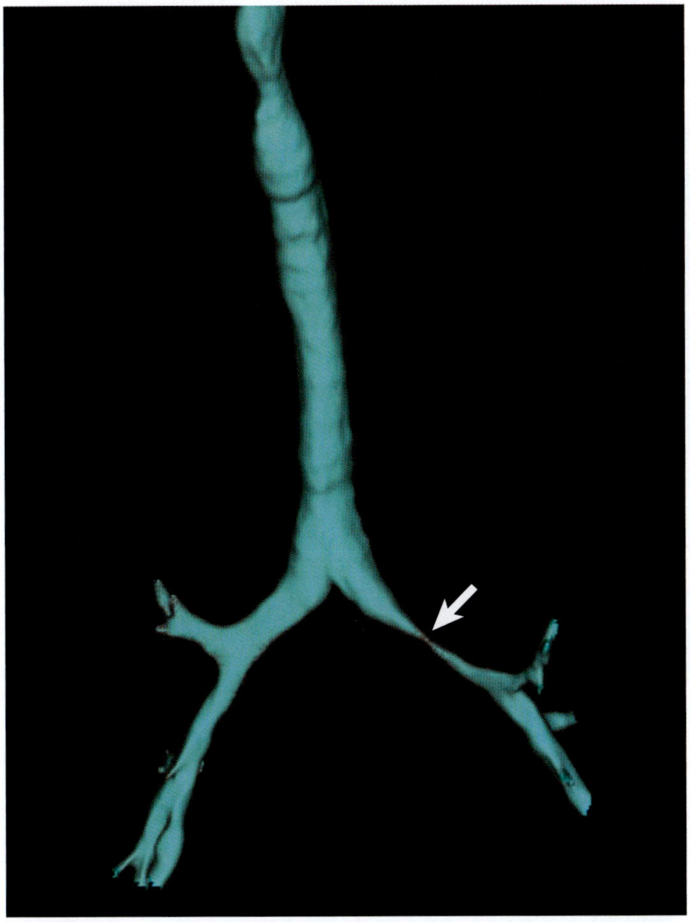

Fig. 56.16 Tracheal and bronchial luminal narrowing in relapsing polychondritis. External three-dimensional rendering CT image demonstrates mild diffuse luminal narrowing of the trachea and severe stenosis of the left main bronchus *(arrow)*.

complications such as pneumonia and atelectasis. However, in patients with advanced disease, careful inspection of the airway on radiographs may reveal tracheal calcification and narrowing.

CT is the main imaging tool in the evaluation of patients with known or suspected relapsing polychondritis. It is highly sensitive for detection of tracheal wall thickening, calcifications, and narrowing. Paired inspiratory–dynamic expiratory CT is the preferred imaging method for the assessment of tracheobronchomalacia.

MRI is less sensitive than CT and is more susceptible to artifact from respiratory motion. However, MRI may aid in the distinction between fibrosis and inflammation and is a potential alternative to CT for patients in whom radiation exposure from CT may be a concern.

Differential Diagnosis

FROM CLINICAL DATA

In a patient with airway symptoms and characteristic findings of relapsing polychondritis (e.g., saddle-nose deformity), the diagnosis is relatively easy to establish. However, when airway involvement is isolated, the differential diagnosis for airway symptoms is broad and includes granulomatosis with polyangiitis, postintubation injury, amyloidosis, and neoplastic tracheal involvement.

FROM SUPPORTIVE DIAGNOSTIC TECHNIQUES

When imaging studies depict the presence of characteristic smooth thickening of the anterior and lateral walls of the trachea, a diagnosis of relapsing polychondritis can be made with a high degree of confidence. Although tracheobronchopathia osteochondroplastica also spares the posterior membranous wall of the trachea, it is distinguished from relapsing polychondritis by the presence of discrete nodules arising from the submucosa of the tracheal wall and protruding into the airway lumen. Other causes of tracheal wall thickening and stenoses can generally be distinguished at CT or MRI by circumferential involvement of the airway wall, without sparing of the posterior membranous portion.

When tracheomalacia is the only imaging finding, the differential diagnosis includes other causes of this condition, including COPD, prior intubation, and prior radiation therapy.

Synopsis of Treatment Options

MEDICAL

Pharmacologic options for the general treatment of patients with relapsing polychondritis include nonsteroidal antiinflammatory drugs, corticosteroids, and dapsone.[51,69] Other immunosuppressive medications, such as cyclophosphamide, azathioprine, and methotrexate, are second-line treatment options.[51,69]

High-dose oral prednisone is usually necessary for the treatment of respiratory tract involvement, and intravenous pulse steroids may be useful for the treatment of acute airway obstruction.[50]

SURGICAL

Surgical options include tracheostomy, tracheal stenting, external airway splinting, and tracheal reconstruction.[51,70]

KEY POINTS: RELAPSING POLYCHONDRITIS

- Average age at onset is in the fifth and sixth decades.
- Relapsing polychondritis is characterized by recurrent inflammation of the cartilaginous structures of the external ear, nose, peripheral joints, larynx, trachea, and bronchi.
- Airway involvement occurs in approximately 50% of cases.
- Respiratory complications (pneumonia, respiratory failure) are the leading cause of mortality.
- Common radiologic findings:
  - Increased attenuation of the tracheal wall (spares the posterior wall)
  - Tracheal wall thickening (usually spares the posterior wall)
  - Focal or diffuse tracheobronchial narrowing
  - Tracheobronchomalacia

Tracheomegaly

Etiology

Tracheobronchomegaly, also referred to as Mounier-Kuhn syndrome, is of uncertain etiology. An underlying defect in elastic tissue has been suggested as a potential causative mechanism.[71] An association with Ehlers-Danlos syndrome, Marfan syndrome, and cutis laxa has been described.[71,72] In addition, a familial form has been reported with a possible autosomal-recessive inheritance.[72] However, most cases occur sporadically.

Secondary tracheomegaly may also develop in the setting of long-standing pulmonary fibrosis.[71,73]

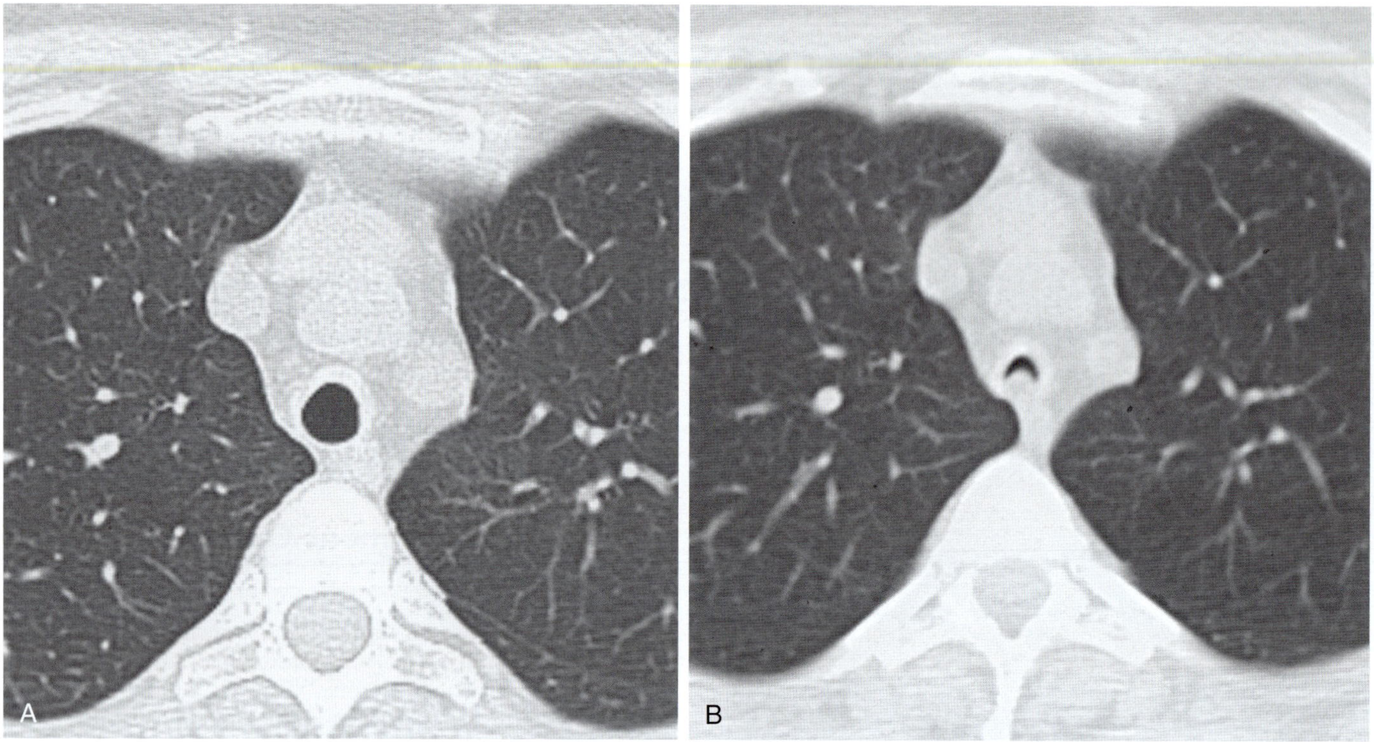

Fig. 56.17 Tracheomalacia in relapsing polychondritis. (A) End-inspiratory CT demonstrates mild luminal narrowing of the trachea with thickening of the anterior and lateral tracheal walls. (B) Dynamic expiratory CT shows >70% cross-sectional area lumen reduction, consistent with tracheomalacia.

Prevalence and Epidemiology

The prevalence of tracheobronchomegaly is unknown. Although once considered extremely rare, it has been recognized with increasing frequency in the past 2 decades, probably as a result of improved visualization of the trachea with CT.[74] There is a male predominance.[71–76]

Acquired tracheomegaly has been estimated to occur in roughly 30% of patients with diffuse pulmonary fibrosis.[73] In this population a potential causative relationship with chronic cough and recurrent respiratory infections has been suggested.[73]

Clinical Presentation

Patients with tracheobronchomegaly typically present in the third and fourth decades.[71–75] The clinical presentation is variable and ranges from minimal to severe respiratory symptoms, including productive cough, copious sputum production, and, rarely, hemoptysis. When tracheobronchomegaly has been complicated by recurrent infections, patients may present with progressive dyspnea and respiratory failure.

In contrast, secondary tracheomegaly is usually an incidental finding on CT scans of patients with long-standing pulmonary fibrosis. Such patients typically present with symptoms related to pulmonary fibrosis, including progressive dyspnea and dry cough.[73]

Pathophysiology

ANATOMY

Severe atrophy of the longitudinal elastic fibers and thinning of the muscularis mucosa allow both the cartilaginous and membranous portions of the trachea and main bronchi to dilate, resulting in increased luminal diameter.[75] Redundant musculomembranous tissue may protrude between the cartilaginous rings, resulting in diverticular protrusions that range in size from several millimeters to several centimeters. When it is diffuse, the condition is referred to as tracheobronchial diverticulosis.[71]

PATHOLOGY

Both the cartilaginous and membranous portions of the trachea and bronchi demonstrate atrophy of muscular and elastic tissue.[72] Recurrent infections may be complicated by bronchiectasis, emphysema, and parenchymal scarring.[72,76]

LUNG FUNCTION

Pulmonary function test results of patients with tracheobronchomegaly typically demonstrate a decrease in expiratory flow rates, an enlarged dead space, and an increased tidal volume.[72]

Increased compliance of the trachea may result in excessive expiratory collapsibility (malacia), which can be detected by bronchoscopy or dynamic expiratory CT scanning.

Manifestations of the Disease

RADIOGRAPHY

On radiographs the diagnosis can be made by measuring the coronal (transverse) and sagittal (anteroposterior) diameters of the trachea. Tracheomegaly is defined in women as tracheal diameter greater than 21 mm (coronal) and 23 mm (sagittal) and in men as tracheal diameter greater than 25 mm (coronal) and 27 mm (sagittal).[75] Bronchomegaly is defined in women by diameters of right and left bronchi greater than 19.8 and 17.4 mm, respectively, and in men by diameters greater than 21.1 and 18.4 mm, respectively.[75] A corrugated or undulated appearance of the tracheal wall may be visible on the lateral chest radiograph. This appearance is due to the presence of outpouchings between the cartilaginous rings of the trachea.

COMPUTED TOMOGRAPHY

Dilation of the internal lumen of the airway is easily visualized on axial CT scans (Figs. 56.18 and 56.19). Although not necessary for diagnosis, external 3D renderings may help demonstrate the distribution of the dilated airways. An undulated appearance of the wall of the trachea and main bronchi is commonly observed on CT (Fig. 56.20). Discrete diverticula may be visualized as tubular blind-ended outpouchings arising from the tracheal and bronchial walls (Fig. 56.21). Tracheal diverticula are a frequent manifestation of tracheobronchomegaly in association with Mounier-Kuhn syndrome. However, they are not usually observed in secondary tracheomegaly that arises in the setting of longstanding, diffuse pulmonary fibrosis.

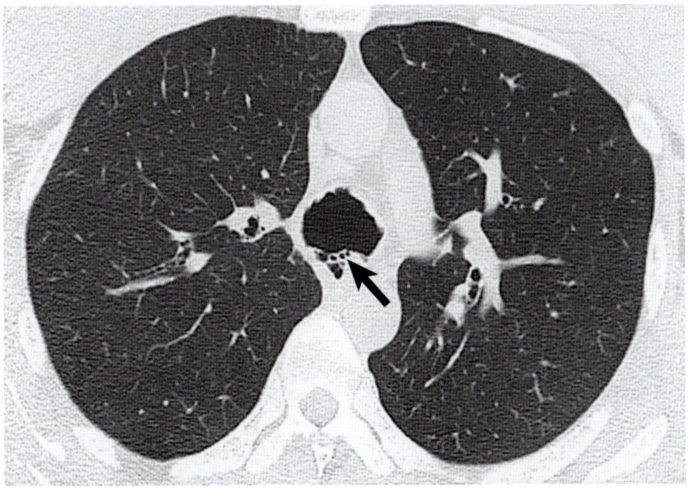

Fig. 56.18 Tracheobronchomegaly. Axial CT image at the level of the carina demonstrates an enlarged trachea with an undulating anterior wall and several small diverticula *(arrow)* arising from the posterior wall.

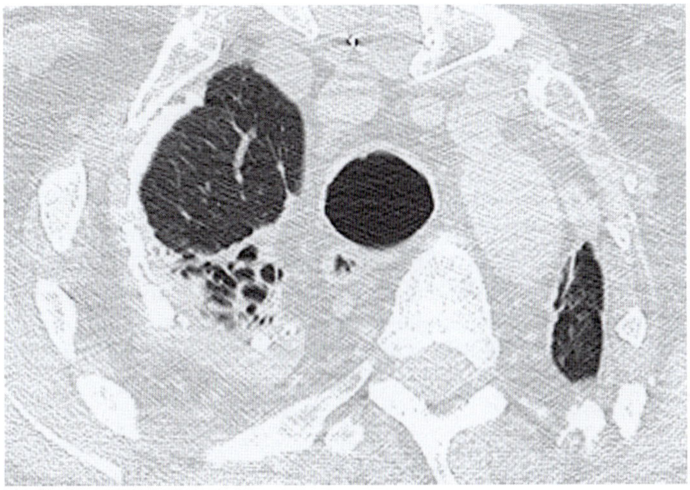

Fig. 56.19 Secondary tracheomegaly due to lung fibrosis. Axial CT image at the lung apices demonstrates enlarged tracheal diameter of 3 cm. Note fibrosis with traction bronchiectasis at the right lung apex.

MAGNETIC RESONANCE IMAGING

Dilation of the internal lumen of the airway and tracheal diverticula may be visualized on MRI.

IMAGING ALGORITHMS

Chest radiography generally suffices for the detection of tracheobronchomegaly and thus serves as the first-line imaging

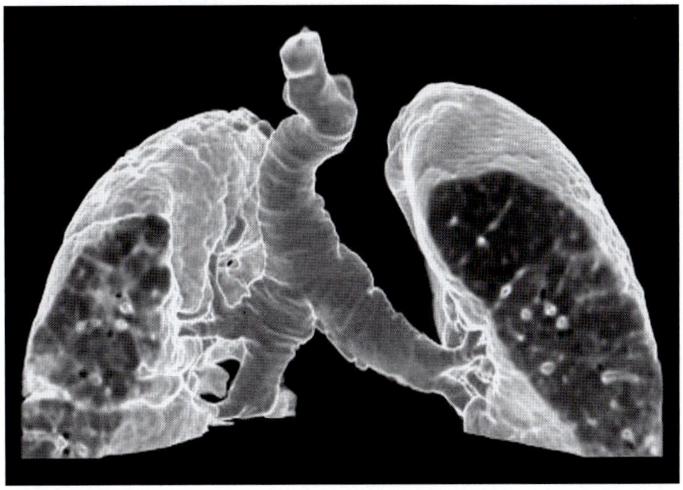

Fig. 56.20 Tracheobronchomegaly. Three-dimensional external rendering of the central airways demonstrates diffuse tracheobronchomegaly.

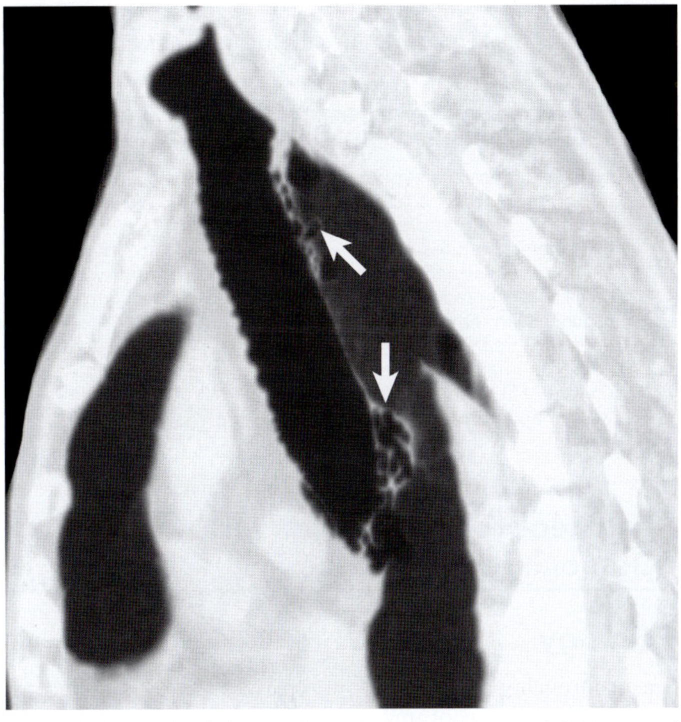

Fig. 56.21 Tracheal diverticulosis. Sagittal reformatted CT image of the trachea demonstrates multiple tubular, air-filled structures *(arrows)* arising from the posterior trachea, representing diverticulosis. Also note the tracheomegaly and corrugated contour of the anterior wall.

study. CT provides more detailed information about the tracheal wall and displays characteristic undulations and diverticula of the airway wall with greater detail than radiographs do. CT is also more sensitive than radiography for the detection of complications, including bronchiectasis, emphysema, and pulmonary fibrosis. Dynamic expiratory CT may be helpful for detecting excessive expiratory collapse (malacia). MRI may be considered an alternative to CT in young patients for whom radiation exposure may be a potential concern.

Differential Diagnosis

FROM CLINICAL DATA

There are no specific clinical features that will differentiate this condition from isolated bronchiectasis or chronic bronchitis.

FROM SUPPORTIVE DIAGNOSTIC TECHNIQUES

The diagnosis can be made with confidence on radiography, CT, or MRI by demonstration of enlargement of the internal lumen of the trachea accompanied by a corrugated contour of the airway wall.

Synopsis of Treatment Options

MEDICAL

Treatment is conservative and includes chest physiotherapy for assistance with clearing of secretions and antibiotics for treatment of pulmonary infections.[71]

SURGICAL

Tracheoplasty or stent placement may be considered in selected patients with tracheobronchomegaly and severe tracheomalacia.

KEY POINTS: TRACHEOBRONCHOMEGALY

- Tracheal dimensions should routinely be assessed on chest radiographs and CT scans of patients with recurrent infections and chronic sputum production.
- Key imaging features of tracheobronchomegaly are increased luminal diameter and corrugated appearance of airway walls.
- Tracheobronchomegaly may be complicated by tracheomalacia, bronchiectasis, emphysema, and fibrosis.
- Secondary tracheomegaly may be observed as an incidental finding on imaging studies of patients with long-standing pulmonary fibrosis. In this condition the wall of the trachea is smooth, and diverticula are usually absent.

Tracheobronchopathia Osteochondroplastica

Etiology

Tracheobronchopathia osteochondroplastica (TBO) is an uncommon, benign disease of unknown etiology.[33,77–80] Various causes or associations have been postulated, including chronic inflammatory or degenerative processes, chemical irritation, amyloidosis, infection, and hereditary factors.[77,78] Two theories of histogenesis have been proposed: (1) enchondrosis or exostosis from the tracheal cartilaginous rings and (2) cartilaginous and osseous metaplasia of elastic tissue in the internal elastic fibrous membrane of the tracheal wall.[77]

Prevalence and Epidemiology

Its prevalence at routine bronchoscopy is well below 1%.[33]

Clinical Presentation

The clinical presentation is variable. The disorder is typically diagnosed during the fifth and sixth decades and has a 3:1 male predilection.[33] TBO may be an incidental finding in an asymptomatic patient or may present with a variety of respiratory symptoms, including dyspnea on exertion, cough, wheezing, recurrent infections, and hemoptysis.[77]

Pathophysiology

ANATOMY

TBO is characterized by multiple submucosal osteocartilaginous nodules that project into the tracheal lumen.

PATHOLOGY

At histopathologic examination the nodules are recognized as submucosal osteocartilaginous growths. The mucosal surface is usually intact, and a connection between the nodule and the perichondrium of the tracheal cartilaginous ring is frequently identified.[33]

Manifestations of the Disease

RADIOGRAPHY

In advanced cases chest radiographs may demonstrate tracheal narrowing with a scalloped and nodular configuration.[33,77] Calcification may also be identified radiographically, especially on the lateral radiograph.[78]

COMPUTED TOMOGRAPHY

CT is the imaging modality of choice for this condition.[77] It demonstrates a characteristic pattern of calcified nodules arising from the anterior and lateral walls of the trachea and protruding into the lumen, which may result in diffuse luminal narrowing (Figs. 56.22 and 56.23). The individual nodules typically range in size from 3 to 8 mm.[79] Thickening of the tracheal cartilage is also typically visible at CT.[33,77,79,80] Similar to relapsing polychondritis, there is sparing of the noncartilaginous posterior membranous wall. A saber-sheath configuration (sagittal to coronal diameter ratio >2) of the trachea, which is most commonly associated with COPD, is also frequently observed in patients with TBO.[77]

Differential Diagnosis

FROM CLINICAL DATA

There are no distinguishing clinical features of this condition.

FROM SUPPORTIVE DIAGNOSTIC TECHNIQUES

The identification of calcified nodules arising from the anterior and lateral walls of the trachea at CT or bronchoscopy is considered diagnostic of this condition.[33,78] TBO can be distinguished from entities such as amyloidosis and infectious tracheitis that have circumferential tracheal involvement. Although relapsing polychondritis has a distribution similar to that of TBO, it characteristically manifests with calcified wall thickening without discrete intraluminal nodules. Moreover, relapsing polychondritis is frequently associated with tracheomalacia, whereas TBO is not usually associated with increased expiratory collapsibility.

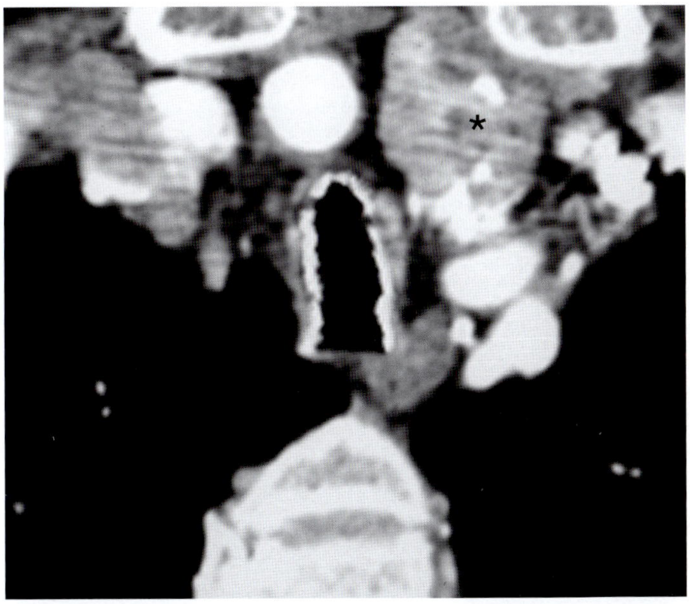

Fig. 56.22 Tracheobronchopathia osteochondroplastica. Axial CT image above the aortic arch demonstrates diffuse thickening and calcification of the tracheal cartilage with nodularity that spares the posterior wall. Also note the saber-sheath configuration of the tracheal lumen. A calcified thyroid nodule *(asterisk)* is incidentally noted. *(Courtesy Michael Gotway, MD.)*

Synopsis of Treatment Options

MEDICAL

Treatment is usually supportive and conservative. There is currently no medical therapy to treat this condition or to prevent the growth of new nodules.[33]

SURGICAL

There is no standard interventional therapy. Treatment options for advanced cases include laser resection, radiation therapy, surgical resection, and stent placement.[77] Interventional therapy is usually tailored for individual cases.

KEY POINTS: TRACHEOBRONCHOPATHIA OSTEOCHONDROPLASTICA

- Diagnosis is typically made during the fifth and sixth decades.
- There is a 3:1 male predilection.
- It is often an incidental finding in an asymptomatic patient but may result in variable respiratory symptoms.
- Identification of calcified nodules arising from the anterior and lateral walls of the trachea is diagnostic and is best visualized with CT.

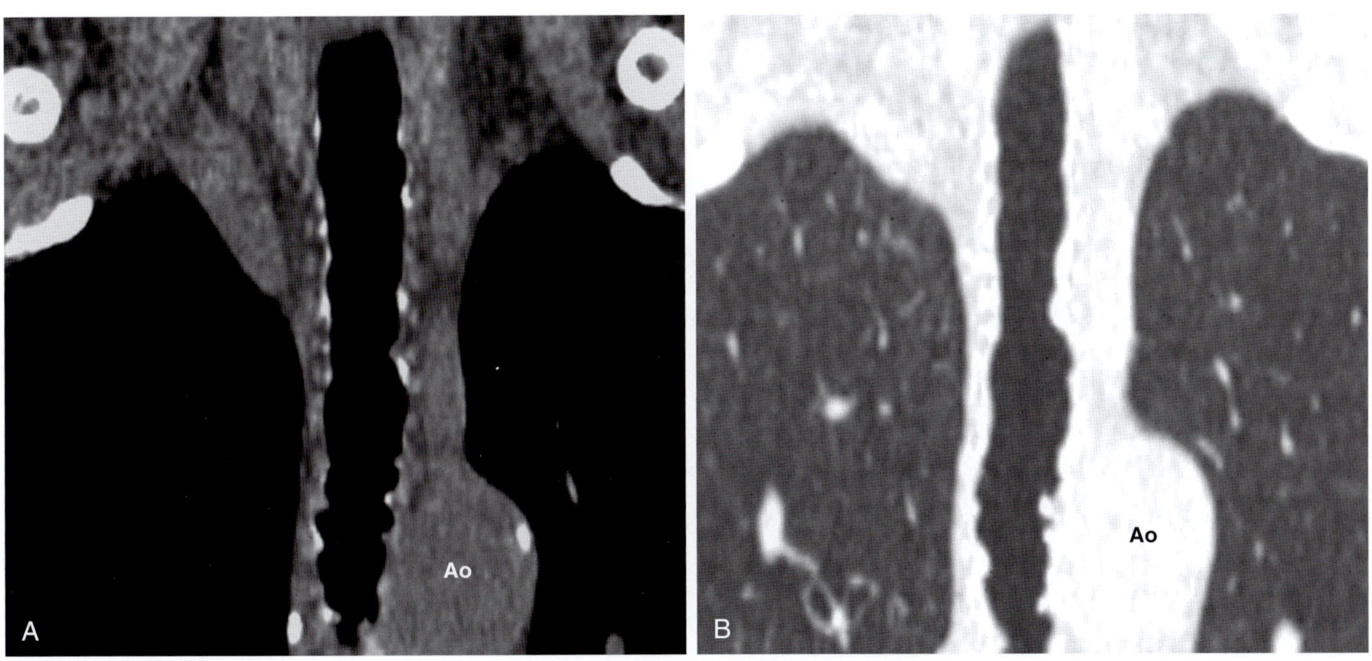

Fig. 56.23 Tracheobronchopathia osteochondroplastica. (A) Coronal CT image shows thickening, nodularity, and calcification of the tracheal cartilage. (B) Coronal CT image at lung windows better demonstrates the marked nodularity of the tracheal wall. *Ao*, Aortic arch.

SUGGESTED READINGS

Kligerman S, Sharma A. Radiologic evaluation of the trachea. *Semin Thorac Cardiovasc Surg*. 2009;21(3):246–254.

Little BP, Duong P-AT. Imaging of diseases of the large airways. *Radiol Clin N Am*. 2016;54(6):1183–1203.

Prince JS, Duhamel DR, Levin DL, et al. Nonneoplastic lesions of the tracheobronchial wall: radiographic findings with bronchoscopic correlation. *Radiographics*. 2002;22:S215–S230.

Ridge CA, O'Donnell CR, Lee EY, Majid A, Boiselle PM. Tracheobronchomalacia: current concepts and controversies. *J Thorac Imaging*. 2011;26(4): 278–289.

The full reference list for this chapter is available at ExpertConsult.com.

57 Bronchiectasis and Other Bronchial Abnormalities*

BRENT P. LITTLE

Bronchiectasis

Etiology

Diseases of the airways are surprisingly common in clinical practice, and imaging tests have a central role in the evaluation of the patient. Bronchiectasis is an important yet, in historic terms, a surprisingly neglected disorder characterized pathologically by abnormal permanent dilatation of the bronchi, leading to significant morbidity and mortality.[1–3] The causes and associations of bronchiectasis are diverse and summarized in Box 57.1. However, the relative impact of the various etiologic factors, such as infection, has changed over time, and there is considerable variation dependent on geographic and ethnic factors.[4–7] The availability of effective antimicrobial therapy and the policy of widespread childhood immunization in many countries have had a significant impact, leading not only to a decrease in the prevalence of postinfectious bronchiectasis but also to a decline in overall mortality.

In the developed world, including the United States and many countries in Europe, postinfectious bronchiectasis is now less of a clinical problem; the more common causes include cystic fibrosis and immunologic deficiencies, which may be primary (as seen in patients with panhypogammaglobulinemia or more selective immunoglobulin subclass defects) or secondary to immunosuppression (as may be seen in the context of hematologic malignant disease or human immunodeficiency virus–related disease).[8–11] In stark contrast, infections such as tuberculosis continue to account for the majority of patients with bronchiectasis in developing countries.[6,12] Defects of mucociliary clearance (either congenital, as in primary ciliary dyskinesia, or acquired), mechanical obstruction (intrinsic or extrinsic), and congenital abnormalities (such as intralobar sequestration) are among the less common but recognized causes of bronchiectasis.[13] However, a cause for bronchiectasis may not be identified in 30% to 70% of patients.[9,11,14] Another complicating factor in the evaluation of patients with bronchiectasis is that in a small proportion of cases, more than one causative factor may be identified.[9]

Prevalence and Epidemiology

The true prevalence of bronchiectasis is unknown. Because it has long been the paradigm of an "orphan" lung disease,[15] reliable published data on the prevalence of bronchiectasis have been frustratingly difficult to come by. One of the fundamental problems has stemmed from the relatively widespread misconception that bronchiectasis is no longer a significant clinical entity. The corollary is that the index of clinical suspicion for a diagnosis of bronchiectasis has been low, and physicians often attribute the symptoms and signs of bronchiectasis to other respiratory diseases (e.g., smoking-related chronic bronchitis) that are perceived to be more common.

Nevertheless, the prevalence of bronchiectasis is known to be remarkably high in select populations; for instance, high rates of bronchiectasis are known to be a problem in indigenous Australians[16] and also native Alaskans.[5] Similarly, bronchiectasis unrelated to cystic fibrosis is strikingly prevalent in parts of New Zealand, where there is an estimated overall prevalence of 1 in 3000 in children younger than 15 years and a staggering prevalence of 1 in 625 for children of Pacific ancestry.[7] These data in contrast to the comparatively low prevalence of bronchiectasis in Finnish children of a similar age.[17] Finally, in most large series of patients with bronchiectasis, a consistent finding has been the preponderance of female patients.[1,6,18,19]

Clinical Presentation

Pulmonologists generally agree that the once dramatic clinical presentation of bronchiectasis (the classic patient with cough and large volumes of purulent and frequently foul-smelling sputum production) is now uncommon.[13] In its place, there is a more insidious form of bronchiectasis in which patients give a typical story of so-called wheezy bronchitis during childhood and chronic purulent rhinosinusitis[9,13]; just less than half of those patients with bronchiectasis will also report an antecedent history of pneumonia or another respiratory tract infection.[9] There is then often something of a "remission" in the teenage years, only to be followed, typically after a viral respiratory tract infection, by the more classic symptoms associated with bronchiectasis—namely, chronic cough and mucopurulent sputum production. Many patients also complain of breathlessness, intermittent hemoptysis, pleuritic chest pain, weight loss, and fatigue.[6,11,13,18] The findings on physical examination are nonspecific and include early to midinspiratory crackles and wheezing.[6,20] Digital clubbing is seen in up to one-quarter of patients with bronchiectasis.[6]

Pathophysiology

ANATOMY

With successive generations of bronchial branching, there is a progressive diminution of airway caliber; a lack of tapering is abnormal. The bronchial tree is composed of the large (bronchi) and small (bronchioles) airways. The traditional distinction is based on the presence or absence of cartilage in the wall; airways reinforced by cartilage and typically greater than 1 mm in diameter are termed

*The editors and publisher would like to thank Drs. Nestor L. Müller and C. Isabela Silva Müller for contributing material on this topic to the prior edition of this work. It has served as the foundation for the current chapter.

BOX 57.1 CAUSES AND ASSOCIATIONS OF BRONCHIECTASIS

Idiopathic
Congenital
- Cystic fibrosis
- Mounier-Kuhn syndrome (tracheobronchomegaly)
- α1-Antitrypsin deficiency
- Williams-Campbell syndrome
- Intralobar sequestration

Postinfectious or postinflammatory
- Bacterial, mycobacterial, viral, protozoal
- Swyer-James (MacLeod) syndrome
- Aspiration of gastric contents
- Inhalation of toxic fumes

Immunodeficiency
- Primary: selective immunoglobulin deficiency, panhypogammaglobulinemia
- Secondary: malignant neoplasia, chemotherapy

Mechanical airway obstruction
- Inhaled foreign bodies
- Neoplastic
- Broncholithiasis
- Bronchostenosis

Defective mucus transport
- Primary ciliary dyskinesia
- Secondary ciliary dyskinesia
- Young syndrome

Immunologic
- Allergic bronchopulmonary aspergillosis
- After heart-lung, lung, or bone marrow transplantation

Miscellaneous associations
- Middle lobe syndrome
- Rheumatoid arthritis
- Sjögren syndrome
- Systemic lupus erythematosus
- Ulcerative colitis
- Yellow nail syndrome
- Celiac disease
- Human immunodeficiency virus infection

bronchi, whereas those without cartilage and typically less than 1 mm in diameter are termed *bronchioles*.[21] Although larger airways are conducive to maximum rate of airflow, a rapid increase in total cross-sectional diameter at the level of the small airways facilitates gas exchange across the alveolar-capillary membrane.[22–24]

PATHOLOGY

The vicious circle hypothesis for the pathogenesis of bronchiectasis, first advocated by Cole and colleagues,[13] is the most widely accepted. The theory is based on the premise that there is initial damage to or disruption of the process of normal mucociliary clearance. This may have been as a result of a viral respiratory infection or a genetic susceptibility, as is the case in patients with cystic fibrosis. The inability to clear mucus permits the "normal" oropharyngeal flora, including *Haemophilus influenzae, Pseudomonas aeruginosa,* and *Streptococcus pneumoniae*, to persist within the airways. The organisms lead to further epithelial damage, reducing mucociliary clearance and encouraging further colonization. An inflammatory host response also contributes to further airway damage and dilatation of the airways. With time, there is loss of the elastin layer in the bronchial wall and destruction of cartilage. Some data, based on serial observations by use of computed tomography (CT), suggest that the vicious circle theory may need some refinement, particularly in the pediatric population, because bronchial dilatation diagnosed by high-resolution CT is not always irreversible or progressive.[25,26]

Three different patterns of bronchiectasis are recognized: cylindrical, varicose, and cystic.[27] In cylindrical bronchiectasis, there is relatively uniform bronchial dilatation, and the implication is that this is perhaps the least severe morphologic type. This should be contrasted with varicose bronchiectasis, in which there are focal narrowings along otherwise dilated airways, and cystic bronchiectasis, which, as the term suggests, indicates grossly dilated airways that have a cystic appearance. Although these morphologic subtypes of bronchiectasis are generally identifiable on high-resolution CT, the clinical utility of making these distinctions is questionable.

LUNG FUNCTION

The classic physiologic defect in bronchiectasis is airflow obstruction, which in some patients is partially reversible.[28,29] The obstructive defect has been variably attributed to the presence of coexistent emphysema,[30] airway hyperreactivity or asthma,[31] constrictive bronchiolitis,[32] and expiratory large airway collapse.[33] However, CT studies suggest that areas of decreased attenuation, possibly reflecting constrictive bronchiolitis at the pathologic level, and severity of bronchial wall thickening are the best correlates of obstructive physiology.[34–36] In some patients with bronchiectasis, there is an associated restrictive ventilatory defect, possibly related to patchy peribronchial fibrosis (presumably consequent on inflammation) and atelectasis.[29]

Manifestations of the Disease

RADIOGRAPHY

The chest radiograph is generally the first radiologic test requested by the pulmonologist when a diagnosis of bronchiectasis is suspected. However, radiography has low sensitivity and specificity in the diagnosis (Fig. 57.1). However, before the advent of CT and before the conception of the high-resolution CT technique, pulmonologists and radiologists were necessarily reliant on chest radiography, followed in many cases by the then gold standard, but now obsolete, investigation of bronchography, in patients with suspected bronchiectasis (Fig. 57.2). In the frequently quoted study by Gudbjerg,[37] the conclusion was that a mere 10% of patients with bronchiectasis would have a normal chest radiograph. However, although this would have been true at the time, the study was published more than 50 years ago, and as discussed before, the clinical manifestations of bronchiectasis have changed. Moreover, many of the radiographic signs described by Gudbjerg (e.g., linear markings, bronchial wall thickening, and patchy or confluent shadows) are nonspecific. This was clearly illustrated by the later study from the Brompton Hospital that compared chest radiographic diagnoses of bronchiectasis with bronchography and confirmed the highly insensitive nature of chest radiography, also showing considerable disagreement between two experienced pulmonary radiologists simply for confirming the presence or absence of individual features of bronchiectasis.[38]

When identified, bronchial dilatation is the key radiographic feature of bronchiectasis. Thus the observer may see poorly defined ring shadows (reflecting the dilated bronchus with peribronchial inflammation when it is seen end-on) or "tram-line" opacities (denoting the nontapering airway), depending on the

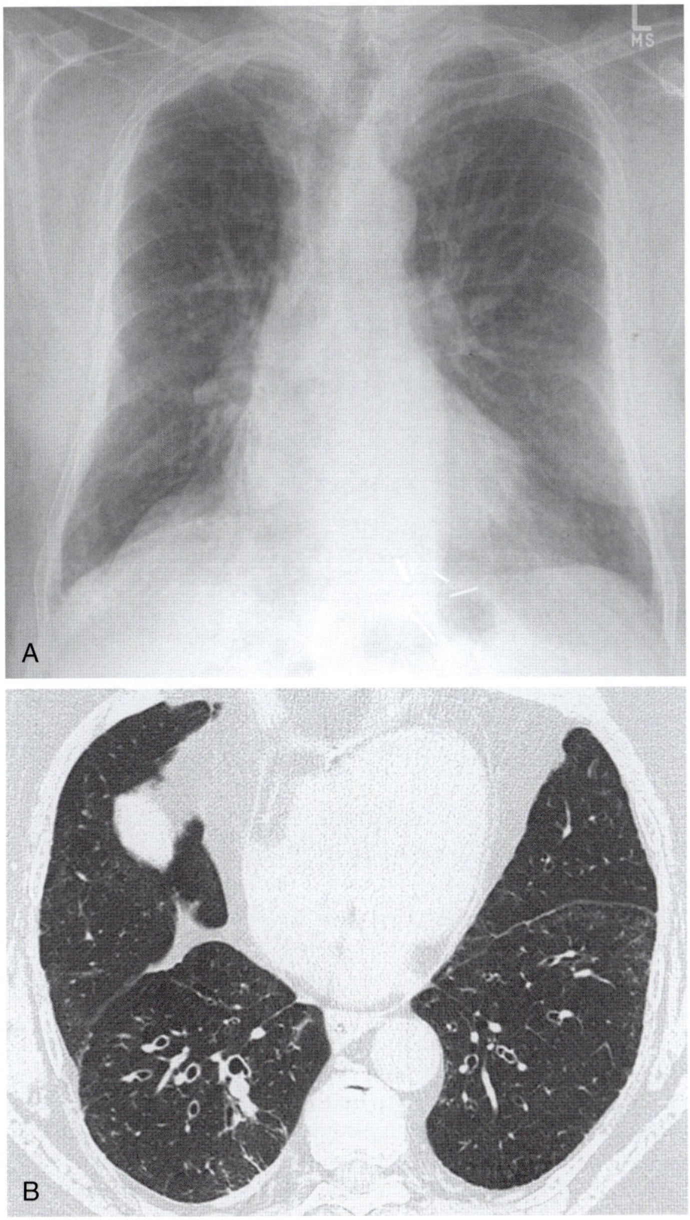

Fig. 57.1 Bronchiectasis evident only on CT. (A) Chest radiograph shows no abnormality. (B) High-resolution CT image shows dilatation of subsegmental bronchi (in relation to adjacent pulmonary artery) characteristic of bronchiectasis.

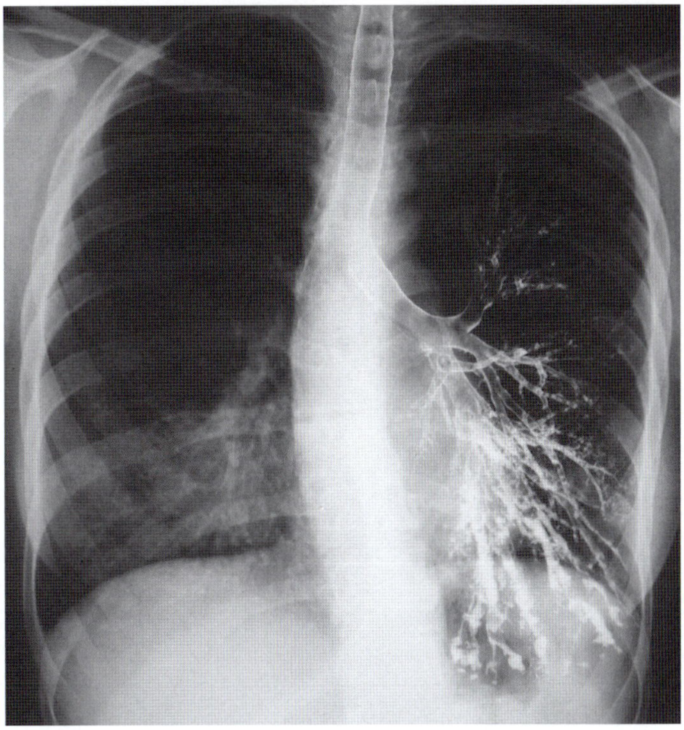

Fig. 57.2 Bronchiectasis on bronchography. Bronchogram shows normal diameter and tapering of the left upper lobe and lingular bronchi and cylindrical and varicose left lower lobe bronchiectasis. *(Courtesy Dr. Reynaldo T. Rodrigues, Federal University of São Paulo, São Paulo, Brazil.)*

orientation of the individual airway with respect to the x-ray beam (Fig. 57.3). With more severe disease, obvious thin-walled cysts, with or without air-fluid levels, may be apparent (Fig. 57.4).

The other recognized features of bronchiectasis on chest radiographs include tubular and branching opacities caused by plugging of dilated airways with mucus, volume loss or hyperexpansion, and foci of subsegmental atelectasis. These are ancillary radiographic signs and must not be regarded as diagnostic of bronchiectasis.

COMPUTED TOMOGRAPHY

In the era before the development of the thin-section CT technique, data on the value of CT in diagnosis of bronchiectasis were disappointing, with sensitivities in the range of 66% to 79%.[39–41] However, with the realization that spatial resolution could be improved significantly by reducing slice collimation, the reported sensitivities for the CT diagnosis of bronchiectasis improved, with sensitivities approaching 100% using thin-section (1–1.5 mm) imaging.[42,43]

A factor to be considered in review of the airways on thin-section CT is the window setting because, in the context of a diagnosis of bronchiectasis, this may have a significant influence on the assessment of luminal diameter.[44–46] In their experimental study, Webb and colleagues[46] showed that for airways surrounded by air, a window centered at −450 Hounsfield units (HUs) provided the most accurate measurement of wall thickness. Indeed, at this window mean, the window width had an imperceptible effect on the evaluation of wall thickness. When the window center was set lower than −450 HUs, wall thickness was overestimated, and the converse was true when the setting was higher.[46]

Computed Tomographic Features of Bronchiectasis

CT signs of bronchiectasis were first described by Naidich and colleagues[47] in 1982, albeit on non–high-resolution CT (10-mm collimation) images. The features identified by these investigators have, with some modifications, largely been validated in subsequent series. Although bronchial dilatation is the key morphologic abnormality, bronchial wall thickening, patchy areas of decreased parenchymal attenuation and vascularity (termed *mosaic attenuation*), plugging of large and small airways, volume loss, crowding of airways, and, in some patients with idiopathic disease, thickening of interlobular septa can be seen in association with bronchiectasis.[39,41–43,48,49]

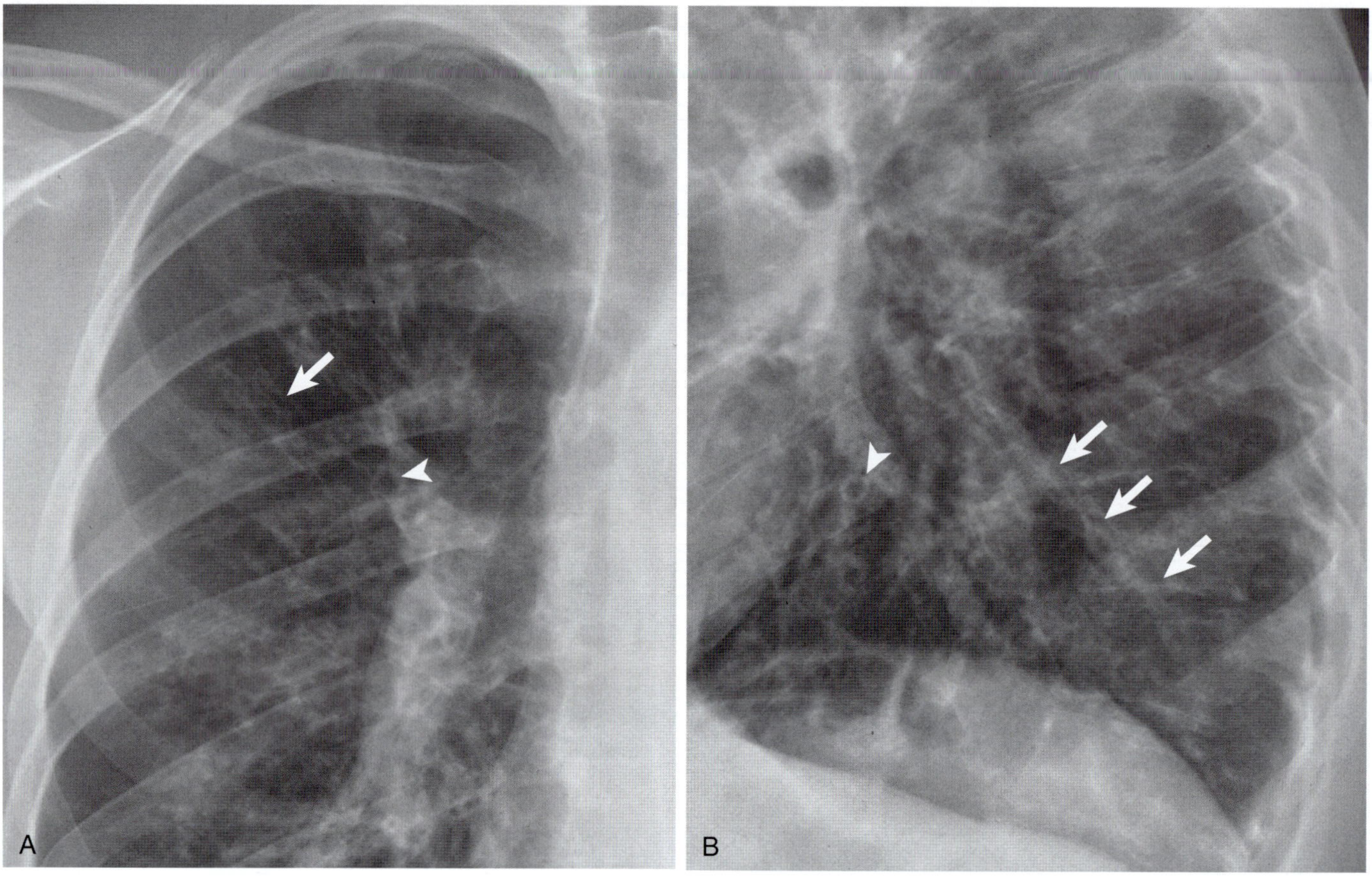

Fig. 57.3 Radiographic signs of bronchiectasis in cystic fibrosis. Magnified views of frontal (A) and lateral (B) chest radiographs demonstrate multiple ring shadows *(arrowheads)* and tram-line opacities *(straight arrows)* consistent with bronchiectasis.

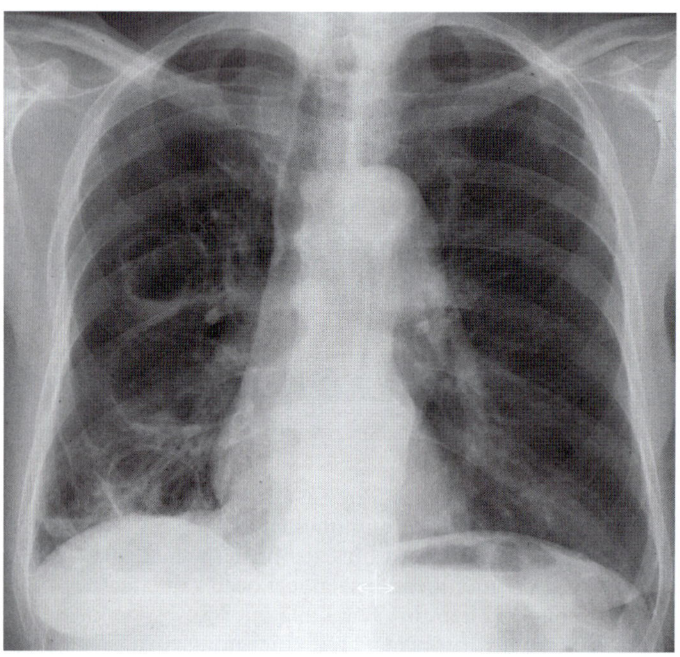

Fig. 57.4 Cystic bronchiectasis on chest radiography. Chest radiograph shows multiple thin-walled cystic opacities in the right lung. Although it is less conspicuous, there is evidence of disease in the left lower lobe.

Bronchial Dilatation. Bronchiectasis is abnormal permanent dilatation of the airways, with or without associated thickening of the walls of the airways. In the normal state the internal diameter of the airway is roughly equal to the transverse diameter of the accompanying pulmonary artery; a bronchoarterial ratio greater than 1 should generally be regarded as abnormal.[50] The CT appearance of bronchiectatic airways depends on the orientation of abnormal bronchi relative to the plane of section. Thus, for airways that are perpendicular to the imaging plane, the radiologist will look for a dilated airway next to a dot representing the normal adjacent pulmonary arterial branch, an appearance that has been likened to a signet ring (Fig. 57.5). In contrast, for bronchi that lie in the plane of section, as in the middle lobe and lingula, the radiologist should look for an absence of normal tapering (Fig. 57.6).

The identification of airway dilatation in patients with severe (varicose or cystic) bronchiectasis does not usually pose a challenge.[51] However, the majority of patients with bronchiectasis now present with mild disease, and the recognition of less severe (cylindrical) bronchial dilatation is certainly problematic. A spurious increase in the bronchoarterial ratio may be seen because the accompanying pulmonary artery can divide before the airway.[52] In this way, the bronchial diameter will appear to be increased compared with the homologous arterial branch. Another consideration is that a bronchoarterial ratio greater than 1 is not always abnormal because it may be seen in up to one-fifth of healthy subjects.[48] Furthermore, it has been shown that there is

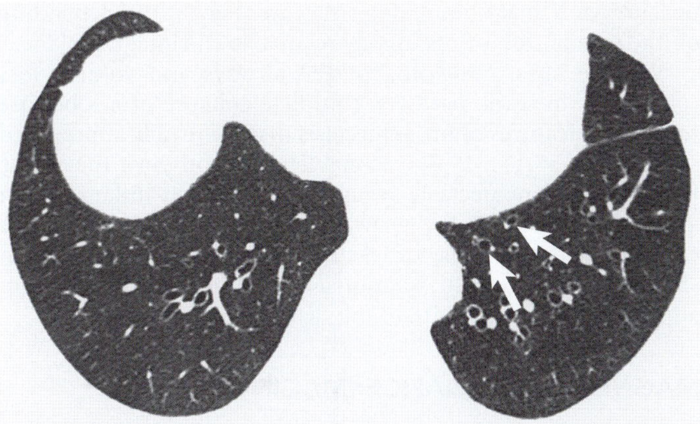

Fig. 57.5 Bronchiectasis: "signet ring" on CT. High-resolution CT shows several bronchi with a luminal diameter greater than the adjacent pulmonary artery. This appearance of a dilated airway and the normal-size adjacent pulmonary artery in patients with bronchiectasis has been likened to a signet ring *(arrows)*.

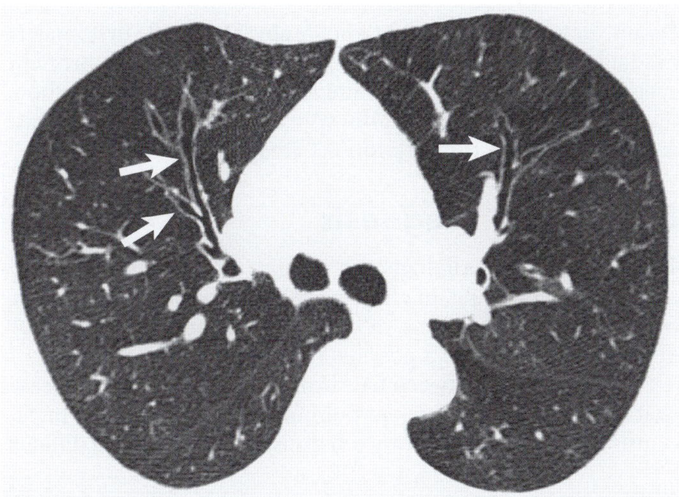

Fig. 57.6 Bronchiectasis: lack of normal bronchial tapering. High-resolution CT image shows bilateral upper lobe bronchiectasis *(arrows)* as denoted by the lack of tapering of the bronchi after they bifurcate.

a normal but progressive increase in the internal diameter of the airways with age, with a bronchoarterial ratio exceeding 1 in just more than 40% of asymptomatic subjects older than 65 years.[53] Finally, altitude may have a bearing on the relationship between airways and their adjacent pulmonary arteries; 50% of healthy subjects had evidence of bronchial dilatation by conventional CT criteria in one study performed in Colorado.[54] Another study confirmed higher bronchoarterial ratios at high altitude compared with sea level.[50] Although the exact mechanisms are not clear, it is conceivable that the increase in bronchoarterial ratio at altitude might be due to vasoconstriction associated with hypoxia,[55] coupled possibly with the phenomenon of hypoxic bronchodilatation.[56]

Kim and colleagues[48] looked for features on CT that would differentiate normal subjects from patients with surgically proven bronchiectasis. This study showed that, in contrast to an increased bronchoarterial ratio and lack of tapering, the visualization of airways within 1 cm of the costal or paravertebral pleura and the identification of airways abutting the mediastinal pleura were more discriminatory, being seen in 81% and 53%, respectively, of the patients with bronchiectasis but in none of the normal subjects.

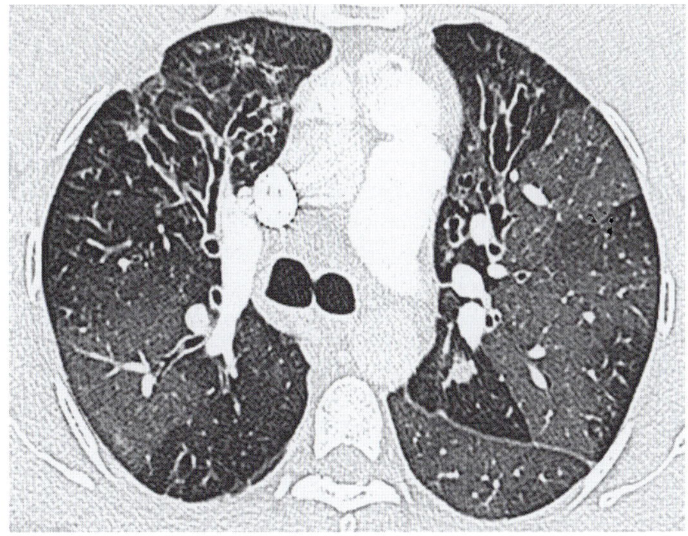

Fig. 57.7 Varicose bronchiectasis in cystic fibrosis. High-resolution CT image shows varicose bronchiectasis in both upper lobes. Note striking mosaic attenuation from small airways disease.

Ancillary Computed Tomographic Features of Bronchiectasis

Although dilatation of bronchi is the cardinal morphologic manifestation of bronchiectasis, there are a number of ancillary signs on CT. A diagnosis of bronchiectasis cannot be made on the basis of these ancillary CT features in the absence of bronchial dilatation. These additional signs of bronchiectasis are discussed briefly.

Bronchial Wall Thickening. Thickening of the bronchial wall commonly accompanies bronchiectasis on CT[47] and is likely to reflect an inflammatory component. As has already been mentioned, appreciation of wall thickening is subject to technical factors; window settings that are too narrow can lead to an overestimation of bronchial wall thickness. Interpretation of bronchial wall thickening is also hampered by the lack of consensus on what constitutes normal wall thickness at CT. In an attempt to address this, Remy-Jardin[57] considered bronchi to be thick walled if the wall of any individual airway was at least twice as thick as that of a normal airway. However, the obvious drawback is the assumption that a normal comparable bronchus will be visible; naturally, this cannot be guaranteed when bronchiectasis is severe and widespread. An alternative definition of wall thickening is internal diameter of the airway lumen less than 80% of its external diameter.[58] This definition is useful but only when bronchial dilatation is relatively mild; plainly, if the dilatation is marked (as in cystic bronchiectasis), wall thickening will be underestimated.

Mosaic Attenuation. Patchy areas of decreased attenuation, within which there is a reduction in the number or caliber of pulmonary vessels, are not only common but also a functionally important finding on CT in patients with bronchiectasis (Fig. 57.7).[34–36] The extent of areas of decreased attenuation on expiratory CT does not correlate with indices of gas transfer such as diffusing lung capacity for carbon monoxide, suggesting that areas of mosaic attenuation are due to associated constrictive bronchiolitis.[34,35]

Regions of air-trapping on expiratory CT tend to be most prevalent in lobes with either extensive or cystic bronchiectasis or in association with large mucous plugs and plugging within the centrilobular bronchioles.[34] However, an additional intriguing finding is the presence of areas of decreased attenuation in some lobes without overt bronchiectasis (Fig. 57.8).[34] On this basis, it has been hypothesized that constrictive bronchiolitis may be the key initial pathologic lesion in bronchiectasis.[34]

Airway Plugging. Inflammatory mucous secretions may fill the ectatic bronchi, resulting in tubular and nodular opacities representing bronchi seen along their long axis and short axis, respectively. Care must be taken not to miss bronchiectasis in these cases (Fig. 57.9). Mucous secretions within the distal airways and inflammatory thickening of the bronchiolar walls may produce a tree-in-bud pattern, which manifests as Y- or V-shaped opacities or a linear branching structure (Fig. 57.10), depending on the orientation of the airway relative to the imaging plane.[59]

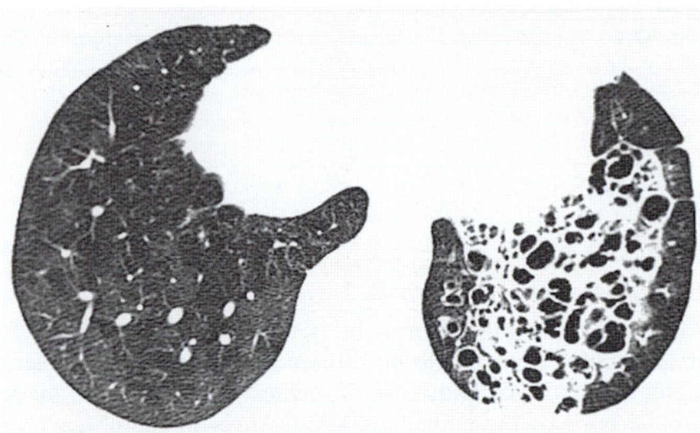

Fig. 57.8 Bronchiectasis and small airways disease. High-resolution CT image shows cystic bronchiectasis in the left lower lobe. No bronchiectasis is seen in the right lower lobe, but there is mosaic attenuation consistent with constrictive bronchiolitis.

Volume Loss. Crowding of the airways and volume loss (including, in some patients, complete collapse of a lobe) are recognized features of bronchiectasis that are readily appreciated at CT (Fig. 57.11). It is reasonable to hypothesize that these features of bronchiectasis are a consequence of inflammation and fibrosis around the airways. However, this is not to be confused with the entity of traction bronchiectasis; as the term suggests, this refers to tractional dilatation of airways from adjacent fibrotic interstitial lung diseases (see later).[60]

MAGNETIC RESONANCE IMAGING

Magnetic resonance imaging (MRI) has a limited role in the diagnosis of bronchiectasis (Fig. 57.12), and the clinical utility of such tests for routine clinical management of patients with bronchiectasis remains debatable.

IMAGING ALGORITHMS

Despite its constraints, chest radiography is often the first imaging modality obtained for the evaluation of patients with bronchiectasis. However, given the limited sensitivity and the likelihood that the majority of patients now present with less severe disease, many will require thin-section CT imaging.[52]

Differential Diagnosis

The challenge for radiologists in making a diagnosis of bronchiectasis is twofold: first, in ensuring that the diagnosis is not being overcalled, because of one of the potential mimics, and second, in trying to determine a possible cause of bronchiectasis.

The distinction between true bronchiectasis and lung diseases characterized by cysts, such as pulmonary Langerhans cell histiocytosis and lymphangioleiomyomatosis, may be rendered difficult,

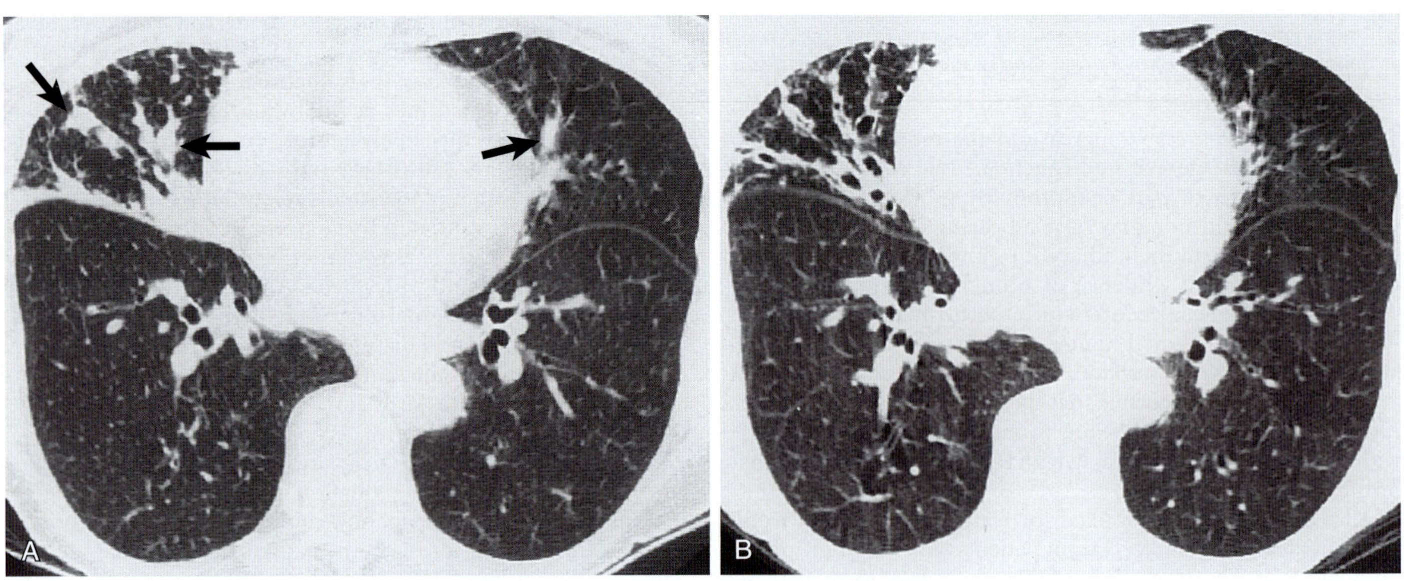

Fig. 57.9 Mucus-filled bronchi. (A) High-resolution CT image shows tubular and nodular *(arrows)* opacities in the right middle lobe and lingula. (B) High-resolution CT performed after expectoration of the mucus shows that the opacities represented ectatic bronchi filled with secretions. In this case, bronchiectasis was a result of previous tuberculosis. *(From Müller NL, Fraser RS, Colman NC, Paré PD.* Radiologic Diagnosis of Diseases of the Chest. *Philadelphia: WB Saunders; 2001.)*

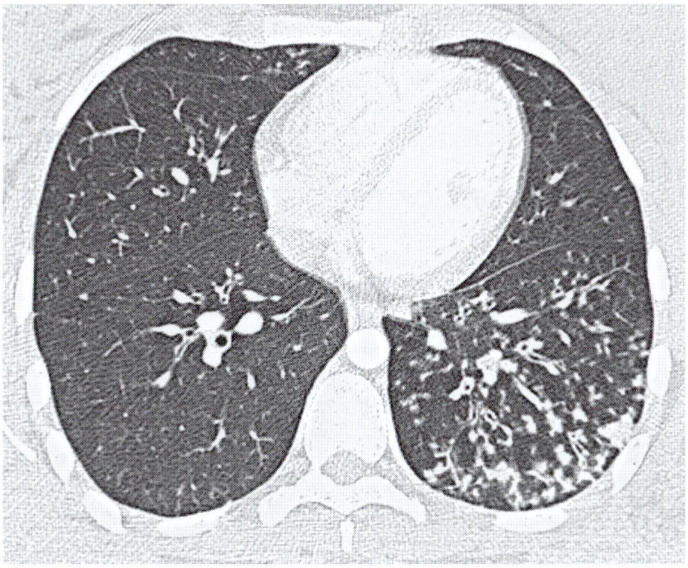

Fig. 57.10 Mucoid impaction in bronchiectasis. High-resolution CT image shows numerous V- and Y-shaped branching opacities and a tree-in-bud pattern in the left lower lobe.

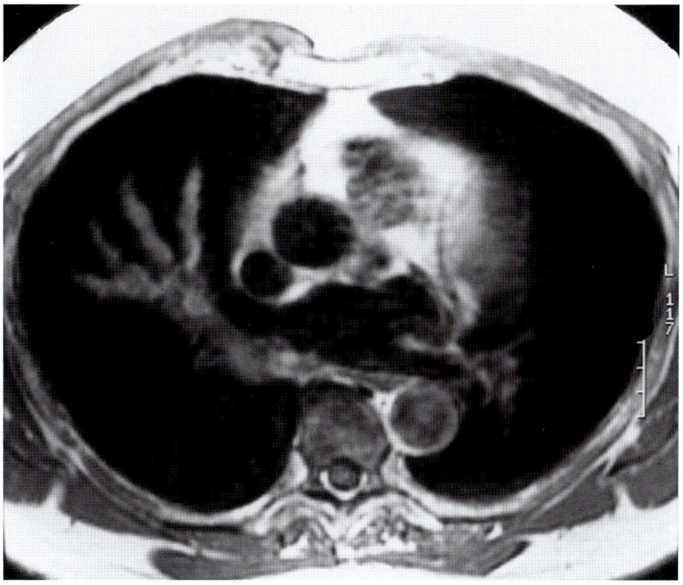

Fig. 57.12 Mucus-filled bronchi on MRI. T1-weighted MRI shows branching opacity in the right middle lobe consistent with mucoid impaction. Note mucus filling the bronchus intermedius.

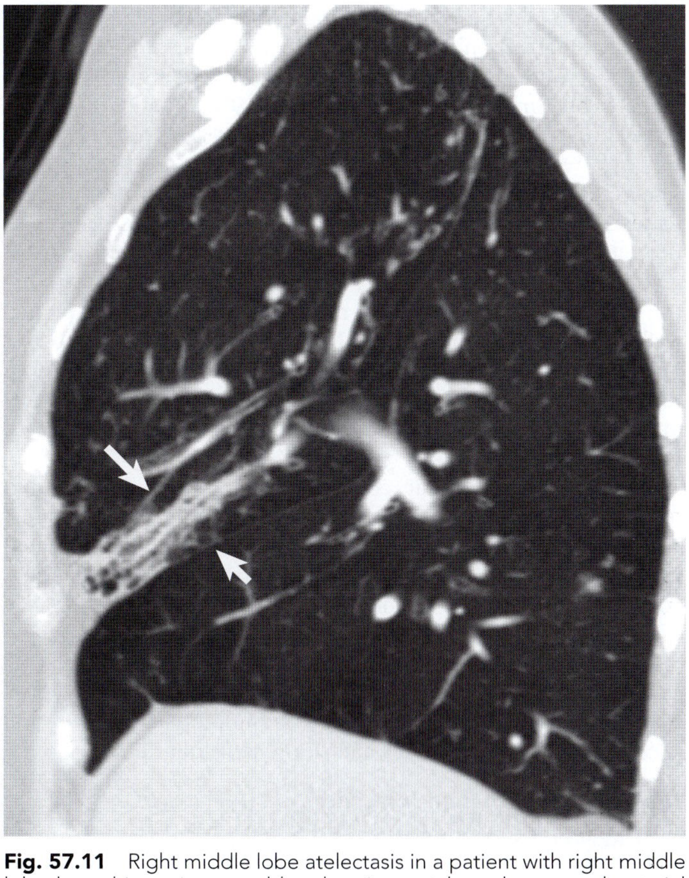

Fig. 57.11 Right middle lobe atelectasis in a patient with right middle lobe bronchiectasis caused by chronic nontuberculous mycobacterial infection. Sagittal CT image shows varicose bronchiectasis and volume loss of the right middle lobe. The minor fissure is displaced inferiorly and posteriorly *(long arrow)*, and the right major fissure is displaced anteriorly and superiorly *(short arrow)*.

particularly if they are severe. In practice, the experienced radiologist will take care to check adjacent sections; plainly, dilated airways will demonstrate continuity, whereas in diseases characterized by intrapulmonary cysts, such continuity will not be seen. Finally, mention must be made again of the term *traction bronchiectasis,* which is occasionally a source of confusion to physicians on radiologic reports (Fig. 57.13).[60] It seems likely that such dilatation of airways, a relatively common finding in patients with interstitial fibrosis, is due to the radial traction on the airways by thickened alveolar attachments in areas of fibrosis.[21,61,62] The important clinical point for the pulmonologist, of course, is that patients with this finding do not present with the clinical picture of patients with true bronchiectasis.

The craniocaudal and axial distribution of abnormalities may help narrow the differential diagnosis of a particular case of bronchiectasis. Bronchiectasis in cystic fibrosis is more common in the upper zones.[63–65] Similarly, allergic bronchopulmonary aspergillosis is generally regarded as a central and upper zonal disease,[66] whereas bronchiectasis that is related to aspiration, immunodeficiency, α1-antitrypsin deficiency, or iatrogenic causes appears to have a predilection for the lower zones. Finally, it might reasonably be expected that bronchiectasis occurring after pneumonia would be relatively localized, occurring in the area affected by the pneumonia. However, consideration of both imaging findings and clinical scenario may lead to a more accurate diagnosis than imaging alone.[67,68]

Specific Causes of Bronchiectasis

Cystic Fibrosis

ETIOLOGY, PREVALENCE, AND EPIDEMIOLOGY

Cystic fibrosis (CF) is an autosomal-recessive hereditary disease. It is the most common lethal genetically transmitted disease in white individuals; the estimated incidence is about 1 per 2000

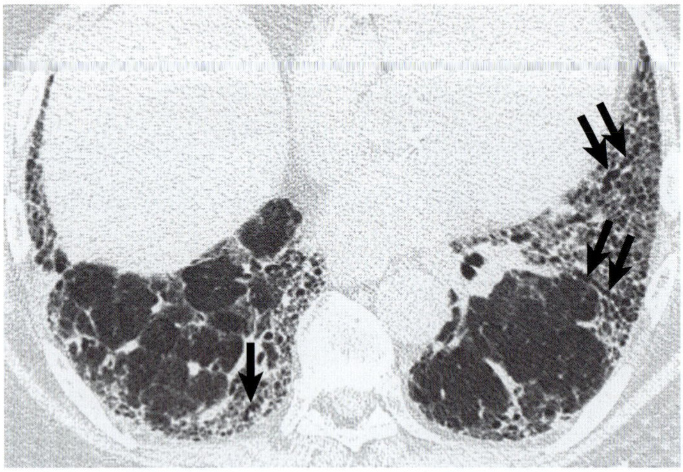

Fig. 57.13 Traction bronchiectasis and bronchiolectasis in idiopathic pulmonary fibrosis. High-resolution CT image shows peripheral predominant reticulation, architectural distortion, and honeycombing. Note associated dilatation and beading of bronchi and bronchioles (traction bronchiectasis and traction bronchiolectasis) *(arrows)*.

to 3500 live births.[69,70] CF is uncommon in nonwhites. There is no sex preponderance. The diagnosis is made before age 5 years in about 80% of cases, during adolescence in 10%,[71] and during adulthood in 10% of cases.[72] The fundamental abnormality consists of the production of abnormal secretions from exocrine glands, such as the salivary and sweat glands, and the pancreas, large bowel, and tracheobronchial tree. The major clinical manifestations are obstructive pulmonary disease, which is found in varying degrees of severity in almost all patients, and pancreatic insufficiency, present in 80% to 90%.[69,70] CF is the most common cause of pulmonary insufficiency in the first 3 decades of life.[73]

CLINICAL PRESENTATION

The pulmonary manifestations of CF include recurrent respiratory infections associated with productive cough, wheezing, and dyspnea. The infection is predominantly caused by bacteria, such as *Pseudomonas aeruginosa*, *Staphylococcus aureus*, and *Haemophilus influenzae*, although viruses, mycoplasma, and fungi are occasionally responsible. The presence of *Burkholderia cepacia* is usually associated with advanced disease.[72] Common complications include hemoptysis and pneumothorax. Most patients eventually progress to respiratory insufficiency accompanied by pulmonary arterial hypertension and cor pulmonale.

PATHOPHYSIOLOGY

Pathology

The earliest pathologic lesion of CF is obstruction of bronchioles and small bronchi by abnormal mucus, which is followed by airway inflammation and infection.[74] Pulmonary disease in patients with CF typically progresses from bronchiolitis and bronchitis to bronchiectasis owing to chronic infection and airway obstruction by the inspissated mucus.[70] Focal emphysema and bullae also can be seen. Histologic examination typically reveals chronic inflammation and fibrosis of the bronchial wall, partial or complete luminal occlusion by purulent material, focal epithelial ulceration, and cartilage destruction.[75]

Lung Function

Pulmonary function tests show progressive airway obstruction and air-trapping, with decreased forced expiratory volume at 1 second, increased vital capacity, and increased residual volume.[75]

MANIFESTATIONS OF THE DISEASE

Radiography

The earliest manifestations of CF consist of round or poorly defined linear opacities measuring 3 to 5 mm in diameter that are located within 2 to 3 cm of the pleura.[76] Less common early manifestations include thickened bronchial walls without bronchial dilation, usually seen as ring shadows, and mild hyperinflation.[76] Progression of disease is characterized by increases in bronchial diameter, bronchial wall thickness, lung volume, and number and size of peripheral nodular opacities and by the development of mucoid impaction and focal areas of consolidation (Figs. 57.14 and 57.15).[76] Bronchiectasis, bronchial wall thickening, and mucous plugging are particularly frequent and are evident in almost all adult patients.[77] The chest radiographic abnormalities have been incorporated into numerous semiquantitative scoring schemes that are believed to be of value in predicting prognosis and directing therapy.[78,79]

Recurrent foci of consolidation occur in most patients, and lobar or segmental atelectasis occurs in many. Hilar enlargement may be due to lymph node enlargement or dilation of the central pulmonary arteries secondary to pulmonary arterial hypertension (see Fig. 57.15).[79] Pneumothorax occurs in 3% to 19% of patients.[70,80]

Computed Tomography

The main manifestation of CF is bronchiectasis, which is present in virtually all adult patients (Fig. 57.16; see Fig. 57.14).[81–83] Bronchiectasis usually involves all lobes but tends to be most severe in the upper lobes.[82,84] The bronchiectasis may be cylindrical, varicose, or cystic.[81] Other common findings are bronchial wall thickening, peribronchial interstitial thickening, and mucous plugging.[81,83] Consolidation or atelectasis can be seen in 80% of cases.[81] Cystic or bullous lung lesions also can be seen and typically predominate in the subpleural regions of the upper lobes (see Fig. 57.16).[81]

Branching or nodular centrilobular opacities (tree-in-bud pattern) are frequently present and may be an early sign of disease.[85] They reflect the presence of bronchiolar dilation with associated mucous impaction, infection, or peribronchiolar inflammation. Focal areas of decreased attenuation and vascularity on inspiratory CT and air-trapping on expiratory CT are common.

Hilar or mediastinal lymph node enlargement and pleural abnormalities may be present, largely reflecting chronic infection. Pulmonary artery dilation resulting from pulmonary hypertension is common in patients who have long-standing disease.

Magnetic Resonance Imaging

MRI may be used as an alternative tool to assess parenchymal and functional abnormalities and to monitor treatment in patients with CF. Although MRI has lower spatial resolution than CT and plays a limited role in the assessment of airway disease, it has the advantage of no radiation exposure, an important consideration in these young patients. MRI may be useful in the follow-up of patients with CF (Fig. 57.17) and could be used to screen for early liver disease, given the increased life expectancy of CF patients in recent years.

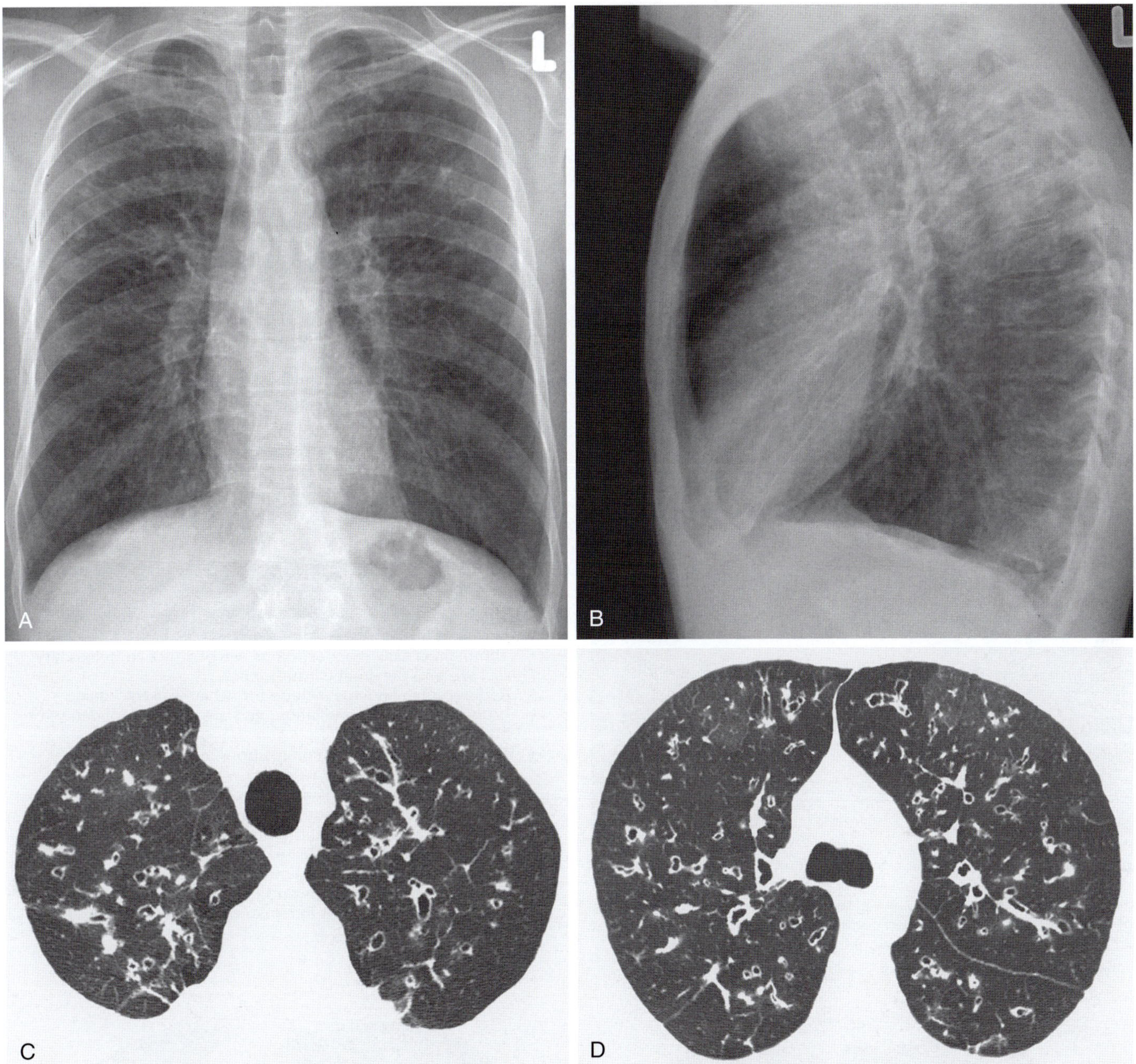

Fig. 57.14 Cystic fibrosis, radiographic and high-resolution CT findings. Posteroanterior (A) and lateral (B) chest radiographs show poorly defined nodular and linear opacities mainly in the upper lobes. Mild hyperinflation with increase in the retrosternal airspace is noted. High-resolution CT scans at the level of the lung apices (C) and tracheal carina (D) show extensive bilateral bronchiectasis and areas of decreased attenuation and vascularity (mosaic attenuation).

Imaging Algorithms

The chest radiograph is the main imaging modality used in the initial evaluation and follow-up of patients with CF. High-resolution CT can show abnormalities in patients who have early CF and normal chest radiographs. In one study of 38 patients who had mild CF with normal pulmonary function, chest radiographs were normal in 17 (45%), showed mild bronchial wall thickening in 17, and showed mild bronchiectasis in 4 (10%).[86] On high-resolution CT in this group, bronchiectasis was present in 77% of all patients and in 65% of patients with normal chest radiographs; only 3 patients had a normal high-resolution CT scan.[86]

When performing repeated high-resolution CT scans in young patients, the risk of radiation has to be considered and the radiation dose minimized. Axial high-resolution chest CT with interspace gaps can be performed at a much lower dose than volumetric scans. When volumetric CT is required, it is recommended that this be performed with low milliamperage (40 mA) and low kilovoltage.

DIFFERENTIAL DIAGNOSIS

The radiologic findings of CF may mimic those of other causes of bronchiectasis, such as allergic bronchopulmonary aspergillosis and postinfectious bronchiectasis. The most characteristic features of bronchiectasis in CF are bilateral symmetric distribution and upper lobe predominance. In one study, bronchiectasis in CF involved mainly the upper lobes in 79% of patients and was usually bilateral and fairly symmetric, whereas the bronchiectasis in the other conditions, such as prior tuberculosis, was most frequently unilateral or asymmetric.[84]

Although the diagnosis of CF may be suggested by a positive family history, persistent respiratory disease, clinical evidence of pancreatic insufficiency, or fatty (or less common cystic) replacement of the pancreas on imaging, confirmation requires a positive sweat test or identification of two abnormal copies of the CF gene. Incorporation of molecular biologic techniques into rapid, cost-efficient, and specific diagnostic tests for most CF genotypes is now possible by using the multiplex polymerase chain reaction.[87]

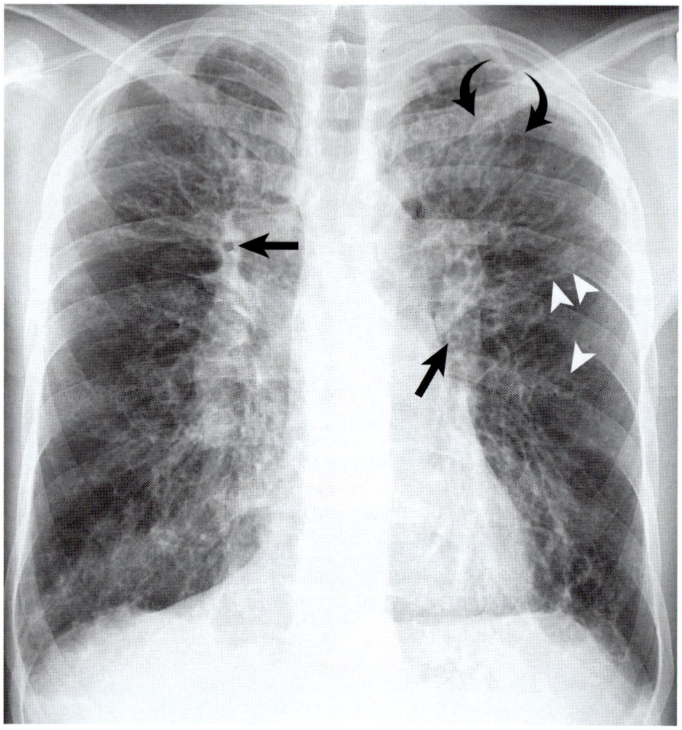

Fig. 57.15 Cystic fibrosis, radiographic findings. Posteroanterior chest radiograph shows marked bronchial wall thickening *(straight arrows)* and extensive varicose *(arrowheads)* and cystic *(curved arrows)* bronchiectasis. Note hyperinflation and enlarged central pulmonary arteries consistent with pulmonary arterial hypertension.

SYNOPSIS OF TREATMENT OPTIONS

Therapy typically includes antibiotics, physiotherapy, and replacement of pancreatic enzymes. Once a disease with a life expectancy confined to the adolescent years, now most patients reach adulthood. The median survival of CF patients has increased significantly over the past few decades to almost 41 years in the United States and approximately 51 years in Canada.[88]

KEY POINTS: CYSTIC FIBROSIS

- The estimated incidence is 1 per 2000–3500 live births in whites; it is uncommon in nonwhites.
- The main clinical manifestations are obstructive pulmonary disease and pancreatic insufficiency.
- Radiographic findings include bronchial wall thickening, bronchiectasis, hyperinflation, and areas of consolidation or atelectasis.
- The main CT manifestation is upper lobe–predominant bronchiectasis.
- Other common findings are bronchial wall thickening, peribronchial interstitial thickening, mucous plugging, branching or nodular centrilobular opacities (tree-in-bud pattern), focal areas of decreased attenuation and vascularity on inspiratory CT, and expiratory air-trapping.
- Judicious use of CT scans and certain CT dose-reduction techniques is important in minimizing radiation exposure in CF patients.

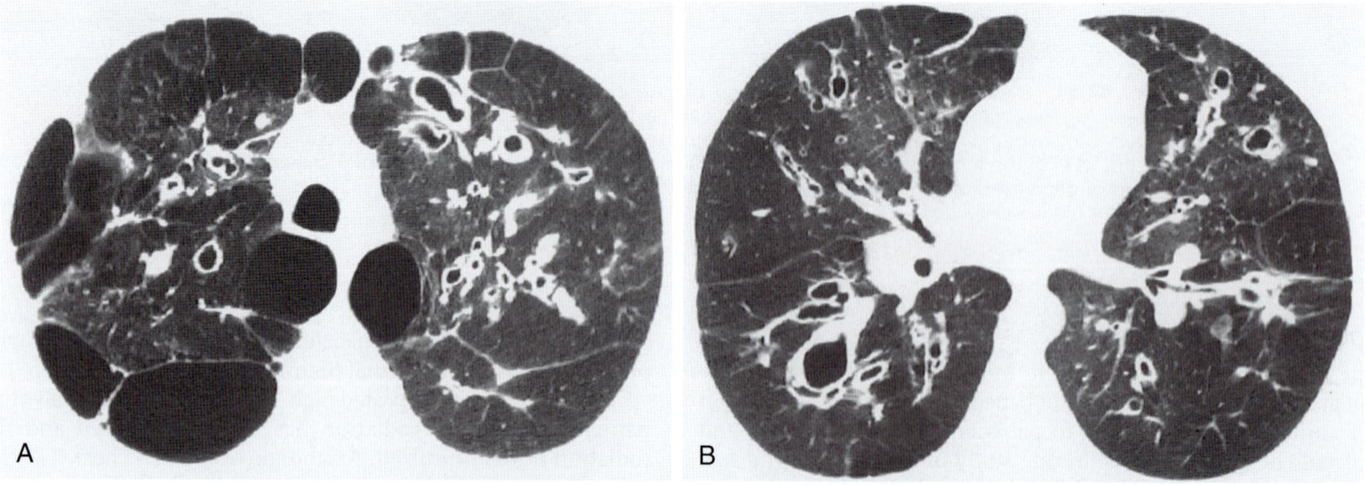

Fig. 57.16 Cystic fibrosis, high-resolution CT findings. (A) High-resolution CT scan at the level of the lung apices shows extensive bronchiectasis and bullous changes. (B) High-resolution CT scan at the level of the inferior pulmonary veins shows bilateral varicose and cystic bronchiectasis and areas of decreased attenuation and vascularity.

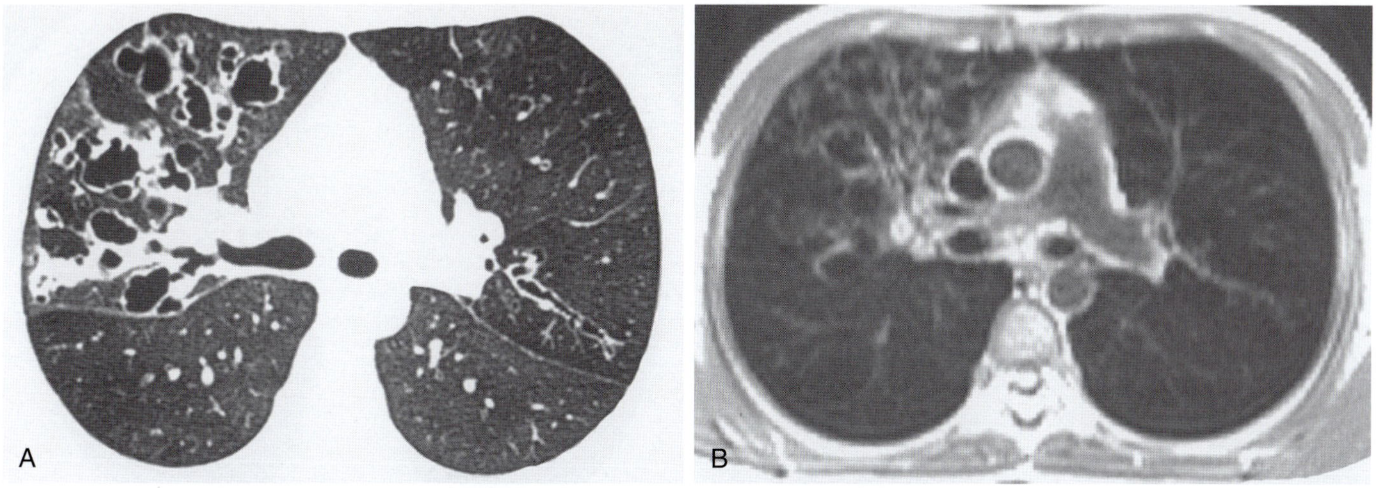

Fig. 57.17 Cystic fibrosis. Comparison between high-resolution CT and MRI findings in a child. (A) High-resolution CT scan shows right upper lobe cystic and varicose bronchiectasis. Cylindrical and varicose bronchiectasis is evident in the left upper lobe. Note mosaic lung attenuation. (B) T1-weighted MR image obtained at a similar level as in (A) shows bronchiectasis in the right upper lobe. Milder areas of bronchiectasis in the left upper lobe and findings of small airway disease are not apparent on the MR image. *(Courtesy Dr. Pedro Daltro, Clínica de Diagnóstico Por Imagem, Rio de Janeiro, Brazil.)*

Primary Ciliary Dyskinesia (Dyskinetic Cilia Syndrome)

ETIOLOGY, PREVALENCE, AND EPIDEMIOLOGY

The term *primary ciliary dyskinesia* refers to a group of autosomal-recessive disorders associated with defective ciliary structure and function, also known as dyskinetic cilia syndrome.[89] The structurally abnormal cilia move ineffectively and predispose to sinusitis, recurrent pulmonary infections, and bronchiectasis. Situs inversus totalis or, less commonly, heterotaxy syndrome is seen in about 50% and 12% of patients, respectively.[90–92] Men have reduced fertility as a result of decreased motility of the spermatozoa.[90,91] Although primary ciliary dyskinesia has an autosomal-recessive pattern of inheritance, the variety of ultrastructural defects associated with the clinical syndrome suggests considerable genetic heterogeneity.[93,94] The incidence of the syndrome in white individuals is estimated to be 1 in 12,500 to 40,000; a higher prevalence has been reported in Japan.[95,96]

CLINICAL PRESENTATION

The age of presentation ranges from 4 months to 51 years.[97,98] The clinical manifestations include infertility, chronic rhinitis, sinusitis, otitis, and recurrent lower respiratory tract infections. The most common bacterial organism found in sputum is *H. influenzae*, but *Pseudomonas* isolates also are common.[89] Half of patients have Kartagener syndrome, defined by the triad of situs inversus totalis, bronchiectasis, and either nasal polyps or recurrent sinusitis.[89] Morbidity in primary ciliary dyskinesia is predominantly related to chronic suppurative airway disease secondary to chronic infection.

PATHOPHYSIOLOGY

Pathology

Ultrastructural abnormalities in primary ciliary dyskinesia seen on electron microscopy include a lack of outer dynein arms, absent or short radial spokes, absent or defective inner dynein arms, absent or disoriented central microtubules, and transposition of peripheral microtubules.[99,100] A combination of structural defects is often present.[101]

Lung Function

Many patients develop mild to moderate airflow obstruction.[102]

MANIFESTATIONS OF THE DISEASE

Radiography

Radiographically, abnormalities progress from bronchial wall thickening to bronchiectasis, hyperinflation, segmental atelectasis, and consolidation.[103] In one study of 30 patients ranging from newborn to 26 years old, radiographic abnormalities were evident in all patients.[103] Findings usually have a lower zone distribution, but radiologic features may resemble the features of bronchiectasis from a variety of other causes; when present, the combination of lower zone–predominant bronchiectasis and situs inversus is nearly pathognomonic for the diagnosis (Fig. 57.18).

Computed Tomography

High-resolution CT typically shows extensive central or diffuse bilateral bronchiectasis in adults (Fig. 57.19).[92] Associated endobronchial mucous plugging, tree-in-bud opacities, and centrilobular nodules are common. Although bronchiectasis can be widespread, in approximately 50% of patients, it involves predominantly or exclusively the lower lobes.[104] In pediatric patients, high-resolution CT shows bronchiectasis in 56% of patients.[92] Pectus excavatum is seen in 9% of patients.[92]

DIFFERENTIAL DIAGNOSIS

The diagnosis of primary ciliary dyskinesia usually is made by assessing ciliary motility in bronchial wall or nasal biopsy specimens or in semen samples or by electron microscopy that shows abnormal ciliary morphology.[89,90]

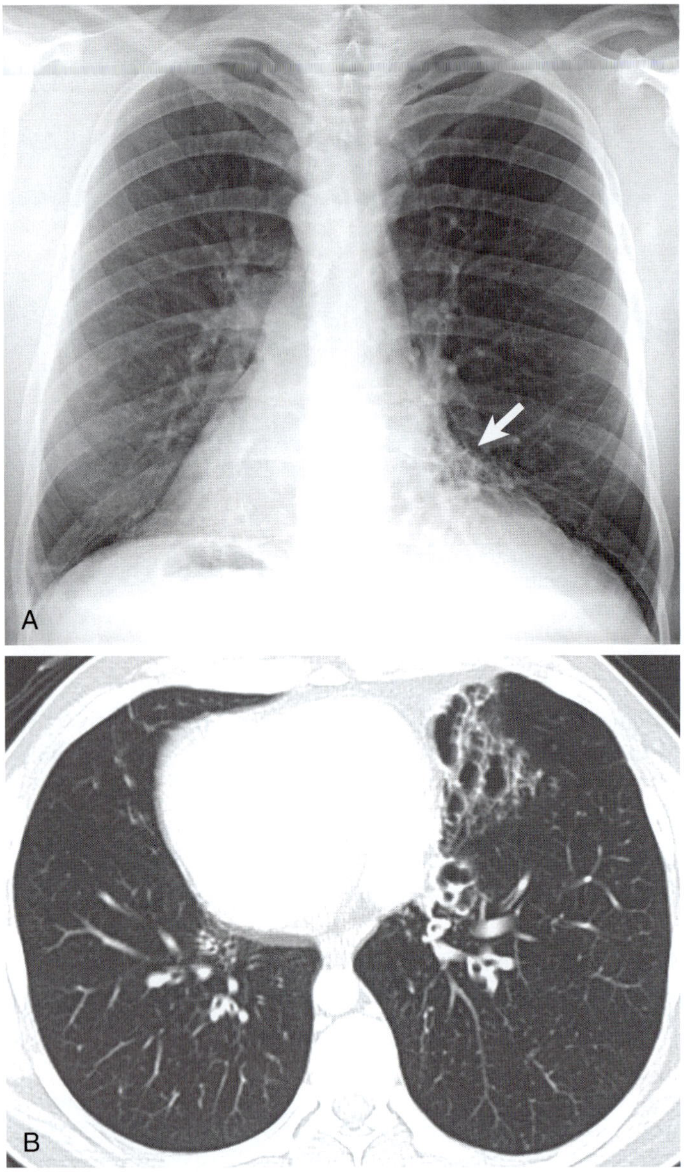

Fig. 57.18 Kartagener syndrome. (A) Posteroanterior chest radiograph shows situs inversus totalis, bronchial wall thickening, and bronchiectasis in the left middle lobe *(arrow)*. (B) CT image through the lower lungs in the same patient shows bronchial wall thickening and cystic and varicoid bronchiectasis, particularly within the left middle lobe.

SYNOPSIS OF TREATMENT OPTIONS

Treatment consists mainly of antibiotics and physiotherapy.[97] Patients usually have a normal life expectancy.[97]

KEY POINTS: PRIMARY CILIARY DYSKINESIA

- Primary ciliary dyskinesia refers to a group of autosomal-recessive disorders associated with defective ciliary structure and function.
- The clinical manifestations include chronic rhinitis, sinusitis, otitis, recurrent lower respiratory tract infections, and infertility.
- Approximately 50% of patients have situs inversus totalis, and 12% have heterotaxy syndrome.
- Radiographic and CT findings include bronchiectasis, bronchial wall thickening, hyperinflation, tree-in-bud opacities, segmental atelectasis, and consolidation.

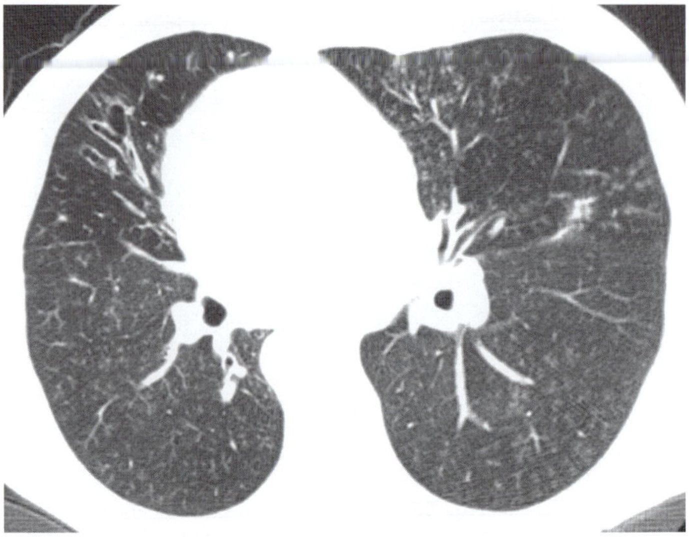

Fig. 57.19 Kartagener syndrome. CT image shows bronchial wall thickening and scattered tree-in-bud opacities bilaterally. Note right lingular cylindrical bronchiectasis.

Allergic Bronchopulmonary Aspergillosis

ETIOLOGY, PREVALENCE, AND EPIDEMIOLOGY

Allergic bronchopulmonary aspergillosis (ABPA) is a condition characterized by chronic airway inflammation and airway damage resulting from persistent colonization and sensitization by *Aspergillus fumigatus* and related species.[105] ABPA is seen almost exclusively in patients with asthma or CF. The estimated prevalence ranges from 2% to 25% in patients with CF and from 1% to 8% in patients with asthma.[106] The pathogenesis of ABPA is unclear, but it is believed that genetic factors and T-cell reactivity to *Aspergillus* play important roles.[105,106]

CLINICAL PRESENTATION

ABPA is frequently first suspected clinically by the presence of peripheral blood eosinophilia and pulmonary opacities in patients who have asthma or CF.[106] The patients may be asymptomatic or present with worsening of asthma, increased cough and wheezing, and expectoration of brown mucous plugs.[106] Physical examination in ABPA is often normal, except for underlying manifestations of asthma or CF.

PATHOPHYSIOLOGY

Pathology

At histology, segmental and proximal subsegmental bronchi are dilated and distended with mucus that contains numerous eosinophils; cell debris consisting of degenerate eosinophils with associated Charcot-Leyden crystals; and scattered, typically fragmented fungal hyphae.[107,108]

MANIFESTATIONS OF THE DISEASE

Radiography

The typical radiographic pattern consists of homogeneous branching opacities, usually involving the upper lobes and almost always in the central segmental bronchi, rather than peripheral

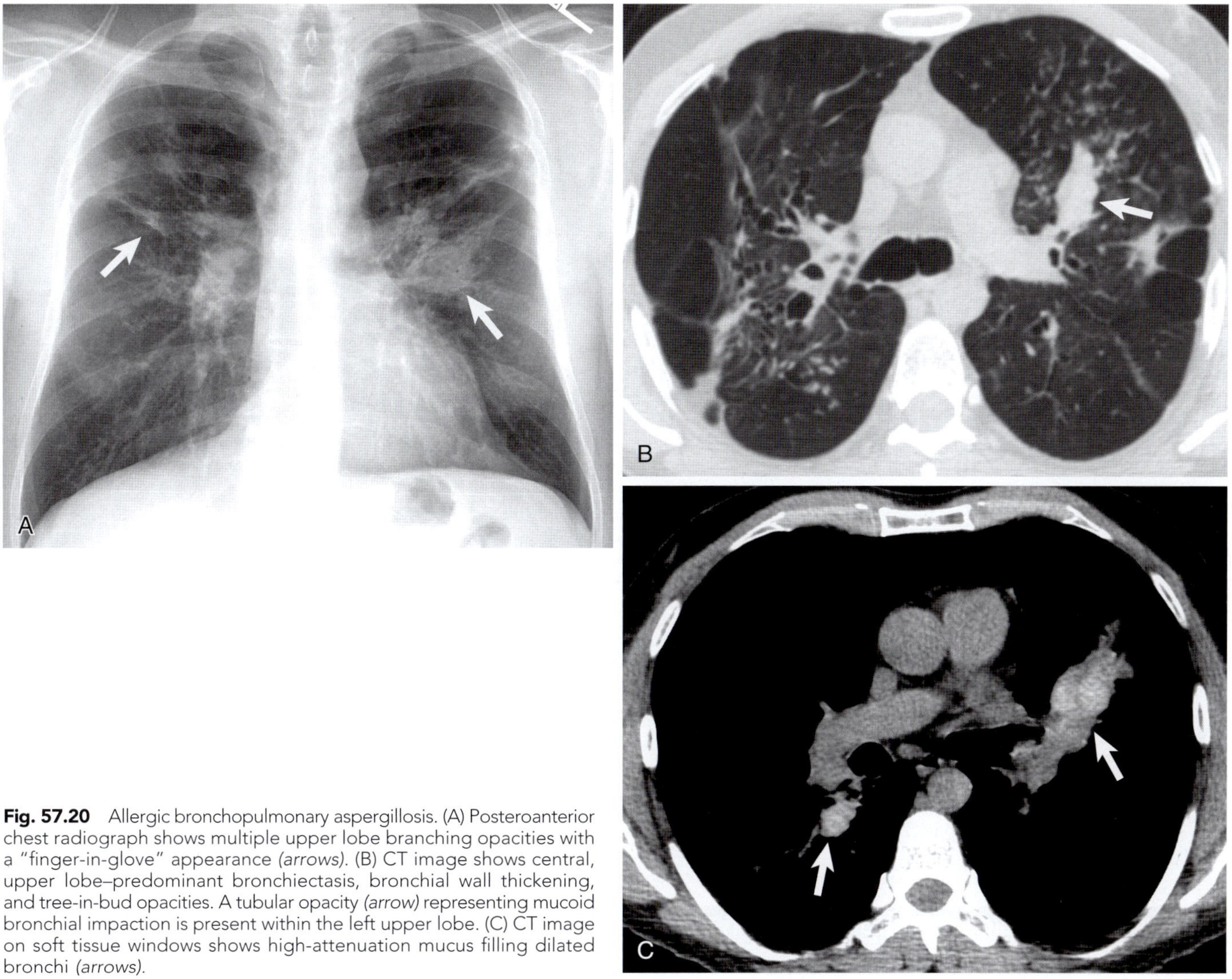

Fig. 57.20 Allergic bronchopulmonary aspergillosis. (A) Posteroanterior chest radiograph shows multiple upper lobe branching opacities with a "finger-in-glove" appearance *(arrows)*. (B) CT image shows central, upper lobe–predominant bronchiectasis, bronchial wall thickening, and tree-in-bud opacities. A tubular opacity *(arrow)* representing mucoid bronchial impaction is present within the left upper lobe. (C) CT image on soft tissue windows shows high-attenuation mucus filling dilated bronchi *(arrows)*.

branches.[109] These bifurcating opacities have been described as having a gloved-finger, an inverted Y or V, or a cluster-of-grapes appearance (Fig. 57.20). The opacities tend to be transient, but they may persist unchanged for weeks or months or may enlarge.

Computed Tomography

The characteristic CT manifestations of ABPA consist of bronchiectasis and mucoid impaction involving mainly the segmental and subsegmental bronchi of the upper lobes (Fig. 57.21; see also Fig. 57.20).[110–112] Other common findings include centrilobular nodules and a tree-in-bud pattern; the latter reflects the presence of dilated bronchioles filled with mucus (see Fig. 57.20).[108] In approximately 30% of patients, the mucous plugs have high attenuation, presumably because of the presence of calcium salts (see Fig. 73.20), which is highly specific for the diagnosis.[113]

Although bronchiectasis and mucoid impaction tend to be bilateral and involve mainly the central regions of the upper lobes, they may be unilateral, be patchy, or involve mainly the lower lobes.[104]

Because ABPA occurs almost exclusively in asthmatics, the presence of central bronchiectasis and mucoid impaction in these patients is highly suggestive of the diagnosis. Patients with asthma have an increased prevalence of bronchiectasis, however, and may have filling of the ectatic bronchi with secretions without having ABPA. In one study the authors retrospectively assessed the accuracy of CT in the diagnosis of ABPA in asthmatic patients; bronchiectasis, centrilobular nodules, and mucoid impaction were all more common in ABPA than in patients with asthma alone.[112] As noted by others, patients who had ABPA consistently had more severe and extensive disease compared with asthmatics, especially when present in three or more lobes.[112]

DIFFERENTIAL DIAGNOSIS

Diagnostic criteria include the presence of underlying asthma or CF, peripheral blood eosinophilia, immediate cutaneous reactivity to *A. fumigatus* antigen, precipitation antibodies against *A. fumigatus* antigen, elevated total serum immunoglobulin E levels, and radiographic or CT findings of central bronchiectasis or mucous impaction.[106] Confidence in diagnosis depends on the numbers and types of abnormalities that are identified and the presence of characteristic histologic findings on specimens obtained by bronchoscopy and positive sputum culture for *Aspergillus* species.[114]

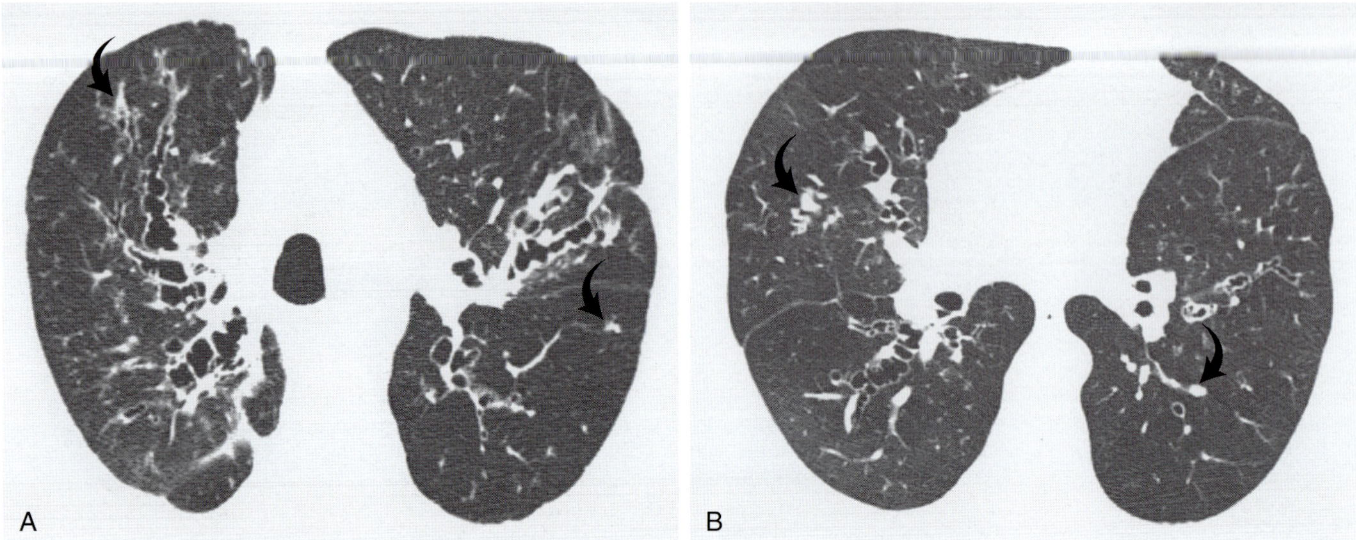

Fig. 57.21 Allergic bronchopulmonary aspergillosis in an asthmatic. (A) High-resolution CT scan through the upper lobes shows severe bilateral bronchiectasis and marked bronchial wall thickening. Mucoid impaction *(arrows)* is noted. (B) High-resolution CT scan at the level of the lower lobe bronchi shows central bronchiectasis, areas of decreased attenuation and vascularity, and mucoid impaction *(arrows)*. *(From Silva CI, Colby TV, Müller NL. Asthma and associated conditions: high-resolution CT and pathologic findings.* AJR Am J Roentgenol. *2004;183:817–824.)*

SYNOPSIS OF TREATMENT OPTIONS

Treatment includes optimal therapy of the underlying asthma or CF and oral corticosteroids.[106] Antifungal agents, such as itraconazole, may be helpful in some patients but are not curative.[106]

KEY POINTS: ALLERGIC BRONCHOPULMONARY ASPERGILLOSIS

- Allergic bronchopulmonary aspergillosis is frequently first suspected clinically by the presence of peripheral blood eosinophilia and pulmonary opacities in patients who have asthma or cystic fibrosis.
- The typical radiographic pattern consists of homogeneous branching gloved-finger opacities.
- The characteristic CT manifestations consist of bronchiectasis and mucoid impaction involving mainly the segmental and subsegmental bronchi of the upper lobes.
- In about 30% of patients, the mucoid impaction has high attenuation on CT.

Tracheobronchomegaly (Mounier-Kuhn Syndrome)

ETIOLOGY, PREVALENCE, AND EPIDEMIOLOGY

Tracheobronchomegaly (Mounier-Kuhn syndrome) is a rare condition characterized by dilation of the tracheobronchial tree that tends to involve the trachea and main bronchi[115] but that may extend from the larynx to the periphery of the lungs (see Chapter 56).[116] Tracheobronchomegaly is more common in men, and most cases are congenital.[115] It has been described in association with other congenital abnormalities of the trachea, Ehlers-Danlos syndrome, and cutis laxa.[115] An acquired form of the condition has been reported as a complication of diffuse pulmonary fibrosis,[117] in association with ankylosing spondylitis,[118] and, occasionally, in rheumatoid arthritis.[119] Most patients are in their third or fourth decade of life at diagnosis (age range, 18 months to 76 years).[120]

CLINICAL PRESENTATION

The increased compliance of the trachea in tracheobronchomegaly results in abnormal flaccidity and easy collapsibility during forced expiration and coughing. The inefficient cough mechanism leads to retention of mucus with resultant recurrent pneumonia and bronchiectasis.[121]

PATHOPHYSIOLOGY

Pathology

The pathologic features consist of marked dilation of the trachea and main bronchi owing to absence of the longitudinal elastic fibers and thinning of the muscular layer of the airway walls.[115,122] Most patients have mucosal herniation between the tracheal rings resulting in tracheal diverticulosis.[122] Other common findings are bronchiectasis and emphysema. Dynamic imaging of the airways shows marked ballooning of the trachea and main bronchi on inspiration and collapse on expiration.[115] This renders the cough mechanism ineffective and, together with the retention of secretions, predisposes to recurrent infection.

MANIFESTATIONS OF THE DISEASE

Radiography

The calibers of the trachea and major bronchi are increased, and the air columns have an irregular corrugated appearance caused by the protrusion of mucosal and submucosal tissue between the cartilaginous rings, an appearance that has been termed

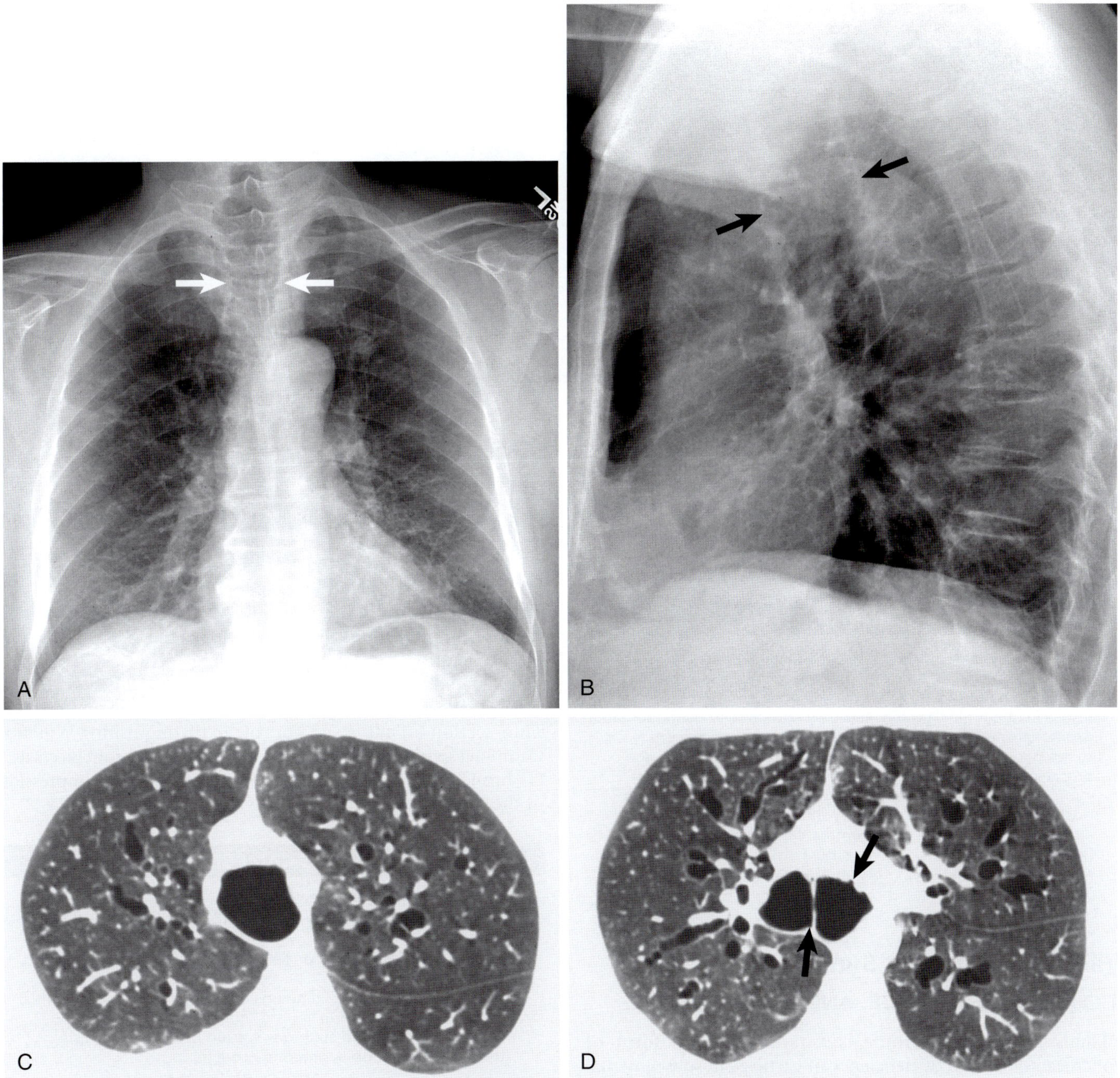

Fig. 57.22 Tracheobronchomegaly (Mounier-Kuhn syndrome): radiographic and CT findings. Posteroanterior (A) and lateral (B) chest radiographs show a marked increase in the caliber of the trachea *(arrows)* and main bronchi. High-resolution CT scans of another patient at the level of the trachea (C) and main bronchi (D) show tracheomegaly and increased caliber of main bronchi and intraparenchymal bronchi. The dilated intraparenchymal bronchi have thin walls, which is distinct from the bronchial wall thickening typically seen in patients who have bronchiectasis. Minimal bilateral bronchial diverticulosis is present (D, *arrows*).

tracheal diverticulosis (Fig. 57.22).[115] This appearance often is visualized best in lateral projection. In women the upper limits of normal of transverse and sagittal diameters of the trachea are 21 mm and 23 mm, respectively, and 19.8 mm and 17.4 mm for the right and left mainstem bronchi, respectively.[115] In men these measurements are 25 mm and 27 mm for the transverse and sagittal tracheal diameters, respectively, and 21.1 mm and 18.4 mm for the right and left mainstem bronchi, respectively; patients with tracheobronchomegaly usually have tracheal and main bronchial diameters significantly exceeding these upper limits.[115]

Computed Tomography

The tracheal and bronchial dilation is well seen on CT (see Fig. 57.22).[116,123] CT also frequently reveals dilation of the intrapulmonary bronchi (see Fig. 57.22).[116,124] As distinct from patients with other causes of bronchiectasis, the dilated bronchi

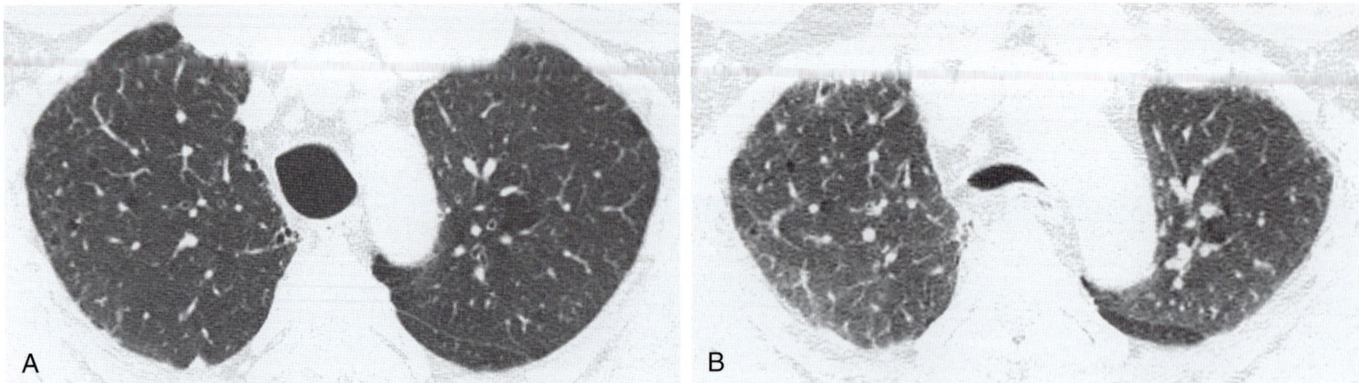

Fig. 57.23 Tracheomegaly: collapse on expiration. (A) Inspiratory CT scan shows an increased caliber of the trachea. Incidental note is made of mild emphysema. (B) Expiratory CT shows abnormal reduction in caliber with "frown" configuration typical of tracheomalacia.

of patients who have tracheobronchomegaly typically have thin walls.[116] Dynamic CT and expiratory CT show ballooning of the airways on inspiration and collapse on expiration typical of tracheobronchomalacia (Fig. 57.23).

KEY POINTS: TRACHEOBRONCHOMEGALY (MOUNIER-KUHN SYNDROME)

- Tracheobronchomegaly is a rare congenital abnormality characterized by marked dilation of the trachea and bronchi. The increased compliance of the trachea in tracheobronchomegaly results in abnormal flaccidity and easy collapsibility during forced expiration and coughing. The inefficient cough mechanism leads to retention of mucus with resultant recurrent pneumonia and bronchiectasis.
- Typically there is an irregular corrugated appearance of the posterior tracheal wall caused by the protrusion of mucosal and submucosal tissue between the cartilaginous rings (tracheal diverticulosis), which is best visualized on the lateral radiograph or sagittal CT reformatted images.

Williams-Campbell Syndrome

ETIOLOGY, PREVALENCE, AND EPIDEMIOLOGY

Williams-Campbell syndrome is a rare congenital form of bronchiectasis caused by deficiency of cartilage in subsegmental bronchi.[125] The condition shows familial clustering and may be associated with other congenital abnormalities.[126] Affected individuals usually are identified in infancy because of repeated chest infections and evidence of bronchiectasis. Occasionally, Williams-Campbell syndrome is first recognized in an adult.[127]

CLINICAL PRESENTATION

The clinical manifestations consist of repeated chest infections since early childhood.

PATHOPHYSIOLOGY

Pathology

Pathologic examination of the lungs in an adult who underwent bilateral lung transplantation showed absence of cartilage in the walls of the medium to small airways, resulting in cystic bronchiectasis.[125]

MANIFESTATIONS OF THE DISEASE

Radiography

The radiographic findings include bronchial wall thickening and cystic spaces (Fig. 57.24).

Computed Tomography

The thin-section CT findings are characteristic and consist of varicose and cystic bronchiectasis limited to the fourth-generation, fifth-generation, and sixth-generation bronchi (i.e., distal to the first-generation segmental bronchi) (see Fig. 57.24).[127–129] Expiratory CT shows collapse of the bronchi and distal air-trapping.[127,130] Thin-section CT plays a major role in distinguishing Williams-Campbell syndrome from other causes of cystic bronchiectasis.[131] CT bronchoscopy shows absence of the cartilage ring impressions in the bronchial wall consistent with cartilage deficiency.[130]

KEY POINTS: WILLIAMS-CAMPBELL SYNDROME

- Williams-Campbell syndrome is a rare congenital form of bronchiectasis caused by a deficiency of cartilage in the subsegmental bronchi.
- Clinical manifestations consist of repeated chest infections since early childhood.
- The high-resolution CT findings are characteristic and consist of cystic bronchiectasis limited to the fourth-generation, fifth-generation, and sixth-generation bronchi (i.e., distal to the first-generation segmental bronchi).

SYNOPSIS OF TREATMENT OPTIONS

Medical

The treatment of the specific cause of bronchiectasis, when it is identifiable (e.g., immunoglobulin replacement in patients with immunoglobulin deficiencies, recombinant human deoxyribonuclease in cystic fibrosis), may be important. Associated conditions, such as chronic rhinosinusitis, are treated.

The mainstays of therapy, when a definite underlying cause cannot be established, include effective clearance of airway secretions (physiotherapy and mucolytics) and vigorous treatment of exacerbations caused by infection.

Surgical

Surgery for bronchiectasis is essentially restricted to patients with troublesome symptoms that are refractory to conventional medical therapy and then only to those with localized (single-lobe) disease.

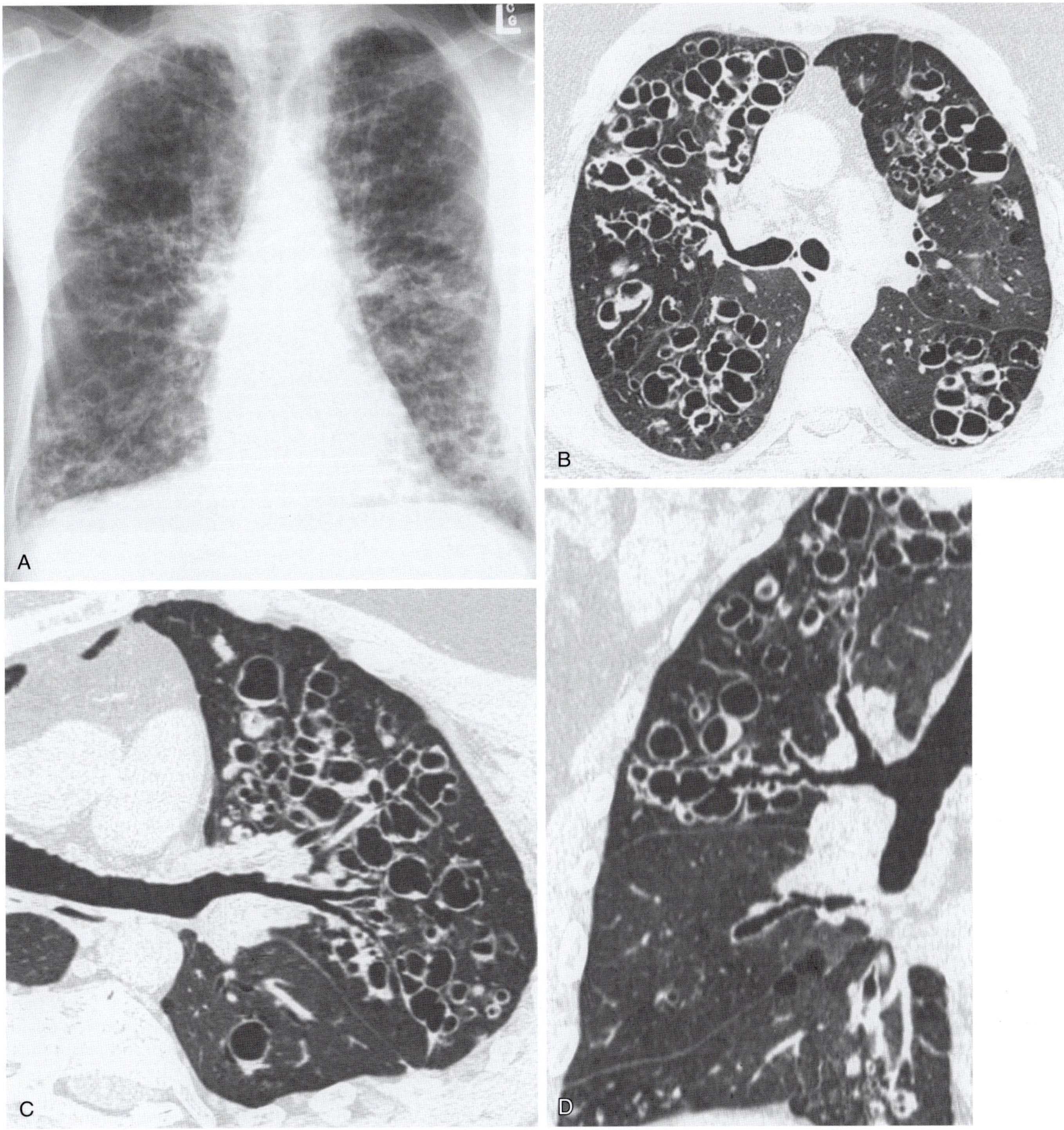

Fig. 57.24 Williams-Campbell syndrome. (A) Chest radiograph shows multiple bilateral thin-walled cysts and pulmonary hyperinflation. (B) High-resolution CT scan shows extensive cystic bronchiectasis. Several ectatic bronchi contain fluid levels. Anterior segmental bronchus of right upper lobe is normal, and bronchiectasis starts at subsegmental bronchi (fourth-sixth order). Curved axial reformation (C) of left lung and coronal reformation (D) of right lung show typical distribution of bronchiectasis distal to the segmental bronchi.

Broncholithiasis

Etiology

Broncholithiasis is a disorder characterized by either the presence of calcified or ossified material within the lumen of bronchi or the distortion of the tracheobronchial tree by calcified peribronchial nodes but without obvious erosion into the lumen. In most cases the finding of broncholiths is due to the extrusion of calcified material from adjacent lymph nodes and erosion into the airways; the calcification in lymph nodes is usually the consequence of chronic necrotizing granulomatous infection, including tuberculosis, histoplasmosis, and rarely actinomycosis.[132–137] In

KEY POINTS: BRONCHIECTASIS

- The true prevalence of bronchiectasis is difficult to predict, but it is known to be higher in specific populations.
- Plethora of causes: Postinfectious bronchiectasis remains a major etiologic factor in developing countries, whereas cystic fibrosis and hypogammaglobulinemia are important causes in Western nations. There is no identifiable cause of bronchiectasis in a significant proportion of patients.
- Clinical features include productive cough, recurrent infection, breathlessness, and intermittent hemoptysis.
- High-resolution CT is the optimal test for diagnosis as radiography is insensitive. The cardinal CT sign is bronchial dilatation.
  - Specific findings: bronchoarterial diameter ratio >1 (highly sensitive but limited specificity), lack of bronchial tapering, bronchus visualized within 1 cm of costal pleura or abutting the mediastinal pleura.
  - Important ancillary CT findings include bronchial wall thickening, mosaic attenuation, airway plugging, and volume loss.

occasional patients the luminal calcification is secondary to the calcification of a foreign body or the migration of calcific material from a more distant source (e.g., a calcified pleural plaque) through a fistulous communication. A rare association with silicosis has also been reported.[138]

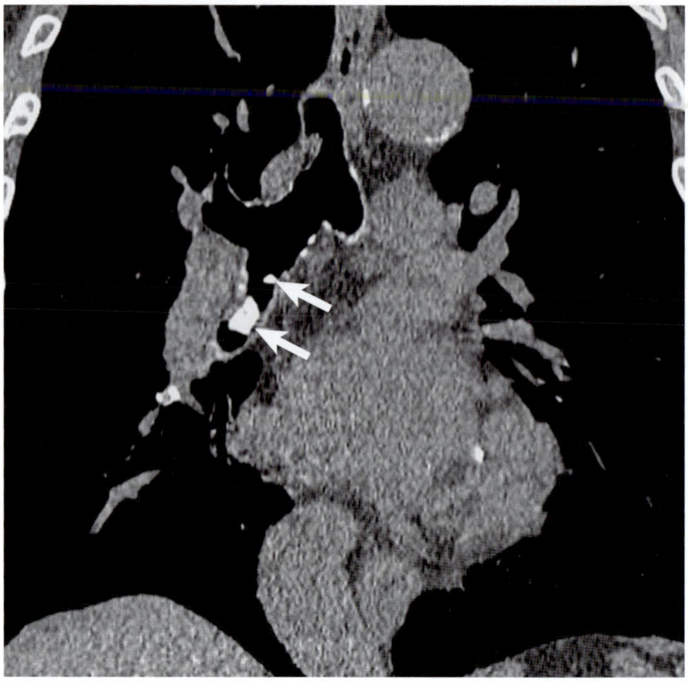

Fig. 57.25 Broncholithiasis from prior tuberculosis. A coronal reformatted image in the soft tissue window demonstrates calcified nodules *(arrows)* in the bronchus intermedius compatible with broncholiths.

Prevalence and Epidemiology

Despite the relatively widespread worldwide prevalence of granulomatous infections, broncholithiasis remains a rare entity. The peak incidence is in the sixth decade, although there is a broad overall age range. There is no gender predilection.

Clinical Presentation

The common symptoms of broncholithiasis are hemoptysis, which in rare instances might be catastrophic, and cough, which is usually nonproductive.[139,140] However, breathlessness, chest pain, and, because of obstructive effects, symptoms resulting from recurrent infections are also reported.[139] Lithoptysis (literally, the expectoration of calcific material) is a characteristic symptom but infrequently reported by patients.[139,141] Rarely, broncholithiasis masquerades as asthma with wheeze as the dominant feature.[139,142]

Pathology

The basic pathogenetic mechanism is thought to be the extrusion and subsequent erosion of dystrophic calcific material from lymph nodes into adjacent structures. The calcification typically affects the tracheobronchial tree, but erosion into the lung parenchyma and mediastinum is known to occur[143]; this may be complicated by the formation of a mediastinal abscess or a fistulous communication.[144,145]

Manifestations of the Disease

RADIOGRAPHY

The radiographic findings in broncholithiasis may be divided into those resulting from the primary pathologic process itself—namely, the presence of calcified foci—and those that are a consequence of erosion and obstruction. As regards the former, there is evidence of either central hilar, the more common scenario, or peripheral calcification.[146,147] A useful clue to the diagnosis, when serial radiographs are available, is the movement of a previously noted focus of calcification in its relationship to an adjacent airway.[148] Depending on the severity and duration of obstruction, there may be segmental atelectasis, lobar atelectasis, or recurrent consolidation from pneumonia[146,149–152]; in rare patients broncholithiasis may be responsible for the so-called middle lobe syndrome.[153]

COMPUTED TOMOGRAPHY

Thin-section, multiplanar CT is the best noninvasive technique for the diagnosis of broncholithiasis (Fig. 57.25).[146,154,155] In one study of patients with proven broncholithiasis, there was calcified endobronchial material in 10 of 15 subjects and peribronchial calcification with airway distortion in 5.[146] Of interest, there was no evidence of an associated soft tissue density mass in any case, contrasting with findings of fibrosing mediastinitis, another condition that may be secondary to histoplasmosis or tuberculosis. CT was also able to demonstrate the effects of obstruction, such as bronchiectasis and atelectasis.

IMAGING ALGORITHMS

The chest radiograph and thin-section CT are the mainstays of the imaging diagnosis of broncholithiasis. A demonstration on serial radiographic examinations of the change in position of a previously noted calcified focus (e.g., at the hilum) is certainly a strong suggestion of the diagnosis. However, in most cases CT is required for confirmation, especially when therapy is being considered.

Differential Diagnosis

There are a number of diagnostic pitfalls and mimics of broncholithiasis of which the radiologist should be aware. These have been elegantly described and illustrated in a review by Seo and colleagues[154] and include calcified balls of fungal hyphae; endobronchial tumors, such as carcinoid, that may rarely calcify[156]; tracheobronchial amyloidosis; tracheobronchopathia osteochondroplastica; and hypertrophy of the bronchial artery with protrusion into the lumen of the airway.

Synopsis of Treatment Options

MEDICAL

Regular observation with no intervention may be considered in some patients with "uncomplicated" disease. Bronchoscopic removal of partially eroded or free broncholiths may be considered in some patients but is used sparingly in many cases because of the risk of hemorrhage. Fragmentation of intraluminal broncholiths may be performed by bronchoscopically delivered laser (Nd-YAG or holmium) energy.

SURGICAL

Surgical resection (segmentectomy, lobectomy, and pneumonectomy) may be considered in some patients. Indications for surgery include the development of significant complications (massive hemoptysis, mediastinal abscess, fistulas) and the failure of previous bronchoscopic broncholith removal (bronchoscopic broncholithectomy).

KEY POINTS: BRONCHOLITHIASIS

- Broncholithiasis is a rare disorder with a peak incidence in the sixth decade of life that is most commonly related to previous granulomatous infection.
- Broncholithiasis occurs when there is extrusion of and subsequent erosion into an airway of calcific material, typically from an adjacent lymph node.
- The typical symptoms are cough and hemoptysis; lithoptysis is uncommon.
- CT findings: endobronchial broncholiths and peribronchial calcification.
- Treatment options include observation, bronchoscopic removal or laser therapy, and surgical resection of affected lobes.

Chronic Bronchitis

Etiology

Chronic bronchitis, one of the traditional syndromes of chronic obstructive pulmonary disease (COPD), has been defined in clinical terms. A diagnosis was traditionally made when there was a history of chronic sputum expectoration (on most days) for 3 months of the year for 2 consecutive years.[157–159] Pulmonary emphysema is one of the other classic syndromes of chronic airflow limitation. However, although it is perhaps convenient to think of these conditions as discrete entities, the concept is now regarded as somewhat outdated; the reality is that emphysema and features of chronic bronchitis frequently coexist, and the "catch-all" term *COPD* is of value.[160–162]

The dominant cause of chronic bronchitis, by far, is cigarette smoke, and there is a clear, demonstrable relationship between a smoking history and the frequency of chronic bronchitis.[163] However, factors other than smoking tobacco that have a putative role in the development of chronic bronchitis and COPD have been identified and include a history of childhood infection, socioeconomic status, occupation, air pollution, age, gender, and possibly climate.[162,164–168]

Prevalence and Epidemiology

As might be expected in a condition whose definition is entirely based on clinical criteria, precise estimates of the prevalence of chronic bronchitis are not forthcoming; symptoms are, by their very nature, subjective and prone to variation over time.[169] Nevertheless, given the worldwide prevalence of smoking in both industrialized and developing countries, it can safely be assumed that chronic bronchitis is very common, affecting 20% of adults in one study.[170]

Clinical Presentation

By definition, patients with chronic bronchitis complain of cough productive of sputum, and symptoms are typically first reported after subjects have smoked for some years. Acute exacerbations are common and are usually from lower respiratory tract infections.

Pathophysiology

PATHOLOGY

In chronic bronchitis there is a background of chronic inflammation that causes lung damage. The key pathologic finding in chronic bronchitis is the presence of enlarged mucous glands and goblet cell hyperplasia. Chronic airway remodeling can occur, leading to the "fixed" airway obstruction that is so characteristic a feature of COPD.[171]

LUNG FUNCTION

The results of lung function tests in patients with "pure" chronic bronchitis (i.e., without associated emphysema) may be entirely normal.[167] Episodic declines in lung function may be seen and might be attributed to airway hyperreactivity during infections.

Manifestations of the Disease

RADIOGRAPHY

The majority of patients with chronic bronchitis have no abnormality on chest radiography.[172] In those with findings, bronchial wall thickening and a general sense of an increase in lung markings, sometimes referred to as "dirty" or "busy" lungs in reports of old, are common (Fig. 57.26). However, the exact pathologic meaning of these radiographic features is difficult to predict. Although some older studies of chest radiographs reported hyperinflation in chronic bronchitis, the inclusion of patients with significant emphysema may have been responsible for this finding.[173]

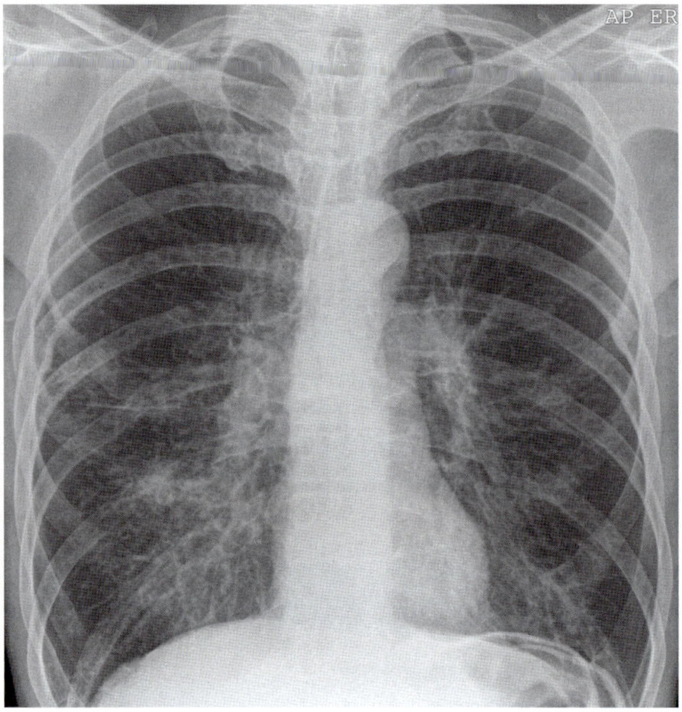

Fig. 57.26 Chronic bronchitis. Chest radiograph shows a generalized increase in lung markings and bronchial wall thickening in the lower zones. An ill-defined opacity in the right lower lung was subsequently proven to be a lung cancer.

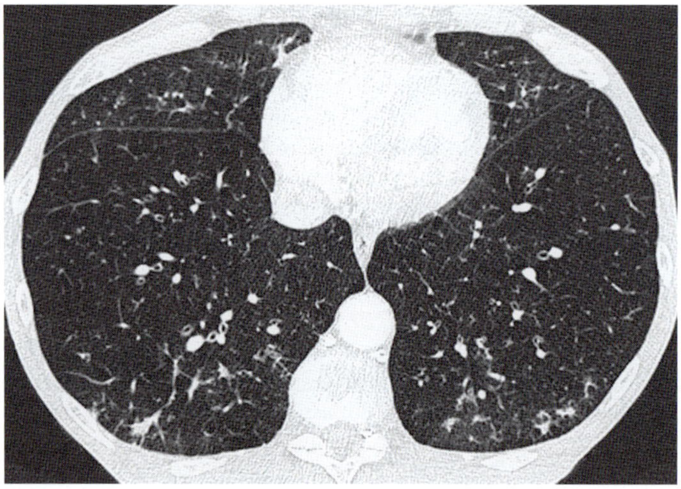

Fig. 57.27 Chronic bronchitis in a long-term smoker. High-resolution CT image shows thick-walled (but not bronchiectatic) subsegmental airways in both lower lobes. There is mild mosaic attenuation suggesting small airways involvement.

COMPUTED TOMOGRAPHY

Bronchial wall thickening and endobronchial mucous plugging are readily depicted but nonspecific features on thin-section CT (Fig. 57.27).[57,174] In the study by Remy-Jardin and colleagues,[57] there was evidence of wall thickening in one-third of smokers. However, there was also evidence of thick-walled bronchi in just less than 20% of normal controls. In some smokers there are signs of small airway involvement with focal areas of mosaic attenuation on inspiratory CT scans and air-trapping on expiratory CT scans.[175]

IMAGING ALGORITHMS

Imaging has a limited role in the evaluation of chronic bronchitis. The chest radiograph perhaps has the greatest value in the detection of infection and in the exclusion of alternative diagnoses.[162] CT should have little if any role in the routine evaluation of patients with chronic bronchitis. A possible exception is the "difficult" case in which the exclusion of other entities (e.g., bronchiectasis) that might manifest with similar chronic respiratory symptoms is important.

Differential Diagnosis

The major differential diagnosis to be considered is that of asthma, a distinction that is potentially problematic, particularly when asthma is chronic and associated with a component of fixed airflow obstruction.[162] Other considerations that may cause bronchial wall thickening on CT include bronchiectasis, constrictive bronchiolitis, diffuse panbronchiolitis, and congestive heart failure.

Synopsis of Treatment Options

MEDICAL

Smoking cessation is the most important aspect of the management of patients with chronic bronchitis and COPD. Influenza vaccination is recommended. Bronchodilator therapy, sometimes with corticosteroids, is prescribed for patients with symptomatic chronic bronchitis or COPD. A pulmonary rehabilitation program improves exercise tolerance and provides symptomatic benefit. Treatment is also directed to the management of acute exacerbations, generally resulting from infection.

KEY POINTS: CHRONIC BRONCHITIS

- Chronic bronchitis is a clinical diagnosis based on a history of chronic sputum expectoration (on most days) for 3 months of the year for 2 consecutive years.
- Imaging plays a limited role in the evaluation of these patients, except to exclude other findings such as bronchiectasis. The major CT findings include bronchial wall thickening and endobronchial mucous plugging.

SUGGESTED READINGS

Bruzzi JF, Remy-Jardin M, Delhaye D, et al. Multi-detector row CT of hemoptysis. *Radiographics*. 2006;26:3–22.

Gibson PG. Allergic bronchopulmonary aspergillosis. *Semin Respir Crit Care Med*. 2006;27:185–191.

Milliron B, Henry TS, Veeraraghavan S, Little BP. Bronchiectasis: mechanisms and imaging clues of associated common and uncommon diseases. *Radiographics*. 2015;35:1011–1030.

Rosen MJ. Chronic cough due to bronchiectasis: ACCP evidence-based clinical practice guidelines. *Chest*. 2006;129(suppl):122S–131S.

Virnig C, Bush RK. Allergic bronchopulmonary aspergillosis: a US perspective. *Curr Opin Pulm Med*. 2007;13:67–71.

The full reference list for this chapter is available at ExpertConsult.com.

58 Asthma*

JONATHAN H. CHUNG | CHRISTOPHER M. WALKER

Asthma is an inflammatory disease characterized by increased airway reactivity and by airflow obstruction that is at least partially reversible and results in recurrent episodes of wheezing, breathlessness, and cough.[1]

Etiology

Asthma can be divided into two main categories: extrinsic and intrinsic. Extrinsic asthma occurs in patients who are atopic, a term used to refer to the genetic predisposition to respond to antigenic challenge with excessive immunoglobulin E (IgE) production. The inheritance is complex but usually incomplete, and evidence of it is much greater if both parents are atopic. Although patients with extrinsic asthma are invariably atopic, atopy itself is not synonymous with asthma. Atopy occurs in more than 30% of the population, whereas the incidence of asthma is generally less than 10%. In addition to atopy and elevated blood levels of IgE, extrinsic asthma is characterized by high incidences of eczema and rhinitis, onset during the first 3 decades of life, seasonal symptoms, and a tendency for remission in later life.[2] Intrinsic asthma occurs in patients in whom atopy or specific external triggers of bronchoconstriction cannot be identified.[3] Affected patients are characterized by being older than patients with extrinsic disease and by having no or a less convincing family history of asthma or atopy, an absence of elevated blood levels of IgE or positive skin or bronchial response to allergen challenge, increased numbers of blood and sputum eosinophils, decreased responsiveness to therapy, and a tendency to persistent and progressive disease resulting in fixed airflow obstruction.[2]

Prevalence and Epidemiology

Asthma is a common disease, and there is good evidence that its prevalence and the prevalence of other allergic disorders is increasing worldwide.[1] The reasons for this increase are unclear. Estimates of prevalence vary by definition, geography, ethnicity, and age. The prevalence of asthma in most countries with available statistics ranges from approximately 5% to 25% in children and 2% to 12% in adults.[1] The highest prevalences are found in the United Kingdom, Australia, and New Zealand (≈12% each) and in Tristan da Cunha, a group of remote islands in the South Atlantic Ocean in which 56% of the population has asthma.[1] Concomitant sinusitis is common, occurring in 47% to 76% of asthma cases.[4]

The prevalence of asthma is highest in childhood and decreases during adolescence and adulthood. The prevalence before the age of 10 years is higher in boys than in girls; after that, it is higher in females.[2] Females are also more likely to visit the emergency department and to be admitted for acute severe asthma.[5]

Asthma is the most common chronic lung disease and an important health problem worldwide.[6] In the United States, it accounts for nearly 2 million emergency department visits, 500,000 hospitalizations, and 5000 deaths each year.[7] Data from Australia, Canada, and Spain indicate that acute asthma accounts for 1% to 12% of all adult emergency department visits.[6] In a study in France, 7% of adult patients with acute asthma who presented to the emergency department were transferred to an intensive care unit.[8]

Clinical Presentation

The diagnosis of asthma is based largely on a history of periodic paroxysms of dyspnea, alternating with intervals of complete or nearly complete remission. Cough can be a prominent symptom and occasionally the only symptom.[6] The onset of acute asthma (asthma attack) is characterized by gradual increase in shortness of breath, cough, and wheezing and by a decrease in expiratory airflow. The exacerbations may progress during hours, days, or weeks.[6] Physical findings include hyperventilation, inspiratory and expiratory rhonchi and wheezes, decreased breath sounds, and prolonged expiration.[2] Cough and wheezing are the result of bronchial inflammation and bronchoconstriction. Contraction of airway smooth muscle, edema, and hypersecretion also affect the bronchioles and result in small airway closure.[1] To compensate, the patient breathes at a higher lung volume to increase outward retraction of the airways, thereby helping to maintain airway patency. The more severe the airflow limitation, the greater the tendency for airway closure to occur and the higher the lung volume must be to keep airways open. The combination of hyperinflation and airflow limitation markedly increases the work of breathing.[1]

Acute asthma attacks may range from mild to life-threatening. In a study of 3772 patients with acute asthma who presented at various emergency departments in France, 975 (26%) had life-threatening attacks, 1834 (49%) had severe exacerbations without life-threatening features, and 963 (26%) had mild to moderate exacerbations.[8] The overall admission rate was 54%, and mean hospital stay was 6 days. Three patients died in the hospital.[8]

Pathophysiology

The basic pathophysiologic abnormality that determines the functional and symptomatic status of an asthmatic patient is airway narrowing, which can occur by four mechanisms: (1) airway smooth muscle contraction, (2) edema and congestion of the airway wall, (3) plugging of the airway lumen by mucous and inflammatory exudate, and (4) airway wall remodeling.[1] Airway remodeling is a heterogeneous process leading to changes in connective tissue deposition and to altered airways structure.[9] For the most part, it is difficult to determine in a given patient

*The editors and publisher would like to thank Drs. C. Isabela Silva Müller and Nestor L. Müller for contributing material on this topic to the prior edition of this work. It has served as the foundation for the current chapter.

what proportion of airway obstruction is caused by each of these mechanisms. However, it may reasonably be concluded that when obstruction is rapidly reversible after the inhalation of smooth muscle relaxants, the pathogenesis is smooth muscle contraction. On the other hand, when obstruction responds during a period of days to steroids and other therapeutic interventions, it is probably caused predominantly by edema and mucous plugging.[2]

Asthma is a chronic inflammatory disorder of the airways associated with airway hyperresponsiveness, an exaggerated bronchoconstrictor response to a wide variety of exogenous and endogenous stimuli that results in acute episodes of dyspnea and wheezing.[1] These include environmental allergens, respiratory viral infections, exercise, analgesics, air pollution, weather changes, cigarette smoke, occupational sensitizing agents, indoor allergens, and irritants, such as household sprays and paint fumes.[1,10–22] Specific antigens can provoke asthmatic attacks in sensitized persons. These individuals frequently suffer from other allergic manifestations, such as hay fever and eczema. Potential antigens are innumerable.

Exercise-induced asthma can be considered to be present when airway narrowing accompanies moderate or vigorous exercise.[11] Rather than being a separate form of asthma, exercise-induced asthma should be considered a trigger for airway narrowing in patients who have asthma. In fact, it occurs in 70% to 80% of patients with asthma who exercise at 80% to 90% of their maximal workload for 6 to 8 minutes.[12]

The association of asthma and gastroesophageal reflux is common; various investigators have estimated the concordance to be 30% to more than 80%.[16] There is evidence that gastroesophageal reflux can induce asthma and that asthma can cause a worsening of gastroesophageal reflux. It is possible that gastroesophageal reflux triggers airway narrowing in susceptible persons by reflex bronchoconstriction secondary to stimulation of afferent nerves in the esophagus or pharynx or by direct aspiration of a small amount of esophageal contents.[17]

PATHOLOGY

On histologic examination, asthma is characterized by the presence of chronic inflammation of the airways that involves mainly the medium-sized and small bronchi.[23] The bronchi are thickened because of a combination of edema and an increase in smooth muscle and in the size of the mucous glands (Fig. 58.1).[23] Bronchiolar abnormalities include wall thickening, mucostasis, and constrictive bronchiolitis (Fig. 58.2).[23] Between clinical episodes, the bronchioles may be nearly normal, as viewed in tissue from asthmatics taken for other reasons.[23]

Histologic changes in the bronchial and bronchiolar walls involve the epithelium, lamina propria, muscularis mucosae, and submucosa.[24] The constellation of abnormalities is referred to as airway wall remodeling and consists of changes in the composition, quantity, and organization of the cellular and molecular constituents of the airway wall as a consequence of chronic injury and repair.[25] Collagen deposition in the subepithelial layer, as well as in the adventitia, may underlie the decreased airway distensibility that may be seen in asthmatic patients.[26] An increase in smooth muscle is also a characteristic feature; it is the result of both hyperplasia and hypertrophy and is most pronounced in subjects who die of the disease.[27] Eosinophils are the most characteristic and numerous inflammatory cells in the airway wall; however, there may also be increases in lymphocytes, macrophages, neutrophils, and mast cells.[1,28]

LUNG FUNCTION

Measurements of airflow limitation, its reversibility, and its variability are important in the diagnosis and management of asthma.[1]

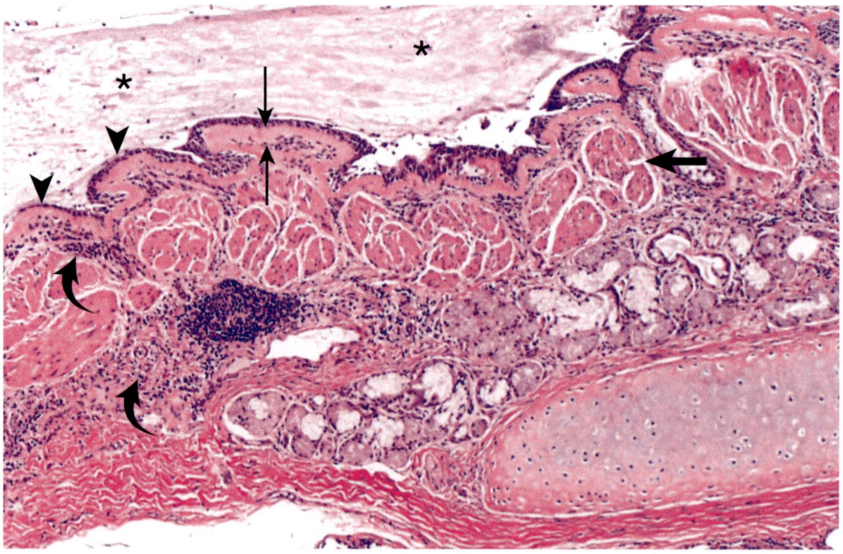

Fig. 58.1 Bronchial abnormalities in asthma. Photomicrograph of autopsy specimen obtained in a 10-year-old boy with fatal status asthmaticus reveals bronchus with luminal mucous plug *(asterisks)*, thinning of surface mucosa *(arrowheads)*, submembranous fibrosis (so-called basement membrane thickening, *vertical straight arrows*), muscle hypertrophy *(horizontal straight arrow)*, and inflammatory infiltrate *(curved arrows)* that is rich in eosinophils. *(From Silva CI, Colby TV, Müller NL. Asthma and associated conditions: high-resolution CT and pathologic findings.* AJR Am J Roentgenol. *2004;183: 817–824.)*

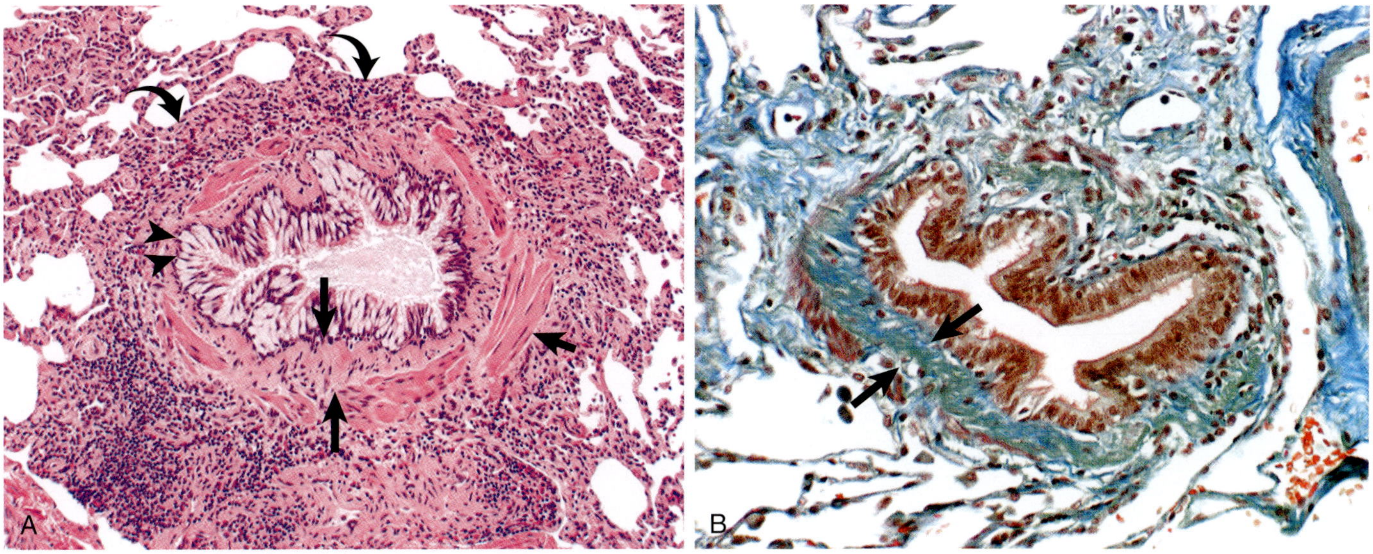

Fig. 58.2 Bronchiolar abnormalities in asthma. (A) Photomicrograph of histopathologic specimen obtained in a 10-year-old boy with fatal status asthmaticus shows a small bronchiole (outside diameter, 0.5 mm from adventitia to adventitia) with muscle hypertrophy *(short straight arrow)*, submucosal and submembranous fibrosis *(long straight arrows)*, and inflammatory infiltrate *(curved arrows)* rich in eosinophils. Goblet cell metaplasia (more typically seen in bronchi of patients with asthma) is prominent and seen as pale swollen cells *(arrowheads)* replacing much of the columnar ciliated epithelium. The extent of submembranous and submucosal fibrosis (structural remodeling) indicates mild constrictive bronchiolitis. (B) Photomicrograph of histopathologic specimen (trichrome stain, intermediate magnification) obtained in a 48-year-old woman with a long history of asthma shows a bronchiole with submucosal thickening that was caused by fibrous tissue *(arrows)* and resulted in luminal narrowing. These findings are characteristic of mild constrictive bronchiolitis. *(From Silva CI, Colby TV, Müller NL. Asthma and associated conditions: high-resolution CT and pathologic findings.* AJR Am J Roentgenol. *2004;183:817–824.)*

The main measurements used for the evaluation of these patients are forced expiratory volume in 1 second (FEV1), forced vital capacity, the ratio of FEV1 to forced vital capacity, and peak expiratory flow.[1] A 12% or greater improvement in FEV1 or 15% or greater improvement in peak expiratory flow spontaneously, after inhalation of a bronchodilator, or in response to a trial of glucocorticosteroid therapy favors a diagnosis of asthma.[1]

Diffuse airway narrowing is the basic functional abnormality of symptomatic asthma; the resulting increase in resistance leads to decreased flow, hyperinflation, gas trapping, and ultimately an increase in the work of breathing. It is most easily detected and quantified by measurements of maximal expiratory flow. The increase in airway resistance is also associated with hyperinflation, as manifested by an increase in functional residual capacity and, to a lesser extent, total lung capacity.[29]

As an asthmatic episode resolves, there is improvement in expiratory flow (peak expiratory flow and FEV1) and vital capacity and a decrease in functional residual capacity. The single-breath diffusing lung capacity for carbon monoxide is often elevated in both stable and acute asthma.[30] The most plausible explanation for this apparent paradox is the transient increase in pulmonary capillary blood volume that is a result of the more negative inspiratory intrathoracic pressure secondary to obstruction of the airways.[2]

Most patients experiencing an acute attack have some degree of hypoxemia as a result of ventilation-perfusion mismatch.[2] There is not a close relationship between measures of airway obstruction and gas exchange in asthma.[31] However, in severe acute attacks, partial pressure of oxygen in arterial blood generally drops to less than 60 mm Hg, FEV1 is less than 1 L, and peak flow is less than 60 L/min.[2] As the severity and duration of obstruction increase, patients become exhausted, their respiratory muscles fatigue, and values of partial pressure of carbon dioxide in arterial blood rise into the hypercapnic range.[2]

Manifestations of the Disease

RADIOGRAPHY

The most common radiographic abnormalities in patients who have asthma are hyperinflation and bronchial wall thickening (Figs. 58.3 and 58.4); less frequent manifestations are prominence of the hila, increased central lung markings, and peripheral oligemia (Fig. 58.5).[32] The prevalence of these abnormalities is influenced by several factors, including the age at onset, the severity of asthma, and the presence of other diseases or complications of asthma.[33]

Pulmonary hyperinflation is manifested as an increase in the depth of the retrosternal space, an increase in lung height, and flattening of the diaphragm (see Fig. 58.3). Thickening of the airways occurs in both segmental and subsegmental bronchi and can be seen either as ring shadows viewed end-on or as "tram-line" opacities viewed en face. Prominence of the main pulmonary artery and its hilar branches with rapid tapering is indicative of transient precapillary pulmonary arterial hypertension secondary to hypoxia. Additional vascular findings include diffuse narrowing and blood flow redistribution into the upper lobes, the latter in the absence of other signs of postcapillary hypertension, and a paucity of vessels in the outer 2 to 4 cm of the lungs.

Despite the observations just outlined, the chest radiograph has a limited role in the diagnosis of asthma. It is often normal, even during an acute attack; moreover, when it is abnormal, the

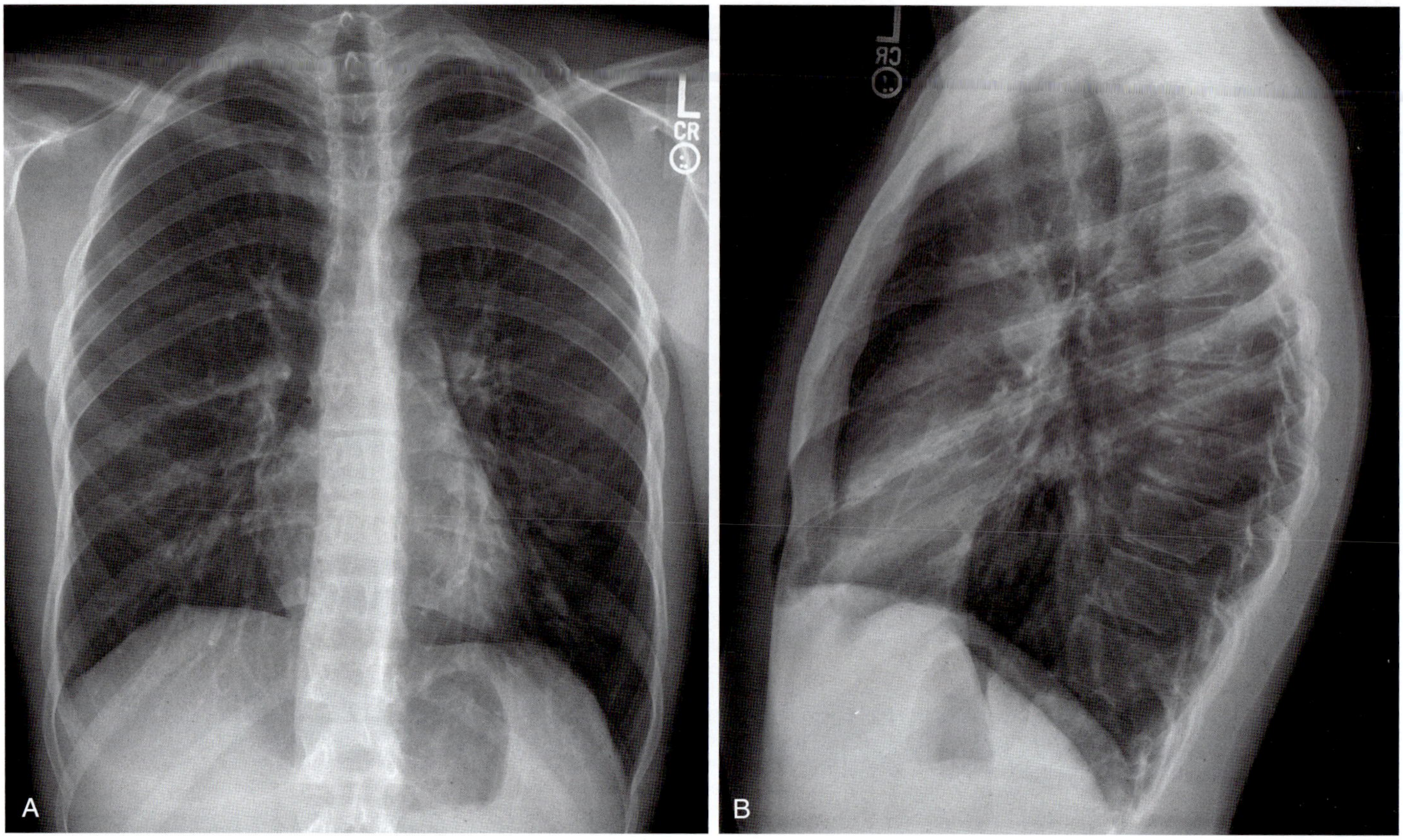

Fig. 58.3 Radiographic manifestations of acute asthma. (A) Posteroanterior chest radiograph shows increased lung volumes and reduction of the peripheral vascular markings. (B) Lateral view demonstrates increased retrosternal airspace.

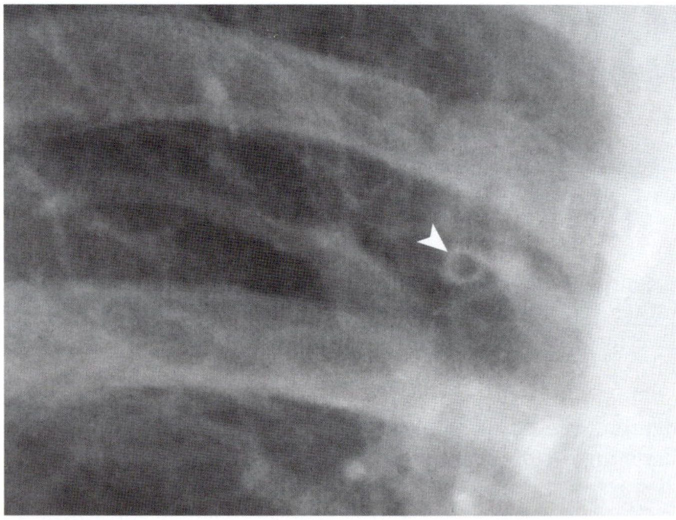

Fig. 58.4 Radiographic manifestations of asthma. A detailed view of the right lung from a frontal radiograph shows bronchial wall thickening *(arrowhead)*, a nonspecific finding that may be seen in asthma.

findings are nonspecific.[34] The two main indications for chest radiography are to exclude other conditions that cause wheezing—particularly emphysema, left-sided heart failure, and obstruction of the trachea or major bronchi by tumor or foreign body—and to identify complications.[35,36] Complications of asthma that may be seen on radiography or computed tomography (CT) include pneumonia, atelectasis (Fig. 58.6), pneumomediastinum (Fig. 58.7), pneumothorax, and occasionally pneumorrhachis (i.e., air within the spinal canal).[1,37]

COMPUTED TOMOGRAPHY

Thin-section CT findings include thickening and narrowing of the bronchi (Fig. 58.8), endobronchial mucous plugging, bronchial dilatation, patchy areas of decreased attenuation and vascularity, and air-trapping.[23] The bronchial wall thickening and luminal narrowing reflect the presence of bronchial wall edema and the increase in smooth muscle and in the size of the mucous glands (see Fig. 58.1). The bronchial abnormalities seen on CT can be quantified subjectively and objectively and have been shown to increase with increasing severity of disease.[25,38] The prevalence of bronchial thickening on high-resolution CT in patients with asthma reported in different studies ranges from 16% to 96% and may be seen in up to 19% of normal controls.[38–41] The wide variability is presumably related to different populations of patients and the subjectivity of the finding. Park and colleagues[38] identified bronchial wall thickening in 17 of 39 (44%) asthmatic patients compared with only 4% of normal controls. Bronchial wall thickening was more prevalent among patients with severe airflow obstruction (83% of patients with FEV1 less than 60% predicted) than in patients with mild obstruction (35% of patients with FEV1 greater than 60%).

Although the majority of bronchi of patients with asthma have normal or decreased internal diameter, approximately 31% to 77% of adult patients with uncomplicated asthma have one

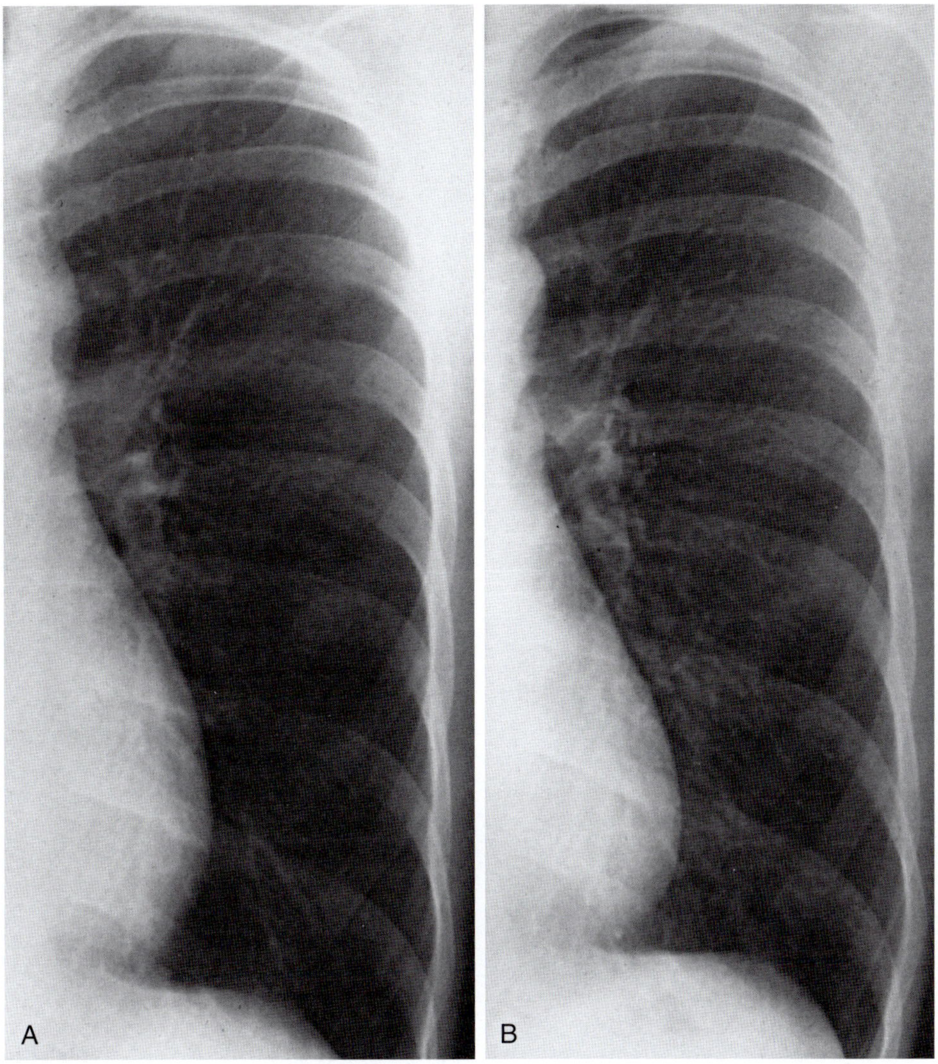

Fig. 58.5 Peripheral oligemia in acute asthma. (A) A detailed view of the left lung from a posteroanterior chest radiograph of a young man during an episode of acute bronchospasm reveals moderate hyperinflation. The vasculature in the outer 2–3 cm of lung is inconspicuous and barely visible, thus creating a subpleural shell of oligemic lung. (B) A repeat study 1 year later during remission shows less hyperinflation; the pulmonary vessels now taper normally, and most are visible well into the lung periphery. *(From Müller NL, Fraser RS, Colman NC, Paré PD.* Radiologic Diagnosis of Diseases of the Chest. *Philadelphia: WB Saunders; 2001.)*

or more bronchi that are dilated (Fig. 58.9).[38,39,41] The bronchiectasis seen in patients with uncomplicated asthma typically is cylindrical, and the bronchoarterial ratio is usually less than 1.5.[40] Follow-up studies suggest that the bronchial dilatation seen in asthmatic patients is not reversible.[42]

High-resolution CT manifestations of bronchiolar abnormalities in patients with asthma include areas of decreased attenuation and vascularity, air-trapping, and small centrilobular opacities.[23] Areas of decreased attenuation and vascularity are seen on high-resolution CT scans performed at end inspiration in approximately 20% of patients with asthma (Fig. 58.10).[38–40] A more common finding is the presence of air-trapping on high-resolution CT images obtained after maximal expiration (Fig. 58.11). In the study by Park and colleagues,[38] air-trapping involving a total volume equivalent to one pulmonary segment or more was seen in 50% of asthmatic patients compared with 14% of healthy subjects. Although the extent of air-trapping increases during an acute attack, air-trapping is also often present in stable patients. This presumably reflects the presence of chronic inflammation and muscle hypertrophy of the small airways or, in some patients, development of constrictive bronchiolitis.

Prominent centrilobular structures or small centrilobular opacities have been reported in 10% to 20% of patients with asthma.[39,40] These presumably reflect the presence of mucostasis in bronchioles or peribronchiolar inflammation (Fig. 58.12; see also Fig. 58.2).

Parenchymal abnormalities in asthma include hyperinflation, emphysema, and occasionally cystic spaces.[23] Emphysema is uncommon in asthmatic nonsmokers; when it is present, it is usually mild and secondary to cicatricial peribronchiolar fibrosis.[43] Rarely, cystic changes may result from overinflation distal to chronic inflammatory bronchiolitis (Fig. 58.13).[23]

Text continued on p. 742

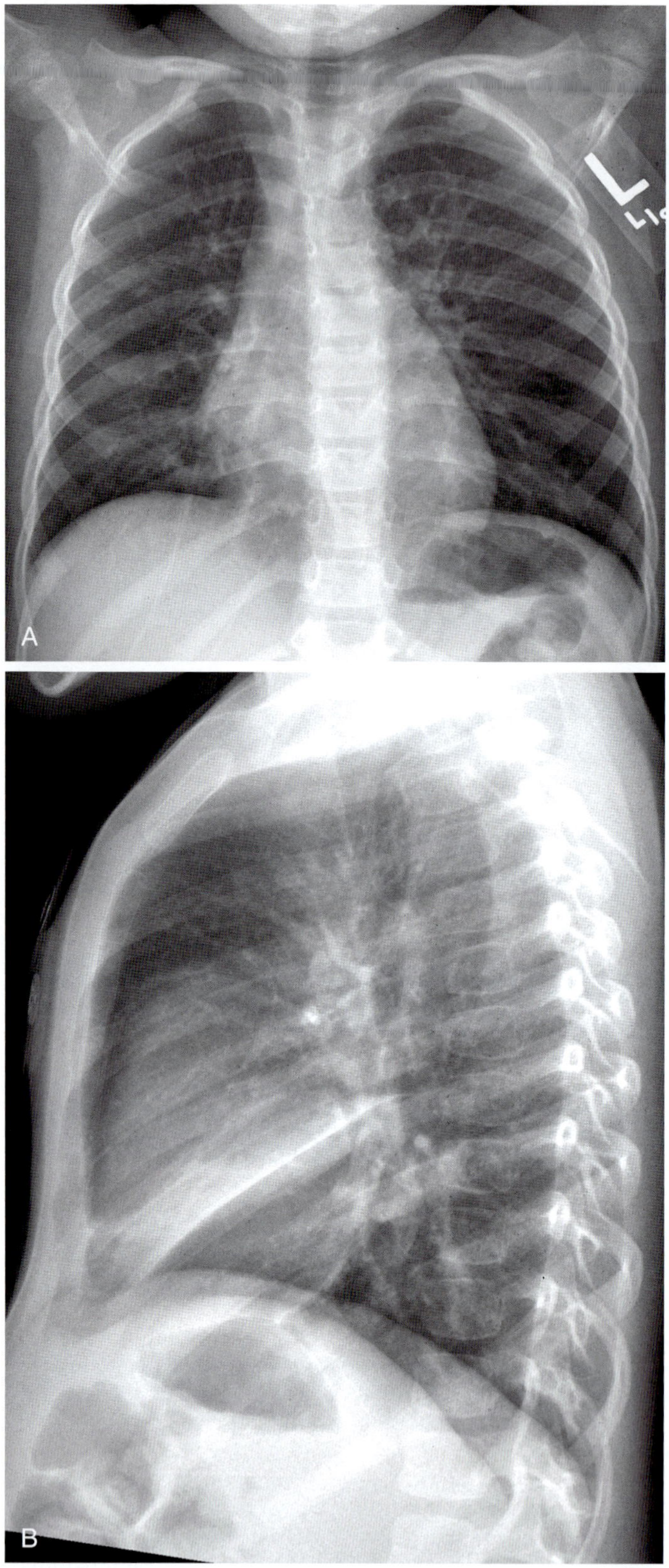

Fig. 58.6 Right middle lobe collapse in acute asthma affecting a pediatric patient. Frontal (A) and lateral (B) chest radiographs show right middle lobe atelectasis.

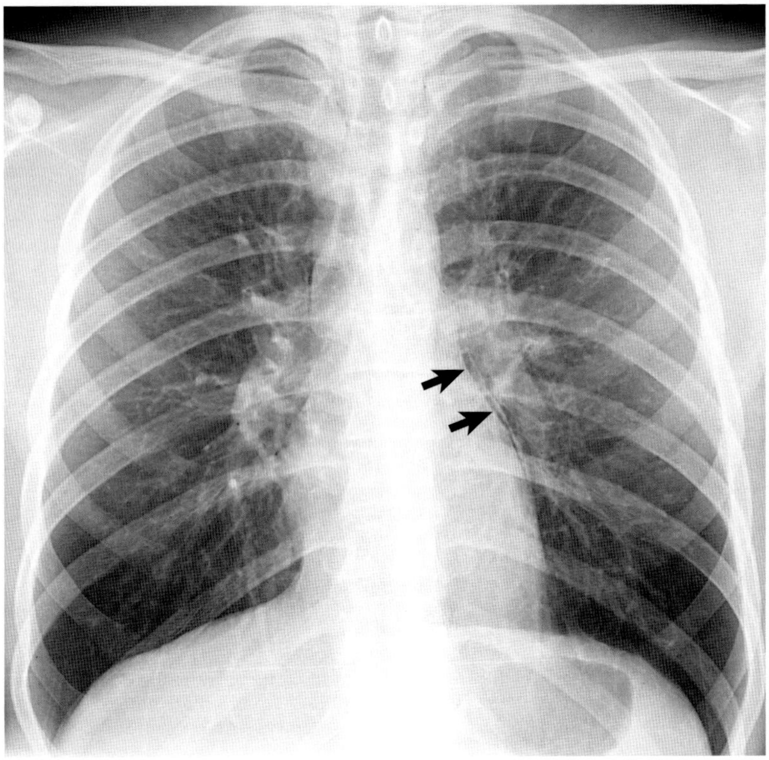

Fig. 58.7 Pneumomediastinum in acute asthma. Posteroanterior chest radiograph in a young man with acute asthma demonstrates hyperinflation and pneumomediastinum *(arrows)*.

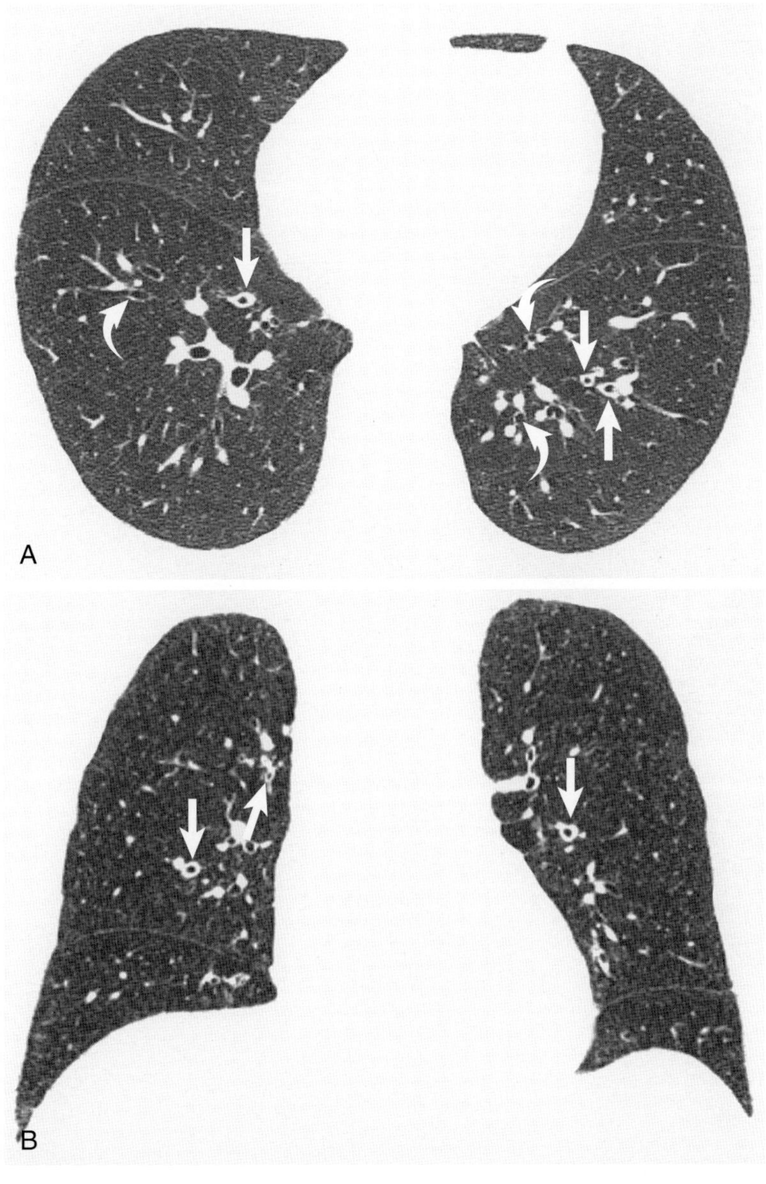

Fig. 58.8 Bronchial wall thickening in chronic asthma in a nonsmoker. (A) High-resolution CT at the level of the lower lobes shows several bronchi with thickened walls *(straight arrows)*. Also noted are several normal-appearing bronchi *(curved arrows)*. (B) Coronal reformatted image shows bronchial wall thickening *(straight arrows)* in the middle and upper lung zones.

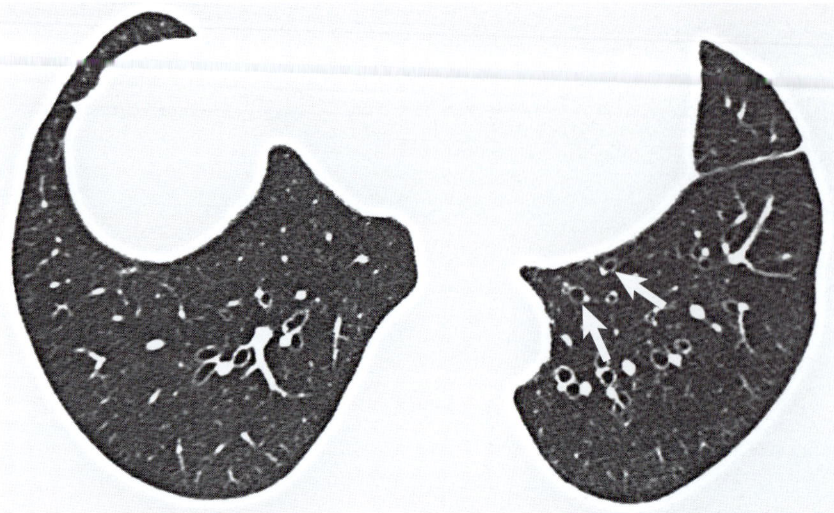

Fig. 58.9 Bronchiectasis in chronic asthma. High-resolution CT at the level of the lower lobes shows left lower lobe bronchiectasis *(arrows)*, areas of decreased attenuation and vascularity in the left lower lobe, and volume loss.

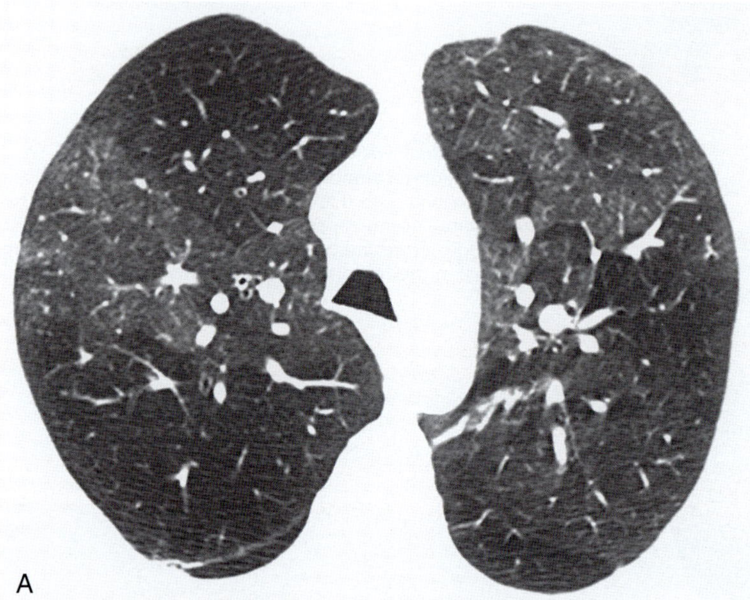

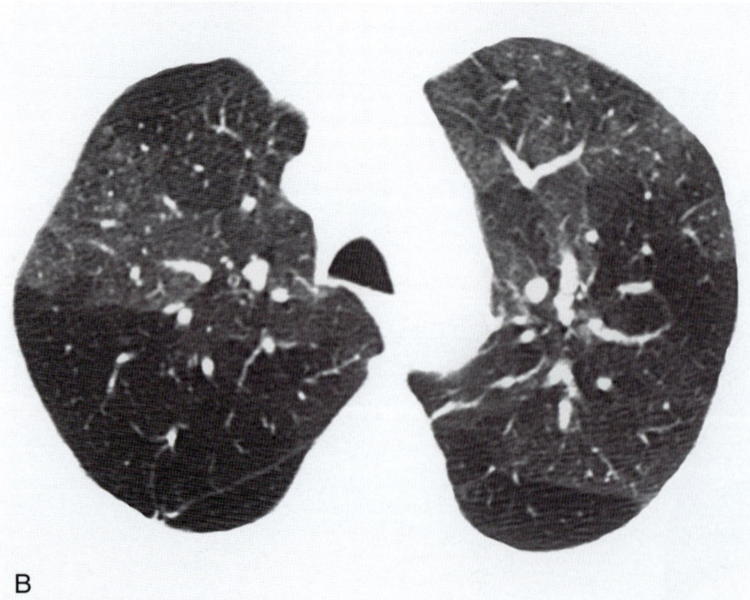

Fig. 58.10 Mosaic attenuation and expiratory air-trapping in severe chronic asthma. (A) High-resolution CT performed at end inspiration shows extensive bilateral areas of decreased attenuation and vascularity with blood flow redistribution to normal lung, resulting in a mosaic attenuation pattern. (B) High-resolution CT performed after maximal expiration demonstrates extensive air-trapping.

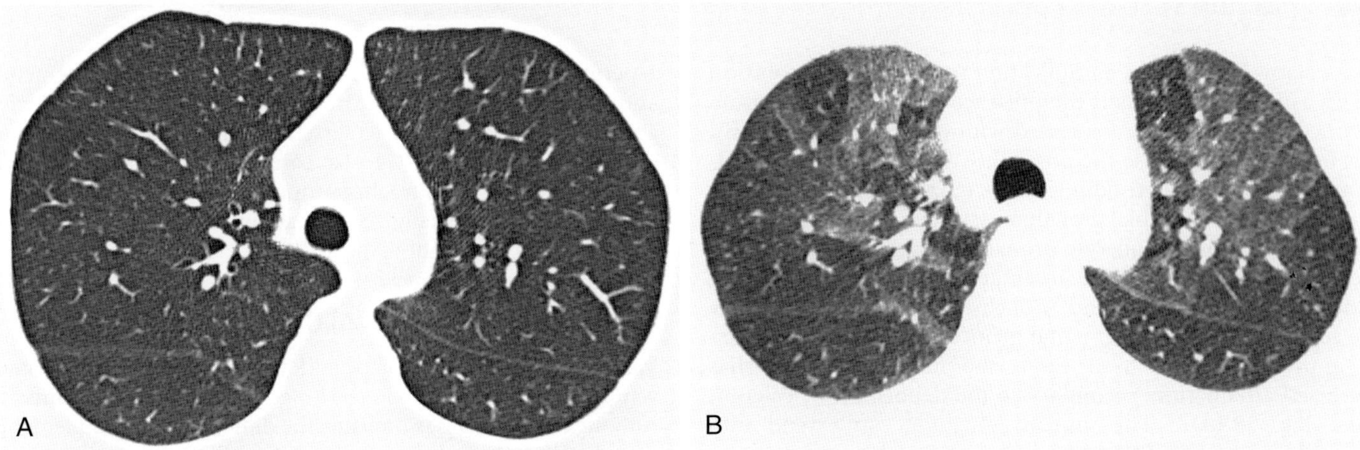

Fig. 58.11 Air-trapping in asthma. (A) High-resolution CT performed at end inspiration shows subtle areas of decreased attenuation and vascularity. (B) High-resolution CT performed after maximal expiration demonstrates extensive air-trapping.

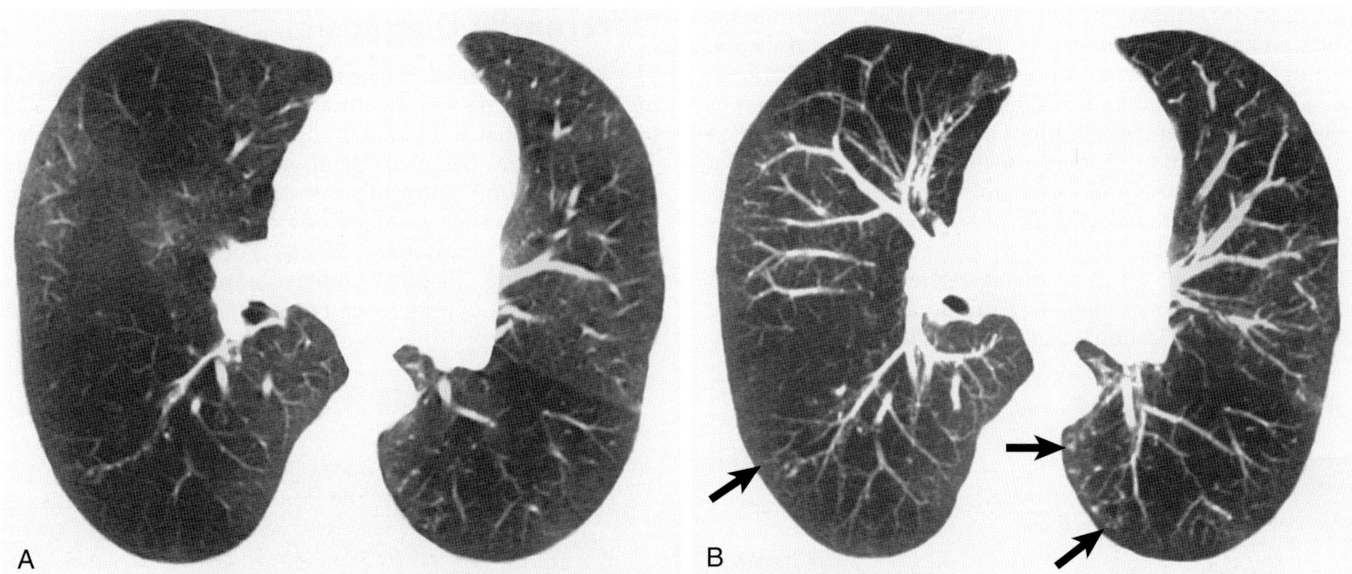

Fig. 58.12 Asthma: CT findings. (A) High-resolution CT image demonstrates extensive areas of decreased attenuation and vascularity consistent with constrictive bronchiolitis and a few small nodular opacities in the peripheral regions of the lower lobes. (B) Maximum-intensity projection image better demonstrates that the peripheral nodular opacities have a centrilobular distribution *(arrows)*. The centrilobular nodules presumably reflect the presence of mucostasis or peribronchiolar inflammation.

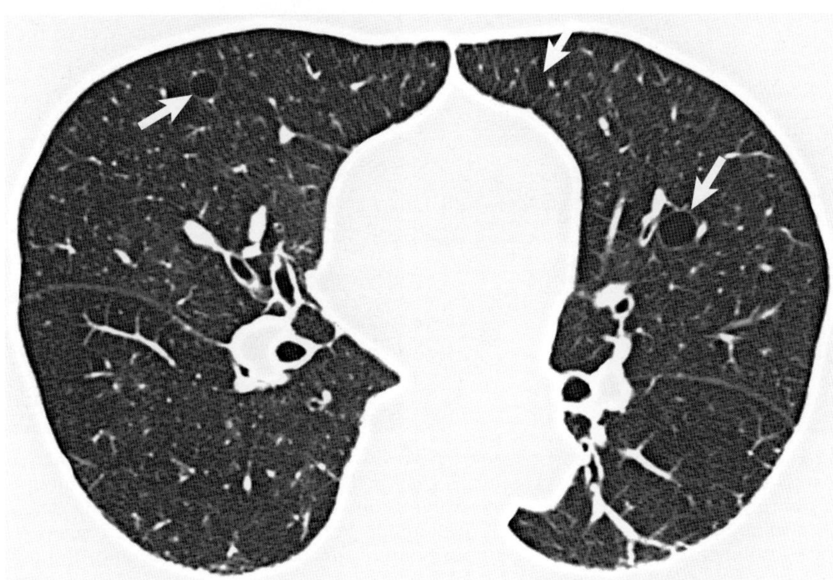

Fig. 58.13 Cysts in chronic asthma in patient never a smoker. High-resolution CT shows bilateral thin-walled cysts *(arrows)* and localized areas of decreased attenuation and vascularity.

A relatively common complication seen on high-resolution CT in asthmatic patients is the presence of mucoid impaction. If mucoid impaction is associated with central bronchiectasis, this finding should raise the possibility of allergic bronchopulmonary aspergillosis, a condition characterized by hypersensitivity reaction to endobronchial growth of *Aspergillus fumigatus*.[23] The CT manifestations of allergic bronchopulmonary aspergillosis include homogeneous tubular, finger-in-glove, or branching endobronchial opacities and bronchiectasis involving mainly the segmental and subsegmental bronchi of the upper lobes.[23] In approximately 30% of cases, the impacted mucus has increased attenuation, secondary to the deposition of calcium salts (Fig. 58.14).[44] The mucous plugging can extend into bronchioles, resulting in centrilobular nodules and tree-in-bud opacities. Obstructive atelectasis may also be seen but is uncommon (see Fig. 58.14). Studies have shown that abnormalities suggestive of allergic bronchopulmonary aspergillosis as opposed to asthma include bronchiectasis, centrilobular nodules, and mucoid impaction.[45,46] The bronchiectasis in allergic bronchopulmonary aspergillosis tends to be central and varicoid (Fig. 58.15) as opposed to the cylindrical bronchiectasis seen in simple asthma. Other complications that are seen with increased prevalence in asthmatic patients, such as chronic eosinophilic pneumonia and eosinophilic granulomatosis with polyangiitis (formerly Churg-Strauss syndrome), are reviewed in Chapters 37 and 46, respectively.

The main role of CT is in the assessment of tracheal and bronchial abnormalities that may mimic asthma and in the assessment of complications such as allergic bronchopulmonary aspergillosis. The value of CT in the diagnosis of endotracheal and endobronchial tumors that may mimic asthma clinically and that may be difficult to visualize on the radiograph is well known (Fig. 58.16).[47,48] CT also can play a major role in distinguishing asthma from tracheobronchomalacia (see Chapter 56), a condition that is being recognized with increasing frequency as a potential mimic of asthma.[36,49]

OTHER IMAGING MODALITIES

Various research tools have been developed that attempt to assess ventilation and perfusion to the lungs in the setting of asthma.[50–54] Although early data is promising, the difficulties with implementation, high costs, and uncertainty of additional benefit of these tools in the clinical setting must be addressed before any new modality can be considered outside the research realm.

Differential Diagnosis

The main differential diagnosis of asthma in patients presenting with wheezing and shortness of breath is airway obstruction by tumor, inhaled foreign body, or tracheobronchomalacia. The differential diagnosis of airway wall thickening includes acute and chronic bronchitis, constrictive bronchiolitis, inflammatory diseases such as sarcoidosis, inflammatory bowel disease, and interstitial pulmonary edema. The differential diagnosis of air-trapping includes other causes of small airways disease, such as hypersensitivity pneumonitis and constrictive bronchiolitis.

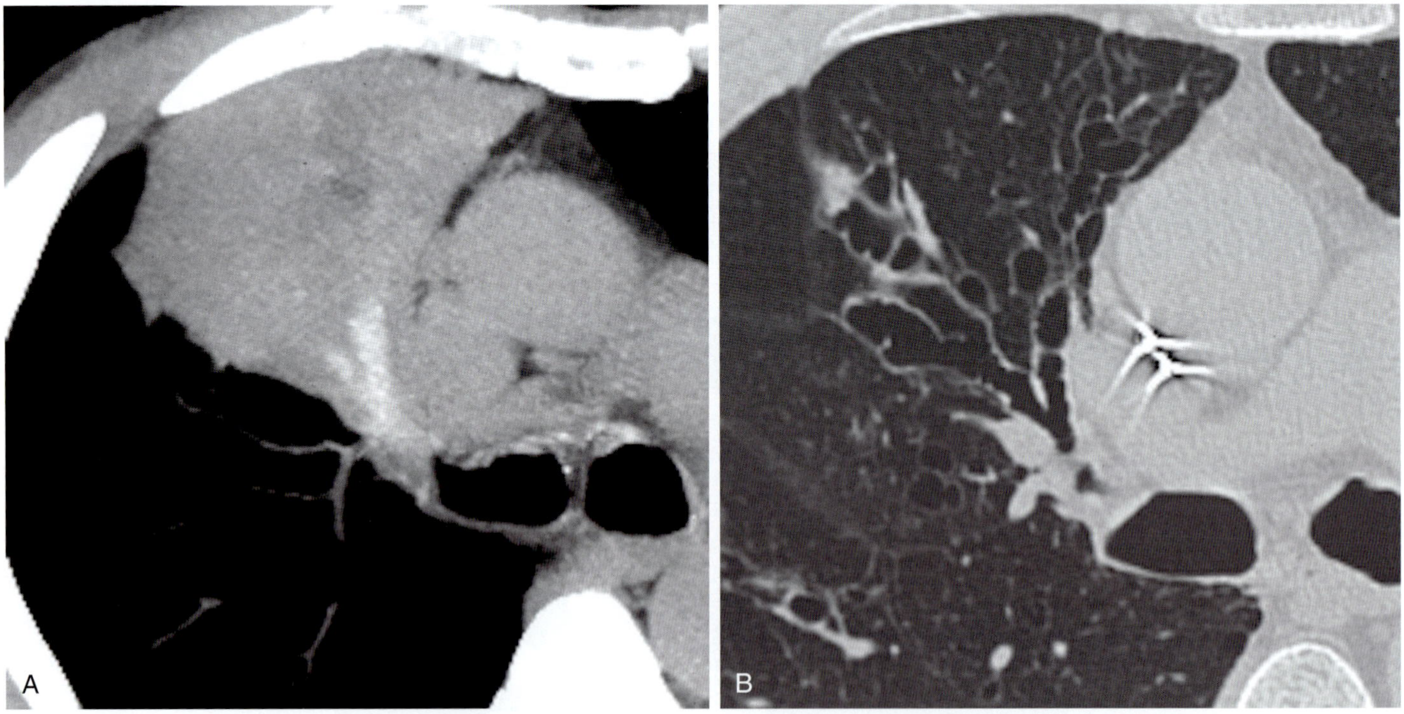

Fig. 58.14 Allergic bronchopulmonary aspergillosis. (A) Axial maximum-intensity projection image from chest CT shows consolidation and atelectasis within the anterior segment of the right upper lobe resulting from hyperdense mucous plugging within bronchiectatic airways, essentially diagnostic of allergic bronchopulmonary aspergillosis. (B) Axial image from a follow-up chest CT scans 6 months later shows resolution of right upper lobe opacity and bronchial mucous plugging; the underlying bronchiectasis is now clearly visible.

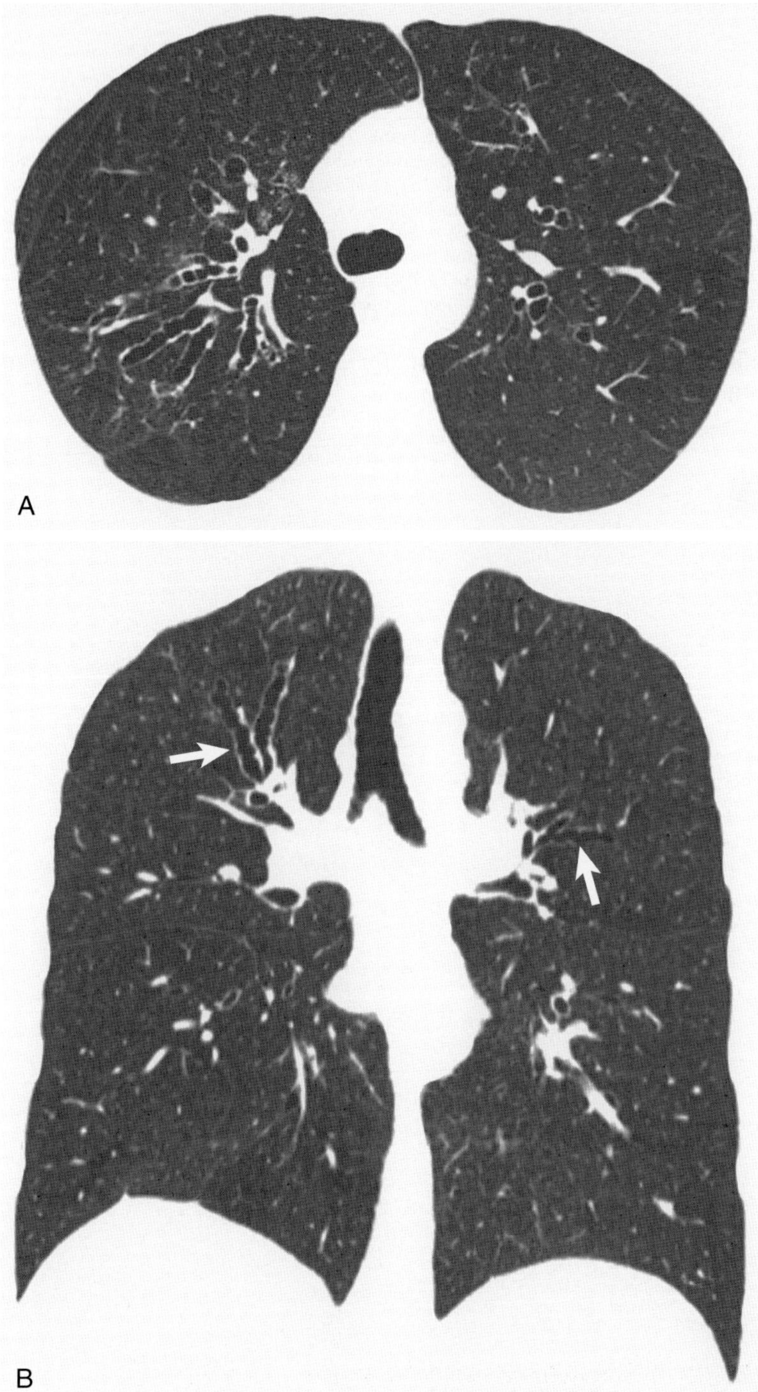

Fig. 58.15 Allergic bronchopulmonary aspergillosis. (A) High-resolution CT image shows extensive varicose bronchiectasis in the upper lobes. (B) Coronal reformatted image demonstrates the upper lobe and central distribution of the bronchiectasis *(arrows)*.

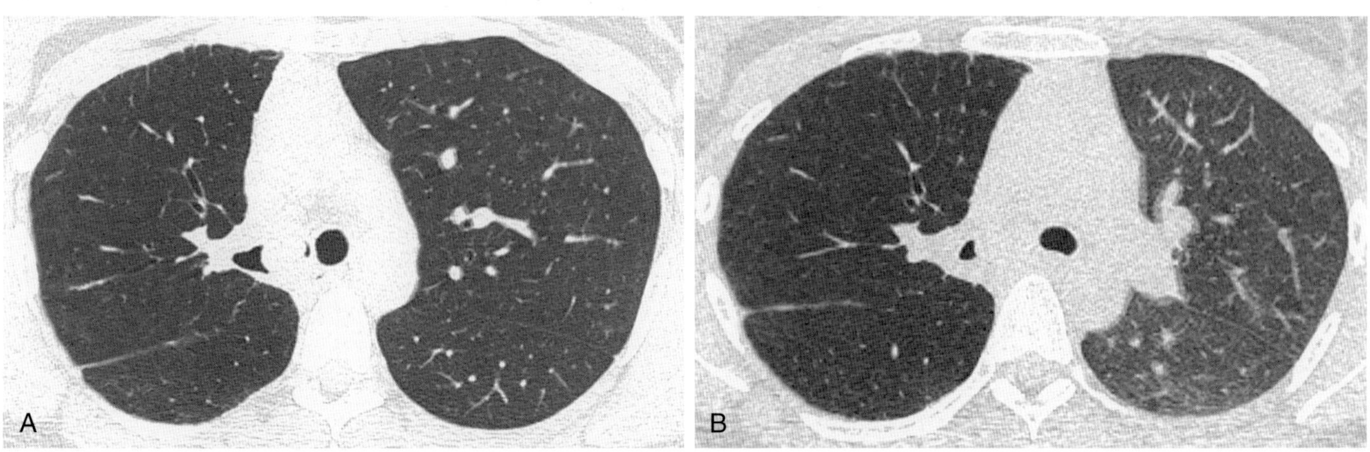

Fig. 58.16 Endobronchial atypical carcinoid tumor in patient who presented with history of "asthma." (A) Inspiratory high-resolution CT image shows endoluminal tumor in right main bronchus. Note decreased size of right lung and diffuse decrease in attenuation and vascularity compared with the left lung. (B) Expiratory CT image demonstrates marked air-trapping within the right lung.

Synopsis of Treatment Options

Treatment of acute asthma usually consists of supplemental oxygen, rapid-acting inhaled β_2-agonists, and, particularly in moderate and severe attacks, oral or intravenous glucocorticosteroids.[1] Subcutaneous or intramuscular injection of epinephrine (adrenaline) may be used in the treatment of severe acute exacerbations of asthma if β_2-agonists are not available.[1] However, it has greater risk of adverse side effects, particularly in hypoxic patients. Long-term control of asthma consists of treatment with inhaled corticosteroids, leukotriene modifiers, long-acting β-agonists, and combination inhalers.

KEY POINTS

- Asthma is a chronic inflammatory disorder of the airways associated with an exaggerated bronchoconstrictor response to a wide variety of stimuli, resulting in recurrent episodes of dyspnea and wheezing. The most important inciting cause is indoor allergens (house dust).
- Pathologic features: thickening of the airway walls by a combination of edema and an increase in smooth muscle and in the size of the mucous glands.
- Imaging findings
  - Chest radiography: often normal or near-normal; may show hyperinflation and bronchial wall thickening.
  - Thin-section CT: thickening and narrowing of the bronchi with mucous plugging, bronchiectasis, patchy areas of decreased attenuation and vascularity, air-trapping; centrilobular nodules are uncommon.
  - The main role of imaging is to exclude other conditions that cause wheezing—particularly, obstruction of the trachea or main bronchi by tumor or foreign body—and to identify complications, including pneumonia, atelectasis, pneumomediastinum, pneumothorax, and allergic bronchopulmonary aspergillosis.

SUGGESTED READINGS

Kligerman SJ, Henry T, Lin CT, Franks TJ, Galvin JR. Mosaic attenuation: etiology, methods of differentiation, and pitfalls. *Radiographics.* 2015;35(5):1360–1380.

Richards JC, Lynch D, Koelsch T, Dyer D. Imaging of asthma. *Immunol Allergy Clin North Am.* 2016;36(3):529–545.

Silva CI, Colby TV, Müller NL. Asthma and associated conditions: high-resolution CT and pathologic findings. *AJR Am J Roentgenol.* 2004;183:817–824.

Trivedi A, Hall C, Hoffman EA, Woods JC, Gierada DS, Castro M. Using imaging as a biomarker for asthma. *J Allergy Clin Immunol.* 2017;139(1):1–10.

The full reference list for this chapter is available at ExpertConsult.com.

59 Bronchiolitis*

SHERIEF GARRANA | CHRISTOPHER M. WALKER | JONATHAN H. CHUNG

Bronchiolitis refers to a wide variety of inflammatory and fibrotic disease processes affecting the small airways.[1–3] Bronchiolitis is common and may be the primary manifestation in various clinical settings (e.g., infections, connective tissue diseases (CTDs), inhalational injuries, cigarette smoking, drug reactions, and transplantation). Bronchiolitis, however, frequently occurs in association with large airway disease and in association with parenchymal and interstitial lung disease (Table 59.1). In this chapter the discussion is limited to conditions that primarily affect the bronchioles. Bronchiolitis associated with large airway disease and with diffuse parenchymal and interstitial lung diseases, such as hypersensitivity pneumonitis and organizing pneumonia, is discussed elsewhere.

Bronchiolitis is the most common form of small airways disease. Multiple classification systems have been proposed, some of which are based on the clinical features along with the presumed etiology and the pulmonary or systemic diseases with which it is associated, some on computed tomography (CT) findings and others on histologic features. Histologic classification into cellular (proliferative) or constrictive (fibrotic) bronchiolitis is valuable as it correlates most directly with the imaging features of small airways disease.[2–5] Given the nonspecific nature of histologic findings, interpretation in the context of the clinical and radiologic findings is crucial.[2] Therefore, in this chapter, we use a classification system based on histologic features in the clinical and radiologic contexts (Table 59.2).

Anatomic Features of the Small Airways and Secondary Pulmonary Lobule

Small airways by definition are airways having a diameter of less than 2 mm.[6] Those include membranous bronchioles, respiratory bronchioles, and alveolar ducts. Membranous bronchioles measure between 0.5 and 1 mm in diameter and are characterized by the absence of cartilage. They are lined by ciliated columnar epithelium and nonciliated Clara cells, surrounded by a layer of smooth muscle, which diminishes distally, and a layer of adventitia. Few goblet cells and seromucinous glands may be present. Terminal bronchioles, the final generation of membranous bronchioles, mark the end of the conducting division of airflow in the lungs and give rise to respiratory bronchioles, which are the beginning of the respiratory division where gaseous exchange occurs.[2,3,6,7] Respiratory bronchioles can arise from terminal bronchioles or from other respiratory bronchioles and then branch into multiple alveolar ducts, alveolar sacs, and alveoli. An acinus is formed by a terminal bronchiole—with its first-order respiratory bronchioles, their branching alveolar ducts, alveolar sacs, and alveoli—and is a functional unit of the lung in which all airways participate in gas exchange.

Bronchioles maintain their mechanical support, structure, and patency through a complex network of elastic fibers attaching bronchioles to each other and to neighboring alveoli. This network is particularly important for maintaining small airway patency during expiration. Collateral ventilation occurs via small accessory channels connecting various portions of the distal small airways. Canals of Lambert provide direct connections between some membranous bronchioles and adjacent alveoli, channels of Martin provide direct interbronchiolar connections, and pores of Kohn provide interalveolar connections.[3,6,7]

The secondary pulmonary lobule (SPL) is the smallest functioning subunit of lung. It consists of 3 to 10 acini enclosed by an interlobular septum of connective tissue and measures 1 to 2.5 cm.[6,8,9] The bronchioles and their accompanying pulmonary artery branches are located near the center of SPLs, and the pulmonary veins are located in the interlobular septa. Thorough understanding of these anatomic features is imperative for accurate radiologic interpretation (Figs. 59.1 and 59.2). Normal bronchioles cannot be identified on CT because of size limitations. The smallest intralobular structures visible on CT are intralobular pulmonary arteries measuring approximately 0.2 mm in diameter, which corresponds to the tip of the terminal bronchiole and the first-generation respiratory bronchiole (Fig. 59.3).[6] Therefore the centrilobular portion is recognized as an area around the tip of the visible pulmonary artery on CT.[10]

Imaging of Small Airways Disease

Conventional radiography is often insensitive for detecting small airways disease, particularly in the early and localized phases of disease. Over the past several decades, technologic advances in CT have revolutionized imaging of the small airways. High-resolution volumetric datasets allow the generation of high-quality, multiplanar, and three-dimensional images. Low-dose volumetric expiratory high-resolution computed tomography (HRCT) is invaluable in detecting small airway obstruction.[11] When used in conjunction, inspiratory and expiratory techniques provide the most reliable assessment of both the extent and severity of disease. Interpretation of characteristic radiologic findings in the appropriate clinical context is often sufficient for clinical diagnosis and initiation of treatment without biopsy confirmation, thus avoiding unnecessary invasive procedures. CT has also become a reliable, noninvasive method for assessing response to therapy without the need for repeated biopsy.[6,7,11]

Magnetic resonance imaging (MRI) has also undergone significant progress over the past decade with efforts to overcome the limitations of other imaging modalities. Technical advances in hardware, sequencing, and contrast media have significantly improved the quality of morphologic and functional MRI assessment of airway pathology. Although MRI utility in the evaluation

*The editors and publisher would like to thank Drs. C. Isabela Silva Müller and Nestor L. Müller for contributing material on this topic to the prior edition of this work. It has served as the foundation for the current chapter.

TABLE 59.1 BRONCHIOLITIS ASSOCIATED WITH LARGE AIRWAY, PULMONARY PARENCHYMAL, AND INTERSTITIAL DISEASE

Bronchiolitis Associated With Large Airways Disease	Bronchiolitis Associated With Parenchymal and Interstitial Lung Disease
Chronic bronchitis/ chronic obstructive pulmonary disease	Hypersensitivity pneumonitis
Asthma	Respiratory bronchiolitis–associated interstitial lung disease
Bronchiectasis	Desquamative interstitial pneumonia
	Lymphoid interstitial pneumonia
	Organizing pneumonia

TABLE 59.2 HISTOLOGIC CLASSIFICATION OF BRONCHIOLITIS INTO CELLULAR (PROLIFERATIVE) OR CONSTRICTIVE (FIBROTIC) BRONCHIOLITIS

Cellular Bronchiolitis	Constrictive Bronchiolitis
Infectious bronchiolitis	Postinfectious
Aspiration bronchiolitis	Transplantation
Respiratory bronchiolitis	Connective tissue diseases
Follicular bronchiolitis	Inhalational lung diseases
Diffuse panbronchiolitis	Diffuse idiopathic pulmonary neuroendocrine cell hyperplasia
	Miscellaneous

of small airways disease is still being researched, it has proven valuable in several other clinical settings, particularly with obstructive airway diseases, including cystic fibrosis.[11]

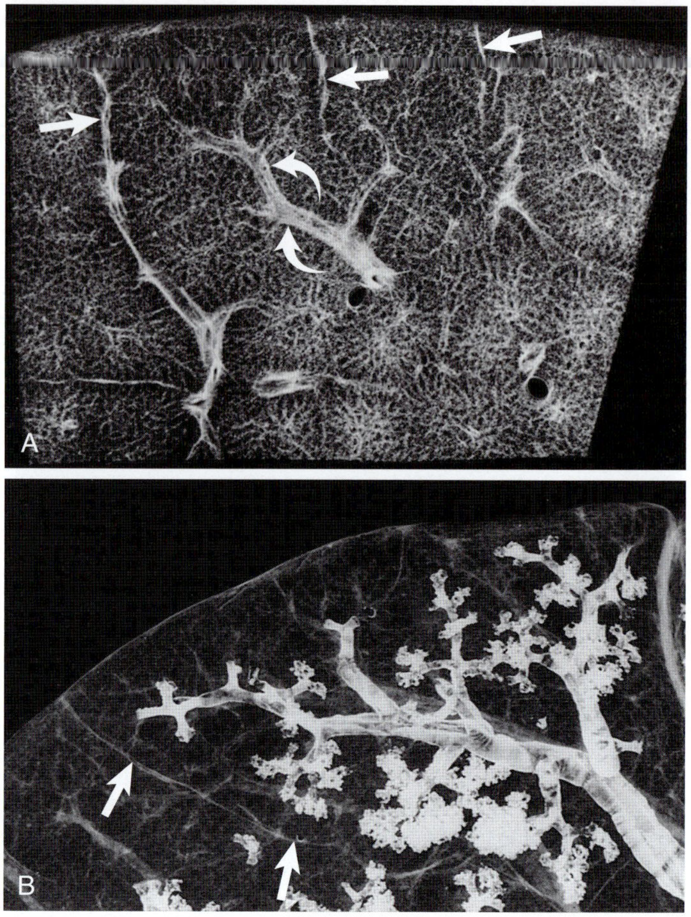

Fig. 59.1 Normal pulmonary lobule: anatomy of the bronchioles and secondary pulmonary lobules (SPLs). (A) Radiograph of a 1-mm-thick lung slice shows interlobular septa *(straight arrows)* marginating the SPLs. The lobular and terminal bronchioles *(curved arrows)* and adjacent pulmonary arteries can be seen to course near the center of the pulmonary lobule. (B) Radiograph of specimen with bronchioles filled with barium shows the pattern of centrilobular branching lines and nodular opacities that can be expected from bronchiolar and peribronchiolar inflammation. The bronchioles and alveolar ducts are located a few millimeters away from the pleural surface and interlobular septa *(arrows)*. *(Courtesy Dr. Harumi Itoh, Department of Radiology, Fukui Medical University, Fukui, Japan. From Müller NL, Fraser RS, Colman NC, Paré PD.* Radiologic Diagnosis of Diseases of the Chest. *Philadelphia: WB Saunders; 2001.)*

DIRECT AND INDIRECT SIGNS ON COMPUTED TOMOGRAPHY

Although normal bronchioles cannot be visualized, bronchiolar diseases may result in direct and indirect signs on CT.[4,12] Direct signs occur resulting from bronchiolar secretions, wall thickening, or peribronchiolar inflammation and include centrilobular nodules, branching centrilobular opacities (tree-in-bud), and occasional small centrilobular lucencies resulting from bronchiolectasis (Fig. 59.4).[4,12] Centrilobular opacities can be recognized because they are centered 3 mm or more from the periphery of the secondary lobule—that is, from the interlobular septa, pleura, and large pulmonary vessels. Indirect signs include areas of decreased attenuation and vascularity (mosaic attenuation) on inspiratory CT and areas of air-trapping on expiratory CT (Fig. 59.5).[4,7,12] The presence of both direct and indirect signs on CT is sensitive and specific for diagnosing small airways disease (Table 59.3).[3,4,6,8]

TABLE 59.3 DIRECT AND INDIRECT COMPUTED TOMOGRAPHY MANIFESTATIONS OF SMALL AIRWAYS DISEASE

Direct Signs	Indirect Signs
Centrilobular nodules (solid and/ or ground-glass attenuation)	Mosaic attenuation (inspiratory CT)
Tree-in-bud opacities	Air-trapping (expiratory CT)
Bronchiolectasis	

CT, Computed tomography.

Accurate interpretation of direct and indirect signs on CT can be challenging, Indirect signs, in particular, warrant further elaboration. By definition, mosaic attenuation is an imaging pattern on inspiratory CT with differing lung attenuation as a result of variable aeration and vascular perfusion, resulting in a heterogeneous parenchymal appearance. It is associated with a broad differential diagnosis, most commonly with diseases affecting the small airways, pulmonary vasculature, alveoli, and interstitium, alone or in combination.[7] Parenchymal lung disease is the most common cause of mosaic attenuation, seen in approximately 50% of cases, followed by small airways disease constituting nearly 33% of cases.[7,13,14] Mild mosaic attenuation can be seen in up to 20% of normal patients. Parenchymal heterogeneity is gradient dependent, with the more dependent portions of the lung being of slightly higher attenuation. Perfusion heterogeneity, with increased perfusion and attenuation more centrally than peripherally, may also be seen.[7,15,16]

Concurrent expiratory imaging for evaluation of air-trapping is the best method for differentiating between the different causes of mosaic attenuation. In a normal expiratory CT, lung attenuation

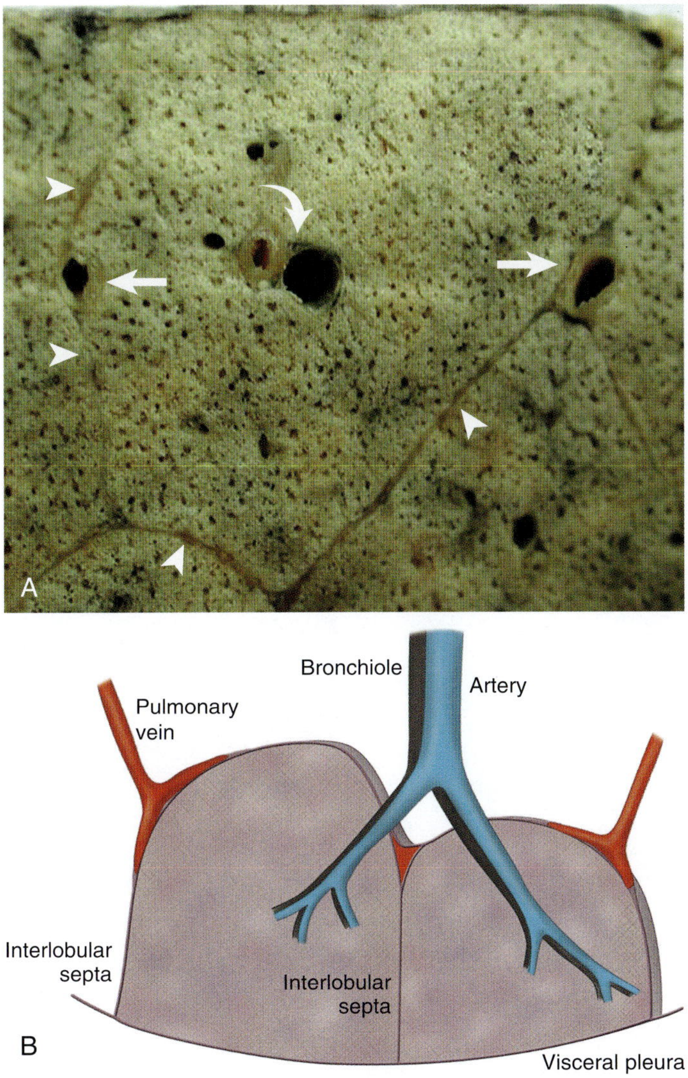

Fig. 59.2 Normal pulmonary lobule. (A) Lung specimen shows secondary lobule surrounded by connective tissue septa *(arrowheads)*. The lobular bronchiole and pulmonary artery *(curved arrow)* are located in the center of the lobule, and the draining pulmonary veins *(straight arrows)* are located in the interlobular septa. (B) Schematic representation shows normal anatomy of two adjacent pulmonary lobules. *(A, Courtesy Dr. Reynaldo T. Rodrigues, Federal University of São Paulo, São Paulo, Brazil.)*

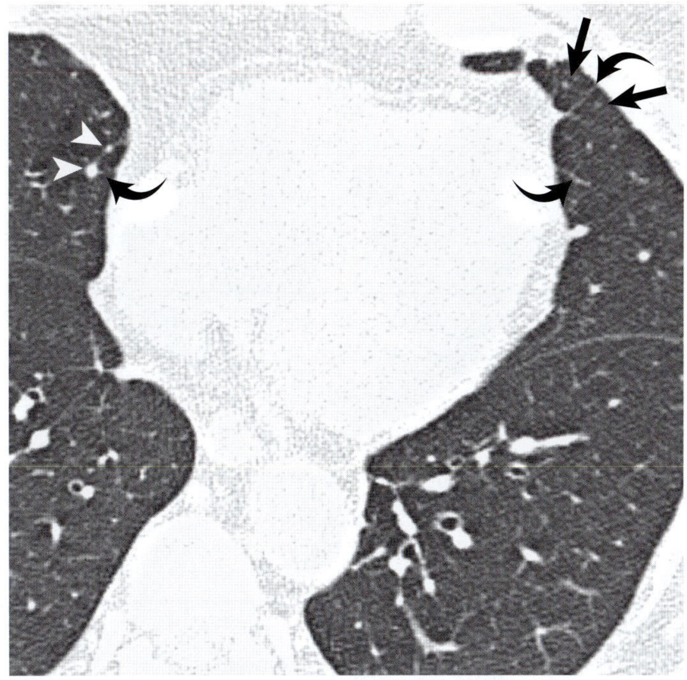

Fig. 59.3 Normal lobules and vessels on high-resolution CT (HRCT). HRCT shows normal interlobular septa *(curved arrows)*. Two pulmonary veins *(arrowheads)* can be seen as focal opacities within interlobular septa in the right middle lobe. The nodular opacity *(straight arrows)* in the center of the lobule corresponds to the lobular artery. The adjacent lobular bronchiole is not seen because its wall is too thin to be identified on CT.

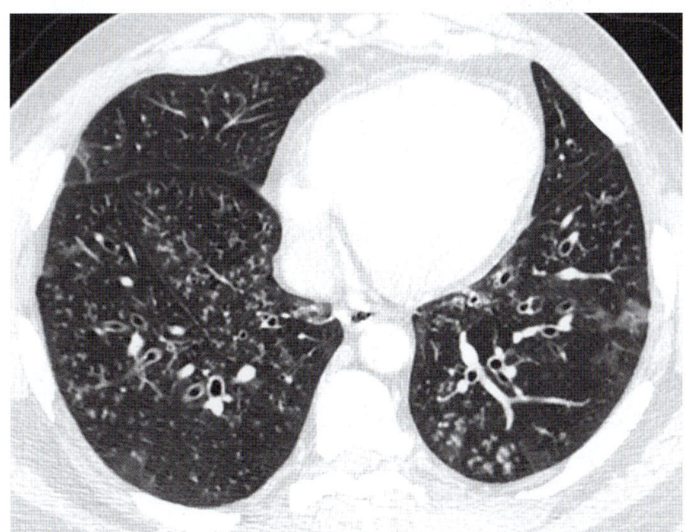

Fig. 59.4 Direct signs of bronchiolitis in a patient with recurrent infection. Axial CT shows several direct signs of small airways disease with centrilobular nodules, tree-in-bud opacities, and peripheral centrilobular lucencies consistent with bronchiolectasis. Cylindrical bronchiectasis is also noted more centrally.

increases as the proportion of air to tissue decreases with expiration of air. The Fleischner Society defines air-trapping as "parenchymal areas with less than normal increase in attenuation and lack of volume reduction" as seen on end expiration CT scans (see Fig. 59.5B).[17] These areas appear as polygonal regions of low attenuation adjacent to areas of lung that have the normal increased attenuation with expiration. A simple measure of the degree of air-trapping is subdivision into mild (25%), moderate (25%–50%), and severe (50%) air-trapping, based on a subjective estimation of the total lung volume of air-trapped lung.[18] If air-trapping is present on expiratory CT with concurrent mosaic attenuation on inspiratory CT, then small airways disease is the most likely culprit, with the hyperlucent foci representing the diseased portions of the lung (Fig. 59.6).[7] In fact, small airways disease is the most common cause of mosaic attenuation where the hyperlucent lung is the abnormal finding. As with inspiratory imaging, a similar physiologic gradient of parenchymal heterogeneity is seen on expiratory imaging. Additionally, areas of lobular air-trapping can be seen in 40% to 80% of normal patients on CT. Several studies have shown mild, moderate, and sometimes even extensive air-trapping in individuals with normal pulmonary function tests.[19,20]

The specific clinicopathologic forms of bronchiolitis are discussed in the following sections.

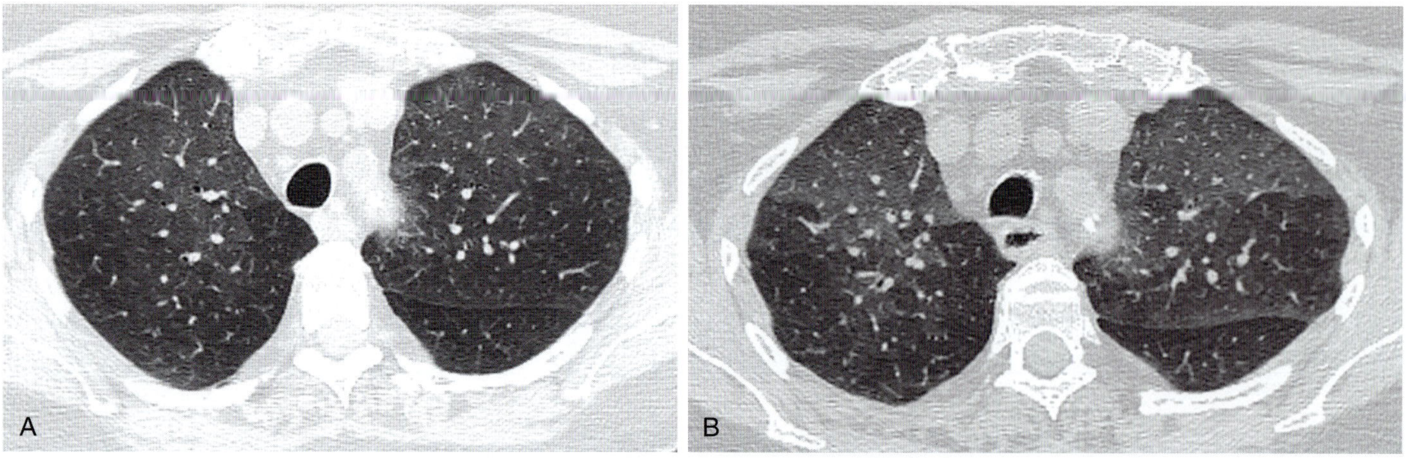

Fig. 59.5 Indirect signs in a patient with constrictive bronchiolitis. (A) Image acquired at full inspiration, as indicated by the cylindrical tracheal contour, demonstrates a heterogeneous parenchymal appearance (mosaic attenuation pattern) with decreased vascular caliber peripherally in the hypoattenuated lung. (B) Concurrent expiratory phase imaging shows exaggerated segmental hypoattenuation in the dependent portions of the lung, consistent with air-trapping.

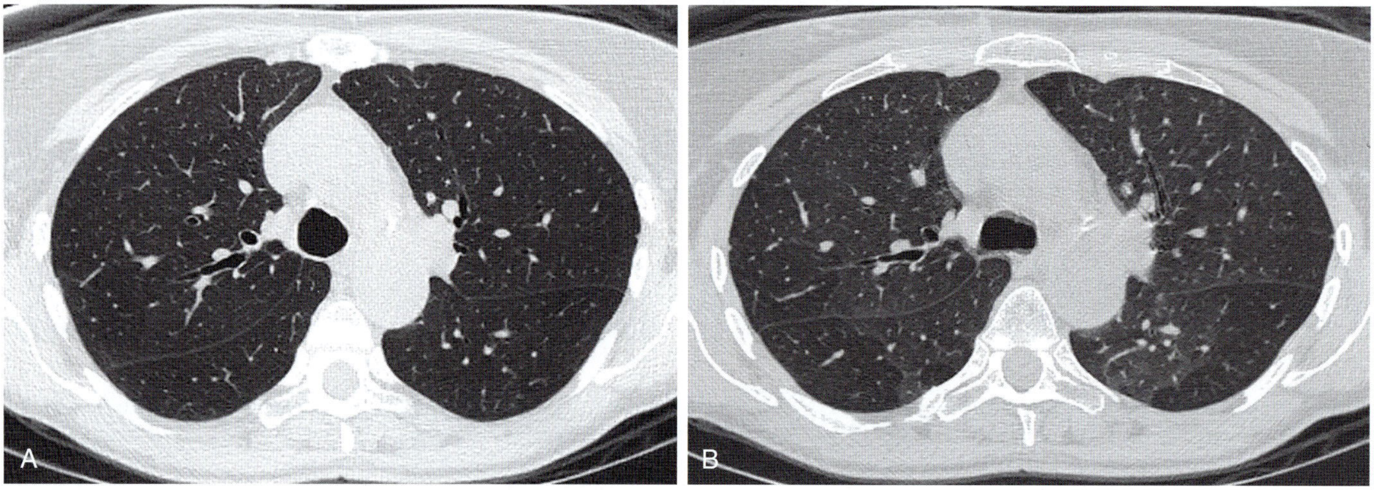

Fig. 59.6 Indirect signs of constrictive bronchiolitis in hematopoietic stem cell transplantation. (A) Inspiratory CT acquired just above the carina demonstrates relatively normal appearance to the lung parenchyma. (B) Expiratory CT demonstrates widespread low attenuation within the lungs and small vascular caliber within the hypoattenuated lung, consistent with air-trapping and hypoxic oligemia.

KEY POINTS: COMPUTED TOMOGRAPHY FINDINGS OF BRONCHIOLITIS

- Direct signs
  - Cause: bronchiolar secretions, bronchiolar wall thickening, peribronchiolar inflammation
  - Manifestation: centrilobular nodules, tree-in-bud opacities, bronchiolectasis
- Indirect signs
  - Cause: small airway obstruction
  - Manifestations: mosaic attenuation on inspiratory CT, air-trapping on expiratory CT

Cellular Bronchiolitis

INFECTIOUS BRONCHIOLITIS

Etiology

Acute infectious bronchiolitis is most common and severe in children, most often caused by viruses (e.g., adenovirus, respiratory syncytial virus), followed by *Mycoplasma* pneumonia. Less common etiologies include *Chlamydia,* bacteria, and fungi, particularly *Aspergillus* in immunocompromised patients.[12,21,22]

Clinical Presentation

Infants and young children usually present with symptoms of an upper respiratory tract infection, followed by dyspnea, tachypnea, and fever approximately 2 to 3 days later; cyanosis and extreme weakness may be seen in severe cases. Adults are probably infected with respiratory viral infections as often as infants are; however, the severity and consequences of infection in otherwise healthy individuals are usually much less, likely because their small airways contribute less to total pulmonary resistance.[23] Nonetheless, severe and sometimes fatal disease can occur.

Pathophysiology

Histologically, inflammatory cells (mainly neutrophils) are present within the airway walls and in inflammatory exudate and mucus in the airway lumens (Fig. 59.7).[12] These findings account for the direct signs on CT.[12] Bronchiolar epithelial necrosis may occur in severe cases.[24] Biopsy is rarely required for diagnosis.

Manifestations of the Disease

Radiography. Conventional radiography in infants and children may demonstrate bronchial wall thickening (peribronchial cuffing) and peribronchial (central) areas of consolidation.[25] Other findings include hyperinflation (caused by partial small airway obstruction) and patchy bilateral consolidations (indicating progression to bronchopneumonia).[26] In adults findings are often subtle, manifesting as multifocal nodular or reticulonodular opacities. As with children, progression to bronchopneumonia results in patchy bilateral consolidations (Fig. 59.8).[27,28]

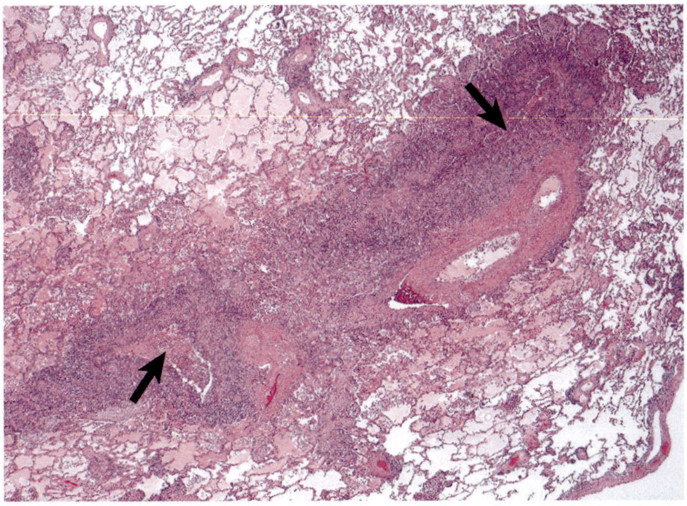

Fig. 59.7 Infectious bronchiolitis: histologic findings. Low-power view shows severe bronchiolitis with an intense lymphoplasmacytic infiltrate in the bronchiolar wall and around the airway. The bronchiolar lumen *(arrows)* contains neutrophils. *(Courtesy Dr. Andrew Churg, Department of Pathology, University of British Columbia, Vancouver, Canada.)*

Computed Tomography/High-Resolution Computed Tomography. Characteristic CT findings include small well-defined centrilobular nodules and tree-in-bud opacities, which can be patchy and unilateral or asymmetric and bilateral. While tree-in-bud opacities, in particular, are highly suggestive of endobronchial spread of small airways infection, they can also been seen with noninfectious etiologies (e.g., aspiration, cystic fibrosis, follicular bronchiolitis).[29–31] Progression to bronchopneumonia results in 5- to 10-mm-diameter airspace nodules and patchy lobular, subsegmental, or segmental ground-glass opacities and consolidations (Fig. 59.9).

Differential Diagnosis

Similar histologic and CT findings may be seen with aspiration or with CTDs, inflammatory bowel disease, and allergic bronchopulmonary aspergillosis.[2,10,29,30,32–34] Acute infectious and/or aspiration bronchiolitis (AB) frequently occur in the setting of preexisting bronchiectasis.[2]

ASPIRATION BRONCHIOLITIS

Etiology, Prevalence, and Epidemiology

AB refers to chronic inflammation of the bronchioles secondary to chronic and recurrent aspiration of gastric and other foreign material. The disease primarily affects individuals with oropharyngeal dysphagia and other patients at high risk for aspiration (elderly, neurologic disorders, dementia). AB may also manifest acutely in certain clinical scenarios, such as in patients presenting

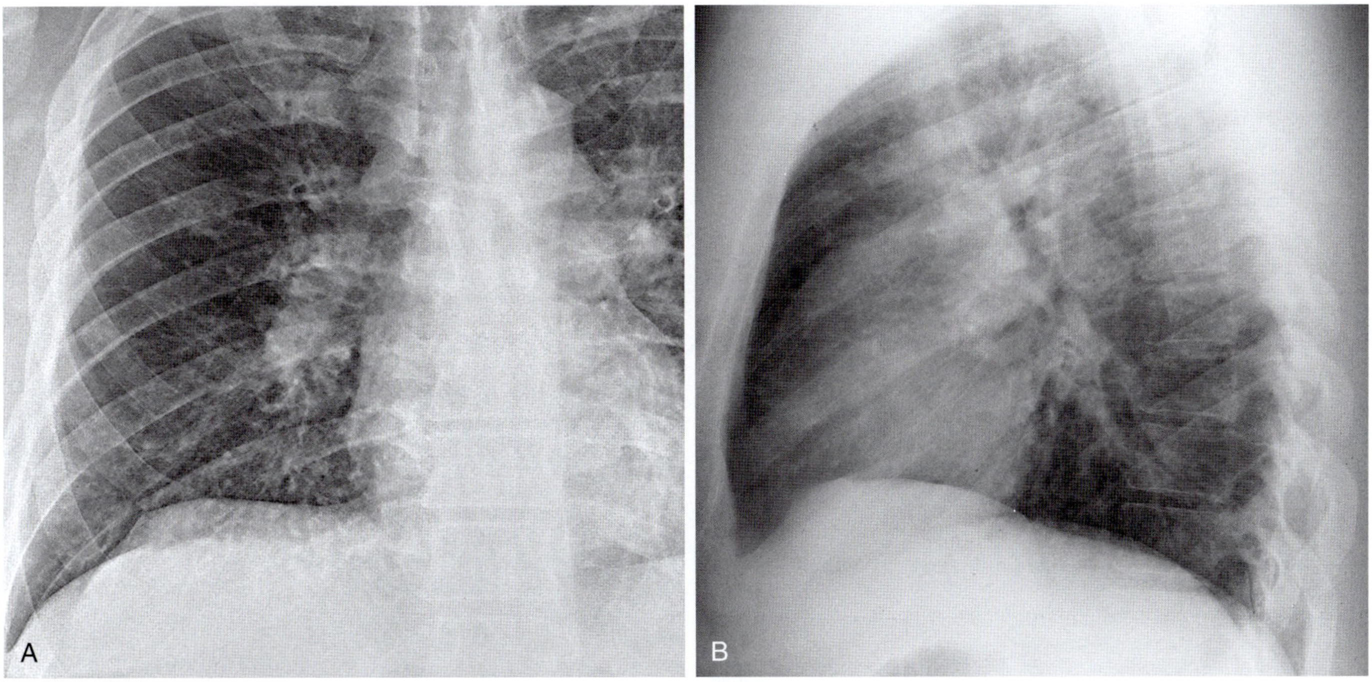

Fig. 59.8 Chest radiograph findings in an adult with respiratory syncytial virus infectious bronchiolitis. (A) Coned posteroanterior and (B) lateral chest radiographs show bilateral multifocal hazy and reticulonodular opacities and peribronchial cuffing.

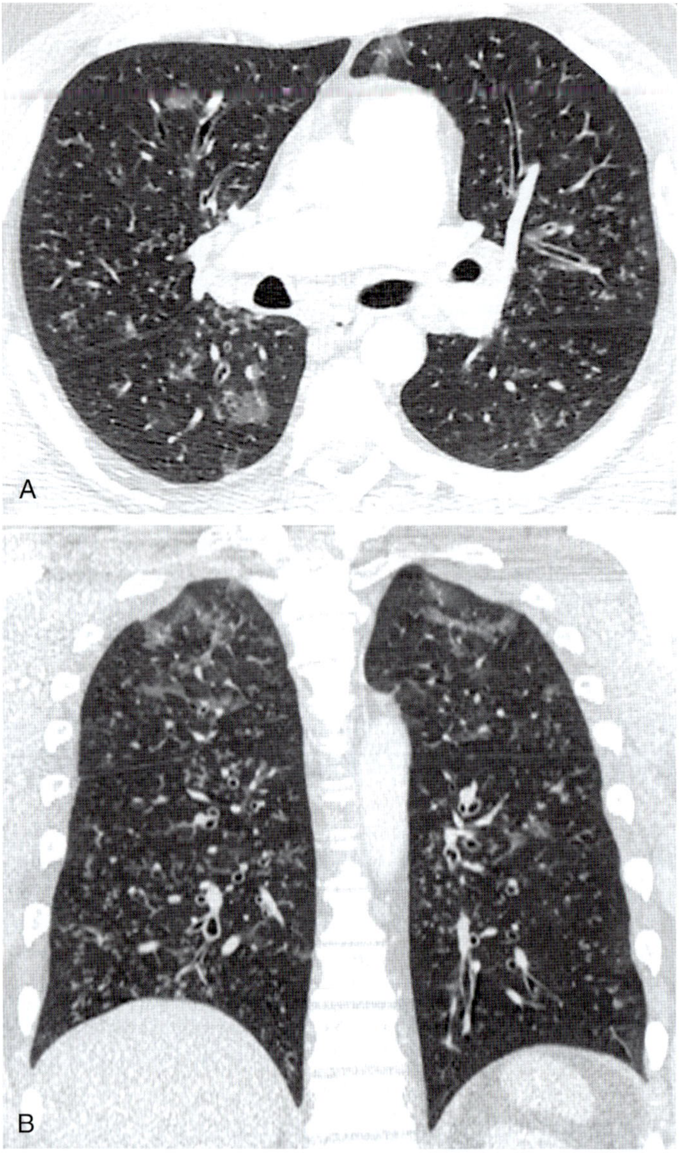

Fig. 59.9 CT findings in respiratory syncytial virus bronchiolitis. (A) Axial CT shows multifocal bilateral centrilobular nodules, tree-in-bud opacities, and a few patchy areas of ground-glass opacity. (B) Coronal CT better demonstrates the diffuse distribution of the disease process, with coalescing upper lobe lobular ground-glass opacities, consistent with developing bronchopneumonia.

KEY POINTS: INFECTIOUS BRONCHIOLITIS

- Etiology
  - Viruses, *Mycoplasma*, bacteria (early bronchopneumonia), and fungi (particularly *Aspergillus*)
- Symptoms
  - Often severe in infants; usually mild in adults
- Radiographic findings
  - Children: peribronchial cuffing, hyperinflation
  - Adults: bilateral nodular/reticulonodular opacities
  - Patchy bilateral consolidations indicating bronchopneumonia
- Computed tomography/high-resolution computed tomography
  - Centrilobular nodules, tree-in-bud opacities, patchy ground-glass opacities, or consolidations
  - Tree-in-bud opacities highly suggestive of small airways infection

with drug overdose–related respiratory depression, acute trauma, or altered mental status resulting from strokes or seizures.[3,35]

Clinical Presentation

Patients usually present with signs of persistent airway disease, such as increased secretions and sputum production, productive cough, wheezing, and dyspnea, all of which are exacerbated by oral intake.[32,35]

Pathophysiology

Histologic findings are very similar to infectious bronchiolitis, with bronchial and bronchiolar inflammation, bronchial wall thickening, and inflammatory exudate and mucus in the airway lumens.

Manifestations of the Disease

Radiography. Conventional radiographic findings are nonspecific and manifest as unilateral or bilateral small nodular and/or patchy opacities with or without lung hyperinflation (Fig. 59.10).

Computed Tomography/High-Resolution Computed Tomography. As with infectious bronchiolitis, diffuse small centrilobular nodules and tree-in-bud opacities are present, which can be patchy and unilateral or asymmetric and bilateral. Patchy lobular consolidations are often present and frequently progress to confluent segmental or lobar consolidations. A distinguishing feature of aspiration is the pattern of distribution within the lungs, which is dependent on patient positioning at time of aspiration. Bedridden patients who remain in a supine position will often present with disease affecting the posterior dependent segments of the upper and lower lobes, hospitalized patients who remain in a midline semiupright position will present with lower lobe–predominant disease, and patients who spend most of their time lying on their right or left side will present with disease involving the right-dependent lung or left-dependent lung, respectively (see Fig. 59.10).[3,22,32]

KEY POINTS: ASPIRATION BRONCHIOLITIS

- Etiology
  - Aspiration of gastric and/or other foreign material
- Symptoms
  - Persistent airway disease and productive cough exacerbated by oral intake
- Radiographic findings
  - Unilateral or bilateral nodular or patchy opacities, +/– hyperinflation
  - Frequent patchy bilateral consolidations indicating bronchopneumonia
- Computed tomography/high-resolution computed tomography
  - Centrilobular nodules, tree-in-bud opacities, patchy ground-glass opacities or consolidations
  - Distribution dependent on patient positioning at time of aspiration

RESPIRATORY BRONCHIOLITIS

Etiology, Prevalence, Epidemiology, and Clinical Presentation

Respiratory bronchiolitis (RB) is predominantly a smoking-related entity, which can occur rarely in nonsmokers or with other inhalational exposures, such as asbestos, nonasbestos dusts, and various fumes.[36] RB is present histologically in virtually all smokers and by definition is not associated with symptoms or functional

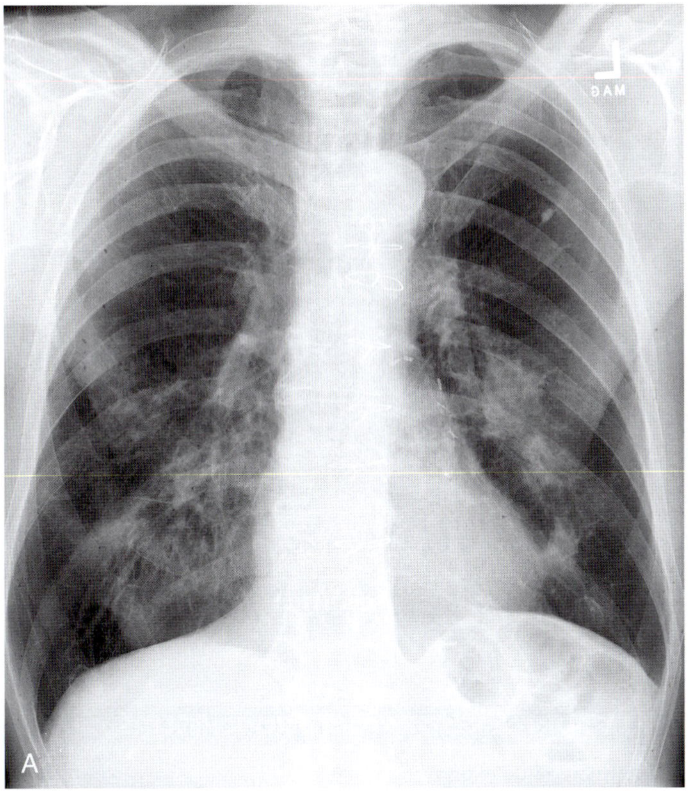

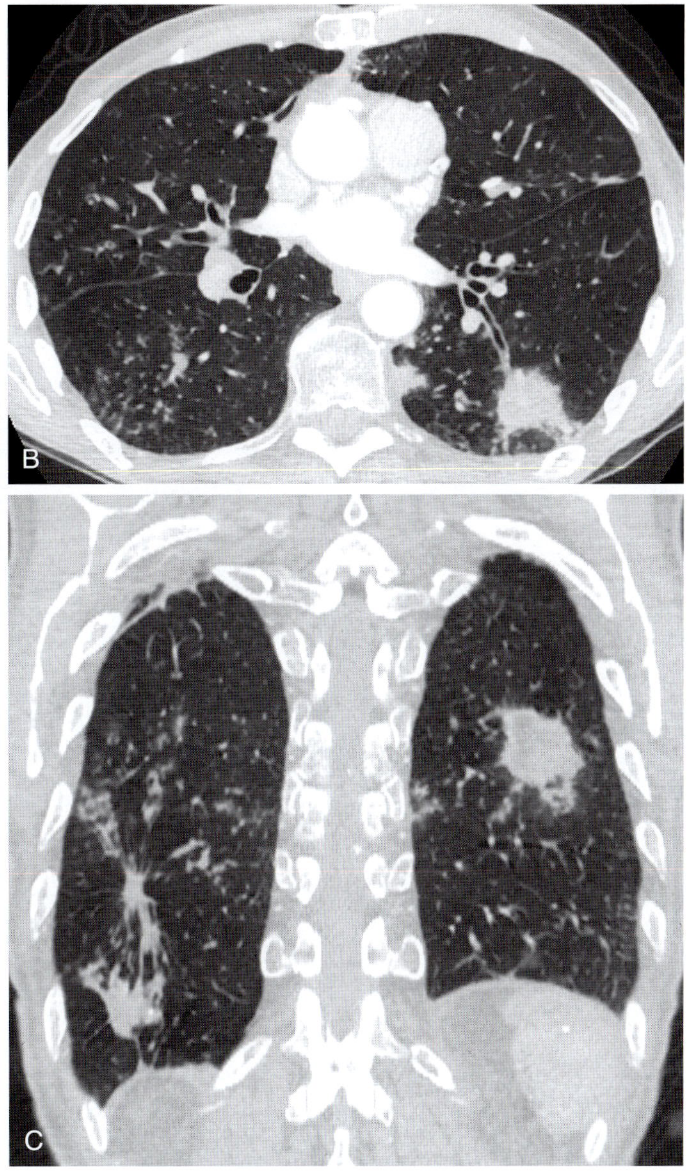

Fig. 59.10 Aspiration pneumonia: radiographic and CT findings. (A) Frontal radiograph shows left greater than right middle– and lower lung zone–predominant consolidations and reticulonodular opacities. (B) Axial CT confirms the radiographic findings, showing bilateral centrilobular nodules, tree-in-bud opacities, patchy ground-glass opacities, and left lower lobe nodular opacities. (C) Coronal CT demonstrates the positional-dependent distribution, with nodular opacities developing predominantly in the dependent posterior and lateral basal segments of the lower lobes, a characteristic finding frequently seen with aspiration pneumonia.

impairment. When involvement is symptomatic or leads to functional decline, the process is referred to as RB-associated interstitial lung disease, discussed separately in further detail (see Chapter 34).[37]

Pathophysiology

RB is characterized histologically by intraluminal and peribronchiolar accumulation of macrophages that contain a finely granular yellow-brown cytoplasmic pigment referred to as smoker's macrophages (Fig. 59.11).[37–39] Other common findings include chronic peribronchiolar mononuclear cell infiltration, mild inflammation, airspace enlargement with fibrosis, and diffuse hyaline-like acellular fibrotic thickening of alveolar septa.[8,21,40] The intensity of macrophage pigmentation and peribronchiolar fibrosis correlates with the number of pack-years smoked.[38] Emphysema is almost always present.[37]

Manifestations of the Disease

Radiography. RB rarely results in any demonstrable abnormality on chest radiography. Subtle upper lung zone–predominant lucencies (representing emphysema), peribronchial cuffing, and small poorly defined nodular or patchy opacities may be present in some patients.

Computed Tomography/High-Resolution Computed Tomography. CT is usually normal or may show mild centrilobular and/or paraseptal emphysema.[41] When present, findings include small, multifocal, poorly defined ground-glass centrilobular nodules; patchy ground-glass opacities; and mosaic attenuation (Fig. 59.12).[42,43] Findings most commonly are upper lung zone predominant, however, and may be diffuse in some patients. Several studies have shown that smoking cessation does not always lead to complete resolution of the radiologic and pathologic features of RB, with the extent of disease often remaining similar among current smokers and ex-smokers, even years after smoking cessation.[36,38,42,43]

Differential Diagnosis

The differential diagnosis for RB on CT includes hypersensitivity pneumonitis (HP), follicular bronchiolitis (FB), infectious bronchiolitis, cholesterol granulomas, pulmonary capillary

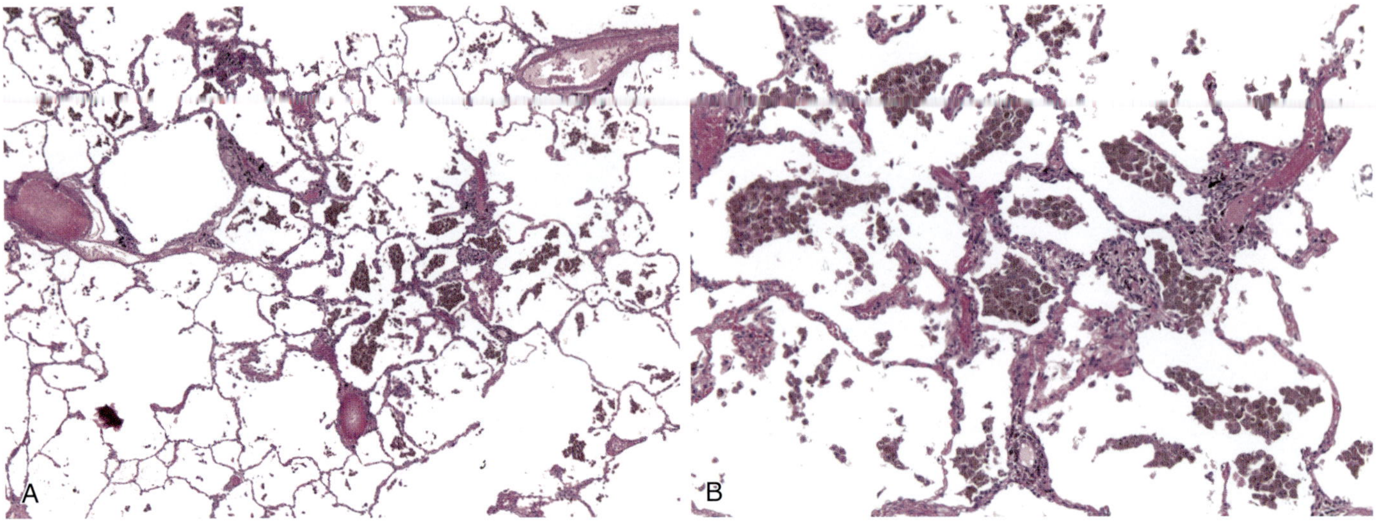

Fig. 59.11 Respiratory bronchiolitis: histologic findings. (A) Histologic specimen shows peribronchiolar airspace clusters of pigmented (smoker's) macrophages. The appearance is characteristic of respiratory bronchiolitis. (B) Magnified view better demonstrates the typical appearance of the pigmented macrophages. *(Courtesy Dr. John English, Department of Pathology, Vancouver General Hospital, Vancouver, Canada.)*

hemangiomatosis, and occasionally pneumoconioses.[8,9] Significant radiologic overlap may be seen with cases of RB and the subacute inflammatory phase of HP, which includes centrilobular ground-glass nodules, patchy ground-glass opacities, and mosaic attenuation on inspiratory CT. Although CT manifestations may be diffuse in both conditions, RB tends to produce a more upper lung zone–predominant pattern when compared with HP. Conversely, focal/lobular air-trapping is more commonly seen with HP on expiratory CT.[8,44] Thus an upper lung zone–predominant or diffuse imaging pattern with concurrent findings of emphysema favors the diagnosis of RB, although diffuse parenchymal involvement with areas of lobular air-trapping favors subacute HP. However, as RB and HP are clinically and histologically distinct entities, a multidisciplinary approach integrating clinical history, histology, and imaging findings is imperative for accurate diagnosis. Recent studies have shown that the combination of smoking history, typical CT findings, and lack of lymphocytosis on bronchoalveolar lavage is highly suggestive of RB.[8,45] Furthermore, cigarette smoking has been shown to have a protective effect against the development of HP. For example, in a study of 400 consecutive patients with various interstitial lung diseases, only 6% of 116 patients with a final diagnosis of hypersensitivity pneumonitis were smokers, compared with 20% of the 284 remaining patients.[46] Cholesterol granulomas and pulmonary capillary hemangiomatosis are two entities seen in the setting of pulmonary hypertension that may also manifest with centrilobular ground-glass nodules. Of importance, these entities should be considered when centrilobular ground-glass nodules are seen in conjunction with known pulmonary hypertension or an enlarged pulmonary trunk on CT.

KEY POINTS: RESPIRATORY BRONCHIOLITIS

- Etiology/definition
  - Accumulation of pigmented macrophages in the lumen of respiratory bronchioles and adjacent alveoli
  - Almost always associated with smoking
- Symptoms
  - By definition, not associated with symptoms or functional impairment
- Radiographic findings: usually normal
- Computed tomography/high-resolution tomography
  - Often normal or showing only emphysema
  - Poorly defined centrilobular nodules, patchy bilateral ground-glass opacities, predominantly in the upper lobes or diffuse

PULMONARY LYMPHOID HYPERPLASIA (FOLLICULAR BRONCHIOLITIS)

Etiology

Pulmonary lymphoid hyperplasia or FB is characterized by peribronchial and peribronchiolar inflammation secondary to the abundance of lymphoid follicles.[47] Several clinical conditions are associated with FB, which are identical to those seen with lymphoid interstitial pneumonia, most commonly in association with CTDs (particularly rheumatoid arthritis [RA] and Sjögren syndrome), immunologic disorders (Hashimoto thyroiditis, pernicious anemia, autoimmune hemolytic anemia, chronic active hepatitis, primary biliary cirrhosis, and myasthenia gravis), congenital or acquired immunodeficiency diseases (common variable immunodeficiency, human immunodeficiency virus/acquired immune deficiency syndrome), systemic hypersensitivity reactions, infection, allergy (including asthma), bone marrow transplantation, and as a reactive process distal to bronchiectasis or in association with middle lobe syndrome.[3,47–49]

Clinical Presentation

FB occurs most frequently among middle-aged adults, presenting with progressive dyspnea and cough. Less common symptoms include fever, weight loss, and recurrent pneumonia. Pulmonary function tests may reveal an obstructive, restrictive, or mixed pattern. FB may occasionally be seen in children.

Pathophysiology

FB is characterized histologically by the presence of abundant lymphoid follicles in bronchiolar walls and, to some extent, along

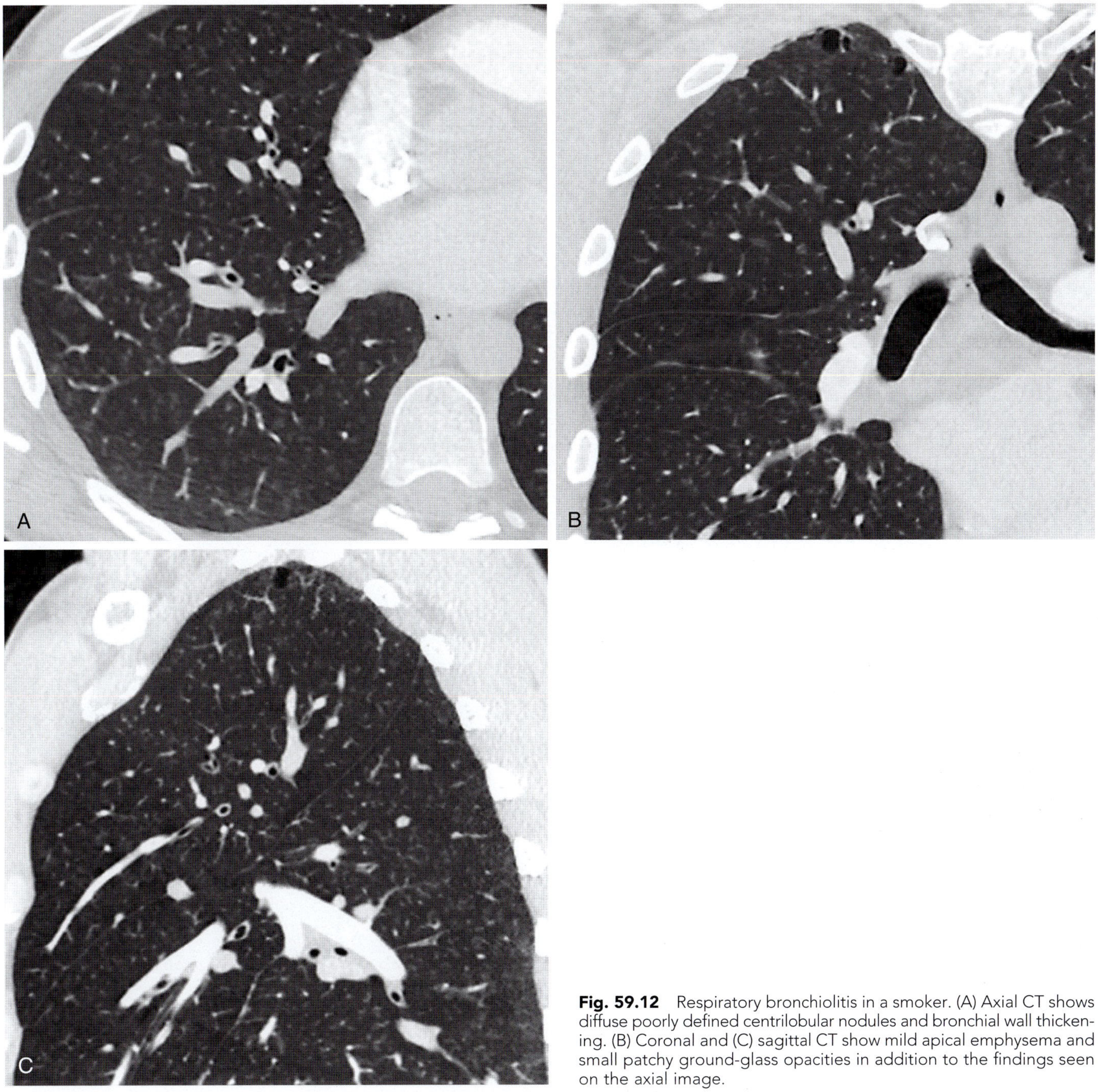

Fig. 59.12 Respiratory bronchiolitis in a smoker. (A) Axial CT shows diffuse poorly defined centrilobular nodules and bronchial wall thickening. (B) Coronal and (C) sagittal CT show mild apical emphysema and small patchy ground-glass opacities in addition to the findings seen on the axial image.

bronchi, interlobular septa, and pleura.[47] Obstructive pneumonia may sometimes occur as a result of airway compression.[49]

Manifestations of the Disease

Radiography. FB findings on radiography tend to be subtle, and in many cases the chest radiograph may be normal. When findings are present, they usually manifest as bilateral reticular or reticulonodular opacities (Fig. 59.13).[3,22,47]

Computed Tomography/High-Resolution Computed Tomography. Typical FB results in small diffuse and poorly defined centrilobular nodules. Other less common and variable findings include peribronchial and subpleural nodules, patchy ground-glass opacities, bronchial wall thickening, and mosaic attenuation. Expiratory CT may show lobular areas of air-trapping. In one study CT showed bilateral centrilobular nodules (100%), patchy ground-glass opacities (75%), peribronchial nodules (42%), and subpleural nodules (25%) (see Fig. 59.13).[3,50]

DIFFUSE PANBRONCHIOLITIS

Etiology, Prevalence, and Epidemiology

Diffuse panbronchiolitis is a progressive form of cellular bronchiolitis associated with chronic inflammation of the respiratory bronchioles and paranasal sinuses.[51] Etiology and pathogenesis remain unknown; however, the disease has been recognized almost exclusively in Asia, particularly in Japan. This distribution is

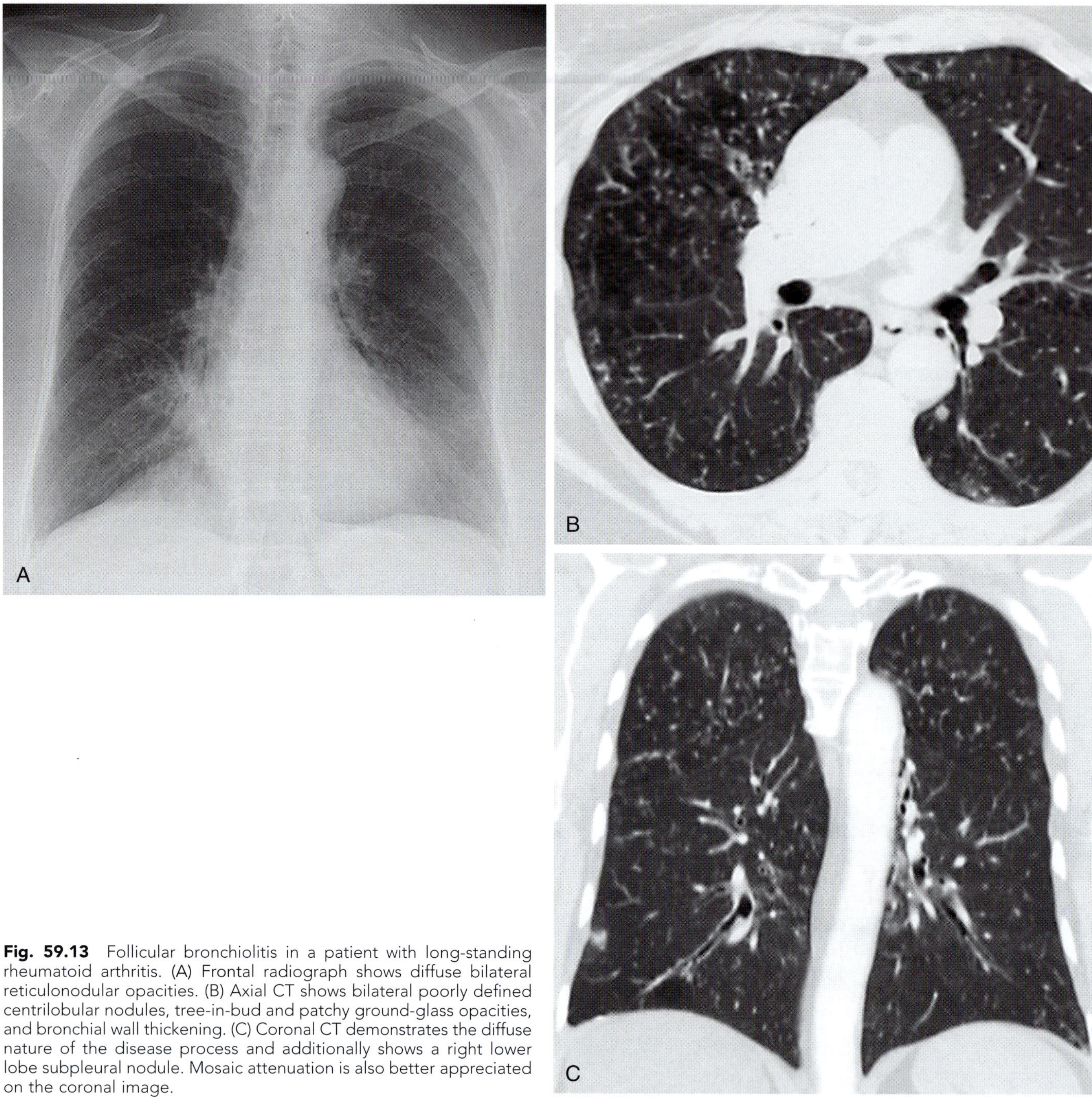

Fig. 59.13 Follicular bronchiolitis in a patient with long-standing rheumatoid arthritis. (A) Frontal radiograph shows diffuse bilateral reticulonodular opacities. (B) Axial CT shows bilateral poorly defined centrilobular nodules, tree-in-bud and patchy ground-glass opacities, and bronchial wall thickening. (C) Coronal CT demonstrates the diffuse nature of the disease process and additionally shows a right lower lobe subpleural nodule. Mosaic attenuation is also better appreciated on the coronal image.

KEY POINTS: PULMONARY LYMPHOID HYPERPLASIA (FOLLICULAR BRONCHIOLITIS)

- Etiology
  - Peribronchial and peribronchiolar inflammation resulting from abundance of lymphoid follicles
  - Associated with multiple clinical conditions: CTDs, most commonly rheumatoid arthritis, immunologic disorders, immunodeficiency, systemic hypersensitivity, infection, hematopoietic stem cell transplantation
- Symptoms
  - Progressive dyspnea and cough
  - Less commonly, fever, weight loss, recurrent pneumonia
- Radiographic findings
  - Often normal
  - Bilateral nodular or reticulonodular opacities
- Computed tomography/high-resolution tomography
  - Poorly defined small bilateral centrilobular nodules
  - Patchy bilateral ground-glass opacities
  - Peribronchial nodules/bronchial wall thickening
  - Subpleural nodules
  - Mosaic attenuation on inspiratory CT; lobular air-trapping on expiratory CT

believed to be highly associated with genetic predisposition located between human leukocyte antigens A and B loci.[52] The average age of onset is approximately 40 years; male-to-female ratio is approximately 2 : 1.[53]

Clinical Presentation

Diffuse panbronchiolitis manifests insidiously with productive cough and progressive dyspnea, worse on exertion. Features of chronic sinusitis are also typical. *Pseudomonas aeruginosa* frequently colonizes the respiratory tract of affected individuals. Pulmonary function tests reveal a marked obstructive and mild restrictive pattern.[22,54]

Pathophysiology

Histologically, mononuclear inflammatory cells (predominantly lymphocytes, plasma cells, and foamy histiocytes) are found within the walls of respiratory bronchioles, alveolar ducts, and, to a lesser extent, adjacent alveoli.[55] Mucus and aggregates of neutrophils may be seen within the airway lumen. The late stage of the disease is frequently complicated by *Pseudomonas aeruginosa* colonization, which is associated with a significantly worse prognosis. In one study the 10-year survival rate for those infected with the organism was only 12%, compared with 73% for those who remained uninfected.[56]

Manifestations of the Disease

Radiography. Chest radiography may show small diffuse nodular or reticulonodular opacities, peribronchial cuffing, and mild to moderate hyperinflation.

Computed Tomography/High-Resolution Computed Tomography. CT often shows diffuse small centrilobular nodules, tree-in-bud opacities, mosaic attenuation, bronchiolectasis, and bronchiectasis.[57] The presence of these findings correlates to the stage of the disease; the earliest manifestation consists of centrilobular nodules, followed by tree-in-bud opacities, bronchiolectasis, and eventually bronchiectasis. Cystic bronchiectasis may be seen in the late stage (Fig. 59.14).[58]

Treatment Options

The majority of patients respond to low-dose macrolide therapy (erythromycin, clarithromycin).[59] The beneficial effect of macrolides has been well established and is related to their antiinflammatory activity and is independent of their bactericidal effect.[60]

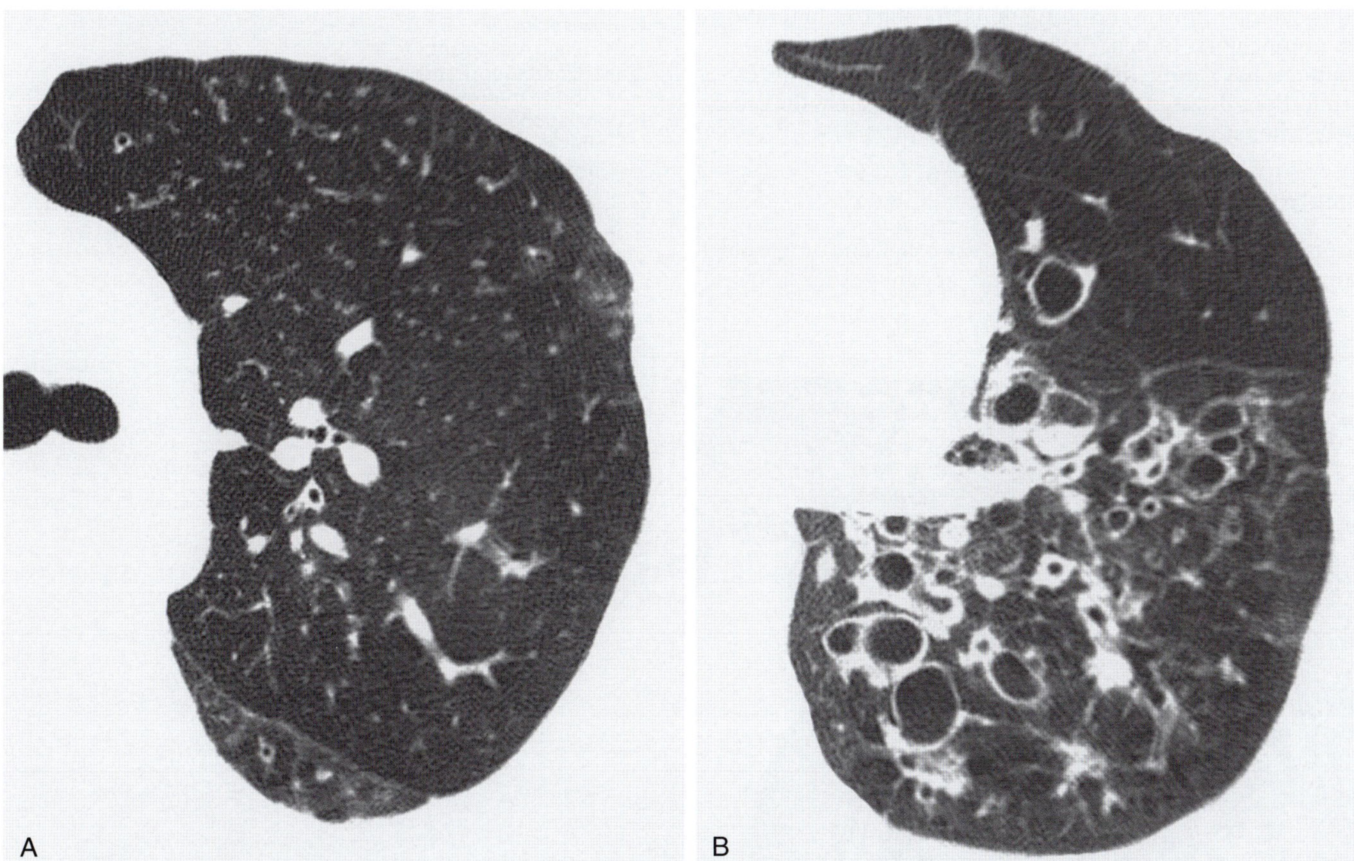

Fig. 59.14 Diffuse panbronchiolitis: high-resolution CT findings. (A) View of the left upper lobe from a high-resolution CT scan shows extensive areas of decreased attenuation and vascularity, mild bronchiectasis, and a few centrilobular nodules and branching opacities. (B) View of the left lung at the level of the inferior pulmonary vein shows varicose and cystic bronchiectasis in the left lower lobe and lingula. Also noted is diffuse decreased attenuation and vascularity in the lingula. *(Courtesy Dr. Noriyuki Tomiyama, Department of Radiology, Osaka University Graduate School of Medicine, Osaka, Japan.)*

KEY POINTS: DIFFUSE PANBRONCHIOLITIS

- Etiology
  - Unknown etiology
  - Characterized by accumulation of foamy macrophages in the walls of respiratory bronchioles and alveolar ducts
  - Occurs almost exclusively in Asia, particularly in Japan
  - Average age at onset is approximately 40 years; 2:1 male-to-female ratio
- Symptoms
  - Cough and progressive dyspnea
  - Chronic sinusitis
- Radiographic findings
  - Small diffuse nodules or reticulonodular opacities
  - Mild to moderate hyperinflation
- Computed tomography/high-resolution computed tomography
  - Diffuse small centrilobular nodules
  - Tree-in-bud opacities
  - Mosaic attenuation on inspiratory CT
  - Bronchiolectasis
  - Bronchiectasis

Constrictive Bronchiolitis

ETIOLOGY, PREVALENCE, AND EPIDEMIOLOGY

Constrictive bronchiolitis (CB), also known as obliterative bronchiolitis or bronchiolitis obliterans, is characterized by peribronchiolar fibrosis, resulting in narrowing or obliteration of the bronchiolar lumen.[2,36] Various pulmonary and systemic conditions have been linked to CB, most commonly CTDs, postinfectious diseases, and transplantation.[60–62] Rarely, the cause may be idiopathic (Box 59.1).[3]

CLINICAL PRESENTATION

Patients typically present with a chronic dry cough and progressive dyspnea. Symptoms may first become apparent after a lower respiratory tract infection.[3] Additional associated symptoms may include chest pain, respiratory distress, and cyanosis. The disease is usually chronic and insidious; however, in rare cases, rapid progression may occur.[2,3] In many cases CB is first detected on CT in asymptomatic patients or patients with symptoms secondary to associated conditions, such as bronchiectasis or asthma.

PATHOPHYSIOLOGY

Characteristic histologic findings include submucosal accumulation of mucopolysaccharide proteins and submucosal and peribronchiolar fibrosis (Fig. 59.15).[2,36] The fibrosis surrounds rather than fills the airway lumen, resulting in extrinsic compression and eventually complete obliteration of the bronchiolar lumen. The areas of bronchiolar fibrosis are typically patchy,

BOX 59.1 SPECIFIC ETIOLOGIES ASSOCIATED WITH CONSTRICTIVE BRONCHIOLITIS

- Postinfectious
  - Viruses (e.g., adenovirus, respiratory syncytial virus, influenza, parainfluenza)
  - *Mycoplasma*
- Connective tissue diseases (e.g., rheumatoid arthritis, Sjögren syndrome)
- Transplant
  - Lung transplant
  - Heart-lung transplant
  - Bone marrow transplant
- Inhalational lung diseases (e.g., nitrous oxide, nitrous dioxide, sulfur dioxide, ammonia, chlorine, phosgene, hot air)
- Diffuse idiopathic pulmonary neuroendocrine cell hyperplasia
- Inflammatory bowel disease
- Paraneoplastic autoimmune multiorgan syndrome
- Drugs (e.g., penicillamine, gold, cocaine, lomustine)
- Idiopathic

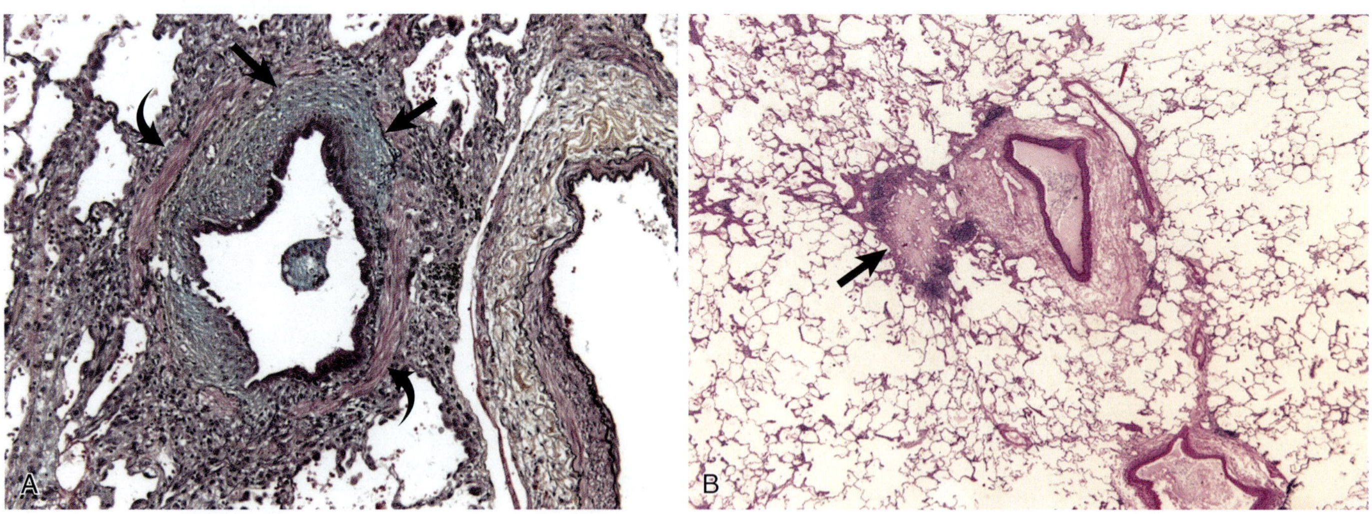

Fig. 59.15 Constrictive bronchiolitis: histologic findings in two patients. (A) Histologic specimen (Movat pentachrome stain) shows narrowing of the bronchiole caused by deposition of acid mucopolysaccharide ground substance proteins *(straight arrows)* in the lamina propria and mild peribronchiolar fibrosis *(curved arrows)*. (B) Histologic specimen (hematoxylin-eosin stain) demonstrates complete obliteration of the bronchiolar lumen *(arrow)* by eosinophilic fibrosis. Also noted are lymphoid aggregates surrounding the obliterated airway, suggestive of connective tissue disease. *(Courtesy Dr. John English, Department of Pathology, Vancouver General Hospital, Vancouver, Canada.)*

even in severely affected patients, and therefore the diagnosis can be missed if lesions are inadequately biopsied.[60]

MANIFESTATIONS OF THE DISEASE

Radiography

The chest radiograph is often normal in patients with mild to moderate disease. When findings are present, they primarily manifest as hyperinflation and peripheral attenuation/decrease of vascular markings (Fig. 59.16). Additional findings may also include peribronchial cuffing, bronchiectasis, and nodular or reticulonodular opacities.[63–65]

Computed Tomography/High-Resolution Computed Tomography

The main manifestation of CB is mosaic attenuation on inspiratory CT with concurrent moderate to severe air-trapping on expiratory CT in 40% to 80% of patients.[14,66] Several studies have shown that the end-expiratory CT finding of air-trapping has a higher sensitivity for detecting constrictive bronchiolitis, as inspiratory CT findings may be subtle and easily missed (Fig. 59.17).[67–69] Contrast between normal and abnormal lung may be enhanced by using CT postprocessing techniques, such as minimum-intensity projection reconstructions, which are particularly useful when clinical suspicion for CB is high and CT findings appear normal (Fig. 59.18).[70,71]

Additional findings include central and peripheral bronchiectasis, bronchiolectasis, and bronchial wall thickening, seen in 20% to 90% of patients (Fig. 59.19).[14,62,72] Small centrilobular nodules and tree-in-bud opacities representing thick-walled bronchioles with or without intraluminal debris may occasionally be seen.[66,73]

The extent of air-trapping must be taken into consideration when interpreting expiratory CT. As discussed earlier, a simple measure of the degree of air-trapping is subdivision into mild (<25%), moderate (25%–50%), and severe (>50%) air-trapping based on a subjective estimation of the total lung volume of air-trapped lung.[18] Air-trapping is frequently seen in asymptomatic subjects with normal pulmonary function, particularly in elderly patients and smokers.[15,74] Lobular air-trapping involving fewer than three adjacent SPLs can be seen in 40% to 80% of normal patients on CT, and several studies have shown mild, moderate, and sometimes even extensive air-trapping in individuals with normal pulmonary function tests.[19,20] Integrating inspiratory and expiratory CT findings provides the highest sensitivity and specificity for a diagnosis of CB.

DIFFERENTIAL DIAGNOSIS

A presumptive diagnosis of CB can often be made with a high degree of confidence by using a multidisciplinary approach, combining clinical history (including pulmonary function testing), histology (when available), and typical CT/HRCT findings. Other causes of chronic airway obstruction with similar imaging findings to CB, including emphysema, chronic bronchitis, asthma, and hypersensitivity pneumonitis, must be excluded before a presumptive diagnosis of CB is made.

When abnormal air-trapping is present on expiratory CT, indicating obstructive airway pathology, both bronchial dilation and mosaic attenuation on inspiratory CT have been shown to be sensitive and specific findings in identifying CB and differentiating it from other diseases that cause airway obstruction.[66,75] Mosaic attenuation occurring as an indirect sign of small airways

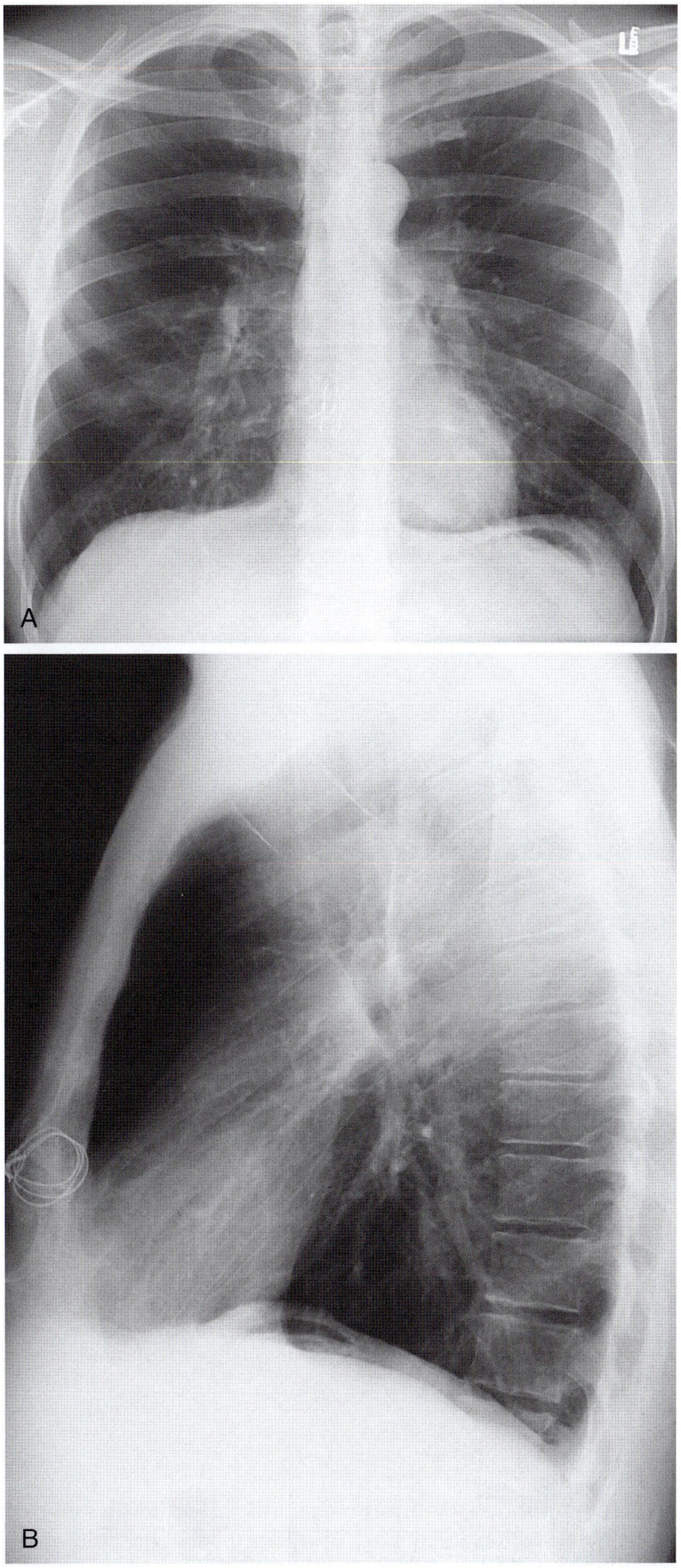

Fig. 59.16 Radiographic findings of constrictive bronchiolitis associated with bilateral lung transplantation. (A) Posteroanterior chest radiograph shows hyperinflation and marked attenuation of the peripheral vascular markings. (B) Lateral view demonstrates an increased retrosternal clear space.

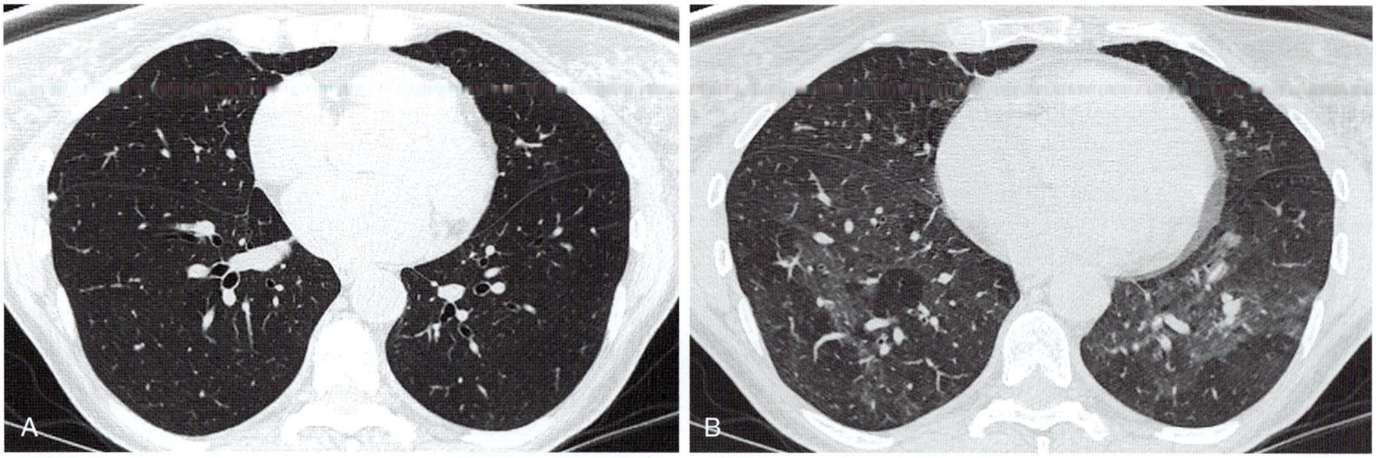

Fig. 59.17 CT findings of constrictive bronchiolitis in a hematopoietic stem cell transplant recipient. (A) Inspiratory CT shows subtle bilateral areas of decreased attenuation and perfusion, resulting in parenchymal heterogeneity, which could be easily missed. (B) Expiratory CT shows extensive bilateral air-trapping.

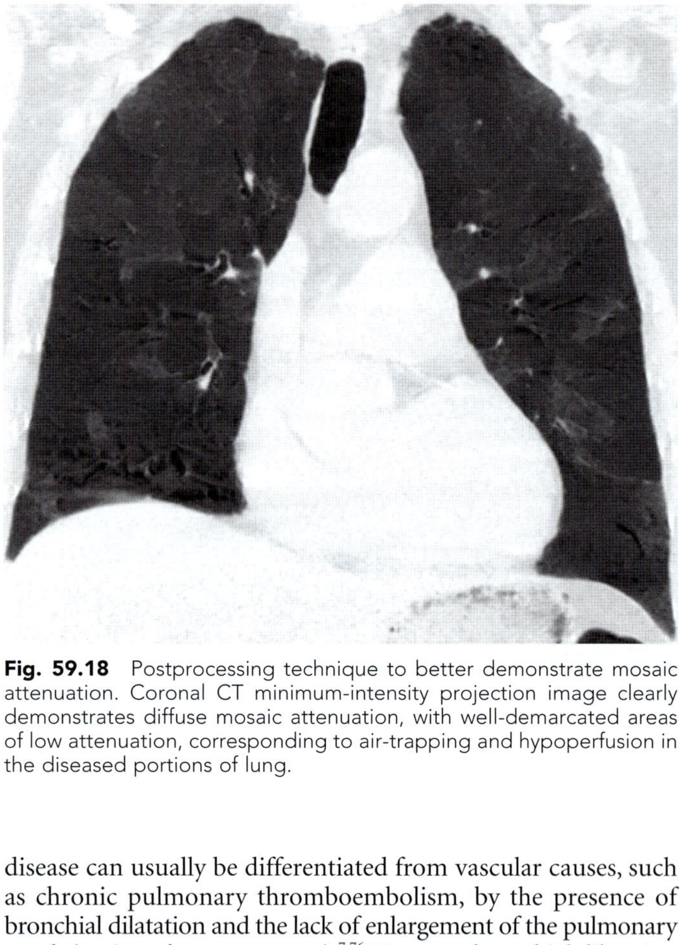

Fig. 59.18 Postprocessing technique to better demonstrate mosaic attenuation. Coronal CT minimum-intensity projection image clearly demonstrates diffuse mosaic attenuation, with well-demarcated areas of low attenuation, corresponding to air-trapping and hypoperfusion in the diseased portions of lung.

disease can usually be differentiated from vascular causes, such as chronic pulmonary thromboembolism, by the presence of bronchial dilatation and the lack of enlargement of the pulmonary trunk (main pulmonary artery).[7,76] However, bronchial dilatation may also occur in patients with chronic pulmonary thromboembolism,[7,77] and there are no reliable differentiating features between mosaic attenuation resulting from CB or from other small airways diseases. Furthermore, air-trapping can also be seen in up to 60% of patients with acute or chronic pulmonary thromboembolism.[78]

Lung biopsy is required for a definitive diagnosis of CB. Patchy disease distribution results in frequent misdiagnosis when transbronchial biopsy specimens are obtained.[79] Even on surgical biopsy specimens, subtle changes or completely scarred bronchioles may be missed on routine hematoxylin-eosin stains.[80] Optimal assessment requires the use of elastic tissue stains.[80]

TREATMENT OPTIONS

CB is essentially irreversible.[61] Corticosteroids and immunosuppressive medications may slow disease progression in some cases.[61] Lung transplantation or lung volume reduction surgery is sometimes considered for patients with persistent severe obstructive symptoms and impairment in lung function.[81]

Specific Causes of, and Underlying Diseases Associated With, Constrictive Bronchiolitis

INFECTION

Childhood infection is a uncommon cause of constrictive bronchiolitis, usually occurring in children younger than 8 years.[3,82] Typical infections are viral, particularly after adenovirus infection (Fig. 59.20).[62,83,84] *Mycoplasma pneumoniae*, and rarely measles, have also been implicated.[21,85] An estimated 1% of patients with acute viral bronchiolitis develop CB.[86] The condition usually does not become apparent until adulthood, and patients are usually asymptomatic or have mild to moderate clinical findings. Some patients may develop features of Swyer-James-MacLeod (SJM) syndrome (discussed in further detail later in this chapter). CB may also be seen in patients with cystic fibrosis, likely sequelae of recurrent pulmonary infection.[3,12] Overall, the majority of patients have a good prognosis; however, severe and sometimes fatal disease may occur.[62,87–89]

TRANSPLANTATION

Lung and Heart-Lung Transplantation

CB is the leading cause of morbidity and mortality in patients with lung and heart-lung transplantation (Fig. 59.21). It is a late complication, occurring at least 3 months after transplantation (median, 16–20 months), and is considered a manifestation of

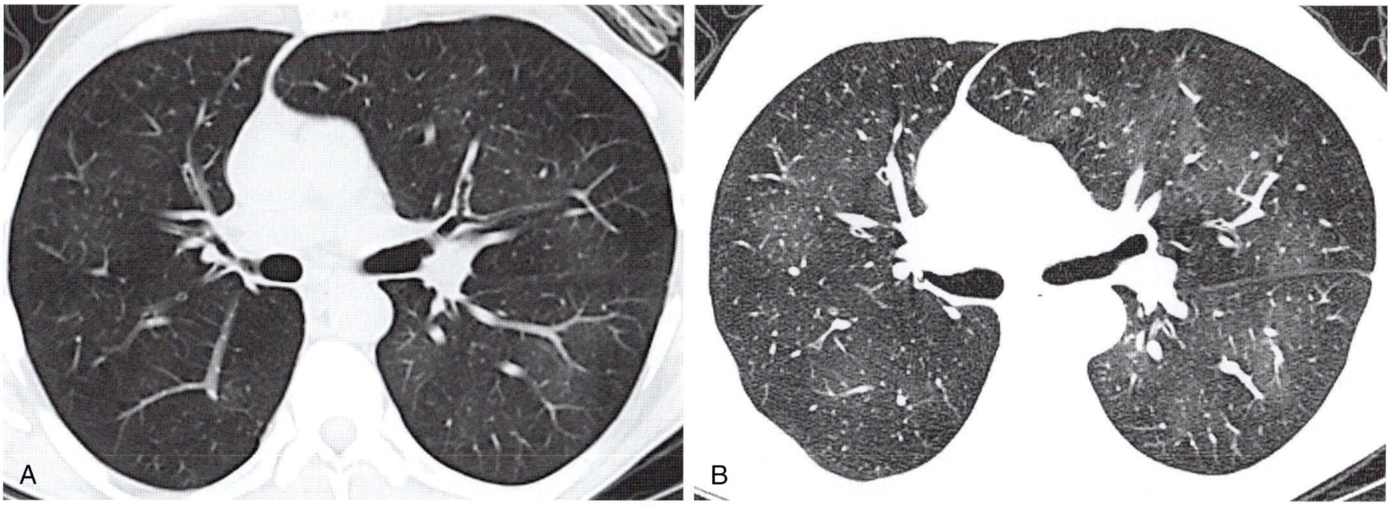

Fig. 59.19 CT findings of constrictive bronchiolitis in a stem cell transplant patient. (A) Inspiratory CT shows subtle bilateral mosaic attenuation and central bronchial wall thickening. (B) Expiratory CT shows extensive bilateral air-trapping.

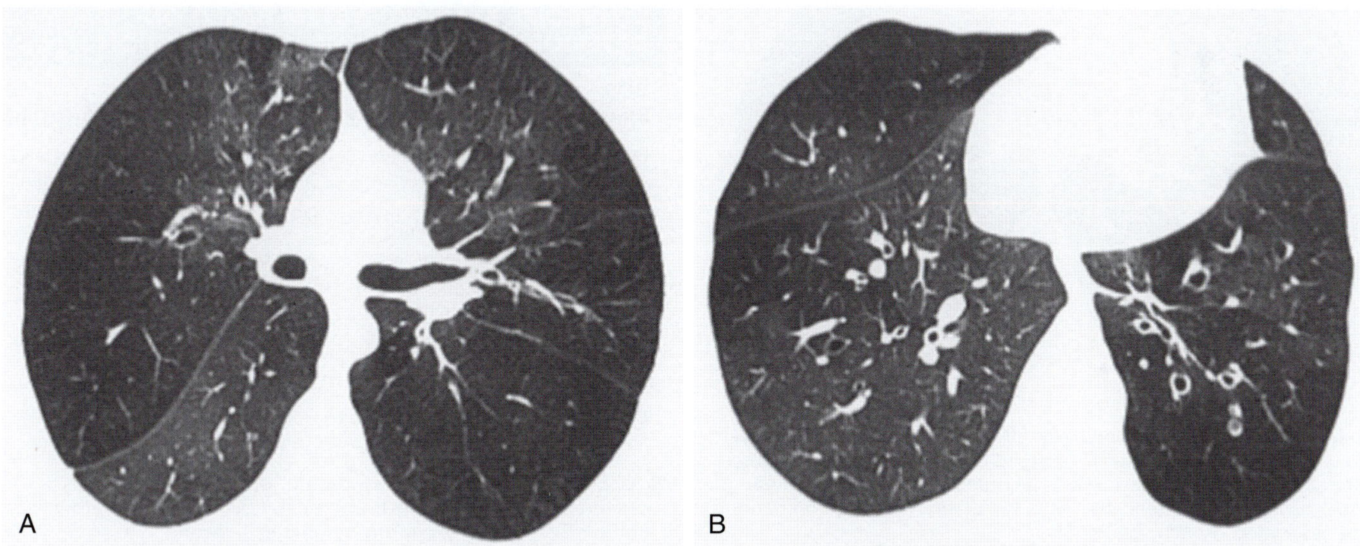

Fig. 59.20 Postinfectious constrictive bronchiolitis after severe childhood viral infection during infancy. (A) High-resolution CT (HRCT) image at the level of left main bronchus shows extensive bilateral areas of decreased attenuation and vascularity with blood flow redistribution (mosaic attenuation). (B) HRCT image at the level of the lung bases shows areas of decreased attenuation and vascularity mainly in the right middle and left lower lobes. Also note left lower lobe bronchiectasis.

chronic allograft dysfunction or chronic rejection.[3,90–92] The prevalence of CB after lung transplantation is approximately 20% at 1 year and 50% at 3 to 5 years, with a reported 5-year survival of approximately 30% to 40% after disease onset.[90,93–96] Acute rejection is the most important risk factor, especially when severe and/or recurrent.[3,91,92] Infection, especially cytomegalovirus pneumonia, is also a common risk factor.[97] The International Society for Heart and Lung Transplantation has established the concept of bronchiolitis obliterans syndrome (BOS) and a staging system based on deterioration of pulmonary function, to quantify the severity of airflow obstruction.[98] A clinical diagnosis of BOS requires a decline of 20% or more in FEV1 during the post-transplant period, after other causes of graft dysfunction have been excluded (Table 59.4). The category of potential BOS, or stage BOS 0-p, remains controversial regarding its prognostic utility.[92,99]

Air-trapping on expiratory CT is the most sensitive and accurate radiologic indicator of CB after transplantation; however, it has been shown to be relatively insensitive in the diagnosis of early CB and detecting early-stage BOS.[14,19,67,99–102] The severity of CT findings, such as bronchial dilatation, bronchial wall thickening, mosaic attenuation, and air-trapping, have only been shown to have a weak correlation with BOS severity.[3,103]

Hematopoietic Stem Cell Transplantation

CB is the most common noninfectious late pulmonary complication of hematopoietic stem cell transplantation, with a prevalence of approximately 5% and typically developing more than 100 days (median, 400–450 days) after transplantation (Fig. 59.22).[90,91,104,105] CB is more commonly reported in cases of allogeneic transplantation; however, it has also been reported in patients who received autologous transplants. The prevalence in allogeneic hematopoietic stem cell transplant patients is approximately 9%, with some studies reporting values up to 48%. Reported 5-year survival ranges between 10% and 27% after disease onset.[91] The pathogenesis is thought to be secondary to the graft-versus-host effect.[90] Major risk factors include old age, chronic graft-versus-host disease, and methotrexate therapy.[3,91] CT findings are identical to CB seen with lung and heart-lung transplant recipients.

CONNECTIVE TISSUE DISEASES

CTDs as a group are considered the most common cause of CB and most frequently seen with RA, usually affecting women in their fifth or sixth decade of life, and with long-standing disease.[106,107] Less commonly, CB may be seen with Sjögren syndrome,[108] systemic lupus erythematosus,[109] scleroderma (systemic sclerosis),[7,110–112] and mixed CTD.[7] CB in association with CTD varies in severity and natural course, with most patients showing slow progression of disease. CB is rarely the sole manifestation of RA.[34,106,107,113] Penicillamine therapy and, less commonly, gold therapy have been implicated as potential causative agents of CB in some patients with RA.[113–115]

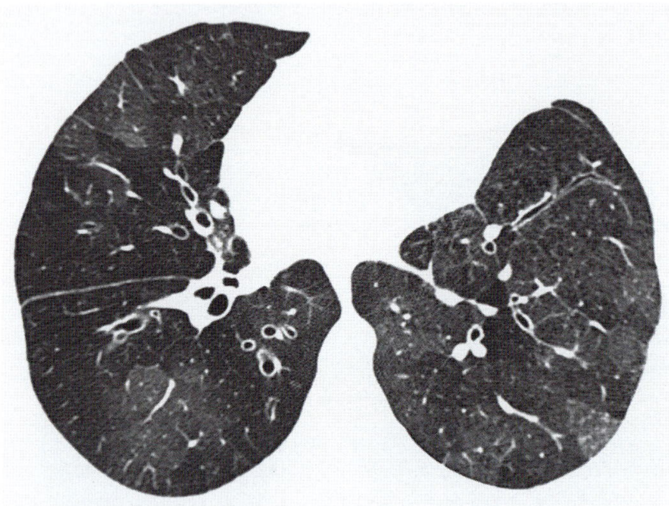

Fig. 59.21 Constrictive bronchiolitis after lung transplantation: mosaic attenuation on high-resolution CT (HRCT). HRCT image shows extensive bilateral areas of decreased attenuation and vascularity and areas of normal or increased attenuation and vascularity (mosaic attenuation). Note associated bronchiectasis.

DIFFUSE NEUROENDOCRINE CELL HYPERPLASIA, CARCINOID TUMORLETS, AND CARCINOID TUMORS

Diffuse idiopathic pulmonary neuroendocrine cell hyperplasia (DIPNECH) is an increasingly recognized condition characterized by extensive proliferation of neuroendocrine cells as clusters or linear arrays of cells along the bronchial and bronchiolar basement membrane.[116] Approximately 50% of patients with DIPNECH and multiple pulmonary carcinoid tumorlets may develop

TABLE 59.4 BRONCHIOLITIS OBLITERANS SYNDROME STAGING SYSTEM BASED ON DETERIORATION OF PULMONARY FUNCTION

BOS Stage	Disease Severity	Pulmonary Function Testing
BOS 0	No constrictive bronchiolitis	FEV1: >90% of baseline and FEF25–75: >75% of baseline
BOS 0-p	Potential constrictive bronchiolitis	FEV1: 81%–90% of baseline and FEF22–75: ≤75% of baseline
BOS 1	Mild constrictive bronchiolitis	FEV1: 66%–80% of baseline
BOS 2	Moderate constrictive bronchiolitis	FEV1: 51%–65% of baseline
BOS 3	Severe constrictive bronchiolitis	FEV1: ≤50% of baseline

BOS, Bronchiolitis obliterans syndrome; *BOS 0-p*, bronchiolitis obliterans syndrome stage 0-potential; *FEF*, forced expiratory flow (rate); *FEV1*, forced expiratory volume in 1 second.

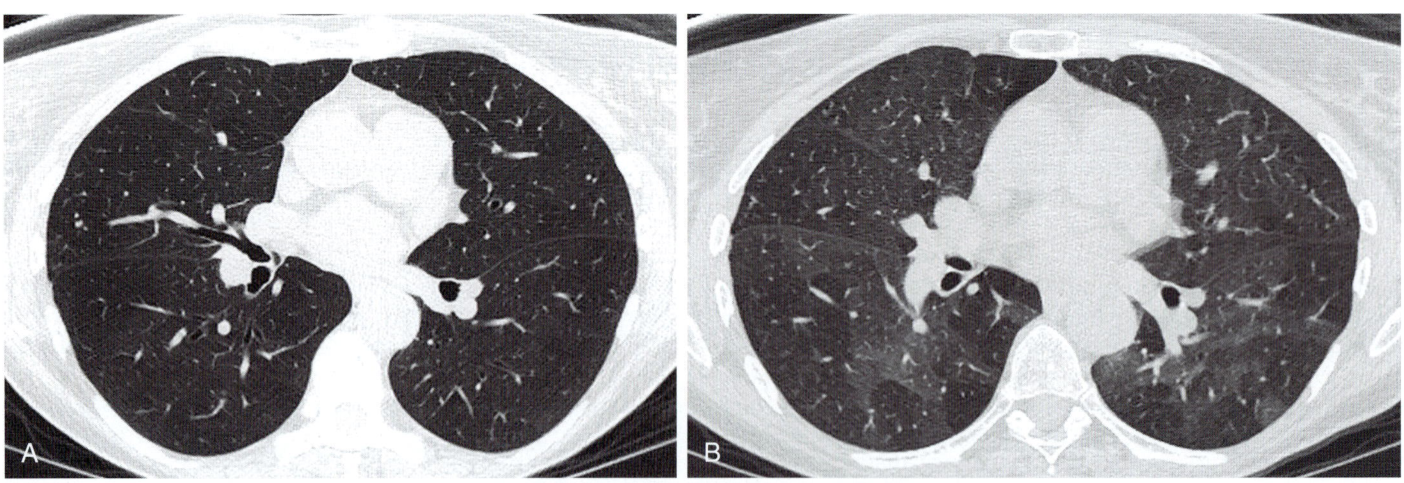

Fig. 59.22 Air-trapping in constrictive bronchiolitis after stem cell transplantation. (A) High-resolution CT image shows subtle areas of decreased attenuation and vascularity. (B) Expiratory CT image demonstrates extensive bilateral air-trapping.

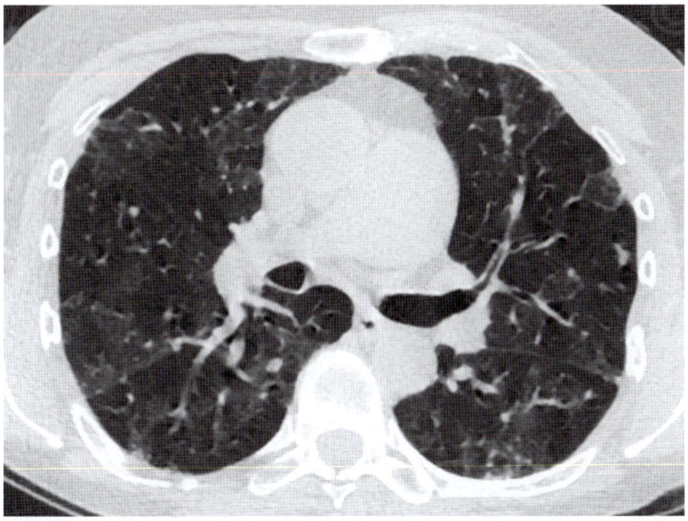

Fig. 59.23 Constrictive bronchiolitis in diffuse idiopathic neuroendocrine cell hyperplasia. Expiratory CT shows multifocal bilateral nodules and micronodules, bronchial wall thickening, and geographic areas of air-trapping.

symptomatic constrictive bronchiolitis.[117,118] CB in these patients is likely due to a combination of intraluminal obstruction by hyperplastic neuroendocrine cells and peribronchiolar fibrosis from peptide secretory products.[116] Characteristic histologic findings include submucosal bronchial and bronchiolar wall fibrosis in both regions with, and regions away, from tumorlets/neuroendocrine hyperplasia.[116] Clinically symptomatic patients are usually women ranging from 50 to 70 years of age.[116,117,119] Chest radiograph may demonstrate multiple pulmonary micronodules, and CT usually shows multifocal pulmonary micronodules with or without mosaic attenuation on inspiratory CT and air-trapping on expiratory CT (Fig. 59.23).[117] Bronchiectasis, bronchial wall thickening, and atelectasis have also been described.[117,118,120]

Bronchiolitis Related to Toxic Gases, Fumes, and Dust

A variety of inhaled agents, including toxic fumes (e.g., diacetyl exposure), smoke, toxic gases (e.g., nitric oxide, nitric dioxide, sulfur dioxide, chlorine, hydrochloric acid, phosgene), inorganic agents (e.g., silica, asbestos), and organic agents are associated with CB.[121] Several studies have shown various occupational lung diseases manifesting as severe CB. One specific example involves workers exposed to flavoring vapors in North American food processing industries. "Popcorn worker's lung," first reported by Kreiss and colleagues[122] in 2000, refers to CB resulting after exposure to diacetyl vapors, a ketone with butter flavoring used in popcorn manufacturing plants.[122,123] Multiple additional studies have since validated the etiologic association between diacetyl exposure and CB, including case series in former employees, cross-sectional epidemiologic studies in current employees, explorative exposure studies, and a few animal exposure studies.[123,124]

The best understood disease process, commonly known as "silo filler's disease," occurs with the inhalation of nitric oxide (NO) and nitrogen dioxide (NO_2), which are byproducts from the anaerobic fermentation of silage. The earliest phase of silo filler's lung is characterized clinically by the abrupt onset of cough, dyspnea, weakness, and a choking or globus sensation.[23] Pulmonary edema can develop within 4 to 24 hours but usually abates without residual lung damage, if the patient survives. The second phase of disease is typically an asymptomatic period, lasting 2 to 5 weeks. The third phase becomes apparent up to 5 weeks after the initial exposure and is characterized by progressive dyspnea caused by CB.[23] Although some studies have shown that exposure to low concentrations of NO_2 in humans is rarely problematic, moderate to severe exposure often results in a rapid onset of acute bronchiolitis; diffuse alveolar damage has also been documented in some patients.[21,125] The majority of patients fully recover; however, some will continue on to develop CB.[21]

Airway abnormalities and pulmonary parenchymal disease are common complications of smoke inhalation. Smoke consists of gases and a suspension of carbon particles coated with combustible products, such as organic acids and aldehydes, in hot air. Acute bronchiolitis from smoke inhalation often resolves but may occasionally progress to CB. Direct heat exposure can cause severe tissue damage to airway mucosa, particularly seen in burn victims.[126,127] CT plays a main role in the assessment of late complications, demonstrating findings such as tracheal stenosis, bronchiectasis, and bronchiolectasis. Mosaic attenuation on inspiratory CT and air-trapping on expiratory CT are frequently seen (Fig. 59.24).

Miscellaneous Causes of Constrictive Bronchiolitis

SAUROPUS ANDROGYNUS

Sauropus androgynus is commonly found in Malaysia, Indonesia, southwest China, and Vietnam. Consumption of juice prepared from the uncooked leaves of the vegetable *S. androgynus,* which is alleged to help weight control, has a known association with constrictive bronchiolitis.[128–130] The patients usually have a poor prognosis and present with rapidly progressive shortness of breath and persistent cough 3 to 4 months after ingestion of blended vegetable juice, with moderate to severe airflow obstruction.[128–131] They typically do not respond to bronchodilator therapy or corticosteroids.

INFLAMMATORY BOWEL DISEASE

Inflammatory bowel disease (IBD) typically involves the intermediate-sized central bronchi. Rarely, the small airways can be involved.[132,133] Chest radiographs are usually normal but may sometimes show hyperinflation, peripheral pulmonary vascular attenuation, and poorly defined reticular or reticulonodular opacities. Typical CT findings include findings of intermediate and small airway involvement and may show central and peripheral bronchiectasis, bronchiolectasis, and bronchial wall thickening, small solid centrilobular nodules that are often related to mucoid impaction, small ground-glass nodules, and mosaic attenuation. Expiratory CT shows air-trapping.[132,133] Correlation with a known history of IBD and evaluation of concurrent involvement of the large- and intermediate-sized airways are important diagnostic clues differentiating IBD as the etiologic cause for small airways disease.

PARANEOPLASTIC AUTOIMMUNE MULTIORGAN SYNDROME

Paraneoplastic autoimmune multiorgan syndrome is a severe autoimmune disorder secondary to an underlying benign or malignant tumor. Mortality rates may be as high as 90% when

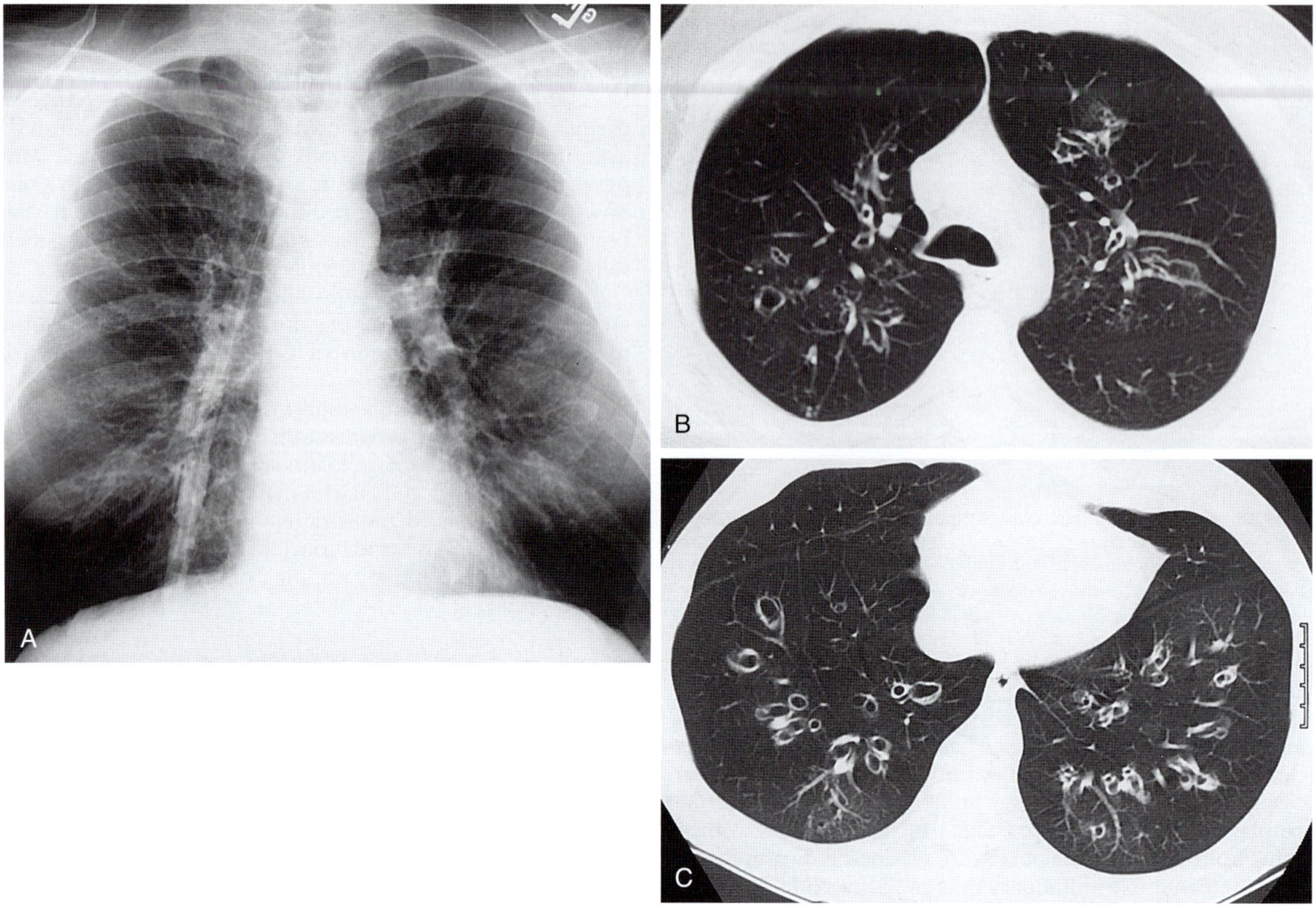

Fig. 59.24 Constrictive bronchiolitis and bronchiectasis years after smoke inhalation. (A) Posteroanterior chest radiograph shows increased lung volume, bronchiectasis, and decreased peripheral vascular markings. (B) and (C) High-resolution CT show extensive bronchiectasis and areas of decreased attenuation and vascularity as a result of constrictive bronchiolitis. *(Courtesy Dr. Christopher Griffin, Department of Radiology, Veterans Affairs Hospital, Portland, Oregon. From Müller NL, Fraser RS, Colman NC, Paré PD.* Radiologic Diagnosis of Diseases of the Chest. *Philadelphia: WB Saunders; 2001.)*

malignancy is involved.[134,135] The most commonly associated neoplasms are non-Hodgkin lymphoma, chronic lymphocytic leukemia, Castleman disease, retroperitoneal sarcomas, and Waldenström macroglobulinemia. The disease process is characterized by immunoglobulin-mediated destruction acantholysis (destruction of intercellular desmosomal protein connections) affecting the skin and mucous membranes, including the mucosa of the large and small airways.[134,135] Respiratory failure occurs in approximately 30% of patients and is usually secondary to CB.[134] Patients often present with progressive dyspnea, deterioration of pulmonary function and hypoxia, and eventually death. Chest radiograph findings are usually normal. CT findings are typical for severe CB. Prognosis is poor when airway involvement is present, and patients are usually nonresponsive to immunosuppressive therapy.[134]

Swyer-James-Macleod Syndrome

ETIOLOGY, PREVALENCE, EPIDEMIOLOGY, AND CLINICAL PRESENTATION

Swyer-James-MacLeod syndrome (SJM) is an uncommon condition characterized radiographically by a hyperlucent lobe or lung and functionally by normal or reduced total lung capacity and presence

KEY POINTS: CONSTRICTIVE BRONCHIOLITIS

- Etiology/definition
  - Characterized by submucosal and peribronchiolar fibrosis with resulting bronchiolar narrowing or obliteration of the bronchiolar lumen.
  - Most common causes are previous infection, connective tissue diseases (mainly rheumatoid arthritis), transplantation (mainly lung and stem cell transplantation), inhalational lung disease, and miscellaneous conditions, such as *Sauropus androgynous* ingestion, inflammatory bowel disease, paraneoplastic pemphigus, and drug-related (gold and penicillamine).
- Clinical symptoms
  - Dry cough and progressive dyspnea
- Radiographic findings
  - Often normal
  - May show central peribronchial cuffing, decreased peripheral vascular markings, and hyperinflation
- Computed tomography/high-resolution tomography
  - Mosaic attenuation on inspiratory CT
  - Air-trapping on expiratory CT; needs to involve more than 25% of the lung to be considered abnormal
  - Bronchiectasis

of expiratory air-trapping.[136,137] The syndrome falls along the spectrum of postinfectious constructive bronchiolitis. Patients are typically young adults who are either asymptomatic or complaining of mild dyspnea, with a history of prior childhood viral infection. In some cases the disease is recognized, or at least suspected, in childhood when chest radiography is performed for evaluation of recurrent respiratory infections. Most cases of SJM, therefore, probably begin as an acute bronchiolitis that eventually progresses to constrictive bronchiolitis, characterized by fibrous obliteration of the airway lumen. The peripheral parenchyma is largely unaffected and remains inflated because of collateral ventilation with resultant air-trapping. However, destructive changes characteristic of emphysema also supervene in some cases.[138]

PATHOPHYSIOLOGY

The main histologic abnormalities are those of CB, characterized by submucosal accumulation of mucopolysaccharide proteins and submucosal and peribronchiolar fibrosis.[139] Other common findings include bronchiectasis and a variable degree of lung parenchymal destruction.[138]

MANIFESTATIONS OF THE DISEASE

Radiography

Inspiratory radiography performed at total lung capacity typically shows a marked difference in radiolucency of both lungs, or the affected and unaffected lobes, caused by decreased perfusion. The ipsilateral hilum is also diminutive but is present (Fig. 59.25). The expiratory chest radiograph shows persistent hyperlucency/air-trapping in the involved lobe or lung.

Computed Tomography/High-Resolution Computed Tomography

Similar to radiography, inspiratory CT shows hyperlucency, decreased vascularity, normal or decreased size of the involved lung or lobe, and air-trapping on expiratory CT (Fig. 59.26). These findings are also frequently seen in the contralateral lung, although one lung is usually more severely affected, leading to the false sense of unilateral involvement on radiography. Unilateral or bilateral bronchiectasis is not uncommon.[140,141]

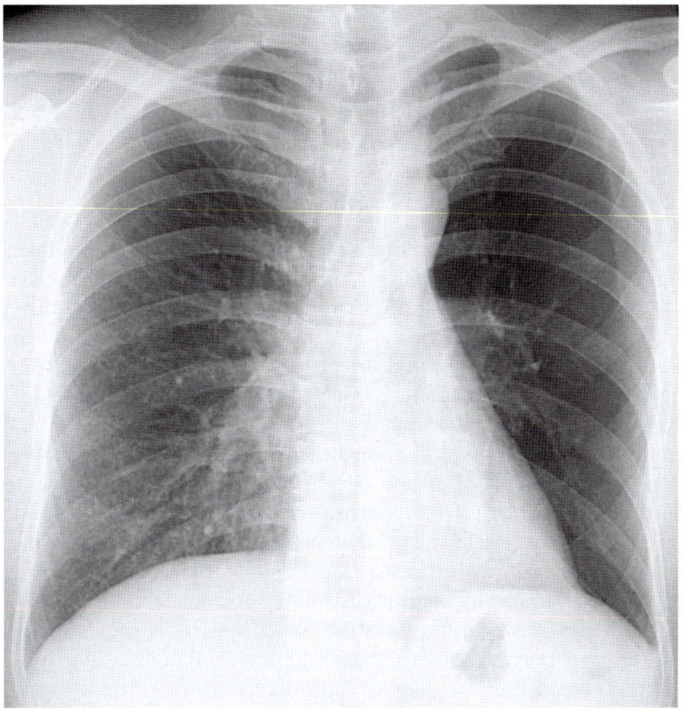

Fig. 59.25 Swyer-James-MacLeod syndrome. Chest radiograph shows hyperlucency and decreased vascularity of the left lung as well as a small left hilum. The mediastinum is shifted to the left, consistent with decreased left lung volume.

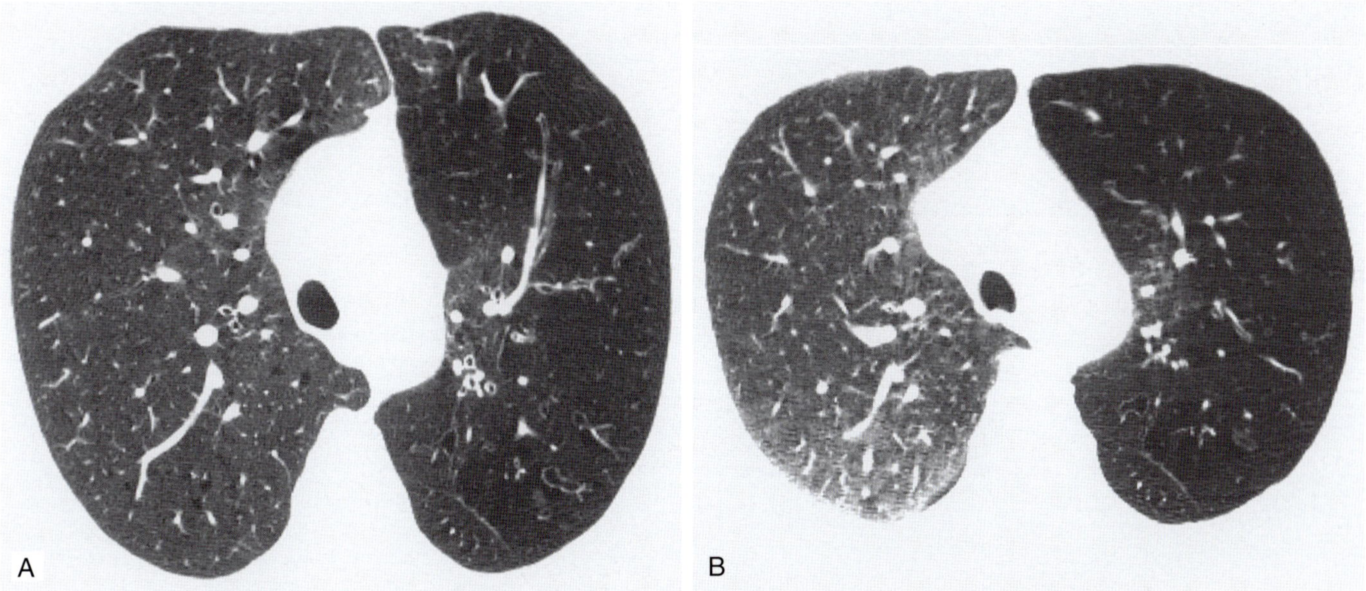

Fig. 59.26 Swyer-James-MacLeod syndrome. (A) High-resolution CT shows decreased attenuation and vascularity of the left lung with associated bronchiectasis and mild volume loss leading to ipsilateral shift of the mediastinum and anterior junction line. (B) Expiratory CT image at the same level shows air-trapping in the left lung. The mediastinum and anterior junction line are now in the midline.

KEY POINTS: SWYER-JAMES-MACLEOD SYNDROME (UNILATERAL HYPERLUCENT LUNG OR LOBE)

- Etiology/definition
  - Characterized radiologically by a hyperlucent lobe or lung and functionally by normal or reduced total lung capacity and presence of expiratory air-trapping
  - Usually sequela of childhood viral infection resulting in constrictive bronchiolitis
- Symptoms
  - Majority are asymptomatic; occasionally, dyspnea or recurrent infections may occur
- Radiographic findings
  - Hyperlucency
  - Decreased vascularity
  - Normal or decreased size of the involved lobe or lung
  - Expiratory chest radiograph shows air-trapping
- Computed tomography/high-resolution computed tomography
  - Hyperlucency and decreased vascularity of the involved lung or lobe on inspiratory CT
  - Air-trapping on expiratory CT
  - Bronchiectasis (in the majority of cases)

DIFFERENTIAL DIAGNOSIS

The diagnosis of SJM can often be made on the chest radiograph, given the marked difference in radiolucency between the affected and unaffected areas. Although the ipsilateral hilum is diminutive, it is still present, which makes it a feature of value in the differentiation from proximal interruption of a pulmonary artery (pulmonary artery agenesis). The presence of expiratory air-trapping is essential for accurate diagnosis of SJM, as it is a reflection of airway obstruction and is invaluable in differentiating the syndrome from other conditions that may give rise to unilateral lung or lobar hyperlucency. An important diagnostic dilemma may arise if the patient presents with the radiographic triad of low lung volume, expiratory air-trapping, and diffusely decreased vascularity resulting from hypoxic vasoconstriction—a triad that makes differentiation of SJM syndrome from an underlying partially obstructive endobronchial neoplasm impossible. CT can then be used to definitively confirm the presence or absence of an obstructing ipsilateral endobronchial lesion. Sequelae of bronchopulmonary dysplasia or chronic lung disease of prematurity may also manifest with similar, but often more extensive, findings of diffuse patchy hypoattenuating lung parenchyma. An important clue to this diagnosis is the history of prematurity with long-term ventilation at birth.

SUGGESTED READINGS

Abbott GF, Rosado-de-Christenson ML, et al. Imaging of small airways disease. *J Thorac Imaging*. 2009;24:285–298.

Elicker BM, Jones KD, et al. Multidisciplinary approach to hypersensitivity pneumonitis. *J Thorac Imaging*. 2016;31:92–103.

Kligerman S, Franks TJ, et al. Clinical-radiologic-pathologic correlation of smoking-related diffuse parenchymal lung disease. *Radiol Clin North Am*. 2016;54:1047–1063.

Kligerman AJ, Henry T, et al. Mosaic attenuation: etiology, methods of differentiation, and pitfalls. *Radiographics*. 2015;35:1360–1380.

Miller WT Jr, Chatzkel J, et al. Expiratory air-trapping on thoracic computed tomography: a diagnostic subclassification. *Ann Am Thorac Soc*. 2014;11(6):874–881.

Winningham PJ, Martínez-Jiménez S, Rosado-de-Christenson ML, Betancourt SL, Restrepo CS, Eraso A. Bronchiolitis: a practical approach for the general radiologist. *Radiographics*. 2017;37(3):777–794.

The full reference list for this chapter is available at ExpertConsult.com.

60 Emphysema*

STEPHEN B. HOBBS

Definition and Etiology

Emphysema is defined as a "condition of the lung characterized by abnormal, permanent enlargement of the airspaces distal to the terminal bronchiole, accompanied by destruction of their walls."[1] Because emphysema decreases the elastic recoil force that drives air out of the lung and thereby reduces maximal expiratory airflow, the disease is clinically classified as one of the chronic obstructive pulmonary diseases (COPDs).[2] In morphologic appearance, two main subtypes of emphysema exist. The centrilobular (or centriacinar) form of emphysema results from dilatation or destruction of the respiratory bronchioles and is the type of emphysema most closely associated with cigarette smoking.[1] The panlobular, or panacinar, form of emphysema is associated with α1-antitrypsin deficiency and results in an even dilatation and destruction of the entire acinus.[1] It has been suggested that one or the other of these two subtypes predominates in severe disease and that the centrilobular subtype is associated with more severe small airways obstruction.[3] There is a relation between the severity of emphysema and the pack-years of cigarette smoking, but this relation is weak. Indeed, only 40% of heavy smokers develop substantial lung destruction resulting from emphysema. On the other hand, emphysema can occasionally be found in individuals with normal lung function who have never smoked.[4]

Prevalence and Epidemiology

The overall prevalence and epidemiology of emphysema are almost impossible to determine for three major reasons. First, the prevalence of emphysema strongly depends on regional factors, such as smoking habits, social standards, and environmental air pollution. Given that these factors largely vary, the prevalence of emphysema will show equally varying features, even in relatively small geographic areas. Second, emphysema becomes clinically evident in advanced disease, whereas mild or moderate disease can remain clinically silent. There are no screening programs dedicated to emphysema, although lung cancer screening with low-dose computed tomography (CT) may incidentally detect it, and a substantial number of individuals with emphysema will remain undiagnosed during their lifetime if no comorbidity exists that can bring to light emphysema as an incidental finding. Third, emphysema is clinically classified as a chronic obstructive lung disease.[5] In this group of diseases the clinical findings may overlap with airways disorders. Furthermore, epidemiologic data exist for COPD as a group of diseases but not for the individual diseases such as emphysema.[6,7] According to the Centers for Disease Control and Prevention, as of 2015 there are 36.5 million people who smoke cigarettes in the United States (1.1 billion smoke worldwide).[8,9] Smoking is the leading cause of preventable death in the United States, accounting for more than 480,000 deaths per year.[10]

Clinical Presentation

In many cases the clinical manifestations of emphysema are entirely nonspecific. In early stages, patients are often asymptomatic, and emphysema may be detected as an incidental finding on a CT examination performed for other purposes.[11] In more advanced cases symptoms may overlap with symptoms caused by coexisting airway abnormalities and can therefore be difficult to attribute to the existence of emphysema. Patients with moderate to advanced disease, however, often complain of cough, either dry or productive, with increased frequency in the morning hours. Depending on the severity of the disease, breathlessness can occur either under exertion or at rest. Patients with severe emphysema can be susceptible to pulmonary infections that can occur at increased frequency or heal with increased delay.

Pathophysiology

PATHOLOGY

The definition of emphysema clearly refers to the acinus as a basic lung structure.[12] The acinus is defined as the lung parenchyma that subtends from the terminal membranous bronchiole and consists of three generations of respiratory bronchioles, alveolar ducts, saccules, and alveoli.[13] As opposed to the secondary pulmonary lobule, the acinus is not grossly identifiable. The terms *centrilobular* and *panlobular* are derived from their gross distributions within the secondary pulmonary lobule as defined by Miller.[14,15] Because of the central location of the terminal bronchioles, the terms *centriacinar, centrilobular, panacinar,* and *panlobular* are roughly equivalent, and both terms are commonly used interchangeably.[13]

The use of animal models and, particularly, genetically modified animals has produced extensive information about the pathogenesis of emphysema.[16–23] The concept of a protease-antiprotease imbalance has been expanded but continues to include the inflammatory cascade, with involvement of the interleukins with Th1 cytokines and both serine proteases and metalloproteases.[22] Neutrophils and macrophages have been joined by CD4-positive and CD8-positive T lymphocytes as important effector cells. The presence of apoptosis in emphysematous lungs has introduced a concept of disordered lung maintenance and repair, and there has been a suggestion of an immune basis for lung destruction.[2,13,16]

PATHOLOGIC SUBTYPES OF EMPHYSEMA

Centrilobular Emphysema

Centrilobular emphysema is characteristically found in cigarette smokers. Causes of centrilobular emphysema or bullae besides

*The editors and publisher would like to thank Dr. Alexander A. Bankier for contributing material on this topic to the prior edition of this work. It has served as the foundation for the current chapter.

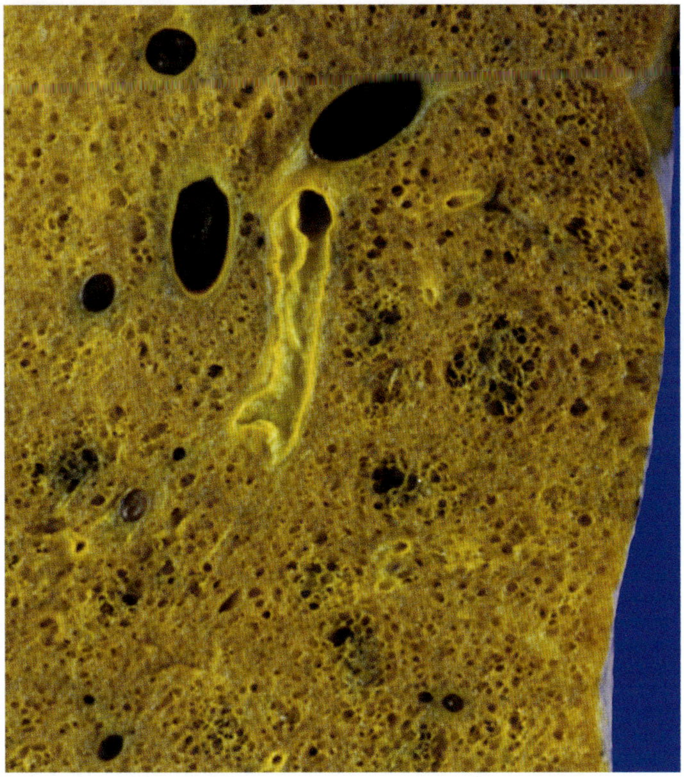

Fig. 60.1 Centrilobular emphysema. Low-power view of a lung specimen shows focal areas of enlargement of the airspaces near the center of the secondary lobules. *(Courtesy Dr. John English, Department of Pathology, Vancouver General Hospital, Vancouver, Canada.)*

cigarette smoking include human immunodeficiency virus (HIV), Salla disease, Marfan syndrome, and Menke syndrome.[24] On gross specimen, centrilobular emphysema is usually more common and more severe in the upper lung zones. In the upper lobe the posterior and apical segments are commonly affected; in the lower lobe the superior segment is more involved. Assessment of the secondary pulmonary lobule will demonstrate the central position of destruction, with sharply demarcated emphysematous areas separated from the acinar periphery by intact alveolar ducts and sacs of normal size (Fig. 60.1). In more severe lesions the destruction will advance toward the periphery of the lobule, which can make the differentiation between centrilobular and panlobular emphysema difficult.[13]

On microscopy airspace enlargement can be associated with a distorted respiratory bronchiole to form the classic centrilobular emphysema lesion. With increasing severity, isolated strands of alveoli can be seen. They are a useful indicator of the presence of emphysema. Collections of macrophages within the airspaces or adjacent to the bronchiole are common (representing respiratory bronchiolitis; see Chapter 34), and pigment can be seen both within the macrophages and in the bronchiolar fibrous tissue.[13]

Panlobular Emphysema

On gross specimen, panlobular emphysema can be difficult to detect. In normal lungs the smaller alveoli can be clearly distinguished from the alveolar ducts and respiratory bronchioles; in panlobular emphysema, this distinction becomes lost because alveoli lose their sharp angles, enlarge, and eventually lose their contrast in size and in shape with the ducts. The lung architecture thus can appear simplified, with formation of small box-like structures. In more severe disease the abnormal enlargement becomes more obvious, even though the destruction is relatively uniform within the individual lobules (Fig. 60.2).[13] On microscopic examination the uniformity of the enlargement throughout the lobules persists (see Fig. 60.2). Airspaces adjacent to the venous septa are similar in size to those adjacent to the airways. Subtle signs of inflammation can be present.[13]

Panlobular emphysema is highly associated with α1-antitrypsin deficiency. Less likely causes of this pattern include hypocomplementemic urticarial vasculitis syndrome, intravenous methylphenidate abuse (so-called Ritalin lung), and some elastin abnormalities, such as cutis laxa and Ehlers-Danlos.[24]

Other "Subtypes" of Emphysema

Paraseptal Emphysema. This emphysematous destruction pattern is located in the periphery of the lung adjacent to the pleura or along interlobular septa. It is thus mainly subpleural in location and bound by the interlobular septa. It may occasionally occur as an isolated finding. However, it is usually seen in association with either severe centrilobular or panlobular emphysema. Paraseptal emphysema can be one of the many causes of spontaneous pneumothorax. Although the exact pathogenesis is unclear, the relationship between paraseptal emphysema and thin and tall body habitus has led to the suggestion that this subtype of emphysema is due to the effects of gravitational pull on the lungs, with a greater negative pleural pressure at the lung apices.[13]

There is some evidence that smoking of marijuana cigarettes may be more highly associated with paraseptal emphysema than regular cigarettes. Some malnutrition syndromes can also cause paraseptal emphysema related to underlying elastase injury.[24] Vanishing lung syndrome (Fig. 60.3), also referred to as giant bullous emphysema, is a rare syndrome characterized by severe paraseptal emphysema and large bullae formation, with the bullae occupying at least one-third of a hemithorax and compressing the adjacent parenchyma. Disease can be unilateral but is more frequently bilateral, and spontaneous pneumothorax is frequent. The disease classically affects young male smokers, but there are few case reports with a possible hereditary component and some possible additional associations with marijuana use and HIV. Bullectomy can result in significant improvements in pulmonary function, but further decline 3 to 4 years after surgery is typical.[27–29]

Paracicatricial Emphysema. Lung destruction, and therefore emphysema, is commonly found adjacent to areas of scarring, which explains the term attributed to this alteration. Because the destruction has no particular position within the lobule, it was also termed *irregular* emphysema. Per definition, it is limited in extent and of little clinical relevance, with patient symptomatology generally attributed to the primary pulmonary diagnosis causing the emphysema, such as pulmonary fibrosis or sarcoidosis.[13]

PHYSIOLOGY

The destruction of pulmonary parenchyma by emphysema creates a decreased mass of functioning lung tissue and thereby decreases the amount of gas exchange that can take place. As lung tissue is destroyed, it loses its elastic recoil and its volume expands. When destruction and expansion occur in a nonuniform manner, the most affected lung tissue can crowd the relatively spared lung tissue and prevent adequate ventilation of the latter. Eventually, obstruction of the small airways can occur, with obstruction being caused by a combination of reversible bronchospasm and

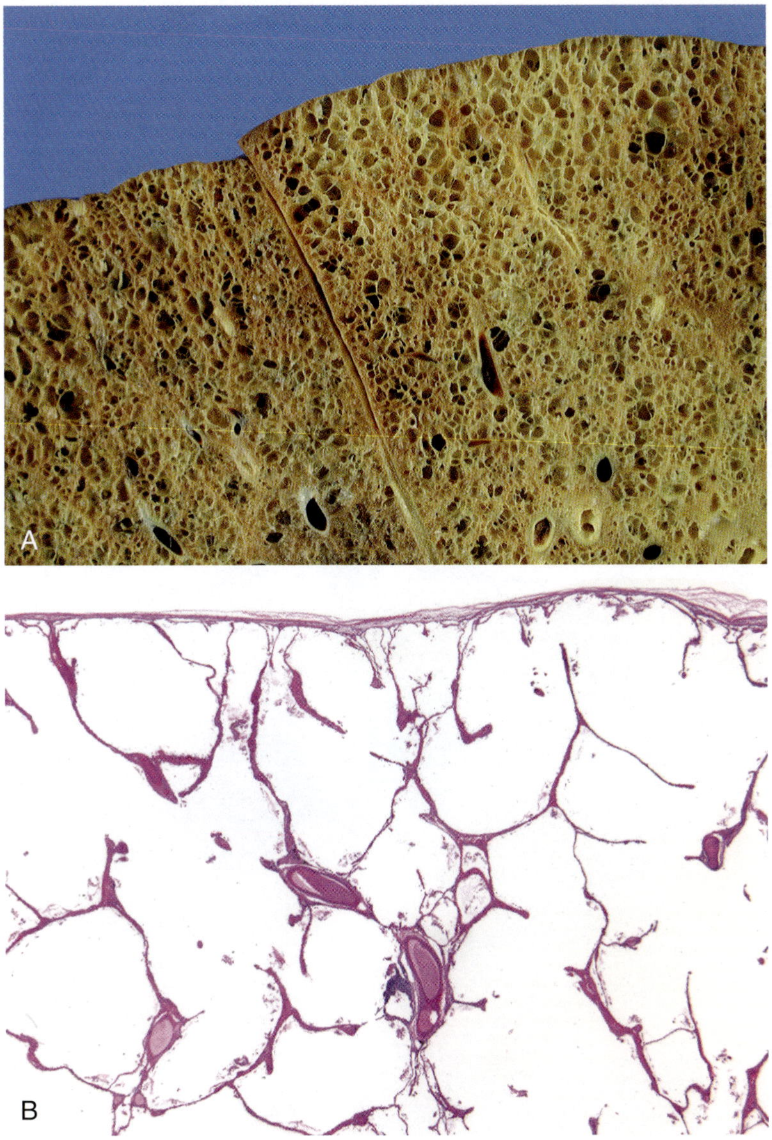

Fig. 60.2 Panlobular emphysema. (A) Low-power view of a lung specimen demonstrates severe uniform enlargement of the airspaces. (B) Histologic specimen shows uniform diffuse enlargement and destruction of the alveoli throughout the acinus. *(Courtesy Dr. John English, Department of Pathology, Vancouver General Hospital, Vancouver, Canada.)*

irreversible loss of elastic recoil by adjacent lung parenchyma. The suitability of a patient for a given treatment will largely depend on the relative contributions of lung destruction, lung recoil, and small airways obstruction to the overall physiologic and clinical impairment of the patient.[30]

In patients with emphysema, the forced expiratory volume in 1 second (FEV1), the forced vital capacity (FVC), the forced expiratory volume as a percentage of vital capacity (FEV/FVC%), the forced expiratory flow (FEF25%–75%), and the maximum expiratory flow at 50% and 75%, respectively, of exhaled vital capacity (Vmax50% and Vmax75%, respectively) will all be reduced. All of these parameters reflect functional obstruction, whether this is caused by alteration of the airway itself or by loss of radial traction resulting from emphysema. The FVC is reduced because the airways close prematurely at an abnormally high lung volume, which is at the source of an increased residual volume.[31,32]

On the other hand, the total lung capacity, the functional residual capacity, and the residual volume are typically increased. In severe disease the expiratory flow-volume curve is grossly abnormal. Flow is strikingly reduced as the airways collapse, and flow limitation by dynamic compression occurs. A scooped-out appearance of the curve is often seen. Flow is greatly reduced in relation to lung volume and ceases at high lung volume because of premature airway closure. Simultaneously, the inspiratory flow-volume curve may be nearly normal. As elastic recoil of the lung is reduced in emphysema, the pressure-volume curve is displaced up and to the left. This probably reflects the disorganization and perhaps loss of elastic tissue as a result of destruction of alveolar walls.[31,32]

Manifestations of the Disease

RADIOGRAPHY

The only direct sign of emphysema on radiographs is the presence of bullae (see Fig. 60.3). However, because of the limited contrast resolution of the chest radiograph, these focal areas of increased lucency can be difficult to detect.[33] Indirect signs of lung destruction caused by emphysema include the focal absence of pulmonary vessels and the reduction of vessel caliber with tapering toward the lung periphery. Abnormalities of the vascular pattern are

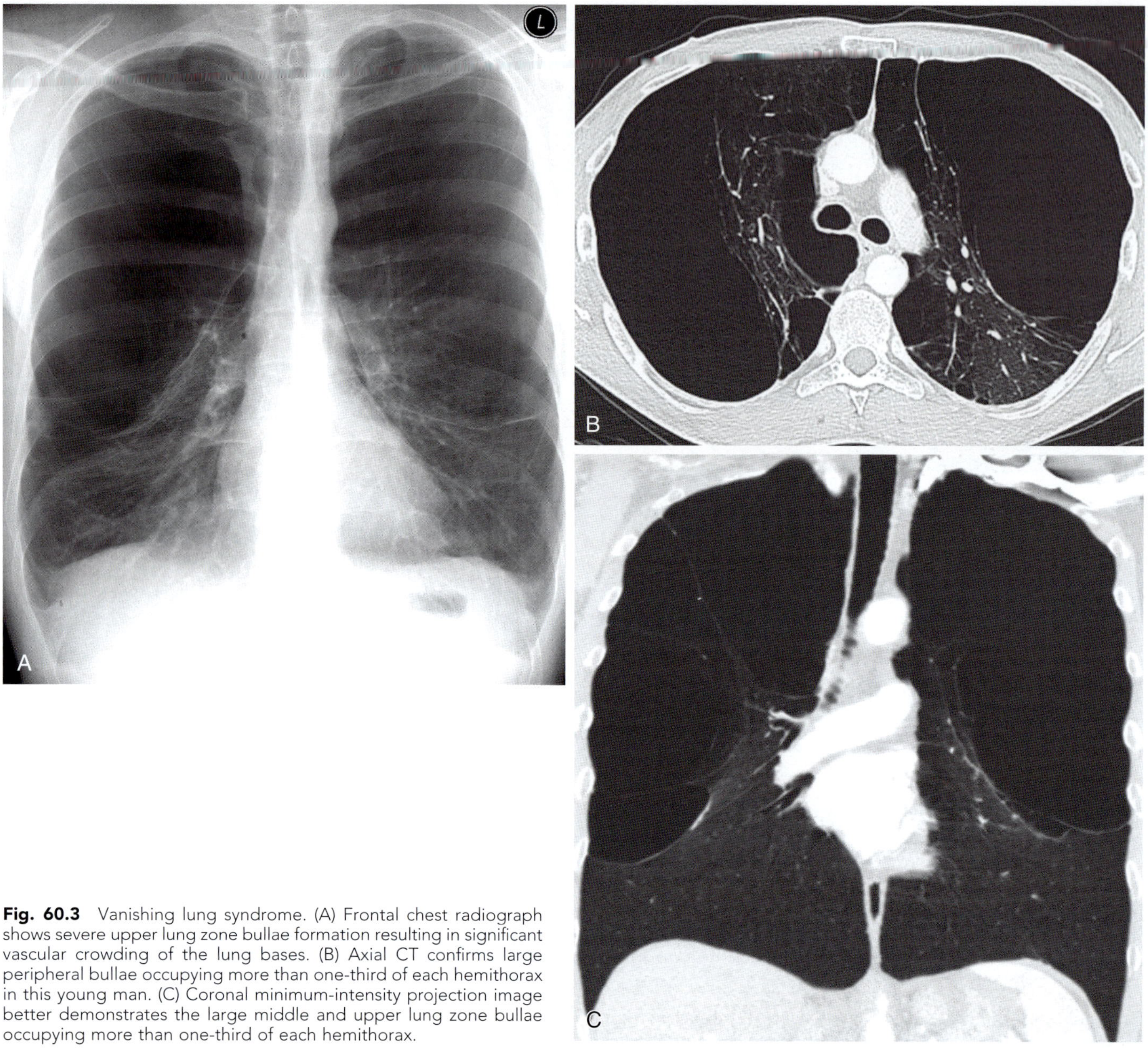

Fig. 60.3 Vanishing lung syndrome. (A) Frontal chest radiograph shows severe upper lung zone bullae formation resulting in significant vascular crowding of the lung bases. (B) Axial CT confirms large peripheral bullae occupying more than one-third of each hemithorax in this young man. (C) Coronal minimum-intensity projection image better demonstrates the large middle and upper lung zone bullae occupying more than one-third of each hemithorax.

indeed highly suggestive of emphysema, but their sensitivity is low. These findings have a sensitivity of only 40% in detecting emphysema.[34] Findings related to hyperinflation of the lungs include flattening of the diaphragm and an increased retrosternal space on the lateral view (Figs. 60.4 and 60.5). These findings are more common than abnormalities of the vascular pattern, but their specificity is also low.[34] The combined signs of hyperinflation and vascular alterations have been shown to allow the diagnosis of emphysema in 29 of 30 autopsy-proven, symptomatic patients but in only 8 of 17 autopsy-proven, asymptomatic patients.[35]

Taking the above into consideration, limitations of radiography in the assessment of emphysema include its low specificity, its low sensitivity in the evaluation of mild disease, its considerable interobserver variability in the interpretation of findings, and its inability to quantify the severity of emphysema.[12,33–35]

COMPUTED TOMOGRAPHY

Computed tomography is superior to chest radiography in the detection of emphysema and in the assessment of its distribution and extent. On CT emphysema is characterized by the presence of areas of low attenuation that contrast with the surrounding lung parenchyma with normal attenuation (Fig. 60.6).[14,36] Mild to moderate centrilobular emphysema is characterized by the presence of multiple rounded and small areas of low attenuation that have diameters of several millimeters and usually have upper lung zone predominance (Fig. 60.7). The lesions have no walls, as they are limited by the surrounding lung parenchyma. Sometimes, the lesions may appear to be grouped around the center of secondary pulmonary lobules (Figs. 60.8).[14,37] Panlobular emphysema is characterized by a uniform destruction of the secondary pulmonary lobule. This leads to widespread and relatively homogeneous patterns of low attenuation.[14,38] Panlobular

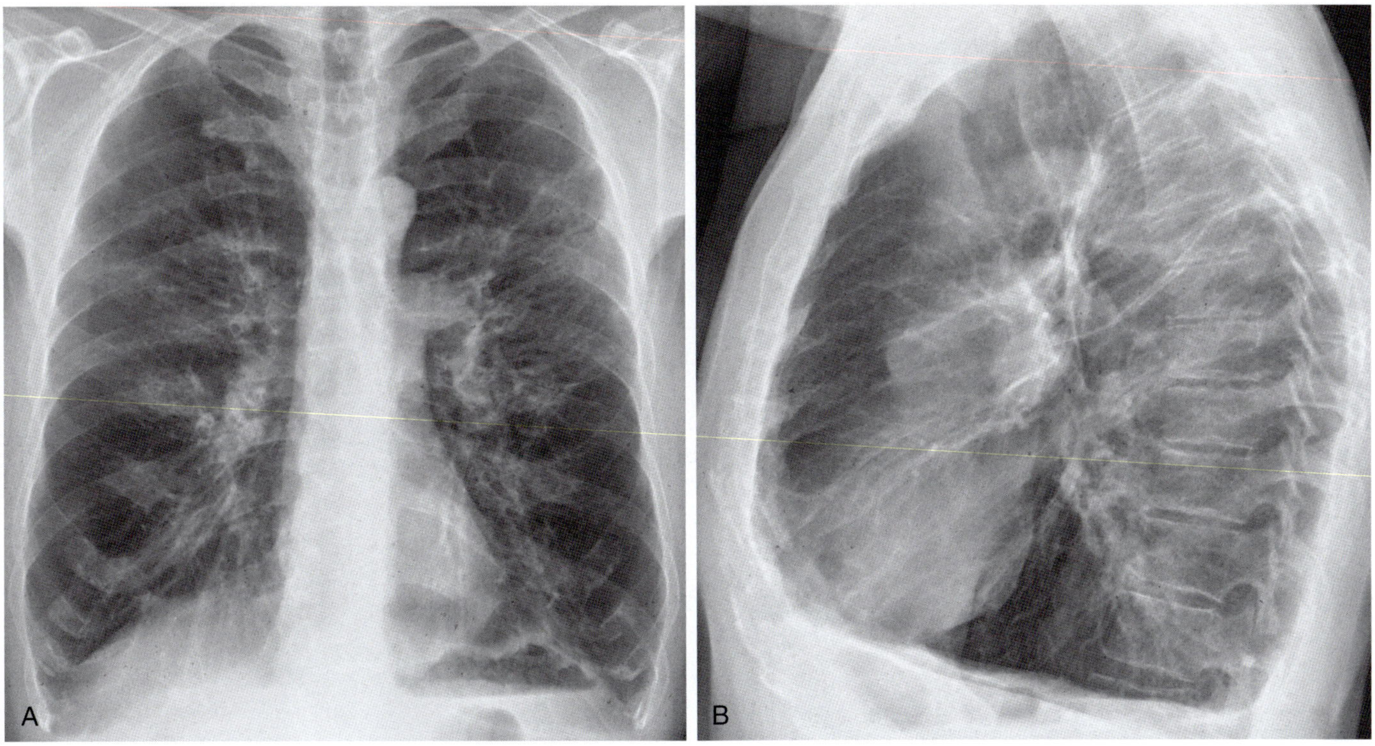

Fig. 60.4 Severe panlobular emphysema. Frontal (A) and lateral (B) chest radiographs show increased intrathoracic volume and flattened diaphragm resulting from overinflation. Simultaneously, transparency of the lung is increased, lung structure is rarified, and increased interstitial markings are shown.

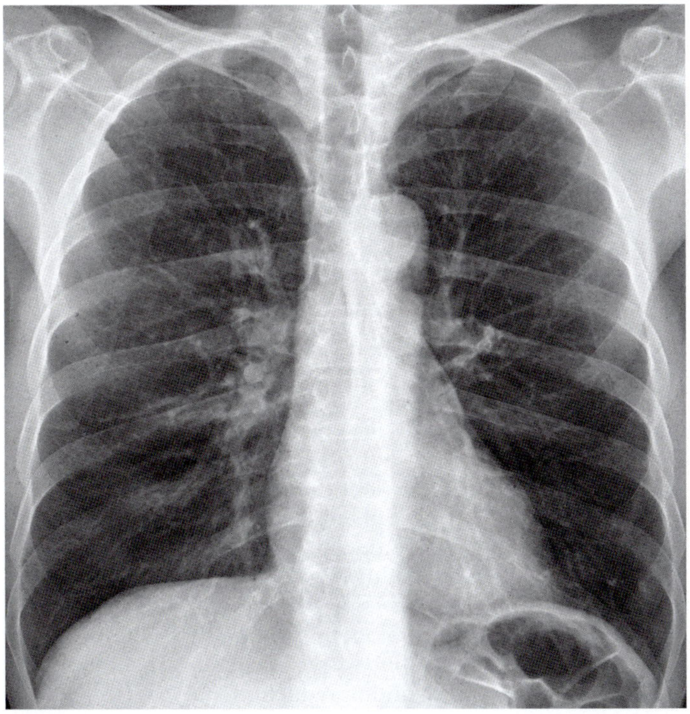

Fig. 60.5 Centrilobular emphysema: radiographic findings. Transparency of the lung parenchyma is nearly normal. In the lung apices, deviation of vascular structures and subtle curvilinear opacities suggest the presence of emphysema and bullae.

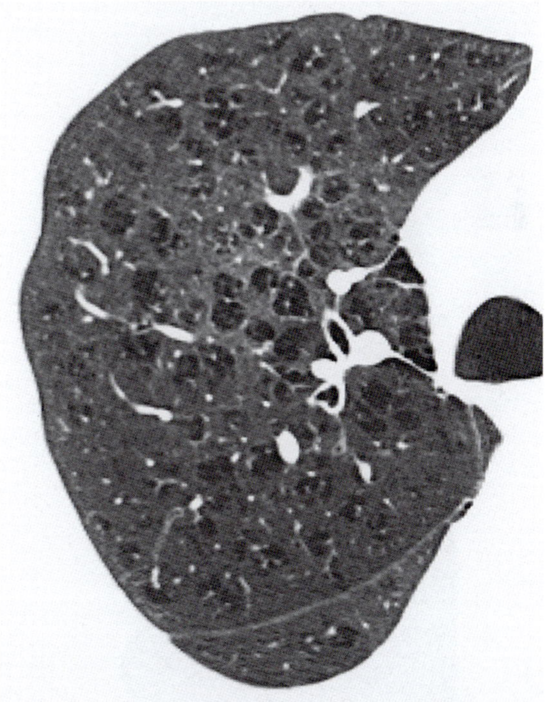

Fig. 60.6 Centrilobular emphysema: classic CT findings. CT image targeted to the right lung shows well-defined "holes" in the centrilobular portions of the secondary pulmonary lobule surrounding small vessels. Note the lack of visible walls.

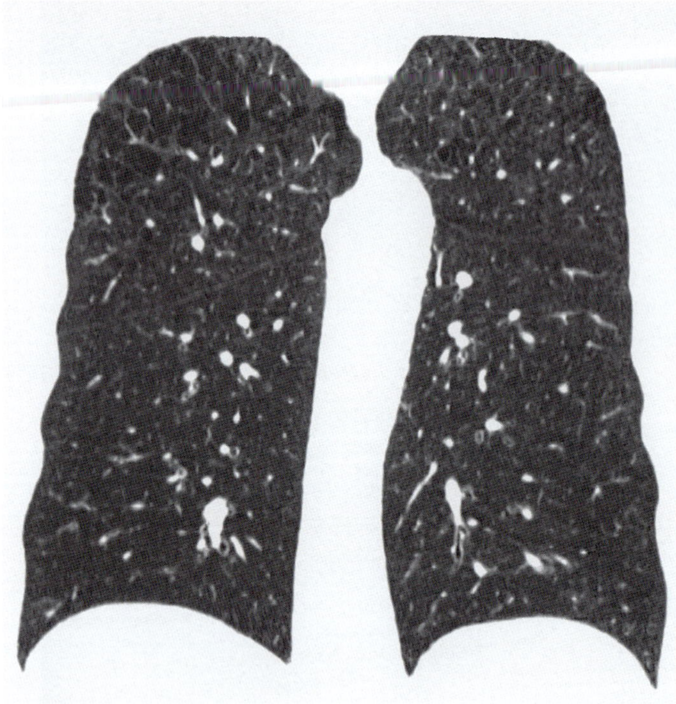

Fig. 60.7 Centrilobular emphysema: coronal reconstruction. Coronal reformatted CT image shows apical predominant emphysema.

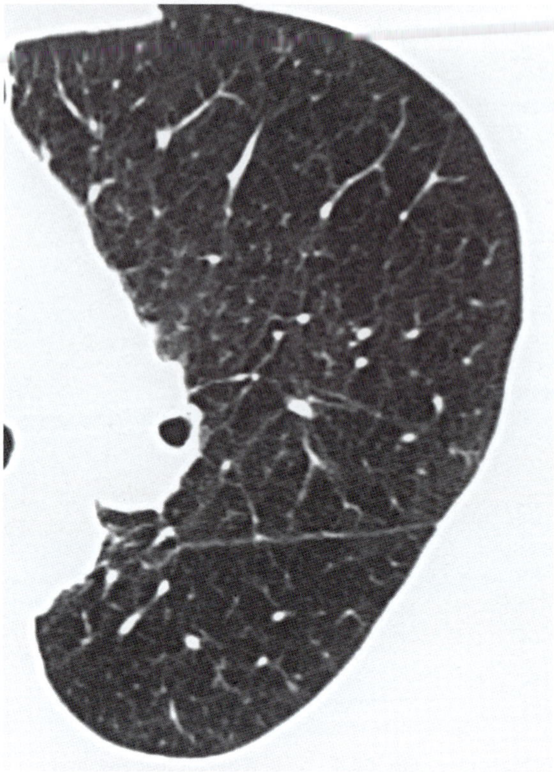

Fig. 60.9 Moderate panlobular emphysema. High-resolution CT section through the left upper lobe shows areas of hypoattenuation with effacement of the lung structure. Structures suggestive of secondary pulmonary lobules can barely be detected.

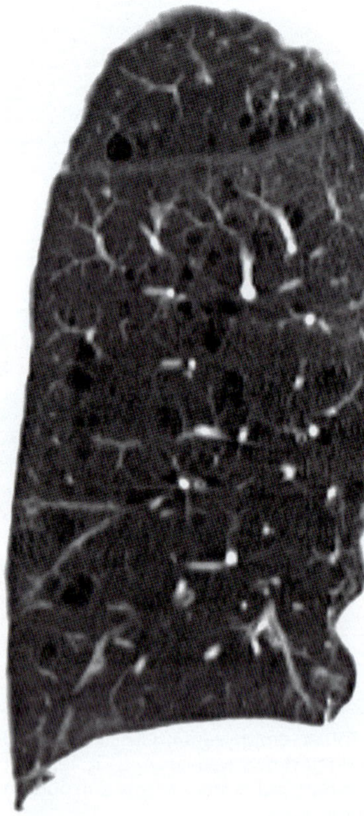

Fig. 60.8 Moderate centrilobular emphysema: coronal reconstruction of high-resolution CT image of the right lung. Although emphysematous lesions can be seen in the entire lung, emphysema predominates in the upper lobe and the uppermost parts of the lower lobe.

emphysema can involve the entire lung in a homogeneous manner or show lower lung zone predominance (Figs. 60.9 and 60.10). On CT, paraseptal emphysema is seen as single or multiple bullae adjacent to the pleura or along interlobular septa (Fig. 60.11). It may be an isolated finding or be associated with centrilobular or panlobular emphysema (Fig. 60.12).

The assessment of mild emphysema can further benefit from the use of minimum-intensity projection technique (Fig. 60.13). This technique uses dedicated software that identifies only areas of lung parenchyma with the lowest attenuation values and simultaneously suppresses normal lung and pulmonary vessels. The technique is based on "slabs" of contiguous high-resolution CT sections through a sample of lung tissue. Comparing minimum-intensity projection and 1-mm high-resolution CT sections, a study has found that the minimum-intensity projection technique is more sensitive for the detection of subtle emphysema.[39]

Of note, the distribution of emphysema in the craniocaudal plane is an important point to recognize and include in the radiology report. Lung volume reduction surgery (LVRS) is a good treatment option for patients with end-stage emphysema and preserved exercise tolerance. CT characterization of the distribution of disease is critical for preoperative evaluation of surgical candidacy. Those patients with a majority of the emphysema in the upper lungs, so-called nonhomogeneous distribution, benefit from LVRS. Those patients with a more diffuse distribution, so-called homogeneous distribution, do not benefit from surgical resection.

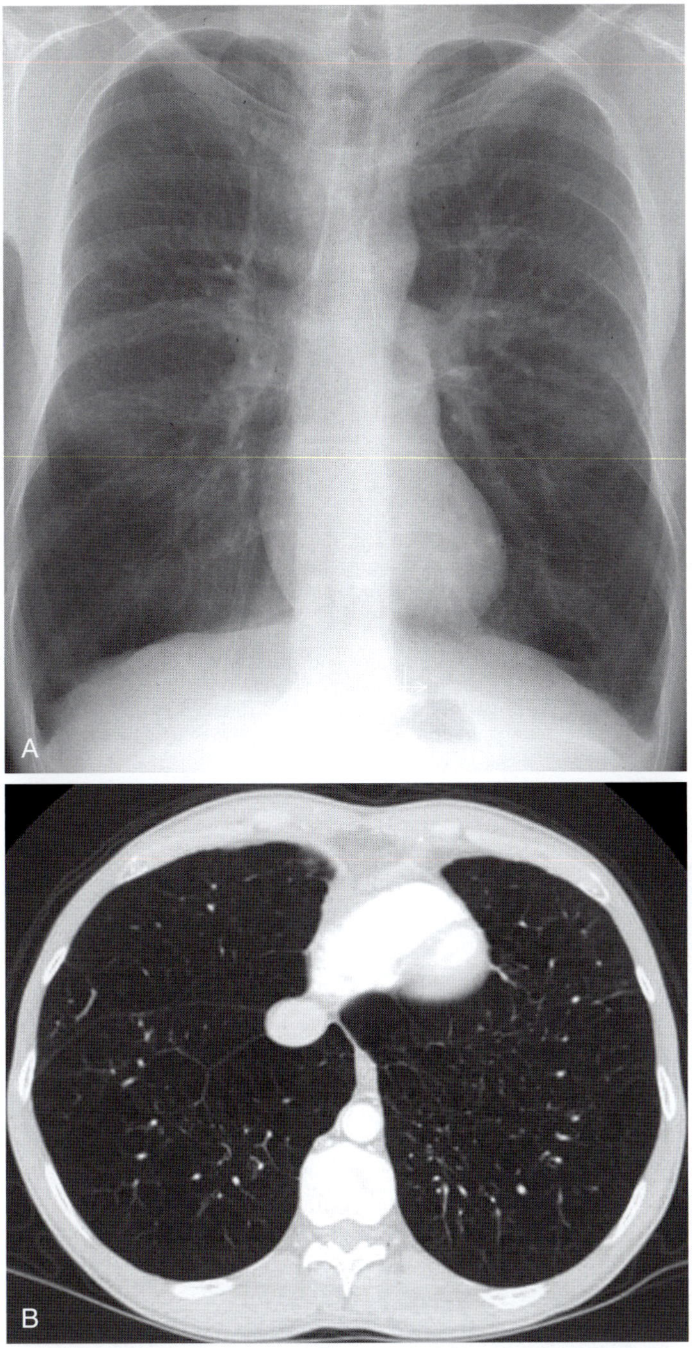

Fig. 60.10 Advanced panlobular emphysema in a patient with α1-antitrypsin deficiency. (A) Frontal chest radiograph showing hyperinflation with greatest lucency resulting from a vessel attenuation in the lower lung zones. (B) High-resolution CT image through the lower lobes shows extensive emphysematous destruction affecting the entire secondary pulmonary lobule. The lack of lung structures gives the resulting areas of hypoattenuation a relatively homogeneous appearance.

Objective Computed Tomographic Quantification of Emphysema

The inherent limitations of subjective visual scoring, the characteristic CT morphology of emphysema, and the digital nature of the CT data set have raised considerable interest in the use of CT as an objective tool for quantification of pulmonary emphysema.[40] Three main approaches have been used to quantify emphysema objectively with CT: first, the use of a threshold density value below which emphysema is considered to be present (threshold technique); second, the assessment of a range of densities present in a CT section and displayed as a distribution curve (histogram technique); and third, the measurement of the overall CT density of the lung parenchyma.

In 1988 Müller and colleagues[41] used a commercially available CT program called Density Mask (General Electric Medical Systems, Milwaukee, WI) that highlights pixels within a given attenuation range and automatically calculates the area of highlighted pixels. In their study the highest correlation was observed with attenuation values lower than −910 Hounsfield units (HU), and as consequence, this threshold was recommended for the identification of emphysema. This work has been built upon by several others, and a more frequently used cutoff for this technique is now −950 HU, which provides better sensitivity and specificity, with thresholds below this value underestimating emphysema and thresholds above it overestimating emphysema.

All of these CT techniques for quantifying emphysema remain in the research stage and are not yet in general use outside of academic medical centers and trials.

Tissue Characterization

Quantifications of pulmonary emphysema by computer-assisted methods are based on mathematic approaches, called metrics, that may be used to describe the heterogeneity of the spatial distribution of the attenuation values within the reconstructed image.[42] These metrics include simple parameters, such as the mean lung density to areas of low attenuation based on a single or a range of density.[42] Textural analyses are more complex metrics. There is considerable interest in these techniques. For example, Ginsburg and colleagues[43] showed that a texture-based approach could differentiate between the lungs of never-smokers, smokers without visual emphysema, and smokers with emphysema. As such, textural analysis may be able to differentiate the very early stages of smoking-related lung injury before the development of emphysema.

Comparison Between Computed Tomographic Quantification and Pulmonary Function Tests

Although pulmonary function tests may be short- and long-term reproducible tests, they represent global measurements of lung function of more than 10 million airways that contribute unequally to airflow.[44] They are of limited value in the measurement of the obstruction of airways, particularly small airways that are predominantly affected in emphysema,[44] and autopsy studies have shown that up to one-third of the lung can be destroyed by emphysema before respiratory function becomes impaired.[45] The insensitivity of pulmonary function tests to diagnose mild emphysema was confirmed by Sanders and colleagues,[46] who found that features of emphysema were visually detected on CT scans in 69% of smokers with normal diffusing lung capacity for carbon monoxide with or without associated obstructive deficit. These authors concluded that CT may be more sensitive than pulmonary function tests in detecting mild emphysema.

The lack of sensitivity of pulmonary function tests for the detection of pulmonary emphysema can be explained by two reasons related to pulmonary zones in which ventilatory disorders are not assessed by conventional pulmonary function tests. First, the total airflow resistance of all respiratory bronchioles contributes little to the total airflow resistance of the lung.[44]

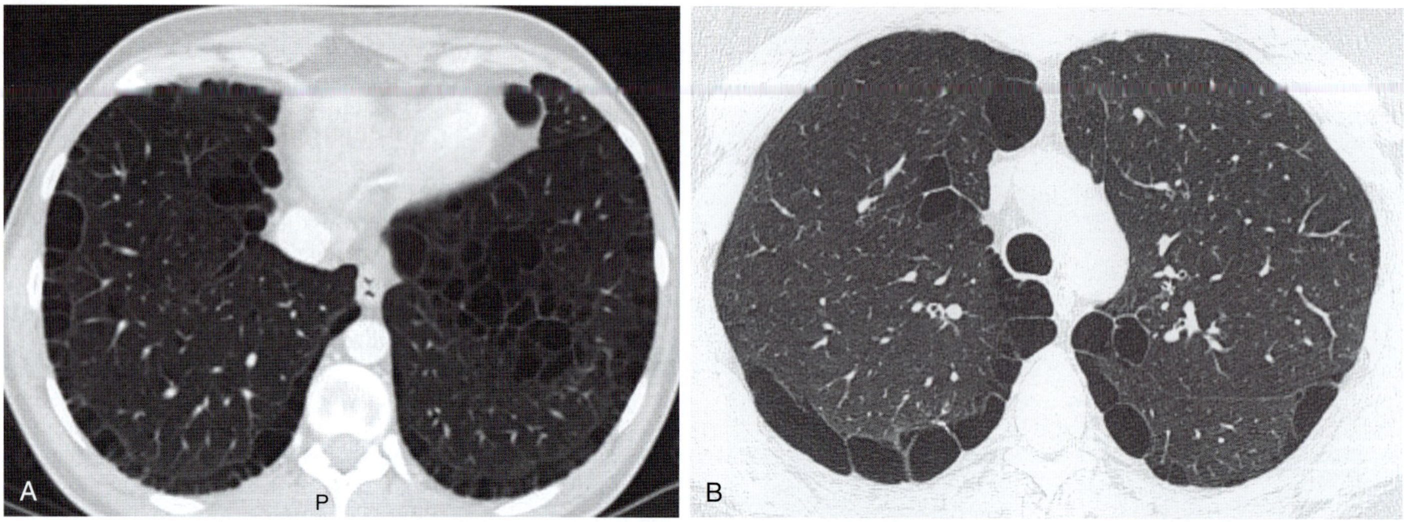

Fig. 60.11 Paraseptal emphysema: typical CT findings in two patients. (A) CT image through the lower lungs shows paraseptal emphysema and blebs adjacent to the pleura and along interlobular septa. (B) CT image at the level of the aortic arch shows multiple bullae adjacent to the pleura, typical of paraseptal emphysema.

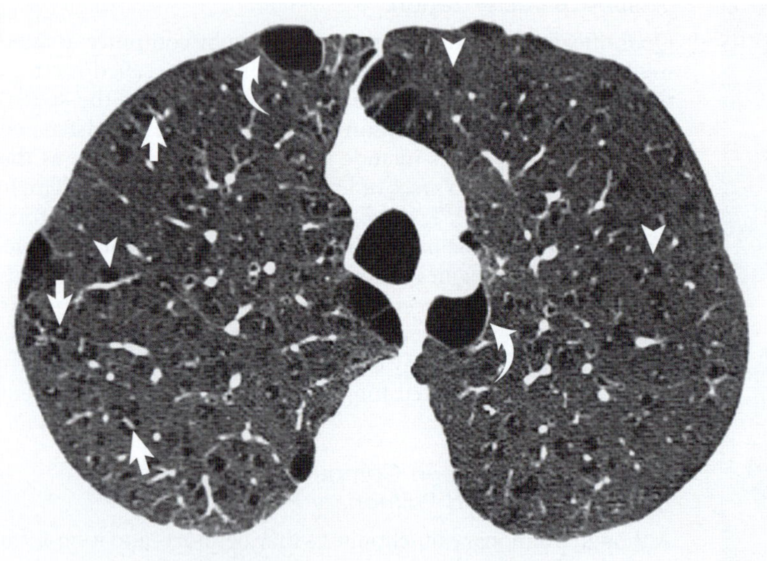

Fig. 60.12 Centrilobular and paraseptal emphysema. High-resolution CT image shows centrilobular emphysema *(arrowheads)* with preserved centrilobular core structures *(small arrows)*. In subpleural location, paraseptal emphysema is seen *(curved arrows)*.

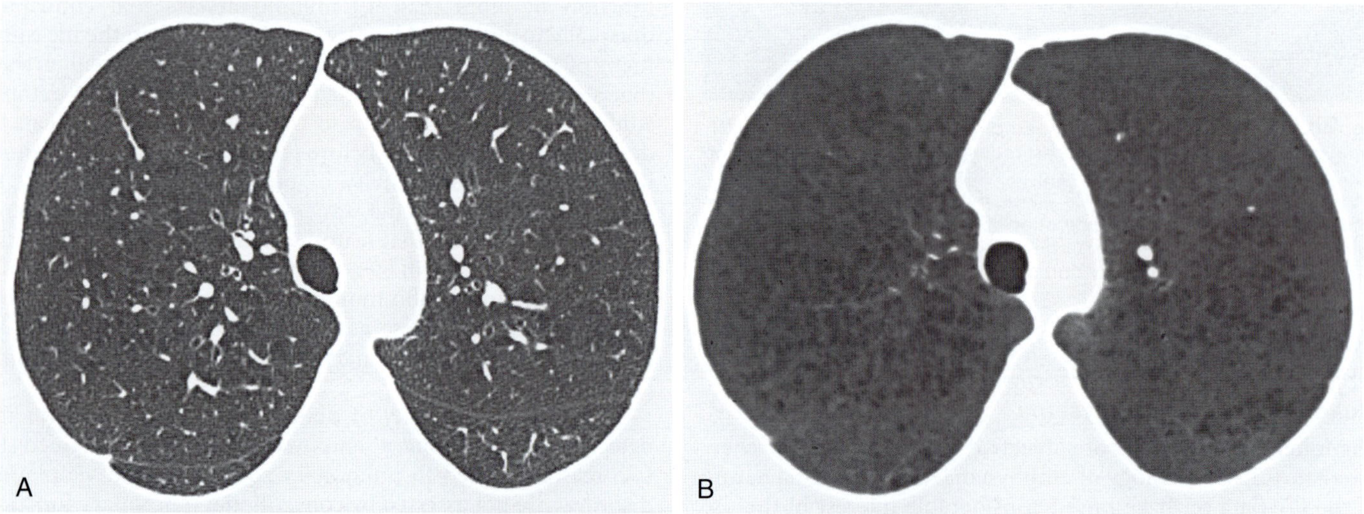

Fig. 60.13 Minimum-intensity projection images to diagnose subtle emphysema. (A) CT image shows subtle centrilobular emphysema in the upper lobes. (B) Lesions are much better seen on the minimum-intensity projection image.

Despite the high airflow resistance through one single respiratory bronchiole, the parallel connection of a large number of bronchioles leads to a wide total cross-sectional area and dramatically reduces the airflow resistance.[47] Second, the upper lung zone has a relatively high ventilation-perfusion ratio compared with the lower lung zone. Thus, in the relatively underventilated upper lung zone, emphysema produces less measurable pulmonary dysfunction than in the lower zone.

MAGNETIC RESONANCE IMAGING

Conventional magnetic resonance imaging (MRI) of the lung parenchyma is difficult to perform. Hyperpolarized helium-3 (^{3}He)-enhanced MRI is still an investigational technique whereby the airspaces are visualized after the inhalation of polarized helium. Using this technique, it has been demonstrated that the apparent diffusion coefficient values in the lungs of patients with clinical symptoms of emphysema are increased relative to those in subjects without emphysema,[48] and there is some evidence suggesting that regional emphysematous changes can be identified by such MRI techniques at an early stage when there are no clinical symptoms.[48,49] More recently, developments in diffusion-weighted MRI by use of hyperpolarized xenon-129 gas, which is substantially less expensive than ^{3}He and more readily available, are also encouraging.[49]

IMAGING ALGORITHMS

If concomitant signs of hyperinflation are absent, the chest radiograph in patients with mild disease may be normal. Even the changes in patients with moderate disease can be so subtle that they are overlooked on chest radiographs. Patients with suspected emphysema because of either a smoking history or a known α1-antitrypsin deficiency should therefore proceed to CT early in the course of their disease.

CT should be performed in typical full-suspended inspiration. The intravenous administration of contrast material and expiratory CT sections are not required in the evaluation of emphysema, but expiratory CT may be useful for evaluating other causes of small airways disease that could be present.

Differential Diagnosis

CENTRILOBULAR EMPHYSEMA

Given the distinct morphologic features and the distribution of the disease, correctly diagnosing centrilobular emphysema is not difficult in typical cases. Panlobular emphysema shows more homogeneous patterns of destruction than centrilobular emphysema with regard to the secondary pulmonary lobule. The panlobular emphysema craniocaudal distribution is also more uniform to lower lung predominance. It is important to recognize that severe centrilobular emphysema may demonstrate a confluent pattern that is identical to panlobular emphysema. However, because of the strong association of panlobular emphysema with α1-antitrypsin deficiency, the use of *panlobular* as a descriptor should be reserved for those cases where the radiologist specifically wants the referring clinician to consider α1-antitrypsin deficiency as a possible underlying etiology rather than merely severe smoking-related emphysema. In addition, α1-antitrypsin deficiency is associated with liver cirrhosis and hepatocellular carcinoma, so a careful evaluation of the hepatic parenchyma for evidence of these is important in suspected cases. Rarer complications of α1-antitrypsin deficiency include panniculitis and vasculitis.

Pulmonary Langerhans cell histiocytosis is another smoking-related disorder. Other than in centrilobular emphysema, the "holes" seen here are preceded by nodules that evolve to cysts. The disease, however, can have an upper lung zone distribution that is similar to the one seen in centrilobular emphysema. Cysts in the lung parenchyma can be lined by fibrous tissue or bronchiolar epithelium. This always gives them a visible "wall," which distinguishes them from the lesions seen in centrilobular emphysema. The same is true for the large group of entities summarized as "cystic lung lesions," such as lymphangioleiomyomatosis or lymphocytic interstitial pneumonia; all of these have walls, but lesions in centrilobular emphysema do not.

PANLOBULAR EMPHYSEMA

In panlobular emphysema the differential diagnosis can be more difficult than in centrilobular emphysema. As mentioned earlier, the distribution of disease in the craniocaudal plane tends to be more uniform to lower lung predominance.

Similar to centrilobular emphysema, the cystic lung diseases can be considered in the differential but would demonstrate more definable walls.

Panlobular emphysema may be difficult to distinguish from constrictive bronchiolitis. Both conditions may result in diffuse areas of decreased attenuation and vascularity. The main distinguishing features are parenchymal destruction and vascular distortion in panlobular emphysema; absence of these features is characteristic of constrictive bronchiolitis.

PARASEPTAL EMPHYSEMA

It is usually easy to identify paraseptal emphysema on CT and to distinguish it from other lung diseases. The main differential diagnosis is with honeycombing in patients who have ground-glass opacities superimposed on areas of paraseptal emphysema. The areas of low attenuation in paraseptal emphysema tend to be larger (1 cm or more) and have thinner walls (1 mm or less) than areas of honeycombing. Furthermore, areas of honeycombing tend to be associated with volume loss and other signs of fibrosis, such as reticulation and traction bronchiectasis. Finally, the craniocaudal distribution of paraseptal emphysema tends to be upper lung zone predominant, and honeycomb cysts tend to be lower lung zone predominant.

Synopsis of Treatment Options

MEDICAL

- Smoking cessation can substantially slow or even stop the progression of pulmonary emphysema.
- Antibiotic administration aims to prevent pulmonary infection.
- Corticosteroids or bronchodilators are used mainly in patients with coexisting small airways disease.
- Pulmonary rehabilitation aims to improve functional exercise capacity and health-related quality of life and to reduce the use of health care resources.
- α1-Antitrypsin substitution, sometimes called augmentation, is available.

KEY POINTS

CENTRILOBULAR EMPHYSEMA

- Strongly associated with cigarette smoking
- Well-defined "holes" in the centrilobular portions of the secondary pulmonary lobule
- Well-defined margins between normal and emphysematous lung create an inhomogeneous appearance
- Anatomic borders of the secondary pulmonary lobule are preserved
- Predominantly involves upper lung zones
- Differential diagnoses include panlobular emphysema, pulmonary Langerhans cell histiocytosis, and "cystic" lung lesions

PANLOBULAR EMPHYSEMA

- Strongly associated with α1-antitrypsin deficiency
- Ill-defined absence of lung parenchyma
- Ill-defined margins between normal and emphysematous lung create a homogeneous appearance
- Anatomic borders of the secondary pulmonary lobule are not preserved
- Homogeneously distributed, occasionally with lower lung zone predominance
- Differential diagnoses include severe centrilobular emphysema, constrictive bronchiolitis, and cystic lung diseases, such as pulmonary Langerhans cell histiocytosis, lymphocytic interstitial pneumonia, and lymphangioleiomyomatosis

SURGICAL

- Endobronchial valves: This intervention consists of the endoscopic implantation of endobronchial valves to collapse distal parts of the lung and to improve respiratory mechanics.
- Bullectomy aims to increase the intrathoracic volume occupied by lung tissue participating in gas exchange by resection of one or more bullae, which by definition do not participate in gas exchange.
- In lung volume reduction surgery, the most emphysematous part of the lung is resected to improve the respiratory mechanics and the expansion of the remaining lung tissue.
- Lung transplantation is reserved for advanced cases of emphysema.

SUGGESTED READINGS

Edwards RM, et al. Imaging of small airways and emphysema. *Clin Chest Med*. 2015;36(2):335–347, x.

Lee P, et al. Emphysema in nonsmokers: alpha 1-antitrypsin deficiency and other causes. *Cleve Clin J Med*. 2002;69(12):928–929, 933, 936 passim.

Lynch DA, Al-Qaisi MA. Quantitative computed tomography in chronic obstructive pulmonary disease. *J Thorac Imaging*. 2013;28(5):284–290.

Matsuoka S, et al. Quantitative CT assessment of chronic obstructive pulmonary disease. *Radiographics*. 2010;30(1):55–66.

Milanese G, et al. Lung volume reduction of pulmonary emphysema: the radiologist task. *Curr Opin Pulm Med*. 2016;22(2):179–186.

Takahashi M, et al. Imaging of pulmonary emphysema: a pictorial review. *Int J Chron Obstruct Pulmon Dis*. 2008;3(2):193–204.

The full reference list for this chapter is available at ExpertConsult.com.

61 Asbestos-Related Disease*

STEPHEN B. HOBBS

Etiology

Asbestos is the general term given to a group of magnesium silicate minerals that have in common a tendency to separate into fibers.[1] The fibers are resistant to heat and acid, thus the name *asbestos,* which is derived from the Greek meaning inextinguishable (*a-*, "not," and *sbestos,* "extinguishable"). Because asbestos is not combustible, has great tensile strength, and is durable, it has been widely used in insulation materials, brake pads and linings, floor tiles, electric wiring, paints, and cements.

Asbestos can be divided mineralogically into two major groups: the serpentines, of which the only member of commercial importance is chrysotile (white asbestos); and the amphiboles, which include amosite (brown asbestos), crocidolite (blue asbestos), and tremolite (a common contaminant of chrysotile). Chrysotile fibers are typically curved, whereas the amphiboles are straight. These physical properties and chemical differences are responsible for the varying uses of asbestos and for their ability to cause disease. Chrysotile is more easily cleared from the lung than the amphiboles, has a weaker fibrinogenic and carcinogenic potential, and is the only type of asbestos fiber that is still widely used. The current products are mainly cements, friction materials, and plastics.[2]

Prevalence and Epidemiology

The widespread use of asbestos in the first 7 decades of the 20th century resulted in an epidemic of asbestos-related illness that continues into the 21st century in spite of a major decline in use after documentation of its major hazards, particularly for amphibole asbestos fibers (crocidolite and amosite) in the 1970s and 1980s.[1] Although the use of asbestos has now been banned in many Western countries, the prevalence of asbestos-related pulmonary and pleural complications has been increasing.[3] For example, surveys in the United States and in Europe have shown a doubling of the prevalence of asbestos-related pleural complications, including mesothelioma, between the early 1970s and 2000.[3] Similarly, whereas mortality rates for the other pneumoconioses decreased between 1968 and 2000, the mortality of asbestosis increased steadily, and it is now the most frequently recorded pneumoconiosis on death certificates.[4] It has been estimated that 8 to 9 million people in the United States have had occupational exposure to asbestos and that such exposure will eventually result in 300,000 deaths.[5] These complications are still occurring because the interval between initial exposure and subsequent biological consequences of asbestos exposure is variable, ranging from approximately 1 year for some cases of pleural effusion to more than 40 years for mesothelioma.[3]

The four main settings in which asbestos-related disease is seen in the Western world are

1. The historical legacy of asbestos exposure affecting older workers
2. The current risk experienced by the work force engaged in certain occupations managing the remaining asbestos hazard, such as building and facility maintenance
3. Asbestos abatement operations for removal of insulation and other asbestos-containing products
4. Renovation and demolition of structures containing asbestos[1]

Most asbestos in North America today exists in building and machinery insulation and old products, such as appliances. New products that may contain asbestos today in the United States include friction surfaces (brake pads), roofing materials, vinyl tiles, and imported cement pipe and sheeting.[1] It is estimated that asbestos is currently still a hazard for approximately 1.3 million workers in the construction industry in the United States and for workers involved in maintenance of buildings and equipment.[1] The risk of asbestos exposure is considerably higher in countries where it continues to be used.[1] Currently, the majority of asbestos is mined in Russia, with other mining operations existing in China, Brazil, and Kazakhstan.[6] Until 2011 Quebec, Canada, operated two asbestos mines, but those mines are now closed despite a 2012 legislative attempt to restart one of the mines.

Clinical Presentation

Most patients who have asbestos-related pleuropulmonary disease are asymptomatic. Patients with asbestosis, chronic airflow obstruction, or diffuse pleural fibrosis may present with shortness of breath.[7] The onset of dyspnea in asbestosis is typically insidious, beginning with dyspnea on exertion.[1] The dyspnea related to asbestosis is generally progressive, even in the absence of continued dust exposure. In patients who have asbestosis, shortness of breath seldom occurs sooner than 20 to 30 years after initial exposure.[7] A nonproductive cough is also commonly present.[1] Pleuritic chest pain may accompany the development of benign asbestos effusion or mesothelioma. Benign asbestos effusions are generally less than 500 mL in volume, are often serosanguineous, and may persist for 2 weeks to 6 months.[7] They are recurrent in 15% to 30% of cases. The presence of pleural effusion or diffuse pleural thickening should raise the possibility of mesothelioma.

*The editors and the publisher would like to thank Drs. C. Isabela Silva Müller and Nestor L. Müller for contributing material on this topic to the prior edition of this work. It has served as the foundation for the current chapter.

Pathophysiology

The pathogenesis of asbestos-related pleuropulmonary disease is complex and incompletely understood. Fiber dose, dimension, and chemical composition may all influence fibrogenicity and carcinogenicity; longer, thinner, more durable fibers (amphiboles) are the most important.[8] Factors related to the host, including pulmonary clearance, immunologic status, and exposure to other noxious substances, such as cigarette smoke, are also important in determining the nature and severity of the reaction to inhaled fibers.[7]

Asbestos fibers are deposited at airway bifurcations and in respiratory bronchioles and alveoli.[1] They migrate into the interstitium, in part through an uptake process involving type I alveolar epithelial cells. Once they reach the interstitium, the asbestos fibers cause an alveolar macrophage-dominated alveolitis, inflammation in the surrounding interstitium, and inflammation followed by fibrotic change in the respiratory bronchioles that extends into the adjacent alveolar tissue.[1]

PATHOLOGIC CHARACTERISTICS

Asbestos-Related Pulmonary Abnormalities

Asbestosis. The earliest pulmonary abnormality seen in association with asbestos exposure consists of fibrosis in the walls of respiratory bronchioles (Fig. 61.1). This process, however, is pathogenetically distinct from pulmonary parenchymal fibrosis and may be seen in patients with a history of exposure to mineral dust other than asbestos.[7,9] Peribronchiolar fibrosis is probably better considered a form of asbestos airway disease separate from asbestosis.[9,10] Asbestosis itself is defined as diffuse interstitial pulmonary fibrosis caused by the inhalation of excessive amounts of asbestos fibers. The interstitial fibrosis involves mainly the lower zones; the worst disease is generally seen closest to the pleura, with relative sparing of the central portions of the lung.[11] The microscopic appearance varies from a slight increase in interstitial collagen to complete obliteration of normal lung architecture and the formation of thick fibrous bands and honeycombing. The microscopic diagnosis of asbestosis is based on the presence of two findings: diffuse interstitial fibrosis, which in advanced cases is identical to that seen in usual interstitial pneumonia, and asbestos bodies, fibers of asbestos to which the lung has added an iron-protein coating (Figs. 61.2 and 61.3).[11] The development of asbestosis requires heavy exposure to asbestos and therefore is seen mainly in asbestos miners and millers, asbestos textile workers, and asbestos insulators. Fibrosis of adjacent visceral pleura is common and often accompanied by parietal pleural adhesions.[11] Asbestosis is commonly associated with prolonged exposure, usually over 10 to 20 years, and the degree of fibrosis is dose dependent.[1] Transport of the asbestos fibers to the pleural surface along lymphatic channels or by direct penetration results in pleural inflammation and fibrosis.[1]

Rounded Atelectasis. Rounded atelectasis, also known as folded lung, consists of a more or less spherical focus of collapsed parenchyma in the periphery of the lung.[7] The overlying pleura is invariably fibrotic and shows one or more invaginations 1 mm

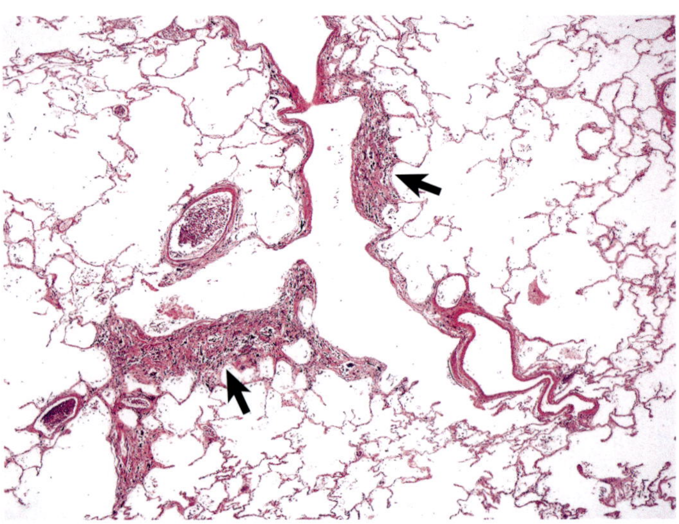

Fig. 61.1 Asbestos-induced peribronchiolar fibrosis. Histologic specimen shows thickening of airway wall *(arrows)* resulting from peribronchiolar fibrosis and pigmented dust. *(Courtesy Dr. Andrew Churg, Department of Pathology, University of British Columbia, Vancouver, Canada.)*

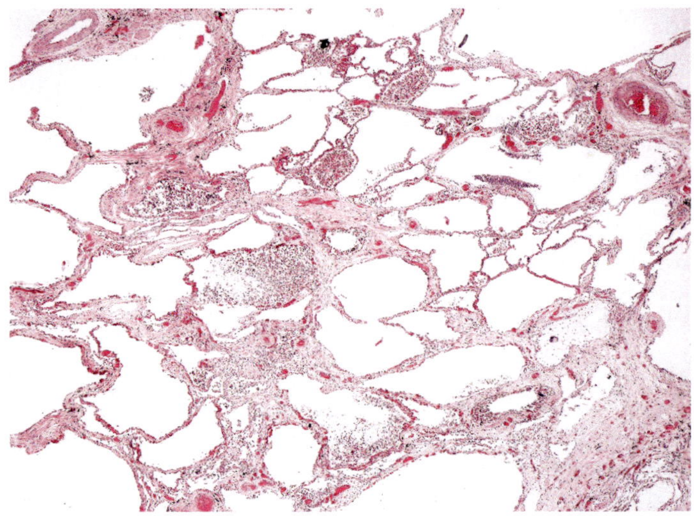

Fig. 61.2 Asbestosis. Low-power view shows diffuse fibrosis. *(Courtesy Dr. Andrew Churg, Department of Pathology, University of British Columbia, Vancouver, Canada.)*

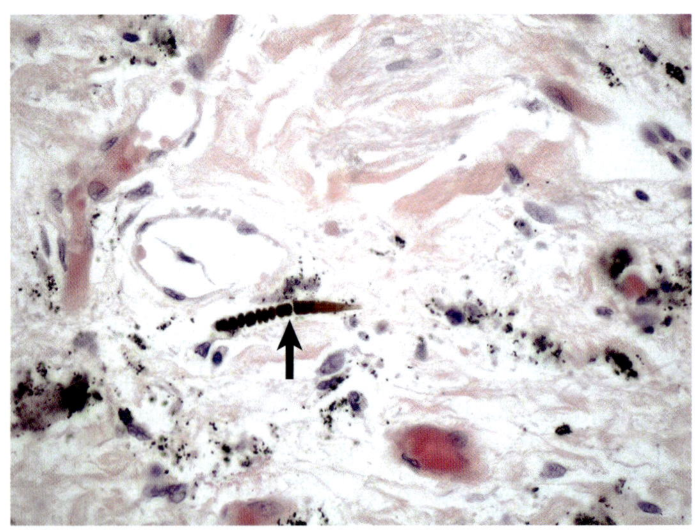

Fig. 61.3 Asbestos body. Pathologic specimen from same case as in Fig. 61.1 shows typical beaded appearance and gold color of asbestos body *(arrow)*. *(Courtesy Dr. Andrew Churg, Department of Pathology, University of British Columbia, Vancouver, Canada.)*

to 3 cm in length into the adjacent lung. Although rounded atelectasis is not related solely to asbestos, the majority of cases are associated with it. The lesion is believed to develop secondary to infolding of thickened visceral pleura with atelectasis of the intervening lung parenchyma.[1] Rounded atelectasis may be multiple and bilateral.

Lung Cancer. Asbestos exposure is associated with an increased risk of lung cancer, and this risk is markedly increased in smokers (supraadditive effect—an effect greater than the sum of either risk alone).[12] Amphiboles, particularly crocidolite, are more potent than chrysotile in inducing lung cancer (between 10 and 50 times greater potency).[13] The risk of lung cancer in commercial chrysotile is believed to be largely determined by the varying content of tremolite.[14] The mechanism of carcinogenesis is unclear. The latent period is variable. Some cases occur less than 10 years after exposure, but the majority of cases occur much later.[2] In a study of 3383 asbestos-exposed workers, 63 (1.9%) had pulmonary carcinoma; the mean latency period for the development of carcinoma was 45.8 ± 9.4 years, and the mean age of patients was 67.6 ± 8.4 years.[15] Asbestos-related cancers can occur anywhere in the lungs and be of any cell type.

Although it is clear that asbestos exposure is associated with an increased incidence of lung cancer, it is controversial whether asbestos-related lung cancer arises only in the presence of pulmonary fibrosis. The various epidemiologic studies assessing the carcinogenic role of asbestos in the presence and absence of fibrosis were recently reviewed, and the conclusion of the reviewers was that the evidence is not conclusive and that the "question of whether or not asbestos-related lung cancer in man arises only in the presence of pulmonary fibrosis may be unanswerable epidemiologically."[16]

Asbestos-Related Pleural Abnormalities

Pleural Plaques. These are the most common form of asbestos-related pleuropulmonary disease.[1] They are usually first seen 20 to 30 years after exposure.[2] Pleural plaques consist of well-defined, pearly white foci of firm fibrous tissue, usually 2 to 5 mm thick and up to 10 cm in diameter.[7] The major determinant of the thickness of the pleural plaques is duration from first exposure.[1] The plaques may have a smooth surface or show fine or coarse nodularity and can be round, elliptical, or irregularly shaped. Histologic examination typically shows them to consist of dense, almost acellular collagen with a basket-weave pattern (Fig. 61.4).[7,10] Pleural plaques are usually limited to the parietal pleura, although they may occasionally be seen in the interlobar fissures. Approximately 10% to 15% of pleural plaques calcify.[2,17] Calcification is seldom evident in workers with a less than 30-year interval from time of first exposure.[3] The calcification may be punctate, linear, or coalescent.

Pleural Effusion. Although only a small percentage of individuals exposed to asbestos develop a benign pleural effusion (3%), this is the most common asbestos-related abnormality seen within the first 20 years after exposure.[18] The effusion is exudative and often hemorrhagic.[1] It may occur as early as 1 year after exposure or much later.[19] Although usually asymptomatic, acute pleural effusions caused by asbestos may also be exuberant, with fever and severe pleuritic pain. Acute pleuritis is thought to underlie many cases of diffuse pleural thickening, with studies demonstrating diffuse pleural thickening in patients with prior benign asbestos effusion in 31% to 80% of patients.[19,20]

Diffuse Pleural Thickening. Diffuse pleural thickening extends continuously over a portion of the visceral pleura and therefore is quite different in appearance from the circumscribed parietal pleural plaque. It may be extensive and cover the whole lung and obliterate lobar fissures; it ranges from less than 1 mm up to 1 cm or more in thickness. Adhesions to the parietal pleura are common. The thickening may extend for a few millimeters into the lung parenchyma and into the lobular septa. These features do not constitute asbestosis.[1] Diffuse pleural thickening is seen in 9% to 22% of asbestos-exposed workers with pleural disease.[1] The frequency of diffuse pleural thickening increases with time from first exposure and is believed to be dose related.[1] Diffuse pleural thickening frequently develops after benign asbestos-related pleural effusion.[19] Less commonly, it may be caused by extension of interstitial fibrosis to the visceral pleura, consistent with the pleural migration of asbestos fibers.[1] Both circumscribed (pleural plaques) and diffuse pleural thickening may be present in the same hemithorax.

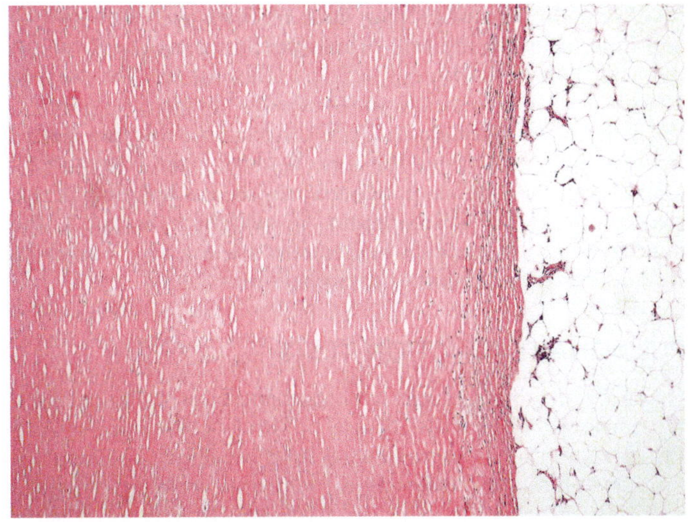

Fig. 61.4 Pleural plaque. Histologic specimen shows acellular collagen and basket-weave pattern characteristic of pleural plaque. *(Courtesy Dr. Andrew Churg, Department of Pathology, University of British Columbia, Vancouver, Canada.)*

Mesothelioma. There is a strong association between asbestos exposure and the development of malignant mesothelioma; the majority of cases of mesothelioma are related to asbestos exposure.[21] The risk of mesothelioma is much greater after exposure to amphiboles, particularly crocidolite (blue asbestos), than after exposure to chrysotile (white asbestos).[22] Although it was initially believed that the risk of mesothelioma from exposure to chrysotile was due to contamination with the amphibole tremolite, similar to other lung cancers, current evidence suggests that chrysotile itself may cause malignant mesothelioma, although the risk is much lower than for amphiboles.[22,23] Mesothelioma has occurred in three main cohorts of asbestos-exposed individuals: workers exposed to asbestos during its mining or milling; workers exposed in the manufacture and use of asbestos products, such as plumbers, carpenters, and installers of asbestos insulation; and persons who were exposed to asbestos unknowingly and incidentally.[22] The last group accounts for 20% to 30% of current cases of malignant mesothelioma in industrialized countries.[22]

The incidence of mesothelioma has markedly increased during the past 30 years, currently being as common in men as carcinomas of the liver, bone, and bladder in many industrialized countries.[21] In countries no longer using asbestos, the incidence of mesothelioma is now expected to start decreasing. However, in developing countries that have recently used asbestos or continue to use it, the rate of mesothelioma may continue to increase.[24] The risk of mesothelioma is almost zero for the first 10 to 15 years after first exposure to asbestos but increases progressively thereafter throughout life.[21] Although the role of asbestos in the development of mesothelioma has been extensively studied, and several explanations have been proposed as to how asbestos may result in the development of malignant disease,[21] the pathogenesis of mesothelioma remains unclear. See Chapter 74 for additional discussion of mesothelioma.

PULMONARY FUNCTION TESTS

Patients with asbestosis may have restrictive lung function, mixed restrictive and obstructive disease, or airflow obstruction alone.[7] When restriction is present, total lung capacity, vital capacity, residual volume, and diffusing capacity are decreased, but good ventilatory function is maintained.[25] Many patients, however, show some degree of airway obstruction as a result of asbestos-induced bronchiolar fibrosis.[25] In addition, emphysema is evident on computed tomography (CT) scans in about 50% of workers who have early asbestosis, a figure double that of those who do not.[26]

Restrictive lung function in asbestos workers may result from asbestosis or from asbestos-related pleural disease.[25] The lung restriction (i.e., the decrease in vital capacity) is much more marked in patients who have diffuse pleural thickening than in those who have only plaques.[27,28] This effect is unrelated to the radiographic extent of pleural thickening; a reduction in vital capacity with little more than costophrenic angle blunting can be similar to that with extensive involvement.[29]

Manifestations of the Disease

RADIOGRAPHY

Interpretation According to the International Classification of Radiographs of the Pneumoconioses

The chest radiograph is an important tool for the detection of asbestos-related pleural and parenchymal abnormalities and to assess the progression of ensuing disease. For it to be useful in epidemiologic studies, however, it is essential that an acceptable classification of the extent of involvement be followed and a standard nomenclature be used. The most widely used schema is the International Labour Office (ILO) International Classification of Radiographs of Pneumoconioses, which was revised most recently in 2011.[30] The objective of this classification is to codify the radiographic changes associated with the pneumoconioses in a simple and reproducible manner such that international comparability of pneumoconiosis statistics has some validity. Because this schema uses radiographic descriptors that are somewhat different from those generally used throughout this book, a short glossary of terms relevant to the interpretation of radiographs of asbestos-exposed workers and other pneumoconiosis patients follows.

Small Rounded Opacities. These opacities are well-circumscribed nodules ranging in diameter from barely visible to up to 10 mm. The qualifiers *p, q,* and *r* subdivide the predominant opacities into three diameter ranges: *p,* up to 1.5 mm; *q,* 1.5 to 3.0 mm; and *r,* 3 to 10 mm.

Small Irregular Opacities. This term is used to describe a pattern that elsewhere in this book has been designated *linear* or *reticular*—in other words, a net-like pattern. Although the nature of these opacities is such that establishment of quantitative dimensions is considerably more difficult than with rounded opacities, three categories have been created: *s,* width up to 1.5 mm; *t,* width exceeding 1.5 mm and up to 3.0 mm; and *u,* width exceeding 3 mm and up to 10 mm.

To record shape and size, two letters must be used. If the reader of the radiograph thinks that all or virtually all opacities are one shape and size, this is noted by recording the symbol twice, separated by an oblique stroke (e.g., *q/q*). If another shape or size is appreciated, this is recorded as the second letter (e.g., *q/t*). The designation *q/t* means that the predominant small opacity is round and of size *q,* but in addition there are a significant number of small irregular opacities of size *t.* In this way, any combination of small opacities can be recorded.

Profusion. This term refers to the number of small opacities per unit area or zone of lung. There are four basic categories: category 0, small opacities absent or less profuse than in category 1; category 1, small opacities definitely present but few in number (normal lung markings are usually visible); category 2, numerous small opacities (normal lung markings are generally partly obscured); and category 3, very numerous small opacities (normal lung markings are usually totally obscured). These categories can be further subdivided by use of a 12-point scale to describe a continuum of changes from complete normality to the most advanced category or grade: 0/– 0/0 0/1; 1/0 1/1 1/2; 2/1 2/2 2/3; 3/2 3/3 3/+. When this scale is used, the radiograph is first classified into one of the four categories 0, 1, 2, or 3. If the category above or below is considered a serious alternative during the process, it is recorded (e.g., a radiograph in which profusion is considered to be category 2 but for which category 1 was seriously considered would be graded 2/1). If no alternative is considered (i.e., the profusion was definitely category 2), it would be classified 2/2. A subdivision is also possible within category 0. If the absence of small opacities is particularly obvious, profusion should be recorded as 0/–. Such a category might be seen in a healthy nonsmoking adolescent. The ILO standard radiographs are the final arbiters of opacity profusion and take precedence over any application of a verbal description of profusion. Thus this reading should always be done side by side with the ILO standard radiographs.[30]

A separate classification for large opacities (>1 cm in diameter) exists whereby A denotes one or more opacities greater than 1 cm but smaller than 50 mm; B denotes one or more opacities greater than A, combined area less than the right upper zone; and C denotes one or more opacities whose combined area is greater than the area of the right upper zone.

Other Findings. Pleural abnormalities are also assessed with respect to location, width, extent, and degree of calcification. Finally, other abnormal features of the chest radiograph can be noted. All of these abnormalities are more completely illustrated and described in the Guidelines for the Use of the ILO International Classification of Radiographs of Pneumoconioses.[30]

There is little doubt that expert readings are superior to nonexpert readings in the detection of disease and avoidance of "overreading."[31] However, use of the radiograph as a definitive tool for the diagnosis of pneumoconiosis in any given individual is limited by a significant prevalence of small opacities sufficient for "diagnosis" in nonexposed working populations, as well as by a significant degree of interreader and intrareader variability.[32,33]

Asbestos-Related Pulmonary Abnormalities

Asbestosis. The initial radiographic manifestation of asbestosis consists of bilateral small irregular linear opacities (reticular pattern, *s* and *t* opacities in the ILO classification) in the lower lung zones.[1] With progression of disease, the distribution and extent or profusion of opacities increases and may spread to the middle and upper lung zones (Fig. 61.5). Fibrosis in the right middle lobe and lingula may result in obscuration of the heart border ("shaggy heart sign"). Extensive fibrosis was more common in the past, with more patients currently having only mild fibrosis. In a study of 3383 asbestos-exposed workers referred for independent medical evaluation, most subjects (79%) had an ILO score below 1/1.[15]

The extent of parenchymal abnormalities (ILO classification profusion score) correlates strongly with functional impairment, particularly reduction in diffusing capacity and ventilatory capacity, and with mortality risk.[1,34] In the assessment of radiographs of asbestos-exposed individuals, a critical distinction is made between radiographs that are suggestive but not presumptively diagnostic (0/1) and those that are presumptively diagnostic but not unequivocal (1/0). This dividing point is generally taken to separate radiographs that are considered to be "positive" for asbestosis (1/0 or higher profusion score) from those that are considered to be "negative" (0/1 or less).[1]

A chest radiograph showing the characteristic findings of asbestosis in the presence of a compatible history of exposure is adequate for the diagnosis; further imaging is not required.[1] However, the chest radiograph has limited sensitivity and specificity in cases of mild fibrosis and may not provide sufficient additional information, such as degree of progression from prior imaging, for use in a given clinical case.[1]

Rounded Atelectasis. The characteristic radiologic manifestation of rounded atelectasis is a rounded or oval, subpleural opacity associated with loss of volume and curving of adjacent pulmonary vessels and bronchi into the edges of the opacity (the "comet tail sign"; Fig. 61.6).[35] The opacity typically abuts an area of pleural thickening or a pleural effusion. The abnormality may occur anywhere in the lungs, but it is most common in the middle and lower lung zones (see Fig. 61.6).[36] In one review of 89 cases of rounded atelectasis in 74 patients, the lower lobes were affected in 33 cases (45%), the lingula in 33 (45%), the middle lobe in 16 (22%), and the upper lobes in 7 (9%).[36] Rounded atelectasis may be unilateral or bilateral and usually measures 2 to 7 cm in diameter.

Most cases of rounded atelectasis are associated with asbestos exposure; however, some have been described in association with other causes of pleural thickening or effusion.[36] The lesion may develop and progress during a few months or several years. In a series of 74 patients, it occurred on a background of benign asbestos effusion in 9 and slowly increasing pleural thickening in 13; in the remaining 52 patients, it was a new finding, with earlier radiographs showing only plaques or being normal.[36]

Asbestos-Related Pleural Abnormalities

Pleural Plaques. Pleural plaques are the most common radiologic manifestation of asbestos-related disease.[1] The characteristic findings on the chest radiograph consist of focal pleural opacities that have irregular margins when seen in profile and sharp, often foliate borders when seen en face (Fig. 61.7).[1] The typical distribution of plaques on chest radiographs is the posterolateral chest wall between the 7th and 10th ribs, the lateral chest wall between the 6th and 9th ribs, the dome of the diaphragm (virtually diagnostic), and the paravertebral pleura (Fig. 61.8).[2,17] The plaques may be bilateral and symmetric or bilateral and asymmetric and less commonly appear unilateral on the chest radiograph.[37] They may be smooth or nodular and can measure as much as 1 cm in thickness. Although noncalcified pleural plaques are the most common radiographic manifestation of asbestos-related disease, they are more striking when calcified, a finding that is seen in 10% to 15% of cases (Figs. 61.9 and 61.10).[2,17] Although calcified plaques may be seen at any location, they are most common in relation to the diaphragm. The prevalence of pleural plaques is related to duration from first exposure; they are rare before 20 years.[1] Calcification of pleural plaques is similarly related to duration and is more common 30 years after first exposure (see Fig. 61.10).[1]

Although detection of plaques radiographically is highly specific for a history of asbestos exposure, its sensitivity is relatively poor. Only 50% to 80% of cases of documented pleural thickening demonstrated by autopsy or thin-section CT are detected on the chest radiograph (Fig. 61.11).[1]

Diffuse Pleural Thickening. Diffuse pleural thickening is seen in 9% to 22% of asbestos-exposed workers with pleural disease.[1] The latency period ranges from 10 to 40 years or more. Diffuse pleural thickening is manifested radiologically as a generalized, more or less uniform increase in pleural width (Fig. 61.12). Diffuse thickening of the visceral pleura is not sharply demarcated and is often associated with fibrous strands ("crow's feet") extending into the parenchyma.[1] Both circumscribed and diffuse pleural thickening may be present in the same hemithorax. The frequency of diffuse pleural thickening increases with time from first exposure and is believed to be dose related.[1] The abnormality is generally considered to be present when there is a smooth, uninterrupted pleural density extending over at least a fourth of the chest wall on the chest radiograph. The ILO classification recognizes pleural thickening as diffuse "only in the presence of and in continuity with an obliterated costophrenic angle."[30] Localized subpleural parenchymal fibrosis is often present without diffuse interstitial fibrosis. Calcification of the pleura occurs with the passage of time and may involve the interlobar fissures.[1]

Separating diffuse pleural thickening from extrapleural fat is important but sometimes difficult.[1] Extrapleural fat pads typically result in bilateral, symmetric "apparent pleural thickening" with gradually tapering or indistinct edges that does not extend into the costophrenic angles. These fat pads also typically occur in the midthoracic wall, between the fourth and eighth ribs, and do not have adjacent parenchymal linear opacities. Differentiation of fat from pleural plaques may be difficult on the radiograph but is readily made on CT (Fig. 61.13).

Pleural Effusion. Benign pleural effusion occurs in approximately 3% of asbestos-exposed individuals and is the most common asbestos-related abnormality seen within the first 20 years after exposure.[18] In one review of 73 benign asbestos-related pleural effusions in 60 patients, the mean latency time from the first exposure to asbestos was 30 years, with a range of 1 to 58 years.[38] The effusion may be asymptomatic or associated with fever and pleuritic chest pain. It may be unilateral or bilateral, persist for months, or recur on the same or the opposite side.[38] The most comprehensive report of the prevalence of asbestos-related pleural effusion was a study of 1135 exposed workers and 717 control subjects in whom benign asbestos effusion was defined by (1) a history of exposure to asbestos; (2) confirmation of the presence of effusion by radiography, thoracentesis, or both; (3) absence of other nonneoplastic disease that could have caused the effusion; and (4) absence of malignant tumor within 3 years.[18] According to these criteria, 34 benign effusions (3%)

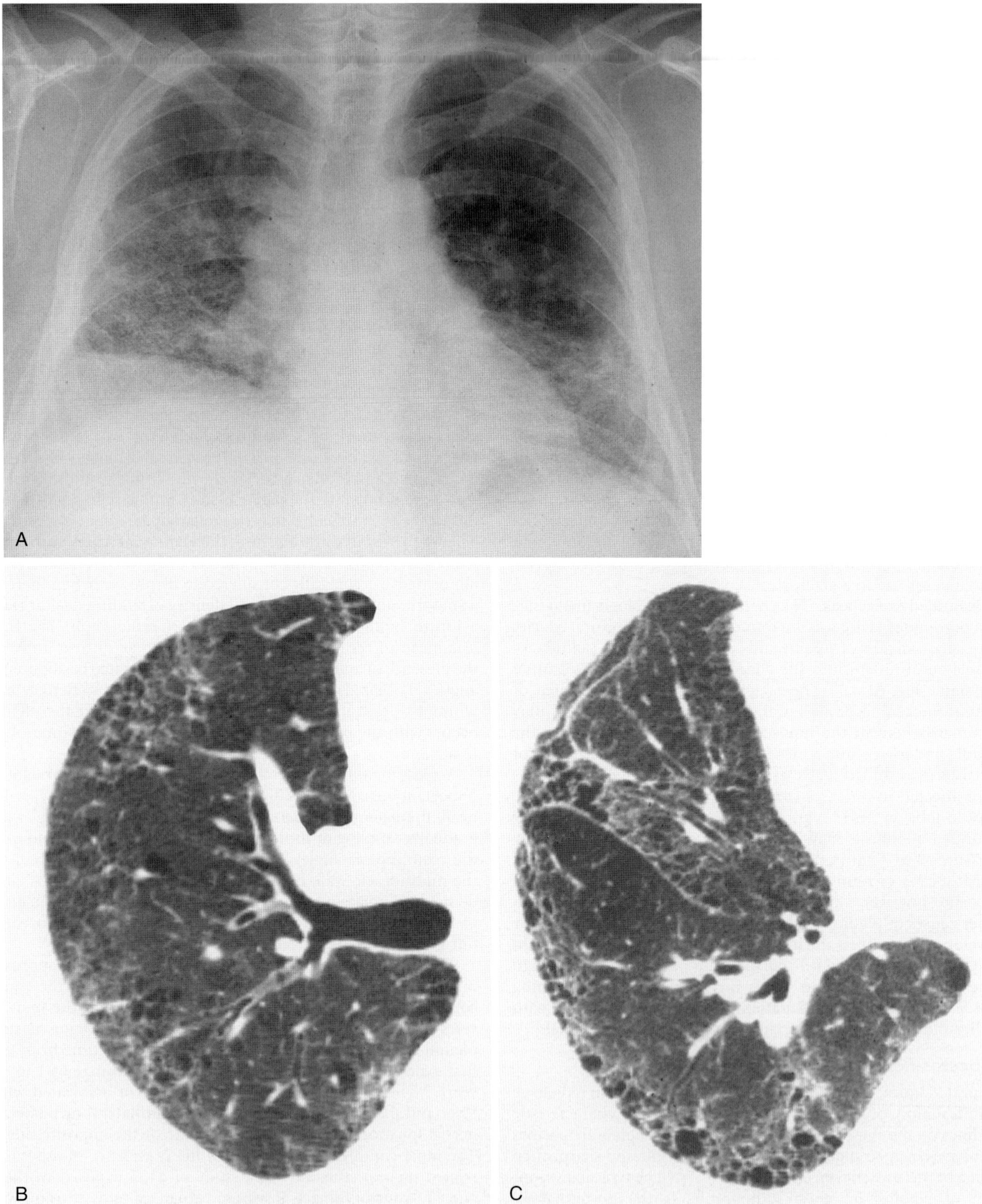

Fig. 61.5 Asbestosis: radiographic and CT findings. Chest radiograph (A) shows extensive bilateral reticulation and hazy increased opacity mainly in the lower lobes. Also note enlargement of the hilar pulmonary arteries consistent with pulmonary arterial hypertension. Magnified views of the right lung from high-resolution CT at the level of the right upper lobe bronchus (B) and right inferior pulmonary vein (C) demonstrate reticulation, minimal ground-glass opacities, and honeycombing, mainly in the subpleural and lower lung zones. Also note emphysema.

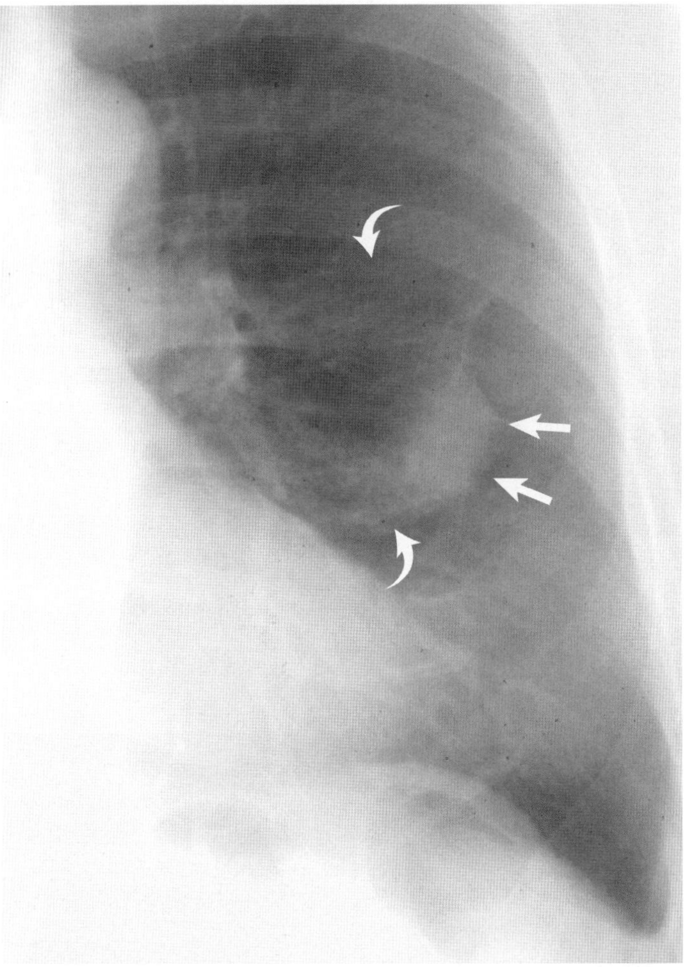

Fig. 61.6 Rounded atelectasis: radiographic features. Magnified view of the left lung from a posteroanterior chest radiograph shows an oval opacity. The lateral margins *(straight arrows)* are well defined (where the opacity abuts the lung), and the medial margins are poorly defined (where the opacity abuts the pleura). Pulmonary vessels *(curved arrows)* can be seen to curve toward the opacity (comet tail sign).

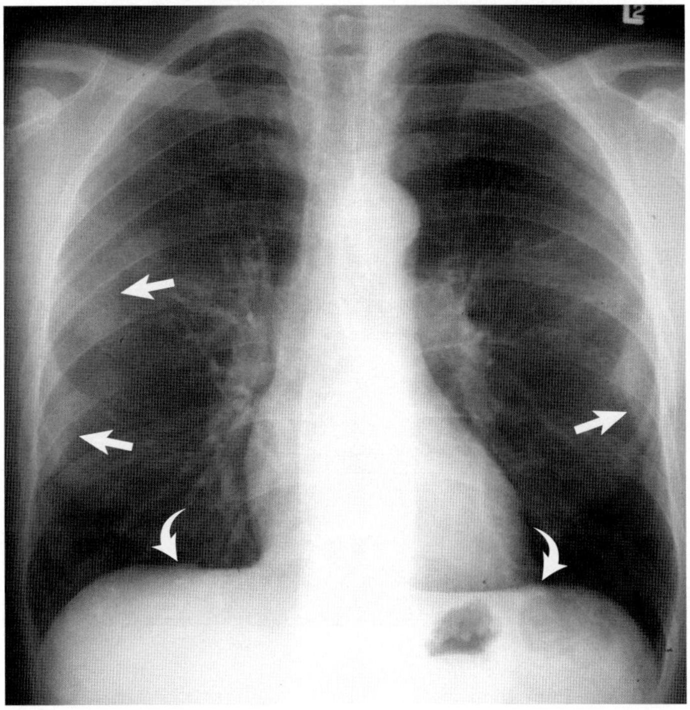

Fig. 61.7 Pleural plaques: radiographic findings. Posteroanterior chest radiograph shows multiple focal pleural opacities along the chest wall *(straight arrows)* and diaphragm *(curved arrows)* characteristic of pleural plaques.

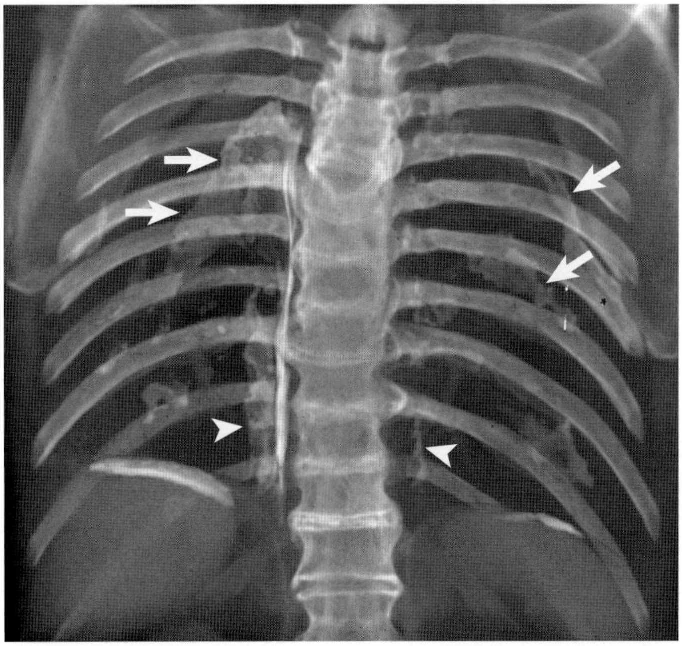

Fig. 61.8 Pleural plaques: characteristic distribution. Volume-rendered image from thin-section CT demonstrates calcified plaques along the ribs *(arrows)*, diaphragm, and paravertebral region *(arrowheads)*. Also noted is more extensive linear pleural calcification along the right paravertebral region.

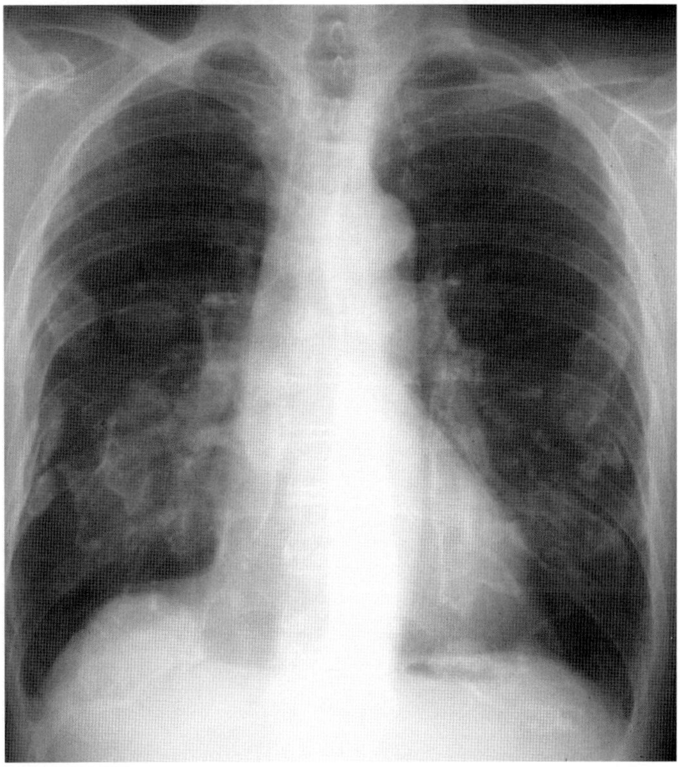

Fig. 61.9 Calcified pleural plaques. Posteroanterior chest radiograph shows numerous bilateral calcified pleural plaques.

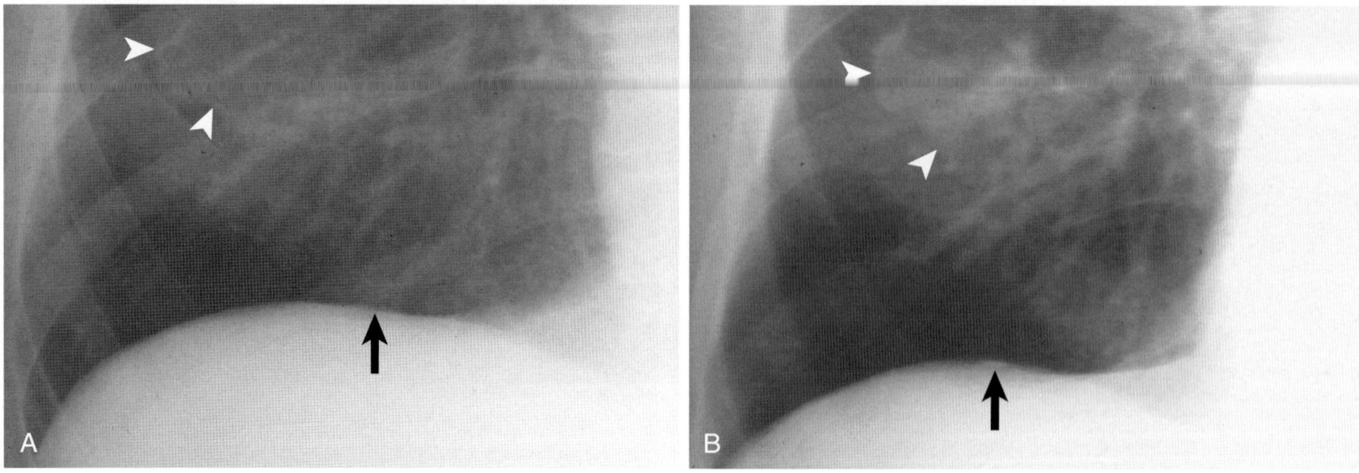

Fig. 61.10 Pleural plaques: development of calcification. (A) View of the right lower chest from a frontal radiograph shows noncalcified pleural plaques along anterior ribs *(arrowheads)* and right hemidiaphragm *(arrow)*. (B) View from chest radiograph obtained 18 years later demonstrates calcification of the plaques along the anterior ribs *(arrowheads)* and right hemidiaphragm *(arrow)*.

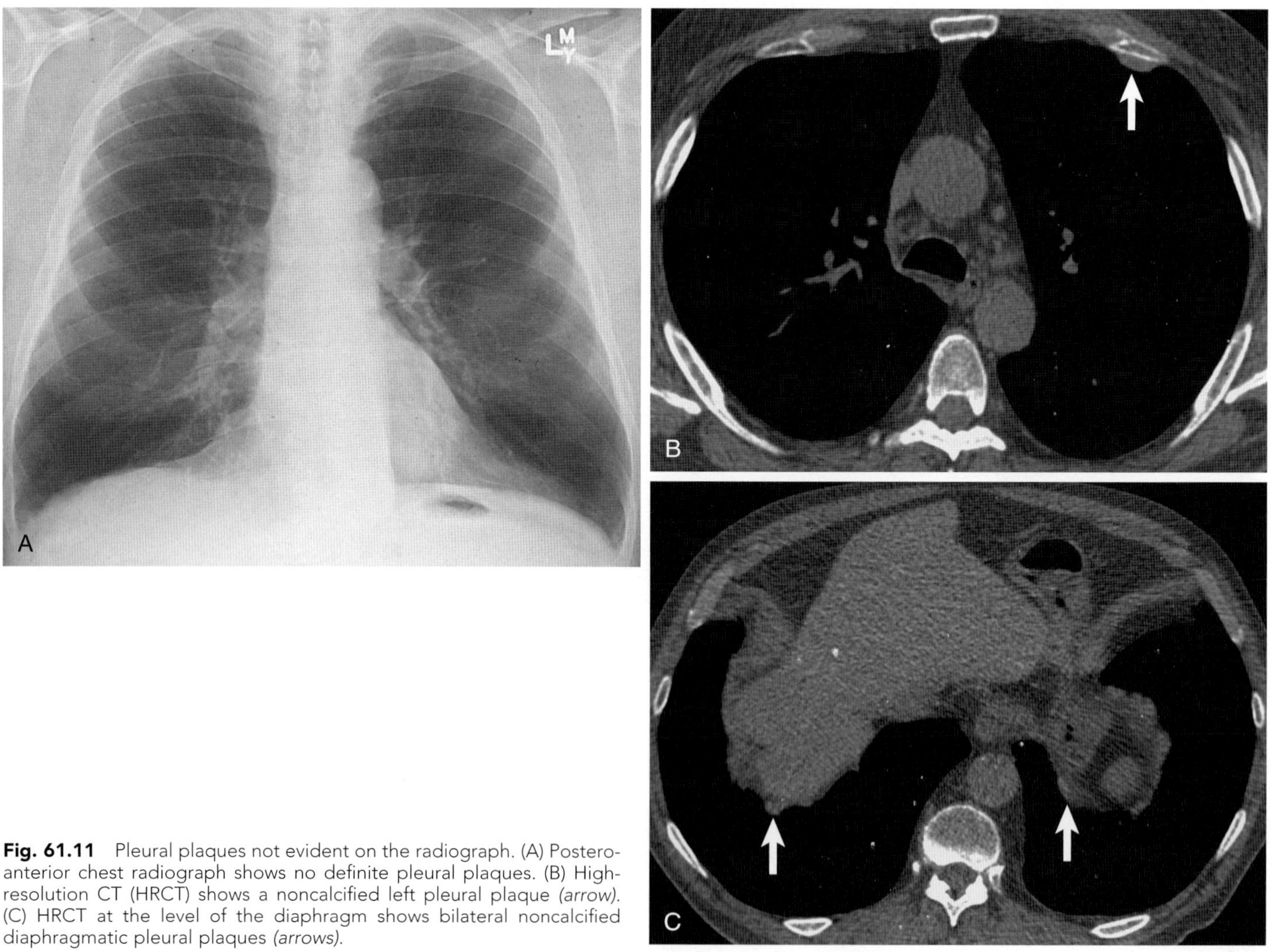

Fig. 61.11 Pleural plaques not evident on the radiograph. (A) Posteroanterior chest radiograph shows no definite pleural plaques. (B) High-resolution CT (HRCT) shows a noncalcified left pleural plaque *(arrow)*. (C) HRCT at the level of the diaphragm shows bilateral noncalcified diaphragmatic pleural plaques *(arrows)*.

were identified in the exposed workers versus none in the control subjects. The likelihood of the presence of effusion was dose related. The latency period was shorter than for other asbestos-related disorders, effusion being the most common abnormality detected during the first 20 years after exposure. Most effusions were small, 28% recurred, and 66% were asymptomatic.[18] Asbestos-related pleural effusion may resolve completely or result in residual pleural thickening that may be mild, resulting in blunting of the costophrenic angle, or diffuse.[1,19]

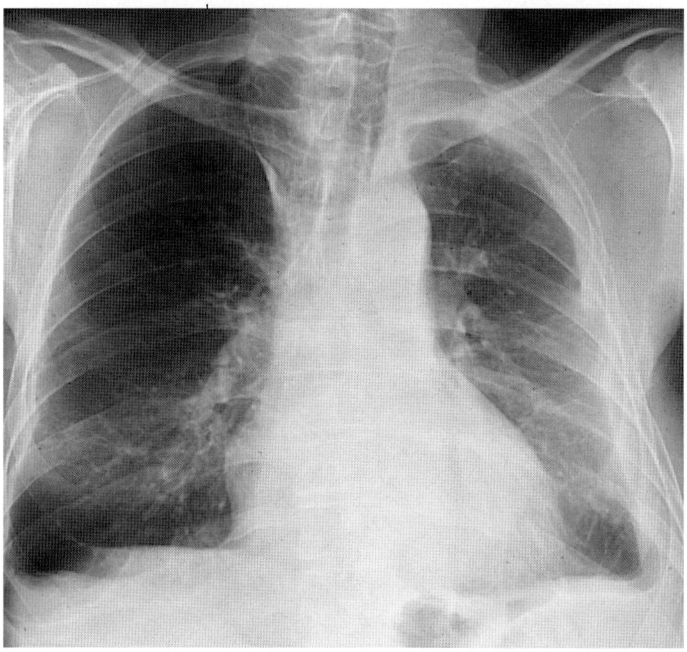

Fig. 61.12 Diffuse pleural thickening: radiographic findings. Chest radiograph shows diffuse left pleural thickening. The pleural thickening along the lateral chest wall is seen in profile as a broad band of homogeneous increased opacity; the thickening along the posterior chest wall is seen en face as a hazy increased opacity over the left lower hemithorax.

Mesothelioma. The radiologic features of mesothelioma are discussed in Chapter 74.

COMPUTED TOMOGRAPHY

Asbestos-Related Pulmonary Abnormalities

Asbestosis. The most common high-resolution CT (HRCT) manifestations of asbestosis are intralobular linear opacities (reticular pattern), irregular thickening of the interlobular septa, nondependent ground-glass opacities, subpleural small rounded or branching opacities, subpleural curvilinear opacities, and parenchymal bands (Figs. 61.14 and 61.15).[39–41] The abnormalities involve mainly the peripheral and dorsal regions of the lung bases. Ground-glass opacities are defined as areas of increased attenuation that do not obscure the underlying vascular margins. Nondependent ground-glass opacities in asbestos-exposed persons may reflect the presence of mild alveolar wall fibrosis beyond the resolving power of CT, inflammation, or edema.[42] Dependent ground-glass opacities are commonly seen, particularly in patients with chronic obstructive pulmonary disease, and represent atelectasis rather than asbestos-related disease. Ground-glass opacities immediately adjacent to thick pleural plaques also usually represent compressive atelectasis rather than fibrosis or inflammation. Small, round (dot-like), and branching subpleural opacities are the earliest asbestos-related pulmonary abnormality evident on HRCT.[41] Typically, they are visible a few millimeters from the pleural surface in a centrilobular location (Fig. 61.16). They reflect the earliest pulmonary abnormality seen in association with asbestos exposure—that is, fibrosis in

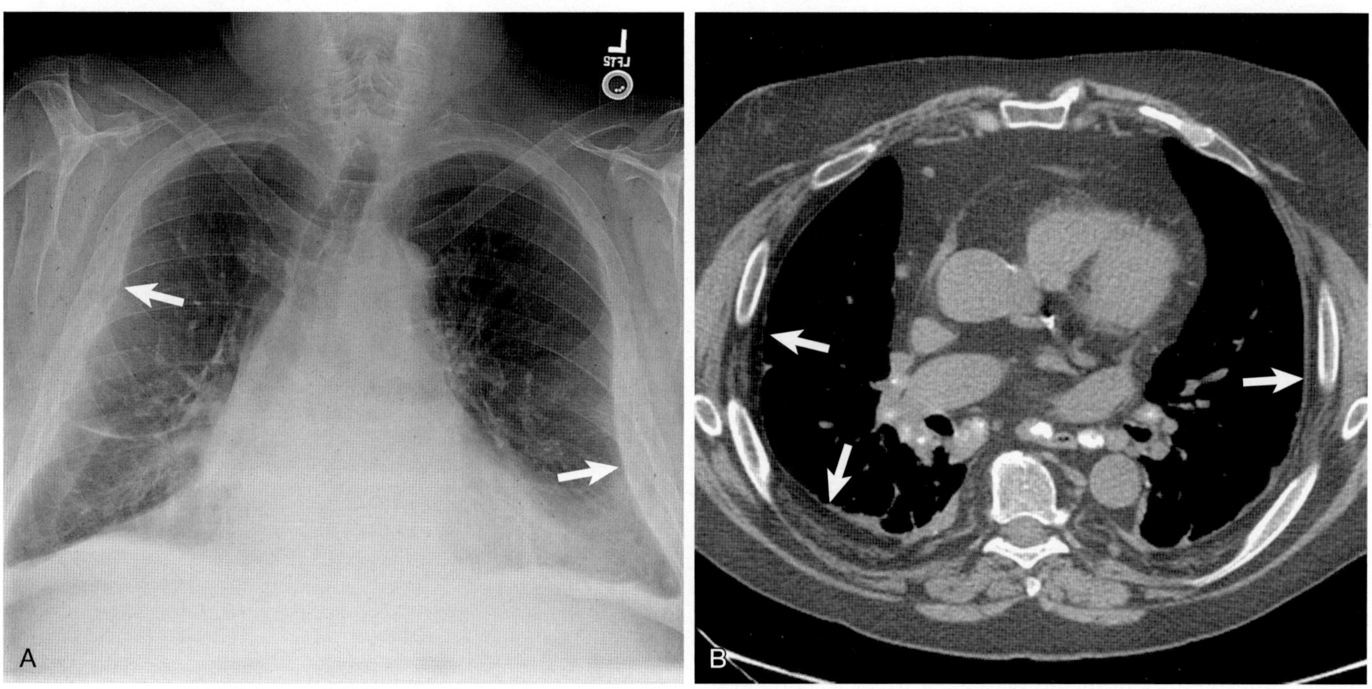

Fig. 61.13 Extrapleural fat mimicking diffuse pleural thickening. (A) Posteroanterior radiograph shows apparent extensive bilateral pleural thickening *(arrows)*. (B) Axial CT scan demonstrates that the apparent pleural thickening is due to abundant extrapleural fat *(arrows)*. Unlike diffuse pleural thickening, extrapleural fat is generally symmetric, does not involve the costophrenic angles, and does not have adjacent lung fibrosis.

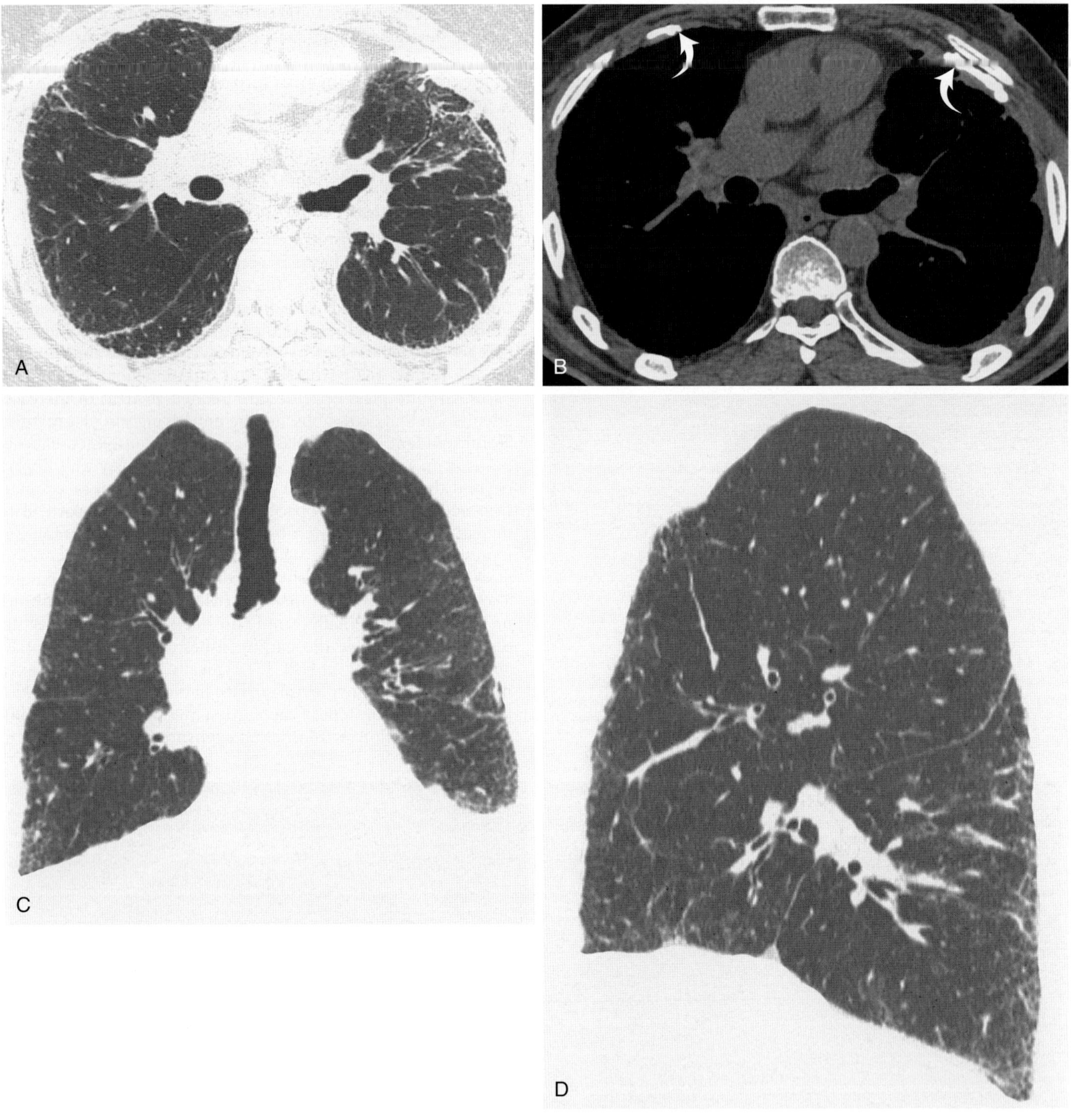

Fig. 61.14 Asbestosis: high-resolution CT (HRCT) findings. (A) HRCT image performed with the patient supine shows bilateral, predominantly subpleural intralobular lines and irregular thickening of interlobular septa. Also noted are nondependent ground-glass opacities and architectural distortion in the anterolateral aspect of the left upper lobe. (B) Soft tissue windows show calcified bilateral pleural plaques *(arrows)* and diffuse irregular left pleural thickening. Coronal (C) and sagittal (D) reformatted images demonstrate predominant subpleural distribution of the fibrosis.

the walls of respiratory bronchioles (see Fig. 61.1).[41] Subpleural dot-like and branching opacities are often evident on CT in patients with normal radiographs and have been shown to progress to subpleural fibrosis.[41] Subpleural curvilinear opacities are areas of increased attenuation of variable length located within 1 cm of the pleura and parallel to the inner chest wall (Fig. 61.17).[43] Most measure 5 to 10 cm in length. They are seen most commonly in early disease; they may reflect atelectasis adjacent to pleural plaques or fibrosis.[41,42] Parenchymal bands are linear opacities measuring 2 to 5 cm in length that course

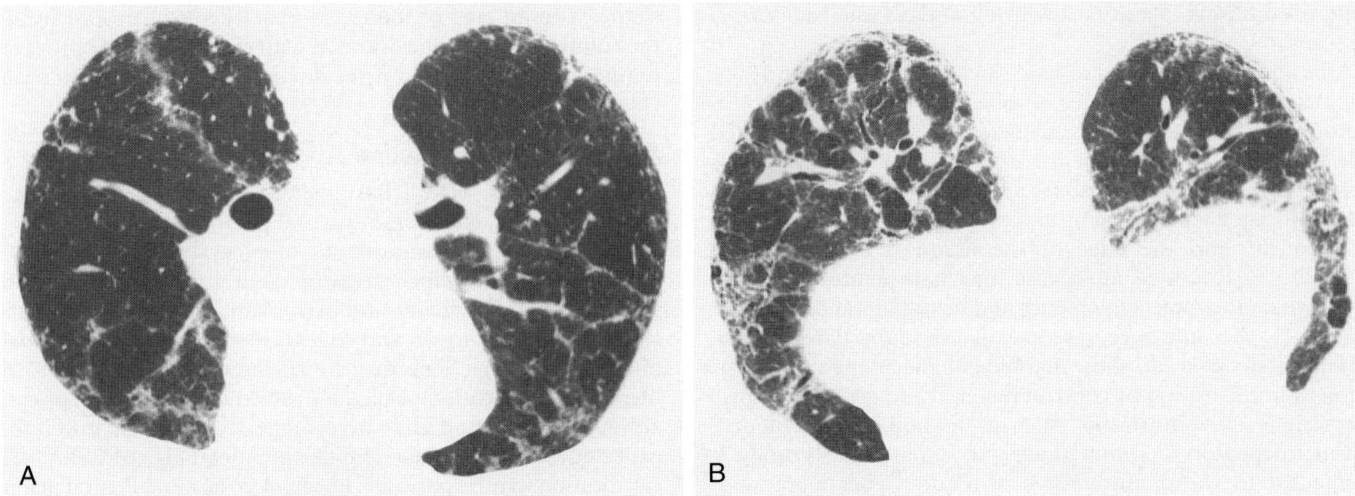

Fig. 61.15 Asbestosis with severe fibrosis: high-resolution CT (HRCT) findings. (A) and (B) HRCT images performed with the patient prone show bilateral, predominantly subpleural intralobular lines and irregular thickening of interlobular septa with associated architectural distortion and mild subpleural honeycombing. Also noted are nondependent ground-glass opacities. The HRCT findings resemble those of idiopathic pulmonary fibrosis.

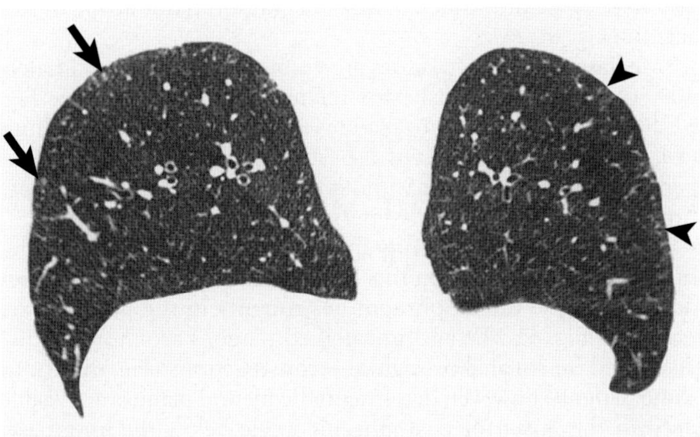

Fig. 61.16 Subpleural nodules in early asbestos-related lung disease. High-resolution CT image with the patient prone shows small, round (dot-like) subpleural opacities *(arrows)* and traction bronchiolectasis *(arrowheads)*. They reflect the earliest pulmonary abnormality seen in association with asbestos exposure—that is, fibrosis in the walls of respiratory bronchioles. *(Courtesy Dr. Jorge Kavakama, São Paulo, Brazil.)*

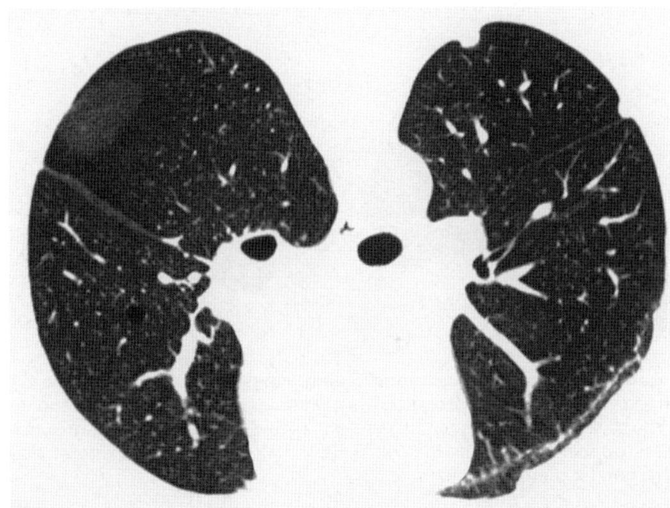

Fig. 61.17 Subpleural curvilinear opacity. High-resolution CT with the patient prone shows curvilinear opacity and ground-glass opacities in the dependent lung adjacent to a pleural plaque. Although subpleural curvilinear opacities may represent fibrosis, there is no evidence of fibrosis in this patient; the curvilinear opacity and the dependent ground-glass opacities are due to atelectasis. *(Courtesy Dr. Jorge Kavakama, São Paulo, Brazil.)*

through the lung and usually abut an area of pleural thickening (Fig. 61.18).[44] Pathologic correlation has shown them to correspond to foci of peribronchovascular or interlobular septal fibrosis associated with distortion of the parenchymal architecture.[42] The bands are more common in asbestosis than in other causes of pulmonary fibrosis; for example, in one study they were present in 79% of patients who had asbestosis, compared with 11% of patients who had idiopathic pulmonary fibrosis.[45] As in other causes of interstitial pulmonary fibrosis, architectural distortion of secondary lobules and irregular thickening of interlobular septa are commonly seen in asbestosis. With progression of fibrosis, irregular linear opacities and honeycombing predominate.[46,47] At all stages the abnormalities involve predominantly the subpleural regions of the lower lung zones.[42,47] The fibrosis is frequently associated with thickening of the adjacent visceral pleura (see Fig. 61.14). Asbestosis tends to progress over time even after cessation of exposure (Fig. 61.19).[48]

Similar to other cases of possible fibrosis, dependent atelectasis may mimic or obscure early fibrosis, and it is essential that CT scans in these patients be obtained in the supine and prone positions or only in the prone position.[46,49] CT also allows detection of parenchymal abnormalities not evident on the chest radiograph.[39,40,44] In a review of the HRCT findings and pulmonary function test results of 169 asbestos-exposed workers who had normal chest radiographs (ILO profusion score below 1/0), CT abnormalities consistent with asbestosis were found in 57; these patients had significantly lower vital capacity and carbon monoxide diffusing capacity than did the workers who had normal CT scans.[40]

Asbestos-related pleural disease can be seen in 95% to 100% of patients who have evidence of asbestosis on HRCT.[39,40,44]

Rounded Atelectasis. The characteristic findings of rounded atelectasis on CT consist of a round or oval opacity that is peripheral in location and abuts an area of pleural thickening and is associated with crowding and curving of pulmonary vessels and bronchi into the edge of the lesion (comet tail sign; Fig. 61.20).[50] Rounded atelectasis may have acute or obtuse angles where it contacts the pleura and be unilateral or bilateral (Fig. 61.21). Because it represents collapsed lung parenchyma, rounded atelectasis can show marked enhancement after intravenous administration of contrast material and generally shows direct signs of volume loss, such as fissural displacement.[51] Optimal depiction of rounded atelectasis, particularly when it is adjacent to the diaphragm, may require assessment with multiplanar reconstructions.

In the majority of cases the diagnosis of rounded atelectasis can be confidently made by CT on the basis of the characteristic features listed earlier. However, atypical cases with an irregular shape, with an area of increased opacity out of proportion for the volume loss, or not associated with curving of adjacent vessels require close follow-up or needle biopsy to rule out carcinoma (Fig. 61.22).

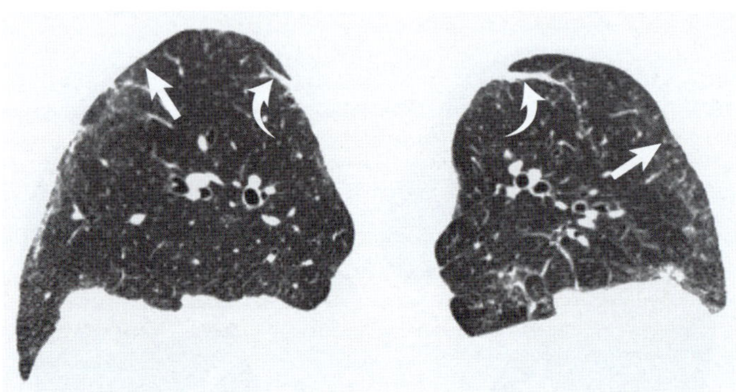

Fig. 61.18 Parenchymal bands in early asbestosis. High-resolution CT image with the patient prone shows bilateral parenchymal bands *(curved arrows)*, small round opacities *(straight arrows)*, nondependent ground-glass opacities, and minimal reticulation. Also noted are bilateral diaphragmatic pleural plaques.

Asbestos-Related Pleural Abnormalities

Pleural Plaques. HRCT has greater sensitivity than chest radiography for the detection of pleural plaques (see Fig. 61.11).[39,44] The characteristic manifestation of pleural plaques on HRCT consist of circumscribed areas of pleural thickening separated from the underlying ribs and extrapleural soft tissues by a thin layer of fat (Figs. 61.23 and 61.24). Pleural plaques are usually bilateral, although they may be asymmetric. According to the literature, calcification of plaques is seen in 10% to 15% of cases, although many find that percentage to be much lower than expected based on their clinical practice (Fig. 61.25).[2,17] The calcification may be punctate, linear, or coalescent. Pleural plaques are easiest to recognize internal to visible rib segments because only the pleura, extrapleural fat, and endothoracic fascia pass internal to ribs, and these are too thin in most normal patients to be recognized on CT.[52] Pleural plaques measuring as little as 1 to 2 mm in thickness can be readily diagnosed in this location. Pleural thickening is also easy to identify in the paravertebral region because of the lack of any normal soft tissue stripe in this region (Fig. 61.26).

Mediastinal pleural plaques are visible on CT in approximately 40% of patients with asbestos-related pleural disease (see Fig. 61.26).[39,44] Less commonly, plaques may involve the pericardium (Fig. 61.27). On occasion, asbestos exposure may result in pericardial fibrosis with or without associated effusion or calcification and, rarely, constrictive pericarditis.[53,54]

Pleural plaques frequently involve the diaphragmatic pleura, but uncalcified plaques in this location can be difficult to detect on CT because the diaphragm lies roughly in the plane of the scan (see Fig. 61.24), and uncalcified plaques are more readily visualized on coronal or sagittal reconstructions (Fig. 61.28). In some patients, however, diaphragmatic pleural plaques are visible deep in the posterior costophrenic angle below the lung base; in this location the pleural disease can be localized with certainty to the parietal pleura because only parietal pleura is present

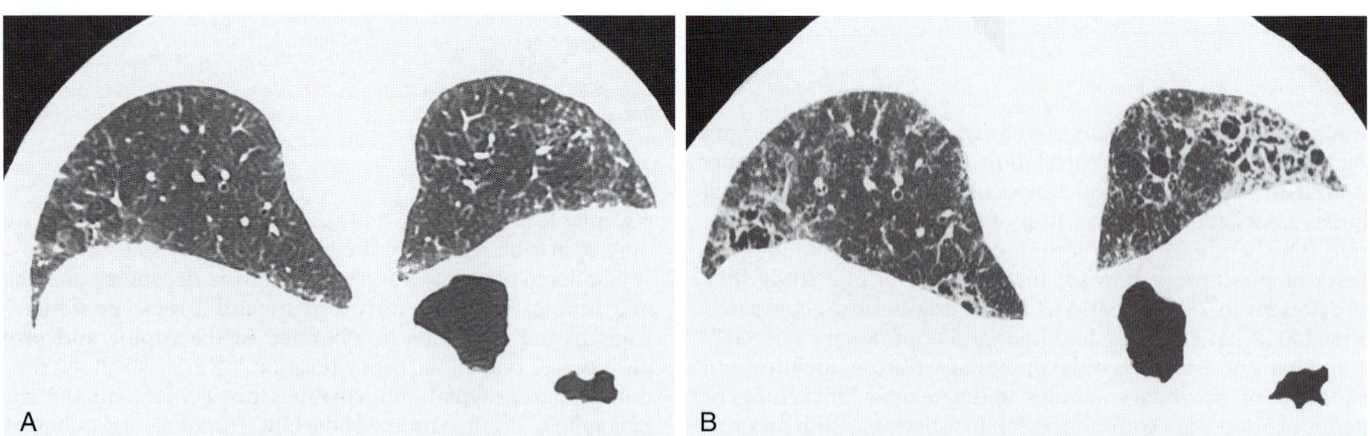

Fig. 61.19 Asbestosis: progression of fibrosis over time. (A) High-resolution CT (HRCT) image with the patient prone shows reticulation, traction bronchiectasis, and early honeycombing in the left lower lobe. Mild fibrosis is present in the right lung base. (B) Follow-up HRCT image 5 years later demonstrates marked progression of the fibrosis. *(Courtesy Dr. Jorge Kavakama, São Paulo, Brazil.)*

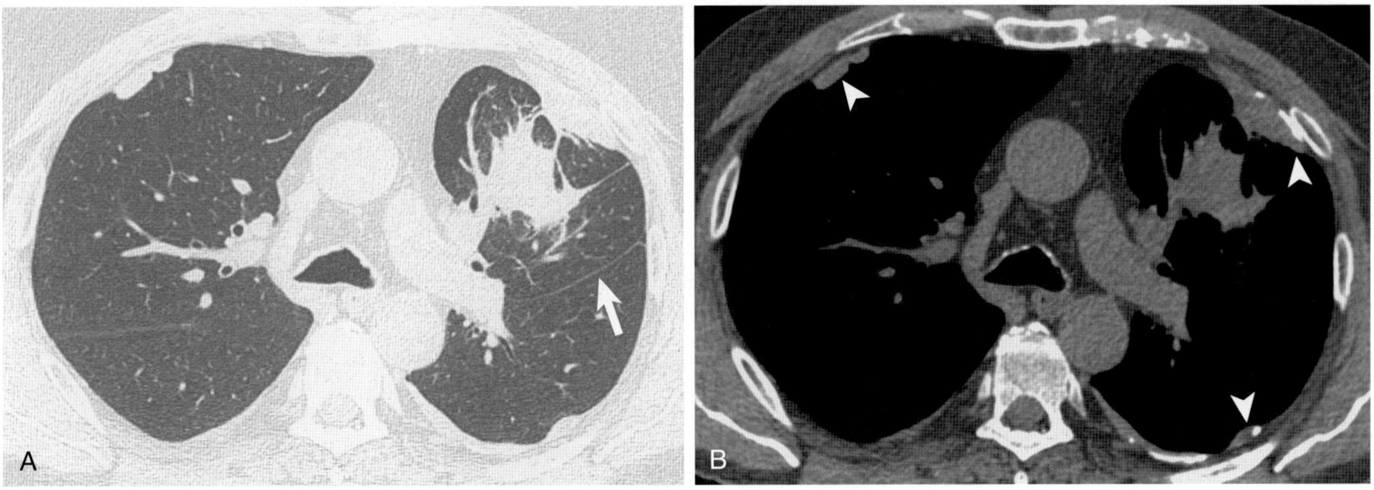

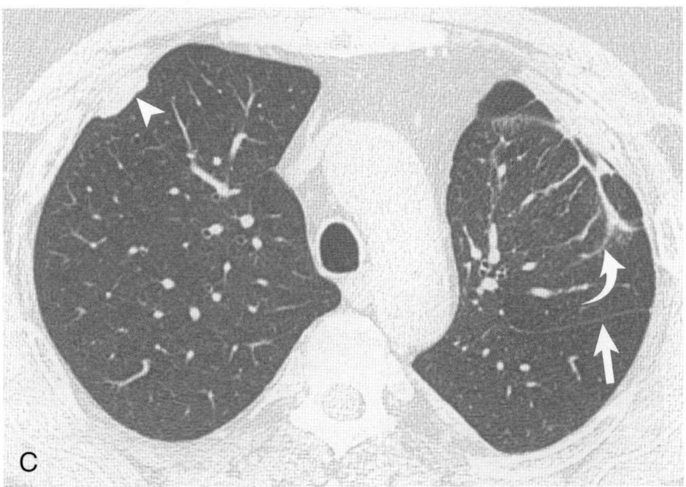

Fig. 61.20 Rounded atelectasis. (A) High-resolution CT (HRCT) image shows irregular mass in the left upper lobe with band-like opacities extending toward an area of pleural thickening. Also note volume loss of the left upper lobe causing curvilinear anterior displacement of the left major fissure *(straight arrow)*. (B) Soft tissue windows demonstrate bilateral calcified and noncalcified pleural plaques *(arrowheads)*. (C) HRCT image at a more cephalad level shows pulmonary vessels *(curved arrow)* curving toward the area of pleural thickening. Also noted are superior and anterior displacement of the left major fissure *(straight arrow)* and a right pleural plaque *(arrowhead)*.

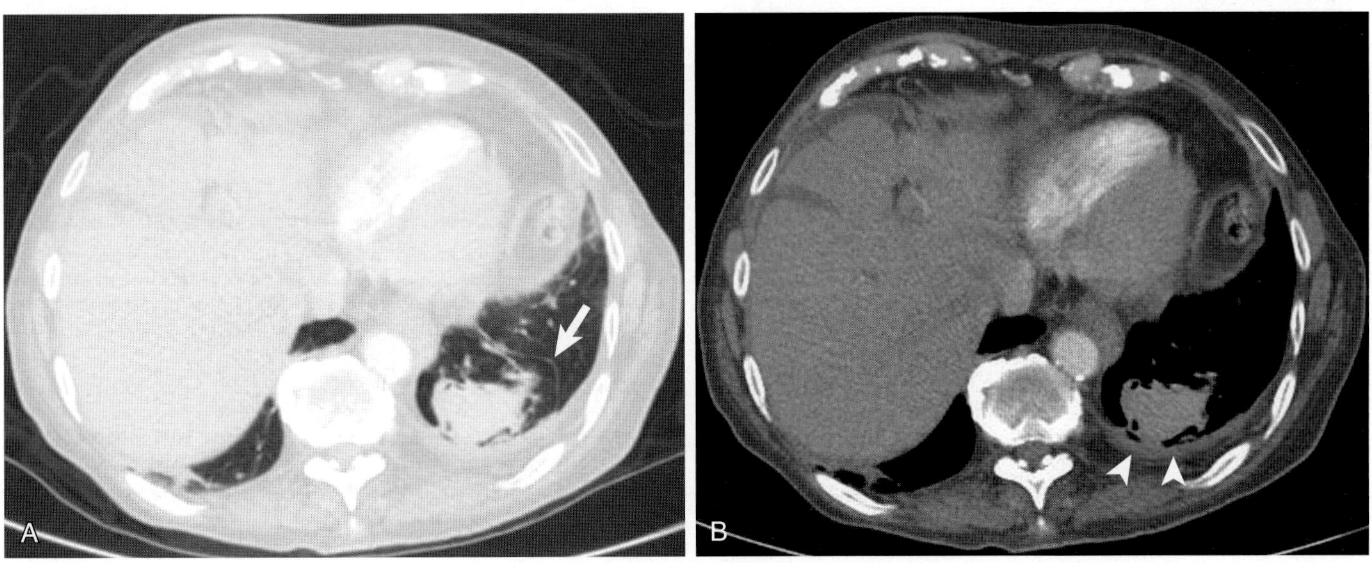

Fig. 61.21 Rounded atelectasis. (A) CT image in a patient with previous asbestos exposure shows a left lower lobe mass with pulmonary vessels curving toward it, consistent with rounded atelectasis. Note the severe degree of left lower lobe volume loss with deviation of the left major fissure posteriorly *(arrow)*. (B) Soft tissue windows demonstrate pleural thickening adjacent to the mass *(arrowheads)*.

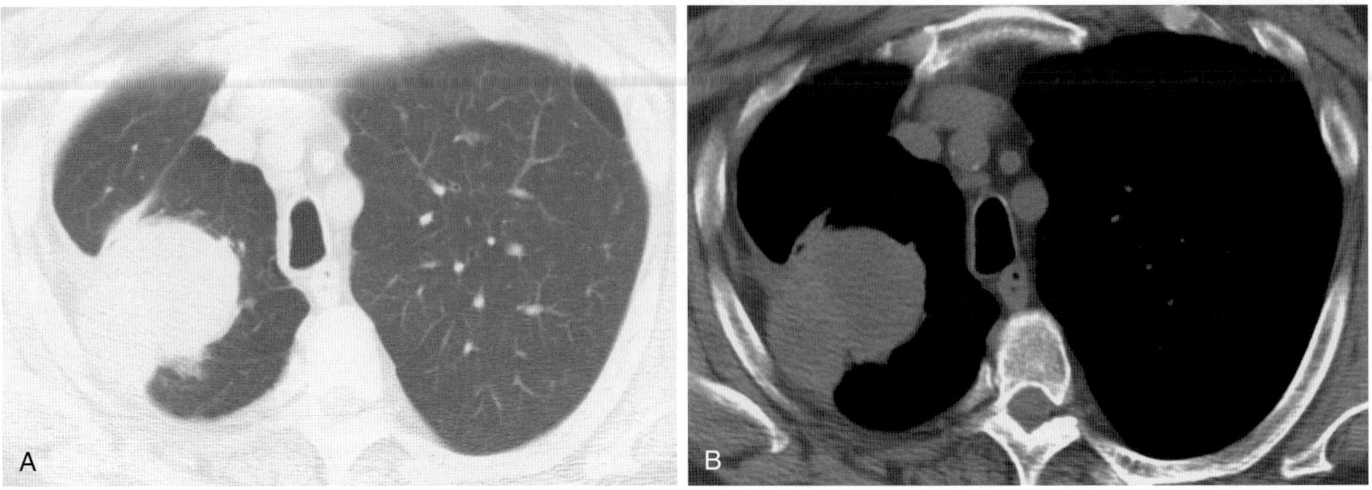

Fig. 61.22 Lung cancer mimicking rounded atelectasis. (A) CT images show right upper lobe mass abutting an area of pleural thickening. Note that the vessels curve toward the edges of the mass and that there is associated right upper lobe volume loss. (B) Soft tissue windows confirm that the mass abuts an area of pleural thickening. The presence of extrapleural fat at this level suggests that the pleural thickening is long standing. Although some of the features are consistent with rounded atelectasis, the size of the mass is out of proportion to the degree of volume loss. A completely collapsed lung occupies only approximately 10% of its original volume. Lung biopsy confirmed the presence of a pulmonary carcinoma. Desmoplastic reaction to a bronchogenic malignancy can mimic the volume loss seen in rounded atelectasis.

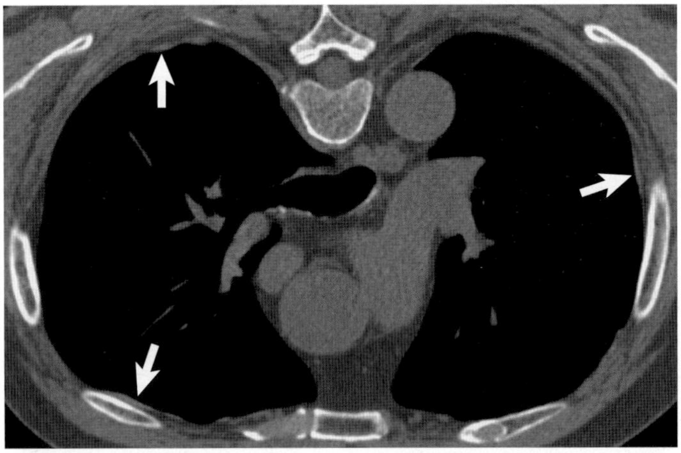

Fig. 61.23 Pleural plaques: high-resolution CT (HRCT) findings. HRCT image shows characteristic appearance of pleural plaques as sharply circumscribed focal areas of pleural thickening *(arrows)* separated from the underlying ribs and extrapleural soft tissues by a thin layer of fat.

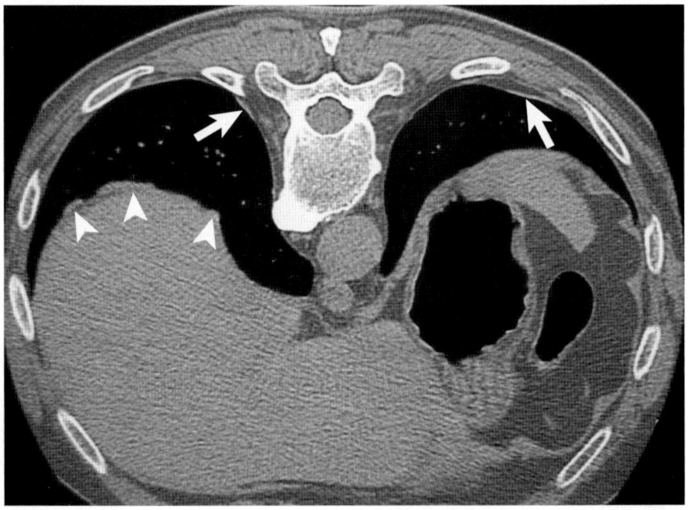

Fig. 61.24 Diaphragmatic and costal pleural plaques. High-resolution CT image shows parietal pleural plaques along the intercostal spaces and paravertebral region *(arrows)* and along the right hemidiaphragm *(arrowheads)*. *(Courtesy Dr. Jorge Kavakama, São Paulo, Brazil.)*

below the lung base. Rarely, pleural plaques may involve an interlobar fissure, localizing the plaque to the visceral pleural surface (Fig. 61.29).

Diffuse Pleural Thickening. Diffuse pleural thickening is defined on CT by the presence of a sheet of thickened pleura at least 5 cm in lateral dimension and 8 cm in craniocaudal dimension (Fig. 61.30).[55] As mentioned previously, the ILO classification recognizes pleural thickening as diffuse "only in the presence of and in continuity with an obliterated costophrenic angle."[30] In one study of 100 asbestos-exposed workers, 7 had diffuse pleural thickening evident on CT.[55] Diffuse pleural thickening related to asbestos exposure may calcify (see Fig. 61.30). The calcification is usually focal and mild but occasionally may be extensive (Fig. 61.31).

On HRCT the margin between an area of diffuse pleural thickening and the adjacent lung is frequently irregular as a result of parenchymal fibrosis, in contrast to the usually sharply circumscribed margins of pleural plaques.[56] The abnormality is generally associated with contralateral pleural abnormalities, either diffuse pleural thickening or plaques.[57] Diffuse thickening rarely involves the mediastinal pleura, although it frequently affects the parietal pleura abutting the paravertebral gutters (Fig. 61.32).[57,58] The absence of mediastinal pleural involvement can be assessed readily on CT scan and is often helpful in distinguishing benign from malignant pleural thickening; in a study of 19 patients, only 1 of 8 with fibrothorax had thickening

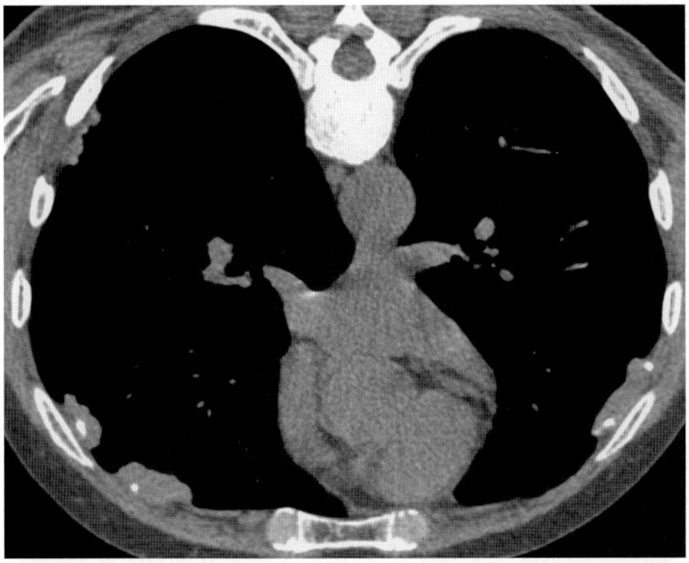

Fig. 61.25 Calcified pleural plaques. High-resolution CT image shows bilateral calcified and noncalcified pleural plaques.

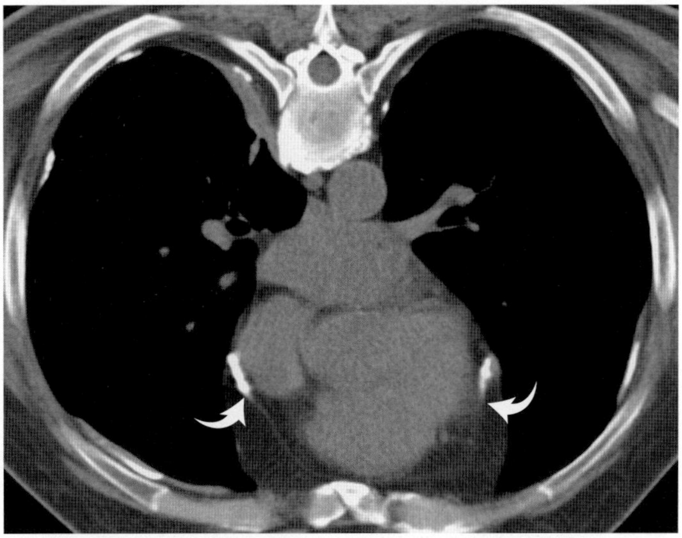

Fig. 61.27 Pericardial plaques. High-resolution CT image shows foci of thickening and calcification *(arrows)* of the pericardium consistent with pericardial plaques. Also noted are calcified and noncalcified paravertebral and costal pleural plaques.

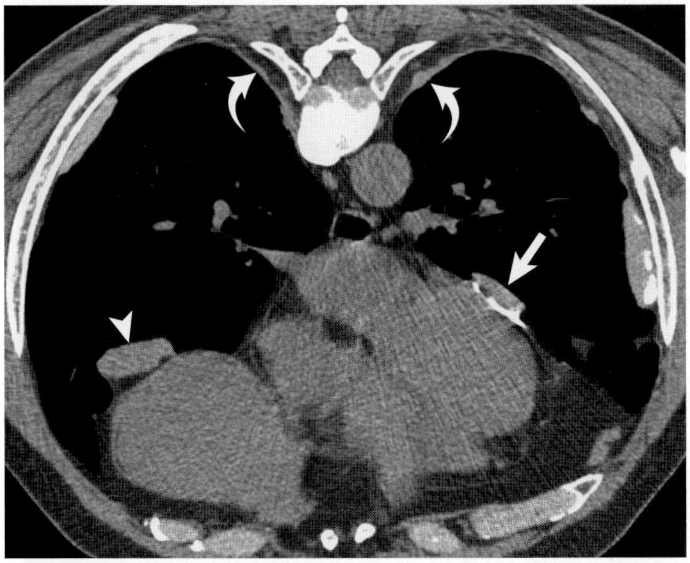

Fig. 61.26 Paravertebral and mediastinal pleural plaques. High-resolution CT image shows paravertebral *(curved arrows)*, mediastinal *(straight arrow)*, diaphragmatic *(arrowhead)*, and costal pleural plaques.

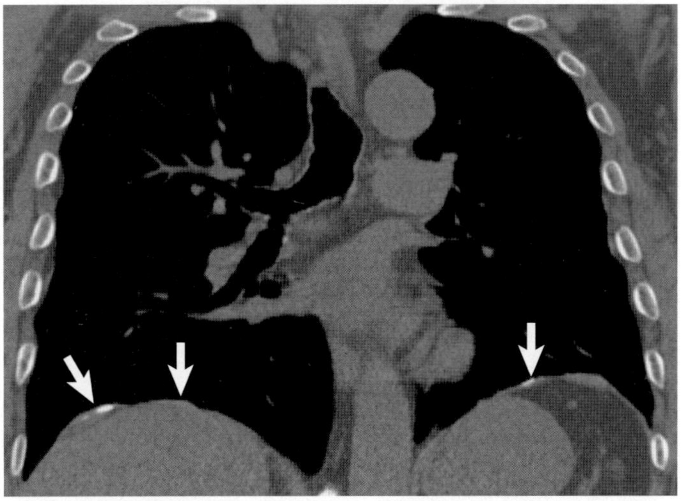

Fig. 61.28 Diaphragmatic pleural plaques. Coronal reformatted CT image shows bilateral calcified and noncalcified diaphragmatic pleural plaques *(arrows)*.

of the mediastinal pleura, compared with 8 of 11 with mesothelioma.[57]

There is a significant correlation between the presence and severity of pleural disease and the presence and severity of asbestosis.[44] In one study HRCT findings of parenchymal fibrosis were visible in 14% of exposed patients who did not have evidence of pleural thickening, in 56% of those with focal plaques, and in 88% of those with diffuse pleural thickening.[59] However, pleural thickening and plaques commonly occur in the absence of pulmonary fibrosis,[60] and asbestosis can sometimes be seen in the absence of visible pleural plaques,[59] although this is more unusual.

Pleural Effusion. Disease in some individuals with a history of asbestos exposure is manifested as pleural effusion. The effusion is exudative and often hemorrhagic (Fig. 61.33).[1]

Mesothelioma. The CT findings of mesothelioma are discussed in Chapter 74.

IMAGING ALGORITHMS

Individuals with a history of exposure to asbestos but no manifestations of disease, and for whom the time since initial exposure is 10 years or more, may be monitored with chest radiographs and pulmonary function tests every 3 to 5 years to identify the onset of asbestos-related disease.[1] Individuals with a history of exposure to asbestos are also at risk for asbestos-related malignant neoplasms, but guidelines for periodic health surveillance for lung cancer or mesothelioma do not yet exist for these patients.[1]

The sensitivity of the chest radiograph for identifying asbestosis at a profusion level of 1/0 (in the ILO classification system) has

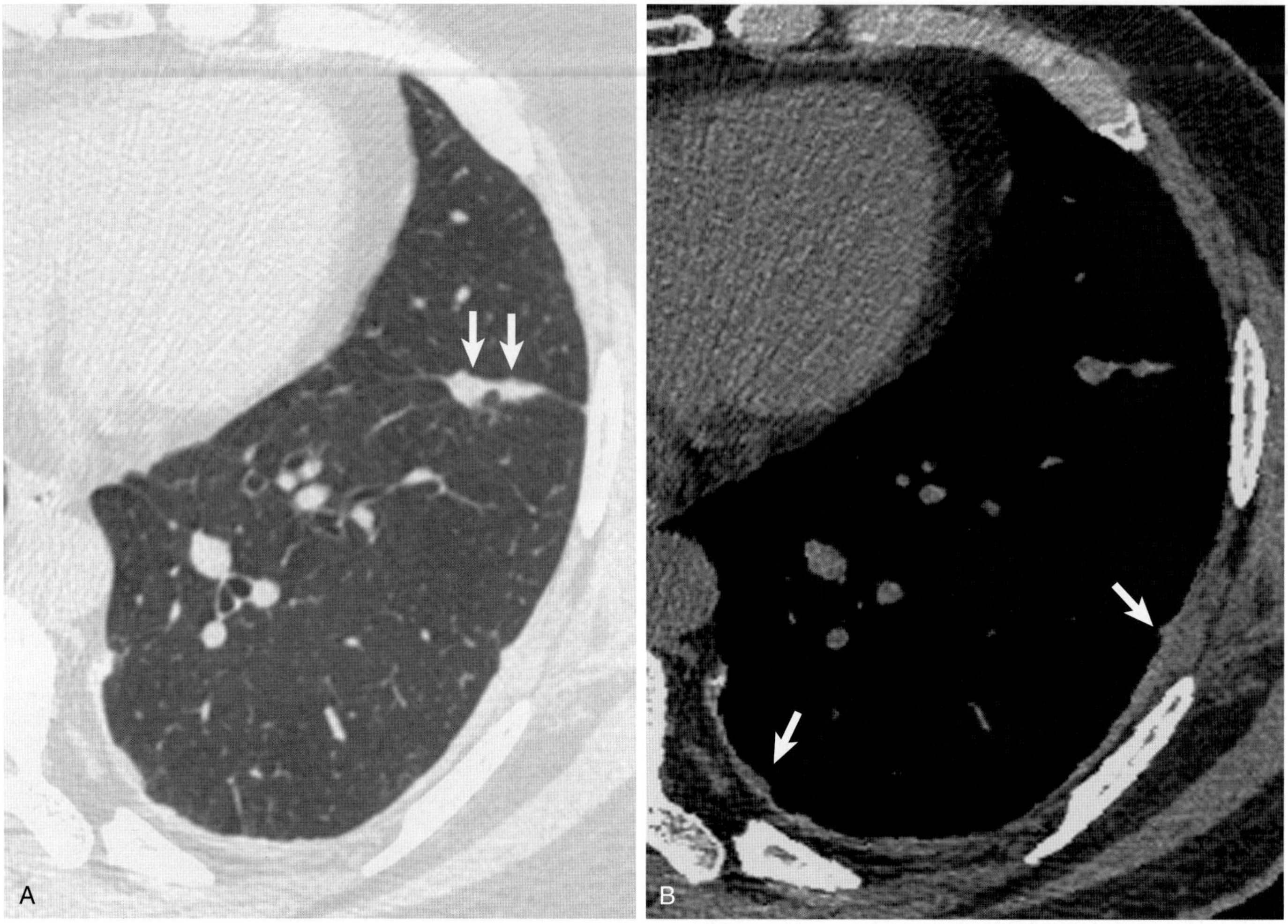

Fig. 61.29 Pleural plaque in left major fissure. (A) View of the left lung from high-resolution CT shows focal nodular thickening *(arrows)* of the left major fissure consistent with pleural plaque. (B) Soft tissue windows confirm presence of pleural plaque and demonstrate extensive thickening of the left costal and paravertebral pleura *(arrows)*.

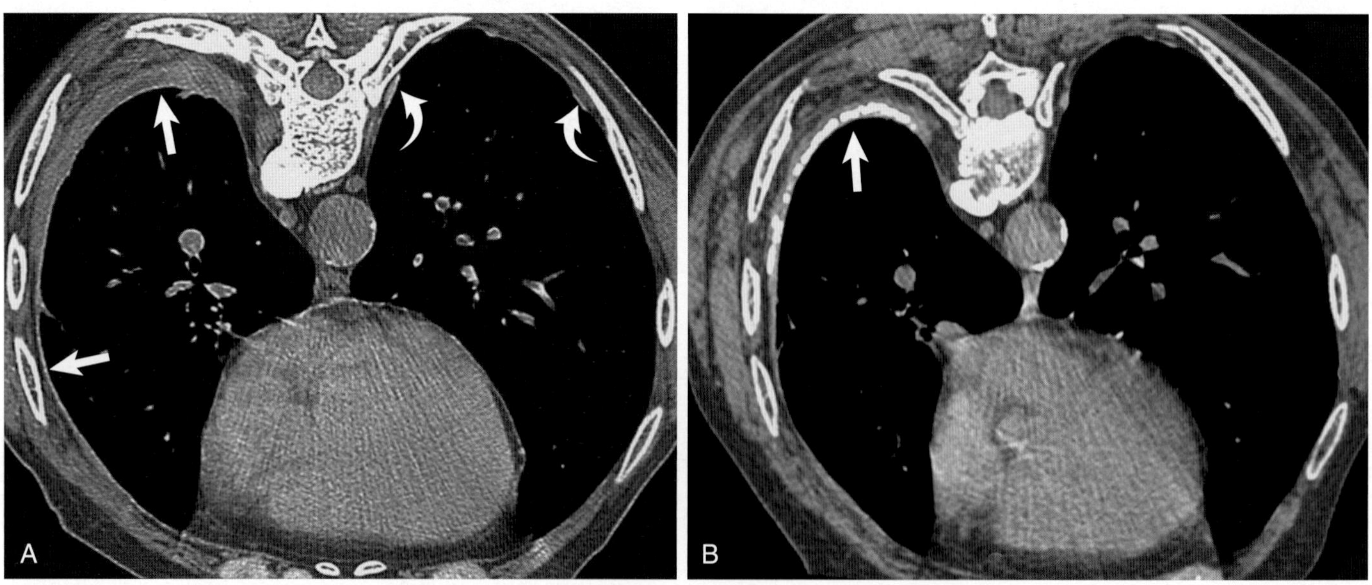

Fig. 61.30 Diffuse pleural thickening: CT findings. (A) CT image in a patient with previous asbestos exposure shows diffuse pleural thickening *(straight arrows)* on the right and pleural plaques *(curved arrows)* on the left. (B) CT image obtained 6 years later shows extensive calcification *(arrow)* of the diffuse pleural thickening. *(Courtesy Dr. Jorge Kavakama, São Paulo, Brazil.)*

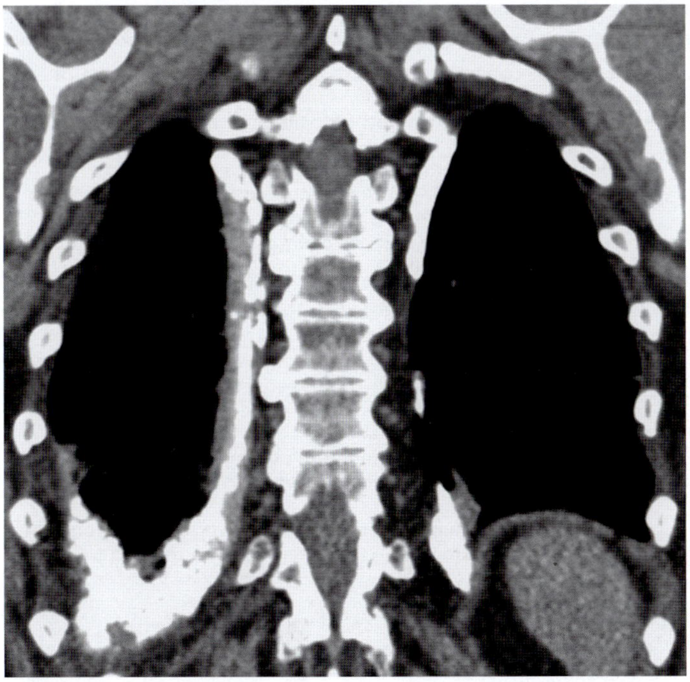

Fig. 61.31 Calcified diffuse pleural thickening. Coronal reformatted CT image in a patient with previous asbestos exposures shows diffuse right pleural thickening and calcification and calcified left paravertebral pleural plaques.

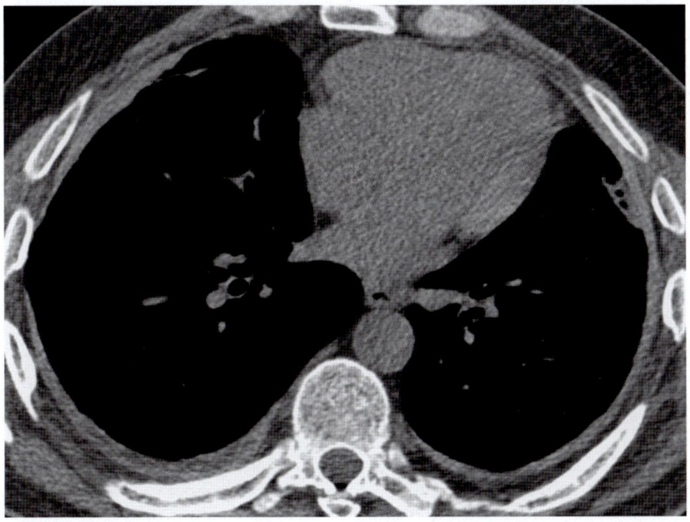

Fig. 61.32 Diffuse pleural thickening. CT image in a patient with previous asbestos exposure shows diffuse bilateral pleural thickening involving the paravertebral pleura and costal pleura but sparing the mediastinal pleura. Sparing of the mediastinal pleura is helpful in distinguishing benign from malignant pleural thickening.

been estimated at or slightly below 90% and the corresponding specificity at 93%.[1] HRCT plays an important role, particularly when experienced readers disagree about the presence or absence of abnormalities on the radiograph, when the radiographic findings are equivocal, when the radiograph is normal but the patient has functional impairment, and when extensive overlying pleural abnormalities do not allow a clear interpretation of the lung parenchyma.[1] HRCT is much more sensitive than chest radiography in the detection of asbestosis,[61,62] although even a normal HRCT scan cannot completely exclude asbestosis.[46] HRCT is also much more sensitive than chest radiography in the detection of pleural plaques and also has greater specificity, allowing distinction of pleural thickening from extrapleural fat.

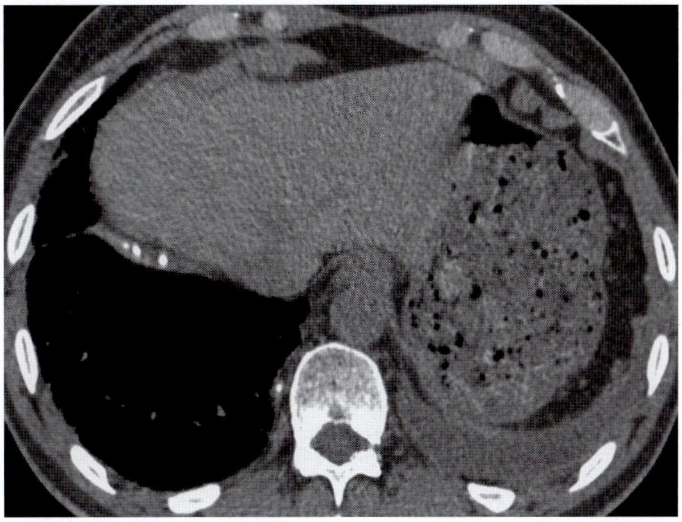

Fig. 61.33 Benign pleural effusion. CT image shows calcified right pleural plaques and small left pleural effusion. The presence of calcified plaques suggests that the first exposure to asbestos in this patient occurred more than 30 years previously. The presence of pleural effusion after such a long latency time should raise the possibility of mesothelioma. Diagnosis of benign asbestos-related pleural effusion was based on clinical history, lack of evidence of mesothelioma at the time of the effusion, spontaneous resolution, and lack of recurrence on follow-up. Benign asbestos-related pleural effusions have been reported to occur 1–58 years after asbestos exposure.

Differential Diagnosis

The diagnosis of asbestosis requires the presence of pulmonary fibrosis and history of exposure of sufficient duration, latency, and intensity to be causal.[1] The latency period is influenced by the duration and intensity of exposure. Under current conditions of exposure in North America, the latency period is often 2 decades.[1] The abnormal chest radiograph and its interpretation remain the most important initial factor in establishing the presence of pulmonary fibrosis,[1] given the strong link of ILO classification to occupational lung disease compensation systems.[1] When the chest radiograph or lung function abnormalities are indeterminate, HRCT scanning is often helpful in demonstrating the presence of fibrosis and pleural changes highly suggestive of asbestos exposure.[1] Clinically and radiologically, asbestosis resembles other interstitial lung diseases, particularly idiopathic pulmonary fibrosis. The differential diagnosis is based mainly on the history of asbestos exposure and on the radiologic demonstration of pleural abnormalities consistent with asbestos exposure. In some cases definitive diagnosis may require lung biopsy.

The main differential diagnosis of rounded atelectasis is with pulmonary carcinoma (see Fig. 61.22). Although this differential diagnosis can be made on CT in the majority of cases, these patients often require follow-up. Rounded atelectasis is typically static or grows very slowly. The most reliable feature in distinguishing rounded atelectasis from carcinoma is the convergence of bronchovascular markings around the edges of the atelectasis. In one study the authors compared the CT findings of 12 cases

KEY POINTS: ASBESTOS-RELATED PULMONARY AND PLEURAL DISEASE

- It has been estimated that 8–9 million people in the United States have had occupational exposure to asbestos and that such exposure will eventually result in 300,000 deaths.
- The chest radiograph plays an important role in the detection of asbestos-related pleural and parenchymal abnormalities and in the assessment of progression of disease. However, the radiograph is falsely normal in 15%–20% of patients with asbestosis and in 20%–50% of patients with pleural plaques.
- Asbestosis
  - The latency period is usually more than 20 years (average, 40 ± 10 years).
  - Degree of fibrosis is dose dependent.
  - The chest radiograph is normal in 15%–20% of cases.
  - High-resolution CT (HRCT) including prone positioning is the optimal imaging modality.
  - HRCT demonstrates a reticular pattern with subpleural curvilinear opacities and parenchymal bands in the lower lungs.
  - The majority of patients with asbestosis will also have pleural plaques or diffuse pleural thickening evident on CT.
- Rounded atelectasis
  - Estimated latency times are 10–40 years.
  - Diagnosis can usually be made on CT as a rounded or oval opacity with significant volume loss abutting focal pleural thickening.
  - Curving of adjacent pulmonary vessels and bronchi into the edges is frequently seen (comet tail sign).
  - It enhances markedly with intravenous administration of contrast material.
  - Usually, uptake is equal to or less than mediastinal blood pool on fluorodeoxyglucose–positron emission tomography imaging.
  - Follow-up is often required to confirm stability.
- Lung cancer
  - Asbestos-related carcinoma likely accounts for 2%–3% of all lung cancer deaths.
  - The latency time is 10 years to more than 60 years (mean, 46 years).
  - It is most common in patients with radiologic evidence of asbestosis.
  - There is greater likelihood of location in the lower lobe.
- Pleural plaques
  - Most common manifestation of asbestos exposure.
  - Usually first seen 20–30 years after exposure.
  - Calcified plaques are seldom evident until more than 30 years after exposure and are likely much more common than reported in the literature.
  - Circumscribed focal areas of pleural thickening, separated from the underlying ribs and extrapleural soft tissues by a thin layer of fat.
- Diffuse pleural thickening
  - Occurs in 9%–22% of asbestos-exposed workers with pleural disease.
  - The latency period is 10–40 years.
  - Smooth, uninterrupted pleural thickening extending for at least 5 cm in lateral dimension and 8 cm in craniocaudal dimension.
  - Fibrothorax frequently involves the paravertebral region, but mediastinal pleural thickening occurs in less than 15% of cases.
- Pleural effusion
  - Occurs in approximately 3% of asbestos workers.
  - It is the most common asbestos-related abnormality seen within the first 20 years after exposure.
  - The latency period is large, 1–58 years after exposure.
  - Usually small; may be unilateral or bilateral, persist for months, or recur.
- Mesothelioma (see Chapter 74)
  - Risk is almost zero for the first 10–15 years after the first exposure but increases progressively thereafter.
  - The mean latency time is 46 ± 12 years.
  - Unilateral sheet-like or lobulated pleural thickening in approximately 80%–90% of cases.
  - Thickening of the mediastinal pleura in approximately 85% of cases.

of rounded atelectasis with 12 cases of "look-alike" masses. Of all the features examined, the presence of converging bronchovascular markings discriminated best between rounded atelectasis and look-alikes, but the sensitivity was only 83% and the specificity 92%.[63] Furthermore, cancer has been shown to develop within an area of rounded atelectasis.[64] In patients with nondiagnostic CT findings, further evaluation may be obtained with needle biopsy or fluorodeoxyglucose–positron emission tomography (FDG-PET) scanning. In one study of 10 cases of rounded atelectasis seen in 9 patients, all lesions were negative on FDG-PET (i.e., FDG uptake similar or less than mediastinal blood pool).[65]

Bilateral pleural plaques are almost invariably associated with asbestos exposure.[1] However, isolated plaques and diffuse pleural thickening may be associated with tuberculosis, trauma, and hemothorax.[1] The main differential diagnostic consideration in patients with pleural effusion or diffuse pleural thickening is mesothelioma, which is typically progressive and more likely to be symptomatic at the time of detection. On occasion, when fibrosis and mesothelial proliferation are exuberant, the distinction may be difficult clinically, radiologically, and histologically. The manifestations of mesothelioma are discussed in Chapter 74.

SUGGESTED READINGS

Champlin J, et al. Imaging of occupational lung disease. *Radiol Clin North Am.* 2016;54(6):1077–1096.

Cox CW, et al. State of the art: imaging of occupational lung disease. *Radiology.* 2014;270(3):681–696.

Norbet C, et al. Asbestos-related lung disease: a pictorial review. *Curr Probl Diagn Radiol.* 2015;44(4):371–382.

The full reference list for this chapter is available at ExpertConsult.com.

62 Silicosis and Coal Workers' Pneumoconiosis*

STEPHEN B. HOBBS

Etiology

Silicosis and coal workers' pneumoconiosis (CWP) are occupational lung diseases; silicosis is caused by continued exposure to excessive amounts of respirable silica, and CWP is caused by exposure to carbonaceous material (anthracosis). Respirable crystalline silicate and coal dust embed in the lungs, causing granulomatous and fibrotic changes that lead to radiographic and pathologic abnormalities. Silica is a naturally occurring mineral that is mainly composed of silicon dioxide (SiO_2). It exists in two forms: crystalline silica, which causes silicosis, and amorphous silica, which is not toxic. The three most common forms of crystalline silica are quartz, cristobalite, and tridymite, but quartz is the most common form of inhaled silica.

The diagnosis of silicosis and CWP is based on the typical radiographic appearance of diffuse nodules or reticulonodular pattern in the presence of a strong occupational exposure to silica and coal dust. The guidelines for the use of the ILO (International Labour Organization) International Classification of Radiographs of Pneumoconiosis were recently updated in 2011 to include criteria for the interpretation of digital images and is the most widely accepted classification of the extent of involvement of the pneumoconioses and one in which the presence or absence of pneumoconiosis is established in workers exposed to mineral dust, including silica.[1] The ILO system uses a step-by-step method to evaluate chest radiographs, which are compared with standard reference film-screen or digital radiographs available from the ILO, with standard nomenclature to describe the shape, size, location, and abundance of opacities.

Prevalence and Epidemiology

Workers engaged in occupations such as tunneling, mining, sandblasting, and quarrying are inevitably exposed to silica owing to its ubiquity in the earth's crust. Other workers engaged in occupations that predispose to silica exposure include jade polishers,[2–4] foundry and pottery workers,[5–7] glass and silica brick workers,[5] goldworking jewelers,[8] and electric cable manufacturers.[9] More newly recognized causes of silica exposure, resulting in accelerated silicosis and silicoproteinosis, include sandblasting in denim clothing and manufacturing engineered stone countertops containing quartz.[10–12] Environmental silica arises as a result of crystalline silica becoming airborne in arid, windy conditions or during agricultural, urban, or construction activities. Inhalation of environmental silica and mixed dust has led to lung fibrosis.[13]

Hnizdo and Sluis-Cremer[14] showed the relationship between exposure to silica and silicosis. The cumulative exposure for the entire cohort in their study was about 2 mg/m^3 per year over an average exposure period of 25 years. No silicosis occurred when the cumulative exposures were less than 0.9 mg/m^3 per year. In contrast, the cumulative risk of silicosis was approximately 25% at a cumulative exposure of 2.7 mg/m^3 per year and 77% at the highest observed cumulative exposure level of 4.5 mg/m^3 per year. This dose-response relationship between the duration of exposure to the quartz-containing dust and the prevalence of silicosis also has been observed by other investigators.[15,16] The effects of smoking on the prevalence of silicosis were illustrated in a cross-sectional survey of 3258 workers in a Dutch fine-ceramic industry, in which the prevalence of silicosis among heavy smokers with 20 years' or more exposure to quartz-containing dust was 50% higher than in light smokers and nonsmokers.[16]

The prevalence and incidence of silicosis worldwide are difficult to determine because of variable industrial practices and work safety standards. The National Institute for Occupational Safety and Health estimated that in 1983 approximately 2.3 million workers at 238,000 work sites were exposed to silica dust.[17] It was more recently estimated that 59,000 workers may be at risk of developing some degree of silicosis, with 250 deaths per year being attributed to silica exposure.[18] Approximately 1500 cases of silicosis are diagnosed annually in the United States; silicosis was cited as the primary or contributing cause of death in 13,744 deaths between 1968 and 1990 in the United States.[19] There has been a trend of decreasing annual death rates correlating with a decreased incidence since a peak during World War II. Specifically, deaths decreased from 1157 in 1968 to 301 in 1988 in the United States,[19] although the prevalence rates in developing nations remain significantly higher. In Colombia and India, respectively, 1.8 million and 1.69 million workers are estimated to be exposed to and at risk of developing silicosis. Workers in India who are involved in quarrying shale sedimentary rocks have a 55% prevalence rate of silicosis, whereas 50% of Latin American miners older than 55 years develop silicosis.[20] A study in Northern Thailand of 266 mortar and pestle workers documented a 21.1% prevalence rate for silicosis.[15] In a separate study involving workers from 33 stone-grinding factories in Thailand, 31 of the factories (93.6%) were found to have levels of total or respirable dust exceeding acceptable levels.[21] The prevalence of silicosis was 9%.

CWP occurs after exposure to coal dust for longer than 20 years on average, but some cases have been reported with less than 10 years of exposure. The severity and prevalence of CWP are related to the duration of exposure, the amount of coal dust inhaled, and the carbon content (rank) of the coal dust. Higher concentrations of coal dust exposure are associated with higher prevalence of CWP. Similarly, a high rank of coal dust, such as anthracite, increases the risk of CWP.[22] The prevalence of CWP

---

*The editors and the publisher would like to thank Dr. Clara G. Ooi for contributing material on this topic to the prior edition of this work. It has served as the foundation for the current chapter.

varies from country to country, within different regions of a country, and from mine to mine. The overall prevalence of CWP in the United States was reported to be 30% in an interagency study in the 1960s. Although this percentage may be decreased in more recent years as a result of federal legislation that mandated substantially lower dust levels in coal mines,[23] some recent studies have demonstrated areas of increased prevalence of progressive massive fibrosis (PMF) among underground U.S. coal miners despite exposure after implementation of those federal dust regulations.[24–26] Currently, it is estimated that 2% to 12% of U.S. coal miners develop category 2 or greater disease after a 40-year working life, with an estimated prevalence of PMF of 1% to 7%.[27,28] In comparison, the predicted prevalences for CWP and PMF in British coal miners are 9% and 0.7%, respectively.[29]

Clinical Presentation

SILICOSIS

The three main clinical presentations of silicosis are acute silicosis (silicoproteinosis), accelerated silicosis, and classic silicosis, and they are determined primarily by the intensity and the length of exposure to silica. Silicoproteinosis (acute silicosis) is an acute and progressive form of silicosis that often results in death from respiratory failure. This variant of silicosis can develop within a few weeks or months of exposure to very high concentrations of silica and is associated with occupations such as sandblasting, surface drilling, tunneling, silica flour milling, and quartzite milling.[30–35] The lungs show a ground-glass appearance similar to that of pulmonary edema and alveolar proteinosis. The lesion may consolidate into appearances more characteristic of PMF over a short time. Workers usually present with rapidly progressive dyspnea, cough, and weight loss and develop cyanosis and respiratory failure. Death usually occurs within a short time despite intensive treatment. It has been proposed that acute silicosis occurs in workers exposed to freshly fractured silica dust and that surface Si* and SiO* radicals generated during fracturing play an important role in the rapid onset of this variant of silicosis.[36,37]

With accelerated silicosis, the exposure time after which the disease becomes clinically evident is much shorter than classic silicosis, ranging from 5 to 10 years of exposure, with the rate of disease progression noticeably faster. The symptom of breathlessness occurs 1 year after exposure, with the patient's condition rapidly deteriorating to hypoxic respiratory failure and death within 5 years.[38,39] High concentrations of dust in a relatively confined space are thought to predispose an individual to this form of silicosis, which is common in certain occupations, such as sandblasting, stone masonry, and other crushing operations.[40,41] Except for this aggressive time course, the radiographic, clinical, and pathologic features of this entity are nearly indistinguishable from classic silicosis.

Long-term exposure to low concentrations of silica is associated with a slow progressive nodular infiltration in both lungs, predominantly in the upper lung zones. Classic silicosis is the most common presentation whereby patients remain asymptomatic until after 10 to 20 years of continuous silica exposure, by which time radiographic abnormalities are evident. In contrast to other inhalational occupational lung diseases, lung changes in silicosis often progress even after the individual has been removed from the causative environment.[42,43] Although most patients are asymptomatic initially, dyspnea on exertion and then at rest is common. A relationship between severity of dyspnea and radiographic abnormalities has been documented.[44,45] The lung lesions are usually progressive and may result in PMF. PMF is the result of the coalescence and agglomeration of several smaller nodules together with increased profusion and enlargement of nodules. According to the Silicosis and Silicate Disease Committee, a PMF lesion is defined as a lesion greater than 2 cm in diameter, in contrast to the 1 cm or larger radiographic size established by the ILO. Cavitation and extensive destruction of the lung parenchyma, including bronchioles and blood vessels, are common in PMF and may signify superimposed infection from anaerobic bacteria or tuberculosis.

With progressive lung damage, pulmonary hypertension and right heart failure eventually supervene. Emphysema is common in silicosis and has been considered the major cause of cor pulmonale and disability by some investigators.[46] Additionally, risk of other cardiovascular diseases is increased, including stroke,[47] peripheral vascular disease,[48] and congestive heart failure.[49] Pneumothorax can complicate silicosis and occurs more frequently among patients with accelerated or acute silicosis. Other conditions that may complicate silicosis include Caplan syndrome, tuberculosis, carcinoma, and connective tissue disease. The two most serious complications, lung cancer and tuberculosis, may affect the prognosis and natural history of the underlying disease. Chronic silica inhalation is associated with a threefold increased risk of mycobacterial infections (silicotuberculosis). The risk increases with more severe disease in terms of nodular profusion and PMF[50]; this predisposition depends on the prevalence of tuberculosis in the population from which the workers originate.[51]

Rheumatoid pneumoconiosis (Caplan syndrome) was initially identified in CWP but is now known to occur in silicosis as well,[52] although rarely. The incidence of this disease ranges from 0.48% to 0.74% and is characterized by rapidly developing large opacities (1–5 cm) located mostly in the periphery of the lungs, often with only mild silicosis.[52]

The association between silicosis and lung cancer has been documented in several studies and recognized as an occupational carcinogen by the International Agency for Research on Cancer since 1996.[53–55] The risk is greatest for workers with established silicosis.[56–58]

The strength of the association between silicosis and connective tissue disease varies with the type of connective tissue disorder. The risk of developing systemic sclerosis particularly in workers with high exposure to silica dust is well established, although such causal associations between silicosis, rheumatoid arthritis, and systemic lupus erythematosus are less widely reported.[59–61]

COAL WORKERS' PNEUMOCONIOSIS

Inhalation of coal mine dust can lead to the development of several disease entities, including CWP, bronchitis, emphysema, Caplan syndrome, and silicosis.[62,63] The two most common patterns of disease found in coal miners are simple CWP and complicated CWP. With increasing duration of coal dust exposure, CWP may progress to complicated CWP, in which the nodules coalesce to form black, rubbery parenchymal masses usually in the upper posterior lungs, resulting in PMF. Progression from simple CWP to PMF has been related to radiographic severity of disease, coal mine dust–exposure level, and total dust burden, with the average transition from simple CWP to complicated CWP occurring over 12.2 years.[25]

CWP is usually asymptomatic, and most chronic pulmonary symptoms in coal miners are attributed to other lung conditions, such as industrial bronchitis from coal dust or coincident emphysema from smoking. The main symptom even in nonsmokers is chronic cough, which persists even after patients leave the workplace. PMF causes progressive dyspnea with production of black sputum (melanoptysis) when the PMF lesion liquefies and ruptures into the airways.[64,65] As with silicosis, PMF lesions often progress to pulmonary hypertension with right ventricular and respiratory failure.[66]

An association between CWP and features of rheumatoid arthritis is well described. It is unclear whether CWP predisposes miners to developing rheumatoid arthritis, whether rheumatoid arthritis takes on a unique form in patients with CWP, or whether rheumatoid arthritis alters the response of miners to coal dust. Multiple rounded nodules in the lung appearing over a relatively short time (Caplan syndrome) represent an immunopathologic response related to rheumatoid diathesis. In contrast to lesions caused by PMF, which congregate in the upper lobes, these new lesions (known as Caplan lesions) tend to coalesce in the lung periphery. Histologically, the lesions resemble rheumatoid nodules, but they have a peripheral region of more acute inflammation.

As in silicosis, patients with CWP are at an increased risk of developing active tuberculous and nontuberculous mycobacterial infections. Weak associations have been reported between CWP and progressive systemic sclerosis and stomach cancer.[67–69] Cumulative dust exposure has been shown to have a significant relationship with increased mortality from cancers of the digestive system. It has been suggested that nitrosation of ingested coal dust in the acidic gastric environment could result in the production of carcinogenic products, which may lead to the higher incidence of gastric cancer in coal miners.[70]

Silicosis in coal miners is usually found in conjunction with simple CWP and rarely as an isolated form of pneumoconiosis. It is difficult to distinguish between silicosis and CWP on chest radiography. The prevalence of silicosis in coal miners can be reliably determined only in autopsy studies. In the National Coal Workers' Autopsy Study from 1972 to 1996, pathologic evaluations of 4115 autopsy cases found 23% of coal miners with pulmonary silicosis and 58% with lymph node silicosis.[71]

Pathophysiology

PATHOLOGY

The pathogenesis of most pneumoconioses is a result of chronic inflammation that involves phagocytosis of the inhaled dust by alveolar and tissue macrophages and its deposition in the lung interstitium.[72–76] Free particulate silica that is not ingested by macrophages enters the perivascular lymphatic channels to be translocated to the draining mediastinal lymph nodes as free particles or within macrophages.[72–74,77,78] Inflammatory cytokines, such as tumor necrosis factor-α and interleukin-1, also are released by damaged epithelial cells and macrophages. These inflammatory mediators destroy the lung parenchyma by attracting other inflammatory cells (macrophages, neutrophils, and lymphocytes), resulting in alveolitis. In vivo and in vitro studies have shown that these silica-exposed macrophages release fibroblast growth factors that facilitate the accumulation of fibroblasts and fibroblast products, which induce inflammatory and fibrogenic reactions in the interstitium, alveoli, and lymph nodes.[78–86] Various growth factors stimulate fibroblast and type II pneumocyte activity. Collagen and fibronectin production rapidly increase and eventually lead to fibrosis. Animal models have shown that even after the exposure to silica ceases, dust-laden macrophages continue to produce inflammatory mediators, such as interleukin-1β and tumor necrosis factor-α, propagating the inflammation-fibrosis cycle.[87]

Silicoproteinosis

Silicoproteinosis is characterized by pulmonary edema, interstitial inflammation, and the presence of surfactant protein similar to that seen in alveolar proteinosis filling the alveolar spaces.[88] The exudate in the alveoli is eosinophilic, with a fine granular appearance. Silicotic nodules are sparse and poorly demarcated, or absent, probably because they form shortly after exposure.[89,90] Collagen deposition and fibrosis are rarely seen in silicoproteinosis.[91]

Accelerated Silicosis

Accelerated silicosis is similar in many respects to acute silicosis, exhibiting an exudative alveolar lipoproteinosis associated with chronic inflammation. In addition, accelerated silicosis is associated with fibrotic granulomas containing collagen, reticulin, and numerous silica particles. The granulomas consist of numerous mononuclear cells, fibroblasts, and collagen fibers, with a predisposition for circular orientation showing the characteristics of immature silicotic nodules.[92] The alveolar septa are lined with hypertrophic and hyperplastic alveolar type II epithelial cells with increased numbers of lamellar bodies.

Classic (Nodular) Silicosis

Nodular silicosis is characterized by the presence of small rounded nodules 3 to 6 mm in diameter.[88,93] The nodules of silicosis are well defined and located in the perivascular and peribronchiolar interstitium and the paraseptal and subpleural interstitium, and they are preferentially distributed in the upper lobes. Adjacent vessels and bronchioles may become involved and destroyed by these nodules, with occlusion of their lumen. Hilar and mediastinal lymph nodes are enlarged and pigmented, similar to that found in the silicotic nodule. Calcification also is a frequent finding.

Progressive Massive Fibrosis

Conglomeration of the nodules frequently occurs to form large masses of PMF, usually in the upper lobes where nodular profusion is greatest. The lower lobes are less frequently involved. PMF lesions sometimes cross the interlobar fissure to form elongated masses from the lung apex to the lower lobe. PMF usually is associated with adjacent emphysema and composed histologically of hyalinized collagen without the concentric lamellar appearance found in silicotic nodules. Cavitation occurs as a consequence of infection by anaerobic organisms, ischemia, or tuberculosis. Although conglomeration usually occurs in a heavily dust-laden lung with a high profusion of nodules, its development does not always parallel nodular profusion.

Rheumatoid Pneumoconiosis

Nodules of rheumatoid pneumoconiosis are similar to necrobiotic nodules found in rheumatoid arthritis and can be classified as either classic or silicotic type.[52] The former correspond to the original cases described by Caplan and are large nodules characterized by uniform necrosis and associated with little background pneumoconiotic nodules. The silicotic type consists of multiple smaller nodules, with the necrotic area retaining some characteristics of a silicotic nodule.

Mixed Dust Fibrosis

Although the radiographic characteristics of mixed dust fibrosis have not been a subject of interest in recent literature, this entity is frequently described in pathology textbooks and is of some clinical importance within the context of lung damage in exposed silica workers.[88,93] Exposure to high content (>18% of total dust deposited in lung) of free crystalline silica results in classic silicosis, whereas mixed dust fibrosis develops in the presence of low silica content (<18% of total dust deposited in lung),[94] particularly with simultaneous inhalation of other minerals, such as nonfibrous silicate (e.g., mica, kaolin, coal, talc, fuller's earth). These nonfibrous silicates augment the strong fibrotic effect of crystalline silica.[88] Instead of the well-defined, whorled appearance found in the silicotic nodule, the lesions in mixed dust fibrosis are characterized by irregular-shaped fibrotic nodules, often called stellate nodules, and a predilection of the fibrotic lesion to extend into the surrounding pulmonary interstitium.

COAL WORKERS' PNEUMOCONIOSIS

The pathology of CWP is distinct from that of silicosis.[22] Although both lesions tend to surround respiratory bronchioles, there is no collagen deposition or hyalinization in CWP lesions. The histologic hallmark of simple CWP is the black coal dust macule, which represents focal deposition of coal dust and pigment-laden macrophages, usually around respiratory bronchioles. As the macules enlarge, they coalesce with other macules to form a discrete network of interstitial fibrosis that results in dilation of respiratory bronchioles, forming focal areas of emphysema.[92] These areas of focal emphysema can accrue to large volumes without causing significant respiratory impairment.

With increased exposure to coal mine dust, nodular lesions develop at the bifurcations of respiratory bronchioles against a background of macules, mostly in the upper lobes. Compared with the nonpalpable macules, these nodules are firm and palpable and can be classified according to their size as micronodules (≤7 mm diameter) and macronodules (8 mm–2 cm).[62] Microscopically, the nodules are composed of heavily coal dust–laden macrophages interlaced with collagen fibers oriented in a haphazard manner. The margins of the nodules may be round, irregular, or stellate. The fibrous stroma is composed of mature and immature collagen and reticulin.

With chronic dust exposure, the nodules of simple CWP coalesce to produce black, rubbery parenchymal fibrous masses resulting in complicated CWP or PMF. These PMF lesions usually are sited in the posterior aspects of the upper lobes and may encroach on and destroy vascular supply and airways or may cavitate. Microscopically, PMF lesions appear as coal dust–laden, irregular or round, well-demarcated fibrotic masses of collagen bundles and haphazardly laid hyalinized collagen fibers intertwined with reticulin. Lesions also may appear as amorphous collagenization or clusters of nodules. As with silicosis, there is a tendency for PMF to progress with or without further exposure.[95] Despite its similarities with conglomerate silicosis, however, the development of PMF in coal workers is unrelated to silica content of the coal.

LUNG FUNCTION

Lung function impairment is not a prerequisite for the diagnosis of pneumoconiosis, which rests on a reliable history of sustained occupational exposure to inhaled dust and a chest radiograph that is abnormal according to the ILO's International Classification of Radiographs of Pneumoconiosis. Lung function evaluation should be used only to quantify clinical disability, particularly for compensation purposes. Lung function impairment in silicosis and CWP may be confounded by the effects of cigarette smoking. Lung function may be normal in the early stages of silicosis or CWP. When present, the lung function impairment may be restrictive, obstructive, or a combination of both. Reduction in diffusing capacity may also be observed.

Manifestations of the Disease

RADIOGRAPHY

Silicosis and CWP are virtually indistinguishable radiologically. The chest radiograph remains the foremost imaging modality by which silicosis and CWP are diagnosed, and disease progression is monitored. However, as an imaging tool, the chest radiograph is relatively insensitive and nonspecific, which can result in underestimation or overestimation of the extent of disease. In addition, a normal chest radiograph does not rule out interstitial fibrosis. Despite these limitations, the ease of performing the study combined with its cost-effectiveness makes radiography almost indispensable.

In the ILO radiographic classification, the radiographic opacities are characterized by their size and shape. Small, rounded opacities are described as "p," "q," or "r" according to their size ("p," < 1.5 mm; "q," 1.5–3 mm; "r," 3–10 mm) (Fig. 62.1), whereas irregular opacities of similar size are denoted as "s" (<1.5 mm), "t" (1.5–3 mm), and "u" (3–10 mm).[1] Profusion of nodules is a measure of the concentration of small opacities per unit area or zone of lung, determined from comparison of the patient's chest radiograph with standard radiographs provided by the ILO.

There are 12 categories of profusion, which represent a continuum of changes ranging from normal to severe profusion.[96,97] These can be grouped into four broad categories based on the degree of obscuration of vascular lung markings by the nodules: category 0 (0/–, 0/0, 0/1), when small opacities are absent or less than category 1; category 1 (1/0, 1/1, 1/2), when small opacities are present in small numbers with normal lung markings; category 2 (2/1, 2/2, 2/3), when numerous small opacities are present, and when lung markings are partially obscured; and category 3 (3/2, 3/3, 3/+), when very numerous small opacities totally obscure normal vascular markings (see Fig. 62.1). Patients with scores 1/0 or greater are considered to have pneumoconiosis. A separate classification for large opacities (>1 cm in diameter) exists whereby A denotes one or more opacities greater than 1 cm but smaller than 50 mm; B denotes one or more opacities greater than A, combined area less than the right upper zone; and C denotes one or more opacities whose combined area is greater than the area of the right upper zone.

Silicosis

The nodules of simple silicosis are well defined and small (1–10 mm in diameter) and found diffusely in the lungs with posterior and upper lung zone predominance (Fig. 62.2; see Fig. 62.1).[98] Nodule calcification is evident in 20% of cases on the chest radiograph, although the incidence is higher on computed tomography (CT). PMF lesions are commonly found at the upper lung zones with smooth or irregular borders, initially at the outer two-thirds of the lung with slow migration toward

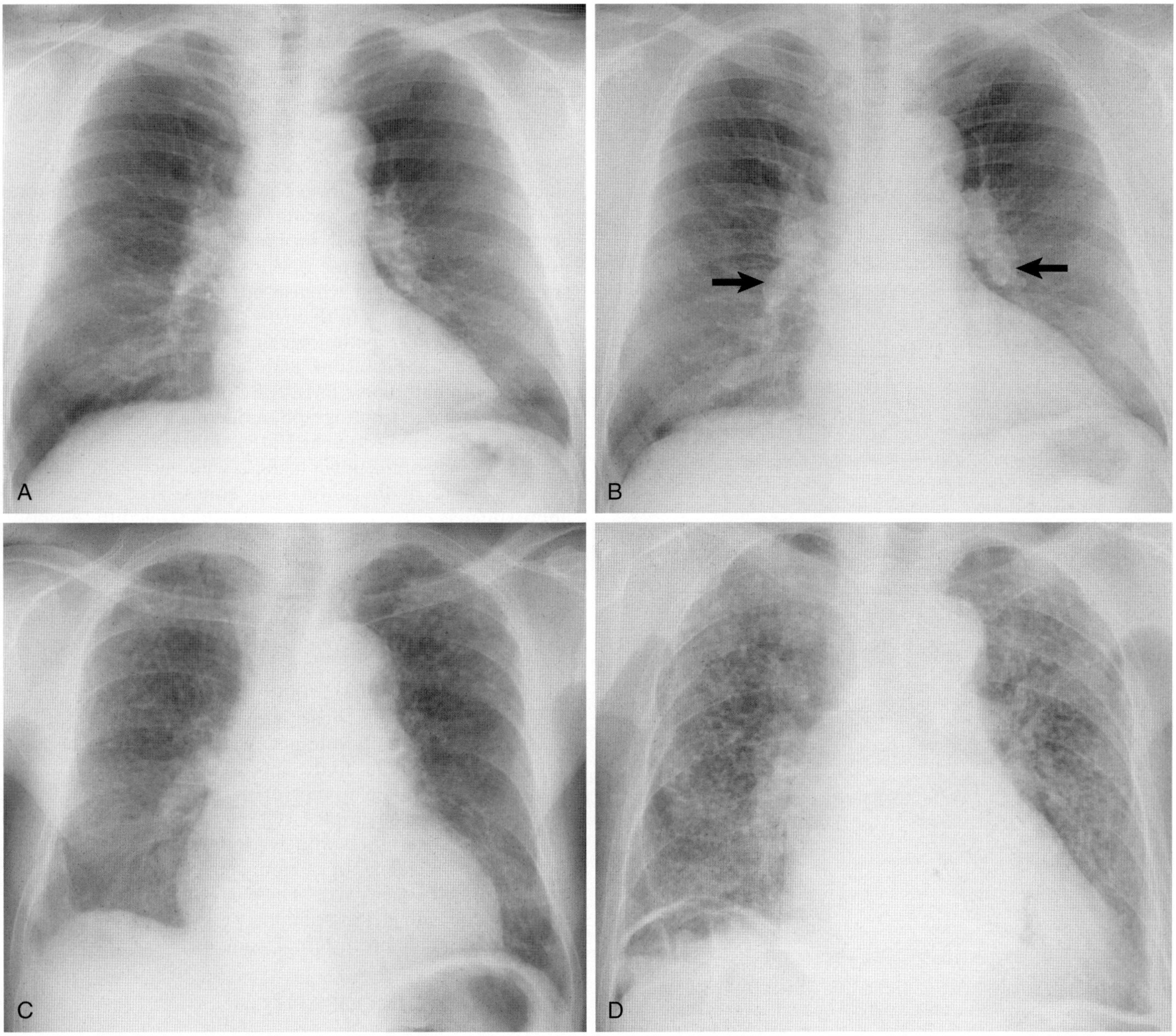

Fig. 62.1 Chest radiographs depicting examples of different nodular size and profusion according to International Labour Office classification in workers with silicosis. (A) Posteroanterior chest radiograph showing small nodules predominantly in the upper lung zones. The nodule size and profusion are p/p and 1/1. (B) Posteroanterior chest radiograph showing nodular profusion category of 2/2. Note eggshell calcification of enlarged hilar lymph nodes *(arrows)*. (C) Posteroanterior chest radiograph shows multiple nodules in both lungs. The nodule profusion category is 2/2, with "r" size nodules. (D) Posteroanterior chest radiograph shows more severe nodular profusion of category 3/3.

the hilum over time (Figs. 62.3 and 62.4). PMF has been described to have an angel's wing appearance on chest radiographs. Punctate, linear, or massive calcifications of the PMF lesions may be found.[99] Classically, paracicatricial emphysema is interposed between the PMF lesion and the pleura accompanied by volume loss in the upper lobes. The presence of paracicatricial emphysema and lung volume loss helps to distinguish unilateral PMF from lung cancer. With increasing severity of PMF and shrinkage of the upper lobes, nodularity is noticeably reduced in the rest of the lung (see Fig. 62.4).[100]

Accelerated silicosis has similar radiographic features as the classic form of silicosis except for its earlier onset and rapid rate of progression, which is truncated to a period of 5 to 10 years (Fig. 62.5). Silicoproteinosis is a variant characterized by rapid and progressive involvement of the lungs, which, based on older case reports, may manifest with extensive bilateral ground-glass opacities similar to the findings in alveolar proteinosis (Fig. 62.6). However, more recent work suggests this more frequently manifests with dependent consolidation, often containing foci of calcification, diffuse solid centrilobular nodules, or more patchy ground-glass opacities.[101,102] The rate of progression ranges from a few months to 1 to 2 years, usually culminating in death in a few years.[33,103]

Rheumatoid pneumoconiosis (Caplan syndrome) manifests as multiple diffuse, well-defined nodules ranging from 5 mm to

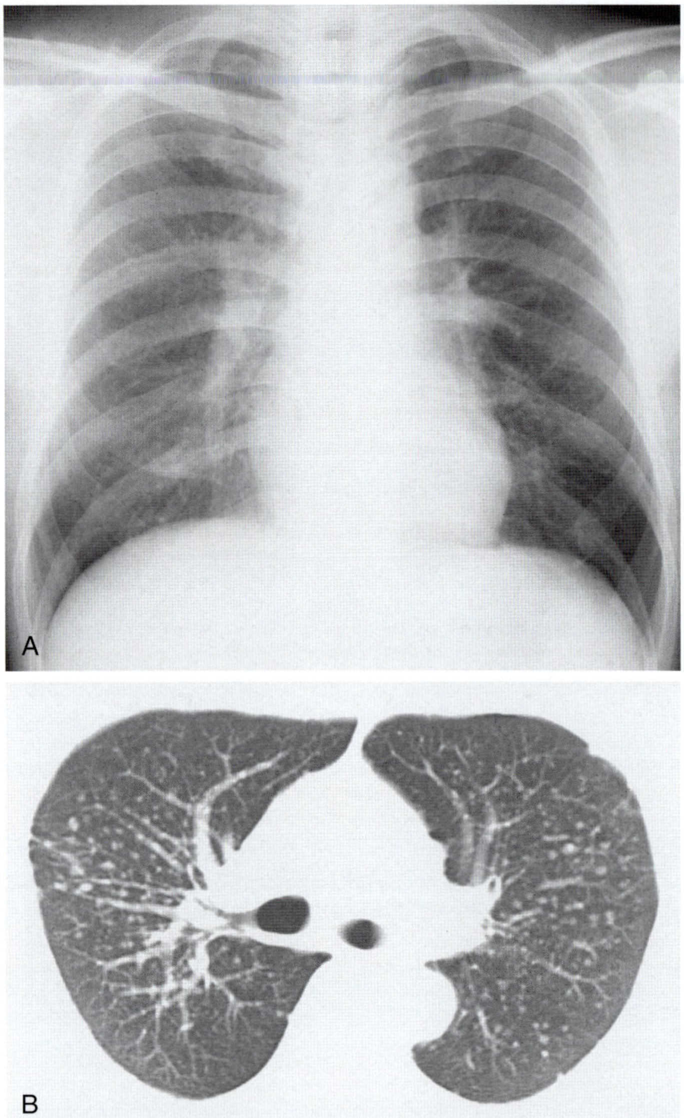

Fig. 62.2 Simple silicosis in a construction site worker. (A) Posteroanterior chest radiograph showing multiple small diffuse nodules with some lower lung zone sparing. (B) Axial CT scan showing well-defined nodules, 2–5 mm, predominantly in centrilobular and subpleural regions, so-called perilymphatic distribution.

5 cm distributed with peripheral predominance (Fig. 62.7). Characteristically, these nodules appear suddenly within a few months during the follow-up of patients. It may be impossible to distinguish silicotic-type nodules of rheumatoid pneumoconiosis from silicotic nodules.

Lymph node involvement in silicosis reflects the pathogenesis of the disease, and hilar lymphadenopathy on the chest radiograph is common. Eggshell calcifications of lymph nodes have become synonymous with silicosis since they were first described more than half a century ago and are mainly referable to the hilar lymph nodes (Fig. 62.8; see Fig. 62.1), although abdominal lymph nodes also have been described to bear eggshell calcifications.[104–106] Their presence in coal and metal miners has been attributed to the concomitant exposure to silica.[105]

Radiographic progression in silicosis is associated with the following risk factors: duration and concentration of silica exposure,[7,32,67,99] initial nodular profusion on chest radiograph,[7,32,43,67,100] simple and complicated disease,[7,32,43,67] tuberculous infection,[107] age at initial radiograph,[32,43] race,[32,43] and time interval between radiographs.[32,43]

Coal Workers' Pneumoconiosis

Radiographically, simple CWP cannot be distinguished from silicosis with any confidence. The nodules are small and round (1–5 mm) and tend to be more ill defined and granular in appearance compared with the homogeneous density of silicotic nodules. The radiographic opacities of simple CWP range in size from 0.001 to 1 cm, whereas opacities in complicated CWP are greater than 1 cm in diameter.[108] In general, there is good correlation between pathologic grading of disease severity and the radiographic profusion, with large opacities showing correlation with pathologic PMF.[108] Before an abnormality can be detected on a chest radiograph, moderate to severe pathologic abnormality has to be present. PMF lesions occur predominantly in the periphery of the upper lobes, as with silicosis, but occasionally are found in the lower lung zones. They are found in approximately 30% of miners with bilateral diffuse nodular opacities.[109,110] Over time, the PMF lesions migrate to the hila, leaving an area of emphysema between the mass and the pleura. When unilateral, the PMF lesions can be mistaken for carcinoma, particularly when there is no obvious associated nodularity elsewhere in the lungs.[111]

Approximately 10% to 20% of exposed miners can develop an atypical variety of CWP in which the radiographic features consist of small irregular opacities (reticular pattern) in the lower zones, decreased lung volumes, traction bronchiectasis, and honeycombing, similar to the appearance of asbestosis or usual interstitial pneumonia. In this variant of CWP, the typical small, rounded opacities of simple CWP may not be present elsewhere in the lungs. Coal miners who develop this form of lung fibrosis have a greater incidence of carcinoma than those with the simple small, rounded opacity type. These irregular opacities also tend to correspond with greater pulmonary impairment than increasing chest radiographic profusion of nodules.

COMPUTED TOMOGRAPHY

Until more recently, the ILO radiographic classification was the only classification system used for the grading of pneumoconiosis. The superiority of CT, particularly high-resolution CT (HRCT) over the chest radiograph, in evaluating interstitial and parenchymal lung disease is well established.[112–115] Because HRCT is considered superior to chest radiography in imaging and diagnosing subtle disease in silicosis and CWP, such as early confluence of nodules and emphysema,[44,98,112] there is a need for a standardized, reproducible, and internationally accepted CT classification system for the pneumoconioses in the English language, similar to the ILO classification for the chest radiograph. A multicenter study involved an international panel of experts who applied a coding sheet for CT lung appearances developed by a task group on Diagnostic Radiology in Occupational and Environmental Diseases.[116,117] This coding sheet is a descriptive classification of CT appearances of parenchymal and pleural abnormalities found in occupational- and environmental-related diseases. In this system, not only the presence of each abnormality found in each lung zone and the pleura is described, but also the severity and extent of silicotic nodules, PMF, diffuse interstitial fibrosis (i.e.,

Text continued on p. 804

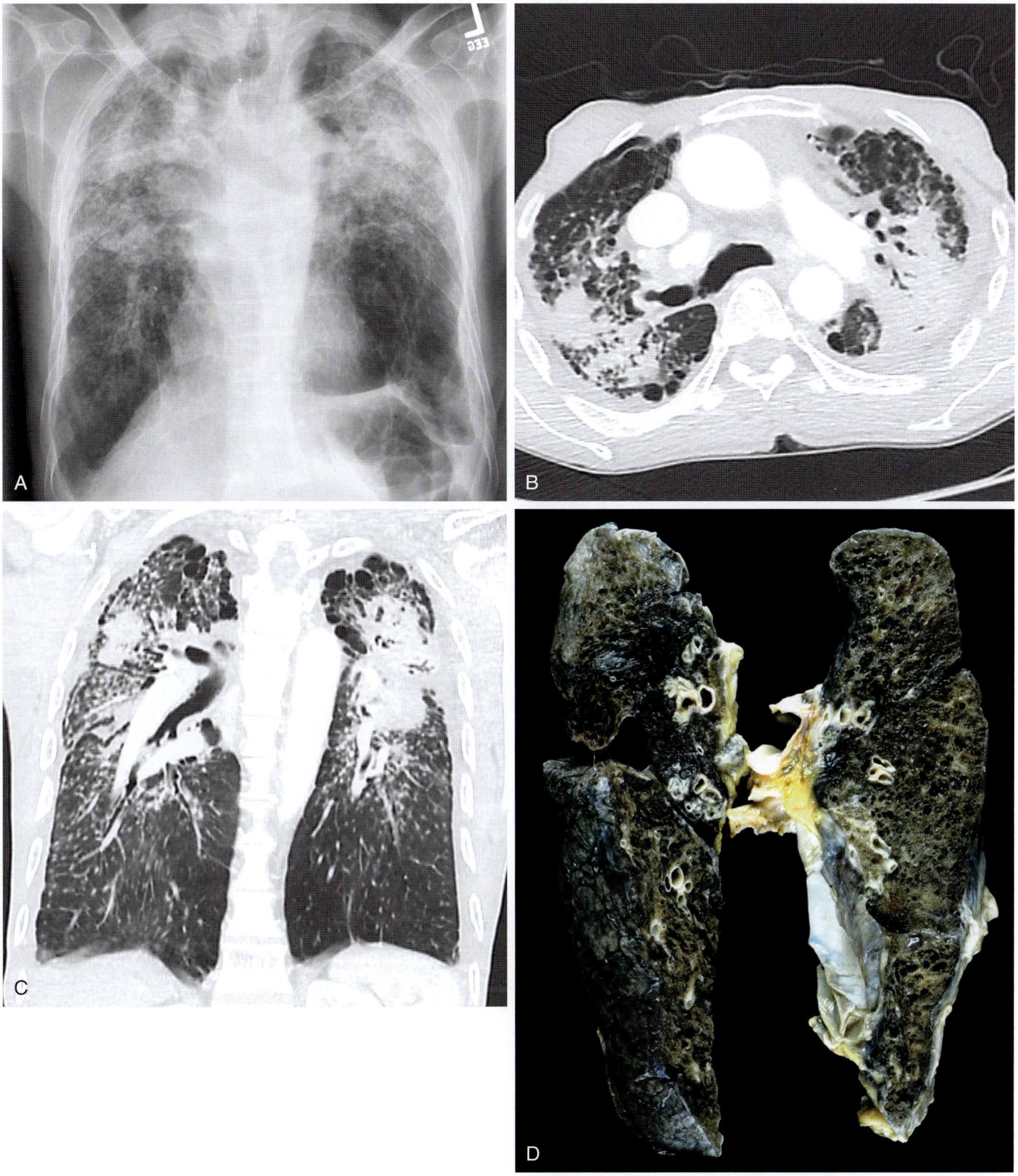

Fig. 62.3 Complicated silicosis with progressive massive fibrosis. (A) Posteroanterior chest radiograph shows large opacities in the upper lung zones with upward retraction of the hila compatible with complicated silicosis. Note bilateral hilar lymphadenopathy. (B) Axial CT scan shows bilateral mass-like opacities with irregular shapes, suggesting progressive massive fibrosis (PMF) with adjacent mild paracicatricial emphysema. (C) Coronal CT image shows marked upper lung zone distribution of nodules and masses. The left lung mass involves both the left upper and left lower lobe by crossing the left major fissure. (D) Gross lung specimen in coronal section from a different patient showing black-pigmented PMF in the right upper lung zone that is contiguous with enlarged right hilar lymph nodes. There is moderate centrilobular emphysema but sparse silicotic nodules.

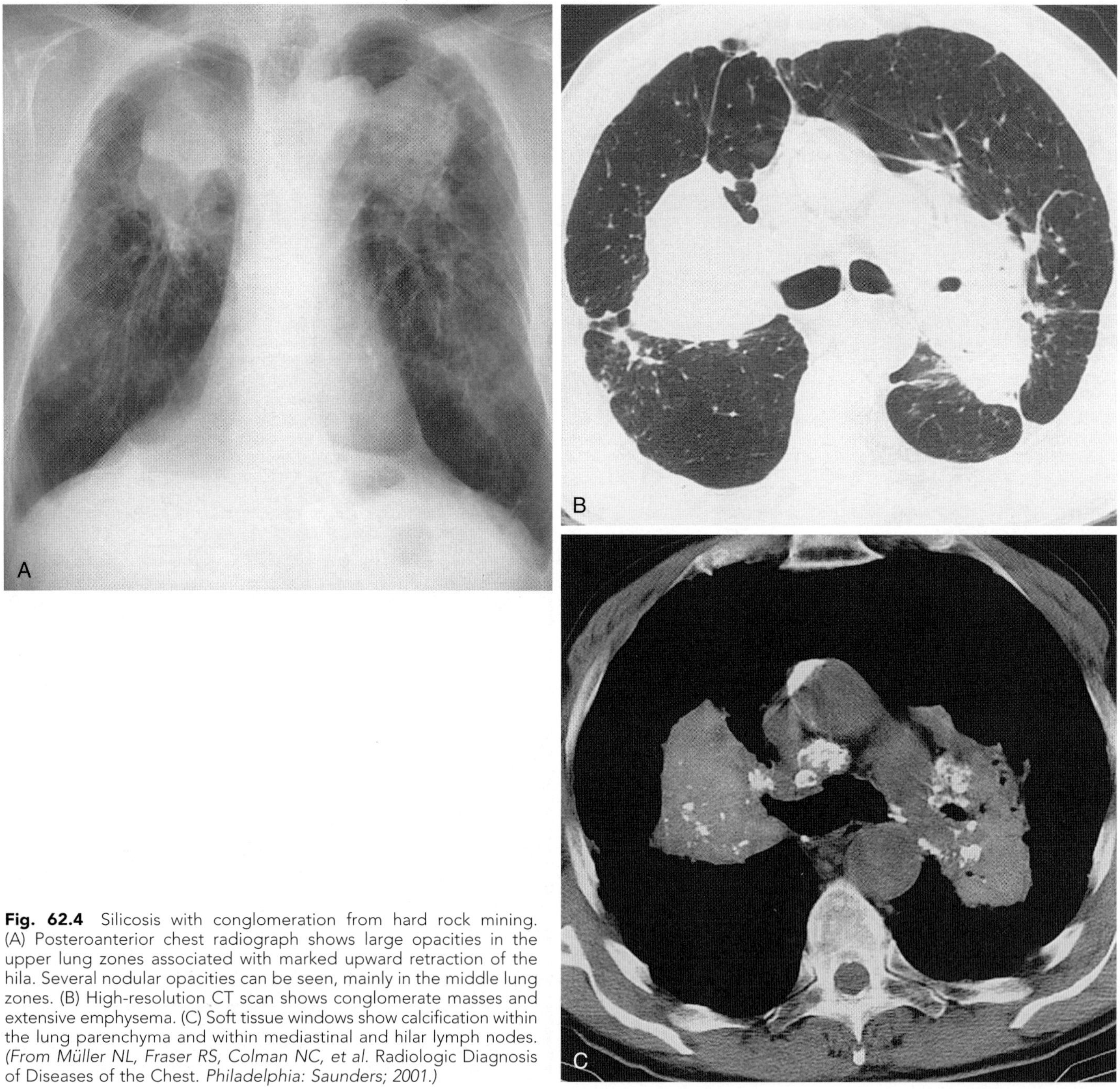

Fig. 62.4 Silicosis with conglomeration from hard rock mining. (A) Posteroanterior chest radiograph shows large opacities in the upper lung zones associated with marked upward retraction of the hila. Several nodular opacities can be seen, mainly in the middle lung zones. (B) High-resolution CT scan shows conglomerate masses and extensive emphysema. (C) Soft tissue windows show calcification within the lung parenchyma and within mediastinal and hilar lymph nodes. *(From Müller NL, Fraser RS, Colman NC, et al.* Radiologic Diagnosis of Diseases of the Chest. *Philadelphia: Saunders; 2001.)*

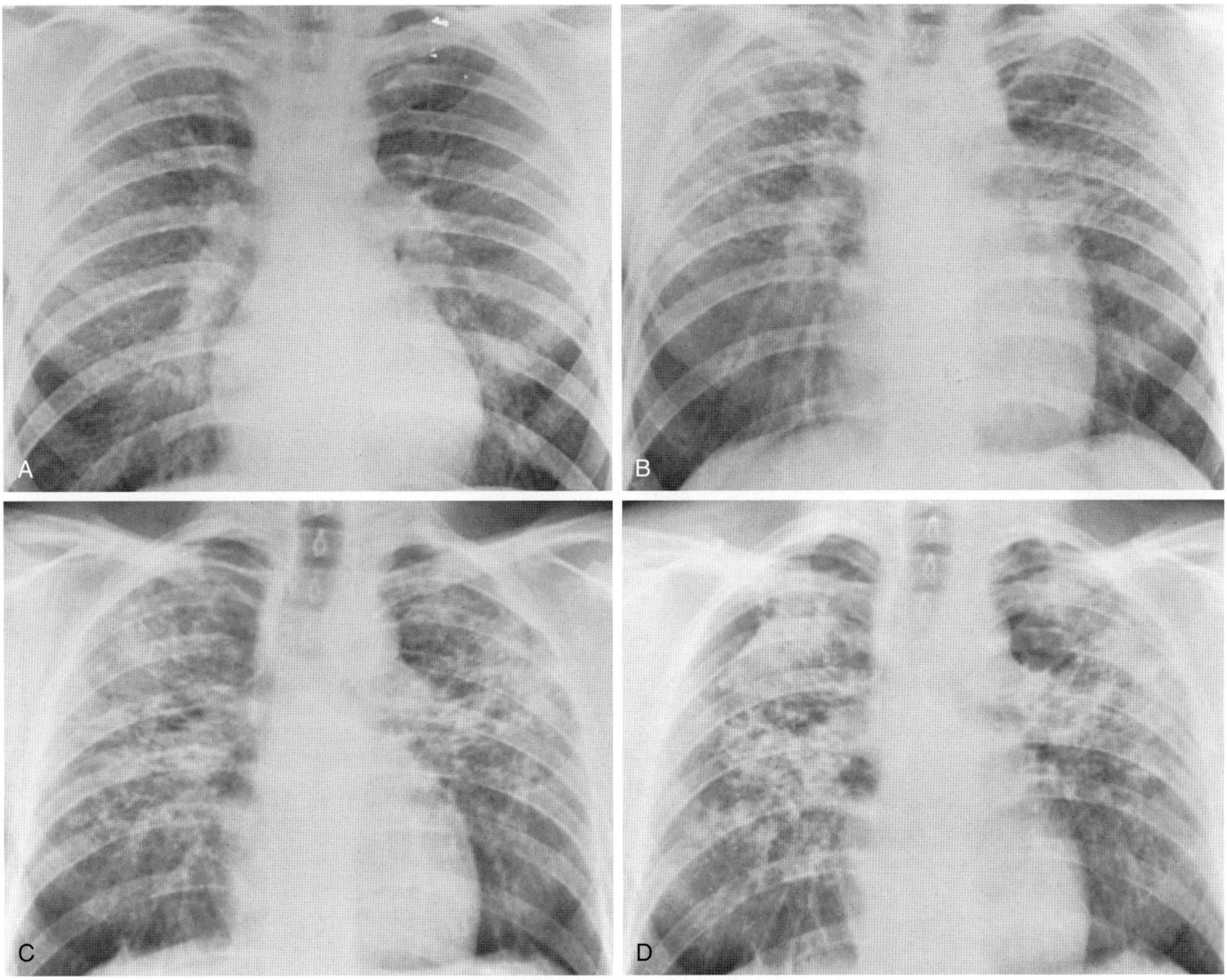

Fig. 62.5 Silicosis showing rapid progression. (A) Radiograph of a 27-year-old sandblaster shows diffuse, predominantly irregular opacities more prominent in the upper lung zones; hilar lymph nodes are enlarged. (B) Two years later, lung volume had reduced, particularly in the upper lung zones (note upward displacement of both hila). The opacities in the upper lungs were showing early coalescence. (C) Three years later, large opacities had developed in the upper lung zones. (D) Seven years after the patient was originally seen, the opacities had become much larger. Note the sharply defined lateral margin of the large opacity on the right. *(From Müller NL, Fraser RS, Colman NC, et al.* Radiologic Diagnosis of Diseases of the Chest. *Philadelphia: Saunders; 2001.)*

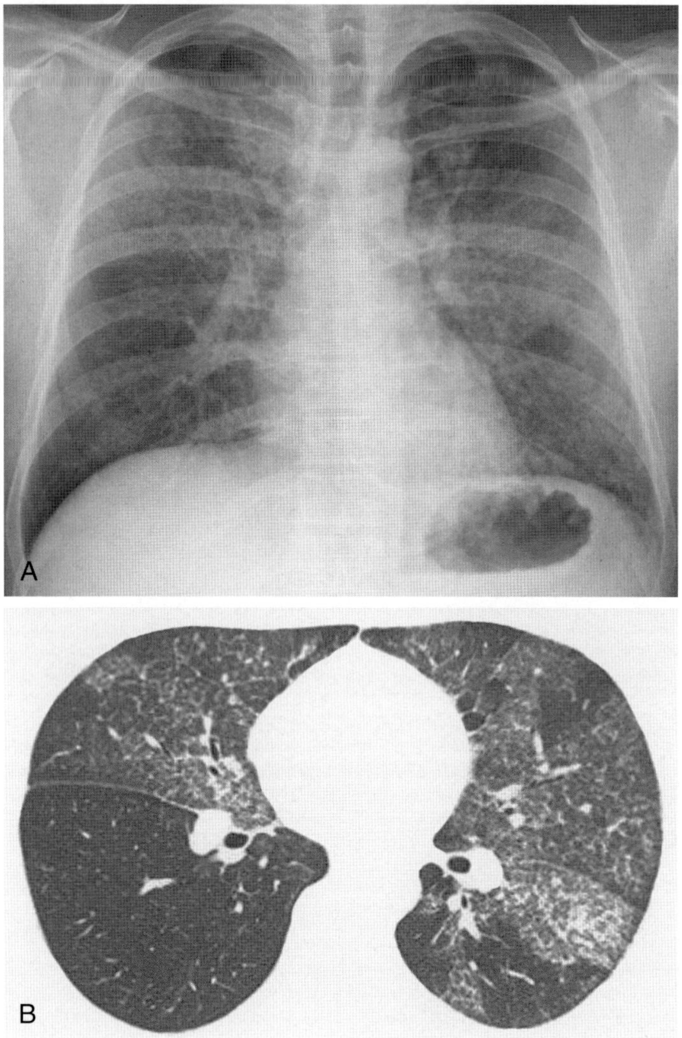

Fig. 62.6 Silicoproteinosis in a man exposed to silica dust as a mason's apprentice. (A) Chest radiograph shows extensive bilateral hazy increased opacity. (B) High-resolution CT (HRCT) scan at the level of the lower lung zones shows bilateral ground-glass opacities and superimposed intralobular lines and smooth thickening of the interlobular septa resulting in a "crazy paving" pattern. The radiographic and HRCT findings resemble those of alveolar proteinosis. *(Courtesy Dr. Jeffrey P. Kanne, Madison, WI.)*

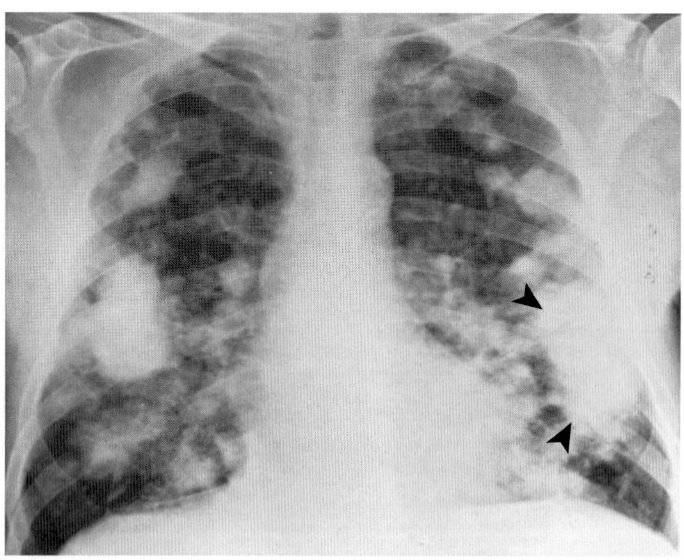

Fig. 62.7 Caplan syndrome. Posteroanterior chest radiograph shows fairly well-circumscribed nodules and masses ranging in diameter from 1 to 5 cm, scattered randomly throughout both lungs with no notable anatomic predilection. No cavitation is apparent, and there is no evidence of calcification. This patient, a 56-year-old man, had been a coal miner for many years and in recent years had developed arthralgia, which proved to be due to rheumatoid arthritis. Diagnosis was established via percutaneous needle aspiration on the large mass situated in the lower portion of the left lung *(arrowheads)*. Inky black fluid was aspirated. *(From Müller NL, Fraser RS, Colman NC, et al.* Radiologic Diagnosis of Diseases of the Chest. *Philadelphia: Saunders; 2001.)*

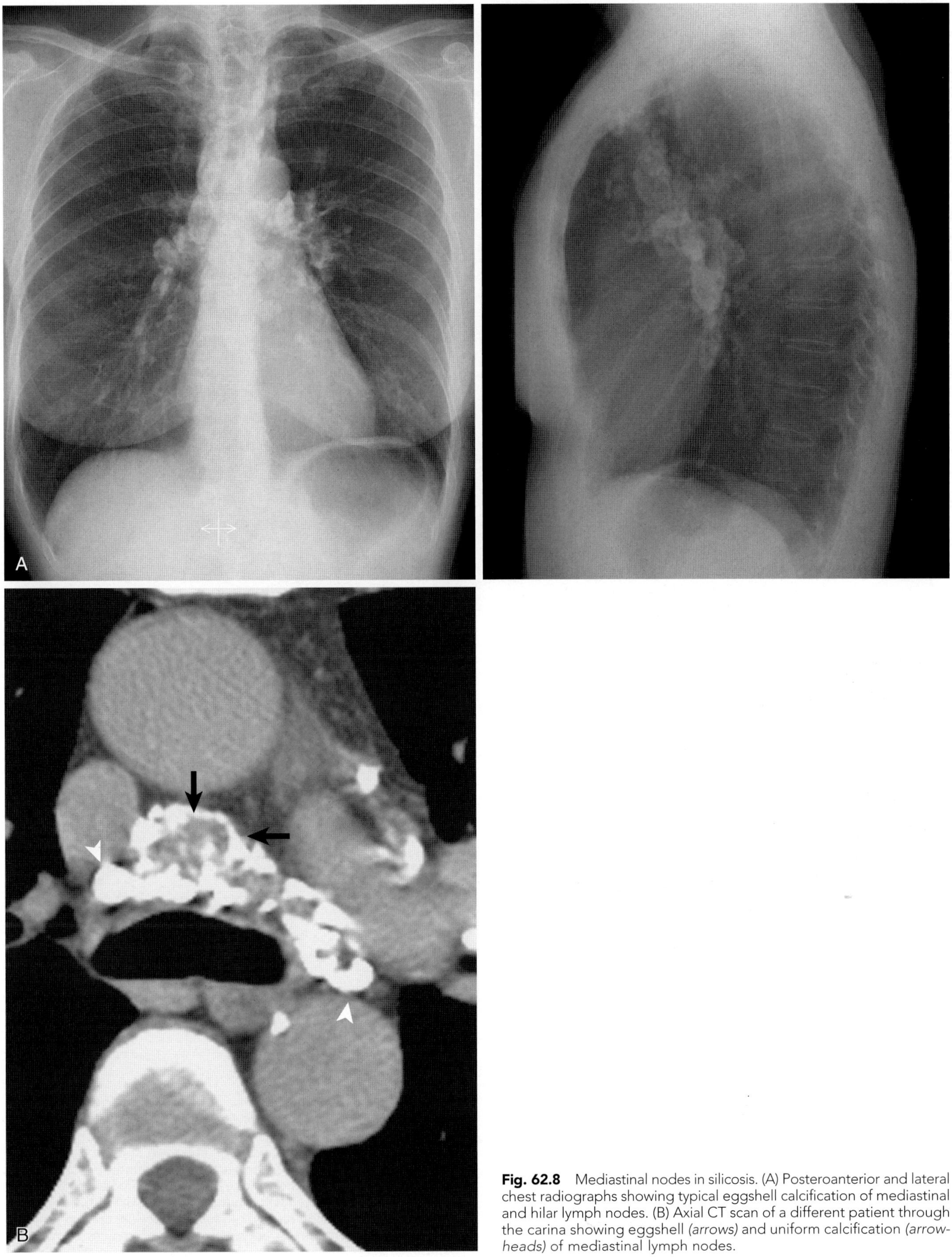

Fig. 62.8 Mediastinal nodes in silicosis. (A) Posteroanterior and lateral chest radiographs showing typical eggshell calcification of mediastinal and hilar lymph nodes. (B) Axial CT scan of a different patient through the carina showing eggshell *(arrows)* and uniform calcification *(arrow-heads)* of mediastinal lymph nodes.

reticular and ground-glass opacities), and emphysema are quantified based on the reference images. The establishment of a reproducible CT classification system would standardize the reporting and documentation of abnormalities found in the CT evaluation of pneumoconiosis. Several studies have demonstrated that upward of 40% of cases will have their initial radiographic classification changed after performing CT either from normal to simple silicosis or silicosis to PMF.[44,112,118,119]

On CT and HRCT the silicotic nodules are well defined, range from 2 to 5 mm, and are found predominantly in the perilymphatic distribution (combination of centrilobular and subpleural distribution) (see Fig. 62.9). The nodular pattern in early disease may be more centrilobular and is often easier to appreciate using maximum-intensity projection (MIP) reconstructions. Usually diffuse and bilateral with posterior lung dominance, the nodules in milder cases may be confined to the upper lung zones with sparing of the lower zones. Silicosis and CWP are distinct diseases with differing histologic features resulting from the inhalation of different inorganic dusts. The radiographic and HRCT appearances of both diseases are quite similar, however, and often indistinguishable. The nodules of simple CWP are similar to the nodules seen in silicosis and are small with upper zone predominance. One important difference is that calcification is more frequently seen in the lung disease of silicosis patients than CWP. On HRCT, CWP with "p" lesions appears as small branching lines or ill-defined punctate attenuation (Fig. 62.10). In some cases small areas of low attenuation with a central dot can be seen. These areas are thought to represent either irregular fibrosis surrounding respiratory bronchioles or dust macules on dilated respiratory bronchioles. Lesions classified as "q" and "r" types are well circumscribed, round, or contracted nodules.[120] Subpleural micronodules are frequent findings and may be associated with

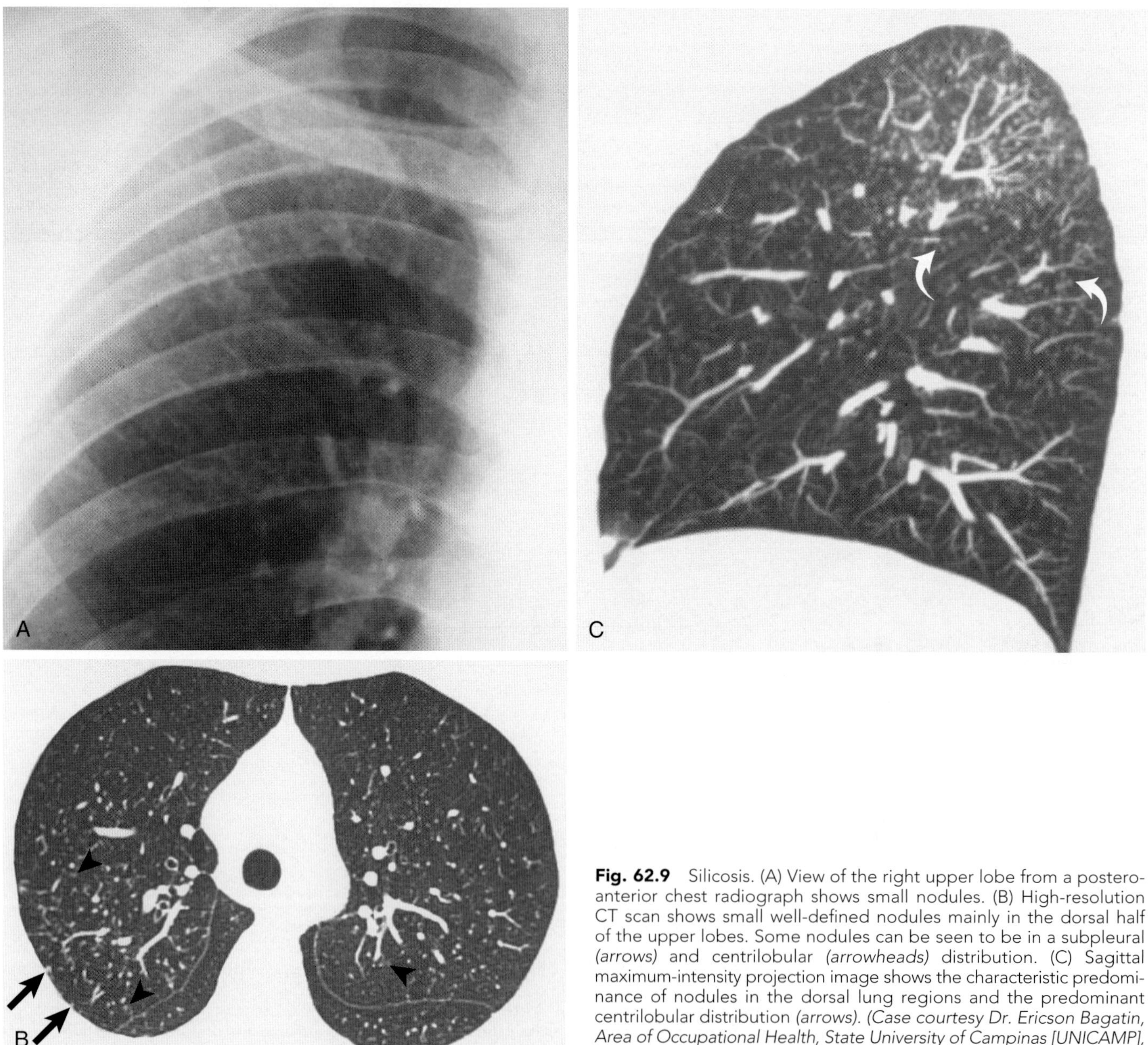

Fig. 62.9 Silicosis. (A) View of the right upper lobe from a posteroanterior chest radiograph shows small nodules. (B) High-resolution CT scan shows small well-defined nodules mainly in the dorsal half of the upper lobes. Some nodules can be seen to be in a subpleural *(arrows)* and centrilobular *(arrowheads)* distribution. (C) Sagittal maximum-intensity projection image shows the characteristic predominance of nodules in the dorsal lung regions and the predominant centrilobular distribution *(arrows)*. *(Case courtesy Dr. Ericson Bagatin, Area of Occupational Health, State University of Campinas [UNICAMP], Campinas, São Paulo, Brazil.)*

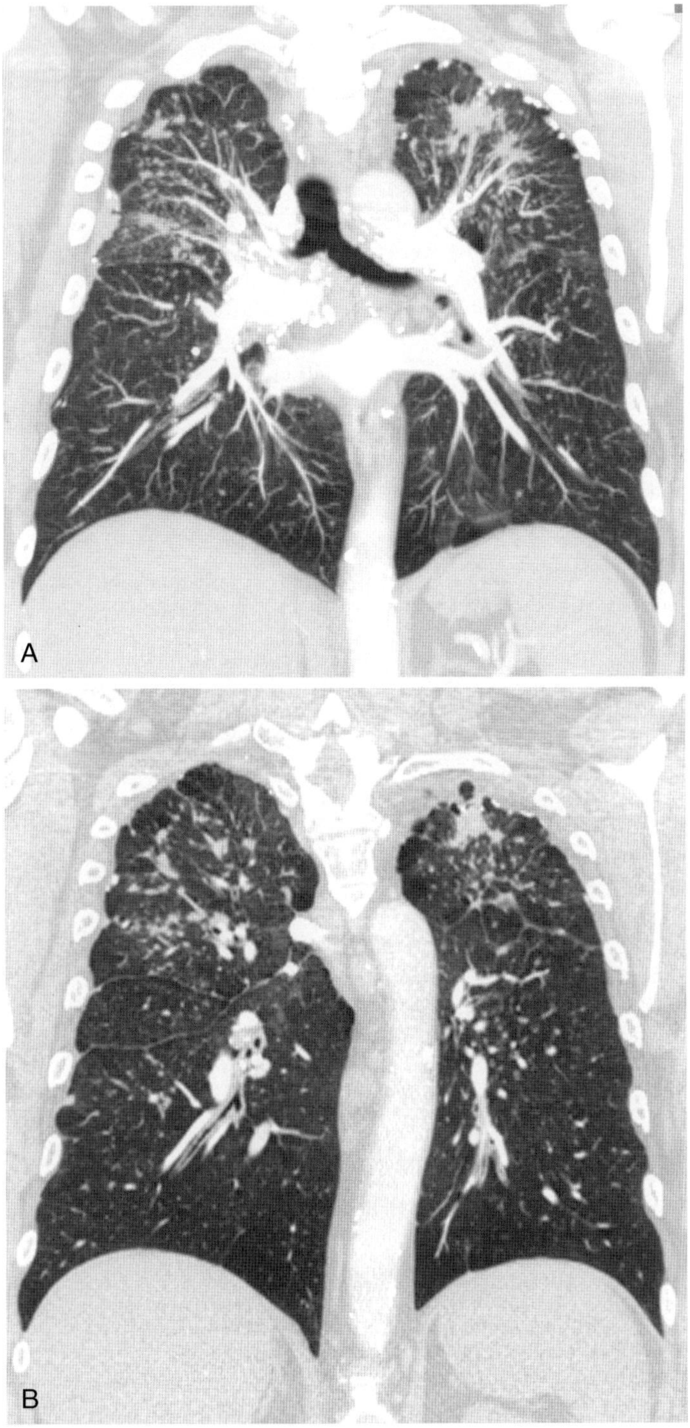

Fig. 62.10 Coal workers' pneumoconiosis. CT findings. (A) Coronal maximum-intensity projection (MIP) image shows small nodules in both lungs. Subpleural nodules mimicking pleural plaques are evident posteriorly. (B) On coronal CT scan the nodules are more difficult to distinguish from vessels and are often easier to detect with MIP reconstructions. The nodular and branching opacities have a centrilobular distribution. The subpleural pseudoplaques are defined better on the CT image.

localized thickening of visceral pleura as a result of fibrosis. Pseudoplaques, which are said to resemble asbestos-related pleural plaques, form when these subpleural nodules coalesce into linear areas of increased attenuation.[121]

Conglomerate masses or PMF appears as mass-like consolidation, usually with irregular margins and associated with adjacent paracicatricial emphysema and lung parenchymal architectural distortion (Fig. 62.11; see Figs. 62.3 and 62.4). The PMF lesions usually are found in the apical and posterior segments of the upper and lower lobes. Cavitation of the PMF lesions occurs as a result of ischemic necrosis or tuberculous infection (Fig. 62.12). When present, calcification may be punctate, curvilinear, or massive[120] (see Fig. 62.11) and was reported in 72% of sandblasters in one study.[122] The smooth, sharply defined flattened lateral border of the PMF lesion adjacent to a zone of emphysematous lung (see Fig. 62.12) helps differentiate PMF from lung carcinoma, which is normally rounded and irregular.

Paracicatricial emphysema (see Fig. 62.11) has been observed to be more prominent in patients with silicosis compared with CWP.[123] There is still debate about whether centrilobular emphysema found in silicosis is due to silica dust, exposure to other dust, such as coal and asbestos, or concomitant smoking.[112,124,125] Some studies have reported that emphysema in silicosis occurs independently of smoking,[119,126,127] whereas other investigators believe that silicosis without PMF does not contribute to emphysema.[112,119,124,125,128]

Hilar and mediastinal lymph nodes are generally enlarged and may calcify, but calcification is more frequently seen in silicosis. In a study of silicosis, hyperdense lymph nodes were present in a third of lymph node stations, most frequently in the subcarinal region. The predominant type of calcification was the uniformly dense calcified lymph node (53.4%) (Fig. 62.13), followed by the speckled variety (26.4%). Central, eccentric, and eggshell calcification (see Fig. 62.8) were rare (4.3%, 7.7%, and 5.2%, respectively).[129]

HRCT appearances of silicoproteinosis has until recently been described only in occasional case reports that suggested findings similar to pulmonary alveolar proteinosis (see Fig. 62.6).[91] However, more recent studies have suggested that the crazy paving pattern is unusual for silicoproteinosis, with more frequent findings including dependent consolidation, often with areas of calcification (83% of patients in one study). The presence of centrilobular nodules is common as well, and patchy ground-glass opacities can be seen.[101,102]

On CT the rheumatoid pneumoconiotic nodules are well defined and may cavitate and calcify. It may be impossible, however, to distinguish silicotic-type nodules of rheumatoid pneumoconiosis from other silicotic nodules.

MAGNETIC RESONANCE IMAGING

The applications of magnetic resonance imaging (MRI) in pneumoconiosis have not been extensively evaluated with studies producing variable results for PMF lesion characterization on T1-weighted, T2-weighted, and contrast-enhanced MRI.[130,131] The difference in signal characteristics, particularly on T1-weighted images, may be attributable to the variable amount of mineral dusts, such as coal, silica, and others, in PMF of CWP, which produce shortening of T1 relaxation of protons, hence the high signal on T1-weighted images found in PMF lesions in CWP.

MRI features of lung cancer occurring in a patient with PMF[132] have been described as a high–signal intensity area separate from the fibrotic mass, which appeared as a low–signal intensity area, on T1-weighted and T2-weighted images. MRI, especially with gadolinium enhancement, may be potentially useful in differentiating lung cancer from the fibrous tissue in the PMF lesions. Other uses of MRI include MR angiography and MRI perfusion of the

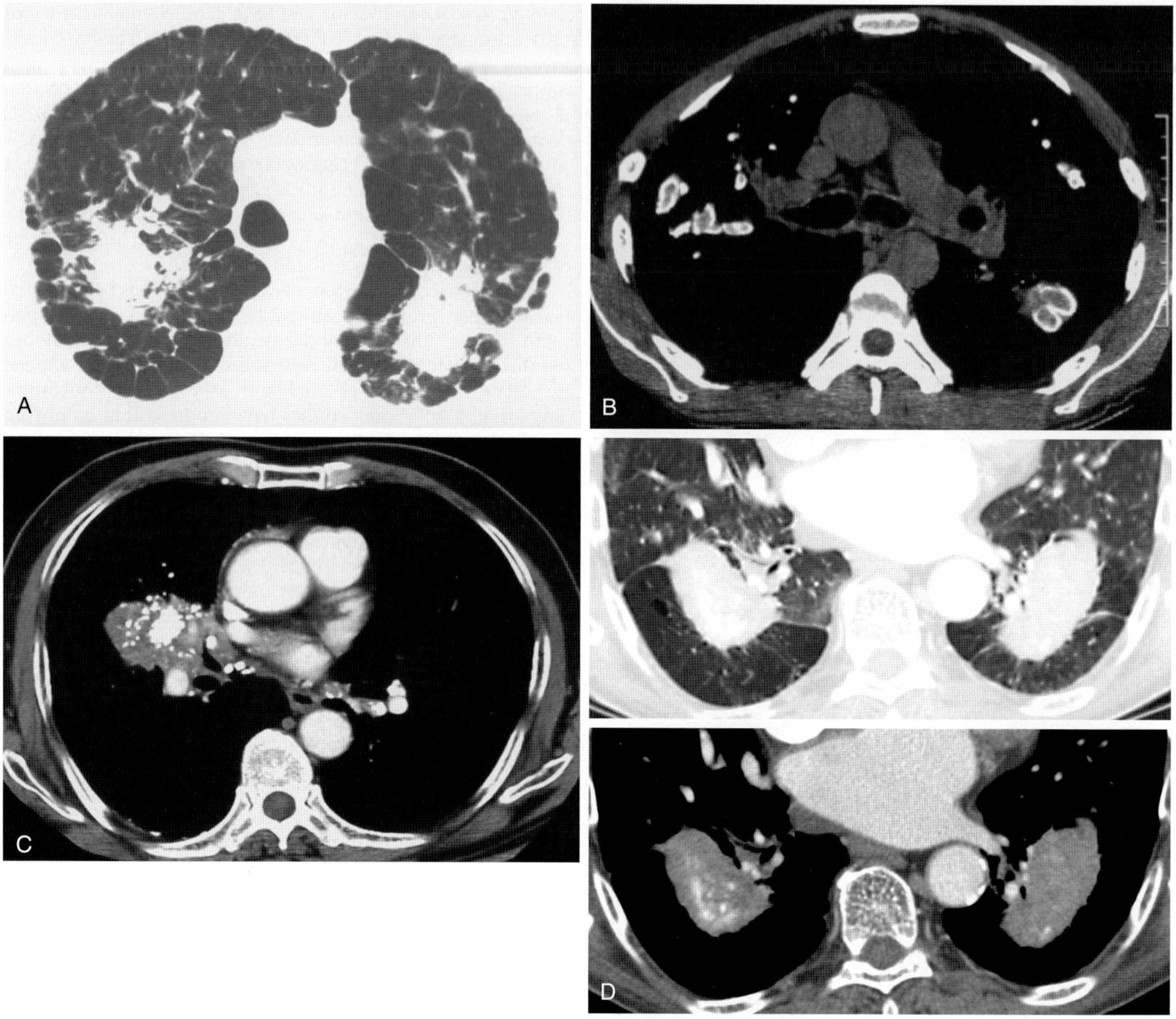

Fig. 62.11 CT scans showing examples of progressive massive fibrosis (PMF). (A) High-resolution CT scan showing masses in the upper lobes with paracicatricial emphysema and well-defined small centrilobular nodules. (B) Axial CT scan through the upper lobes in another patient with complicated silicosis showing curvilinear calcification of PMF lesions. (C) Axial contrast-enhanced CT scan through the right middle lobe of a patient with unilateral PMF with punctate and nodular calcification. Also noted are calcified bilateral hilar lymph nodes. (D) Composite image with axial CT scan in lung window *(top image)* and soft tissue window *(bottom image)* shows bilateral masses that cross the major fissures and contain calcifications. There is paracicatricial emphysema surrounding the masses.

lung to image complications of silicosis that involve the central vessels, such as pulmonary artery stenosis.[133]

POSITRON EMISSION TOMOGRAPHY/ COMPUTED TOMOGRAPHY

The utility of PET-CT in silicosis has not been thoroughly investigated, but increased uptake has been described in PMF lesions and in enlarged mediastinal and hilar lymph nodes (Fig. 62.14).[134,135] In the clinical setting of concomitant lung cancer arising in a silicosis patient, this may cause diagnostic problems resulting in false-positive results. Increased uptake in silicotic mediastinal lymph nodes has been reported in a patient with established lung cancer, with false upgrading of tumor stage.[136] However, the masses that are atypical for PMF, history of high-risk malignancy elsewhere, or a change in clinical status should prompt consideration for biopsy of metabolically active lesions.[137]

IMAGING ALGORITHMS

The chest radiograph provides a quick and easy method of diagnosing silicosis and CWP and should be performed first. The chest radiograph is insensitive, however, in the detection of early silicosis or CWP, subtle conglomeration of nodules, and subtle emphysema. In these circumstances a thin-section CT scan of the thorax should be performed with MIP reconstructions.

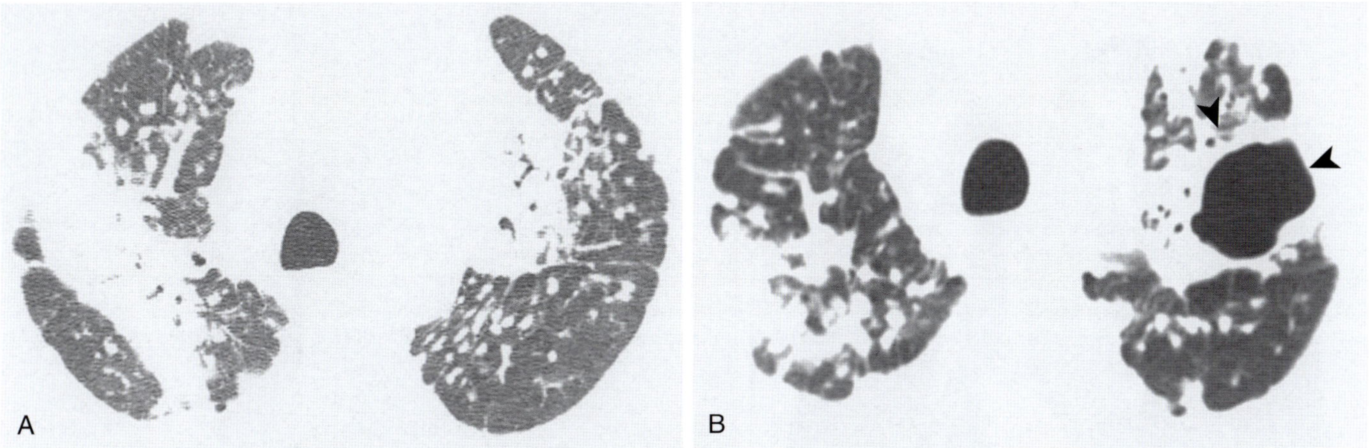

Fig. 62.12 Silicotuberculosis in a patient with complicated silicosis. (A) High-resolution CT (HRCT) scan through the upper lobes shows bilateral lung masses compatible with progressive massive fibrosis amid small silicotic nodules. (B) Follow-up HRCT scan in lung window shows cavitation *(arrowheads)* within the left progressive massive fibrosis lesion. A cavitary nodule in a patient with known silicosis should be considered tuberculosis until proven otherwise.

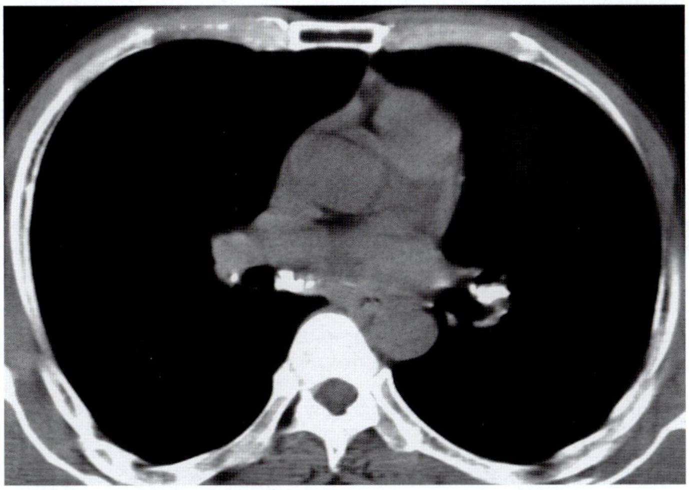

Fig. 62.13 Dense nodal calcification in silicosis. CT scan shows densely calcified lymph nodes.

MRI, particularly with gadolinium enhancement, may be potentially useful in differentiating lung cancer from fibrous tissue in PMF lesions on a case-specific basis. MR angiography and MRI perfusion of the lung are other MRI techniques that may be used to image complications, such as pulmonary artery stenosis.

The clinical utility of PET-CT in silicosis and CWP is limited and, like MRI, should only be used in select patients, including cases with suspected lung cancer.

Differential Diagnosis

Differential diagnostic findings on chest radiograph and CT are as follows:

Differential diagnoses for bilateral hilar and mediastinal lymphadenopathy include
- Primary tuberculosis
- Sarcoidosis
- Fungal infections such as histoplasmosis and coccidioidomycosis
- Lymphoma
- Metastatic nodal disease

Differential diagnoses for multiple lung nodules include
- Sarcoidosis
- Fungal infections
- Miliary tuberculosis
- Simple silicosis
- Simple coal workers' pneumoconiosis (CWP)
- Mixed dust pneumoconiosis

Differential diagnoses for progressive massive fibrosis include
- Complicated silicosis
- Complicated CWP
- Sarcoidosis
- Talcosis

Differential diagnoses for acute silicoproteinosis include
- Alveolar proteinosis
- Pulmonary edema
- Acute interstitial pneumonia
- Lipoid pneumonia
- Infections including *Pneumocystis*

CLASSIC SIGNS

SILICOSIS

- Well-defined centrilobular and subpleural nodules (perilymphatic pattern)
- Diffuse distribution with posterior and upper lung zone predominance
- Progressive massive fibrosis found at the apical and posterior segments of the upper lobes and superior segment of the lower lobes
- Hilar and mediastinal lymph node enlargement
- Calcification of nodes common on CT (50%)

COAL WORKERS' PNEUMOCONIOSIS

- Small nodular opacities
- Ill-defined margins
- Perilymphatic distribution with upper lung zone predominance
- Calcification of nodules is less common than in silicosis
- Mediastinal and hilar lymph node enlargement
- Subpleural nodules adjacent to visceral pleura (pseudoplaques)

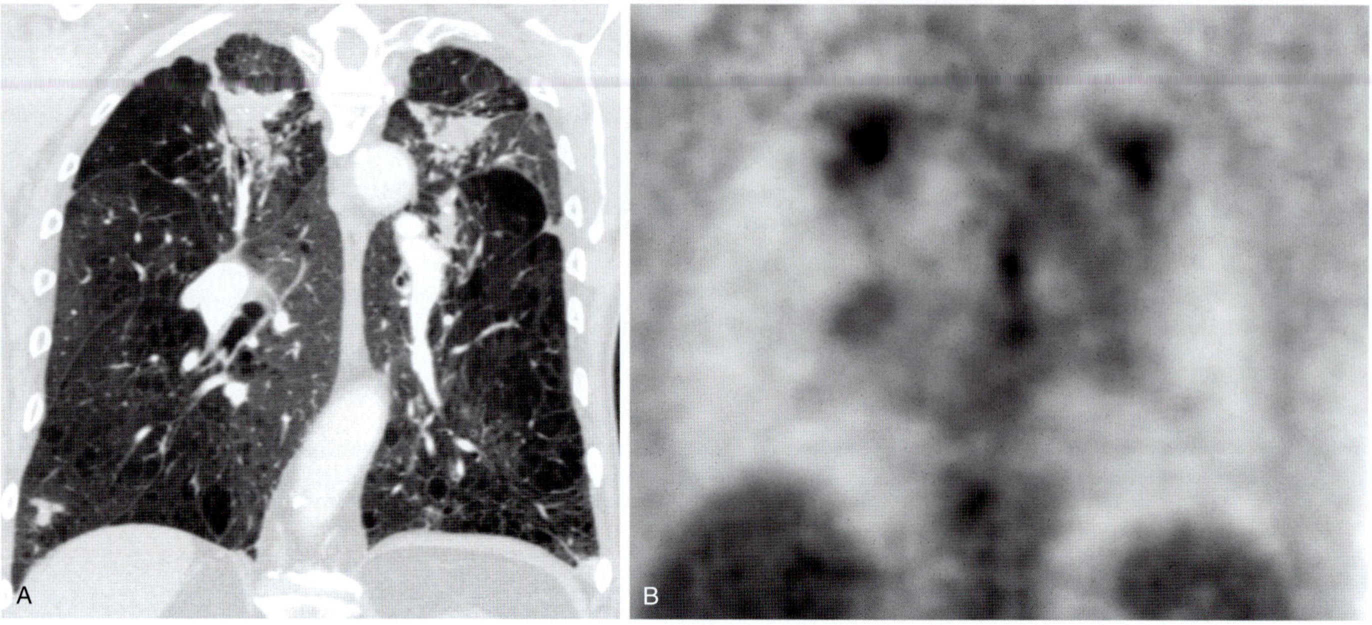

Fig. 62.14 Complicated silicosis with increased uptake on positron emission tomography–computed tomography (PET-CT). (A) Coronal CT scan shows bilateral progressive massive fibrosis (PMF) lesions with extensive emphysema and a few silicotic nodules around the PMF lesions. (B) Coronal fluorodeoxyglucose-PET image shows increased uptake in both upper lobe PMF lesions. The uptake in the upper lobe lesions is indistinguishable from that of lung cancer.

KEY POINTS

- Silicosis and coal workers' pneumoconiosis (CWP) are occupational lung diseases caused by continual exposure to silica and coal dust.
- Radiologic manifestations include diffuse perilymphatic nodules (centrilobular and subpleural nodules), which may calcify and may coalesce into large masses (Progressive massive fibrosis or PMF).
- Emphysema is usually due to cigarette smoking, but it may be seen in occupational dust inhalational exposure, even in nonsmokers.
- Lung function impairment is related to the degree of nodulation, PMF, and emphysema.
- Complications of silicosis and CWP include connective tissue disease, Caplan syndrome, lung carcinoma, pulmonary hypertension, right heart failure, tuberculosis, and peripheral vascular disease.
- The chest radiograph is the foremost imaging modality used in the initial evaluation and follow-up of patients with suspected or proven silicosis or CWP.
- CT is superior to chest radiography in detecting early silicosis and CWP, emphysema, and conglomeration of nodules (early PMF).
- CT is helpful in the assessment of patients with silicosis or CWP and suspected pulmonary complications, such as tuberculosis or pulmonary carcinoma.
- Positron emission tomography–CT may show false-positive fluorodeoxyglucose uptake in patients with PMF without malignancy.

SUGGESTED READINGS

Chong S, Lee KS, Chung MJ, et al. Pneumoconiosis: comparison of imaging and pathologic findings. *Radiographics*. 2006;26:59–77.

Cox CW, et al. State of the art: imaging of occupational lung disease. *Radiology*. 2014;270(3):681–696.

Fujimura N. Pathology and pathophysiology of pneumoconiosis. *Curr Opin Pulm Med*. 2000;6:140–144.

International Labour Office. *Guidelines for the Use of ILO International Classification of Radiographs of Pneumoconiosis. Occupational Safety and Health Series No. 22*. Geneva: International Labour Office; 2011.

The full reference list for this chapter is available at ExpertConsult.com.

63 Uncommon Pneumoconioses*

STEPHEN B. HOBBS

The most common pneumoconioses are silicosis, coal workers' pneumoconiosis, and asbestosis (see Chapters 61 and 62). There are numerous rare pneumoconioses related to variable occupational dust exposures. Hard metal lung disease, aluminum pneumoconiosis, talc pneumoconiosis, welders' pneumoconiosis, and chronic beryllium disease are discussed here. The high-resolution computed tomography (HRCT) findings of these uncommon pneumoconioses vary and are relatively nonspecific; however, there are predominant and characteristic findings for each type of pneumoconiosis. The most common HRCT finding of pneumoconiosis consists of centrilobular nodular and branching linear opacities, consistent with a bronchiolocentric process. Interstitial fibrosis may be manifested as reticulation, traction bronchiectasis, honeycombing, or more confluent areas of high attenuation. Similar to the other pneumoconiosis, HRCT has higher sensitivity and specificity than chest radiography in evaluating pleuroparenchymal abnormalities and is often helpful in detecting the early parenchymal changes in each type of pneumoconiosis.

Hard Metal Lung Disease

ETIOLOGY, PREVALENCE, AND EPIDEMIOLOGY

Hard metal is an alloy of tungsten carbide in a matrix of cobalt to which small amounts of titanium, nickel, chromium, niobium, vanadium, or molybdenum may be added. Hard metal is heat resistant and is as indestructible as diamond. Hard metal lung disease is a rare form of occupational lung disease that can occur in workers engaged in the manufacture, use, or maintenance of tools composed of hard metal. Cobalt is generally considered the main cause of hard metal lung disease, hence also the term *cobalt lung*.[1] Some experimental studies have shown that biological reactivity to a mixture of cobalt and tungsten carbide is much greater than that to cobalt alone.[2] Hard metal lung disease is more likely to occur in poorly regulated workplaces, but because its low prevalence in exposed workers and/or the lack of correlation with the intensity or duration of exposure, the existence of a possible genetic susceptibility to hard metal disease has been suggested.[3–5]

CLINICAL PRESENTATION

Exposure to hard metal may result in three main respiratory complications: asthma, hypersensitivity pneumonitis, and/or pulmonary fibrosis. Hard metal workers occasionally develop symptoms of asthma that are similar in their clinical manifestations to other forms of occupational asthma. The typical symptoms of cough, wheeze, dyspnea, chest tightness, and rhinitis occur after approximately 4 to 6 hours at the workplace. The clinical manifestations of hypersensitivity pneumonitis resulting from cobalt are similar to the manifestations observed in other forms of hypersensitivity pneumonitis. In the more insidious forms of hard metal disease, the symptoms are those of any other fibrotic lung diseases, with cough, gradual shortness of breath, and weight loss. Cyanosis and finger clubbing are present in the more advanced stages of the disease.[1,6] The disease can be fatal and sometimes rapidly progressive.[7]

PATHOLOGIC FINDINGS

The general and nonspecific pathologic features of hard metal interstitial lung disease include infiltration of the interstitium with lymphocytes and plasma cells, hyperplasia of the alveolar epithelium, and occasionally cellular accumulation within the alveolar lumen (desquamative interstitial pneumonia). The lesions are bronchiolocentric, and the distribution is patchy. There are occasional descriptions of granulomas in the lungs of hard metal workers with interstitial lung disease.

The most characteristic finding in hard metal lung disease is the presence of multinucleated giant cells in the interstitium and alveolar airspaces (Fig. 63.1). These cells may contain large numbers of nuclei and have been described as "bizarre" or "cannibalistic" on account of the presence of inclusions, which contain apparently phagocytosed cellular material (giant cell interstitial pneumonia).[1,6]

IMAGING FINDINGS

Radiography

The most common radiographic abnormality consists of small irregular opacities, predominantly in the middle and lower lung zones (Figs. 63.2 and 63.3; see Fig. 63.1). Other findings include small nodular opacities and diffuse reticulonodular or ground-glass opacities, particularly in subacute presentations. The chest radiograph may appear normal despite the presence of symptoms and functional impairment. During attacks of hard metal lung disease, a fine diffuse reticulonodular pattern can be seen.

Computed Tomography

The HRCT appearance of hard metal interstitial lung disease varies and may mimic sarcoidosis,[8] nonspecific interstitial pneumonia (NSIP),[9,10] or usual interstitial pneumonia (UIP).[11]

The findings of panlobular and multilobular ground-glass opacities or consolidation correspond histopathologically to areas of interstitial thickening caused by inflammatory cell infiltration and intraalveolar accumulation of macrophages and multinucleated giant cells. The findings of parenchymal distortion, traction

*The editors and the publisher would like to thank Dr. Masanori Akira for contributing material on this topic to the prior edition of this work. It has served as the foundation for the current chapter.

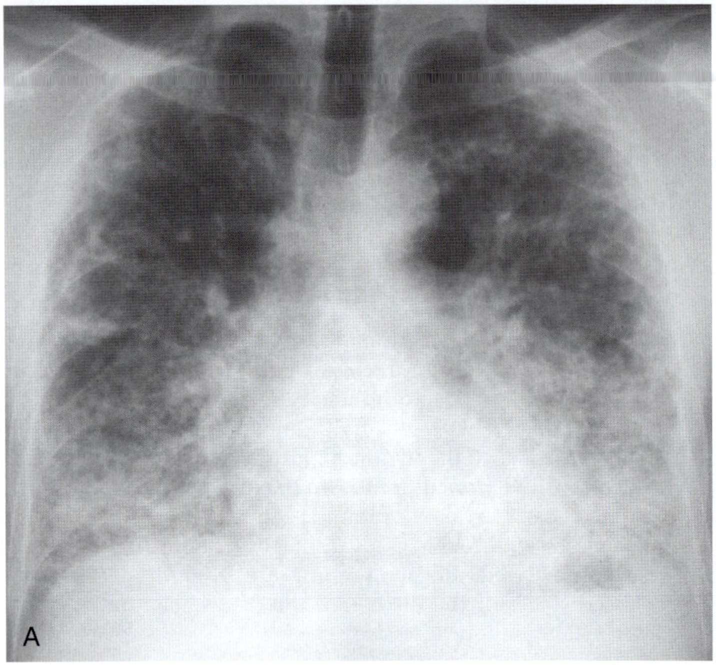

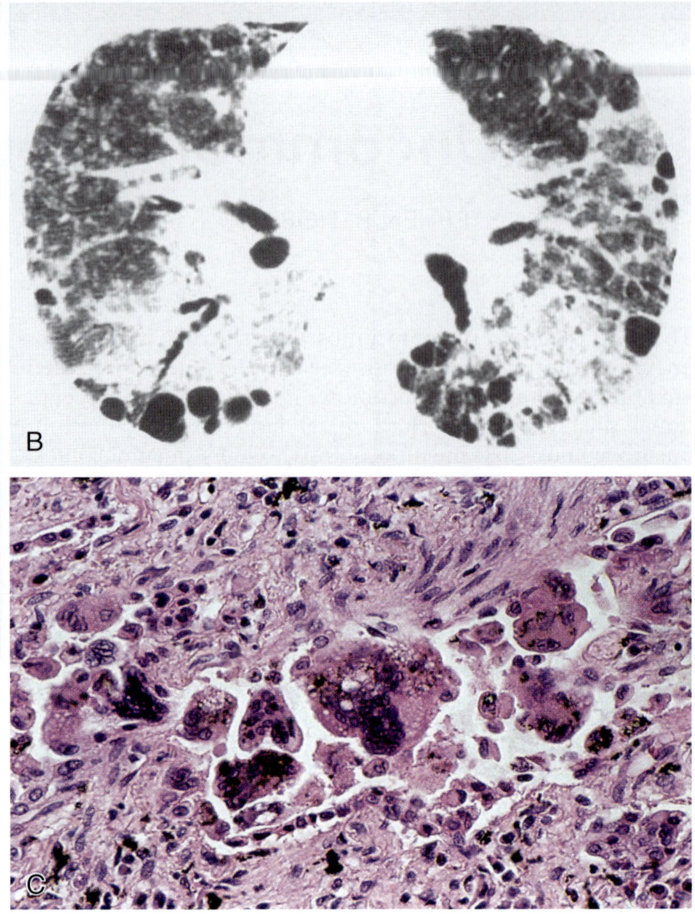

Fig. 63.1 Hard metal interstitial lung disease. (A) Posteroanterior chest radiograph reveals coarse reticular pattern and patchy ground-glass opacities involving predominantly the peripheral lung regions and lower lung zones. (B) High-resolution CT scan shows extensive bilateral ground-glass opacities, foci of consolidation, centrilobular nodules, mild reticulation, traction bronchiectasis, and several bullae. (C) Histologic specimen of the lung obtained at autopsy shows bizarre multinucleated giant cells along with interstitial inflammation and fibrosis in the alveolar airspaces.

bronchiectasis, and reticulation correspond histopathologically to areas of diffuse interstitial fibrosis and fibrosis around bronchovascular structures.[12] Depending on the severity of the giant cell interstitial pneumonia, the findings may range from ground-glass opacities to dense consolidation (see Figs. 63.1, 63.2, and 63.3). In a fatal case of hard metal disease, which was characterized by a large amount of intraalveolar accumulation of macrophages and multinucleated giant cells within a few years of initial exposure, consolidation with lobular distribution was found.[13]

Imaging Algorithm

Chest radiography is the imaging modality used in the initial assessment and follow-up of patients with hard metal lung disease. Further evaluation of the lung parenchyma can be obtained with CT. HRCT may be useful in detecting the early parenchymal changes in these patients.

DIFFERENTIAL DIAGNOSIS

The differential diagnosis includes all other types of interstitial pneumonias, drug-induced lung disease, sarcoidosis and other granulomatous lung disease that mimics sarcoidosis, hypersensitivity pneumonitis, and other pneumoconioses. As with any occupational disease, the cornerstone of the diagnosis is a comprehensive and detailed work history. Tungsten particles usually can be shown by energy-dispersive x-ray spectroscopy, and their presence confirms the diagnosis because tungsten is never identified as a background atmospheric contaminant in the general population. Particles of cobalt also may be found, but they are less common because cobalt is soluble in tissue fluid.[14] A pathologic diagnosis of giant cell interstitial pneumonia is pathognomonic for hard metal lung disease. The presence of multinucleated cannibalistic giant cells in bronchoalveolar lavage (BAL) fluid also is diagnostic for hard metal lung disease, even without a surgical lung biopsy specimen.[1] Concentrations of cobalt in the blood and urine may correlate well with levels of exposure, when measured within a few days after exposure.[6]

SYNOPSIS OF TREATMENT OPTIONS

Asthmatic symptoms and hypersensitivity pneumonitis usually can be easily controlled by eliminating exposure and appropriately treating the hypersensitivity reaction. In hard metal interstitial lung disease, the progression of the disease depends on the time of diagnosis and the continuation of the exposure. Apart from exposure cessation, no medical treatment has proven to be beneficial. In the early stage of disease, improvement and even complete remission may be obtained if the exposure ceases completely. The use of corticosteroids or cyclophosphamide has been reported; however, no controlled studies are available regarding the treatment of hard metal interstitial lung disease.[1,6,15] Lung transplantation has been performed in patients with hard metal lung disease, and recurrence was observed in the transplanted lung.[16]

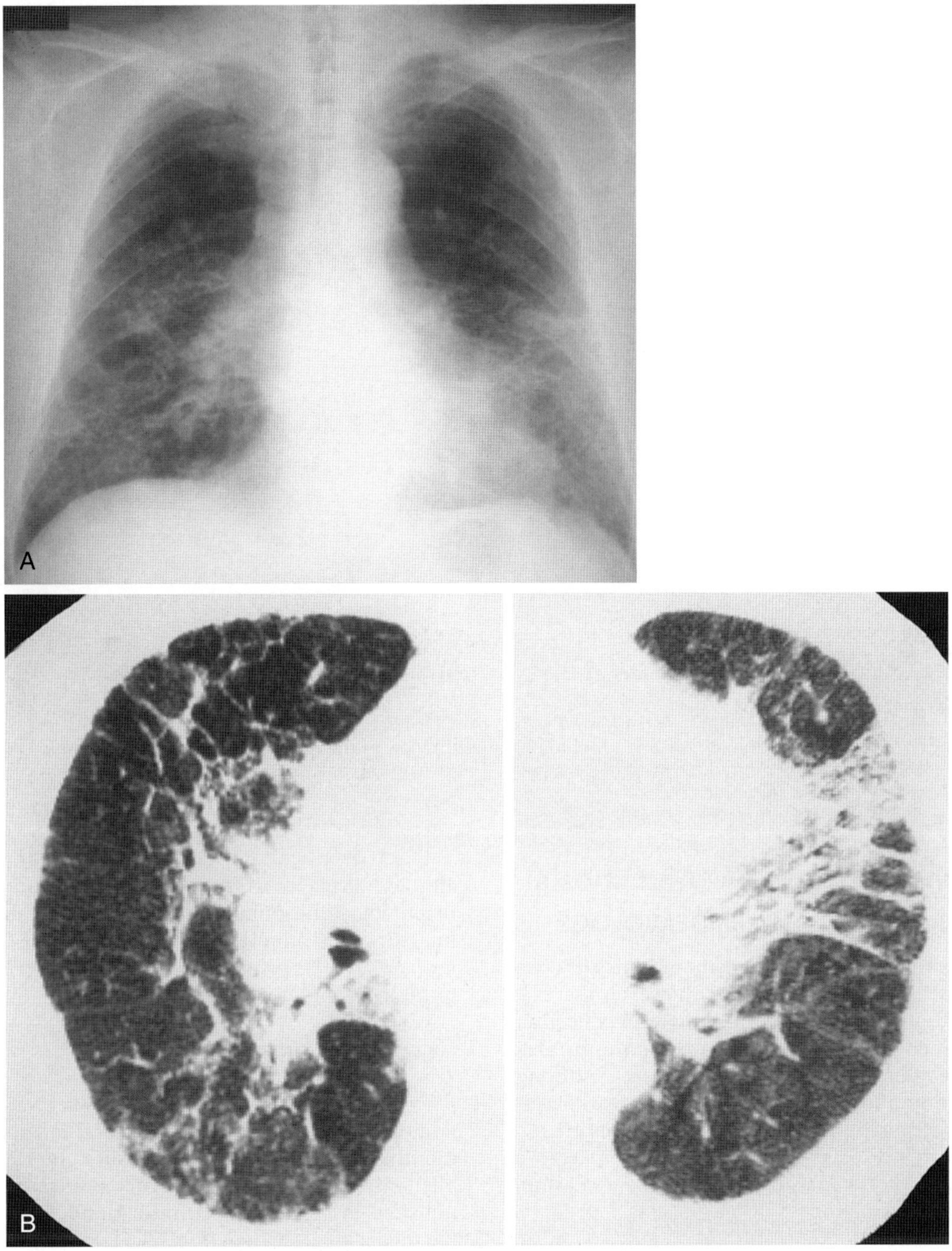

Fig. 63.2 Hard metal interstitial lung disease. (A) Chest radiograph shows reticulonodular pattern in the middle and lower lung zones. (B) High-resolution CT scan shows ground-glass opacities, areas of consolidation, mild reticulation, and traction bronchiectasis.

KEY POINTS: HARD METAL LUNG DISEASE

- Cobalt is the main cause of hard metal lung disease.
- Three main respiratory effects are asthmatic reactions, hypersensitivity pneumonitis, and pulmonary fibrosis.
- The most characteristic pathologic finding is the presence of "bizarre" or "cannibalistic" multinucleated giant cells, which are often also present in bronchoalveolar lavage fluid.
- Common radiologic findings include the following:
    - Panlobular and multilobular ground-glass opacities or consolidation corresponding histopathologically to areas of intraalveolar accumulation of macrophages and multinucleated giant cells
    - Parenchymal distortion, traction bronchiectasis, and reticulation corresponding histopathologically to areas of interstitial fibrosis

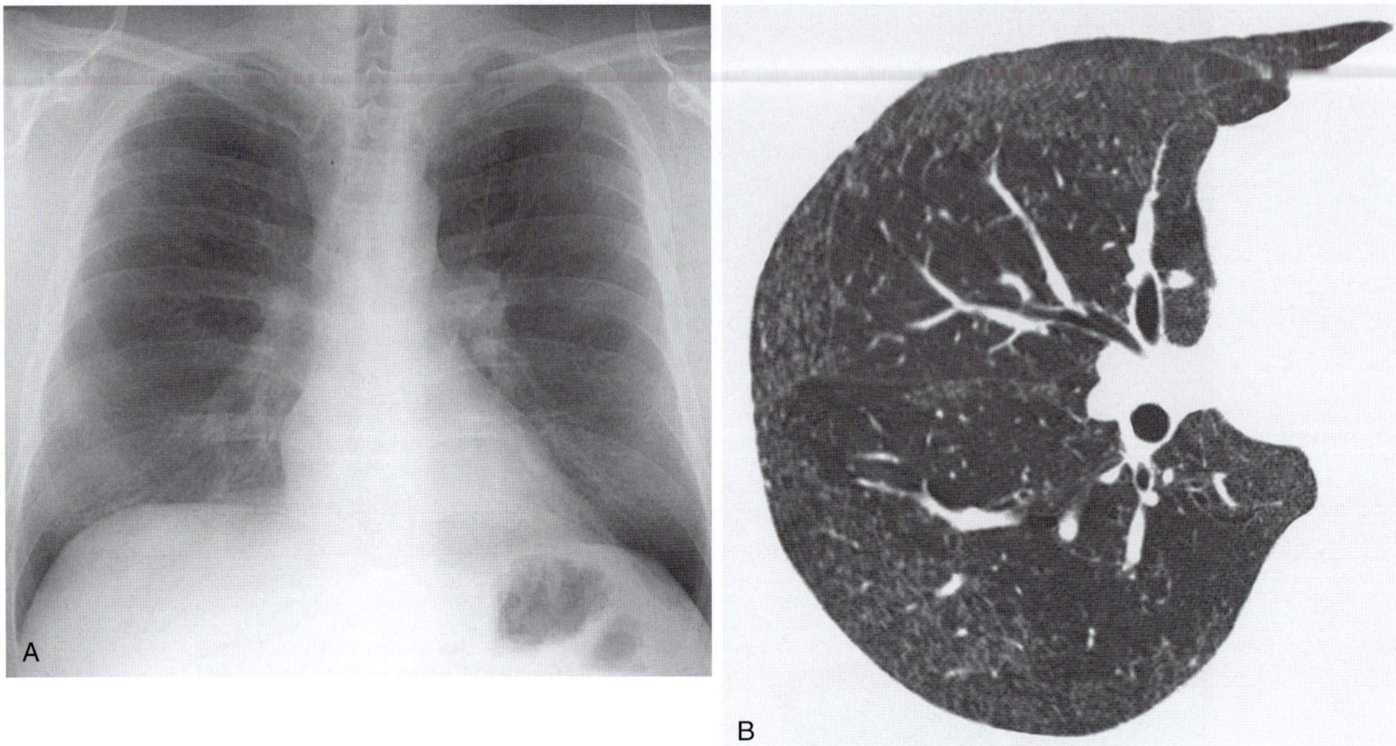

Fig. 63.3 Hard metal interstitial lung disease. (A) Chest radiograph shows hazy opacity and fine nodular pattern in the middle and lower lung zones. (B) View of the right lung from a high-resolution CT scan reveals fine nodular opacities in the peripheral lung regions.

Aluminum Pneumoconiosis (Aluminosis)

ETIOLOGY, PREVALENCE, AND EPIDEMIOLOGY

Exposure to aluminum, alumina, and potroom fumes has been associated with diffuse interstitial fibrosis; however, the exact etiologic agent of aluminum-induced fibrosis is uncertain. Stearin-coated, mineral oil–coated, and bare aluminum metal all may be equally effective in producing fibrosis.[17] Although exposure to aluminum metal and its oxides in the workplace is common, pneumoconioses attributable to these agents are rare, ranging from 1% to 8% of exposed employees.[18,19] Work in aluminum smelters is associated with the development of asthma and chronic airflow obstruction.

CLINICAL PRESENTATION

Clinical symptoms in patients with pulmonary fibrosis usually consist of cough and dyspnea on exertion. Pulmonary function test results are consistent with a restrictive disease process with reduced lung volumes and decreased diffusing capacity of lung for carbon monoxide.[20]

PATHOLOGIC FINDINGS

Histologic examination of lung tissue samples shows subpleural and interstitial fibrosis with scar emphysema and spotted granulomatous pneumonitis with giant cells (Fig. 63.4). Energy-dispersed x-ray analysis shows high interstitial concentrations of aluminum.[17] Diffuse interstitial fibrosis attributable to aluminum exposure is usually most severe in the upper lung zones, although it may be diffuse. Such a distribution is distinct from that of idiopathic pulmonary fibrosis or asbestosis. Desquamative interstitial pneumonia, granulomatous lung reaction, and pulmonary alveolar proteinosis have been described after exposure to fumes from aluminum welding.[21]

IMAGING FINDINGS

Radiography

Radiographic abnormalities may become apparent after a few months or several years of exposure. Typical findings include bilateral hazy opacities or small nodular opacities more pronounced in the upper or middle lung zones and widening of the mediastinal shadow (Fig. 63.5). Emphysematous changes in the basal lung and displacement of the hila upward or backward, indicating pulmonary contracture, characterize advanced cases.[22,23] The reticulation and honeycombing sometimes may be diffuse (see Fig. 63.4).[18] Aluminum-associated pulmonary fibrosis is associated with a high frequency of secondary spontaneous pneumothorax.[22]

Computed Tomography

HRCT findings of aluminum pneumoconiosis vary and may mimic silicosis, sarcoidosis, respiratory bronchiolitis, and hypersensitivity pneumonitis. Less commonly, findings are similar to NSIP and UIP. The findings include nodular opacities, reticulation, and upper lung fibrosis.[21] The nodular pattern consists either of well-defined nodules 2 to 5 mm in diameter, identical to those of silicosis, or of ill-defined centrilobular nodules diffusely distributed throughout both lungs, similar to those seen in hypersensitivity pneumonitis.

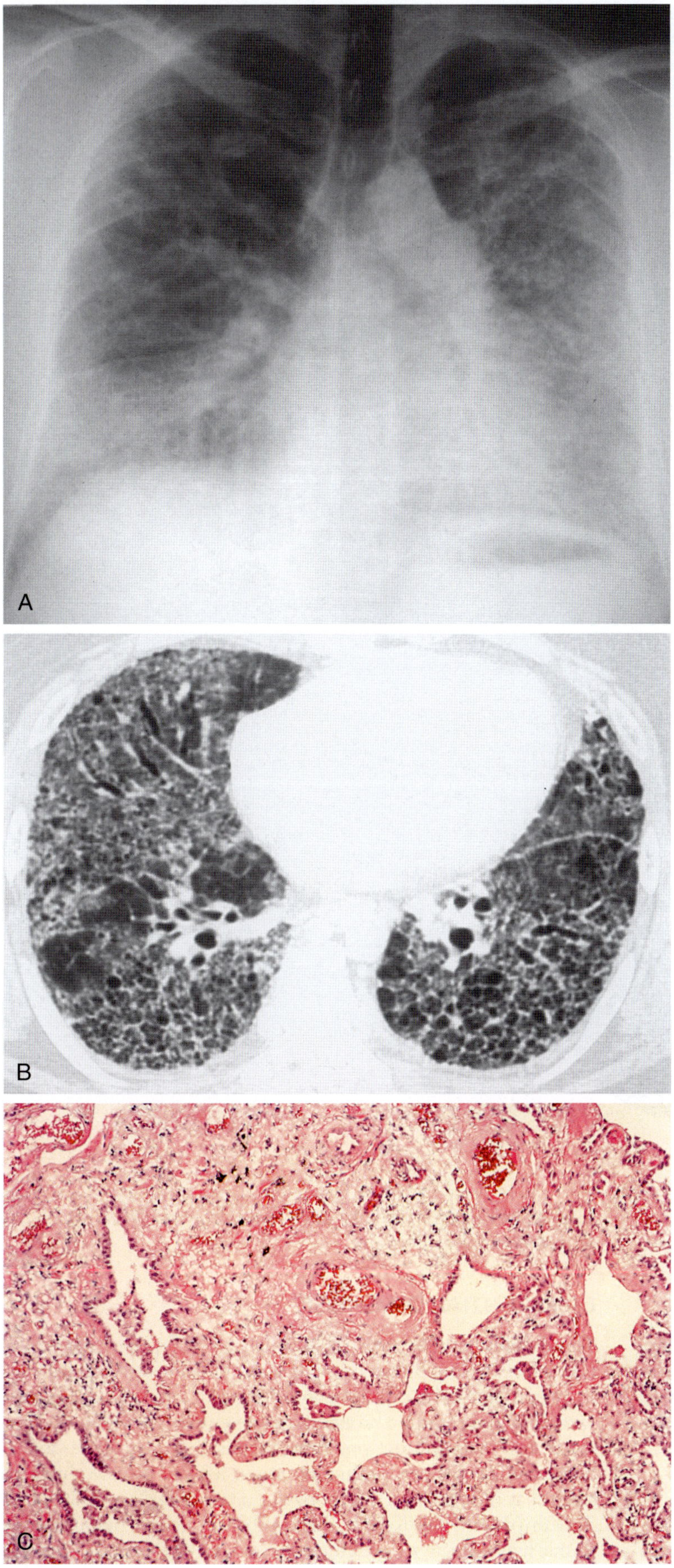

Fig. 63.4 Aluminum pneumoconiosis. (A) Chest radiograph shows extensive bilateral reticulonodular pattern. (B) High-resolution CT scan reveals extensive reticulation, traction bronchiectasis, traction bronchiolectasis, and honeycombing. (C) Histologic specimen of the lung obtained at surgical lung biopsy shows interstitial fibrosis with an interstitial mononuclear infiltrate.

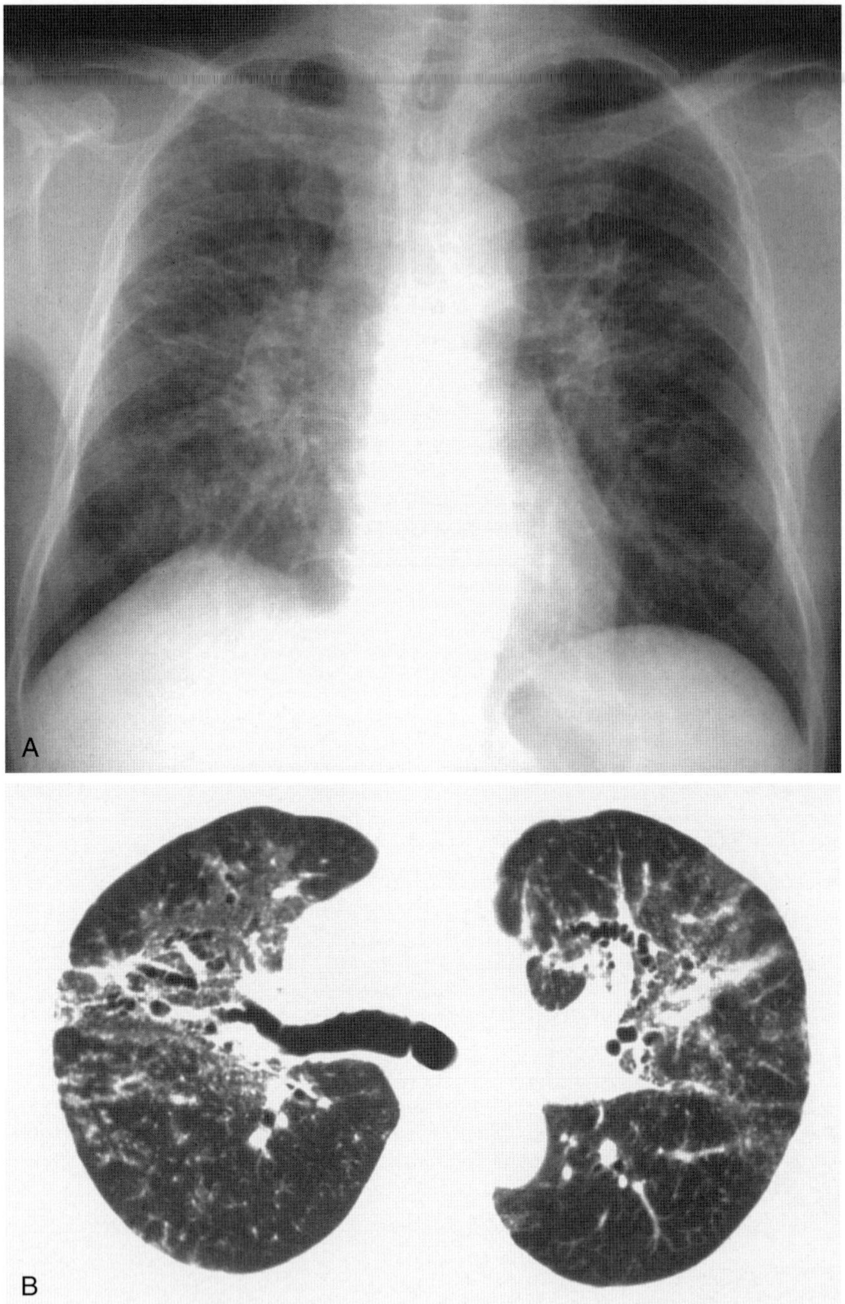

Fig. 63.5 Aluminum pneumoconiosis. (A) Chest radiograph shows ground-glass opacities mainly in the upper and middle lung zones. Mild upward displacement of the hila is also noted. (B) High-resolution CT scan shows ground-glass opacities mainly in the central lung regions, a few small nodular and irregular linear opacities, and traction bronchiectasis.

Aluminum pneumoconiosis in the early stages may be associated with normal chest radiographs and the presence of small, ill-defined, rounded centrilobular opacities mainly in the upper lobes.[17]

The presence of fibrosis results in a reticular pattern and honeycombing (see Fig. 63.4). The distribution is predominantly upper lung or diffuse, different from that of idiopathic pulmonary fibrosis. Ground-glass opacities also are seen, with or without traction bronchiectasis (see Fig. 63.5). A case with increased attenuation of mediastinal lymph nodes has been described, resulting from histologically proven aluminum storage.[24]

Imaging Algorithm

Chest radiography is the main imaging modality used in the initial assessment and follow-up of patients with aluminum pneumoconiosis. HRCT has higher sensitivity and specificity than chest radiography and may show abnormalities in patients with a normal radiograph.[17]

DIFFERENTIAL DIAGNOSIS

The differential diagnosis includes all other types of interstitial pneumonias, drug-induced lung disease, sarcoidosis, hypersensitivity pneumonitis, and other pneumoconioses. Ground-glass opacities with or without traction bronchiectasis resemble NSIP. Honeycombing is seen in aluminum pneumoconiosis, but the distribution of honeycombing is predominantly upper lung or diffuse, different from that of idiopathic pulmonary fibrosis. Small, rounded, and ill-defined centrilobular opacities in the early stages of aluminosis mimic hypersensitivity pneumonitis, coal workers' pneumoconiosis, silicosis,[25] or respiratory bronchiolitis. Large opacities with shrinkage in both upper lungs resemble silicosis or sarcoidosis. Biological monitoring of plasma and urine reveals higher exposure to aluminum in affected workers.

SYNOPSIS OF TREATMENT OPTIONS

The approach of choice is complete removal from exposure to the offending substance in the workplace. No medical treatment has proven beneficial. The prognosis for severe forms of lung fibrosis is poor because the disease can continue to progress after the end of exposure.

KEY POINTS: ALUMINUM PNEUMOCONIOSIS (ALUMINOSIS)

- Prevalence is less than 10% in individuals exposed at the workplace.
- Clinical symptoms include dyspnea on exertion, cough, and spontaneous pneumothorax.
- Common radiologic findings include the following:
  - Nodular, reticular, ground-glass opacities with or without traction bronchiectasis
  - Predominantly upper lung zones or diffuse
  - High-resolution CT findings in early stages: small, rounded, and ill-defined centrilobular opacities mainly in the upper lung zones

Talc Pneumoconiosis

ETIOLOGY, PREVALENCE, AND EPIDEMIOLOGY

Talc is a pure hydrous magnesium silicate with an ideal chemical composition of 63.5% silicon dioxide, 31.7% magnesium oxide, and 4.8% water, but in practice, substitutions of ions may occur in the mineral lattice or the talc may be contaminated by other minerals. Findings related to talc exposure can be separated into four principal categories: three forms by inhalation and one by intravenous (IV) administration. The first form is caused by talc mined with high–silica content mineral and is called *talcosilicosis.* Findings in this form are identical to the findings of silicosis. Talcoasbestosis, the second form, closely resembles asbestosis and is produced by crystalline talc, generally inhaled with asbestos fibers. The third form, pure talcosis, caused by inhalation of pure talc, may result in acute or chronic bronchitis, interstitial inflammation, or fibrosis. The fourth form, resulting from IV administration of talc, usually is associated with the IV use of crushed oral medications and production of vascular granulomas.[26,27] Pure talc also may cause acute onset of pulmonary symptoms when extremely large quantities are aspirated. Such exposure may be accidental and has been documented most often in infants who inhale cosmetic talc.[27] Talc is used to promote pleural adhesions in the treatment of spontaneous pneumothorax and recurrent pleural effusions. Pleural instillation of pure talc may result in pleural thickening and fibrosis and may cause significant pulmonary disease if the talc enters the lung.[27] Overall rates of talc-related pneumoconiosis in exposed populations ranges from 10% to 27%.[28,29]

CLINICAL PRESENTATION

The predominant symptoms are dyspnea and cough. Cyanosis and finger clubbing are seen in advanced cases. Cough is either dry or productive of only small amounts of tenacious mucus.

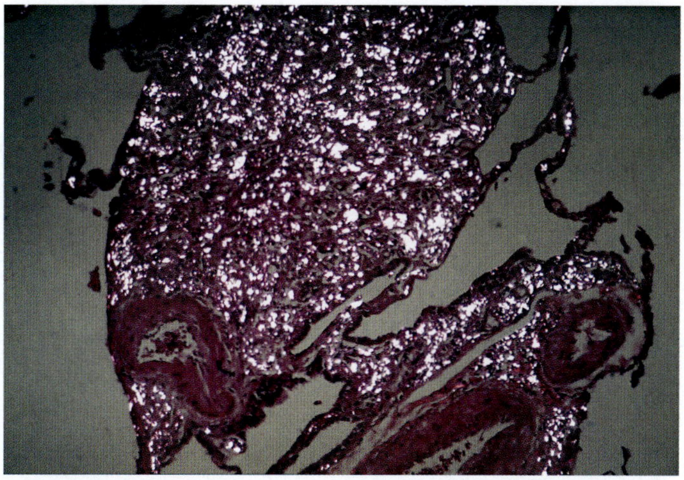

Fig. 63.6 Talc pneumoconiosis. Photomicrograph of an autopsied lung specimen examined under polarized light shows strongly birefringent dust particles.

Clinically, talc pneumoconiosis is initially symptom free, but as it progresses, it may resemble a mild form of asbestosis, and it is accompanied by a reduction in lung volumes and diffusing capacity.[30] Progressive disease can occur in the absence of continued exposure, leading to progressive dyspnea, weight loss from labored breathing and hypoxia, and cor pulmonale with eventual right-sided heart failure.

PATHOLOGIC FINDINGS

The pathologic findings in talc pneumoconiosis include diffuse interstitial fibrosis, ill-defined fibrotic nodules, and foreign-body granulomas associated with dense accumulations of birefringent talc dust particles (Fig. 63.6).[31] Pulmonary diseases caused by inhalation of talc dust result in different histologic findings from intravenously administered talc in IV drug users. When the lesions are located in the lumen or wall of the blood vessel, or there is evidence of marked pulmonary arterial hypertension in association with the presence of foreign material, the evidence for vascular origin is strong.[32] In advanced stages talcosis in IV drug users results in large perihilar conglomerated masses that contain large numbers of particles, giant cells, and extensive fibrosis and that resemble the massive fibrosis seen in inhalational talcosis, sarcoidosis, or silicosis.

IMAGING FINDINGS

Radiography

The various types of talc can produce several distinctive radiographic appearances: nodular, linear, and conglomerate fibrosis. The nodular pattern consists of opacities 3 to 5 mm in diameter, identical to those of silicosis. These changes sometimes favor the middle lung zones but may be distributed throughout all zones (Fig. 63.7). Conglomeration of nodules may result in large opacities similar to those of silicotic conglomerations or coal workers' progressive massive fibrosis, which may show evidence of cavity formation.[33]

A diffuse linear interstitial pattern also may occur that resembles the findings in asbestosis. Bilateral pleural plaques in the lateral parts of the lower thorax and diaphragmatic plaques with calcification are sometimes seen. Pure talc, when it causes

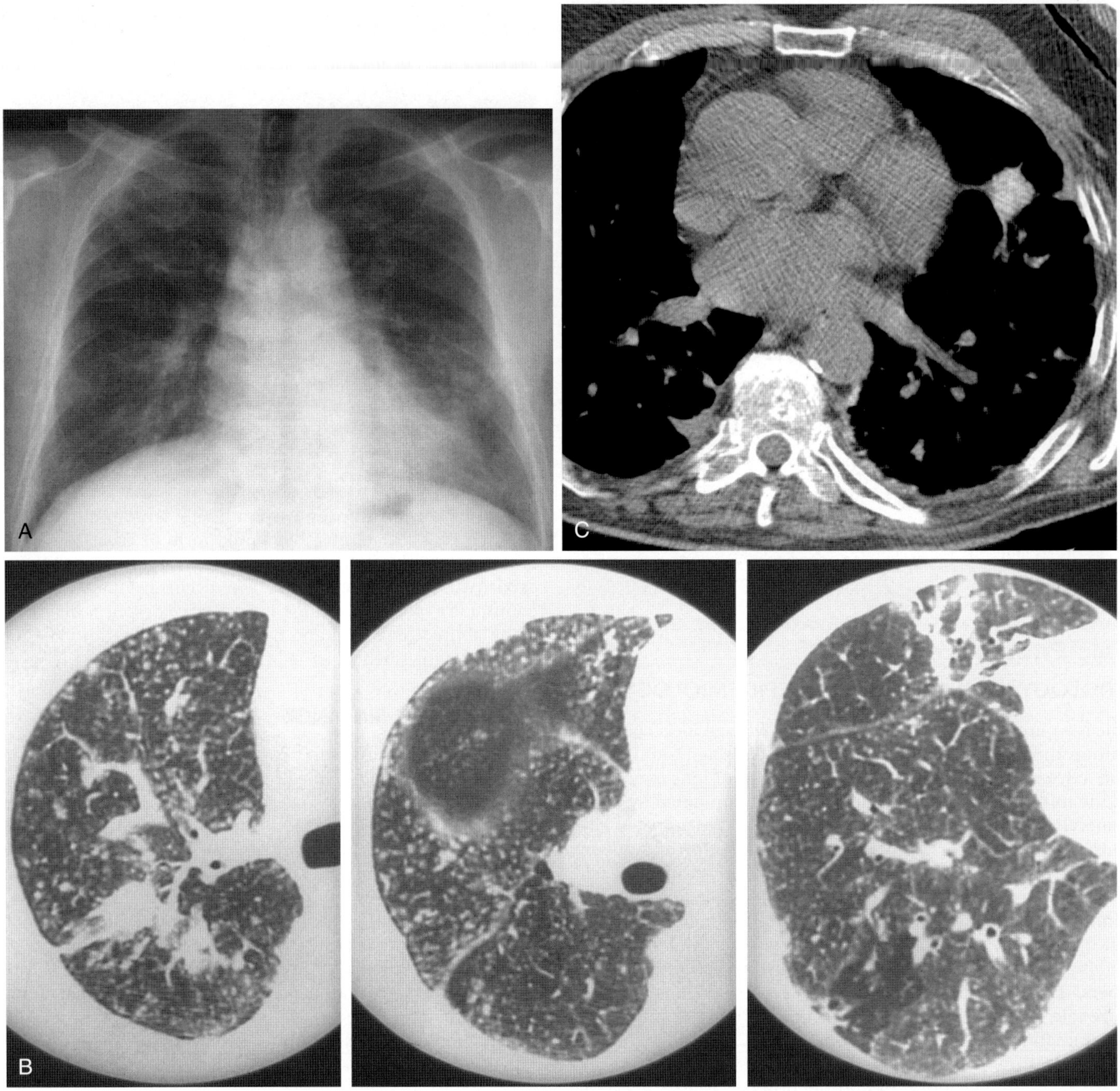

Fig. 63.7 Talc pneumoconiosis. (A) Chest radiograph shows poorly defined small nodular opacities diffusely distributed throughout both lungs. Confluent opacities are also noted. (B) Views of the right lung from high-resolution CT scans at three different levels show small centrilobular nodules in all lung zones. Focal large opacity in the right upper lobe is noted. Incidental note is made of mild right middle and lower lobe consolidation. (C) Axial CT scan in a different patient reveals a left upper lobe nodule containing high-attenuation talc material.

pneumoconiosis, leads to a mixture of rounded and irregular opacities, which appear in the middle zones and are often perihilar in distribution.[28]

The radiographic findings of IV administration of talc include small nodular opacities that may progress to large masses or mass-like areas of consolidation. The large mass densities resemble those of massive pulmonary fibrosis in silicosis and anthracosis; however, they may appear far closer to the hilum than in the latter diseases (see Chapter 62). Lymph node enlargement is common.[34,35]

Computed Tomography

HRCT manifestations of pulmonary talcosis caused by the inhalation of talc consist of small centrilobular and subpleural nodules and conglomerated masses containing focal areas of high attenuation (see Fig. 63.7).[36,37] Other frequent findings include septal lines, subpleural lines, ground-glass opacities, and lobular areas of low attenuation. Lymph node enlargement containing focal areas of high attenuation consistent with talc deposition also is seen.[37] HRCT findings in patients with

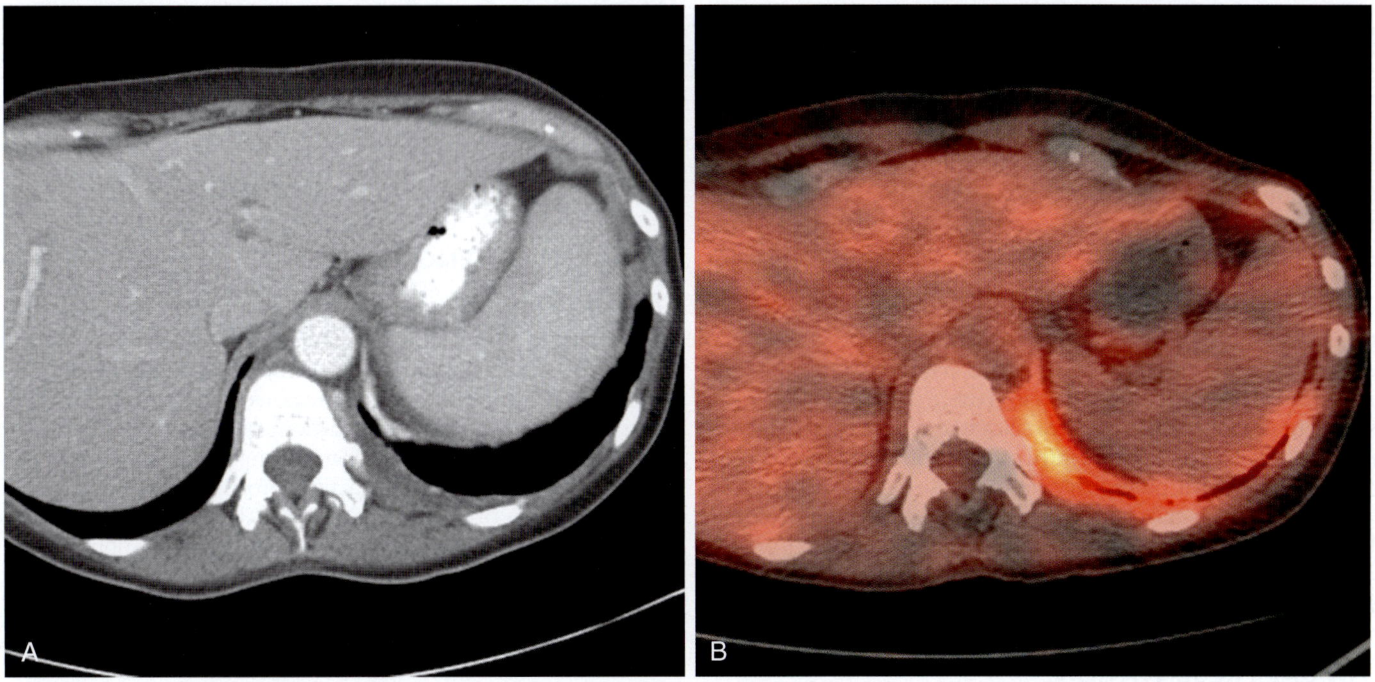

Fig. 63.8 Talc pleurodesis with increased fluorodeoxyglucose (FDG) uptake. (A) Axial CT image shows left pleural thickening containing focal areas of high attenuation owing to talc accumulation. A small left pleural effusion is noted. (B) Fused image from an FDG–positron emission tomography–CT study shows intense uptake corresponding to talc deposits.

pulmonary talcosis resulting from chronic IV drug abuse include diffuse small nodules or ground-glass opacities (sometimes tree-in-bud), perihilar conglomerate masses with areas of high attenuation, and lower lobe panacinar emphysema (see Chapter 52).[34,35] Lower lobe panacinar emphysema is more common in methylphenidate (Ritalin) abusers than in other drug abusers.[35]

Positron Emission Tomography

Talc pleurodesis produces high-density areas of pleural thickening on CT (Fig. 63.8) owing to talc deposits and increased fluorodeoxyglucose uptake on positron emission tomography that can persist indefinitely.[38,39]

Imaging Algorithm

Chest radiography is the main imaging modality used in the initial assessment and follow-up of patients with talc pneumoconiosis. Further evaluation of the parenchyma can be obtained with CT. CT is more sensitive in detecting pleural plaques and lymph node enlargement with areas of high attenuation.

DIFFERENTIAL DIAGNOSIS

Diagnosis is made on the history of adequate exposure and on the radiologic findings. When the exact composition of inhaled dust is unavailable, mineralogic analysis of BAL fluid can be useful in the diagnosis of talc pneumoconiosis.[40]

In talcoasbestosis the main differential diagnosis is with other conditions that may result in reticulation with basilar predominance. These include all other types of interstitial pneumonias. The existence of pleural plaques suggests talcoasbestosis, but pleural plaques are seen in workers exposed to talc contaminated with asbestos and workers free of asbestos exposure.[29] In talcosilicosis and pure talcosis the main differential diagnosis includes sarcoidosis and other infectious and noninfectious granulomatous lung disease.

SYNOPSIS OF TREATMENT OPTIONS

As with silicosis and asbestosis, there is no specific treatment for inhalational talc pneumoconiosis. Steroids may be used empirically in respiratory failure associated with recent IV exposure, and spontaneous radiographic and clinical improvement has been noted in a few such cases.[41] The carcinogenicity of inhaled talc is controversial. Mortality studies conducted on workers exposed to asbestos-free talc fail to show consistent effects of talc on lung cancer mortality. Lung cancer mortality may be significantly higher in workers exposed to a mixture of talc and silica or talc and asbestos.[42]

KEY POINTS: TALC PNEUMOCONIOSIS

- Talc pneumoconiosis includes inhalational talc pneumoconiosis (talcoasbestosis, talcosilicosis, pure talcosis) and intravenous (IV) talcosis.
- Clinical symptoms include dyspnea, cough, cyanosis, and finger clubbing in advanced cases.
- Common radiologic findings include the following:
  - Small centrilobular and subpleural nodules
  - Conglomerated masses containing focal areas of high attenuation
  - Reticulonodular pattern resembling asbestosis in talcoasbestosis
  - Enlarged mediastinal lymph nodes containing focal areas of high attenuation consistent with talc deposition
  - Lower lobe panacinar emphysema in IV talcosis associated with Ritalin injection

Welders' Pneumoconiosis

ETIOLOGY, PREVALENCE, AND EPIDEMIOLOGY

Exposure to welding fumes is known to be a risk factor for pneumoconiosis, chronic bronchitis, and lung cancer.[43] The principal component of the inhaled dust is iron oxide; the condition also is known as welders' siderosis. Welders' pneumoconiosis was first described by Doig and McLaughlin in 1936.[44] Over the years, welding has evolved from a process that was initially relatively simple, and in which bare iron electrodes were used almost exclusively, into a complex technology in which numerous different electrodes are used. Diffuse pulmonary fibrosis often has been attributed to inhalation of substances other than iron oxide during welding, such as silica or asbestos.[45–47] When free silica is also present, the disease is referred to as silicosiderosis, a form of mixed dust pneumoconiosis. However, interstitial pulmonary fibrosis is seen in some welders without coexisting silicosis.[48] A survey of the chest radiographic abnormalities in 661 British electric arc welders found a 7% prevalence of International Labour Organization radiographic category 0/1 or higher small rounded opacities.[49]

CLINICAL PRESENTATION

Siderosis seldom results in symptoms, although forced expiratory volume in 1 second may be reduced.[50,51]

Arc welders with pulmonary fibrosis may present with dyspnea on exertion and cough and have restrictive physiology on pulmonary function studies.[45–47] In welders' pneumoconiosis, ferritin is elevated in serum or BAL fluid or both.[52]

PATHOLOGIC FINDINGS

The main histologic features of siderosis are iron dust and dust-laden macrophages associated with minimal fibrosis (macules) (Fig. 63.9). Visual inspection of the lung specimen usually reveals macules that vary from red to brown, gray, or black. Microscopically, the dust macules appear as colored spots in the centers of the lobules. Similar collections of dust frequently extend along the interlobular septa and pleural lymphatics. Many of the particles appear as rounded ferruginous bodies with round or polygonal black cores. The term *ferruginous body* refers to a mineral particle to which pulmonary macrophages have added an iron protein coat.[53] Dense nodular fibrosis also is sometimes seen and has been attributed to concomitant exposure to silica. Some experimental studies suggest, however, that iron or welding fumes may be able to produce nodular fibrosis also.[54,55]

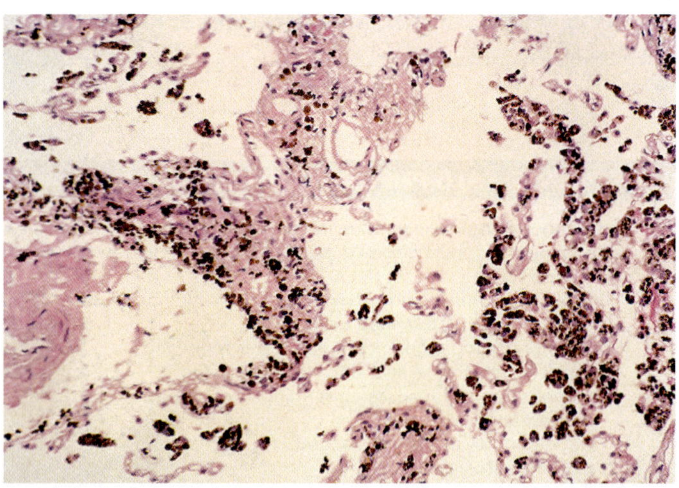

Fig. 63.9 Welders' pneumoconiosis. Histologic specimen of the lung obtained by transbronchial lung biopsy shows a large amount of iron-containing macrophages within alveolar airspaces associated with fibrous tissue around small vessels and airways.

IMAGING FINDINGS

Radiography

The typical chest radiographic manifestations of arc welders' siderosis consist of very fine nodules that are most prominent in the middle third of the lungs in the perihilar regions or in the lower lung zones (Fig. 63.10). The finely nodular shadows on chest radiographs resolve after removal of patients from occupational exposure.[56] The micronodules do not reflect reactive fibrosis but instead, radiopaque accumulations of iron particles that lie within macrophages, aggregated along the perivascular and peribronchial lymphatic vessels. As noted earlier, however, several authors have reported symptomatic welders with evidence of pulmonary fibrosis.[45–47]

Computed Tomography

The most common CT findings in the arc welders are ill-defined micronodules and fine branching linear lines diffusely distributed in the lung (see Fig. 63.10). Most of the micronodules have a centrilobular distribution. Coalescence of micronodules and fine branching lines results in a fine reticular pattern. The micronodules and fine branching lines on CT correspond to dust macules, which are collections of dust-laden macrophages surrounding the small airway and vessels. Emphysema is often seen. In some welders a honeycomb pattern (Fig. 63.11) and ground-glass opacities (Fig. 63.12) also may be found.[52,57,58] In one study small centrilobular nodules were seen on HRCT in 9 of 11 cases (81.8%), emphysematous changes also were found in 3 of the cases (27.3%), and fibrosis was found in 3 of the cases (27.3%).[52] Conglomerated masses with areas of high attenuation indicating organizing pneumonia with siderosis have been reported (Fig. 63.13).[57]

Imaging Algorithm

The chest radiograph is usually the initial imaging modality used in the evaluation of welders' pneumoconiosis. HRCT often shows parenchymal abnormalities in patients with normal radiographs.

DIFFERENTIAL DIAGNOSIS

The HRCT appearance of siderosis mimics that of hypersensitivity pneumonitis. In siderosis, however, mosaic attenuation and ground-glass opacities are less prominent than in hypersensitivity pneumonitis. Other lung diseases that manifest with centrilobular nodules, such as respiratory bronchiolitis, respiratory bronchiolitis–associated interstitial lung disease, follicular bronchiolitis, diffuse panbronchiolitis, and *Mycoplasma* pneumonia, also are included in the differential diagnosis.

KEY POINTS: WELDERS' PNEUMOCONIOSIS

- Generally asymptomatic or minimal symptoms.
- Elevation of ferritin in serum and/or BAL fluid.
- Ill-defined centrilobular nodules corresponding to collections of dust-laden macrophages surrounding the small airways and vessels

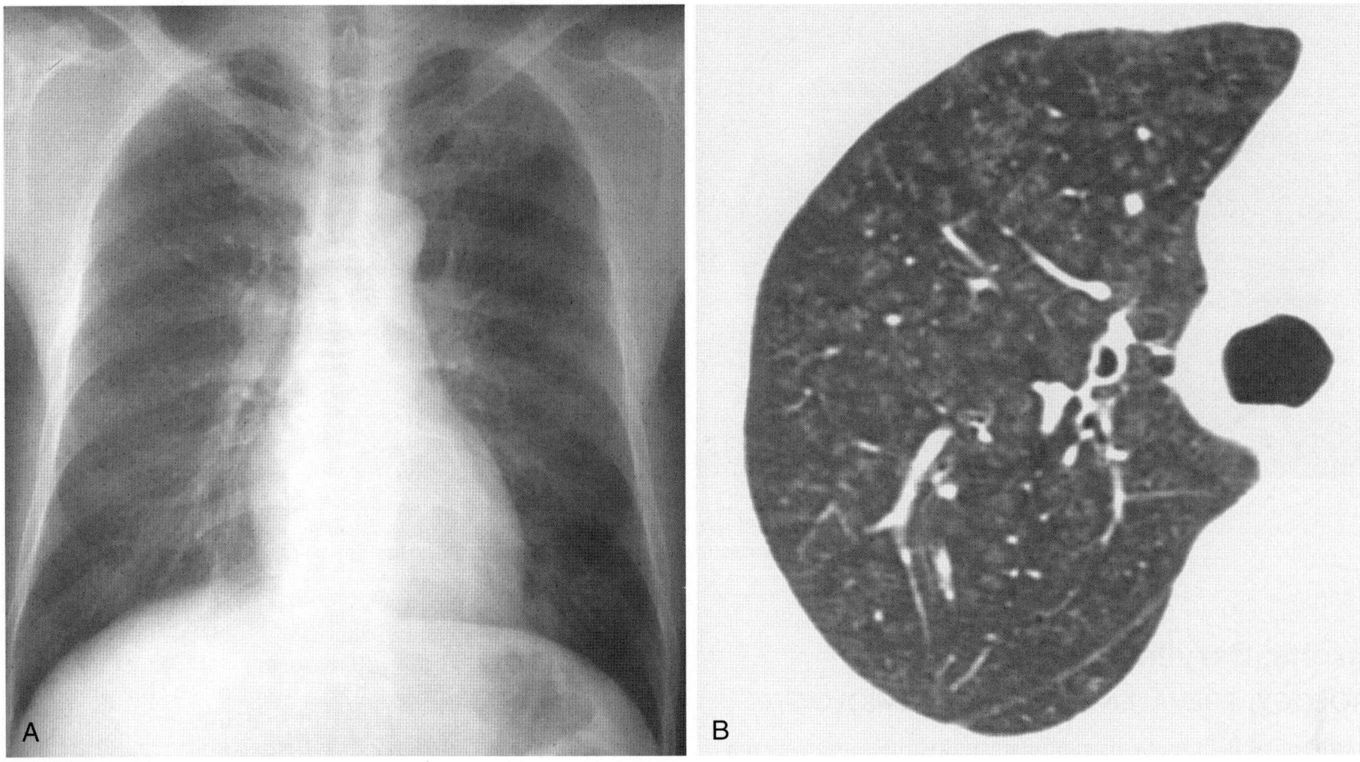

Fig. 63.10 Welders' pneumoconiosis. (A) Posteroanterior chest radiograph reveals fine nodular opacities that are most prominent in the middle third of the lungs. (B) View of the right upper lobe from a high-resolution CT scan shows ill-defined centrilobular micronodules mimicking hypersensitivity pneumonitis.

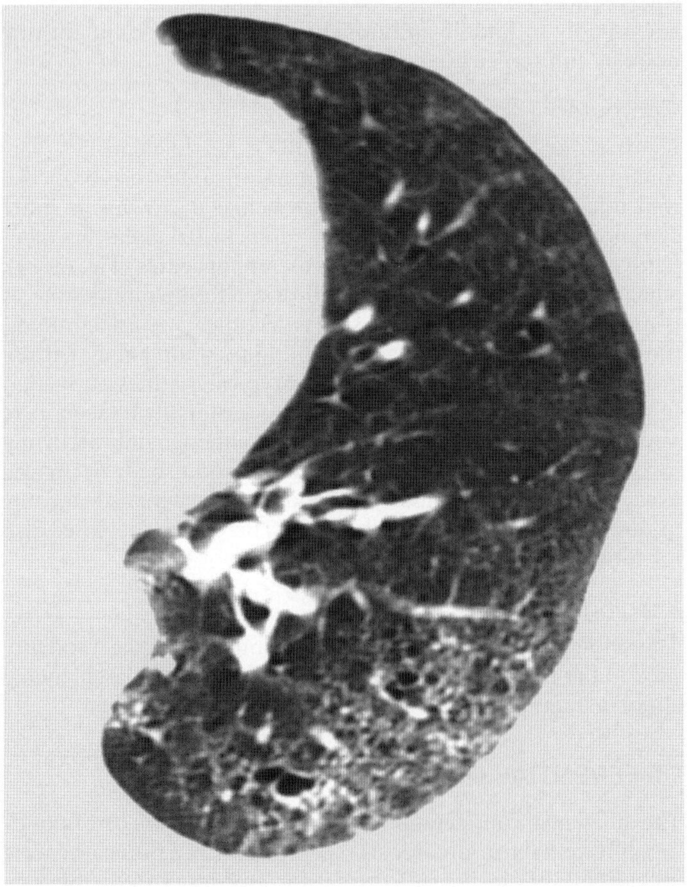

Fig. 63.11 Welders' pneumoconiosis. View of the left lung from a CT scan shows ground-glass opacities, reticulation, traction bronchiectasis, and mild emphysema.

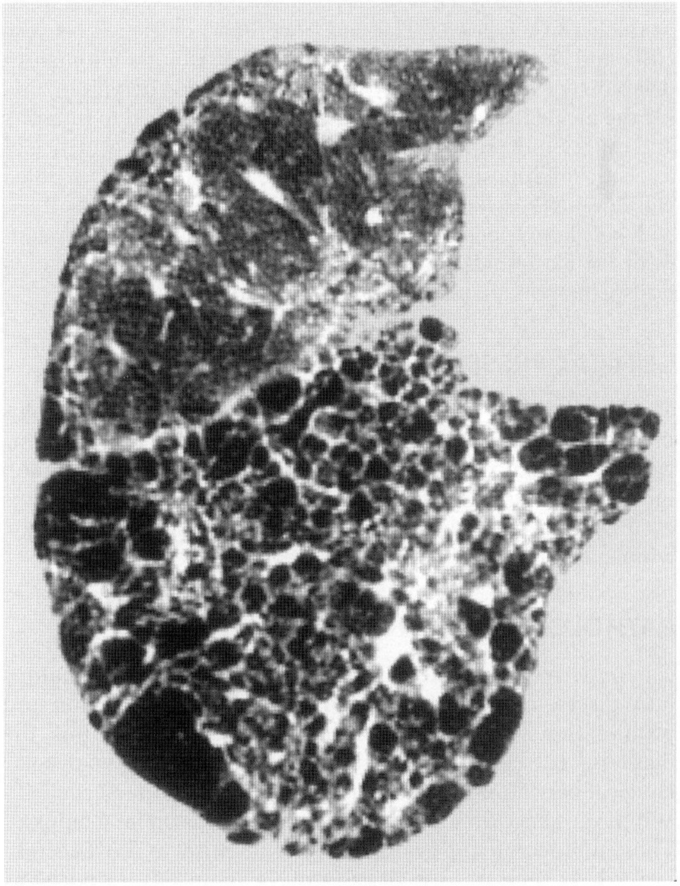

Fig. 63.12 Welders' pneumoconiosis. View of the right lung from a CT scan shows ground-glass opacities, extensive reticulation, and honeycombing. Centrilobular and paraseptal emphysema is noted.

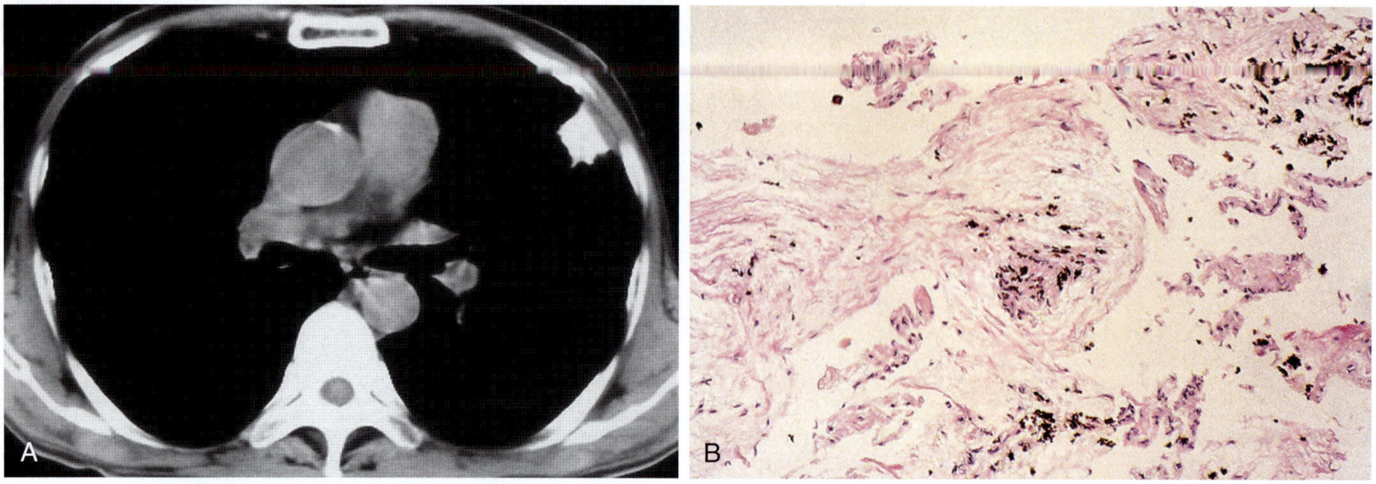

Fig. 63.13 Welders' pneumoconiosis. (A) CT scan shows a high-attenuation subpleural nodule in the left upper lobe. Lung windows (not shown) also showed bilateral small centrilobular nodules. (B) Transbronchial biopsy specimen from the mass reveals organization with siderosis.

Chronic Beryllium Disease

ETIOLOGY, PREVALENCE, AND EPIDEMIOLOGY

Beryllium is a light metal used in many industries but most commonly in nuclear industry applications, aerospace engineering, ceramics, dentistry, and electronic manufacturing. Acute toxicity has virtually disappeared with the advent of industrial control measures to minimize air levels. However, chronic beryllium disease (CBD, sometimes referred to as berylliosis) is still a risk for those working with beryllium.[59] There are two primary differences between CBD and the other pneumoconiosis: (1) It is a granulomatous delayed-type hypersensitivity response to inhaled beryllium, and (2) the incidence and severity are not as clearly linked to intensity and duration of exposure. In addition, there is some evidence of a genetic predisposition.[60] Approximately 10% of patients exposed will develop beryllium hypersensitivity, and about half of those with beryllium hypersensitivity will develop CBD. Treatment options favor corticosteroids, but there is no cure. Methotrexate and lung transplantation are additional considerations.[59]

CLINICAL PRESENTATION

The lungs are the primary organ affected by CBD. Other organs include lymph nodes, skin, salivary tissue, liver, spleen, kidneys, bone, myocardium, and skeletal muscle. Dyspnea is the most common initial presenting symptom, with other physical signs and symptoms occurring late in the disease course, including inspiratory crackles, lymphadenopathy, skin lesions and hepatosplenomegaly.[59]

PATHOLOGIC FINDINGS

The underlying pathology of CBD is that of a granulomatous lung disease caused by a delayed hypersensitivity reaction and proliferation of beryllium-specific T cells. Because of this, the diagnosis is based on a positive blood test or bronchoalveolar lavage of beryllium-specific lymphocyte proliferation test (BeLPT) and the presence of nonnecrotizing granulomas on lung biopsy.[61] These nonnecrotizing granulomas are identical to those seen in sarcoid. As such, almost all cases of CBD are misdiagnosed as sarcoid if a history of beryllium exposure is not obtained to prompt a BeLPT. Screening workers for CBD using blood BeLPT can be performed. Those with a positive screening examination but no lung disease are considered "sensitized" but do not have CBD, despite their lifetime risk for the disease.

IMAGING FINDINGS

Radiography

The radiographic appearance of CBD is identical to sarcoidosis. Appearances range from classic hilar and mediastinal lymphadenopathy to middle and upper lung zone–predominant tiny nodules and upper lung zone fibrosis.

Computed Tomography

As mentioned, the appearance of CBD is nearly identical to sarcoidosis. Airway involvement is commonly manifested as bronchial wall thickening, although severe bronchial narrowing is more common in sarcoidosis. Pulmonary parenchymal disease includes perilymphatic nodules and conglomerate opacities (Fig. 63.14), which can progress to mass-like fibrosis, although frank fibrosis is more common in sarcoidosis. As in other pneumoconioses, the perilymphatic nodules may result in pseudoplaques. Diffuse ground-glass opacities would be an atypical manifestation, and fibrosis in a UIP or NSIP pattern can occasionally be seen. Like sarcoidosis, lymphadenopathy is frequent, although only occurring in 25% of cases (less than in sarcoidosis) and usually occurring in association with lung disease as opposed to the lymphadenopathy in sarcoidosis, which can be isolated. There is an increased risk for lung cancer.[60]

Imaging Algorithm

The chest radiograph is usually the initial imaging modality used in the evaluation of CBD. HRCT often shows parenchymal abnormalities in patients with normal radiographs.

DIFFERENTIAL DIAGNOSIS

The differential considerations should be based on the corresponding differential for sarcoidosis (see Chapter 31). Some advocate including CBD in the differential for any case of possible sarcoidosis to prompt obtaining an adequate exposure history.[60]

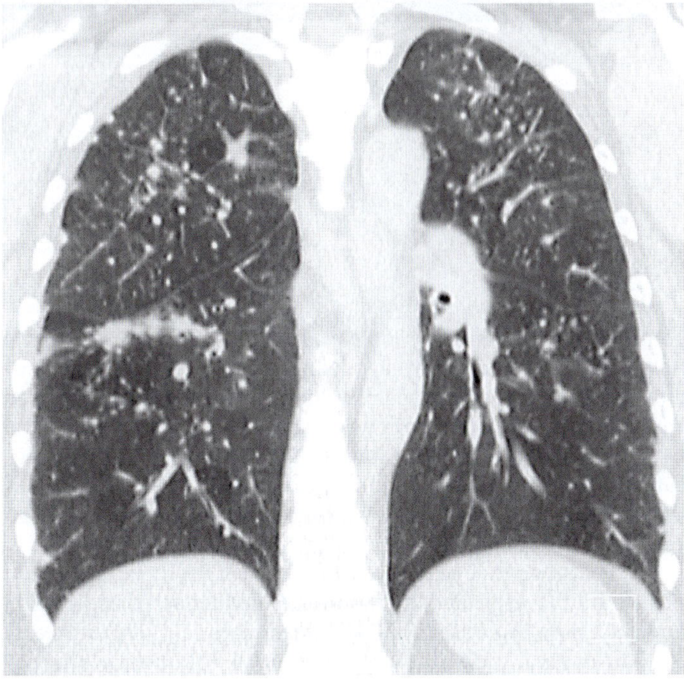

Fig. 63.14 Chronic beryllium disease (CBD). Coronal CT scan shows an identical appearance to sarcoidosis, with upper lung zone–predominant perilymphatic nodules and conglomerate opacities with some mosaic attenuation corresponding to air-trapping on expiration (not shown). Patient's occupational history revealed work in satellite manufacturing, and the patient tested positive to a blood beryllium-specific lymphocyte proliferation test, confirming CBD as the diagnosis.

KEY POINTS: CHRONIC BERYLLIUM DISEASE

- It involves rare exposure to those in the aerospace, nuclear, ceramics, and electronics industries.
- Serum or bronchoalveolar lavage testing of beryllium-specific lymphocyte proliferation test confirms sensitivity to beryllium in those with an exposure history.
- Nonnecrotizing granulomas identical to those seen in sarcoidosis are seen on biopsy.
- Radiographic and CT findings are nearly identical to sarcoidosis.

SUGGESTED READINGS

Chong S, Lee KS, Chung MJ, et al. Pneumoconiosis: comparison of imaging and pathologic findings. *Radiographics*. 2006;26:59–77.

Cox CW, et al. State of the art: imaging of occupational lung disease. *Radiology*. 2014;270(3):681–696.

Culver DA, Dweik RA. Chronic beryllium disease. *Clin Pulm Med*. 2003;10:72–79.

Feigin DS. Talc: understanding its manifestations in the chest. *AJR Am J Roentgenol*. 1986;146:295–301.

Nemery B, Verbeken EK, Demedts M. Giant cell interstitial pneumonia (hard metal lung disease, cobalt lung). *Semin Respir Crit Care Med*. 2001;22:435–448.

Tutkun E, et al. Farewell to an old friend: chest x-ray vs high-resolution computed tomography in welders' lung disease. *Clin Respir J*. 2014;8(2):220–224.

The full reference list for this chapter is available at ExpertConsult.com.

64 Aspiration

TOMÁS FRANQUET

Aspiration refers to the misdirection of contents of the oral or upper gastrointestinal tract that have passed through the trachea and larynx and entered the lung.[1,2] The diagnosis rests mostly on the history of presenting illness, medical history, vital signs, and chest radiograph.[1] Aspiration includes a spectrum of clinical and radiologic manifestations secondary to chemical pneumonitis or bacterial pneumonia that range from asymptomatic focal inflammatory reactions with few or no radiologic abnormalities to severe life-threatening disease.[3]

Pulmonary complications develop when there is a compromise of the usual defenses that protect the lower airways, and aspirated material affects the lower respiratory tract by direct toxic effect, sufficient volume to cause obstruction, or contamination, thus resulting in bacterial infection. The pathogenesis of lung injury depends on the amount and nature of the aspirated material, the frequency of aspiration, and the host's response to the aspirated material.[1] Three different clinicopathologic syndromes have been described: aspiration pneumonia, aspiration pneumonitis, and aspiration of inert fluids or particulate material. In the management of aspiration syndromes, it is important to distinguish aspiration pneumonitis from aspiration pneumonia.[2] Aspiration pneumonia refers to pulmonary infection caused by aspiration of colonized oropharyngeal secretions; aspiration pneumonitis refers to the acute lung injury caused by the aspiration of materials inherently toxic to the lungs: gastric acid, milk, mineral oil, and volatile hydrocarbons.

The most important predisposing factors for aspiration are alcoholism, debilitating diseases, loss of consciousness, structural abnormalities of the pharynx and esophagus, neuromuscular disorders, and deglutition. Aspiration is common in normal persons during sleep or periods of diminished consciousness. Aspiration has been documented in 70% of patients in stupor or coma.[4,5]

Aspiration Pneumonia

ETIOLOGY, PREVALENCE, AND EPIDEMIOLOGY

Aspiration pneumonia results from aspiration of secretions containing a variety of bacteria that are normally present in the oropharynx. Healthy adults have an average of 10 to 100 million bacteria per milliliter of oropharyngeal secretions.[1,6–8]

Although the microbial agent of aspiration pneumonia is variable, 90% of aspiration pneumonias are caused by polymicrobial flora that include enteric gram-negative bacilli, anaerobic bacteria, *Staphylococcus aureus*, *Streptococcus pneumoniae*, and *Haemophilus influenzae*.[9–11] The most common anaerobes are *Prevotella* and *Fusobacterium* species.

Under these circumstances, aspiration material is well tolerated, and the microorganisms neither reach the alveoli nor invade the mucosa of the normal tracheobronchial tree. Pneumonia is more common when host defenses are impaired.[12] Failure of mechanical defenses and defects in phagocytosis or ciliary function, neutropenia, and hypogammaglobulinemia can result in increased frequency or severity of pneumonia. Patients with poor dental hygiene or advanced periodontal disease are at particular risk for development of aspiration pneumonia.[13] In these individuals the amount of bacteria per milliliter of oropharyngeal secretions may increase 100- to 1000-fold.

The pathogenesis of lung injury depends on the amount and nature of the aspirated material, the frequency of aspiration, and the host's response to the aspirated material.[14] During sleep, 50% of normal individuals aspirate small volumes of oropharyngeal secretions,[15] but host defenses prevent lung infections, and the types of microorganisms aspirated are less virulent.[12] The distinction between aspiration pneumonia and other forms of pneumonia is largely based on the clinical characteristics, but clearly overlaps exist.[16,17]

Aspiration pneumonia is a major form of community-acquired pneumonia (CAP) and health care–associated pneumonia (HCAP), occurring as an acute fulminant illness or as a chronic, insidious process.[17,18] As many as 5% to 15% of cases of CAP are related to aspiration.[19,20] Most hospital-acquired infections result from aspiration of pharyngeal contents, and the majority of cases occur without the use of intubation or other respiratory assistance. In these patients the stomach may become colonized with gram-negative bacteria, and aspiration may overwhelm lung defenses, resulting in the development of pneumonia.[21] Intubation and mechanical ventilation may increase the incidence and size of aspirations, with a resultant increase in the development of pneumonia.[14,21] Critical factors in pathogenesis include colonization of the oropharynx with pathogenic microorganisms, aspiration of these organisms from the oropharynx into the lower respiratory tract, and compromise of the normal host defense mechanisms.

Recurrent pneumonias in the neonatal period are often the result of direct lung contamination from a congenital tracheoesophageal fistula.[22] Acute episodes of aspiration are symptomatic, and patients usually present with symptoms of pneumonia or respiratory distress.[23] In adults esophageal fistulas are generally acquired lesions and should be suspected in any patient with any underlying condition predisposing to aspiration.[24–26] They may occur as a complication of intrathoracic malignant neoplasms (60%), infection, or trauma.[26,27]

Fistulous connections between the esophagus and the lung, bronchi, or trachea are exceedingly rare in the absence of predisposing factors.[28] Fistulas may occur in 5% to 10% of patients with advanced esophageal cancer.[29] In such cases radiation therapy is complicated with a high risk of fistula formation.[30,31] Tracheoesophageal fistula in these patients is usually incurable, and once this complication has developed, the prognosis is extremely poor.[29] The clinical presentation is variable. Some patients present with an acute onset, whereas others have a subacute or chronic presentation. Diagnosis is usually made with a fluoroscopic esophagram. However, computed tomography (CT) may be helpful in the diagnosis of fistulous track formation in cases with normal findings on esophagography.[32]

In the past acute aspiration was reported in 7% to 16% of patients undergoing anesthesia.[33] However, in recent years, the frequency of aspiration of gastric contents during anesthesia has decreased considerably, and symptomatic aspiration pneumonia is currently an uncommon complication of anesthesia.[34]

Lentil aspiration pneumonia is a granulomatous pneumonitis caused by aspiration of leguminous material, such as lentils, beans, and peas.[35–37] Predisposing factors, such as neurologic disorders, structural abnormalities of the pharynx and esophagus, emergency surgical procedures, and dementia, are frequent associations.[37] The histologic findings are characteristic and consist of an epithelioid granuloma, with or without central necrosis, in response to durable cellulose content. Repetitive aspiration episodes may result in numerous small bilateral nodules representing inflammation with foreign-body reaction in bronchioles, ducts, and alveolar sacs.[35]

CLINICAL PRESENTATION

The clinical presentation of aspiration pneumonia is variable. Some patients present with an acute onset; others have a subacute or chronic presentation. Acute aspiration is usually associated with cough, wheezing, cyanosis, dyspnea, and tachypnea. Acute aspiration is usually associated with cough, wheezing, cyanosis, dyspnea, and tachypnea; the characteristic clinical manifestations are usually those of an acute pneumonia and consist of fever, leukocytosis, increase in respiratory secretions, and purulent sputum. Less common manifestations include pleuritic chest pain and hemoptysis. However, the signs and symptoms of pneumonia may be milder or even absent in the elderly. Silent aspiration occurs during anesthesia or while a patient is intubated in the intensive care unit.

PATHOLOGIC FINDINGS AND PATHOPHYSIOLOGY

Acute aspiration is not uncommon and represents a common incidental finding at autopsy in debilitated patients dying of other causes. Pathologic changes depend on the amount and nature of the aspirated material and the time after aspiration at which the lungs are examined.[38] The classic pathologic appearance is a necrotizing acute bronchopneumonia in which there is a foreign-body granulomatous reaction to aspirated exogenous material. Histologically, aspiration pneumonia is characterized by the presence of edema, hemorrhage, numerous polymorphonuclear leukocytes, and foreign-body granulomas within alveolar spaces. The process centers around the bronchioles, which can be destroyed and replaced by acute inflammation and necrosis. Multinucleated giant cells are often seen in the surrounding infiltrate.

Complications associated with aspiration pneumonia include abscess formation, necrotizing pneumonia, pleural effusion, and empyema. Lung abscess is defined as an inflammatory mass within lung parenchyma, the central part of which has undergone purulent liquefaction necrosis.[39] The most common cause of lung abscess is aspiration.[40] The most frequently involved regions are the posterior segment of an upper lobe or the superior segment of a lower lobe, especially when aspiration occurs in a supine position.[41]

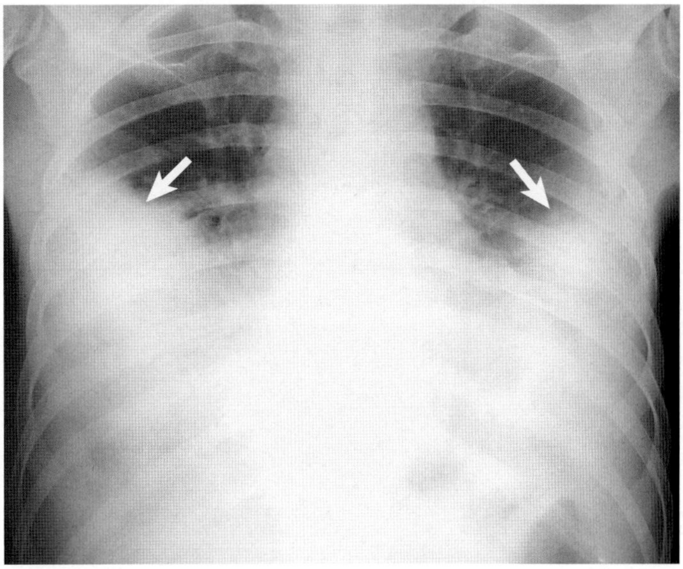

Fig. 64.1 Acute aspiration pneumonia in an alcoholic man. Anteroposterior chest radiograph shows extensive middle and lower lung zone–predominant consolidation *(arrows).*

MANIFESTATIONS OF THE DISEASE

Radiography

The chest radiograph typically demonstrates unilateral or bilateral patchy or confluent consolidation involving mainly the dependent lung regions (Fig. 64.1).[21] The location of pneumonia depends on the position of the patient when aspiration occurs. In recumbent patients diffuse perihilar consolidation reflects pneumonia involving mainly the posterior segments of the upper lobes or superior segments of the lower lobes; in upright patients consolidation is seen mainly in the basal segments of the lower lobes. Consolidations may be simultaneously present in various lobes when a large volume of fluid is aspirated (Fig. 64.2).

Prolonged clinical course or large aspirations may result in severe necrotizing bronchopneumonia or lung abscess formation occurring 8 to 14 days after the initial aspiration event.[42] Lung abscesses consist of single or multiple, often cavitary, nodules or masses usually measuring 2 to 6 cm in diameter. Their internal margins are smooth in 90% of cases and shaggy in 10%.[40] Air-fluid levels are seen in 70% of cases and adjacent parenchymal consolidation in 50% (Fig. 64.3).[40] Lung abscesses may be seen anywhere in the lungs but are most commonly located in the dependent regions (Fig. 64.4). Neither clinical nor radiographic features permit a specific diagnosis of lung abscess.[40]

When aspiration is secondary to congenital tracheobronchial fistulae, the radiologic manifestations are variable, depending on the spread and severity of the aspiration. The most common radiographic pattern is that of bronchopneumonia with patchy airspace opacities.[43] The most useful diagnostic imaging modality is esophagram, and barium is the best contrast agent to use to demonstrate the presence of a fistula (Fig. 64.5).[43] In adults radiographic findings are nonspecific. Diagnosis should be strongly suspected in any patient with a known esophageal carcinoma in whom there is evidence of recurrent pneumonias (Fig. 64.6). Consolidation is usually unilateral but may involve both lungs.

Bronchopleural fistula, defined as a communication between the bronchus or lung parenchyma and pleural space, is a known

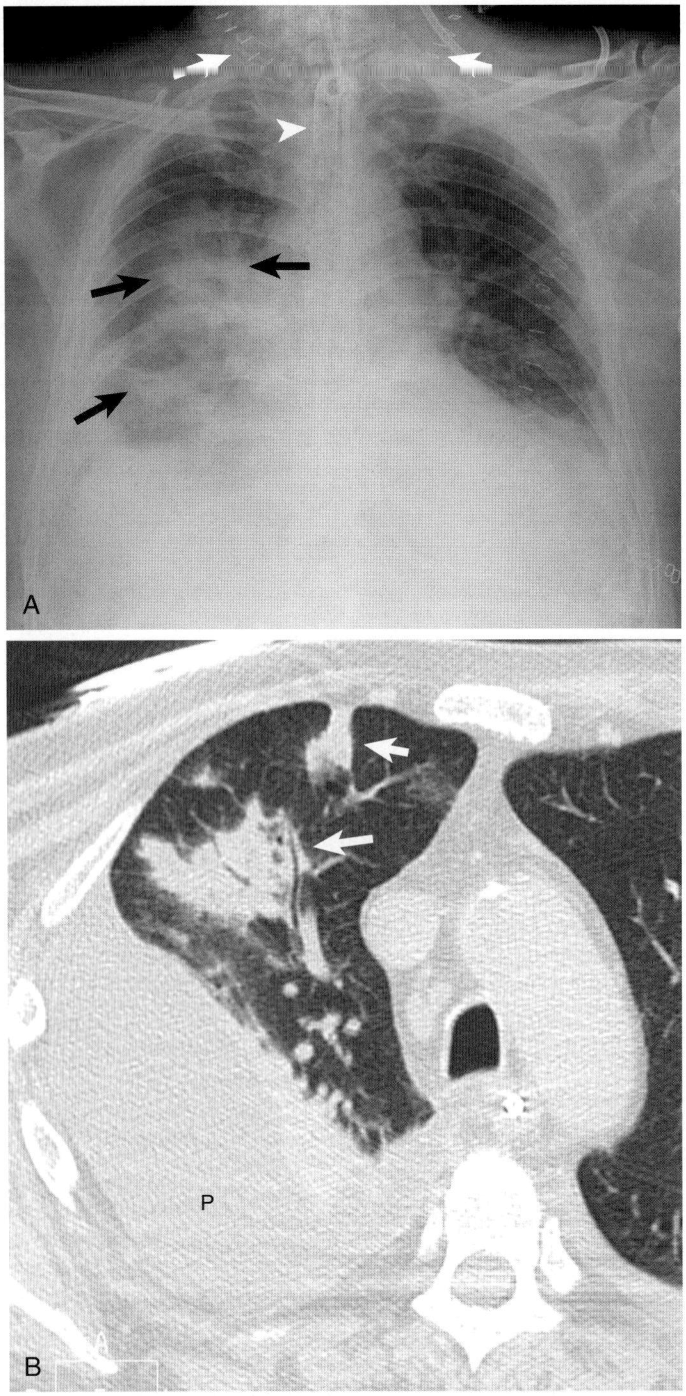

Fig. 64.2 Acute aspiration pneumonia after neck surgery. (A) Anteroposterior chest radiograph shows extensive right lung consolidation *(black arrows)* and right pleural effusion. Note postsurgical metallic staples *(white arrows)* and tracheostomy tube *(arrowhead)*. (B) Corresponding CT shows multifocal areas of consolidation *(arrows)* in the right upper lobe. A large pleural effusion (P) is also seen.

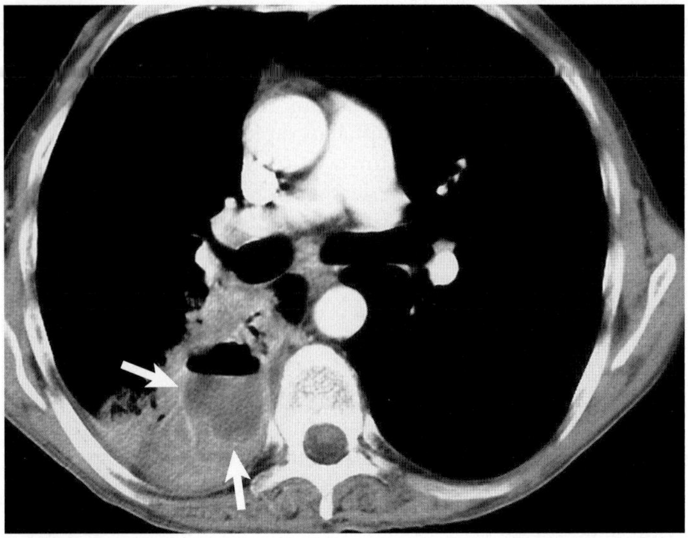

Fig. 64.3 Acute aspiration pneumonia with abscess formation in an alcoholic man. A contrast-enhanced CT shows consolidation in the superior segment of the right lower lobe. An abscess *(arrows)* with an air-fluid level and an irregular poorly defined wall is visible within the consolidation.

complication of necrotizing pneumonia that may accompany aspiration (Figs. 64.7 and 64.8).[44]

Elderly persons may have diminished production of saliva as a result of medications and oral/dental disease, leading to poor oral hygiene and oropharyngeal colonization with pathogenic organisms.[45] A distinct form of infection is caused by *Actinomyces israelii*, an anaerobic bacterium that is normally found in the mouths of patients with poor oral hygiene. Aspiration of infected material results in a localized or lobar pneumonia, usually in the dependent portions of the lung. Although radiologic features include focal or patchy ill-defined consolidations and progressive abscess formation, pulmonary actinomycosis can mimic a broad spectrum of pathologies, from benign infection to lung cancer.[46] If untreated, actinomycosis spreads, invading the chest wall, the mediastinum, or the diaphragm (see Fig. 64.4).

Computed Tomography

Similar to the radiographic findings, CT manifestations of aspiration pneumonia consist of unilateral or bilateral patchy or confluent consolidation and ground-glass opacities involving mainly the dependent lung regions. Other common findings include centrilobular branching structures ("tree-in-bud" opacities) and centrilobular nodules, reflecting cellular bronchiolitis, peribronchiolar inflammation, and interlobular septal thickening.[47] Airspace nodules, ground-glass opacities, and lobular consolidation are seen better by CT than by conventional radiography.[3,48] In patients with infection secondary to aspiration of contaminated secretions, as from periodontal disease, the CT findings may also include multiple rounded opacities surrounded by a halo of ground-glass opacity that may mimic septic emboli. The opacities are usually unilateral but may involve both lungs (Fig. 64.9). These may progress to abscess formation and cavitation.

DIFFERENTIAL DIAGNOSIS

The most useful imaging modalities available for the evaluation of patients with known or suspected aspiration pneumonia are chest radiography and CT. Imaging examinations should always be interpreted with awareness of the clinical findings, including duration of symptoms, presence of fever, cough, and dyspnea, and the degree of leukocytosis.[49,50] Knowledge of the immune status of the patient is helpful in arriving at a short list of most likely causative organisms. In the absence of clinical information, radiologists cannot reliably distinguish between pneumonia and other pulmonary processes.[51]

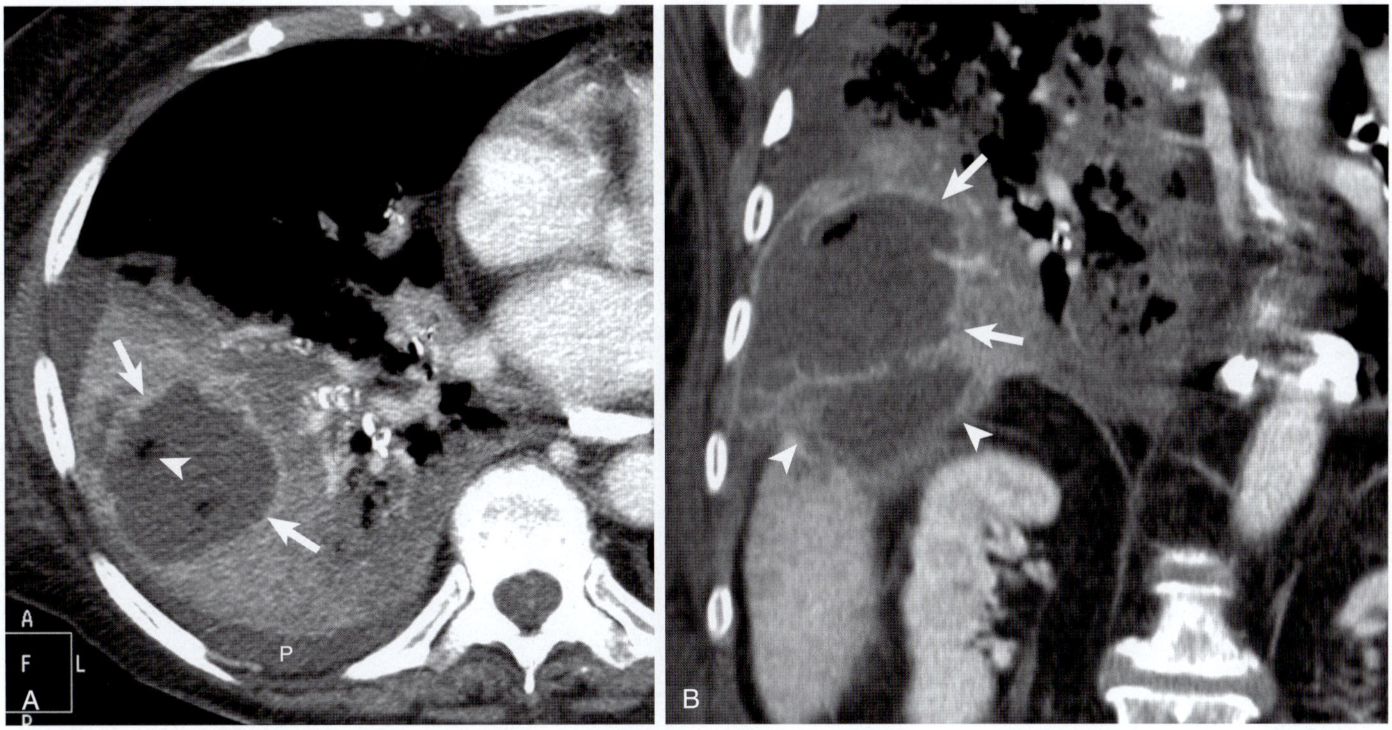

Fig. 64.4 Acute pulmonary actinomycosis and abscess formation. (A) Contrast-enhanced CT obtained after 10 days of aspiration shows extensive right lower lobe consolidation containing a large abscess with ill-defined margins *(arrows)* and small foci of air *(arrowhead)*. Note small associated right pleural effusion (P). (B) Coronal reformatted CT shows a subdiaphragmatic collection *(arrowheads)* close to the hepatic surface. *Actinomyces* infection *(arrows)* often crosses fascial boundaries including the chest wall, diaphragm, and mediastinum.

Although certain radiologic patterns are highly suggestive of pneumonia, chest radiography is of limited value in determining the specific etiology.[52–55] Distinction of localized pneumonia from other pulmonary processes cannot be made with certainty by imaging.[56,57] Diagnosis is equally difficult when pneumonia manifests with diffuse bilateral opacities. Other conditions that also commonly manifest with diffuse bilateral opacities include pulmonary edema and acute respiratory distress syndrome (ARDS).[49,58,59]

Aspiration Pneumonitis

ETIOLOGY, PREVALENCE, AND EPIDEMIOLOGY

Aspiration pneumonitis refers to the acute lung injury caused by the aspiration of materials inherently toxic to the lungs, such as gastric acid, milk, mineral oil, and volatile hydrocarbons.[60] Pneumonitis caused by aspiration of large amounts of gastric contents (Mendelson syndrome) is the most serious aspiration syndrome, with a mortality rate ranging from 30% to 70%. Vomiting with massive pulmonary aspiration of gastric contents is a very frequent phenomenon and is probably one of the most common etiologies of aspiration diseases.[60,61] This syndrome occurs in patients who have a marked disturbance of consciousness, including from a drug overdose, seizures, or a massive cerebrovascular accident.[60] Today, pulmonary aspiration of gastric contents is a rare complication during modern anesthesia.[34]

The magnitude of injury is directly related to the pH and volume of aspirated material. Severe pulmonary damage occurs predominantly when the pH of the aspirate is less than 2.5 and the volume more than 25 mL. Because gastric acid prevents the growth of bacteria, the contents of the stomach are sterile under normal conditions. Colonization of the gastric contents by potentially pathogenic organisms may occur when the pH in the stomach is increased by the use of antacids, histamine H_2–receptor antagonists, or proton-pump inhibitors.[62,63]

Gastrointestinal conditions related with gastric acid aspiration include vomiting, gastroesophageal reflux, achalasia, and hiatal hernia.[64] Acid liquid introduced into the airways is rapidly disseminated throughout the bronchial tree and lung parenchyma, producing a chemical pneumonitis within minutes. The overall mortality rate associated with massive aspiration is approximately 30% and exceeds 50% in those patients with initial shock or apnea, secondary pneumonia, or ARDS.[61] The posterior segments of the upper lobes or superior segments of the lower lobes are most frequently involved when the patient is recumbent.

Aspiration of barium contrast medium is a well-recognized complication that occurs during radiologic examination of the gastrointestinal tract and can have serious consequences in weak and debilitated patients.[65,66] Predisposition to barium aspiration is caused by several factors, including swallowing disorders or recent esophageal surgery. The overall mortality rate associated with massive barium aspiration is approximately 30% and exceeds 50% in those patients with initial shock or apnea, secondary

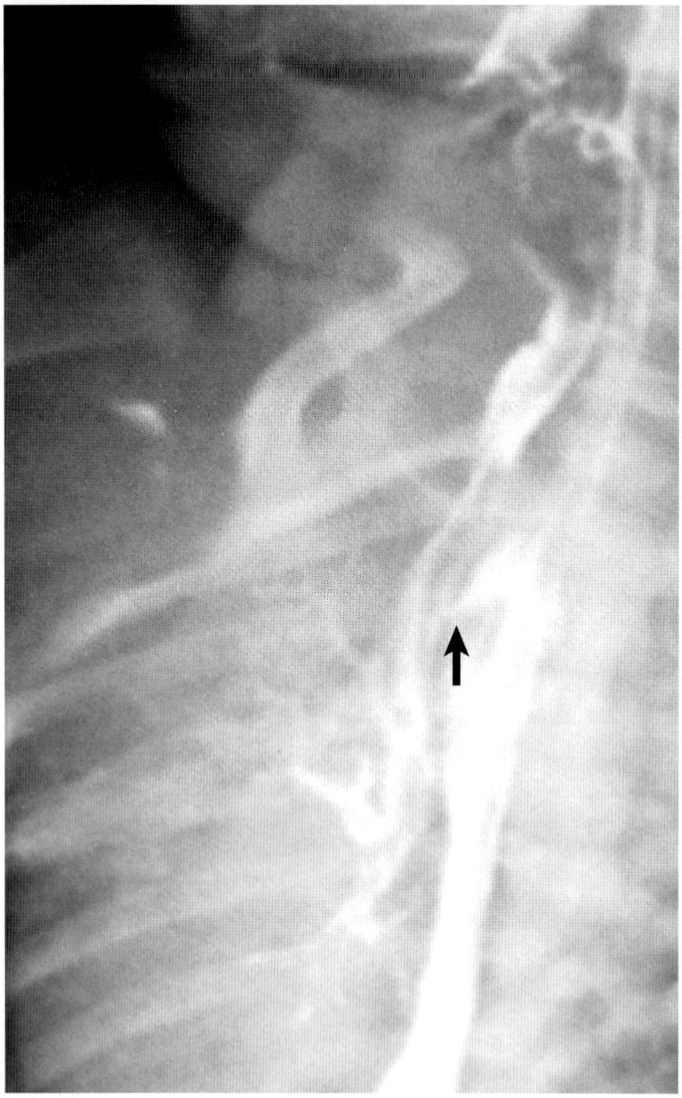

Fig. 64.5 Tracheoesophageal fistula in an infant with respiratory difficulty after feeding. Esophagram shows a fistula *(arrow)* between the trachea and the middle esophageal segment. Note contrast within the right lower lobe bronchi.

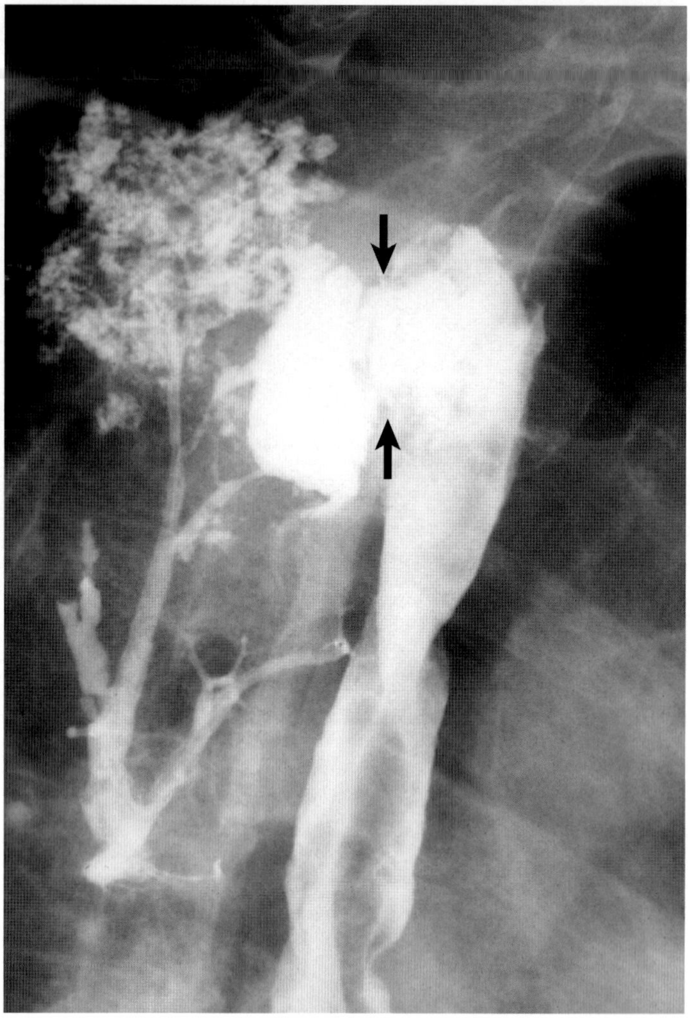

Fig. 64.6 Postradiation pulmonary esophageal fistula in a man with advanced esophageal carcinoma. Esophagram reveals a fistula *(arrows)* between the esophagus and the lung parenchyma. Note the retrograde alveolar filling by contrast material.

pneumonia, or ARDS. Water-soluble nonionic contrast medium may be the cause of significant morbidity but does not cause intense chemical pneumonitis as occurs with aspirated ionic water-soluble contrast media.

Acute aspiration of volatile hydrocarbons may cause a chemical pneumonitis. Most cases of hydrocarbon pneumonia are related to accidental poisoning in children. Adult fire-eaters use liquid hydrocarbons, such as petroleum, for the performance of the flame-blowing part of the show. For flame blowing, the performer blows out a mouthful of liquid hydrocarbon against a burning stick, thus creating an aerosol that catches fire around the stick.[67,68] This entity is rare but easily diagnosed on the basis of clinical history. A relatively common late complication of hydrocarbon aspiration is the development of pneumatoceles.[68]

CLINICAL PRESENTATION

The characteristic clinical presentation of gastric acid pneumonitis is abrupt in onset, with dyspnea, cyanosis or arterial hypoxemia, low-grade fever, rales, and opacities on chest radiography. The clinical course is variable. In a retrospective study of 50 patients with gastric acid pneumonitis, 12% of the patients died shortly after aspiration, 62% had rapid clinical and radiologic improvement (mean time, 4.5 days), and 26% demonstrated rapid improvement but then had clinical and radiographic progression associated with recovery of bacterial pathogens from the sputum and a fatal outcome in more than 60%. Long-term follow-up studies demonstrate either complete recovery or radiographic evidence of pulmonary fibrosis.[69]

PATHOLOGIC FINDINGS

The pathologic changes of chemical lung injury include focal and confluent areas of edema with protein-rich fluid in the alveolar spaces, hyaline membrane formation, and denudation of the alveolar epithelium. Diffuse alveolar damage (i.e., ARDS) after severe acute chemical injury is nonspecific and indistinguishable to that of other etiologies.

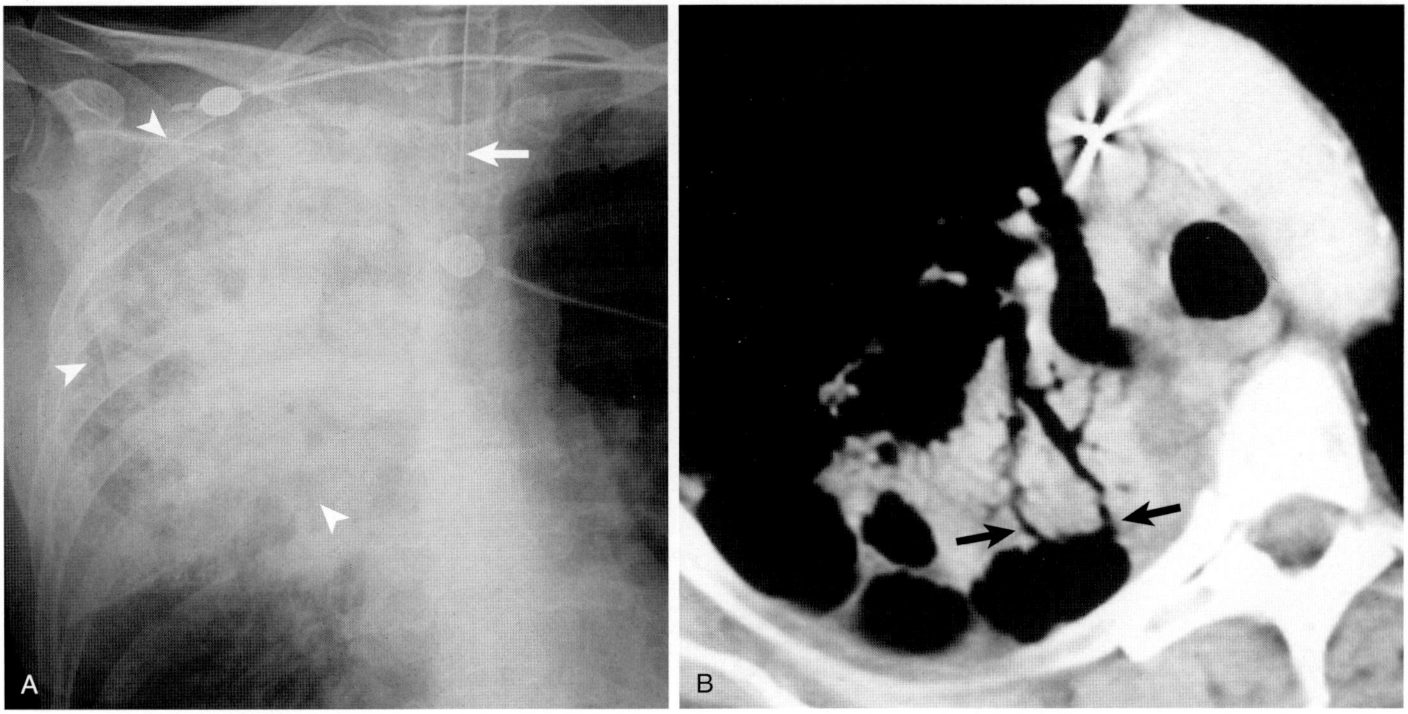

Fig. 64.7 Acute aspiration pneumonia in a man with fever and putrid sputum who aspirated a large amount of vomitus. (A) Anteroposterior chest radiograph shows extensive heterogeneous right upper lobe consolidation *(arrowheads)*. Note endotracheal tube *(arrow)*. (B) Close-up view of the corresponding CT demonstrates multiple bronchopleural fistulas *(arrows)* likely from necrotizing pneumonia.

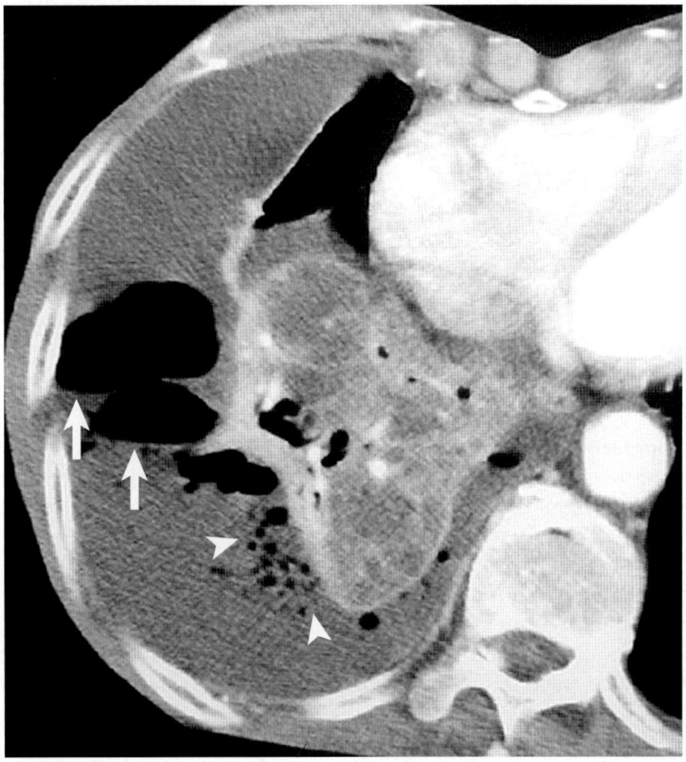

Fig. 64.8 A man with aspiration pneumonia, fever, and chest pain. Contrast-enhanced CT demonstrates right lower lobe heterogeneous consolidation and a large empyema containing air-fluid levels *(arrows)*, scattered air bubbles *(arrowheads)*, and enhancing visceral pleural thickening.

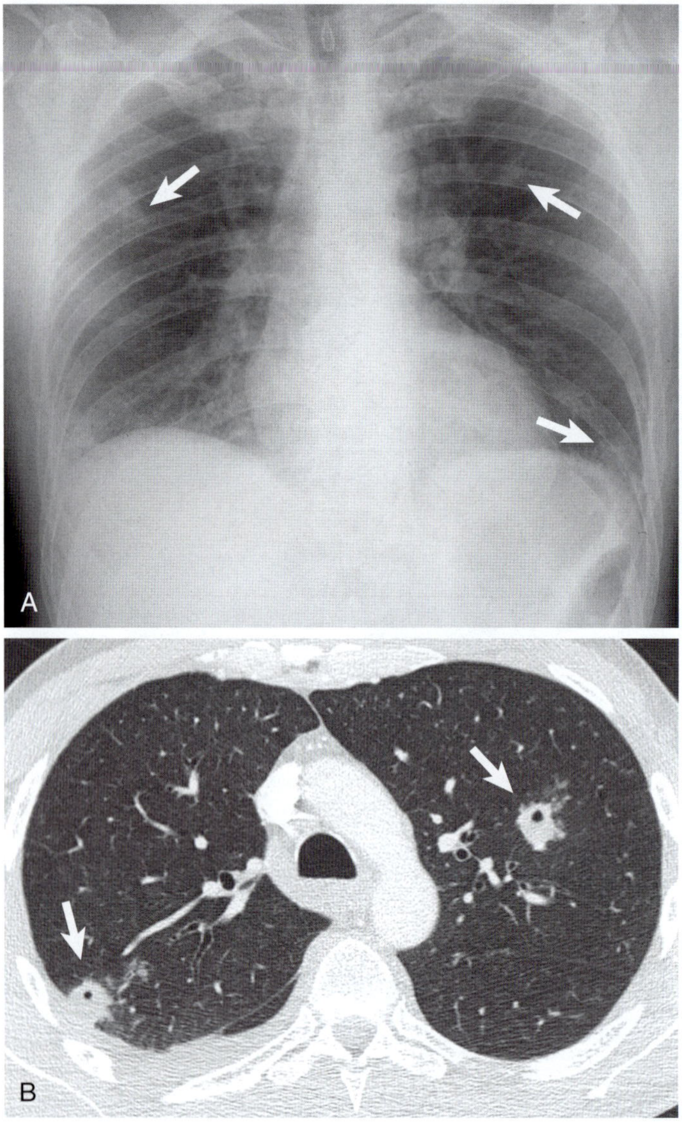

Fig. 64.9 An alcoholic with fever, putrid sputum, and pyorrhea. (A) Anteroposterior chest radiograph shows bilateral ill-defined nodules *(arrows)*. (B) Axial CT demonstrates multiple cavitated nodules *(arrows)*. A small right pleural effusion is also visible.

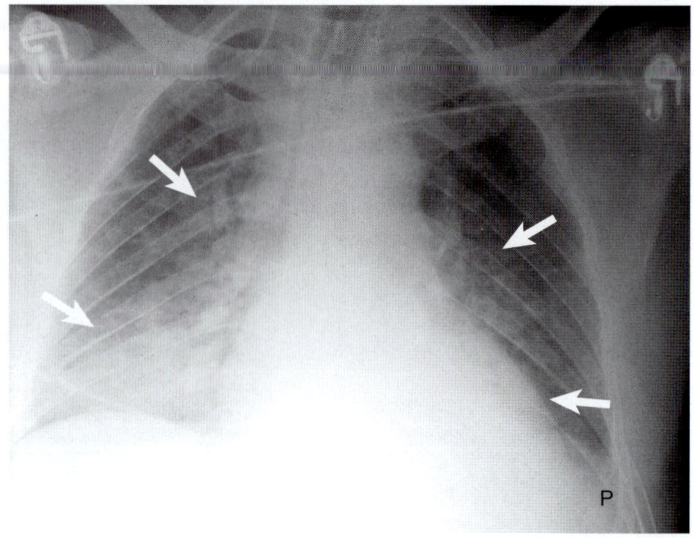

Fig. 64.10 Acute aspiration pneumonia in a woman with intestinal obstruction. Anteroposterior chest radiograph performed 8 hours after aspiration shows extensive bilateral consolidation *(arrows)* and a left pleural effusion (P).

MANIFESTATIONS OF THE DISEASE

Radiography

The characteristic radiographic appearance of acute pure gastric acid aspiration is that of bilateral perihilar ill-defined consolidation. The normal size of the heart and the absence of signs of pulmonary venous hypertension help differentiate this form of edema from that of cardiac origin. (Fig. 64.10). Radiographic changes may worsen for several days in uncomplicated cases, but improvement is generally manifested within the first week after aspiration.[70] Worsening of opacities after initial improvement suggests development of superimposed bacterial pneumonia, ARDS, or pulmonary embolism.[70]

In hydrocarbon aspiration, chest radiograph shows scattered pulmonary opacities that are almost invariably bilateral with middle and lower lung zone predominance.[68] Although consolidations tend to clear over the next few days, formation of pneumatoceles may also occur (Fig. 64.11).[68] Hydrocarbon aspiration may be complicated with the development of a bronchopleural fistula and spontaneous pyopneumothorax.[68]

Aspiration of barium results in a characteristic appearance of high-density material in the dependent lung regions (Fig. 64.12).

Computed Tomography

The CT manifestations of acute aspiration of sterile gastric contents consist of dependent areas of consolidation and ground-glass opacities, frequently associated with poorly defined centrilobular nodules resulting from chemical bronchiolitis and peribronchiolar inflammation. Aspiration of large amounts of gastric acid may result in extensive ground-glass opacities and, commonly, superimposed linear intralobular opacities and smooth septal thickening consistent with diffuse alveolar damage.

Aspiration of Inert and Nontoxic Fluids

ASPIRATION OF WATER (DROWNING)

Drowning has been described as the process of experiencing respiratory impairment from submersion/immersion in liquid.[71] Drowning accidents account for an estimated 7000 to 8000 deaths in the United States annually. It represents a major cause of accidental death at all ages, being the second leading cause of injury-related death in children younger than 10 years and the third leading cause of unintentional injury-related death among adults younger than 60 years.[72–76] Drowning accounts for more than one-half million deaths annually worldwide. This number is probably a gross underestimate because of underreporting.[76]

The acute aspiration of massive quantities of either fresh- or saltwater produces pulmonary edema that radiographically is indistinguishable from pulmonary edema of other etiologies. The clinical significance is more closely related to the volume than to whether the aspirate is freshwater or saltwater.[77,78] However,

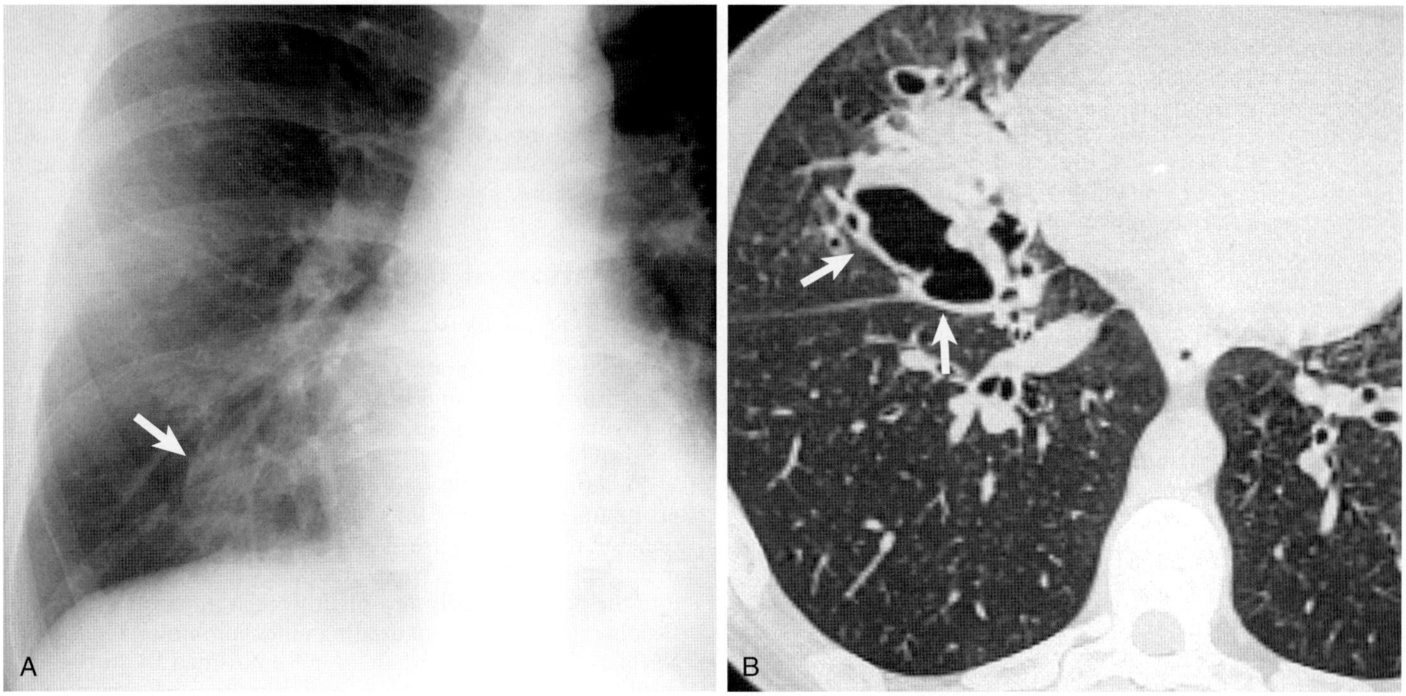

Fig. 64.11 Fire-eaters' lung in a young man after aspiration of petroleum. (A) Close-up posteroanterior chest radiograph during the acute phase shows focal consolidation *(arrow)* in the right lung base consistent with aspiration pneumonia. (B) Follow-up CT 3 weeks later shows a postinflammatory pneumatocele *(arrows)* in the right middle lobe.

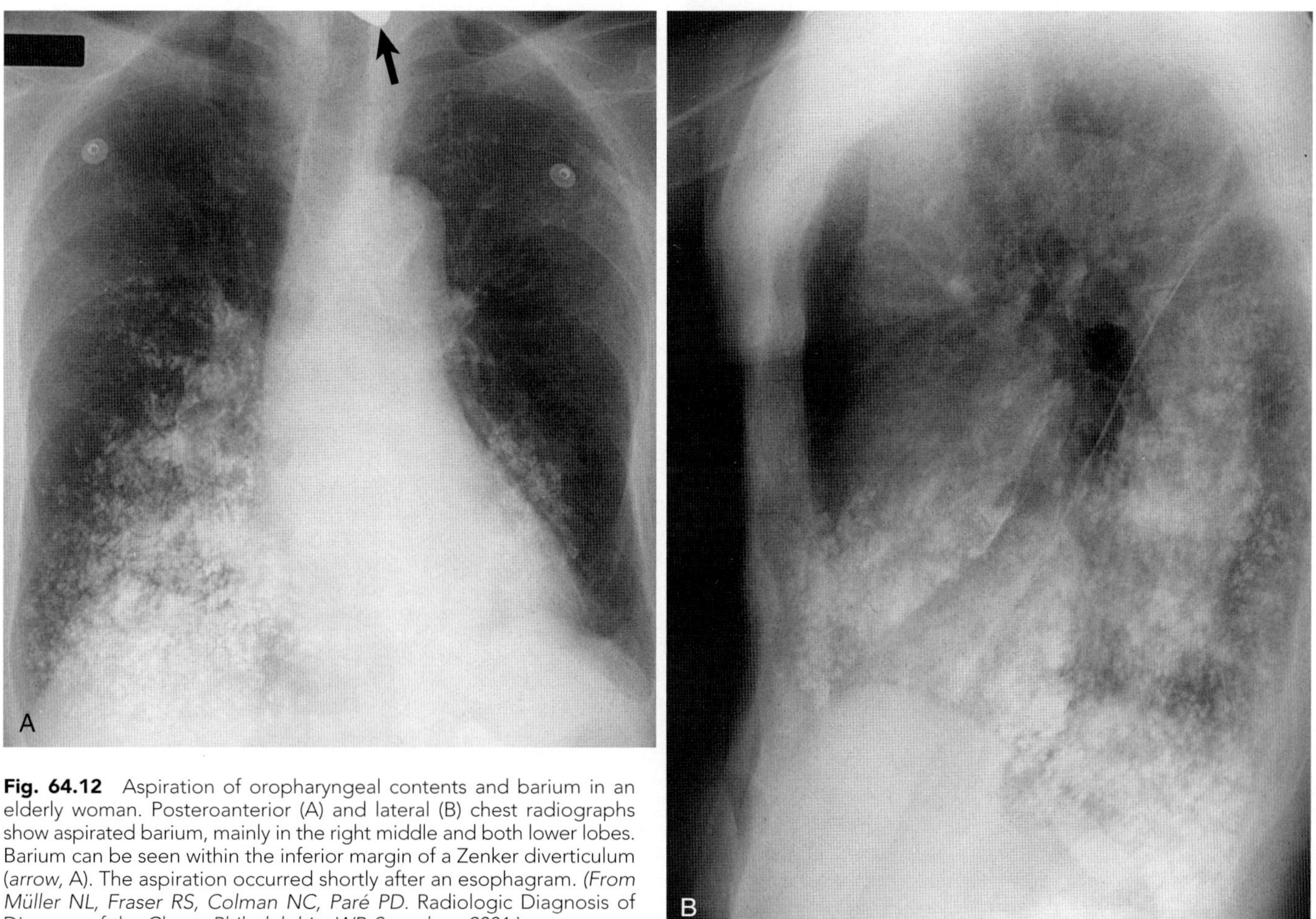

Fig. 64.12 Aspiration of oropharyngeal contents and barium in an elderly woman. Posteroanterior (A) and lateral (B) chest radiographs show aspirated barium, mainly in the right middle and both lower lobes. Barium can be seen within the inferior margin of a Zenker diverticulum (*arrow*, A). The aspiration occurred shortly after an esophagram. *(From Müller NL, Fraser RS, Colman NC, Paré PD.* Radiologic Diagnosis of Diseases of the Chest. *Philadelphia: WB Saunders; 2001.)*

aspiration of water increases the risk of pneumonia, particularly when contaminated.[79] Aspirated seawater causes alveolar edema by exerting an osmotic effect that draws free water into the lungs and by causing irritant damage to alveolar epithelial cells, increasing their permeability. Aspiration of freshwater is thought to cause a loss of surfactant, leading to alveolar instability, but it also causes damage to epithelial and endothelial cells, disrupting the integrity of the gas exchange barrier. Clearance of aspirated fresh water can be very rapid from otherwise normal alveoli.

The radiographic findings in severe near-drowning are alveolar edema with extensive bilateral fluffy densities that tend to coalesce throughout both lungs. However, in mild drowning, chest radiographic findings range from normal to confluent irregular perihilar densities of subsegmental or segmental distribution with peripheral sparing (Figs. 64.13 and 64.14). Pneumonia may complicate the aspiration of fresh- or saltwater and, depending on the water source, may be caused by a variety of microorganisms, including bacteria, fungi, and mycobacteria. The aspiration of mud, sand, and aquatic vegetation has been reported in 60% of episodes; sand bronchograms and sand within the maxillary sinuses and stomach may be seen on CT.[77,80] Hypoxia, pulmonary edema, acidosis, and aspiration comprise the syndrome of near-drowning.

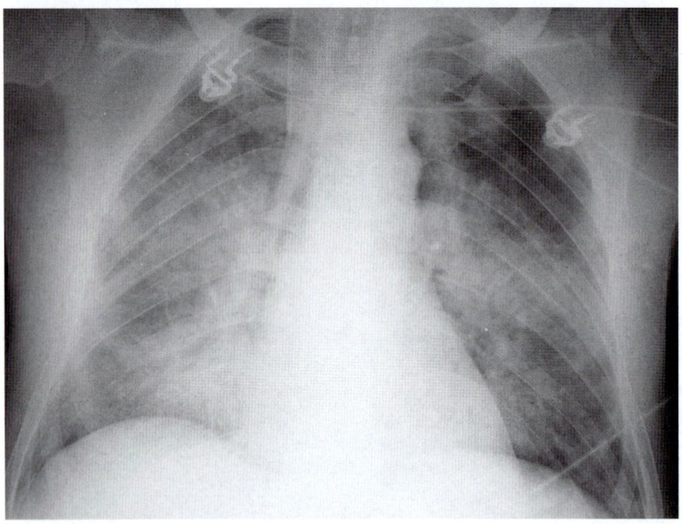

Fig. 64.13 Near-drowning in a middle-aged man. Anteroposterior chest radiograph taken in the intensive care unit shows diffuse bilateral opacities most consistent with pulmonary edema.

Aspiration of Lipids

ETIOLOGY, PREVALENCE, AND EPIDEMIOLOGY

Chronic exogenous lipoid pneumonia is an uncommon pulmonary disorder that results from repetitive aspiration or inhalation of fat-like material of animal, vegetable, or mineral origin into the distal lung.

In adults the most common cause of exogenous lipoid pneumonia is the use of mineral oil for the treatment of constipation and the frequent use of oily nose drops for chronic rhinitis, mainly at bedtime.[81,82] These mineral oil substances introduced into the nose can easily and silently reach the bronchial tree of sleeping patients without exciting reflex inhibition. Once in the alveolar spaces, oily substances are emulsified by lung lipase, resulting in a foreign-body reaction.[81] In the appropriate clinical setting the diagnosis may be supported by bronchoalveolar lavage or transbronchial biopsy or both.

CLINICAL PRESENTATION

In most cases of mineral oil aspiration the patient remains asymptomatic, and the pulmonary lesion is discovered serendipitously.

PATHOLOGY

The characteristic histologic findings consists of numerous lipid-laden macrophages that fill and distend the alveolar walls and interstitium, where they may be associated with accumulation of lipid material, inflammatory cellular infiltration, and variable

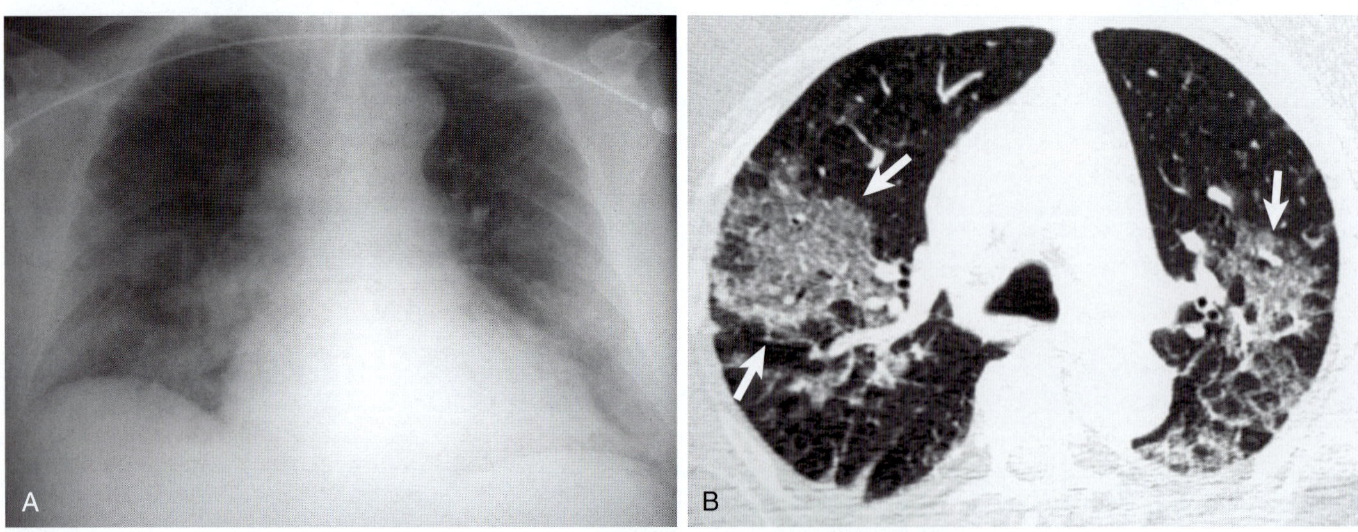

Fig. 64.14 Near-drowning in saltwater. (A) Anteroposterior chest radiograph taken within a few hours of near-drowning shows perihilar- and basal-predominant opacities in keeping with pulmonary edema. (B) Axial CT shows bilateral patchy areas of ground-glass opacity *(arrows)* associated with intralobular lines and septal thickening.

amounts of fibrosis.[81] Lipoid pneumonia in children is usually caused by aspiration of cod liver oil and milk.[83]

MANIFESTATIONS OF THE DISEASE

Radiography

The radiographic findings are nonspecific and include single or multiple areas of consolidation. The appearance may mimic a bronchogenic carcinoma manifesting as a spiculated nodule or mass.

Computed Tomography

CT is the method of choice in establishing the diagnosis of lipoid pneumonia, frequently demonstrating focal areas of fat density (−30 to −120 Hounsfield units) (Figs. 64.15 and 64.16), although many cases do not demonstrate this specific finding (Fig. 64.17).[84–87] On occasion, exogenous lipoid pneumonia may result in a crazy paving pattern on high-resolution CT (HRCT) scans (Fig. 64.18)[81] similar to that seen in other conditions, such as pulmonary hemorrhage, pulmonary edema, infections, alveolar proteinosis,[62] and some types of lung adenocarcinomas.[88]

Aspiration of Foreign Bodies

ETIOLOGY, PREVALENCE, AND EPIDEMIOLOGY

Aspirated foreign bodies are by far the most common cause of intraluminal airway abnormality in children of all ages, although most occurrences are in children younger than 4 years.[3,20,89–91] Most inhaled foreign bodies are food and broken fragments of teeth that frequently lodge in a main or lobar bronchus.[89,90] Clinically, most patients are children with varying degrees of cough and a recent history of foreign-body aspiration. In most cases radiologic manifestations include obstructive lobar or segmental overinflation or atelectasis (Figs. 64.19 and 64.20). Diagnosis requires careful integration of clinical data and radiographic findings, and a definitive diagnosis is usually made by conventional neck and chest radiographs and bronchoscopy.[91] CT is far more sensitive than chest radiography at demonstrating radiolucent foreign bodies.[92,93] In some cases CT may provide additional diagnostic information, showing subtle low-density intrabronchial material that is often the only finding that can help suggest the diagnosis (Fig. 64.21).[92,93] Although aspiration of a foreign body is diagnosed immediately or within 2 to 3 days of the event in the majority of pediatric patients, on occasion the diagnosis may not be made for weeks or sometimes even months.[94] Once a foreign body is within the lung parenchyma, prolonged irritation with intermittent infections may cause massive hemoptysis.[90]

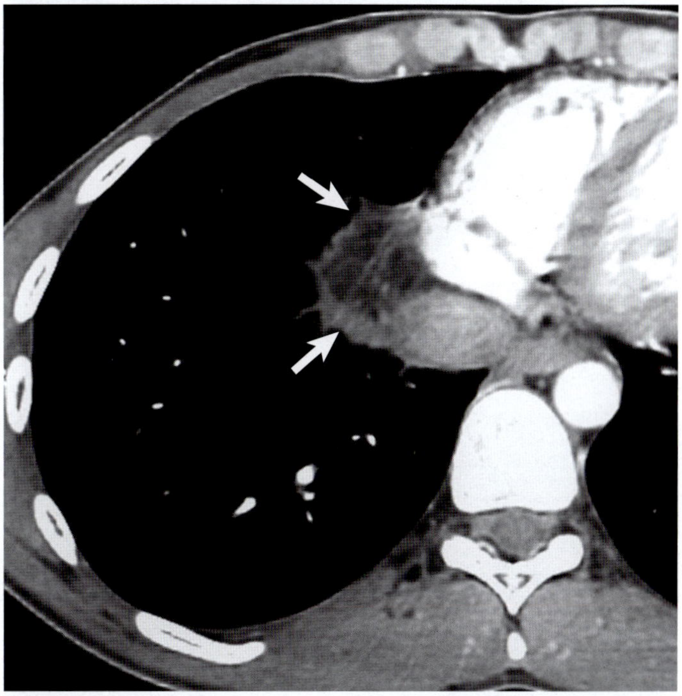

Fig. 64.15 Exogenous lipoid pneumonia in a man with cough. Thin-section CT shows focal consolidation in the middle lobe containing intrinsic fat attenuation *(arrows)*, which is diagnostic of lipoid pneumonia.

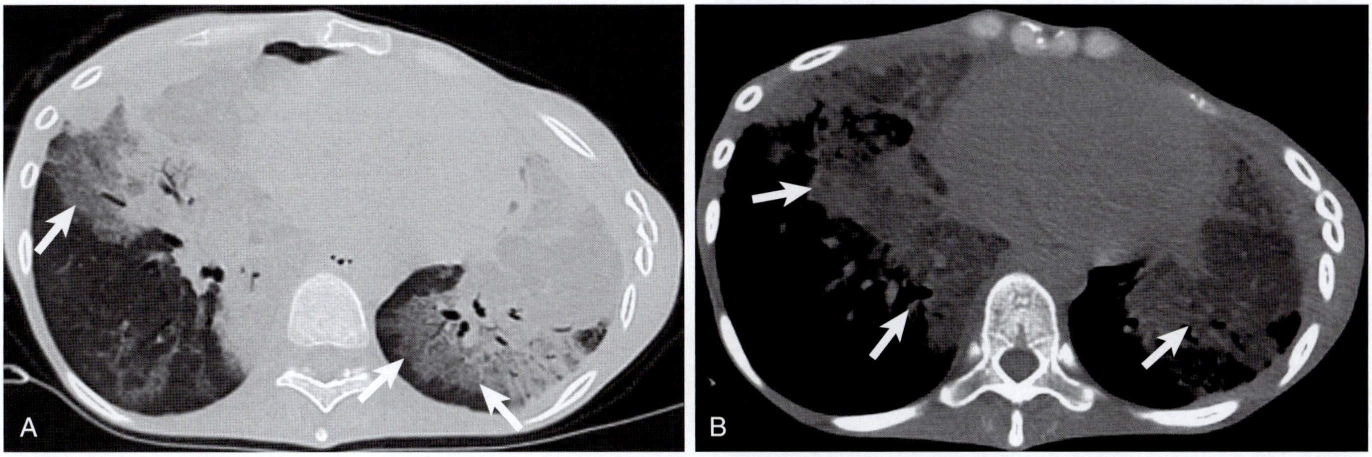

Fig. 64.16 Young woman with a history of chronic laxative use and self-induced vomiting. (A) Axial CT in lung windows shows patchy bilateral ground-glass opacities *(arrows)*, consolidation and thickened interlobular septa in both lower lobes. Ground-glass opacities in conjunction with septal thickening has been termed *crazy paving*. (B) Axial CT in soft tissue windows shows multiple bilateral areas of consolidation with fat attenuation values (−40 Hounsfield units) *(arrows)*. These findings are characteristic of exogenous lipoid pneumonia. *(Courtesy Alberto Hidalgo, MD.)*

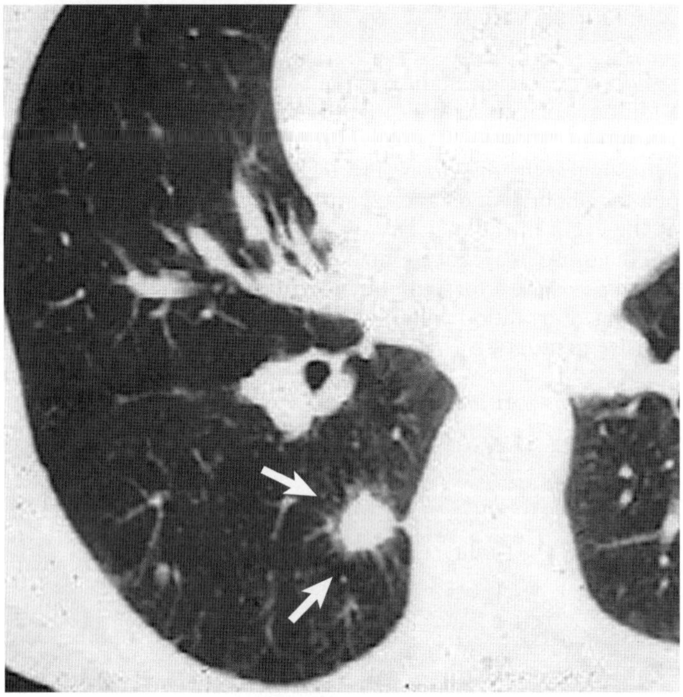

Fig. 64.17 Middle-aged man with hemoptysis. Close-up view of an axial CT shows a spiculated nodule *(arrows)* in the right lower lobe. A bronchogenic carcinoma was suspected. Surgery revealed an exogenous lipoid pneumonia.

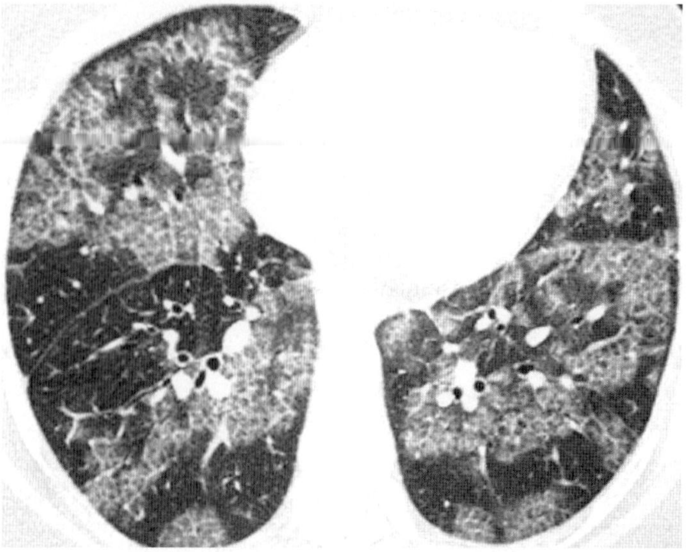

Fig. 64.18 Exogenous lipoid pneumonia in a woman with mild dyspnea. High-resolution CT scan through lung bases shows patchy areas of ground-glass opacities and superimposed fine reticulation resulting in a crazy paving pattern.

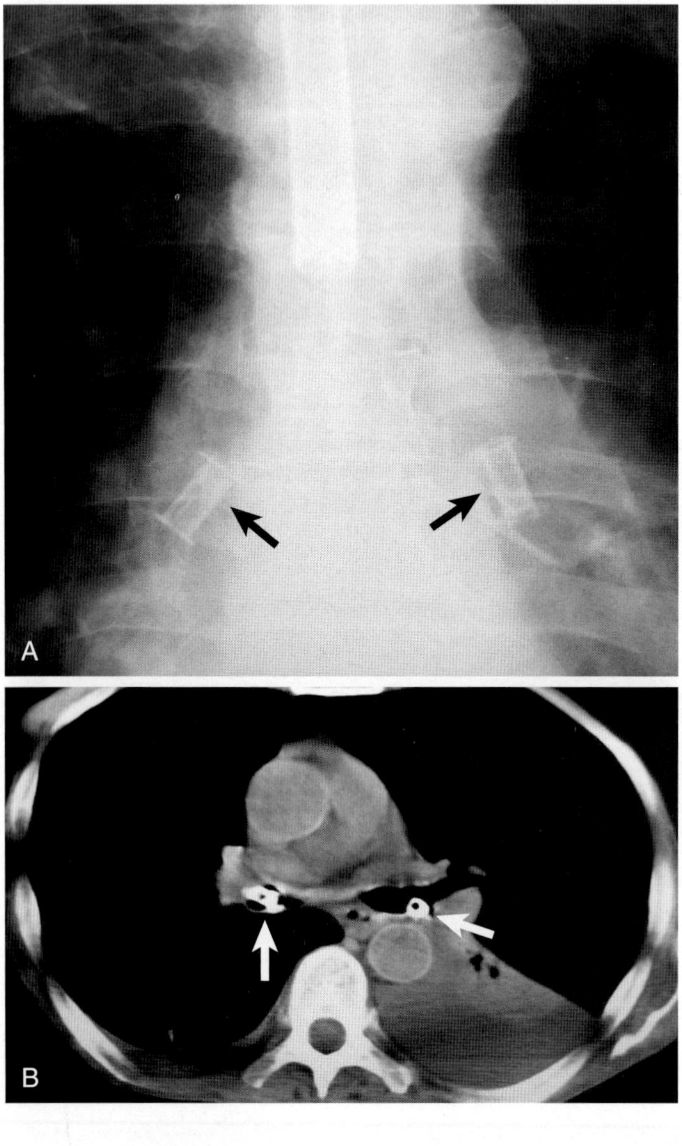

Fig. 64.19 Aspiration of multiple esophageal speech devices in a mentally impaired man who had previously had a radical laryngectomy. (A) A close-up view of the chest radiograph shows two esophageal speech devices *(arrows)* in the bronchus intermedius and left lower bronchus. (B) Noncontrast CT nicely depicts the intrabronchial devices *(arrows)*. Note associated left lower lobe collapse and small pleural effusions.

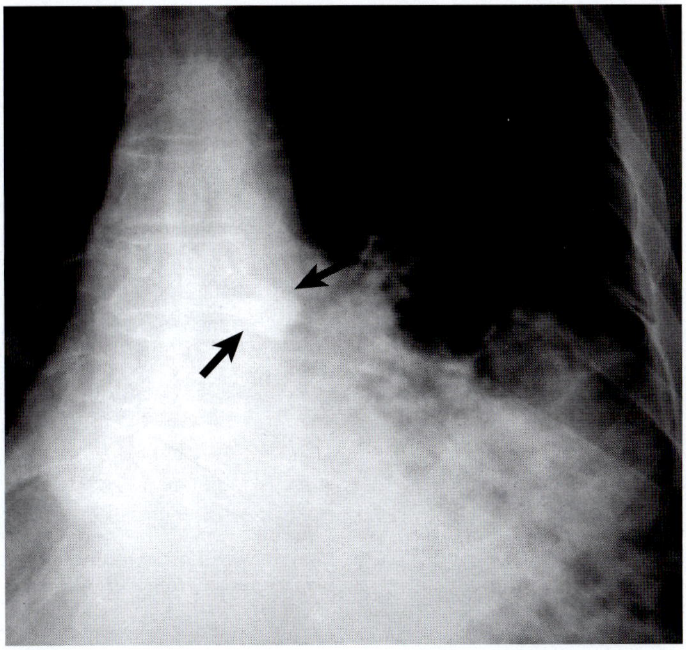

Fig. 64.20 Aspiration of a tooth. This elderly man developed recurrent episodes of infection in the left lower lobe after inadvertent aspiration of a tooth. Close-up view of a chest radiograph shows an endobronchial tooth *(arrows)* and multiple rounded lucencies in the left lower lung representing postobstructive bronchiectasis.

Foreign-body aspiration is unusual in adults and is often overlooked as a cause of airway obstruction.[3] Although the condition is often clinically silent, life-threatening hemoptysis may develop.[3,92] The radiologic manifestations are nonspecific and include a chronic loss of volume in the affected lobe, recurrent pneumonias, and the development of bronchiectasis.[89,90] On occasion the development of a chronic inflammatory reaction around the inhaled material may lead to intrabronchial mass formation. In such cases a foreign body can manifest on chest radiography or CT scans as a centrally located mass with lobar or segmental collapse that mimics a bronchogenic carcinoma.[3]

Aspiration Bronchiolitis

Diffuse aspiration bronchiolitis is a disease entity characterized by chronic inflammatory reaction to recurrent aspirated foreign particles in the bronchioles.[95] Patients with esophageal conditions, such as achalasia, Zenker diverticulum, or esophageal carcinoma, are at risk for aspiration bronchiolitis.[96,97] These patients often develop moderate to marked dilatation of the esophagus with associated symptoms, such as dysphagia, regurgitation, and aspiration. The radiographic findings are nonspecific and include lobar, segmental, or disseminated small nodular shadows. HRCT demonstrates unilateral or bilateral centrilobular nodular and branching opacities (tree-in-bud pattern) (Fig. 64.22) and 5- to 10-mm-diameter poorly defined airspace nodules.[98] On radiographic and pathologic examination, diffuse aspiration bronchiolitis may resemble diffuse panbronchiolitis. Complete healing of bronchiolar inflammation may occur.

Chronic pulmonary microaspiration, defined as the recurrent subclinical aspiration of small droplets of gastric contents or foreign particles into the lungs, may result in a variety of complications, including aspiration pneumonitis, aspiration pneumonia, and aspiration bronchiolitis.[99] CT manifestations consist of centrilobular nodules and ground-glass opacities that tend to involve predominantly the dependent regions.[99] Chronic pulmonary microaspiration must be suspected in those patients with chronic cough and presence of risk factors for aspiration.

Gastroesophageal Reflux and Constrictive Bronchiolitis

A significant number of patients with chronic bronchitis have gastrointestinal reflux,[64] and there is some evidence to suggest an association between reflux and asthma.[50] Intermittent aspiration may cause mucosal injury of bronchioles and possibly result in airflow obstruction. Gastroesophageal reflux and aspiration have been considered predisposing factors to the development of constrictive bronchiolitis (synonym: obliterative bronchiolitis). HRCT findings of constrictive bronchiolitis include focal areas of decreased attenuation and vascularity, bronchial dilatation, and air-trapping.[98] Air-trapping and bronchial dilatation appear to be the most sensitive and specific findings in patients with constrictive bronchiolitis (Fig. 64.23). Given the probable association between hiatal hernias and esophageal dysmotility, the presence of hiatal hernias and diffuse esophageal dilation on imaging should be specifically commented upon in patients with suspicion for recurrent aspiration.

Synopsis of Treatment Options

The most important consideration is prevention. The most important preventive measures in patients with impaired consciousness or other predisposing factors include the semirecumbent position, surveillance of enteral feeding, and avoidance of excessive sedation. Patients with suspected aspiration pneumonia are treated with antibiotics. Aspiration pneumonitis does not require antibiotic treatment. Inhaled foreign bodies usually require removal by bronchoscopy.

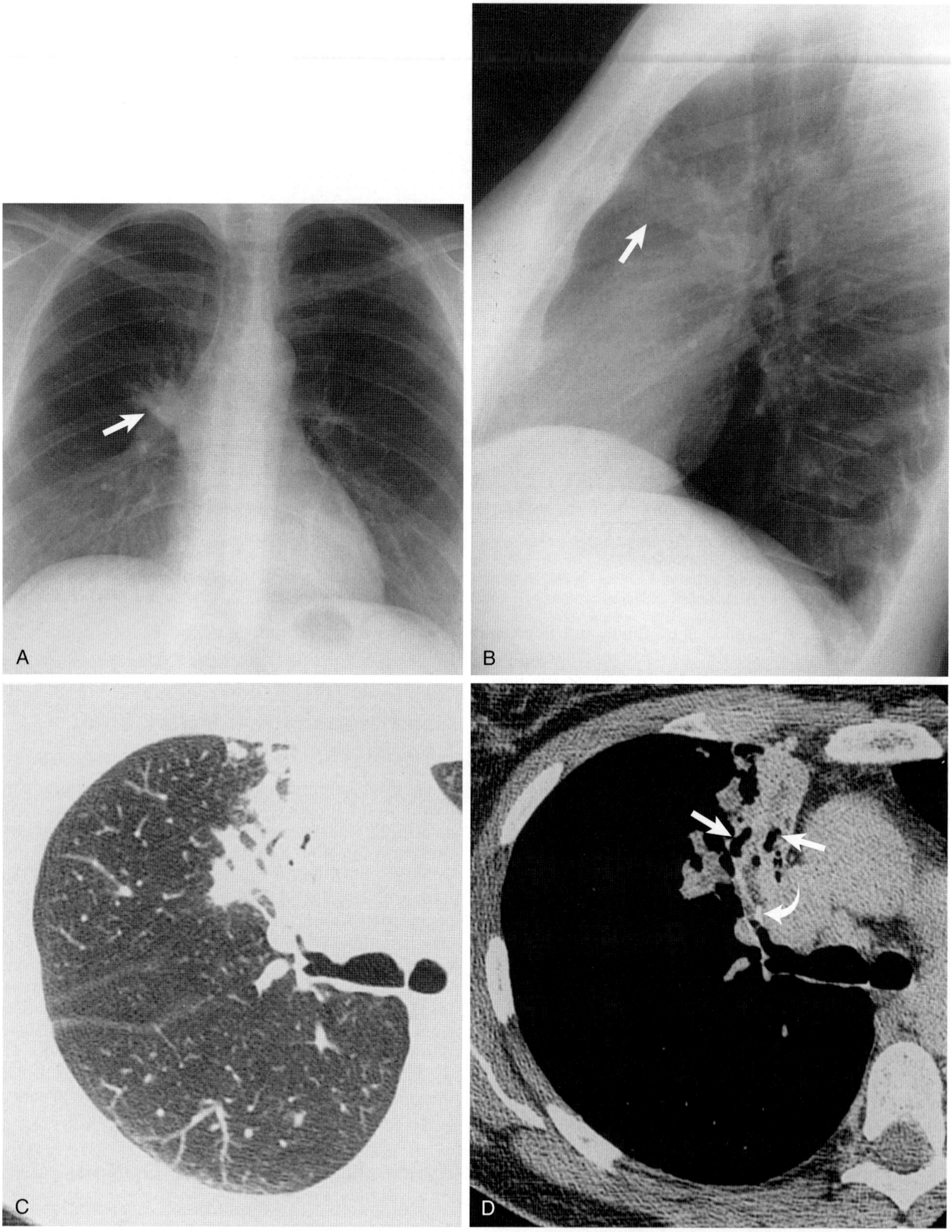

Fig. 64.21 Obstructive pneumonitis caused by foreign-body aspiration in a middle-aged woman. Posteroanterior (A) and lateral (B) chest radiographs show localized consolidation and atelectasis involving the anterior segment of the right upper lobe *(arrows)*. High-resolution CT (C and D) shows evidence of obstructive pneumonitis and bronchiectasis (*straight arrows*, D) in the anterior segment of the right upper lobe. The localized area of high attenuation (*curved arrow*, D) within the bronchial lumen represents an aspirated popcorn kernel. *(From Müller NL, Fraser RS, Colman NC, Paré PD.* Radiologic Diagnosis of Diseases of the Chest. *Philadelphia: WB Saunders; 2001.)*

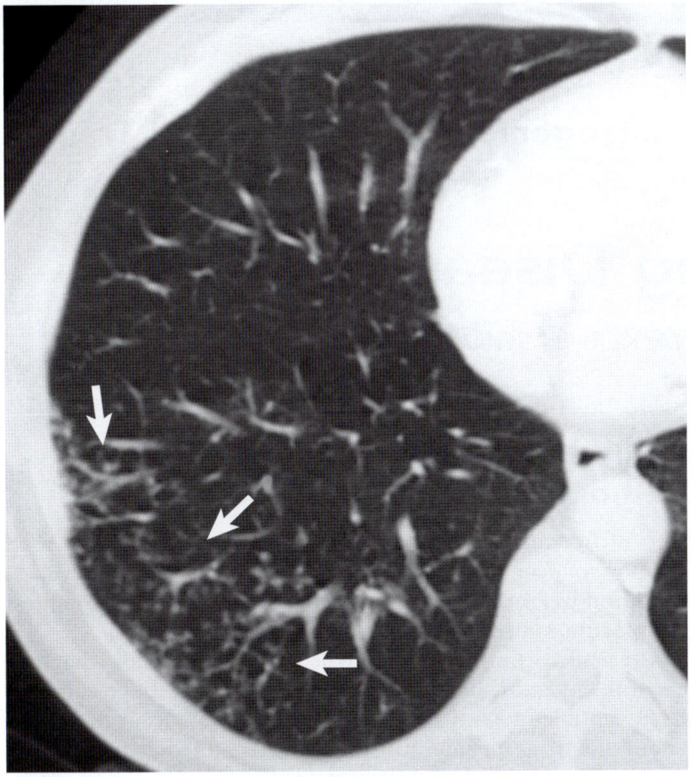

Fig. 64.22 Cellular bronchiolitis in a young woman with recurrent aspiration. High-resolution CT obtained at the level of the lung bases shows centrilobular branching and linear opacities resulting in a "tree-in-bud" appearance *(arrows)*, typical of infectious or aspiration bronchiolitis.

KEY POINTS: PULMONARY ASPIRATION

- Conditions associated with increased risk of pulmonary aspiration include old age (>70 years), alcoholism, loss of consciousness (stroke), structural abnormalities of the pharynx and esophagus, neuromuscular disorders, and deglutition abnormalities.
- Types of aspiration
  - Aspiration pneumonia: pulmonary infection caused by aspiration of colonized oropharyngeal secretions
  - Aspiration pneumonitis (chemical pneumonia): acute lung injury caused by the aspiration of materials inherently toxic to the lungs, such as gastric acid, milk, mineral oil, and volatile hydrocarbons
  - Aspiration of inert and nontoxic fluids: acute lung injury caused by the aspiration of inert fluids, such as water, saline, and barium
  - Aspiration of lipids
  - Aspiration of foreign bodies
- Pulmonary complications caused by aspiration usually involve the posterior segment of the upper lobes or the superior segment of the lower lobes.
- The radiographic findings most commonly consist of patchy areas of consolidation. Abscess or empyema may develop.
- Esophagram is the imaging modality of choice to demonstrate the presence of tracheoesophageal fistula.
- CT is the modality of choice in establishing the diagnosis of exogenous lipoid pneumonia, which can result from aspiration of mineral oil or a related substance.

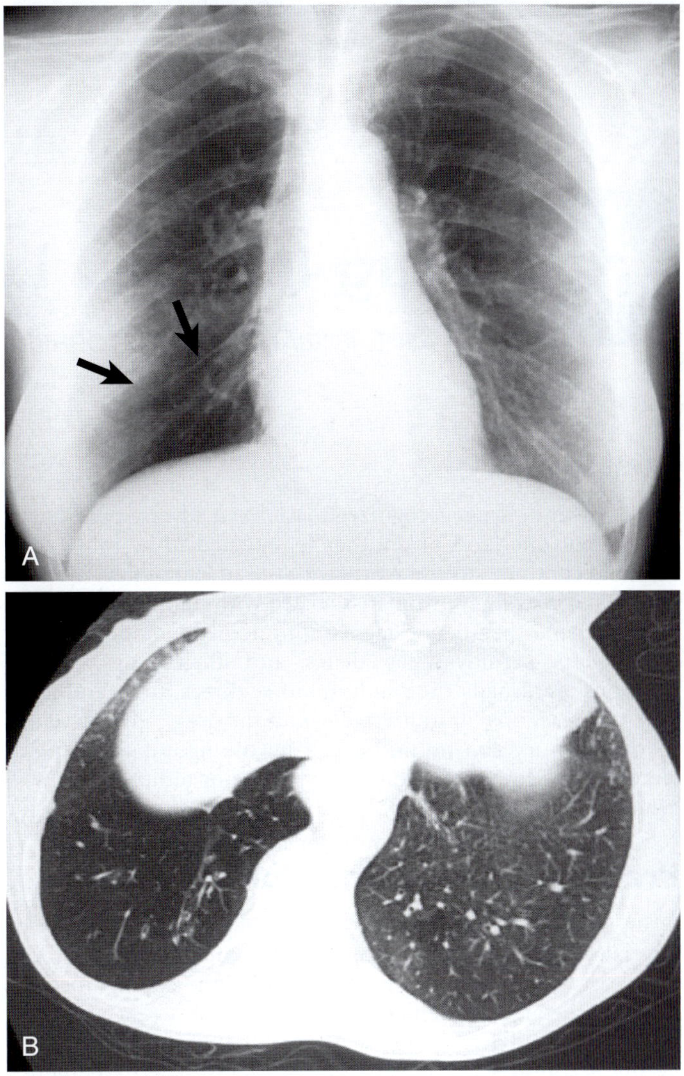

Fig. 64.23 Gastric aspiration and constrictive bronchiolitis in a woman with achalasia. (A) Posteroanterior chest radiograph shows a hyperlucent right lower lung zone with associated loss of volume and a reduced number of lung vessels *(arrows)*. (B) Expiratory CT shows a hyperlucent right lower lobe with a reduced size and number of vessels. These findings correlate with the presence of localized small airway disease (air-trapping).

SUGGESTED READINGS

DiBardino DM, Wunderink RG. Aspiration pneumonia: a review of modern trends. *J Crit Care*. 2015;30(1):40–48.

Franquet T, Gimenez A, Roson N, Torrubia S, Sabate JM, Perez C. Aspiration diseases: findings, pitfalls, and differential diagnosis. *Radiographics*. 2000;20(3):673–685.

Marik PE. Pulmonary aspiration syndromes. *Curr Opin Pulm Med*. 2011;17(3):148–154.

Pereira-Silva JL, Silva CI, Araujo Neto CA, Andrade TL, Müller NL. Chronic pulmonary microaspiration: high-resolution computed tomographic findings in 13 patients. *J Thorac Imaging*. 2014;29(5):298–303.

The full reference list for this chapter is available at ExpertConsult.com.

65 Drug-Induced Lung Disease*

SARAH T. KURIAN | CHRISTOPHER M. WALKER | JONATHAN H. CHUNG

Etiology

The number of drugs recognized to cause an adverse pulmonary reaction of one kind or another is reported to be more than 600[1] and continues to rise yearly with the advent of new medications. Pharmacologic groups associated with pulmonary toxicity include chemotherapeutic agents, antimicrobials, antiinflammatory agents, cardiovascular drugs, and illicit drugs.[2,3] Drug reactions are usually the result of either direct (toxic and idiosyncratic reactions) or indirect effects of the drug.[4,5] The development of injury can be influenced by the age of the patient, concomitant administration of oxygen, prior radiotherapy, and synergism with other drugs.[6]

Prevalence and Epidemiology

Drug therapy is common and may result in a great variety of adverse effects. In 2006 82% of the US population reported use of at least one prescription medication, over-the-counter medication, or dietary supplement in the previous week, and 29% reported use of five or more of these drugs.[7,8] Adverse drug events accounted for 1.7% to 2.5% of estimated emergency department (ED) visits for all unintentional injuries,[9] with 27.3% of these ED visits resulting in hospitalization in 2013 and 2014.[10] Individuals aged 65 years or older were twice as likely than younger individuals to develop adverse drug events.[11] The majority of adverse drug effects are dermatologic, gastrointestinal, and neurologic. Respiratory complications are estimated to account for approximately 54,000 adverse drug events in the United States per year or approximately 7.7% of all adverse drug events.[11] Drug reactions are even more common in inpatients. One English study showed that nearly 1 in 7 hospital inpatients experience an adverse drug reaction.[12] Fatal drug reactions occur in 0.1% of medical inpatients and 0.01% of surgical inpatients.[13] The prevalence of drug-induced lung disease varies considerably among different drugs, ranging from approximately 1 in 100,000 treatments for nitrofurantoin to more than 40% in women who receive nitrosourea-based chemotherapy for the treatment of breast cancer.[14] The estimated prevalence rate of pulmonary reactions for each drug can be found on the Pneumotox website (http://www.pneumotox.com).

*The editors and the publisher would like to thank Drs. C. Isabela Silva Müller and Nestor L. Müller for contributing material on this topic to the prior edition of this work. It has served as the foundation for the current chapter.

Clinical Presentation and Pathophysiology

The most common clinical manifestations of patients with pulmonary drug reaction are cough, dyspnea, fatigue, fever, chest pain, and weight loss. Drug-induced lung disease may manifest as an acute, subacute, or chronic process.

Adverse reactions to drugs can be classified into those that may occur in any individual taking the drug and those that occur only in susceptible individuals.[13] Reactions that may occur in anyone taking the drug include drug side effect, defined as undesirable pharmacologic effect at recommended doses; drug interaction, defined as action of a drug on the effectiveness or toxicity of another one; and drug overdose. These drug reactions are predictable and account for at least 80% of adverse drug reactions.[15] Reactions that occur only in susceptible individuals include drug intolerance, defined as a threshold to the normal pharmacologic action of a drug; drug idiosyncrasy, defined as a genetically determined, qualitatively abnormal reaction to a drug related to a metabolic or enzyme deficiency; and drug allergy, defined as an immunologically mediated reaction, characterized by specificity, transferability by antibodies or lymphocytes, and recurrence on reexposure.[13] An example of an allergic respiratory drug reaction is asthma, most commonly caused by aspirin and nonsteroidal antiinflammatory drugs.[13] Allergic drug reactions, however, account for less than 10% of adverse pulmonary drug reactions.[15] The pathogenesis of most pulmonary drug reactions is unknown.[15]

The histologic findings of pulmonary drug reactions are often nonspecific and mimic those of various acute and chronic lung diseases.[3,16] The most common histologic patterns are diffuse alveolar damage, nonspecific interstitial pneumonia, organizing pneumonia, eosinophilic pneumonia, hypersensitivity pneumonitis, and acute or chronic diffuse alveolar hemorrhage,[4,17,18] Pulmonary damage caused by intravenous injection of crushed oral tablets leading to Ritalin lung and talcosis are discussed in Chapter 52. Drug-related constrictive bronchiolitis is discussed in Chapter 59.

Certain drugs tend to cause a predictable pattern of lung injury (Table 65.1); however, this is not always the case, and patterns of lung injury may overlap (Fig. 65.1).

CHOICE OF IMAGING MODALITY

Thin-section CT more precisely assesses the presence and characterizes the pattern and distribution of parenchymal and airway abnormalities than chest radiography does, and it may demonstrate abnormalities in patients with normal radiographs.[19,20] Padley and colleagues[20] detected abnormal findings on CT in all 23 patients

TABLE 65.1 COMMON DRUGS ASSOCIATED WITH VARIOUS PATTERNS OF LUNG INJURY

Pattern of Injury	Common Drugs
Diffuse alveolar damage	Busulfan, cyclophosphamide, carmustine, bleomycin, paclitaxel, docetaxel, checkpoint inhibitors
Nonspecific interstitial pneumonia (NSIP)	Amiodarone, methotrexate, nitrofurantoin, bleomycin, hydrochlorothiazide, carmustine
Organizing pneumonia	Amiodarone, acebutolol, minocycline, nitrofurantoin, bleomycin, gold salts, cyclophosphamide, methotrexate, penicillamine, phenytoin, carbamazepine, mesalamine, hydralazine, interferon
Eosinophilic pneumonia	Amiodarone, bleomycin, nitrofurantoin, phenytoin, β-blockers, nonsteroidal antiinflammatory drugs, antidepressants, hydrochlorothiazide, minocycline, sulfonamides, sulfasalazine, mesalamine
Hypersensitivity pneumonitis	Methotrexate, cyclophosphamide, mesalamine, fluoxetine, amitriptyline, docetaxel, paclitaxel
Diffuse alveolar hemorrhage	Anticoagulants, amphotericin B, amiodarone, cyclophosphamide, carbamazepine, methotrexate, mitomycin, nitrofurantoin, penicillamine, phenytoin, propylthiouracil

Adapted from Rossi SE, Erasmus JJ, McAdams HP, Sporn TA, Goodman P. Pulmonary drug toxicity: radiologic and pathologic manifestations. *Radiographics.* 2000;20(5):1245–1259.

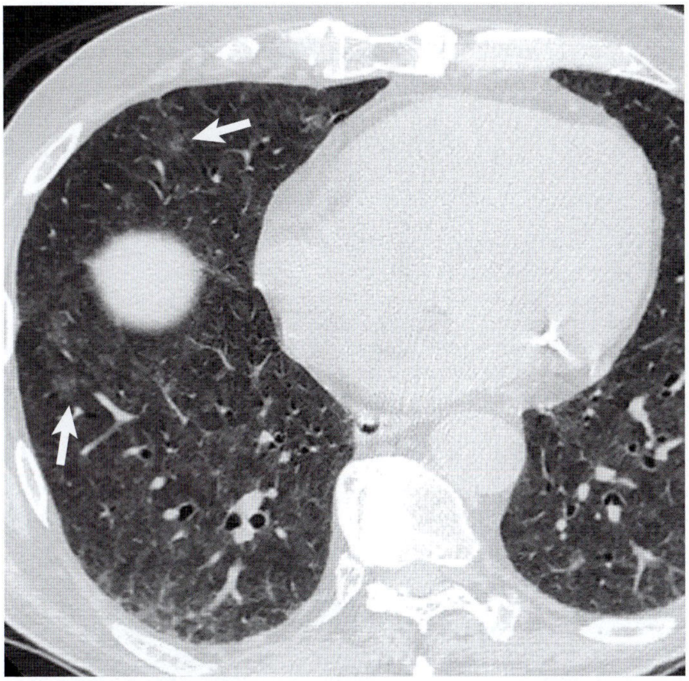

Fig. 65.1 Drug-induced lung injury resulting in a combination of nonspecific interstitial pneumonia and hypersensitivity pneumonitis patterns caused by lenalidomide and bortezomib therapy in a patient with relapsed multiple myeloma. Axial CT at the lung bases demonstrates bilateral ground-glass opacities, tiny (<5 mm) centrilobular ground-glass nodules *(arrows)*, and peripheral reticulation and architectural distortion. Cessation of the drugs resulted in marked clinical improvement with resolution of dyspnea.

with drug-induced lung disease compared with 17 patients (74%) on radiography. CT can also be of value in identifying findings suggestive of an alternative diagnosis and in monitoring response to treatment.[21] In some cases the CT findings closely reflect the histologic findings and are highly suggestive of a particular drug-reaction pattern.[21–23] However, there is considerable overlap between the various patterns on CT. Cleverley and colleagues,[24] in a retrospective study of 20 patients with drug-induced lung disease, found that CT had an accuracy of only 45% in predicting the specific histologic pattern of reaction. In spite of these limitations, thin-section CT is currently the best noninvasive method to assess the presence of drug-induced lung disease and to predict the underlying histologic pattern.[17,25] Thin-section CT is also of value in monitoring the appearance, progression, and resolution of pulmonary damage in these patients.

IMAGING PATTERNS

Drug-induced lung disease typically manifests in five characteristic patterns in the lung. These are diffuse alveolar damage, nonspecific interstitial pneumonia, organizing pneumonia, hypersensitivity pneumonitis, and alveolar hemorrhage. The pathophysiology and imaging features of each entity is discussed herein.

Of note, all patterns of *chronic interstitial pneumonias* have been reported as manifestations of drug reactions; however, desquamative interstitial pneumonia, lymphocytic interstitial pneumonia, and usual interstitial pneumonia are uncommon manifestations of drug-induced lung disease. For example, a fibrotic process that mimics idiopathic pulmonary fibrosis, characterized by the presence of usual interstitial pneumonia on surgical lung biopsy, has been well characterized for nitrofurantoin.[17]

Diffuse Alveolar Damage

Diffuse alveolar damage is the histopathologic finding that corresponds to the clinical entity of acute respiratory distress syndrome (ARDS). Diffuse alveolar damage is one of the most common histologic manifestations of pulmonary drug toxicity and has been observed most commonly as a reaction to chemotherapeutic drugs used in the treatment of malignant neoplasms, particularly busulfan, cyclophosphamide, BCNU, bleomycin, paclitaxel, and docetaxel.[17] Less commonly, it may also be seen in patients receiving amiodarone, aspirin, narcotics, or low-dose cytotoxic agents such as methotrexate.[2,17] Recently, checkpoint inhibitor immunotherapy has been found to cause a generalized pneumonitis that may represent diffuse alveolar damage or nonspecific interstitial pneumonia; the exact histologic pattern of lung injury, however, has not been fully elucidated.[26] Diffuse alveolar damage manifests initially as an acute exudative phase followed by a chronic reparative phase.

The acute phase is characterized by necrosis of type II pneumocytes and alveolar endothelial cells with alveolar and interstitial edema and formation of hyaline membranes.[27] These findings are most prominent in the first week after lung injury. In contrast, the chronic reparative phase is characterized by the proliferation of type II pneumocytes and fibroblasts. In some cases there is progression to end-stage honeycombing.[17]

Histologic features seldom allow distinction of drug reaction from other common causes of diffuse alveolar damage.[17] The exception is busulfan, which is typically associated with marked cytologic atypia.[17]

By radiograph and CT, diffuse alveolar damage mimics ARDS resulting from any other cause, demonstrating bilateral ground-glass opacities and areas of consolidation predominantly involving the dependent lung.[3,24] In the early exudative phase, patchy ground-glass opacities with adjacent areas of lobular sparing are often the predominant finding. The ground-glass opacities rapidly become confluent and may be associated with smooth linear opacities, resulting in a crazy paving pattern, and with dependent areas of consolidation (Fig. 65.2). With further progression of disease the consolidation may predominate. Architectural distortion and traction bronchiectasis are commonly identified in the organizing phase of diffuse alveolar damage. The chronic fibrotic phase may result in extensive reticulation and honeycombing (Fig. 65.3).[17,28]

Nonspecific Interstitial Pneumonia

Nonspecific interstitial pneumonia (NSIP) is a common reaction pattern seen in association with drug toxicity and with other conditions, particularly collagen vascular diseases and hypersensitivity pneumonitis.[29] Drugs most commonly associated with an NSIP pattern include amiodarone, methotrexate, nitrofurantoin, bleomycin, hydrochlorothiazide, and bis-chloroethylnitrosourea (BCNU, also known as carmustine).[3] Less common causes include busulfan, chlorambucil, cyclophosphamide, phenytoin, checkpoint inhibitors, and gold salts.[17] NSIP is characterized histologically by varying proportions of interstitial inflammation and fibrosis that are temporally uniform, with infiltration by mononuclear inflammatory cells, mild interstitial fibrosis, and reactive hyperplastic type II pneumocytes.[27,29]

The CT findings of NSIP related to drug reaction are similar to those described in patients with the idiopathic form or with NSIP secondary to other causes.[3] The abnormalities usually consist of extensive bilateral ground-glass opacities. With progression to fibrosis, there is superimposed reticulation, traction bronchiectasis,

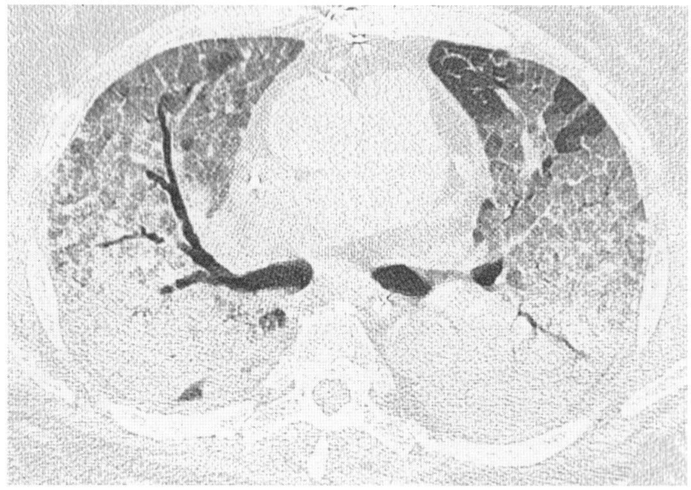

Fig. 65.2 Diffuse alveolar damage caused by amiodarone. Axial CT demonstrates extensive bilateral ground-glass opacities and dependent areas of consolidation. Note focal lobular areas of sparing and smooth lines superimposed on the ground-glass opacities, resulting in a crazy paving pattern. The patient presented with progressive shortness of breath and developed respiratory failure.

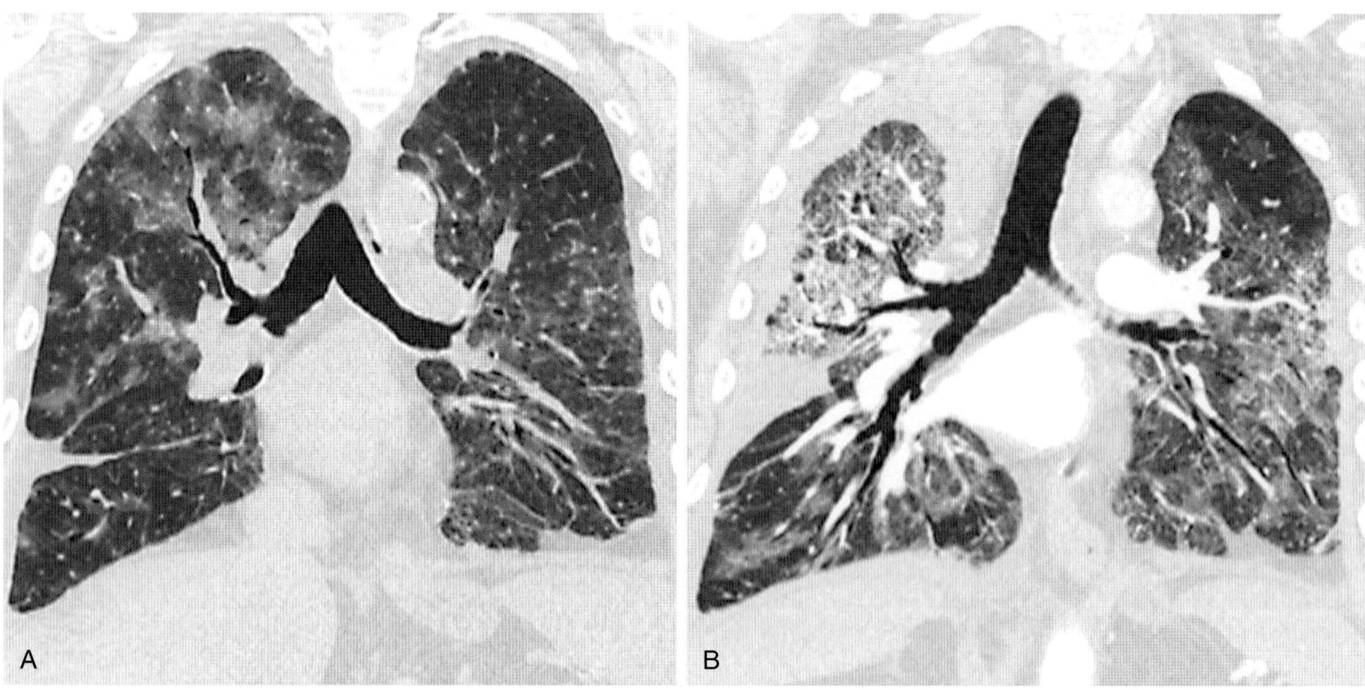

Fig. 65.3 Progression of diffuse alveolar damage. (A) Coronal CT shows the acute exudative phase of diffuse alveolar damage manifesting as bilateral ground-glass opacities and small pleural effusions extending into the right minor and major fissures. (B) Follow-up CT 1 month later shows the chronic reparative phase of diffuse alveolar damage with fibrotic changes, particularly in the right upper lobe. Notice the lower lung volume, reticulation, architectural distortion, and increased pleural fluid.

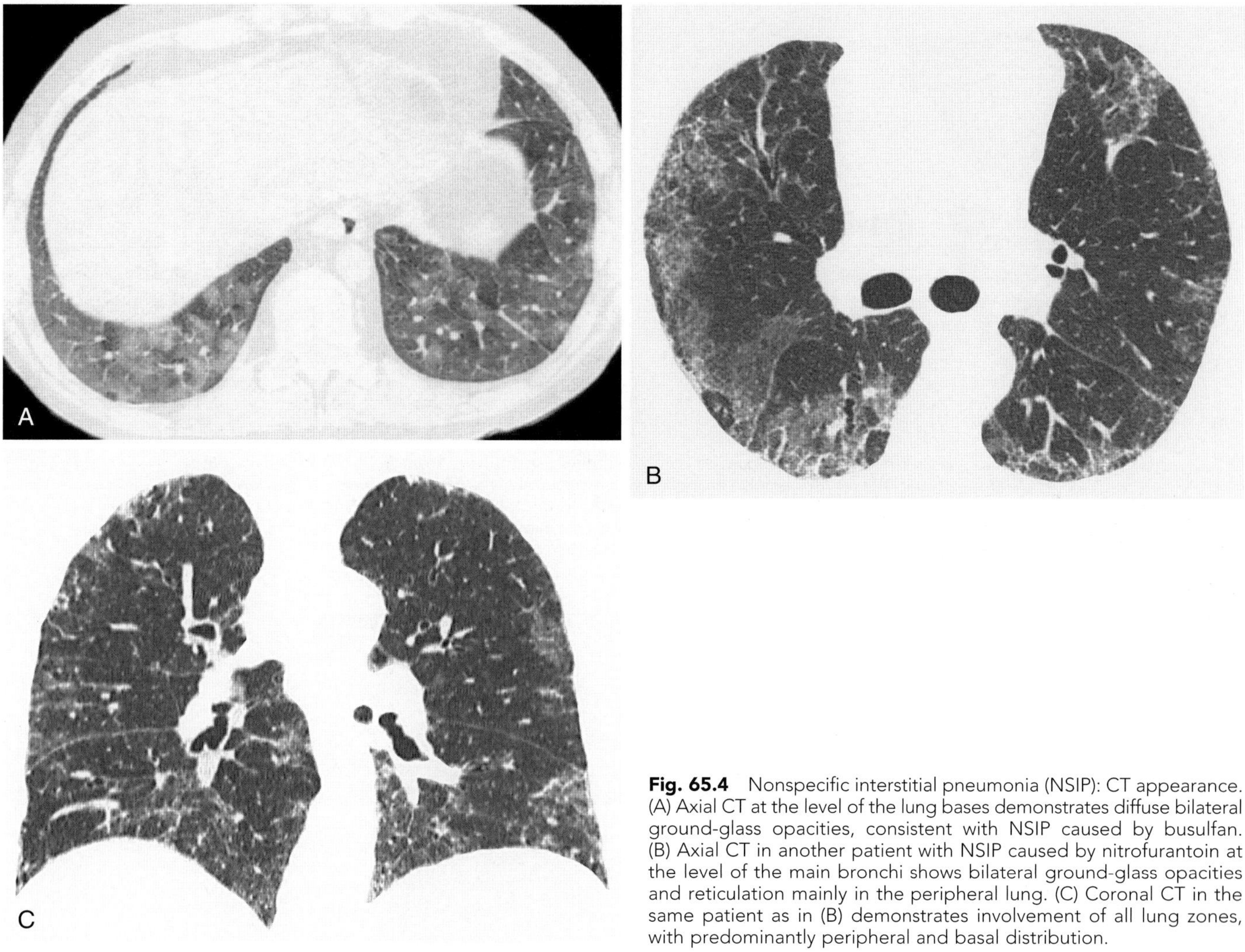

Fig. 65.4 Nonspecific interstitial pneumonia (NSIP): CT appearance. (A) Axial CT at the level of the lung bases demonstrates diffuse bilateral ground-glass opacities, consistent with NSIP caused by busulfan. (B) Axial CT in another patient with NSIP caused by nitrofurantoin at the level of the main bronchi shows bilateral ground-glass opacities and reticulation mainly in the peripheral lung. (C) Coronal CT in the same patient as in (B) demonstrates involvement of all lung zones, with predominantly peripheral and basal distribution.

and bronchiolectasis (Fig. 65.4).[30] A peribronchovascular distribution may also be present, particularly in patients with drug reaction to nitrofurantoin.[20]

Organizing Pneumonia

Organizing pneumonia is a common pattern of lung injury and repair. It may be idiopathic (cryptogenic organizing pneumonia) or be seen in association with a variety of conditions, including infection, drugs, connective tissue disorders, aspiration, hematologic disorders, solid-organ and hematopoietic stem cell transplantation, radiotherapy, and inflammatory bowel disease.[31] Organizing pneumonia is characterized histologically by the presence of buds of organizing granulation tissue in respiratory bronchioles, alveolar ducts, and adjacent alveoli.[29] Organizing pneumonia is an increasingly recognized manifestation of drug reaction and is generally reversible after drug cessation or corticosteroid therapy. The most common drugs that can result in an organizing pneumonia pattern are amiodarone, acebutolol, minocycline, nitrofurantoin, bleomycin, gold salts, cyclophosphamide, methotrexate, penicillamine, phenytoin, carbamazepine, mesalamine, hydralazine, and interferon.[2,32]

The clinical, radiologic, and histologic findings of drug-induced organizing pneumonia resemble those seen in patients with idiopathic organizing pneumonia (cryptogenic organizing pneumonia) and also can overlap with the features of chronic eosinophilic pneumonia (see later).[31,33] Organizing pneumonia classically manifests as patchy or confluent areas of bilateral consolidation predominantly involving the peripheral lung regions.[23] In a study of nine patients with biopsy-proven drug-induced organizing pneumonia, the most common high-resolution CT finding was airspace consolidation in a subpleural or peribronchial distribution, seen in approximately 90% of patients (Fig. 65.5).[31] The consolidation usually had an asymmetric bilateral distribution with no zonal predominance. Ground-glass opacities were identified in 80% of the patients, usually in a bilateral asymmetric and random distribution.[31] Consolidation may distribute in a perilobular pattern, which characteristically outlines the secondary pulmonary lobule involving the adjacent pleura, interlobular septa, paraseptal interstitium, and paraseptal alveoli (Fig. 65.6).[34] Centrilobular nodules are rare.

In patients with an organizing pneumonia pattern secondary to amiodarone, the areas of consolidation may have high attenuation at CT (82–175 Hounsfield units), often accompanied by high attenuation in liver or spleen resulting from deposition of iodine-containing amiodarone metabolites (Figs. 65.7 and 65.8). This pattern is virtually diagnostic of amiodarone toxicity, which

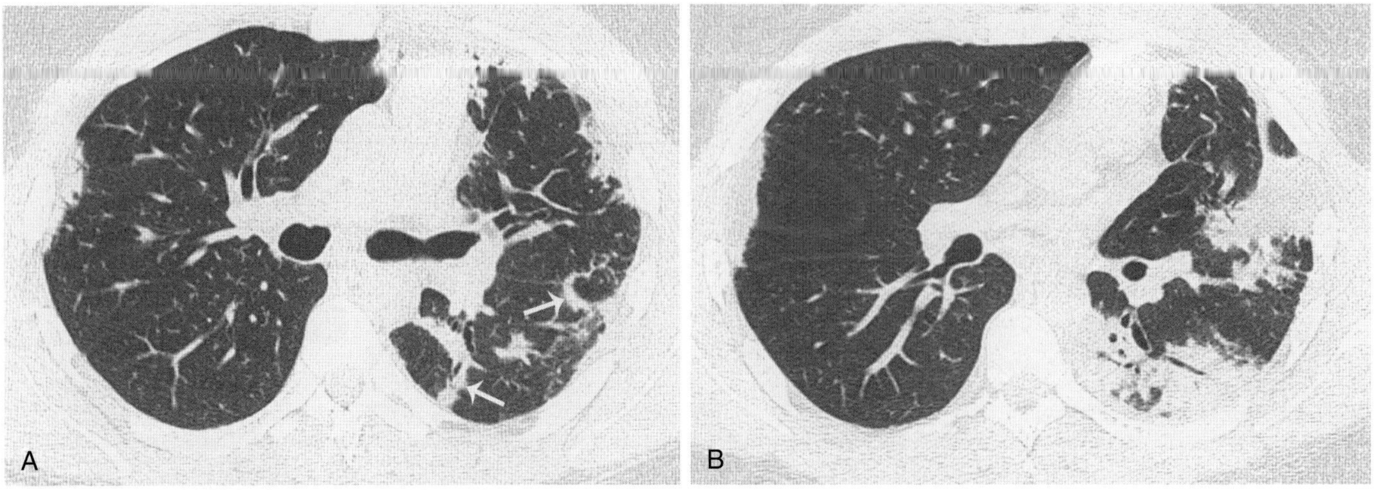

Fig. 65.5 Organizing pneumonia caused by mesalamine used for the treatment of ulcerative colitis. (A) CT at the level of the left upper lobe bronchus shows bilateral areas of consolidation in the peripheral lung regions. Also note perilobular distribution *(arrows)* in the left lower lobe, a characteristic feature of organizing pneumonia. (B) CT at a lower level shows subpleural consolidation in the right lung and peribronchial and peripheral consolidation in the left lung.

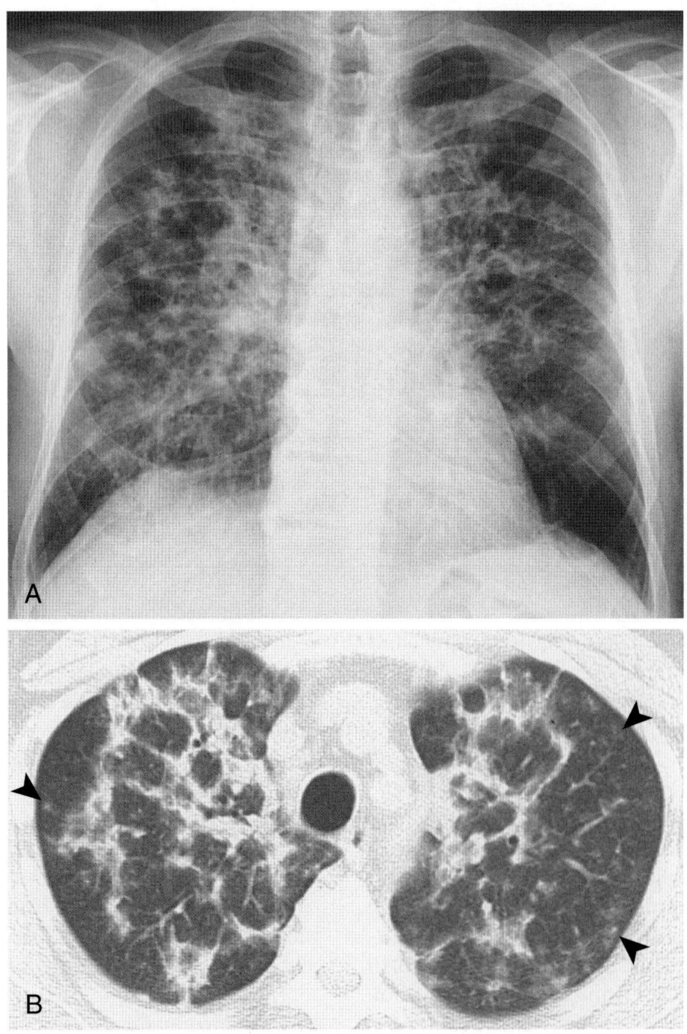

Fig. 65.6 Classic central and perilobular distribution of consolidation in organizing pneumonia caused by mesalamine used for treatment of ulcerative colitis. (A) Chest radiograph shows bilateral irregular nodular opacities and consolidation in a predominantly central distribution. (B) Axial CT demonstrates the classic perilobular distribution of opacities, referring to the polygonal or arcade-like pattern of opacification that occurs around the secondary pulmonary lobule. A few poorly defined centrilobular nodules *(arrowheads)* are also evident.

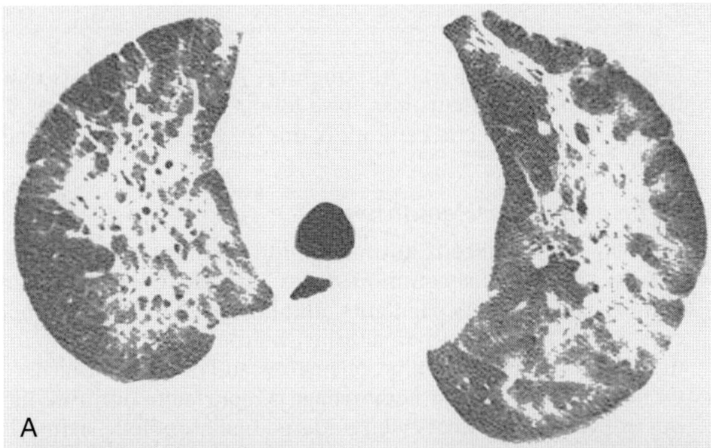

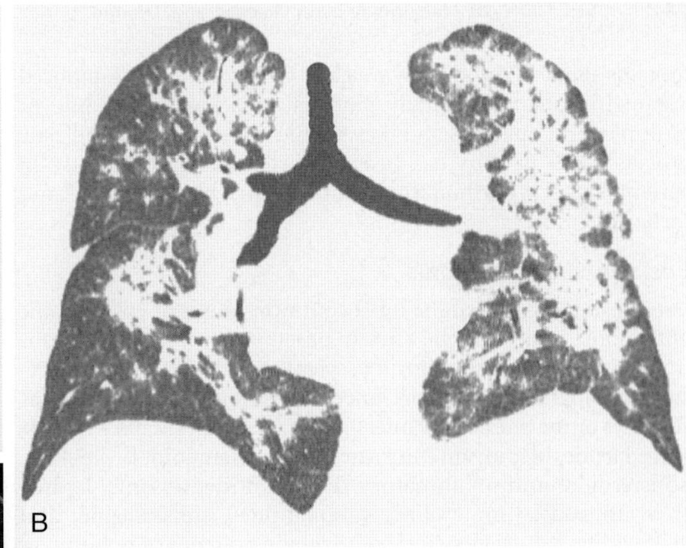

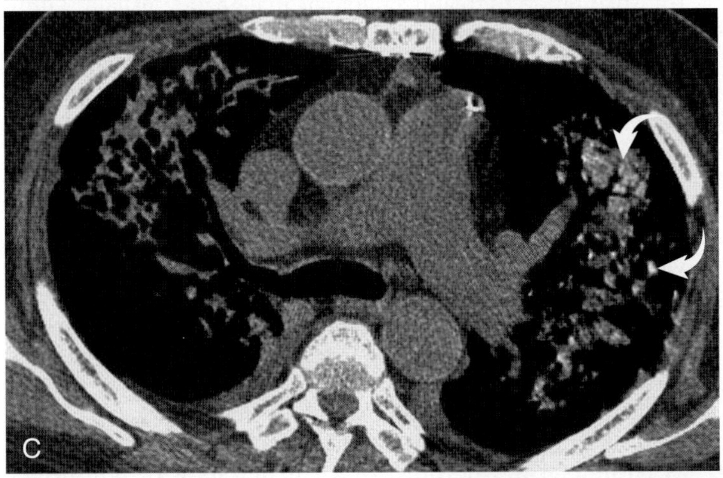

Fig. 65.7 Organizing pneumonia caused by amiodarone. Axial (A) and coronal (B) CT demonstrate extensive bilateral areas of consolidation in a peribronchial distribution. Soft tissue window axial CT at the level of the upper lobes (C) shows areas of high attenuation *(arrows)* characteristic of amiodarone toxicity. Note small bilateral pleural effusions secondary to left-sided heart failure. *(From Silva CI, Müller NL. Drug-induced lung diseases: most common reaction patterns and corresponding high-resolution CT manifestations.* Semin Ultrasound CT MR. *2006;27:111–116.)*

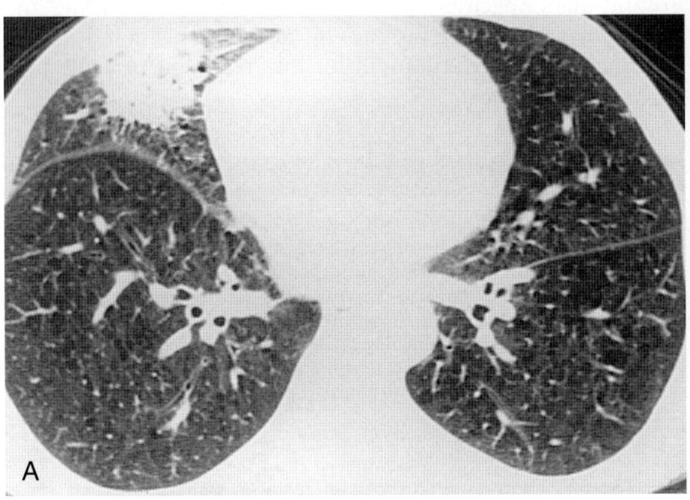

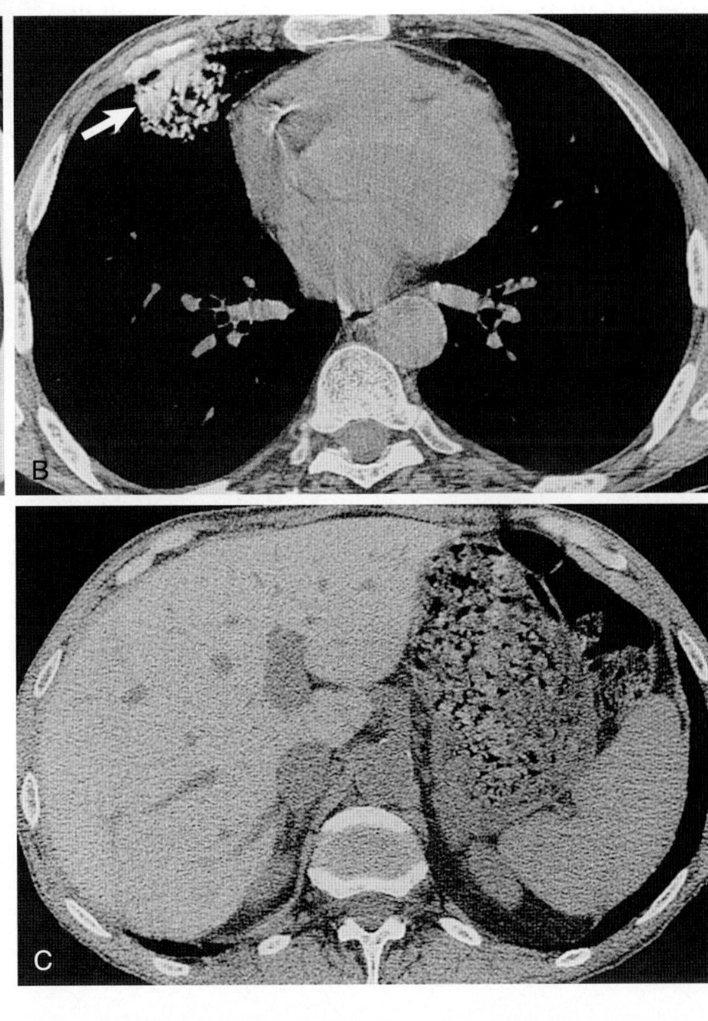

Fig. 65.8 Classic findings of amiodarone toxicity. (A) Axial CT at the level of the inferior pulmonary veins shows a focal area of consolidation in the right middle lobe. (B) Axial CT at the same level with soft tissue windows shows that the consolidation in the right middle lobe *(arrow)* has an attenuation greater than that of chest wall and cardiac muscle. (C) Axial CT through the upper abdomen shows high attenuation of the liver. *(From Müller NL, Fraser RS, Colman NC, Paré PD.* Radiologic Diagnosis of Diseases of the Chest. *Philadelphia: WB Saunders; 2001.)*

contains about 37% iodine by weight.[21] On occasion, drug-induced organizing pneumonia may manifest as a solitary nodule or multiple focal opacities and may mimic infection or a neoplastic process. This pattern has been reported most commonly in patients receiving amiodarone, minocycline, bleomycin,[35,36] and carbamazepine.[37,38]

Eosinophilic Pneumonia

Drug reaction is one of the most common causes of eosinophilic pneumonia, which may be acute in onset or may have an insidious course with progression during several months.[39] It is characterized histologically by the presence of eosinophils in the alveolar airspaces or the pulmonary interstitium.[18] Common causes include amiodarone, bleomycin, nitrofurantoin, phenytoin, β-blockers, nonsteroidal antiinflammatory drugs, antidepressants, hydrochlorothiazide, minocycline, sulfonamides, sulfasalazine, and mesalamine.[2,3,22] Diagnosis is based on the presence of pulmonary opacities and consolidations by imaging; the identification of eosinophilia in peripheral blood, lung biopsy specimen, or bronchoalveolar lavage fluid; and the association with administration of a known drug in the absence of other causes of pulmonary opacities and eosinophilia, such as parasitic infestation, fungal infection, and immunologic or systemic diseases.[3,39] The presence of peripheral eosinophilia is variable in patients with drug-induced eosinophilic pneumonia; it is described in approximately 40% to 86% of patients.[22,40]

With imaging, drug-induced eosinophilic pneumonia looks similar to eosinophilic pneumonias of other causes and organizing pneumonia.[3,22,23] It typically manifests as migratory opacities and consolidation, resembling simple pulmonary eosinophilia (Fig. 65.9), or as chronic bilateral areas of consolidation in a characteristic upper lobe and peripheral distribution. The areas of consolidation most commonly are symmetric and involve mainly the middle and upper lung zones; however, they may be asymmetric and involve any lung region (see Fig. 65.9). Focal areas of ground-glass opacity surrounded by a crescent or ring of consolidation (the reversed halo sign) have been described in 5 of 14 patients with histologic diagnosis of drug-induced eosinophilic pneumonia (see Fig. 65.9).[22] Less common high-resolution CT findings include small nodules, septal thickening, and reticulation.[22,41]

Hypersensitivity Pneumonitis

Hypersensitivity pneumonitis is a relatively uncommon manifestation of drug-induced lung disease.[17] It has been described most commonly with methotrexate, cyclophosphamide, mesalamine, fluoxetine, amitriptyline, docetaxel, and paclitaxel.[19,42] Of interest, tyrosine kinase inhibitors, used in the treatment of chronic myeloid leukemia, have been found to cause interstitial lung disease that mimics hypersensitivity pneumonitis in its subpleural and peribronchovascular distribution of ground-glass opacities and consolidations.[43]

The histopathologic and radiologic features of drug-induced hypersensitivity pneumonitis usually are indistinguishable from those commonly seen in hypersensitivity pneumonitis secondary to immunologic reaction to inhaled organic antigens. Hypersensitivity pneumonitis is characterized histologically by the presence of cellular bronchiolitis, noncaseating granulomas, and bronchiolocentric cellular interstitial pneumonia composed predominantly of lymphocytes.[44]

Hypersensitivity pneumonitis tends to manifest as diffuse bilateral ground-glass opacities or small, poorly defined centrilobular nodules (Fig. 65.10; see Fig. 65.1). Although the literature suggests that the majority of patients also have lobular air-trapping on CT images obtained at end expiration, this is less common in actual clinical practice.[3,24]

Diffuse Alveolar Hemorrhage

Alveolar hemorrhage is an uncommon manifestation of drug toxicity.[17] The most common drugs associated with alveolar hemorrhage are anticoagulants, amphotericin B, amiodarone, cyclophosphamide, carbamazepine, methotrexate, mitomycin, nitrofurantoin, penicillamine, phenytoin, and propylthiouracil.[3,17] Of note, diffuse alveolar hemorrhage is reported to occur in one out of every five patients who undergo hematopoietic stem cell transplantation to treat hematologic malignancy, usually within the first few weeks after transplant.[45]

The radiographic manifestations of alveolar hemorrhage include patchy or confluent ground-glass opacities and bilateral areas of consolidation.[23,46] The opacities usually are widespread but more prominent in the perihilar areas and the middle and lower lung zones; the lung apices and costophrenic angles are usually spared.[46]

The CT findings of pulmonary hemorrhage are nonspecific, with extensive bilateral ground-glass opacities and possible areas of consolidation.[46] The ground-glass opacities may have a patchy distribution or be diffuse. CT scans performed 2 to 3 days after the acute episode show a decrease in the ground-glass opacities and consolidation and presence of small poorly defined centrilobular nodules and, less commonly, interlobular septal thickening.[47]

A variant of diffuse alveolar hemorrhage is the entity known as retinoic acid syndrome, which manifests with nonspecific ground-glass opacities, septal lines, peribronchial cuffing and pleural or pericardial effusion. This rare complication occurs in patients who receive tretinoin for the treatment of acute promyelocytic leukemia.

KEY POINTS

- The clinical, radiologic, and histologic manifestations of pulmonary drug reactions are nonspecific and mimic those of various acute and chronic lung diseases.
- Diffuse alveolar damage (corresponding to the clinical entity acute respiratory distress syndrome), nonspecific interstitial pneumonia, and organizing pneumonia are the most common patterns of drug-induced lung injury.
- Drug reaction is one of the most common causes of eosinophilic pneumonia.
- Diffuse alveolar hemorrhage and hypersensitivity pneumonitis are uncommon manifestations of drug toxicity.
- The only drug reaction that may result in a characteristic appearance on CT is amiodarone lung. Because amiodarone contains about 37% iodine by weight, it typically results in high attenuation where it accumulates, which is usually visualized in the liver and in the lung.
- A complete list of drugs that may result in pulmonary toxicity and the types of reaction associated with various drugs can be found at http://www.pneumotox.com.

DRUGS OF NOTE

Illicit Drugs

Cocaine. Use of cocaine and its derivatives, especially "crack," is a major health problem in both urban and suburban settings. When smoked, the crystalline precipitate of freebase cocaine (crack) reaches the cerebral circulation within 6 to 8 seconds

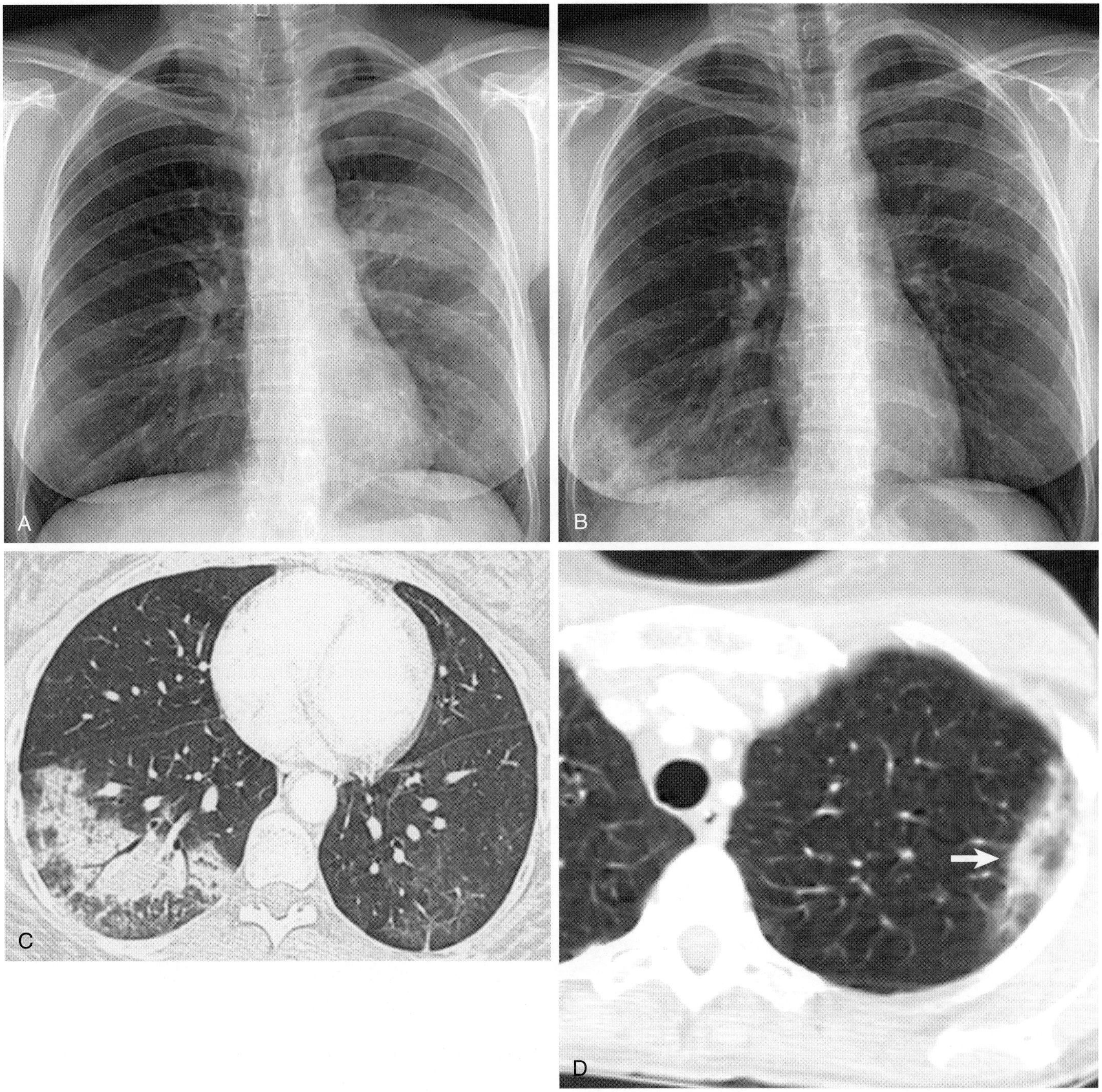

Fig. 65.9 Manifestations of acute and chronic eosinophilic pneumonia. (A) Chest radiograph, from a patient who developed eosinophilic pneumonia during treatment for ulcerative colitis with mesalamine, shows patchy consolidation in the left upper and lower lobes. (B) Chest radiograph 22 days later from the same patient shows resolution of the previous consolidation but development of new consolidation in the left upper and right lower lobes. Fleeting, migratory consolidations are characteristic of acute eosinophilic lung disease. (C) Axial CT from the same patient shows atypical asymmetric distribution and lower lobe involvement. Mild ground-glass opacities and linear opacities are seen in the left lower lobe. (D) Axial CT from a different patient with chronic eosinophilic pneumonia shows left upper lobe consolidation *(arrow)* marginating a central area of ground-glass opacity (so-called reversed halo sign). The reversed halo sign is seen in up to 36% of patients with drug-induced eosinophilic pneumonia.

and causes virtually instantaneous euphoria. This property, along with its ease of administration and wide availability, has made crack cocaine the most frequently abused controlled substance in the United States.[48,49] Use of the drug has been associated with a variety of pulmonary complications, including cardiogenic and permeability pulmonary edema, hemorrhage, airway thermal injury (sometimes complicated by tracheal stenosis or the reactive airways dysfunction syndrome), asthma, chronic obstructive pulmonary disease, pneumothorax, pneumomediastinum, and pneumopericardium.[50,51]

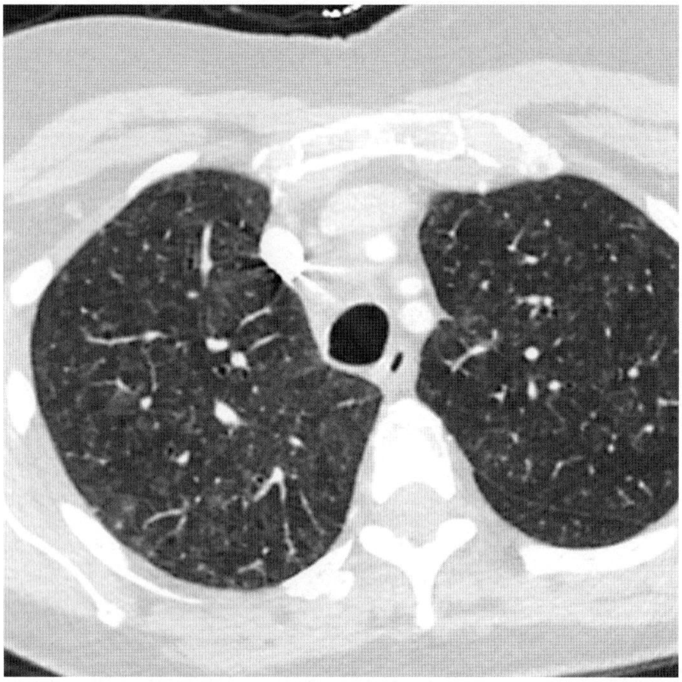

Fig. 65.10 Hypersensitivity pneumonitis caused by docetaxel. Axial CT shows scattered lobular ground-glass opacities and centrilobular ground-glass nodules. Note scattered subtle mosaic attenuation, typical of this condition.

Cocaine-induced cardiogenic pulmonary edema manifests with interlobular septal thickening, pleural effusions, cardiomegaly, and ground-glass opacities or consolidation[51,52]; it generally resolves within 24 to 72 hours regardless of treatment. Cocaine and crack may also cause increased pulmonary capillary permeability edema, which results in bilateral perihilar-predominant ground-glass opacities or consolidation but without septal lines, pleural effusion, or cardiomegaly (Fig. 65.11).[51] Pulmonary hemorrhage results in transient focal or diffuse bilateral ground-glass opacities or consolidation[51,53] that clear rapidly after cessation of use of the responsible agent. Because pulmonary edema and pulmonary hemorrhage are usually radiographically indistinguishable, the development of respiratory failure with bilateral airspace opacities that appear shortly after the use of crack and that clear rapidly after cessation of drug use has been termed *crack lung* (Fig. 65.12).[51,54]

Less common manifestations of cocaine use include fleeting areas of consolidation, resulting in a Löffler syndrome–like appearance, and a pattern of organizing pneumonia.[48] Barotrauma related to cocaine abuse may result in pneumomediastinum (see Fig. 65.12), pneumothorax, or (rarely) hemopneumothorax or pneumopericardium.[55,56] Pneumomediastinum and pneumothorax result from the deep inhalation of cocaine, followed by a Valsalva maneuver and coughing, which may lead to alveolar rupture and subsequent dissection of air into the pulmonary interstitium and mediastinum or into the pleural space.[51,57]

Heroin and Other Opiates. The use of heroin increased considerably in the past 2 decades.[58] From 2001 to 2014 there was a sixfold increase in the total number of deaths caused by heroin overdose in the United States.[59] In some western cities the death toll from heroin overdoses has become the largest category of preventable deaths.[58] The majority of patients with

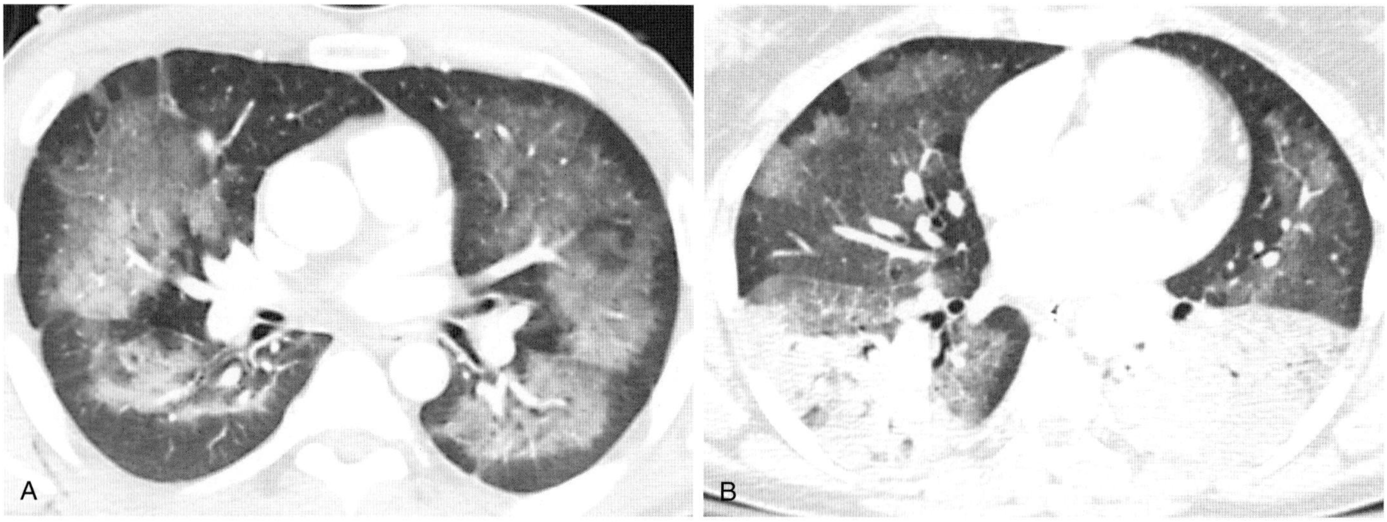

Fig. 65.11 Diffuse alveolar damage caused by cocaine abuse. (A) Axial CT demonstrates perihilar-predominant ground-glass opacities and consolidation. (B) Axial CT from a different patient shows nondependent ground-glass opacities with scattered septal thickening and dependent consolidation, typical of cocaine-induced diffuse alveolar damage. Note the absence of pleural effusions in both examples.

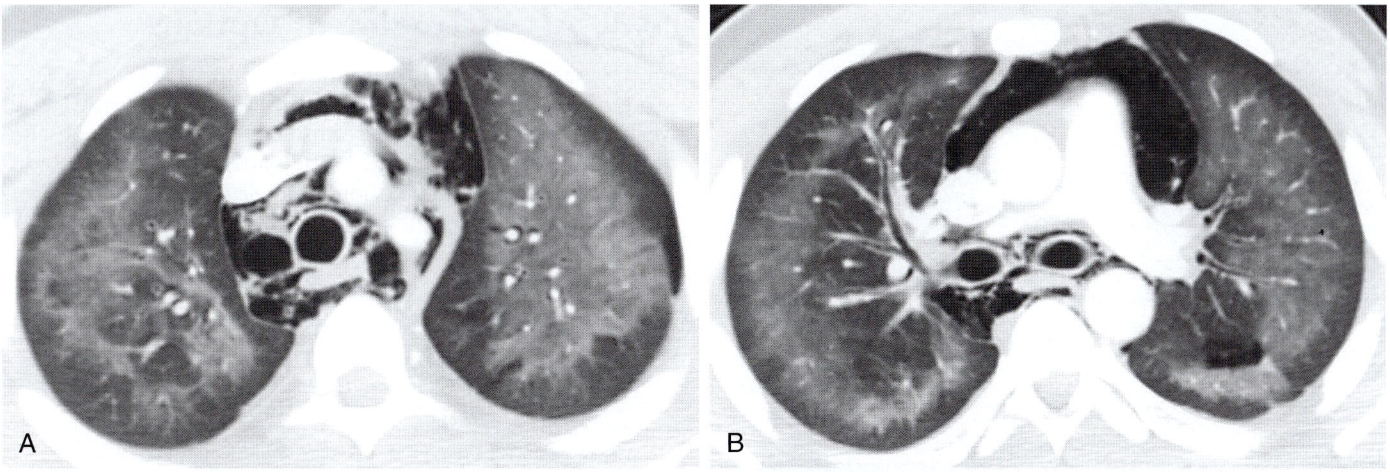

Fig. 65.12 Crack lung. (A) Axial CT at the level of aortic branch vessels and (B) pulmonary trunk shows bilateral ground-glass opacities and extensive pneumomediastinum caused by alveolar rupture and subsequent dissection of air into the pulmonary interstitium and mediastinum. Interstitial air is best appreciated along the left major fissure.

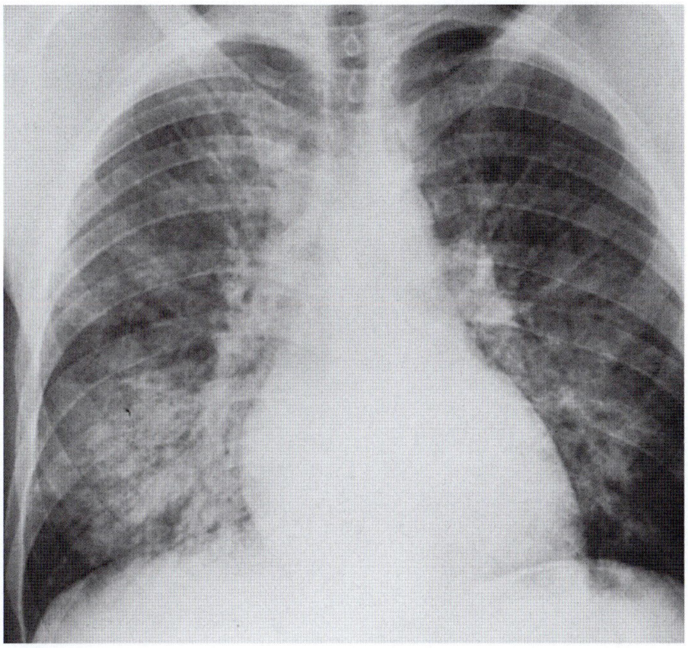

Fig. 65.13 Acute pulmonary edema caused by opiates. Chest radiograph shows perihilar-predominant consolidation typical of acute pulmonary edema. Several hours previously, this 19-year-old man had injected a large dose of meperidine and methadone intravenously. He had an uneventful recovery. *(From Müller NL, Fraser RS, Colman NC, Paré PD.* Radiologic Diagnosis of Diseases of the Chest. *Philadelphia: WB Saunders; 2001.)*

fatal overdose have noncardiogenic pulmonary edema.[58] The diagnosis of heroin or other opiate overdose is made clinically by the presence of altered mental status, decreased respiratory drive, pinpoint pupils, and circumstantial evidence of drug use.[58]

The radiologic findings are those of pulmonary capillary permeability edema and consist of bilateral ground-glass opacities or consolidation, often in a predominantly perihilar distribution (Fig. 65.13).[51] In up to 20% of cases the edema may be unilateral or markedly asymmetric.[58] In such patients the findings can be identical to aspiration pneumonia, a relatively common complication in patients with opiate overdose resulting from depression of the central nervous system. Aspiration pneumonia results in areas of consolidation that affect the dependent lung regions, particularly the superior segments of the lower lobes and the apical and posterior segments of the upper lobes when the aspiration occurs while the patient is recumbent.[51] Because of the relatively vertical orientation of the right main bronchus, the right lung is affected more than the left.

A number of other pulmonary abnormalities can be seen in opiate addicts. Bronchiectasis has been identified in some individuals, presumably related to recurrent infection and aspiration.[60] Unilateral or bilateral pneumothorax, hemothorax, hemopneumothorax, and pyopneumothorax have been reported as complications of attempted intravenous injections in the supraclavicular fossa, the so-called pocket shot.[57] Septic emboli, sometimes associated with right ventricular endocarditis, can also be seen. Septic emboli are manifested on chest radiography and CT as multiple nodules and wedge-shaped peripheral opacities measuring approximately 1 to 3 cm in diameter, which are frequently cavitated. The nodules tend to be most numerous in the peripheral lung regions and the lower lobes (Fig. 65.14).[61,62] On occasion, a tricuspid valve vegetation may be visible on contrast-enhanced CT (see Fig. 65.14). Chest wall complications of intravenous drug use include vertebral body osteomyelitis, sometimes with associated epidural abscess, costochondritis, septic arthritis, and necrotizing fasciitis.[51]

Differential Diagnosis

The clinical, radiologic, and histologic manifestations are often nonspecific.[63] Criteria for diagnosis include history of drug exposure, consistent radiologic findings, histologic evidence of lung damage, and exclusion of other common causes of pulmonary injury, such as opportunistic infection, radiation pneumonitis, pulmonary thromboembolism, oxygen administration, and progression of the primary illness.[64] In clinical practice, however, biopsy is seldom performed, and the diagnosis is based primarily on clinical and radiologic findings.

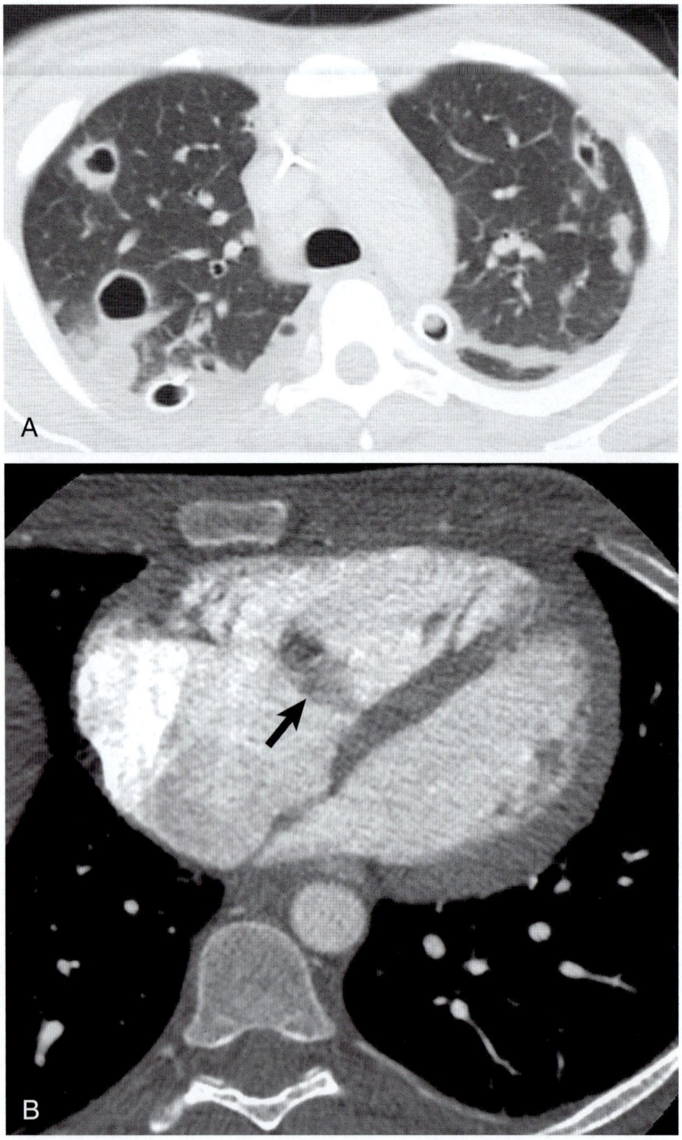

Fig. 65.14 Septic embolism with tricuspid valve vegetation related to intravenous drug use. (A) Axial CT at the level of the upper lobes shows bilateral cavitary and noncavitary randomly distributed pulmonary nodules. Note bilateral chest tubes used for treatment of bilateral pneumothoraces. (B) Axial CT at the level of the heart shows a large mass *(arrow)* surrounding the tricuspid valve compatible with vegetation. *(Figures reproduced with permission from Reddy G, Steiner R, Walker C, eds.* Cardiac Imaging: Case Review Series. *2nd ed. Philadelphia: Elsevier/Saunders; 2013.)*

Synopsis of Treatment Options

In the majority of cases drug-induced lung disease resolves on drug discontinuation. Therefore, clinical status permitting, the suspected drug should be discontinued and the patient observed until improvement occurs.[14] Some patients may require corticosteroid therapy.[14] On occasion, acute drug-induced lung disease may cause deterioration in spite of therapy and result in fatality.

SUGGESTED READINGS

Choi MH, Jung JI, Chung WD, Kim YJ, Lee SE, Han DH, Ahn MI, Park SH. Acute pulmonary complications in patients with hematologic malignancies. *Radiographics.* 2014;34:1755–1768.

Gotway MB, Marder SR, Hanks DK, et al. Thoracic complications of illicit drug use: an organ system approach. *Radiographics.* 2002;22:S119–S135.

Foucher P, Camus P. Pneumotox. Available at: http://www.pneumotox.com.

Myers JL, Limper AH, Swensen SJ. Drug-induced lung disease: a pragmatic classification incorporating HRCT appearances. *Semin Respir Crit Care Med.* 2003;24:445–453.

Silva CI, Müller NL. Drug-induced lung diseases: most common reaction patterns and corresponding high-resolution CT manifestations. *Semin Ultrasound CT MR.* 2006;27:111–116.

Taylor AC, Verma N, Slater R, Mohammed TH. Bad for breathing: a pictorial of drug-induced pulmonary disease. *Curr Probl Diagn Radiol.* 2016;45(6): 429–432.

The full reference list for this chapter is available at ExpertConsult.com.

66 Therapeutic Radiation and Radiation-Induced Lung Disease*

MARCELO F. BENVENISTE | DANIEL R. GOMEZ | BRADLEY S. SABLOFF | JEREMY J. ERASMUS

Radiation therapy is an important modality in the management of patients with intrathoracic malignant neoplasms and primary and secondary chest wall neoplasms. Radiation therapy for these tumors usually results in radiation of the adjacent lung, and radiation-induced lung injury has been reported in association with treatment of lung, breast, esophageal, and thymic neoplasms and in lymphoma and pleural mesothelioma. Adverse effects of radiation therapy on the lung parenchyma—in particular, acute pneumonitis and chronic fibrosis—include ground-glass opacities or consolidation in the acute phase and traction bronchiectasis, volume loss, architectural distortion, and consolidation in the late phase.[1–7]

Improvements in radiation techniques and delivery, including three-dimensional (3D) conformal radiotherapy (3D-CRT), intensity-modulated radiotherapy (IMRT), stereotactic body radiotherapy (SBRT), proton therapy, and altered fractionation schedules, have improved locoregional control and survival in patients with non–small cell lung cancer (NSCLC).[8–18] Of importance, the imaging manifestations of radiation-induced lung disease associated with these newer therapeutic approaches often differ from those seen with conventional radiation therapy.

Knowledge of the expanded spectrum of manifestations of radiation-induced lung disease is important in the management of patients after radiation therapy and is useful in the diagnosis of local recurrence of malignant disease and in differentiating radiation-induced lung disease from infection. In this chapter we review the etiology and clinical and imaging manifestations of radiation-induced lung disease and emphasize unexpected or atypical manifestations that can occur when newer radiation techniques are used.

Etiology

Radiation-induced lung disease rarely occurs with fractionated total doses less than 20 Gy and is commonly present in patients who receive doses greater than 60 Gy.[19–24] A pooled analysis of 24 studies of 1911 patients with both small cell and NSCLC who received chemoradiation showed that the incidence of clinically significant radiation-induced pneumonitis (grade 2–3 according to the Radiation Therapy Oncology Group/European Organization for Research and Treatment of Cancer criteria) was 6% for total doses less than 45 Gy and 12% for doses greater than 55 Gy.[23,25] Although the total dose of radiation delivered is important in the development of radiation-induced lung disease, other radiation technique factors that affect lung injury are the fractions into which the total dose is divided, the dose rate, and the volume of lung irradiated.[19,23,24,26–30] The injury sustained by the lungs tends to decrease as the number of fractions in which the radiation is delivered increases.[22,23]

Improved techniques of radiation therapy and dose escalation can modify the development and extent of lung injury.[8–16] For instance, because the new fractionation strategies are often associated with an increase in radiation dose, there is a tendency to increase acute toxicity. However, by decreasing the treated volume, aggressive hyperfractionated schedules can limit acute radiation-induced injury of adjacent lung.

Various patient factors can increase the degree of injury sustained by the lung after irradiation of a thoracic neoplasm; these include age, low performance status, cigarette smoking, preexisting lung disease, and prior radiation therapy. The effect of neoadjuvant or concurrent chemotherapy on radiation-induced lung injury is not clear; some studies report an increase, whereas others have reported no significant association with pneumonitis.[8,9,24,31–34] In addition, although steroids ameliorate radiation pneumonitis, an abrupt termination of administration can unmask latent radiation injury to the lung.[35] Conversely, cytoprotectants such as amifostine, an organic thiophosphate, have shown promise in reducing the incidence and severity of injury associated with radiation therapy, although they have not been established as standard of care in preventing pulmonary toxicity.[36–39]

Prevalence

Because of the complexity of factors that determine whether a patient with a thoracic malignant neoplasm will receive radiation therapy, including histology, stage, symptoms, and performance status, together with the heterogeneity of treatment options and numerous factors that can influence the degree of injury sustained by the lung after radiation therapy, the true prevalence of radiation-induced lung disease is difficult to ascertain for patients with lymphoma; pleural mesothelioma; and lung, esophageal, breast, and thymic cancers.[40–43] However, radiation-induced lung injury is common in these patients, and subclinical changes in pulmonary function test results occur in an even larger percentage of patients.[24,36,38,44–51]

Of the multiple thoracic malignancies, patients with lung cancer often receive the highest doses of radiation to the largest volume of lung and are accordingly more likely to develop radiation-induced lung disease. On the basis of a reported incidence of 10% to 20%, moderate to severe radiation-induced pneumonitis will probably occur in approximately 15,000 to 25,000 patients with lung cancer in 2016.[23] This incidence is likely underestimated because the nonspecific symptoms of

*The editors and the publisher would like to thank Drs. M. Kara Bucci and Reginald F. Munden for contributing material on this topic to the prior edition of this work. It has served as the foundation for the current chapter.

radiation-induced lung disease can be misattributed to preexisting respiratory or cardiovascular disease.

Radiation Therapy Planning and Treatment Terminology

The goal of radiation therapy planning is to deliver a high dose of radiation to the tumor while sparing the surrounding normal tissue. To enable systematic tumor volume delineation, the International Commission on Radiation Units and Measurements has specified the use of concentric target volume delineations before radiation therapy.[52] The gross tumor volume (GTV) is obtained outlining visible malignancy, including any involved nodes, on imaging studies. Next, a margin around the GTV is added for potential microscopic subclinical disease and is called the clinical target volume. An additional margin is added to the treatment plan to account for possible tumor movement during treatment because of respiratory motion and is called the internal target volume. The final volume treatment plan is the planning target volume and accounts for anticipated differences in patient positioning during the delivery of treatment.

Types of Radiation Therapy Delivery

Sophisticated radiation therapy techniques, such as 3D-CRT, IMRT, and SBRT, allow the delivery of high therapeutic dose to the tumor, decreased radiation dose to adjacent tissue, and improved local tumor control rate.[53–55] In contrast to conventional radiation therapy treatment planning, 3D-CRT uses a 3D image reconstructed from computed tomography (CT) scanning data to determine the target volumes to be treated. A computer planning system is used to design beam arrangements with a variety of orientations that deliver maximal radiation dose to the tumor while limiting exposure to normal structures. In IMRT the combination of powerful computer planning algorithms with multileaf collimators results in a high-precision dose delivered to the tumor with a steep dose fall-off outside the target, which decreases the volume of normal tissue that is radiated.[56] Murshed and colleagues,[57] in a study of 41 patients with advanced-stage NSCLC (stage III–IV), demonstrated a 10% improved target conformity of IMRT when compared with 3D-CRT. SBRT has steep dose gradients, allowing delivery of a highly precise dose conformed to the shape of the tumor. SBRT uses only a few fractions of radiation while delivering a significantly high biologic effective dose (>100 Gy). Because the target volume is small, SBRT is being used more frequently with curative intent in patients with peripheral early-stage NSCLC (Fig. 66.1). In these patients SBRT is used rather than conventional radiation therapy or surgical resection as it achieves local control rates of 80% to 95%[58] and improves overall survival compared with conventional radiation therapy.[59–64]

Recent Innovations in Radiation Therapy

Radiation therapy has improved considerably during the past few decades by refinements of existing techniques and introduction of new technology, including positron emission tomography (PET)-CT using the radiopharmaceutical ^{18}F-deoxyglucose, a D-glucose analog labeled with fluorine-18 (^{18}F-FDG–PET-CT), four-dimensional (4D) treatment planning, and proton therapy.

The increasing use of advanced CRT techniques such as IMRT and SBRT in thoracic radiation oncology makes precise target delineation important as these techniques have a higher likelihood of geographic misses.[65] Use of FDG–PET-CT and 4D treatment planning improves the precision in radiation therapy by increasing the accuracy of tumor delineation and minimizing damage to surrounding structures.[66,67]

FDG–PET-CT improves delineation of the extent of the tumor compared with CT alone when there is associated postobstructive atelectasis. The use of FDG–PET-CT results in less variation in lung cancer contouring compared with CT alone and reduces the risk of geographic misses with SBRT.[68] In addition, because tumor volume delineation by FDG–PET-CT is typically smaller than that defined by CT, this can potentially facilitate dose escalation without increasing side effects.[69–72] Also, the detection of unsuspected nodal metastases by FDG–PET-CT improves the target accuracy for nodal radiation and decreases isolated nodal failures.[73] In addition to assisting with target volume delineation, PET-CT imaging may have an important role in adaptive planning. Adaptive planning is the modification of a radiation treatment plan during the course of therapy to account for changes in the tumor and/or adjacent tissue. The use of FDG–PET-CT has been reported to allow a smaller target volume to be radiated during radiotherapy delivery and to facilitate dose escalation.[74]

The use of 4D imaging in radiation treatment planning introduces the concept of time to the 3D conformal treatment planning and compensates for tumor motion, patient movement, and movement occurring either during a single fraction (intrafraction) or between multiple fractions (interfraction) of radiation.[75] Intrafractional movement can cause significant target deformation resulting from respiratory motion, and interfractional variation can interfere in tumor delineation as tumor and anatomy may change significantly between each treatment session. 4D treatment planning allows an assessment of tumor motion across an entire respiratory cycle, and radiation therapy is delivered accordingly. 4D-CT is currently being used in conjunction with 3D-CRT and IMRT to achieve high-precision radiation dose delivery to the tumor.[75] In addition, in the treatment of lung cancer, using SBRT with 4D-CT imaging allows a significant reduction of target volumes and decreased dose to surrounding tissue when compared with conventional 3D-CT.[76–78] 4D-CT–based planning has also optimized radiation delivery in patients with lung cancer receiving proton therapy.[79] In patients with target volumes that have a large amount of motion (typically >1 cm), two approaches can be used to further reduce the amount of lung treated. The first, *respiratory gating,* allows delivery of radiation only during certain phases of the respiratory cycle while the patient breathes normally. The second, *deep inspiratory breath hold*, has the patient "hold his or her breath" after deep inspiration. Because radiation is delivered when the tumor is in a relatively "fixed" position with either of these approaches, the full extent of the tumor motion does not need to be delineated.

Proton therapy can allow high-dose radiation delivery to the tumor with minimal radiation exposure to the adjacent organs. The advantage of proton therapy relies on the physical characteristics of the proton particles, which deposit nearly all the therapeutic dose at a particular depth (Bragg peak), and this typically results in a negligible exit dose beyond the target. However, in aerated lung, proton beams travel beyond the distal edge of the tumor and can cause damage to adjacent lung tissue. A study assessing dosimetric values for stage I and III NSCLC treated with proton therapy, compared with 3D-CRT and IMRT, has shown that all three techniques provide adequate tumor coverage, but proton therapy delivers lower doses to the adjacent

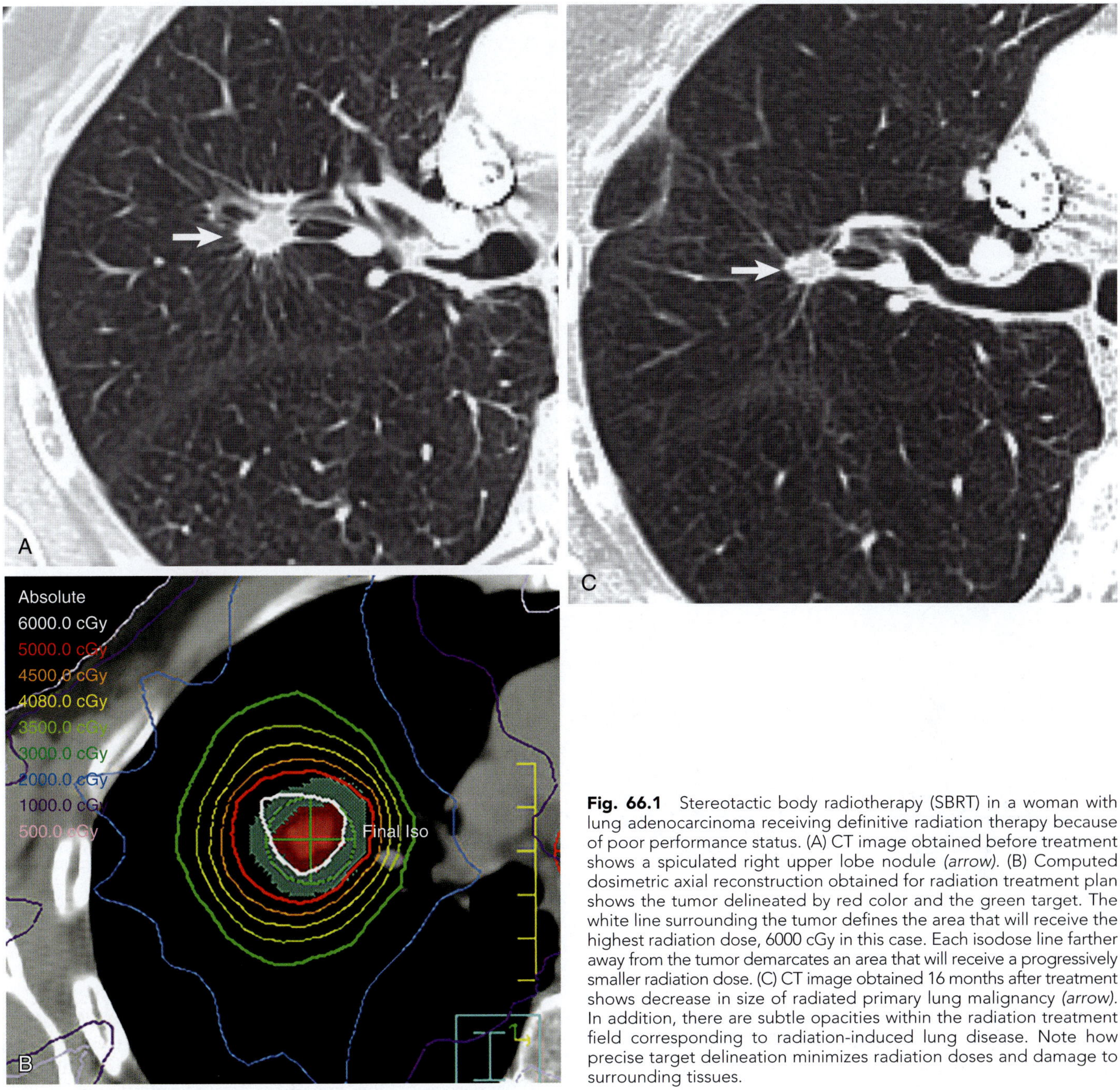

Fig. 66.1 Stereotactic body radiotherapy (SBRT) in a woman with lung adenocarcinoma receiving definitive radiation therapy because of poor performance status. (A) CT image obtained before treatment shows a spiculated right upper lobe nodule *(arrow)*. (B) Computed dosimetric axial reconstruction obtained for radiation treatment plan shows the tumor delineated by red color and the green target. The white line surrounding the tumor defines the area that will receive the highest radiation dose, 6000 cGy in this case. Each isodose line farther away from the tumor demarcates an area that will receive a progressively smaller radiation dose. (C) CT image obtained 16 months after treatment shows decrease in size of radiated primary lung malignancy *(arrow)*. In addition, there are subtle opacities within the radiation treatment field corresponding to radiation-induced lung disease. Note how precise target delineation minimizes radiation doses and damage to surrounding tissues.

lung, esophagus, and spinal cord than the two other techniques.[80] Sejpal and colleagues[81] compared photon and proton-based RT and showed that proton therapy resulted in lower rates of esophagitis and severe pneumonitis than 3D-CRT and IMRT. However, the use of proton therapy in patients with lung cancer is not clearly defined.[82] Currently, proton therapy has been indicated for centrally located tumors adjacent to the heart, spinal cord, and esophagus (Fig. 66.2) as well as tumors close to the brachial plexus.[83] In addition, a recent phase II randomized study from The University of Texas M.D. Anderson Cancer Center highlighted the need for adequate patient selection for this approach. Patients with locally advanced NSCLC were randomized to IMRT or passive scattering proton therapy (proton therapy using 3D-conformal techniques). The coprimary end points were the incidence of radiation pneumonitis and locoregional control, and in this unselected patient population, there was no difference between the two modalities.[84] Further analyses are underway comparing IMRT with intensity-modulated proton therapy (proton therapy incorporating features of inverse planning and with greater conformality than the passive scattering approach), which use selective dose escalation based on normal tissue doses.

Dose and Fractionation

External-beam radiation therapy is an established treatment option for patients with nonresectable locally advanced (stage III) NSCLC. Typically, a standard dose of 60 Gy, given in a single fraction per day, 5 days a week, during 6 weeks is used. The use

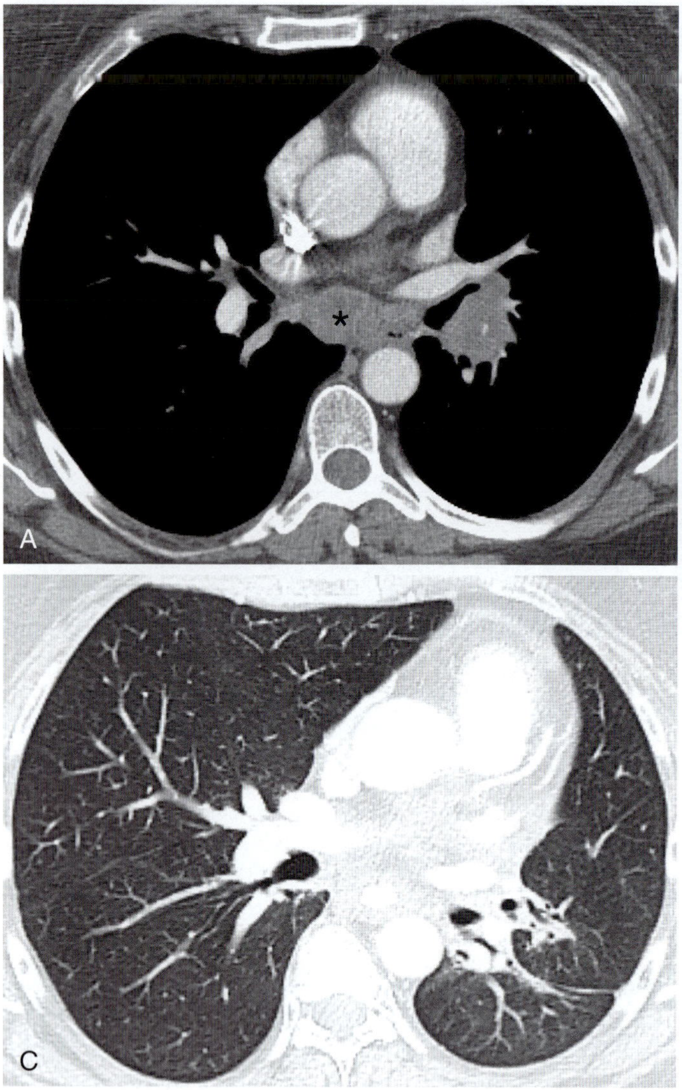

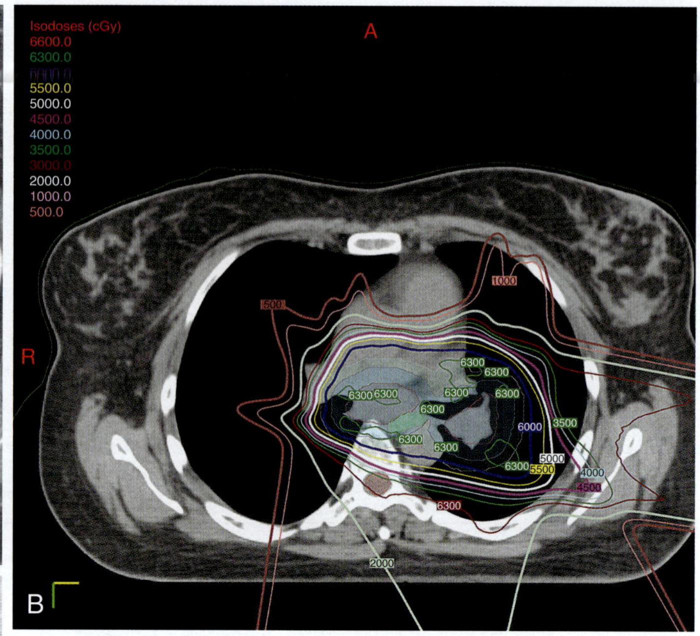

Fig. 66.2 Proton radiation in a woman with lung adenocarcinoma. (A) CT image obtained before treatment shows a left lower lobe mass extending to the left hilar region and subcarinal nodal metastasis *(asterisk)*. (B) Computed dosimetric axial reconstruction obtained for proton radiation plan shows primary lung malignancy and nodal metastatic disease receiving maximal isodose (6600 cGY). (C) CT image obtained 3 years after radiation therapy shows focal lung opacities confined to treatment field and normal adjacent lung.

of this dose has been recently confirmed in a comparison study as 74 Gy in a phase III national trial.[85,86] However, because changing the time interval and the dose of radiation can influence the response of both normal and tumor tissues to radiotherapy and can optimize radiation treatment, different fractionation schedules have also been assessed as treatment options for stage I to III NSCLC.[87] In the hyperfractionation scheme, there is delivery of more than one fraction in 24 hours, using a larger number of fractions per week (between 10 and 25 fractions) and using a dose per fraction of less than 1.8 Gy.[88] Although several hyperfractionation regimens have been tested in randomized trials for NSCLC, it has not been shown to be superior to standard fractionated regimens. Currently, a hyperfractionated schedule is selectively used for patients with NSCLC located near the spinal cord and brachial plexus, as late side effects can occur after high doses with a standard fractionation regimen. However, in the setting of small cell lung cancer, a hyperfractionated regimen of 1.5 Gy delivered twice daily to 45 Gy is one of a limited number of acceptable treatment options and is currently being further assessed in a phase III randomized trial.

In addition, accelerated fractionation can be used. Accelerated fractionation is related to the intensity of the treatment over time in which the rate of dose accumulation is greater than 10 Gy per week. One type of accelerated radiotherapy is called continuous hyperfractionated accelerated radiotherapy (CHART), which combines hyperfractionation and accelerated schemes in a 54-Gy treatment, given in three fractions a day, 1.5 Gy per fraction, during 12 days. Saunders and colleagues[89] compared the CHART scheme with standard radiation therapy and demonstrated improved survival in NSCLC patients.

An alternative to hyperfractionation is hypofractionation, which includes a larger dose per fraction (>3.0 Gy) and fewer fractions, 1 to 4 days a week, and is the basis of SBRT.

Clinical Presentation

The description of classic radiation-induced lung injury has three main phases: (1) an initial latent phase (first 3–4 weeks after completion of therapy); (2) an early phase: acute exudative pneumonitis (3 weeks to 6 months); and (3) a late phase: pulmonary fibrosis (6 months and later).[31,90] Radiation-induced lung disease usually manifests clinically as acute pneumonitis 4 to 12 weeks after completion of radiation therapy, although symptoms occasionally occur as early as 1 month after the beginning of radiation therapy and as late as 6 months after completion of treatment.[22,24] The earlier clinical presentation of acute pneumonitis can occur with the newer treatment regimens that use hyperfractionated accelerated radiation. For instance, in a study evaluating escalated hyperfractionated accelerated radiation therapy in locally advanced NSCLC, acute pneumonitis developed in 40% of the patients, and onset was typically before the completion of treatment (median, 4 weeks after beginning of treatment; range, 3–5 weeks).[16]

In general, clinical symptoms are proportional to the extent of the radiation-induced lung injury and pretreatment pulmonary function of the patient. Symptomatic patients typically present with cough and mild dyspnea, although patients can have severe respiratory compromise.[22,91] In addition, patients can occasionally present with chest pain, fever associated with nonproductive cough, or cough productive of small amounts of blood-tinged sputum.[22,31,91]

Acute radiation-induced pneumonitis manifesting as mild to moderate dyspnea generally resolves with treatment.[24,92] In the 6.7% to 16% of patients with NSCLC who develop severe respiratory distress, morbidity and mortality can be high.[31,36,93,94] In fact, Wang and colleagues[31] reported that severe acute radiation-induced pneumonitis was associated with a mortality rate approaching 50% in the first 2 months after the onset of symptoms. Also, although IMRT after extrapleural pneumonectomy in patients with pleural mesothelioma has not typically been associated with radiation-induced injury in the remaining lung,[95] 6 of 13 patients (46%) in a study developed severe pneumonitis in the contralateral lung 5 to 57 days (mean, 30 days) after completion of therapy, with subsequent demise of all 6 patients.[51]

It is important to be aware that (1) symptomatic radiation-induced pneumonitis does not predict subsequent fibrosis, and (2) the clinical manifestations of acute radiation-induced pneumonitis often cannot be accounted for by the radiation therapy received by the patient (i.e., the dyspnea is more severe than would be expected from the volume of lung irradiated). It is postulated that a hypersensitivity reaction occurs in response to localized lung irradiation and results in an out-of-field pneumonitis.[31,96,97]

In the late phase of radiation-induced lung injury, pulmonary fibrosis localized to the region of the irradiated lung typically develops after 6 months. Most patients with radiation fibrosis are asymptomatic, although dyspnea that varies from minimal to severe can be present. Symptoms are usually minimal if fibrosis is limited to less than 50% of one lung.[91] Chronic respiratory failure and cor pulmonale secondary to fibrosis of a large volume of lung can occasionally occur as late manifestations of radiation-induced lung disease.[22]

Pathophysiology

Radiation-induced lung injury has classically been described as separate phases encompassing acute pneumonitis and fibrosis that occur at different times after radiation therapy. However, radiation-induced lung injury can be viewed as a continuum, with no distinct separation between the temporal sequences of the different phases of injury.[98] In terms of the pathophysiologic process, radiation therapy initiates a sequence of molecular and genetic changes resulting in lung injury.[91,98] The biologic effects of ionizing radiation begin with the overproduction of oxygen free radicals, more generally known as reactive oxygen species.[99,100] Reactive oxygen species result in damage to endothelial cells and exudation of proteinaceous material into the alveoli, desquamation of epithelial cells from the alveolar wall, and infiltration of inflammatory cells.[91,100] Depending on the severity of injury, these pathologic exudative changes may resolve in a few weeks to months or result in an acute radiation pneumonitis.

The continuous overproduction of reactive oxygen species after the initial injury may occur for months or years after the completion of radiation therapy and result in the progressive tissue damage, loss of parenchymal cells, and fibrosis that are histologically typical of late radiation lung injury.[101,102] Uncommonly, radiation-induced lung injury is manifested as organizing pneumonia, most commonly outside the expected radiation field,[103–105] and chronic eosinophilic pneumonia, particularly in patients with history of asthma or atopy.[106]

LUNG FUNCTION

The severity of pneumonitis (grade 1–5) is usually defined clinically by the Southwest Oncology Group standard response criteria or the toxicity criteria of the Radiation Therapy Oncology Group and the European Organization for Research and Treatment of Cancer, according to the absence or presence of dyspnea and cough and the treatment required by the patient.[24,25,91,107] However, unfortunately, these grading systems are to a large extent subjective and difficult to correlate with pulmonary function test results. Fifty percent to 90% of patients experience a decline in pulmonary function test results after radiation therapy, and these tests have been comprehensively evaluated in an effort to predict the incidence and severity of radiation-induced pneumonitis.[24,50,91,108–110] Pulmonary function test results are relatively normal in most patients in the 4 to 8 weeks after completion of radiation therapy.[91] Subsequently, a wide range of changes can occur in pulmonary function in both the acute pneumonitis phase and late fibrotic phase. Decreases have been noted in vital capacity, inspiratory capacity, total lung capacity, residual volume, forced expiratory volume in 1 second, and carbon monoxide diffusing capacity (DLCO).[24,110] DLCO is generally the most severely affected parameter, and the impairment can progress with a reported annual decrease of 3.5% after the first year that follows radiation therapy completion.[24,109–112]

Manifestations of the Disease

GENERAL

The histopathologic response of the lungs to radiation injury is limited and manifested radiologically as two major distinct patterns. To describe these patterns of radiation-induced lung disease, the end of radiation therapy has traditionally been used as a reference point for the temporal sequence of changes because the length of treatment varies, and thus reference from the beginning of treatment would be inconsistent. Typically, acute radiation pneumonitis occurs 4 to 12 weeks after completion of radiation therapy and is followed within 6 to 12 months by radiation-induced fibrosis in the region of the radiation-induced lung injury.[19,28–30,113–116]

The criteria for the diagnosis of radiation-induced organizing pneumonia include radiotherapy within 12 months, symptom

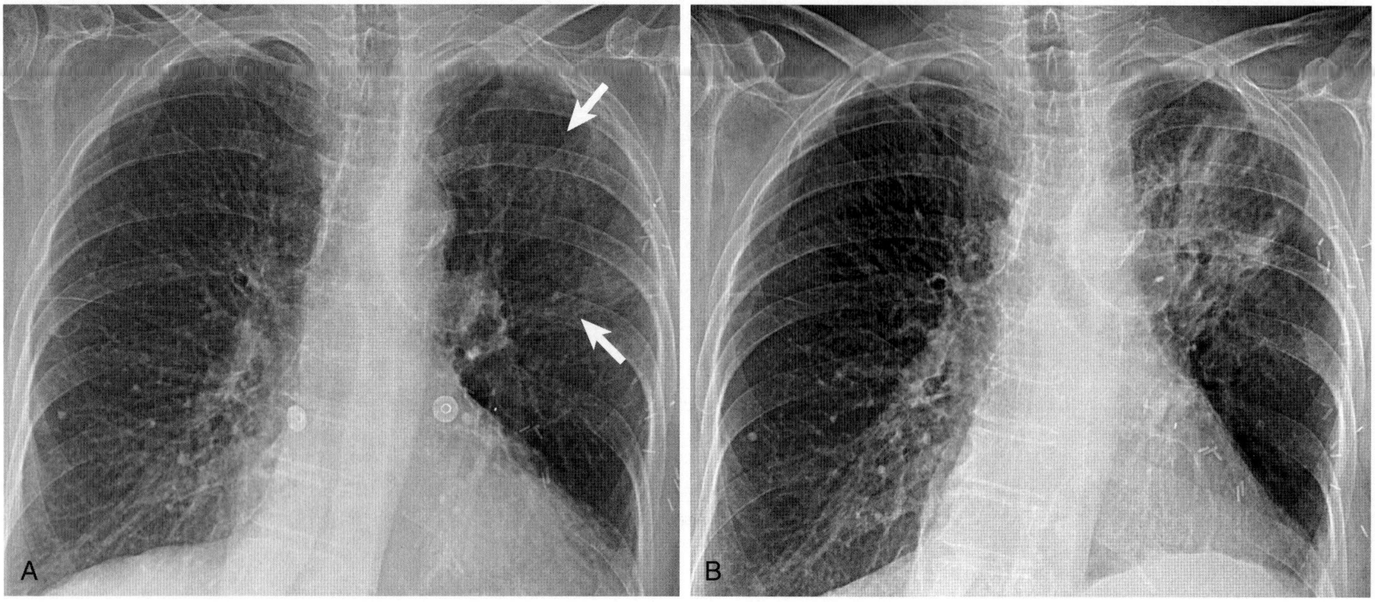

Fig. 66.3 Radiation pneumonitis in a woman with non–small cell lung cancer in the left lung. (A) Chest radiograph obtained 1 month after completion of radiation therapy shows radiation pneumonitis manifesting as increased hazy opacities in left lung *(arrows)* within the radiation field. (B) Chest radiograph obtained several months after completion of radiation therapy shows consolidation, volume loss, and traction bronchiectasis consistent with fibrosis.

duration of at least 2 weeks, pulmonary airspace opacities outside the radiation treatment field on chest radiography or CT, and exclusion of other causes.[105] Diagnostic criteria for radiation-induced chronic eosinophilic pneumonia are similar to those associated with organizing pneumonia but include the presence of blood eosinophilia higher than 1×10^9/L or more than 40% eosinophils in the differential cell count of bronchoalveolar lavage fluid.[106]

RADIOGRAPHY

The acute phase of radiation-induced lung disease initially is manifested radiographically as ground-glass opacities or consolidation in the treatment field (Fig. 66.3). Although radiation pneumonitis usually occurs within the irradiated lung, radiation pneumonitis outside the treatment fields has been reported.[117–123] Ipsilateral pleural effusions can occur after radiation therapy and usually develop at the time of radiation pneumonitis (i.e., within 6 months after completion of therapy).[7,20] Pleural effusions that develop after 6 months, continue to increase in size, or present as large effusions may require thoracentesis for differentiation of benign from malignant disease.

Although the opacities of radiation pneumonitis can gradually resolve without radiologic sequelae when the injury to the lung is limited, in cases of more severe injury, there is usually a progression to fibrosis.[20,124] The majority of fibrosis will occur within the first 12 months, and the development commonly progresses slowly in the 6 to 12 months after completion of therapy and stabilizes within 2 years. Radiation fibrosis is manifested radiologically as a well-defined area of volume loss, linear scarring, consolidation, and traction bronchiectasis. Consolidation usually coalesces and typically has a relatively sharp margin that conforms to the treatment field rather than to anatomic boundaries (Fig. 66.4).[20,27,29,30,124] With the evolution of radiation fibrosis, the demarcation between normal and irradiated lung parenchyma often becomes more sharply defined.

COMPUTED TOMOGRAPHY

CT is more sensitive than chest radiography in detecting radiation-induced lung disease. Ground-glass opacities representing early radiation pneumonitis (Fig. 66.5) can be seen a few weeks after completion of radiation therapy, although the radiograph is often normal.[20,120–122] With some of the newer treatment regimens, opacities can sometimes be observed on CT before or at completion of radiation therapy. On occasion, acute pneumonitis detected on CT can appear nodular and simulate metastatic nodules.[125,126] Typically, the nodules of radiation pneumonitis will be within the lung that underwent radiation therapy and are irregular or poorly marginated (Fig. 66.6). The nodules usually coalesce into areas of consolidation and eventually become a component of the radiation fibrosis. CT is the optimal modality for assessment of the evolution and chronic manifestations of radiation-induced lung injury (Fig. 66.7) and for the detection of locoregional recurrence of malignant disease (see the section on differential diagnosis).

The technique used to deliver radiation will affect the CT manifestations of radiation-induced lung disease. Radiation-induced lung disease varies in shape and distribution with new radiation delivery techniques as the radiation dose is altered according to the location, extent, and type of malignant neoplasm for delivery of a tumoricidal dose while limiting the dose of radiation to adjacent lung. Recognition of imaging manifestations of this treatment can be facilitated with computed dosimetric reconstruction, whereby treatment volumes are superimposed on CT images (Figs. 66.8 and 66.9).[127] In addition, the use of

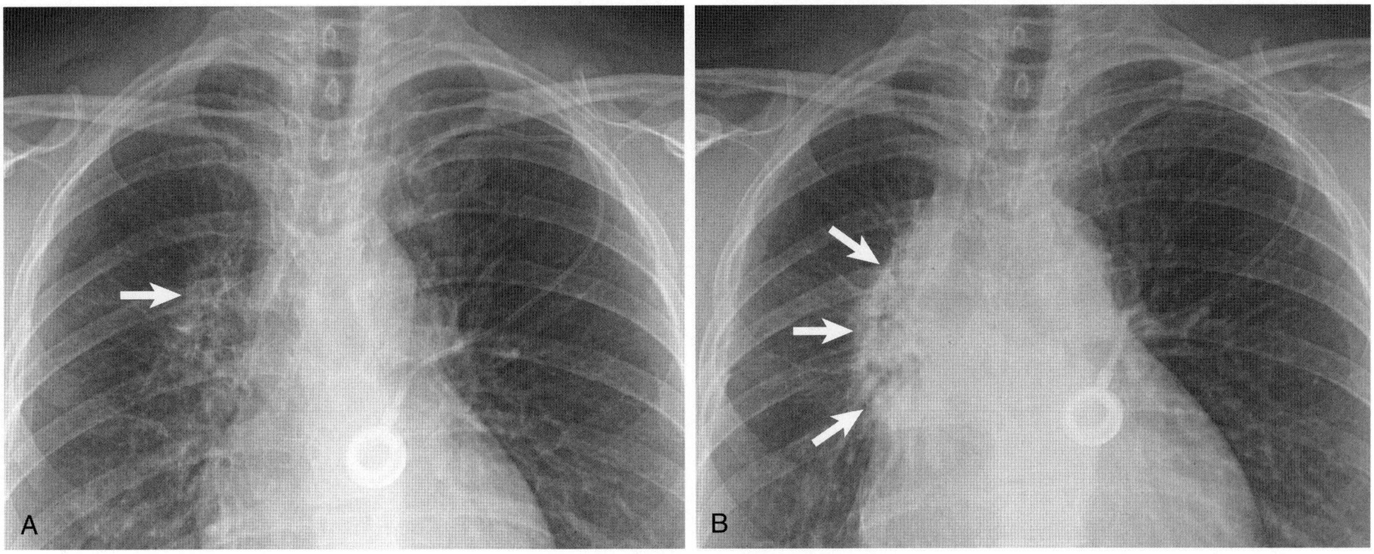

Fig. 66.4 Temporal evolution of radiation-induced lung disease in a woman with non–small cell lung cancer. (A) Chest radiograph obtained after resection of right lung cancer and 5 months after completion of radiation therapy shows radiation pneumonitis manifesting as increased hazy opacity *(arrow)* within radiation field. (B) Chest radiograph obtained 19 months after completion of radiation therapy shows evolution of postradiation findings with consolidation, traction bronchiectasis, and volume loss associated with architectural distortion. Note sharp demarcation between normal and irradiated lung parenchyma *(arrows)*.

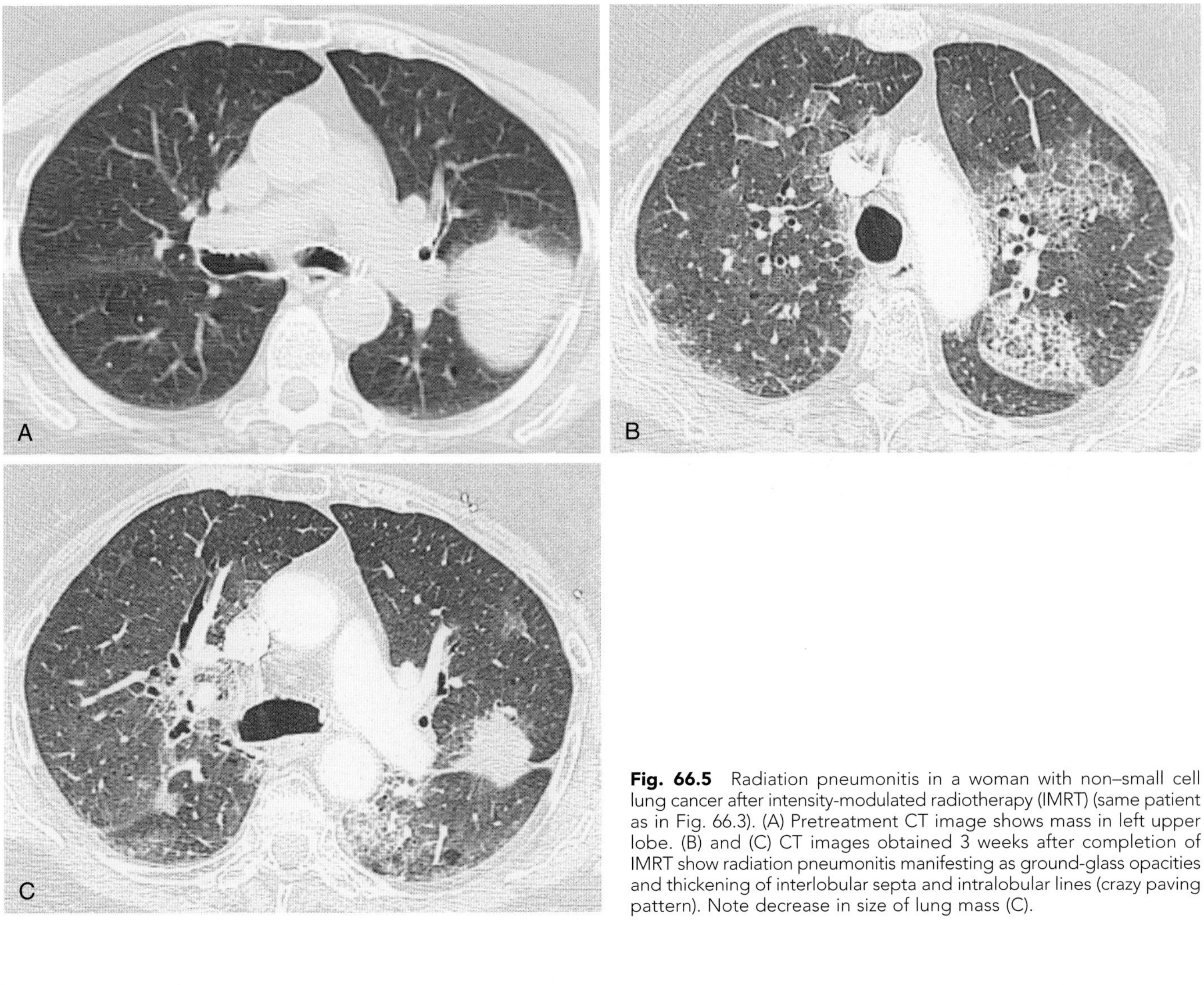

Fig. 66.5 Radiation pneumonitis in a woman with non–small cell lung cancer after intensity-modulated radiotherapy (IMRT) (same patient as in Fig. 66.3). (A) Pretreatment CT image shows mass in left upper lobe. (B) and (C) CT images obtained 3 weeks after completion of IMRT show radiation pneumonitis manifesting as ground-glass opacities and thickening of interlobular septa and intralobular lines (crazy paving pattern). Note decrease in size of lung mass (C).

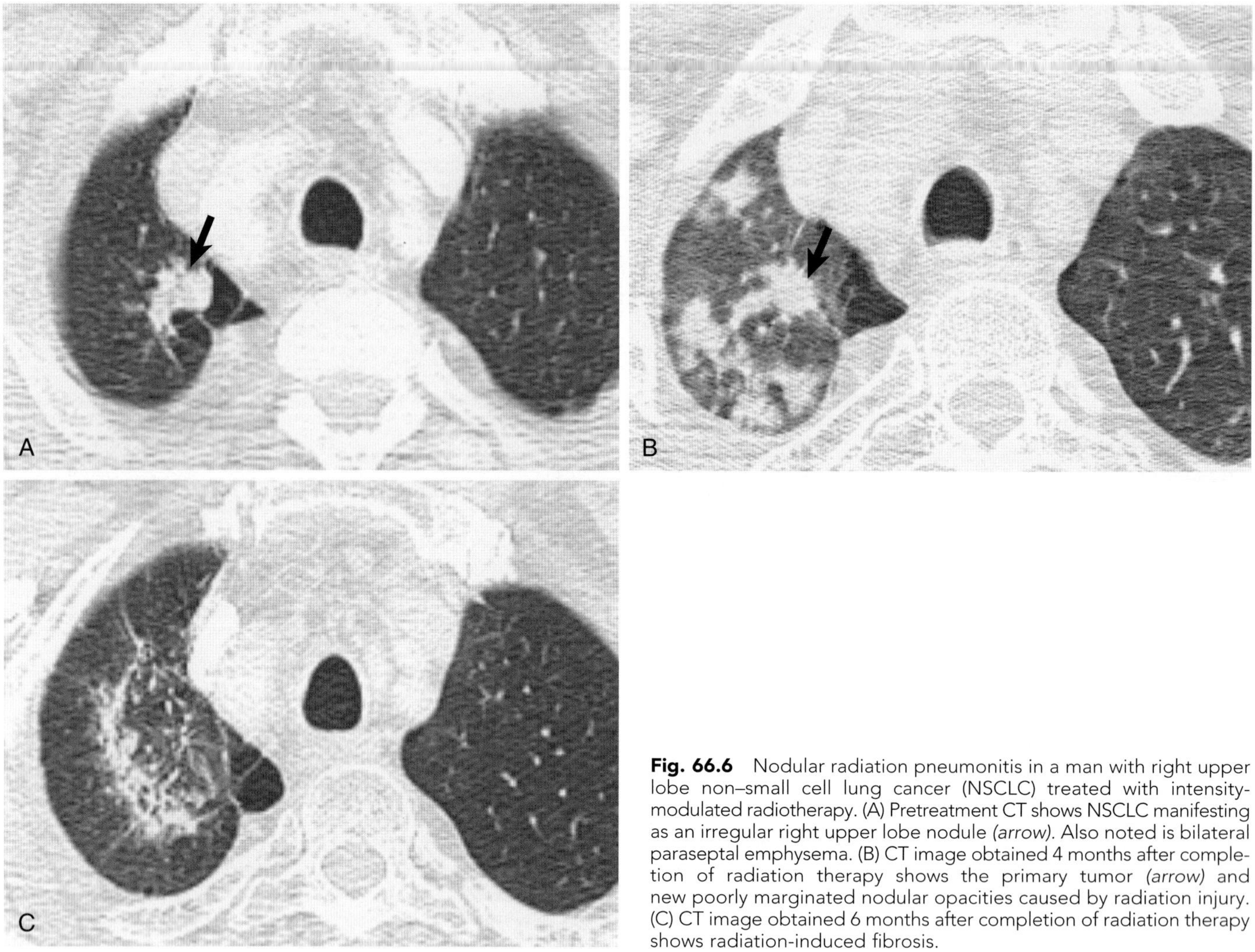

Fig. 66.6 Nodular radiation pneumonitis in a man with right upper lobe non–small cell lung cancer (NSCLC) treated with intensity-modulated radiotherapy. (A) Pretreatment CT shows NSCLC manifesting as an irregular right upper lobe nodule *(arrow)*. Also noted is bilateral paraseptal emphysema. (B) CT image obtained 4 months after completion of radiation therapy shows the primary tumor *(arrow)* and new poorly marginated nodular opacities caused by radiation injury. (C) CT image obtained 6 months after completion of radiation therapy shows radiation-induced fibrosis.

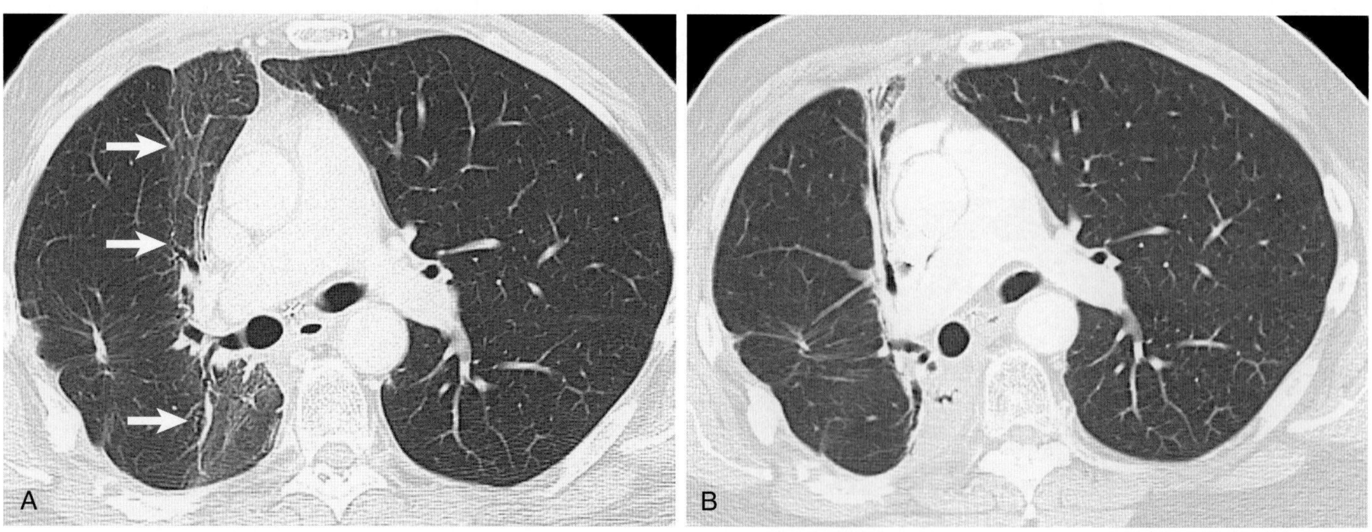

Fig. 66.7 Radiation fibrosis in a man after resection of right lower lobe non–small cell lung cancer and conventional radiation therapy. (A) CT scan obtained 4 months after conventional radiation therapy shows ground-glass opacities in the right lung. Note sharp demarcation between normal lung and ground-glass opacities *(arrows)*. (B) CT scan obtained 10 months after completion of radiation therapy shows opacity with sharp margin, traction bronchiectasis, and volume loss consistent with fibrosis.

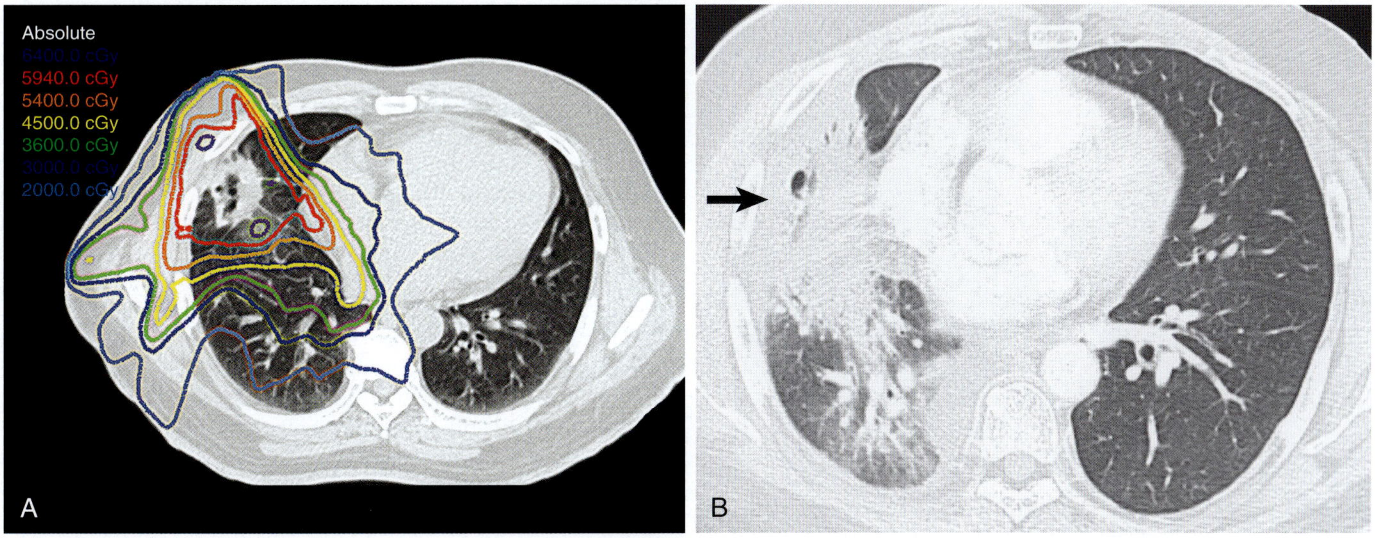

Fig. 66.8 Radiation-induced fibrosis in a man with a history of non–small cell lung cancer treated by intensity-modulated radiotherapy (IMRT). (A) Computed dosimetric reconstruction axial image used for planning IMRT shows a right middle lobe mass. The highest area of radiation (59.4 Gy) is a red line surrounding the region of the mass. Note that with IMRT, the highest dose of radiation is delivered to the tumor, whereas with standard radiation therapy, the highest dose would be at the chest wall. (B) CT image obtained 5 months after completion of radiation therapy shows that areas of consolidation resulting from radiation-induced lung injury *(arrow)* correlate with areas with the highest radiation dose on computed dosimetric reconstruction image used for planning IMRT. Also noted are volume loss and focal consolidation in the right lower lobe. Note loculated pleural fluid adjacent to the vertebral body.

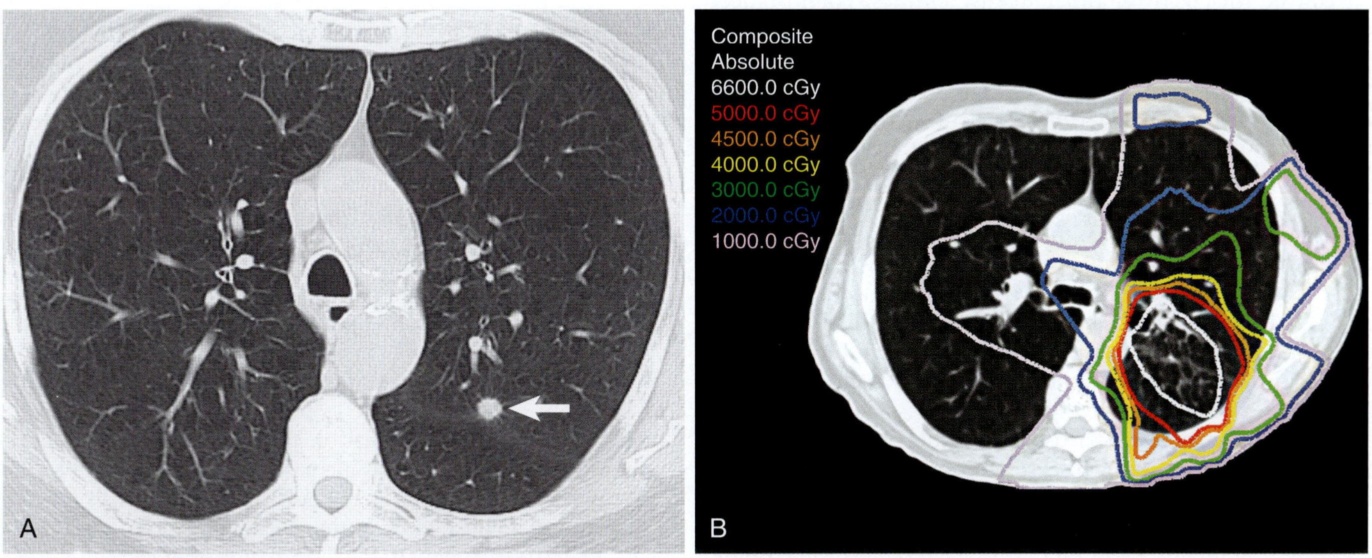

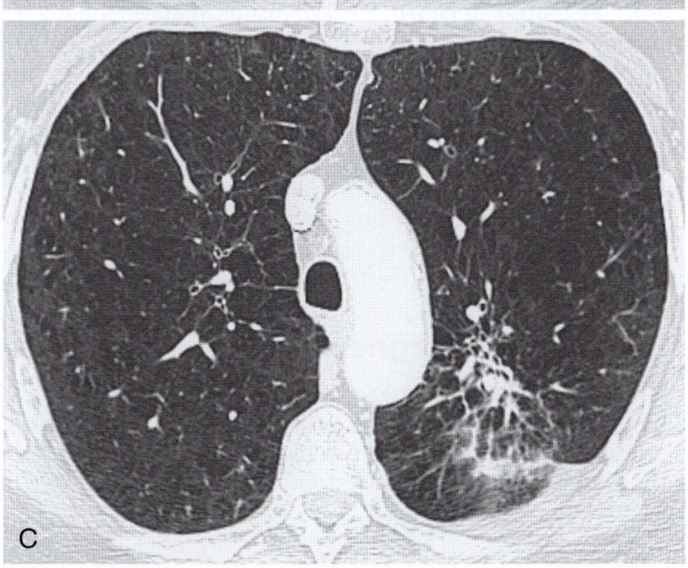

Fig. 66.9 Radiation-induced lung disease in a man with emphysema and stage I non–small cell lung cancer treated with three-dimensional conformal radiotherapy (3D-CRT) because of poor respiratory function. (A) Pretreatment CT image shows a small left upper lobe nodule *(arrow)*. (B) Computed dosimetric reconstruction used for 3D-CRT shows the area of lung receiving the highest radiation dose of 66 Gy delineated by the white line surrounding the location of the nodule. (C) CT image obtained 3 years after completion of radiation therapy shows focal opacity corresponding to the area of the lung receiving the highest radiation dose consistent with radiation-induced fibrosis.

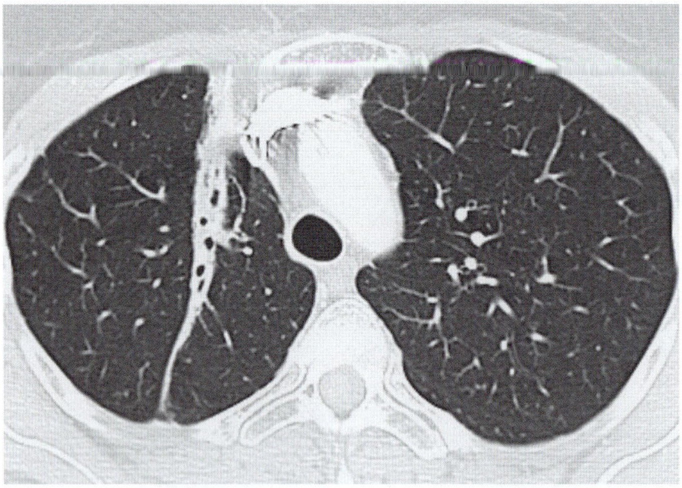

Fig. 66.10 Radiation-induced fibrosis in a woman with non–small cell lung cancer after lung injury resulting from three-dimensional conformal radiotherapy. CT scan obtained 7 years after completion of radiation therapy shows only a linear band of fibrosis with traction bronchiectasis that resembles scar.

the newer methods of delivering radiation can result in lung opacities at unusual locations away from the site of disease that can be mistaken for other disease entities. For instance, when an NSCLC is treated, radiation-induced lung disease can manifest as modified conventional (consolidation, volume loss, and bronchiectasis similar to but less extensive than conventional radiation fibrosis), scar-like (linear opacity in the region of the original tumor (Fig. 66.10), and mass-like patterns (Fig. 66.11). Although diagnostic confusion is unlikely to arise from the modified conventional and scar-like patterns, the mass-like pattern can easily be misinterpreted as malignant neoplasia in the absence of a history of new methods of radiation therapy delivery.[128] In accordance, it is important to be aware that the newer techniques of 3D-CRT, IMRT, SBRT, and proton therapy often distribute dose to unexpected areas, and to avoid diagnostic confusion, the specific isodose patterns associated with each individual patient plan need to be recognized.

It is also important that the typical radiologic manifestations of radiation-induced lung disease associated with traditional radiation treatment fields be recognized. NSCLC typically has treatment fields that encompass the primary tumor with an additional 2-cm margin around the visualized edge of the tumor and a 1-cm margin around regional lymph nodes that are to be treated.[129] Nodal regions that are not grossly involved are no longer electively treated in NSCLC. In patients with small cell lung cancer, two types of radiation field arrangements have typically been used: extensive fields encompassing the hila, the mediastinum, and both supraclavicular areas and limited fields encompassing only the primary tumor and adjacent nodal stations with a high likelihood of neoplastic involvement.[129] In patients with breast cancer, the use of tangential radiation fields can result in radiation-induced lung disease that characteristically is manifested on CT as parenchymal opacities confined to the anterolateral subpleural region of the lung (Fig. 66.12).[122,130] To avoid confusion with infection such as tuberculosis, it is important to know that supraclavicular treatment fields are also occasionally used in breast cancer patients and will often result in apical radiation-induced lung disease (see Fig. 66.12). In patients with esophageal cancer, radiation fields with a 5-cm margin above and below the tumor are generally used. The radiation beams are angled to limit radiation exposure of the spinal cord and result in paramediastinal opacities in the lower lobes. Radiation therapy for head and neck cancer patients often includes the apical aspect of the thorax and results in bilateral apical radiation-induced lung disease. The mantle field used for definitive radiation therapy for Hodgkin or non-Hodgkin lymphomas includes all the major lymph node regions above the diaphragm and results in a classic appearance of radiation pneumonitis and fibrosis in the paramediastinal areas and in the apices (Fig. 66.13).[131,132]

The imaging findings of radiation-induced organizing pneumonia and chronic eosinophilic pneumonia are similar to those seen in patients with the idiopathic forms of these conditions (see Chapters 29 and 37) and may overlap with those of radiation pneumonitis. However, unlike typical radiation pneumonitis, the opacities may be migratory and are typically outside the radiation treatment field (Fig. 66.14).[105,106] The newer methods of delivering radiation can also result in lung opacities at unusual locations away from the site of the treated malignant neoplasm. Therefore parenchymal abnormalities outside the radiation treatment field can be related to radiation pneumonitis, organizing pneumonia, chronic eosinophilic pneumonia, infection, and tumor recurrence.

Pericardial effusions can occur after radiation therapy, are usually small in volume, and are accordingly usually detected by CT rather than by chest radiography. Pericardial effusions usually occur 6 to 9 months after completion of therapy.[133,134] In addition, chronic cardiac complications can occur, and these include chronic pericarditis, cardiomyopathy, myocardial infarction, coronary artery disease, conduction abnormalities, and valvular disease.[134]

COMPUTED TOMOGRAPHY–POSITRON EMISSION TOMOGRAPHY

Integrated CT-PET imaging performed with the radiopharmaceutical ^{18}F-FDG is increasingly used for posttreatment follow-up of various malignancies to facilitate early detection of locoregional recurrence and distant metastases. FDG-PET has been reported to be more accurate than CT in the evaluation of recurrent malignant disease after radiation therapy.[135–144] Acute radiation pneumonitis can manifest as increased FDG activity on PET, and this can persist in regions of radiation-induced fibrosis for up to 18 months.[135] The high negative predictive value of a normal FDG-PET study in patients with radiation-induced lung disease is clinically useful, and focal pulmonary opacities with low FDG uptake can be observed (Fig. 66.15). Focal, intense FDG uptake or FDG uptake that increases over time in the irradiated lung is suggestive of recurrent malignant disease (Fig. 66.16). However, a limitation of PET imaging is that false-positive uptake of FDG is not uncommon early after completion of radiation therapy and can persist. Because radiation pneumonitis can have increased FDG uptake that mimics recurrent disease, FDG-PET imaging is best performed 6 months after radiation therapy completion.

Differential Diagnosis

Patients with thoracic neoplasms treated with radiation can develop radiation-induced lung disease as well as superimposed lung disease. Diagnosis requires a high index of suspicion because the clinical and imaging manifestations of infection and recurrence

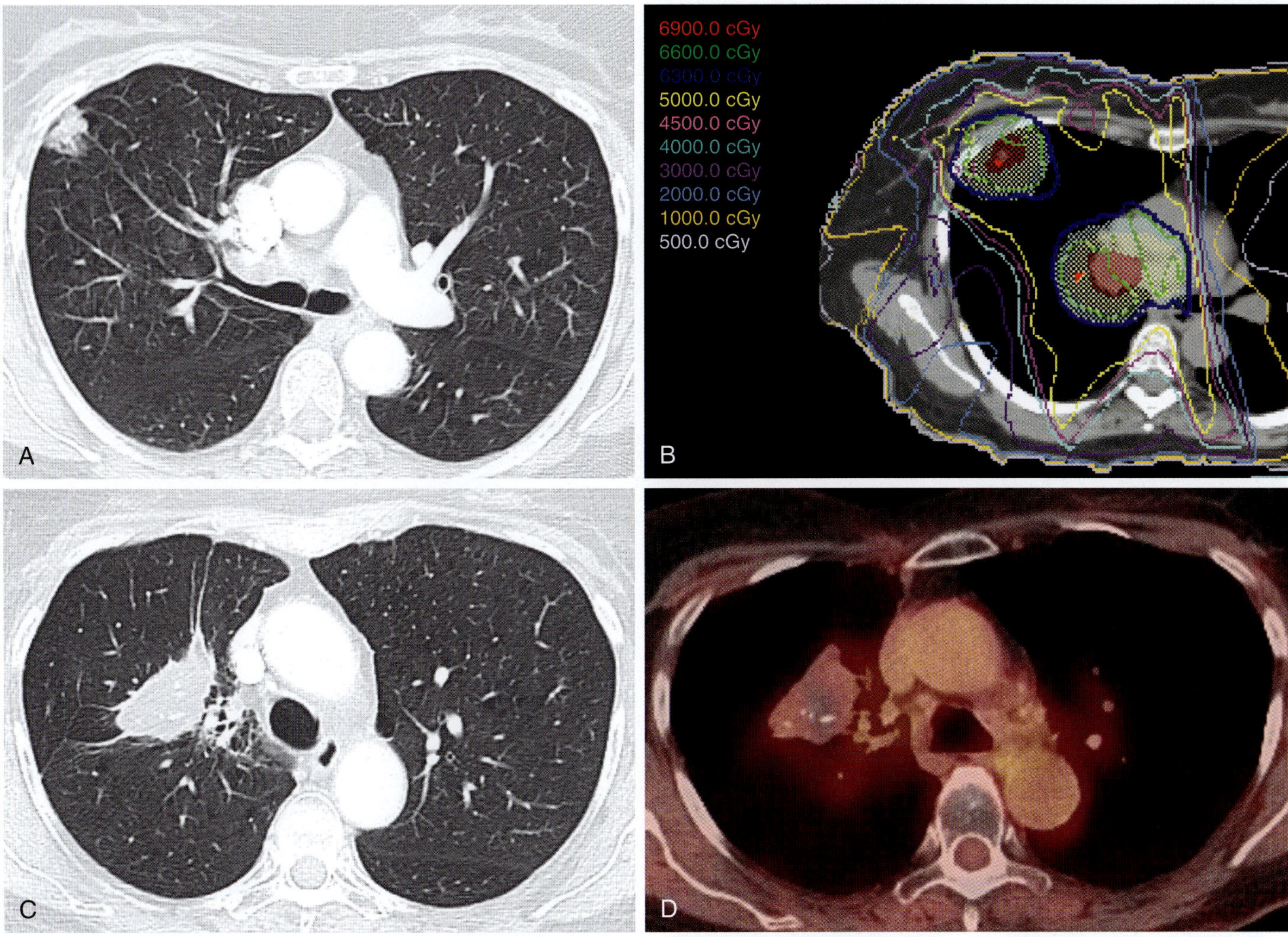

Fig. 66.11 Mass-like pattern of radiation-induced-lung disease in a woman with non–small cell lung cancer after intensity-modulated radiotherapy (IMRT). (A) Pretreatment CT image shows a right upper lobe nodule consistent with a primary lung malignancy. Right hilar adenopathy due to nodal metastatic disease is not shown. (B) Computed dosimetric axial reconstruction used for IMRT planning shows primary lung malignancy and right hilar adenopathy receiving maximal isodoses with sparing of the spinal cord. (C) CT image obtained 6 years after completion of radiation therapy shows mass-like opacity resulting from radiation-induced lung injury. Note how correlation with the radiation treatment plan can prevent misinterpretation of this opacity as malignancy. (D) Integrated positron emission tomography–CT obtained 6 years after completion of IMRT shows low-grade fluorodeoxyglucose uptake in mass-like opacity consistent with focal fibrosis and absence of recurrent malignancy. Note dystrophic calcification within the focal fibrosis.

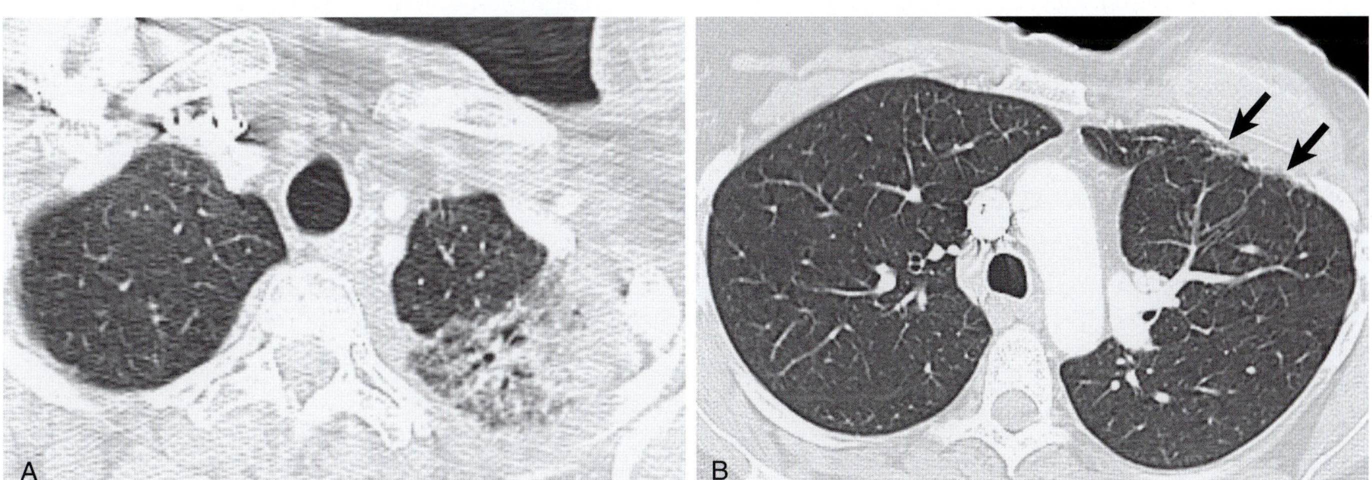

Fig. 66.12 Radiation-induced fibrosis in a woman with left breast cancer treated with tangent fields matched to supraclavicular fields. (A) CT scan obtained 6 years after completion of radiation therapy shows apical fibrosis. (B) CT image more caudad to (A) shows typical pattern of subpleural radiation fibrosis in lung *(arrows)* adjacent to treated chest wall.

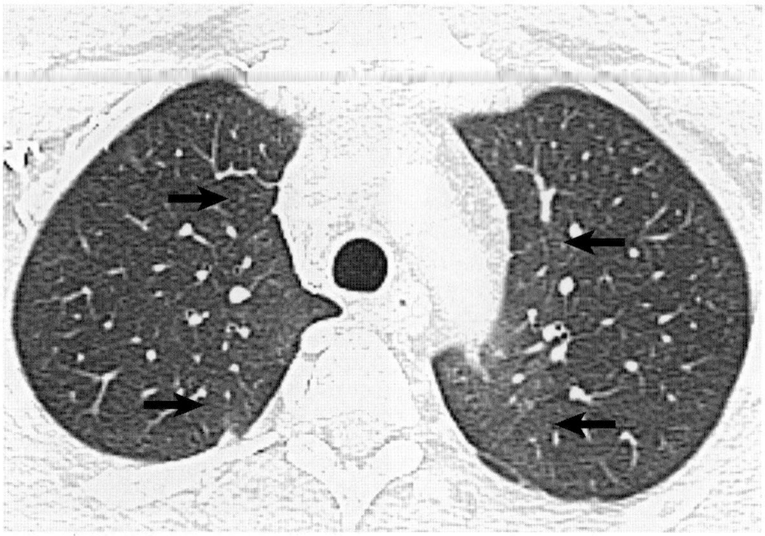

Fig. 66.13 Paramediastinal radiation-induced lung disease in a man with large cell lymphoma. CT image obtained 10 weeks after completion of radiation therapy shows subtle paramediastinal ground-glass opacities *(arrows)* in upper lobes indicative of radiation pneumonitis.

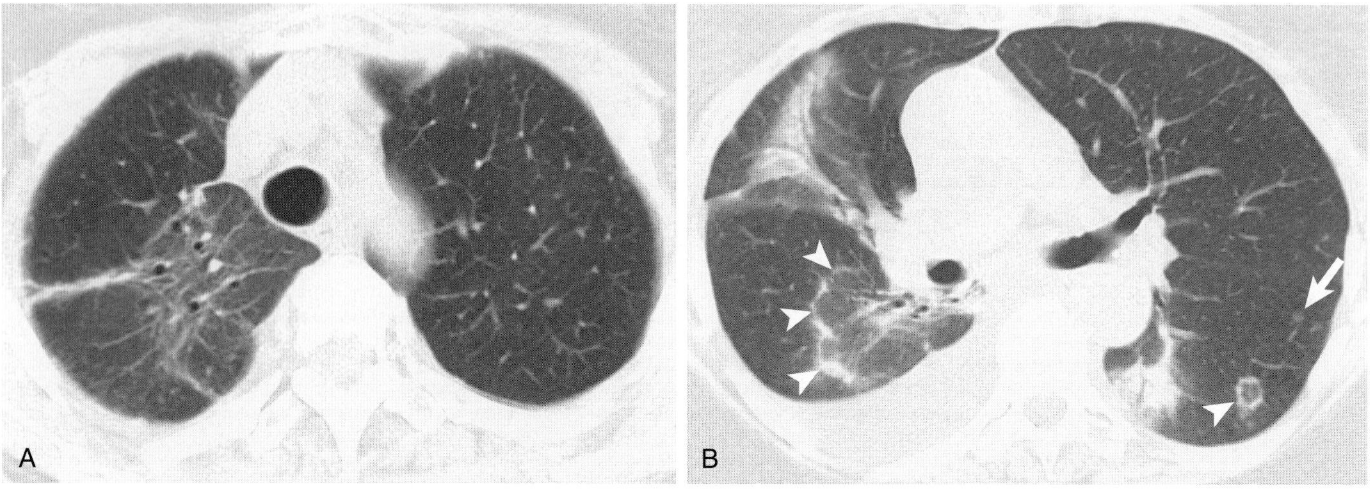

Fig. 66.14 Organizing pneumonia in a woman with early right breast carcinoma treated by conventional radiation therapy. (A) CT image at the level of great vessels shows localized ground-glass opacities and dilated bronchi in the right upper lobe. Note sharp demarcation between normal lung and ground-glass opacities. The findings are similar to those of radiation pneumonia. (B) CT image at the level of bronchus intermedius demonstrates bilateral peribronchial opacities outside the radiation treatment field. Note ring-like consolidation *(arrowheads)* surrounding ground-glass opacity (reversed halo sign) in both lower lobes typical of organizing pneumonia. Also noted is a small nodule *(arrow)* in the left lower lobe and a right pleural effusion.

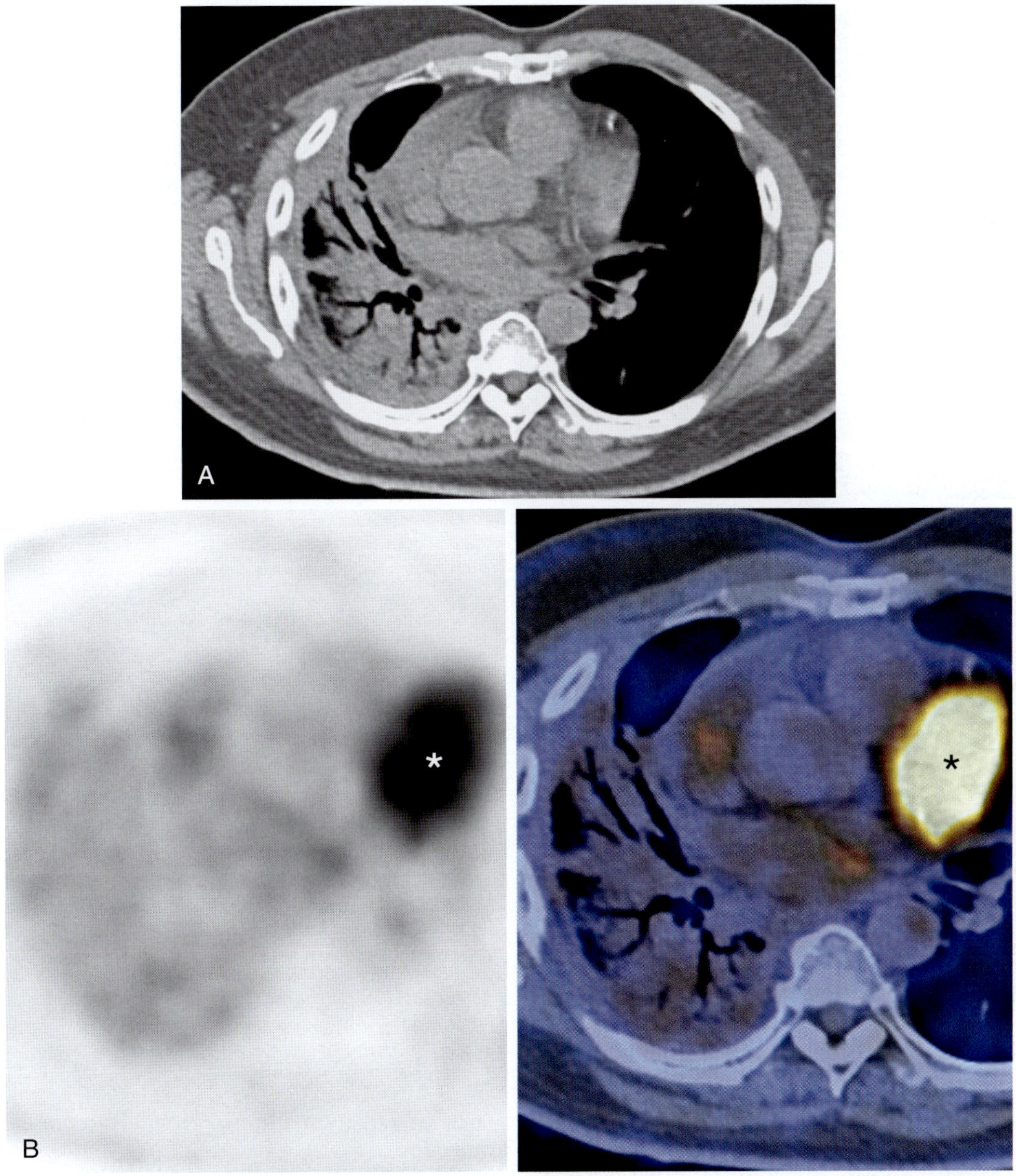

Fig. 66.15 Radiation-induced fibrosis in a man with a history of non–small cell lung cancer treated by intensity-modulated radiotherapy (IMRT). CT (A) and composite image (B) containing positron emission tomography (PET) *(left image)*, and integrated CT-PET *(right image)* 13 months after IMRT show homogeneous low-grade fluorodeoxyglucose (FDG) uptake within an area of radiation fibrosis in the right lung. High negative predictive value of FDG-PET scan allows conservative management. Note physiologic FDG uptake in the myocardium *(asterisks)*.

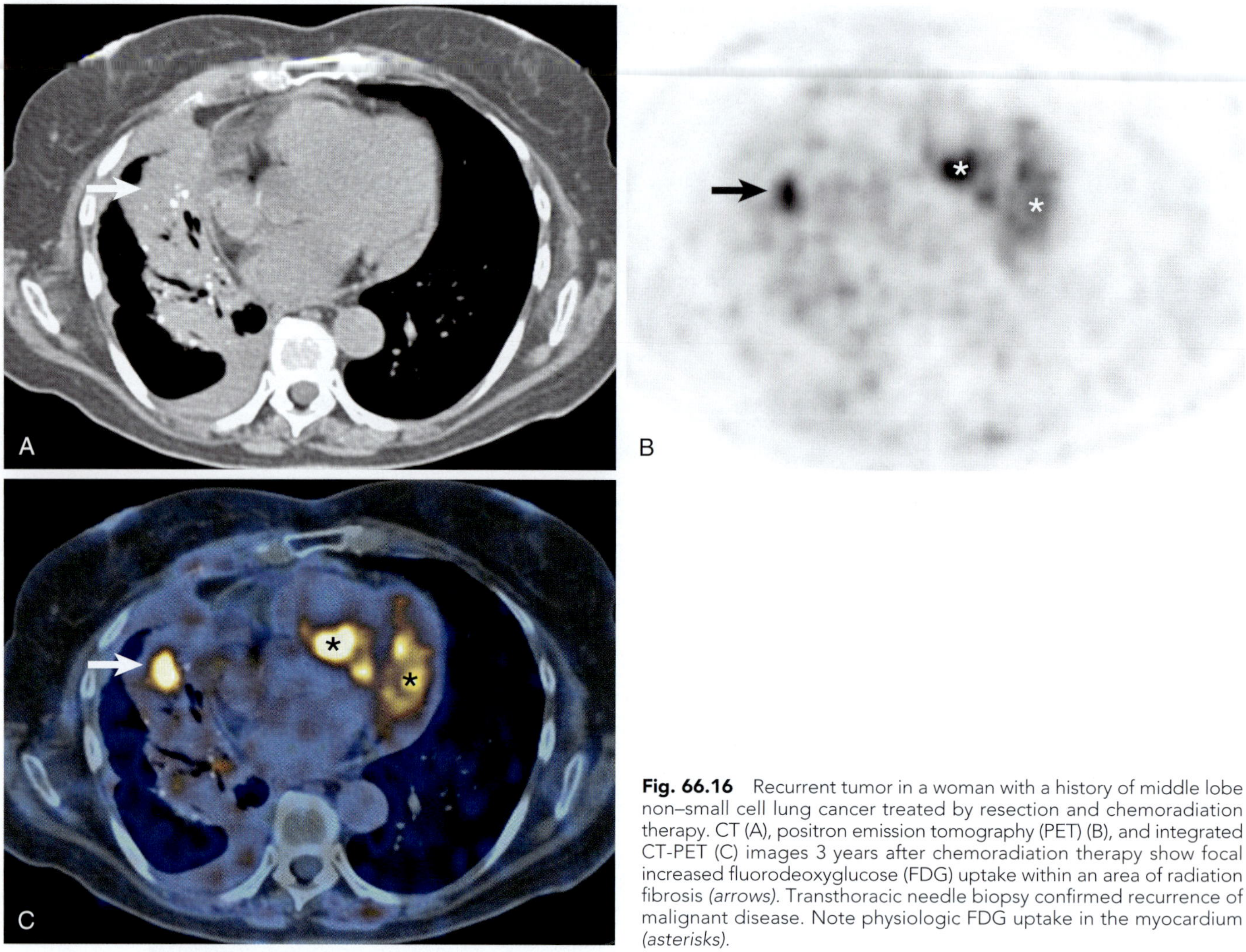

Fig. 66.16 Recurrent tumor in a woman with a history of middle lobe non–small cell lung cancer treated by resection and chemoradiation therapy. CT (A), positron emission tomography (PET) (B), and integrated CT-PET (C) images 3 years after chemoradiation therapy show focal increased fluorodeoxyglucose (FDG) uptake within an area of radiation fibrosis *(arrows)*. Transthoracic needle biopsy confirmed recurrence of malignant disease. Note physiologic FDG uptake in the myocardium *(asterisks)*.

of the underlying neoplasm are often similar.[145] Knowledge of the temporal relationship of the imaging manifestations to radiation therapy completion date, radiation dose administered, and technique used can be useful in suggesting the diagnosis. In general, radiation pneumonitis should be suspected in patients who have received more than 40 Gy of radiation if the imaging findings occur within the radiation treatment fields and within an appropriate time course. When radiologic manifestations atypical for radiation-induced lung disease are observed, the possibility of infection and local recurrence of malignant disease should be considered.[27,125,126,146,147] Infection should be considered if the chest radiograph or CT image shows pulmonary opacities occurring before completion of radiation therapy and/or outside of the radiation treatment fields. Because radiation pneumonitis normally has a more indolent course than an infection, an abrupt onset is suggestive of an infection unless there has been recent discontinuation of steroids.[145] Additional findings can also suggest the presence of infection. For example, radiation-induced lung disease in the lung apices corresponding to supraclavicular radiation fields (Fig. 66.17) may be confused with pulmonary tuberculosis.[20] In these cases CT findings of centrilobular nodules or tree-in-bud opacities are more likely to be due to tuberculosis than to radiation-induced lung disease.[148] Cavitation within an area of radiation fibrosis generally represents superimposed infection.[7]

Local tumor recurrence can be difficult to diagnose during the evolution of radiation-induced lung disease. However, as radiation-induced lung disease stabilizes, alteration in the contour of the fibrosis, particularly the development of convex margin, should suggest tumor recurrence. Multiplanar reformatted images are often helpful in evaluating the size and contour alterations in postradiation opacities detected on axial images. The reformatted images often better delineate the linear configuration, volume loss, or sharp margin of the fibrotic lung. Alternatively, if volume expansion or convex margin is confirmed on multiplanar images, the possibility of recurrent malignancy or superimposed infection should be considered. In addition, filling in of bronchi within radiation-induced fibrosis is abnormal and usually results from local recurrence of malignant disease (Fig. 66.18) or a superimposed infection. Other signs of local recurrence include development of nodules outside of radiation treatment fields, irregularity of central airways, and pleural effusion development more than 12 months after completion of treatment.

The clinical and imaging manifestations of radiation-induced organizing pneumonia and chronic eosinophilic pneumonia may be similar. The differentiation between the two entities is based

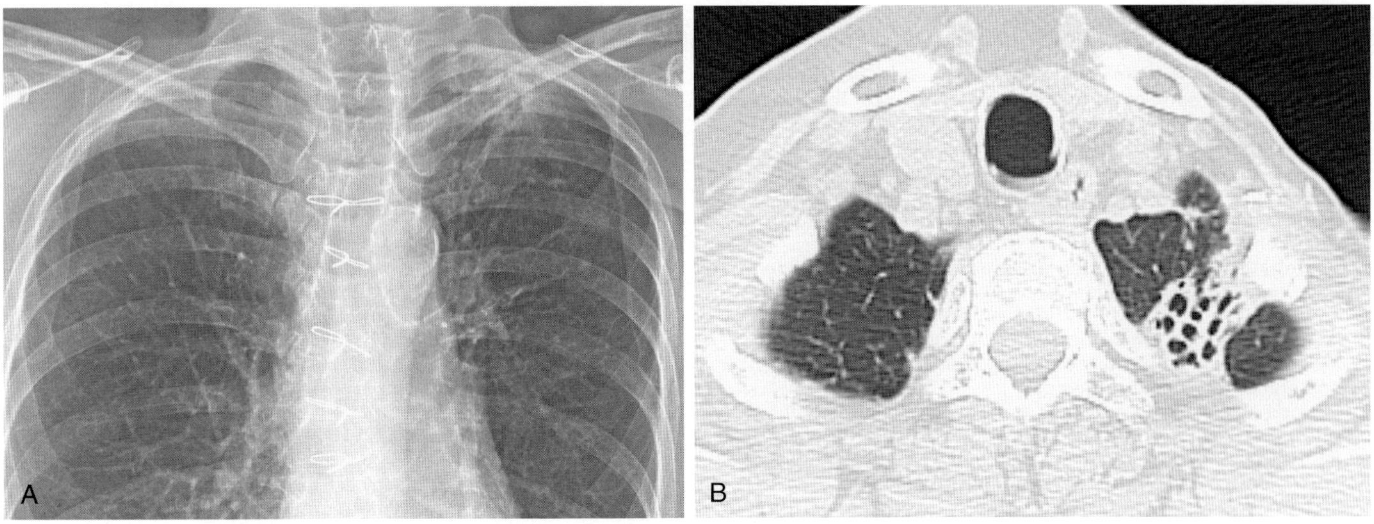

Fig. 66.17 Radiation-induced fibrosis misinterpreted as infection in a woman with chronic cough, weight loss, and history of left breast cancer treated with supraclavicular fields 44 years prior. (A) Chest radiograph shows heterogeneous opacities in the left upper lobe with associated volume loss. (B) CT scan reveals well-marginated atelectatic lung and traction bronchiectasis, findings typical of radiation-induced fibrosis. Sputum cultures were negative for *Mycobacterium tuberculosis* and nontuberculous mycobacterial infection.

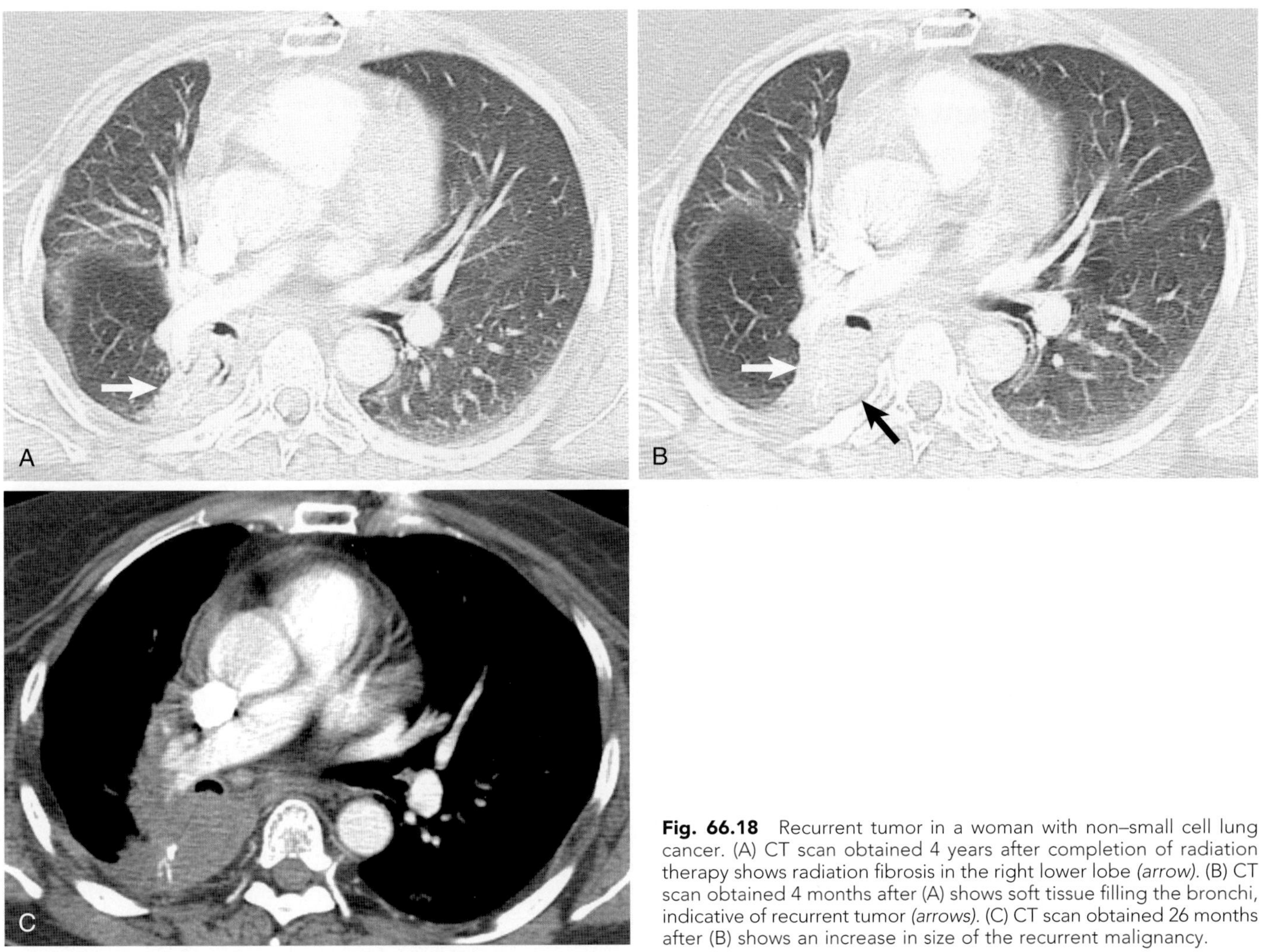

Fig. 66.18 Recurrent tumor in a woman with non–small cell lung cancer. (A) CT scan obtained 4 years after completion of radiation therapy shows radiation fibrosis in the right lower lobe *(arrow)*. (B) CT scan obtained 4 months after (A) shows soft tissue filling the bronchi, indicative of recurrent tumor *(arrows)*. (C) CT scan obtained 26 months after (B) shows an increase in size of the recurrent malignancy.

KEY POINTS

- Radiologic manifestations of radiation-induced lung disease are common, and correlation of imaging findings with the radiation technique, field, and dose, as well as date of radiation completion, is vital in providing the correct diagnosis.
- Acute radiation-induced lung disease typically occurs 4–12 weeks after completion of radiation therapy but can occur before completion of radiation therapy with some of the newer treatment regimens.
- Acute radiation-induced lung disease is manifested as ground-glass opacities or consolidation in the radiation treatment field and can have increased fluorodeoxyglucose (FDG) uptake on positron emission tomography (PET) imaging.
- Ipsilateral pleural effusions develop within 6 months after completion of radiation therapy.
- Fibrosis occurs in the region of acute radiation-induced lung disease 6–12 months after completion of radiation therapy.
- Fibrosis is manifested as consolidation with air bronchograms and sharp borders and is associated with volume loss, architectural distortion, and traction bronchiectasis.
- Fibrosis can progress for 6–12 months after completion of radiation therapy and stabilizes within 2 years.
- Local tumor recurrence can be difficult to diagnose with PET, radiography, and CT during the evolution of radiation-induced lung disease.
- Fibrosis is typically not FDG avid or only mildly FDG avid on PET imaging, although increased FDG uptake can persist for up to 18 months after completion of radiation therapy.
- The high negative predictive value of a normal FDG-PET study in patients with radiation-induced lung disease is clinically useful in excluding recurrence of malignant disease.
- Imaging manifestations of radiation-induced organizing pneumonia and chronic eosinophilic pneumonia are similar to those of idiopathic forms. The parenchymal opacities may occur outside of the port field and be migratory. These features are helpful in distinguishing these entities from radiation pneumonitis.
- After radiation-induced lung disease stabilizes, an alteration in the contour of the fibrosis, particularly development of a convex margin, should suggest tumor recurrence.
- Filling in of bronchi within radiation fibrosis is usually due to local recurrence of malignant disease or superimposed infection.

on the presence of parenchymal and peripheral blood eosinophilia in chronic eosinophilic pneumonia and the typical histologic findings of intraluminal granulation tissue polyps within alveolar ducts and surrounding alveoli associated with chronic inflammation of the surrounding lung parenchyma in organizing pneumonia.[149]

Synopsis of Treatment Options

Corticosteroids are the most commonly used therapy for radiation-induced acute pneumonitis.[22] However, there is no consensus as to when treatment should be initiated, and there are no controlled trials on the efficacy of corticosteroid therapy in patients with acute radiation-induced pneumonitis.[150] In general, corticosteroids are given on the basis of the severity of symptoms, and although they can result in an objective response, pneumonitis may progress with therapy.

SUGGESTED READINGS

Benveniste MF, Welsh J, Godoy MC, Betancourt SL, Mawlawi OR, Munden RF. New era of radiotherapy: an update in radiation-induced lung disease. *Clin Radiol.* 2013;68:e275–e290.

Huang K, Palma DA, IASLC Advanced Radiation Technology Committee. Follow-up of patients after stereotactic radiation for lung cancer: a primer for the nonradiation oncologist. *J Thorac Oncol.* 2015;10:412–419.

Larici AR, del Ciello A, Maggi F, et al. Lung abnormalities at multimodality imaging after radiation therapy for non–small cell lung cancer. *Radiographics.* 2011;31:771–789.

Ulaner GA, Lyall A. Identifying and distinguishing treatment effects and complications from malignancy at FDG PET/CT. *Radiographics.* 2013;33:1817–1834.

Viswanathan C, Carter BW, Shroff GS, Godoy MC, Marom EM, Truong MT. Pitfalls in oncologic imaging: complications of chemotherapy and radiotherapy in the chest. *Semin Roentgenol.* 2015;50:183–191.

The full reference list for this chapter is available at ExpertConsult.com.

67 Blunt Thoracic Trauma*

PHILLIP A. SETRAN | STEVEN L. PRIMACK | CRISTINA S. FUSS

Blunt thoracic trauma is a common indication for hospital admission, with the predominant cause of trauma being motor vehicle collisions. The thorax is the fourth most injured area in unrestrained passengers, but it is the most commonly injured area in individuals who are restrained by a seat belt.[1] Other common causes of blunt thoracic trauma include falls from heights of greater than 10 feet and motor vehicle collisions involving pedestrians/bicyclists. Radiologists must know the typical injuries associated with thoracic trauma to provide the proper diagnosis and contribute to the immediate treatment plan.

The initial screening test in thoracic trauma is the frontal chest radiograph obtained in the trauma bay. After the chest radiograph, computed tomography (CT) is the next most used diagnostic modality, although in the stable patient, cross-sectional imaging is often performed concurrently with radiographs. CT allows evaluation of the airways, pulmonary parenchyma, aorta and great vessels, pericardium, pleura, chest wall, diaphragm, and osseous structures.

The rapid acquisition of data with multidetector helical CT scanners has led to a significant increase in cross-sectional imaging in the setting of trauma.[2,3] The value of multiplanar reformation, as allowed by the current CT scanners, cannot be overemphasized in the trauma setting.

Acute Traumatic Aortic Injury

Acute traumatic aortic injury (ATAI) is a common cause of prehospital mortality, accounting for approximately 15% to 20% of prehospital traumatic deaths.[3] Of individuals with ATAI, 70% to 90% die at the trauma scene.[3] Surviving trauma patients require prompt and accurate diagnosis to allow timely repair of the injury, especially given that 60% may have no overt clinical sign of thoracic trauma.[3] The incidence of ATAI is approximately 1/100,000 per year.[1]

Seven criteria have been described as important clinical predictors for the presence of ATAI.[4] They are age older than 50 years; unrestrained patient; hypotension (defined as systolic blood pressure <90 mm Hg); thoracic injury; abdominopelvic injury requiring emergent laparotomy; concomitant fractures of the lumbar spine, pelvis, or long bones; and major head injury. If more than four of these criteria are present, the likelihood for ATAI is greater than 30%. A more recent evaluation of these criteria found that only four of the seven criteria were predictive of ATAI (abdominopelvic injury, thoracic injury, hypotension, and being unrestrained). Furthermore, the likelihood of ATAI in patients with three or four of these criteria was much lower, at 2%, which may be due to differences in patient populations and injury detection over the years.[5]

ACUTE TRAUMATIC AORTIC INJURY ANATOMY

Most blunt aortic injuries occur at the level of the aortic isthmus just distal to the subclavian artery origin.[3] The aortic isthmus extends from the origin of the subclavian artery to the insertion of the ligamentum arteriosum. The propensity for injury to occur at this location is not completely understood, but multiple mechanisms have been proposed. The osseous pinch mechanism suggests that the isthmus becomes compressed between the spine and the sternum. Shearing stress caused by sudden deceleration with force vectors pointing in opposite directions, centered at the aortic isthmus, is another hypothesis. The sudden increase in intraaortic pressure at the time of trauma, termed the *water hammer effect*, is a third possibility.[3] The fourth theory is the viscous response theory, which states that the velocity of compression is the most important determining factor in internal chest trauma.[1]

The ascending aorta is injured in less than 5% of patients with blunt ATAI who survive transport for further treatment.[3] However, the ascending aorta is injured in approximately 22% of patients examined at autopsy. Ascending aorta injuries are frequently (80%) associated with significant cardiac damage, including valvular damage or pericardial tamponade, a lethal combination of injuries.[6] Traumatic aortic injuries located at the diaphragmatic hiatus account for less than 2% of cases.[7]

A mediastinal hematoma should prompt a close look at its proximity to the aorta and subsequent determination of aortic integrity. Hematoma is invariably present in the setting of aortic rupture but may also occur because of adjacent sternal or thoracic spine fractures or venous injury.

The continuous motion of the heart during cross-sectional scanning leads to motion artifacts of the ascending aorta that can have the appearance of aortic dissection or pseudoaneurysm; these artifacts are present even with current rapid-acquisition multidetector CT scanners. Care should be taken when interpreting the aorta in this area, especially as the ascending aorta is statistically less often injured.

Because the majority of patients with ATAI do not survive to hospitalization, and less than 5% of surviving patients will have an ascending aortic injury, the benefit of gated cardiac CT at initial presentation is limited. Most patients with ATAI are too unstable to undergo prolonged imaging, and thus evaluation of the aorta with standard, nongated CT is generally preferred. Finally, given the additional time and training requirements for technologists to adequately perform gated CT, in most cases only large academic trauma centers will have the resources to provide gated CT at all times of the day. However, in stable patients or those who require additional imaging after their initial presentation, gated CT can be an excellent resource to better evaluate potential ascending aortic injuries.

*The editors and the publisher would like to thank Drs. Nicholas J. Statkus, Joshua R. Hill, and Marc V. Gosselin for contributing material on this topic to the prior edition of this work. It has served as the foundation for the current chapter.

PATHOLOGY

ATAI ranges from intimal hemorrhage to complete transection. A transverse tear is the most common initial event, which can be segmental (55%) or circumferential (45%) and may be partial (65%) or transmural (35%). Spiral/irregular tears are very rare.[8] The adventitia may be injured in up to 40% of cases, and adventitial injury is almost universally fatal because of rapid exsanguination, although in rare cases, temporary tamponade may be achieved by surrounding mediastinal soft tissues.[9] Of those patients who survive and reach the hospital after aortic rupture, 22% die during initial resuscitation, 28% die during or shortly after surgical repair, and 14% develop subsequent paraplegia.[10] Approximately 60% of tears involve the intima and media with an intact adventitia.[6] Although infrequent, aortic dissection occurs in approximately 11% of trauma patients and may be secondary to baseline hypertension, along with subsequent acute increase in intraaortic blood pressure during the insult.[7]

MANIFESTATIONS OF THE DISEASE

Radiography

The chest radiograph is used to evaluate for the presence of a mediastinal hematoma, a finding that can be seen secondary to ATAI, sternal/thoracic spine fracture, or small artery or vein damage within the mediastinum.[11] A mediastinal hematoma may represent free or partial flowing blood, indicative of small mediastinal vessel rupture, versus a contained rupture, the latter being more concerning for an ATAI.

The chest radiograph is most useful for exclusion of ATAI. The negative predictive value of a properly obtained chest radiograph is 98%.[12] However, the positive predictive value is low, only 15%. Mediastinal fat, anomalous vessels, and the thymus can mimic mediastinal hemorrhage on the chest radiograph.[13] Furthermore, technical considerations, such as supine imaging, magnification factors, and rotational factors, can also mimic mediastinal hematoma. The mechanism of injury should dictate the need for CT rather than the presence of a wide mediastinum. A more specific sign for mediastinal hematoma involves comparing the right paratracheal density with the left aortic arch region. When the right paratracheal region is equally dense or denser than the aortic arch, a mediastinal hematoma is more likely present (Figs. 67.1 and 67.2).

Findings indicative of a contained aortic rupture include rightward deviation of a gastric tube (see Fig. 67.1), rightward deviation of the trachea, downward displacement of the left main bronchus, loss of aortic arch definition, increased aortic arch density (see Fig. 67.2), and increased width and density of the descending aorta.[14] Findings indicative of a free- or partial-flowing hematoma include increased right paratracheal density in relation to the aortic arch, loss of aortic arch definition, left apical cap, and widened mediastinum (see Figs. 67.1 and 67.2).[14]

The presence of a mediastinal hematoma is a sensitive but nonspecific finding in the setting of ATAI. The remaining signs have varying levels of specificity, the strongest of which include left apical cap (present in 65%), downward deviation of the left main bronchus (65%), and obscuration and increased density of the descending thoracic aorta (67%).[6]

Computed Tomography

Multidetector helical CT is a very sensitive diagnostic tool for exclusion of ATAI, often quoted as the gold standard for ATAI detection.[15] A morphologically normal aorta with no mediastinal hematoma has a 100% negative predictive value for exclusion of ATAI.[7] The positive predictive value is unclear at this time, however, with equivocal studies (hematoma only) requiring follow-up CT, aortography, or clinical observation.

Minimal aortic injury, defined as lesions only affecting the aortic intima without secondary signs of injury, represent about 10% of all cases of ATAI. Imaging findings suggesting minimal aortic injury include a polypoid intraluminal clot, low-density filling defect, or small intimal tear (Fig. 67.3). Minimal aortic injury is important to recognize, as the treatment is different. Increasing reports show resolution of the injury on follow-up CT using conservative, nonoperative management (see Fig. 67.3).

Direct signs of ATAI that often require surgery or endovascular repair include a change in caliber of the aorta, aortic wall or contour abnormality (pseudoaneurysm) (see Figs. 67.1 and 67.2), contrast extravasation (Fig. 67.4), and dissection.[16] Diffuse circumferential perimural hematoma, which can extend down to the abdominal portion of the aorta, is another important finding (Fig. 67.5). It is important to distinguish ATAI and the congenital variant of a "ductus bump." A ductus bump is a mild, smooth, regular contour change of the aorta in the region of the ligamentum arteriosum and is a normal variant (Fig. 67.6).

Transesophageal echocardiography is another valid option for exclusion of ATAI if there are no contraindications, such as vertebral body fracture or severe maxillofacial injury. The disadvantages of transesophageal echocardiography include the logistical time required to perform the study and the user dependence. If involvement of the ascending aorta is suspected, further evaluation with cardiac-gated computed tomography angiography should be considered.

Text continued on p. 869

CLASSIC SIGNS: RADIOGRAPHIC FINDINGS IN ACUTE TRAUMATIC AORTIC INJURY

SIGNS WITH HIGH SENSITIVITY AND LOW SPECIFICITY

- Mediastinal widening
- Abnormal or indistinct contour of the aorta

SIGNS WITH RELATIVELY HIGH SPECIFICITY AND LOW SENSITIVITY

- Rightward deviation of trachea at level of T4
- Rightward deviation of nasogastric tube at level of T4
- Thickening of right paratracheal stripe
- Negative predictive value of normal radiograph: 98%

CLASSIC SIGNS: COMPUTED TOMOGRAPHY FINDINGS OF ACUTE TRAUMATIC AORTIC INJURY

DIRECT SIGNS

- Irregularity of wall of the aorta
- Pseudoaneurysm
- Abrupt caliber change of aorta
- Intimal flap
- Extravasation of contrast material

INDIRECT SIGNS

- Periaortic hematoma
- Negative predictive value of good-quality normal spiral CT: 100%

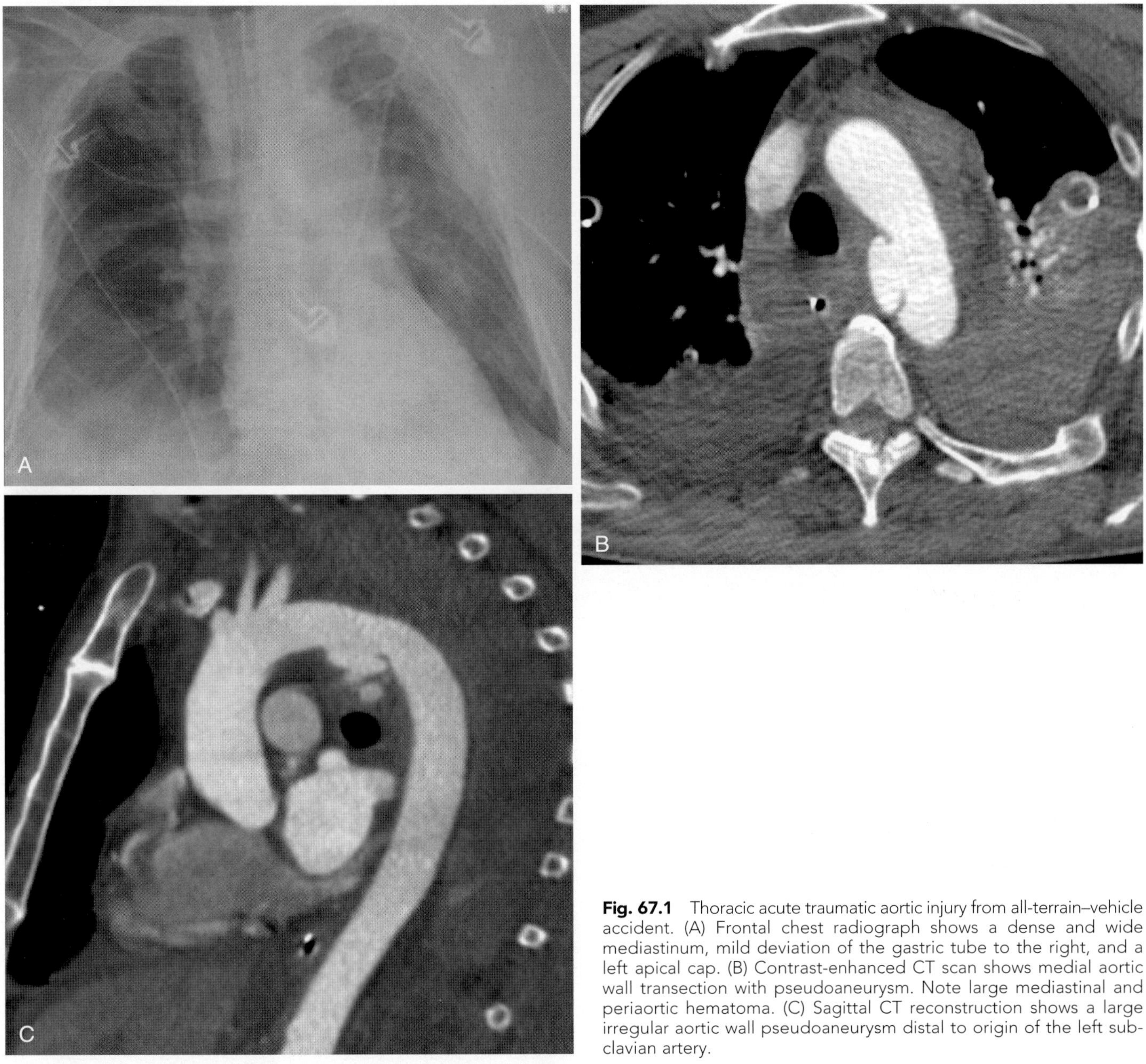

Fig. 67.1 Thoracic acute traumatic aortic injury from all-terrain–vehicle accident. (A) Frontal chest radiograph shows a dense and wide mediastinum, mild deviation of the gastric tube to the right, and a left apical cap. (B) Contrast-enhanced CT scan shows medial aortic wall transection with pseudoaneurysm. Note large mediastinal and periaortic hematoma. (C) Sagittal CT reconstruction shows a large irregular aortic wall pseudoaneurysm distal to origin of the left subclavian artery.

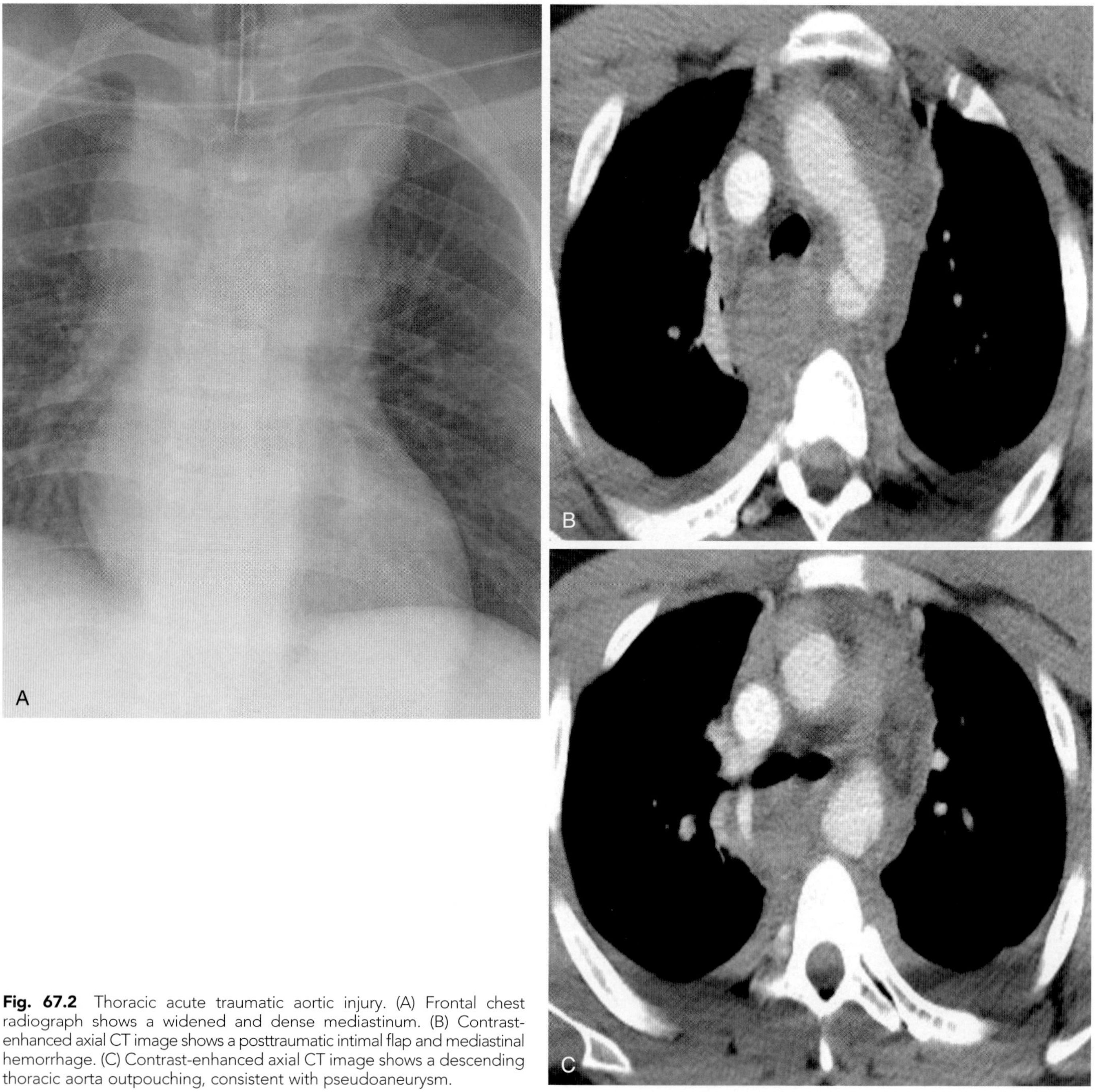

Fig. 67.2 Thoracic acute traumatic aortic injury. (A) Frontal chest radiograph shows a widened and dense mediastinum. (B) Contrast-enhanced axial CT image shows a posttraumatic intimal flap and mediastinal hemorrhage. (C) Contrast-enhanced axial CT image shows a descending thoracic aorta outpouching, consistent with pseudoaneurysm.

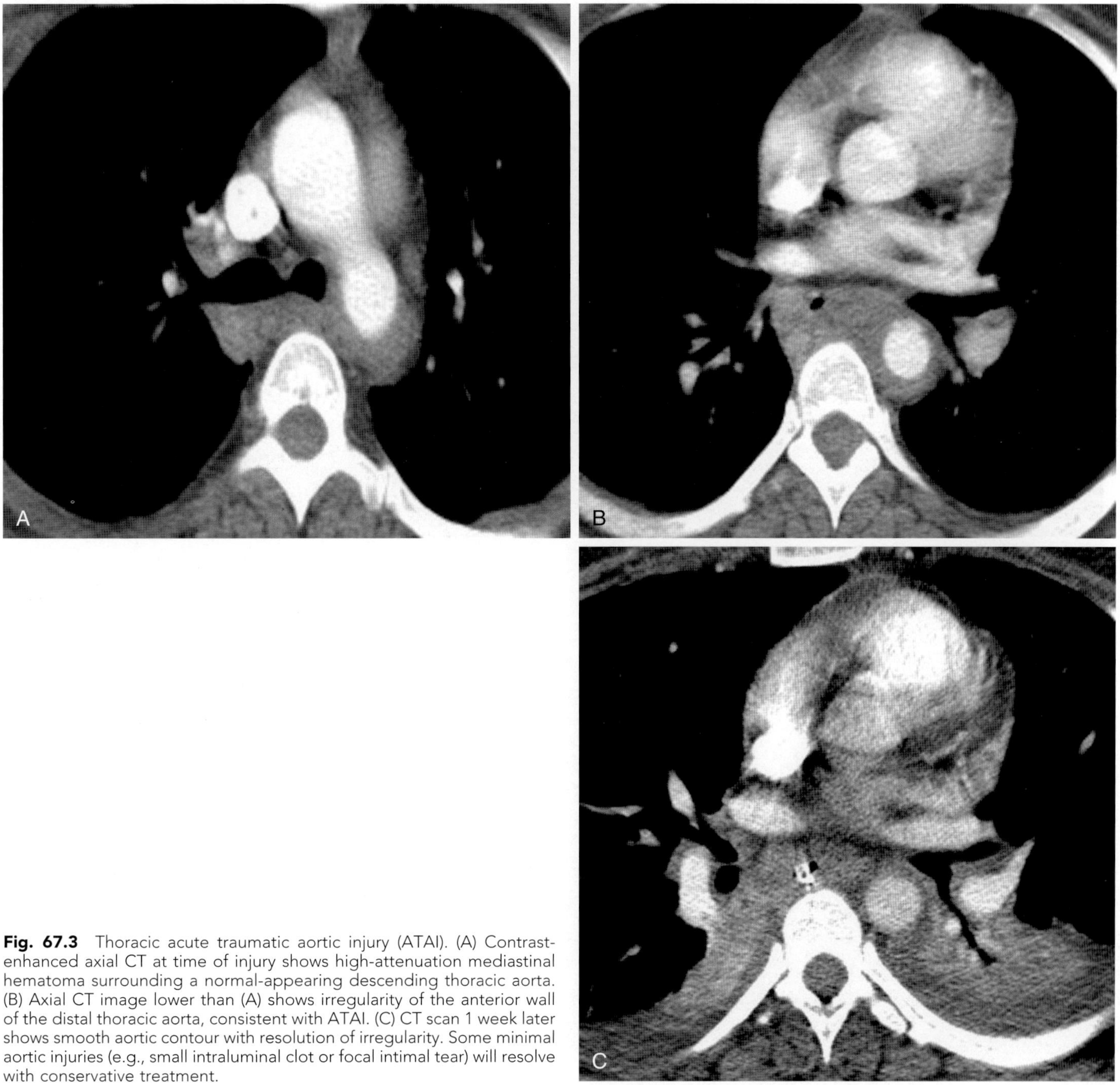

Fig. 67.3 Thoracic acute traumatic aortic injury (ATAI). (A) Contrast-enhanced axial CT at time of injury shows high-attenuation mediastinal hematoma surrounding a normal-appearing descending thoracic aorta. (B) Axial CT image lower than (A) shows irregularity of the anterior wall of the distal thoracic aorta, consistent with ATAI. (C) CT scan 1 week later shows smooth aortic contour with resolution of irregularity. Some minimal aortic injuries (e.g., small intraluminal clot or focal intimal tear) will resolve with conservative treatment.

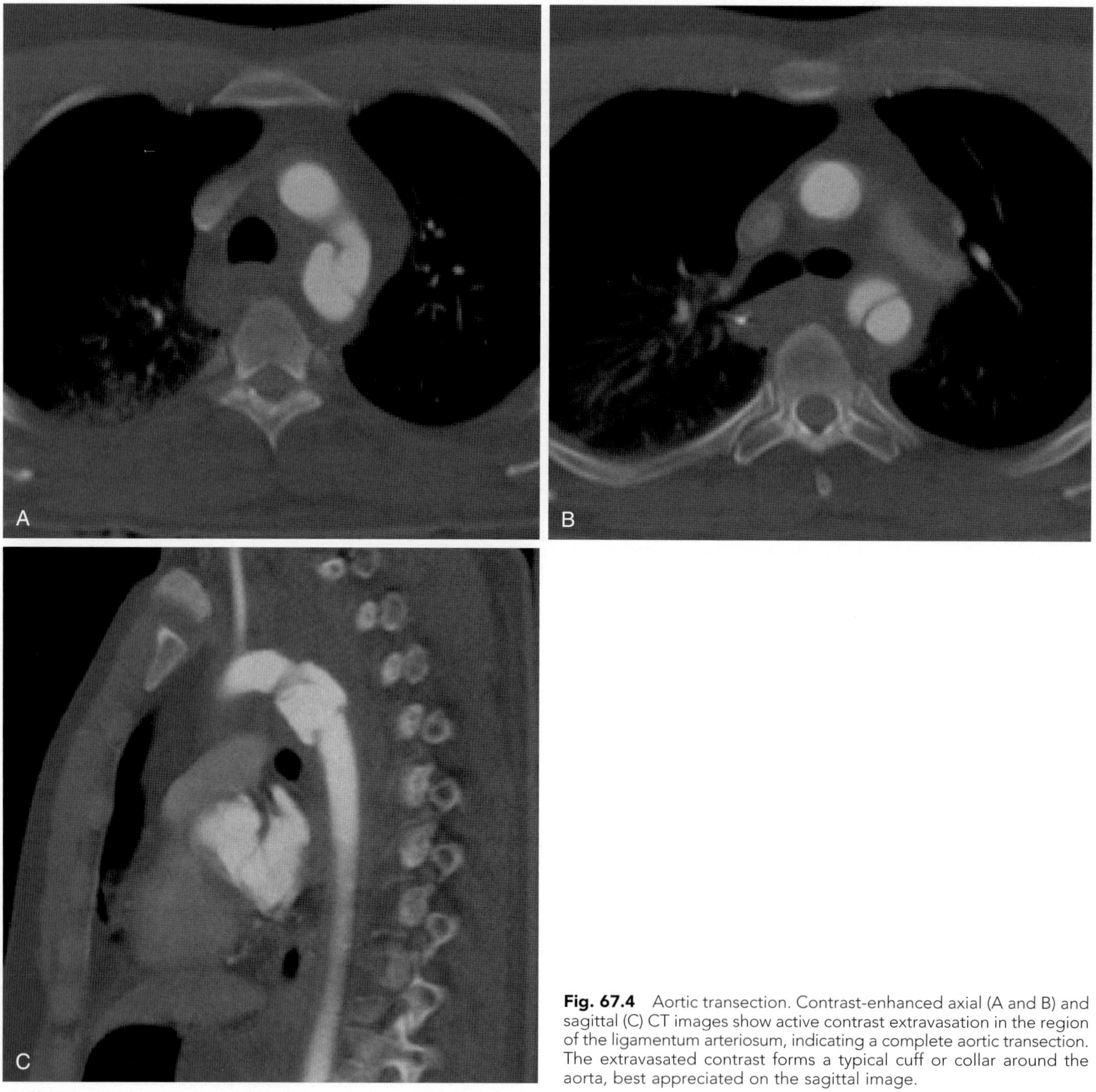

Fig. 67.4 Aortic transection. Contrast-enhanced axial (A and B) and sagittal (C) CT images show active contrast extravasation in the region of the ligamentum arteriosum, indicating a complete aortic transection. The extravasated contrast forms a typical cuff or collar around the aorta, best appreciated on the sagittal image.

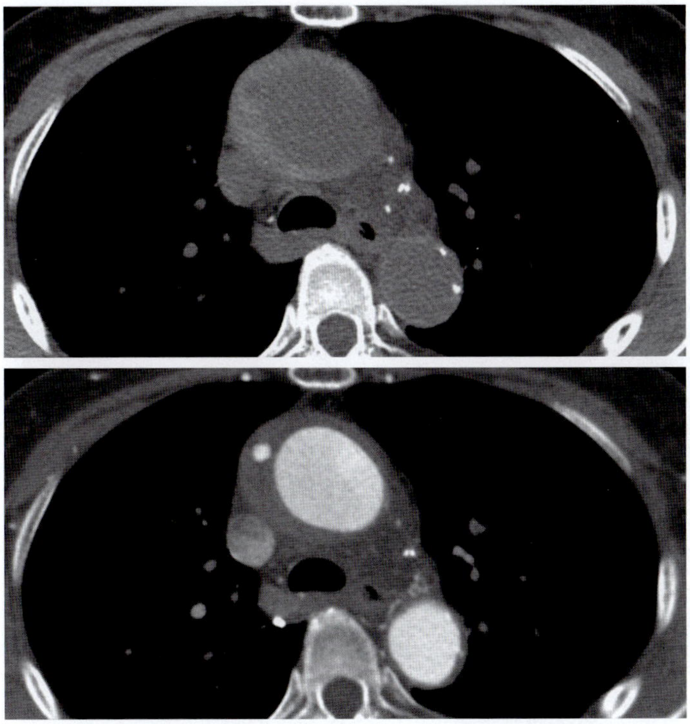

Fig. 67.5 Thoracic acute traumatic aortic injury with perimural hematoma. Composite image with unenhanced axial CT image *(top image)* and contrast-enhanced axial CT image *(bottom image)* shows high attenuation, eccentric thickening of the ascending aortic wall, and a small anterolateral defect containing contrast.

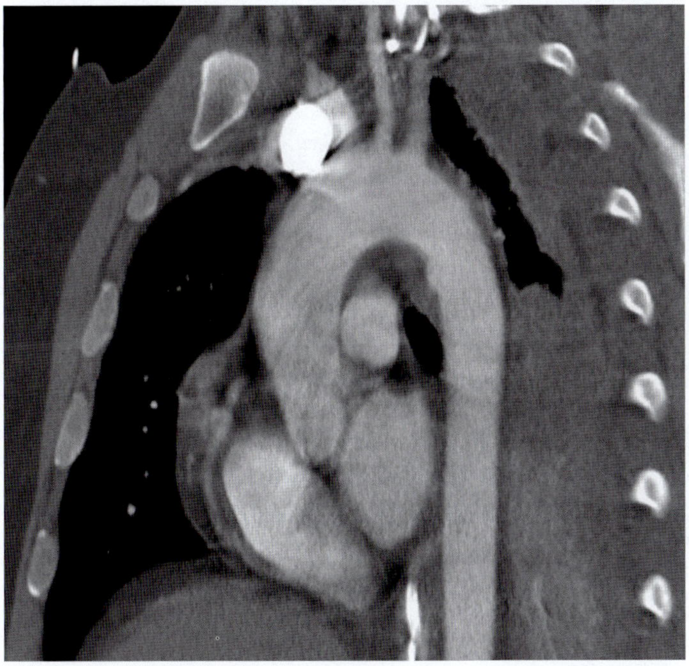

Fig. 67.6 Ductus bump, a normal anatomic variant. Contrast-enhanced sagittal CT image shows a luminal outpouching in the region of the ligamentum arteriosum with smooth, obtuse angles between the outpouching and the aortic wall, consistent with a ductus bump. In contrast, an aortic pseudoaneurysm or transection forms acute angles with the aortic wall (see Figs. 67.1 and 67.4).

Great Vessel and Supraaortic Branch Vessel Injury

The great vessels include the superior and inferior vena cava, pulmonary arteries, pulmonary veins, and aorta. Injury to the great vessels other than the aorta is rare.[17] The supraaortic branch vessels comprise the brachiocephalic artery (right subclavian/right common carotid arteries), left common carotid artery, left subclavian artery, and brachiocephalic veins. Blunt traumatic injury to the supraaortic branch vessels is uncommon. When branch vessel injury is suspected, angiography can be a useful tool to diagnose subtle injury.[17] One case review of 166 aortograms with 24 cases of positive aortic or supraaortic branch vessel injury, performed in high-mechanism thoracic trauma, revealed 4% with isolated injury to the aortic branch vessels and 1% with injuries to the aorta and its branches.[18]

MANIFESTATIONS OF THE DISEASE

Radiography

The screening trauma radiograph is unlikely to aid in the diagnosis of great vessel and supraaortic branch vessel injury. As in ATAI, a mediastinal hematoma may be present (Fig. 67.7).

Computed Tomography

Multidetector CT and possibly subsequent angiography for evaluation of the great and supraaortic branch vessels are the most important diagnostic modalities. Similar to the setting of ATAI, CT may show endoluminal/intimal irregularity compatible with intimal tear. Alternatively, subtle findings, such as asymmetric vascular caliber, localized hematoma (Fig. 67.8), or decreased contrast enhancement, may provide further evidence of vascular injury. Finally, dissection and complete disruption, if present, should reveal the dissection flap and pseudoaneurysm (Fig. 67.9; see Fig. 67.7) that are typically seen with these entities. Although multidetector CT scans are likely to detect a traumatic injury to the supraaortic branch vessel, angiography is still considered the diagnostic gold standard.

Cardiac Injury

Significant cardiac injuries are uncommon in patients with blunt trauma who are seen in the emergency department. Autopsy data indicate that numerous prehospital deaths result from traumatic cardiac or valvular rupture.

Blunt cardiac injury can be divided into cardiac contusion and, more rarely, pericardial or myocardial rupture. The most innocuous and most common of these injuries, cardiac contusion, is usually a clinical diagnosis. Although CT can reveal multiple ancillary signs of cardiac contusion, the presence of normal myocardial enhancement should not be used to rule out cardiac injury.[19] However, cardiac magnetic resonance imaging (MRI) and/or echocardiography may be beneficial if cardiac contusion is suspected to evaluate for wall motion abnormalities. Hemopericardium is visible on nearly all CT scans in cases of pericardial rupture.

PATHOLOGY

Hemopericardium may be the result of cardiac chamber rupture (prehospital death) or damage to the small surrounding pericardial vessels from displaced rib fractures (patient survives to

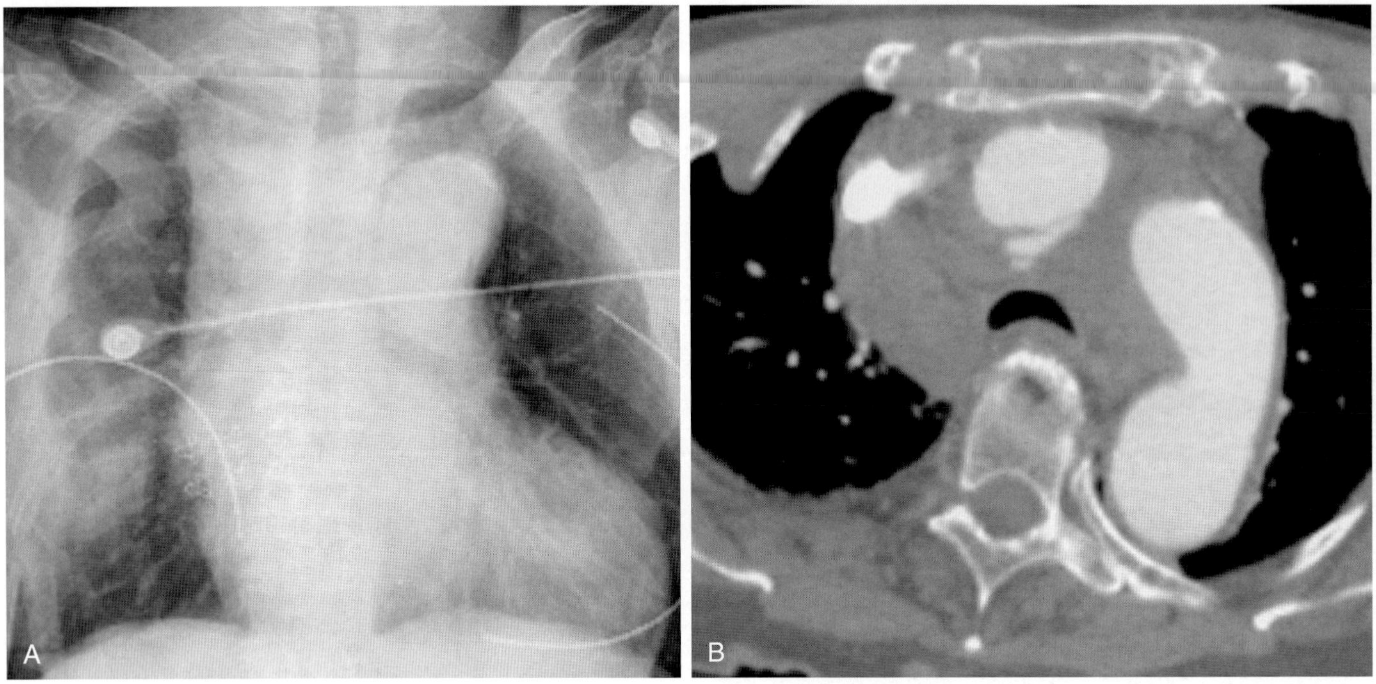

Fig. 67.7 Brachiocephalic artery injury after motor vehicle collision. (A) Frontal chest radiograph shows a dense mediastinum compatible with free-flowing mediastinal hematoma. (B) Contrast-enhanced CT scan shows a large, dense mediastinal hematoma. Note irregular contrast collection just anterior to the trachea representing a pseudoaneurysm off the posterior aspect of the brachiocephalic artery. Of note, the patient has a common aortic arch variant, with single origin of the brachiocephalic and left common carotid arteries and with baseline aneurysmal dilatation unrelated to the trauma.

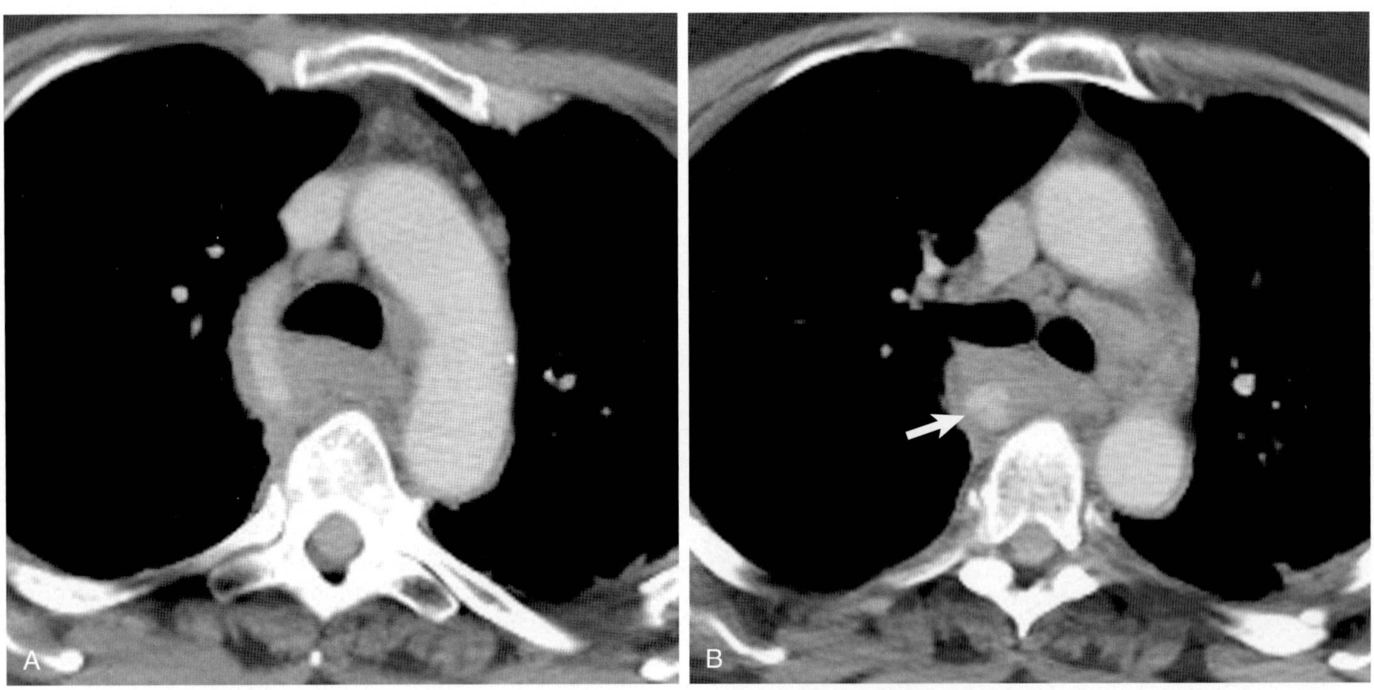

Fig. 67.8 Azygos vein injury. (A) and (B) Axial contrast-enhanced CT images show irregularity of the azygos vein (*arrow*, B) with surrounding hemorrhage, consistent with traumatic laceration, a rarely seen thoracic injury.

hospitalization). Pericardial rupture more commonly occurs on the left side, although it can also occur along its pulmonary or diaphragmatic borders, or both. Such injuries become significant when the heart herniates through the tear, resulting in cardiac filling impedance or coronary vessel occlusion. The proposed mechanism of injury for pericardial rupture likens the injury to a pendulum because the inferior portion of the heart is free floating without significant attachments. In the setting of a lateral deceleration injury, the heart presumably collides with the adjacent pericardium, creating the rupture.[20] Cardiac herniation through

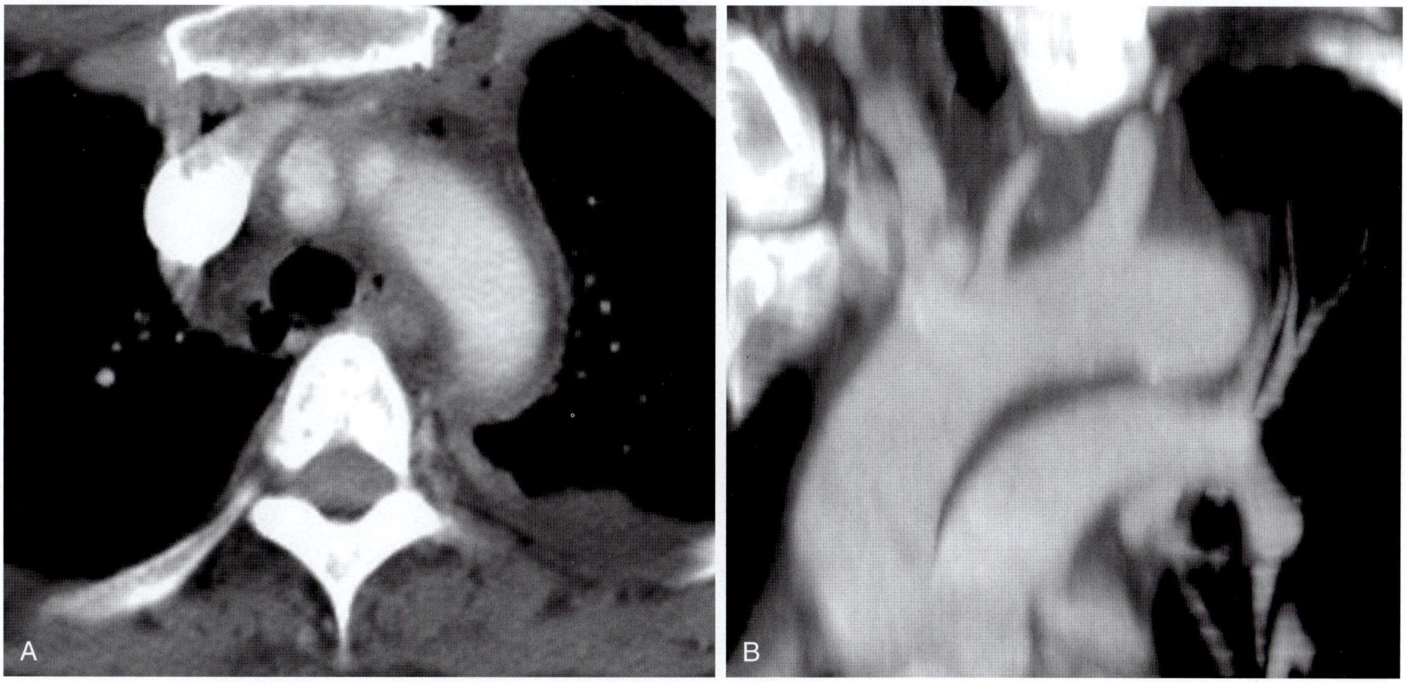

Fig. 67.9 Brachiocephalic artery injury. (A) Axial and (B) oblique sagittal contrast-enhanced CT images show an outpouching at the origin of the brachiocephalic artery, consistent with a traumatic pseudoaneurysm.

a pericardial defect may not be present initially and may occur after the administration or discontinuation of positive-pressure ventilation.[20] The most commonly ruptured cardiac chamber in the autopsy population is the right ventricle, whereas the atria are the most commonly ruptured chambers in individuals who survive to hospitalization.[21]

MANIFESTATIONS OF THE DISEASE

Radiography

Hemopericardium may or may not be evident on chest radiography at presentation and usually manifests with an enlarged cardiac silhouette. Cardiac herniation should be suspected by an unusual position or configuration of the heart.

Computed Tomography

Most patients who have a mechanism of injury to produce hemopericardium are imaged with CT if stable, which reveals a hyperdense fluid collection in the pericardial space (Fig. 67.10). Not all pericardial tears are associated with cardiac herniation; the chest radiograph and CT scan may be unrevealing. The presence of a focal pericardial defect with a collar sign of herniating cardiac tissue is the usual imaging manifestation (Fig. 67.11). The presence of adjacent pneumothorax, pneumomediastinum, or both may complicate the diagnosis because the pericardium may be mistaken for the pleura in these settings.

Finally, pneumopericardium can rarely be seen in the trauma setting. Pneumopericardium, as opposed to pneumomediastinum, conforms more tightly to the cardiac contour and does not extend beyond the superior aortic recess. In addition, pneumopericardium, if significant, may result in compression of the heart with tamponade physiology.

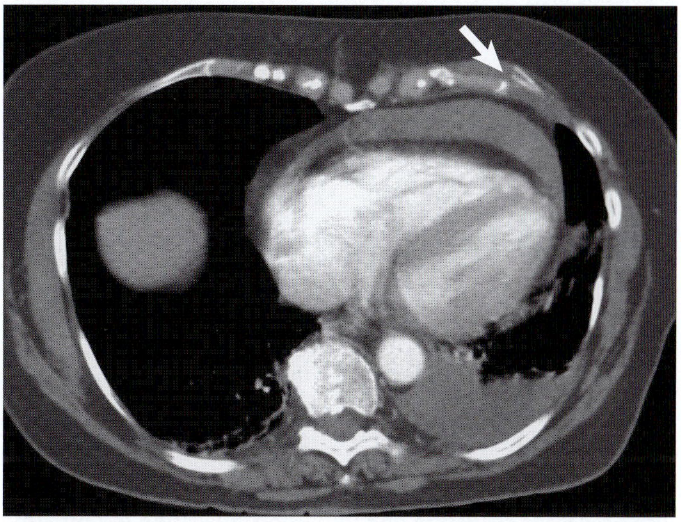

Fig. 67.10 Hemopericardium after head-on motor vehicle collision. Contrast-enhanced CT scan shows hyperdense pericardial fluid compatible with hemopericardium. Note anteriorly displaced left rib fracture *(arrow)*, the likely cause of the hemopericardium and left hemothorax.

Pulmonary Contusion

Pulmonary contusion is seen in 30% to 70% of patients with blunt thoracic injury.[1,22] It is the most common cause of pulmonary parenchymal opacification on chest radiography in blunt thoracic trauma. Short-term morbidity is substantial, and clinical signs and symptoms include hypoxia, mild fever, hemoptysis, and dyspnea. Acute respiratory failure may develop, requiring intubation and mechanical ventilation. Pulmonary contusion is

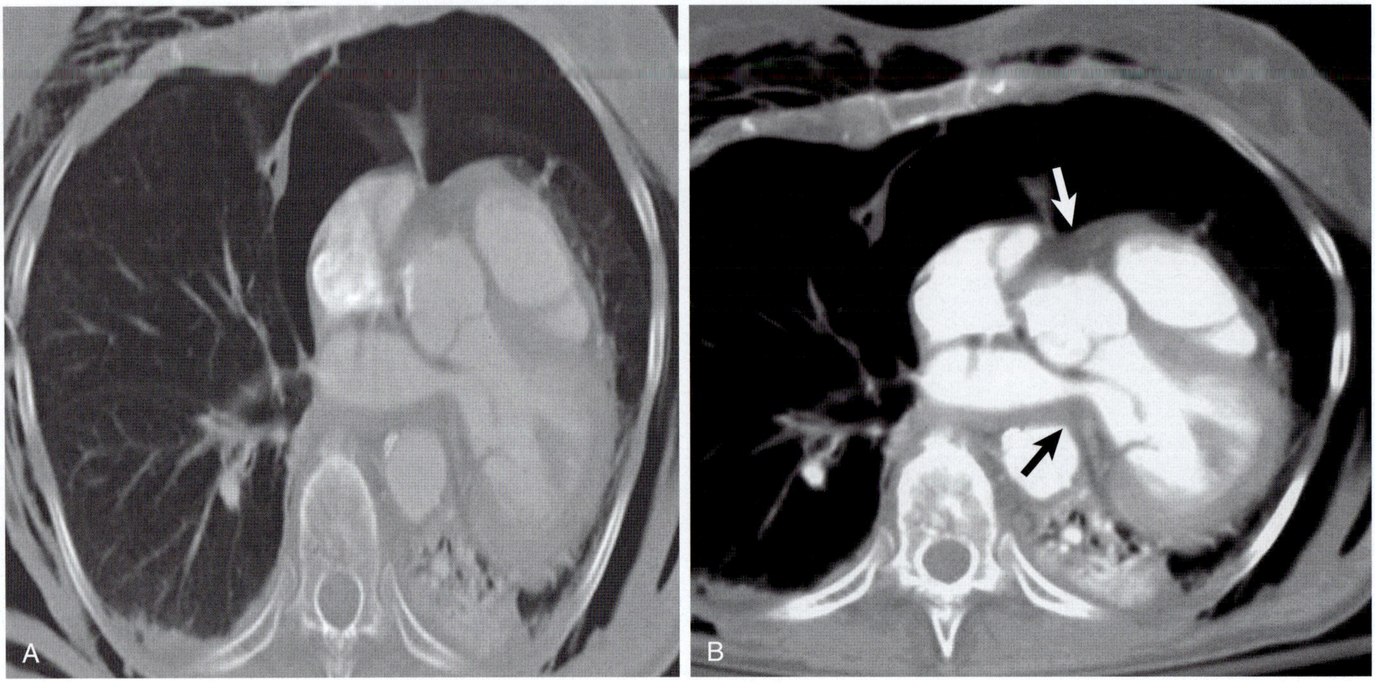

Fig. 67.11 Pericardial rupture and cardiac herniation. Contrast-enhanced axial CT images in lung (A) and soft tissue (B) windows show the cardiac "collar sign" *(arrows)* indicating pericardial tear with concomitant cardiac herniation. The lung windows make the empty pericardial sac more apparent. Extensive soft tissue air is also present.

also associated with long-term respiratory dysfunction in patients with blunt chest trauma.[23] The mortality rate is estimated at 10% to 25%.[24]

MECHANISM OF INJURY

Pulmonary contusion represents pulmonary hemorrhage and edema from disruption of the alveolar capillary membrane.[14] It is often caused by a direct blow to the chest wall, with injury of the adjacent lung. Contrecoup injuries are common, and parenchymal contusion is frequently seen where the lungs have been compressed against the denser heart, liver, chest wall, and spine.[25] In deceleration injuries, such as motor vehicle accidents, the alveolar capillary membrane is disrupted as the lower-density alveoli shear from the higher-density bronchovascular bundles.[14,26,27] Pulmonary contusions may also be the result of rib fracture fragments directly lacerating the lung.

Although rare, disruption of the alveolar capillary membrane also occurs via spallation and implosion. Spallation is a bursting phenomenon that occurs when pressure waves deposit energy at liquid-gas interfaces, such as the blood-air interface of the alveolus. Spallation can occur from a blast injury or a direct blow. Implosion occurs after the transmission of a pressure wave through the alveolus, when there is overexpansion of alveolar gas.[14,26]

MANIFESTATIONS OF THE DISEASE

Radiography

Pulmonary contusions manifest as focal, patchy, or diffuse ground-glass opacities or parenchymal consolidation (Fig. 67.12). These opacities cross segmental and fissural boundaries and are often present at the site of impaction and adjacent to rib fractures. The lung bases are most frequently affected secondary to increased basilar mobility.[14] Air bronchograms are usually absent owing to blood filling the airways.

Progression of pulmonary parenchymal contusion follows a predictable temporal pattern on imaging. Contused lung may not be apparent on initial chest radiography but is usually present within 6 hours after the inciting injury. Conspicuity of pulmonary opacities peaks at 24 to 72 hours and gradually diminishes over 1 week (see Fig. 67.12), although severe contusions may be radiographically evident for 2 weeks. Persistence beyond this duration should prompt consideration of other pulmonary disease commonly seen in trauma patients, such as pneumonia, hydrostatic or noncardiogenic pulmonary edema, and fat embolism syndrome (with concurrent long bone injury). Finally, in the setting of acute trauma, pulmonary contusion may be difficult to differentiate from aspiration pneumonitis (Fig. 67.13) and atelectasis, and these entities are often present concurrently.

CLASSIC SIGNS: RADIOGRAPHIC FINDINGS IN PULMONARY CONTUSION

- Patchy areas of consolidation
- Nonsegmental distribution
- Evident radiographically 0–6 hours after trauma
- Peaks within 24-–48 hours after injury
- Resolves within 3–10 days

Computed Tomography

CT is superior to chest radiography in the detection of pulmonary contusion (Fig. 67.14).[28] In an experimental model using anesthetized dogs, chest radiography detected 38% of pulmonary contusions compared with 100% detected by CT.[29] The clinical indication for CT in the detection and quantification of

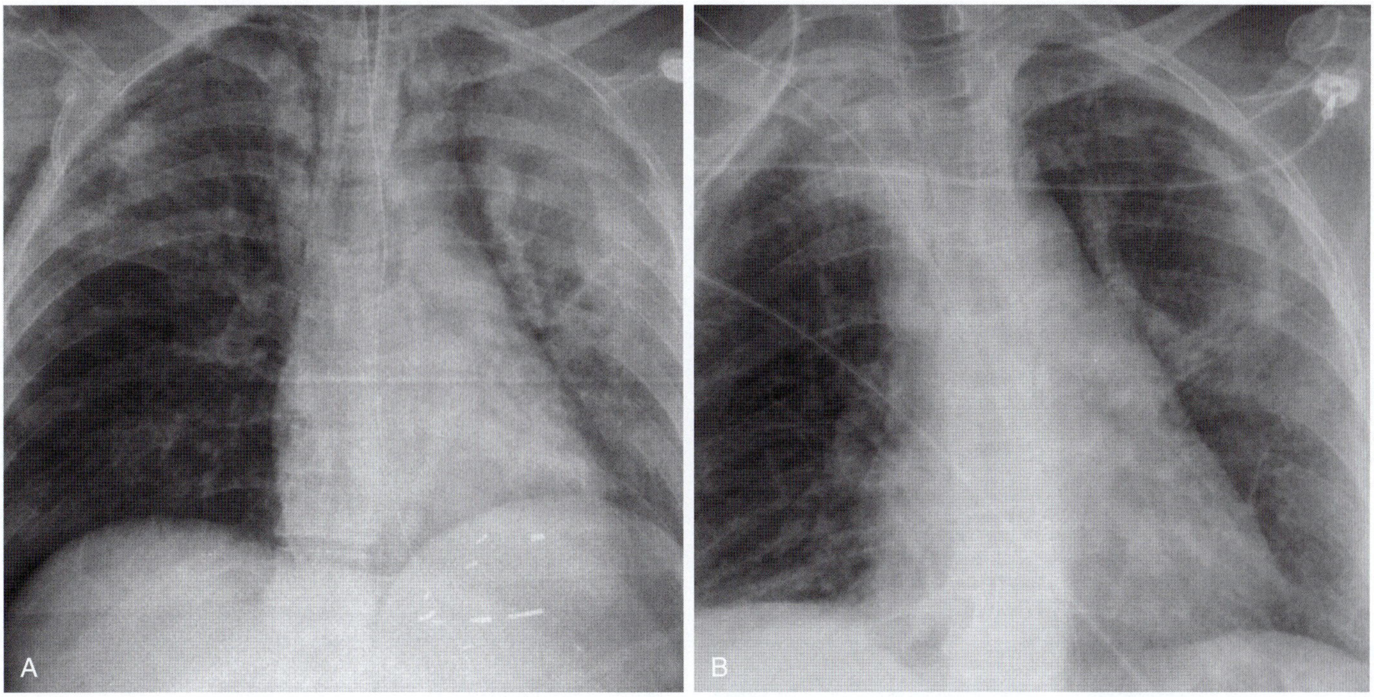

Fig. 67.12 Traumatic pneumatocele and contusions with evolution over time. (A) Initial chest radiograph shows acute injury phase and shows a large, dense oval opacity within the left lung, corresponding to a traumatic pneumatocele filled with blood. Patchy bilateral opacities are compatible with pulmonary contusion. (B) Radiograph acquired 8 days later shows the posttraumatic pneumatocele with nearly resolved hematoma. Of note, some pneumatoceles will remain hyperdense and can be easily mistaken for a pulmonary nodule or mass without the history of trauma.

pulmonary contusion is debatable, however. Quantification of contusion severity has been shown to be of prognostic value in assessing the likelihood of the need for mechanical ventilation and the development of pneumonia and acute respiratory distress syndrome[30]; greater than 80% of patients with 20% or more contused lung progress to acute respiratory distress syndrome.[31] No prospective studies have shown changes in management or outcome, however, with the use of CT solely for the evaluation of pulmonary contusion.[30]

Pulmonary Laceration and Traumatic Lung Cyst

Pulmonary laceration is a tear in the lung parenchyma resulting in a traumatic lung cyst. The cyst may be filled with air (pneumatocele), blood (hematocele or hematoma), or both.

MECHANISM OF INJURY

Shear forces, spallation, and implosion can all cause pulmonary laceration. A rib fracture fragment can puncture the lung, causing a parenchymal tear as well.

MANIFESTATIONS OF THE DISEASE

Radiography

On the initial chest radiograph, pulmonary lacerations are usually obscured by the consolidation related to pulmonary contusion. On occasion, traumatic pneumatoceles may be seen as thin-walled cystic spaces within the areas of consolidation (see Fig. 67.12). As the lung contusion resolves, pulmonary lacerations become visible as thin-walled cystic spaces or as soft tissue masses (pulmonary hematomas).

Radiographic resolution of traumatic lung cysts occurs over weeks to months. Uncommonly, the cysts persist for years. If clot remains in the cavity, these cysts can be mistaken for pulmonary nodules, and air-filled cavities may mimic other forms of cystic lung disease. Knowledge of previous trauma is important in correctly differentiating among these entities.

CLASSIC SIGNS: RADIOGRAPHIC FINDINGS IN PULMONARY LACERATION

- Often initially obscured by pulmonary contusion
- May manifest as traumatic pneumatocele or hematoma
- Pneumatoceles appear as thin-walled cystic spaces with or without air-fluid levels
- Unilocular or multilocular
- Hematomas manifest as soft tissue masses
- May persist for months or, occasionally, years

Computed Tomography

CT is superior to radiography in identifying pulmonary laceration. Four types of intraparenchymal pulmonary lacerations have been described based on CT appearance, mechanism of injury, location of associated rib fracture, and surgical findings.[32] Type 1, the most common type, manifests as pneumatoceles or partially fluid-filled cysts formed after a sudden compressive force causes alveolar rupture. Type 2 results from shear injury of the lower lung near the spine as a compressive force causes the lung to shift across the vertebral column (see Fig. 67.14). Type 3 manifests as lung cysts near the chest wall adjacent to a rib fracture fragment

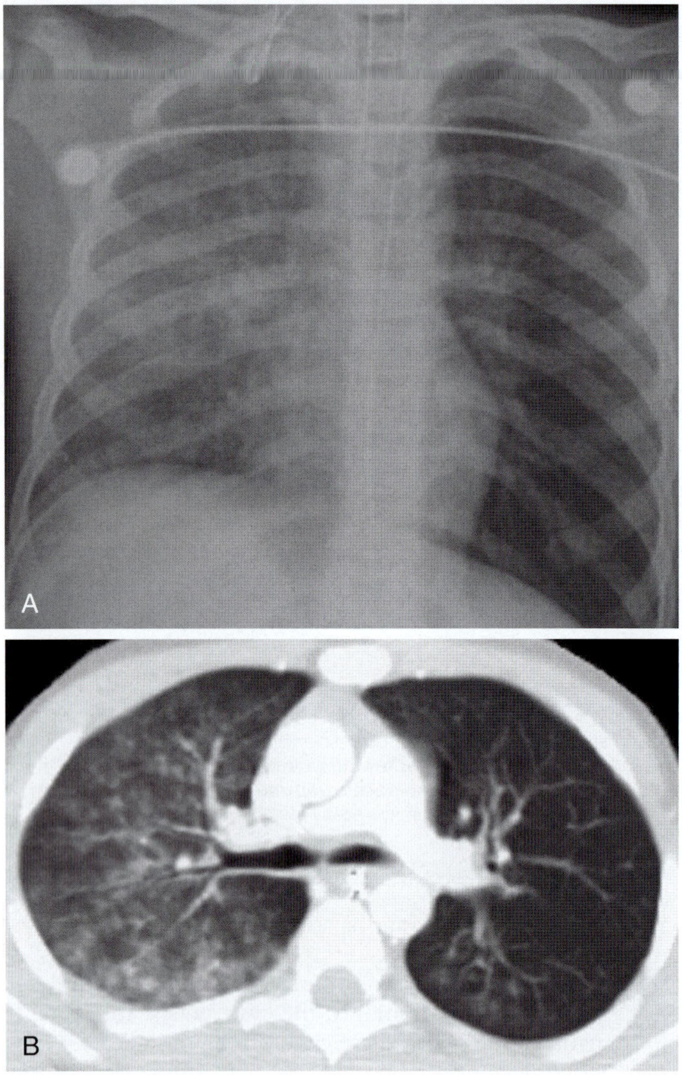

Fig. 67.13 Aspiration after trauma. (A) Frontal chest radiograph shows numerous ill-defined nodular opacities in right middle and upper lung zones. (B) Axial CT scan shows extensive tree-in-bud opacities in the right lung and minimal tree-in-bud opacities in the superior segment of the left lower lobe. In a patient with trauma, these findings are characteristic of aspiration.

that has directly punctured the pulmonary parenchyma. Type 4 occurs when previously formed pleuropulmonary adhesions tear the lung after sudden movement or fracture of the attached chest wall.

Traumatic lung cysts are frequently obscured during initial imaging secondary to surrounding pulmonary contusion and become more apparent as pulmonary contusion resolves (see Fig. 67.14).[28] On imaging, traumatic lung cysts manifest as ovoid structures secondary to the elastic recoil of the lung.[14,25] If blood completely fills the cyst, an ovoid opacity representing pulmonary hematoma or hematocele is seen. When blood partially fills the cavity, an air-fluid level is present (see Fig. 67.14). Multiple small air-filled lung cysts can result in a "Swiss cheese" appearance of the lungs,[27] also called "pulverized lung."[33]

The most common complication associated with a pulmonary laceration is a pneumothorax, and although rare, other complications include infection with formation of a pulmonary abscess and the development of a bronchopleural fistula.

Airway Injury

Tracheobronchial injuries include mucosal tears and complete transection of the airway. These are uncommon injuries, occurring in 1% to 3% of patients with blunt thoracic trauma.[6,25]

MANIFESTATIONS OF THE DISEASE

Radiography

The radiographic manifestations of tracheobronchial injury are usually nonspecific and include pneumomediastinum, pneumothorax, pneumoretroperitoneum, deep cervical air, and subcutaneous air (Fig. 67.15).[34,35] Injuries to the trachea or proximal left main bronchus typically result in pneumomediastinum and not pneumothorax.[35] The fallen lung sign is specific to bronchial fracture. This sign describes the lung "falling" dependently, rather than collapsing centrally toward the hilum in the presence of a pneumothorax. On occasion, air is seen tracking within the bronchial wall, creating the double wall sign.

Tracheal or bronchial tear should be suspected with persistent or increasing soft tissue air, or if pneumothorax persists despite continuous chest tube drainage. Extraluminal position of the endotracheal tube and cuff overinflation may also indicate tracheal injury (see Fig. 67.15).[36]

Approximately 75% of tracheobronchial injuries occur within 2 cm of the carina. Right main bronchus injuries generally occur closer to the carina (usually within 2.5 cm) than injuries to the left main bronchus, and the right main bronchus is injured more frequently than either the trachea or the left main bronchus.

Computed Tomography

CT plays a limited role in the detection of tracheobronchial injuries. Direct visualization of a tear on CT is difficult and best accomplished using thin (<3 mm) collimation (see Fig. 67.15). Complications of tracheobronchial injury include bronchopleural fistula and, rarely, tracheoesophageal fistula. Undiagnosed, untreated tracheal and bronchial injuries may lead to stenosis. These patients have a propensity to develop postobstructive pneumonia and bronchiectasis.[35] A high index of suspicion and liberal use of bronchoscopy are important for the prompt diagnosis of tracheobronchial injury.[36,37]

Hemothorax

Hemothorax occurs in approximately 50% of patients after blunt thoracic trauma. Intrathoracic blood may arise from any surrounding structures, including the lung, mediastinum, thoracic wall, and diaphragm.[27] Hemothoraces may be large and increase rapidly if the bleeding source is arterial. Delayed hemothorax rarely happens, although it is more common in patients with multiple rib fractures and/or flail chest. It manifests as new-onset sharp pleuritic chest pain and dyspnea.[38] On occasion, intraperitoneal blood migrates to the pleural space through congenital or acquired diaphragmatic defects or traumatic rupture of the diaphragm.

MANIFESTATIONS OF THE DISEASE

Radiography

Small hemothoraces may be missed on chest radiography. Blunting of the posterior costophrenic angle requires at least 75 mL of pleural fluid and is best seen on an upright lateral projection.

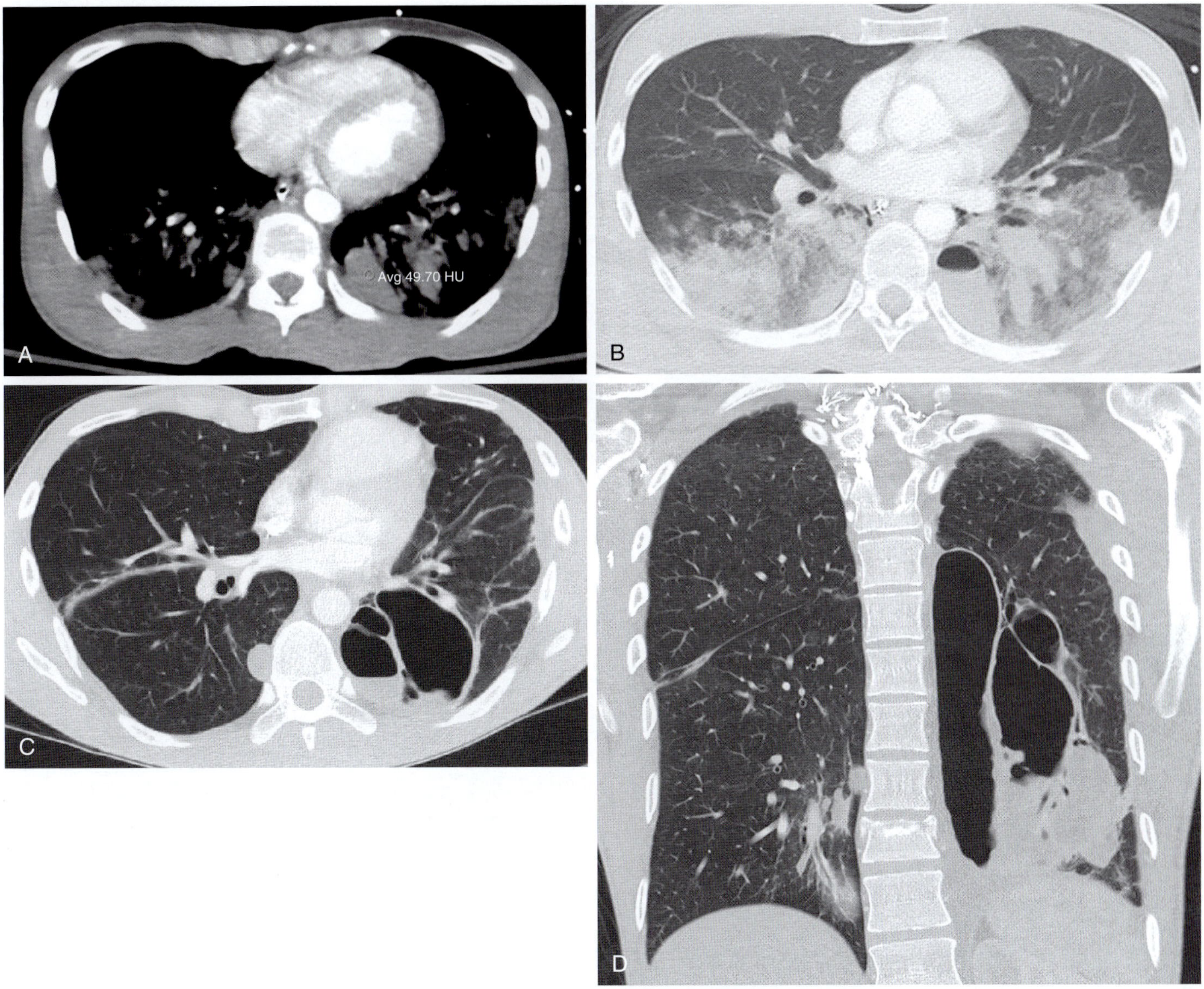

Fig. 67.14 Traumatic pneumatoceles and contusion. Contrast-enhanced axial CT images in soft tissue (A) and lung (B) windows show multiple posterior oval lesions containing air-fluid levels, consistent with traumatic pneumatoceles. The fluid density is consistent with acute blood. Bilateral areas of ground-glass opacities and consolidation represent contusion and possible superimposed aspiration. Contrast-enhanced axial (C) and coronal (D) CT images acquired 3 weeks later show that the hemorrhage within the large left traumatic pneumatoceles is mostly resolved. Note the oblong, vertically oriented morphology of the medial pneumatocele, likely a result of a shearing or contusive force transmitted to the lung via the spinal column. Finally, note the smaller hematopneumatocele in the right lower lobe immediately adjacent to the vertebral body.

On the supine radiograph the apex is the most dependent portion of the pleural space, and fluid should be suspected if an apical cap is seen.[39] Pleural fluid may also manifest as a hazy opacity of the lower or entire hemithorax in a supine or semierect radiograph.

Computed Tomography

CT is much more sensitive and specific than radiography in the detection and characterization of pleural fluid. Hemothorax typically can be differentiated from simple fluid or chyle by its relatively high attenuation values, usually 35 to 70 Hounsfield units, and often heterogeneous appearance (Fig. 67.16).[22] Active bleeding occasionally can be identified by noting contrast extravasation into the pleural space. Fluid-hematocrit levels may also be seen. As the blood clots, loculations develop with the appearance of "fibrin balls" that may mimic pleural tumors.[40]

Pneumothorax

Pneumothorax is a common sequela of blunt chest trauma. Mechanisms include rupture of the alveoli and dissection through the interstitium to the pleural space,[14,22] lung puncture from rib fracture fragments, tracheobronchial injury, and extension of pneumomediastinum through a tear in the parietal pleura. Even

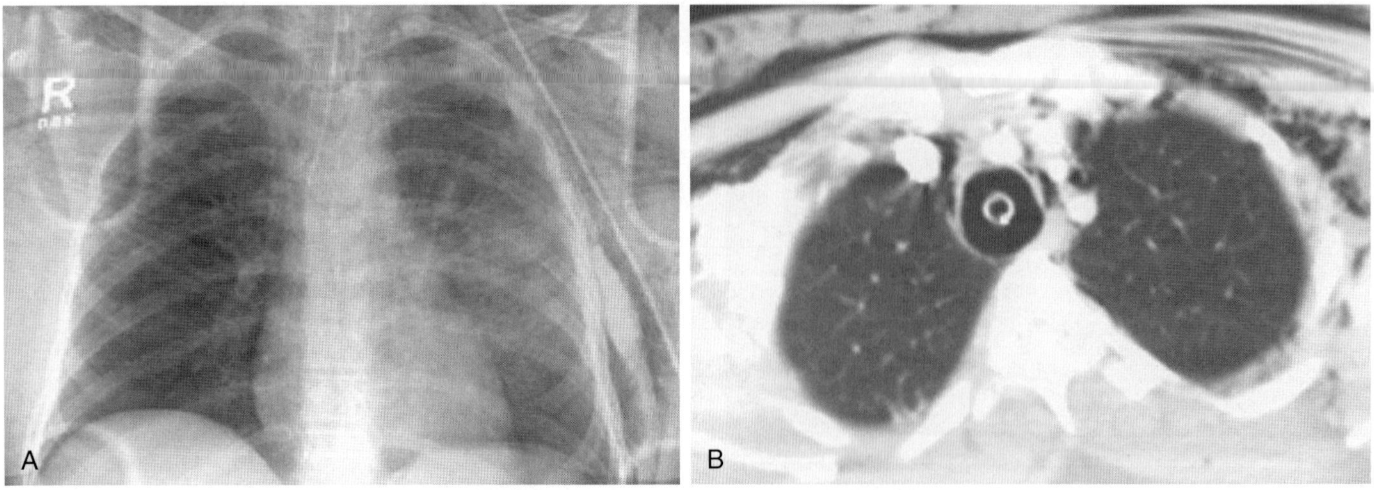

Fig. 67.15 Airway injury and pneumomediastinum after high-velocity motor vehicle collision. (A) Frontal chest radiograph shows extensive chest wall air and abnormally enlarged endotracheal balloon in the midthoracic trachea. The findings taken together indicate tracheal injury. (B) Axial CT scan shows abnormally enlarged endotracheal tube balloon, pneumomediastinum, and chest wall air. The patient was found to have a tear through the posterior membranous portion of the trachea that was believed to be secondary to traumatic intubation, given the unusual location of the injury (i.e., >2 cm from carina).

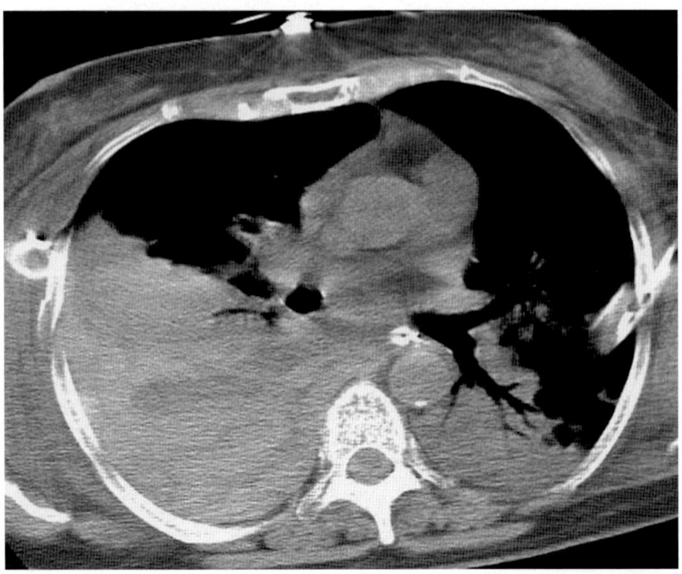

Fig. 67.16 Hemothorax after motor vehicle collision. Axial CT scan shows large right hyperdense pleural fluid collection, consistent with acute hemorrhage. Note the partially visualized right lateral rib fracture and bilateral chest tubes.

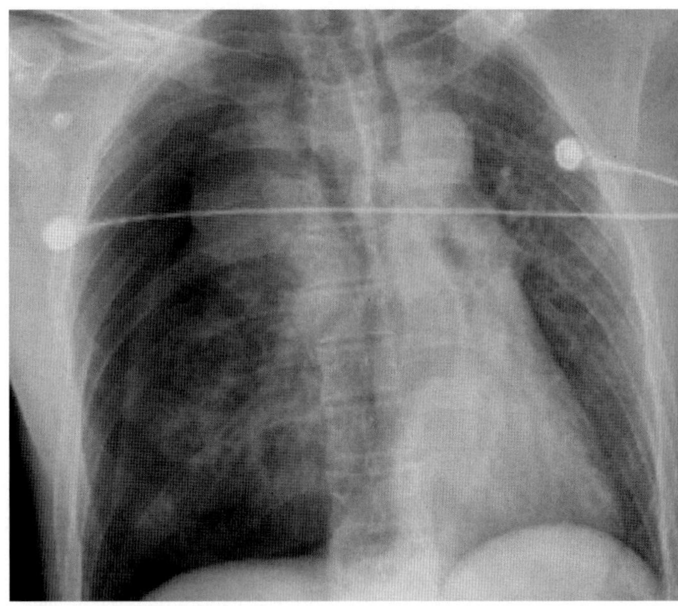

Fig. 67.17 Tension pneumothorax and traumatic lung cysts after motorcycle accident. Frontal chest radiograph shows large right pneumothorax. There is downward displacement of right hemidiaphragm and leftward mediastinal shift, suggesting tension physiology. Note rounded air- and fluid-filled opacities in right lower lung zone compatible with pneumatoceles and parenchymal hematomas. Patchy right lung opacities likely represent coexistent pulmonary contusion.

a tiny pneumothorax can expand rapidly in a patient receiving positive-pressure ventilation.[25]

MANIFESTATIONS OF THE DISEASE

Radiography

On supine radiographs, the anteromedial recess is the least dependent aspect of the pleural space and the site of earliest accumulation of pleural air. Signs of anteromedial pneumothorax include sharp delineation of the mediastinal structures, outlining of the medial diaphragm beneath the heart, and a deep anterior cardiophrenic sulcus. A subpulmonic pneumothorax manifests as a hyperlucent upper abdominal quadrant, deep lateral costophrenic sulcus (Fig. 67.17), and visualization of the anterior costophrenic sulcus and inferior surface of the lung.[41] The classic radiographic finding of pneumothorax is a thin visceral pleural line seen when air is present within the lung and pleural space. Subcutaneous air coupled with rib fractures indicates the presence of pneumothorax even if pleural air is radiographically occult.

Pneumothorax is associated with partial or complete lung collapse. Tension pneumothorax is a life-threatening condition that occurs when intrathoracic pressure exceeds atmospheric pressure. Although tension pneumothorax is a clinical diagnosis, the most specific radiographic finding suggesting tension physiology is depression or inversion of the hemidiaphragm.[14,42] Although increased intrathoracic pressure on the affected side can cause the mediastinum to shift to the contralateral side, mild mediastinal shift is often present in the absence of tension physiology.

Computed Tomography

CT is much more sensitive than radiography in the detection of pneumothorax and should be used in mechanically ventilated patients. Of pneumothoraces detected on CT, 30% were missed on supine and semirecumbent chest radiographs.[14,41]

Pneumomediastinum

Pneumomediastinum is present in 10% of patients with blunt thoracic injury and is most commonly secondary to the Macklin effect.[43] This is the process by which air dissects along bronchovascular bundles after alveolar rupture and spreads to the mediastinum. Mediastinal air may also arise from the extension of subcutaneous or deep cervical air. Direct extension of retroperitoneal air to the mediastinum occurs via periesophageal and periaortic fascial planes and at the level of the sternocostal attachment of the diaphragm.[14,44] Esophageal injury is a rare cause of pneumomediastinum in the setting of blunt thoracic trauma.

MANIFESTATIONS OF THE DISEASE

Radiography

Pneumomediastinum can be identified on the chest radiograph by visualization of lucency along the pericardium and lateral mediastinum outlined laterally by the visceral and parietal pleura linings.[14] Pneumomediastinum may be difficult to differentiate from medial pneumothorax; this can best be done by searching for other manifestations of the two entities. In a child elevation of the thymus by mediastinal air may be seen and is termed the *thymic sail sign*. The ring around the artery sign is seen when air surrounds the pulmonary artery or its branches and is best visualized on the lateral projection.[44] The tubular artery sign is present when mediastinal air outlines the medial side of an arterial branch and normal lung outlines the lateral side. Extraluminal air next to a major bronchus results in clear visualization of the bronchial wall—the double bronchial wall sign. Air posterior and inferior to the pericardium yields the continuous diaphragm sign in which the entire diaphragm is visualized.

Pneumopericardium may mimic pneumomediastinum, and differentiation on radiography relies on identification of the pericardial sac or appreciation of air confined to the limits of the pericardium. The Mach band effect is an error in perception that creates the appearance of a lucency surrounding a convex border, such as the heart. This perceived lucency may result in an incorrect diagnosis of pneumomediastinum. The absence of a nearby opaque pleural line suggests the Mach effect rather than pneumomediastinum as the etiology of the pericardial lucency.

Pneumomediastinum typically resolves with time, and serious complications, such as tension pneumomediastinum, are rare. Failure of resolution or lack of improvement should raise the suspicion for tracheobronchial injury.

Traumatic Diaphragmatic Injury

Traumatic diaphragmatic injury is a tear in the diaphragm resulting from penetrating or blunt injury. Penetrating diaphragmatic injury is twice as common as blunt injury. Diaphragmatic rupture occurs in 0.8% to 8% of all patients with major blunt trauma.[13] Detection of diaphragmatic injury requires a high index of suspicion because masking of the injury by pleural fluid or pulmonary contusion may delay diagnosis. In addition, diaphragmatic injury is associated with other major traumatic injuries, including pneumothorax, hepatic and splenic lacerations, and pelvic fractures, which may distract from identification of diaphragmatic injury.[45]

MECHANISM OF INJURY

Penetrating diaphragmatic injury results from direct trauma that produces a small tear in the diaphragm (usually <1 cm in length). Penetrating injury results from shootings, stabbings, and, less commonly, iatrogenic causes such as a malpositioned chest tube. Stabbings and shootings usually result in left-sided diaphragmatic damage, presumably because most assailants are right-handed and facing their victims.[46]

Blunt trauma causes an increase in intrathoracic pressure that ruptures the hemidiaphragm. Shearing injury may occur when a lateral blow distorts the chest wall.[45] Diaphragmatic tears associated with blunt trauma are usually 10 cm or greater. Injury is most frequently left sided (75%)[46] owing to the protective cushioning effect of the liver. Relative difficulty in detection of right-sided injury may contribute to its underdiagnosis and underrepresentation in the literature.

MANIFESTATIONS OF THE DISEASE

Radiography

The chest radiograph, although a useful screening tool, is insensitive in the detection of diaphragmatic rupture. Although serial radiographs can increase sensitivity by 12%,[14] overall sensitivity ranges from 17% to 64%. Radiographic signs of diaphragmatic injury include obscuration of the hemidiaphragm, elevation of the hemidiaphragm, and contralateral shift of the mediastinum.[45] The most specific radiographic finding is the presence of gas-containing stomach or bowel within the thorax (Fig. 67.18). Termination of a nasogastric tube within the left hemithorax is another specific finding (see Fig. 67.18).

CLASSIC SIGNS: RADIOGRAPHIC FINDINGS IN DIAPHRAGMATIC TEAR

- Visualization of herniated stomach or bowel in chest
- Extension of nasogastric tube above level of diaphragm
- Irregularity of diaphragmatic contour
- Elevated hemidiaphragm in the absence of atelectasis
- Contralateral shift of the mediastinum
- Radiographic findings have low sensitivity

Computed Tomography

CT is the imaging modality of choice in the evaluation of patients with blunt chest trauma and suspected diaphragmatic injury. The sensitivity of cross-sectional CT images in detecting diaphragmatic rupture is 70% to 90%.[10] Thin-collimation and

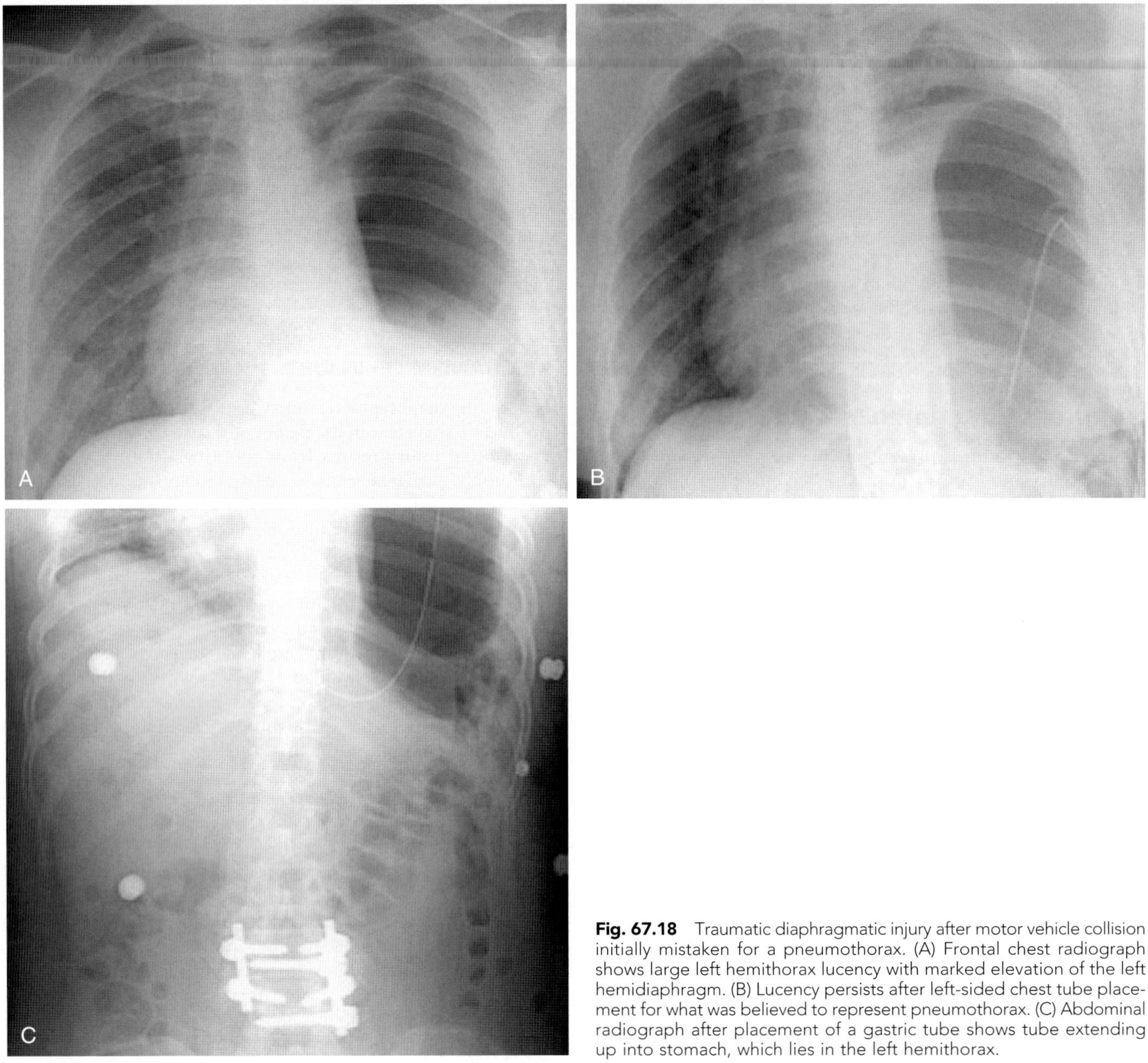

Fig. 67.18 Traumatic diaphragmatic injury after motor vehicle collision initially mistaken for a pneumothorax. (A) Frontal chest radiograph shows large left hemithorax lucency with marked elevation of the left hemidiaphragm. (B) Lucency persists after left-sided chest tube placement for what was believed to represent pneumothorax. (C) Abdominal radiograph after placement of a gastric tube shows tube extending up into stomach, which lies in the left hemithorax.

thin-reconstruction images (1- to 2-mm-thick slices) are recommended if diaphragmatic injury is suspected. Sagittal and coronal reformations have been shown to increase sensitivity[47] and confidence of interpretation.

A constellation of CT findings have been evaluated for the detection of diaphragmatic rupture. The most frequently cited are direct discontinuity or focal defect of the diaphragm (Fig. 67.19), intrathoracic herniation of abdominal viscera, the collar sign, and the dependent viscera sign (Fig. 67.20).[48] Visualization of a focal discontinuity of the diaphragm is 73% to 82% sensitive and 90% specific for diaphragmatic injury (see Figs. 67.19 and 67.20).[49,50] The Bochdalek hernia with a focal defect in the posterolateral hemidiaphragm can mimic traumatic rupture and accounts for most false-positive findings.

Intrathoracic herniation has a sensitivity of 55% to 75%[48,50,51] and a specificity of 100%. Waist-like constriction of herniated abdominal contents at the level of diaphragmatic rupture creates the collar sign, best depicted on coronal and sagittal reformations (see Fig. 67.20). With helical CT, the collar sign has a sensitivity of 63% and a specificity of 100%.[37] The dependent viscera sign has a sensitivity of 55% to 90%.[48,50,51] This sign describes the dependent position of the stomach, spleen, and bowel that has herniated into the thorax (see Fig. 67.20). Other signs suggestive of diaphragmatic injury include irregularity of the diaphragm (Fig. 67.21), thickening of the diaphragm (Fig. 67.22), segmental nonrecognition of the diaphragm (see Fig. 67.19), and elevated abdominal organs.[51]

Magnetic Resonance Imaging

Although CT is the imaging modality of choice for the detection of diaphragmatic injury, cardiac and respiratory-gated MRI may be of use in a stable patient when radiographic and CT findings are nondiagnostic. On MRI a tear is seen as a focal discontinuity of the T1 and T2 hypointense diaphragm.

Thoracic Skeletal or Chest Wall Trauma

Fracture localization in thoracic trauma is a simple process. It is the search for secondary adjacent injury that should be the main diagnostic objective.

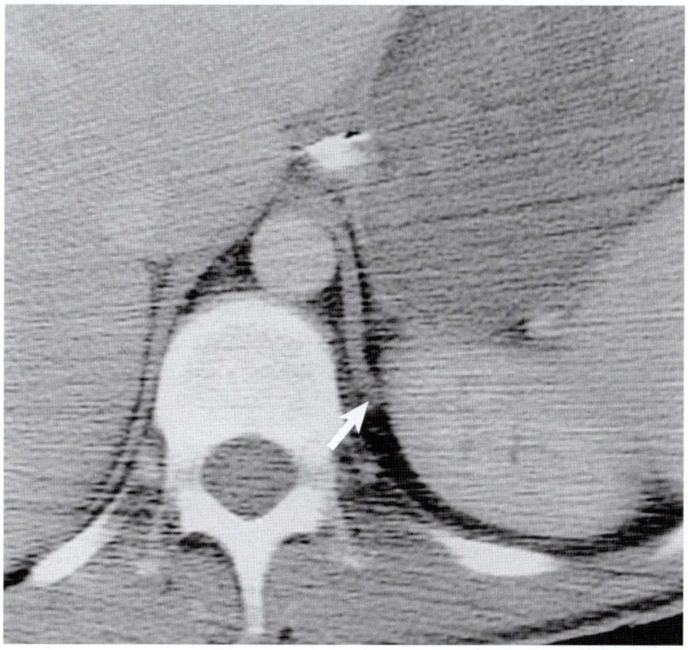

Fig. 67.19 Traumatic rupture of the left hemidiaphragm diagnosed 10 days after a motor vehicle accident and subsequently confirmed at surgery. Contrast-enhanced CT scan shows abrupt discontinuity of the left hemidiaphragm *(arrow)* at the level of the medial arcuate ligament. *(From Müller NL, Fraser RS, Colman NC, et al.* Radiologic Diagnosis of Diseases of the Chest. *Philadelphia: Saunders; 2001.)*

CLASSIC SIGNS: COMPUTED TOMOGRAPHY FINDINGS IN DIAPHRAGMATIC TEAR

- Sharp discontinuity of hemidiaphragm
- Herniation of omental fat or abdominal viscera
- Waist-like narrowing of herniated viscera (collar sign)
- Lack of visualization of hemidiaphragm
- Sensitivity of CT: 70%–90%
- Specificity of CT: 90%
- Accuracy improved with thin sections and multiplanar reconstructions

Rib fractures occur in 60% of patients with blunt thoracic trauma[33] but usually do not occur in restrained passengers in collisions at speeds of less than 30 miles (<50 km) per hour.[1] Rib fractures are more common in elderly individuals, given the less elastic properties of the skeleton. The most commonly fractured ribs are the fourth through the ninth ribs.[6]

First, second, and third rib fractures are associated with a significant mechanism of injury, occurring with aorta or great vessel injury in 14% and tracheobronchial injuries in 2% of cases.[6,52] Fractures of the 10th, 11th, and 12th ribs are associated with renal, splenic, and hepatic injuries. In children rib fractures indicate a significant mechanism of injury and are associated with a higher mortality rate.[1] Sternal fractures are seen predominantly in restrained passengers and occur in 8% of individuals with a significant mechanism of injury.[6] Thoracic spine fractures occur in 3% of blunt trauma patients and are associated with a high percentage of secondary neurologic impairment.[33]

Flail chest is a clinical diagnosis in which mismatched inspiratory and expiratory mechanics impair ventilation. Segmental fractures of four or more contiguous ribs should alert the clinician to the possibility of a flail chest.

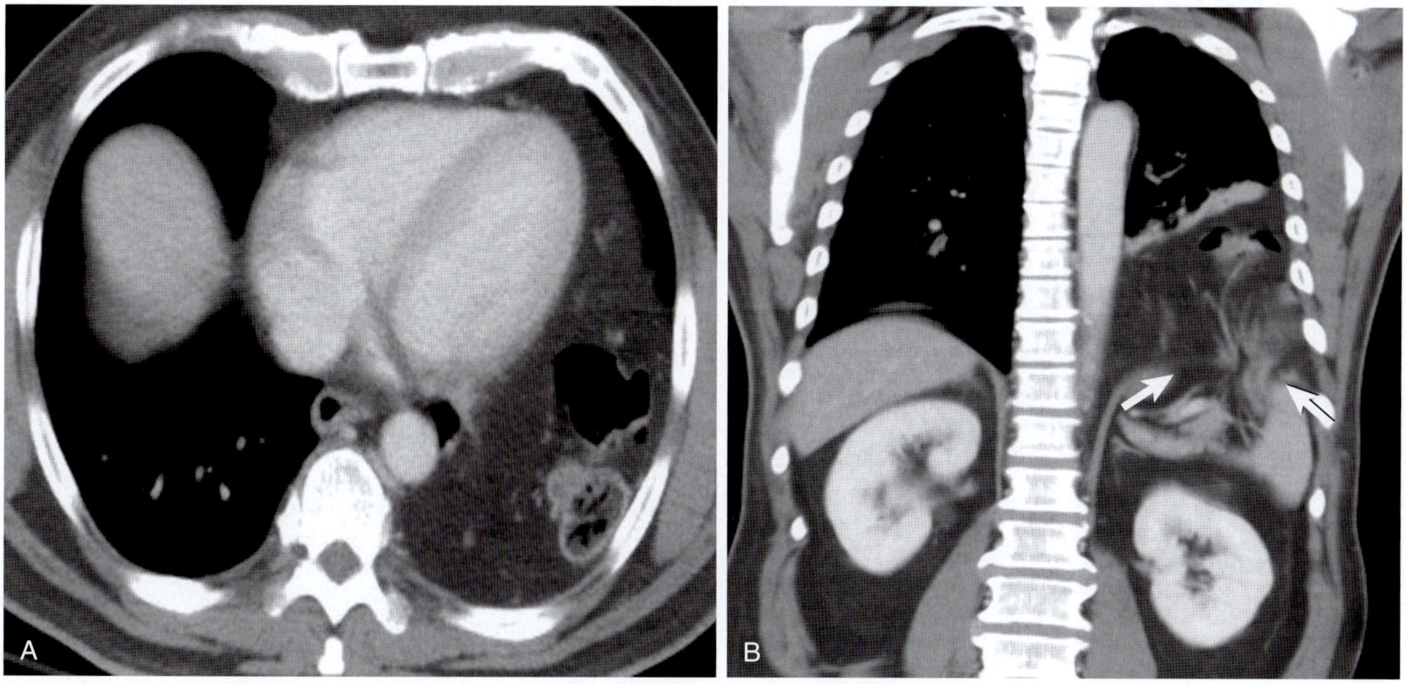

Fig. 67.20 Chronic diaphragmatic injury with dependent viscera and collar signs. Contrast-enhanced axial (A) and coronal (B) CT images show herniation of visceral fat and part of the stomach into the left thoracic cavity (dependent viscera sign). Collar sign (*arrows,* B) of the mesentery is evident on the coronal image.

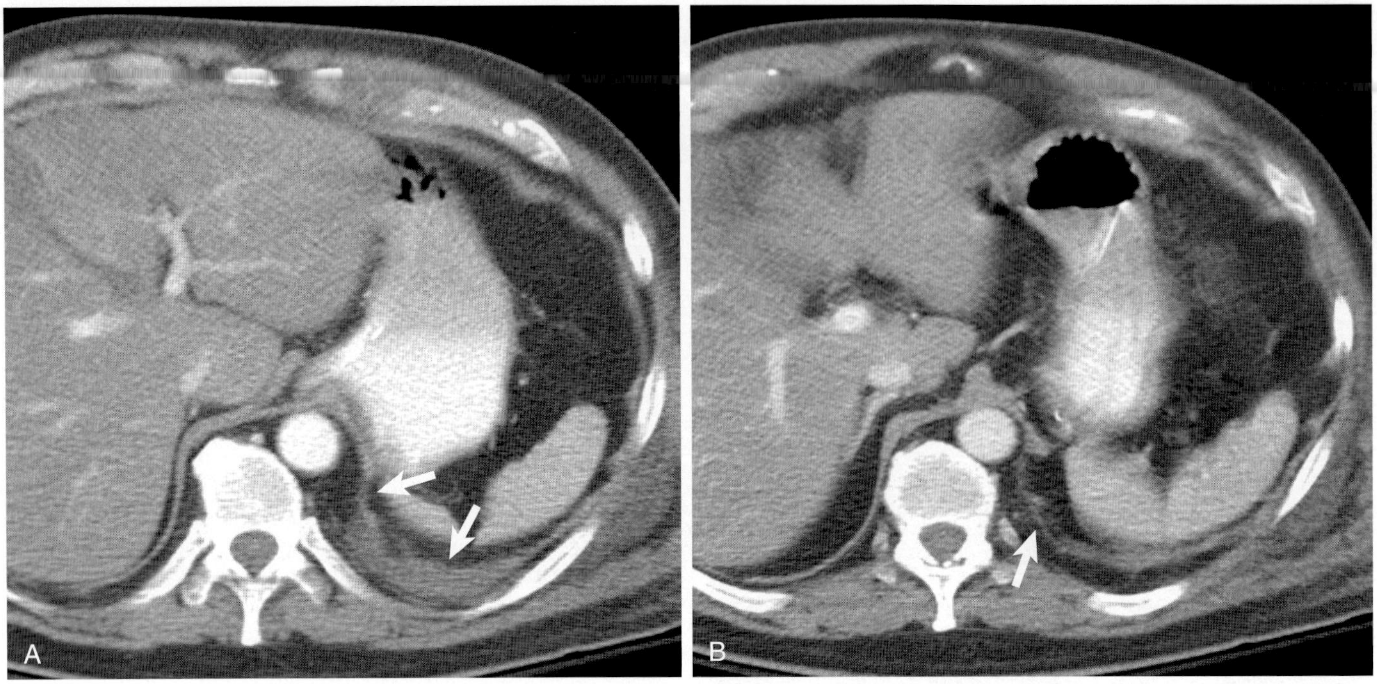

Fig. 67.21 Traumatic diaphragmatic injury. (A) and (B) Axial contrast-enhanced axial CT images show elevation and irregularity of the left hemidiaphragm *(arrows)* with surrounding hyperdense fluid, consistent with acute traumatic diaphragmatic injury and adjacent hemothorax.

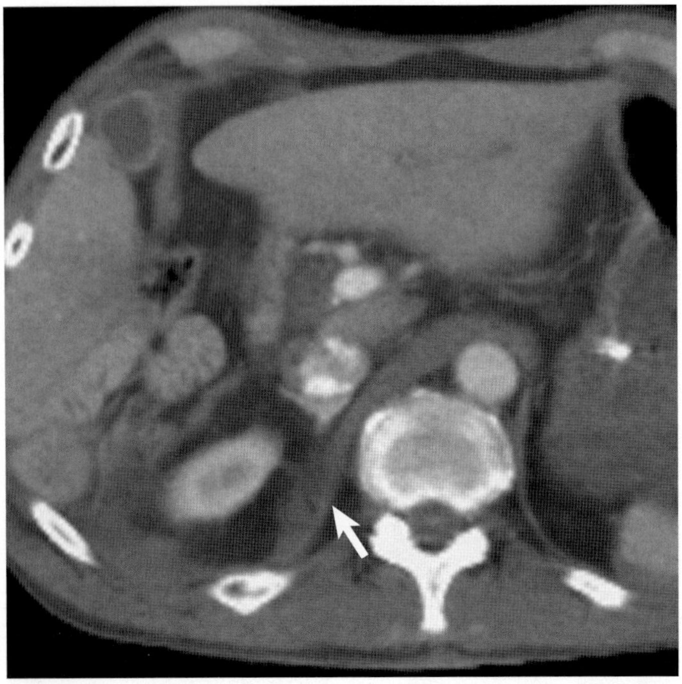

Fig. 67.22 Traumatic diaphragmatic injury. Axial CT scan shows an asymmetrically thickened right medial hemidiaphragm crus *(arrow)* with adjacent fat stranding. The patient had a large right hemidiaphragm rupture repaired surgically.

The sternoclavicular joints and sternum are important sites to evaluate for fracture or dislocation because injury in these locations can cause adjacent mediastinal hematoma that may raise concern for ATAI if the fracture is not identified. Anterior sternoclavicular dislocation is the most common type of dislocation, whereas posterior sternoclavicular dislocation, although less common, is associated with an increased risk of tracheal, esophageal, and great vessel impingement or injury.[6] Although the mechanism associated with sternal fractures increases the risk of cardiac injury, there is no association with ATAI.

Thoracic spine fractures are most common in the thoracolumbar region. Wedge compression and burst fractures secondary to hyperflexion and axial load mechanisms are the predominant fracture types.[33] Thoracic spine fractures may result in significant neurologic impairment (62% with fracture or dislocation injuries) because the spinal cord occupies a larger percentage of the available space in the canal than in the more spacious cervical and lumbar spinal regions.[2] In addition, a limited blood supply is present, which, when injured, has little collateral reserve and predisposes to ischemic insult.

MANIFESTATIONS OF THE DISEASE

Radiography and Computed Tomography

Clavicle fractures are nearly always seen on radiography. Many rib fractures can be diagnosed with radiography; however, CT is more sensitive (Figs. 67.23; see Figs. 67.10 and 67.16). Two different morphologies of rib fractures exist: buckling of the cortex and a fracture gap. Particular attention should be paid to buckling of the cortex-type rib fractures, which are often missed. Peripheral opacities that parallel the chest wall represent extrapleural hematomas adjacent to rib fractures (Fig. 67.24). Extrapleural hematoma, just as the name implies, is extrapleural bleeding that does not communicate with the pleural space and results from damaged intercostal vessels, muscles, and open fractures.[1] Extrapleural hematoma manifests on CT as a hyperdense biconvex or nonconvex lesion that displaces extrapleural fat inward, which is referred to as the "extrapleural fat sign." The

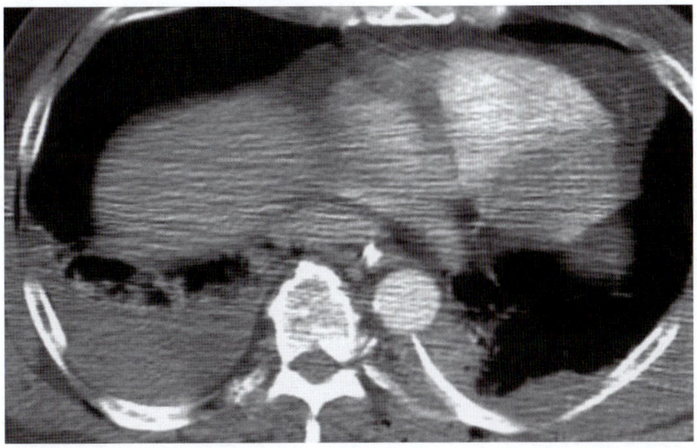

Fig. 67.23 Rib fracture. Axial contrast-enhanced CT scan shows displaced left posterior rib fracture abutting the posterior wall of the descending thoracic aorta. The patient went on to surgical fixation of the rib fracture, given the proximity to the aorta.

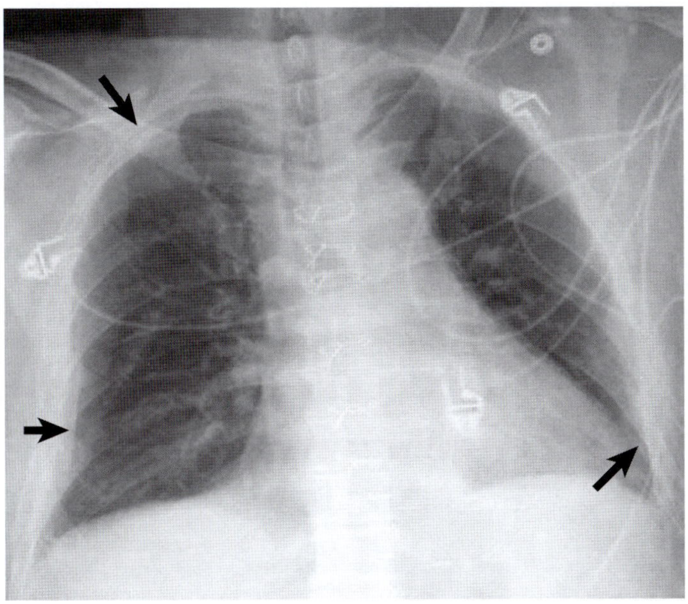

Fig. 67.24 Rib fractures and extrapleural hematoma. Frontal chest radiograph in a trauma patient who has multiple bilateral rib fractures not easily appreciated on radiography. Note isolated, peripheral opacities *(arrows)* that parallel the chest wall, representing extrapleural hematomas adjacent to rib fractures.

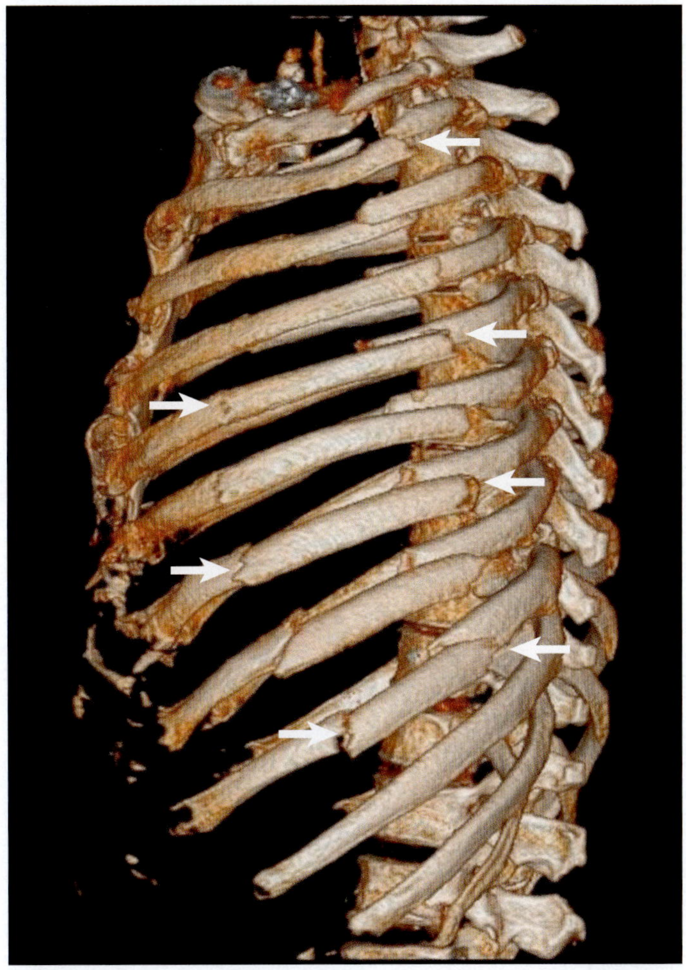

Fig. 67.25 Rib fractures with flail chest after falling from a tree. Three-dimensional reformatted CT image shows multiple contiguous displaced rib fractures *(arrows)*, some of which are segmental. This patient had flail chest clinically. Three-dimensional reformatted images are useful to the surgeon for surgical planning.

possibility of a flail chest should be considered whenever a large extrapleural hematoma is seen.[52] Three-dimensional reformatted images are often helpful in visualizing rib trauma in the setting of a flail chest and aid the surgeon in surgical planning (Fig. 67.25). The anterior rib costal cartilage is uncommonly fractured in blunt trauma. These types of fractures are most easily seen on maximum-intensity projection images or coronal reconstructions using a soft tissue window. The fracture manifests as a central cleft or focus of air within the middle substance of the costal cartilage.

Scapular fractures indicate a significant mechanism of injury and can be seen on 57% of initial chest radiographs.[52] Approximately 50% of patients with a scapular fracture have a pneumothorax.[52] Ipsilateral subclavian, axillary, or brachial artery injury may be present in 11% of patients with scapular fracture.[1]

Thoracic spine fractures are not easily seen on the frontal radiograph; 10% to 30% of fractures are missed.[52] Paraspinal hematoma and an indistinct or dense descending aorta are indirect signs of vertebral body injury. Thoracic spine fractures often occur along with sternal fractures.[33] The rule of 2s is a rough rule of thumb to aid in the diagnosis of spinal fractures: There should be no variance greater than 2 mm between interspinous distance, interpediculate distance, and width of facet joints. In addition, the posterior height of the vertebral body should be no more than 2 mm more than the anterior height on sagittal/lateral imaging.[53]

Sternal fractures are rarely seen on frontal radiographs but, similar to rib fractures, are easily seen on sagittal CT images, although they can be easily missed on axial images (Figs. 67.26 to 67.28). Sternoclavicular dislocations are difficult to visualize radiographically and are more commonly identified on CT (Fig. 67.29). A careful search for tracheal, esophageal, and great vessel impingement or injury should be preformed in a patient with a posterior sternoclavicular joint dislocation.

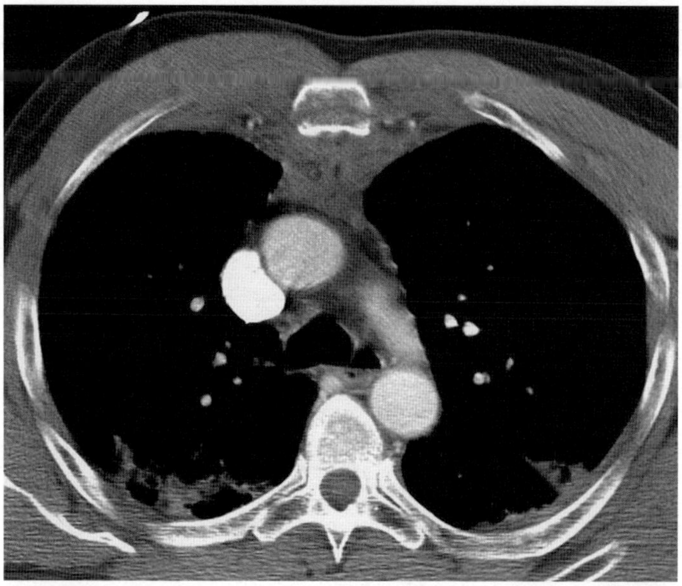

Fig. 67.26 Sternal fracture. Contrast-enhanced CT axial image shows a coronally oriented fracture through the sternum with an adjacent mediastinal hematoma. With sternal injuries or costochondral separation, it is important to exclude active extravasation from adjacent internal mammary arteries, especially if a hematoma is present.

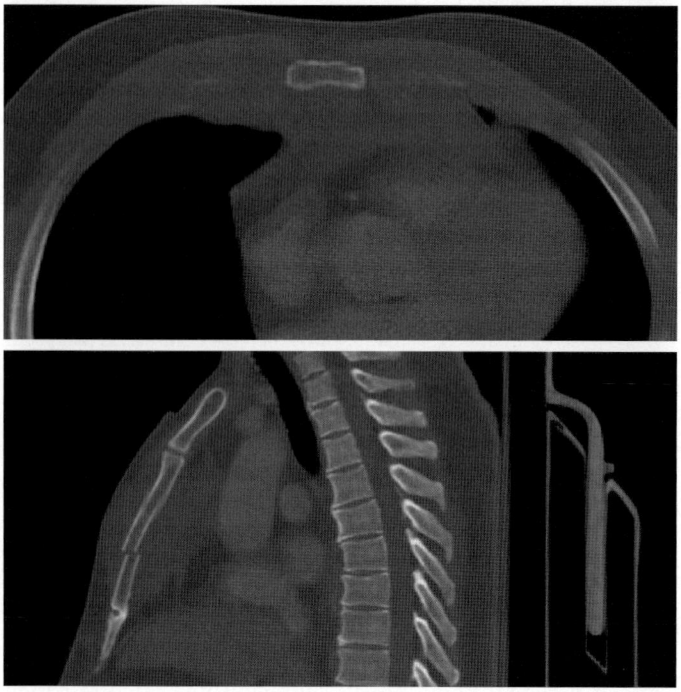

Fig. 67.27 Sternal fracture. Composite image with axial *(top image)* and sagittal *(bottom image)* CT images shows a transversely oriented fracture through the midsternum with adjacent mediastinal hematoma. The fracture is subtle on the axial image but clearly apparent on the sagittal image, demonstrating the usefulness and importance of multiplanar imaging, especially in detecting sternal fractures.

KEY POINTS

- The main value of the chest radiograph in trauma patients is in showing evidence of mediastinal hematoma and in ruling out a large pneumothorax.
- A normal chest radiograph has a 98% negative predictive value in ruling out acute traumatic aortic injury (ATAI).
- CT is the imaging modality of choice in the assessment of patients with clinical or radiographic findings suggestive of ATAI, vertebral fracture, pulmonary laceration, or diaphragmatic tear after blunt chest trauma.
- Ideally, CT should be performed using thin collimation (1 mm), thin reformations (1–2 mm), and overlapping images for multiplanar reformations.
- A morphologically normal aorta on a good-quality, contrast-enhanced multidetector CT scan in a patient with no mediastinal hematoma has a 100% negative predictive value for exclusion of ATAI.
- CT with multiplanar reformations provides optimal visualization of thoracic spine fractures and superior assessment of suspected sternal fractures.

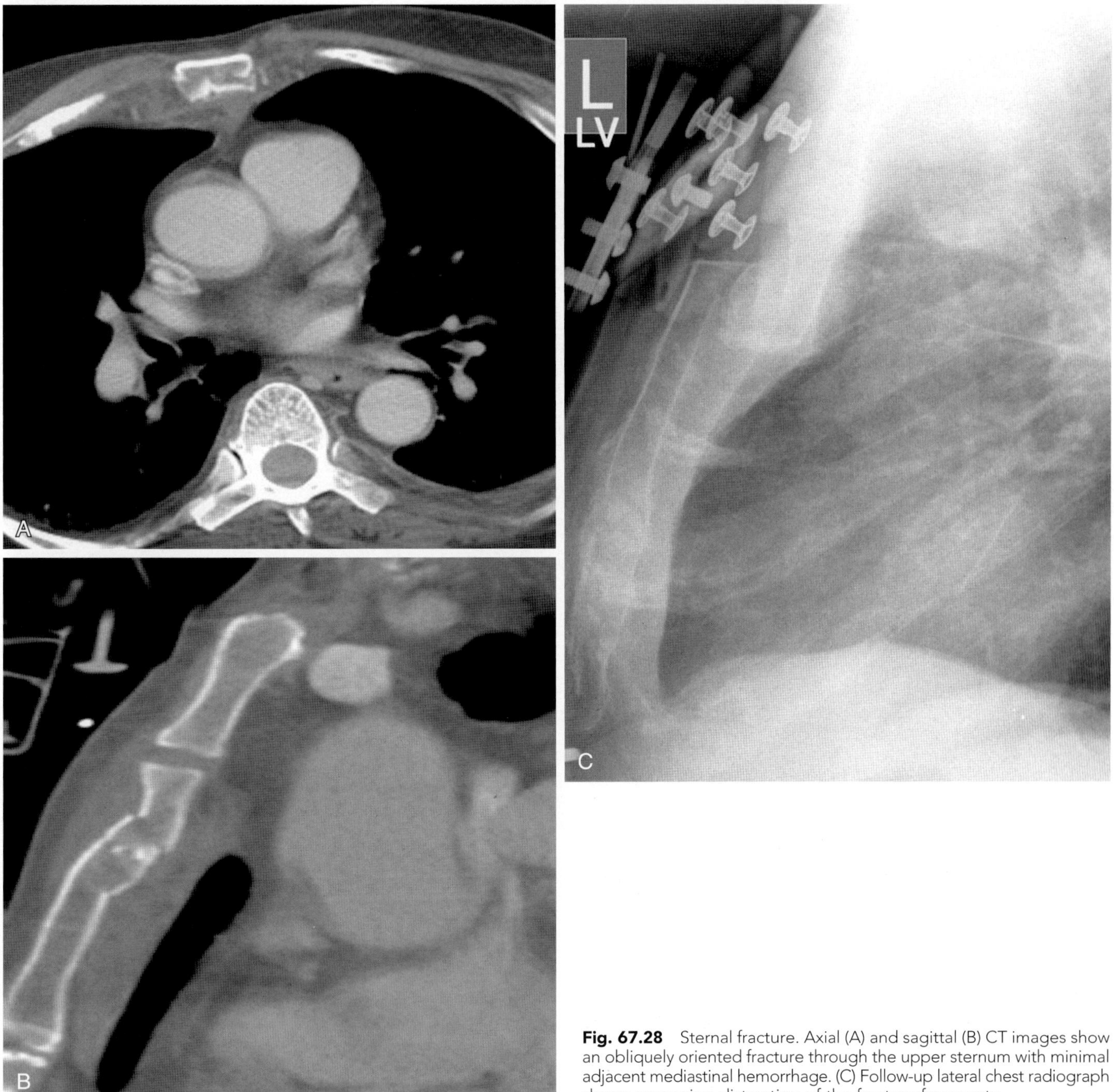

Fig. 67.28 Sternal fracture. Axial (A) and sagittal (B) CT images show an obliquely oriented fracture through the upper sternum with minimal adjacent mediastinal hemorrhage. (C) Follow-up lateral chest radiograph shows worsening distraction of the fracture fragments.

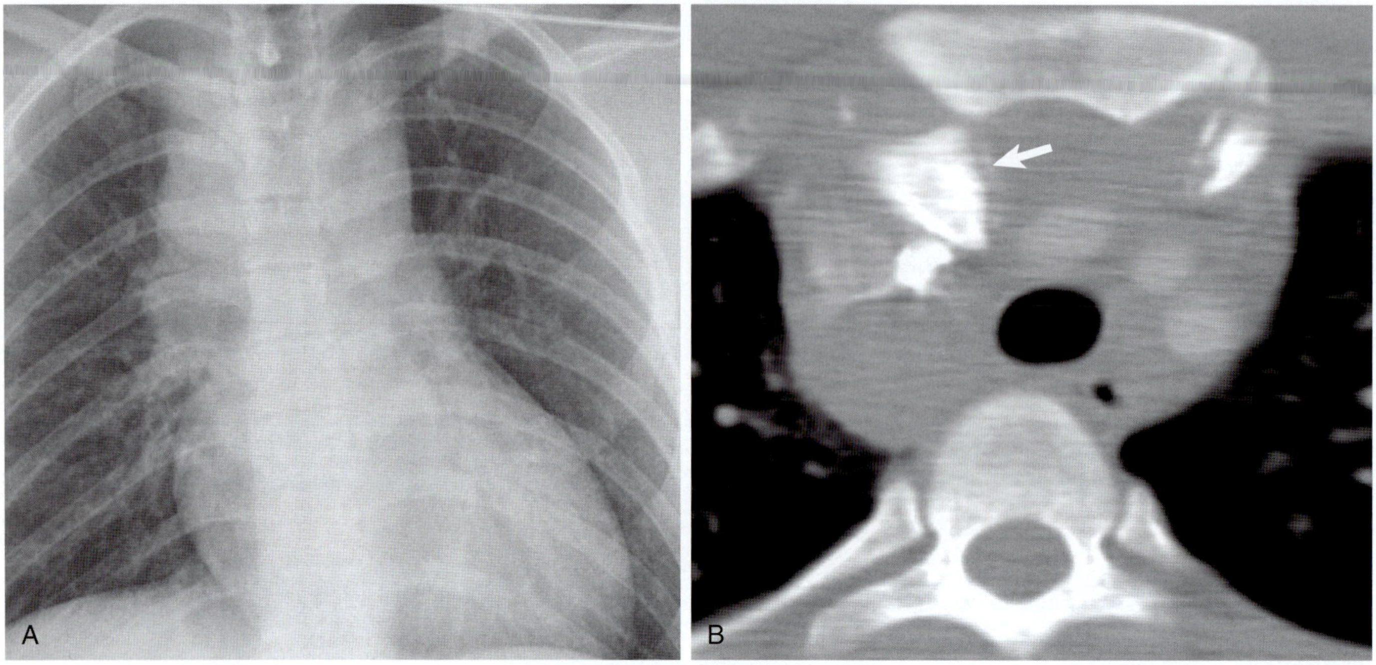

Fig. 67.29 Posterior sternoclavicular dislocation. (A) Frontal radiograph shows a dense, widened mediastinum after trauma, concerning for acute traumatic aortic injury. (B) Axial contrast-enhanced CT image shows extensive mediastinal hemorrhage with a posterior right sternoclavicular joint dislocation *(arrow)*. No traumatic injury of the great vessels, supraaortic branch vessels, or aorta was present.

SUGGESTED READINGS

Alkadhi H, Wildermuth S, Desbiolles L, et al. Vascular emergencies of the thorax after blunt and iatrogenic trauma: multi-detector row CT and three-dimensional imaging. *Radiographics*. 2004;24:1239–1255.

Miller LA. Chest wall, lung, and pleural space trauma. *Radiol Clin North Am*. 2006;44:213–224.

The full reference list for this chapter is available at ExpertConsult.com.

68 Postoperative Complications*

MYLENE T. TRUONG | CAROL C. WU | CHARLES S. WHITE

A spectrum of cardiopulmonary diseases can be treated surgically. Surgical procedures in the thorax include lung resection, lung transplantation, cardiovascular and mediastinal surgery, as well as pleural and cavitary space reduction procedures. This chapter reviews the surgical procedures, indications, and imaging findings in the postoperative setting, both expected and unexpected, including potential complications. In the intensive care unit, postoperative findings, such as malposition of support lines and tubes, and cardiopulmonary diseases, such as pulmonary edema, pneumonia, pneumothorax, pleural and pericardial fluid collections, and pulmonary embolism, are described in other chapters.

Thoracotomy and Chest Wall Surgery

DESCRIPTION

Thoracotomy is defined as a surgical incision into the chest. In posterolateral thoracotomy a large transverse incision along the lateral aspect of the chest via the fifth intercostal space transects the latissimus dorsi. This incision starts at the anterior axillary line, continues posteriorly beneath the tip of the scapula, and then extends caudally to terminate between the spine and the medial border of the scapula. Typically, in patients older than 40 years, the ribs at the incision site are resected at the costovertebral angle to prevent rib fractures. A thoracoabdominal incision involves a posterolateral incision via the seventh or eighth intercostal space with extension of the incision anteriorly through the costal arch and into the abdomen. In axillary thoracotomy or mini-thoracotomy, a linear incision from the anterior axillary line inferomedially to the midhemithorax avoids the division of several muscles, most importantly the latissimus dorsi. In anterior or anterolateral thoracotomy the incision starts at the midaxillary line and follows the inframammary fold to terminate in the parasternal location. A median sternotomy involves a midline incision from the suprasternal notch to the xiphoid process. In limited anterior thoracotomy the incision length is restricted generally to less than 10 cm.[1] "Clamshell" incision combines bilateral anterolateral thoracotomies with transverse sternotomy. Video-assisted thoracoscopic surgery (VATS) consists of the use of a fiberoptic camera and surgical instruments placed via three to five intercostal incisions along the anterior and posterior axillary lines.[2,3] More recently, uniportal VATS using a single incision for access rather than multiple incisions has been developed without incurring additional perioperative complications.[4] Advances in robotic technology have led to the amalgamation of robotic surgical techniques with the VATS procedure, now known as robot-assisted thoracic surgery (RATS).

*The editors and the publisher would like to thank Dr. Thomas O. Flukinger for contributing material on this topic to the prior edition of this work. It has served as the foundation for the current chapter.

Chest wall surgery aims to resect the lesion with margins wide enough to eradicate the disease, while at the same time leaving a defect that can be closed effectively. The two goals of chest wall reconstruction are to cover the defect and to restore chest wall rigidity. Tissue defect coverage is most commonly accomplished with the use of flaps. A soft tissue flap may contain bone, fascia, muscle, fat, or a combination of those. A flap can be transferred from a donor site to a recipient site (free flap), with surgical development of a new vascular supply, or it can be rotated into position, with its vascular supply maintained through a pedicle connected to the donor site. Free flaps require delicate microsurgical technique to ensure adequate perfusion. Pedicle flaps are more commonly used in thoracic tumor resections because the surgical procedure is less complex and postoperative perfusion is more reliable. Flap nomenclature includes the type of tissue transferred, the distance to be transferred (local or distant), and the numbers and types of pedicles. Myocutaneous and omental flaps are most commonly used in thoracic surgery. Omental flaps are usually brought to the thorax in the retrosternal location via a surgical defect in the anterior diaphragm.[3,5] To restore chest wall rigidity, prosthetic material (meshes, metals) or autogenous tissue, such as fascia lata, may be used. Important characteristics of effective synthetic material include rigidity, malleability, inertness (to allow ingrowth of fibrous tissue), and radiolucency (to allow easier imaging reassessment).[6]

INDICATIONS, CONTRAINDICATIONS, PURPOSE, AND UNDERLYING MECHANISMS

Median sternotomy allows wide access for anterior mediastinal surgery and is the incision of choice for open-heart surgery. A posterolateral thoracotomy is the standard approach for lung resection and surgery involving the esophagus, posterior mediastinum, and aorta. The thoracoabdominal incision is used in esophageal surgery. An axillary thoracotomy is commonly used for pulmonary lobar resection; an anterior thoracotomy is commonly used for open-lung biopsies and in some esophageal surgeries. A limited anterior thoracotomy is used in minimally invasive cardiac surgery.[1] Clamshell incision is primarily used in bilateral lung transplantation. In the past clamshell thoracotomy was also used to allow access to both lungs in the resection of bilateral primary or metastatic malignancies, which is now frequently achieved by VATS. VATS has become increasingly popular for both diagnostic and therapeutic procedures.[3,7]

Chest wall resection is most commonly indicated for chest wall tumors, either primary or metastatic. Between 5% and 8% of lung cancers involve the parietal pleura and chest wall, requiring complete resection of the affected chest wall.[3,5] Other common indications for chest wall resection include radiation necrosis, severe infections, and trauma.[5] To fix chest wall defects at the resection site, chest wall reconstruction is indicated for all full-thickness skeletal defects that have the potential of paradoxical chest wall motion.[6] Chest wall reconstruction is also performed to correct chest wall deformities, most often congenital, such as pectus excavatum and cleft sternum, where failed midline fusion and resultant separation of the sternum leaves the heart and great vessels unprotected.[3,5]

Indications for intrathoracic flaps include repair of tracheoesophageal fistulas; buttressing of tracheal, bronchial, and esophageal anastomoses; repair of esophageal perforations; repair of bronchopleural fistulas; filling of tissue defects; reinforcement of the chest wall; and space obliteration after treatment of postpneumonectomy empyema. Omental flaps deliver a reliable blood supply and are commonly used to fill the residual space left from muscle flaps and for treatment of poststernotomy mediastinitis and chronic deep tissue infections.[5]

EXPECTED APPEARANCE ON RELEVANT MODALITIES

On initial postoperative imaging, skin staples are noted in the operative site. Titanium staples used in current automated staplers minimize artifacts on computed tomography (CT) and magnetic resonance imaging.[3,8] In the first few weeks after thoracotomy, CT can identify minimal soft tissue swelling and subcutaneous air in the operative site. In the long term, CT may also show atrophy of denervated muscles at the incision site.[9] Imaging after chest wall resection and reconstruction can demonstrate mild to marked musculoskeletal distortion, depending on the type and extent of surgery, and large reconstructions can cause mediastinal shift.[10]

After median sternotomy, four to seven stainless steel sternal wires are visible in a vertical configuration. Imaging of the sternum can also show gaps, step-offs (ventral-dorsal misalignment), and impaction (overriding of sternal halves). Although little or no sign of healing of the sternum is expected on imaging in the first few postoperative months, by 1 year, healing is visualized as a continuum of cortical bone over the sternotomy site. Minor sternal irregularities can persist.[11] Within the first week after sternotomy, air can be visible on radiography as subcutaneous linear lucencies in the chest and neck or as small focal air pockets in the mediastinum or retrosternal space, which is best visualized on lateral radiography. Retrosternal air can persist for weeks.[12] Retrosternal soft tissue thickening and mediastinal widening resulting from small amounts of fluid in the mediastinum or pericardium are also commonly seen within the first postoperative week. These expected radiographic changes in the early postoperative period after sternotomy may confound identification of mediastinitis.[11,13–15]

Intrathoracic flaps often produce changes in the contour of the heart and mediastinum on radiography. The omental flap frequently appears as a soft tissue opacity in the retrosternal or perihilar region.[2,16,17] On CT the omental graft typically has linear opacities representing omental vessels and increased attenuation of the fat caused by edema, resulting in a "smoky" appearance. The omental flap can be followed from the abdominal cavity through the anterior diaphragm to its final intrathoracic location.[2,18] The thymic and mediastinal fat pad flaps typically appear as fat-attenuation tissue adjacent to the proximal airways on CT, although thymic tissue also may have a component of soft tissue attenuation, depending on the age of the patient.

Intrathoracic muscle flaps have a soft tissue component and, when used in the oncologic setting, can be confused with tumor recurrence if their characteristic features are not recognized. Muscle flaps can have various appearances on imaging because of the vascular pedicles and muscle configurations in characteristic locations. Anterior serratus and latissimus dorsi flaps are usually identified in the posterolateral chest and can mimic empyema. A rectus abdominis muscle flap is generally seen in the inferior retrosternal region. Unilateral pectoral flaps produce a difference in opacity between the hemithoraces on chest radiography. Intercostal muscle flaps are most often identified in the paraspinal region or azygoesophageal recess and typically arise from the posterolateral chest wall.[2,18] On CT intercostal flaps have a curvilinear shape with a component of fat attenuation and linear calcification, presumably from remnants of periosteum.[19,20] Flaps can atrophy because of muscle denervation and disuse and show fatty infiltration over time on CT. Gore-Tex, methyl methacrylate, and stainless steel mesh are often used in flap surgery for chest wall defects and are identified on CT as high-attenuation linear opacities of variable thickness beneath muscle flaps.[5,18]

POTENTIAL COMPLICATIONS AND RADIOLOGIC APPEARANCE

Complications of chest wall surgery include flail chest, winged scapula, fistula formation, incisional dehiscence, wound infection, seroma, and flap failure, as well as lung and bowel herniation.[5,21]

Dehiscence, the premature opening of any surgical site, is due to poor wound healing (Fig. 68.1). Dehiscence can result from or precipitate wound infection. Risk factors include diabetes, advanced age, obesity, and trauma during the postoperative period. A sizable dehiscence can be identified radiographically as a gap between approximated tissues that may progressively widen over time. A midsternal stripe (midline vertical radiolucency) that widens over time should also raise suspicion. Reorientation of sternal wires on chest radiography is noted in up to 90% of patients with dehiscence. Sternal wire displacement is the single best radiologic sign of dehiscence, allowing early detection. However, a repeat sternotomy may also lead to reorientation of sternal wires. Fractured and displaced wires

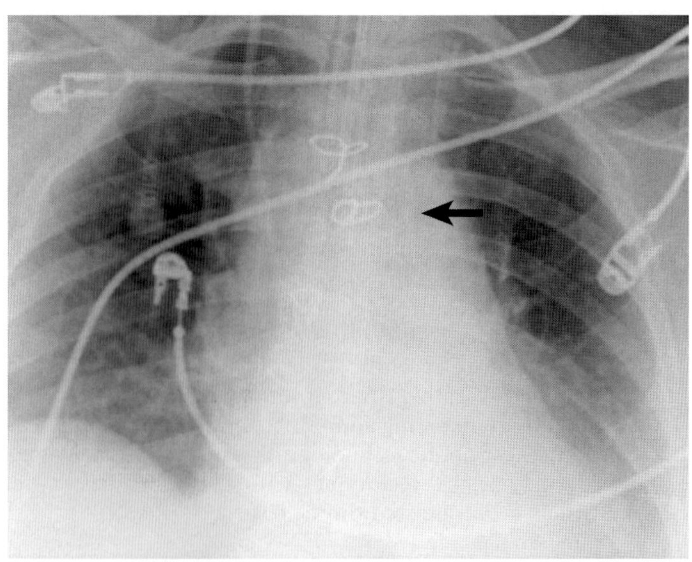

Fig. 68.1 Sternal dehiscence after coronary bypass graft surgery. Frontal chest radiograph demonstrates misaligned wires with leftward displacement of the second wire from the top *(arrow)*.

may migrate into the parasternal soft tissues or, rarely, elsewhere in the thorax.[22,23]

Wound infection after chest wall surgery and thoracotomy includes both soft tissue and bone infections. Wound infection occurs in almost 5% of chest wall reconstructions as prosthetic mesh is an excellent substrate for bacterial growth.[3,5] Soft tissue infection and osteomyelitis after sternotomy are important clinical problems. CT findings of sternal infection include parasternal soft tissue stranding, sinus tracts, sternal erosions, and abscess formation. CT sinography can be performed to assess sinus tract depth and to show any mediastinal communication. Early sternal osteomyelitis is difficult to differentiate from expected minor sternal irregularities after surgery and may not become fully apparent until it has reached a late stage.[10,11]

Seroma is a localized serous fluid collection in the operative site. It is a common problem in the immediate postoperative period and is identified after procedures involving mesh and Silastic implants.[5] On CT seroma appears as a fluid attenuation ovoid collection. Seroma is visualized on ultrasonography as an anechoic fluid collection. Seroma typically resolves after repeated aspiration or spontaneously within a few weeks but may persist and develop a serosal lining that prevents dead space closure and proper wound healing.[5,24]

Flap failure can be partial or complete. Partial flap failure involves loss of function in only a part of the flap. Flap hemorrhage and infection can lead to partial flap failure and can appear radiographically as an increase in flap size. Total flap failure occurs almost exclusively after complete vascular pedicle disruption, leading to flap necrosis.[5,24] Lung herniation through the intercostal space is a rare complication caused by lack of chest wall integrity. Lateral and oblique radiographs may show lung parenchyma protruding outside the osseous thorax. CT is more sensitive and clearly shows the location and extent of the hernia (Fig. 68.2). Lung herniation is typically benign but may rarely cause lung strangulation.[7,25] Bowel herniation may occur after any surgery with an omental flap because the procedure creates a potential passageway for bowel loops through the anterior diaphragm. Herniation is usually a straightforward diagnosis manifested radiographically by loops of bowel extending into the thorax.[10,26]

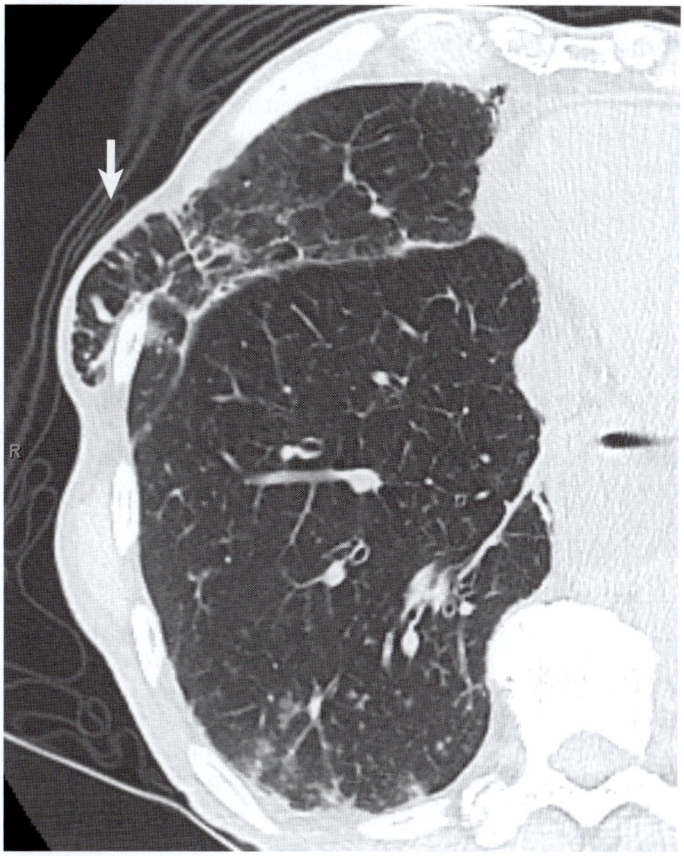

Fig. 68.2 Lung herniation in a man who had undergone right thoracotomy for esophagectomy 16 years earlier. In the preoperative evaluation for a renal mass, chest CT shows herniation of a portion of the lateral segment of the right middle lobe *(arrow)* into the right lateral chest wall.

Pulmonary Resection

DESCRIPTION

Pulmonary resection involves removal of lung parenchyma, ligation of the vessels supplying the targeted lung section, and resection of the associated bronchi at the most proximal location through thoracotomy, VATS, or RATS. In some cases pulmonary resection procedures may also include resection of parts of the chest wall, diaphragm, pericardium, and associated vasculature.

Wedge resection or nonanatomic sublobar resection consists of the removal of a small wedge-shaped piece of lung tissue, usually through VATS. Segmentectomy is the anatomic resection of the lung based on the segmental vessels and airways and can be performed through a limited thoracotomy or VATS. Lobectomy involves the resection of an entire lobe of the lung, its surrounding visceral pleura, and associated airways and pulmonary vasculature. It can be performed via open thoracotomy, VATS, or RATS. A variant of the lobectomy involves a sleeve resection of the bronchus. The proximal and distal edges of the remaining bronchus are reattached with an end-to-end anastomosis.

Pneumonectomy, performed through a posterolateral thoracotomy, VATS, or RATS, consists of resection of an entire lung along with its visceral pleura and includes hilar dissection and ligation of the ipsilateral main bronchus, pulmonary artery, and superior and inferior pulmonary veins. Pneumonectomy can be intrapericardial or extrapericardial, depending on whether the hilum is dissected inside or outside the pericardial sac. The mainstem bronchial stump after pneumonectomy is typically covered with adjacent tissue (pleura, omentum) to decrease the likelihood of an air leak.[3,8,27] In contrast, extrapleural pneumonectomy consists of the resection of the parietal pleura, ipsilateral diaphragm, and pericardium, in addition to the lung and visceral pleura.[3,27]

Lung volume reduction surgery involves the resection of emphysematous upper lobe lung tissue, most often by wedge resection. Lung volume reduction surgery can be performed through a median sternotomy or VATS and is typically performed bilaterally. Bullectomy and blebectomy consist of the removal of lung bullae or blebs, respectively. A giant bullectomy refers to the resection of a single dominant lung bulla; an apical bullectomy involves the resection of lung bullae located in the lung apices. The major difference between a bleb and bullae is that a bleb is a collection of air within layers of visceral pleura rather than within the lung parenchyma. Bullectomy and blebectomy are usually accomplished through wedge resection as part of VATS.

INDICATIONS, CONTRAINDICATIONS, PURPOSE, AND UNDERLYING MECHANISMS

Wedge resection is used for indeterminate pulmonary nodules, pulmonary metastases, and stage I lung cancers in selected patients unable to tolerate larger resection, including older patients and those with reduced cardiopulmonary function. Wedge resection is also used, instead of an anatomic resection, in those with additional subsolid lesions concerning for adenocarcinomas and those with prior lung resection, to help preserve lung parenchyma and pulmonary function.[28] Wedge resections, usually of more than one lobe, are also used to obtain tissue for pathologic diagnosis in individuals with diffuse lung disease. Segmentectomy is primarily indicated for patients with suppurative pulmonary lesions, such as tuberculosis and bronchiectasis, but it is also used in selected lung cancer patients. Sleeve resection is used to treat tumors involving the junction of lobar bronchi in the right upper lobe, left upper lobe, and left lower lobe. Lobectomy is the surgical resection of choice for early stage non–small cell lung cancer. Pneumonectomy is indicated for cancer that is centrally located, adherent to hilar structures, or crosses a fissure. Pneumonectomy is occasionally performed for extensive inflammatory disease.[3,27] Completion pneumonectomy can be performed when lung cancer recurs within a previously surgically treated lung. In contrast, extrapleural pneumonectomy is primarily reserved for pleural mesothelioma. Lung volume reduction surgery is used as palliative surgery for selected patients with severe debilitating pulmonary emphysema despite optimal medical management.[3,7] A giant bullectomy is indicated if a bulla occupies more than 30% of a lung, causes dyspnea, and overlies normal lung parenchyma. Apical bullectomy and blebectomy can be performed to treat pneumothorax resulting from bulla or bleb rupture that causes clinical symptoms.[3,29]

EXPECTED APPEARANCE ON RELEVANT MODALITIES

After pulmonary resection, imaging shows characteristic staple lines at the operative site. Focal atelectasis, edema, and hemorrhage at the resection margin manifest as an area of increased opacity or density. This density typically decreases and resolves within days to weeks. Over time, granulation tissue manifesting as soft tissue can occur at the resection margin. The pleural space initially fills with fluid and over time closes by a number of compensatory mechanisms. These mechanisms include expansion of remaining lung, narrowing of intercostal spaces, elevation of the diaphragm, mediastinal shift, and inward displacement of the chest wall. The degree to which these changes occur is related to the extent of pulmonary resection and to the patient's underlying cardiovascular disease.[2,27]

After wedge resection and segmentectomy, there is typically complete obliteration of the pleural space within several days by the expansion of the ipsilateral lung. After lobectomy, the pleural space is obliterated within 1 week, primarily through ipsilateral lung expansion and rotation, although minor diaphragmatic elevation and mediastinal shift also contribute. At times, a small amount of fluid in the pleural space may persist and radiographically mimic lobar collapse in the lobectomy site. The remaining lung will show compensatory hyperinflation with increased radiolucency and more widely spaced vascular markings. A small postlobectomy pneumothorax or hydrothorax is frequently visible on chest radiography in the immediate postoperative period.[8,13,27,30] The juxtaphrenic peak sign, a small triangular opacity projecting superiorly over the medial half of the diaphragm or near its highest point is a finding that occurs in about half of patients after upper lobectomy. Its prevalence increases gradually during the weeks after lobectomy, and it is more common on the right.[30,31]

Initially after surgery, the postpneumonectomy space contains mostly air and a small amount of fluid. During the first postoperative week, between one-half and two-thirds of the hemithorax gradually fills with fluid, and air is slowly resorbed (Fig. 68.3). Complete opacification of the hemithorax through compensatory methods typically occurs within 3 to 7 months but may occur in weeks.[13,32,33] In contrast, after extrapleural pneumonectomy the surgical space may fill faster, as quickly as 1 week, because of the absence of fluid resorption after excision of the pleura.[13,32] The air-fluid level slowly rises, and although a small volume of air may persist at the apex without clinical significance; the postpneumonectomy space is typically obliterated within weeks to months. Over time, up to one-third of postpneumonectomy patients have complete pleural fluid resorption, leaving mediastinal structures and thickened fibrous tissue. In the remaining two-thirds, imaging demonstrates a variably sized fluid collection. The trachea and mediastinal structures remain in the midline in the early postoperative period and then gradually shift during the course of weeks to months toward the side of surgery. The degree of shift depends primarily on the compliance of the contralateral lung. Those with a residual fluid collection generally have less mediastinal shift.[33,34] Stump thrombosis is an in situ thrombus encountered incidentally on late postoperative surveillance CT in the residual pulmonary artery stump after pneumonectomy (Fig. 68.4). It occurs in approximately 10% of postpneumonectomy cases and is more common in the right pulmonary artery stump.[35] Stump thrombosis can also uncommonly occur after lobectomy. Management of this condition with anticoagulation remains controversial.

After lung volume reduction surgery, the chest radiograph shows a higher position and greater curvature of the diaphragm and a decrease in diameter of the middle to lower anteroposterior rib cage. The diameter of the transverse rib cage shows little or no decrease in size.[8,36] CT studies have demonstrated that the intrathoracic trachea typically decreases in length and increases in axial area during the course of several months after lung volume reduction surgery.[37]

POTENTIAL COMPLICATIONS AND RADIOLOGIC APPEARANCE

Air leaks are an important clinical complication after pulmonary resection, particularly when highly friable emphysematous lung has undergone surgical manipulation (Fig. 68.5). After lung volume reduction surgery, invagination of visceral pleura can result in triangular fluid and air collections in the pleural space and lead to atypical manifestations of pneumothorax, pleural effusions, and pulmonary abnormalities. In particular, subpulmonic pneumothorax is a unique and frequent occurrence after lung volume reduction surgery.[3,8,29]

After pulmonary resection, an unexpected contralateral or absence of expected ipsilateral mediastinal shift after surgery may indicate an underlying pathologic process. For example, absence of mediastinal shift to the left after left pneumonectomy may indicate an expansion of the pneumonectomy space by air, blood, chyle, or fluid. Underlying bronchopleural fistula, empyema,

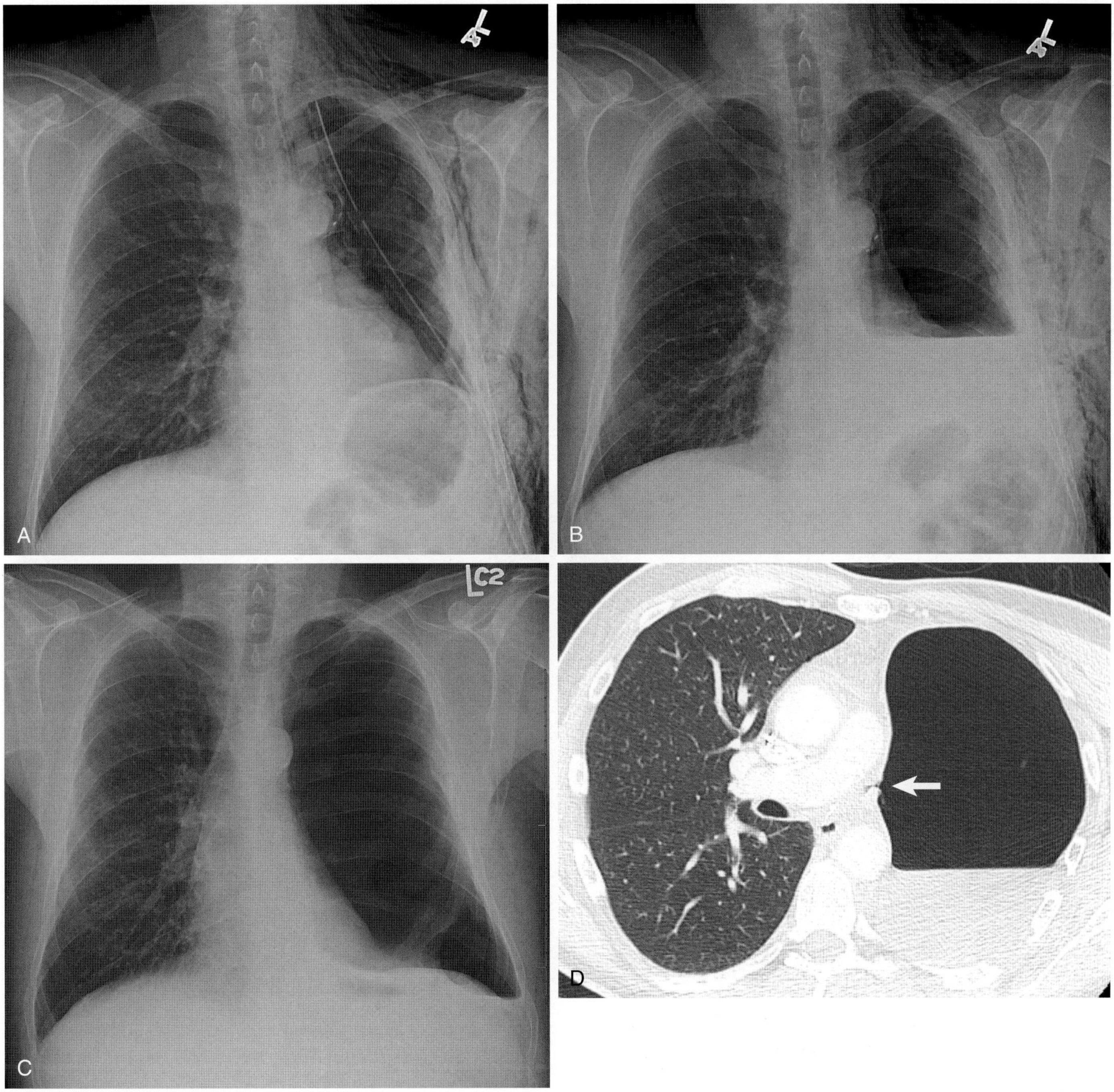

Fig. 68.3 Bronchopleural fistula in a man with central left upper lobe lung cancer who had undergone left pneumonectomy. On postoperative day 1, the expected finding of air in the left pneumonectomy space is noted (A). On postoperative day 3 (B), the pneumonectomy space gradually fills with fluid. An air-fluid level is noted. However, on postoperative day 20, the patient developed shortness of breath and fatigue. Chest radiograph (C) shows an increase in the amount of air in the left pneumonectomy space under tension with contralateral shift of the heart and mediastinum and flattening of the left heart border, suspicious for an air leak. CT (D) shows communication between the left main bronchus and the left pneumonectomy space consistent with bronchopleural fistula *(arrow)*.

and/or tumor growth should be considered (Fig. 68.6). An additional sign of volume expansion is a change from the normal convex curve of the mediastinum to a concave curve on the affected side. This sign is most commonly seen with empyema. Alternatively, volume loss in the contralateral lung, such as pulmonary fibrosis, which prevents compensatory hyperinflation and atelectasis, can sometimes account for lack of expected shift of the mediastinum to the side of lung resection. CT is the modality of choice to identify the pathologic process underlying abnormal mediastinal shifts.[7,8,38]

Bronchopleural fistula after pulmonary resection is a communication between the bronchial stump and the pleural space, resulting from dehiscence at the bronchial stump. This complication typically occurs within the first 2 weeks after surgery, although it

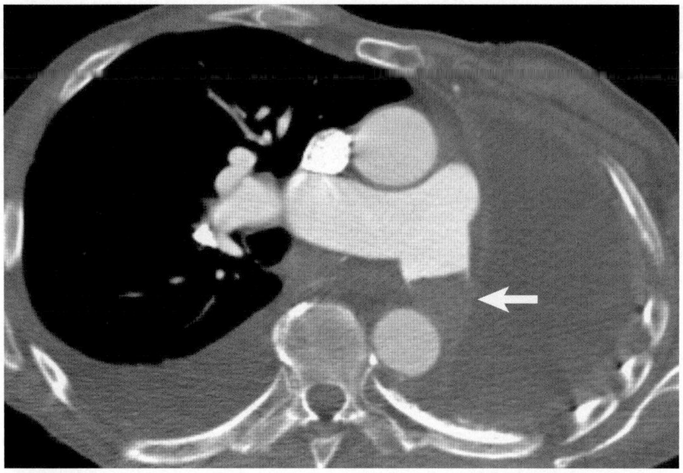

Fig. 68.4 Pulmonary artery stump thrombus in a man with mesothelioma who had undergone left extrapleural pneumonectomy 2 years earlier. Contrast-enhanced CT shows thrombus *(arrow)* in the left pulmonary artery stump.

may occur months later. The reported incidence of bronchopleural fistula that follows pulmonary resection varies but averages around 5% to 8%, 3% to 6%, and 0.5% to 1% after extrapleural pneumonectomy, pneumonectomy, and lobectomy, respectively.[3,39–42] Risk factors for bronchopleural fistula include inflammatory disease, preoperative radiation therapy, residual malignancy at the bronchial stump, diabetes, and resection involving the right lung.[3,39,40,43]

Bronchopleural fistula (BPF) leads to pneumothorax, and a late appearance predisposes patients to infection of the pleural space, resulting in empyema (Fig. 68.7). On chest radiography a decrease in the air-fluid level greater than 2 cm in the post-pneumonectomy space is a sensitive indicator of BPF. Other indicators of BPF include the development of a new air-fluid level and the expansion of a loculated pleural air collection in the operative site. CT with thin-section images on the order of 1 to 2 mm can sometimes demonstrate the fistulous connection from the bronchial stump to the pleural space (see Fig. 68.3). Indirect signs such as small bubbles of air around the bronchial stump may also suggest BPF.

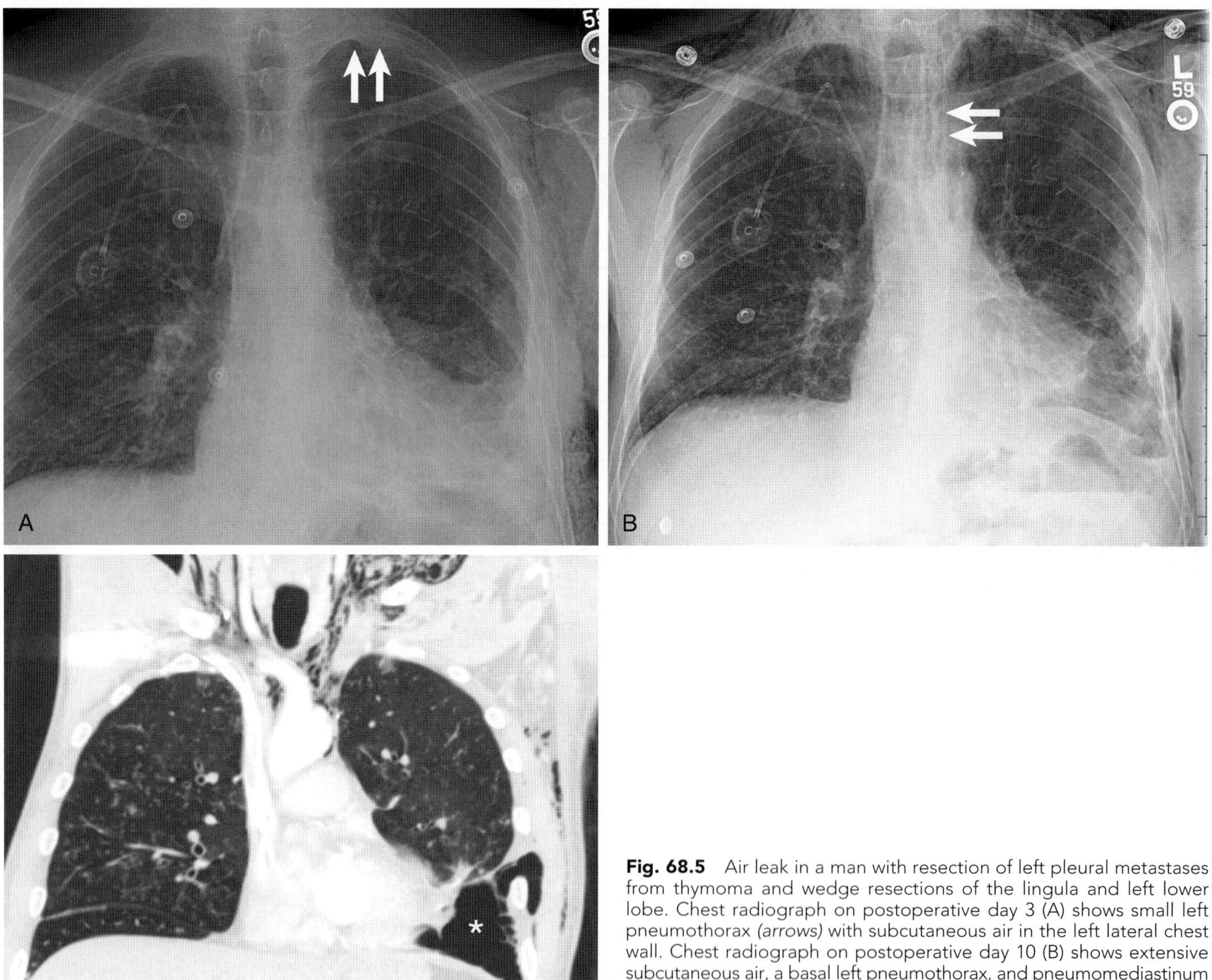

Fig. 68.5 Air leak in a man with resection of left pleural metastases from thymoma and wedge resections of the lingula and left lower lobe. Chest radiograph on postoperative day 3 (A) shows small left pneumothorax *(arrows)* with subcutaneous air in the left lateral chest wall. Chest radiograph on postoperative day 10 (B) shows extensive subcutaneous air, a basal left pneumothorax, and pneumomediastinum *(arrows)*. CT (C) shows air leak from the left pleural space *(asterisk)* adjacent to the site of the wedge resection in the lingula, extending into the subcutaneous soft tissues of the left lateral chest wall. Air tracks superiorly to the neck and into the superior mediastinum.

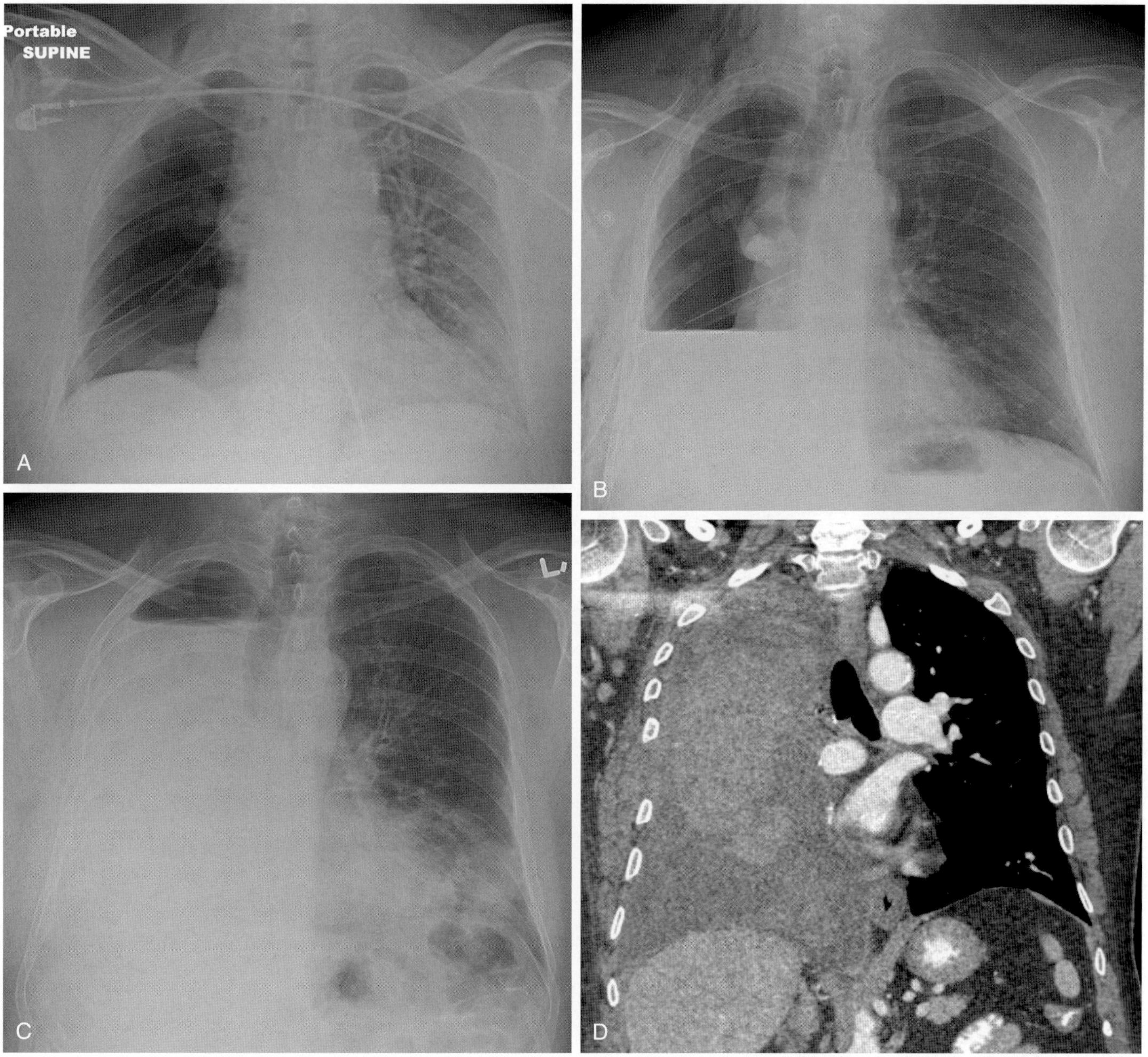

Fig. 68.6 Hemothorax in a man with right upper lobe lung cancer who had undergone pneumonectomy. Expected filling of the right pneumonectomy space is noted on serial radiographs at day 1 (A), day 2 (B), and day 18 (C). However, 1 month postoperatively, he experienced shortness of breath, and laboratory results showed a drop in hematocrit. CT chest (D) showed heterogeneous hyperattenuation of the right pneumonectomy fluid, consistent with hemothorax. The patient was treated with video-assisted thoracoscopic surgery evacuation of the hemothorax.

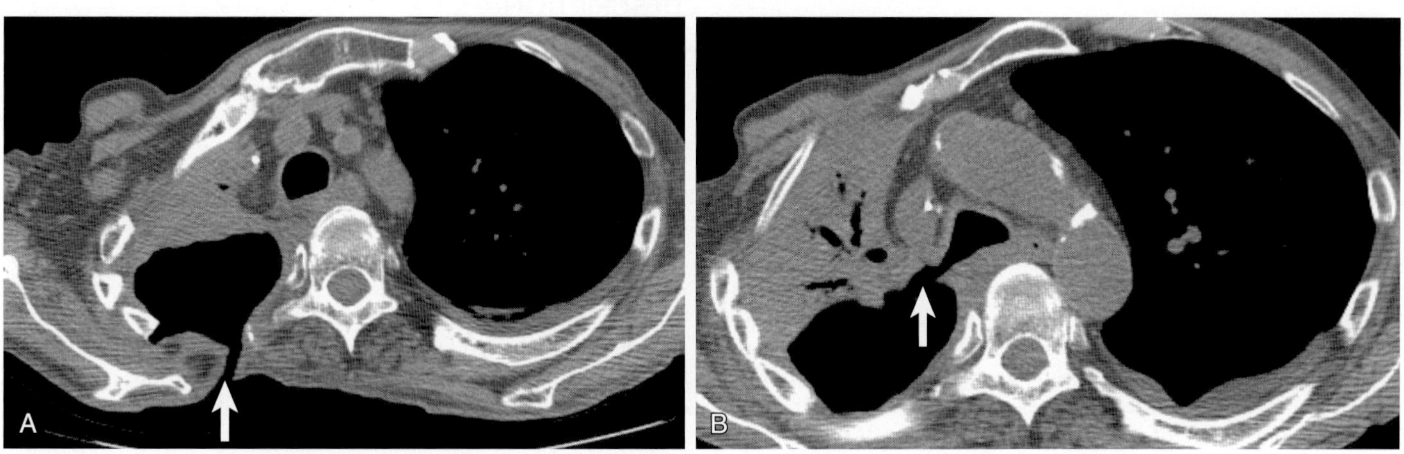

Fig. 68.7 Bronchopleural fistula in a man with non–small cell lung cancer treated with chemoradiation therapy. Because of empyema, an Eloesser procedure was performed with right thoracoplasty and chest wall resection (*arrow* in A). Note the communication between the right mainstem bronchus and the right posterior pleural space (*arrow* in B).

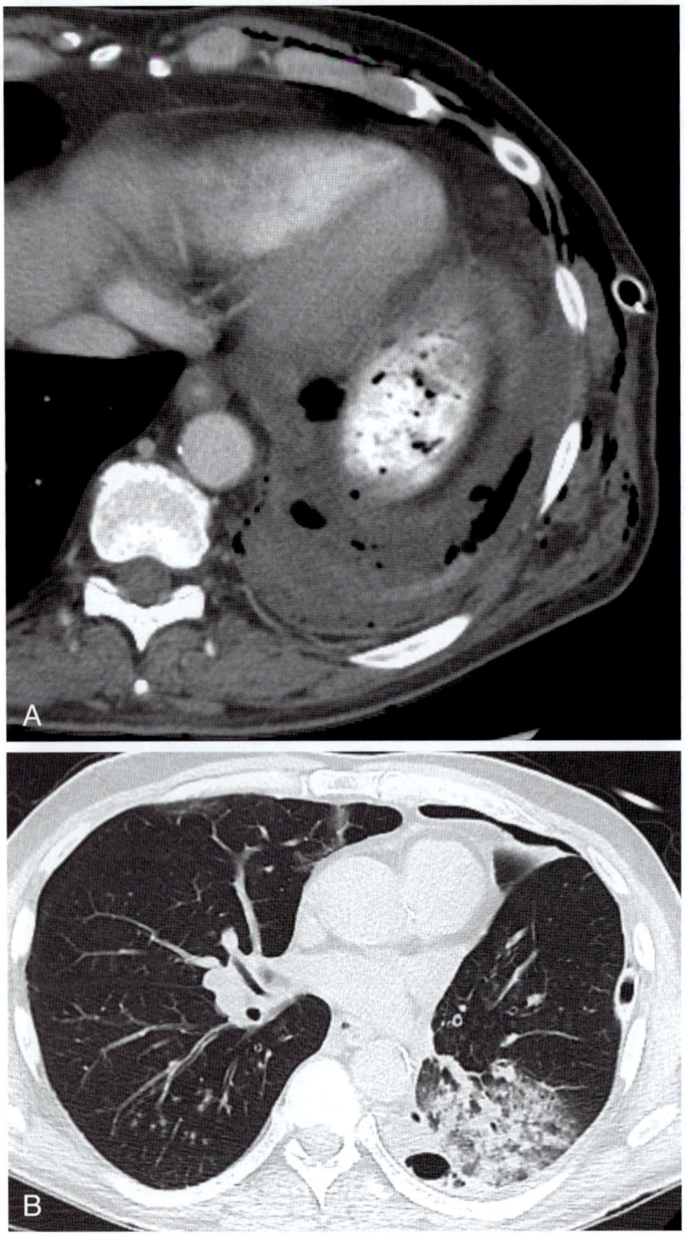

Fig. 68.8 Empyema 5 days post–left upper lobectomy for lung cancer. CT (A) shows loculated left pleural effusion with enhancing rind. In the left lower lobe, consolidation and ground-glass opacities are consistent with pneumonia (B).

Empyema can be identified on radiography in the early postoperative period by rapid fluid filling of the pneumonectomy space and contralateral shift of the mediastinum. CT shows expansion of the pneumonectomy space with fluid, which can be complex, with intermediate attenuation and with mass effect on the adjacent heart and mediastinum. CT also frequently demonstrates irregular thickening of the parietal pleura with enhancement after administration of intravenous contrast (Fig. 68.8).

Postpneumonectomy syndrome is an uncommon complication with marked ipsilateral mediastinal shift resulting in compression of the contralateral mainstem bronchus that typically occurs in children and young adults months to years after pneumonectomy (Fig. 68.9). The syndrome is almost exclusively seen after right pneumonectomy. CT of postpneumonectomy syndrome usually demonstrates a marked rightward and posterior displacement of the mediastinum with counterclockwise rotation of the heart and great vessels. CT also shows left lung hyperinflation with significant displacement of the left lung into the anterior right hemithorax. As the trachea and left mainstem bronchus are rotated to the right, they are stretched and compressed by both the aortic arch and left pulmonary artery anteriorly and by the descending aorta and vertebral column posteriorly. Symptoms include stridor caused by airway narrowing and recurrent infection caused by impaired clearance of secretions. This can be treated by placing tissue expanders or breast implants into the pneumonectomy space to reposition the mediastinum toward midline.[44,45]

Lobar torsion is a rare and serious complication after lobectomy in the early postoperative period that arises from rotation of a remaining lobe on its bronchovascular pedicle. The resultant compression of pulmonary vasculature can lead to pulmonary infarction and death. The earliest radiographic finding is lobar atelectasis that is due to bronchial compression in the twisted lobe. Vascular compression quickly leads to lobar congestion, which is visualized on chest radiography as a rapidly expanding opacity in the affected lobe. On CT the torsed lobe demonstrates increased volume and consolidation and decreased enhancement because of poor arterial flow. Additional CT findings include tapering and obliteration of the proximal pulmonary artery and associated bronchus and a component of ground-glass opacity in the affected lobe.[27,46,47] Right middle lobe torsion after right upper lobectomy is most common (Fig. 68.10).[21,48]

Cardiac herniation is an extremely rare but potentially lethal complication after pneumonectomy, with an intrapericardial approach in which the pericardial defect is not closed adequately. The heart herniates through this defect into the empty hemithorax (Fig. 68.11). It occurs within the first 24 hours postoperatively. Without prompt recognition, the mortality rate is nearly 50%.[7,38] Chest radiography is diagnostic of right-sided herniation, demonstrating displacement of the heart into the right side of the chest. An early sign of right-sided herniation is a focal convex bulge of the right border of the heart, representing early herniation of the right atrium, termed the snow cone sign. In contrast, left-sided herniation is difficult to diagnose on the posteroanterior radiograph, and the only reliable finding for diagnosis is a posteriorly displaced heart on the lateral chest radiograph. Cardiac herniation is easily recognized on CT by shift of the heart into the hemithorax.[7,21,27,38]

Lung Transplantation

DESCRIPTION

Lung transplantation involves extraction of the donor lung, resection of the recipient's lung, and implantation of the donor lung. Extraction of the donor lung involves separation of pleural attachments, harvesting of the pulmonary veins along with a left atrial cuff, and division of the pulmonary bronchus and artery. Unlike other pneumonectomies, transplant recipient pneumonectomy is performed with a more distal ligation of the pulmonary artery, immediately beyond the first upper lobe branch. Implantation comprises three anastomoses performed in the posterior-to-anterior anatomic order: bronchus, pulmonary artery, and pulmonary veins-left atrium. Flaps of intercostal muscle, pericardium, or omentum are sometimes used to wrap the end-to-end bronchial anastomoses in an attempt to reduce the incidence of bronchial dehiscence. Some surgeons use a "telescoping" technique when there is bronchial size discrepancy that involves insertion

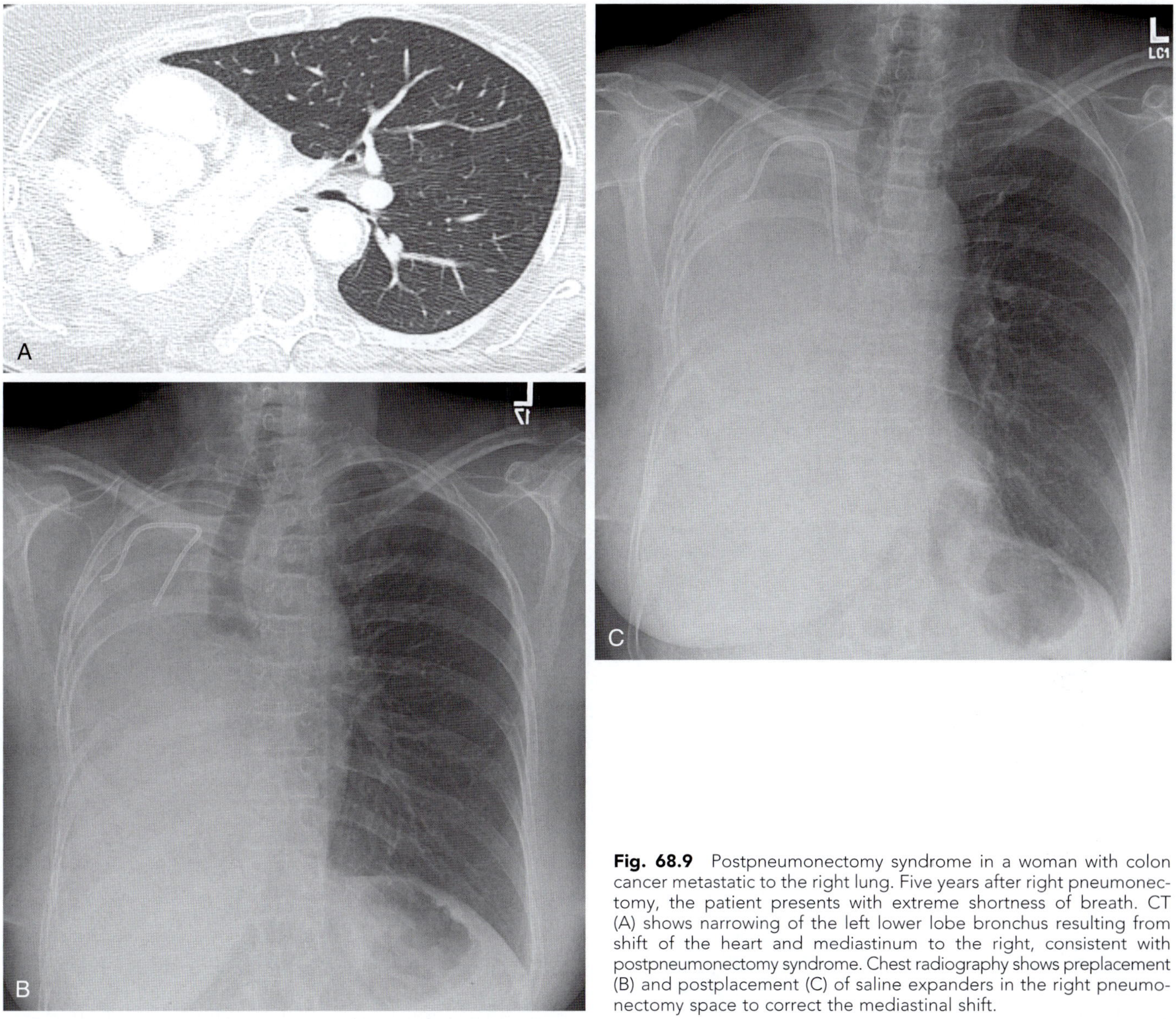

Fig. 68.9 Postpneumonectomy syndrome in a woman with colon cancer metastatic to the right lung. Five years after right pneumonectomy, the patient presents with extreme shortness of breath. CT (A) shows narrowing of the left lower lobe bronchus resulting from shift of the heart and mediastinum to the right, consistent with postpneumonectomy syndrome. Chest radiography shows preplacement (B) and postplacement (C) of saline expanders in the right pneumonectomy space to correct the mediastinal shift.

of the smaller bronchus into the larger bronchus, followed by suturing at the external margin of the overlap. When bronchial size is the same, end-to-end anastomosis is performed. Infrequently, in an attempt to reduce the incidence of bronchiolitis obliterans syndrome and bronchial dehiscence, bronchial circulation reconstruction is performed and involves connection of the donor bronchial arteries to the recipient internal thoracic arteries (internal mammary arteries). Single-lung transplantation is typically performed through a posterolateral thoracotomy; bilateral transplantation is performed through a clamshell incision. Living-related lobar transplantation consists of lower lobe harvested from two living related donors, followed by implantation into the respective hemithoraces of a relative, typically a child.[3,7,49]

INDICATIONS, CONTRAINDICATIONS, PURPOSE, AND UNDERLYING MECHANISMS

Lung transplantation is a treatment option for severe end-stage pulmonary and vascular diseases, including chronic obstructive pulmonary disease, idiopathic pulmonary fibrosis, cystic fibrosis, primary pulmonary hypertension, and, rarely, pulmonary fibrosis associated with collagen vascular disease, sarcoidosis, lymphangioleiomyomatosis, and pulmonary Langerhans cell histiocytosis. Pulmonary emphysema, including α1-antitrypsin deficiency, is the most common primary disease, accounting for about half of transplantation recipients. Double-lung transplantation is the procedure of choice for cystic fibrosis because of propensity for chronic bacterial pneumonia or colonization.[3,50]

EXPECTED APPEARANCE ON RELEVANT MODALITIES

In the early postoperative period, imaging shows chest tubes in both the apex and base, small pleural effusions, and mild pulmonary edema because of the positive fluid balance. At the bronchial anastomotic site, CT often demonstrates a small amount of peribronchial air, and if telescoping has been performed, a small anterior endoluminal flap is also frequently visualized.[3,49,51]

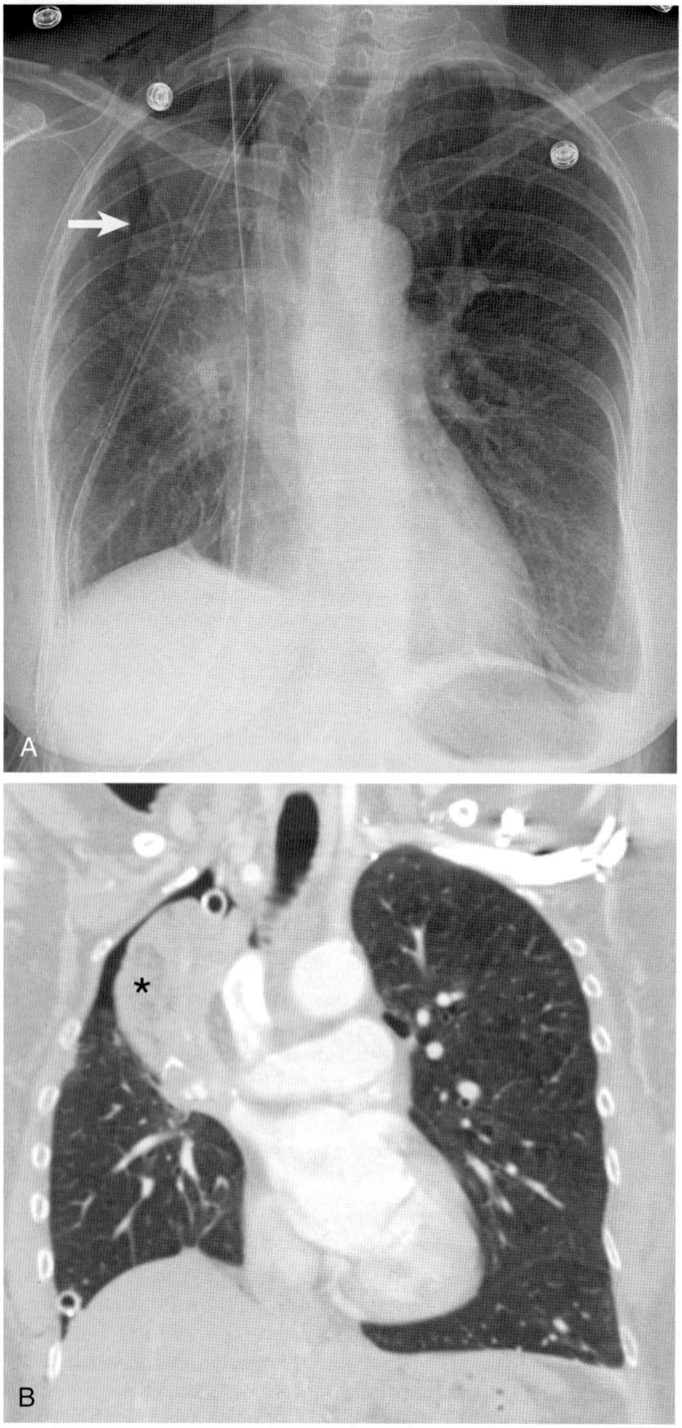

Fig. 68.10 Lobar torsion after robotic-assisted sleeve right upper lobectomy for non–small cell lung cancer. Chest radiograph on postoperative day 1 (A) shows opacity in the right upper hemithorax adjacent to the mediastinum *(arrow)*. CT chest with intravenous contrast (B) shows obliteration of the right middle lobe pulmonary artery and bronchus and reversed halo sign with central ground-glass opacity *(asterisk)* surrounded by dense consolidation, consistent with infarction. The patient was taken back to the operating room, and right middle lobectomy was performed for lobar ischemia.

POTENTIAL COMPLICATIONS AND RADIOLOGIC APPEARANCE

The diversity of complications of lung transplantation is attributed to the complexity of the surgical technique, the severity and chronicity of the underlying pathology, and the need for immunosuppressive therapy. Complications related to lung transplantation include primary graft dysfunction (PGD), graft rejection, bronchial dehiscence, bronchiolitis obliterans syndrome (BOS), upper lung fibrosis, and posttransplantation lymphoproliferative disorder (PTLD).

Primary graft dysfunction, also known as reimplantation edema, reperfusion edema, and primary graft failure, occurs in 11% to 100% of lung transplantation patients.[52,53] Because of increased capillary permeability and alveolar damage caused by a combination of pulmonary ischemia, pulmonary denervation, organ preservation, surgical trauma, and lymphatic disruption in the transplanted lung, interstitial and alveolar edema of the allograft occurs when reperfusion begins. PGD is characterized by declining pulmonary function clinically.[3,49] PGD occurs within the first 48 to 72 hours postoperatively and typically peaks around day 4, slowly resolving within 3 weeks. On radiography PGD commonly manifests with a noncardiogenic pulmonary edema pattern that includes reticulonodular opacities in the perihilar and basilar regions of the middle and lower lungs[2,51,54] and may mimic infection or fluid overload. It is therefore a diagnosis of exclusion. On CT septal thickening with patchy or confluent opacities are frequently observed. Although it is a common postoperative finding, reperfusion edema causing complete lung opacification or worsening after 5 days may represent another complication, such as acute rejection or infection, and requires further evaulation.[21,50,54]

Acute graft rejection occurs in nearly all transplant patients and is often recurrent. Once diagnosed, it is usually well controlled with corticosteroids, but it may lead to graft failure. Acute rejection occurs within the first week through the first year after transplantation but most often occurs in the first 3 to 6 months.[21,46,54] As in reperfusion edema, radiologic findings are nonspecific, and timing of presentation postoperatively is important for diagnosis. The most common radiologic findings are ground-glass and interstitial opacities, pleural effusions, septal thickening, and "perihilar haze" or "flare." These changes occur primarily in the middle and lower lobes. However, up to 50% of patients have no radiologic findings, and it is difficult to differentiate acute rejection from other pathologic processes, particularly infection. Therefore transbronchial biopsy is the gold standard for diagnosis.[2,46,49,51]

Airway anastomotic complications include bronchial dehiscence, bronchial stenosis, bronchomalacia, as well as bronchovascular, bronchopleural, and bronchomediastinal fistula. These complications occur in approximately 15% of patients after lung transplantation.[50,54] Chest radiography is of limited value in identifying bronchial anastomotic complications, but unexplained pneumothorax or pneumomediastinum may suggest bronchial dehiscence. Dehiscence is an early complication, typically occurring 2 to 4 weeks postoperatively; stricture and bronchomalacia are late complications typically occurring 2 to 9 months postoperatively.[55] Risk factors for bronchial anastomotic dehiscence include donor bronchi ischemia, postoperative infection, acute rejection, prolonged mechanical ventilation, and donor-recipient bronchial size discrepancy. Dehiscence is primarily due to local ischemia caused by a combination of bronchial blood supply

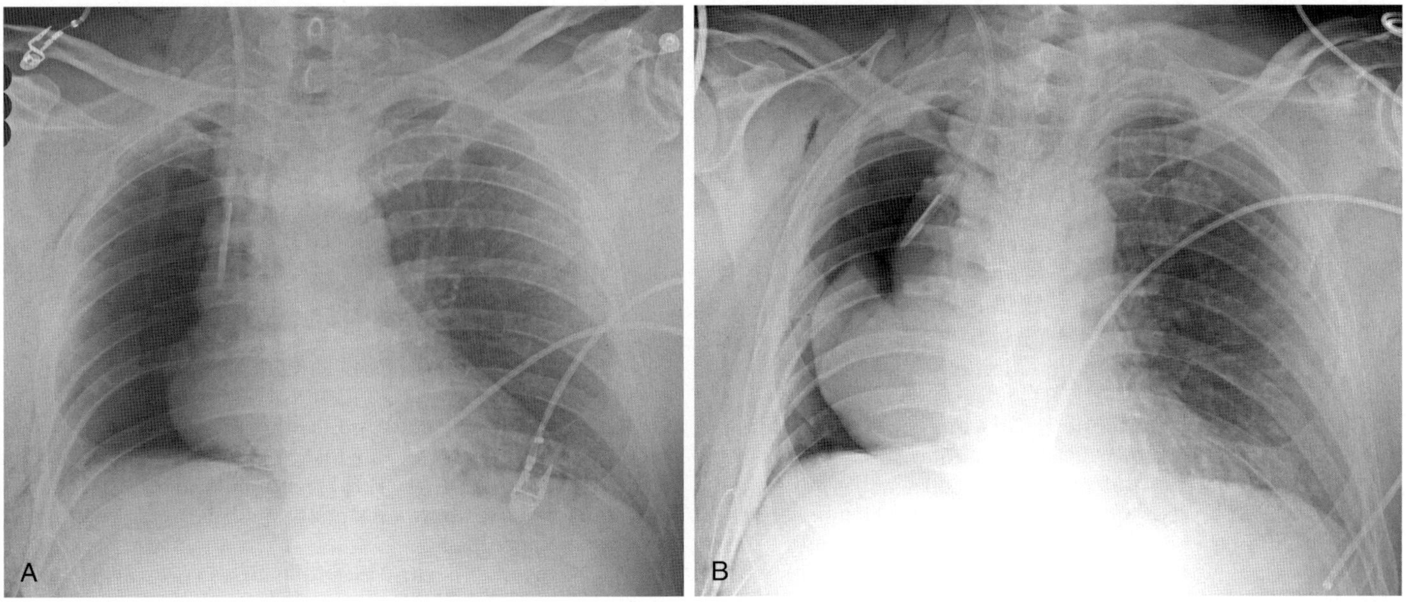

Fig. 68.11 Cardiac herniation in a man with right mesothelioma status post–right extrapleural pneumonectomy with en bloc resection of the diaphragm and pericardium. Postoperative day 1 chest radiograph (A) shows air in the right pneumonectomy space. The next day he became hypotensive, and chest radiograph (B) shows shift of the heart into the right pneumonectomy space. At emergent surgery the heart had herniated superiorly above the pericardial reconstruction at the opening for the aorta and superior vena cava. The hernia was reduced, and a Dacron patch was placed.

disruption and tension on the bronchial suture line. On CT a bronchial wall defect at the anastomotic site is the most sensitive and specific sign of dehiscence. Diagnosis is facilitated by multiplanar reconstructions and minimum-intensity projection images. Although perianastomotic air is often present in the early postoperative period, new air or an increase in air is a sensitive sign of dehiscence, especially if it is localized to the omental flap.[16] In addition, the presence of a posterior endoluminal flap should raise the possibility of dehiscence.

Bronchial stenosis is present in up to 10% of patients and can be demonstrated on CT as bronchial narrowing at the anastomotic site.[46,49,50,54] Bronchial stenosis can also be seen, although less frequently (5% of patients), after pulmonary sleeve wedge resection.[27,54] Bronchomalacia involves the deterioration of bronchial elastic and connective tissue, resulting in airway collapse on expiration. It is identified on dynamic chest CT by a greater than 50% reduction, with some authors now suggesting a 70% reduction threshold in airway lumen diameter on expiration.

Bronchiolitis obliterans syndrome (BOS) is the hallmark of chronic lung rejection. Developing 6 to 18 months postoperatively, BOS refers to the deterioration of graft function, with a progressive decline in forced expiratory volume in 1 second for which there is no other cause, such as infection, acute rejection, or anastomotic complications. BOS is thought to occur through immunologically mediated injury that begins with lymphocytic bronchiolitis and progresses to cause small airway scarring and obliteration.[3,7,46] BOS incidence increases with time after transplantation and with increased episodes of acute rejection and cytomegalovirus infection. BOS occurs in a majority of lung transplant recipients surviving at least 3 years.[21,49] BOS is the principal factor limiting long-term survival and accounts for 40% and 35% of deaths in adult and pediatric patients, respectively, after lung transplantation. Chest radiography is typically normal early in the disease; but late in the disease, it may show decreased peripheral vascular

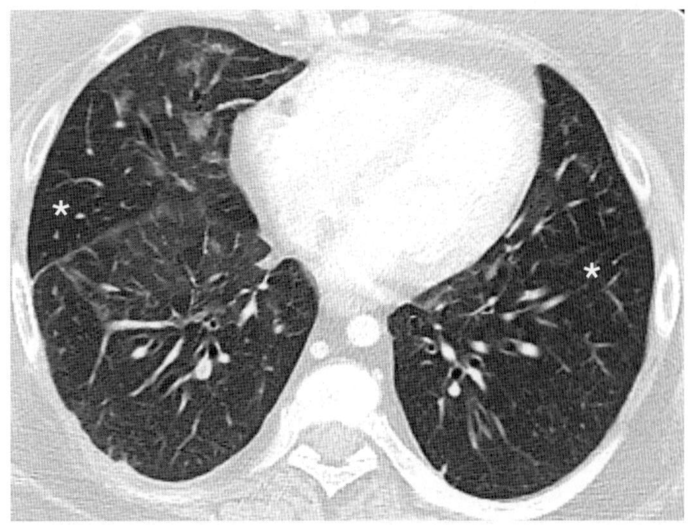

Fig. 68.12 Bronchiolitis obliterans syndrome in a woman with heart and double-lung transplants 10 months earlier for pulmonary hypertension who presents with shortness of breath. CT shows cylindrical bronchiectasis, ground-glass opacities, and areas of relative hypoattenuation *(asterisks)*. Transbronchial biopsy showed acute and chronic rejection and constrictive bronchiolitis.

markings, slight volume loss, and subsegmental atelectasis.[46,49] On chest CT decrease of lung attenuation and vascularity occurs in more than 80% of patients.[54,56,57] Expiratory CT demonstrates air trapping and is useful for the early diagnosis of BOS.[57,58] Other common CT findings are bronchiectasis and bronchial wall thickening (Fig. 68.12).[3,49,54]

Another manifestation of chronic rejection is pleuroparenchymal fibroelastosis (PPFE), which is referred to as restrictive allograft syndrome (RAS) in the transplant population, which is characterized by upper lobe–predominant progressive fibrosis (see Chapters 36 and 70). Histologically, visceral pleural thickening with collagenous fibrosis, subpleural elastosis, and intraalveolar collagenous fibrosis is observed.[59,60] On imaging RAS initially presents as irregular bilateral apical pleural thickening. Over time, findings such as reticulonodular opacities in upper lung zones with associated volume loss, resulting in elevation of the hila and decrease in the anteroposterior diameter of the apex, can be observed. As the disease progresses the reticulonodular opacities extend more inferiorly, and bullae or cysts can be seen in the lung apices.[61]

PTLD is a spectrum of diseases ranging from polyclonal lymphoid hyperplasia to aggressive high-grade lymphoma. Postulated to be caused by proliferation of Epstein-Barr virus–infected donor B lymphocytes, PTLD is much more common in patients seronegative for Epstein-Barr virus before transplantation. PTLD most frequently develops 2 months to 1 year postoperatively and has a prevalence of 2% to 10% and a mortality rate of 40% to 90%.[62] The most common radiologic manifestations include pulmonary nodule(s) or mass(es) with or without hilar and mediastinal lymphadenopathy. On CT the nodules may be surrounded by ground-glass opacity. Other radiologic findings include pleural effusions, septal thickening, and nonspecific consolidation.[2,21,49,50]

Cardiovascular Surgery

DESCRIPTION

Median sternotomy is the most frequently used incision in performing coronary artery bypass grafting (CABG), cardiac valve replacement or repair, and proximal aortic surgery. For access to the descending thoracic aorta, a left thoracotomy is typically used. Minimally invasive techniques with hemisternotomy or mini-thoracotomy are increasingly used, with benefits of decreased blood loss, shorter length of hospital stay, and less postoperative pain.[63] Cardiopulmonary bypass, a standard part of many cardiovascular surgical procedures, involves the extracorporeal transfer of blood through a mechanical circuit for cooling, filtration, and oxygenation. A cardioplegia solution is also typically added to decrease cardiac motion. CABG involves the surgical placement of a conduit from a proximal arterial location to a site distal to an obstructive coronary lesion. The saphenous vein graft (SVG) and the left internal mammary artery (LIMA) are the most commonly used conduits. The saphenous vein graft typically has its proximal attachment to the ascending aorta. The left internal mammary artery typically has its proximal attachment to the subclavian artery and attaches distally to the left anterior descending coronary artery or its branches. Other conduit vessels include the basilic and cephalic veins, as well as the gastroepiploic, radial, and inferior epigastric arteries. After harvest of the conduit vessel and start of cardiopulmonary bypass, the aorta is clamped and the conduit sutured into position.[64,65]

Open surgical and thoracic endovascular aortic repair (TEVAR) techniques are used to treat aortic diseases, including aneurysms, acute and chronic dissection, intramural hematoma, penetrating ulcers, traumatic transections, and pseudoaneurysms. In aortic aneurysm surgical repair, the aneurysmal sac is incised, and a synthetic graft is placed inside. The graft is sutured proximally and distally to normal vessel, and the aneurysmal sac is typically trimmed and sutured around the graft, creating a perigraft space. In aortic dissection surgical repair, the aorta is resected, and the false lumen is obliterated proximally and distally by suture closure of the intima and adventitia. This is followed by tubular interposition of a synthetic graft. An alternative to surgery for the treatment of both aortic aneurysm and dissection, TEVAR is the deployment of a stent-graft composed of an endostent covered by a synthetic graft material within the diseased aorta.[64,66] Hybrid procedures, branched and fenestrated endografts, and percutaneously introduced aortic valves have emerged as viable alternatives to traditional surgeries.

INDICATIONS, CONTRAINDICATIONS, PURPOSE, AND UNDERLYING MECHANISMS

Standard indications for CABG include triple-vessel and left main coronary artery disease. Other indications include two-vessel disease in the proximal left anterior descending coronary artery and circumflex artery or in patients with reduced ejection fraction or angina refractory to medical treatment. Valve surgeries are indicated in selected patients with stenosis, regurgitation, or infective endocarditis.

Indications for thoracic aortic aneurysm repair include a growth rate of more than 1 cm per year, aneurysms causing symptoms, and aneurysms greater than 5.5 and 6.5 cm in size for ascending and descending aneurysms, respectively. Dissections originating in the ascending aorta (type A) are considered surgical emergencies. The surgical indication for dissections not involving the ascending aorta (type B) is an associated aneurysmal size greater than 5 cm or the development of complications, including rupture, aneurysm formation, persistent pain, refractory hypertension, and organ ischemia.[64,67] The safety and effectiveness of stent-graft technology now allow less invasive treatment of aortic disease in selected patients who do not have a standard surgical indication.[66] TEVAR has become accepted as the treatment of choice for complicated type B aortic dissection.[68]

EXPECTED APPEARANCE ON RELEVANT MODALITIES

Early postoperative radiographs after CABG typically demonstrate mediastinal drains with radiopaque markers in the anterior mediastinum and posterior pericardium.[14,15] The cardiomediastinal silhouette is typically widened with contour haziness as a result of edema and bleeding.[14] A left internal mammary artery pedicle results in additional widening of the midmediastinum and is easily detected by a row of surgical clips in the graft distribution. Nearly all post-CABG patients have some degree of interstitial pulmonary edema evident on chest radiography. However, by the third postoperative day, the edema usually resolves, and the cardiomediastinal silhouette returns to its preoperative appearance. Atelectasis and small pericardial and pleural effusions are common in the early postoperative period and often persist for weeks. Atelectasis and pleural effusion are most common in the left hemithorax. Transient phrenic nerve paresis resulting in temporary hemidiaphragmatic elevation has been described in some patients after cardiopulmonary bypass hypothermia with local ice-slush application (so-called phrenic frostbite).[14,15] The location of the saphenous vein graft attachments to the aorta can sometimes be identified on the chest radiograph by small wire circles around the ostia or by small washer-like markers. Although catheter angiography remains the gold standard for CABG graft assessment, advances in electrocardiogram-gated cardiac CT allow the noninvasive assessment of bypass graft patency with high diagnostic accuracy.[12,65,69]

After aortic surgery, the stent-graft appears as a woven interlacing metal structure on chest radiography. On CT it appears as studded metallic opacities within the aortic wall. Air bubbles can be visible in the aneurysmal sac on early postoperative CT. Follow-up CTs have demonstrated semicircular thin thrombi within the inner circumference of the stent in up to 19% of cases. These thrombi have no clinical significance.[70] The diseased portion of the aorta (aneurysmal sac and false lumen in aneurysm and dissection, respectively) is covered and excluded from the systemic circulation. Over the course of months, the aneurysmal sac and false lumen thrombose to either be completely obliterated or to persist as a small thrombosed aortic attachment.[70,71]

CT commonly demonstrates a small amount of perigraft air during the first postoperative week after synthetic aortic conduit placement. Early postoperative CT also demonstrates a mixture of water and soft tissue attenuation around the outside of the graft, representing a combination of residual fluid, hematoma, and fibrous tissue. As this perigraft collection diminishes, CT commonly demonstrates a thin ring of fat attenuation around the graft.[71,72] Rarely, CT may show small outpouchings of the aorta near the graft anastomotic sites after repair of aortic dissection. These outpouchings represent small diverticula where reappositions of the true and false lumina have failed and reperfused with blood.[72,73] Lifelong clinical and imaging surveillance is mandatory after TEVAR because late treatment failure may develop even years after the initial procedure.

Surgical felt is commonly used to reinforce anastomotic and aortic cannulation sites during cardiac and aortic surgeries. Felt appears as a high-attenuation ring around the graft anastomotic sites or as a small high-attenuation "pledget" at sites of cannulation and should not be confused for vascular calcification (Fig. 68.13).[74] If the aortic root is replaced during surgery, the site of coronary artery reattachment to the graft often demonstrates a contrast-enhancing bulge that can mimic a pseudoaneurysm.[75] Oversewn graft side branches can also appear as a focal outpouching mimicking pseudoaneurysm (Fig. 68.14).[74]

POTENTIAL COMPLICATIONS AND RADIOLOGIC APPEARANCE

Complications after CABG include massive air embolism, sternal wound infection, hemomediastinum, and acute lung injury. Graft

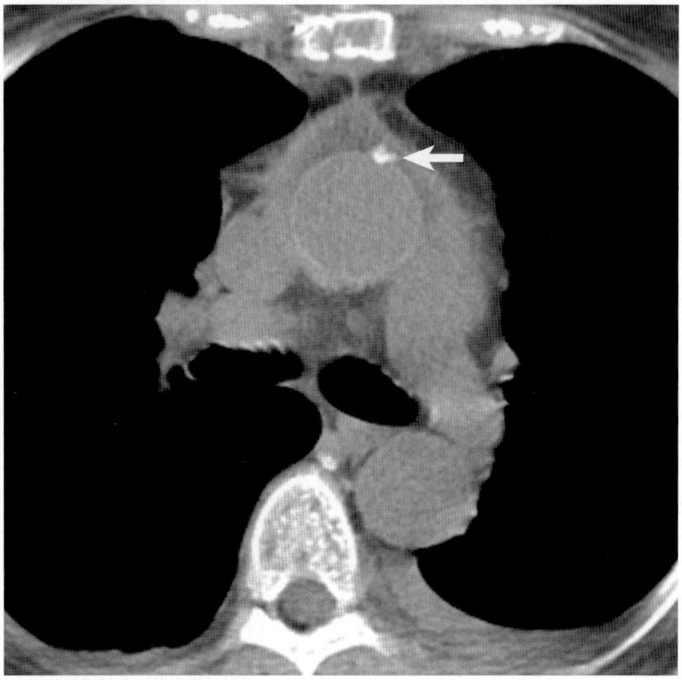

Fig. 68.13 Felt pledgets. CT shows high-attenuation felt pledget material *(arrow)* anterior to the aorta.

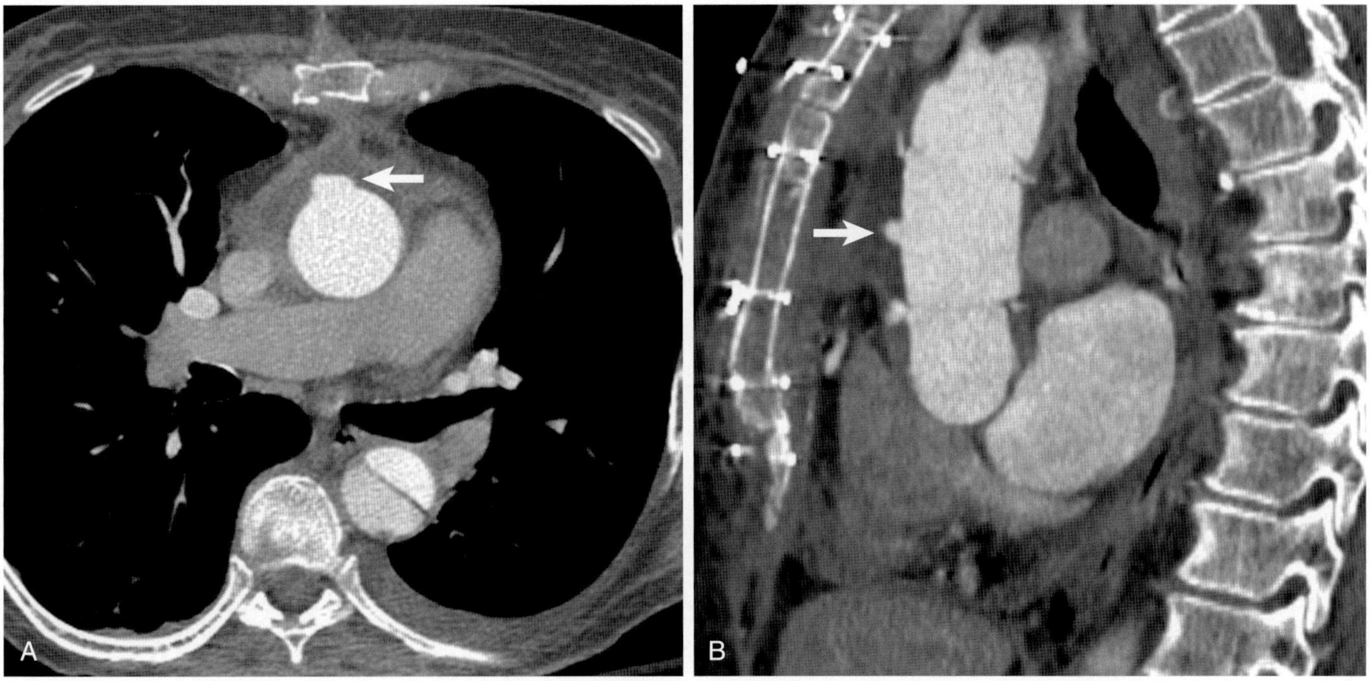

Fig. 68.14 Oversewn graft side branch. Axial (A) and sagittal (B) CT images show a focal outpouching *(arrows)* within the middle portion of the interposition graft consistent with an oversewn graft side branch. This may be mistaken for a pseudoaneurysm. Note descending thoracic aortic dissection.

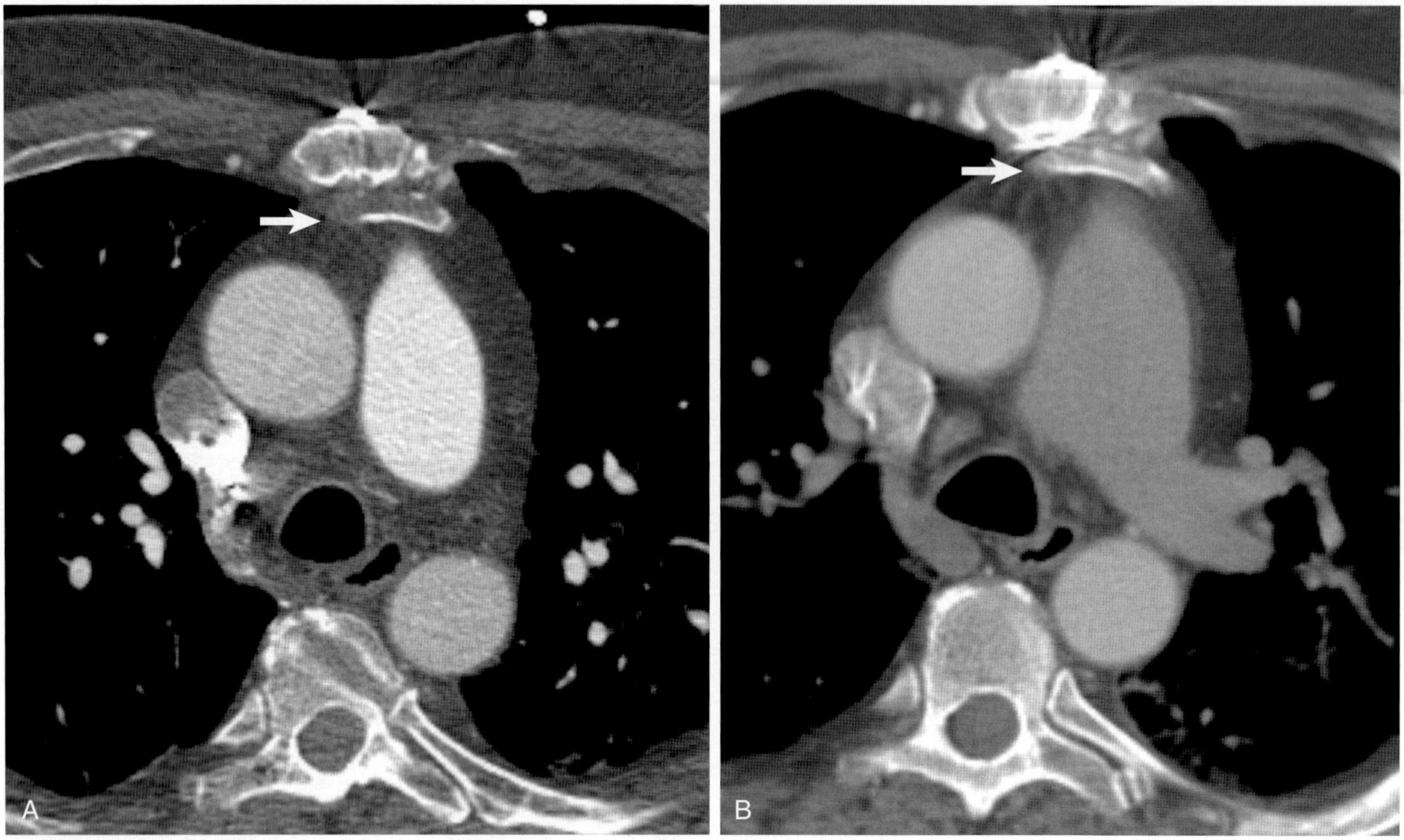

Fig. 68.15 Saphenous vein graft thrombus in a man who had coronary artery bypass graft surgery 22 years earlier who presents with chest pain and shortness of breath. CT (A) shows occlusion of the saphenous venous graft *(arrow)* supplying the left circumflex artery. The patient underwent percutaneous transluminal coronary angioplasty and thrombectomy, and stents were placed in the saphenous vein graft to the obtuse marginal branch. CT 2 weeks later (B) shows patency of the graft with stent placement *(arrow)*.

complications are divided into early (<1 month) and late (≥1 month) complications. Thrombotic occlusion of the grafted vessel is the most common early complication related to technical problems at the site of the anastomoses or during harvesting.[76] Late complications include atherosclerotic graft stenosis related to the high pressure of the arterial circulation, potentially leading to occlusion. The "string sign" (or string phenomenon) refers to diffuse narrowing of a grafted vessel, reported in LIMA grafts.[77] Graft occlusion is more frequent in venous than in arterial grafts. The nubbin sign, typically seen with SVG, refers to the proximal occlusion of a graft, near its anastomosis on the anterior portion of the ascending aorta, with contrast opacification of a short proximal segment.[78] Partial SVG occlusion can be visualized on CT as vessel narrowing from thrombosis or atherosclerotic plaque (Fig. 68.15).

SVG dilatation can be due to true aneurysms or pseudoaneurysms, with the former being more common than the latter by a 6:1 ratio.[79] True aneurysms of SVG are due to atherosclerosis, occurring as a late complication arising years after CABG, with a risk of thrombosis or thromboembolism, fistula, rupture, and myocardial infarction. In contrast, pseudoaneurysm may occur as an early or late complication after CABG and is most common at the site of graft anastomosis. Factors leading to pseudoaneurysm include surgical technique, vascular suture rupture, vein weakness in the valve areas, progressive atherosclerosis and wound infection. On chest radiography SVG dilatation appears as mediastinal opacities along various aspects of the heart border, depending on the site of the graft anastomosis.[79] For example, SVG dilatation connected to the left anterior descending or left circumflex coronary artery would appear as an opacity along the left upper cardiac border on radiography. SVG aneurysm is visualized on CT as an enhancing, round mass connected to the graft lumen that contains a variable amount of thrombus.[65]

Pericardial complications after CABG include pneumopericardium, hemopericardium, constrictive pericarditis, and postpericardiotomy syndrome. Although mediastinal widening is normal after cardiac surgery, mediastinal widening beyond 60% to 70% from preoperative size may be indicative of a pathologic process, although variations of mediastinal width often occur because of difference in projection and depth of inspiration. Pathologic mediastinal widening is typically caused by air, blood, or other fluid in the pericardial sac and with rapid or massive accumulation can lead to cardiac tamponade.[12,14,80] Pneumopericardium is visualized radiographically as a sharp outline of air contouring the heart.[80] On chest radiography hemopericardium and pericardial effusion cause loss of detail in the mediastinal contour and a widened subcarinal angle. An increased lucency of the margin of the cardiac silhouette (differential density sign) and an increased size of the pericardial stripe on lateral chest radiography (also known as the Oreo-cookie sign or the epicardial fat pad sign) are also signs of pericardial effusion. CT demonstrates an enlarged pericardial space with water or blood attenuation in pericardial effusion and hemopericardium, respectively.[12,13,81] Common findings of constrictive pericarditis on CT include pericardial calcification, a narrowed tubular right ventricle, and a sigmoid ventricular septum. Pericardial thickening of 4 mm or more is the hallmark sign of constrictive pericarditis.[12,81] Postpericardiotomy syndrome is an autoimmune process occurring 2 weeks to 6 months after pericardiotomy. On chest radiography postpericardiotomy syndrome most commonly manifests as concomitant pericardial and bilateral pleural effusions, often with basilar opacities.[12,13]

Complications specific to the use of synthetic aortic grafts and stent-grafts include pseudoaneurysm, perigraft hematoma, aortic perforation, endoleak, and graft infection.[7,21,64] On CT a pseudoaneurysm is visualized as an enhancing outpouching from the aortic anastomotic site. A low-attenuation component representing thrombosis may involve part or all of the pseudoaneurysm and predispose it to infection. When infected, the pseudoaneurysm often demonstrates septa and fluid collections.[66,71] Thrombotic graft occlusion is rare and identified on CT as a low-attenuation mass within the graft lumen. A perigraft hematoma is visualized on CT as a homogeneous low-attenuation collection with sharp margins that lacks septa and gas.[72] Aortic stent-grafts have a number of potential complications, including migration, kinking, and fracture, which can be detected on chest radiography. Aortic perforation may occur either during stent-graft insertion or after erosion of the aortic wall by stent-graft struts. Chest radiography can demonstrate a rapidly enlarging periaortic hematoma or hemothorax.[66,82]

Endoleak is defined as persistent blood flow within the sac outside the stent-graft and is classified into types I to V according to the source of blood flow: type I, leak at the attachment site; type II, leak from a branch artery; type III, graft defect; type IV, graft porosity; and type V, endotension. Recently, with technologic advances in endovascular treatment, type IV and type V endoleaks have been considered historical phenomena and are no longer observed.[68] Early or primary endoleaks occur in the first 30 days after an endovascular procedure, whereas those that fail to seal within 30 days are called persistent or secondary endoleaks and represent the main failure of endovascular treatment.[83] Causes include stent-graft misplacement, lumen size mismatch, and incomplete expansion. The characteristic finding of an endoleak is the appearance of contrast material inside the aneurysmal sac on CT angiography (Fig. 68.16). As calcifications of the aneurysmal sac can mimic contrast material extravasation, non–contrast CT is useful for diagnosis. Small leaks may not be visualized on CT and may be suggested only by failure of the aneurysmal sac to decrease in size after stent-graft placement. A small endoleak is observed on delayed CT by late extravasation of contrast material into the aneurysmal sac because of slow perigraft flow of circulating "pools" of contrast material.[72,73,82]

Graft infection is a serious complication that can lead to complete graft failure. Perigraft air manifesting after the first few postoperative weeks is a highly sensitive indicator of infection (Fig. 68.17). Similarly, expanding perigraft soft tissue, particularly if there is a fluid or high-attenuation component, is highly suggestive of infection. Infectious fluid collections are typically irregular in shape, septated, and in close proximity to the graft. A more subtle finding of infection on CT is haziness of the graft margins with adjacent soft tissue and loss of perigraft fat attenuation.[72]

Mediastinal Surgery

DESCRIPTION

Mediastinal surgical procedures target the esophagus, trachea, and other mediastinal structures. Esophageal resection is performed through either a transthoracic or transcervical approach. Ivor-Lewis esophagectomy involves an abdominal incision with gastric mobilization. A right-sided thoracotomy then allows esophageal mobilization and resection, gastric pull-up through the esophageal hiatus, and midthoracic anastomosis. A transcervical (or transhiatal) esophagectomy uses an anterior cervical incision and a supraumbilical abdominal incision. The surgeon uses both openings to mobilize and to resect the esophagus and to pull up the stomach for cervical anastomosis.[3,84,85] These procedures are increasingly performed using minimally invasive thoracoscopic or robotic techniques.[86,87] Esophageal bypass surgery involves the

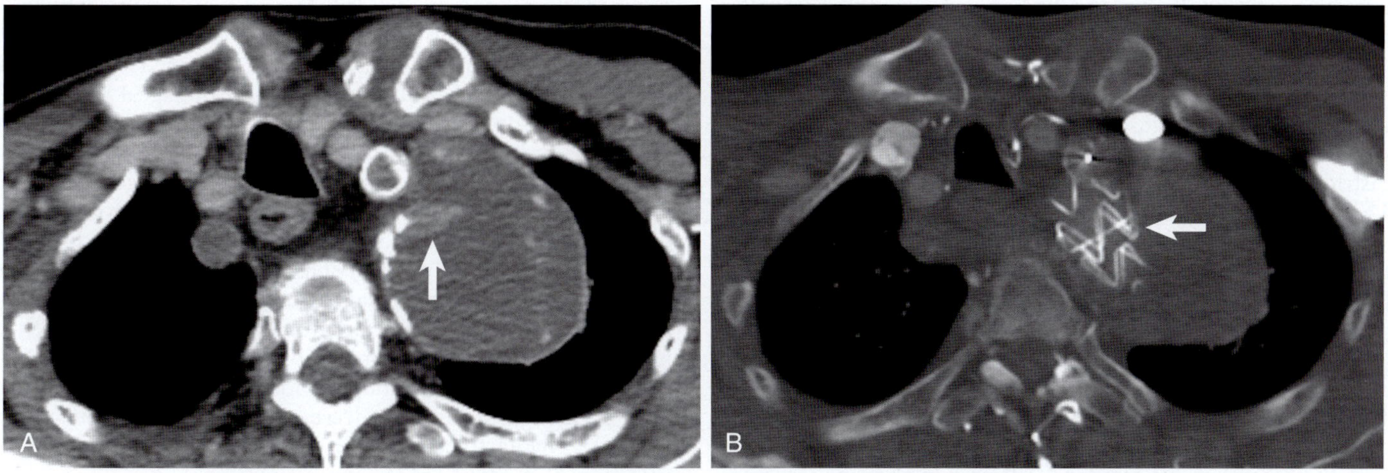

Fig. 68.16 Endovascular leak in a man who had endovascular repair of thoracic aortic aneurysm. On delayed-phase imaging, CT (A) shows a blush within the thrombosed portion of the saccular aortic aneurysm, consistent with type III endoleak *(arrow)*. CT (B) shows the superior aspect of the aortic stent *(arrow)*.

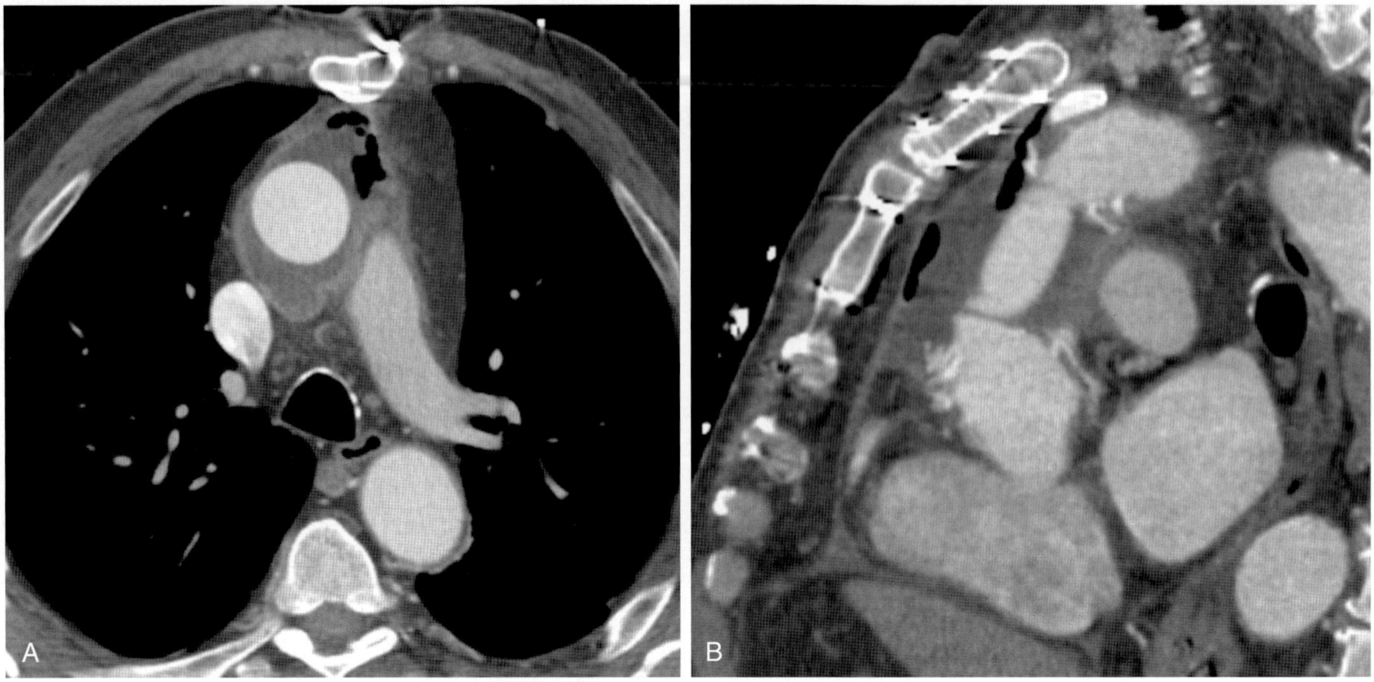

Fig. 68.17 Perigraft infection. Axial (A) and sagittal (B) contrast-enhanced CT shows a rim-enhancing fluid- and air-containing collection surrounding the ascending aortic graft.

construction of a conduit interposed between the cervical esophagus and a selected inferior anastomotic point. The surgery is performed through cervical and abdominal incisions. The stomach is the preferred conduit because it has a reliable blood supply and requires only a single anastomosis. The colon is used as the conduit when the stomach is not available, and the jejunum is used if neither stomach nor colon is available. Colonic and jejunal conduits each require three anastomoses. The anterior mediastinum is the anatomic space of choice for conduit placement, and the native esophagus is typically left in situ.[3,84,85]

Myotomy and pneumatic dilation are used to increase the caliber of an area of narrowed esophagus. Myotomy is typically performed laparoscopically. It involves complete division of the circular muscle within the stenotic area, most often the esophagogastric junction. Pneumatic dilation consists of placement of a dilator containing a deflated balloon into the esophagus with repeated dilatation to disrupt the surrounding muscle layer.[3,84]

Fundoplication involves the creation of an intraabdominal segment of the esophagus, reduction of any existing hiatus hernia, approximation of diaphragmatic crura, and wrapping of the gastric fundus around the abdominal esophagus (fundoplication). There are a variety of fundoplication procedures, and they differ mostly by the degree to which the esophagus is wrapped. Fundoplication is increasingly performed laparoscopically (Nissen, Hill, Guarner procedures), although thoracotomy is still used (Belsey Mark IV procedure).[3,84]

Access to the different mediastinal compartments for biopsy or resection is accomplished through a variety of approaches. The Chamberlain procedure is used to access the anterior mediastinum through an anterior parasternal mediastinotomy over the second costal cartilage. Anterior mediastinal access is also obtained through a horizontal transcervical incision, complete or partial upper sternotomy, or VATS. A transcervical incision is used for standard cervical mediastinoscopy (Fig. 68.18). The middle mediastinum and posterior mediastinum are most commonly reached through posterolateral thoracotomy or VATS.[3,7,21]

INDICATIONS, CONTRAINDICATIONS, PURPOSE, AND UNDERLYING MECHANISMS

Esophageal resection is indicated for the management of both benign and malignant conditions but is most commonly performed for the treatment of esophageal carcinoma. A transthoracic resection with right thoracotomy is preferred for the resection of carcinomas of the middle two-thirds of the esophagus because it avoids interference with the aortic arch. A left thoracotomy approach is typically reserved for tumors of the distal esophagus, gastroesophageal junction, and gastric cardia. Transcervical esophagectomy is used primarily for cervicothoracic esophageal tumors and neuromotor conditions not amenable to other treatments. Esophageal bypass surgery is reserved as a palliative measure in some cases of nonresectable esophageal cancer.[3,84,85]

Pharyngoesophageal myotomy is used to treat upper esophageal sphincter dysfunction and as part of the treatment of Zenker diverticulum. Heller myotomy of the lower esophageal sphincter and pneumatic dilation can be performed to treat lower esophageal constriction, most commonly resulting from motor disorders (achalasia, diffuse esophageal spasm). Pneumatic dilation can also be used for esophageal strictures.[3,84] Fundoplication is indicated in patients with nonresponsive gastroesophageal reflux and those with severe complications resulting from reflux or hiatal hernias. Nissen fundoplication is commonly performed with a Heller myotomy to decrease the rate of postmyotomy reflux.[3,84] Mediastinal access is also needed for the biopsy or resection of mediastinal lesions.

Median sternotomy is the standard incision for primary malignant neoplasms of the anterior mediastinum, including thymomas. A partial upper sternotomy may be used for

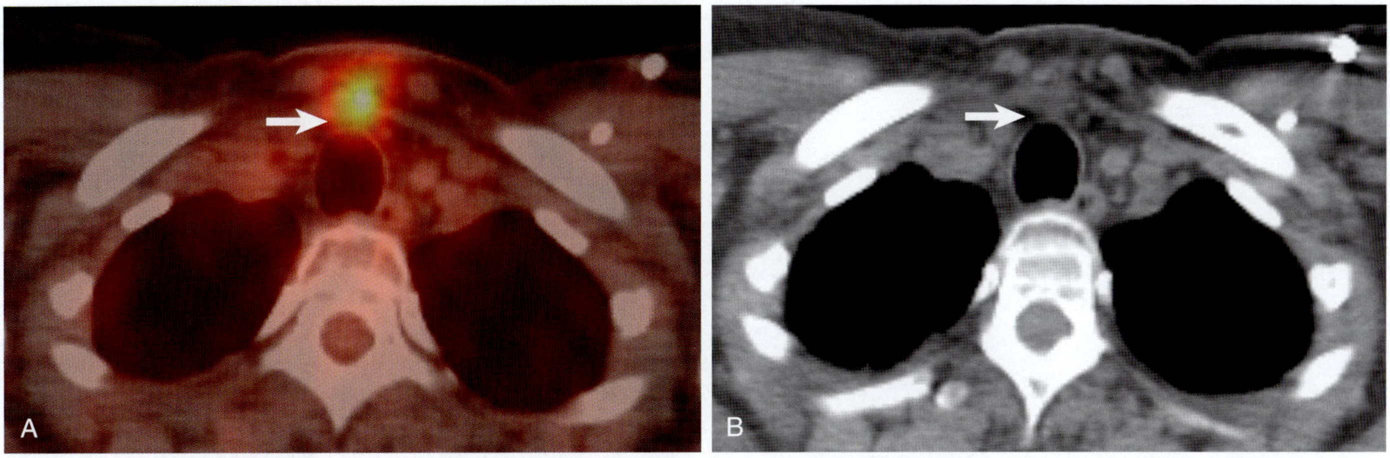

Fig. 68.18 Mediastinoscopy in a woman with right upper lobe lung cancer. Positron emission tomography (A) and CT (B) show focus of increased fluorodeoxyglucose uptake in the pretracheal space that correlates to an area of increased soft tissue with stranding of the mediastinal fat, consistent with the track of mediastinoscopy performed 3 days earlier *(arrows)*. Knowledge of this potential pitfall is important to avoid misinterpretation as nodal disease.

noninvasive anterior mediastinal tumors. Transcervical is the approach favored for thymectomy in selected myasthenia gravis patients and for resection of symptomatic mediastinal cysts (pericardial, pleural) and the upper trachea. This incision is combined with a partial or complete median sternotomy in some cases of thymectomy for myasthenia gravis and for the resection of invasive upper tracheal lesions. Lower tracheal lesions are resected through a posterolateral thoracotomy. Common indications for tracheal resection are tumors within or invading the trachea and tracheal stenosis, most commonly resulting from prolonged use of a tracheostomy or endotracheal tube.[3,7,21]

The Chamberlain procedure is used for biopsy of anterior mediastinal lesions and aortopulmonary window and paraaortic lymph nodes in stations 5 and 6.[3,7] Mediastinoscopy is usually performed to sample paratracheal and anterior subcarinal lymph nodes. In recent years mediastinal lymph node sampling is increasingly achieved through endobronchial ultrasound–, endoscopic ultrasound–guided techniques, and VATS.[88]

EXPECTED APPEARANCE ON RELEVANT MODALITIES

After esophagectomy, metallic clips, staples, and sutures indicate the anastomotic location on CT and chest radiography. Routine postoperative esophagrams show the characteristic esophageal wall indentation of the intrathoracic anastomotic site.[85] The anastomosis after a transthoracic esophagectomy is typically located at the level of the thoracic inlet. The gastric pull-up manifests as a widened mediastinum with intrathoracic air on chest radiography. On CT a partially collapsed stomach is typically visualized in the right posterior mediastinum anterior to the vertebral body. In contrast, a colonic conduit is located in the anterior mediastinum (Fig. 68.19).[85,89]

Imaging studies after fundoplication show evidence of the gastric wrap below the diaphragm. An esophageal stent, commonly placed after pneumatic dilation and for inoperable cancer palliation, manifests as a tubular metallic density within the inner wall of the esophagus on imaging.[84,89]

Mild mediastinal widening from gas or fluid is not uncommon after mediastinal operations, including thymectomy and tracheal resection. However, mediastinal air or fluid that persists or increases beyond the first few postoperative weeks should raise concern for a pathologic process.[7,8]

POTENTIAL COMPLICATIONS AND RADIOLOGIC APPEARANCE

Complications after surgery in the mediastinum include chylothorax resulting from injury of the thoracic duct, aspiration pneumonitis, recurrent laryngeal nerve damage, mediastinitis, mediastinal abscess (Fig. 68.20), and mediastinal hemorrhage (Fig. 68.21).[7]

Esophageal perforation, a complication seen in 1% of stent placements and 5% of dilations, can occur in any mediastinal surgery. The high incidence is usually due to concomitant esophageal disease.[7,90] The most common site of perforation is immediately above the gastroesophageal junction. Specific signs include subcutaneous air in the neck and upper thorax, left hydropneumothorax, and pneumomediastinum, particularly in the left costovertebral angle (V sign of Naclerio).[7,46,90,91] Esophagram typically allows diagnosis of perforation on the basis of contrast material extravasation. In patients with atypical symptoms, or if the esophagram is normal in a patient with suspicious symptoms (10% false-negative rate), CT is often performed because of its high sensitivity. CT findings of perforation include extraluminal air, paraesophageal fluid or contrast material, and esophageal wall thickening.[84,90,91]

Important anastomotic site complications after esophagectomy are leak and stricture. With an incidence of 10%, the anastomotic leak rate is higher with cervical than thoracic anastomosis but shows no difference between stapled and hand-sewn anastomosis.[92–96] Anastomotic leak can occur early (2–3 days) as a result of surgical failure or late (3–7 days) resulting from ischemia at or just below the anastomosis secondary to necrosis of the proximal gastric conduit. The diagnosis of an anastomotic leak is usually made on esophagography. Fluoroscopy has a higher

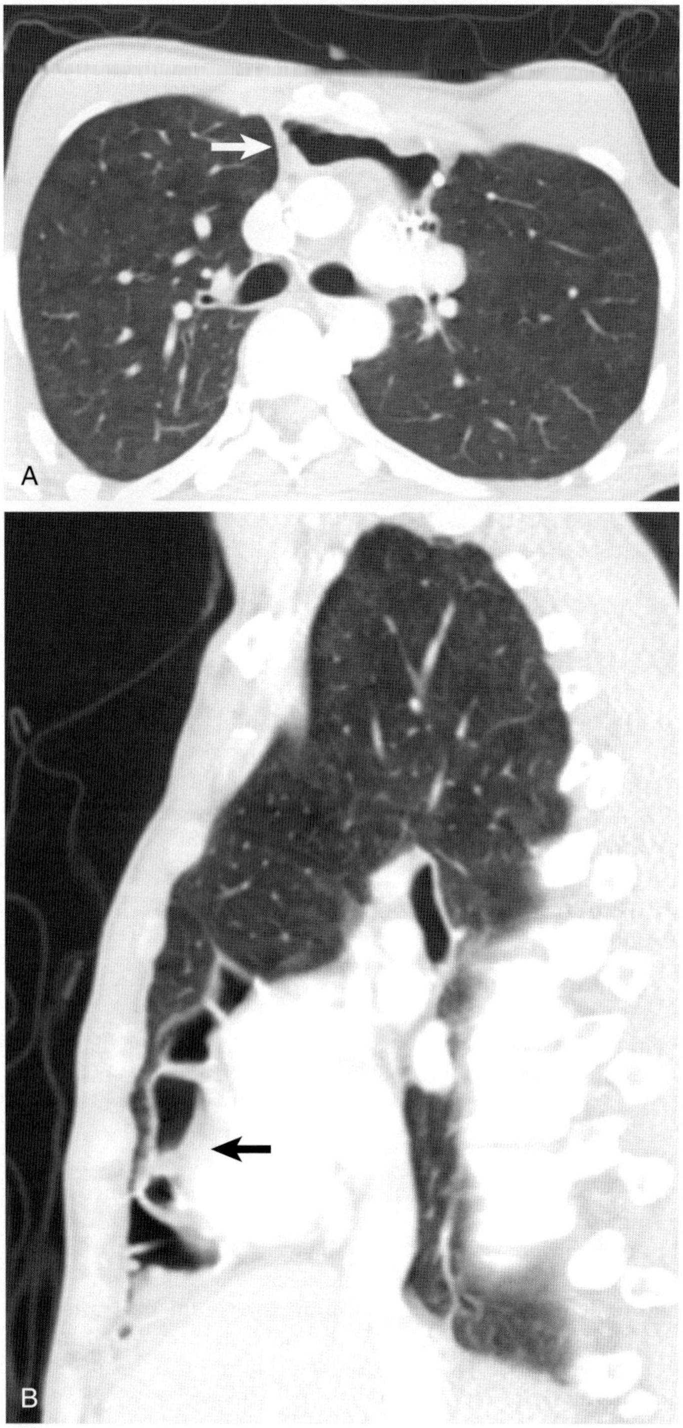

Fig. 68.19 Colonic interposition in a man with esophageal stricture who had undergone esophagectomy. CT shows the interposed colon *(arrow)* in the anterior mediastinum on axial (A) and sagittal (B) images.

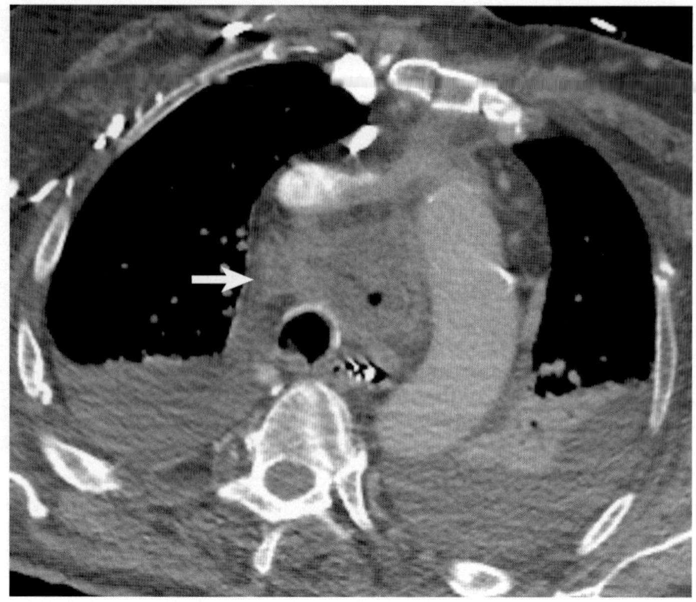

Fig. 68.20 Mediastinal abscess in a man who presents with fever 6 days postresection of the retrosternal thyroid goiter via cervical incision and median sternotomy. CT chest with intravenous contrast shows a mediastinal fluid collection with enhancing rim in the pretracheal space with pockets of air, consistent with mediastinal abscess *(arrow)*.

specificity for the diagnosis of anastomotic leak compared with CT; however, CT is more sensitive and is useful to evaluate the extent of the leak (Fig. 68.22) and associated complications, including mediastinitis, pneumomediastinum, mediastinal abscess, and empyema. Most leaks close spontaneously.[84,92] Failure of the conduit is a devastating and potentially fatal complication occurring in 0.5% to 3.2% of cases.[97] The most common cause of conduit failure is vascular compromise caused by twisting of the conduit or constriction at the diaphragmatic hiatus or at the esophagogastric anastomosis. Overdistention of the conduit can also lead to ischemia; thus gastric decompression, particularly in the early postoperative period, is crucial. The proximal aspect of the stomach is the most common site of necrosis.[98] Gastric necrosis should be suspected in the setting of an enlarging leak or failure of conservative management of the leak. Endoscopy is more sensitive and specific than CT for the detection of early gastric necrosis. CT findings of gastric necrosis include gastric wall thickening out of proportion to lumen distention and lack of conduit enhancement.

Anastomotic stricture after esophageal resection is common, occurring in around one-third of patients.[93,99] In many cases the stricture is severe enough to cause significant dysphagia. Although anastomotic strictures are generally identified on postoperative esophagram, a CT scan may be the first study to show a significant stricture and is valuable in defining sequential morphologic changes in the stricture.[84,93,99] Chronic inflammation related to the stricture itself or dilatation procedures can result in false-positive ^{18}F-fluorodeoxyglucose (FDG) uptake and mimic recurrent malignancy.

After esophagectomy, fistula formation can occur, the most common being esophagopleural and tracheoesophageal fistula. In esophagopleural fistula, imaging demonstrates either pleural effusion or hydropneumothorax on the affected side. CT can demonstrate oral contrast material in the pleural space as confirmation and, sometimes, even the esophagopleural fistulous connection itself.[84,85] Airway-esophageal or airway-gastric fistula can occur both early and late in the postoperative course and is suspected in the setting of cough after oral intake or recurrent aspiration with radiographic evidence of excess air in the esophagus or stomach. Diagnosis can be made by demonstration

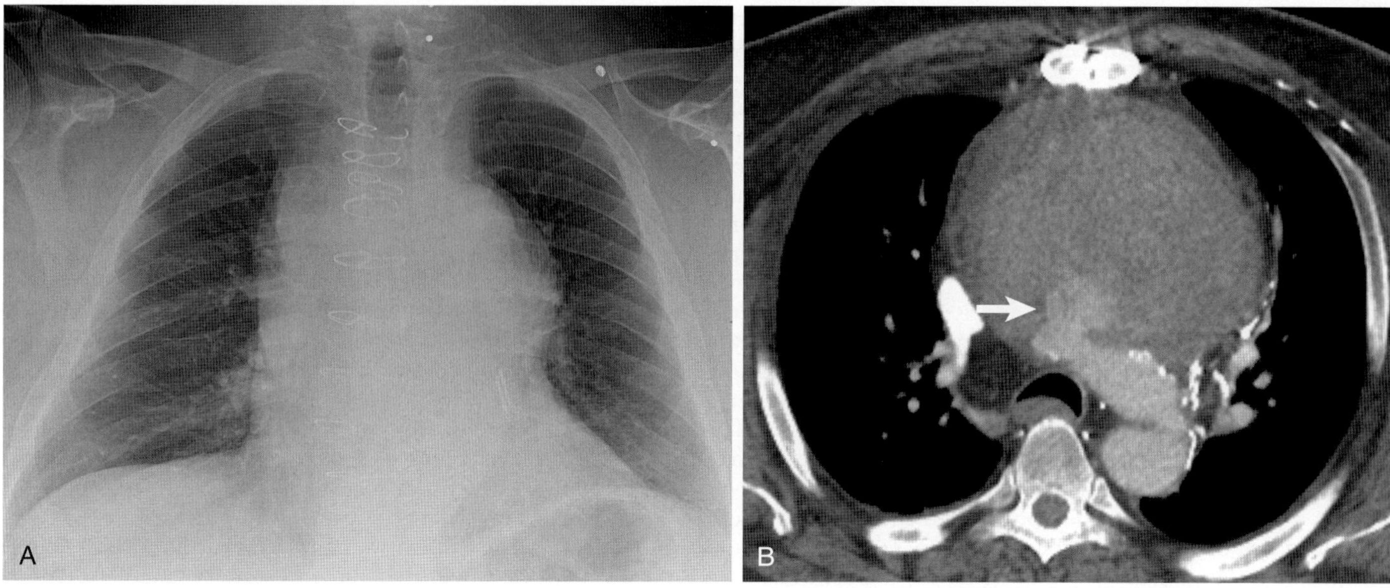

Fig. 68.21 Mediastinal hematoma in a man who had undergone aortic valve replacement and coronary artery bypass grafting procedure 2 years earlier. He presents with chest pain. Chest radiograph (A) shows widened mediastinum. Chest CT with intravenous contrast (B) shows anterior mediastinal hematoma resulting from ascending aortic pseudoaneurysm with active extravasation *(arrow)*.

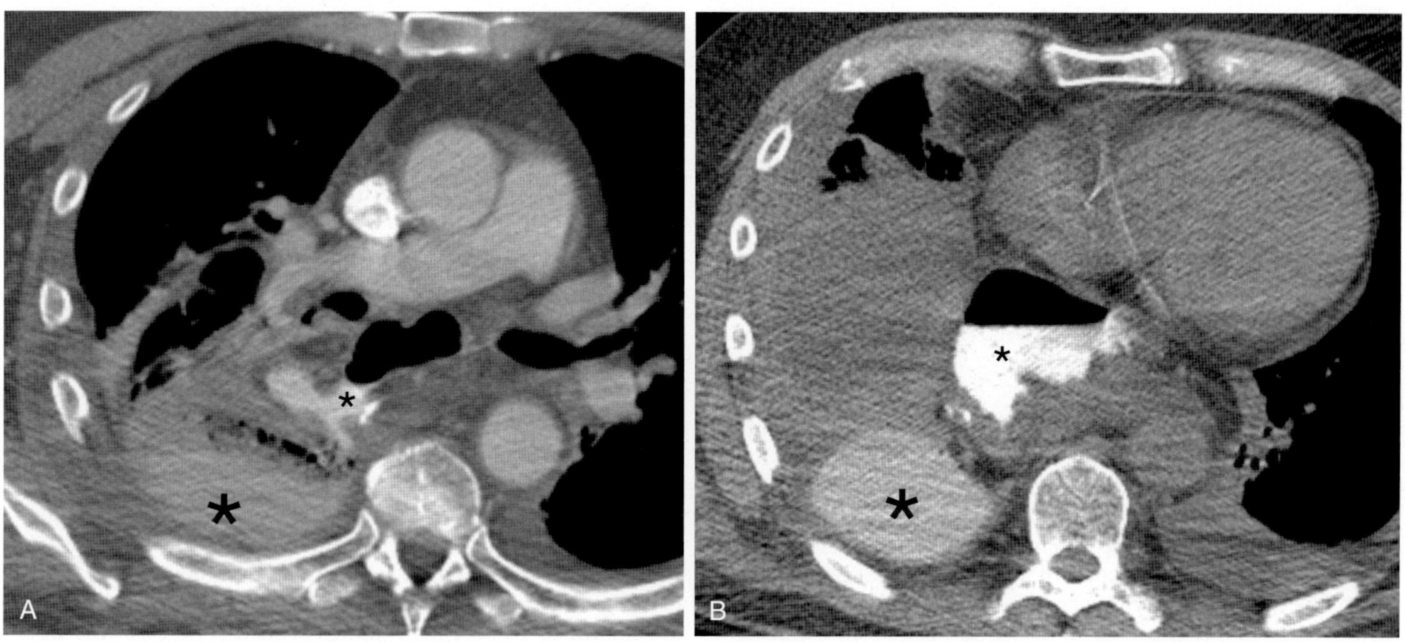

Fig. 68.22 Esophageal leak in a man with esophageal cancer 9 days post–Ivor Lewis esophagectomy with right upper quadrant abdominal pain and fever. CT (A and B) shows oral contrast in the gastric pull-up *(small asterisk)* and the right pleural space *(large asterisk)*, consistent with esophageal anastomotic leak.

of oral contrast material in the trachea on prone esophagography,[47,84] or by visualization of fistulous connection on endoscopy or CT.[100,101]

Paraesophageal herniation of a variable amount of abdominal contents through the esophageal hiatus into the thorax can be an early or late complication of esophagectomy. It is most common after Nissen fundoplication if there is "slipping" of the esophageal wrap down to the gastric body and superior displacement of the stomach. With gastric herniation, the cardia and lower esophagus remain below the diaphragm.[3,84] Herniation of the bowel or pancreas can also occur and is most frequent after esophageal resection with new conduit formation. On radiography the herniated bowel typically manifests as a retrocardiac pseudomass with an air-fluid level, usually left sided and medial in location. There is a risk of strangulation of herniated viscera. The stomach may also undergo volvulus, increasing the likelihood of strangulation. Gastric volvulus is identified on chest radiography as a "beak" at the gastroesophageal junction or a double air-fluid level above and below the diaphragm, representing the antrum and fundus, respectively. Barium esophagography reveals an "upside-down" appearance of the herniated stomach, and the presence of a Schatzki or B ring 2 cm or more above the diaphragmatic hiatus is used to confirm the diagnosis.[3,84,102]

After tracheal resection, anastomotic site complications include dehiscence, stenosis, and malacia. Tracheal dehiscence, a rare complication with high mortality rate, is heralded by subcutaneous air, at times with concomitant pneumomediastinum, pneumothorax, or empyema.[3,7,21,47] Tracheal stenosis is considered significant when there is a reduction of luminal diameter of more than 50% on CT. Similarly, tracheomalacia is considered significant when there is a reduction of luminal diameter of more than 70% on expiratory CT. Volumetric CT reconstructions allow precise measurements of the tracheal lumen and the longitudinal extent of the stenosis. CT is considered the best technique for serial reassessment.[7,47]

Pleural and Cavitary Space Reduction Surgery

DESCRIPTION

Pleurodesis is a procedure that produces dense adhesions between the visceral and parietal pleura through the induction of inflammation and scarring. The inflammation may be induced by talc or other chemicals introduced into the pleural space or by mechanical abrasion of the pleural surfaces.[3,103] The procedure can be performed via thoracoscopy or tube thoracostomy. Thoracoplasty involves the resection of a portion of the chest wall to reduce the thoracic cavity that physically compresses underlying tissue. It commonly involves the segmental resection of 7 to 10 ribs.[3,5] Historically, extrapleural plombage was a procedure in the 1930s to 1950s that placed material, most commonly Lucite spheres or a paraffin wax "pack," into the extrapleural space to collapse tuberculous cavitary lung lesions.[3,104] Similarly, artificial pneumothorax created by injection of air into the pleural cavity every 2 to 4 weeks, continued for 2 to 4 years, is an old procedure to collapse the lung affected by tuberculous infection.[105]

An Eloesser flap thoracostomy window involves an inversed U-shaped skin incision, partial resection of underlying ribs, insertion of the skin flap into the chest wall cavity, and sewing of the flap to the base of the empyema cavity. The procedure creates a drainage pathway for the pleural space.[106,107]

INDICATIONS, CONTRAINDICATIONS, PURPOSE, AND UNDERLYING MECHANISMS

Pleurodesis often accompanies bullectomy or blebectomy, and the combination has become an effective treatment of spontaneous and recurrent pneumothoraces. Other indications for pleurodesis include malignant and benign pleural effusion refractory to medical treatment.[7,103]

Thoracoplasty, artificial pneumothorax, oleothorax (injection of paraffin oil into the pleural space), and extrapleural plombage were used to treat cavitary upper lobe lesions caused by tuberculosis by collapsing the involved portion of the lung until the introduction of effective antituberculosis therapy in the 1950s. Currently, the indication for thoracoplasty is to obliterate excessive dead space associated with chronic empyema infection, particularly post–lung resection.[108] Extrapleural plombage, oleothorax, and artificial pneumothorax procedures are now rarely performed.[3,5,109]

The Eloesser procedure or open-window thoracostomy is used to treat severe chronic empyema that failed more conservative management in patients who are not suitable candidates for or failed decortication.[106]

EXPECTED APPEARANCE ON RELEVANT MODALITIES

After pleurodesis, pleural thickening and loculated pleural effusions are present in the majority of patients. Talc deposits in the pleura appear as focal areas of high attenuation on CT that can be linear or nodular in configuration. Talc incites an inflammatory reaction that can show increased ^{18}F-FDG uptake on positron emission tomography even years or a decade after the procedure (Fig. 68.23). Pleural nodules, representing the accumulation of fibrotic granulation tissue produced from pleural inflammation, are of variable sizes and tend to remain stable over time and may enhance on CT with administration of intravenous contrast.[3,110,111] Hyperattenuation and FDG avidity can also be observed along the lymphatic drainage pathway for the parietal pleura, including the anterior peridiaphragmatic, paracardiac, internal mammary, and peri–inferior vena cava lymph nodes.[112] These imaging findings can complicate evaluation of pleural metastases in patients who have undergone pleurodesis for malignant pleural effusion. Increase in size of pleural nodules or intrathoracic lymph nodes over time should raise suspicion for recurrence or progression of underlying malignancy.

Thoracoplasty produces a significant chest wall deformity that can mimic massive trauma. On radiography there is collapse of the upper and lateral chest wall, volume loss in the lung, ipsilateral mediastinal shift, and pleural thickening with or without calcification (Fig. 68.24).[3,7,8] On chest radiography Lucite balls are identified as air-filled, tightly packed spheres in the upper thorax. Over time, Lucite balls become rigidly fixed by a process of hyalinization and fibrosis manifesting radiographically as thin soft tissue density surrounding each sphere. A paraffin pack from oleothorax is identified radiographically as a single, large, oval structure of fat density in the upper thorax. Over time, it develops a pseudocapsule rim that often becomes calcified.[3,8,104,109]

An Eloesser window usually appears en face as an elliptic radiolucency and in profile as a downward-sloping chest wall defect on chest radiograph. Opacity created by gauze used to pack the cavity is seen within the cavity.[113] The chest wall defect extending into the pleural space with or without packing materials is clearly delineated on CT (see Fig. 68.7).

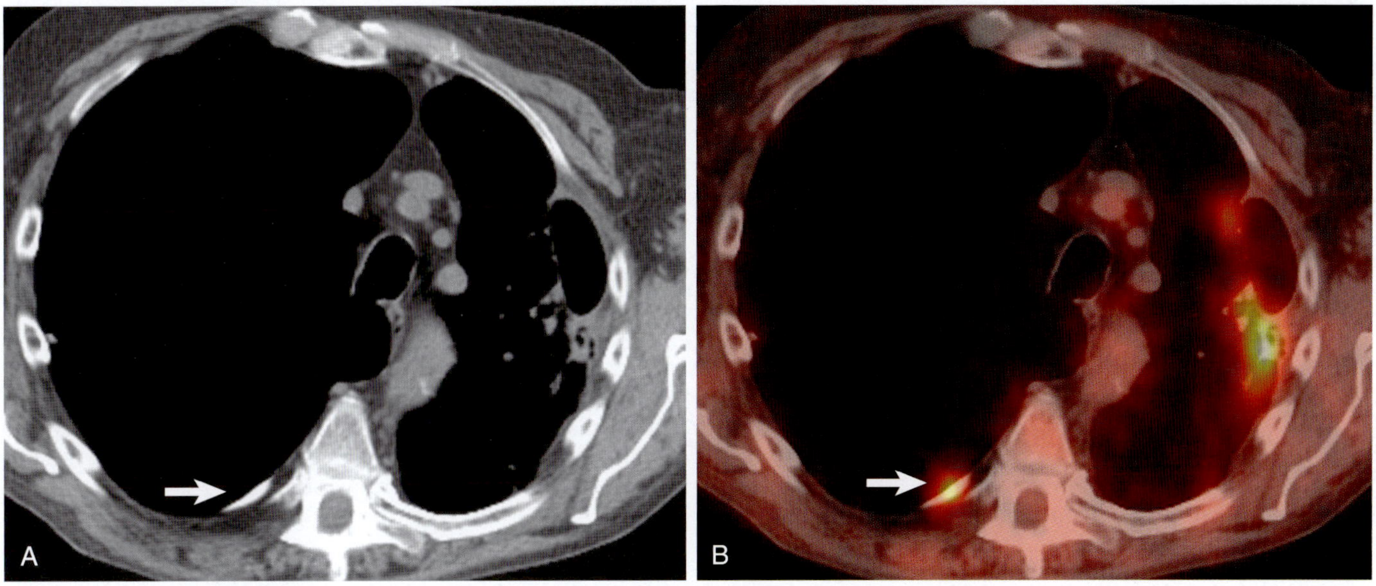

Fig. 68.23 Talc pleurodesis in a man with left upper lobe lung cancer and persistent spontaneous right pneumothorax. CT (A) and fused CT–positron emission tomography (PET) (B) 3 weeks later show the fluorodeoxyglucose-avid left upper lobe primary tumor. High-attenuation material in the right posterior pleura is consistent with talc (*arrow* in A). Talc incites an inflammatory reaction in the pleura that is FDG avid on PET (*arrow* in B) even years after the procedure and should not be misinterpreted as pleural metastasis.

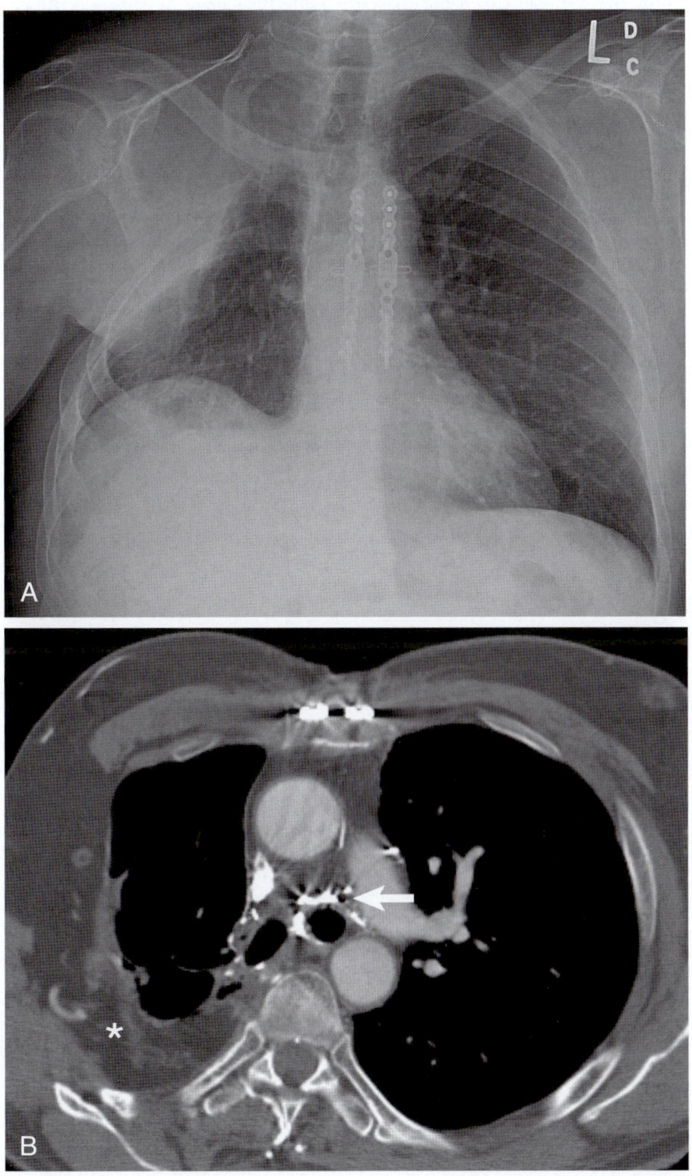

Fig. 68.24 Thoracoplasty in a man with right upper lobectomy for lung cancer. He developed empyema and required thoracoplasty and muscle flap coverage for repair. Because of an abscess in the sternomanubrial junction, he had partial sternectomy and reconstruction with titanium plates. Chest radiograph (A) shows volume loss in the right lung resulting from thoracoplasty of right second, third, and fourth ribs. CT (B) shows serratus anterior muscle flap *(asterisk)* and sternal titanium plates. Note collateral vessels adjacent to the left main bronchus *(arrow)* resulting from partial stenosis or thrombosis of the left subclavian vein.

KEY POINTS

- Knowledge of postoperative findings for common thoracic surgeries and their expected evolution over time can help radiologists avoid misinterpretation of normal findings as pathologic processes.
- Most postoperative complications occur in the first 2 postoperative weeks. Prompt detection of these complications by the radiologist can facilitate appropriate management and improve clinical outcome.
- The most common complications after thoracic surgery are atelectasis, pneumonia, pleural and pericardial fluid collections, pulmonary edema, and pneumothorax. Some thoracic surgeries are also associated with complications more specifically related to the procedures.
- Sites of tissue anastomosis (airway, esophageal, aortic) are prone to postoperative complications.

POTENTIAL COMPLICATIONS AND RADIOLOGIC APPEARANCE

Complications after pleurodesis include tachycardia, pain, fever, and dyspnea. Empyema, hypotension, and acute respiratory distress syndrome have also been reported.[114]

Thoracoplasty may result in severe rotoscoliosis that is visualized radiographically as extensive upper thoracic spinal bowing toward the operative side.[3] Infection is the underlying cause of most complications of extrapleural plombage. Lucite sphere dispersion and fluid in the plombage space are radiographic signs of infection. Soft tissue breakdown by infection or local foreign-body reaction leads to Lucite sphere migration and paraffin wax extrusion. Erosion of nearby structures can result in a number of complications, such as hematoma, lung infection, and bowel obstruction.[3,104,109] Chronic pyothorax with loculated pleural fluid often occurs and persists with artificial pneumothorax procedures. In rare cases chronic inflammation associated with the pyothorax can lead to the development of non-Hodgkin B-cell lymphoma in the pleural cavity, typically occurring more than 20 years after the procedures.[105,115] Pyothorax-associated lymphoma manifests as pleural soft tissue mass with or without chest wall involvement adjacent to the margin of a coexistent empyema cavity on imaging.[116]

Conclusion

Postoperative complications differ according to the type of surgery and the time elapsed since surgery. The radiologist must be vigilant in evaluating postoperative chest radiographs as findings related to complications are often subtle. CT is the preferred imaging modality for the evaluation of unexplained radiographic abnormalities and clinical signs and symptoms. Awareness of normal and abnormal imaging findings is key to accurate interpretation of postoperative studies.

SUGGESTED READINGS

Alpert JB, Godoy MC, Degroot PM, et al. Imaging the post-thoracotomy patient: anatomic changes and postoperative complications. *Radiol Clin North Am*. 2014;52(1):85–103.

Chae EJ, Seo JB, Kim SY, et al. Radiographic and CT findings of thoracic complications after pneumonectomy. *Radiographics*. 2006;26(5):1449–1468.

Christensen JD, Seaman DM, Washington L. Imaging of complications of thoracic and cardiovascular surgery. *Radiol Clin North Am*. 2014;52(5):929–959.

El-Sherief AH, Wu CC, Schoenhagen P, Little BP, Cheng A, Abbara S, Roselli EE. Basics of cardiopulmonary bypass: normal and abnormal postoperative CT appearances. *Radiographics*. 2013;33(1):63–72.

Gladish GW, Rice DC, Sabloff BS, et al. Pedicle muscle flaps in intrathoracic cancer resection: imaging appearance and evolution. *Radiographics*. 2007;27(4):975–987.

Jokerst C, Sirajuddin A, Mohammed TL. Imaging the complications of lung transplantation. *Radiol Clin North Am*. 2016;54(2):355–373.

Kim SH, Lee KS, Shim YM, et al. Esophageal resection: indications, techniques, and radiologic assessment. *Radiographics*. 2001;21:1119–1137.

Ng YL, Paul N, Patsios D, et al. Imaging of lung transplantation: review. *AJR Am J Roentgenol*. 2009;192(suppl 3):S1–S13, quiz S14–S19.

Riley P, Rooney S, Bonser R, Guest P. Imaging the post-operative thoracic aorta: normal anatomy and pitfalls. *Br J Radiol*. 2001;74:1150–1158.

Valente T, Rossi G, Rea G, et al. Multidetector CT findings of complications of surgical and endovascular treatment of aortic aneurysms. *Radiol Clin North Am*. 2014;52(5):961–989.

The full reference list for this chapter is available at ExpertConsult.com.

69 Chest Radiography in the Intensive Care Unit*

ANUPAMA BRIXEY | MATTHEW BENTZ | STEVEN L. PRIMACK

Chest radiography is the primary imaging modality used in the intensive care unit (ICU), given its portability, rapid image acquisition, and immediate bedside return of information on the preview screen. Of consequence, it is of utmost importance that both radiologists and intensivists are adept in reading these studies.

Portable ICU radiographs are obtained in an anteroposterior (AP) view in which the x-ray beam traverses the patient anterior to posterior at a standard distance of 40 inches, compared with 72 inches for a posteroanterior (PA) view. This decreased distance contributes to greater magnification and decreased sharpness of images. Furthermore, the majority of ICU radiographs are obtained in the supine or semiupright position because of patient immobility. This often results in low lung volumes, which presents an additional challenge in interpretation.

Digital radiography has improved the quality of radiographs by allowing postprocessing manipulation of images, such as window leveling, magnification, inversion, and so forth, to enhance contrast, reduce noise, and improve image blur.[1] It has also improved image acquisition in the ICU by allowing immediate review of the radiograph at the bedside by both the technologist and intensivist. This gives the technologist the ability to quickly obtain a repeat acquisition if there is either a technical or positioning error noted on the preview screen. In addition, if there are dramatic abnormalities noted on the preview image, such as a large pneumothorax, the intensivist can initiate treatment sooner.

Over the past several years, multiple studies dedicated to evaluating the clinical benefit of routine daily chest radiographs (CR) in ICU patients have been performed.[2,3] A meta-analysis by Oba and Zaza in 2009, comprising eight trials and 7078 ICU patients, found that there were no increased adverse outcomes in patients who did not undergo routine daily chest radiographs versus patients who did. Furthermore, patients who had radiographs only for specific clinical indications received an average of 0.4 to 4.4 CRs during their ICU stay, compared with 2.4 to 10.5 CRs for the routine daily group.[2] According to the 2014 American College of Radiology Appropriateness Criteria, "routine daily chest radiographs are not indicated for patients admitted to the ICU." Radiographs should be obtained on admission and thereafter only in response to a specific clinical indication or after insertion of an external device, such as an endotracheal tube.

Owing to the severity of disease and frequent need for insertion of external devices, ICU patients more often than not have abnormal chest radiographs and are at risk for ICU-related complications. Common thoracic pathologic processes in the ICU include atelectasis/mucus plugging with lung collapse, aspiration, pneumonia, pulmonary edema, pleural disease, and iatrogenic complications. Acute respiratory distress syndrome (ARDS) is a more severe pathologic process that also occurs in ICU patients, but incidence and mortality have steadily declined. Each of these major processes will be discussed in further detail in this chapter.

Atelectasis

Atelectasis is the most common cause of a lung opacity in an ICU patient. When an entire lobe is atelectatic, this is described as lobar collapse. There are six recognized mechanisms of atelectasis: gravity dependent, obstructive (resorptive), passive, compressive, adhesive, and cicatricial.[4] Gravity-dependent small airway collapse is commonly seen in postoperative patients as a result of shallow breathing and small airway collapse. However, atelectasis in ICU patients is often multifactorial and frequently results in the presence of more than one type of atelectasis on a radiograph.[5] Obstructive atelectasis results from obstruction of a large- or medium-sized airway, which causes resorption of air distally and results in lobar collapse. Compressive atelectasis, also referred to as relaxation atelectasis by some radiologists, is the result of an intrathoracic space-occupying process (most commonly pleural effusions in ICU patients) that prevents air from entering the alveoli. Passive atelectasis is also frequently encountered, given the prevalence of pneumothoraces in ICU patients. In this setting the lung is not directly in contact with the chest wall, so the lung maintains its innate tendency to passively collapse instead of being forced open by the chest wall with each breath. Adhesive atelectasis is secondary to decreased surfactant and is commonly seen in ARDS patients or in premature neonates. Finally, cicatricial atelectasis is a chronic form of atelectasis as a result of scarring or lung fibrosis and is not seen de novo in ICU patients.

RADIOGRAPHY

The left lower lobe is the most common site of atelectasis (66%), followed by the right lower lobe (22%) and right upper lobe (11%).[6] When atelectasis is linear or plate-like (i.e., subsegmental atelectasis), it is often located in the gravity-dependent lower lobes (Figs. 69.1 and 69.2). Although atelectasis is most commonly subsegmental in ICU patients, it may involve complete pulmonary segments or lobes (Fig. 69.3). Direct signs of atelectasis, such as displacement of interlobar fissures or crowding of vessels/bronchi may prove useful in determining the location of atelectasis. On occasion, atelectasis can be ill-defined and appear similar to a layering pleural effusion. In recumbent patients radiographic evidence of volume loss may not be as evident.

In lobar atelectasis the presence or absence of air bronchograms is useful to determine the potential effectiveness of airway clearance techniques. If air bronchograms are present, the atelectasis

*The editors and the publisher would like to thank Dr. Peder E. Horner for contributing material on this topic to the prior edition of this work. It has served as the foundation for the current chapter.

is most likely related to small airways collapse, and an inspiratory flow device, such as an incentive spirometer, may be useful in opening the collapsed alveoli. If air bronchograms are absent in lobar atelectasis, however, mucoid impaction is the most likely etiology, and airway clearance techniques, such as chest physiotherapy or acapella devices, have a high likelihood of providing clinical benefit.[7] Noninvasive airway clearance techniques are just as effective in clearance of airway secretions as fiberoptic bronchoscopy; therefore bronchoscopy is generally reserved only for intractable cases.[8]

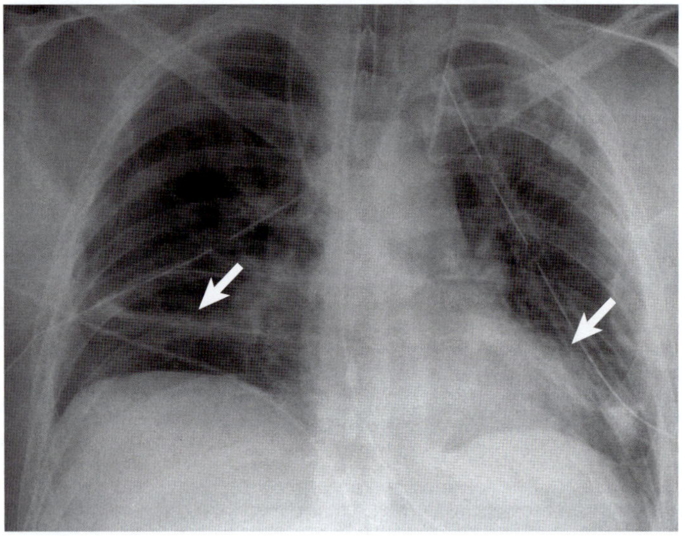

Fig. 69.1 Linear (discoid) subsegmental atelectasis. Anteroposterior chest radiograph shows multiple tubes and lines and bibasilar discoid opacities *(arrows)* with vascular crowding consistent with subsegmental atelectasis.

COMPUTED TOMOGRAPHY

Computed tomography (CT) findings are similar to those seen on radiographs. Atelectasis is characterized on CT by increased density with volume loss and crowding of bronchi and vasculature, often within a defined anatomic distribution (e.g., subsegmental, segmental, or lobar) (see Fig. 69.2B). An obstructing mucus plug may be identified proximal to the collapsed lung (see Fig. 69.3C). Intravenous contrast can aid in distinguishing atelectasis from consolidation: Atelectasis should enhance greater than skeletal muscle, whereas consolidation often enhances either similar to or less than skeletal muscle (Fig. 69.4). It is important to note that vessels enhance in both conditions and should not be confused for parenchymal enhancement.

Aspiration

Aspiration commonly occurs in critically ill patients, given that the risk of aspiration increases with decreased level of consciousness.[9] Aspiration and its consequences can be thought of as a spectrum of clinicopathologic injury: aspiration of inert/nontoxic substances, aspiration pneumonitis, and aspiration pneumonia.[10]

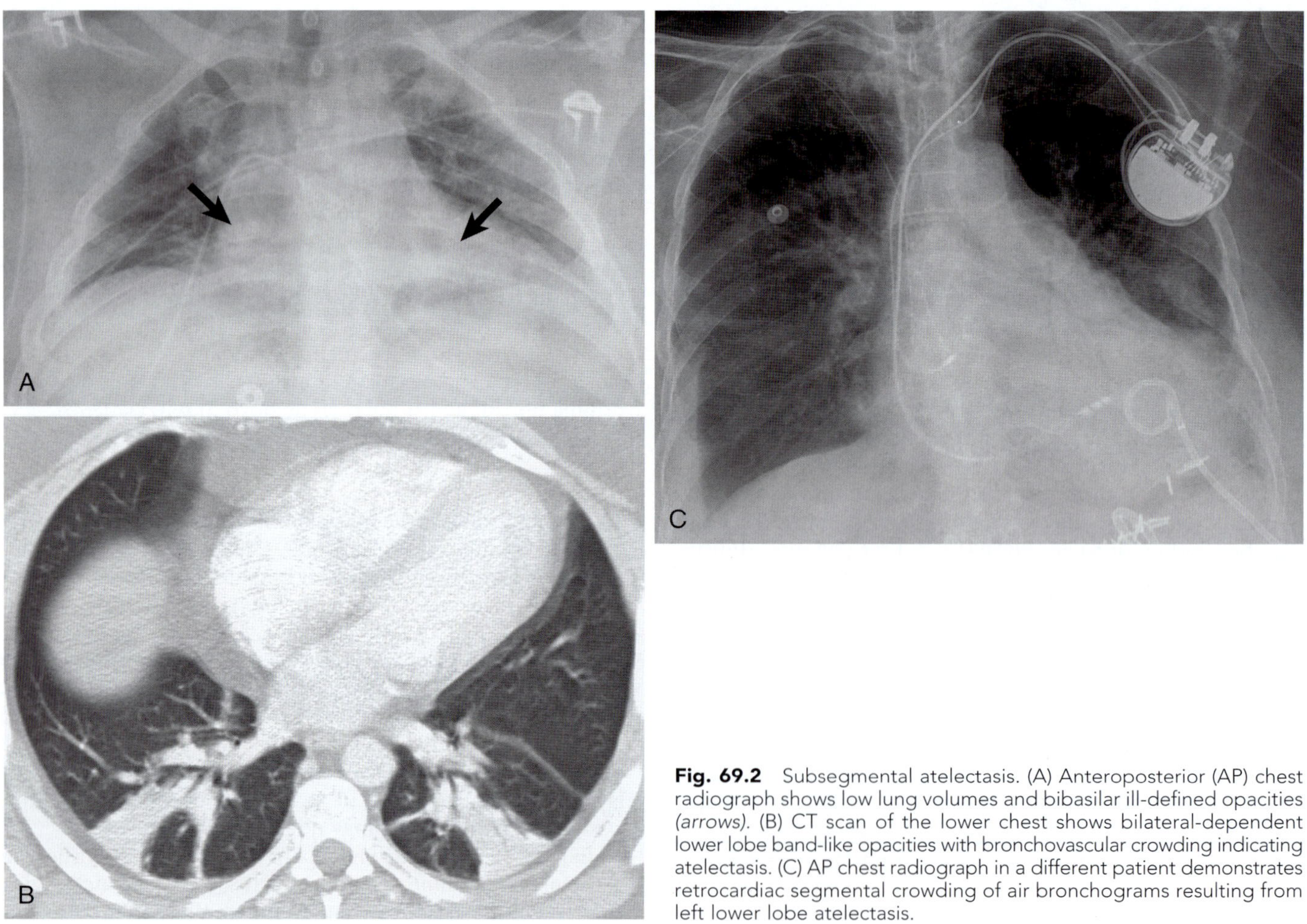

Fig. 69.2 Subsegmental atelectasis. (A) Anteroposterior (AP) chest radiograph shows low lung volumes and bibasilar ill-defined opacities *(arrows)*. (B) CT scan of the lower chest shows bilateral-dependent lower lobe band-like opacities with bronchovascular crowding indicating atelectasis. (C) AP chest radiograph in a different patient demonstrates retrocardiac segmental crowding of air bronchograms resulting from left lower lobe atelectasis.

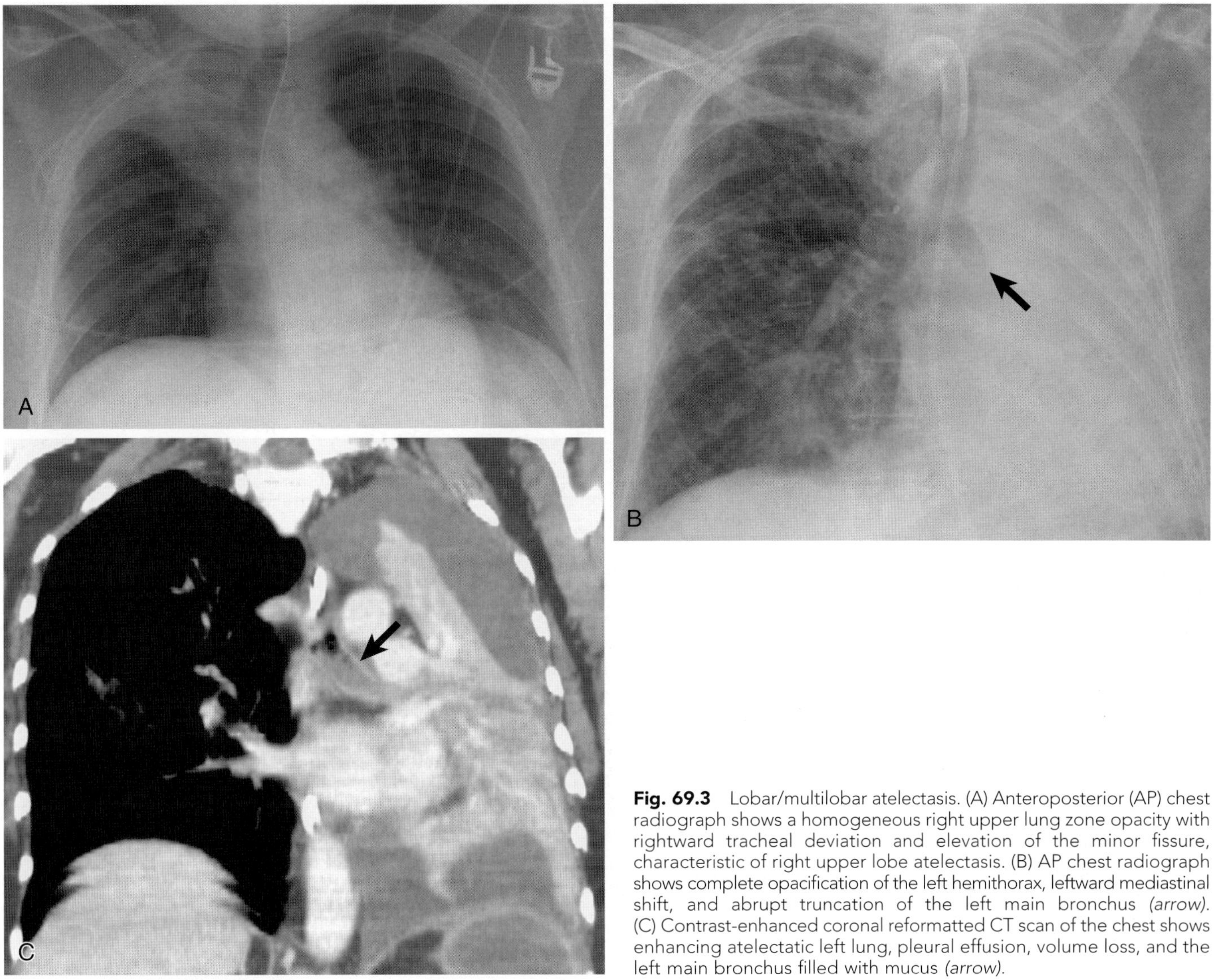

Fig. 69.3 Lobar/multilobar atelectasis. (A) Anteroposterior (AP) chest radiograph shows a homogeneous right upper lung zone opacity with rightward tracheal deviation and elevation of the minor fissure, characteristic of right upper lobe atelectasis. (B) AP chest radiograph shows complete opacification of the left hemithorax, leftward mediastinal shift, and abrupt truncation of the left main bronchus *(arrow)*. (C) Contrast-enhanced coronal reformatted CT scan of the chest shows enhancing atelectatic left lung, pleural effusion, volume loss, and the left main bronchus filled with mucus *(arrow)*.

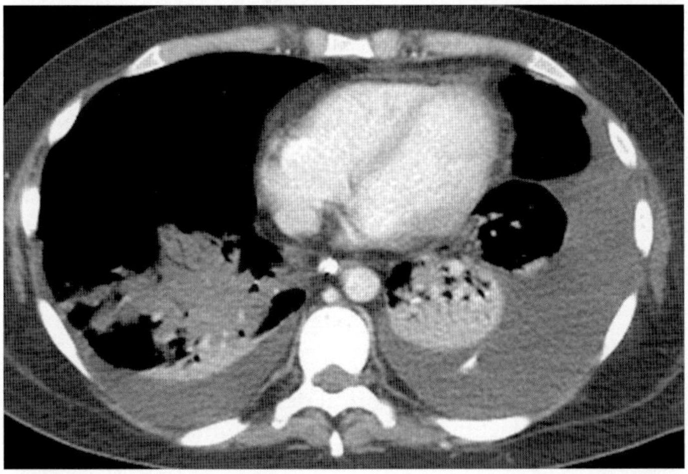

Fig. 69.4 Enhancing atelectasis. CT scan of the chest demonstrates enhancement within the left lower lobe consistent with atelectasis. Nonenhancing right lung is secondary to necrotizing pneumonia. Moderate left and small right pleural effusions are also present.

Within the ICU, distinguishing aspiration pneumonitis from aspiration pneumonia based on clinical symptoms is imperative because pneumonitis typically does not require treatment, whereas aspiration pneumonia usually requires antibiotics. Severe aspiration events can lead to acute respiratory failure, sepsis, or ARDS. The severity of aspiration-related lung injury is related to the volume and type (i.e., inert substances vs. sterile gastric acid vs. oropharyngeal secretions colonized by bacteria) of aspirate.[11] It is important to remember that an intubated patient with an inflated endotracheal tube cuff can still aspirate around the endotracheal cuff. In addition, gastric contents often become colonized by bacteria in ICU patients, given that all mechanically ventilated patients are placed on stress-ulcer prophylaxis (histamine 2–receptor antagonists or proton-pump inhibitors), which raises the gastric pH. This predisposes ICU patients to the development of aspiration pneumonia after aspiration of gastric contents.[12]

RADIOGRAPHY

Aspiration may manifest as a focal or multifocal consolidative pattern (Fig. 69.5). Poorly defined nodules in a small airway distribution also are commonly identified (Fig. 69.6), resulting in

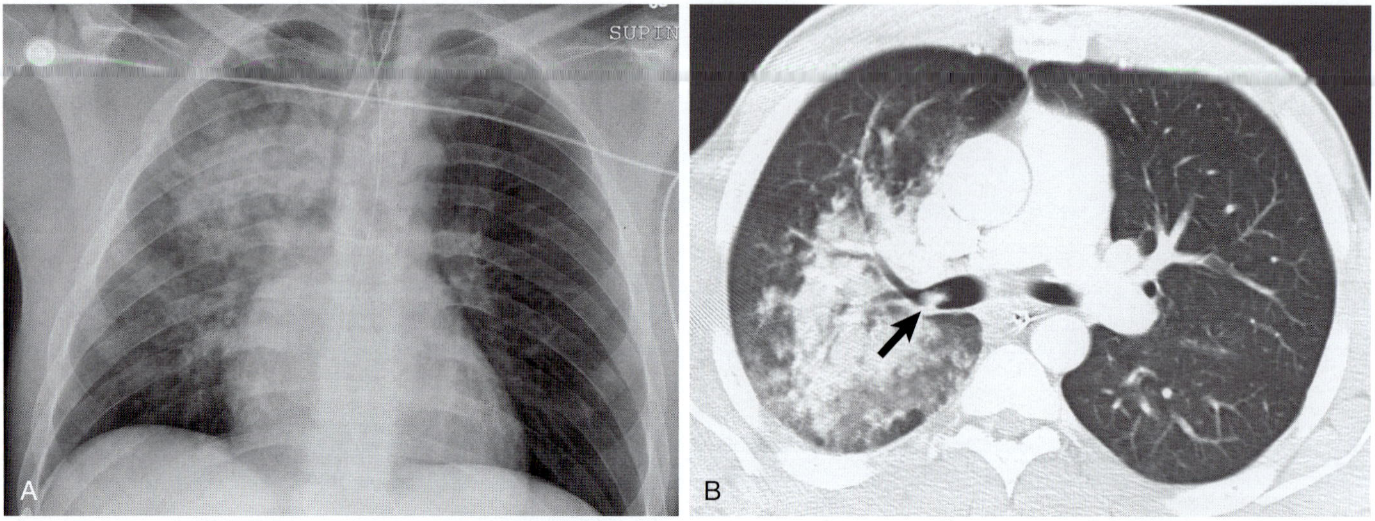

Fig. 69.5 Aspiration, consolidative pattern. (A) Anteroposterior chest radiograph shows right upper lung zone consolidation. (B) CT scan shows right upper lobe posterior segmental consolidation and centrilobular nodules. Note aspirated debris in the right upper lobe bronchus *(arrow)*.

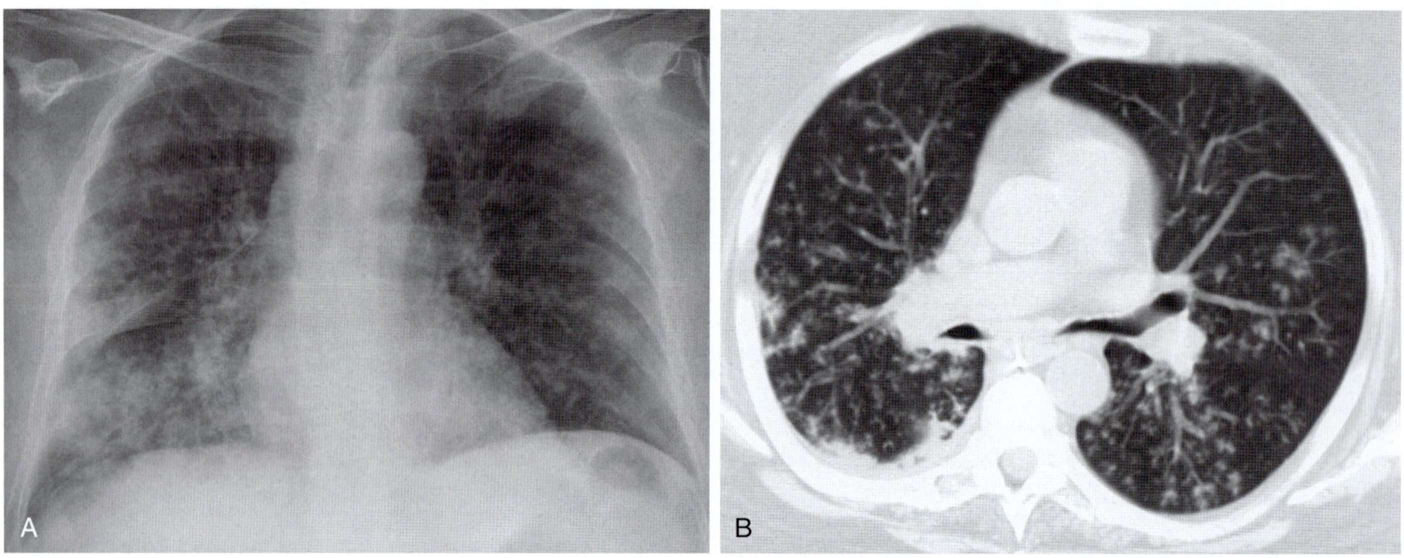

Fig. 69.6 Aspiration, tree-in-bud pattern. (A) Anteroposterior chest radiograph shows bilateral 3- to 5-mm ill-defined nodular opacities. (B) CT scan of chest shows predominantly posterior bilateral nodules with tree-in-bud opacities.

a tree-in-bud appearance often seen on CT. Airway thickening, bronchiolar impaction, and volume loss also are frequently identified. Although the radiographic appearance of aspirated material varies, the chest radiograph may be normal in 10% of cases.[13]

Aspiration pneumonitis may progress over the first day but usually begins to clear within a few days (Fig. 69.7). Progression of consolidation with persistent/worsening clinical symptoms suggests the development of pneumonia. In a recumbent patient, aspiration is typically located in the posterior segments of the upper lobes, the superior segments of the lower lobes, and the posterior basilar segments of the lower lobes. This distribution results in a central predominance on a supine AP radiograph.

COMPUTED TOMOGRAPHY

CT findings are similar to the radiographic findings of consolidative or tree-in-bud opacities in a dependent distribution (see Figs. 69.5B and 69.6B). CT is more sensitive, however, in depicting the tree-in-bud pattern, the extent of aspiration, and the exact distribution. In addition, CT can show small airway filling and obstruction (see Fig. 69.5B). It also better identifies complications such as lung abscess.

Pneumonia

There are multiple subcategorical definitions of pneumonia in ICU patients. Pneumonia in patients admitted from home or developing within the first 48 hours of hospital admission is defined as community-acquired pneumonia. If this patient has been hospitalized within the past 90 days, resides in a skilled nursing facility, or has received antibiotics/chemotherapy/wound care within 30 days, then it is classified as health care–associated pneumonia. Pneumonia that develops in a patient greater than 48 hours after admission is defined as nosocomial pneumonia

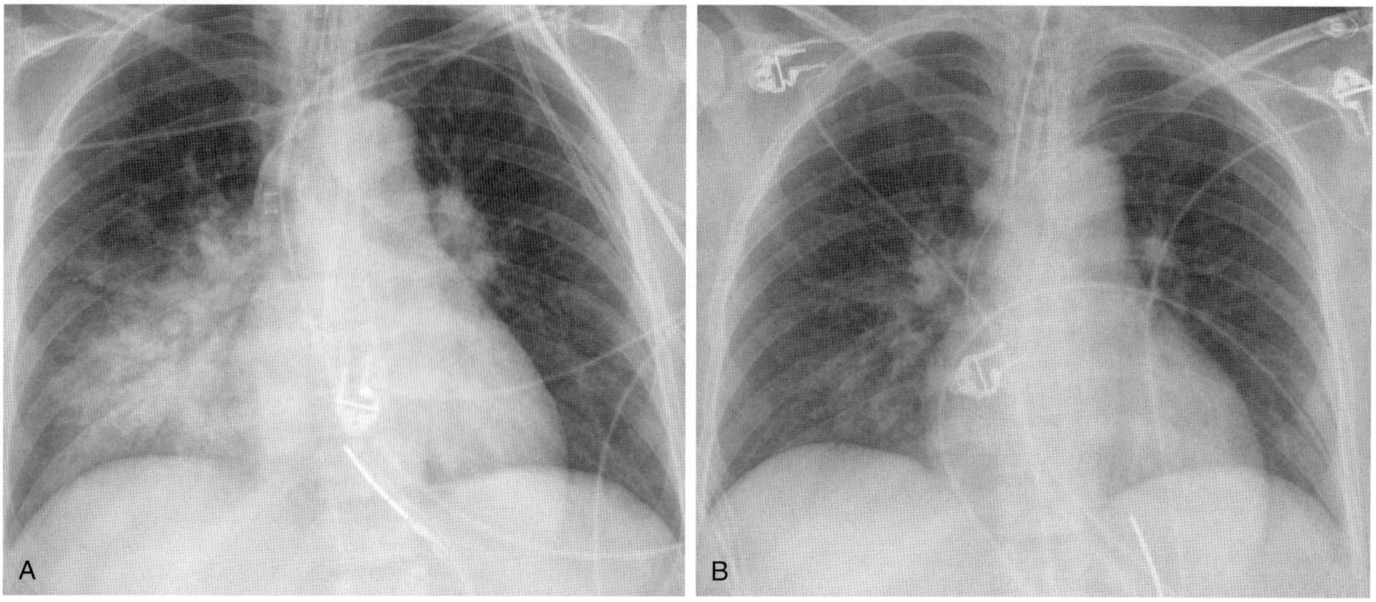

Fig. 69.7 Aspiration pneumonitis, temporal change. (A) Anteroposterior (AP) chest radiograph shows right perihilar and lower lung zone consolidation. (B) AP chest radiograph 2 days later shows marked improvement.

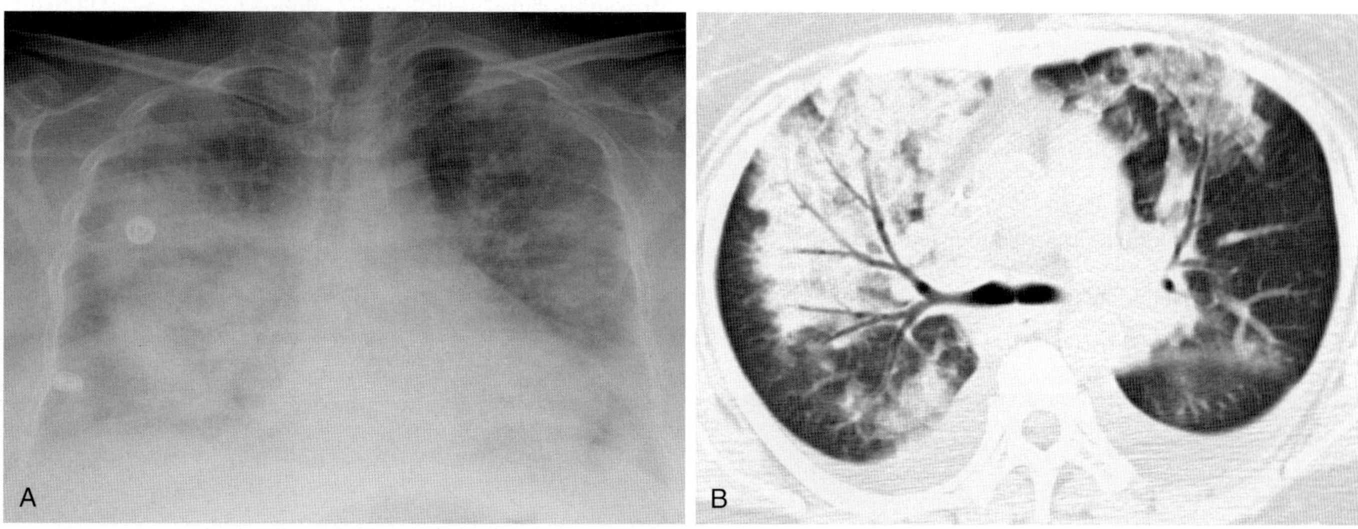

Fig. 69.8 Multifocal bacterial bronchopneumonia. (A) Anteroposterior chest radiograph shows multifocal dense consolidation, worse on the right. (B) CT scan confirms bilateral and asymmetric distribution of consolidation and air bronchograms. Bilateral pleural effusions also are noted.

and is most commonly seen in the ICU. When nosocomial pneumonia occurs in patients receiving mechanical ventilation for greater than 48 hours, it is termed ventilator-associated pneumonia (VAP). Accurately diagnosing pneumonia in the ICU requires a combination of predefined clinical symptoms, radiographic abnormalities, and laboratory analysis of respiratory secretions. According to the study by Alp and colleagues,[14] the incidence of nosocomial pneumonia in the ICU was 6.8% using the established criteria by the Centers for Disease Control and Prevention. Of these nosocomial pneumonias, 75.5% were VAPs.

RADIOGRAPHY

The chest radiograph typically shows patchy areas of consolidation or poorly defined opacities that are often multifocal (Fig. 69.8). Air bronchograms are helpful for the diagnosis of pneumonia but also occur with atelectasis. In contrast to atelectatic air bronchograms, pneumonia-related air bronchograms are not characterized by volume loss and "crowding" of the bronchi. Cavitation can occur and is a more specific finding of pneumonia when present. Radiographic changes in pneumonia typically develop more slowly than in atelectasis, aspiration, or pulmonary edema. Although pneumonia is commonly present in patients with ARDS, the chest radiograph has been found to be only 57% accurate in differentiating pneumonia without ARDS from non–pneumonic-induced ARDS.[15]

COMPUTED TOMOGRAPHY

Radiographs alone are generally adequate to evaluate pneumonia, but CT can be an asset in evaluating potential complications of pneumonia, such as developing cavitation or in determining the extent and character of parapneumonic effusions. In the setting of new ill-defined opacities on a background of preexisting consolidation, CT better differentiates the potential etiology of multifocal opacities and whether they stem from one or more than one process. Contrast-enhanced studies of pneumonia often show only mild or no enhancement of the involved parenchyma; however, hypoenhancement of parenchyma should raise concern for necrotizing pneumonia (see Fig. 69.4).

Pulmonary Edema

Pulmonary edema is a common cause for admission to critical care units and frequently develops during an ICU stay. Patients present with dyspnea and tachypnea and are often found to be hypoxic. Pulmonary edema can be subdivided into hydrostatic or increased permeability based on the mechanism of development.

Hydrostatic Pulmonary Edema

Hydrostatic pulmonary edema develops most commonly as a result of increased pulmonary venous pressures resulting from left-sided heart failure, renal failure/insufficiency, or hypervolemia.

RADIOGRAPHY

The classic findings of hydrostatic pulmonary edema include a widened vascular pedicle and pulmonary vascular congestion.[16,17] Peribronchial cuffing, subpleural interstitial edema manifesting as fissural thickening, and vascular indistinctness are present in early interstitial pulmonary edema. As the pulmonary capillary pressure increases, interlobular septal thickening develops along with ground-glass opacities (Fig. 69.9). Eventually, consolidative opacities develop. The findings are usually bilateral and symmetric. However, in acute mitral regurgitation, there is frequently right upper lobe predominance (Fig. 69.10). Underlying chronic lung disease, such as emphysema, can also lead to an asymmetric distribution of pulmonary edema because of lack of involvement of areas occupied by bullae (Fig. 69.11). In cardiogenic pulmonary edema, dependent consolidation and cardiomegaly are often present. Pleural effusions may be bilateral or unilaterally on the right. In contrast, in hydrostatic (noncardiogenic) pulmonary edema the consolidation is usually diffuse or peripheral (Fig. 69.12), septal lines are uncommon, and heart size is normal.

COMPUTED TOMOGRAPHY

Early findings of hydrostatic pulmonary edema, such as ground-glass opacities, airway thickening, and interlobular septal thickening, are better depicted on CT. Ground-glass opacities on CT tend to have a gravity-dependent distribution. Small pleural effusions are seen earlier on CT than on radiographs, and CT more accurately defines the location and extent of consolidation, when present (Fig. 69.13).

Increased-Permeability Pulmonary Edema

Increased-capillary permeability pulmonary edema is synonymous with nonhydrostatic and noncardiogenic pulmonary edema. Etiologies include pulmonary causes (e.g., aspiration pneumonitis, bacterial pneumonia, thoracic trauma) and extrapulmonary causes (e.g., sepsis, neurogenic pulmonary edema, extrathoracic trauma, pancreatitis, and drug toxicity).

RADIOGRAPHY

The typical radiographic appearance consists of extensive bilateral airspace opacities (Figs. 69.14 and 69.15). The distribution is

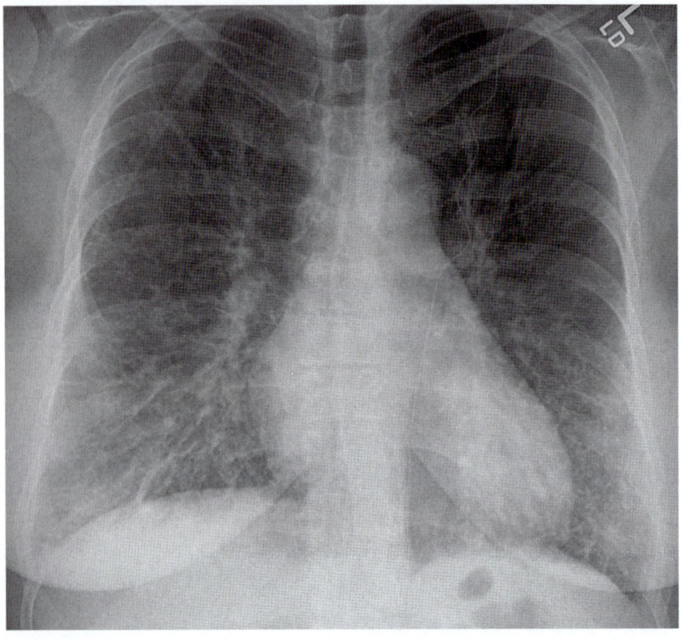

Fig. 69.9 Hydrostatic pulmonary edema. Anteroposterior chest radiograph in a postpartum woman shows bilateral, symmetric, pulmonary vascular enlargement, indistinctness, and septal thickening.

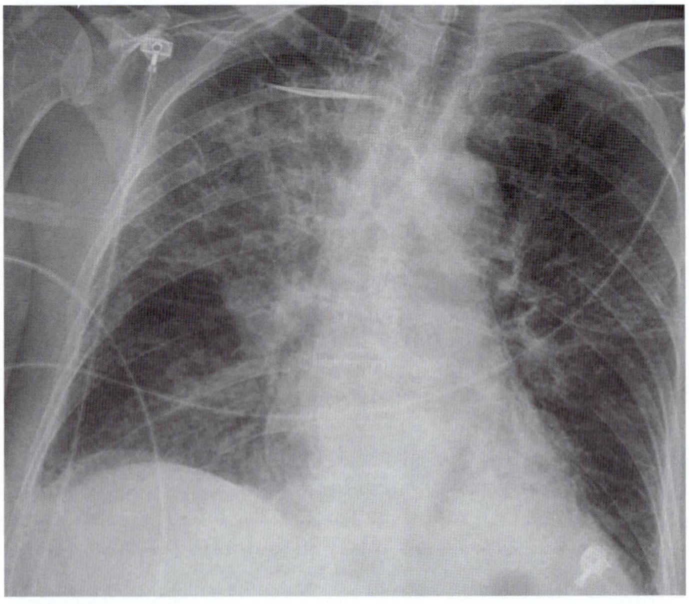

Fig. 69.10 Acute mitral regurgitation. Anteroposterior chest radiograph shows right upper lobe distribution of poorly defined opacities, vascular indistinctness, and septal thickening characteristic of pulmonary edema secondary to acute mitral regurgitation.

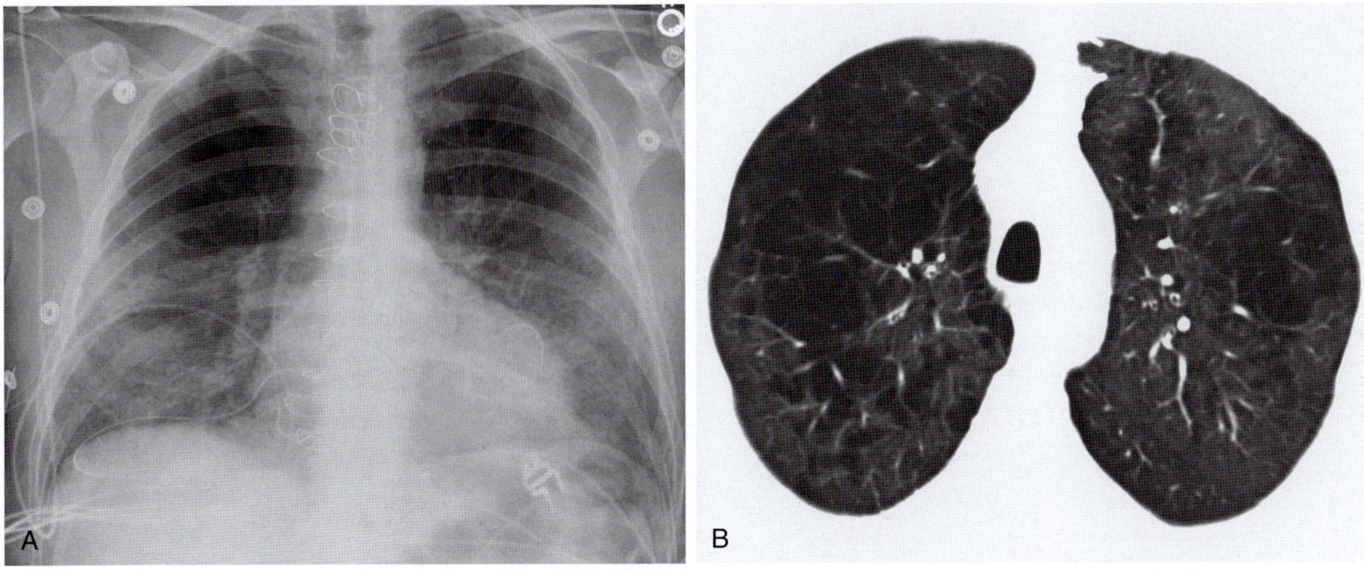

Fig. 69.11 Hydrostatic pulmonary edema and emphysema. (A) Anteroposterior chest radiograph shows bilateral hazy opacities within the lower lung zones and left upper lung zone. (B) CT scan shows upper lobe–predominant emphysema that explains the asymmetric and uncharacteristic distribution of radiographic findings.

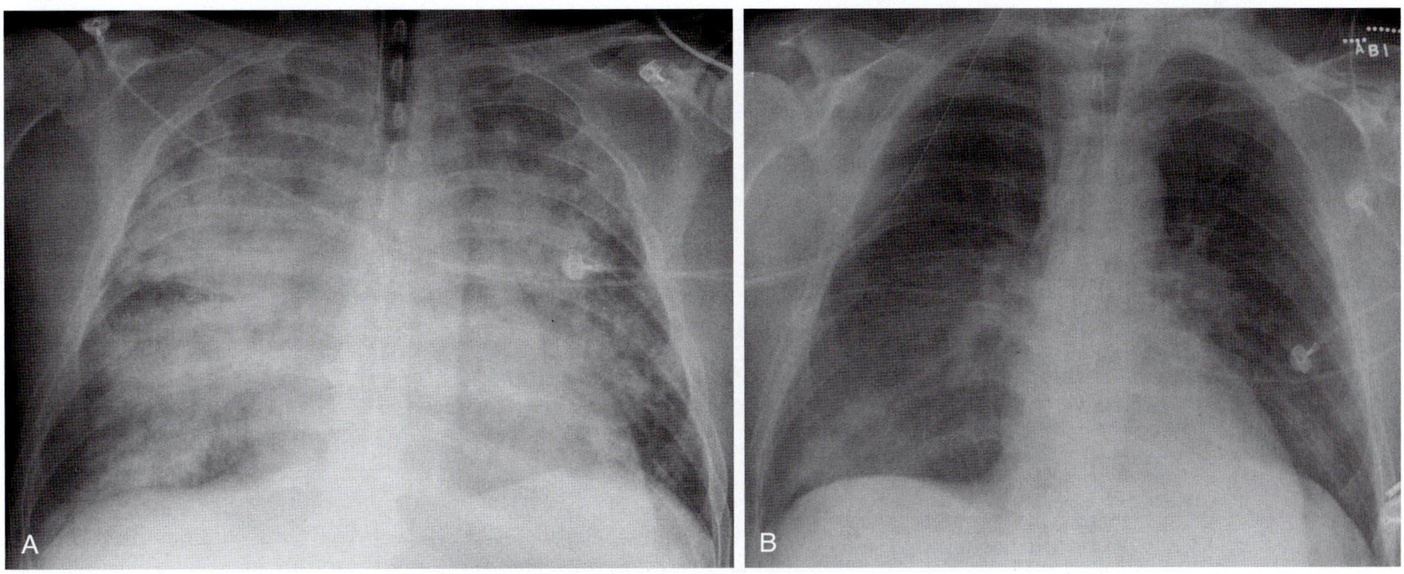

Fig. 69.12 Acute renal failure–related hydrostatic pulmonary edema. (A) Anteroposterior (AP) chest radiograph shows bilateral perihilar consolidation, enlarged cardiac silhouette, and a wide vascular pedicle. (B) Follow-up AP chest radiograph 3 days later shows interval right internal jugular venous dialysis-catheter placement and marked improvement of parenchymal abnormalities.

usually initially patchy but rapidly progresses to a diffuse distribution. The distribution of opacities from pulmonary causes tends to be more asymmetric and patchy, whereas that of extrapulmonary causes tends to be symmetric, diffuse, and homogeneous. Air bronchograms are commonly identified. Septal lines are uncommon. The vascular pedicle, heart size, and pulmonary vascular size are usually normal.

Radiographically distinguishing hydrostatic from increased permeability pulmonary edema can be difficult. The most useful distinguishing feature is that increased permeability pulmonary edema has a much higher incidence of a patchy peripheral distribution than hydrostatic pulmonary edema.[16,17] Although a widened vascular pedicle, pulmonary vascular engorgement, and pleural effusions are more commonly identified in hydrostatic pulmonary edema, these findings also may be present with noncardiogenic pulmonary edema. Furthermore, the two entities frequently coexist, which further complicates interpretation.

Acute Respiratory Distress Syndrome

ARDS is a disease process that represents an advanced form of increased-permeability (noncardiogenic) pulmonary edema. In 2011 the European Society of Intensive Care medicine revised the definition of ARDS based on limitations of the widely used 1994 definition. With the new criteria, ARDS is defined as acute onset (within 1 week) of respiratory symptoms, presence of

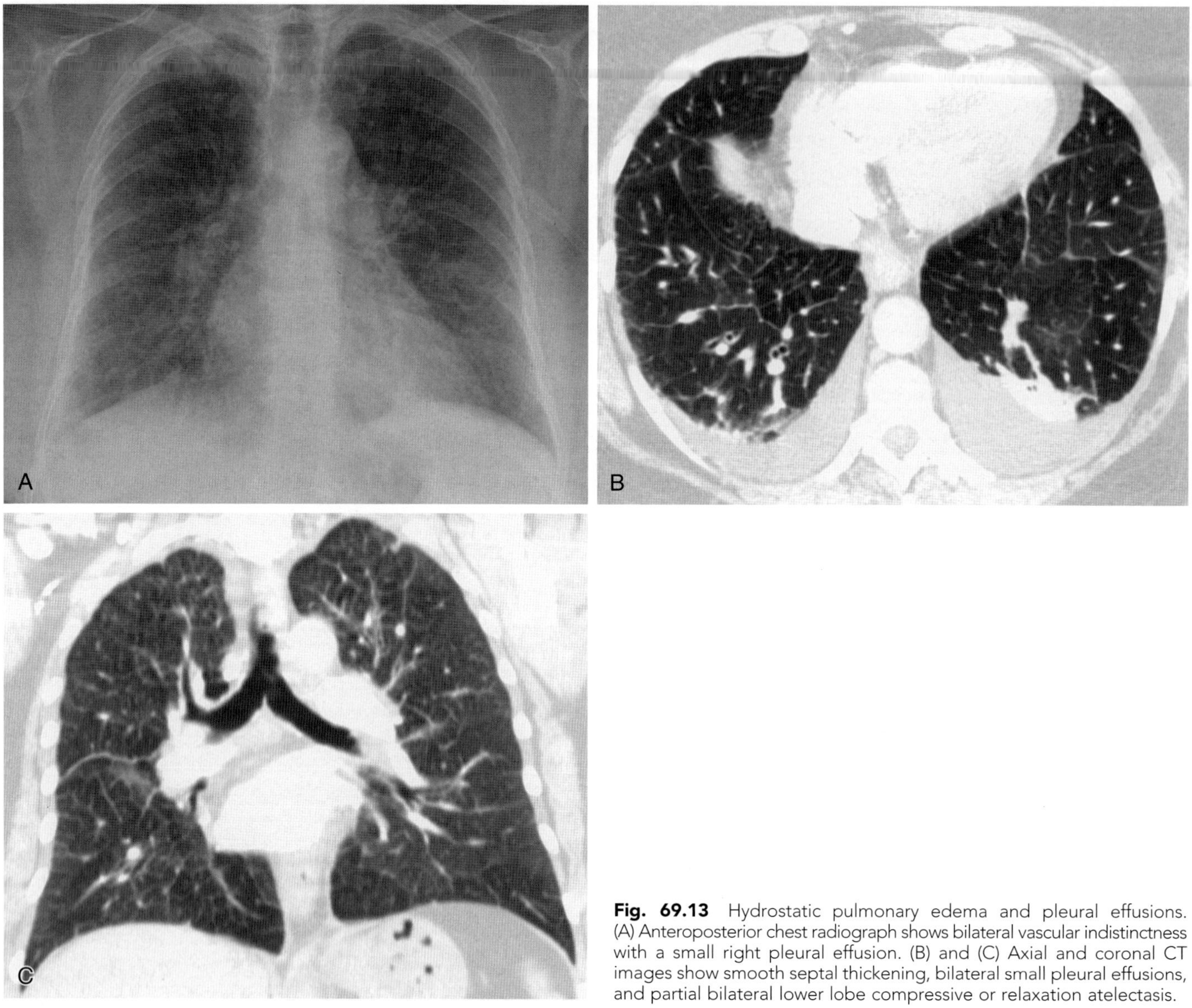

Fig. 69.13 Hydrostatic pulmonary edema and pleural effusions. (A) Anteroposterior chest radiograph shows bilateral vascular indistinctness with a small right pleural effusion. (B) and (C) Axial and coronal CT images show smooth septal thickening, bilateral small pleural effusions, and partial bilateral lower lobe compressive or relaxation atelectasis.

bilateral parenchymal opacities, respiratory failure not explained by hydrostatic edema, and a partial pressure of oxygen in arterial blood/forced inspiratory oxygen (PaO_2/FiO_2) ratio less than 300 mm Hg. ARDS can be further classified as mild/moderate/severe based on the actual PaO_2/FiO_2 ratio, and the previously used term *acute lung injury* has been discarded.[18]

The specific site of injury is the alveolar-capillary membrane. The capillary endothelium becomes permeable, allowing transcapillary migration of proteinaceous fluid and inflammatory cells, such as neutrophils, into the interstitium. Injury also affects the alveolar basement membrane, which becomes denuded. The repair process results in hyaline membrane formation and diffuse alveolar damage.[19] Causes for development of ARDS may be due to direct pulmonary injury (i.e., pneumonia or aspiration) but are often systemically induced (i.e., sepsis, trauma, pancreatitis).

RADIOGRAPHY

Radiographically, patchy ground-glass and consolidative opacities are present within the first 24 hours, and the findings become diffuse within 3 days (Fig. 69.16). Lung volumes are decreased, and air bronchograms are commonly identified. The diagnosis of ARDS requires the presence of new bilateral opacities, and the most common imaging pattern is that of increased permeability pulmonary edema.

COMPUTED TOMOGRAPHY

CT provides important information about the extent and severity of ARDS and resultant complications, such as pneumothorax and pneumonia. ARDS is the prototype of increased permeability pulmonary edema, so the hallmark CT findings demonstrate this pattern. The consolidative opacities are often in a dependent distribution and tend to spare the apices (see Fig. 69.16).[20] Pulmonary causes of ARDS result in relatively asymmetric, patchy, ground-glass, and consolidative opacities. In contrast, extrapulmonary etiologies of ARDS generally primarily manifest as symmetric extensive ground-glass opacities. Patchy foci of relatively normal-appearing parenchyma are often present. CT identifies early indicators of barotrauma, such as small pneumothoraces,

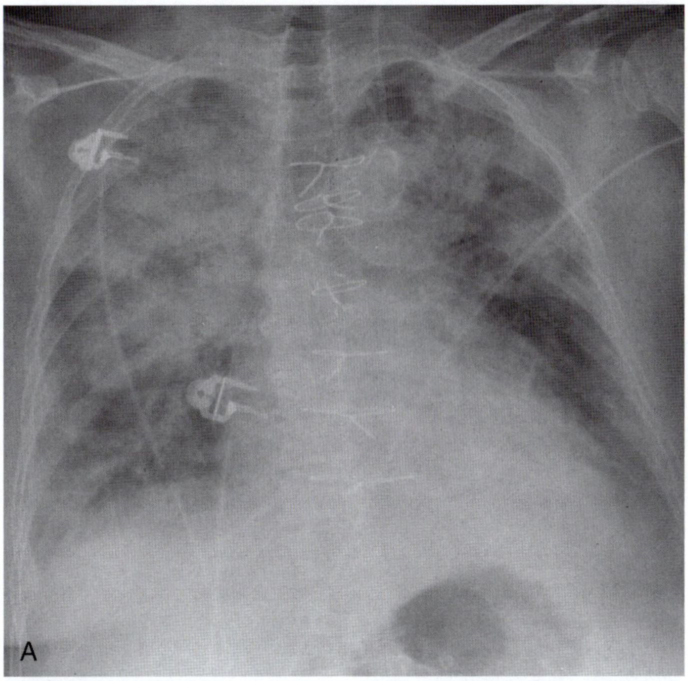

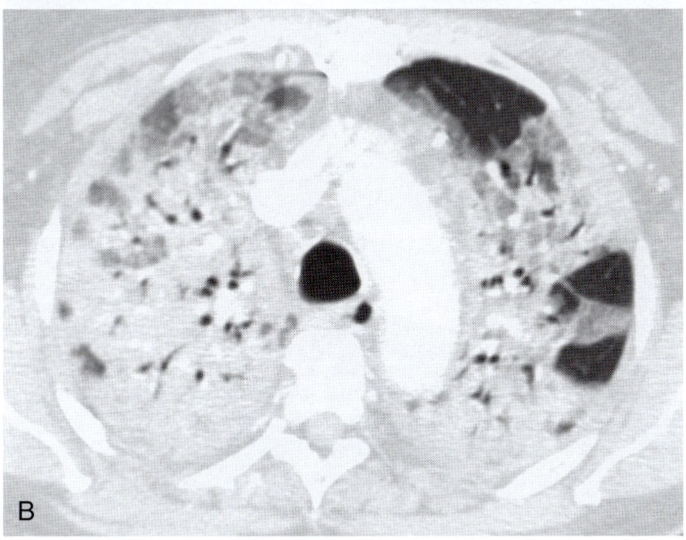

Fig. 69.14 Postoperative noncardiogenic pulmonary edema. (A) Anteroposterior chest radiograph shows bilateral asymmetric patchy consolidation with upper lung zone predominance. (B) CT scan shows bilateral asymmetric dense consolidation and ground-glass opacities.

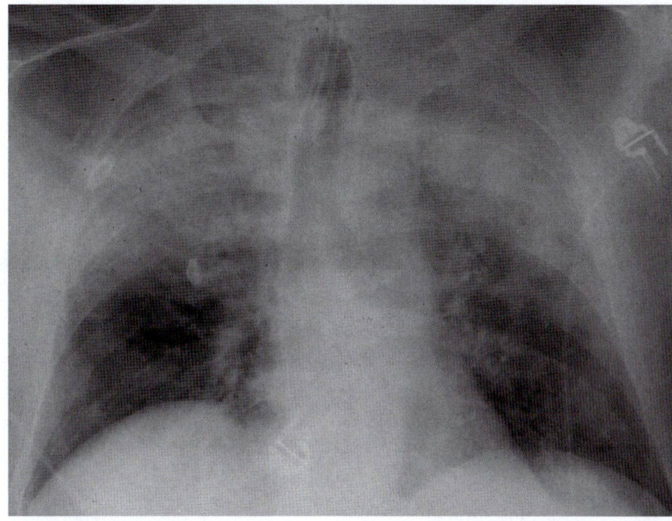

Fig. 69.15 Transfusion-related acute lung injury. Anteroposterior chest radiograph obtained 5 hours after blood transfusion shows extensive bilateral consolidation with upper lung zone predominance requiring intubation.

pneumomediastinum, or pneumatoceles, which may be obscured on a portable AP radiograph. Patients who enter the recovery phase of diffuse alveolar damage often show replacement of ground-glass and consolidative opacities with reticular opacities, traction bronchiectasis, and fibrosis (Fig. 69.17). Bronchiectasis was reported in 92% of affected lobes in one study.[21]

Pleural Processes

PNEUMOTHORAX

Pneumothorax, defined as air between the visceral and parietal pleura, commonly occurs in ICU patients. Etiologies include trauma, complication from central line placement/thoracentesis, barotrauma from positive pressure ventilation, and occasionally pulmonary infections. Given that pneumothoraces manifest atypically in ICU patients and that delayed diagnosis of pneumothorax is more likely to lead to tension pneumothorax in intubated patients,[22] being familiar with the radiographic manifestations of pneumothorax in ICU patients is extremely important.

Radiography

Pneumothoraces are difficult to detect in recumbent patients because the intrapleural air collects anteriorly across the chest. Therefore the classic visceral pleural line may not be identified.

Radiographic findings in a recumbent patient include a medial or lateral deep sulcus sign or increased lucency over the diaphragm because 38% and 26% of pneumothoraces in supine patients occur in anteromedial and subpulmonic regions, respectively (Figs. 69.18 and 69.19).[23] Decubitus radiographs or bedside ultrasound can be performed to confirm the presence or absence of a pneumothorax in difficult cases.

A common pitfall in the diagnosis of pneumothorax in an ICU patient is a skin fold. The skin fold manifests as an edge or interface rather than the line of the visceral pleura. Pulmonary vessels are often seen peripheral to the skin fold, indicating that this does not represent a visceral pleural line (Fig. 69.20).

Patients with ARDS have an increased incidence of pneumothorax resulting from poor lung compliance and elevated mean airway pressures while on mechanical ventilation. However, because of the increased stiffness of the lungs, there is often little shift of the mediastinum. Although diagnosis of a tension pneumothorax is based on clinical findings, the chest radiograph usually suggests the diagnosis. Depression of the hemidiaphragm is the most reliable sign for diagnosing a tension pneumothorax (Fig. 69.21). It is crucial to detect a small basilar pneumothorax in a mechanically ventilated patient because most (60%–96%) pneumothoraces in ventilated patients progress to tension.[24] Therefore the inferior-most aspect of the costophrenic angles ideally should be visualized on every radiograph in a supine mechanically ventilated patient.

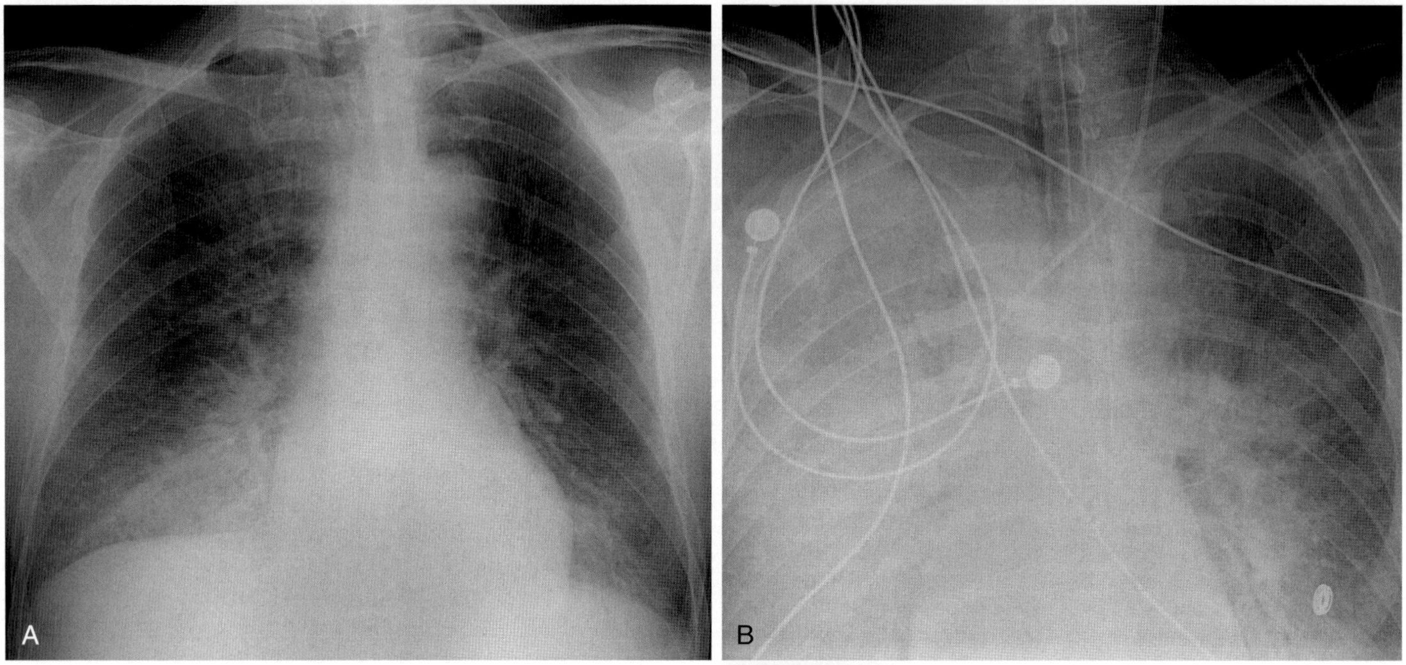

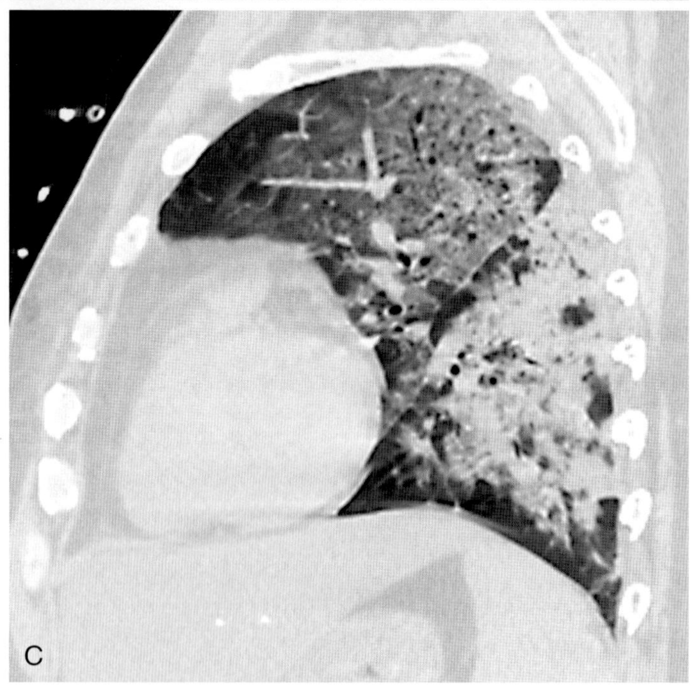

Fig. 69.16 Diffuse alveolar damage/acute respiratory distress syndrome (ARDS). (A) Anteroposterior (AP) radiograph shows right greater than left lower lobe consolidation compatible with pneumonia. (B) Subsequent AP chest radiograph shows interval endotracheal intubation and marked progression of diffuse right greater than left consolidation typical of diffuse alveolar damage with ARDS. Asymmetric opacities with ARDS typically occur with pulmonary causes, whereas symmetric opacities are more typical of nonpulmonary causes of diffuse alveolar damage. (C) Sagittal reformatted CT from a different patient with ARDS shows characteristic ventrodorsal and cephalocaudal gradient of ground-glass opacity and consolidation. *(Reproduced with permission from Gutschow S, Walker C. Acute thoracic conditions in the intensive care unit. In: Shepard J-A.* Thoracic Imaging: The Requisites. *3rd ed. St. Louis: Elsevier; 2018.)*

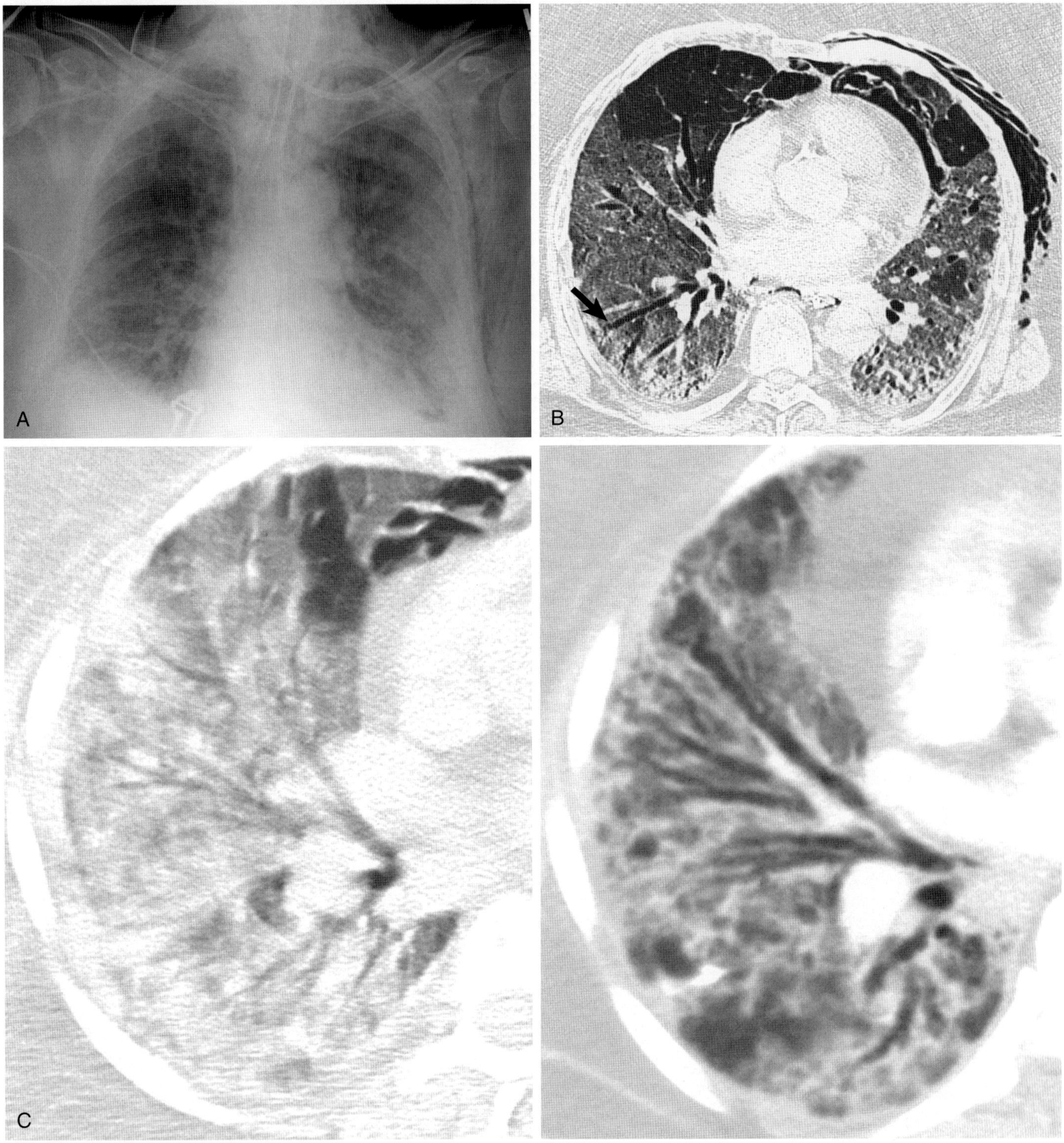

Fig. 69.17 Acute respiratory distress syndrome developing after vascular surgery. (A) Anteroposterior chest radiograph shows extensive bilateral hazy opacities, pneumomediastinum, left chest wall and neck soft tissue gas, an endotracheal tube, right subclavian catheter, and a feeding tube. (B) CT scan in the same patient shows extensive dependent ground-glass opacities, stretching and dilation of bronchi *(arrow)*, pneumomediastinum, and left chest wall soft tissue gas. Note sharp demarcation between normal and abnormal lung parenchyma. (C) Composite image from a different patient demonstrating acute ground-glass opacities of acute respiratory distress syndrome *(left image)*, followed by development of fibrotic changes and traction bronchiectasis 2 weeks later *(right image)*.

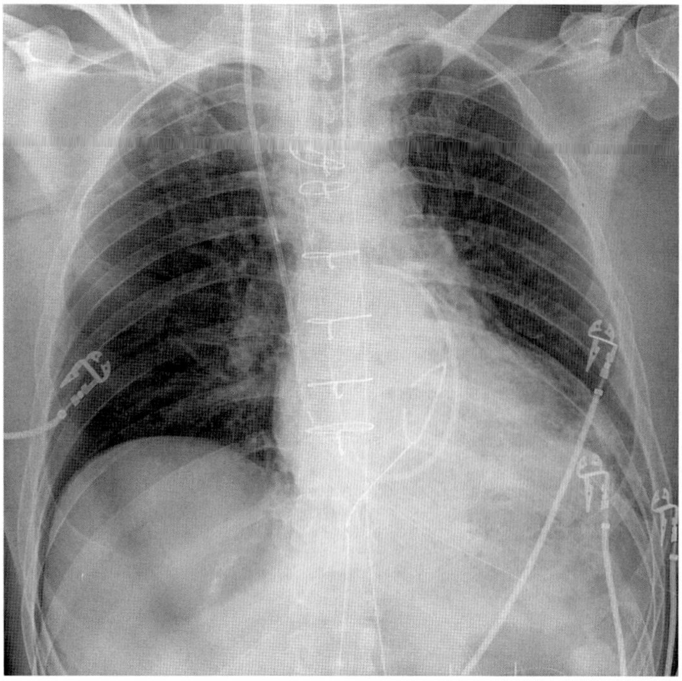

Fig. 69.18 Pneumothorax, lateral deep sulcus sign. Anteroposterior radiograph shows a right deep sulcus sign and lucency overlying the liver in keeping with subpulmonic pneumothorax. The visceral pleural line is faintly visualized laterally. *(Reproduced with permission from Gutschow S, Walker C. Acute thoracic conditions in the intensive care unit. In: Shepard J-A.* Thoracic Imaging: The Requisites. *3rd ed. St. Louis: Elsevier; 2018.)*

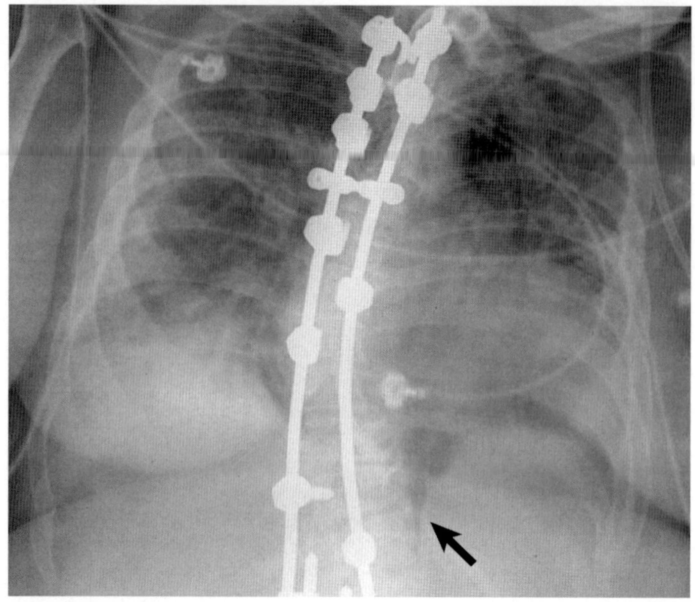

Fig. 69.19 Pneumothorax, medial deep sulcus sign. Anteroposterior chest radiograph shows a lucency extending into the medial left costophrenic sulcus *(arrow).*

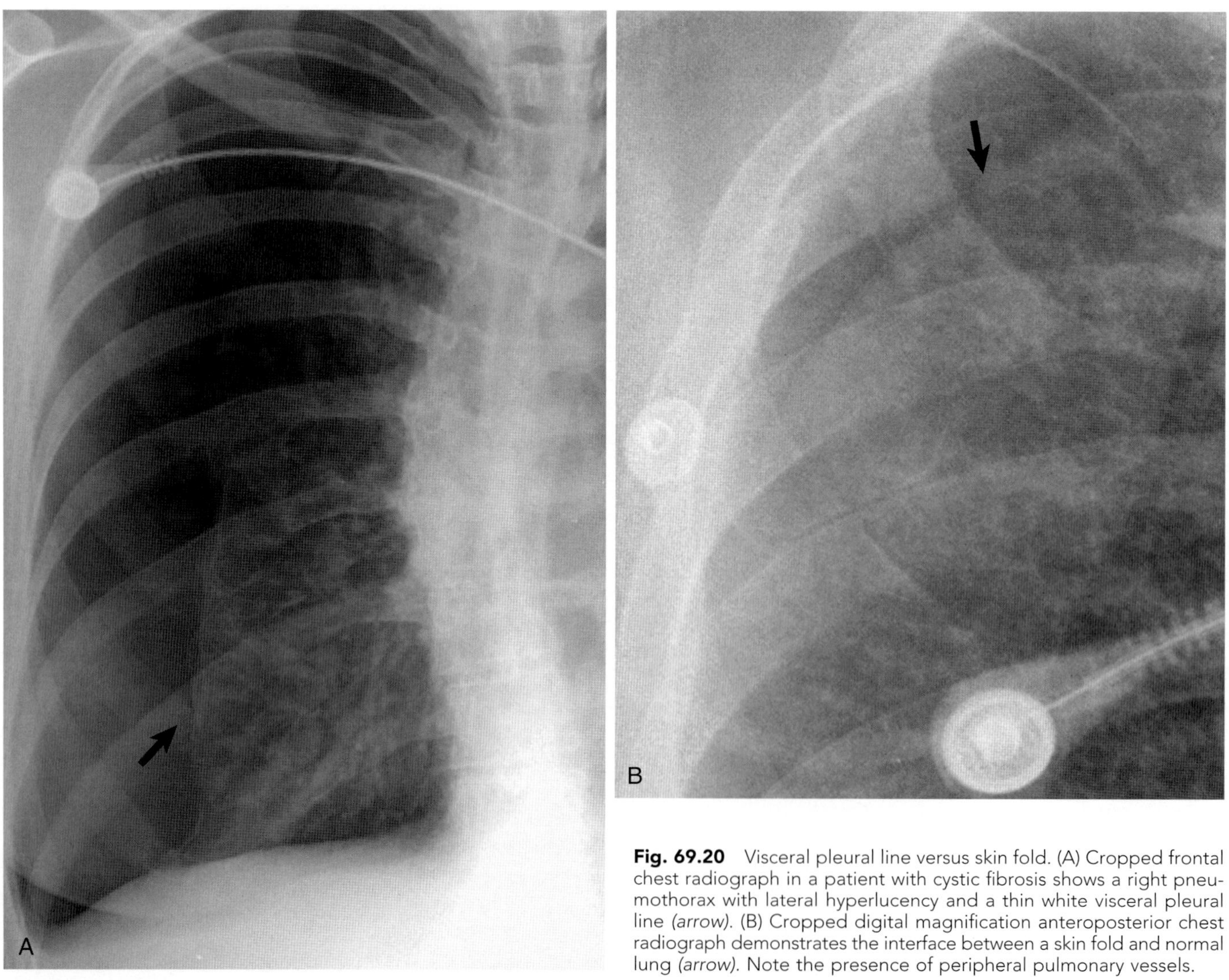

Fig. 69.20 Visceral pleural line versus skin fold. (A) Cropped frontal chest radiograph in a patient with cystic fibrosis shows a right pneumothorax with lateral hyperlucency and a thin white visceral pleural line *(arrow)*. (B) Cropped digital magnification anteroposterior chest radiograph demonstrates the interface between a skin fold and normal lung *(arrow)*. Note the presence of peripheral pulmonary vessels.

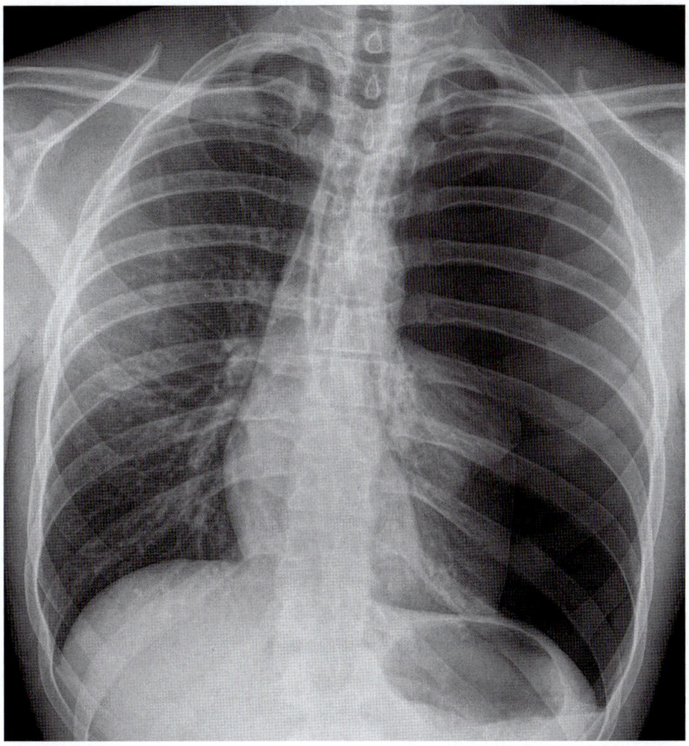

Fig. 69.21 Tension pneumothorax. Anteroposterior radiograph reveals a large left pneumothorax with contralateral mediastinal and tracheal shift. Note left rib interspace widening and left hemidiaphragm depression, all findings that raise the possibility of tension physiology, which was confirmed clinically. *(Reproduced with permission from Gutschow S, Walker C. Acute thoracic conditions in the intensive care unit. In: Shepard J-A.* Thoracic Imaging: The Requisites. *3rd ed. St. Louis: Elsevier; 2018.)*

Ultrasonography

Given that radiography commonly misses small pneumothoraces in supine critically ill patients, ultrasound is often obtained as the follow-up examination of choice when a pneumothorax is suspected but not detected by radiography and the patient is too unstable to obtain a CT scan. In a study by Lichtenstein and colleagues,[25] three dynamic and static sonographic signs were used in the evaluation of pneumothorax (absence of lung sliding, the A line sign, and the lung point) and found that in the diagnosis of occult pneumothorax, thoracic sonography decreased the need for evaluation by CT.

PLEURAL EFFUSION

Small collections of pleural fluid are common in ICU patients. When small and bilateral, these collections most often represent transudative effusions secondary to hypervolemia in the setting of renal failure, cardiomyopathy, cirrhosis, or aggressive fluid resuscitation. Alternatively, a large unilateral effusion is often an exudative effusion secondary to infection, hemothorax, or malignancy. Transudative effusions can resolve with diuresis, whereas exudative effusions often require drainage and treatment of the underlying disease.

Radiography

It has been reported that effusions can be detected on supine chest radiographs with an accuracy of 67% to 95%.[26] Small effusions are often identified by characteristic blunting or

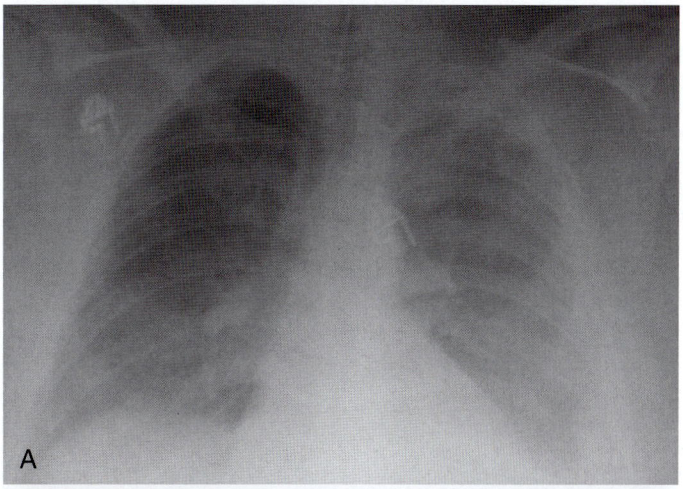

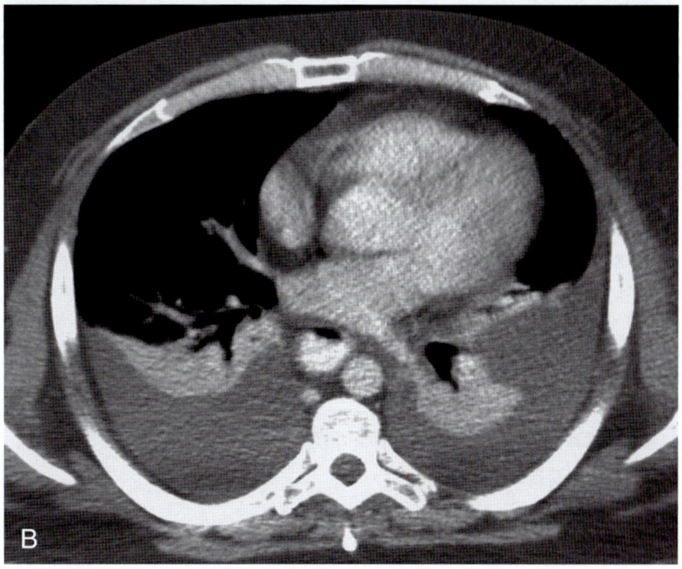

Fig. 69.22 Pleural effusions. (A) Supine anteroposterior chest radiograph shows bilateral (left greater than right) hazy "veil-like" opacities. (B) Contrast-enhanced CT scan shows bilateral large layering pleural effusions without pleural enhancement, suggesting transudative effusions. The volume of pleural fluid is often underestimated on supine radiographs.

obscuration of the costophrenic angles. Larger effusions in a supine patient are recognized by haziness or a veil-like opacity (Fig. 69.22). Effusions also may track over the lung apex or into a fissure. Loculated pleural fluid appears as a homogeneous opacity with a convex border. Lateral decubitus radiographs (affected side down) may help determine whether a pleural fluid collection is loculated or free flowing. The volume and complexity of pleural fluid are often underestimated on supine radiographs (Fig. 69.23).

Ultrasonography

Ultrasound has become the preferred method in the ICU with which to evaluate and sample pleural effusions.[27] Echogenic effusions and presence of fibrinous septations are diagnostic for exudative effusions.

Computed Tomography

CT is useful in evaluating loculated pleural fluid collections that may require surgical intervention, paramediastinal pleural

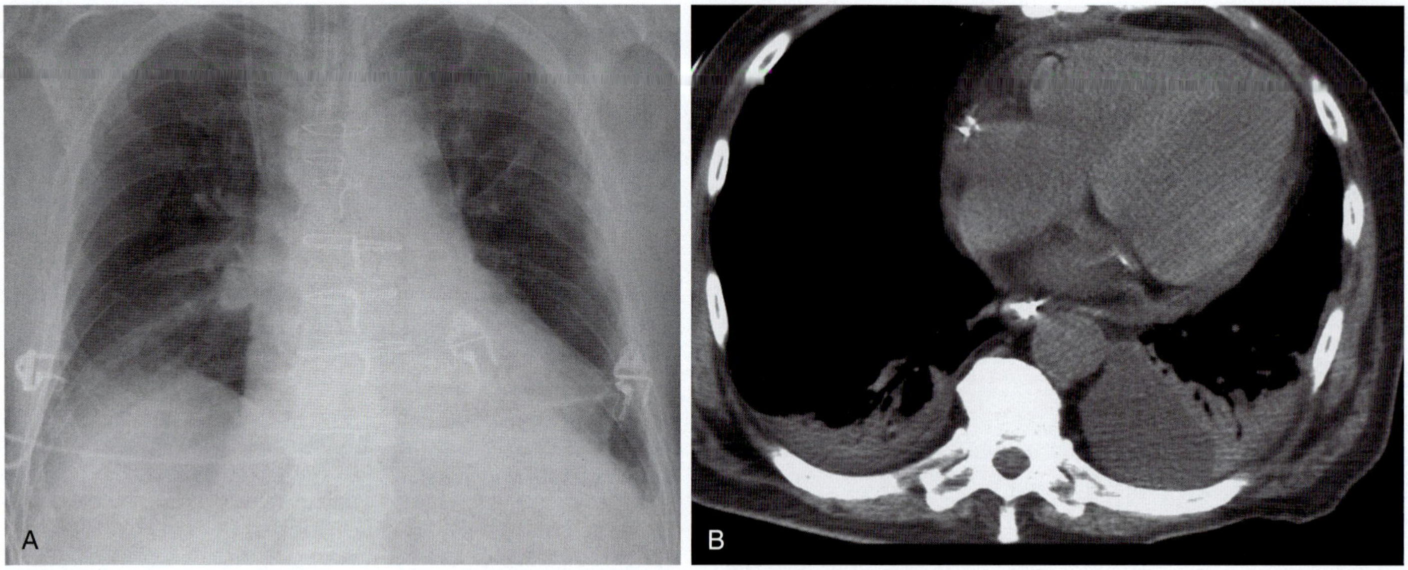

Fig. 69.23 Loculated retrocardiac pleural effusion. (A) Anteroposterior chest radiograph shows bibasilar and retrocardiac opacities, consistent with atelectasis. (B) Nonenhanced CT scan of the chest in the same patient reveals loculated left medial pleural fluid collection and bilateral-dependent atelectasis. A small right pleural effusion is also evident.

collections that may require CT-guided tube thoracostomy placement, and in differentiating pleural from parenchymal disease. With intravenous contrast media, exudative effusions usually demonstrate enhancement of the visceral pleura (Fig. 69.24). Increased density of the fluid suggests a hemothorax.

Support Equipment and Iatrogenic Complications

It is crucial on each ICU radiograph to accurately assess the location of support equipment for early recognition of potential complications. Because support equipment can migrate or become dislodged, it is just as important to carefully evaluate the location of all invasive devices on follow-up radiographs as it is on the initial radiograph. Specific tools for assessing endotracheal tubes, intravascular catheters, orogastric or nasogastric tubes, chest tubes/mediastinal drains, and ventricular assist devices are discussed in detail later.

Endotracheal Tubes

The tip of the endotracheal tube ideally should be situated below the clavicular heads but at least 2 cm above the carina when the neck is in neutral position. If the neck is flexed, the tube can migrate 2 cm caudally, whereas extension of the neck can cause 2 cm of cephalad migration. If an endotracheal tube is advanced too far, it typically extends into the right main bronchus (Fig. 69.25), which may result in left lung and right upper lobe collapse.

The balloon cuff should be assessed on every radiograph to ensure that it is not overinflated (Fig. 69.26). A balloon cuff-to-tracheal lumen ratio greater than 1.5 has a high likelihood of causing long-term tracheal complications, such as tracheal stenosis (see Fig. 69.26B and 69.26C).[28] Acute complications of endotracheal tube placement include inadvertent esophageal placement, aspiration of gastric contents, dislodging of teeth or fillings (with subsequent bronchial aspiration), and pneumothorax.[29] Pneumomediastinum occasionally can be identified after uncomplicated tracheostomy tube placement (Fig. 69.27).

Intravascular Catheters

Central venous catheters are most commonly inserted into the internal jugular or subclavian veins. The tip of the central venous catheter should be located between the origin of the superior vena cava (SVC; located below the anterior first rib on the chest radiograph) and the right atrium.[30] However, Cadman and colleagues[31] found that central venous catheter tips located within the upper one-third of the SVC were 16 times more likely to thrombose than were catheters with tips in the lower one-third of the SVC. Placement of a central venous catheter too distally, as in the right atrium, is more likely to cause arrhythmias, such as atrial fibrillation. Therefore catheter tip placement in the lower SVC or at the superior cavoatrial junction is ideal.

Aberrant placement of central venous catheters includes placement into normal smaller branch veins or anomalous veins, such as a persistent left SVC (Fig. 69.28). Other important aberrant placements to consider are intraarterial and extravascular placements, including within the pleural space. As a general rule, if the course of a catheter is not clearly within the expected course of a vein, aberrant placement should be considered. On AP chest radiographs a subclavian venous catheter should always course below or posterior to the clavicle. If a radiograph shows a catheter coursing above the clavicle, one should consider the possibility of subclavian artery or extravascular placement (Figs. 69.29 and 69.30), either of which can be confirmed or excluded by transducing a central venous pressure or secondarily by obtaining a blood gas from the catheter. Post–device placement radiographs should always be assessed for signs of pneumothorax, hemothorax, or increased mediastinal density suggesting a mediastinal hematoma (Fig. 69.31).

Pulmonary artery (Swan-Ganz) catheters are occasionally placed for evaluation of pulmonary capillary wedge pressure and cardiac output. The tip should be located in the main, right,

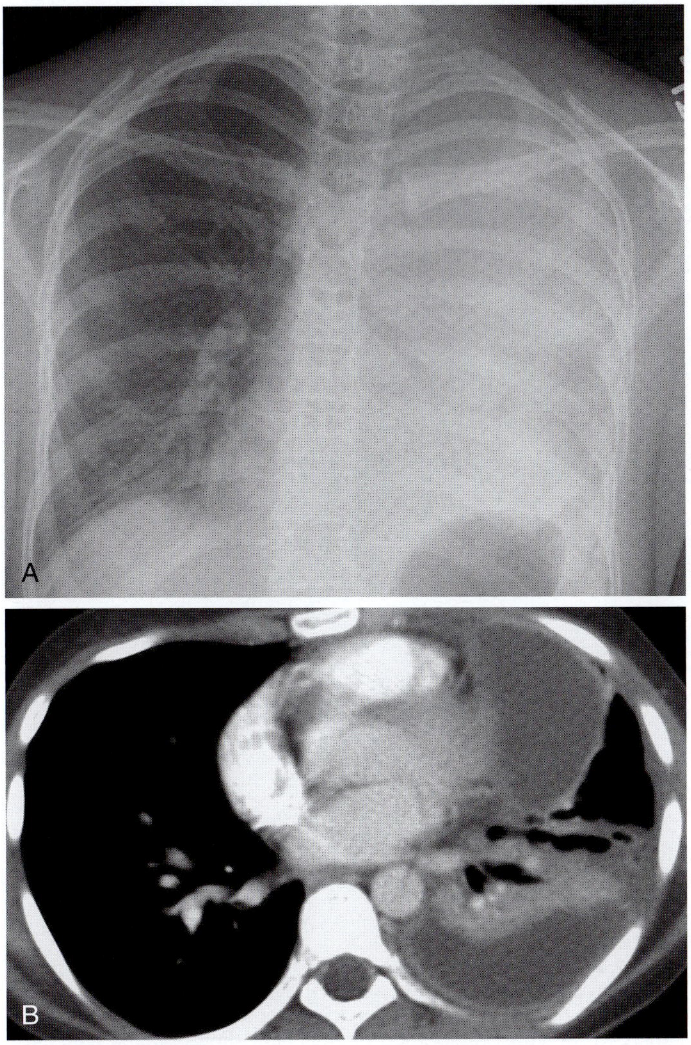

Fig. 69.24 Empyema and bronchopleural fistula. (A) Frontal chest radiograph in a patient with recent pneumonia shows complete opacification of the left hemithorax. (B) Contrast-enhanced CT scan of the chest shows a large multiloculated left pleural effusion with gas and abnormal parietal pleural enhancement, consistent with postpneumonic bronchopleural fistula and empyema.

or left pulmonary artery and should not be distal to the proximal interlobar pulmonary artery. Approximately 24% of these catheters are malpositioned on the initial chest radiograph and need to be repositioned.[32] Additional complications of pulmonary artery catheter placement include arrhythmias, intracardiac knotting, pulmonary artery thrombosis, pulmonary artery rupture, cardiac perforation, and pulmonary hemorrhage (Fig. 69.32).

Intraaortic balloon pumps are used to treat cardiogenic shock. These devices increase coronary perfusion and decrease cardiac afterload. The balloon inflates during diastole and deflates in systole, which causes a sudden drop in afterload resulting in increased stroke volume and coronary perfusion. The tip should be in the upper descending thoracic aorta, approximately 1 to 2 cm distal to the origin of the left subclavian artery (Fig. 69.33). If the tip is too proximal, it may extend into a great vessel and occlude the vessel. If the tip is too distal, the inferior portion of the balloon may obstruct the renal arteries, and it may not function appropriately to decrease afterload and increase coronary

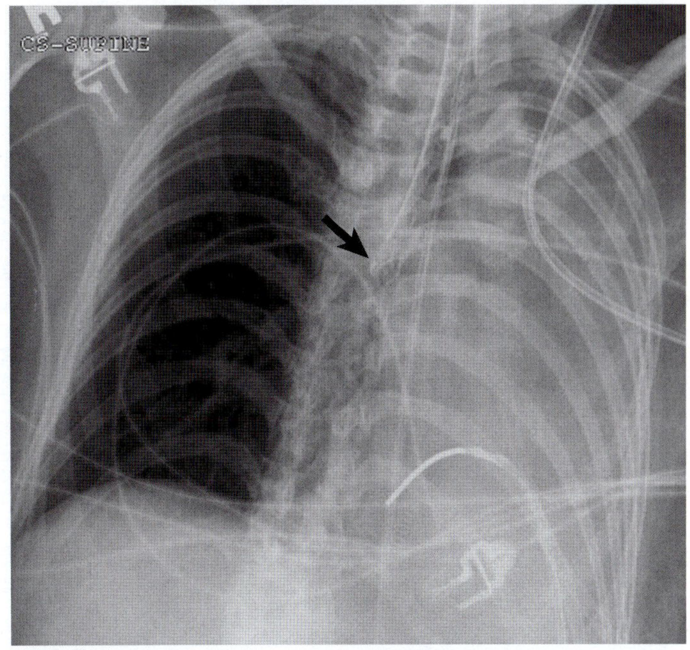

Fig. 69.25 Right main bronchial intubation. Anteroposterior chest radiograph shows the endotracheal tube tip within the right main bronchus *(arrow)*, resulting in left lung collapse with associated leftward mediastinal shift.

perfusion. A tip greater than 5 cm below the aortic arch or below T5 to T6 is highly predictive of major complications.[33]

Extracorporeal membrane oxygenation (ECMO) provides short-term support for patients in cardiopulmonary (venoarterial) or respiratory (venovenous) failure.[34] In both types, percutaneous cannulas are placed within large central veins to divert blood for oxygenation. In central venoarterial ECMO, venous blood is diverted via a central catheter in the right atrium and returned to the ascending aorta through an arterial cannula (Fig. 69.34). In venovenous ECMO, blood is diverted through a cannula placed in the femoral or internal jugular vein and is returned to the same vein through a dual-lumen system or returned to a different vein via a separate catheter (see Fig. 69.34B). Common complications of ECMO cannulation catheters are similar to those of typical central venous catheters, although arterial dissection, thrombosis, and pseudoaneurysm are additional considerations for venoarterial ECMO catheters.

Orogastric, Nasogastric, and Feeding Tubes

Gastric and feeding tubes are commonly used for suction, feeding, and pharmaceutical administration in the ICU. A feeding tube is best differentiated from a nasogastric or orogastric tube by its larger size and weighted tip (Fig. 69.35). A post–placement radiograph is the standard of care because malplacement can have dire consequences. The gastric or feeding tube should follow the midline or immediate paramedian course of the esophagus within the posterior mediastinum to the diaphragm. It is important that the most proximal side-hole of the gastric tube, which is located several cm proximal to the tip, be placed below the gastroesophageal junction; otherwise, food and caustic medications will be delivered into the esophagus. Feeding tube tips should be within the distal stomach or proximal duodenum.

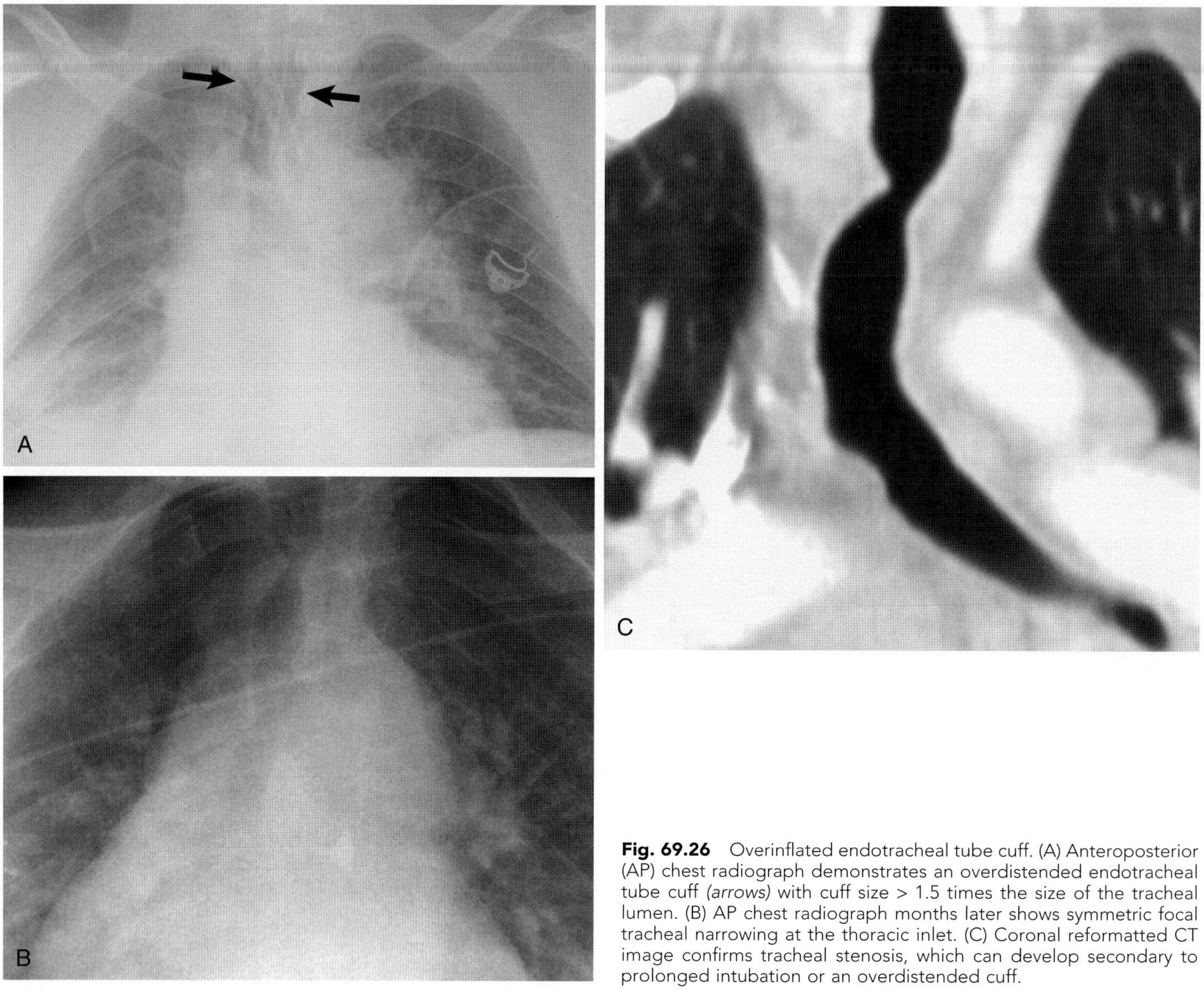

Fig. 69.26 Overinflated endotracheal tube cuff. (A) Anteroposterior (AP) chest radiograph demonstrates an overdistended endotracheal tube cuff *(arrows)* with cuff size > 1.5 times the size of the tracheal lumen. (B) AP chest radiograph months later shows symmetric focal tracheal narrowing at the thoracic inlet. (C) Coronal reformatted CT image confirms tracheal stenosis, which can develop secondary to prolonged intubation or an overdistended cuff.

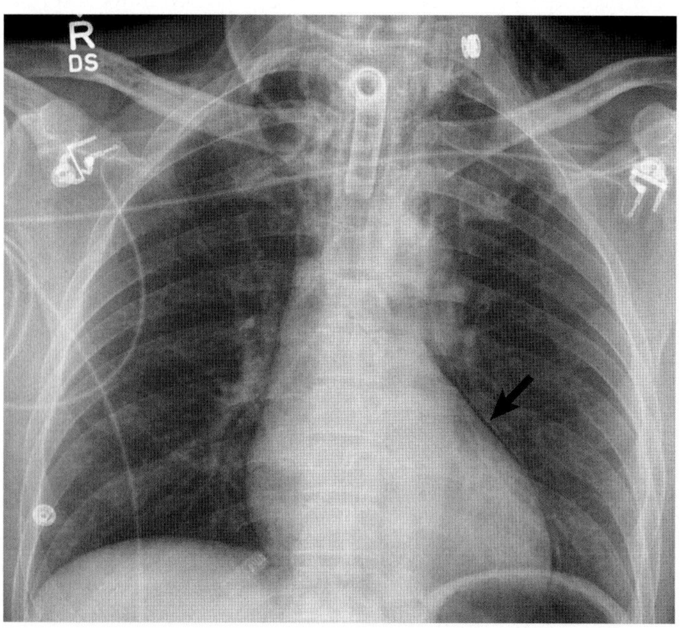

Fig. 69.27 Tracheostomy tube with pneumomediastinum. Anteroposterior chest radiograph shows development of pneumomediastinum *(arrow)* and soft tissue gas in the neck after placement of a tracheostomy tube.

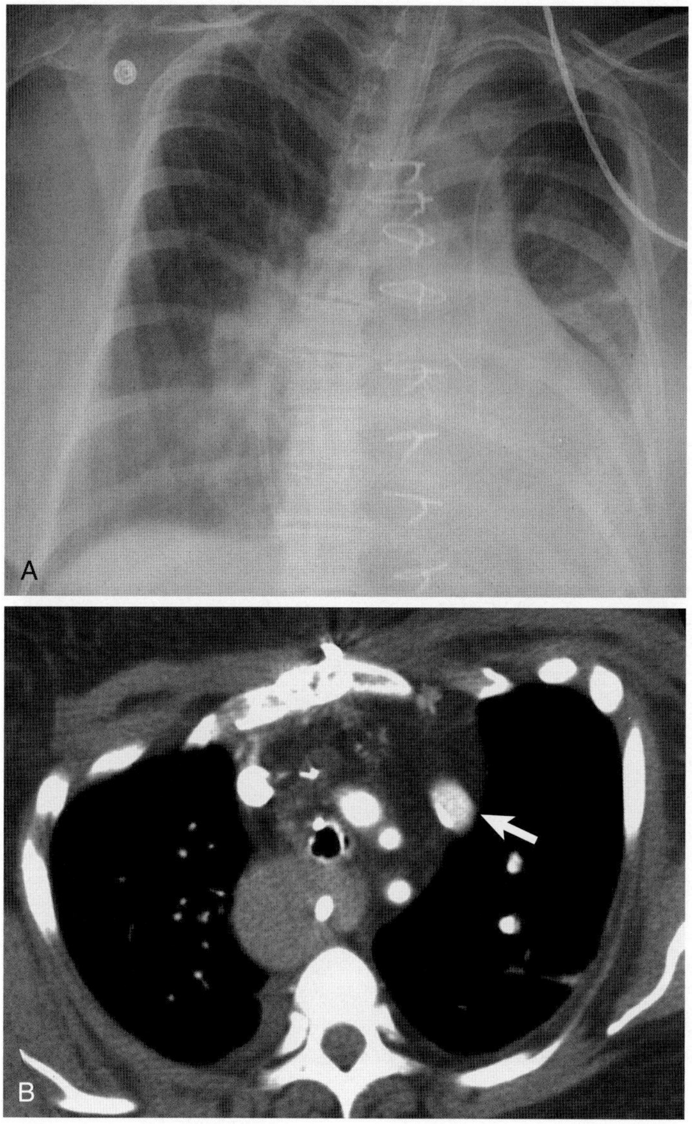

Fig. 69.28 Peripherally inserted central catheter (PICC) placement into persistent left superior vena cava (SVC). (A) Anteroposterior chest radiograph shows PICC placement into the left mediastinum, presumed to be within a persistent left SVC. (B) Contrast-enhanced CT scan of the chest obtained for other reasons confirms PICC within a persistent left SVC *(arrow)*.

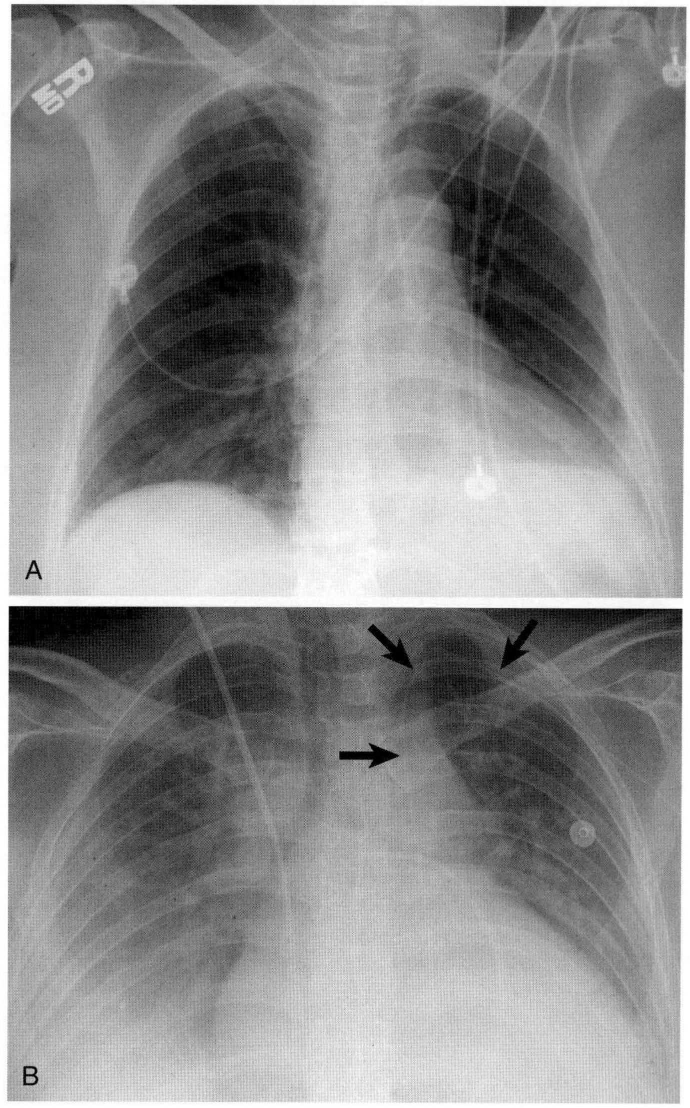

Fig. 69.29 Intraarterial catheter placement. (A) Anteroposterior (AP) chest radiograph after line placement shows right neck catheter coursing leftward within the mediastinum and projecting within the aorta. Waveform and blood gas analysis confirmed intraarterial placement through the carotid artery with the catheter tip in the aorta. (B) AP chest radiograph after left peripherally inserted central catheter placement shows that the catheter extends above the clavicle *(arrows)* consistent with course through the subclavian artery and catheter tip in the descending thoracic aorta.

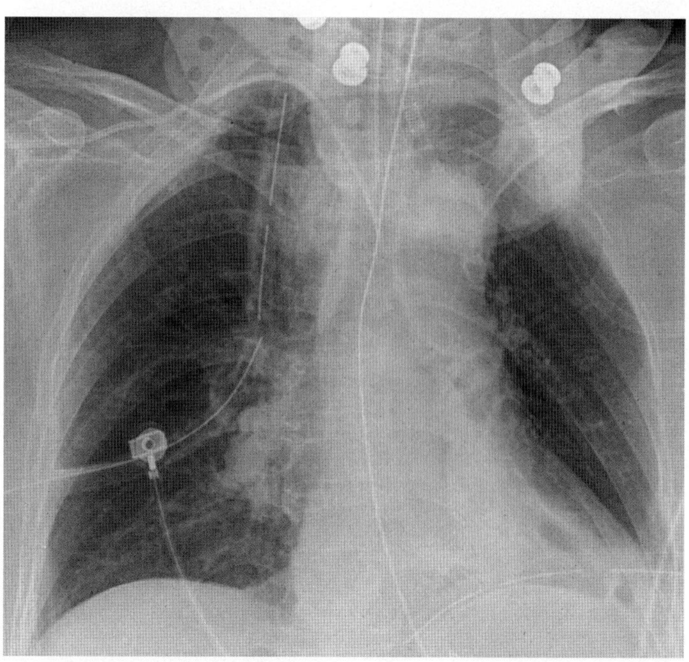

Fig. 69.30 Subclavian arterial line placement. Anteroposterior chest radiograph shows a right subclavian catheter, which courses superior to the clavicle and leftward within the mediastinum. Waveform and blood gas analysis confirmed intraarterial placement.

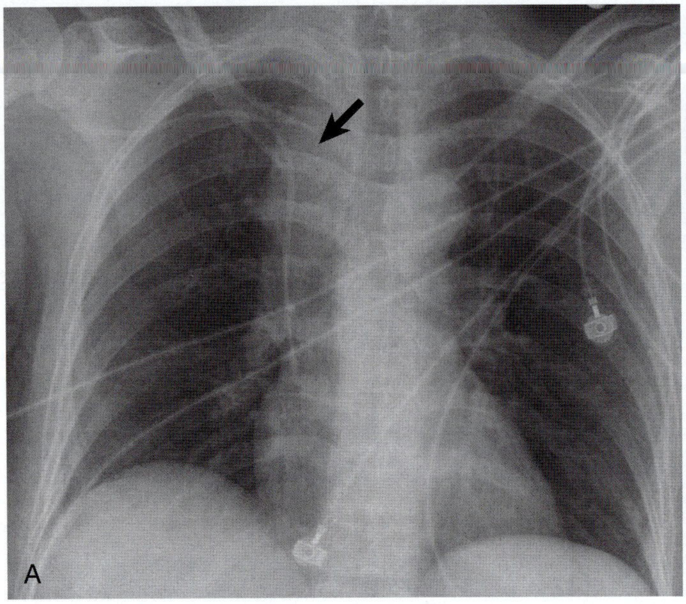

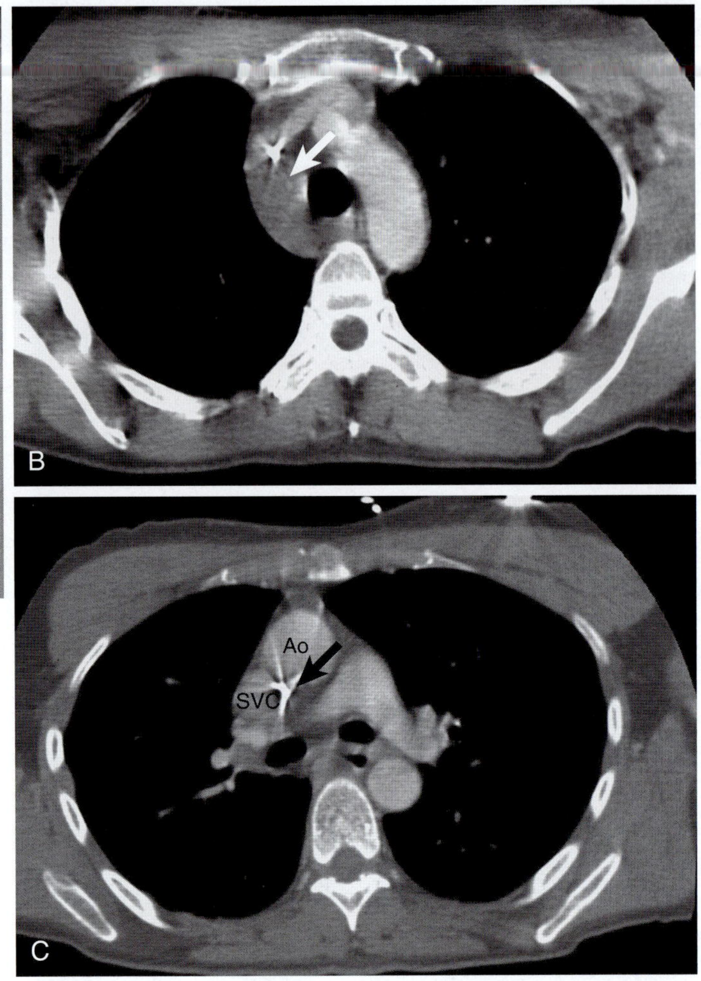

Fig. 69.31 Extravascular catheter placement. (A) Frontal chest radiograph shows right subclavian approach catheter projecting over SVC and increased density of right paratracheal stripe *(arrow)*, concerning for mediastinal hematoma. (B) and (C) Axial contrast-enhanced CT scans of chest show mediastinal hematoma *(white arrow)* and extravascular catheter placement *(black arrow)*. *Ao*, Aorta; *SVC*, superior vena cava.

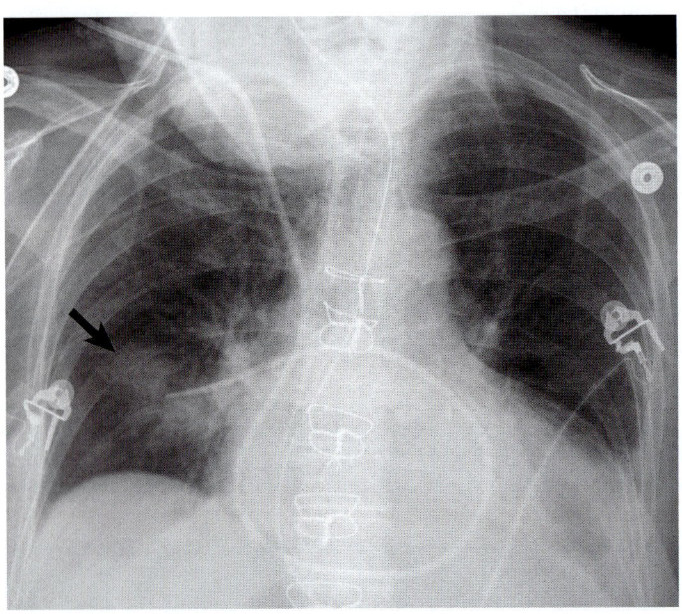

Fig. 69.32 Pulmonary artery catheter–related pulmonary hemorrhage. Anteroposterior chest radiograph in a patient with hematemesis shows pulmonary catheter with tip within distal right lower lobe pulmonary artery branch and surrounding opacity *(arrow)* representing hemorrhage.

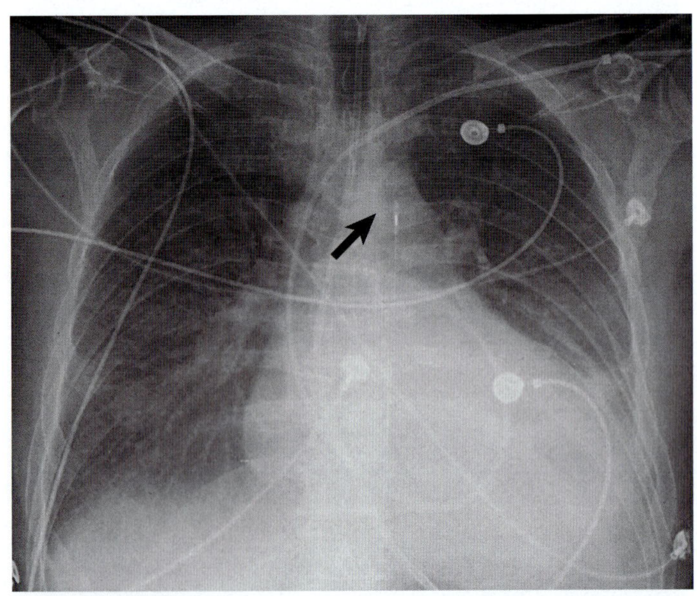

Fig. 69.33 Normal intraaortic balloon pump. Frontal chest radiograph shows normal position of an intraaortic balloon pump tip *(arrow)* in the proximal descending thoracic aorta distal to the left subclavian artery origin.

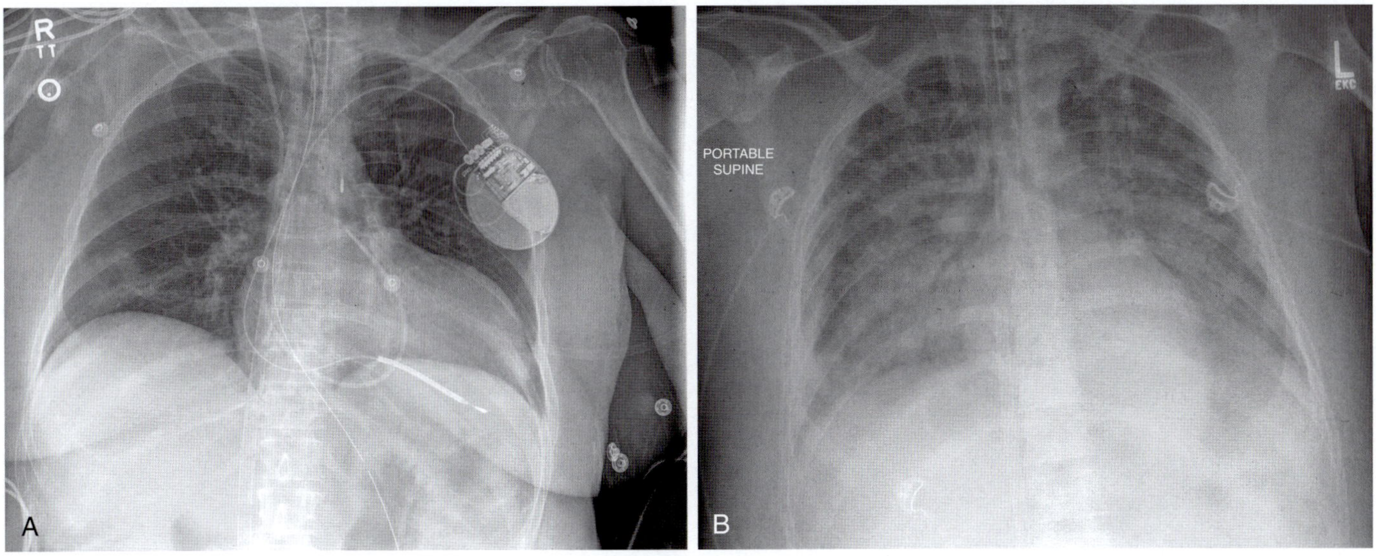

Fig. 69.34 Extracorporeal membrane oxygenation (ECMO) cannulation catheters. (A) Anteroposterior (AP) chest radiograph of a patient with cardiomyopathy on venoarterial ECMO in which the femoral catheter traversing the right atrium and terminating in the superior vena cava diverts venous blood away from the body. Oxygenated blood is pumped into the body via an arterial catheter located in the femoral artery (not pictured). (B) AP chest radiograph in a separate patient with acute respiratory distress syndrome on venovenous ECMO shows a right internal, jugular venous catheter and a separate femoral catheter in which blood is pumped out of the body through one catheter, oxygenated, and then returned to the body through the second catheter.

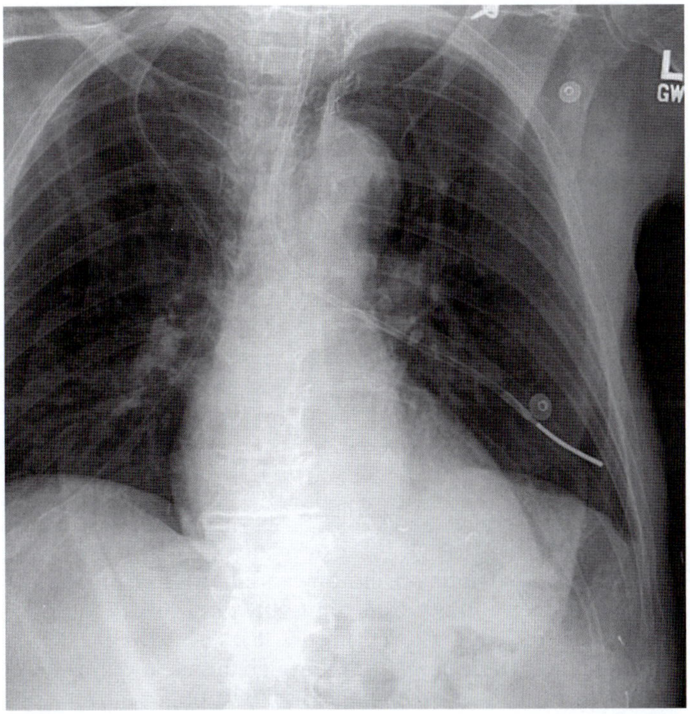

Fig. 69.35 Left lower lobe feeding tube placement. Anteroposterior chest radiograph shows placement of a feeding tube within a distal left lower lobe bronchus.

There is no increased risk of aspiration in tubes placed in the stomach over those placed in the small bowel.[34] Tubes may be coiled within the oropharynx, esophagus, or stomach. Tracheal or bronchial placement can occur and is potentially lethal if nutrition is administered (see Fig. 69.35). If a feeding tube enters the pleural space, it can result in a pneumothorax, which becomes apparent after the tube is extracted.

Chest Tubes/Mediastinal Drains

Tube thoracostomy is most commonly performed in the ICU for evacuation of a pneumothorax or pleural effusion. Because air rises, ideal positioning in the setting of a pneumothorax is an apically directed tube. Placement of inferiorly directed tubes just above the hemidiaphragm is typically performed for removal of pleural fluid (hydrothorax, hemothorax, empyema, etc.) because most fluid collections are gravity dependent. If a loculated fluid collection is being drained, the tip will ideally be placed centrally into the collection for effective evacuation. The most common complication of tube thoracostomy is malposition. It is important that the proximal side-hole or "sentinel eye" (demarcated by an interruption of the radiopaque stripe) be placed within the inner margin of the ribs to allow effective evacuation and to prevent air or fluid from entering the soft tissues of the chest wall (Fig. 69.36). Placement of a chest tube within a fissure can also lead to ineffective evacuation and is often suspected when the tube is noted to take a horizontal course.[29] The dreaded complication of tube thoracostomy is placement into the lung parenchyma, mediastinum, or through the diaphragm and into the liver/spleen (see Fig. 69.36B and C). Mediastinal drains are

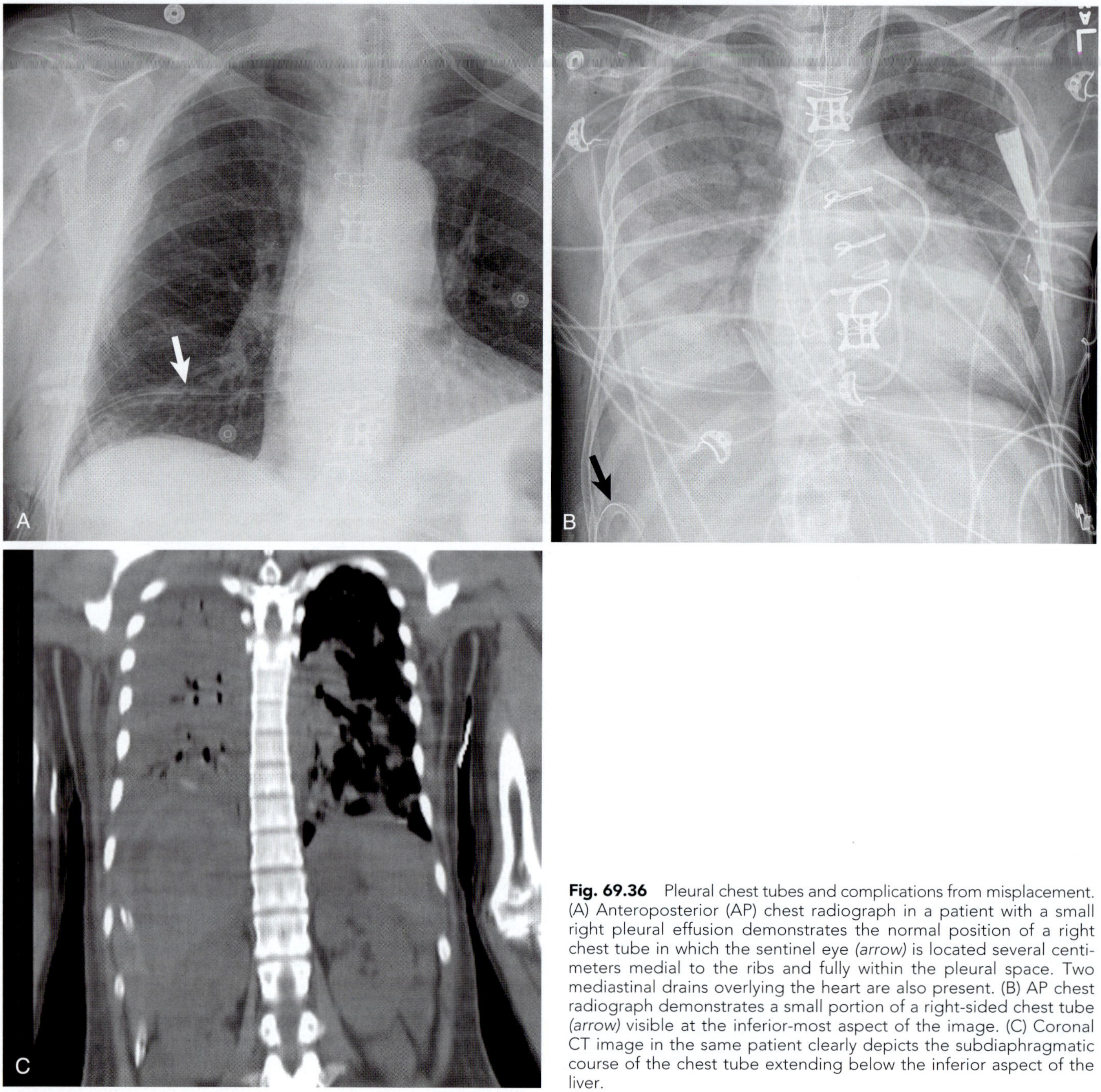

Fig. 69.36 Pleural chest tubes and complications from misplacement. (A) Anteroposterior (AP) chest radiograph in a patient with a small right pleural effusion demonstrates the normal position of a right chest tube in which the sentinel eye *(arrow)* is located several centimeters medial to the ribs and fully within the pleural space. Two mediastinal drains overlying the heart are also present. (B) AP chest radiograph demonstrates a small portion of a right-sided chest tube *(arrow)* visible at the inferior-most aspect of the image. (C) Coronal CT image in the same patient clearly depicts the subdiaphragmatic course of the chest tube extending below the inferior aspect of the liver.

routinely inserted postcardiac surgery to aid in clearance of blood from the mediastinum and to prevent cardiac tamponade. Their appearance is similar to chest tubes, but they may be of a smaller caliber and overlie the heart or mediastinum (Fig. 69.37).

Ventricular Assist Devices

Surgically or percutaneously implanted ventricular assist devices (VADs) are placed in patients with cardiomyopathy as either a bridge to transplant, a bridge to recovery, or for long-term "destination therapy" in those who are ineligible for transplant.[30] VADs can be used to perform the work of the left ventricle (LVAD), right ventricle (RVAD), or bilateral ventricles (BVAD). Blood is diverted into an inflow cannula located in the left ventricular apex and is pumped into the outflow cannula connected to the ascending aorta (Fig. 69.38). The drive line, which provides power to the device, exits through the left lower quadrant of the abdomen and is a common portal of entry for microorganisms.[35] Hemorrhage is the most common complication of LVAD placement (Fig. 69.39). On a chest radiograph, bleeding at the cannula insertion site can be suspected by mediastinal/pericardial enlargement or abnormal contour and density of the mediastinum.[36] Other common complications of VAD placement include infection, thrombosis, and cannula obstruction.

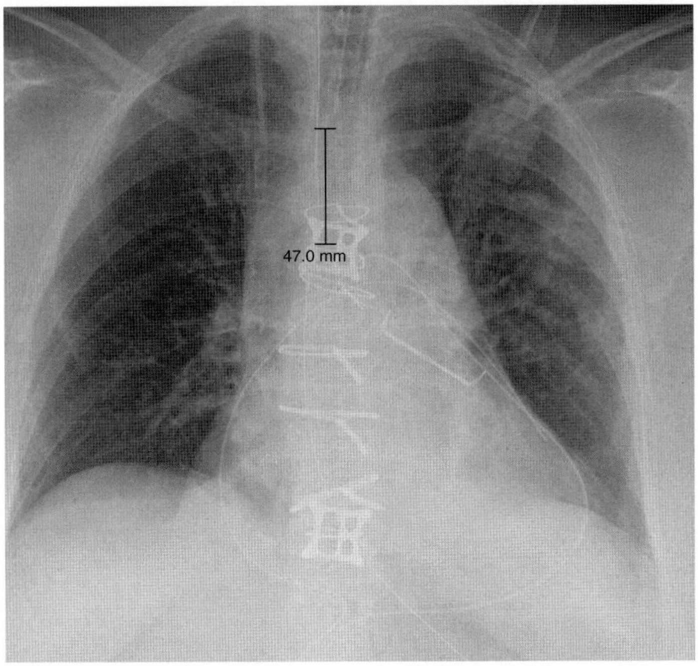

Fig. 69.37 Mediastinal drains. Anteroposterior chest radiograph shows three mediastinal drains overlying the heart. Note the smaller caliber relative to pleural chest tubes (shown on prior figure).

KEY POINTS

- Daily chest radiographs are no longer indicated for intensive care unit (ICU) patients. Radiographs should be obtained on admission after insertion of an external device, such as an endotracheal tube, or for a specific clinical indication.
- If air bronchograms are absent in lobar atelectasis, mucoid impaction is the most likely etiology.
- Volume loss, crowding of vessels or air bronchograms (if present), and intense enhancement help differentiate atelectasis from consolidative processes, such as pneumonia.
- Aspiration manifests as dependent areas of consolidation or tree-in-bud opacities. Aspiration pneumonitis typically resolves spontaneously within 24–48 hours, whereas aspiration pneumonia persists.
- Hydrostatic pulmonary edema is initially characterized by pulmonary vascular indistinctness, subpleural interstitial thickening, septal thickening, cardiomegaly, and pleural effusions. Ground-glass and consolidative opacities develop as the edema progresses.
- Increased permeability pulmonary edema is characterized by extensive ground-glass opacities and consolidation; findings are diffuse when induced by an extrapulmonary cause and patchy when induced by a pulmonary insult.
- Radiographic findings of pneumothorax in a recumbent patient include a deep sulcus sign or increased lucency over the hemidiaphragm.
- Pneumothoraces in patients on mechanical ventilation are at high risk for rapid expansion and/or progressing to tension physiology, necessitating prompt diagnosis and treatment. Short-term follow-up imaging is indicated in patients not receiving tube thoracostomy.
- Pleural effusions in a supine patient are most often recognized on radiographs as a veil-like opacity. Ultrasound is now the preferred method with which to evaluate pleural effusions in ICU patients.
- The position of all support equipment should be assessed on every radiograph, including follow-up imaging, because of the possibility of malplacement as well as the risk of migration/dislodgment, which can result in major complications.

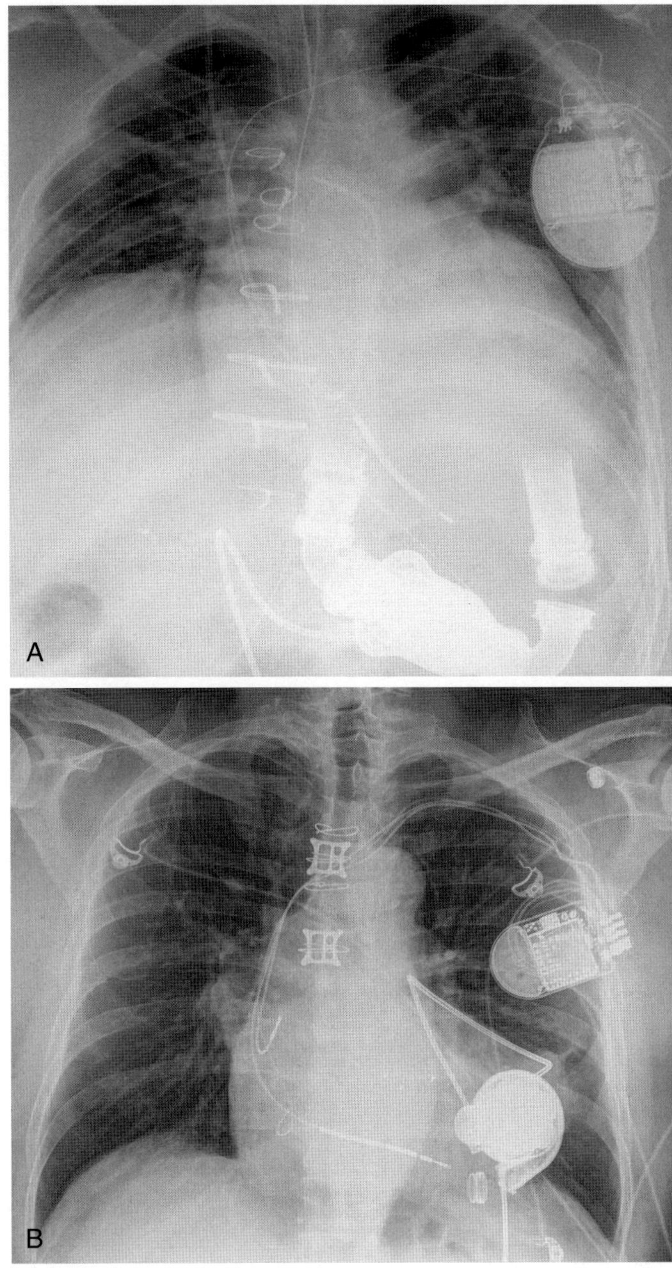

Fig. 69.38 Left ventricular assist devices (LVADs). (A) Anteroposterior (AP) chest radiograph shows a second-generation HeartMate II LVAD (Thoratec, Pleasanton, CA) in which the small inflow cannula is located at the left ventricular apex and the longer outflow cannula extends toward the ascending aorta. The distal-most portion of the outflow cannula that inserts into the ascending aorta is not radiopaque and is therefore not seen. (B) AP chest radiograph shows the HeartWare third-generation LVAD (Medtronic, Minneapolis, MN), which contains an integrated inflow and outflow cannula and is implanted in the pericardial sac (unlike second-generation LVADs), avoiding the need for abdominal surgery and resultant intraabdominal complications.

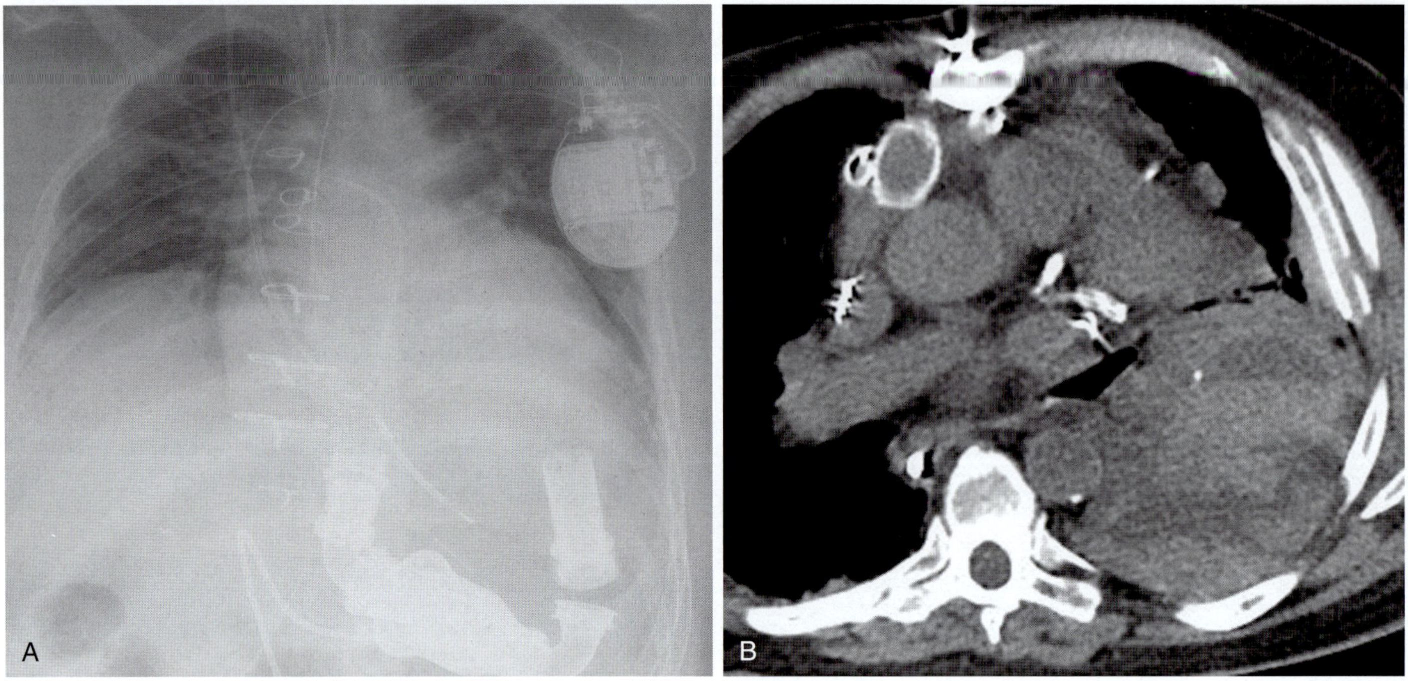

Fig. 69.39 Hemorrhage from left ventricular assist device (LVAD) placement. (A) Anteroposterior chest radiograph after LVAD implantation shows an abnormal contour to the left ventricular apex and a new left pleural effusion, which was suspected to represent hemothorax. (B) Chest CT confirms the presence of a large hemothorax that required surgical evacuation.

SUGGESTED READINGS

Godoy MC, Leitman BS, de Groot PM, et al. Chest radiography in the ICU: part 1, evaluation of airway, enteric, and pleural tubes. *AJR Am J Roentgenol*. 2012;198(3):563–571.

Godoy MC, Leitman BS, de Groot PM, et al. Chest radiography in the ICU: part 2, evaluation of cardiovascular lines and other devices. *AJR Am J Roentgenol*. 2012;198(3):572–581.

Ketai LH, Godwin JD. A new view of pulmonary edema and acute respiratory distress syndrome. *J Thorac Imaging*. 1998;13(3):147–171.

Marik PE. Aspiration pneumonitis and aspiration pneumonia. *N Engl J Med*. 2001;344(9):665–671.

Ranieri VM, Rubenfeld GD, Thompson BT, et al. Acute respiratory distress syndrome: the Berlin definition. *JAMA*. 2012;307(23):2526–2533.

The full reference list for this chapter is available at ExpertConsult.com.

70 Noninfectious Lung and Stem Cell Transplantation Complications

BRENT P. LITTLE

Lung Transplantation Complications

Lung transplantation can prolong life in a variety of diseases that cause progressive respiratory failure. As of 2015, more than 55,000 adult lung transplantations and almost 4000 heart-lung transplantations had been performed worldwide, more than 3500 a year.[1,2] The most common indications for lung transplantation in adults have been chronic obstructive pulmonary disease (COPD), pulmonary fibrosis and other interstitial lung diseases (ILDs), and bronchiectasis (most commonly cystic fibrosis); more recently, idiopathic interstitial pneumonias have become the leading cause for lung transplantation.[1] In children cystic fibrosis is the most common disease for which lung transplantation is performed and was the indication in more than 50% of all cases of transplantation in the period 1999 to 2013, and in more than 70% of children older than 6 years.[3] The International Society for Heart and Lung Transplantation maintains guidelines for selection of appropriate candidates; general considerations include a high risk of death within 2 years without lung transplantation and high likelihoods of surviving in the perioperative period and at 5 years after transplantation.[4]

Survival after lung transplantation has significantly increased over the past 20 years.[1] However, transplantation complications still cause significant morbidity and mortality. As of 2013, 1-year survival was 88%, and 5-year survival was 55% for recipients aged 12 years and older.[5] One major center found a 31% rate of hospital readmission in adult lung transplantation within 1 month after discharge; 67% of patients were readmitted within 1 year, usually for pulmonary, infectious, or pleural complications.[6] Chronic complications, such as chronic transplant rejection, also remain a significant cause of long-term mortality.

Surgical Anatomy

Although single-lung transplantation can be performed in selected cases of pulmonary fibrosis, double-lung transplantation is more widely used for cases of COPD and bronchiectasis. Both single- and double-lung transplantation involve harvesting and meticulous hilar dissection of the donor lungs, with sequential creation of bronchial, arterial, and left atrial cuff anastomoses to the recipient.[7] Single-lung transplantations are performed through a lateral thoracotomy, whereas double-lung transplantations use a transverse (clamshell) thoracosternotomy, with an incision extending horizontally across the chest and sternum from axilla to contralateral axilla.[7,8] Bronchial artery anastomoses are usually not performed, and systemic bronchial revascularization usually takes place over several weeks. As the transient interruption of systemic bronchial arterial supply is thought to be a potential mechanism of bronchial complications, such as stenosis and dehiscence, as well as possibly increasing the rate of the bronchiolitis obliterans syndrome (BOS), a technique of en bloc double-lung transplantation with direct bronchial arterial revascularization has been used by a minority of groups.[9]

Time Course of Complications

The dismal outcomes in the early era of lung transplantation were predominantly due to complications in the first postsurgical month. Airway ischemia with dehiscence was a particular problem before establishment of the sequential double-lung transplantation technique.[8] Although survival rates have markedly improved, significant risks of morbidity and mortality still plague the early postsurgical period.[10] The most common reported causes of death in the first 30 days are noncytomegalovirus (CMV) infections (19%), graft failure (25%), multiorgan failure (12%), cardiovascular causes (12%), and technical failures (11%).[1] The readmission rate for lung transplant recipients within the first month is significantly higher than after treatment for myocardial infarction and complex vascular surgery.[11]

In the intermediate and chronic posttransplantation periods, infections remain an important cause of morbidity and mortality; in addition to bacterial infections, respiratory viruses such as cytomegalovirus and adenovirus, pneumocystis, and fungal infections become more common.[12] Chronic rejection (now called chronic lung allograft dysfunction) is a major concern in the late posttransplantion period and is a leading source of morbidity and mortality after the first year.

Types of Lung Transplantation Complications

PLEURAL COMPLICATIONS

Prevalence and Clinical Considerations

Pleural complications, such as pneumothorax, hemothorax, chylothorax, and empyema, comprise a large percentage of complications in the first month after transplantation, affecting approximately 22% of patients.[13] Pneumothorax is the most common pleural problem, comprising almost 50% of pleural complications in one study.[13] Pneumothoraces can occur as a result of undersizing of donor lungs, as expansion of the donor lung can take days or weeks to complete. Small air leaks can also be a cause and may spontaneously resolve. Most cases of pneumothorax are managed through watchful waiting or thoracostomy tube placement.[13] The presence of a persistent or increasing pneumothorax despite thoracostomy placement can suggest the presence of a bronchopleural fistula, which can occur in bronchial anastomotic dehiscence.

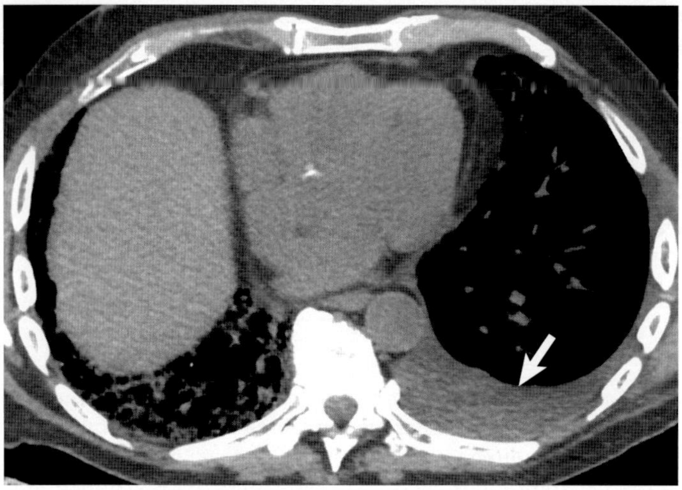

Fig. 70.1 Pleural effusion. CT image at the lung bases shows a small left pleural effusion *(arrow)* occurring shortly after left lung transplantation. Note native right lung fibrosis.

Pleural effusions are common in the first few days of lung transplantation, typically developing in the first hours after transplantation (Fig. 70.1). Effusions are usually exudative, with high red blood cell and neutrophil content, and resolve or decrease in size by day 9 after surgery.[14] An empyema occurred in 27% of patients with pleural fluid in one study; 25% were bacterial in origin, whereas 60% were attributable to fungal organisms, such as *Candida albicans*. An elevated neutrophil count in pleural fluid of greater than 21% was 70% sensitive and 79% specific for pleural infection in the study.[15] The development of an empyema is associated with an increase in risk of death.

Hemothorax and chylothorax can manifest in the first few hours or days after transplantation, and are uncommon occurrences, usually heralded by a rapid accumulation of pleural fluid or increased thoracostomy tube drainage. Hemothorax may be caused by surgical injury of an intercostal, bronchial, or other artery and can require surgical exploration or embolization. Injury to the thoracic duct can result in chylothorax, for which ligation of the thoracic duct may be required.[13]

Imaging Manifestations

Radiography. Small pleural effusions are commonly seen at radiography in the first few days after transplantation, but typically begin to decrease in size within the first week. Small pneumothoraces are also very common and usually resolve spontaneously. However, persistent or worsening pleural air or fluid can be crucial to recognition of a significant pleural complication.

Rapid development or sudden increase in size of a postsurgical pleural fluid collection is concerning for the possibility of a hemothorax or chylothorax (Fig. 70.2). Pleural fluid sampling is usually diagnostic, confirming blood or chyle. Persistent or new pleural fluid may suggest empyema; fluid loculation or pleural gas may occur, but are not always present, and may be difficult to discern at portable supine radiography. A new or increasing pneumothorax may suggest a significant air leak or bronchopleural fistula resulting from bronchial dehiscence.

Computed Tomography. Although not first-line imaging for patients in the immediate postsurgical period, computed tomography (CT) can be used as a supplement to radiography. CT is highly sensitive for the detection of pneumothoraces and pleural fluid collections and can aid in the assessment of fluid loculation (Fig. 70.3; see also Fig. 70.1). Detection of high-attenuation pleural fluid confirms hemothorax (see Fig. 70.2). The presence of pleural thickening and/or enhancement with the "split pleura sign" can suggest empyema (Fig. 70.4), although these findings can also occur in the chronic setting, resulting from pleuroparenchymal inflammation without active infection.

KEY POINTS: PLEURAL COMPLICATIONS

- Pleural complications are common in the first month after lung transplantation.
- Pneumothoraces are most common, may be due to a size discrepancy between donor and recipient or air leak, and are usually treated conservatively with thoracostomy tubes and surveillance.
- Pleural effusions are common and usually develop within the first hours after transplantation.
- Empyemas may occur in almost one-third of patients with pleural fluid and are often bacterial in etiology; loculation and pleural thickening are imaging clues.
- A rapidly developing pleural fluid collection in the early postsurgical period suggests the possibility of hemothorax or chylothorax. High-attenuation blood products at CT confirm hemothorax.

PRIMARY GRAFT DYSFUNCTION

Prevalence and Clinical Considerations

Primary graft dysfunction (PGD) is known by a variety of names, including posttransplantation edema, reperfusion edema, and implantation response. PGD is a form of acute lung injury with noncardiogenic alveolar edema occurring within 72 hours of lung transplantation, representing a complex inflammatory reaction to ischemia/reperfusion injury. Free radicals, cytokines, neutrophils, macrophages, and other immune modulators have been implicated in this condition.[16] PGD is defined and graded based on the presence of bilateral airspace opacities on radiographs, a decreased ratio of partial pressure of oxygen in arterial blood/forced inspiratory oxygen (FiO_2), and the absence of alternative causes. Significant PGD is classified as grade 3 (severe) and defined as a ratio less than 200.[17]

Overall, the condition occurs in up to 30% of recipients at some time during the first 72 hours after transplantation.[18] Risk factors for the condition include a history of smoking by the donor, pulmonary hypertension, use of cardiopulmonary bypass, recipient history of sarcoidosis, increased FiO_2 during lung reperfusion, and single-lung transplantation.[19] PGD occurs in as many as 60% of single-lung transplantations, in which about half of patients in one study developed radiographic findings within 3 hours of transplantation.[20]

PGD is associated with a significant increase in 90-day mortality and is associated with a higher incidence of chronic rejection and hospital readmission.[18,21] All grades of PGD predispose to chronic rejection in the form of bronchiolitis obliterans, resulting in a decrease in long-term survival.[22] PGD may predispose to bronchial complications; in one study recipients with PDG in the first 72 hours after surgery were more than twice as likely to experience bronchial dehiscence, stenosis, bronchomalacia, and hemoptysis, possibly a correlate of direct ischemic/reperfusion bronchial injury.[23] Undersizing of the donor lung may increase the incidence of PGD, possibly through a mismatch in donor and recipient pulmonary arterial sizes that leads to high reperfusion pressures; one study found a 39% decrease in odds of PGD

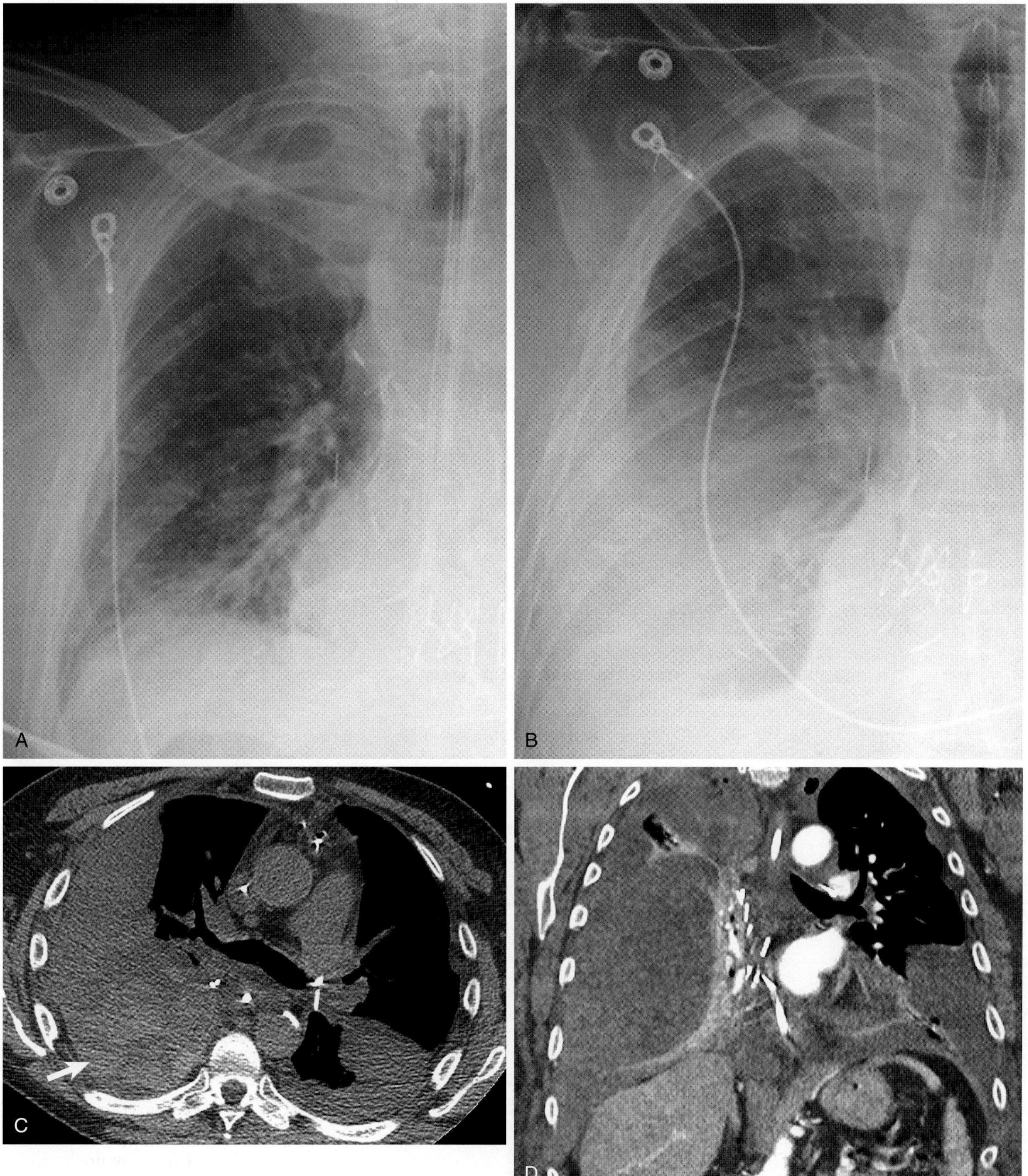

Fig. 70.2 Hemothorax manifesting as a rapidly developing pleural fluid collection in the early postsurgical period after lung transplantation. Radiographs approximately 1 week after surgery (A) and 1 day later (B) show rapid development of a large right pleural fluid collection. Axial (C) and coronal (D) CT images show a large right pleural fluid collection; high-attenuation material within the pleural fluid confirms hemothorax (*arrow* in C).

in cases in which oversized lungs were used.[24] Despite several possible medical therapies, supportive care remains the most common treatment.

Imaging Manifestations

Radiography. The chest radiograph typically reveals bilateral airspace opacities that usually appear from 24 to 72 hours after transplantation, often with a perihilar and basilar predominance (Fig. 70.5). Some studies of single-lung transplantations have found development of opacities as early as 3 hours after transplantation in approximately 50% of recipients.[20] The opacities may worsen over the course of hours to days but in general show improvement or resolution by postoperative day 5 to 10.[25] The radiographic appearance is nonspecific and can also be seen in cardiogenic edema, pneumonia, hyperacute rejection, and venous obstruction.[18]

Computed Tomography. CT is generally not typically used for primary evaluation of PGD but usually shows bilateral diffuse ground-glass opacities and/or consolidation. The appearance can be similar to diffuse alveolar damage, cardiogenic edema, and some infections. The opacities improve or resolve within the first week after transplantation.

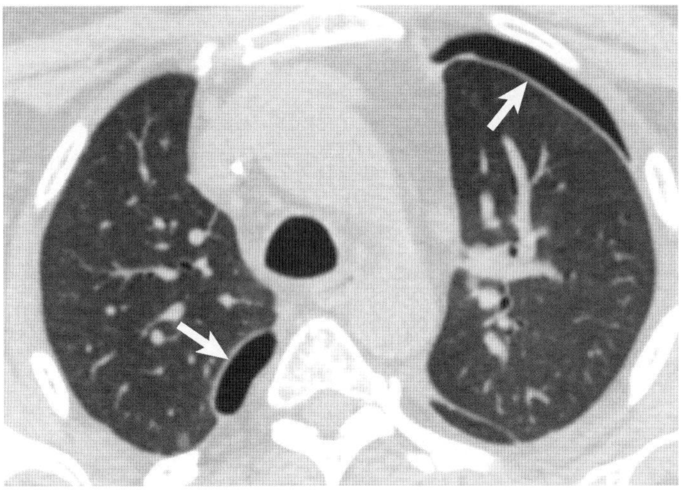

Fig. 70.3 Pneumothorax. CT image shows small bilateral pneumothoraces *(arrows)* in a patient approximately 2 weeks after bilateral lung transplantation. The left pneumothorax resolved spontaneously, but the right pneumothorax persisted and was due to bronchial anastomotic dehiscence.

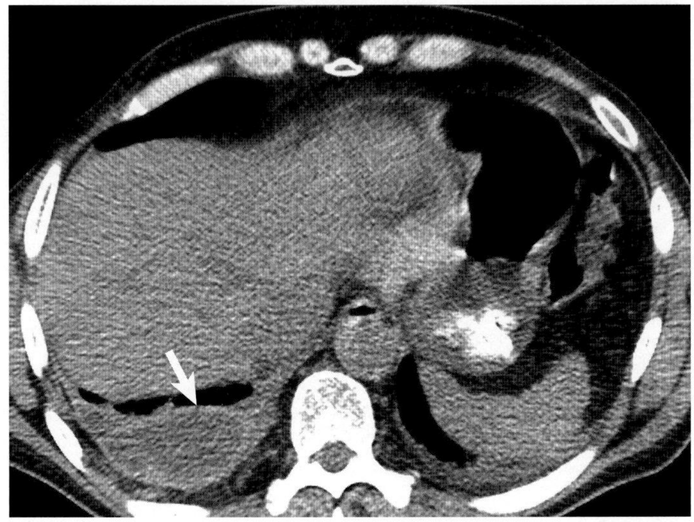

Fig. 70.4 Empyema several months after bilateral lung transplantation. CT image shows a small loculated right pleural effusion with pleural thickening *(arrow)*, representing an empyema.

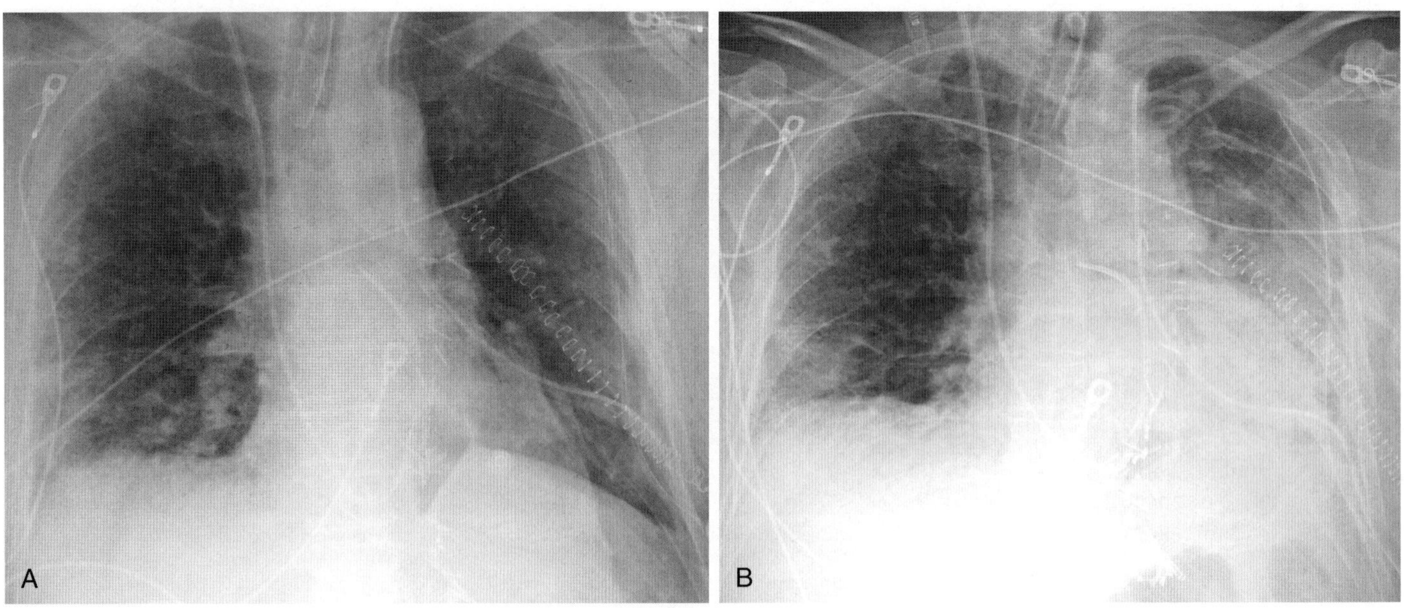

Fig. 70.5 Primary graft dysfunction in a patient with unilateral left lung transplantation. (A) Radiograph 1 day after lung transplantation is clear. (B) Radiograph on day 2 shows airspace opacities in the left lung in the setting of worsening hypoxemia. The airspace opacities improved over the next few days, and no infection was identified.

KEY POINTS: PRIMARY GRAFT DYSFUNCTION

- Primary graft dysfunction (PGD) is an acute lung injury that occurs within 72 hours after transplantation.
- PGD occurs in up to 30% of recipients and is associated with both a higher risk of early postsurgical mortality and an increase in incidence of chronic complications, including chronic lung allograft rejection.
- Imaging shows diffuse airspace opacities developing 24–72 hours after transplantation, with improvement or resolution after 5–10 days.
- Treatment is generally through supportive care.

REJECTION

Prevalence and Clinical Considerations

Rejection is classified as hyperacute, acute, or chronic. These conditions have distinctly different times of onset, durations, mechanisms, and outcomes.

Hyperacute rejection is an attack on the donor allograft by preformed recipient antibodies and occurs either during surgery or in the first few postsurgical hours, usually with devastating results and complete graft failure.

Acute rejection is an acute lung injury syndrome that develops over the course of hours or days; although most common in the first year after transplantation, it can occur at any time after transplantation. Symptoms include fever, dyspnea, cough, and hypoxia. Pulmonary function tests (PFTs) can show a decline in forced expiratory volume in 1 second (FEV1) and vital capacity.[26] At histology, acute cellular rejection is characterized by a perivascular monocellular infiltrate.[27] Acute rejection occurs in approximately 35% of recipients within 1 year of transplantation.[2] Although episodes of acute rejection do carry a small risk of mortality, the condition usually responds to steroids or is self-limiting and accounts for less than 4% of all deaths within the first month after transplantation.[12] However, episodes of acute rejection can hasten the onset of or worsen the severity of chronic rejection. Acute rejection can be diagnosed and graded at transbronchial biopsy according to a standard grading system, but a large degree of interobserver variation in scoring of rejection has been noted in a large study.[28]

Acute fibrinous and organizing pneumonia (AFOP) is a form of OP with deposition of fibrin within alveoli and occurs in a small subset of patients after lung transplantation. It may occur in the first year or even first week after transplantation and may mimic acute cellular rejection. Acute and subacute forms have been noted, and the acute form may be mistaken for acute cellular rejection or infection.[29] AFOP may respond rapidly to corticosteroid treatment, but a fulminant acute course may fail to respond to any therapy, with a mortality rate as high as 90%.[30]

Chronic rejection rarely develops before the first few months after transplantation, but is the major cause of long-term and overall mortality in lung transplantation.[31] Chronic rejection causes shortness of breath and progressive respiratory insufficiency. Although previously BOS was traditionally nearly synonymous with the concept of chronic lung transplant rejection, the term *chronic lung allograft dysfunction* (CLAD) is now widely used in appreciation of subtypes of chronic rejection. CLAD refers to both BOS and the more recently described restrictive allograft syndrome (RAS). RAS carries a poorer prognosis than BOS; BOS patients live on average 3 to 5 years after diagnosis, while those affected by RAS have a mean survival between 6 and 18 months.[32] Some studies have also documented a chronic form of AFOP as a form of CLAD, also with a poorer prognosis than BOS.[33] Definitive medical treatment for CLAD is lacking, and the only effective eventual therapy is retransplantation in appropriate cases.[34] A variety of factors can hasten the development of CLAD, including respiratory viral infections, episodes of acute rejection, and aspiration.[35,36]

BOS is the most common subtype of chronic rejection, and may affect up to half of patients surviving after the first year of transplantation.[26] The condition shows a progressive pattern of small airway obstruction with air-trapping and chronic respiratory insufficiency. The condition can be diagnosed by a decline in FEV1 greater than 20% below the average of two baseline measurements after lung transplantation. Transbronchial biopsy can also diagnose BOS, but interpretation can be variable. Some studies point to different outcomes based on histology; one study found that histology of true constrictive bronchiolitis was associated with a 3-year survival of 60%, whereas the so-called lymphocytic bronchiolitis subtype survival was 91%.[37]

RAS has been recently appreciated as a subtype of chronic rejection and produces a predominantly restrictive pattern of progressive decline in respiratory function. RAS may account for up to 25% of all CLAD cases.[38] Histopathology shows a pattern similar to idiopathic pleuroparenchymal fibroelastosis, with a peripheral distribution of abnormal collagen deposition, fibroblastic foci, and thickening of the alveolar septal network.[39] RAS has been defined as a decline in FEV1 greater than 20% and a decline in total lung capacity greater than 10% below posttransplantation baseline.[31] The fibrosis in RAS tends to be upper lobe predominant. Although patients with RAS tend to have a worse prognosis than in BOS,[32] subtypes of the condition have been described at CT (described later), and may portend different prognoses, with graft survival in a slow-onset subtype averaging 33.5 months and in a more rapid-onset group averaging 6.4 months.[31]

Imaging Considerations

Radiography. Portable radiography is the most common imaging modality used in the early posttransplantation period. Both hyperacute and acute rejection usually manifest with diffuse airspace opacities within the transplanted lung(s), often worse in the perihilar regions and lung bases (Fig. 70.6). The radiographic appearance is generally indistinguishable from other causes of airspace opacities, including pulmonary edema, primary graft dysfunction, and infection. AFOP may similarly manifest with bilateral airspace opacities, sometimes with a basilar and peripheral distribution.[30] Distinguishing among these possibilities relies on the time course of development and supportive clinical data. Hyperacute rejection produces progressive opacities that arise within the first few hours of transplantation, whereas PGD usually has onset after 24 hours and begins to improve within 5 days (see Fig. 70.5). Acute rejection is more common after the first week and has peak prevalence within the first year.

Radiographs have a limited role in the evaluation of chronic rejection and can be normal, especially in cases of BOS. However, hyperinflation, bronchial wall thickening and, at times, bronchiectasis can be seen in BOS, whereas low lung volumes with upper lobe nodularity, consolidation, architectural distortion, and traction bronchiectasis are more typical of RAS (Fig. 70.7).

Computed Tomography. CT is seldom performed in the setting of hyperacute rejection. Although generally first suspected at radiography, acute rejection typically shows bilateral ground-glass opacities, consolidation, and septal thickening with a basilar

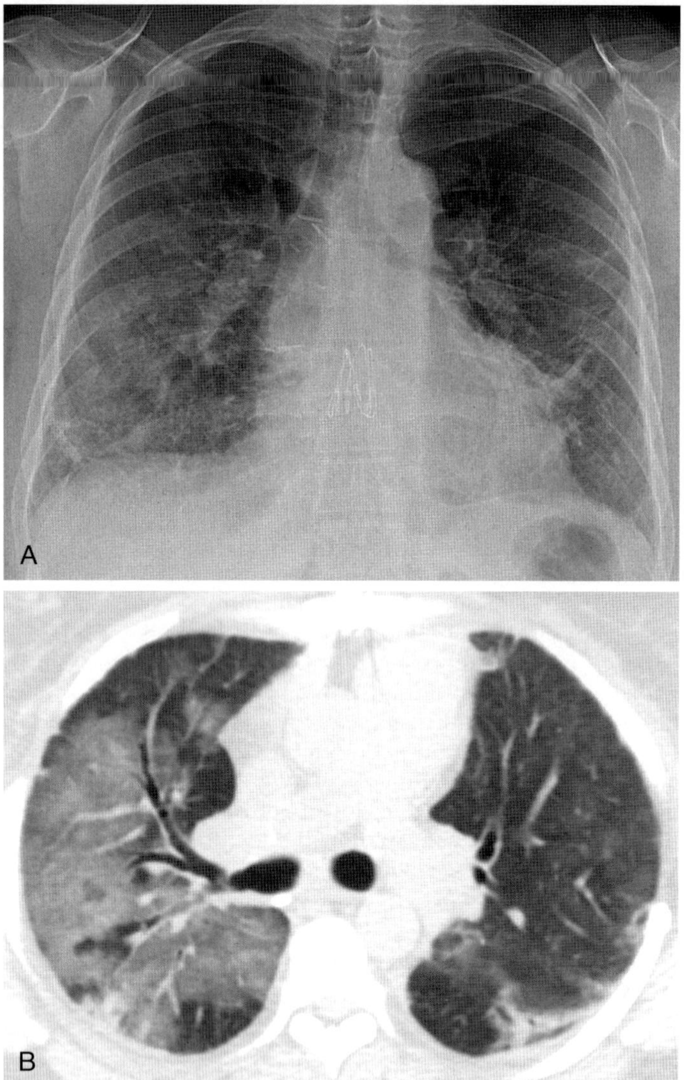

Fig. 70.6 Acute cellular rejection in a patient with dyspnea and hypoxemia several months after lung transplantation. (A) Radiograph shows bilateral patchy airspace opacities. (B) CT image shows bilateral ground-glass opacities, with greater involvement of the right lung.

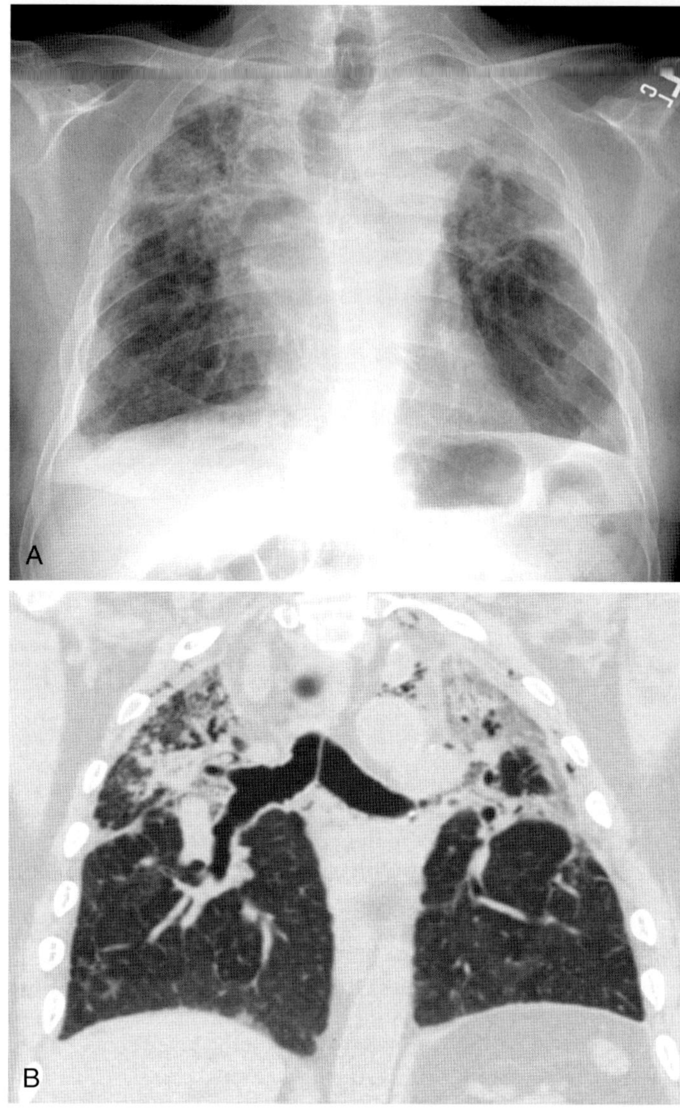

Fig. 70.7 Restrictive allograft syndrome in a patient approximately 2 years after bilateral lung transplantation. (A) Radiograph shows upper lobe volume loss, architectural distortion, and patchy opacities. (B) CT image shows upper lobe peripheral reticulation, architectural distortion, and traction bronchiectasis.

predominance.[27] In AFOP CT may show basilar-predominant consolidation, ground-glass opacities, and reticulation.[30]

For evaluation of chronic rejection, thin-slice CT is the preferred imaging modality, as it is much more sensitive in detection and characterization of CLAD. A helical series is acquired at full inspiration with an additional axial acquisition performed at maximal expiration to assess for air-trapping. Mosaic attenuation—the presence of alternating low- and high-attenuation areas of lung—is common in BOS (Fig. 70.8). Areas of low-attenuation lung correspond to air-trapping and do not significantly increase in attenuation at expiration. Areas of higher-attenuation lung correspond to more normally aerated lung and increase in attenuation at expiration. A true mosaic attenuation pattern is seen in most cases, with smaller vessel diameters in areas of low attenuation caused by hypoxemic vasoconstriction. However, although these findings can suggest BOS, the degree of mosaic attenuation may not correlate with the BOS stage and degree of obstructive physiology at PFTs.[40] Although mosaic attenuation with air-trapping is often the earliest finding of BOS, helpful secondary findings include bronchial wall thickening and bronchiectasis, which in one study correlated better with airflow limitation than did mosaic attenuation (see Fig. 70.8).[40]

RAS usually shows an upper lobe–predominant pattern of fibrosis at CT that can be identical to idiopathic pleuroparenchymal fibroelastosis. Peripheral reticulation, architectural distortion, traction bronchiectasis, nodules, and consolidation are possible findings (see Fig. 70.7). One study proposed two different CT subtypes of RAS; a "mild" subtype gradually developed upper lobe–predominant nodules, reticulation, and volume loss, with a delayed onset of graft failure; the other group showed sudden onset of upper lobe consolidation and volume loss, with a poorer prognosis and median graft survival of only 6.4 months.[31] Three-dimensional CT volumetry reveals a difference in lung volumes among subtypes of CLAD, with recipients with BOS having no significant decrease in lung volumes but those with RAS showing

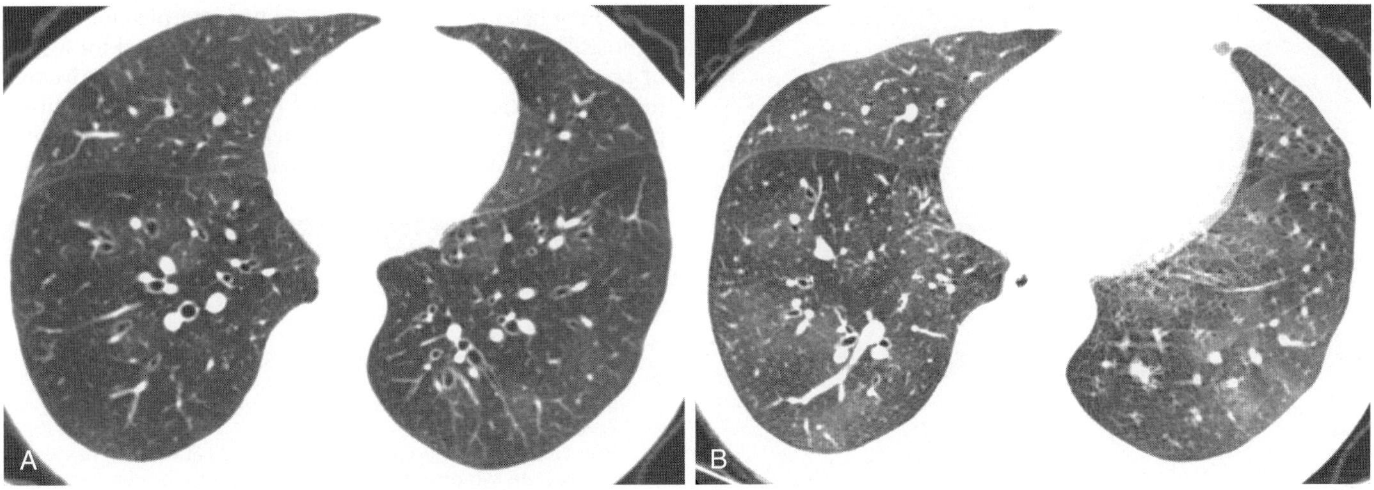

Fig. 70.8 Bronchiolitis obliterans syndrome in a patient after bilateral lung transplantation. (A) Inspiratory series shows bilateral mosaic attenuation, bronchial wall thickening, and mild bronchiectasis. (B) Expiratory series shows accentuation of the mosaic attenuation pattern. The low-attenuation areas of the lung fail to show a normal increase in attenuation, confirming air-trapping.

an almost 25% reduction in volume by CT.[38] One study examined the CTs of patients at CLAD onset and found a higher incidence of consolidation and ground-glass opacity in patients who eventually developed RAS, the restrictive phenotype of CLAD, than in those who developed primarily BOS.[41]

KEY POINTS: REJECTION

- Hyperacute rejection is rare and usually manifests during surgery or within the first few hours after transplantation.
- Acute rejection is most common in the first year after transplantation but can occur at any time. Mortality is uncommon, but episodes of acute rejection can hasten the development and increase the severity of bronchiolitis obliterans. Diffuse airspace opacities are common.
- Acute fibrinous and organizing pneumonia may occur in the first year after transplantation and can mimic acute rejection. Imaging findings include bilateral ground-glass opacities and patchy consolidation.
- Chronic lung allograft dysfunction is a major cause of long-term and overall mortality and comprises both bronchiolitis obliterans syndrome (BOS) and restrictive allograft syndrome.
- BOS is the most common subtype of chronic rejection and is a major cause of morbidity and mortality after the first year. A mosaic attenuation pattern with air-trapping, bronchiectasis, and bronchial wall thickening are typical CT features.
- Restrictive allograft syndrome is a more recently characterized form of chronic rejection that has restrictive physiology and a worse prognosis than BOS. Imaging features include upper lobe–predominant volume loss, reticulation, architectural distortion, pleural thickening, and traction bronchiectasis.

AIRWAY COMPLICATIONS

Prevalence and Clinical Considerations

The incidence of significant airway complications has been reported as between 2% and 33%.[42] A study of 232 lung transplantations found that longer recipient bronchus length, telescoping anastomotic technique, and prolonged donor ventilation were associated with increased airway complications.[43] Another study of 270 lung transplantation patients found that primary graft dysfunction within 72 hours of transplantation, lung infection in the first month, diabetes, and COPD were independent risk factors for airway complications.[23] Patients may present with unexplained hypoxemia, obstructive PFTs, or atelectasis or postobstructive pneumonia in the involved lobes.[12]

Bronchial dehiscence is an uncommon but potentially devastating complication. In the early perioperative period, dehiscence can arise from ischemia resulting from interruption of the bronchial arterial blood supply during transplantation; other potential contributors include immunosuppressive medications, infection, acute rejection, and donor-recipient bronchial size mismatch.[44,45] In the intermediate or late period, infection is a more common cause. Fistulas, most commonly to the pleura or esophagus, can rarely occur.[46]

Bronchial stenosis is usually a late complication, occurring more than 3 months after transplantation, usually resulting from granulation tissue, infection, or bronchial ischemia. *Aspergillus* is a known common offending organism.[42] The most common site of bronchial stenosis is the bronchial anastomosis, but nonanastomotic stenosis can also occur. Although nonanastomotic stenosis can occur in any bronchus, the most common sites are the bronchus intermedius and the right middle lobe bronchus; severe stenosis of the former has been called "vanishing bronchus intermedius syndrome."[47]

Bronchomalacia can occur at the site of a bronchial stenosis or in isolation. Bronchial collapse at expiration is the key to the diagnosis.

Imaging Considerations

Radiography. Radiography is used to exclude other sources of respiratory symptoms in lung transplantation patients and is seldom helpful in evaluation of suspected airway complications. In cases in which bronchial dehiscence leads to a bronchopleural fistula, a pneumothorax or pneumomediastinum may occasionally be detected at radiography.[46] Lobar atelectasis can also uncommonly be seen, usually in cases of severe bronchial stenosis.

Computed Tomography. Thin-slice CT with multiplanar reformats is used for detection and characterization of post-transplantation airway complications. Bronchial dehiscence may

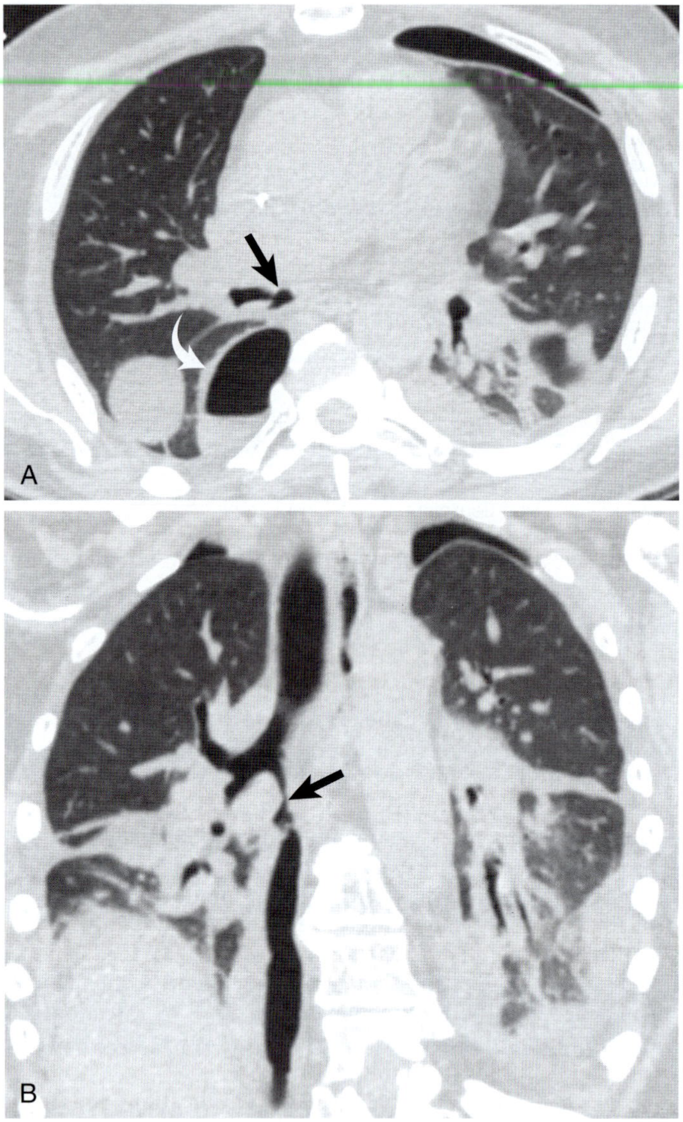

Fig. 70.9 Bronchial dehiscence in a patient several weeks after bilateral lung transplantation. (A) Axial CT image shows irregularity of the right bronchial anastomosis, with a focal air collection communicating with the bronchus *(arrow)*; there is a loculated right pneumothorax *(curved arrow)*. (B) Coronal CT image shows communication of the bronchial anastomosis with a pleural air collection at the site of the dehiscence, representing a bronchopleural fistula *(arrow)*.

be detected as a visible bronchial discontinuity, often with adjacent extraluminal air, pneumothorax, or other evidence of air leak (Fig. 70.9).[46] In one study of CT findings of bronchoscopically proven dehiscence, a bronchial wall discontinuity was 100% sensitive and 94% specific for dehiscence, and an extraluminal air collection was 100% sensitive and 72% specific for the complication.[48] Bronchial stenosis usually manifests as a focal area of bronchial narrowing; bronchial wall thickening or irregularity can occur, and occasionally air-trapping distal to the anastomosis can be seen. Excessive bronchial collapse (>70%) at expiratory series suggests bronchomalacia and can be associated with stenosis or other evidence of bronchial injury.

Treatment

A variety of airway stents can be used for the treatment of bronchial stenosis, dehiscence, and bronchomalacia. In addition, endobronchial ablation or balloon bronchoplasty can be performed for bronchial stenosis.[46] Primary surgical repair may be required for a subset of cases of bronchial dehiscence refractory to conservative treatment.[45] Medical therapy can also play a role, with antibiotic prophylaxis in the setting of bronchial injuries and positive-pressure ventilation for tracheomalacia.[49]

KEY POINTS: AIRWAY COMPLICATIONS

- Airway complications occur in up to 33% of lung transplantation patients.
- Bronchial dehiscence is uncommon and usually occurs in the early period after transplant; infection and ischemia are potential causes. CT shows focal mediastinal air collections adjacent to the dehiscence, usually showing a bronchial connection.
- Bronchial stenosis is usually a late complication and may cause obstructive symptoms. Anastomotic stenosis is most common, but nonanastomotic stenosis may occur at any site, most commonly in the bronchus intermedius and right middle lobe bronchus. CT shows focal bronchial narrowing.
- Bronchomalacia may occur in isolation or at the site of a stenosis. Bronchial collapse at expiration on CT is diagnostic.
- Treatment includes conservative treatment, ablation or bronchoplasty, and less commonly, primary surgical repair.

VASCULAR COMPLICATIONS

Prevalence and Clinical Considerations

Primary anastomotic vascular complications are uncommon but can carry significant clinical implications and a poor prognosis. *Venous or arterial stenosis* can occur, thought to be due to donor-recipient size mismatch, vascular twisting or kinking at an anastomosis, granulation tissue, or thrombus formation.[50] In one study venous or arterial stenosis was found in 1.75% of transplant vascular anastomoses.[51] Another series found at least one vascular stenosis in 1.8% of lung transplantation patients; the stenosis typically occurred in the early period, with a mean of 9 days after transplantation surgery.[50] Patients can present with unexplained hypoxemia or pulmonary hypertension.[45]

Venous thrombosis at the anastomotic site is an uncommon finding at CT but was identified in 15% of lung transplantation patients in one echocardiography study, possibly because CT is not as frequently performed in the early postoperative period.[52] Venous thrombosis can result in allograft failure or stroke, and larger thrombus size and degree of resulting vein stenosis correlated with poor outcome.[52] Complete thrombosis can lead to hemorrhagic venous infarction of a lobe.[53]

Pulmonary embolism (PE) is the most frequent vascular complication in lung transplantation patients, with an overall incidence in one meta-analysis of approximately 4%, similar to that of PE in patients after other major thoracic surgeries. Half of events occurred within the first 30 days after surgery; 11% of patients with PE died within 1 year, with 75% of deaths within the first month, usually also accompanied by infection or rejection.[54] The incidence in single-lung transplantations is higher (12%), with 92% of events involving the allograft.[54] Some studies have found a higher incidence of lung infarction (37.5%) in transplantation patients, likely because of compromised bronchial arterial blood supply.[55]

Imaging Considerations

Radiography. Radiographs may help exclude other sources of respiratory symptoms but are often normal. Significant pulmonary vascular abnormalities, such as complete pulmonary vein thrombosis, may manifest with focal edema within the affected lobe.

Computed Tomography. Thin-section CT with contrast is most commonly used for primary evaluation of vascular complications after lung transplantation. Timing for pulmonary arterial enhancement can be used for evaluation of pulmonary arterial anastomoses and for pulmonary emboli. CT can demonstrate stenosis as a focal narrowing of a pulmonary artery or vein, usually at the anastomotic site.[56] Pulmonary venous thrombosis is an uncommon finding at CT but can be detected as a focal filling defect within a pulmonary vein, usually near the anastomosis (Fig. 70.10).

Magnetic Resonance Imaging. Magnetic resonance imaging (MRI) may have a limited role in diagnosis of vascular complications in lung transplantation patients, especially in those in whom an allergy to iodinated contrast may preclude evaluation with CT. However, CT is typically first-line imaging, as pulmonary and bronchial complications are well characterized at CT.

Conventional Angiography. Catheter angiography can be used to confirm vascular abnormalities diagnosed at cross-sectional imaging and may be helpful in cases in which CT or MRI is compromised by artifact or motion. In addition, angiography is performed in conjunction with angioplasty and guides endovascular stent placement.[57]

Ventilation-Perfusion Scan. Ventilation-perfusion scintigraphy is primarily used for evaluation of possible pulmonary embolism and can be used as an alternative to CT angiography, especially in the setting of an allergy to iodinated contrast medium.

Treatment

Anticoagulation is used in the treatment of pulmonary emboli or venous thrombosis. Angioplasty can be used for dilation of pulmonary arterial or venous stenosis. A variety of endovascular stents have been successful in the treatment of stenoses in conjunction with angioplasty.[56,57] Surgery may be indicated in some cases of venous or arterial stenosis.[51]

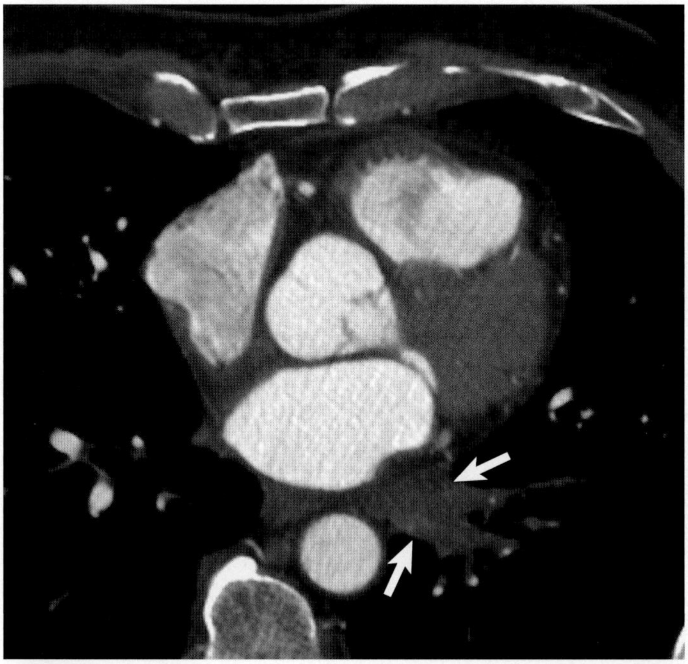

Fig. 70.10 Pulmonary vein thrombosis. Axial CT image shows complete thrombosis of the left inferior pulmonary vein *(arrows)*. Although resulting from radiofrequency ablation for atrial fibrillation in this case, this complication can occur at the venous anastomosis after lung transplantation.

KEY POINTS: VASCULAR COMPLICATIONS

- Pulmonary emboli are the most common lung transplantation complication; pulmonary infarcts may be more common in transplantation patients because of an interruption of bronchial arterial supply.
- Venous or arterial stenosis may occur because of granulation tissue, kinking, or twisting at an anastomosis.
- Venous thrombosis is uncommonly seen at CT but can lead to pulmonary hemorrhage or venous infarct.

DISEASE RECURRENCE AND MALIGNANCY

Prevalence and Clinical Considerations

Recurrence of primary disease occurred in 1% of transplantations in a multicenter study of 1394 patients.[58] However, this percentage is dramatically higher in diffuse lung diseases. In a study of transplantations for diffuse lung disease, sarcoidosis accounted for 9 of 26 (35%) cases of recurrence. Other recurrences included pulmonary Langerhans cell histiocytosis, alveolar proteinosis, lymphangioleiomyomatosis, talc granulomatosis, and diffuse panbronchiolitis. The overall recurrence rate for these six diffuse lung diseases combined was 27%, and the imaging appearance upon recurrence was often different from the morphology of the original disease.[58]

Malignancies such as primary lung cancer, lymphoproliferative disease, and Kaposi sarcoma can occur in lung transplantation patients; other malignancies, including breast, cervical, and tongue cancer, have also been reported.[59,60] Immunosuppressive medications, activity of specific viral infections, and a decrease in innate antitumor surveillance may be responsible for the elevated cancer rate compared with the general population.[61] Most malignancies arise de novo, but a small percentage are considered donor related; in the case of lung cancer, the number of donor-related malignancies may be underestimated.[61] In a study of more than 18,000 adult lung transplant recipients in the United Network for Organ Sharing database, the incidence of cancers other than skin cancer was 1.4% at 1 year and 7.9% at 5 years, a rate threefold higher than the general US population, with lung cancer (26.2%) and lymphoproliferative disease (20%) comprising most malignancies.[61]

Posttransplantation lymphoproliferative disease (PTLD) refers to a histologically heterogeneous group of disorders ranging from polyclonal proliferation of lymphoid cells, B-cell or T-cell lymphoma, or classic Hodgkin lymphoma.[62,63] PTLD usually has onset within the first year after transplantation and afflicts 2.8% to 6.1% of patients 1 year after lung transplantation.[64,62] Although intrathoracic PTLD is most common in the early period after transplantation, an extrathoracic presentation can occur, usually after the first year. Patients can present with lymph node enlargement and tenderness, cough, dyspnea, and systemic symptoms, such as fever, sweats, and fatigue.[63] Epstein-Barr virus (EBV) and transplant immunosuppressive regimens are thought to contribute to the development of the disease; EBV-negative pretransplantation status and subsequent seroconversion are thought to be contributors to the development of PTLD.[63]

Imaging Considerations

Radiography. Radiographs may show findings in keeping with recurrent disease of a particular type, such as upper lobe–predominant nodules or volume loss in sarcoidosis. In malignancies and PTLD, radiographs may show a solitary nodule or mass, several nodules or masses, or less commonly, lymphadenopathy. However, CT is the primary method of evaluating recurrent disease in lung transplantation patients.

Computed Tomography. In recurrent disease CT may show findings suggestive of the disease and may provide the first evidence of recurrence (Fig. 70.11). The pattern of disease at recurrence may not follow the original imaging manifestations.[58]

Posttransplantation malignancies, such as lung cancer, may be detected as a new pulmonary nodule or mass, consolidation, or lymph node enlargement. PTLD most commonly manifests as multiple (or less commonly, solitary) pulmonary nodules or masses (Fig. 70.12). Other manifestations include thoracic lymph node enlargement or septal or pleural thickening.[64,62] Extrathoracic PTLD involvement may manifest as abdominal, pelvic, or neck lymph node enlargement.[63]

Fluorodeoxyglucose–Positron Emission Tomography. Fluorodeoxyglucose–positron emission tomography (FDG-PET) imaging is an essential modality for staging of malignancy and may be used as part of evaluation of malignancies in lung transplantation patients. In addition, PET may be used for staging of PTLD, as masses, nodules, and lymph node involvement are usually FDG-PET positive, and PET may suggest sites of disease not suspected on the basis of CT alone.[65]

Treatment

Treatment of recurrent disease includes therapies specific to the conditions. Retransplantation may be considered in a subset of cases. Treatment of malignancies such as lung cancer may involve surgery, radiation, and/or chemotherapy. PTLD in the early postoperative period may be treated with antiviral drugs and a decrease in dose of immunosuppressive drugs; advanced disease may require chemotherapy and/or radiation.[64]

Noninfectious Complications of Hematopoietic Stem Cell Transplantation

Hematopoietic stem cell transplantation (HSCT) is used for the treatment of a variety of hematologic malignancies, nonmalignant

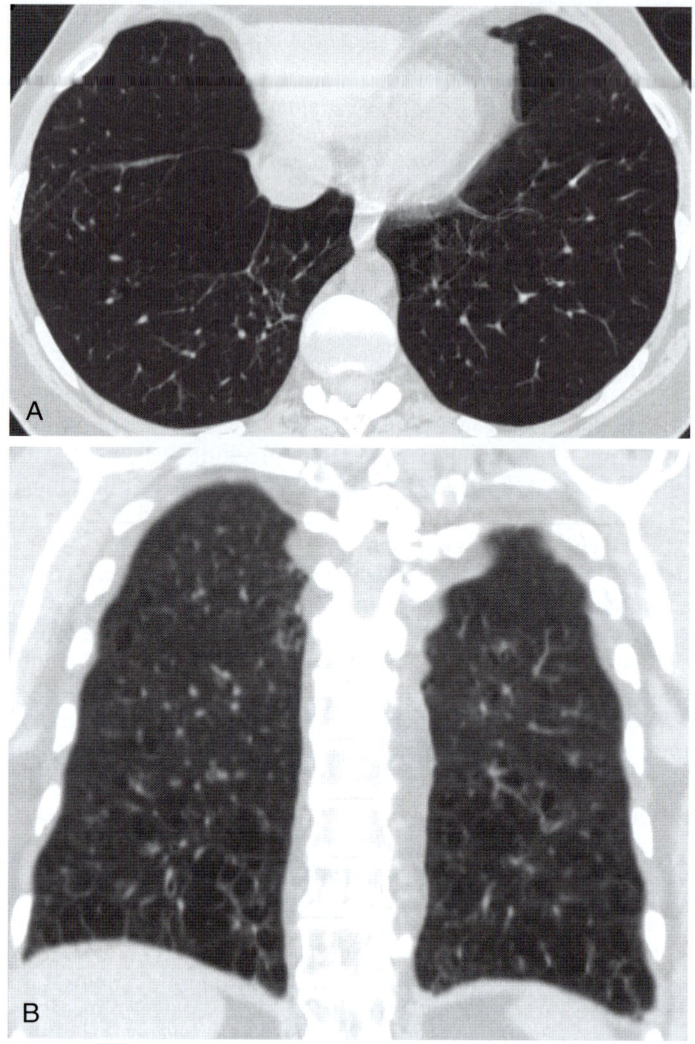

Fig. 70.11 Recurrence of emphysema in lung transplantation for α1-antitrypsin deficiency. (A) Axial CT image shows a typical appearance of lower lobe panacinar emphysema. (B) Coronal CT image several years after bilateral lung transplantation shows recurrence of emphysema in the basilar lower lobes.

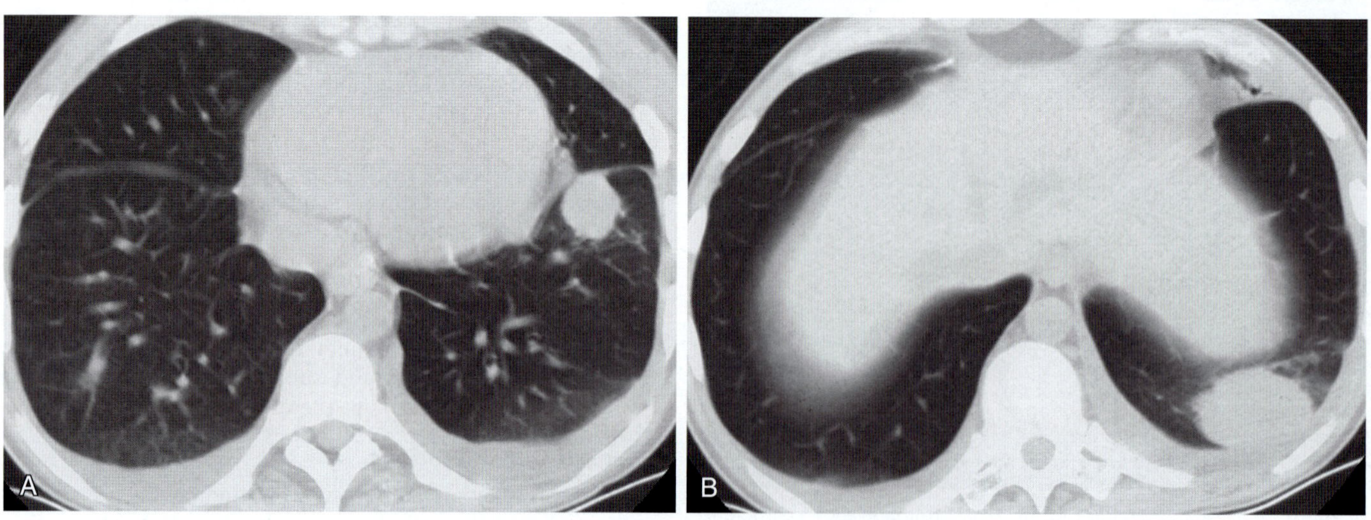

Fig. 70.12 Posttransplantation lymphoproliferative disease after bilateral lung transplantation. Axial CT images (A) and (B) show nodules within the lower lobes and a mass in the left lower lobe. Pleural effusions are also present bilaterally.

KEY POINTS: DISEASE RECURRENCE AND MALIGNANCY

- Recurrence of primary disease occurs in a small minority of all lung transplantations but in up to 27% in cases of diffuse lung disease. Sarcoidosis recurrence is most commonly reported. Patterns of recurrence at imaging often differ from primary presentation.
- Malignancies are more common in lung transplantation patients than in the general population and include primary lung cancer, lymphoproliferative disease, Kaposi sarcoma, and others.
- Posttransplantation lymphoproliferative disease affects a minority of lung transplantation patients and can manifest with multiple or solitary pulmonary nodules or masses, lymph node enlargement, and septal or pleural thickening.

blood cell aplasias, and some solid tumors; because of new indications and wider use of the procedure in existing indications, the number of surviving patients who have had HSCT has grown to almost 500,000 worldwide.[66] After a conditioning regimen that includes combinations of chemotherapy and often radiation designed to eliminate malignant cells or dysfunctional marrow cells, cells from either the patient's own body (autologous transplantation) or from a histocompatible-related donor (allogeneic transplantation) are given to "rescue" the recipient.[67]

Infectious or noninfectious pulmonary complications occur in almost half of patients after HSCT; only noninfectious complications will be covered here.[68] Although those who are free of primary disease at 2 to 5 years have a subsequent greater than 80% survival rate at 10 years, the incidence of chronic disease is high; the most common causes of death in the chronic setting include infection, graft-versus-host disease (GVHD), lung diseases, and recurrent or secondary malignancies.[66]

Early Complications: Pulmonary Edema, Diffuse Alveolar Hemorrhage, and Periengraftment Respiratory Distress Syndrome

Several diffuse pulmonary complications may arise in the early period after HSCT, usually occurring within 30 days after transplantation.

Pulmonary edema may occur in the setting of volume overload resulting from fluids and blood products administered during conditioning and shortly after transplantation and may be accompanied by dyspnea, crackles, and hypoxemia.[69]

PERIENGRAFTMENT RESPIRATORY DISTRESS SYNDROME

Periengraftment respiratory distress syndrome (PERDS) refers to acute lung injury in the early posttransplantation period and has also been referred to as "periengraftment syndrome."[70] The condition is a noncardiogenic edema that arises from capillary leakage, with average onset 7 days after HSCT. Patients may present with dyspnea, fever, and skin rash; mortality of approximately 20% is reported.[70]

Diffuse alveolar hemorrhage (DAH) has been reported in 2% to 21% of HSCT patients and has a high mortality rate, with onset usually within the first 30 days after transplantation. Presentation can include dyspnea, hypoxemia, and cough.[70] Diagnosis relies on evidence of pneumonitis, blood and/or hemosiderin-laden macrophages in bronchoalveolar lavage fluid, and absence of findings of infection.[69] Hemoptysis is present in a minority (<20%) of cases.[71] DAH and diffuse alveolar damage in acute lung injury often occur together.

Imaging Considerations

Pulmonary edema from volume overload, PERDS, and DAH may have similar appearances at imaging. Chest radiographs typically show diffuse bilateral hazy airspace opacities and/or consolidation, often with a perihilar predominance. CT shows bilateral ground-glass opacities and/or consolidation, and centrilobular ground-glass opacity may also be present (Fig. 70.13).[70] In pulmonary edema, septal thickening and pleural effusions may be a clue to the diagnosis (Fig. 70.14) but can also be seen in other conditions.

Treatment

Treatment of PERDS and DAH usually involves high-dose corticosteroids. Most patients with DAH require mechanical ventilation and intensive care support, whereas a minority of patients with PERDS require ventilation.[69] Pulmonary edema

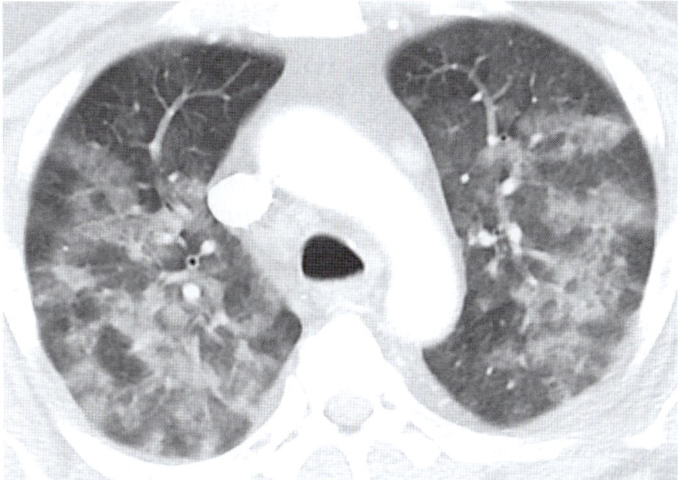

Fig. 70.13 Diffuse pulmonary hemorrhage. Axial CT image shows patchy bilateral ground-glass opacities, an appearance that can be seen in diffuse alveolar hemorrhage after stem cell transplantation.

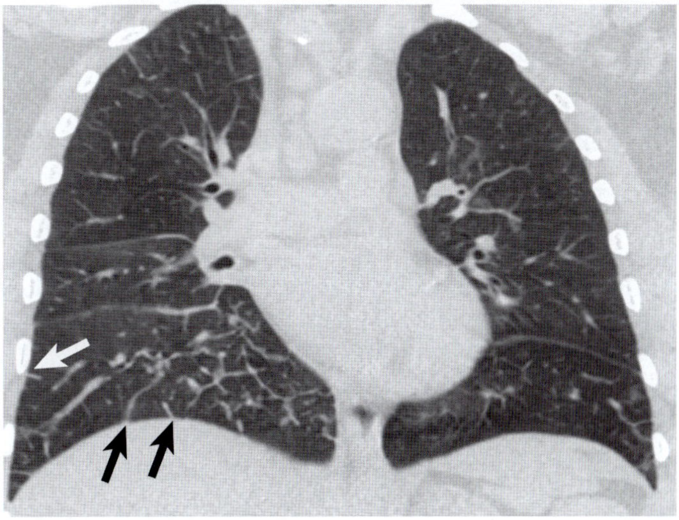

Fig. 70.14 Pulmonary edema after stem cell transplantation. Coronal CT image shows bilateral smooth interlobular septal thickening *(arrows)*, thickening of the interlobar fissures, and a small amount of perihilar ground-glass opacity.

resulting from volume overload may be self-limiting or may require reduction in fluids, diuretics, or supportive care.

CHRONIC GRAFT-VERSUS-HOST DISEASE AND BRONCHIOLITIS OBLITERANS SYNDROME

Prevalence and Clinical Considerations

Chronic graft-versus-host disease (cGVHD) is an immune-mediated inflammatory disease affecting approximately 30% to 70% of hematopoietic stem cell transplantation patients and is a significant cause of morbidity and mortality. GVHD can affect multiple organ systems or, less commonly, a single organ and can occur as early as 1 year after transplantation or as late as decades after the procedure.[72] *BOS* is the pulmonary manifestation of cGVHD and is the most common chronic lung disease after HSCT, with an incidence of 5.5%.[73] As in lung transplantation, the condition is characterized by a progressive bronchiolar and peribronchiolar fibrosis that causes bronchiolar obstruction and air-trapping.[74] Patients typically present with chronic dyspnea, cough, and occasionally wheezing. Diagnosis can be made by transbronchial or open lung biopsy but is most frequently made by clinical findings, PFTs, and suggestive CT features. In the setting of an additional organ system finding of GVHD, a clinical diagnosis of BOS can be made by satisfying these criteria[72]:

- FEV1/forced vital capacity ratio <0.7 or in 5th percentile of predicted
- FEV1 <75% of predicted with >10% decline in less than 2 years
- Absence of infection by imaging and/or laboratory testing
- At least one supportive finding of air-trapping:
  - Air-trapping at expiratory CT or ancillary findings of small airway disease
  - Elevated residual volume >120% of predicted

Imaging Considerations

As in lung transplantation, the primary imaging finding of BOS after stem cell transplantation is air-trapping at thin-section CT. A mosaic attenuation pattern can be seen on inspiratory series, with lobular or regional areas of low-attenuation lung that fail to show a normal increase in attenuation at expiration (see Fig. 70.8). Expiratory CT is more sensitive for detection of mosaic attenuation and air-trapping than inspiratory CT alone. Additional findings of bronchiolitis obliterans can include bronchiectasis, bronchial wall thickening, and small airway (centrilobular) nodules.[72] In a small number of cases the "thoracic air leak syndrome" may develop in the setting of BOS and manifests with persistent pneumomediastinum and interstitial emphysema.[75]

Treatment

Systemic corticosteroids (prednisone) are the most frequent treatment for GVHD/BOS but many have limited effect.[73,76] Azithromycin, fluticasone, and montelukast may provide some benefit for airflow limitation and may have a steroid-sparing effect. Supportive care with pulmonary rehabilitation may increase quality of life and decrease symptoms. Lung transplantation may be used in severe cases.[75]

OTHER MANIFESTATIONS OF LATE-ONSET IDIOPATHIC PNEUMONIA SYNDROME

Prevalence and Clinical Considerations

Although BOS as a manifestation of cGVHD is the most common late-onset idiopathic pneumonia syndrome (IPS), many other lung diseases occur after HSCT. In the largest study of late-onset idiopathic pneumonia syndrome (LOIPS), 2.4% of patients developed LOIPS after HSCT, with a median time from transplantation of 11.3 months. Most common symptoms were dyspnea (88%), fever (50%), and cough (60%). Although many patients improved with therapy, 33% of patients died.[76]

OP is a late complication of HSCT characterized by loose plugs of connective tissue within small airways and interstitial inflammation at histopathology.[77] The condition is the most widely recognized ILD associated with HSCT, affecting 2% of patients, with median onset of approximately 150 days after transplantation in one large series.[68] Patients present with low-grade fever, dyspnea, and nonproductive cough, with symptoms that do not respond to empirical antibiotic therapy. Risk factors for the development of OP include allogeneic graft origin, history of acute GVHD, CMV infection, and radiation conditioning for transplantation.[68] As in other conditions and in cryptogenic OP, OP in stem cell transplantation patients responds well to corticosteroids.[77] Although patients can relapse after steroid taper, the death rate is very low, with no deaths attributable to OP in the study by Jinta and colleagues.[68]

Many other diffuse lung diseases can manifest after HSCT as part of IPS, including nonspecific interstitial pneumonia (NSIP), diffuse alveolar damage (DAD), lymphoid interstitial pneumonia (LIP), and eosinophilic pneumonia. Pleuroparenchymal fibroelastosis (PPFE) has also been rarely described.[75]

Imaging Considerations

In OP radiography can show patchy airspace opacities, often bilateral and multifocal.[68] CT is often performed for characterization of often nonspecific radiographic findings. The most common CT features of OP after stem cell transplantation are ground-glass opacity, consolidation, and linear opacities. Although peripheral or peribronchovascular consolidation can occur, as in many cases of cryptogenic OP or OP in other diseases, one series found a greater prevalence of ground-glass opacity, linear opacities, and upper lobe predominance than in OP from other causes.[77] CT may also show peripheral consolidation with central ground-glass opacities representing the CT halo or atoll sign (Fig. 70.15). Many patients have residual abnormalities at CT, including

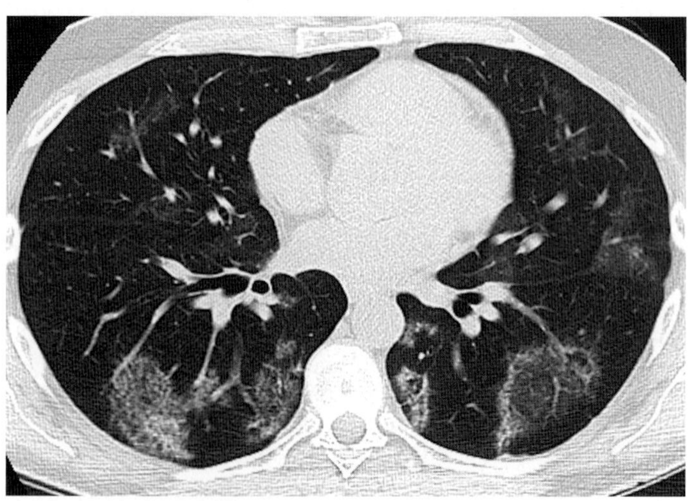

Fig. 70.15 Organizing pneumonia after stem cell transplantation. Axial CT image shows bilateral focal ground-glass opacities with peripheral consolidation (the "atoll" or "reverse halo" sign).

band-like opacities, traction bronchiectasis, and fibrosis that can resemble fibrotic nonspecific interstitial pneumonia.[77,78]

The range of additional diffuse lung diseases associated with HSCT may manifest with ground-glass opacity and/or consolidation (e.g., eosinophilic pneumonia, NSIP, and DAD). LIP may manifest with thin-walled cysts, nodules, and ground-glass opacity. PPFE manifests as upper lobe volume loss, traction bronchiectasis, architectural distortion, and pleural thickening.[75]

In a study of 40 patients with LOIPS, 55% of patients had predominantly consolidation on thin-section CT, and 45% had predominantly ground-glass opacity; the patients with predominantly consolidation tended to have a better survival than those with ground-glass opacity, although this difference fell short of statistical significance.[76]

Treatment

In contrast to many patients with BOS, patients with other types of LOIPS may show either complete resolution or significant improvement of PFTs with steroid therapy, including those with predominantly OP, NSIP, or eosinophilic pneumonia.[73] PPFE typically has a progressive course that is refractory to drug therapy.

PULMONARY HYPERTENSION AND OTHER VASCULAR DISEASES

Incidence and Clinical Considerations

Pulmonary hypertension is an uncommon complication in HSCT, with a reported incidence of 2.4%; patients can present with dyspnea and hypoxemia, and progression to right ventricular failure and death can occur.[73] Pulmonary venoocclusive disease and transplant-associated microangiopathy have also been reported.

Imaging Considerations

Right heart catheterization is the gold standard for the diagnosis of pulmonary hypertension, and echocardiography can be used to estimate pulmonary arterial pressures. The condition may be suspected at CT or MRI when pulmonary artery enlargement is present. A main pulmonary artery greater than 32.5 mm or a diameter larger than the adjacent ascending aorta may prompt further evaluation for the possibility of the condition. In addition, pulmonary hypertension has been associated with BOS in both lung transplantation and HSCT, and findings of mosaic attenuation with air-trapping, bronchial wall thickening, and bronchiectasis may prompt consideration.[79]

Treatment

Therapies for pulmonary hypertension include supplemental oxygen, phosphodiesterase-5 inhibitors, and other medical therapy.[80]

IMAGING ALGORITHMS

Radiography is typically the first imaging examination performed for the evaluation of acute disease in stem cell transplantation patients. Many infections can be detected as nodules or diffuse or focal pulmonary airspace opacities. Acute syndromes, such as pulmonary edema and capillary leak syndrome, can manifest as diffuse airspace opacities. However, CT is usually pursued in the setting of acute symptoms with normal or indeterminate findings at radiography, and thin-section CT is the first modality pursued in cases of suspected chronic lung disease and in surveillance for BOS. For suspected chronic lung disease, most centers obtain an inspiratory thin-section volumetric CT and an expiratory axial acquisition, obtained at a fraction of the dose of the helical series.

KEY POINTS: HEMATOPOIETIC STEM CELL TRANSPLANTATION

- Infectious or noninfectious pulmonary complications occur in almost half of patients after hematopoietic stem cell transplantation (HSCT).
- Early complications of HSCT include pulmonary edema, periengraftment respiratory distress syndrome, and diffuse alveolar hemorrhage and usually manifest with bilateral airspace opacities at radiography or CT.
- Bronchiolitis obliterans syndrome (BOS) is the pulmonary manifestation of chronic graft-versus-host disease and affects 5.5% of HSCT patients. Pulmonary function tests show obstructive physiology, and mosaic attenuation with air-trapping is typically seen at CT.
- Other types of late-onset idiopathic pneumonia syndrome after HSCT include organizing pneumonia, nonspecific interstitial pneumonia, diffuse alveolar damage, lymphoid interstitial pneumonia, and eosinophilic pneumonia. Consolidation and ground-glass opacity are common findings at CT.
- Pulmonary hypertension occurs in a small minority of HSCT patients and has been associated with BOS. Although right heart catheterization and echocardiography establish the diagnosis of pulmonary hypertension, enlargement of the pulmonary arteries may suggest the diagnosis at radiography, CT, or MRI.

SUGGESTED READINGS

Choi YW, Rossi SE, Palmer SM, DeLong D, Erasmus JJ, McAdams HP. Bronchiolitis obliterans syndrome in lung transplant recipients: correlation of computed tomography findings with bronchiolitis obliterans syndrome stage. *J Thorac Imaging*. 2003;18(2):72–79.

Inamoto Y, Lee SJ. Late effects of blood and marrow transplantation. *Haematologica*. 2017;102(4):614–625.

Krishnam MS, Suh RD, Tomasian A, et al. Postoperative complications of lung transplantation: radiologic findings along a time continuum. *Radiographics*. 2007;27(4):957–974.

Park CH, Paik HC, Haam SJ, et al. HRCT features of acute rejection in patients with bilateral lung transplantation: the usefulness of lesion distribution. *Transplant Proc*. 2014;46(5):1511–1516.

Tejwani V, Panchabhai TS, Kotloff RM, Mehta AC. Complications of lung transplantation: a roentgenographic perspective. *Chest*. 2016;149(6):1535–1545.

Schlemmer F, Chevret S, Lorillon G, et al. Late-onset noninfectious interstitial lung disease after allogeneic hematopoietic stem cell transplantation. *Respir Med*. 2014;108(10):1525–1533.

The full reference list for this chapter is available at ExpertConsult.com.

71 Pneumothorax

ASHISH GUPTA | JEAN M. SEELY

Pneumothorax is the presence of air between the parietal and visceral pleura in the pleural cavity. It is caused most frequently by trauma or blunt or penetrating injury, which may be accidental or iatrogenic. If it is not caused by trauma, it is referred to as spontaneous; this may be primary (not associated with an underlying cause) or secondary to preexisting significant pulmonary disease. Pneumothorax may also occur after pneumomediastinum, with air-tracking into the pleural space.

Primary Spontaneous Pneumothorax

Etiology

A primary spontaneous pneumothorax occurs when air collects in the pleural space of a healthy individual without preceding trauma and without underlying lung disease. The etiology of primary spontaneous pneumothorax is a matter of debate. Traditionally, it is thought to result from the rupture of a small, thin-walled air-containing space (emphysema-like changes [ELCs]) within or deep to the visceral pleura into the pleural cavity. By convention ELCs are defined as blebs, when smaller than 1 cm in diameter, and bullae, which are larger than 1 cm in diameter (Figs. 71.1 and 71.2). On pathology examination, pleural blebs are defined as emphysematous spaces occurring within the substance of the pleura[1]; bullae are in direct contact with the parenchyma.[2] It is likely that most air-containing spaces associated with pneumothorax are, in fact, bullae. Smoking is an important risk factor for primary spontaneous pneumothorax. The lifetime risk for development of pneumothorax in smoking men is 12% compared with 0.1% in nonsmoking men.[3,4] One study showed that smoking increased the relative risk of a first spontaneous pneumothorax approximately 9-fold among women and 22-fold among men, and that there is a striking dose-response relationship between smoking and the occurrence of spontaneous pneumothorax.[3] Small airway inflammation (respiratory bronchiolitis) associated with smoking is likely responsible for the increased risk of pneumothorax in smokers.[5] Cannabis smoking has also been linked with accelerated development of apical peripheral bullous disease, predisposing for pneumothorax, in the absence of parenchymal changes elsewhere in the lungs.[6]

Prevalence and Epidemiology

Primary spontaneous pneumothorax occurs most commonly in patients between 18 and 40 years of age.[7,8] The male-to-female ratio is about 4:1 to 5:1.[9] The incidence of primary spontaneous pneumothorax is estimated to be approximately 7.4 to 18 per 100,000 per year for men and 1.2 to 6 per 100,000 per year for women.[3,10] It has been observed that the typical person who presents with a primary spontaneous pneumothorax has an asthenic body habitus, being taller and thinner than the average person.[11] An increased pleural pressure gradient between apex and base of lung is likely responsible for the increased risk in taller individuals.[12]

FAMILIAL

More than 10% of patients with primary spontaneous pneumothorax report a family history of the disease, thought to be by autosomal-dominant inheritance.[13,14] Other modes of inheritance have been suggested: more than one gene, with some cases inherited as an X-linked recessive disorder and others as an autosomal-dominant trait with incomplete penetrance. Recently, mutations in the gene encoding folliculin have been identified in individuals with familial spontaneous pneumothorax.[13] Mutations in this gene were known previously to cause Birt-Hogg-Dubé syndrome (Fig. 71.3), an autosomal-dominant inherited disease characterized by benign skin tumors, diverse types of renal cancer, pulmonary cysts, and spontaneous pneumothorax.[13] The presence of thin-walled cysts in basilar and subpleural locations of the lung is a feature of this disease.[13] The location of these cysts contrasts with the apical distribution of other more well-recognized causes of spontaneous pneumothorax, such as emphysematous bullae and idiopathic blebs.[15] About 80% of patients with Birt-Hogg-Dubé syndrome manifest pulmonary cysts, and between 11% and 32% of patients develop pneumothorax.[13] When large, the cysts may be multiseptated.[16] A significant fraction of families with familial spontaneous pneumothorax have mutations in the folliculin gene; this should be considered a forme fruste of Birt-Hogg-Dubé syndrome.[13,17]

An intrinsic abnormality of connective tissue resulting in an increased tendency to bulla or bleb formation is also important. For example, spontaneous pneumothorax is a well-known complication in patients with Marfan syndrome—an autosomal-dominant disease with a frequency of spontaneous pneumothorax of 4.4%–11%, Ehlers-Danlos syndrome, homocystinuria, mitral valve prolapse, and α1-antitrypsin deficiency.[13]

Pathophysiology

The cause of primary spontaneous pneumothorax is debatable.[18–21] Although patients with primary spontaneous pneumothorax do not have clinically apparent lung disease, subpleural bullae are found in 76% to 100% of patients during video-assisted thoracoscopic surgery[22–24] and in virtually all patients during thoracotomy.[21,25,26] Even among nonsmokers with a history of pneumothorax, 81% have bullae, also called ELCs.[9] Whereas it has generally been assumed that these bullae on the visceral pleura leak, causing the pneumothorax, there is a lack of evidence of actual rupture of the bullae at thoracoscopic surgery.[21,27] Furthermore, simple surgical removal of the bullae does not prevent recurrence of spontaneous pneumothorax.[18,21] It is more likely that small airway disease plays an important role, whereby inflammation-induced obstruction of the small airways increases alveolar pressure, which results in leaking of air into the lung interstitium. The air then moves to the hilum, causing pneumomediastinum (Hamman syndrome),[28] or ruptures into the pleura, causing a pneumothorax.[21] Some authors have suggested that the porosity of the visceral pleura is increased in patients with spontaneous pneumothorax.[29]

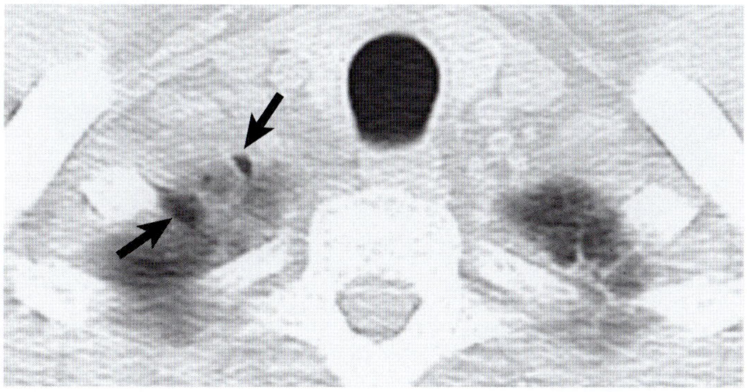

Fig. 71.1 Blebs in a young man with history of spontaneous pneumothorax. CT demonstrates two 5-mm lucencies in the right lung apex, consistent with blebs *(arrows)*.

ANATOMY OF THE PLEURA

The outer surface of the lung and the inner surface of the protective thoracic cage are covered by an elastic, serous, and lubricating membrane to form the pleural cavity. This is almost like inserting a sealed wet and stretchable plastic bag between the lung and the thoracic wall and diaphragm to decrease friction.[30]

The anatomy of the pleura is complex.[31] It covers the upper surface of the diaphragm and extends, in front, as low as the costal cartilage of the 7th rib; at the side of the chest, it extends to the lower border of the 10th rib on the left and to the upper

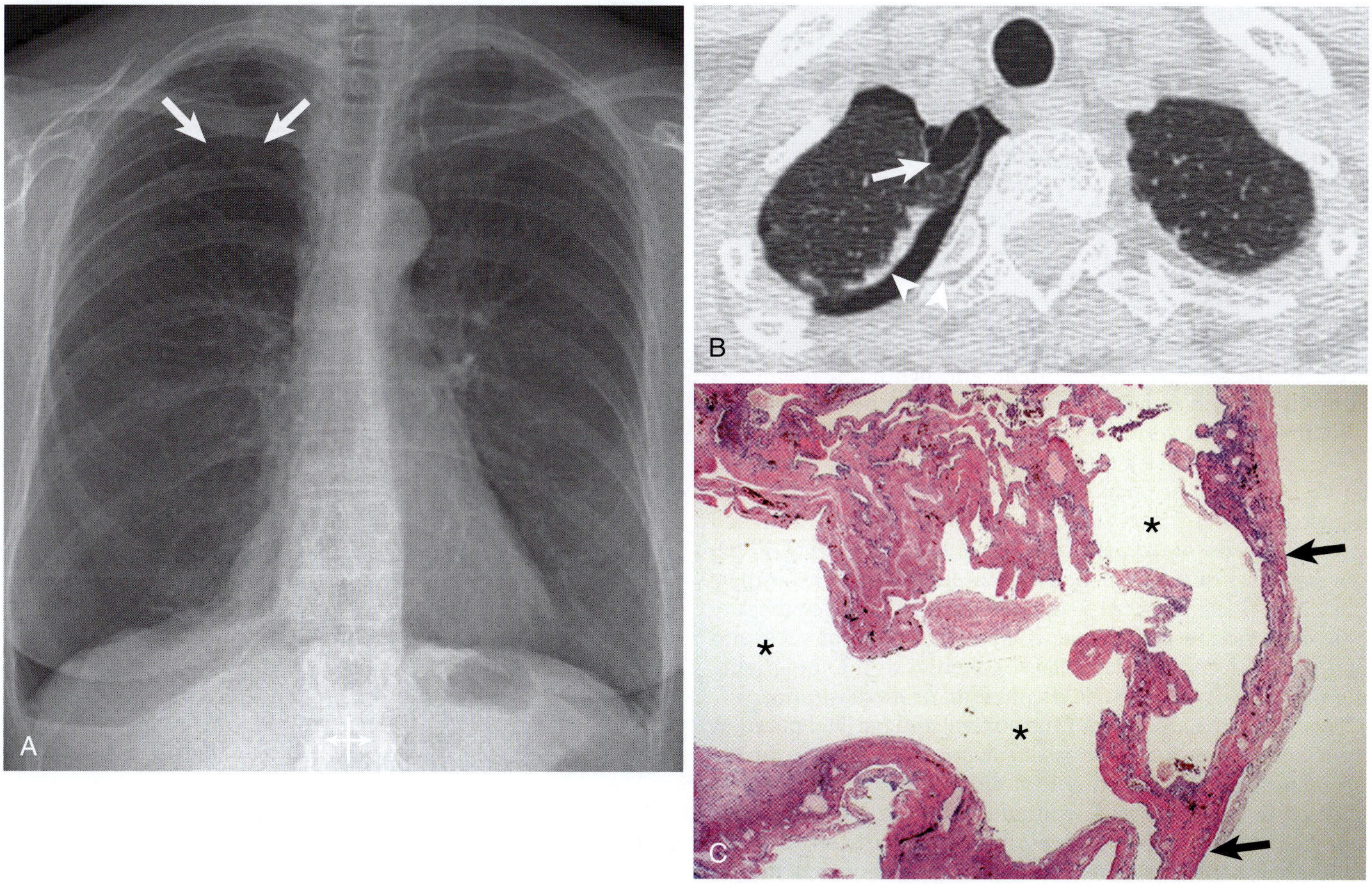

Fig. 71.2 Bulla and pneumothorax. (A) Posteroanterior chest radiograph in inspiration demonstrates a moderate right pneumothorax with apical bullae *(arrows)* outlined by air within the pleural space. A tiny right pleural effusion is seen in the costophrenic angle. (B) Thin-section CT of the lung apices in another patient who presented with a recurrent spontaneous right pneumothorax shows a bulla *(arrow)* and the pneumothorax displacing thickened, fibrotic visceral pleura *(arrowheads)*. (C) Pathology slide: emphysematous bulla. At bullectomy, a large emphysematous space *(stars)* is seen in direct contact with the intact visceral pleura *(arrows)*.

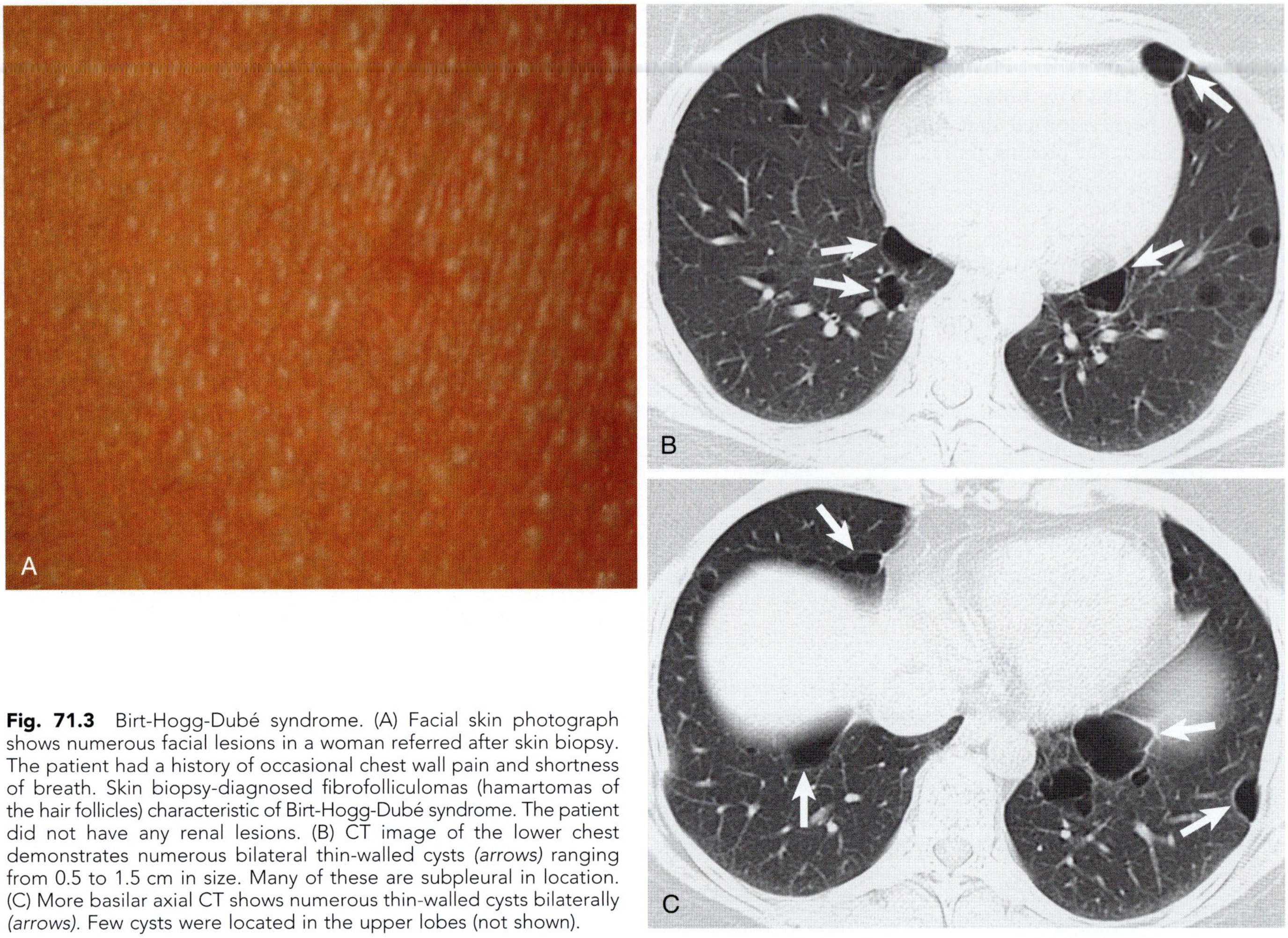

Fig. 71.3 Birt-Hogg-Dubé syndrome. (A) Facial skin photograph shows numerous facial lesions in a woman referred after skin biopsy. The patient had a history of occasional chest wall pain and shortness of breath. Skin biopsy-diagnosed fibrofolliculomas (hamartomas of the hair follicles) characteristic of Birt-Hogg-Dubé syndrome. The patient did not have any renal lesions. (B) CT image of the lower chest demonstrates numerous bilateral thin-walled cysts *(arrows)* ranging from 0.5 to 1.5 cm in size. Many of these are subpleural in location. (C) More basilar axial CT shows numerous thin-walled cysts bilaterally *(arrows)*. Few cysts were located in the upper lobes (not shown).

border of the same rib on the right; and behind, it reaches as low as the 12th rib and sometimes even to the transverse process of the first lumbar vertebra.

The normal pleura is a thin translucent membrane and consists of five layers. These may be difficult to distinguish by light microscopy. These layers are (1) the mesothelium, flattened mesothelial cells joined primarily by tight junctions (Fig. 71.4); (2) a thin layer of submesothelial connective tissue; (3) a superficial elastic tissue layer; (4) a second loose subpleural connective tissue layer rich in arteries, veins, nerves, and lymphatics; and finally, (5) a deep fibroelastic layer adherent to the underlying lung parenchyma, chest wall, diaphragm, or mediastinum.[1]

The lymphatic anatomy of the visceral and parietal pleura is important in the homeostasis of pleural fluid volume in the normal individual. The amount of fluid in the pleural cavity is regulated by the hydrostatic-osmotic pressure relationship and pleural-lymphatic drainage. Excess fluid, large particles, and cells in the pleural cavity are removed through preformed stomas assisted by respiratory movements. These naturally occurring pores exist in the caudal portions of the peripheral parietal and lower mediastinal parietal pleura.[1,32] Most of the fluid that accumulates abnormally in the pleural space is derived from the lung through the visceral pleura and absorbed primarily through the parietal pleura.[1]

The normal volume of pleural fluid in the adult is proportional to body weight (0.1–0.2 mL/kg).[1] The normal pleural fluid has a protein concentration of approximately 1.5 g/dL.[33] The pleural fluid has a few cells under normal conditions, including rare macrophages, mesothelial cells, and lymphocytes.[1] The entire surface area of the pleura in an adult man is 2000 cm^2.[25]

The parietal pleura derives its blood supply from branches of the intercostal arteries.[30] The mediastinal pleura is supplied by the pericardiophrenic artery, whereas the diaphragmatic parietal pleura derives its blood supply from the superior phrenic and musculophrenic arteries. The visceral pleura derives most of its blood supply from the bronchial arterial system.[1]

Clinical Presentation

Most episodes of primary spontaneous pneumothorax occur while the patient is at rest.[34] All patients have ipsilateral pleuritic chest pain or acute dyspnea.[21] Chest pain may be minimal or severe. Symptoms usually resolve within 24 hours, even if the pneumothorax remains untreated and does not resolve.[21] Patients with a small pneumothorax (<15% of the hemithorax) may have normal findings on physical examination. Patients with a larger pneumothorax may have decreased movement of the chest wall, a positive "coin test" result, diminished fremitus, or decreased to absent breath sounds on the affected side. The Hamman sign, initially reported in 1937 as a sign of pneumomediastinum, is now thought to be more likely associated with left-sided pneumothorax.[35] The sign results from the presence of gas in close contact with the heart, characterized by a peculiar crunching, bubbling, popping, or crackling sound that varies with the phase of the cardiac cycle and is best heard in the left lateral decubitus position.[35]

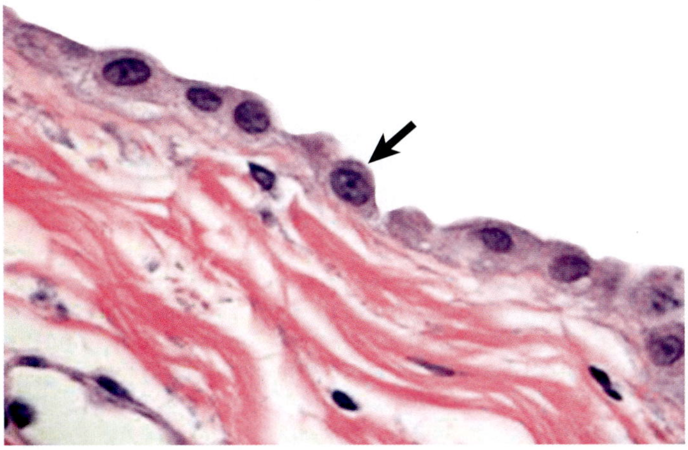

Fig. 71.4 Pathology slide: normal visceral pleura. Mesothelial cells *(arrow)* and vascular layer of the visceral pleura are shown on this pathology slide. Note the cuboidal shape of the mesothelial cells.

Manifestations of the Disease

RADIOGRAPHY

Upright Chest Radiograph

The most helpful sign is a thin pleural line (<1 mm thick) parallel to the chest wall (Fig. 71.5), with no lung markings projecting beyond it. Because the lung is partly collapsed by the pneumothorax, it might be anticipated that its density would be increased and that this altered density, compared with that of the normal lung, should be sufficient to suggest the diagnosis; in fact, this is often not the case. First, as the lung progressively collapses with the increasing size of the pneumothorax, blood flow through it diminishes; therefore the ratio of air to tissue and blood is not altered, and the overall density of the collapsing lung is not changed.[36] Second, lung density is reduced in the region of pneumothorax because of the presence of air both anterior and posterior to it.[37]

When pneumothorax is strongly suspected clinically but is not identified, gas in the pleural space may be detected on radiography by one of two methods: (1) chest radiograph in the erect position in full expiration, with the reason for this being that reducing the negative pleural pressure increases the relative size of the pleural space and thus allows easier detection of pneumothoraces, and (2) chest radiograph in the lateral decubitus position, with the involved side up, with the rationale being that air will be more visible over the lateral chest wall than at the apex. Compared with the erect chest radiograph, the lateral decubitus view is more sensitive. A study comparing inspiratory

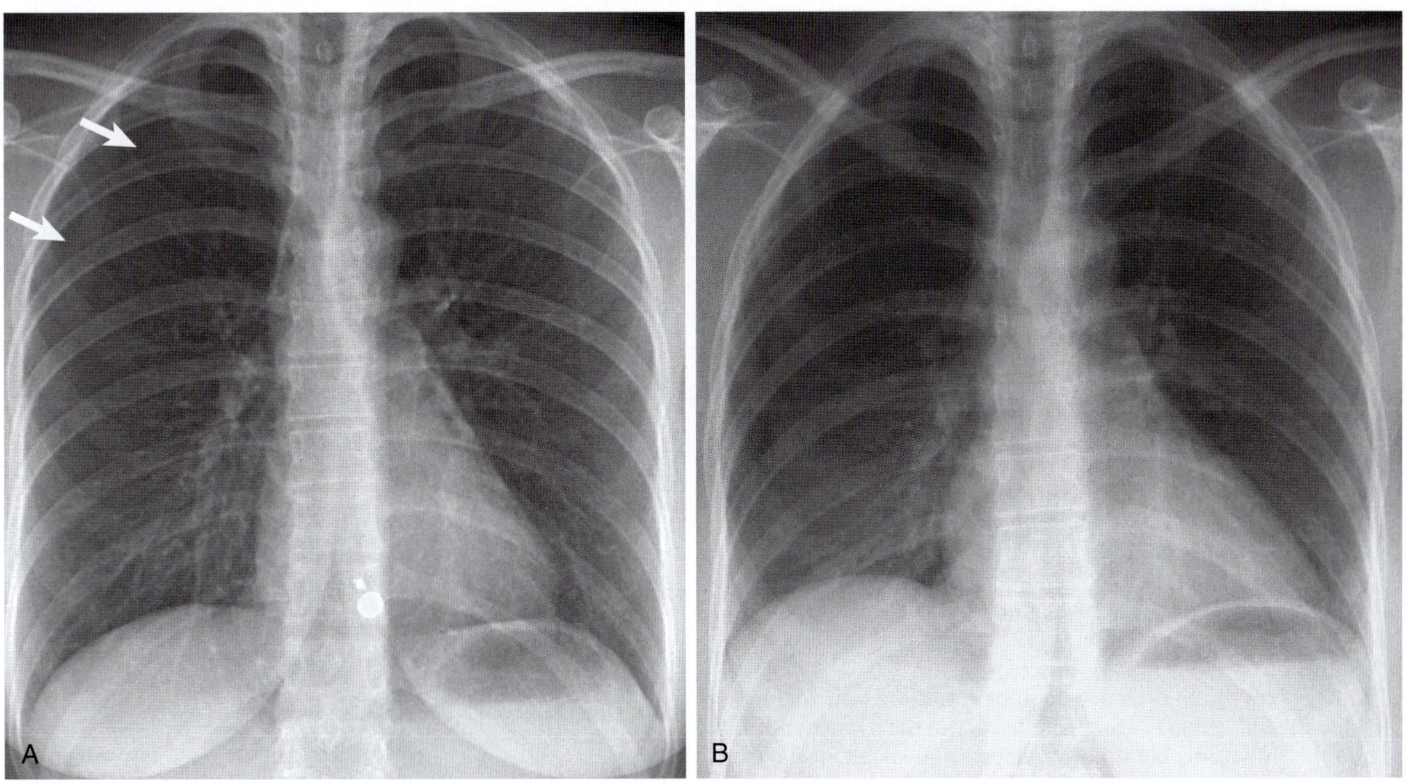

Fig. 71.5 Primary spontaneous pneumothorax in a nonsmoker. (A) Posteroanterior chest radiograph in full inspiration demonstrates a thin white line of the visceral pleura *(arrows)* from a small right pneumothorax. (B) Chest radiograph in expiration better demonstrates the right pneumothorax. Thin-section CT (not shown) demonstrated a small apical bleb.

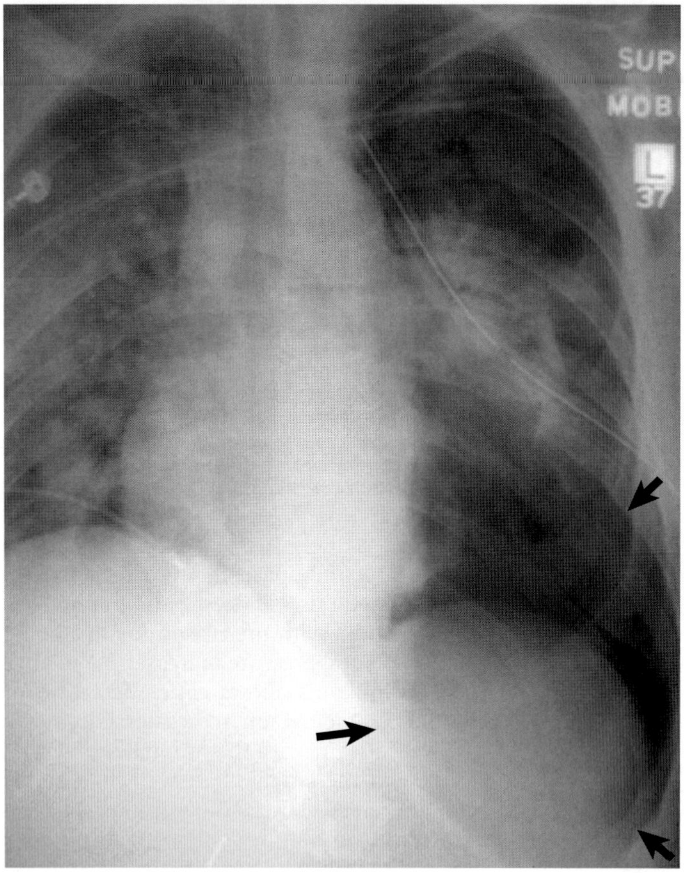

Fig. 71.6 Chest radiography: deep sulcus sign. Supine chest radiograph demonstrates a large, left anterior pneumothorax causing the deep sulcus sign *(arrows)*. The left chest tube was not functioning.

and expiratory upright films found that both were equally sensitive for pneumothorax detection.[38] Given the limitations of expiratory films, inspiratory films are recommended as the initial examination of choice for pneumothorax detection.

Supine Chest Radiograph

In the supine patient, the main finding is the deep sulcus sign (Fig. 71.6), a very deep radiolucent costophrenic sulcus. Note that the most nondependent portion of the pleural space in a supine patient is the inferior lateral hemithorax. It is important that the lateral costophrenic angles be included on the radiograph, as failure to diagnose pneumothorax may be life threatening because of the risk of tension.[39] The supine view is much less sensitive for pneumothorax and grossly underestimates the true size of a pneumothorax. In one study of trauma patients, more than 50% of pneumothoraces were missed on the supine chest radiograph compared with computed tomography (CT).[40] In a cadaver study the lateral decubitus film was most sensitive (88%), followed by the erect radiograph (59%), with the least sensitive being the supine view (37%).[41]

Other clues to the presence of a pneumothorax on a supine view are the following: relative hypolucency in the hypochondrial region or the entire hemithorax, depression of an ipsilateral hemidiaphragm, double-diaphragm appearance, sharp delineation of the cardiomediastinal and diaphragmatic borders, increased visualization of the mediastinal fat pads (floating cardiac pad sign),[42] lobulated appearance of mediastinal fat pad,[43] visible inferior border of the collapsed lower lobe or the heart, band of air in the minor fissure, and visible lateral edge of the right middle lobe.[44]

In suspected pneumothorax, if only a single chest radiograph is taken, it should be done upright, on inspiration. When a pneumothorax is suspected in a supine patient, confirmation can be readily obtained with a lateral decubitus view. CT may also be useful and has been shown to identify 50% to 64% of occult pneumothoraces in the trauma setting.[45]

Cause of Pneumothorax on the Chest Radiograph

Aside from the presence of a pneumothorax, the radiograph is often normal.[46] However, apical blebs or bullae (see Fig. 71.2), apical scarring, and diffuse emphysema may be identified.[47] In a study of 116 patients with surgically treated pneumothorax, parenchymal abnormalities were found in 68% and pleural thickening in 4%.[47] The most common abnormalities were apical bullae, seen in 44% of patients.[47] A study of chest radiographs of 100 patients presenting with first episode of primary spontaneous pneumothorax, followed for 57 months, revealed an increased likelihood of recurrence in the presence of certain radiographic abnormalities, including pleural thickening, blebs/bullae, pleural irregularities, and pleural adhesions.[48] Another study found an increased likelihood of recurrence of pneumothorax after surgery in patients with a residual apical space on postoperative radiographs.[49]

COMPUTED TOMOGRAPHY

Several studies have shown that thin-section CT is a reliable method of detecting blebs and bullae in patients with spontaneous pneumothorax.[19,46,50–53] The most common parenchymal abnormality associated with spontaneous pneumothorax is emphysema, which may be readily diagnosed on thin-section CT (Fig. 71.7). If emphysema is not present, most patients will have an isolated bulla or bleb (see Fig. 71.2).[9,46,47] In one study evidence of emphysema was seen on CT in 16 of 20 (80%) patients with spontaneous pneumothorax.[46] In another investigation localized areas of emphysema were identified in 22 of 27 (81%) lifelong nonsmokers who had a previous spontaneous pneumothorax.[9] The emphysema involved mainly the upper lobes and the peripheral rather than the central lung regions. The role of thin-section CT in predicting recurrence of pneumothorax is controversial. Some studies have found a significant relationship between the presence of blebs and bullae at CT after a first episode of primary spontaneous pneumothorax and the development of an ipsilateral recurrence or a contralateral episode of pneumothorax.[54] Some researchers have questioned its role in preoperative assessment and predicting recurrence.[55,55a] A CT-based scoring system (dystrophic severity score) has been proposed based on size, number, and distribution of apical air-containing lesions. This score has been shown to predict ipsilateral recurrence and contralateral pneumothorax after the first episode in patients treated conservatively.[56]

ULTRASONOGRAPHY

Ultrasonography is a sensitive and reliable method for diagnosis of a pneumothorax.[40,57–60] Findings of pneumothorax on ultrasound have been well described, such as the absence of visceral pleural sliding movements during respiration—called disappearance of the "gliding sign," absence of comet tail artifacts in the supine patient, absence of lung pulse—lung sliding resulting from transmitted cardiac pulsations, and identification of lung point—identification of the edge of pneumothorax by reappearance of the normal respiratory pattern (lung sliding and B lines).[61,61a,62,62a] The presence of B lines (echogenic vertical lines moving with respiration, reaching the lower portion of field without fading), lung sliding, and lung pulse are helpful in ruling out pneumothorax. Among these factors, lung point is reported to be 100% specific when identified.[63]

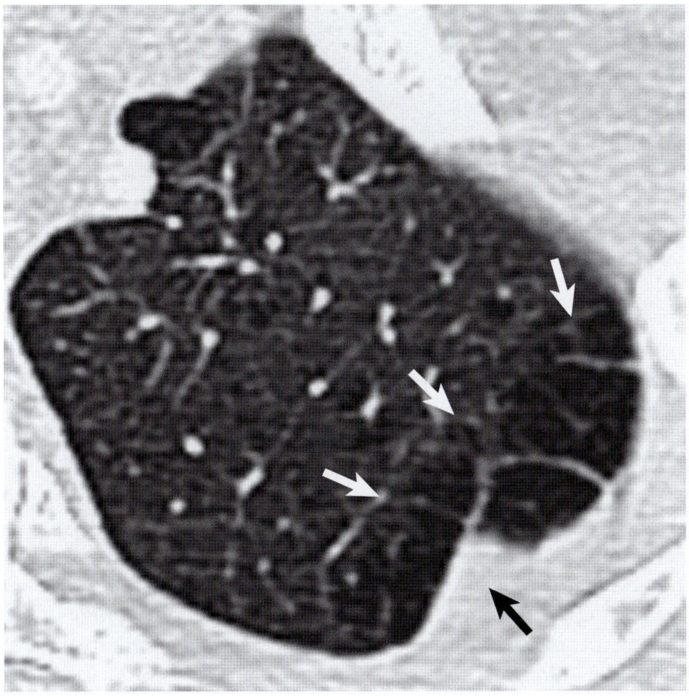

Fig. 71.7 Emphysema in a patient with history of secondary spontaneous pneumothorax. Thin-section CT image demonstrates paraseptal emphysema *(white arrows)* adjacent to an area of localized pleural thickening *(black arrow)*.

In a study of 183 patients after percutaneous needle biopsy, pneumothorax was identified in 46 patients (25%) by CT, in 44 by ultrasonography, and in 19 by chest radiography. The sensitivity of ultrasonography was 95.7%, and its specificity was 100%.[57] Most investigations of pleural ultrasound otherwise have been limited to the trauma setting. Several meta-analyses comparing ultrasound with chest radiography, in the acute care setting, have shown the superiority of ultrasound for the diagnosis of pneumothorax.[48,64,65] Ultrasound can also allow semiquantitative assessment of pneumothorax size by assessing the position of the lung point.[66]

Differential Diagnosis

The thin white line of the visceral pleura in pneumothorax must be distinguished from the black line of a skin fold, which is accentuated by the Mach effect (Fig. 71.8). Skin folds are usually seen to pass outside the chest cavity, are straight or only minimally curved, and usually do not run parallel to the chest wall as with a true visceral pleural line.[67] The superolateral portion of the major fissures is a shadow identified in the upper hemithorax that appears as a curvilinear opacity of a curving edge, seen close to the lateral chest wall in proximity to the sixth posterior rib (Fig. 71.9). This was reported in about 15% of cases in a study of 1068 normal subjects and is attributed to extrapleural fat intruding into the major fissure.[68] A large bulla may sometimes be mistaken for a pneumothorax; it is critical to differentiate this from pneumothorax (Fig. 71.10). Sometimes internal lung markings are visible in a bulla. A clue to bullous lesions is that those abutting the chest wall have a concave appearance. If there is any doubt, CT of the chest should be obtained. A huge bronchogenic cyst has also been mistaken for a pneumothorax.[69] The scapula may sometimes be mistaken for a pneumothorax, but once considered, it can be traced in continuity with the rest of the bone. Hair, extraneous monitoring or support lines, and even the subcostal groove of the rib may mimic a pneumothorax.[67] On occasion, pneumomediastinum may be confused with pneumothorax.[70]

In the erect individual a pneumothorax is first evident near the apex of the chest (see Figs. 71.2 and 71.5); subpulmonic

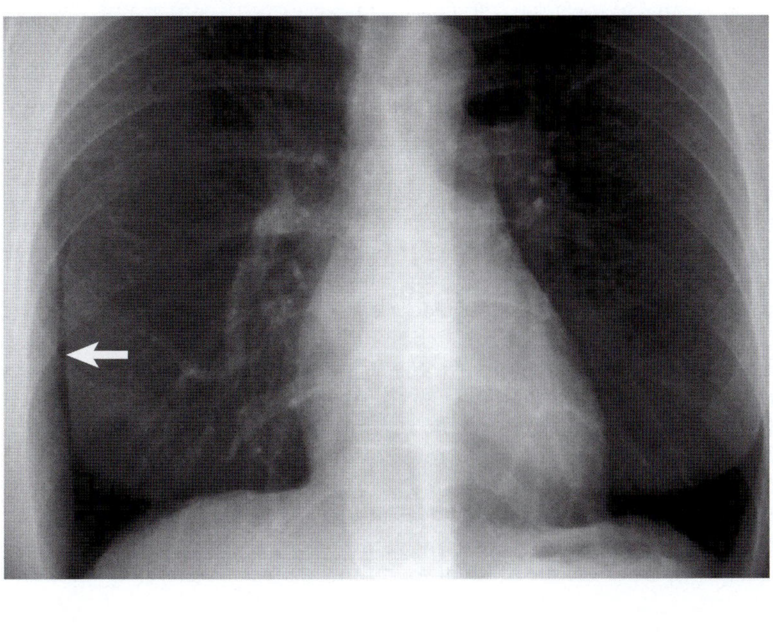

Fig. 71.8 Chest radiography: skin fold. Magnified view from a chest radiograph shows a prominent skin fold overlying the lower right hemithorax, creating a thick black Mach line *(arrow)*, which is distinct from the white visceral pleural line of a pneumothorax.

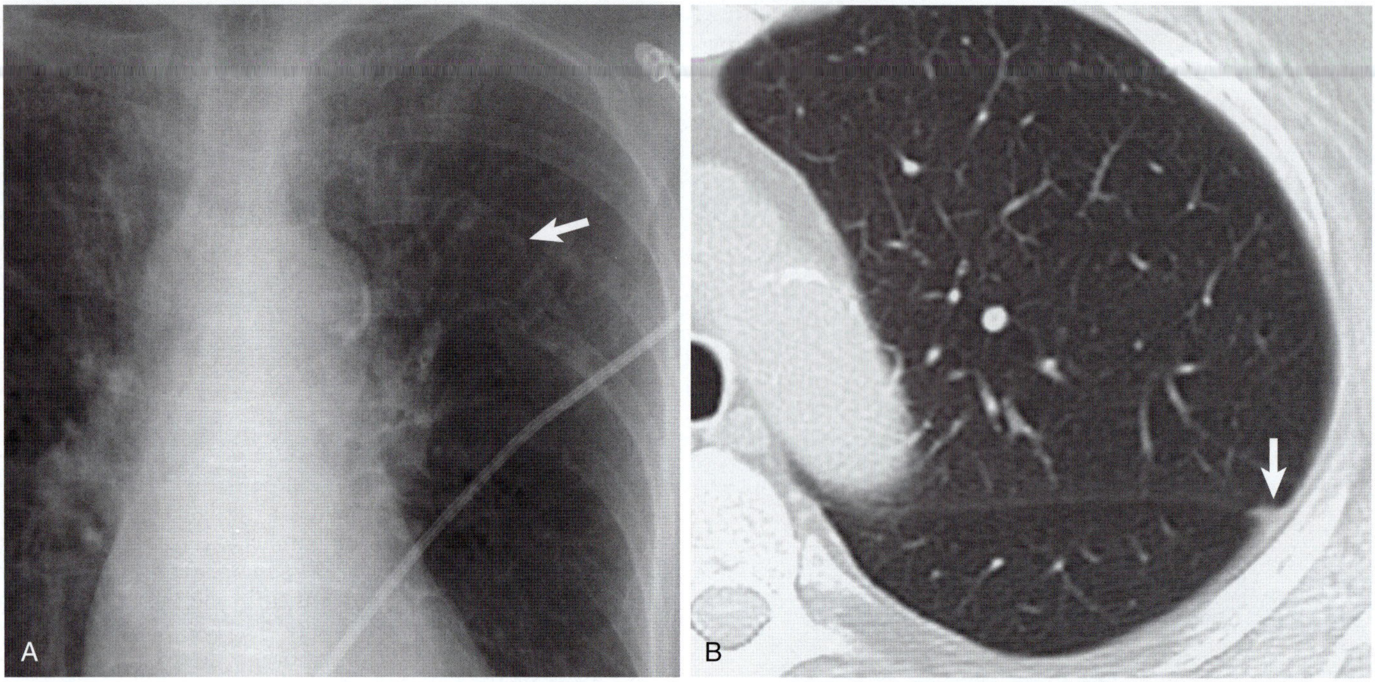

Fig. 71.9 Normal superolateral major fissure. (A) Frontal chest radiograph demonstrates a thin white line in the left upper lung coursing in the expected region of the major fissure *(arrow)*. This is distinguished from pneumothorax by the presence of lung markings superior and lateral to the line and by the typical location of the fissure. (B) Axial CT image shows the extrapleural fat intruding into the left major fissure *(arrow)*.

pneumothoraces have been reported occasionally (Fig. 71.11).[71] Free air under the diaphragm, colonic interposition (Chilaiditi syndrome) if it is right sided (Fig. 71.12), and gastric distention on the left[72] have been confused with a subpulmonic pneumothorax. Lateral decubitus views may help differentiate these entities from pneumothoraces.

CLASSIC SIGNS

- White visceral pleural line
- Absence of lung markings beyond white line of visceral pleura
- Deep sulcus sign (supine radiograph)
- Prominent mediastinal fat tags

TENSION PNEUMOTHORAX

Tension pneumothorax is a potentially fatal medical emergency that requires high degree of suspicion, immediate recognition, and treatment because affected patients rapidly become severely hypoxic and acidotic and often die.[73] It is mostly seen in the setting of trauma, emergency resuscitation, or in ventilated patients. Its pathophysiology is trapping of inspired air in the pleural space, presumably on the basis of a bronchopleural ball-valve mechanism, leading to tension.[36] Definitions for tension physiology differ in patients with a pneumothorax. Tension may be defined by mediastinal shift on the chest radiograph, by hemodynamic compromise, or by increased intrapleural pressure that remains positive throughout the respiratory cycle.[74] The last definition is preferred as the more objective definition and clearly explains the hiss of air heard on thoracic needle decompression of tension pneumothorax. Clinical presentation depends on the ventilatory status of patients. Patients with unassisted breathing present with predominantly respiratory signs and symptoms and seldom with hemodynamic compromise. On the other hand, patients on ventilator-assisted breathing frequently present with sudden hemodynamic compromise and cardiac arrest.[75]

Radiologic findings that may suggest tension physiology in the setting of pneumothorax include mediastinal shift, ipsilateral flattening of the heart border, hemidiaphragm depression, increased rib separation, and increased thoracic volume.[74] Mediastinal shift is not a reliable finding because it may occur in the absence of tension physiology (Fig. 71.13).[74] Mediastinal mobility is observed more commonly in younger patients.[76] The majority of patients with mediastinal shift do not have tension pneumothorax. In a study of 176 patients presenting to the emergency department, 30 patients had radiologic evidence of mediastinal shift, whereas only 2 had clinical signs of tension pneumothorax.[77] Tachycardia, hypotension, and cyanosis should suggest a tension pneumothorax.[21] The use of chest radiography for the diagnosis of tension pneumothorax can be problematic; it has been associated with a fourfold increase in mortality in two studies of ventilated patients who waited 30 minutes to 8 hours for the chest radiograph.[78,79] If the patient is hemodynamically unstable (e.g., partial pressure of oxygen <92%, blood pressure <90 mm Hg, respiratory rate >10, decreased level of consciousness), immediate chest decompression must always precede a chest radiograph.[74] However, in the awake, stable patient, a chest radiograph is the first test of choice.

Tension pneumothorax is treated with high-concentration oxygen and emergency needle decompression, followed by chest tube insertion.[80] Needle decompression is typically performed in the second to third intercostal space in the midclavicular line by a large-bore (10–16 gauge) needle. A recent meta-analysis recommends a catheter of at least 6.44 cm in length to ensure that 95% of the patients would have penetration of the pleural space at the site of needle decompression and therefore a successful

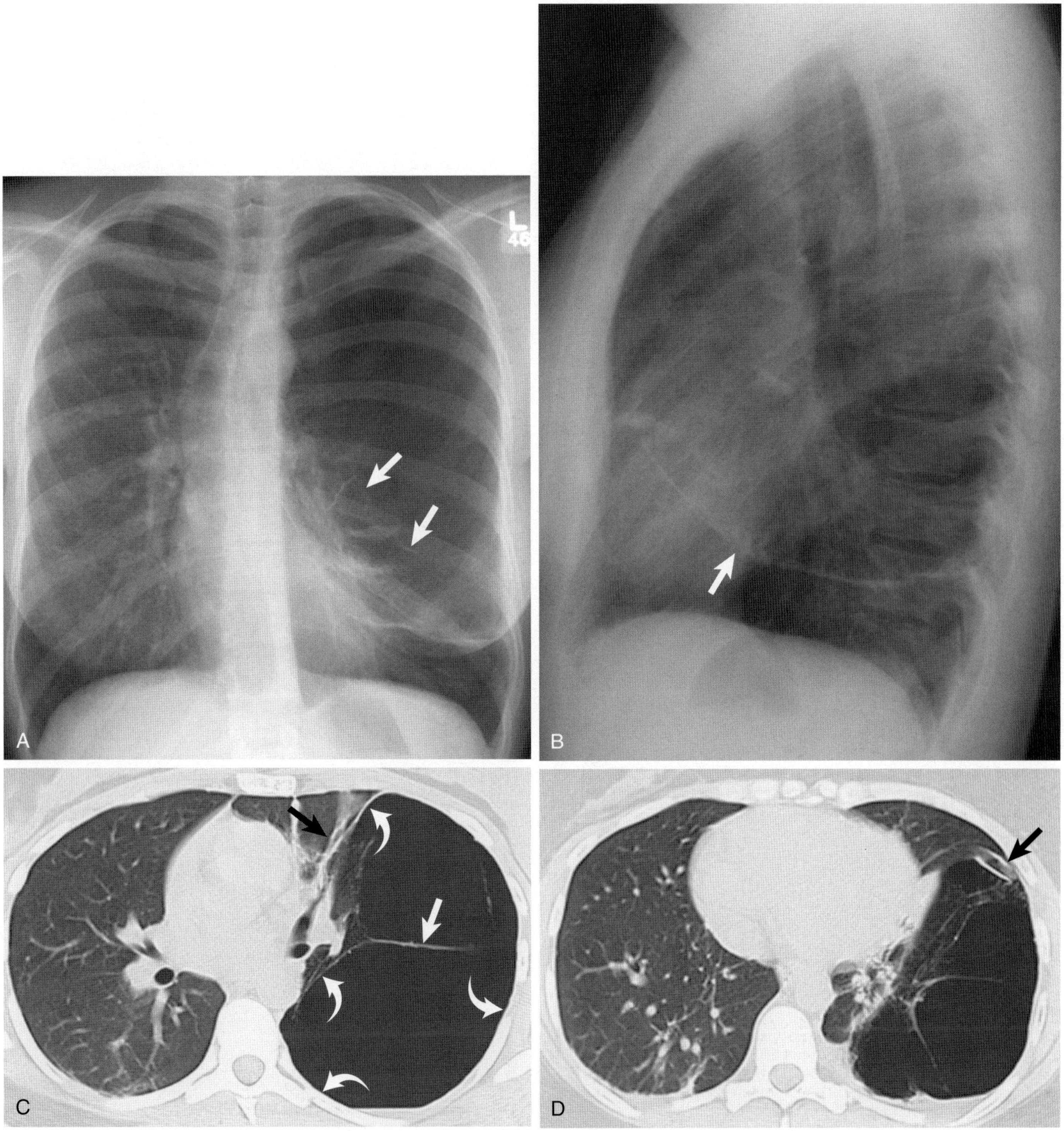

Fig. 71.10 Giant bulla. (A) Posteroanterior chest radiograph shows a hyperlucent left hemithorax. There is a faint white line *(arrows)* that is concave with respect to the chest wall, consistent with a large bulla, not a pneumothorax. (B) Lateral chest radiograph better demonstrates the thin curvilinear white line *(arrow)* indicating the inferior margin of the large left bulla. This was not appreciated by the emergency department staff, and a left-sided chest tube was mistakenly placed into the lung. (C) CT shows the huge bulla *(curved white arrows)*, contralateral mediastinal shift, and compressive atelectasis of the left upper lobe *(black arrow)*. Note the thin-walled septation within the bulla *(straight white arrow)*. (D) CT obtained at a more caudad level shows the chest tube *(black arrow)* within the lung. The bulla extended the full length of the hemithorax, from apex to hemidiaphragm. At resection, it was found to be a large bulla that had a broad base attachment to the left lower lobe, probably the result of an old infection.

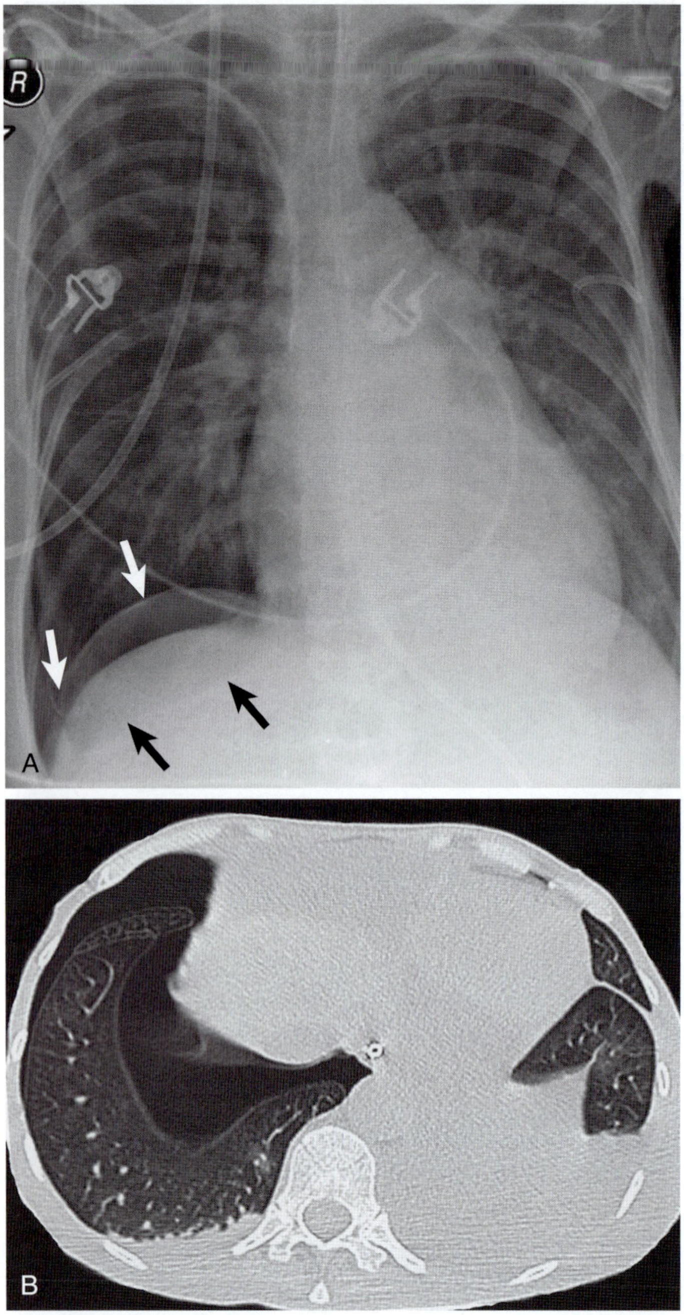

Fig. 71.11 Subpulmonic pneumothorax. (A) Supine chest radiograph shows a thin white line *(white arrows)* associated with the deep sulcus sign *(black arrows),* in keeping with basal or subpulmonic pneumothorax. (B) CT demonstrates the large right basal pneumothorax with air in the anterior, least dependent portion of the chest just above the hemidiaphragm.

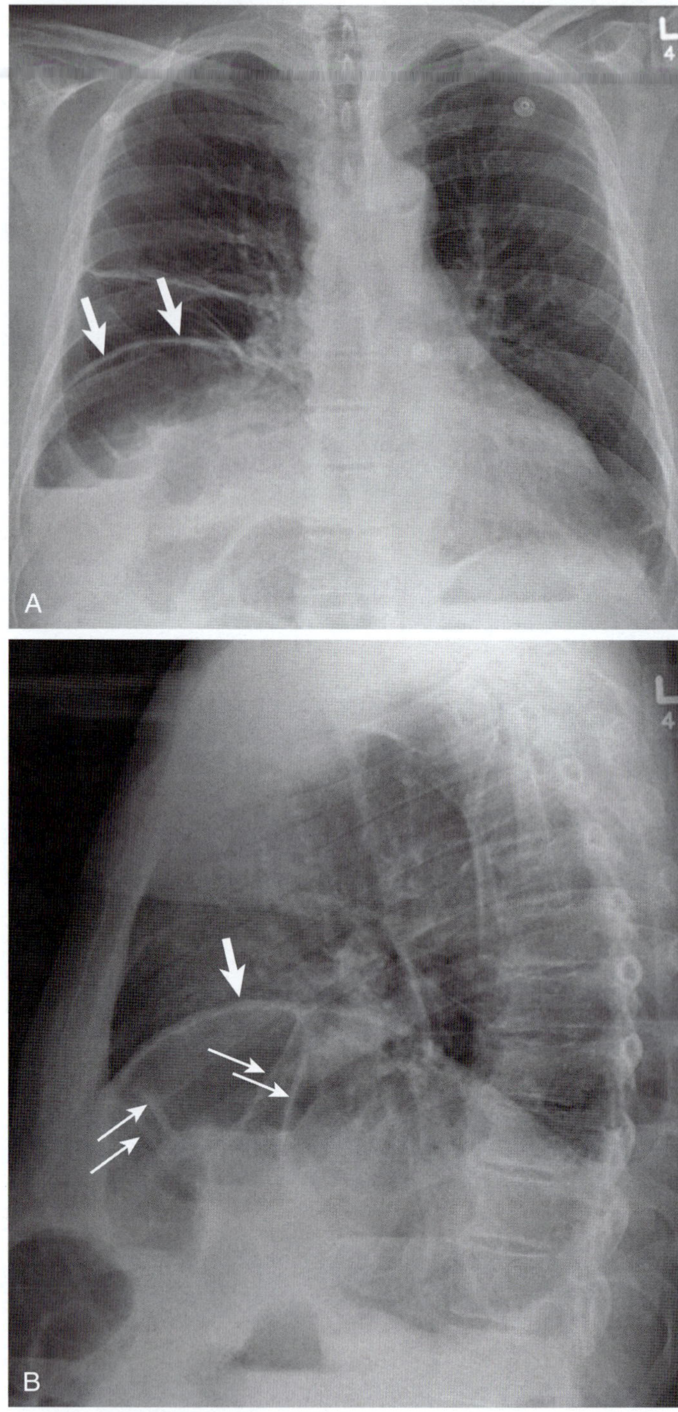

Fig. 71.12 Colonic interposition. (A) Upright portable chest radiograph demonstrates a thick white line overlying a lucent area at the base of the right hemithorax, simulating a basal pneumothorax *(arrows).* (B) Lateral radiograph demonstrates multiple haustrations *(thin arrows)* within the gas collection, in keeping with colonic interposition (Chilaiditi syndrome). The thick white line *(thick arrow)* represents the elevated right hemidiaphragm.

procedure.[81] Diagnosis is confirmed by egress of air through the needle in most of the respiratory cycle.[80]

Secondary Pneumothorax

Etiology, Prevalence, and Epidemiology

The annual incidence of secondary spontaneous pneumothorax is 6.3 per 100,000 population in men and 2.0 per 100,000 in women.[10] The incidence varies over time, as with the acquired immune deficiency syndrome (AIDS)-related *Pneumocystis jirovecii* pneumonia of the 1980s and 1990s.[83] Many cases are associated with the formation of subpleural bullae or cystic spaces related to emphysema or interstitial fibrosis; rupture of one of these is likely

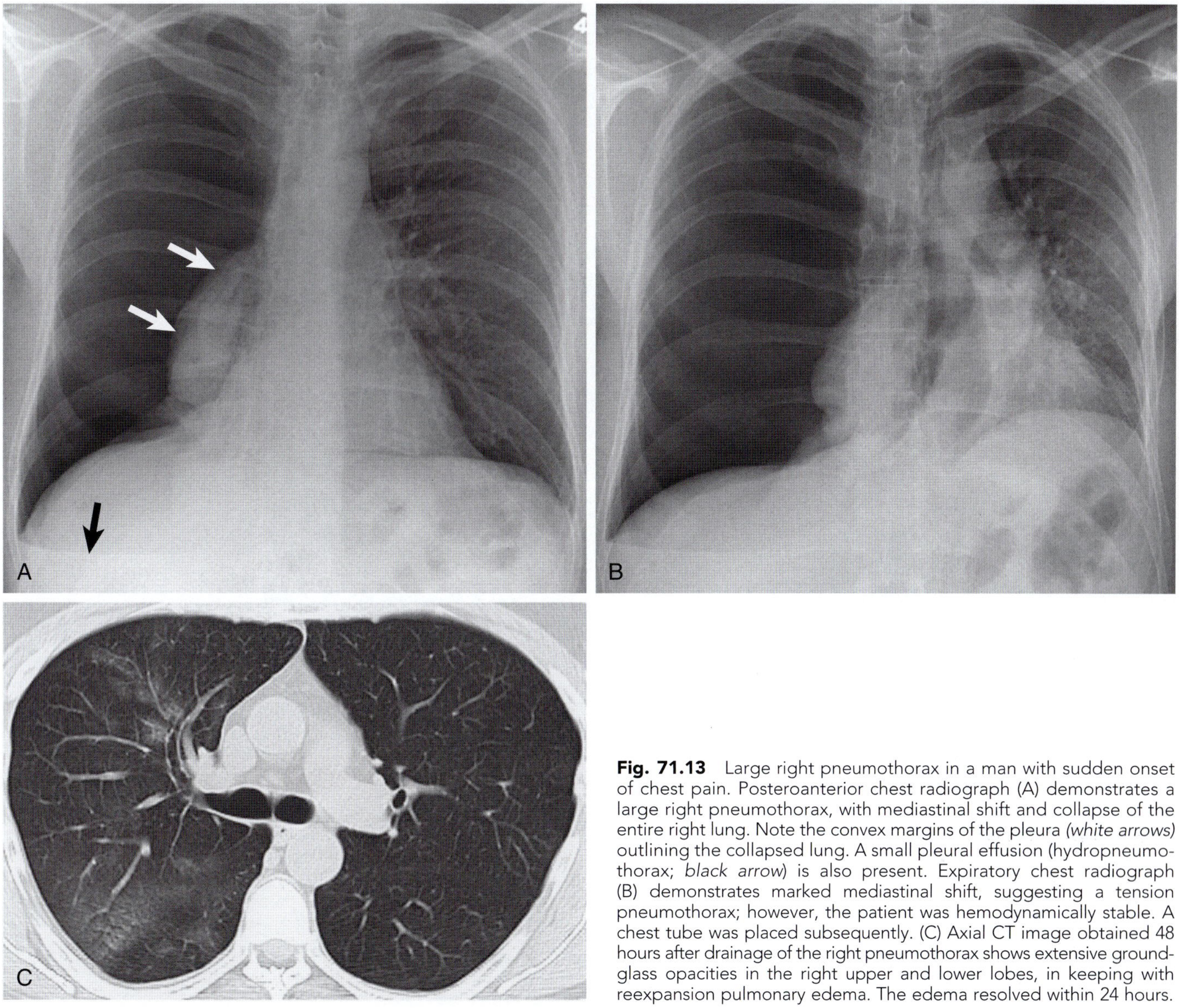

Fig. 71.13 Large right pneumothorax in a man with sudden onset of chest pain. Posteroanterior chest radiograph (A) demonstrates a large right pneumothorax, with mediastinal shift and collapse of the entire right lung. Note the convex margins of the pleura *(white arrows)* outlining the collapsed lung. A small pleural effusion (hydropneumothorax; *black arrow*) is also present. Expiratory chest radiograph (B) demonstrates marked mediastinal shift, suggesting a tension pneumothorax; however, the patient was hemodynamically stable. A chest tube was placed subsequently. (C) Axial CT image obtained 48 hours after drainage of the right pneumothorax shows extensive ground-glass opacities in the right upper and lower lobes, in keeping with reexpansion pulmonary edema. The edema resolved within 24 hours.

to be the immediate cause of pneumothorax (Fig. 71.14). As opposed to primary pneumothorax, the patient's height and body habitus are not as important in the etiology of the secondary form.[84] The most common cause of secondary pneumothorax is chronic obstructive pulmonary disease (COPD); with increasing age, the incidence of secondary spontaneous pneumothorax also increases.[10] In addition to COPD and AIDS, many other underlying lung diseases, such as cystic fibrosis, aggressive or cavitating pneumonia, interstitial pulmonary fibrosis, and cystic lung diseases, such as pulmonary Langerhans cell histiocytosis and lymphangioleiomyomatosis, may cause secondary pneumothorax (Box 71.1).[18,67] In women, who are less commonly affected by secondary pneumothorax, specific causes are catamenial pneumothorax and pneumothorax from lymphangioleiomyomatosis.[85]

Pneumothorax frequently is the presenting event that leads to the diagnosis of lymphangioleiomyomatosis in affected patients (Fig. 71.15).[86] The reported incidence of pneumothorax in women with lymphangioleiomyomatosis is 39% to 76% on the basis of a review of nine studies; the largest study showed an incidence of 66%.[86] Many patients average 2.6 pneumothoraces before the diagnosis of lymphangioleiomyomatosis is established.[86] In pulmonary Langerhans cell histiocytosis, pneumothorax precedes or complicates the clinical course of 25% of patients (Fig. 71.16).[21] Pneumothorax is a rare manifestation of sarcoidosis, usually occurring late in the course of the disease. There are sporadic reports of cases of pneumothorax as the initial manifestation of sarcoidosis.[87–90] In these patients thoracotomy showed extensive pleural infiltration by noncaseating granulomas.[88,90] High-resolution CT scans showed cavitated subpleural nodules and subpleural bullae in one case.[88]

Pathophysiology

The mechanism of bulla or cyst rupture in secondary spontaneous pneumothorax is probably multifactorial. Local airway obstruction caused by pneumonia, mucus plugs, or bronchoconstriction is

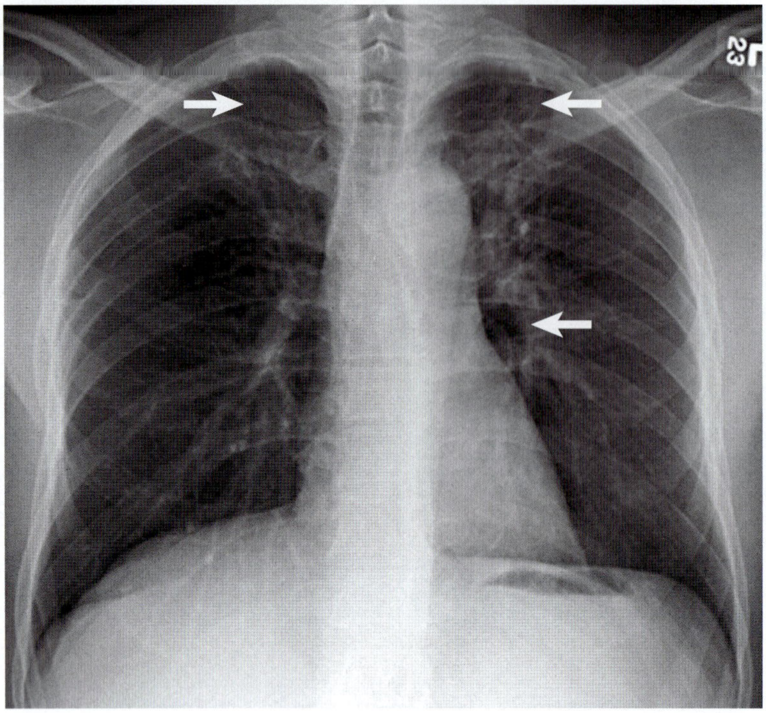

Fig. 71.14 *Pneumocystis jirovecii* pneumatoceles. Chest radiograph in a human immunodeficiency virus–positive man with a prior history of *P. jirovecii* pneumonia demonstrates bilateral upper lobe scarring with volume loss and subpleural cysts *(arrows)*. This patient is at risk for the development of pneumothorax from rupture of one of the subpleural cysts.

BOX 71.1 ETIOLOGY: SECONDARY SPONTANEOUS PNEUMOTHORAX

- Developmental disease
  - Congenital pulmonary airway malformation
- Connective tissue disease
  - Lymphangioleiomyomatosis
  - Tuberous sclerosis
  - Neurofibromatosis
  - Marfan syndrome
  - Ehlers-Danlos syndrome
  - Mitral valve prolapse
- Infection
  - Fungal pneumonia (especially *Pneumocystis jirovecii* pneumonia in patients with acquired immune deficiency virus [AIDS])
  - Bacterial pneumonia
  - Miliary tuberculosis
  - Hydatid disease
- Neoplasms
  - Primary lung cancer
  - Carcinoid tumor
  - Mesothelioma
  - Metastatic disease (carcinoma, sarcoma, germ cell tumors)
- Drugs and toxins
  - Chemotherapy for malignant disease
  - Paraquat poisoning
  - Hyperbaric oxygen therapy
  - Radiation therapy
  - Aerosolized pentamidine therapy for AIDS
- Immunologic disease
  - Granulomatosis with polyangiitis
  - Idiopathic pulmonary hemorrhage
  - Idiopathic pulmonary fibrosis
  - Langerhans cell histiocytosis
  - Sarcoidosis
  - Rheumatoid arthritis
  - Ankylosing spondylitis
  - Polymyositis or dermatomyositis
  - Scleroderma
- Chronic obstructive pulmonary disease
  - Asthma
  - Emphysema
  - Cystic fibrosis
- Pneumoconiosis
  - Silicoproteinosis
  - Berylliosis
  - Bauxite pneumoconiosis
- Vascular disease
  - Pulmonary infarction
  - Metabolic disease
  - Pulmonary alveolar proteinosis
- Intraabdominal disease
  - Gastropleural fistula
  - Colopleural fistula

Modified from Müller FS, Fraser RS, Colman NC, Paré PD. *Radiologic Diagnosis of Diseases of the Chest*. Philadelphia: WB Saunders; 2001.

likely to be important. When alveolar pressure exceeds the pressure of the interstitium of the lung, as may occur in patients with COPD and airway inflammation after coughing, air from the ruptured alveolus moves into the interstitium, then centripetally along the bronchovascular bundle to the hilum of the ipsilateral lung; if the rupture occurs at the hilum and air moves through the mediastinal pleura into the pleural space, pneumothorax results (the Macklin effect; Fig. 71.17).[91,92] An alternative mechanism for secondary spontaneous pneumothorax occurs when air from a ruptured alveolus moves directly into the pleural

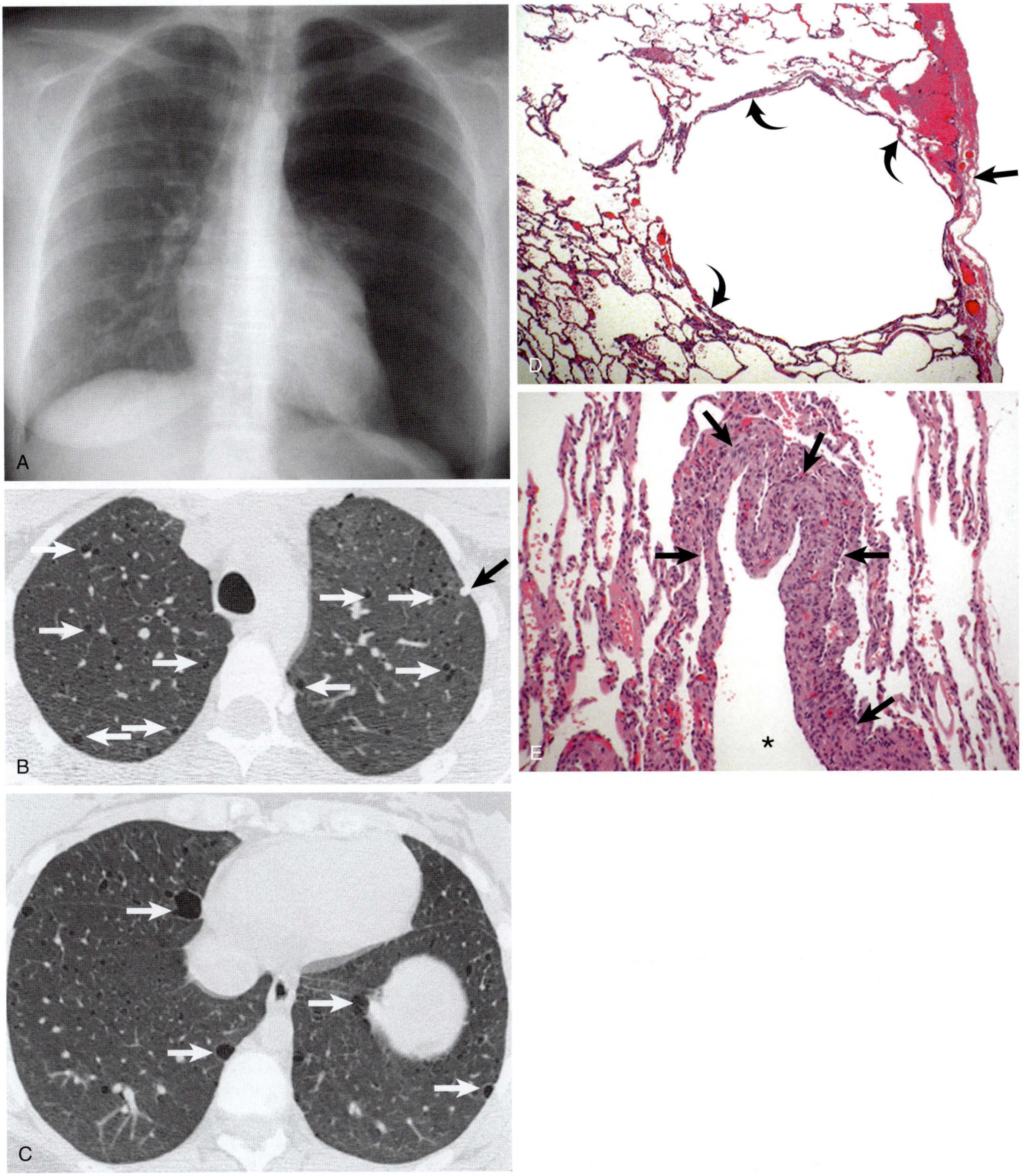

Fig. 71.15 Lymphangioleiomyomatosis. (A) Posteroanterior chest radiograph shows a large left pneumothorax. There is no sign of interstitial lung disease. (B) High-resolution CT demonstrates thin-walled cysts scattered throughout the upper lobes *(white arrows)*, with no pulmonary nodules. The left pneumothorax has been drained by a small chest tube *(black arrow)*. (C) CT image obtained at the level of the costophrenic sulci demonstrates cysts *(white arrows)* within the lung bases. The findings are characteristic of lymphangioleiomyomatosis. (D) An image of the pleura from pathologic examination resected at left pleurectomy shows a cyst *(curved arrows)* that abuts the visceral pleura *(straight arrow)*. (E) Another pathology section demonstrates the spindle cell (smooth muscle) proliferation *(arrows)* surrounding one of the subpleural cysts *(star)*, in keeping with a diagnosis of lymphangioleiomyomatosis.

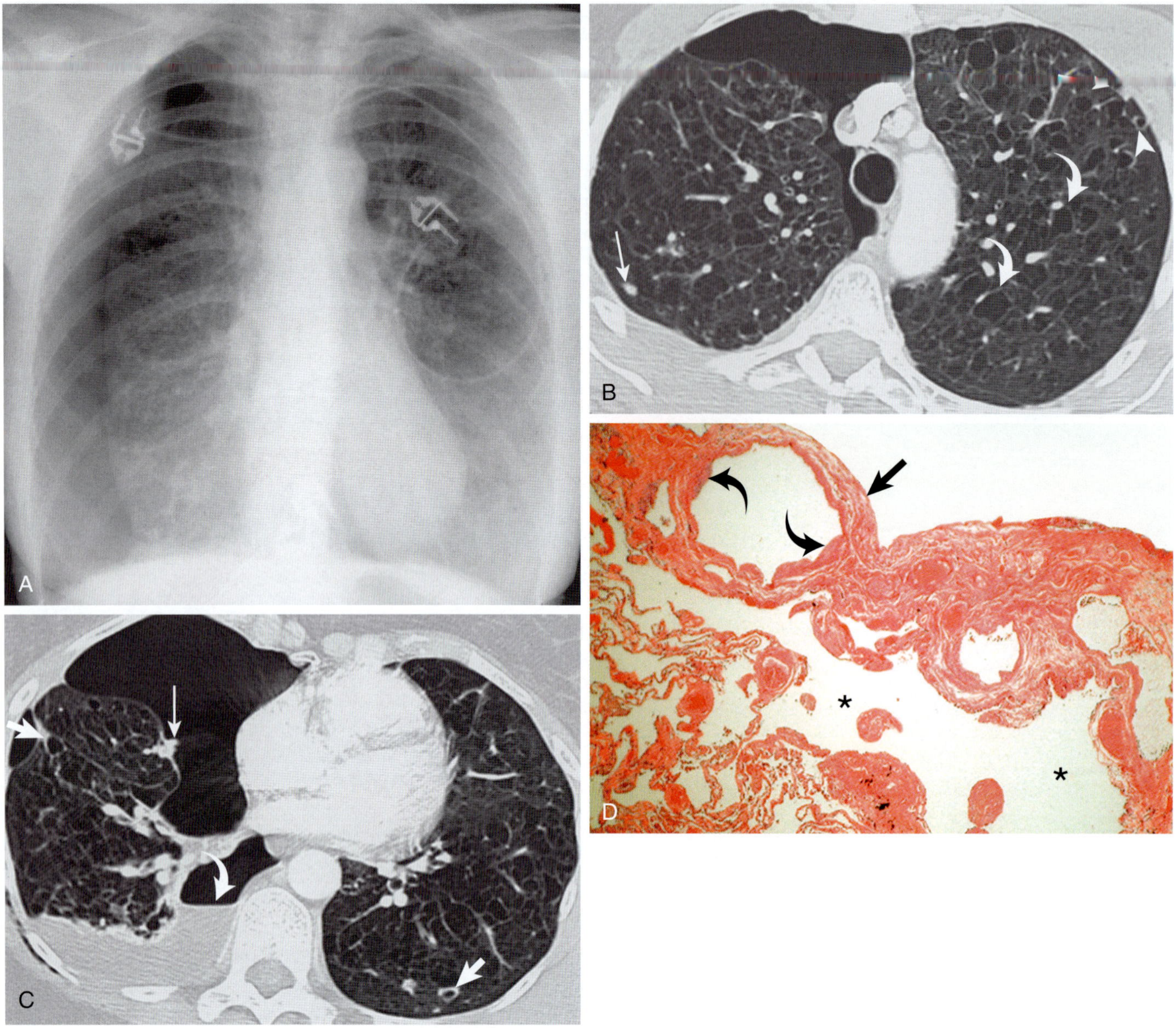

Fig. 71.16 Langerhans cell histiocytosis in a heavy smoker. (A) Frontal chest radiograph shows a large, spontaneous right pneumothorax and an interstitial pattern of opacification sparing the lung bases. (B) Thin-section CT demonstrates a right pneumothorax, extensive emphysema *(curved arrows)*, several small nodules *(thin arrows)*, and a thin-walled cavitary nodule *(arrowhead)*. (C) CT image more caudally shows large right pneumothorax with a moderate-sized pleural effusion (hydropneumothorax; *curved arrow*). A subpleural nodule in the right middle lobe transgresses the right pleural space *(thin arrow)*. Two other cavitary nodules *(thick arrows)* are identified. The patient had a persistent air leak requiring pleurectomy and wedge resection of the right upper and middle lobes. (D) Pathology slide demonstrates a cyst *(curved arrows)* along the visceral pleura *(straight arrow)*. Emphysematous changes are clearly identified *(stars)*. Fibrotic stellate nodules were identified elsewhere (not shown), consistent with Langerhans cell histiocytosis.

space as a result of necrosis of the lung, as with *P. jirovecii* pneumonia.[21]

CATAMENIAL PNEUMOTHORAX

Catamenial (Greek for *monthly*) pneumothorax is an underdiagnosed condition, affecting females in the reproductive age group, which is part of thoracic endometriosis syndrome (catamenial pneumothorax, catamenial hemothorax, catamenial hemoptysis, and lung nodules) and refers to the development of recurrent pneumothorax at the time of menstruation. Possible mechanisms include spontaneous rupture of blebs; migration of air directly through the vagina, uterus, and fallopian tubes into the peritoneal cavity, then into the pleural space through fenestrations in the diaphragm; erosion of visceral pleura by endometrial deposits, which may spread to the pleura through fenestrations in the diaphragm; or alveolar rupture caused by prostaglandin-induced bronchiolar constriction or by a check-valve mechanism exerted

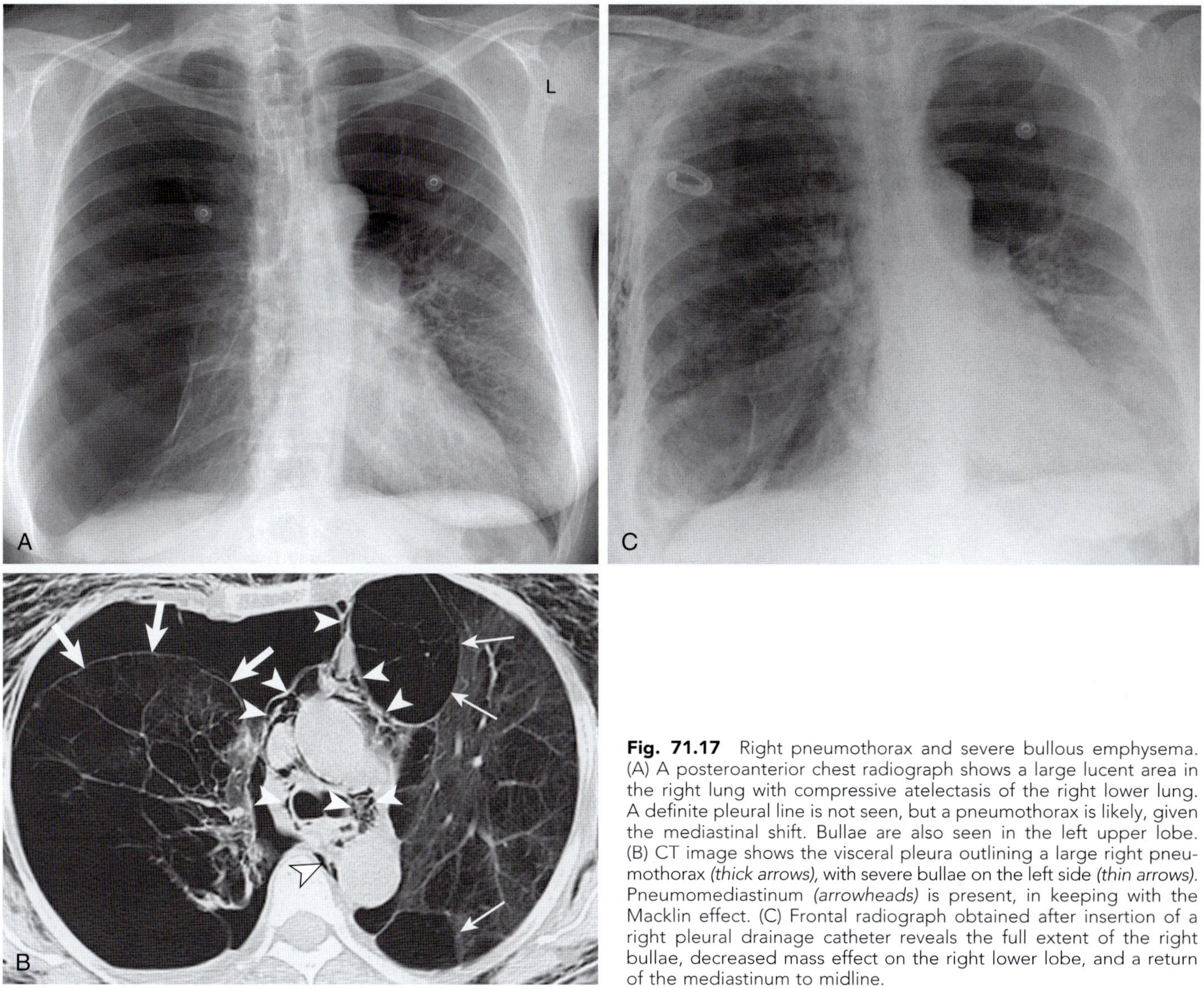

Fig. 71.17 Right pneumothorax and severe bullous emphysema. (A) A posteroanterior chest radiograph shows a large lucent area in the right lung with compressive atelectasis of the right lower lung. A definite pleural line is not seen, but a pneumothorax is likely, given the mediastinal shift. Bullae are also seen in the left upper lobe. (B) CT image shows the visceral pleura outlining a large right pneumothorax *(thick arrows)*, with severe bullae on the left side *(thin arrows)*. Pneumomediastinum *(arrowheads)* is present, in keeping with the Macklin effect. (C) Frontal radiograph obtained after insertion of a right pleural drainage catheter reveals the full extent of the right bullae, decreased mass effect on the right lower lobe, and a return of the mediastinum to midline.

by bronchiolar endometrial implants.[93] The most likely theory, "retrograde menstruation," or regurgitation of endometrial tissue through the fallopian tubes, followed by migration to pleura through diaphragmatic holes, is supported by the finding that normal peritoneal flow moves up the right paracolic gutter to the right hemidiaphragm.[94] Furthermore, diaphragmatic fenestrations are more common on the right, likely explaining the preponderance of cases on this side.[95] There has also been good documentation of pneumoperitoneum occurring at the same time as the pneumothorax.[96]

Rarely, endometriosis may be disseminated through the hematogenous route, by which uterine endometrial tissue literally "metastasizes" to the lung through the venous system that drains the uterus.[97] In this instance the result is the appearance of pulmonary nodules or deposits that are clinically manifested by hemoptysis, not by pneumothorax or hemothorax.

The diagnosis of catamenial pneumothorax is not made by eliciting a history of endometriosis; less than one-third of catamenial pneumothoraces have been reported to be associated with pelvic endometriosis.[98] Instead, a recurrent history of shoulder or chest pain within 72 hours of the onset of menses in a woman of reproductive age should elicit the diagnosis. Eighty-five percent to 90% of cases occur on the right (Fig. 71.18), 5% on the left, and 5% bilaterally.[99]

Catamenial pneumothorax is an uncommon cause of pneumothorax, accounting for 1% to 5.6% of cases of spontaneous pneumothorax.[85,100] However, a prospective study of 32 women found that with a careful history, catamenial pneumothorax accounted for 25% of the spontaneous pneumothoraces.[98] In all these patients the following diaphragmatic abnormalities were found at surgery: holes (one patient), endometrial implants (three patients), and both (four patients). Visceral pleural endometriosis was found in one patient.

Clinical Presentation

In patients with underlying lung disease, dyspnea is always present with secondary spontaneous pneumothorax and is usually severe,

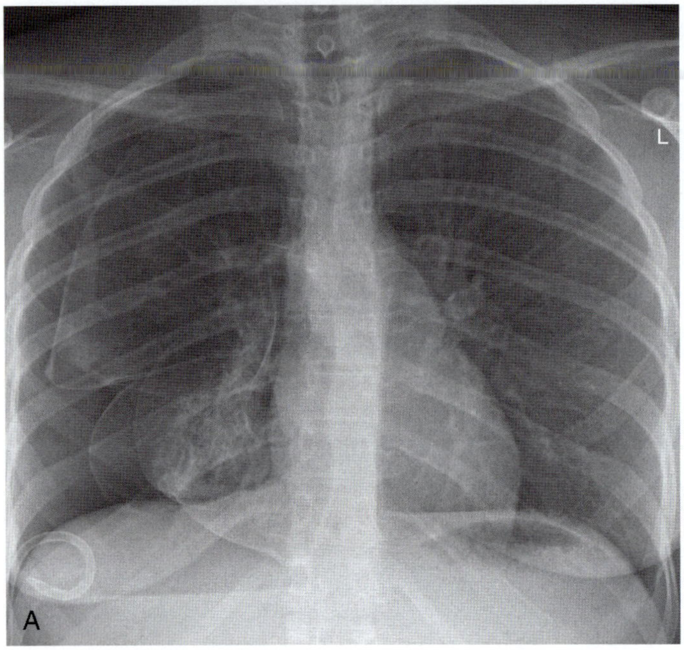

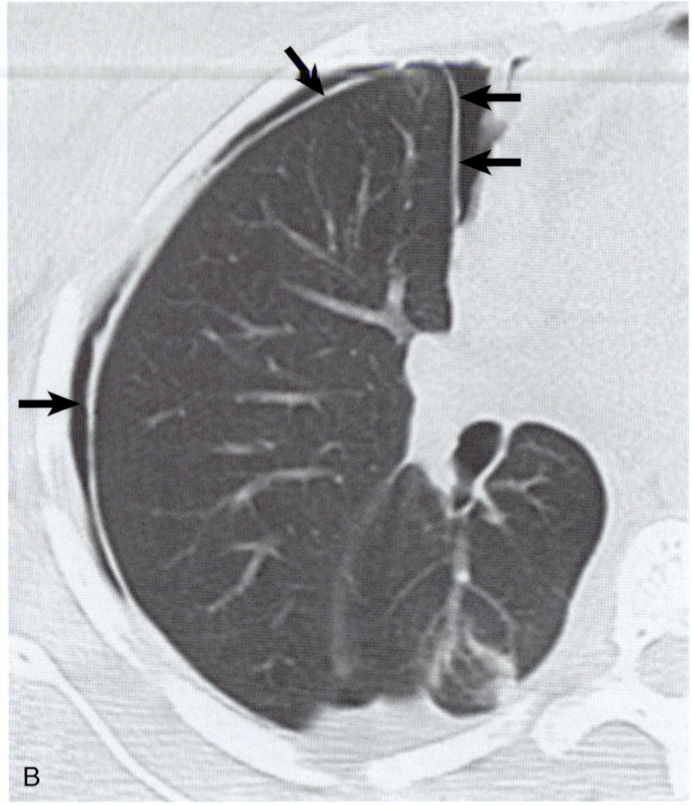

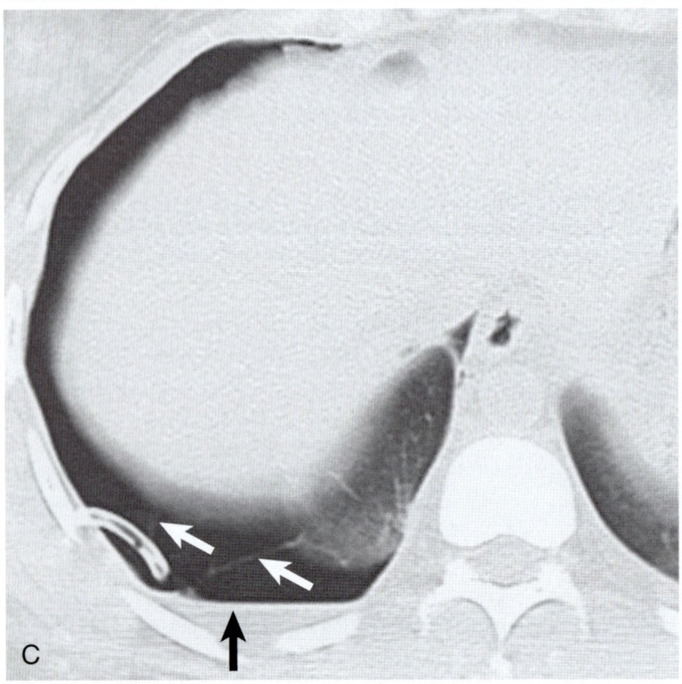

Fig. 71.18 Catamenial pneumothorax. (A) Posteroanterior chest radiograph shows a moderate right hemopneumothorax, still present despite placement of a small pigtail catheter. (B) CT scan demonstrates smooth visceral pleural thickening *(arrows)* involving the entire right lung. (C) CT image more inferiorly demonstrates a hemopneumothorax *(black arrow)* and pleural adhesions *(white arrows)* related to recurrent pneumothoraces and pleural effusions. Despite catheter drainage, there was a persistent air leak, requiring decortication and pleurectomy. At pathologic examination, the visceral pleural peel contained lymphoid cells, hemosiderin deposits, and multiple areas of fibrosis. No endometrial cells were identified in the pleura, but they were found in the pleural fluid. The patient also had hemorrhagic ascites and pelvic endometriosis.

even with a small one.[21,87,101] Most patients have ipsilateral chest pain.[102] Severe hypoxemia or hypotension can occur and be life threatening.[21,87,101] Symptoms do not resolve spontaneously, as they do in primary pneumothorax.

Manifestations of the Disease

RADIOGRAPHY

As with primary pneumothorax, a thin white pleural line parallel to the chest wall may be seen. However, in some cases this may be difficult to differentiate from the wall of a bulla. The diagnosis and treatment of pneumothorax in patients with cystic lung disease may be difficult when the chest radiograph alone is relied on (see Fig. 71.17). The complex appearance of the lungs themselves or partial adherence of the lung to the chest wall resulting from prior surgery or inflammation, or both of these factors, may result in an unusual configuration of the pneumothorax or may mask it altogether.[103]

COMPUTED TOMOGRAPHY

When the diagnosis of a pneumothorax on chest radiography is uncertain, chest CT is recommended.[44] CT is more sensitive than chest radiography for distinguishing apical bullae from pneumothorax.[50] Air is identified in the pleural space, separating the lung

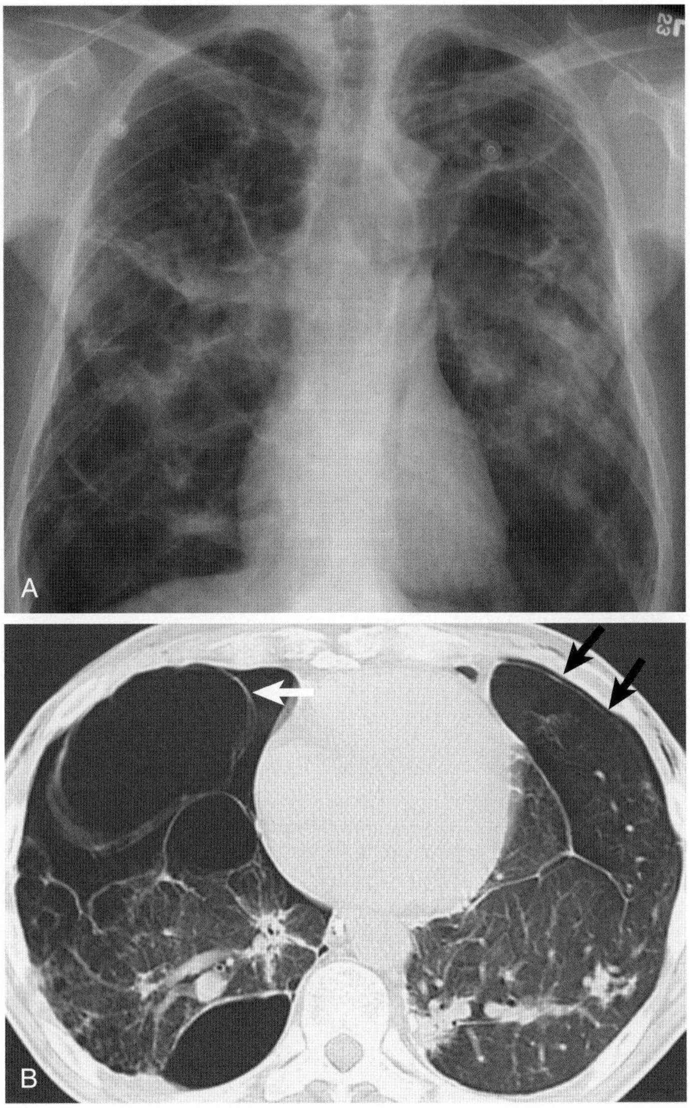

Fig. 71.19 Bilateral pneumothoraces and sarcoidosis. (A) A posteroanterior chest radiograph demonstrates numerous large cystic areas in the lungs and fibrosis in the upper lobes, in keeping with known end-stage sarcoidosis. A small drainage catheter is seen in the left lower hemithorax, for treatment of a left pneumothorax. The patient complained of new right-sided chest pain. A right pneumothorax was suspected but could not be confirmed on the radiograph. (B) CT reveals bilateral pneumothoraces, demonstrating the double-wall sign *(black arrows)* on the left. On the contralateral side, a right pneumothorax outlines a large bulla *(white arrow)*.

from the chest wall. It is critical to differentiate pneumothorax from large bullae or cystic lung disease (see Figs. 71.10 and 71.17). A helpful sign is visualization of air external to the bulla, called the double-wall sign.[44] This sign occurs when air is outlining both sides of the bulla wall, parallel to the parietal pleura (Fig. 71.19). Other signs in patients with giant bullous emphysema include compressed or consolidated lung, nonanatomic hyperlucency, and immediate symptomatic relief and lung expansion at chest tube placement.[104] One potential pitfall in the appreciation of the double-wall sign of pneumothorax occurs when two large bullae are adjacent to one another. This situation can produce an apparent double-wall sign, mimicking pneumothorax. However, careful scrutiny of multiple images will show the absence of air in the pleural space and that the bulla wall is not parallel to the chest wall or parietal pleura.[44]

With other diseases resulting in secondary pneumothoraces, such as lymphangioleiomyomatosis, sarcoidosis, and pulmonary Langerhans cell histiocytosis, the diagnosis of interstitial lung disease may be made with thin-section CT. In patients with secondary pneumothorax, CT may help in management of pneumothorax recurrence, during management of a persistent air leak,[103] and in planning of a surgical intervention.[105]

In patients with suspicion of catamenial pneumothorax, CT is often performed to rule out alternative diagnoses. Findings are often nonspecific and include the presence of unilateral, mostly right-sided pneumothorax or hemopneumothorax.[106] The presence of the associated pneumoperitoneum and low-attenuation diaphragmatic implants on contrast-enhanced study are helpful to suggest the diagnosis. Magnetic resonance imaging (MRI) may show pleural effusion with T1 hyperintensity because of the presence of blood products. Pleural and diaphragmatic implants can also be seen with high T1 and T2 signal. Restricted diffusion on diffusion-weighted imaging has also been reported in pleural deposits.[107–110]

IATROGENIC PNEUMOTHORAX

In most series iatrogenic causes now outnumber other causes of secondary pneumothorax.[10,111,112] With more sophisticated medical procedures and treatment for the critically ill patient, iatrogenic damage to the thorax has become increasingly common. An important cause of iatrogenic trauma to the lung is increasing use of positive-pressure ventilation. Experimental evidence shows that the lung can be damaged with interstitial emphysema at peak pressures as low as 40 cm water.[113] The placement of catheters, chest tubes, endotracheal tubes, and feeding tubes (Fig. 71.20), as well as pacemaker leads and counterpulsation balloons, may cause serious complications. Follow-up chest radiography after these procedures is therefore important.[113] In one study of 106 patients with iatrogenic pneumothoraces identified during 5 years, the most common cause of an iatrogenic pneumothorax was transthoracic needle aspiration,[40] followed by thoracentesis,[34] subclavian venipuncture,[27] and positive-pressure ventilation.[9,111] There were 90 cases of spontaneous pneumothorax at this institution during the same period. The authors concluded that the incidence of iatrogenic pneumothorax exceeded that of spontaneous pneumothorax and that there is substantial morbidity and some mortality from iatrogenic pneumothorax.[111]

The largest study to date is from the Agency for Healthcare Research and Quality in the United States, which analyzed 7.5 million discharge summaries from 994 short-term acute care hospitals across 28 states in 2000.[112] Excluding the iatrogenic pneumothoraces occurring after procedures that intentionally puncture the lung, such as lung biopsies, the study found that 0.67 per 1000 hospitalized patients were at risk for accidental iatrogenic pneumothorax. The high-risk procedures identified were vascular (noncardiac) catheterization (25%), thoracentesis (25%), respiratory intubation (21%), placement and adjustment of cardiac pacemakers (12%), operations on the larynx and bronchus (each 7%), operations in the abdominal cavity (gastrectomy, 5%; nephrectomy, 3%), bronchoscopy (8%), and percutaneous skin and breast biopsies (5%; Fig. 71.21).[112] Affected patients stayed in the hospital for an average of 4.4 days more, at a cost of more than US$18,000, and had a 6% higher risk of death in the hospital.[112]

The relative incidence rates of the various iatrogenic causes of pneumothorax are summarized in Table 71.1.

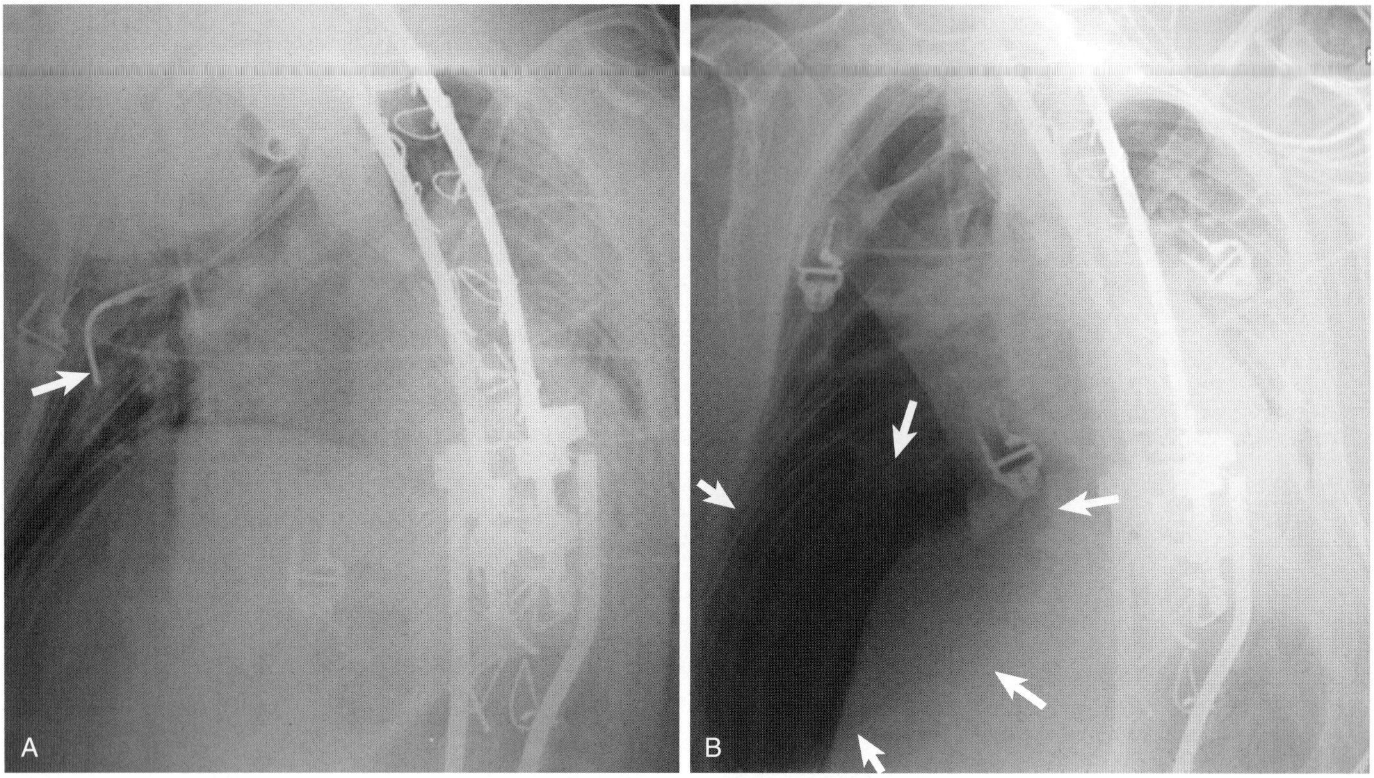

Fig. 71.20 (A) Malpositioned feeding tube. Portable chest radiograph of a patient in the intensive care unit for respiratory failure demonstrates a feeding tube *(arrow)* within the right lower lobe bronchus. (B) Portable chest radiograph obtained 6 hours later shows that the feeding tube has been removed. A large right pneumothorax is seen, as evident by the deep sulcus sign *(arrows)*.

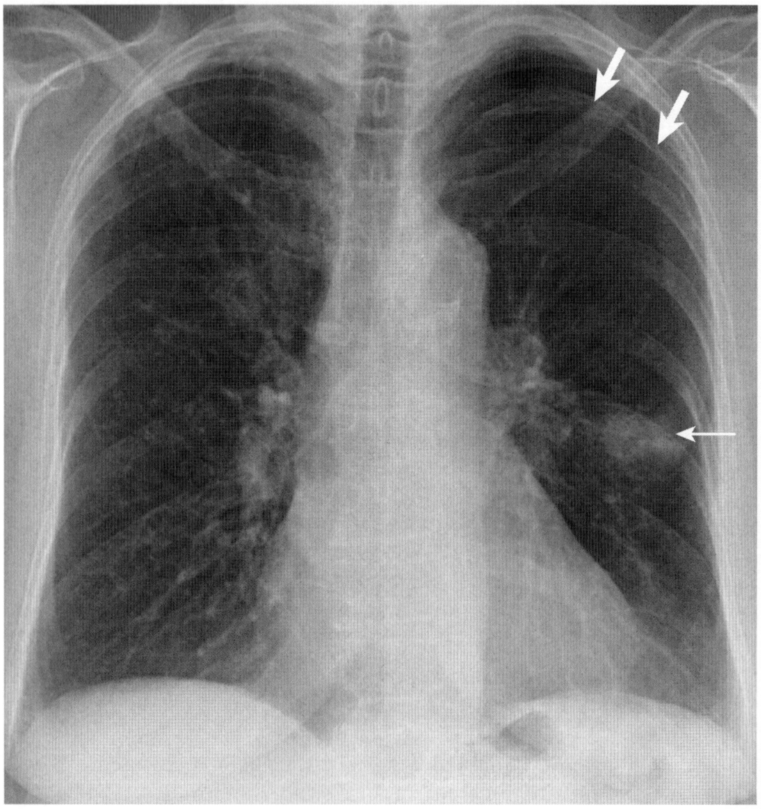

Fig. 71.21 Pneumothorax after lung biopsy. Posteroanterior chest radiograph shows the thin white line *(thick arrows)* of the visceral pleura outlined by an apical left pneumothorax. The patient had undergone an image-guided biopsy of the left lower lobe nodule *(thin arrow)* 30 minutes earlier. The pneumothorax was stable over serial radiographs, and the patient was asymptomatic; no tube drainage was required.

TABLE 71.1 IATROGENIC CAUSES OF PNEUMOTHORAX

	Incidence Rate (%)
BIOPSY PROCEDURES	
Transthoracic needle biopsy	25–35
Transbronchial biopsy	1–6
Colonoscopy	0.2–0.5
Liver biopsy	0.3
Breast biopsy	0.01–3
Axillary node biopsy	Case reports
THERAPEUTIC PROCEDURES	
Coronary artery bypass grafting, awake patient	6–19
Thoracentesis	2.3–12.1
Central venous catheterization	1–12
Percutaneous nephrolithotomy	2
Nephrectomy	1.3
Cardiac pacemaker placement or revision	1.1
Electromyographic electrode insertion	1.1
Tracheostomy	0.3
Feeding tube insertion	0.2
Positive-pressure ventilation	0.1
Gastrectomy	0.06
Acupuncture	Case reports

BILATERAL PNEUMOTHORAX

Most bilateral pneumothoraces are related to bilateral spontaneous pneumothoraces. However, patients with pleuropleural communications or a single pleural cavity can develop bilateral pneumothoraces from unilateral pathology. This rare condition is called "buffalo chest," as the North American buffalo has a single pleural cavity. In humans these communications can be iatrogenic after major cardiothoracic surgery, such as heart-lung or double-lung transplantation, or rarely, congenital.[114,114a,114b]

Bilateral pneumothoraces have been described from iatrogenic causes,[115] acupuncture,[116] treated lung cancer metastases,[117] mesothelioma,[118] osteosarcoma metastases,[119] Hodgkin disease,[120] angiosarcoma metastases,[121,122] and benign causes, such as lymphangioleiomyomatosis,[123] cystic fibrosis,[124] Langerhans cell histiocytosis,[120] hydatid cysts,[125] miliary tuberculosis,[126] chronic graft-versus-host disease,[127] and emphysema.[126] Most patients (34%) have pulmonary disease related to disorders of cells of mesenchymal origin.[120] The main determinant of prognosis is underlying lung disease.[120] There are several case reports of fatal bilateral pneumothoraces.[128,129] In one study, 2 of 40 patients died, resulting in a mortality rate of 5% (see Fig. 71.19).[130]

PNEUMOTHORAX EX VACUO OR TRAPPED LUNG

The term *pneumothorax ex vacuo* was originally described for the appearance of pneumothorax in patients with sudden lobar collapse, most commonly of the upper lobe, caused by acute bronchial obstruction.[131–133] The sudden collapse results in an increased negative intrapleural pressure adjacent to the affected lobe, which leads to focal accumulation of gas that originates in ambient tissues and blood (Fig. 71.22). It is analogous to the vacuum phenomenon.[133]

More recently, this term has been used by some authors to also describe development of gas in the pleural space because the lung is unable to expand to fill the thoracic cavity after the evacuation of pleural fluid.[134–136]

Visceral pleural thickening leading to decreased parenchymal compliance is termed *trapped lung* (Fig. 71.23). Trapped lung is defined by the inability of the lung to expand and fill the thoracic cavity because of the restricting "peel."[137] This restriction may be due to a benign inflammatory or fibrotic cortex or to malignant seeding with visceral pleural tumor.

Chest tube insertion in patients with ex vacuo pneumothorax caused by acute bronchial obstruction is not recommended, and treatment should be directed toward relief of bronchial obstruction. Chest tube insertion in asymptomatic patients with pneumothorax after pleural drainage is of unlikely clinical benefit.[138,139] Because of significant impact on patient dyspnea, treatment with decortication in benign disease and pleurectomy in malignant pleural disease is often performed to relieve symptoms.[140]

Synopsis of Treatment Options

The treatment of pneumothorax is evacuation of air from the pleural space and prevention of recurrent pneumothorax. Evacuation of air may be accomplished by manual aspiration with a catheter, insertion of a chest tube, pleurodesis, thoracoscopy through a single insertion port into the chest, video-assisted thoracoscopic surgery, or thoracotomy. Small pneumothoraces may resolve spontaneously. Selection of an approach depends on the size of the pneumothorax, the severity of the symptoms, whether there is a persistent air leak, and whether the pneumothorax is primary or secondary.[21] Typically, spontaneous pneumothoraces may be evacuated by manual aspiration through a small catheter or insertion of a small-bore (<14 Fr) catheter attached to a Heimlich valve or a water-seal device until the lung reexpands against the chest wall and the air leak resolves.[105] Reliable patients may be sent home with a small-bore catheter attached to a Heimlich valve (Fig. 71.24) if the lung has reexpanded after removal of pleural air. Follow-up is typically arranged within 2 days.[105] Secondary pneumothoraces should be treated with chest tube drainage, followed by pleurodesis after the first episode to minimize recurrence.[141]

Complications of chest tube drainage include pain, pleural infection, incorrect placement of the tube, hemorrhage, hypotension,[21] and pulmonary edema[142] resulting from lung reexpansion.

REEXPANSION PULMONARY EDEMA

Reexpansion pulmonary edema is an uncommon complication that occurs when a collapsed lung is rapidly reexpanded by evacuation of air or fluid.[142,143] In the largest series reported, 83% of cases were the result of chronically collapsed lung from a pneumothorax; 83% were on the affected side (see Fig. 71.13), 6.7% bilateral, and a few in the contralateral lung.[142] The onset of reexpansion pulmonary edema occurs as rapidly as 1 hour in 64% of cases and uniformly occurs by 24 hours.[142] Although it is likely that rapid reexpansion by application of negative pressure contributes to reexpansion pulmonary edema, it can occur in more than 33% of cases when reexpansion is allowed without pleural suction. The mortality remains about 20%.[142]

The pathophysiologic mechanism of reexpansion pulmonary edema is unclear, but the common end point in the pathologic process probably results from increased endothelial permeability.[142] The increased permeability of the capillary bed is believed to

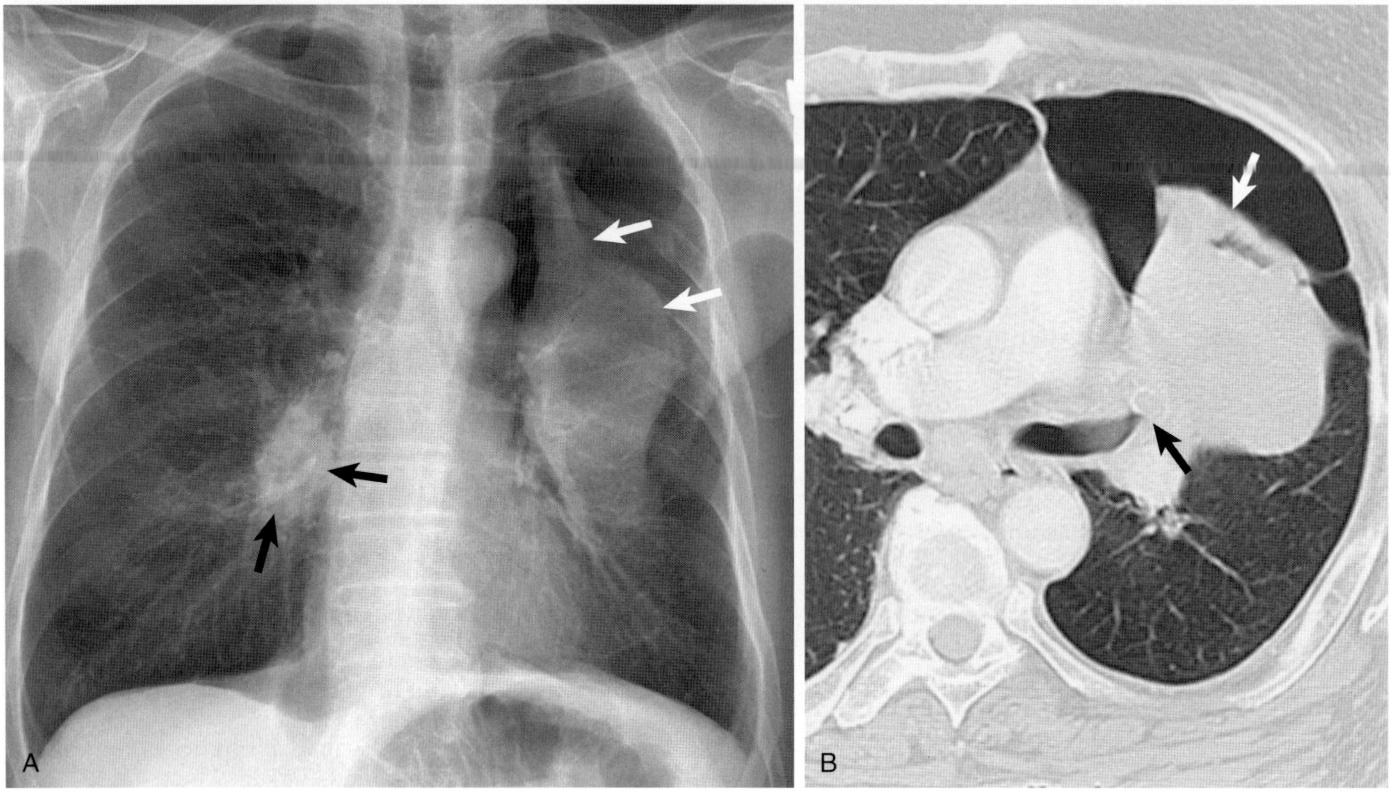

Fig. 71.22 Pneumothorax ex vacuo. (A) A posteroanterior chest radiograph demonstrates a left pneumothorax and left upper lobe collapse *(white arrows)*. Also noted is a right perihilar mass *(black arrows)*. The patient had bilateral squamous cell carcinomas. The left one gradually obstructed the left upper lobe, causing a spontaneous pneumothorax. (B) CT image demonstrates the mass in the left upper lobe, completely obstructing the bronchus *(black arrow)*, with an anterior pneumothorax *(white arrow)*, representing pneumothorax ex vacuo. No other cause of the pneumothorax was found.

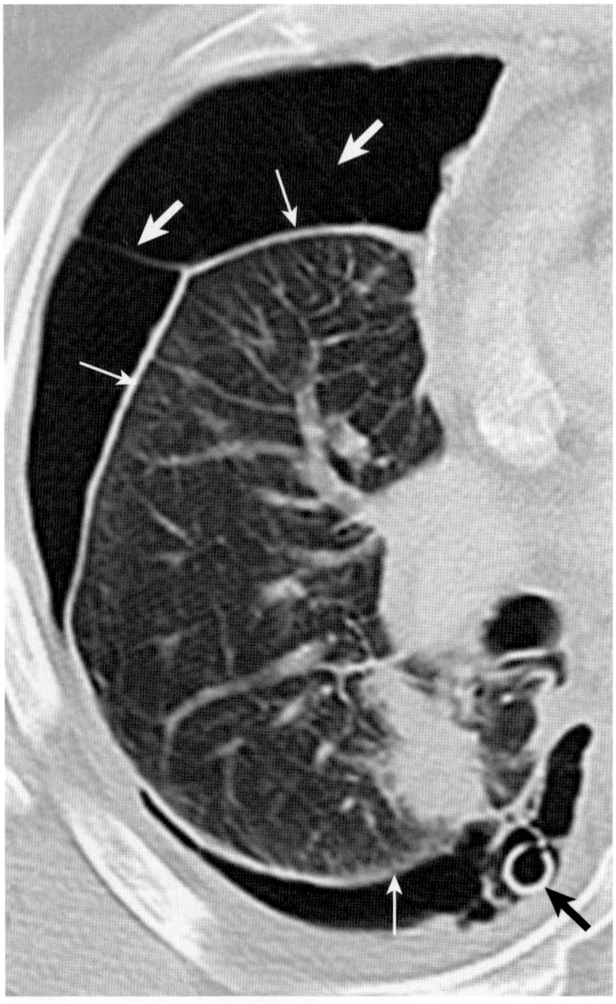

Fig. 71.23 Trapped lung. CT image in a patient with right-sided mesothelioma who had a large pleural effusion drained by chest tube *(black arrow)* demonstrates the large right pneumothorax and pleural adhesions *(thick white arrows)*. The visceral pleura is markedly thickened by tumor *(thin white arrows)*, which prevented the lung from reexpanding, so-called trapped lung. Despite several weeks of drainage, no change in size of the pneumothorax occurred, and when the tube was removed, the space refilled with fluid. Some authors now refer to this phenomenon as pneumothorax ex vacuo.

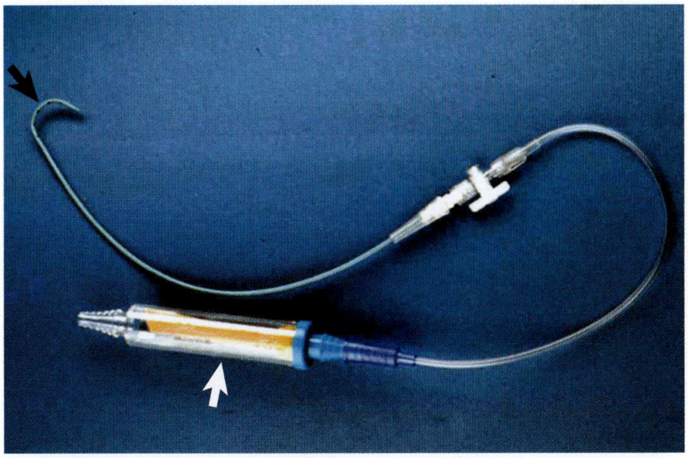

Fig. 71.24 Chest tube. Photograph demonstrates an 8-gauge pigtail catheter attached to a Heimlich valve *(white arrow)*. The five side-holes *(black arrow)* allow fast drainage, and the device is portable and easily managed on an outpatient basis.

result from mechanical injury secondary to vascular distention and increased pulmonary flow that occur during pulmonary reexpansion and reperfusion injury as blood flow returns to the now fully expanded lung. The pathologic mechanism premised to be the basis of reexpansion pulmonary edema is similar to that observed in acute respiratory distress syndrome and post-pneumonectomy pulmonary edema.[143]

The mainstays in therapy for reexpansion pulmonary edema remain oxygenation, a low threshold for mechanical ventilation with positive end-expiratory pressure, diuresis, and hemodynamic support.[142–144] Prostaglandin analogs have been used once the diagnosis was suspected, early in therapy.[142] Reexpansion pulmonary edema usually resolves within 24 to 72 hours.[142,144]

SIZE OF PNEUMOTHORAX

Estimation of the size of a pneumothorax is a contentious issue.[145] It has been well documented that the chest radiograph is a poor method for determining the size of a pneumothorax, whereas the chest CT image shows good correlation with the size of a pneumothorax.[146] Several methods, including the Light index,[147] Collins method,[148] and Rhea method[149] have been proposed. However, to provide physicians with guidelines, the British Thoracic Society divides pneumothoraces into small and large on the basis of the distance from visceral pleural surface (lung edge) to chest wall at the level of the hilum, defining small as less than 2 cm and large as more than 2 cm.[80] A small rim of air around the lung actually translates into a relatively large loss of lung volume, with a 2-cm deep pneumothorax occupying about 50% of the hemithorax. It has been shown that secondary pneumothoraces above this volume are unlikely to respond to simple aspiration and require chest tube drainage.[105] A large pneumothorax is an objective indication for drainage.[67] The American College of Chest Physicians has proposed a different arbitrary system for estimating pneumothorax size. They suggest that small pneumothoraces be defined by distances of less than 3 cm from the apex to the cupola of the lung and large pneumothoraces by distances of more than 3 cm.[105] Regardless of definition of size of pneumothorax, the treating physician is reminded that all pneumothoraces must be treated on the basis of the clinical status of the patient.[151]

RECURRENCE OF PNEUMOTHORAX

Recurrence rates for all spontaneous pneumothoraces are high, on the order of 30%.[7,10,84,152] After a first recurrence, the likelihood of subsequent recurrence increases progressively up to 62% for a second and 83% for a third recurrence.[141] Independent risk factors for recurrence in 122 patients with spontaneous pneumothoraces are pulmonary fibrosis detected on chest radiography, physical characteristics, smoking behavior, and age older than 60 years.[153] The second line of therapy for spontaneous pneumothorax is to prevent recurrence, which can be achieved by instillation of sclerosing agents, such as talc, mechanical pleural abrasion, resection of bullae, and pleurodesis through video-assisted thoracoscopic surgery, or limited thoracotomy. The goal is to achieve symphysis between parietal pleura and visceral pleura and to prevent relapse of pneumothorax.[18] Simply performing bullectomy is not adequate; recurrence rates are much higher than when it is performed along with pleural symphysis.[18]

It is generally accepted that primary pneumothoraces should be treated in case of recurrence, persisting air leak greater than 3 to 5 days, in the presence of hemopneumothorax or bilateral pneumothoraces, and if the patient is in a risky profession (aircraft personnel, divers).[151] With secondary pneumothoraces, treatment is mandatory, even after the first episode. Very often hospitalization is recommended.[105] A thoracoscopic approach with pleurodesis is generally preferred to medical instillation of a sclerosing agent.[141] The conclusion of the 2001 Delphi consensus conference on pneumothorax is that early aggressive intervention is required to avoid mortality and the risk of subsequent pneumothoraces in patients with compromised lung function.[105]

For catamenial pneumothorax, treatment usually involves achieving two goals: closure of the holes in the diaphragm and hormone treatment of the endometriosis. The options for closure of the holes are to perform pleurodesis of the chest, to resect the portion of the diaphragm involved, and to suture closed the individual holes.[155]

HYDROPNEUMOTHORAX

Anytime an air-fluid level is identified in the pleural space, a hydropneumothorax should be suspected (see Figs. 71.2 and 71.13). Loculated hydropneumothoraces may occur as single or multiple collections and may contain many air-fluid levels. Hydropneumothoraces occur relatively infrequently with spontaneous pneumothorax, being seen in less than 5% of cases.[21]

KEY POINTS

- Primary spontaneous pneumothorax is more common in smokers, men, and patients with tall and thin body habitus.
- The most common pulmonary disease leading to secondary pneumothorax is chronic obstructive pulmonary disease. Other common causes are interstitial and cystic lung diseases, particularly pulmonary Langerhans cell histiocytosis and lymphangioleiomyomatosis.
- The majority of secondary pneumothoraces are iatrogenic. The most common causes are transthoracic needle aspiration, thoracentesis, subclavian venipuncture, and positive-pressure ventilation.
- Apical bullae or blebs are seen on the radiograph in approximately 40% and on thin-section CT scan in 80% of patients with primary spontaneous pneumothorax.
- CT can be helpful in determining the underlying cause of pneumothorax and in distinguishing pneumothorax from severe bullous or cystic lung disease.

SUGGESTED READINGS

Baumann MH, Strange C, Heffner JE, et al. Management of spontaneous pneumothorax: an American College of Chest Physicians Delphi consensus statement. *Chest*. 2001;119:590–602.

Tschopp JM, Bintcliffe O, Astoul P, et al. ERS task force statement: diagnosis and treatment of primary spontaneous pneumothorax. *Eur Respir J*. 2015;46:321–335.

MacDuff A, Arnold A, Harvey J, BTS Pleural Disease Guideline Group. Management of spontaneous pneumothorax: British Thoracic Society Pleural Disease Guideline 2010. *Thorax*. 2010;65(suppl 2):ii18–ii31.

O'Connor AR, Morgan WE. Radiological review of pneumothorax. *Br Med J*. 2005;330:1493–1497.

Pereyra MF, Ferreiro L, Valdés L. Unexpandable lung. *Arch Bronconeumol*. 2013;49(2):63–69.

Rierson D, Bueno J. Pneumothorax in the supine patient: subtle radiographic signs. *J Thorac Imaging*. 2016;31(4):W16–W22.

Sahn SA, Heffner JE. Spontaneous pneumothorax. *N Engl J Med*. 2000;342:868–874.

Zhan C, Smith M, Stryer D. Accidental iatrogenic pneumothorax in hospitalized patients. *Med Care*. 2006;44:182–186.

The full reference list for this chapter is available at ExpertConsult.com.

72 Pleural Effusion*

ASHISH GUPTA | JEAN M. SEELY

Etiology, Prevalence, and Epidemiology

Pleural effusion is the accumulation of fluid in the pleural space resulting from disruption of the homeostatic forces responsible for the movement of pleural fluid.[1] Pleural effusions may result from pleural, parenchymal, or extrapulmonary disease. Approximately 1 million people develop this abnormality each year in the United States.[2]

Clinical Presentation

The oncotic pressures on both sides of the parietal and visceral pleura are normally equal, but an inequality exists in the hydrostatic pressures between the systemic circulation that supplies the parietal pleura and the low-pressure pulmonary circulation that supplies the visceral pleura. One fundamental component of the lymphatic anatomy is the existence of naturally occurring pores (stomas) in the caudal portion of the peripheral parietal pleura and lower mediastinal pleura.[3] These pores are capable of transferring particulate matter and cells directly into lymphatic channels for removal. Most of the fluid that accumulates abnormally in the pleural space is derived from the lung through the visceral pleura and absorbed primarily through the parietal pleura.[4]

Transudative effusions are mostly caused by an imbalance of hydrostatic and oncotic forces (Table 72.1). It can also occur because of increased negative pleural pressure (atelectasis) or movement of intraabdominal fluid into the pleural cavity (mostly on the right side) through diaphragmatic pores. These effusions have low protein levels and show low specific gravity. Exudative effusions usually result from pleural diseases or from injury in the adjacent lung and can be due to an increase in capillary permeability, as in pneumonia, or decreased lymphatic drainage, as in mediastinal carcinomatosis (Table 72.2).[5] These effusions typically display high protein and lactate dehydrogenase (LDH) levels and an elevated specific gravity.

Traditionally, exudates are distinguished from transudates by measuring the pleural fluid protein concentration. Exudates have a protein level greater than 30 g/L, and transudates have a protein level less than 30 g/L. Care should be taken in interpreting the pleural protein concentration if the serum total protein level is abnormal. In these cases the distinction is based on the ratio of pleural to serum protein levels and measurement of serum and pleural fluid LDH. The effusion is considered to be an exudate when the pleural fluid protein level divided by serum protein level is greater than 0.5, when pleural fluid LDH divided by serum LDH is greater than 0.6, and when pleural fluid LDH is more than two-thirds the upper limit of normal serum LDH.[2]

Manifestations of the Disease

RADIOGRAPHY

Small pleural effusions are not readily identified on conventional chest radiographs. When approximately 175 mL of fluid accumulates in the pleural space, there may be a noticeable blunting of the lateral costophrenic angle on erect frontal views; however, 525 mL of fluid occasionally may be required before the blunting of the angle is apparent (Box 72.1).[6] A retrospective analysis of 71 patients who had chest computed tomography (CT) scans and posteroanterior and lateral chest radiographs showed that pleural fluid becomes visible on upright lateral radiographs at approximately 50 mL. This occurs in the form of a meniscus in the posterior costophrenic sulcus on the lateral view, whereas in the posteroanterior projection, the meniscus becomes visible at about 200 mL.[7] It is estimated that at least 500 mL of pleural fluid is necessary to obliterate the hemidiaphragm.[7]

Pleural effusions can be entirely overlooked on supine radiographs or can be misdiagnosed as pulmonary consolidation or atelectasis.[8] Pleural fluid is often represented as a hazy opacity of one hemithorax with preserved vascular shadows. Other signs are loss of sharp silhouette of the ipsilateral hemidiaphragm and thickening of the minor fissure. The supine radiograph often underestimates the volume of pleural fluid. A prospective study of supine radiographs in 40 patients with pleural effusions showed that effusions with less than 175 mL are unlikely to be detected by this technique.[8]

Lateral decubitus chest radiographs can be used to detect small, free-flowing pleural effusions.[9] As little as 5 mL of pleural fluid can be detected by elevating the patient's hips and aiming the central beam at the lateral chest wall parallel to the expected fluid level.[10,11]

The appearance of free pleural fluid as a homogeneous opacity with a concave upper border, higher laterally than medially, on erect frontal and lateral radiographs is called the pleural meniscus (Fig. 72.1). The meniscus appearance can be explained by the configuration of free fluid within the pleural space and its relationship to the x-ray beam. As a result of its elasticity, the lung tends to preserve its shape while recoiling from the chest wall. This property of the lung causes the fluid to rise against gravity and surround the lower part of the lung. Because x-ray beams have to traverse a greater depth of fluid at the periphery of the thorax, the upper margin appears higher in the form of a meniscus. The superior margin of the fluid located more medially does not produce a layer of sufficient depth to be visible on the radiograph.

Subpulmonic Effusion

Significant amounts of pleural fluid can accumulate in the subpulmonic region, causing flattening and inversion of the

*The editors and the publisher would like to thank Dr. Anoop P. Ayyappan for contributing material on this topic to the prior edition of this work. It has served as the foundation for the current chapter.

TABLE 72.1 CAUSES OF TRANSUDATIVE PLEURAL EFFUSIONS

Common	Less Common	Rare
Left heart failure	Nephrotic syndrome	Constrictive pericarditis
Cirrhosis	Mitral stenosis	Superior vena cava obstruction
Hypoalbuminemia	Hypothyroidism	Urinothorax
		Meigs syndrome
		Ovarian hyperstimulation syndrome

TABLE 72.2 CAUSES OF EXUDATIVE PLEURAL EFFUSIONS

Common	Less Common	Rare
Malignancy	Pulmonary embolism	Drugs
Parapneumonic effusions	Rheumatoid arthritis	Yellow nail syndrome
	Benign asbestos effusion	
	Dressler syndrome	
	Pancreatitis	

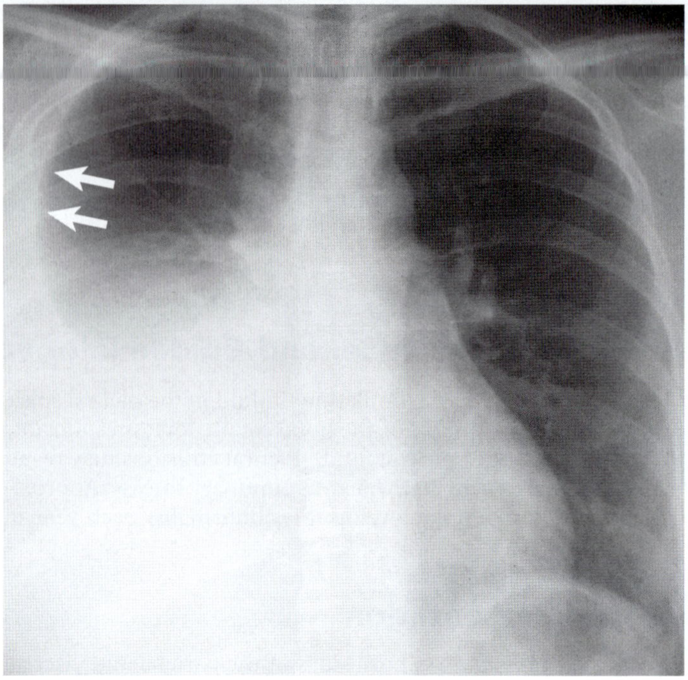

Fig. 72.1 Free pleural effusion. Posteroanterior chest radiograph shows the meniscus sign *(arrows)* in a large right pleural effusion.

BOX 72.1 CLASSIC SIGNS OF PLEURAL EFFUSION

RADIOGRAPHIC SIGNS

Meniscus sign on frontal radiograph (>200 mL)

Blunting of costophrenic sulcus on lateral view (>50 mL)

Subpulmonic effusion: lateral displacement of the apex of the pseudodiaphragm

COMPUTED TOMOGRAPHY SIGNS

Sickle-shaped opacity in most dependent part of the thorax, the posterior costophrenic sulci in supine patient

Fluid attenuation (0–20 Hounsfield units)

hemidiaphragm without significant blunting of the lateral costophrenic angle. In effect, the lung "floats" on a layer of fluid. These effusions are often transudates and can be difficult to diagnose on the posteroanterior radiograph and may require a lateral decubitus view or ultrasound. On erect frontal radiographs the apex of the pseudodiaphragmatic contour in patients with subpulmonic effusion is more lateral than the apex of the normal hemidiaphragm in about 50% of the cases (Fig. 72.2).[12,13] This appearance is accentuated on expiratory views.[13] Decubitus view with the involved side dependent results in the accumulation of the fluid along the lateral wall (see Fig. 72.2). Nonvisualization of the intrapulmonary blood vessels below the level of the hemidiaphragm may be the only evidence of a subpulmonic effusion, but this sign is nonspecific and can be caused by lower lobe airspace disease or ascites.[14–16] The normal distance between the left hemidiaphragm and gastric air bubble is usually less than 1 cm, and an abnormal separation of these two has been described as a helpful sign in the diagnosis of left-sided subpulmonic effusions.[16] In the lateral view, typically the pseudodiaphragmatic contour presents a flat superior surface that slants sharply downward at the major fissure.[13]

The radiographic appearance of interlobar fluid is multifactorial and depends on the shape and orientation of the fissure, location of fluid within the fissure, and direction of the x-ray beam. Fluid in the major fissure usually appears as a sharp curvilinear interface that is lucent medially and more dense laterally in erect frontal radiographs. It has been classically described as the "incomplete fissure sign," implying that the effusion is bound by the edge of the incompleteness of the fissure.[17] This sign may be seen even when the major fissure is complete when the effusion is bound by the lateral border of the lower lobe.[18] An interface lucent laterally and more dense medially is usually due to parenchymal disease in the lower lobe.[17] On the lateral chest radiograph, fluid within the upper part of the major fissures is seen as an arcuate opacity with a "fading off" anterior concave margin and sharp posterior interface.[16] This is due to the usual concave surface and lateral facing of the upper part of major fissures so that fluid in the lateral aspect of the fissure is seen in profile, whereas fluid located medially is seen obliquely.[19] Another interesting appearance is the "middle lobe step," which occurs when fluid accumulates lateral to the middle or lower lobes and extends to the undersurface of the upper lobes.[18] Because incompleteness of the major and minor fissures is a common finding,[19] it is likely that the middle lobe step is due to fluid within the incomplete major and minor fissures.[16,17]

Pleural pseudotumor is due to accumulation of pleural fluid within an interlobar fissure. This can mimic a pleural or parenchymal mass and create diagnostic confusion. It is most often encountered with minor fissure encapsulation in patients with resolving left heart failure. On frontal views the location of the opacity at the site of the fissure and slight tapering of the medial and lateral margins suggest minor fissure encapsulation (Fig. 72.3). Lateral views are usually confirmatory because the long axis of the opacity confirms the position of the distended fissure, and the tapering extremities are seen more clearly in this projection (see Fig. 72.3). These effusions disappear on treatment of the primary cause and are also termed *vanishing tumors* (see Fig. 72.3).

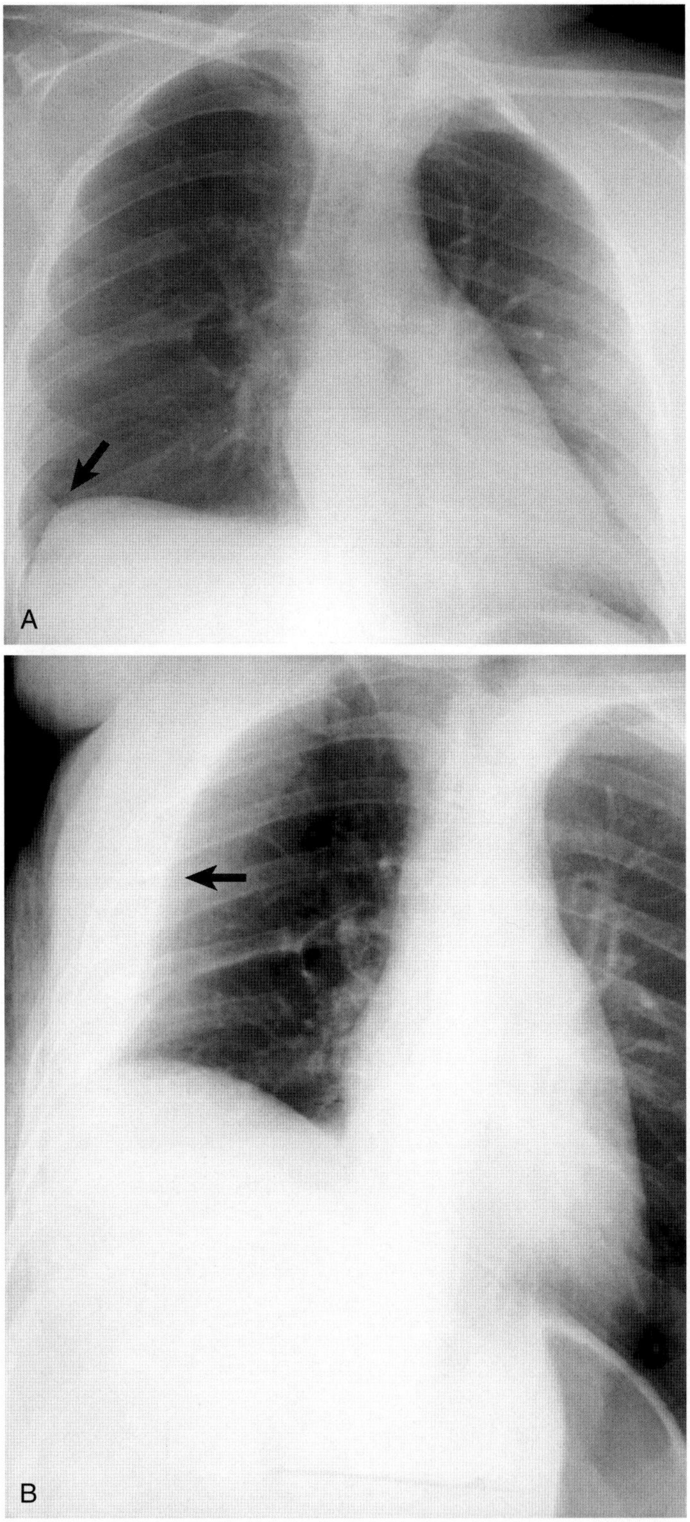

Fig. 72.2 Subpulmonic effusion. (A) Chest radiograph shows that the crest of the pseudodiaphragmatic surface *(arrow)* lies more lateral than the expected location of the apex of an elevated hemidiaphragm. Note the nonvisualization of intrapulmonary blood vessels below the right hemidiaphragm. (B) Right lateral decubitus view shows fluid accumulation *(arrow)* in the dependent hemithorax.

On supine radiographs free pleural effusions produce a hazy density over the hemithorax, caused by the posterior layering of the fluid.[9,10] This results in an increased homogeneous density superimposed over the lungs that does not obscure normal bronchovascular markings or show air bronchograms. The pleural fluid can cap the apex of the lungs on a supine view (Fig. 72.4) because of the relatively small capacity of the apex compared with the base of the thorax and because the superior and lateral aspects of the apex are the most dependent parts of the thorax tangential to a frontal x-ray beam.[16] Apical capping, seen in about 50% of large effusions, is usually not seen in small- or moderate-sized effusions.[8] Blunting of the lateral costophrenic angle can be seen in the supine position when there is sufficient pleural fluid to fill the posterior hemithorax up to or near the level of the lateral costophrenic angle and is seen in 25% of moderate-sized and 41% of large effusions.[8]

COMPUTED TOMOGRAPHY

CT has been shown to be superior to chest radiographs in distinguishing a peripheral parenchymal lesion from a pleural process.[20] On CT a free-flowing pleural effusion produces a sickle-shaped opacity in the most dependent part of the thorax. Free pleural fluid in a supine patient first accumulates in the posterior costophrenic sulci, the most dependent portion of the chest. Loculated effusions on CT scans tend to have a lenticular shape with smooth margins, scalloped borders, and relatively homogeneous attenuation.

Pleural effusions are characterized on CT by attenuation values between those of water (0 Hounsfield units [HU]) and soft tissue (approximately 100 HU), typically in the order of 10 to 20 HU.[21] CT density measurements alone are considered unreliable in differentiating transudates from exudates or in the diagnosis of chylous pleural effusions.[22,22a] The presence of pleural thickening, pleural nodules, loculation of pleural fluid, or increased attenuation of extrapleural fat can be detected using CT, and these ancillary findings occur most commonly with exudative effusions.[23,24] CT scans for pleural effusion should be performed with contrast enhancement because pleural abnormalities are better visualized and more easily distinguished from adjacent parenchymal abnormalities. In our experience, CT in systemic venous phase rather than pulmonary arterial phase is better for assessing for pleural enhancement, thickening, and nodularity. It is also often easier to appreciate pleural thickening and nodularity by reviewing the 5-mm sections rather than the thin-section images.

Distinguishing small pleural effusions from ascites on CT is facilitated by analysis of four signs: the diaphragm sign,[25] the displaced-crus sign,[26] the interface sign,[27] and the bare-area sign (see Box 72.1).[28] Ascites can be readily differentiated from the pleural effusion if the diaphragm is identifiable adjacent to an abnormal fluid collection in the right upper quadrant. On CT fluid "inside" the diaphragm is ascites, whereas fluid "outside" the diaphragm is pleural effusion (diaphragm sign). Pleural effusions displace the crus anteriorly and laterally away from the spine (displaced-crus sign) (Fig. 72.5). The presence of the diaphragm produces an indistinct interface between the pleural effusion and liver, whereas its absence in ascites results in a sharp, well-defined interface (interface sign) (Fig. 72.6). The right lobe of the liver is directly attached to the posterior abdominal wall and the diaphragm without intervening peritoneum. This direct attachment that lacks a peritoneal covering is called the bare

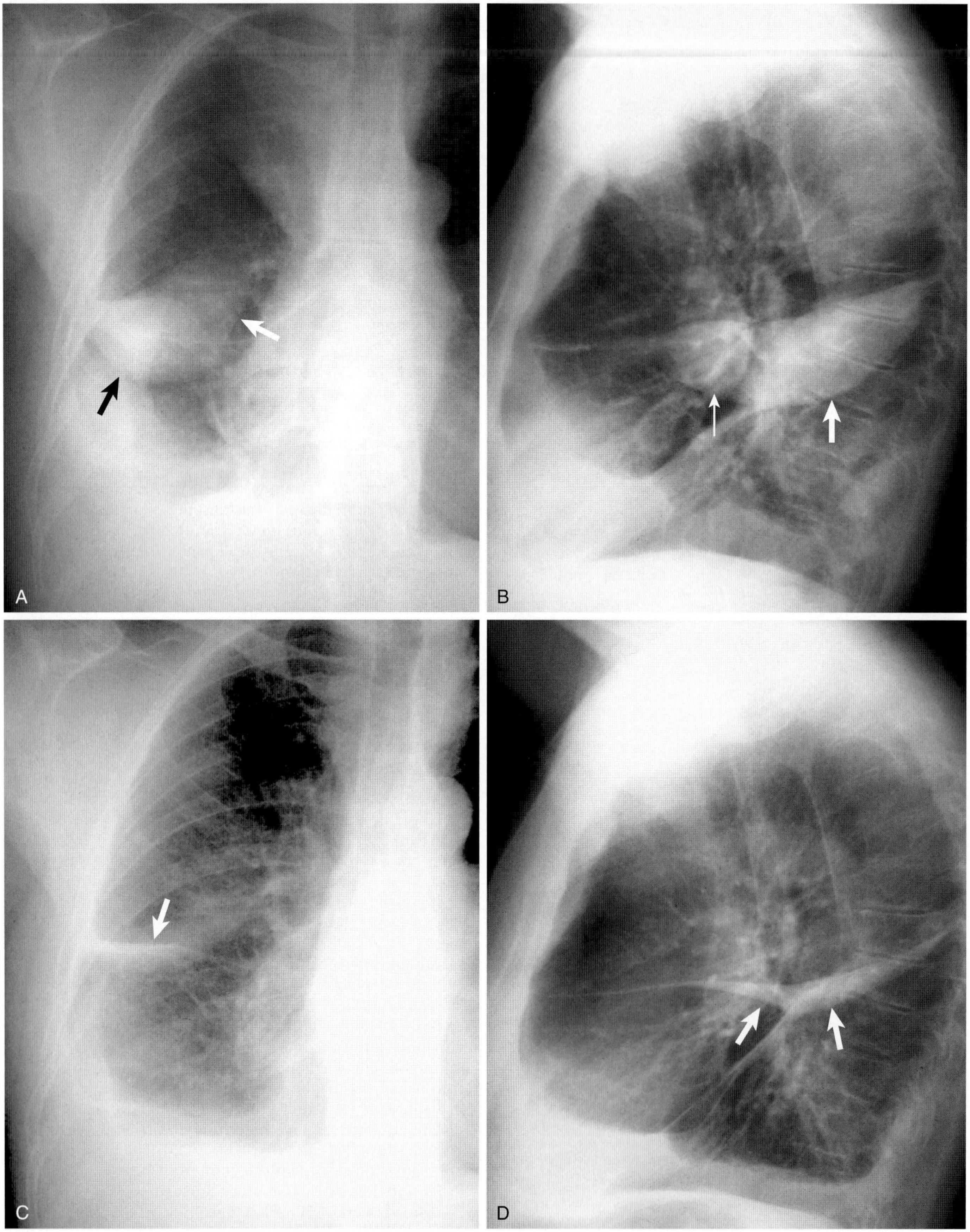

Fig. 72.3 Pleural pseudotumor. (A) Posteroanterior chest radiograph in a patient with left heart failure shows fluid in the minor *(black arrow)* and major *(white arrow)* fissures simulating a mass. There also is free fluid in the right pleural cavity. (B) Lateral chest radiograph shows that the opacity is located within the distended minor *(thin arrow)* and major *(thick arrow)* fissures. (C) Posteroanterior chest radiograph obtained 1 week later shows decrease in interlobar fluid *(arrow)*. (D) Corresponding lateral chest radiograph shows decrease of interlobar fluid *(arrows)* after improvement of cardiac status.

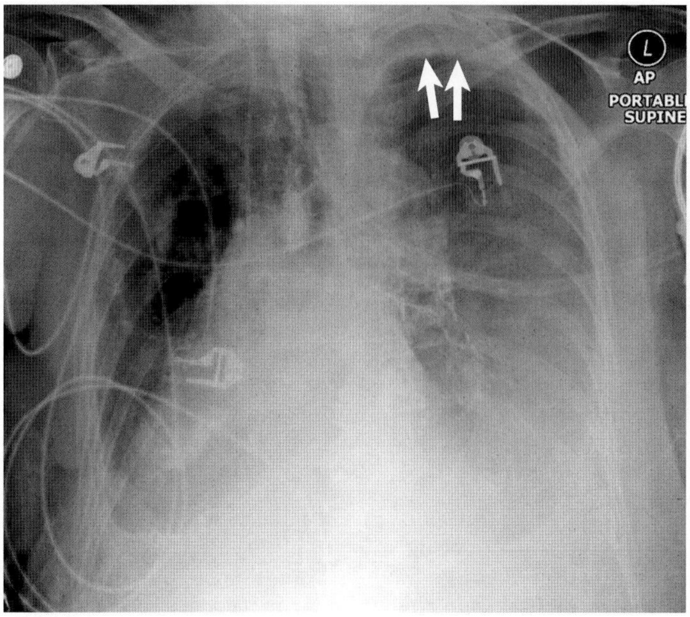

Fig. 72.4 Apical pleural fluid. Supine chest radiograph reveals large left and small right pleural effusions. The larger left effusion produces a hazy increased density in the hemithorax and an apical cap *(arrows)*. The right apical cap was related to previous granulomatous infection and remained stable for years.

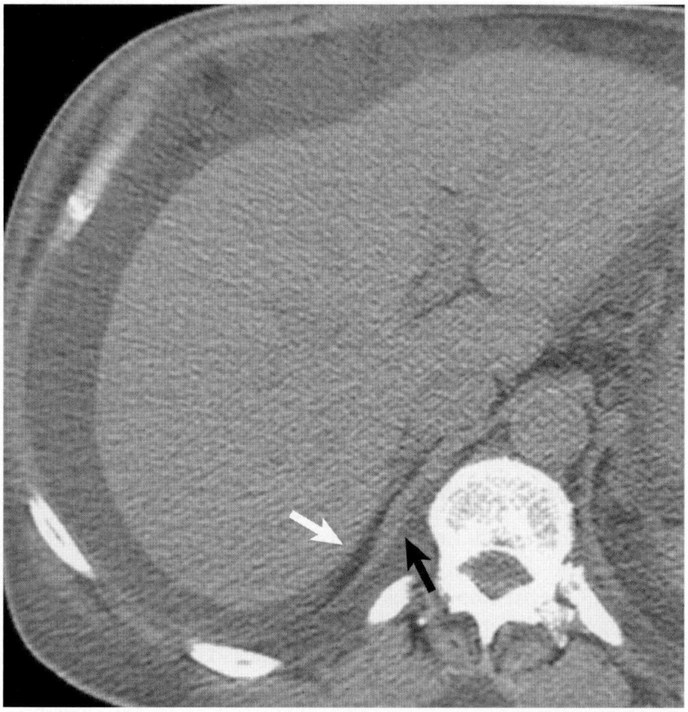

Fig. 72.5 Displaced-crus sign in pleural effusion. CT scan reveals anterior and lateral displacement of right hemidiaphragmatic crus by pleural fluid *(black arrow)* in a patient with bilateral effusions and ascites. Ascites does not extend behind the bare area of the liver *(white arrow)*.

area. Ascites cannot extend behind the liver at the level of the bare area, whereas a pleural effusion can because the posterior sulcus of the right pleural space extends behind the liver (bare-area sign). Fluid behind the liver at the level of the bare area is in the pleural space. When these four signs were compared in a retrospective blinded analysis of 52 patients with right pleural effusion, ascites, or both, it was observed that when effusion and ascites were present, none of the four signs alone could reliably differentiate the fluid collections; however, combined use of the four signs led to correct identification of all the abnormal fluid collections.[29]

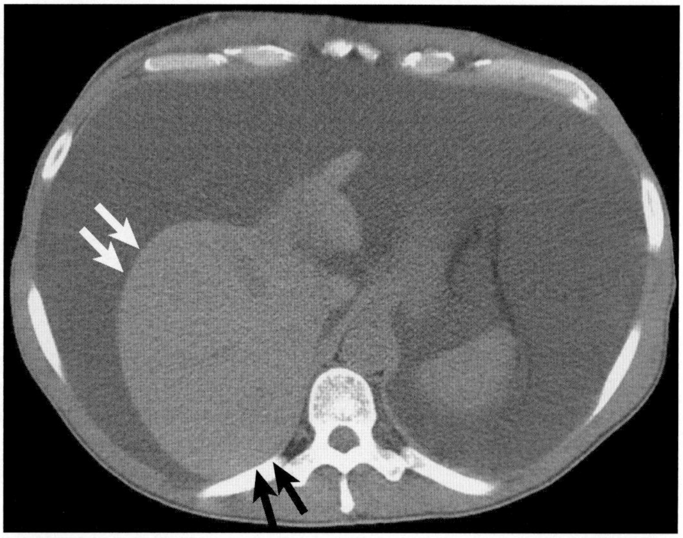

Fig. 72.6 Interface and bare area signs in ascites. CT scan illustrates a distinct interface between ascitic fluid and the liver *(white arrows)*. Ascites does not extend behind the liver at the level of the bare area *(black arrows)*.

MAGNETIC RESONANCE IMAGING

Magnetic resonance imaging (MRI) plays a limited role in the evaluation of pleural effusion. Fluid collections in the pleural cavity show low signal intensity on T1-weighted images and a high relative signal intensity on T2-weighted images because of their water content. Differentiation of transudates from exudates is unreliable on conventional MRI; however, a study using diffusion-weighted MRI showed that application of diffusion gradients to analyze pleural fluid can differentiate between these two with a sensitivity of 91% and specificity of 85%.[30] Subacute or chronic hemorrhage in the pleural space can be recognized by very high signal intensity on T1-weighted and T2-weighted images. In subacute or chronic hematomas, a concentric ring sign, consisting of an outer dark rim composed of hemosiderin and bright signal intensity in the center because of the T1 shortening effects of methemoglobin, can be observed.[22]

ULTRASONOGRAPHY

Ultrasound is a reliable method for detecting small pleural effusions and for guiding thoracentesis. Most pleural effusions, whether free flowing or loculated, are hypoechoic with a sharp echogenic line that delineates the visceral pleura and lung. An anechoic effusion can be a transudate or exudate (Fig. 72.7). Complex septated, complex nonseptated, or homogeneously echogenic effusions are always exudates (Fig. 72.8).[31] Fibrinous septations are better visualized on ultrasound than on CT scans. Ultrasound has the added advantage of being portable, allowing bedside imaging with the patient in a sitting or recumbent position.

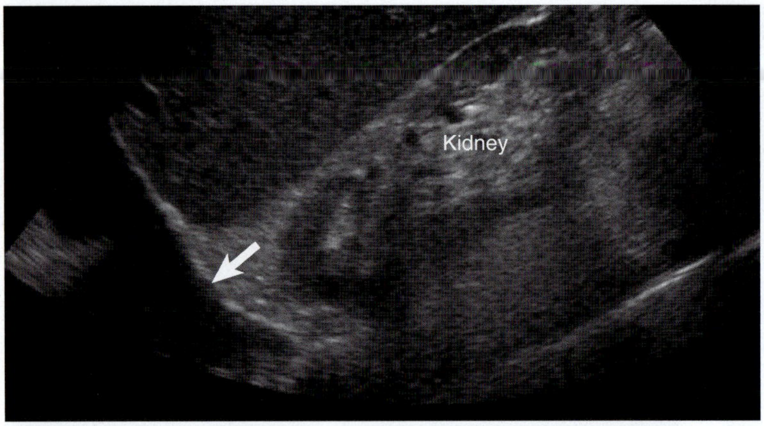

Fig. 72.7 Right pleural effusion. Sagittal ultrasound image of the right upper quadrant shows an anechoic fluid collection above the right hemidiaphragm consistent with a pleural effusion *(arrow)*.

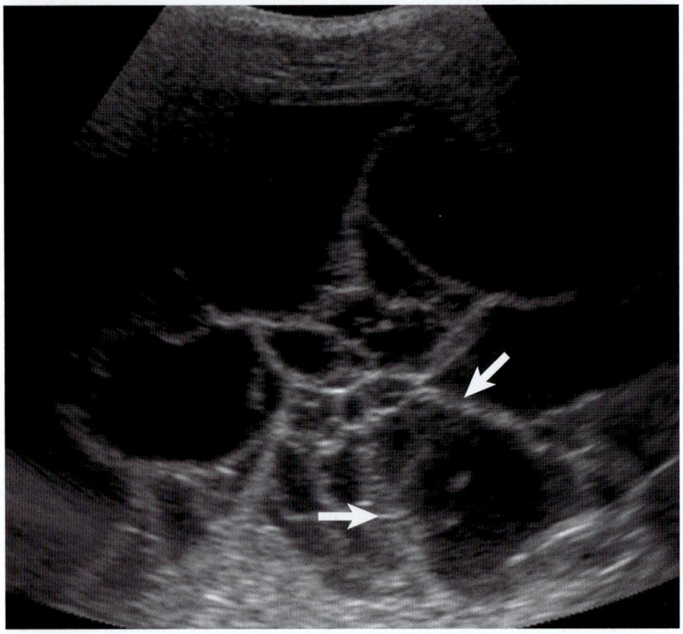

Fig. 72.8 Empyema. Ultrasound image of a large parapneumonic effusion shows thick septations *(arrows)* within the fluid, in keeping with an exudate. Frank pus was aspirated during thoracentesis.

POSITRON EMISSION TOMOGRAPHY/ COMPUTED TOMOGRAPHY

Positron emission tomography (PET) using fluorodeoxyglucose (FDG) has been shown to be an accurate diagnostic tool in differentiating benign from malignant pleural effusions in patients with malignant disease with sensitivity of 88% to 100% and specificity of 67% to 94%.[32–35] A retrospective review of PET-CT studies in 32 patients with primary extrapleural malignancy and pleural effusion revealed that PET was more sensitive than CT alone in identifying pleural involvement, and the presence of concomitant pleural abnormalities is the most accurate sign of malignancy when assessing the nature of pleural effusion (Fig. 72.9).[36] Focal increased uptake within the posterior portion of the fluid, presumably resulting from an uptake in malignant cells accumulating in the dependent location, a relatively infrequent finding in patients with malignant pleural effusion, is considered highly specific for malignancy.[36]

False-positive uptake of FDG by the pleura can result from pleural infection or from inflammation after talc pleurodesis; interpretation of the PET findings should take into account the results of pleural fluid analysis and the patient's recent medical history.[37] A negative PET result can be useful, however, by confirming the absence of pleural metastatic disease, particularly when the results of thoracentesis also are negative.

Differential Diagnosis

Differential diagnoses from clinical data and other supportive diagnostic techniques are listed in Box 72.2.

TRANSUDATIVE EFFUSION

Left heart failure accounts for most transudative pleural effusions.[2] Effusions in a hepatic hydrothorax, hypoalbuminemia, nephrotic syndrome, constrictive pericarditis, or urinothorax and during peritoneal dialysis also can have the characteristics of a transudate. The development of a transudative effusion indicates that the pleural membrane is normal, and if the underlying problem is corrected, the fluid is reabsorbed without sequelae. Thoracentesis should not be performed for bilateral effusions in a clinical setting strongly suggestive of a pleural transudate unless there are atypical features or they fail to respond to therapy.

EXUDATIVE EFFUSION

Pneumonia, malignancy, thromboembolism, connective tissue diseases, and drugs account for most exudative effusions. Exudative pleural effusions develop when the pleural surface or the local capillary permeability or both are altered. A diagnostic pleural fluid sample should be gathered with a fine-bore (22-gauge) needle and a 50-mL syringe. The sample should be placed in sterile vials and blood culture bottles and analyzed for protein, glucose, LDH, pH, Gram stain, acid-fast bacillus stain, cytology, and microbiologic culture.

INFECTION

Most empyemas occur as a complication of pneumonia or lung abscess, after thoracic surgery, or in association with an intra-abdominal infection. Bacteria such as *Staphylococcus aureus, Streptococcus pneumoniae,* and enteric gram-negative bacilli are the most common etiologic agents. In an infected effusion, a

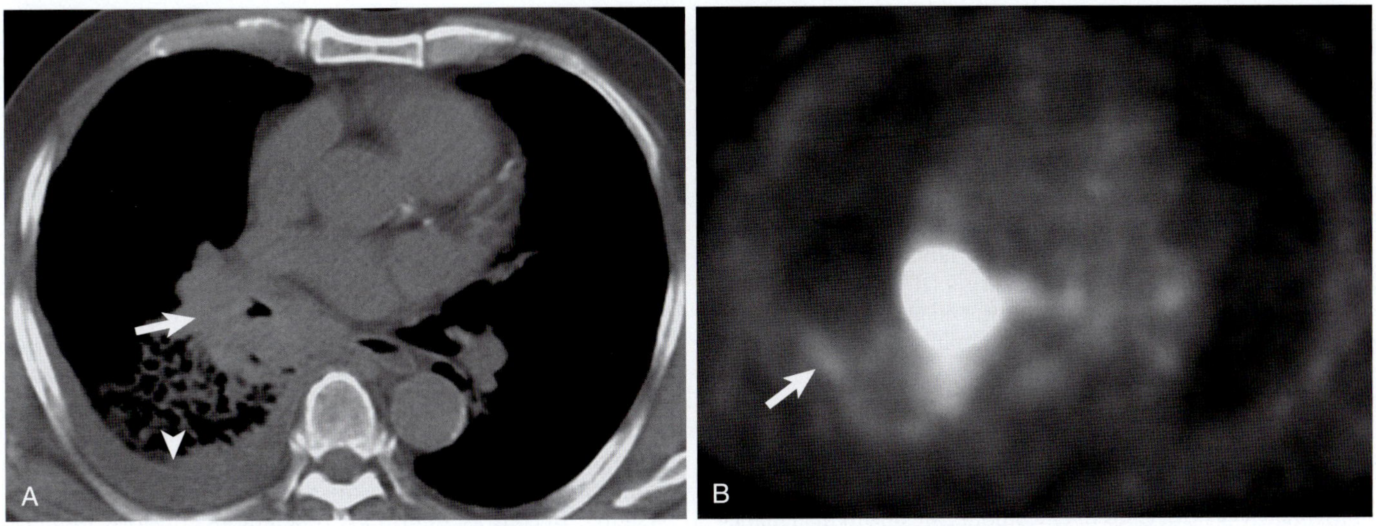

Fig. 72.9 Malignant pleural effusion. (A) CT image shows a mass in the medial aspect of the right lower lobe *(arrow)* with a small ipsilateral pleural effusion *(arrowhead)*. (B) Fluorodeoxyglucose–positron emission tomography image shows markedly increased uptake in the right lower lobe mass and increased uptake in the parietal pleura *(arrow)* suggestive of malignant effusion.

BOX 72.2 ETIOLOGY OF PLEURAL EFFUSION

- Pleuropulmonary infection
  - *Mycobacterium* tuberculosis
  - Nontuberculous bacteria
  - *Actinomyces* and *Nocardia* species
  - Fungi
  - Parasites
  - Viruses and *Mycoplasma*
- Pleuropulmonary malignancy
  - Lung cancer
  - Metastatic disease—to pleura and mediastinal lymph nodes
  - Lymphoma
  - Leukemia
- Connective tissue disease and vasculitis
  - Systemic lupus erythematosus
  - Rheumatoid disease
  - Granulomatosis with polyangiitis
- Pulmonary embolism and infarction
- Asbestos exposure
- Drugs
- Heart failure
- Metabolic and endocrine disease
  - Myxedema[258]
  - Diabetes mellitus
  - Amyloidosis
- Skeletal disease
  - Gorham disease (chylothorax)[259]
  - Langerhans cell histiocytosis
- Liver disease
- Kidney disease
  - Dialysis
  - Urinoma
  - Nephrotic syndrome
  - Acute glomerulonephritis
  - Uremia
- Pancreatic disease
  - Acute pancreatitis
  - Chronic pancreatitis with pleuropancreatic fistula
- Gynecologic tumor
  - Ovary, uterus, fallopian tube
  - Ovarian hyperstimulation syndrome
- Gastrointestinal tract
  - Gastric/duodenal-pleural fistula
  - Diaphragmatic hernia
  - Idiopathic inflammatory bowel disease
- Miscellaneous causes
  - Subphrenic abscess
  - Lymphatic hypoplasia
  - Yellow nail syndrome
  - Dressler syndrome
  - Familial paroxysmal polyserositis
  - Systemic cholesterol embolization[260]
  - Extramedullary hematopoiesis[261]
- Idiopathic[262] causes

pH <7.2 indicates the need for tube drainage. Closed-needle biopsy of the pleura for histologic examination has been recommended for undiagnosed exudative effusions when tuberculosis is a concern. The combination of histology and culture establishes the diagnosis of tuberculosis in 90% of patients.

MALIGNANCY

Malignancy is the second most common cause of pleural effusion after left heart failure in elderly patients. The most frequent causes are pulmonary, breast, ovarian, and gastric carcinomas. Malignant effusions can be diagnosed by pleural fluid cytology alone in about 60% of cases. According to the most recent British Thoracic Society (BTS) guidelines, as much fluid as possible should be sent for cytology from the available diagnostic sample (likely to be 20–40 mL) and, when the initial result is negative but malignancy is suspected, the sending of a higher-volume sample after a second aspiration should be considered. If the initial aspiration is both therapeutic and diagnostic, greater than 60 mL should be sent for cytologic examination.[38] If the first pleural cytology specimen is negative, the test should be repeated. The yield depends on the skill of the cytologist and on tumor type, with a higher diagnostic rate for adenocarcinoma than for mesothelioma, lymphoma, and sarcoma. Percutaneous pleural biopsies are recommended when cytology findings are not diagnostic. The diagnostic yield from pleural biopsy is higher under image guidance, which can identify areas of pleural thickening or nodularity.

CONNECTIVE TISSUE DISEASES AND VASCULITIS

Connective tissue disorders and vasculitis may produce pleural effusion with varying degrees of pleural inflammation. The collagen vascular diseases and vasculitides most commonly associated with pleural effusions are rheumatoid arthritis (RA), systemic lupus erythematosus (SLE), Sjögren syndrome, and granulomatosis with polyangiitis (formerly Wegener granulomatosis). RA is unlikely to be the cause of an effusion if the glucose level in the fluid is greater than 1.6 mmol/L (29 mg/dL).

CHYLOTHORAX

Approximately 50% of cases of chylothorax are due to malignancy (particularly lymphoma); 25% are related to trauma; and the rest are due to tuberculosis, sarcoidosis, and amyloidosis. Pseudochylothorax or cholesterol pleurisy results from the accumulation of cholesterol crystals in a long-standing pleural effusion. It can occur in chronic rheumatoid pleurisy and tuberculosis. If a chylothorax or pseudochylothorax is suspected, pleural fluid should be sent to measure triglyceride and cholesterol levels and to determine the presence of cholesterol crystals and chylomicrons. A true chylothorax shows the presence of chylomicrons and has a high triglyceride level (>1.24 mmol/L). In a pseudochylothorax the cholesterol level is elevated (>5.18 mmol/L), and cholesterol crystals are often seen at microscopy.

Pleural Effusion Caused by Infection

Infectious pleural effusions, most caused by bacterial infections, tend to be exudative in nature. The formation of pleural fluid is attributed to increased capillary permeability and protein leakage as a result of the inflammatory process. In addition, inflammatory exudate on the pleural surface and fibrous thickening of the pleura impede reabsorption of fluid by the lymphatics.

MYCOBACTERIA

Pleural involvement is one of the most common extrapulmonary manifestations of *Mycobacterium tuberculosis* infection. Pleural involvement may be seen at any time in the natural course of the disease but occurs most commonly 3 to 7 months after the primary infection.[39] About 80% of patients with tuberculous pleural effusion have concomitant pulmonary tuberculosis.[40]

Epidemiology

The frequency of tuberculous effusion depends on the prevalence of tuberculosis in the population studied. In developed countries, such as the United States and United Kingdom, pleural involvement is seen in less than 10% of cases of infection with *M. tuberculosis*.[41] In countries where tuberculosis is common, it is the most frequent cause of exudative pleural effusion or empyema.[42–44]

Emergence of the human immunodeficiency virus (HIV) pandemic has had a profound effect on the epidemiology of tuberculosis. One meta-analysis showed significant association between presence of HIV and extrapulmonary tuberculosis.[45] In a prospective study of 1000 patients with pleural effusion in a tertiary care hospital in Spain, of the 42 patients with HIV infection, the most common cause of pleural effusion was tuberculosis.[46] The rate of pleural involvement in HIV-positive patients with tuberculosis can be 40%.[47] Tubercular pleural effusions in HIV-positive patients are also more likely to be bilateral and have associated parenchymal involvement and positive bacteriology when compared with HIV-negative patients.[48]

Pathophysiology

Tuberculous pleural effusions usually occur after a latent period of 3 to 6 months after primary infection and are due to the rupture of the subpleural Ghon focus into the pleural cavity.[2] These primary tuberculous effusions are the result of a delayed-hypersensitivity reaction to bacilli entering the pleural space rather than direct infection. An effusion in reactivation disease is due to direct infection of the pleural space, rather than an immunologic phenomenon, and occurs as a result of the direct spread of bacilli from the cavitary lung lesions, bloodstream, and lymphatic system.[49] In contrast to primary tuberculous effusions, numerous bacilli are secreted into the pleural cavity. Chronic active infection may lead to the formation of a tuberculous empyema. Rupture of a parenchymal cavity into the pleural space can result in a bronchopleural fistula and pyopneumothorax.

Clinical Presentation

The clinical presentation of tuberculous pleural effusion may be acute or insidious. Symptoms include dyspnea, cough, pleuritic chest pain, and malaise.

Manifestations of the Disease

Radiography. Tuberculous pleural effusion in non-HIV–infected patients is almost invariably unilateral and seldom massive. In one retrospective study, only 19 of 113 (17%) tuberculous pleural effusions occupied more than two-thirds of the hemithorax on posteroanterior upright chest radiographs.[50]

Apart from detecting pleural fluid, routine radiographs have a limited role in establishing the diagnosis because parenchymal lesions most often go undetected.[51,52] It is prudent to keep these patients in isolation until a thorough evaluation for the presence of active pulmonary tuberculosis is negative.

Computed Tomography. Patients may develop new pulmonary lesions while on medications for tuberculous pleural effusions. A paradoxical response, affecting 16% of patients in one study, generally occurs 3 to 12 weeks after the beginning of antituberculous therapy, usually regressing without a change in the initial drug regimen.[53–55] In a retrospective review of 16 patients with radiologic evidence of paradoxical response to antituberculous therapy, CT revealed the development of new peripheral pulmonary nodules or masses, which mostly abutted the normal or thickened pleura, subsequently decreasing in size and finally disappearing on continuation of the same antituberculous medication.[56]

Tuberculous pleuritis may progress to chronic persistent pleural effusion or empyema (Figs. 72.10 and 72.11), which may be defined as persistent, grossly purulent pleural fluid containing numerous tubercle bacilli.[57] Tuberculous empyema may manifest as a loculated pleural fluid collection with parenchymal disease and cavitation. In most cases of tuberculous empyema, the final outcome is extensive fibrothorax, easily detected as a thick calcified pleural rind on chest radiographs and CT.[57]

Chronic persistent effusion should be suspected if pleural thickening is greater than 2 cm or when more than one linear shadow is visible running parallel to the inner chest wall on

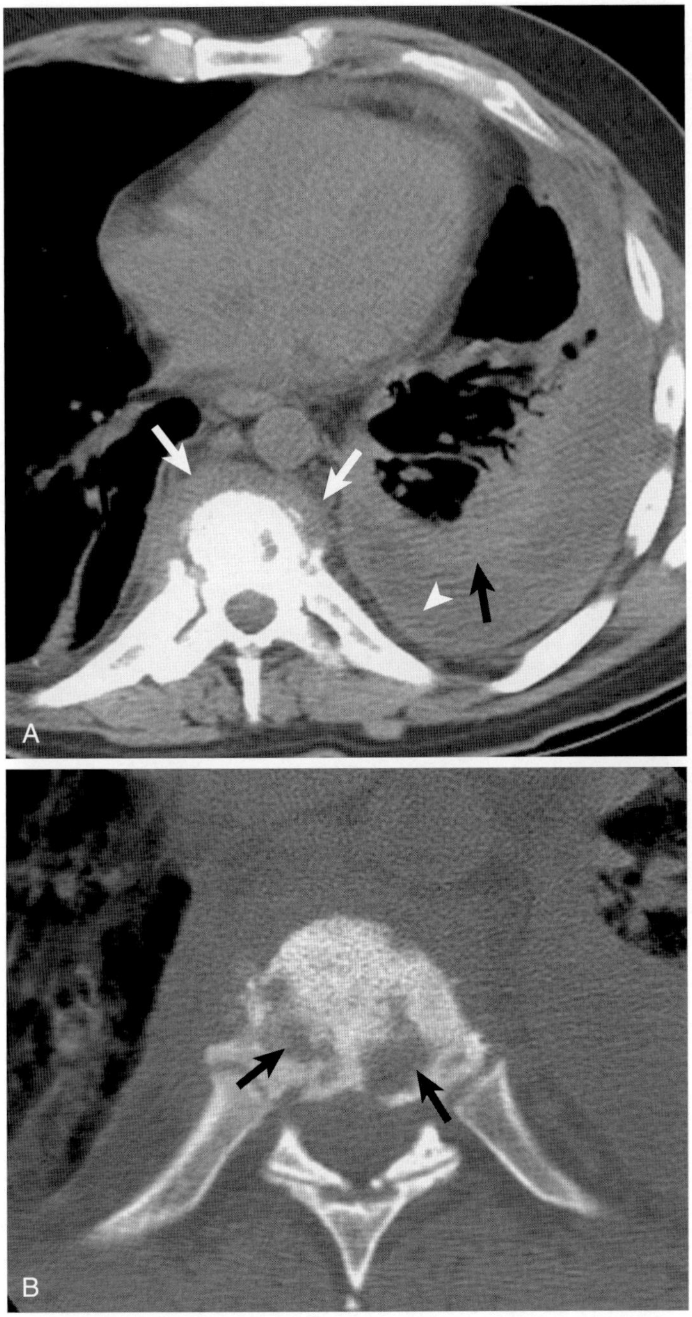

Fig. 72.10 Tuberculous spondylitis and pleural effusion. (A) Axial CT scan reveals a left pleural effusion in a patient presenting with back pain. There is smooth thickening of the parietal pleura *(arrowhead)*, suggestive of an empyema. Visceral pleura *(black arrow)* abutting the consolidated lung also is thickened. Note abnormal paravertebral soft tissue *(white arrows)* resulting from tuberculous spondylitis. (B) CT scan at the same level obtained in bone windows shows lytic destruction of the vertebral body *(arrows)*. Findings are consistent with Pott disease and tuberculous empyema.

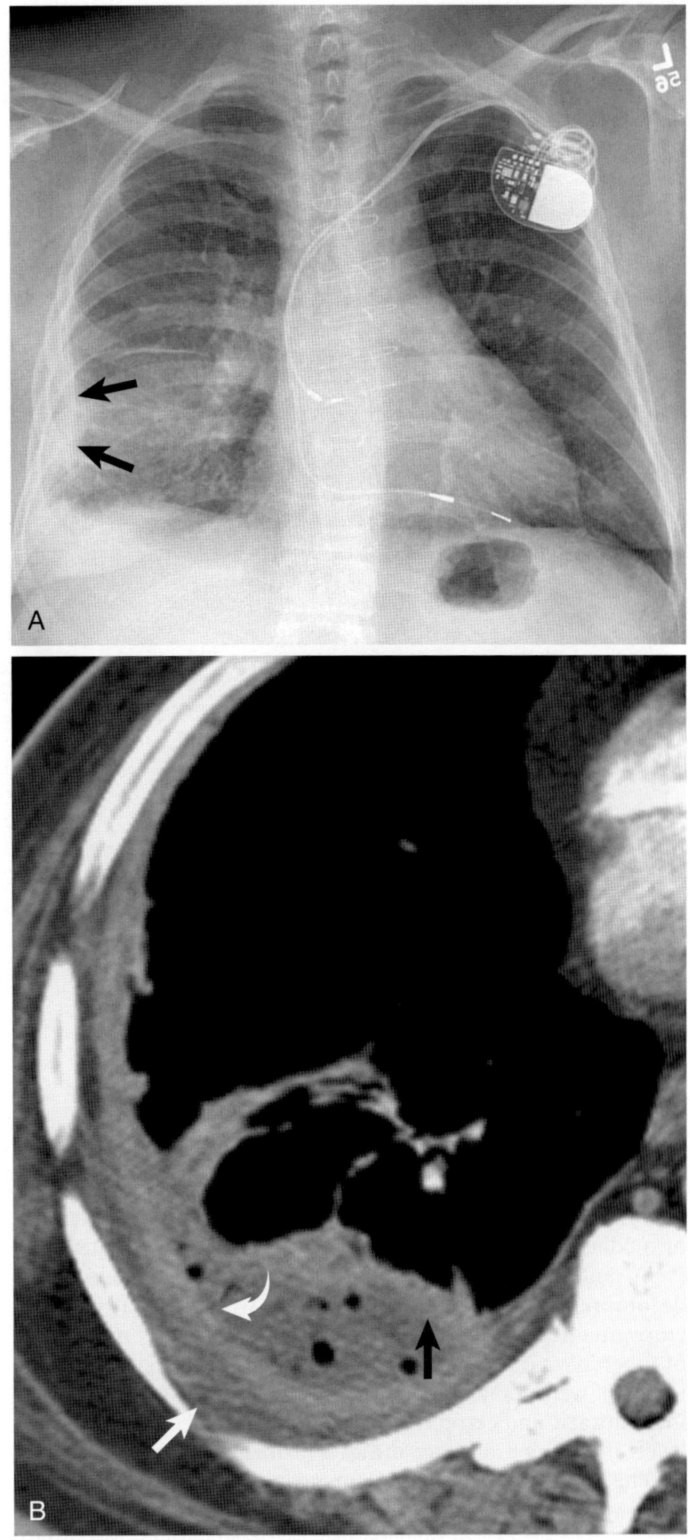

Fig. 72.11 Empyema. (A) Posteroanterior chest radiograph shows blunting of the right costophrenic sulcus and thickening of the pleura laterally *(arrows)*. Hazy increased opacity is seen overlying the lower lung, suggestive of a loculated effusion. (B) Contrast-enhanced chest CT scan shows loculated fluid collection in the right pleural space containing multiple locules of air. The parietal *(curved arrow)* and visceral pleura *(black arrow)* show enhancement and thickening (split pleura sign). Note the stranding of the extrapleural fat *(straight white arrow)*, in keeping with an active inflammatory process.

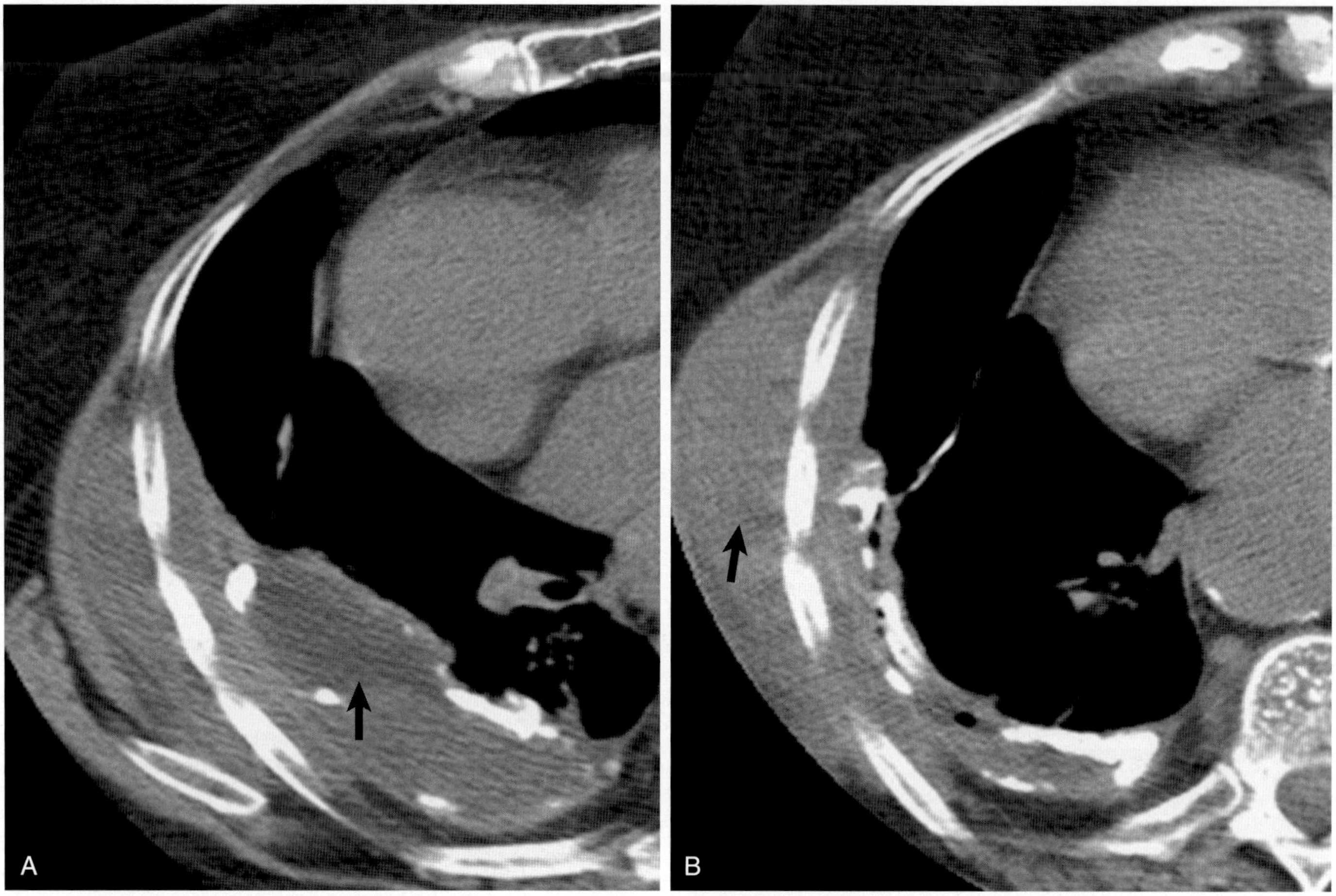

Fig. 72.12 Empyema necessitatis. (A) CT scan shows an old sterile empyema *(arrow)* in a patient with a family history of tuberculosis. Note pleural calcifications indicating long-standing disease. (B) CT scan acquired 6 months later at the same level shows that the right-sided pleural fluid collection has decreased in size, but fluid *(arrow)* now extends into the chest wall, in keeping with empyema necessitatis.

chest radiographs.[58] CT shows a loculated pleural fluid collection in association with pleural thickening and calcification.[59] Pleural thickening caused by tuberculosis can mimic malignancy and can involve pleura in circumferential fashion with involvement of mediastinal pleura, parietal pleural thickness of greater than 1 cm, and nodularity.[60] Chronic tuberculous empyema may decompress through the chest wall, in which case it is called empyema necessitatis, a rare but well-recognized complication of tuberculous empyema.[61] CT findings of empyema necessitatis include well-demarcated, thick-walled fluid collections in intrathoracic and extrathoracic locations (Fig. 72.12).[61] Air-fluid levels in the pleural space indicate bronchopleural fistula.

The occurrence of malignant neoplasm is a relatively rare but important complication of chronic tuberculous empyema. Pathologic cell types of malignancy associated with long-standing empyema include malignant lymphoma, squamous cell carcinoma, mesothelioma, malignant fibrous histiocytoma, sarcoma, and hemangioendothelioma.[62]

Tuberculous pleurisy can result in chyliform (pseudochylous or cholesterol effusion) pleural effusion.[63–65] Fat-fluid or fat-calcium level at CT was described as pathognomonic of tuberculous chyliform effusion, and associated findings included parietal pleural thickening of 4 to 10 mm and curvilinear or nodular pleural calcifications.[65]

Investigations and Differential Diagnosis

Thoracentesis of a primary tuberculous pleural effusion characteristically yields a clear, straw-colored exudate with total pleural fluid protein greater than 3 g/100 mL, pleural fluid LDH greater than 200 U, and pleural fluid–serum LDH ratio greater than 0.5. The fluid is lymphocyte predominant, often exceeding 70% or more of all cellular material, and so during cytologic examination may appear as the only cell type, resulting in an erroneous diagnosis of lymphoma.[66] The glucose content is often low in tuberculous effusions. This finding is not specific for tuberculosis, however; low pleural fluid glucose content also is seen in bacterial pneumonia, rheumatoid disease, and pulmonary carcinoma.

Several studies have shown that a level of adenosine deaminase (ADA) in pleural fluid greater than 40 IU/L can indicate pleural tuberculosis with a sensitivity of 81% to 100% and specificity of 83% to 100%.[67,68] Analysis and determination of the isoenzymes have shown that increases in ADA with tuberculous pleurisy are due to increase in ADA_2. Estimation of pleural fluid ADA_2 levels has a similar sensitivity and a slightly better specificity compared with the pleural ADA in the diagnosis of tuberculous pleuritis.[69] False-positive results can occur in other lymphocytic effusions, such as malignancies and parapneumonic effusions, but are rare.[70,71]

An elevated pleural fluid interferon-γ level also is valuable in diagnosing tuberculous pleural effusions. In a prospective study of 595 pleural effusions, of which 82 (14%) were due to tuberculosis, a cutoff of 3.7 international units (IU)/mL yielded a sensitivity of 98% and a specificity of 98% for diagnosing tuberculosis.[72] In a study comparing the efficacy of different biologic markers for the diagnosis of tuberculous pleuritis, interferon-γ proved to be the most sensitive and specific biologic marker.[73]

Definitive diagnosis of pleural tuberculosis requires the identification of mycobacteria by microscopy or culture of the pleural fluid or tissue. Mycobacterial culture has a higher sensitivity than direct smear for acid-fast bacilli because direct examination requires a concentration of 10,000 bacilli/mL, whereas culture requires the presence of only 10 to 100 organisms/mL. Microscopy and culture of the pleural fluid are negative in many cases and may not exclude tuberculous pleurisy. The incidence of positive culture from pleural fluid is low, having been reported in 15% to 30% of proven cases.[2,51]

In patients with tuberculous effusions, culture of pleural biopsy specimens is positive in 55% to 80% of cases, and in one series a diagnostic sensitivity of 79% and specificity of 100% were achieved when histology and culture were combined.[74] In a study to determine the optimal number of pleural biopsy specimens for the diagnosis of tuberculous pleurisy, it was shown that the sensitivity of percutaneous needle biopsy for diagnosis of tuberculous pleurisy was greatest when more than six specimens were obtained; on average, these contained more than two specimens of parietal pleura.[75] Image-guided pleural biopsy can be useful in obtaining diagnostic tissue in patients who have small effusions.[76] Thoracoscopy can be performed under local anesthesia in patients with pleural effusion and provides a means to visualize directly the pleural abnormalities. Thoracoscopic pleural biopsy has a high diagnostic rate with sensitivity greater than 90% and can be performed easily and safely.[77,78]

The potential of pleural fluid polymerase chain reaction in the diagnosis of tuberculous pleural effusion has been explored, but sensitivities range from 20% to 81%, and specificities range from 78% to 100%, implying a low clinical utility of the test.[79–81]

Treatment

Tuberculous empyema should be managed with intercostal drainage of pus, antituberculous therapy, and the consideration of surgical interventions such as decortication when conservative measures are unsuccessful.

BACTERIA OTHER THAN MYCOBACTERIA

A parapneumonic effusion is an accumulation of exudative pleural fluid secondary to an ipsilateral pneumonia or lung abscess. A complicated parapneumonic effusion or an effusion in which the bacterial cultures are positive requires an invasive procedure, such as tube thoracostomy, for its resolution.[2]

Prevalence and Epidemiology

Parapneumonic effusions occur in some 20% to 40% of the approximately 1 million patients hospitalized yearly with pneumonia in the United States.[82] These effusions are usually serous exudates that resolve spontaneously without specific therapy; approximately 10% become complicated or progress to empyema.[83] Delays in drainage of clinically significant effusions have been associated with increased morbidity and mortality.[84] In a multicenter prospective study of 1906 patients with clinical and radiographic evidence of community-acquired pneumonia, the mortality risk was 6.5 times higher when the effusions were bilateral and 3.7 times higher when the effusion was unilateral.[85]

Bacteriology

The bacteriology of parapneumonic effusions and empyemas is diverse, and significant differences are noted between community-acquired and nosocomial infections. Regardless of the setting, most culture-positive effusions are due to gram-positive aerobic bacteria, most commonly streptococcal species, followed by staphylococci.[86] In the nosocomial setting, gram-negative aerobes, such as *Haemophilus influenzae, Escherichia coli, Pseudomonas,* and *Klebsiella,* also are common causes of pleural infections.[87] The incidence of anaerobic bacterial pleural infection is reported to range from 12% to 34%.[88] The most frequent anaerobic isolates are *Bacteroides* species and *Peptostreptococcus.*[86] On occasion, *Actinomyces, Nocardia,* or fungi such as *Aspergillus* may be the cause of empyema.[86]

Clinical Presentation

The clinical picture in patients with pneumonia is similar whether or not they have pleural infection and parapneumonic effusion. Pleural infection should be suspected in any patient being treated with antibiotics who has nonresolving pneumonia.[89] In contrast to aerobic pleuropulmonary infections that usually manifest as an acute febrile illness, anaerobic infections have a more subacute or chronic presentation, with associated weight loss and anemia.[90]

On occasion, a purulent effusion can occur without pneumonia (primary empyema). This may represent a postpneumonic empyema in which pulmonary consolidations have already resolved or a nonpneumonic empyema, most often iatrogenic and related to thoracic surgery.[86] It also can be secondary to thoracic trauma, esophageal perforation, or transdiaphragmatic spread of abdominal infections.[86]

Rarely, bilateral pleural effusions are present, with one side representing empyema and the other being a noninfected pleural effusion (Fig. 72.13). The Contarini condition is characterized by empyema on one side and contralateral pleural effusion secondary to fluid overload or congestive cardiac failure; the condition was named after the 95th doge of Venice, who died in 1625 with orthopnea, foul-smelling sputum, cardiac arrhythmia, and clear pleural fluid on one side and pus on the other.[91]

Pathophysiology

The progression of parapneumonic effusion can be divided into three stages. The first stage is the exudative stage, in which the accumulation of fluid in the pleural space is most likely the combined result of the pulmonary interstitial fluid traversing the pleura to enter the pleural space and increased permeability of the capillaries in the pleural space.[82] This effusion is free flowing; is not infected; and has normal biochemical characteristics, such as a pH greater than 7.30, glucose level greater than 60 mg/dL, and a slightly elevated LDH level.[88] At this stage, this sterile exudate is also referred to as "simple parapneumonic effusion," and most do not require chest tube drainage.[38]

This effusion may progress to the second stage, which is the fibropurulent stage, in patients with no or ineffective antibiotic therapy. This stage is characterized by the accumulation of fibrin clots and fibrin membranes, resulting in a heavily loculated pleural space. Gram stains and bacterial cultures are usually positive, with the cytology of the pleural fluid usually showing neutrophils greater than 10,000/mL. The metabolic and cytolytic activities in this stage are high, as reflected by low pH values (<7.20), low

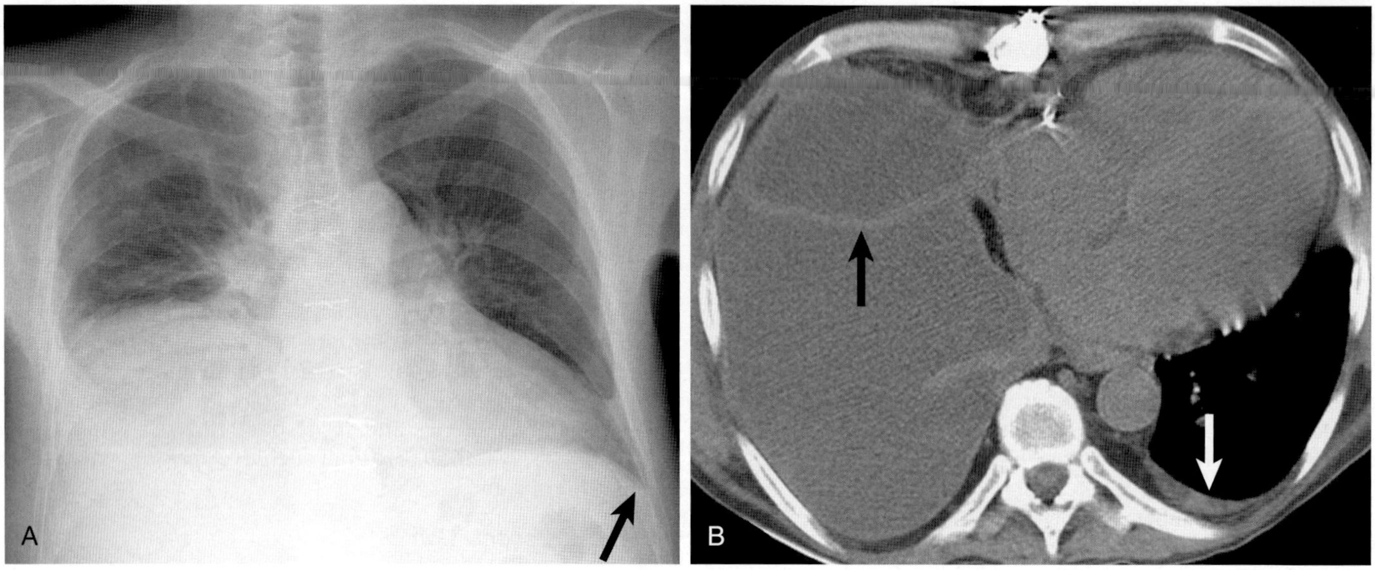

Fig. 72.13 Contarini condition. (A) Posteroanterior chest radiograph shows pulmonary edema and moderate right and small left *(arrow)* pleural effusions. The upper margin of the right effusion has a convex contour consistent with loculation. (B) Nonenhanced CT scan shows a large loculated right pleural effusion displacing the heart contralaterally. Note the smooth costal pleural thickening and large pleural septation *(black arrow)* consistent with empyema. There is a small left-sided pleural effusion *(white arrow)* secondary to cardiac decompensation, consistent with Contarini condition.

glucose level (<35 mg/dL), and high LDH value (>1000 IU/L), consistent with "complicated parapneumonic effusion."[38,88]

If the effusion is not drained at the fibropurulent stage, it can progress to the final organizational stage characterized by fibroblast proliferation, leading to transformation of interpleural fibrin membranes into a web of thick and nonelastic pleural peels. The peel over the visceral pleura prevents the lung from expanding. The further course after such an organization varies. Some individuals exhibit spontaneous healing with resolution of pleural thickening,[92] whereas others progress to lung function deficit and chronic infection of the pleural space, making way for further complications, such as lung abscess, bronchopleural fistula, or empyema necessitatis.[86]

Manifestations of the Disease

Radiography. The evaluation of patients with pneumonia also must include assessment for a parapneumonic effusion. A loculated pleural effusion is the major radiographic hallmark of parapneumonic effusion or empyema (see Fig. 72.11). No other specific radiographic features are seen except, rarely, the presence of gas in the pleural space (pyopneumothorax) or chest wall owing to gas-forming bacteria, such as *Clostridium perfringens* and *Bacteroides fragilis,* or more likely from bronchopleural fistula or recent thoracentesis.

Prompt recognition and precise characterization of a parapneumonic effusion is important because delays in drainage of clinically significant effusions have been associated with increased morbidity and mortality.[84] The detection of pleural fluid on standard radiographs is affected by patient position, which alters the distribution of pleural effusions as previously discussed.

The lateral decubitus view often reveals small effusions that have not been demonstrated by erect chest radiographs. Bilateral decubitus chest radiographs also may help to separate dense consolidation from free-flowing pleural fluid.[86] A decubitus chest radiograph also can guide decision making for thoracentesis. Small free-flowing pleural effusions (<10-mm thickness) in the lateral decubitus view usually resolve with antibiotic therapy alone, and thoracentesis of these effusions is often unnecessary.[93]

Computed Tomography. CT is often used to evaluate pleural or parenchymal complications of pneumonia. It is sensitive in the detection of parapneumonic effusions, depicting multiple loculations in these effusions, and has proved helpful in revealing poor chest tube placement.[94] Empyemas typically have an oval or lentiform shape, exhibit obtuse margins with the pleura, have scalloped contours, and have mass effect on the airways and adjacent lung, displacing them away from the effusion.[95] These help to distinguish them from the more rounded appearance of pulmonary abscesses, which typically form acute angles with the chest wall.[95] There may be several loculated effusions, requiring more than one chest tube for adequate drainage.

A contrast-enhanced chest CT scan that shows parietal and visceral pleural enhancement, and thickening with increased attenuation of the extrapleural fat is highly suggestive of an empyema in the appropriate clinical setting.[96] Enhancement of the pleura in empyema is thought to be caused by the increased vascularity of the inflamed pleura.[96] The presence of fluid between the enhancing thickened pleural layers has been termed the *split pleura sign* (see Fig. 72.11). Although best seen with contrast-enhanced CT, it may be present on noncontrast CT (see Fig. 72.10). If no interventional procedure has been performed, gas bubbles within a pleural fluid collection are virtually diagnostic of an empyema and indicate either infection caused by gas-forming bacteria or more likely the presence of a bronchopleural fistula. Enhancing pleura and thickened parietal pleura are strongly associated with empyema. In a study of empyema, pleural enhancement was present in every patient, and pleural thickening was seen in 92% of patients.[89] In another study a retrospective review of the CT findings in 30 children with parapneumonic effusions in which 21 met the clinical criteria for empyema, pleural enhancement was noted in all children with empyema and 8 children with parapneumonic effusions (89%).[97] Pleural thickening is also more commonly, and to greater extent, seen in patients with empyema than in patients with parapneumonic effusion. Absence of pleural thickening suggests simple parapneumonic effusion.[38]

When parapneumonic effusion or empyema complicates bacterial pneumonia, mediastinal lymph node enlargement can occur. In a retrospective study of 50 patients with parapneumonic effusion or empyema, enlargement of mediastinal nodes greater than 1 cm was present in 18 patients (36%), whereas 13 patients had nodes measuring less than 1 cm (26%), indicating that intrathoracic lymphadenopathy less than 2 cm could be regarded as a normal finding in empyema.[99] In this study no correlation could be established between the presence of enlarged nodes with the length of the illness, stage of the effusion, presence of frank purulence, extent of consolidation, or the size of the effusion.[99] In another study intrathoracic lymphadenopathy occurred in 48% of cases with empyema, suggesting that in patients with smooth pleural thickening and pleural effusion, lymphadenopathy alone should not be used as a criterion to differentiate empyema from malignant or tuberculous pleural effusion.[100]

CLASSIC COMPUTED TOMOGRAPHY SIGNS OF EMPYEMA

- Split pleura sign
- Oblong configuration
- Obtuse angle with adjacent pleura
- Displacement of adjacent lung and airways from pleura

Ultrasonography. A clear-cut distinction between an uncomplicated parapneumonic effusion and an infected effusion cannot be made with confidence using transthoracic sonography alone. Infected fluid may be completely sonolucent without internal echoes. A retrospective study of 50 patients with parapneumonic effusions using sonography found that most of these effusions were septated and echogenic (see Fig. 72.8), and there was no relationship between sonographic features and biochemical parameters or outcome measures.[101] This study also showed that septa may be found in stage I collections, which are frequently known to resolve without tube drainage.[101] When the effusions are small in size, transthoracic ultrasound is useful for guiding thoracentesis or for inserting chest tubes and is especially useful in circumstances that require precise targeting, such as loculated effusions.[86]

Chest ultrasonography is useful for showing early fibrin membranes and septations in the pleural cavity in patients with empyema. In the absence of clear septations on ultrasonography, simple chest tube drainage with or without fibrinolysis is adequate, whereas septated effusions often require mechanical adhesiolysis.[102]

Management

Parapneumonic effusions are classified on the basis of anatomic characteristics of the fluid, the bacteriology of the pleural fluid, and the chemistry of the fluid.[103] Category 1 pleural fluid is a small free-flowing effusion less than 10 mm thick on a decubitus radiograph, CT, or ultrasound. Thoracentesis is not done because the risk of a poor outcome with a category 1 effusion is low. Observation is an acceptable treatment option for this category of effusion.

Category 2 effusion is free flowing and small to moderate in size (>10 mm thick and less than half of the hemithorax). Gram stain and culture of the pleural fluid are negative, and the pleural fluid pH is greater than 7.20. The risk of a poor outcome with category 2 effusions is low. It is recommended that the pleural fluid be analyzed within a short time to determine whether any poor prognostic factors develop that would indicate the need for aggressive drainage.

Category 3 effusions occupy more than half the hemithorax, are loculated, or are associated with thickened parietal pleura. Gram stain or culture is positive. The pleural fluid pH is less than 7.20, or the pleural fluid glucose is less than 60 mg/dL. The risk of a poor outcome with a category 3 effusion is moderate. Category 4 effusions are characterized by pleural fluid that consists of pus, and the risk of a poor outcome is high.

As it is impossible clinically to differentiate simple from complicated parapneumonic effusion in patients with possible pleural infection, BTS guidelines recommend diagnostic pleural fluid sampling under imaging guidance in all patients with a pleural effusion greater than 10-mm depth in association with a pneumonic illness or recent chest trauma or surgery and who have features of ongoing sepsis.[38] If a patient has sufficient pleural fluid to warrant a thoracentesis, a therapeutic rather than diagnostic thoracentesis is recommended.[2] If the fluid reaccumulates and there was no poor prognostic factor at the time of initial thoracentesis, no additional therapy is indicated as long as the patient is doing well. If the fluid reaccumulates, and there were poor prognostic factors present at the time of the initial thoracentesis, a second therapeutic thoracentesis should be performed. If the fluid reaccumulates a second time, a tube thoracostomy should be performed.[2] Chest tube drainage is recommended by BTS in patients with frankly purulent fluid aspirated, identification of organisms on Gram stain and/or culture, pleural fluid pH less than 7.2, or loculated pleural fluid. Along with poor prognostic factors, if the pleural fluid is loculated, more aggressive therapy is indicated, such as tube thoracotomy with fibrinolytics. If complete drainage is not achieved with one or two administrations of fibrinolytics, thoracoscopy should be done. Decortication should be performed without delay if the lung does not reexpand completely with thoracoscopy alone.

FUNGI

Pleural effusions are uncommon in immunocompetent hosts with acute or disseminated histoplasmosis.[104] In a series of 50 patients with acquired immune deficiency syndrome (AIDS) and disseminated histoplasmosis, 5 (10%) patients showed pleural effusions on chest radiographs.[105]

Small pleural effusions may occur in about 20% of patients with acute coccidioidomycosis and is thought to be secondary to direct spread of contiguous parenchymal infection.[133,134] Spontaneous rupture of a coccidioidal pulmonary cavity into the pleural space is known to occur in 1% to 5% of patients with chronic cavitary disease, resulting in a pyopneumothorax.[106]

Effusions caused by *Blastomyces dermatitidis* usually are associated with acute airspace pneumonia.[107] Of a series of 26 patients with pulmonary blastomycosis, 23 (88%) showed radiographic evidence of blastomycotic pleural disease; of these, only 4 patients had pleural effusions (Fig. 72.14), and the patients responded well to amphotericin B therapy.[108]

Pleural effusions are more common in immunosuppressed patients with thoracic cryptococcosis.[109–112] A retrospective study

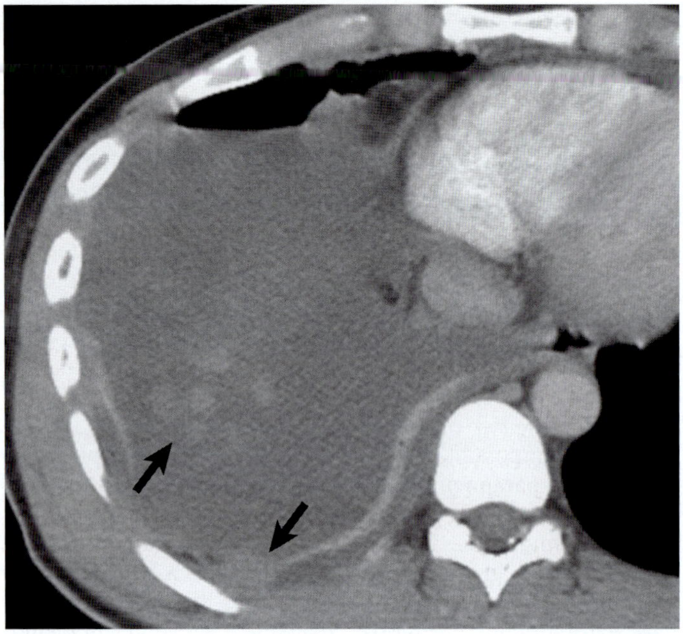

Fig. 72.14 Blastomycosis. Contrast-enhanced CT scan shows a large right pleural effusion with multiple enhancing pleural nodules *(arrows)*. Biopsy specimen and cultures were positive for *Blastomycosis dermatitidis*. The patient was human immunodeficiency virus negative.

comparing 16 immunocompromised patients with 13 immunocompetent patients, all with pulmonary cryptococcosis, reported effusions only in 3 (19%) immunocompromised hosts, whereas none of the immunocompetent patients showed effusions.[112]

Fungal thoracic empyema, most often hospital acquired, is caused mainly by *Candida* species. The major causes of fungal empyema include abdominal infection, bronchopulmonary infection, surgical intervention, and repeated thoracentesis. *Aspergillus* thoracic empyema is uncommon and can have a radiologic appearance of marked pleural thickening bordered by a shaggy inner margin.[113] It is caused by rupture of an aspergilloma cavity or as a complication of a preexisting chronic empyema.

PARASITES

Pleuropulmonary amebiasis is a relatively common condition in developing countries. The liver is the most common extraintestinal site of amebic involvement, followed by the lung. Pulmonary involvement is usually by a direct transdiaphragmatic extension of a hepatic abscess across an obliterated pleural space, resulting in consolidation, abscesses, or bronchohepatic fistula. About 6% to 40% of patients with amebic liver abscesses are known to develop pleuropulmonary complications; a right-sided pleural effusion occurs in about 60% of cases.[114] In addition to a right-sided pleural effusion, radiographs commonly reveal an elevated right hemidiaphragm with an upward hump-like prominence on the right lateral view and a triangular right lower lobe consolidation. The effusions usually are serofibrinous. In contrast to bacterial empyemas, which progress from an early exudative stage to the final organizing stage, amebic empyemas do not show temporal progression, and loculations and septations are only rarely detected on sonography.[114] The pulmonary consolidation may cavitate, providing communication between the bronchial tree and the liver abscess. Expectoration of a fluid having an "anchovy sauce" appearance indicates the development of a bronchohepatic fistula.

Echinococcus *Granulosus*

Pleural effusion is uncommon in hydatid disease but occurs when a pulmonary hydatid cyst ruptures into the pleural space, resulting in a hydropneumothorax. Daughter cysts floating on the surface of the fluid produce irregularities of the fluid surface, creating the water lily sign or the "sign of the camalote."

PLEURAL EFFUSIONS IN PATIENTS WITH ACQUIRED IMMUNODEFICIENCY SYNDROME

Pleural effusions are seen in 7% to 27% of hospitalized patients with HIV infection.[115] The three most common causes of effusions are bacterial pneumonia, tuberculosis, and Kaposi sarcoma. Bacterial pneumonia is the most common condition associated with pleural effusion in HIV-infected patients in the United States, whereas in underdeveloped countries it is tuberculosis.[116,117] Noninfectious pleural effusion in hospitalized patients with AIDS is most often caused by hypoalbuminemia.[116] Patients with HIV usually have small effusions. Bilateral effusions are more common in patients with AIDS-related Kaposi sarcoma and lymphoma.[118]

Asbestos-Related Pleural Effusion

ETIOLOGY, PREVALENCE, AND EPIDEMIOLOGY

Benign asbestos-related pleural effusions are a significant and underrecognized manifestation of asbestos exposure with important sequelae, such as diffuse pleural thickening, which may be associated with functional impairment and for which compensation may be sought.[119]

CLINICAL PRESENTATION

Benign effusion is the most common asbestos-related abnormality during the first 20 years after exposure; typically, there is a latency period of 10 years.[120] The majority of patients are asymptomatic (44%–66%), but some can present with symptoms of acute pleuritis with pain and fever.[120–122] Effusions are mostly unilateral but can sometimes be bilateral, recurrences are frequent, and can be on the same or the contralateral side.[120,122,123]

PATHOPHYSIOLOGY

Benign asbestos-related pleural effusions are exudative but have a variable composition; often the pleural fluid is hemorrhagic, of mixed cellularity, and may have an increased eosinophil count.[121] Asbestos fibers are not usually found in the effusion.[120] Epler and colleagues[120] reported a dose-response relationship with an increased incidence of effusions in individuals with the most severe exposure; prevalence was 7% with severe, 3.7% with indirect, and 0.2% with peripheral exposure.[120] These investigators also suggested an occupational relationship, with the effusions seen most commonly in asbestos pipe coverers and least commonly among shipfitters and welders.[120] The effusions usually resolve spontaneously after 3 to 4 months.[121,124] They may persist or recur, however, over several years. In Epler's study, most effusions were small and recurred in 29% of cases.[120]

DIFFERENTIAL DIAGNOSIS

Benign asbestos-related effusion is defined by (1) exposure to asbestos, (2) confirmation by radiographs or thoracentesis, (3) no other disease related to pleural effusion, and (4) no malignant tumor within 3 years after the onset of the effusion. One case of mesothelioma has been reported 6 years after benign effusion.[120] Asbestos exposure should be sought carefully in patients with "idiopathic" pleural effusion.[120] The presence of pleural plaques is helpful to identify benign asbestos-related pleural effusion, but pleural plaques have a much longer latency period than pleural effusions and are most commonly not present (Fig. 72.15).[119] The presence of "crow feet"—linear parenchymal structures converging on the pleura—and rounded atelectasis is helpful in suggesting the diagnosis; they are seen less frequently in exudative pleural effusions of other causes. The absence of nodular, circumferential, or mediastinal pleural thickening is helpful in suggesting a benign diagnosis.[124]

Pleural Effusion Caused by Neoplasms

Malignancy is the second most common cause of a pleural effusion after left heart failure in patients older than 50 years.[125] In regions with low incidence of tuberculosis, neoplastic diseases are responsible for approximately 70% to 80% of exudative pleural effusions.[126] The pathogenesis of pleural effusion in malignancy is multifactorial.[2] Possible mechanisms include (1) tumor invasion of the pleura, stimulating an inflammatory reaction associated with capillary fluid leak; (2) tumor invasion of the pulmonary or pleural lymphatics and bronchopulmonary, hilar, or mediastinal lymph nodes, hindering the return of lymphatic fluid to the circulation; (3) bronchial obstruction by a carcinoma, creating an increased negative intrapleural pressure and increasing transudation; (4) hypoproteinemia in debilitated patients, leading to increased transudation; (5) infection associated with obstructive pneumonitis, resulting in a parapneumonic effusion; and (6) a drug reaction, radiation therapy, or deposition of immune complexes related to circulating tumor antigens, causing increased pleural capillary permeability.

In men lung cancer is the most common metastatic tumor to the pleura; in women it is breast cancer. Together, the two cancers account for 50% to 65% of all malignant effusions. Pleural effusions from an unknown primary are responsible for 7% to 15% of all malignant effusions.

Usually, patients with primary lung and breast malignancies develop ipsilateral pleural effusions; infrequently, the effusion is bilateral.[127,128] In breast cancer the pathogenesis of ipsilateral effusion is thought to be due to spread of tumor cells from the chest wall to the pleura via the chest wall lymphatics.[129] In ovarian and gastric carcinomas malignant effusions do not show a predilection for the ipsilateral side, which supports the theory of tertiary spread from hepatic metastases.[127]

Pleural metastases do not always result in an effusion; when present, the size of the effusion varies widely.[130] Large and massive pleural effusions are more likely to be malignant (55%).[50,126] In a chart review of 766 patients with pleural effusions, of which 30% were malignant, 49% of large effusions (occupying more than two-thirds of the hemithorax) and 59% of massive effusions (occupying the entire hemithorax) were malignant.[50]

There have been several attempts to differentiate benign and malignant pleural effusions using ultrasound and CT.[13,24,131] In an ultrasound evaluation of 210 patients with exudative pleural effusions, sheet-like pleural thickening and pleural masses greater than 1 cm were seen mostly in malignant effusions.[131] A retrospective analysis of 211 patients with pleural effusions, using contrast-enhanced CT, showed that 52% of malignant effusions did not reveal any pleural finding apart from the effusion, suggesting that absence of pleural thickening does not preclude a neoplasm.[24] In the same study the presence of nodules in the diaphragmatic, mediastinal, and visceral pleura was highly specific (100%) for malignancy (Fig. 72.16), whereas mediastinal and circumferential pleural thickening showed specificities of 97% and 99%, respectively.[24] In another prospective study of 40 patients with suspected malignant effusion, using the

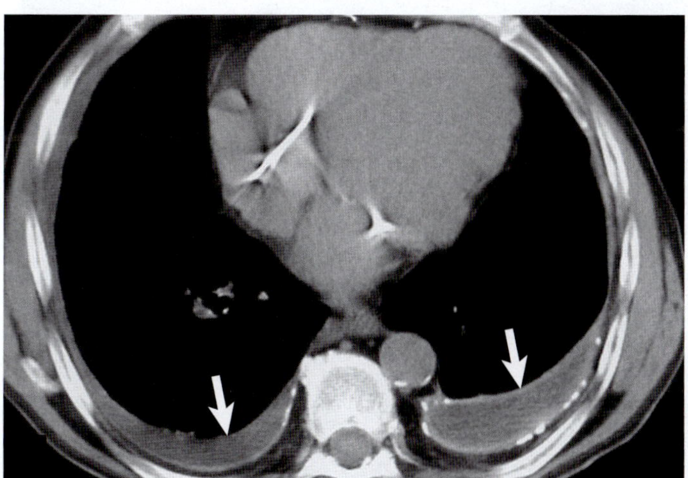

Fig. 72.15 Asbestos-related pleural effusions and thickening. CT scan shows bilateral pleural effusions with parietal and visceral *(arrows)* pleural thickening. The patient had been exposed to asbestos, and the effusions were stable over several years. Bilateral pleural calcification also is present.

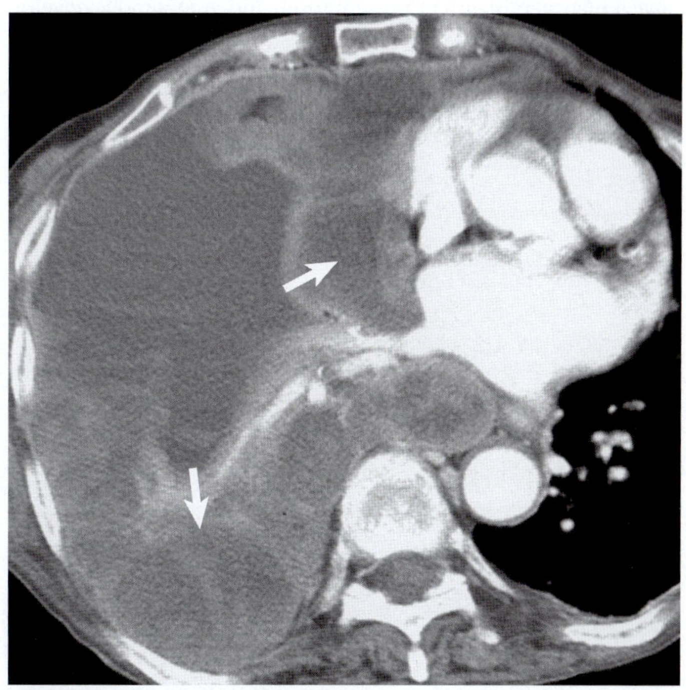

Fig. 72.16 Tension pleural effusion in malignant pleural disease. Contrast-enhanced CT scan shows a large right pleural effusion and associated mass effect, with displacement of the heart into the left hemithorax. Note the multiple large, peripherally enhancing pleural lesions *(arrows)*, involving the mediastinal, diaphragmatic, and costal pleura, in keeping with metastatic pleural disease.

diagnostic criteria of pleural nodularity, irregularity, and thickness greater than 1 cm, CT correctly identified malignancy in 27 of 32 effusions (sensitivity 84%, specificity 100%).[132] In patients with unilateral metastasis to the pleura, the CT findings may be indistinguishable from those of mesothelioma.[124]

Malignant pleural effusion is exudative, and diagnosis is established when malignant cells are identified in pleural fluid or tissue. As a diagnostic procedure, cytologic examination of pleural fluid gives a higher yield than closed pleural biopsy.[133] On analysis of 500 cases of malignant pleural effusions, the yield from pleural fluid cytologic examination was 66%, whereas that of pleural biopsy was 46%.[133] When the two procedures were combined, the yield of a positive diagnosis increased to 73%, making them complementary. When a diagnosis is not arrived at after repeated cytologic examination and closed pleural biopsy, open pleural biopsy or thoracoscopy with biopsy may have to be done to reach a diagnosis. Thoracoscopy with multiple biopsy specimens gives a yield of about 80% to 97% in malignant pleural disease, especially when a biopsy specimen of the visceral pleura is obtained as well.[134] Whenever technically feasible, thoracoscopy is the procedure of choice. Surgical thoracoscopy also may facilitate breaking up loculations and releasing adhesions, aiding lung reexpansion in patients with a trapped lung.

Median survival after diagnosis of a malignant pleural effusion is 3 to 12 months. It depends on the type and stage of the underlying malignancy. Malignant effusions secondary to lung cancers have the shortest survival time, ovarian cancers have the longest survival time, and effusions from an unknown primary have an intermediate survival time.

PULMONARY CARCINOMA

About 5% to 15% of all patients diagnosed with lung cancer have a pleural effusion at presentation, and at least 50% develop one at some time during the course of their disease.[135–137] The presence of pleural effusion in a patient with bronchogenic carcinoma is an ominous sign. In most of these cases, cytology is positive for neoplastic cells, and the patient is classified as having stage IV and M1a disease with an associated 6% to 8% chance of long-term survival (Fig. 72.17).[138] Even the presence of minimal pleural effusion (<10-mm thickness on lateral decubitus chest x-ray or on CT) was found to be independently associated with worse survival, when compared with patients with no effusion, among patients with small cell lung cancer in a recent study.[139]

In lung cancer pleural metastases are more common in adenocarcinoma and can be due to spread by contiguity or by pulmonary artery invasion and embolization.[140] Pleural metastases most commonly involve the visceral pleura; parietal pleural involvement is due to spread from visceral pleura along pleural adhesions or from implantation of exfoliated cells from the visceral pleura.[140]

Pleural effusion associated with lung malignancy tends to be moderate to large in volume and is usually ipsilateral to the primary lesion. When contralateral mediastinal shift does not occur in large or massive effusions, a carcinoma of the mainstem bronchus causing atelectasis should be suspected. A fixed mediastinum secondary to neoplastic node infiltration, extensive neoplastic involvement of the ipsilateral lung, or malignant mesothelioma can result in similar manifestations.[141] A preoperatively detected pleural effusion in a patient with lung malignancy should be further investigated with cytology and, if negative, by video-assisted thoracoscopy.[142]

METASTATIC NONPULMONARY CARCINOMA

The main extrathoracic primary sites associated with malignant pleural effusions are breast, ovary, and stomach,[127] with breast

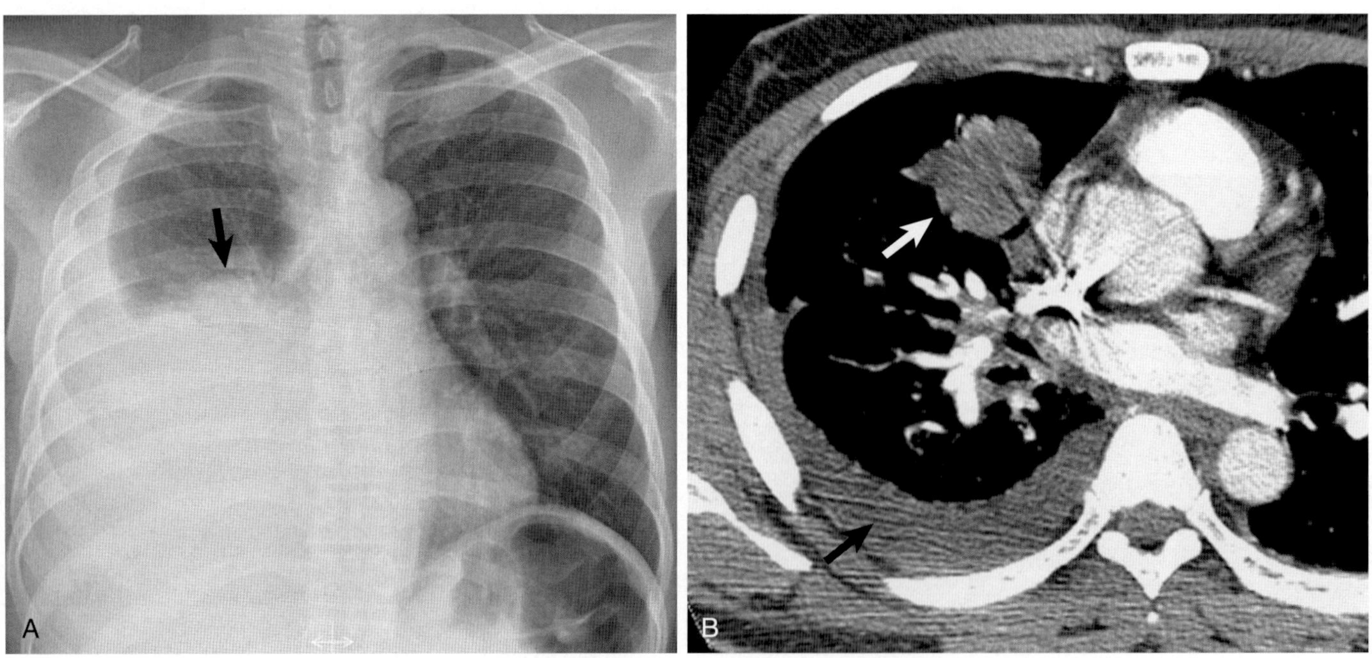

Fig. 72.17 Malignant pleural effusion. (A) Chest radiograph shows large right pleural effusion without contralateral mediastinal shift. Note the lobulated opacity *(arrow)* in the upper lobe. (B) Contrast-enhanced CT scan reveals right upper lobe bronchogenic carcinoma *(white arrow)*. The ipsilateral pleural effusion *(black arrow)* was positive for malignancy on cytology, in keeping with an unresectable tumor.

being the most common. Approximately 50% of all patients with breast cancer develop an effusion at some time during the course of the disease.[143] The effusion is usually unilateral and occurs on the same side as the breast carcinoma.[128,144] Spread of cancer cells from the chest wall to the pleura is usually via chest wall lymphatics.[129] Contiguous spread through the chest wall to the parietal pleura rarely occurs (Fig. 72.18).[130]

Although uncommon, breast cancer can manifest with bilateral effusions and has poor prognostic ramifications.[145] This manifestation of pleural malignancy is often associated with hepatic metastases and hematogenous spread to the pleura.[130]

In a retrospective study of 365 autopsies of patients with breast carcinoma, pleural effusions were more common in patients who had lymphangitic spread (60%) compared with patients who did not (42%), supporting the hypothesis that lymphatic obstruction is important in the pathogenesis of effusion in metastatic breast cancer.[146] The prognosis of patients with breast cancer and pleural involvement is poor, and death usually occurs within a year and often within months.[147]

HODGKIN DISEASE AND NON-HODGKIN LYMPHOMA

Approximately 10% of malignant pleural effusions are caused by lymphoma.[148] Unilateral or bilateral pleural effusion is reported with a frequency of 25% in patients with thoracic Hodgkin lymphoma and 20% in patients with non-Hodgkin lymphoma.[149,150]

Pleural effusion in lymphoma can develop by three mechanisms: (1) pleural infiltration shedding cells into the pleural space, (2) lymphatic obstruction by infiltration of the pulmonary and mediastinal lymph nodes, and (3) obstruction of the thoracic duct, resulting in chylothorax (Fig. 72.19).[151] Direct pleural infiltration is the predominant cause in non-Hodgkin lymphoma, whereas lymphatic, thoracic duct, or venous obstruction seems to be the primary mechanism in Hodgkin disease.[148]

Pulmonary infections, radiation therapy, and chemotherapeutic agents also can cause pleural effusion in lymphoma. Radiation-induced effusions can be due to radiation pleuritis, usually seen 6 weeks to 6 months after radiation therapy, or secondary to lymphatic obstruction from mediastinal fibrosis.[152]

Pleural effusions are uncommon in primary pulmonary lymphoma, being seen in approximately 10% of patients.[153,154] In a retrospective study of 15 patients, multiple bilateral pulmonary nodules were the most common CT manifestation of recurrent lymphoma, whereas small- or moderate-sized pleural effusions were noted in only 5 patients (33%).[155]

Primary effusion lymphoma is an unusual and infrequently occurring B-cell non-Hodgkin lymphoma seen predominantly in HIV-seropositive men, caused by Kaposi sarcoma–associated herpesvirus, manifesting as lymphomatous serous effusion without a contiguous tumor mass.[156] A review of imaging findings of six patients with primary effusion lymphoma revealed bilateral or unilateral pleural effusions with or without pericardial effusion and ascites, mild diffuse serosal surface thickening, and no parenchymal or mediastinal abnormalities.[157]

Pyothorax-associated lymphoma is a non-Hodgkin lymphoma of mostly B-cell phenotype developing in chronic inflammation

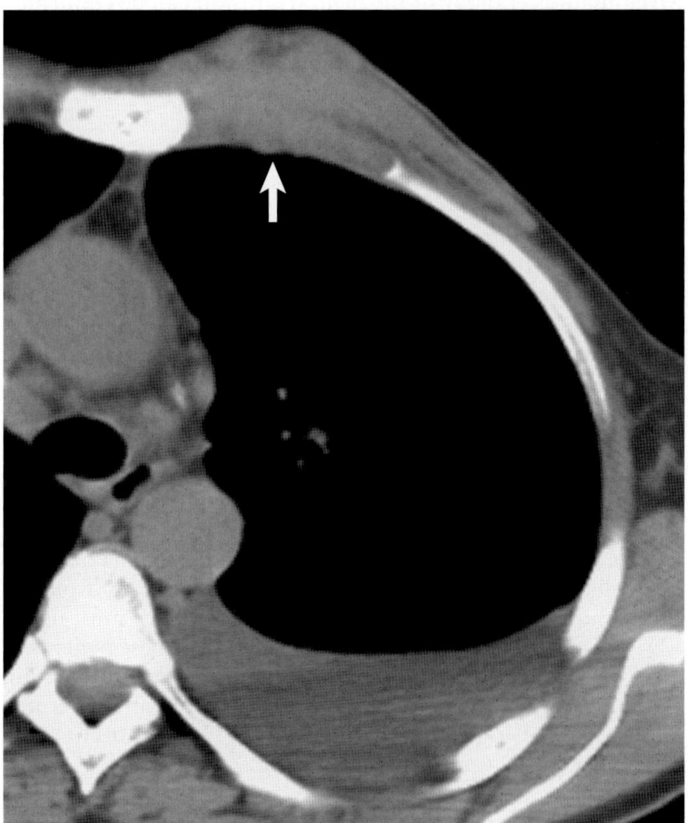

Fig. 72.18 Malignant pleural effusion. CT scan shows large chest wall mass, in keeping with breast carcinoma recurrence. Infiltration of the adjacent pleura *(arrow)* is visible. Cytology confirmed malignant ipsilateral left pleural effusion.

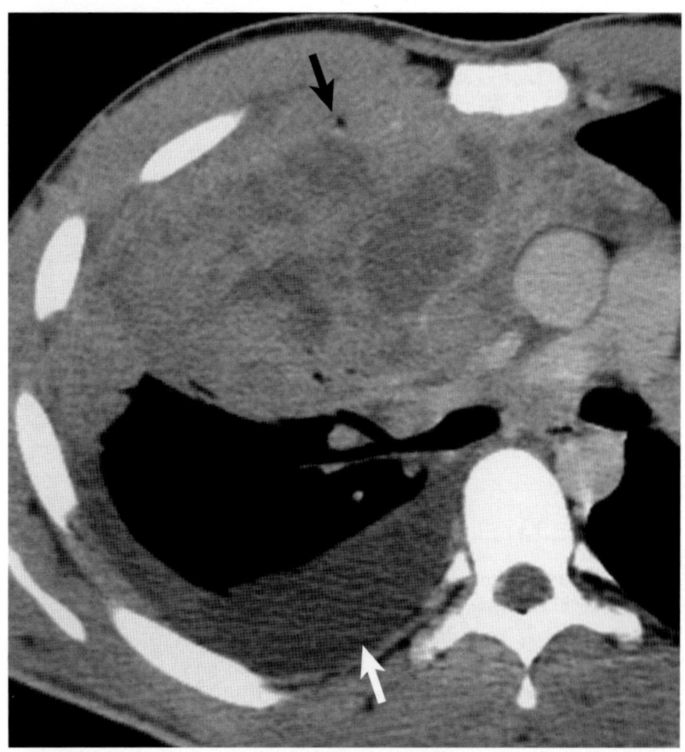

Fig. 72.19 Chylous effusion caused by non-Hodgkin lymphoma. Contrast-enhanced CT scan shows a necrotic mediastinal mass involving the adjacent pleura *(black arrow)* and associated with a moderate pleural effusion *(white arrow)*. The low attenuation of the fluid suggests a chyliform effusion.

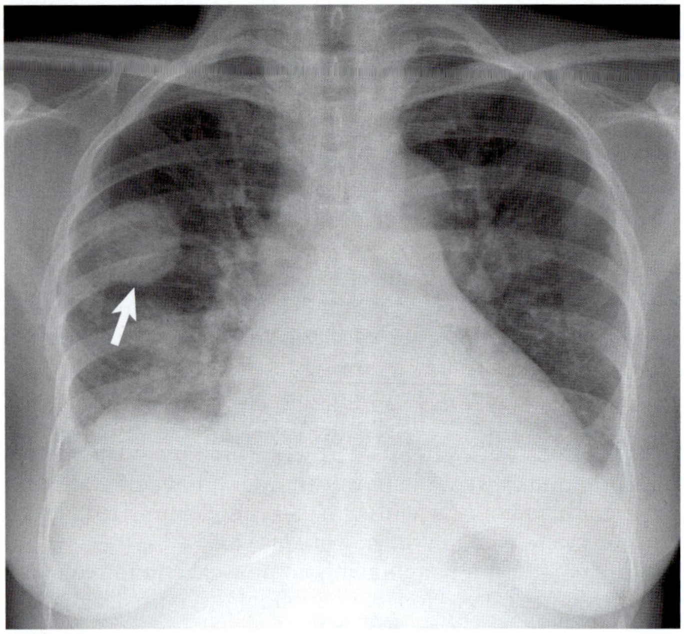

Fig. 72.20 Multiple myeloma with amyloid cardiomyopathy. Posteroanterior chest radiograph shows chest wall lesion *(arrow)*, in keeping with history of multiple myeloma. Note moderate cardiomegaly, pulmonary vascular redistribution, and bilateral small pleural effusions consistent with cardiac failure. The patient had amyloid cardiomyopathy.

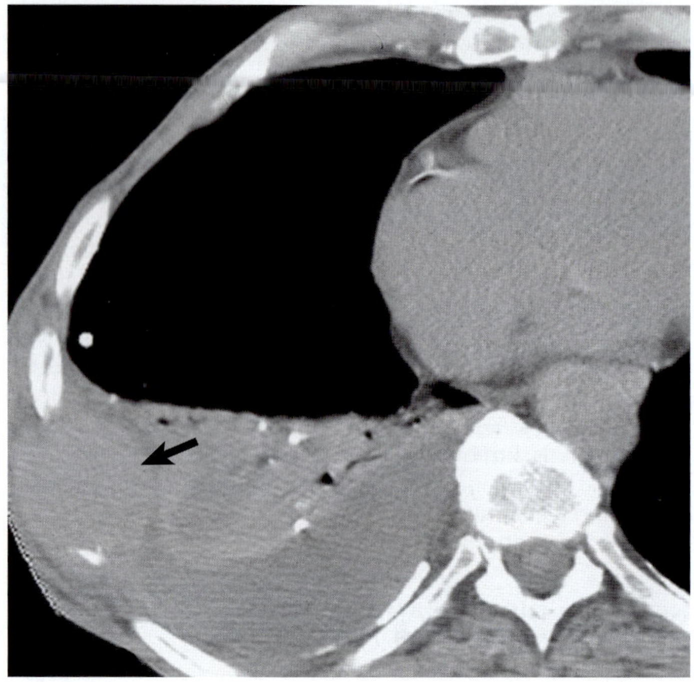

Fig. 72.21 Myelomatous pleural effusion. CT scan shows rib destruction with large soft tissue component *(arrow)* infiltrating the adjacent pleura with ipsilateral effusion. Asbestos-related pleural disease also is evident.

(mostly related to tuberculosis), strongly associated with Epstein-Barr virus infection. In a review of 106 patients with pyothorax-associated lymphoma, there was a marked male predominance (12.3 : 1), and 70% of cases were positive for Epstein-Barr virus.[158] In a series of 112 patients with chronic empyema, the CT findings of a mass in the empyema sac and empyema involvement of the mediastinal pleura were significant predictors of empyema-associated malignancy.[159]

Pleural fluid associated with lymphoma is usually serous or serosanguineous. The diagnosis of lymphoma in pleural fluid specimens can be difficult because the cytologic features of the malignant cells in small cell and mixed small and large cell lymphomas may be indistinguishable from features of reactive lymphoid cells.[160] Cytologically atypical lymphocytes also have been described in tuberculous effusions, resulting in an appearance that can be mistaken for lymphoma.[161] To overcome these diagnostic difficulties, various ancillary studies, such as immunocytochemistry, morphometry, flow cytometry, and cytogenetics/molecular genetics, can be readily performed on effusion specimens and aid in the diagnosis and classification of lymphomas.[162]

MULTIPLE MYELOMA

Pleural effusion can occur in about 6% of patients with multiple myeloma.[163] Because effusions have various etiologies, individualized therapy is necessary. In descending order of occurrence, these etiologies are cardiac failure secondary to amyloidosis (Fig. 72.20), pulmonary embolism, chronic renal failure, second neoplasm, and pleural myelomatous involvement.[163,164] Pleural effusions may occur secondary to pleural myelomatous involvement from adjacent skeletal or parenchymal tumors (Fig. 72.21), direct implantation of the tumor nodules on the pleura, or mediastinal lymph node infiltration. Immunoglobulin A myelomas show a propensity to invade extraosseous structures; 80% of effusions are seen in this type of multiple myeloma.[165] Myelomatous etiology of the pleural effusion can be confirmed by the demonstration of atypical plasma cells in the pleural fluid, detection of a monoclonal protein in pleural fluid electrophoresis, or histologic evaluation of a pleural biopsy specimen.[165]

Pleural Effusion Caused by Cardiac Failure

Transudative pleural effusions are a common finding in patients with hydrostatic pulmonary edema caused by left heart failure (less commonly with right heart failure), particularly when the edema is severe, and are most often bilateral. Unilateral effusion can occur and are more common on the right. A unilateral left-sided pleural effusion and effusion in absence of cardiomegaly should prompt the search for a cause other than heart failure. Associated radiologic evidence of cardiac enlargement, with or without pulmonary venous hypertension, makes the diagnosis obvious in most cases. Treatment with diuretics progressively alters the composition of pleura fluid, in patients with heart failure, with increase in concentration of total protein and LDH, characteristics of an exudate. Calculation of the serum-pleural fluid gradients for protein and albumin may be the most useful way to distinguish transudates from exudates in these patients.[166]

A well-demarcated collection of pleural fluid contained within an interlobar fissure can occur in cardiac failure and is termed *pulmonary pseudotumor.* These vanishing tumors occur most frequently in the minor fissure (see Fig. 72.3).

Pleural Effusion Caused by Pulmonary Thromboembolism

In the appropriate clinical setting, a combination of diaphragmatic elevation, basal pulmonary opacity, and a small pleural effusion on the chest radiograph suggests thromboembolic disease. It has been estimated that pleural effusions occur in 30% to 50% of patients with pulmonary embolism.[167–169] Most patients with pleural effusion resulting from pulmonary embolism present with pleuritic chest pain.[170] Effusions are mostly unilateral, small, and exudative but occasionally can be bilateral. The side of the pleural effusion does not always correlate with the side of pulmonary embolism.[168,171] The effusion can be clear, blood tinged, or bloody on pleural tap. Bloody pleural fluid is characteristic of pulmonary embolism in absence of trauma or malignancy.[172] Most effusions are free but can be loculated in case of delay in diagnosis.[171]

In a review of 230 patients with pulmonary embolism, chest radiograph and CT revealed pleural effusions in 32% and 47% of patients, respectively, and these effusions were unilateral (85%) and small (90%), occupying less than one-third of the hemithorax (Fig. 72.22).[168] In a recent study on a CT-based scoring system, pleural effusion in patients with pulmonary embolism was one of the factors in the final model for predicting all-cause 30-day mortality.[173,174]

Pleural effusions associated with pulmonary infarction often develop and resolve synchronously with the infarct, but in some cases they appear later or clear sooner. Large pleural effusion with presence of radiographic infarct take longer (14–21 days) to resolve than pleural effusions without infarct (7–10 days).[172] Effusions that progress during therapy should be evaluated for recurrent pulmonary thromboembolism, secondary infection, or pleural hemorrhage after anticoagulation (see Fig. 72.22).[175]

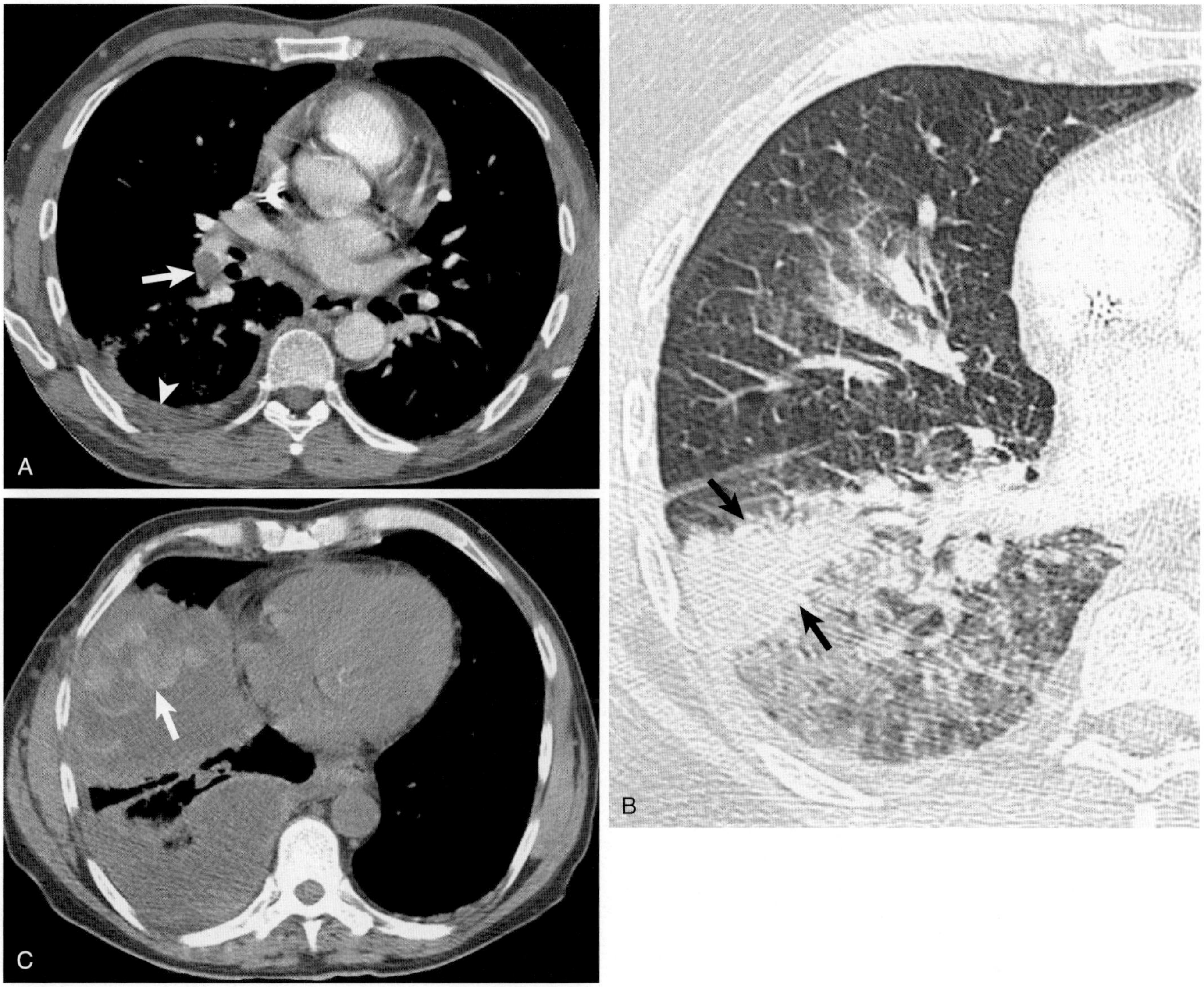

Fig. 72.22 Pleural effusion caused by pulmonary embolism. (A) Contrast-enhanced CT scan shows central filling defect within the right lower lobe pulmonary artery *(arrow)*, consistent with acute pulmonary embolism. A small pleural effusion *(arrowhead)* also is present. (B) CT image in lung window shows a wedge-shaped triangular opacity *(arrows)* with surrounding ground-glass opacity, consistent with a right lower lobe infarct. (C) Noncontrast CT scan shows new large right effusion, containing high-attenuation material *(arrow)* consistent with hemothorax. The patient had been excessively anticoagulated.

Pleural Effusion Caused by Trauma

Blunt chest trauma accounts for 100,000 hospital admissions per year in the United States.[176] Hemothorax is a common manifestation of penetrating and nonpenetrating trauma. On occasion, effusion may be due to accumulation of chyle within the pleural space after injury to the thoracic duct. In a series of 203 patients with chylothorax, the chylothorax in 101 patients (50%) was related to trauma or surgery.[177]

Pleural hemorrhage, if acute, can be identified on CT by the presence of a fluid-fluid level or increased density of the pleural fluid (Fig. 72.23). When blood in the pleural space becomes defibrinated, the fluid is radiologically indistinguishable from an effusion of any other cause.[178] The site of hemorrhage can affect the size of the hemothorax.[178] When bleeding occurs from a systemic vessel, the hemothorax tends to enlarge despite the quantity of blood present, whereas when it occurs from the pulmonary vasculature, the expanding hemothorax compresses the lung, and the resultant pulmonary tamponade may produce hemostasis.[178]

Placement of thoracostomy tubes for chest trauma is often done in an emergency setting. Malpositioning of chest tubes in extrathoracic, intraparenchymal, mediastinal, and intrafissural locations is common, reportedly occurring at frequencies of 26% to 58% and requiring immediate repositioning.[179,180] CT is much more accurate than anteroposterior chest radiographs in showing malpositioned chest tubes.[179–181]

Rupture of the esophagus after closed chest trauma is rare. Occurring with much greater frequency is spontaneous rupture after severe vomiting (Boerhaave syndrome) or as a complication of esophagogastroscopy or gastroscopy. A review of 127 patients with esophageal perforation revealed that iatrogenic perforation secondary to endoscopy or dilation was the most common cause in 50 patients (39%), and the site of the tear was usually in the lower half of the esophagus.[182]

The presence or absence of chest radiographic findings depends on the time interval between the perforation and the study, the site of the tear, and the integrity of the mediastinal pleura.[183] Rupture of the mediastinal parietal pleura results in the rapid development of hydropneumothorax or pyopneumothorax.[184] Pleural effusion is almost always left sided but can occur bilaterally (Fig. 72.24). Absence of pleural rupture causes mediastinal and subcutaneous air to develop rapidly. In 75% of these patients a small sympathetic pleural effusion attributable to mediastinitis develops insidiously.[184] Subcutaneous air never occurs in approximately 40% of patients and does not occur for at least 1 hour after perforation; chest radiographs acquired immediately after an esophageal perforation can be normal and should not exclude the diagnosis of perforation.[184]

In an appropriate clinical setting, air in the mediastinum on a chest CT scan is highly suggestive of an esophageal perforation.[185] Thoracentesis and pleural fluid analysis can establish the integrity of mediastinal pleura. Evidence of a left pleural effusion in a patient with a history and radiologic features suspicious for a traumatic diaphragmatic hernia is highly suggestive of vascular compromise because fluid seldom accumulates in the pleural space in the absence of strangulation (Fig. 72.25).[186]

Chylothorax

Chylothorax is the presence of chyle in the pleural space. The thoracic duct transports chyle from the intestinal lacteals and generally drains it into the left subclavian vein. Chylothorax usually occurs as a result of the leakage of chyle after the disruption or obstruction of the thoracic duct or one of its major divisions.[187]

Chyle is characteristically a milky white, opalescent fluid. The gross appearance of the pleural fluid can be misleading because milky effusions are not always chylous in nature, and not all chylous effusions are milky.[188] A pseudochylothorax or chyliform

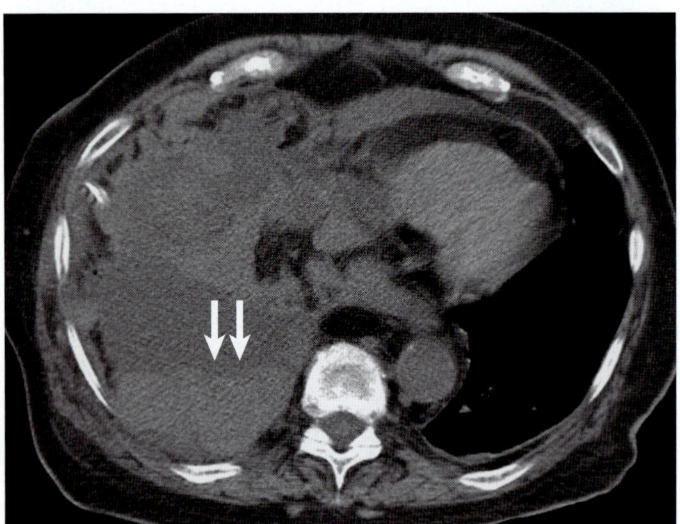

Fig. 72.23 Hemothorax. Noncontrast CT scan shows multiloculated fluid collection with heterogeneous attenuation in right pleural space. The effusion shows high-density areas and fluid-fluid level *(arrows)*, in keeping with a hemothorax. Note cardiac displacement to the left and a small pericardial effusion. The patient had sustained numerous right rib fractures superiorly (not shown) in a motor vehicle accident.

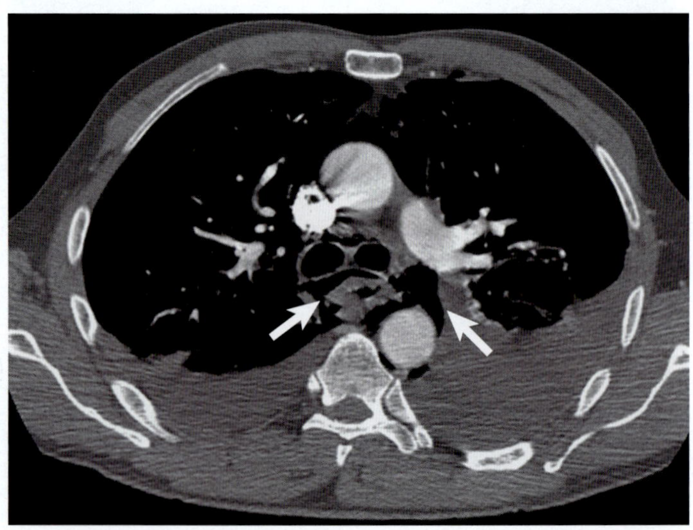

Fig. 72.24 Esophageal perforation in a man with severe chest pain after prolonged vomiting. CT scan shows bilateral pleural effusions (larger on the left) and extensive pneumomediastinum *(arrows)*, predominantly located posteriorly around the esophagus. This is highly suggestive of esophageal rupture (Boerhaave syndrome), which was confirmed on a subsequent esophagogram (not shown).

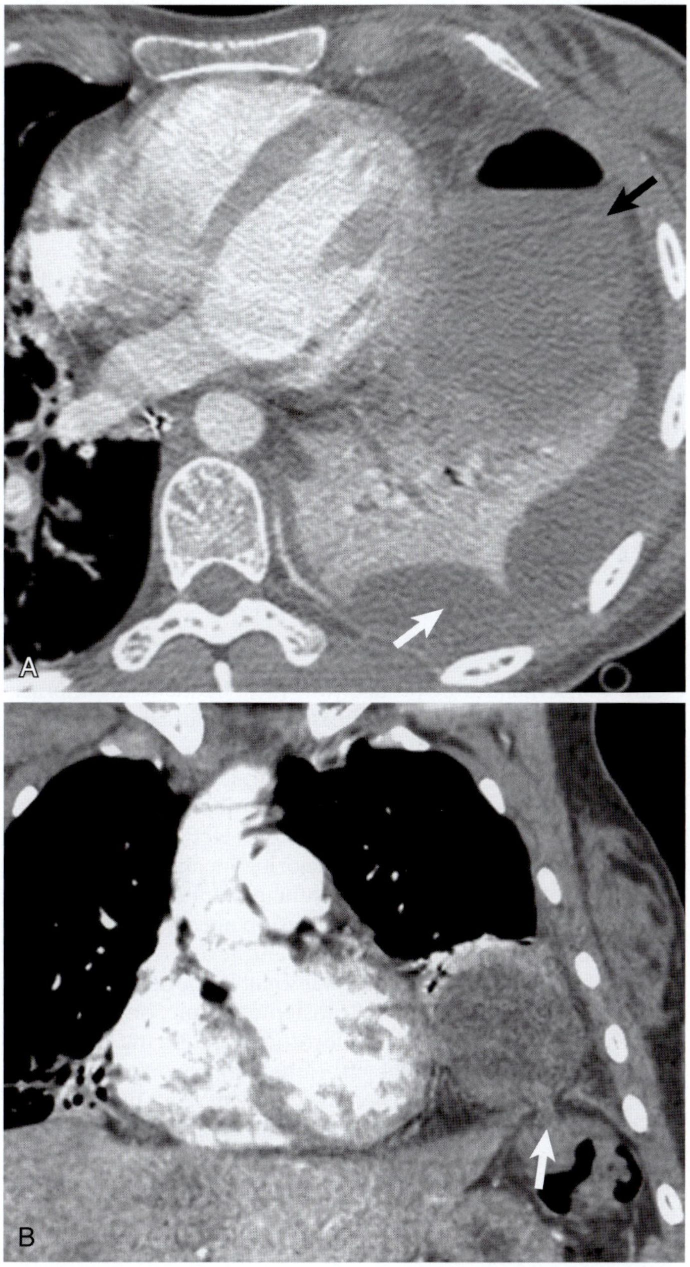

Fig. 72.25 Traumatic diaphragmatic hernia. (A) Contrast-enhanced CT scan shows air-fluid level in nonenhancing bowel *(black arrow)*, which abuts the rib anteriorly, in keeping with diaphragmatic rupture. Moderate left pleural effusion *(white arrow)* and lack of enhancement of bowel strongly suggest infarction. (B) Coronally reconstructed CT scan shows a defect *(arrow)* in the left hemidiaphragm with herniation of the splenic flexure of the colon into the left hemithorax. At surgery, bowel infarction was confirmed, and the diaphragmatic defect was repaired.

effusion is a pleural fluid having a milky appearance usually associated with chronic pleurisy. In contrast to chylothorax, chylomicrons are not present in this fluid, which has a very high content of cholesterol, and the entity has nothing to do with lymphatic vessels or chyle. There are numerous causes of chylothorax (Table 72.3), of which the most common are malignancy (particularly lymphoma) and trauma (especially during surgery), the former being responsible twice as often as the latter.[2] Traumatic

TABLE 72.3 CAUSES OF CHYLOTHORAX

Common	Rare
Malignancy	Lymphangioleiomyomatosis
Lymphoma	Sarcoidosis
Metastatic carcinoma	Obstruction of central veins
Trauma	Amyloidosis
Surgery	
Penetrating injuries	
Tuberculosis	

rupture and resultant chylothorax can be an early or late complication after road traffic accidents.[188] It also is a well-recognized complication of pleuropulmonary surgeries, with an incidence of around 0.7%.[189] Thoracic duct laceration and chylothorax are well-known complications of esophagectomy, with an incidence of 0.6% to 4%.[190,191] Patients with malignancy involving the middle third of the esophagus are at increased risk of developing postoperative chylothorax.[188] Because the thoracic duct crosses to the left of the spine between the fifth and seventh thoracic vertebrae, disruption tends to cause right-sided chylothorax when the lower portion of the duct is affected and left-sided disease when the upper half is involved (Fig. 72.26).

Radiographic findings of chylothorax are similar to those of pleural effusion of nonchylous etiology. The attenuation of chylous effusions at CT varies; it may be low owing to the fat content of the fluid but is usually not because of its high protein content.[64] Lymphangiography is the imaging procedure of choice in the diagnosis and localization of suspected thoracic duct laceration because it may show leakage of contrast material into the pleural space.[192,193]

Chylothorax and pseudochylothorax can be differentiated by lipid analysis of the fluid. On occasion, an empyema can appear milky and may be confused with a chylous effusion. They can be distinguished by bench centrifugation.

Pleural Effusion in Connective Tissue Disease

PLEURAL EFFUSION CAUSED BY IMMUNOLOGIC DISEASE

Pleural pathology in connective tissue disorders is often a reflection of the underlying pulmonary process. Among connective tissue disorders, SLE and RA are the ones most commonly associated with pleural effusions and thickening (Table 72.4). Increased capillary permeability is the fundamental feature of pleural involvement in connective tissue disorders. An immune mechanism seems to be the cause of pleural involvement in RA and SLE, whereas a pleural infiltrative process is thought to be responsible for the capillary leak in Sjögren syndrome, scleroderma, and polymyositis/dermatomyositis.

SYSTEMIC LUPUS ERYTHEMATOSUS

Pleuritic chest pain and pleural effusions are the initial manifestations in about 5% of patients with SLE and occur sometime during the course of SLE in 70% of cases.[194,195] Drug-induced lupus can also involve pleura in similar fashion. Pleural

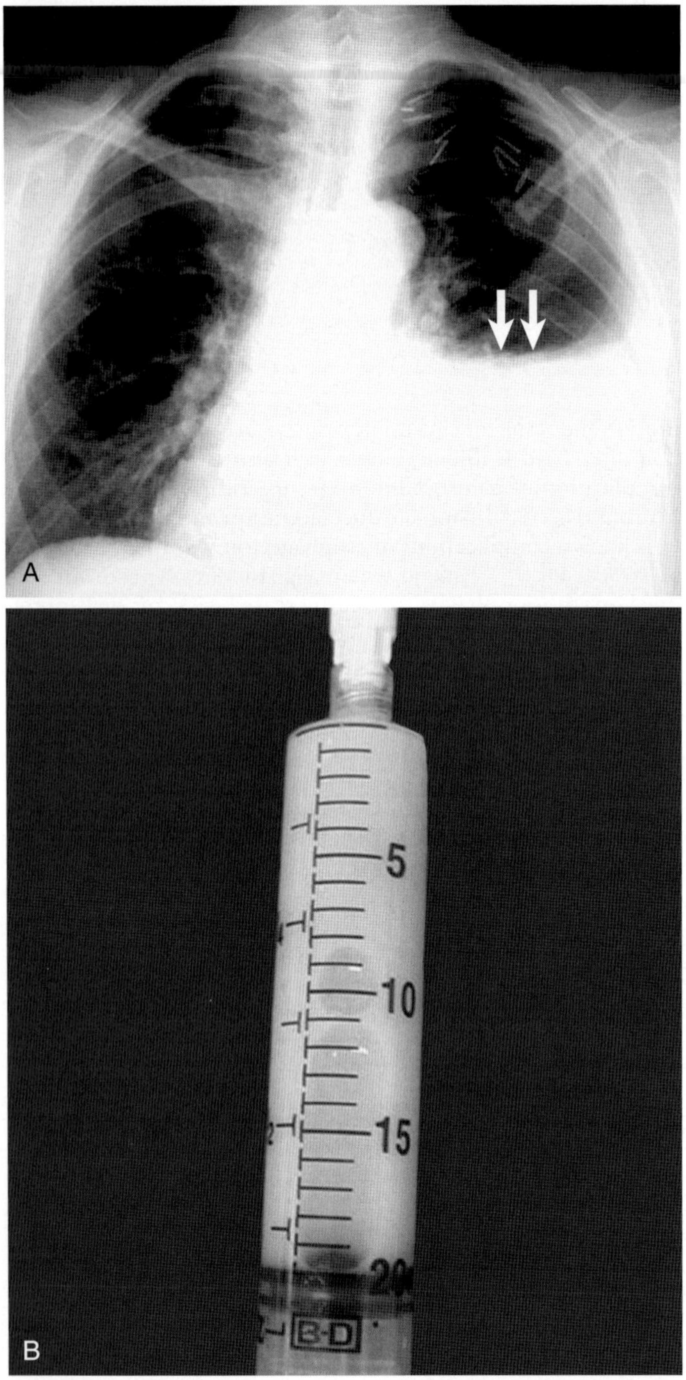

Fig. 72.26 Chylothorax. (A) Portable anteroposterior chest radiograph obtained 3 days after resection of fibrous dysplasia of the first left rib and medial half of the left clavicle shows moderate-sized left pleural effusion *(arrows)*. (B) Photograph of pleural fluid obtained after thoracentesis shows milky white color of a chylous pleural effusion. The thoracic duct had been injured at surgery, just proximal to its insertion into the left subclavian vein.

abnormalities in the form of adhesions, thickening, or effusions have been reported in approximately two-thirds of patients at autopsy and are regarded as the most common intrathoracic manifestation of SLE.[196]

Pleural effusions in patients with SLE can develop from a localized immune response or from other causes, such as primary nephrotic syndrome, pulmonary thromboembolism, and infections.[197] Effusions secondary to lupus pleuritis are usually accompanied by pain and splinting, whereas serous effusions related to kidney disease are painless.

Pleural effusions in SLE are usually small but occasionally can be massive. Pleural effusions are bilateral in 50%, unilateral (equally involving either sides) in 34%, and alternating in 17% of cases.[198] They are generally serous or serosanguineous and are invariably exudative.[195,199]

Enlargement of the cardiopericardial silhouette occurs in 35% to 50% of patients with SLE.[200] When cardiac enlargement is associated with bilateral pleural effusions, the diagnosis of lupus serositis should be strongly considered, particularly in young women. In a series of 34 patients with SLE evaluated using high-resolution CT, interstitial lung disease and airway disease were the most common manifestations, whereas pleural thickening was observed in only 5 patients (15%) and pleural effusions in 3 (9%), indicating that pleural abnormalities may be less common than previously suggested.[201] Pleural biopsy is of limited value because of lack of specificity.

RHEUMATOID DISEASE

Pleural abnormalities are probably the most frequent intrathoracic manifestation of rheumatoid disease, with about 50% of affected patients showing pleural changes at autopsy.[202] Rheumatoid pleurisy can occur with or without pleural effusion. These effusions are observed more frequently in middle-aged men with positive rheumatoid factor despite the fact that RA occurs predominantly in women.[203] The majority of patients with pleural effusion secondary to RA have subcutaneous nodules. Most patients with rheumatoid pleural effusion are asymptomatic but can also present with dyspnea, pain, and fever.[204]

Chest radiographs usually show a small to moderate unilateral pleural effusion, which can be transient, chronic, or relapsing[205] and when chronic may lead to fibrothorax requiring decortication.[206] On thoracentesis the effusions may have an opalescent sheen and milky appearance because of the presence of cholesterol and fat (chyliform effusion) and are exudative with high protein and low glucose levels.[207] Rheumatoid nodules or interstitial lung disease can be seen in 30% of patients with rheumatoid pleurisy.[206] Empyema occurs with increased frequency in these patients owing to necrosis of subpleural rheumatoid nodules, resulting in a pyopneumothorax.

DRESSLER SYNDROME

Dressler syndrome, also known as post–myocardial infarction or postpericardiotomy syndrome, is characterized by chest pain, systemic signs of inflammation (fever, malaise, leukocytosis), and pericardial and pleural effusions. This has been described in many forms of myocardial or pericardial injury, including cardiopericardial surgery, trauma, angioplasty,[208] pacemaker insertion,[209] radiofrequency ablation,[210] and Takotsubo cardiomyopathy.[211] The prevalence of this condition was approximately 1% to 4% in patients with acute myocardial infarction but has been declining because of earlier reperfusion with thrombolysis and angioplasty.[1,212–216]

The postpericardiotomy syndrome can occur after any type of cardiac injury. It is a common postoperative complication occurring in 10% to 40% of individuals who have undergone wide incision of the pericardium.[217] In a review of

TABLE 72.4 PLEURAL EFFUSIONS IN CONNECTIVE TISSUE DISORDERS

Disease	Incidence	Pathogenesis	Fluid Characteristics	Comments
Rheumatoid arthritis Serous effusion	5%	Local immune pleuritis	Exudative; pH and glucose low in 80%	Usually responds to corticosteroids/ immunosuppressive agents
Empyema-like fluid	Uncommon	Necrosis of nodule; massive exudation of white cells	Sterile empyema	May resolve with corticosteroids
Empyema	Uncommon	Bronchopleural fistula	Gram stain/culture positive	Antibiotics/drainage
Cholesterol effusion	Uncommon	Cholesterol from senile cells and granulomas	Milky; high cholesterol content	May require decortication/ pleurodesis
Chylous effusion	Rare	Lymphatic obstruction from amyloidosis	Increased triglycerides	—
Systemic lupus erythematosus	50%	Local immune pleuritis	Exudative	May resolve with corticosteroids
Wegener granulomatosis	5%–55%	Vasculitis and infarction of subpleural parenchyma	Small unilateral exudative effusion	Resolves spontaneously or with corticosteroids/ cyclophosphamide
Sjögren syndrome	<1%	Lymphocytic infiltration of pleura; local immune pleuritis	—	May require pleurodesis
Scleroderma	Rare	Direct pleural involvement by systemic disease	—	No clinical importance
Ankylosing spondylitis	Rare	Subpleural infection/noninfectious inflammation	Small exudative effusion	No clinical importance
Polymyositis/ dermatomyositis	Rare	Lymphocytic or plasma cell infiltration of pleura	Small effusions	No clinical importance
Churg-Strauss syndrome	29%	Inflammation of pleura or pulmonary infarction	Serous: bloody, eosinophilic	May resolve with corticosteroids
Behçet syndrome Effusion	<5%	Superior vena cava obstruction from thrombosis	Transudate	May require pleurodesis
Chylothorax	Rare	Jugulosubclavian confluence thrombosis/thoracic duct rupture	Chylothorax	May require pleurodesis

Adapted from Levine H, Szanto M, Grieble HG, et al. Rheumatoid factor in nonrheumatoid pleural effusions. *Ann Intern Med.* 1968;69:487–492.

postpericardiotomy syndrome, radiographic abnormalities were present in 79%, pleural effusions in 68%, pericardial effusions in 50%, and nonspecific pulmonary opacities in 10%.[217] Pleural effusions were more commonly bilateral (22 patients) than unilateral (4 patients).[217] These abnormalities displayed a dramatic response to steroid therapy, resolving completely within a few days.

Catamenial Pleural Effusion

The presence of endometrial tissue within the thorax is extremely rare. Catamenial pneumothorax was the most common form of thoracic endometriosis, affecting 73% of patients (mean age, 35 years). The other forms of thoracic endometriosis occurred at lesser frequencies: catamenial hemothorax in 14%, catamenial hemoptysis in 7%, and lung nodules in 6%.[218]

The most likely theory, "retrograde menstruation" or regurgitation of endometrial tissue through the fallopian tubes, followed by migration to pleura through diaphragmatic holes, is supported by the finding that normal peritoneal flow is up the right paracolic gutter to the right hemidiaphragm.[219] Diaphragmatic fenestrations are more common on the right, likely explaining the preponderance of cases on this side.[220] The radiographic manifestations are those of pneumothorax or hemothorax; pleural nodules are only rarely visible.[220,221] Catamenial hemothorax has been reported in association with clomiphene therapy for infertility.[222] Of all cases, 85% to 90% occur on the right, 5% occur on the left, and 5% occur bilaterally.[223]

Pleural Effusion Related to Disease of Abdominal Organs

Many intraabdominal and pelvic disorders are associated with pleural effusion. Lymphatic channels are present in the diaphragm that can transport particulate matter and fluid from the peritoneum to the pleural space, the channels on the right being larger.[224] Flow always appears to be away from the peritoneum toward the pleura, never in the reverse direction.[225,226] As seen in catamenial disease, anatomic defects within the diaphragm allow fluid passage.[227] Small pleural effusions are common after abdominal surgery, affecting 49% of patients in one study.[228]

LIVER AND BILIARY TRACT

A large pleural effusion in a patient with cirrhosis and no evidence of primary pulmonary or cardiac disease has been called hepatic hydrothorax.[229] In a review of 200 consecutive patients who had cirrhosis associated with ascites, 12 (6%) were found to have this complication.[230] A right-sided predominance is common; in this series, 9 were right-sided, 2 were bilateral, and 2 were left sided. They may vary in size from small to massive. These effusions almost invariably are associated with ascites, which is the primary source of the transudative effusion. The ascitic fluid in the abdomen enters the pleural cavity via defects in the diaphragm. Therapy is directed at reducing the ascites with diuretics and sodium restriction. Therapeutic thoracentesis brings only temporary relief because fluid rapidly reaccumulates. Tube thoracostomy may drain the pleural fluid and the ascites, resulting in severe hypovolemia, and close monitoring of patients' vital signs and volume of chest tube drainage is important.

KIDNEY

Dialysis

Pleural effusion is seen in approximately 20% to 51% of patients on long-term dialysis.[231,232] The fluid can be exudate or transudate depending on the cause; exudative pleural effusions are frequently serosanguineous or hemorrhagic and contain high levels of protein and LDH.[231,233,234] Most effusions are bilateral, and the most common cause of unilateral and bilateral effusion is volume overload. Other causes include heart failure, parapneumonic effusion, uremic pleuritic, atelectasis, and tuberculous pleurisy.[231]

Hydronephrosis and Urinoma

Urinothorax is a rare complication of an obstructed kidney that results in an ipsilateral pleural effusion caused by retroperitoneal leakage of urine that is thought to enter the pleural space via the diaphragmatic lymphatics.[235] It also has been reported in patients with trauma, malignancy, renal biopsy, and renal transplantation. The pleural fluid smells like urine and resolves when the obstruction is removed.[236] The diagnosis can be confirmed by showing that the pleural fluid creatinine level is higher than the serum creatinine level. The effusion is a transudate and has a low pH.[235]

Nephrotic Syndrome

Pleural effusion is common in patients with the nephrotic syndrome, being seen in 40% of cases.[237] The fluid is a transudate.

Uremia

The pericardium and pleura may become inflamed in patients who have uremia.[233,238,239] Fibrinous pleuritis has been shown in about 20% of uremic patients at autopsy.[239] Spontaneous remission, often with recurrences or constrictive pleural thickening requiring surgical decortication, may occur.[239]

PANCREAS

Acute or chronic pancreatitis is sometimes associated with pleural effusion, often without radiographic evidence of another intrathoracic abnormality. Effusions are predominantly left sided.[240] Chronic pancreatitis is more commonly associated with pleural effusion than is acute disease.[241] The effusion is often recurrent; pancreatic duct disruption may lead to the creation of a pancreaticopleural fistula, with or without pseudocyst formation.[242–245] For patients who fail to benefit from medical therapy, surgery is indicated. The condition is often elusive because respiratory rather than abdominal symptoms usually predominate, and the fistula can be difficult to show radiologically. Confirmation is by showing a high amylase content in the pleural aspirate relative to that in the serum.[245]

OVARY

Ovarian Tumor

A definite association between pleural effusion and benign ovarian tumor was first reported in 1934.[246] This relationship between pleural effusion and ovarian tumors (Meigs-Salmon syndrome) consists of pleural effusion, ascites, and benign tumors of the ovary other than fibromas.[247–250] These benign tumors include tumors of the fallopian tube or uterus and mature teratomas, struma ovarii, and ovarian leiomyomas. This terminology sometimes also includes ovarian or metastatic gastrointestinal malignancies. The importance of Meigs syndrome is that the presence of ascites and pleural effusion does not indicate that a pelvic mass is malignant. The benign tumors in Meigs syndrome are usually fibromas or fibrothecomas and constitute 4% of all ovarian neoplasms.[251]

Ovarian Hyperstimulation Syndrome

Ovarian hyperstimulation syndrome (OHSS) is a rare, potentially life-threatening complication that commonly occurs a few days after induction of follicular rupture after administration of human chorionic gonadotropin when follicular growth is medically induced using either clomiphene citrate or gonadotropins. Prevalence of severe OHSS is reported to range from 0.5% to 5% of fertilizations.[252]

The pathophysiology of OHSS has not yet been completely elucidated. OHSS is characterized by massive ovarian enlargement together with a fluid shift into extravascular compartments owing to increased capillary permeability of the ovarian vessels and other mesothelial surfaces. This results in ascites, pleural or pericardial effusion, oliguria, hemoconcentration, and thromboembolic phenomena.

The most common radiographic findings are bilaterally elevated hemidiaphragms, pleural effusion (bilateral or right-sided), and atelectasis.[252a,252b] Isolated pleural effusion without ascites can occur in OHSS.[253]

SUBPHRENIC ABSCESS

Small pleural effusions are commonly found in association with acute subphrenic infection; in one study of 47 patients, they were found in 37 (79%).[254] Additional findings include elevation of the hemidiaphragm and basal atelectasis or pneumonitis.[254] Air under the hemidiaphragm is a helpful sign when present.

Yellow Nail Syndrome

The yellow nail syndrome is a rare disorder in middle-aged and elderly individuals characterized by the triad of primary lymphedema, recurrent pleural effusion, and yellow discoloration of the nails (Fig. 72.27). It is often associated with pericardial effusion, rhinosinusitis, and bronchiectasis. Pathogenesis is thought to be related to lymphatic obstruction secondary to anatomic or functional abnormalities (or both) in the lymphatic vessels.

Pleural effusions occur in 63% of cases of yellow nail syndrome and are bilateral in 50%.[255,256] The effusions can be small or massive and are sometimes chylous. The underlying mechanism of fluid retention in the pleural space is probably related to lymphatic abnormalities; treatment with diuretics has not proven effective.[256] Large symptomatic effusions are best treated with pleural abrasion, chemical pleurodesis, or parietal pleurectomy.[256] High-resolution CT has been shown to be useful for assessing the extent of the airway disease in this rare disorder. In a small series of four patients, CT showed bronchiectasis, bronchial wall thickening, and bronchial dilation in all cases.[257]

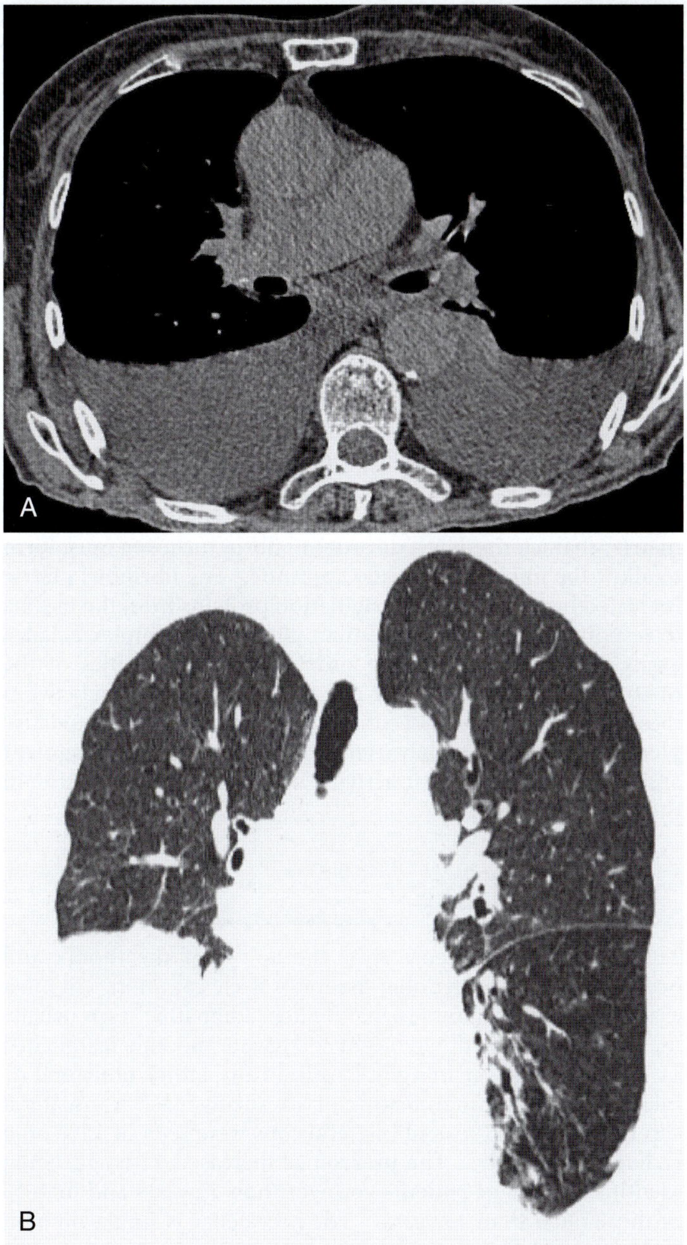

Fig. 72.27 Yellow nail syndrome. (A) CT image shows moderate bilateral pleural effusions. (B) Coronal image shows bilateral pleural effusions and mild cylindrical bronchiectasis in the left lower lobe. The patient had all of the clinical features of yellow nail syndrome.

KEY POINTS

- Exudates have a protein level >30 g/L, and transudates have a protein level <30 g/L.
- Left heart failure accounts for most transudative pleural effusions. Other causes include liver failure, hypoalbuminemia, nephrotic syndrome, constrictive pericarditis, and peritoneal dialysis.
- Pneumonia, malignancy, pulmonary thromboembolism, and connective tissue diseases account for most exudative effusions.
- The lateral decubitus view is the most sensitive radiographic method for detecting small pleural effusions.
- Septated effusions are exudates, and septations are better visualized on ultrasound than on CT.
- Ultrasound-guided pleural aspiration is a safe and accurate method for obtaining pleural fluid and is particularly helpful in small or loculated pleural effusions.
- CT scans for pleural effusion should be performed with contrast enhancement before full drainage of the fluid for better visualization of the pleural abnormalities.
- CT can help differentiate between benign and malignant pleural thickening.
- Positron emission tomography–CT is more sensitive than CT alone in differentiating benign from malignant pleural effusions.
- Image-guided biopsy of pleural thickening or nodularity has a higher yield than blind pleural biopsy or thoracentesis in the diagnosis of malignancy.
- Thoracoscopy should be considered when less invasive tests have failed to provide a diagnosis.

SUGGESTED READINGS

English JC, Leslie KO. Pathology of the pleura. *Clin Chest Med*. 2006;27:157–180.

Hooper C, Lee YCG, Maskell N, BTS Pleural Disease Guideline Group. Investigation of a unilateral pleural effusion in adults: British Thoracic Society Pleural Disease Guideline 2010. *Thorax*. 2010;65(suppl 2):ii4–ii17.

Light RW. Pleural effusions. *Med Clin North Am*. 2011;95(6):1055–1070.

Müller NL. Imaging of the pleura. *Radiology*. 1993;186:297–309.

Qureshi NR, Gleeson FV. Imaging of pleural disease. *Clin Chest Med*. 2006;27:193–213.

Roberts ME, Neville E, Berrisford RG, Antunes G, Ali NJ, BTS Pleural Disease Guideline Group. Management of a malignant pleural effusion: British Thoracic Society Pleural Disease Guideline 2010. *Thorax*. 2010;65(suppl 2):ii32–ii40.

Sahn SA. Pleural effusions of extravascular origin. *Clin Chest Med*. 2006;27:285–308.

The full reference list for this chapter is available at ExpertConsult.com.

73 Benign Pleural Thickening

CAROL C. WU | JEAN M. SEELY

Etiology

Benign pleural thickening caused by fibrosis is the second most common pleural abnormality, the most common one being effusion. Pleural fibrosis has a number of causes and is the outcome of many pleural diseases and a potential complication of every inflammatory condition that affects the lungs.

The pleura show a variety of patterns of fibrosis. These may be either localized (apical caps, pleural plaques) or diffuse.[1] In some respects pleural fibrosis can be considered defective healing.[2] Central to the pathogenesis of pleural fibrosis is inflammation of the pleural cavity. The response of the mesothelial cell to injury and its ability, along with the underlying basement membrane, to maintain its integrity are crucial in determining whether normal healing or pleural fibrosis ensues.[2]

The pleura acts not only as a protective barrier but as an immunologically and metabolically responsive membrane that is involved in maintaining a dynamic homeostasis in the pleural space.[3] The mesothelial cells secrete glycosaminoglycans and other surfactant-like molecules to lubricate the pleural surface in addition to proinflammatory, antiinflammatory, and other immunomodulatory mediators, factors that promote deposition and clearance of fibrin, and growth factors and extracellular matrix proteins to aid in serosal repair.[4] Pleural injury and fibrosis are characterized by disordered fibrin turnover.[4] Interactions among mesothelial and inflammatory cells, cytokines, growth factors, and blood-derived products are important in the pathogenesis of tissue fibrosis.[4] The exact timing of these interactions, as well as genetic factors, may be the difference between resolution of an injury, leading to normal repair and regeneration, and excessive matrix formation with fibrosis and scar formation.[4]

Most of the diffuse forms of visceral or parietal pleural fibrosis result from organization of recurrent effusions. The most common causes are collagen vascular diseases, asbestos exposure, and drugs, especially methysergide, methotrexate, bromocriptine, practolol, and mitomycin.[5]

Pathophysiology

ANATOMY

Pleuritis with associated pleural effusion develops in a number of different diseases. In most cases the pleural inflammation regresses, with or without medication and without sequelae of pleural fibrosis. However, in others, pleural inflammation progresses to pleural fibrosis. In experimental models of pleuritis, the mesothelial cells proliferate and become reactive in response to injury.[2] Reactive mesothelial cells become columnar with increased microvilli and upregulation of the enzymes of the oxidative pathway.[6,7] Fibrinolysis and synthesis of prostacyclins and hyaluronic acid–rich glycoproteins are stimulated in an attempt to remove debris and to repair the mesothelial cell surface, maintaining the integrity of the pleural surface.[8] The degree of mesothelial cell and basement membrane injury and regeneration appears to be the key to whether complete recovery or pleural fibrosis occurs.[2]

For pleural fibrosis to develop, an increase in the extracellular matrix, characterized by a disorder in fibrin turnover, must form to allow the fibrotic process to continue.[2] The fibrinous matrix is created by the release of coagulation proteins from the plasma in response to pleural space inflammation.[2] A complex balance exists between procoagulant and fibrinolytic activities of the mesothelial cells.[9] In exudative pleuritis, local equilibrium between these activities is disrupted, enhancing fibrin deposition. Exudative pleural effusions are characterized by increased procoagulant and depressed fibrinolytic activity, favoring fibrin deposition in the pleural space.[9]

The Apical Cap

Thickening of the pleura over the apices of the thorax and occasionally in the interlobar fissures is fairly common.[10] In most cases the etiology is unknown.[11,12] Such "idiopathic" caps usually measure less than 5 mm in height and have a smoothly marginated or undulating lower margin.[12] Apical caps, either unilateral or bilateral, are a common feature of advancing age.[12] A unilateral cap was seen in 11%, and bilateral caps were seen in 12% on a radiographic study.[11] The prevalence increased with age, being identified in 6% of patients younger than 45 years and in 16% of those older than 45 years.[11] The prevalence is similar in men and women.[11] There is no significant association of apical caps with tuberculosis, emphysema, diffuse interstitial fibrosis, silicosis, or asbestosis.[13]

Pathology

Apical caps consist mainly of extrapleural fat and a combination of parenchymal and to a lesser extent pleural fibrosis.[13] On histologic examination the pleura is thickened by dense, sometimes hyalinized collagen, accompanied in some cases by small foci of mononuclear inflammatory cells. The architecture of the underlying lung parenchyma is preserved, but the airspaces are obliterated by fibrous tissue; elastic tissue in the alveolar septa is typically increased. Focal areas of calcification or ossification can be seen.[11,13] The pathogenesis of the fibrosis is uncertain. In one autopsy study an association with histologic evidence of chronic bronchitis and pulmonary artery narrowing was identified. The investigators suggested that intermittent or continuing low-grade infection combined with relative apical ischemia might be responsible for the fibrosis.[12–14]

Manifestations of the Disease

RADIOGRAPHY

The apical cap is an irregular, nonhomogeneous opacity located at the extreme apex of the lung.[15] The lower border is usually sharply marginated, but it is frequently tented or undulating (Fig. 73.1).[11] The cap opacity is of variable thickness (usually <5 mm in craniocaudal dimension) and of variable transverse diameter.[15] It may be unilateral or bilateral. In patients with a cap related to prior tuberculosis, the apical opacity can measure more than 1 cm in thickness on the radiograph (Fig. 73.2).[16]

COMPUTED TOMOGRAPHY

Extrapleural fat with interspersed vessels accounts for most of the opacity seen on the radiograph (see Figs. 73.1 and 73.2).[16] Extrapleural fat is commonly thicker adjacent to areas of chronic pleural disease, possibly resulting from retraction of the lung from fibrosis.[17] An apical pneumothorax can outline the apical cap (Fig. 73.3).[18] The thin white visceral line will be thickened in this case and is well depicted in the presence of air in the pleural space.

Differential Diagnosis

Other lesions arising in the lung, pleura, or extrapleural space may produce unilateral or bilateral apical caps. These include the following:

- *Neoplasm:* Pancoast (superior sulcus) tumor (Fig. 73.4), lymphoma extending from the neck or mediastinum, metastases, and mesothelioma
- *Infection:* Extrapleural abscesses or tuberculosis extending from the neck
- *Radiation fibrosis:* After treatment for lymphoma, head and neck or breast carcinoma (Fig. 73.5)
- *Hemorrhage:* Extrapleural dissection of blood from a ruptured aorta, fractures of the ribs or spine, or bleeding resulting from subclavian line placement
- *Vascular anomalies:* Coarctation of the aorta with dilated collaterals over the apex, fistula between the subclavian artery and vein
- *Miscellaneous:* Mediastinal lipomatosis with subcostal fat extending over the apices[12]
- *Pleural effusions:* In a supine patient may also simulate an apical cap, as the fluid tracks to the most dependent portion of the pleural space (Fig. 73.6)

KEY POINTS: APICAL CAPS

- Typically bilateral and symmetric
- Measure <5 mm in thickness
- Most commonly idiopathic
- Prevalence increases with age

Pleural Plaques

Etiology, Prevalence, and Epidemiology

Pleural plaques are the most common manifestation of asbestos inhalation[19] (see Chapter 61). Asbestos-induced fibrosis can

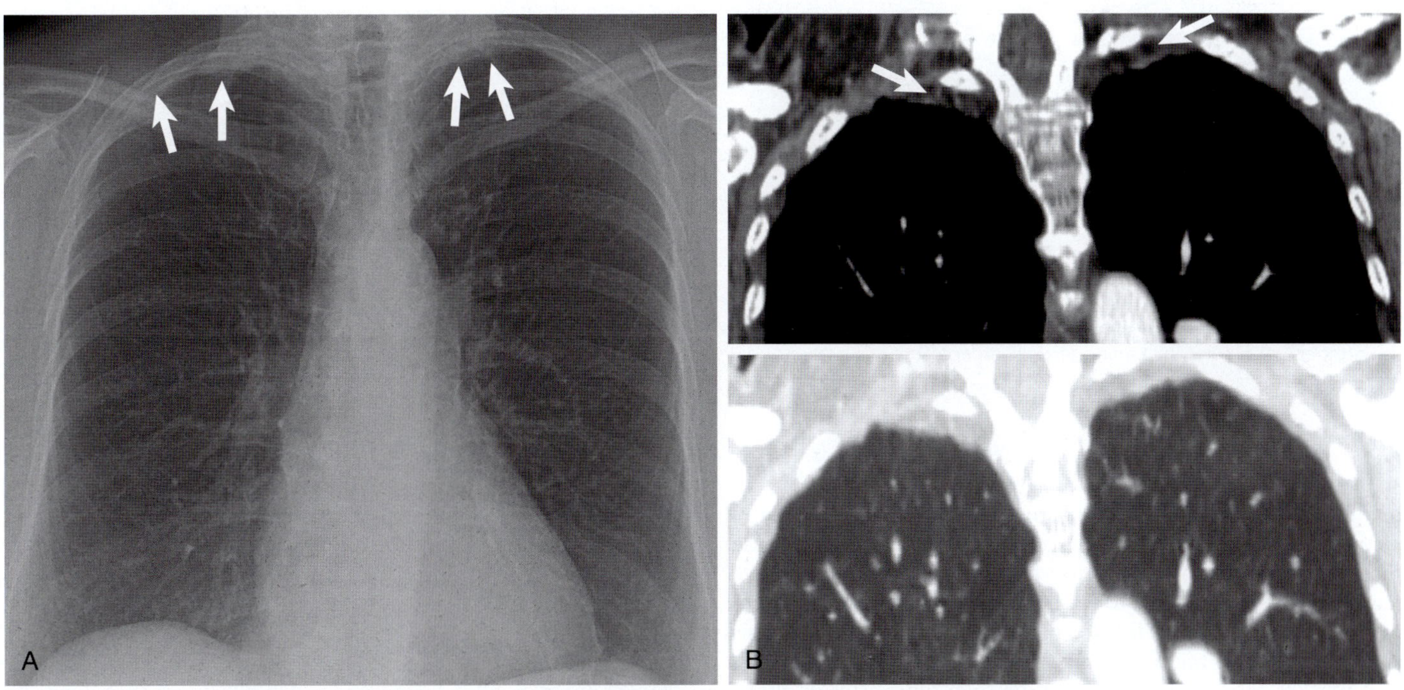

Fig. 73.1 Apical caps. (A) Posteroanterior chest radiograph demonstrates biapical pleural thickening *(arrows)* that has an undulating margin with the lung. This is symmetric bilaterally and measures less than 5 mm in height. (B) Composite image with coronal reformatted CT scans in soft tissue and lung windows shows the radiographic opacity is composed mostly of extrapleural fat *(arrows)* in addition to pleural thickening. The undulating inferior margin of the apical cap is better seen in lung window.

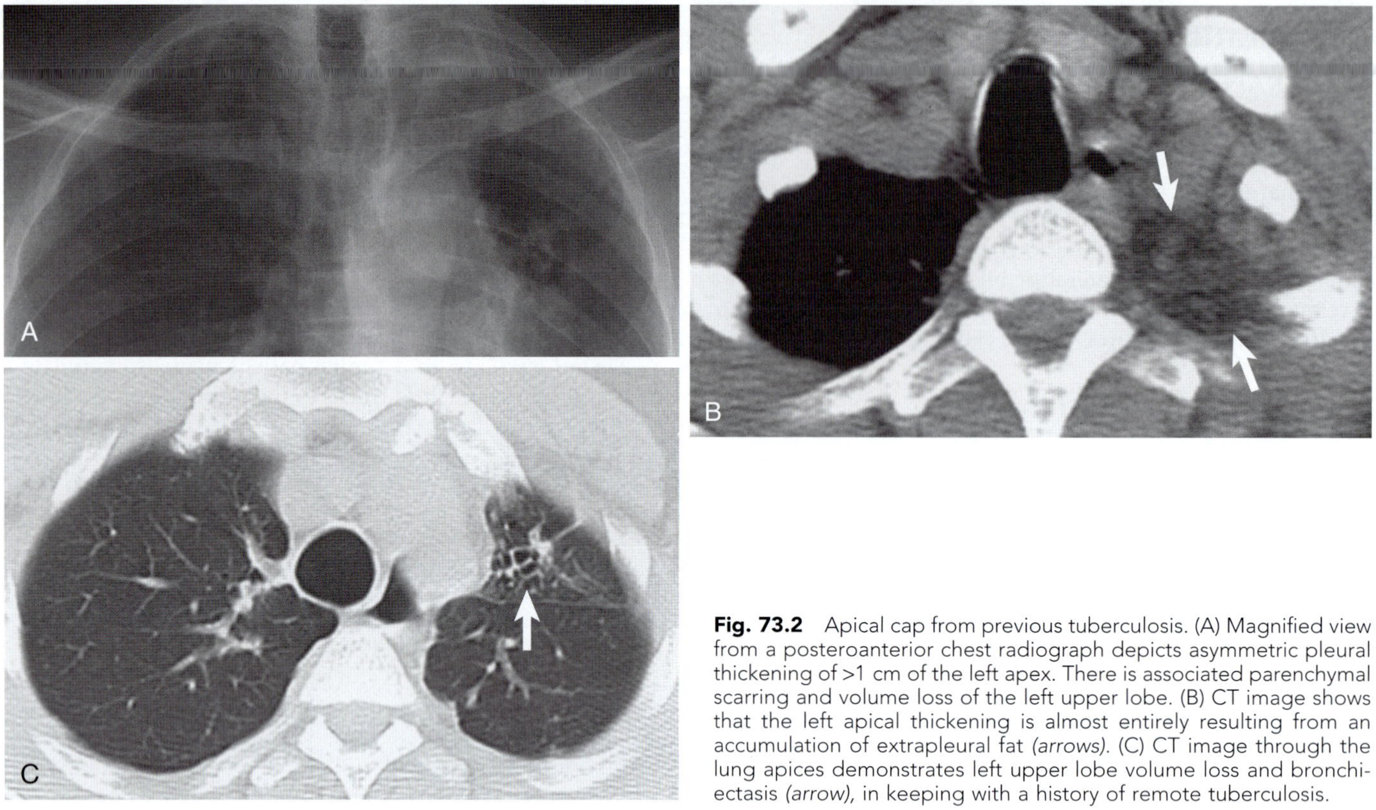

Fig. 73.2 Apical cap from previous tuberculosis. (A) Magnified view from a posteroanterior chest radiograph depicts asymmetric pleural thickening of >1 cm of the left apex. There is associated parenchymal scarring and volume loss of the left upper lobe. (B) CT image shows that the left apical thickening is almost entirely resulting from an accumulation of extrapleural fat *(arrows)*. (C) CT image through the lung apices demonstrates left upper lobe volume loss and bronchiectasis *(arrow)*, in keeping with a history of remote tuberculosis.

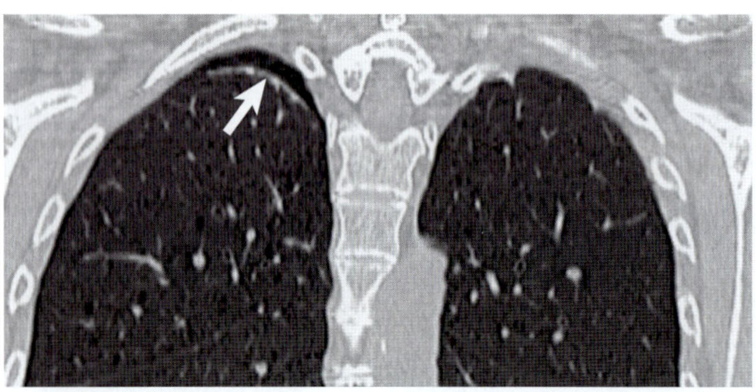

Fig. 73.3 Apical cap and right pneumothorax. Coronal reconstruction of high-resolution CT image shows a small right pneumothorax outlining the right apical pleural thickening *(arrow)*; an apical cap is present only on the right side.

involve the pulmonary interstitium (asbestosis), the parietal pleura (pleural plaques), or the visceral and parietal pleura (diffuse pleural thickening).[20] The pleura appears to be more sensitive than the lung parenchyma to the effects of asbestos fibers. Pleural plaques occur with lower inhaled fiber burdens, whereas asbestosis is associated with higher fiber burdens.[21] Pleural plaques serve as a marker of exposure and may be seen with brief or slight exposure.[22] Although the overall incidence of plaques increases with dose, a linear correlation does not exist between plaque severity and total dust exposure.[23] However, a direct relationship has been found between the intensity of asbestos exposure and total area of pleura involved by the plaques in a postmortem study.[24] Among environmentally exposed individuals, the prevalence ranges from 0.53% to 8%.[25] Studies of occupationally exposed individuals show frequencies of 3% to 14% in dockyard workers and up to 58% among insulation workers.[25,26] However, the previously reported prevalence figures must be considered in the context of the method used to detect pleural plaques.[24]

There is a latency period of 20 to 30 years between asbestos exposure and the development of pleural plaques. Calcification is seen in 15%[27] of patients after a latency period of 30 to 40 years, with calcification of plaques increasing with time from exposure. Diaphragmatic calcification is highly suggestive of previous exposure to asbestos.

There are other less common causes of pleural plaques besides asbestos. Silicosis has been described to cause pleural plaques; however, an autopsy study demonstrated that both visceral pleura and parietal pleura are involved, whereas asbestos plaques typically involve the parietal pleura.[28] Chest trauma (hemothorax), infection (empyema), and artificial pneumothoraces previously used for the treatment of tuberculosis can also cause pleural plaques.[1] In contrast to asbestos-induced pleural plaques, these lesions are usually unilateral and may be upper zonal in distribution.

Clinical Presentation

Plaques are frequently diagnosed incidentally on chest radiographs or computed tomography (CT) scans and have important medicolegal significance.[29] Patients with pleural plaques are generally not symptomatic in the absence of associated pulmonary disease or diffuse pleural fibrosis.

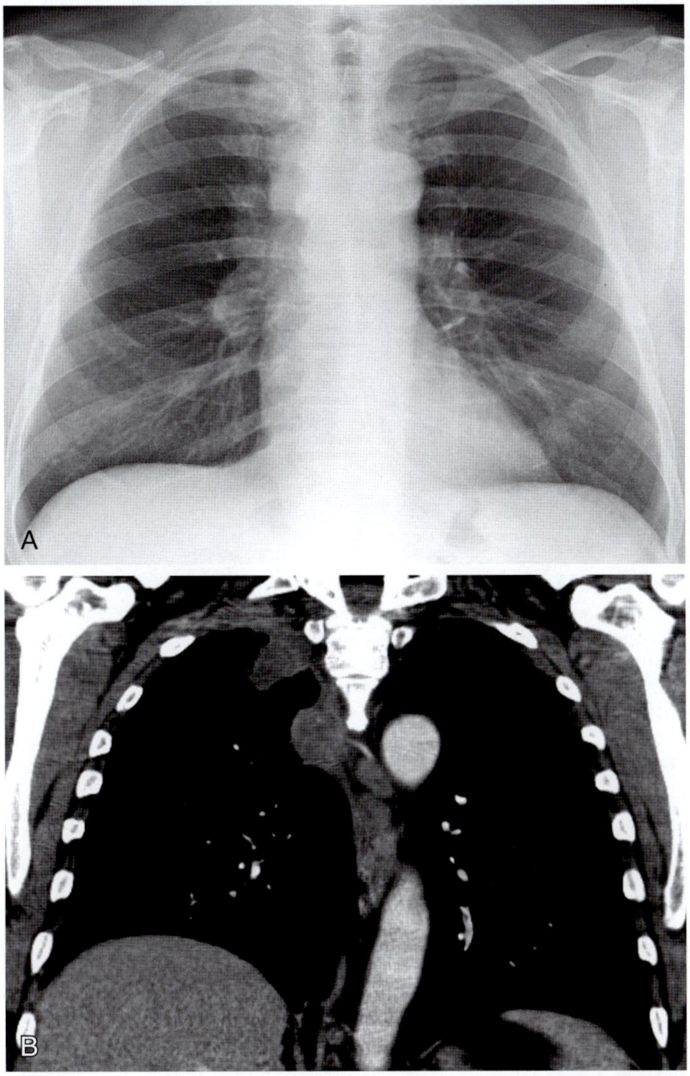

Fig. 73.4 Pancoast tumor. (A) Posteroanterior chest radiograph and (B) coronal contrast-enhanced CT scan show a soft tissue mass in the right lung apex and thickening of the right paratracheal stripe representing lymph node metastases.

Pathophysiology

Whereas microscopic fragments of asbestos fibers have been isolated from pleural plaques, it remains unclear how fibers reach the parietal pleura and if they are responsible for inflammation and fibrosis.[30] Chrysotile fibers, fine, short, and especially fragmented fibers, are better able to reach the pleura and probably account for many of the pathogenetic and anatomic features of asbestos-related disease.[31] Some have proposed that pleural plaques are the direct result of local inflammation of the parietal pleura from asbestos fibers that protrude out of the visceral pleural surface.[32] However, there have been no confirmative pathologic data to support this. The most plausible explanation for plaque pathogenesis is that the asbestos fibers reach the parietal pleura by retrograde lymphatic drainage involving flow from the mediastinal lymph nodes to the retrosternal and intercostal lymphatics.[33] Asbestos fibers may also embolize to the parietal pleura through the costal vascular supply.[33] Plaques are located in the vicinity of stomas in the parietal pleura, so-called Kampmeier foci, where asbestos fibers are resorbed by lymphatic flow.[34]

These stomas are typically located in the lower hemithorax, which is why most plaques tend to occur below the sixth ribs.

PATHOLOGY

Pleural plaques are discrete elevated areas of hyaline fibrosis almost invariably arising from the parietal pleura.[27] They consist of acellular bundles of collagen in an undulating basket-weave pattern and may contain abundant numbers of asbestos fibers, almost exclusively chrysotile fibers, but asbestos bodies (ferruginous bodies containing an asbestos core) are absent.[35,36] The inner side is covered by normal mesothelial cells; on the costal side there may be signs of low-grade inflammation.[37]

Pleural plaques may progress over time, in the absence of continued exposure.[38] Typically, they will increase the amount of calcification over time. There is no evidence that pleural plaques undergo malignant degeneration into mesothelioma.[26,27,39]

Pleural plaques are discrete, elevated, opaque, shiny, rounded lesions (Fig. 73.7).[20] Thin plaques are smooth and gray-white. Thick plaques are ivory colored or gray and may have a smooth or nodular surface.[20] On microscopic examination plaques are seen to be laminated collagenous connective tissue, acellular, with few inflammatory or fibrocystic nuclei (Fig. 73.8); many are covered with a thin layer of regular or well-differentiated mesothelial cells.[20] Elastic staining shows intact lamellae beneath the plaque in continuity with the surrounding normal parietal pleural connective tissue. This suggests that plaques are extrapleural and develop between the pleural connective tissue and the covering layer of mesothelial cells.[32]

Parietal pleural plaques are well-demarcated lesions that most commonly occur between the sixth through ninth ribs in the posterolateral thorax. They occur more frequently in the lower hemithorax. The costophrenic angles and apices are spared. Plaques may be found over the dome of the diaphragm and on the pericardium.[19,40]

LUNG FUNCTION

Pleural plaques are not usually associated with impairment of lung function.[41,42] As pleural plaques are covered by a normal mesothelium and are not associated with adherence between the lung and the chest wall during respiratory movements, the lung can still slide along the chest wall and can fully expand.[43] It has been suggested that when there is an impairment of lung function, it is more likely due to subclinical interstitial fibrosis.[44]

Manifestations of the Disease

RADIOGRAPHY

The earliest manifestation of a pleural plaque on the chest radiograph is as a unilateral or bilateral thin line of soft tissue density under a rib in the axillary region, usually the seventh or eighth rib. Noncalcified pleural plaques are difficult to identify on the chest radiograph except when the x-ray beam is tangential to the plaque. The plaque appears in profile as a sharply marginated dense band of soft tissue ranging from 1 to 10 mm in thickness, paralleling the inner margin of the lateral thoracic

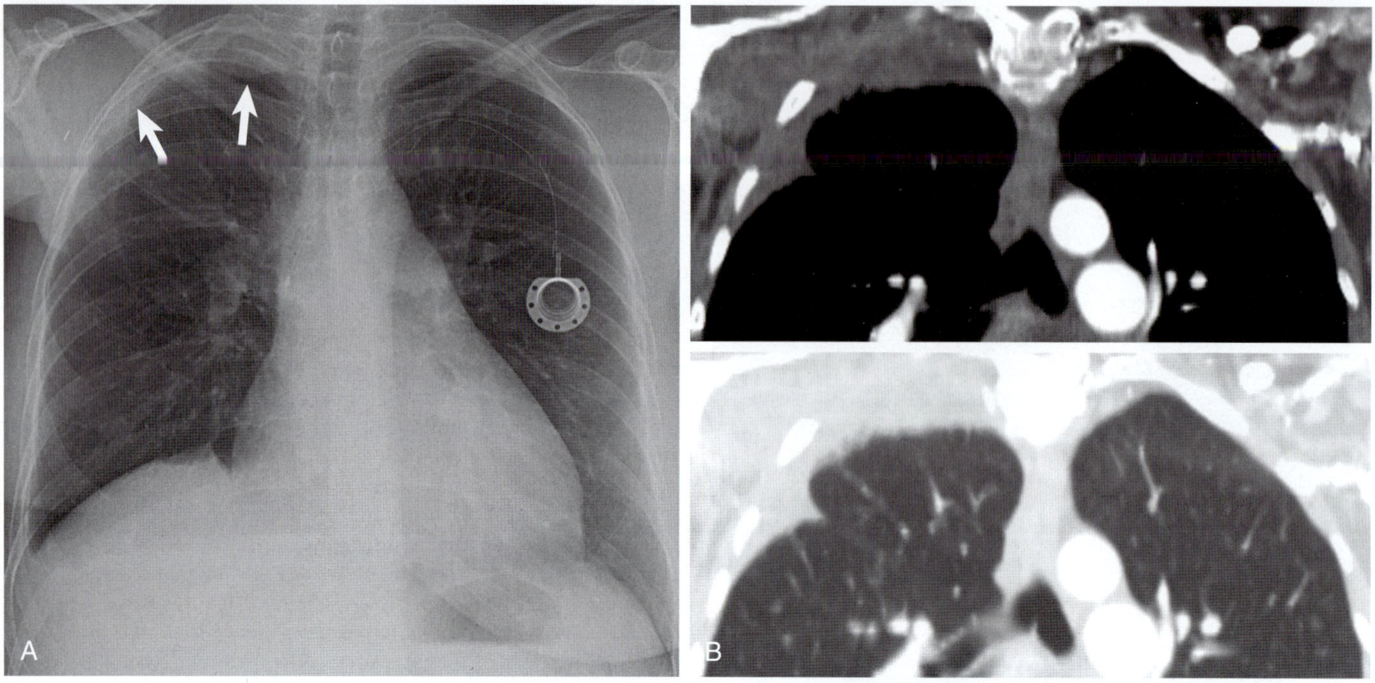

Fig. 73.5 Radiation fibrosis. (A) Posteroanterior chest radiograph demonstrates asymmetric right apical pleural thickening *(arrows)* postradiation therapy for breast cancer. Note is made of a smaller right breast shadow. (B) Composite image with coronal reformatted CT scans in soft tissue and lung windows shows the radiographic opacity is composed of extrapleural fat, pleural thickening, and reticulations from pulmonary fibrosis. Note right upper lobe volume loss.

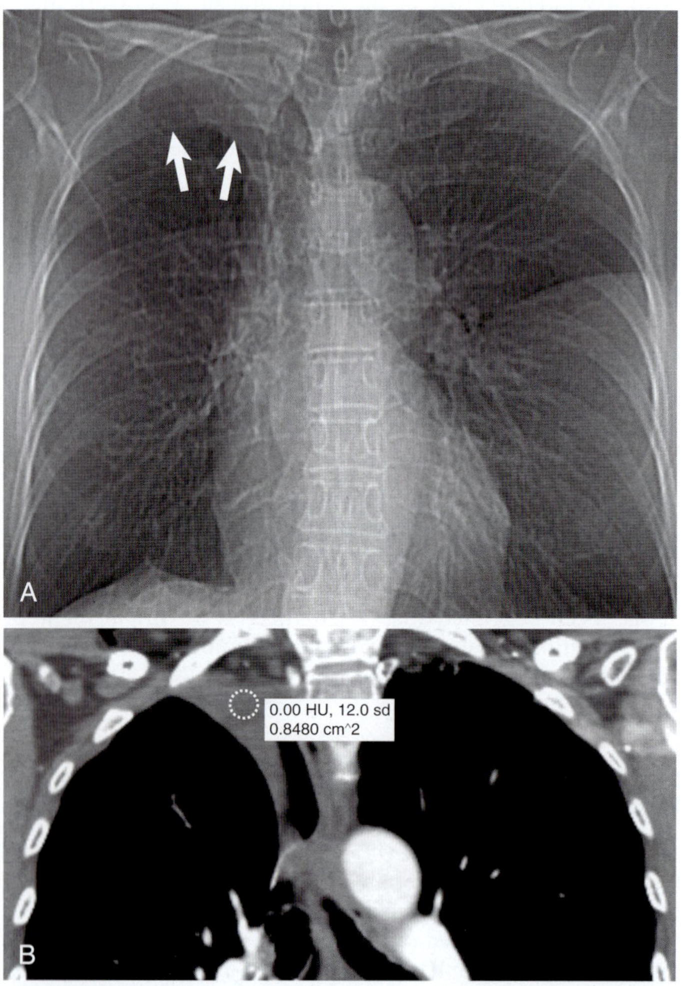

Fig. 73.6 Loculated pleural effusion post right upper lobectomy. (A) Scout view of CT demonstrates right apical opacity mimicking pleural thickening *(arrows)*. (B) Coronal reformatted CT image shows loculated right apical pleural fluid with density of 0 Hounsfield units.

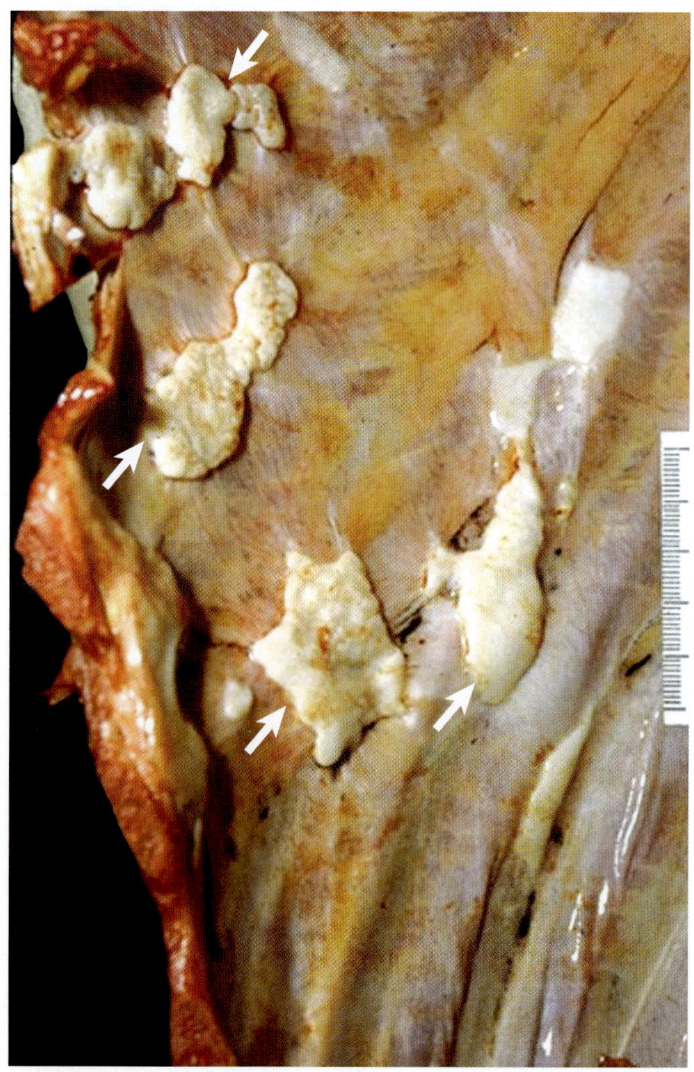

Fig. 73.7 Asbestos-related pleural plaques in an asbestos miner. Autopsy specimen shows numerous pearly white pleural plaques along the costal parietal pleura *(arrows)*.

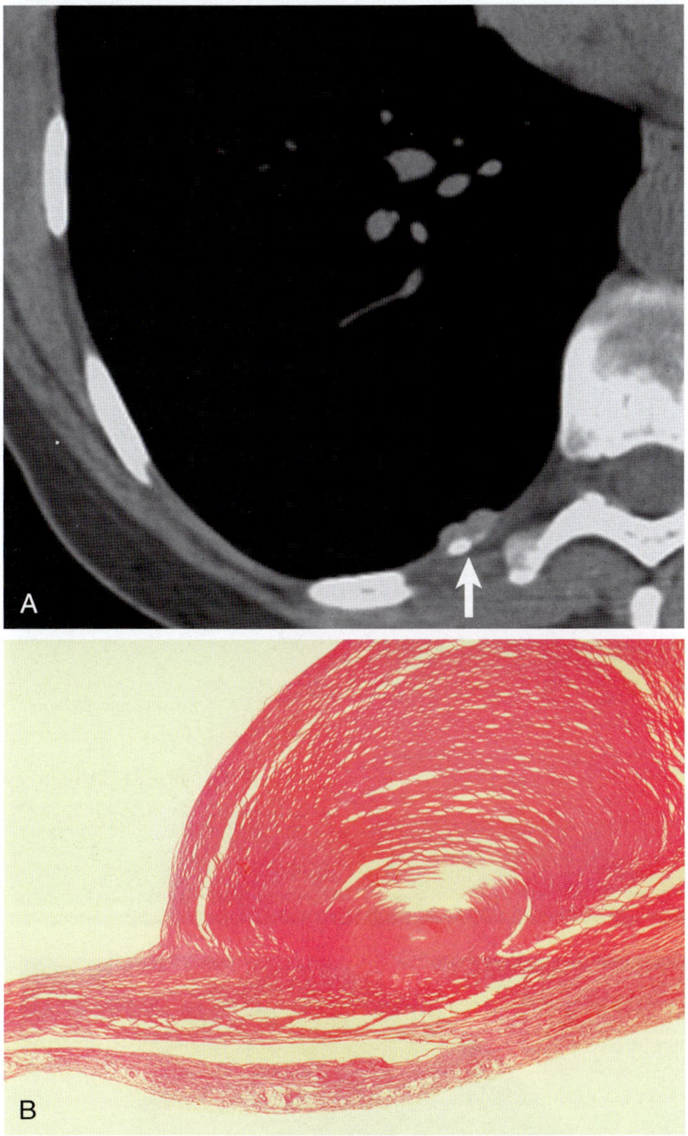

Fig. 73.8 Pleural plaque. (A) Magnified view from a CT image at the level of the right lower lobe shows a single pleural plaque that is partially calcified *(arrow)*. The patient presented with a spontaneous pneumothorax, for which pleurectomy was performed. There was no history of trauma. (B) Pathology section shows the full thickness of the pleural plaque. The collagenous plaque demonstrates the typical acellular basket-weave appearance.

wall. As with any extraparenchymal lesion, pleural plaques viewed en face can be difficult to see. They have a characteristically sharply defined medial edge and an ill-defined lateral margin, the so-called incomplete border sign (Fig. 73.9).[45] The holly leaf sign refers to the radiographic appearance of pleural plaques with irregular thickened nodular edges (Fig. 73.10). The majority of asbestos-related plaques occur in the parietal pleura. Visceral pleural plaque formation is uncommon. The radiographic diagnosis of visceral pleural thickening is not reliable unless it occurs in the interlobar fissures (Fig. 73.11). Recognition of a calcified pleural plaque in a thickened minor fissure[46] or major fissure[47] has been reported. These visceral plaques usually are associated with extensive parietal pleural disease.[48]

The chest radiograph has reported sensitivities of 30% to 80% in the detection of pleural plaques.[27] Detection is dependent on a number of factors, including plaque thickness, size, and position; radiographic technical factors; and the presence of calcification.[49]

The International Labour Office (ILO) classification of pneumoconioses assesses asbestos-induced pleural disease on chest radiography using the posteroanterior projection.[50] Autopsy studies report a high false-negative rate for the radiographic detection of pleural plaques.[40,41]

COMPUTED TOMOGRAPHY

On CT a pleural plaque is defined as a discontinuous soft tissue focal thickening of the pleural surface, with or without foci of calcification.[35,51,52] Plaques typically have edges that are thicker than the central portion (Fig. 73.12; see also Fig. 73.8) and can progress in size, extent, and calcification with time.[49] Pleural plaques are internal to and separated from the ribs by a thin fat layer (Fig. 73.13).[53] This fat layer also separates the thickened pleura from the innermost intercostal muscle, subcostal muscle, and intercostal vein. Intercostal vessels may cause normal extrapleural soft tissues to appear thicker in the paravertebral regions. Paraspinal pleural plaques should be diagnosed only if thickening is visible at multiple levels, extrapleural fat is visible between the pleura and intercostal vessels, thickened pleura is seen to indent the adjacent lung, or there is dystrophic calcification within the plaque.[53]

The characteristic sites for pleural plaques related to asbestos exposure are the posterolateral chest wall between the sixth and ninth ribs, the dome of the diaphragm (Fig. 73.14), and the mediastinal pleura, particularly over or involving the pericardium (Fig. 73.15).[54] Typically, plaques are not present at the apices or the costophrenic angles. Plaques that arise from the visceral pleura are rare and usually found in the lower aspects of the interlobar fissures; they may calcify and are usually associated with extensive parietal pleural plaque formation.[48] The size and number of pleural plaques are variable. Pleural plaques are bilateral in the majority of asbestos-exposed individuals, but they can also be unilateral. Unilateral plaques can also be related to prior hemothorax (Fig. 73.16) or empyema (see Fig. 73.10). According to the literature, calcification of plaques is seen in 10% to 15% of cases, although many radiologists find that percentage to be much lower than expected based on their clinical practice where the majority of pleural plaques are calcified.

Some plaques demonstrate subtle reticular densities in the adjacent lung, giving rise to the term *hairy plaques.*[27] This usually represents compressive atelectasis in asymptomatic patients or potentially subclinical fibrosis in some patients who demonstrate functional impairment but who do not manifest any other evidence of pulmonary asbestosis.

Asbestos-related pleural plaques may grow in the absence of continued exposure.[55] However, by themselves, they have no malignant potential. The plaques simply serve as a risk indicator for malignant pleural disease.

MAGNETIC RESONANCE IMAGING

On magnetic resonance imaging (MRI), most pleural plaques have low signal on T1- and T2-weighted sequences, whereas mesotheliomas are typically T2 hyperintense.[56,57] Plaques are avascular and do not enhance with contrast.

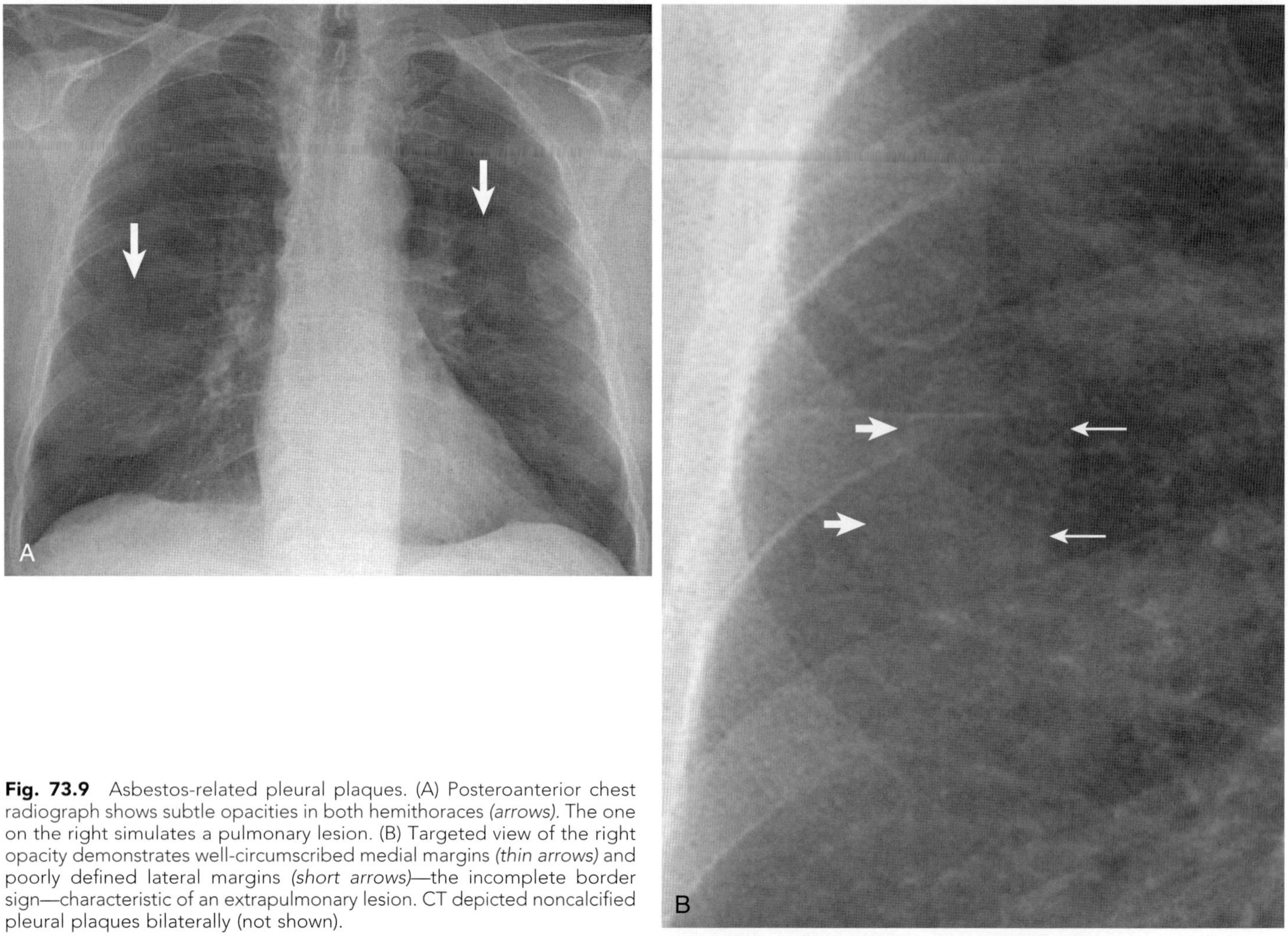

Fig. 73.9 Asbestos-related pleural plaques. (A) Posteroanterior chest radiograph shows subtle opacities in both hemithoraces *(arrows)*. The one on the right simulates a pulmonary lesion. (B) Targeted view of the right opacity demonstrates well-circumscribed medial margins *(thin arrows)* and poorly defined lateral margins *(short arrows)*—the incomplete border sign—characteristic of an extrapulmonary lesion. CT depicted noncalcified pleural plaques bilaterally (not shown).

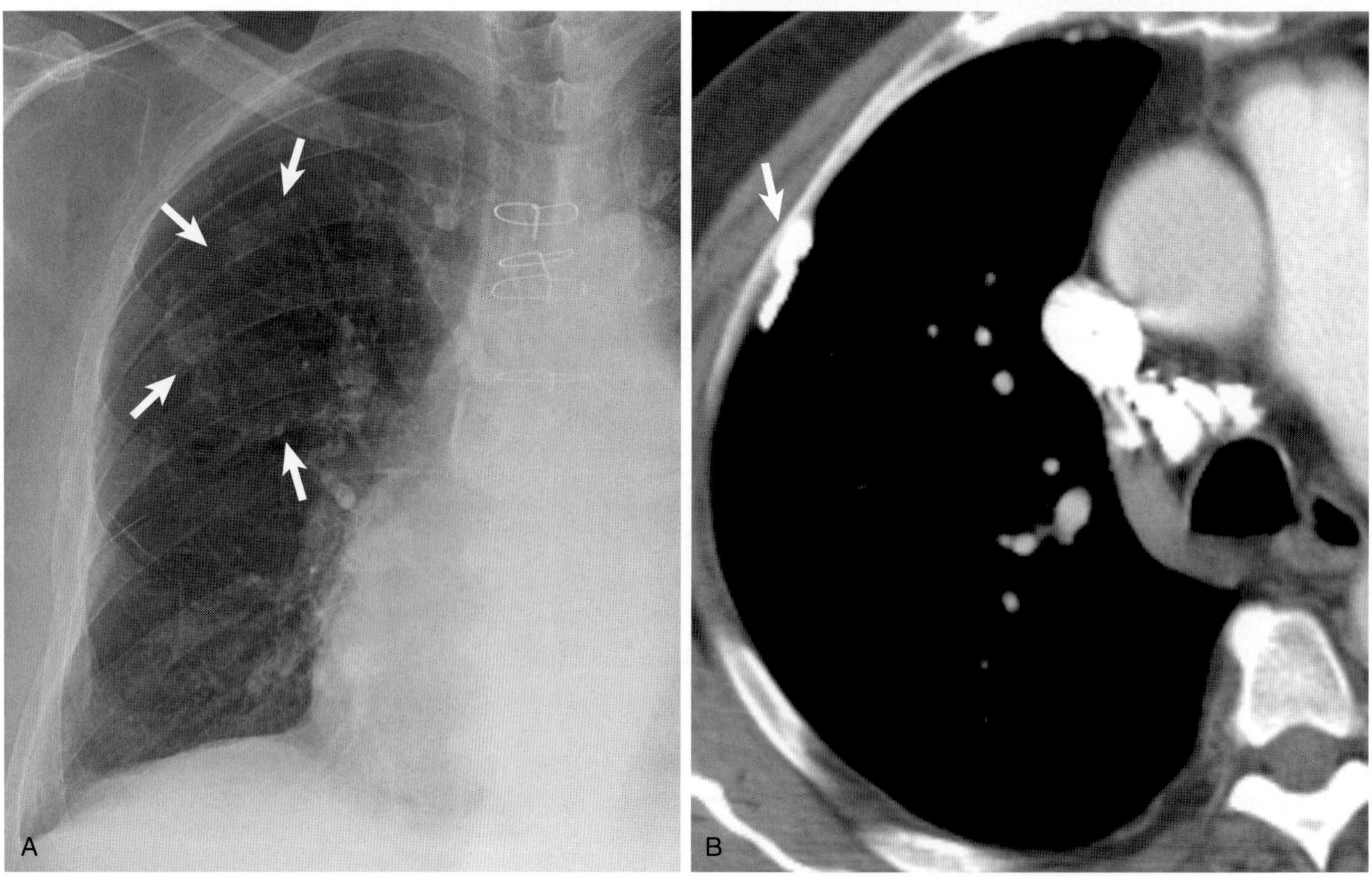

Fig. 73.10 Unilateral calcified pleural plaque. (A) Posteroanterior chest radiograph shows an opacity with dense nodular edge *(arrows)*, consistent with the holly leaf sign. (B) Axial CT image confirms the presence of right calcified pleural plaque *(arrow)* and calcified right lower paratracheal lymph node likely related to prior granulomatous infection.

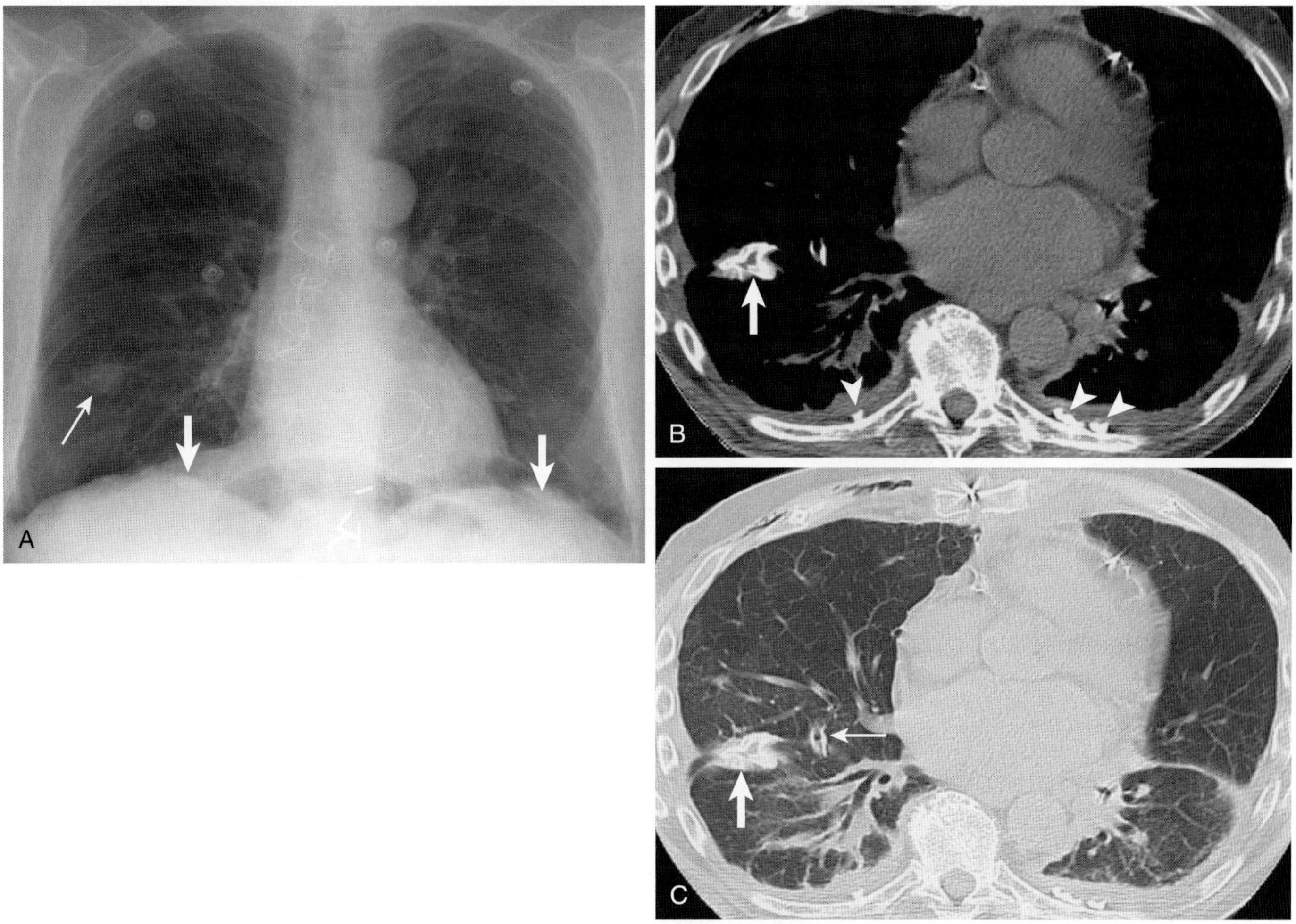

Fig. 73.11 Asbestos-related pleural plaques. (A) Posteroanterior chest radiograph demonstrates a nodular calcific opacity in the lower right hemithorax *(thin arrow),* in the expected location of the interlobar fissure. Calcified diaphragmatic pleural plaques are present bilaterally *(thick arrows),* in keeping with asbestos-related pleural disease. (B) CT image shows the dense calcification of the pleural plaque, located in the major fissure *(arrow).* This represents a visceral pleural plaque, which is unusual. Numerous calcified parietal pleural plaques are also present *(arrowheads).* (C) CT scan of the same level obtained with lung windows confirms the intrafissural location of the visceral pleural plaque *(arrow).* The patient had an unrelated posttraumatic pneumothorax being treated with chest tube drainage *(thin arrow).*

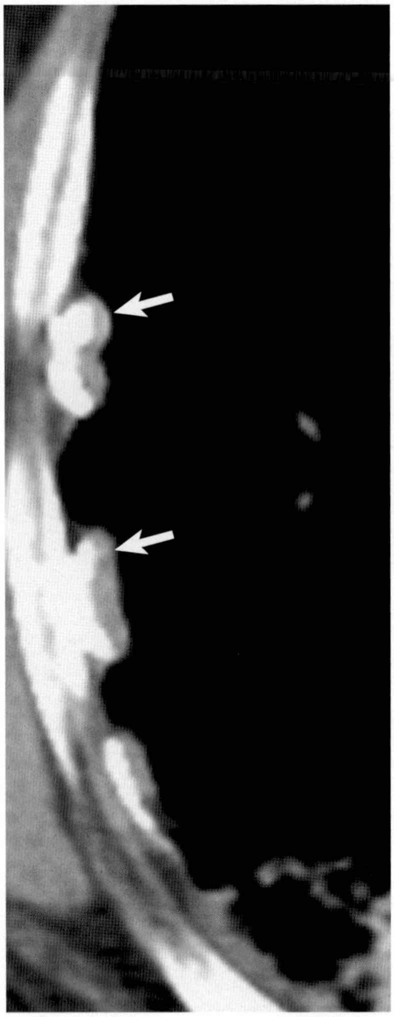

Fig. 73.12 Asbestos-related pleural plaques. CT image shows three right-sided pleural plaques with the typical well-defined discrete margins and thicker edges *(arrows)*.

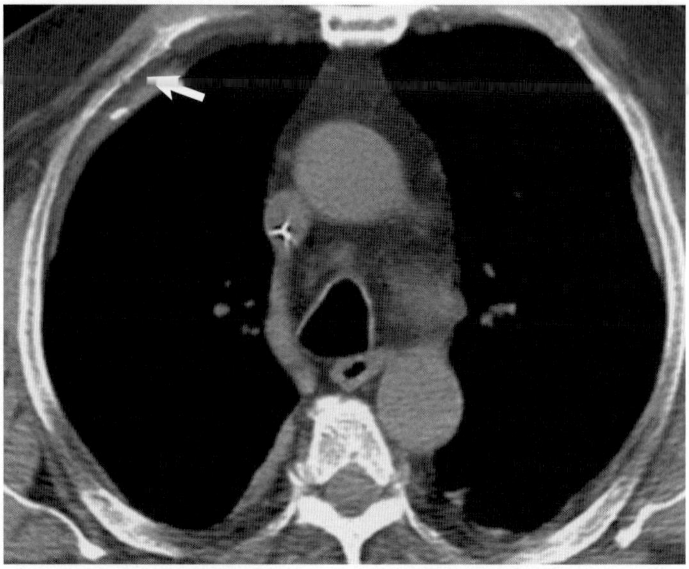

Fig. 73.13 Asbestos-related pleural plaques. CT image shows bilateral noncalcified pleural plaques along the left costal and right paravertebral pleura, with a small amount of calcification in the anterior right costal plaque. A thin layer of fat *(arrow)* separates the partly calcified plaque from the adjacent rib.

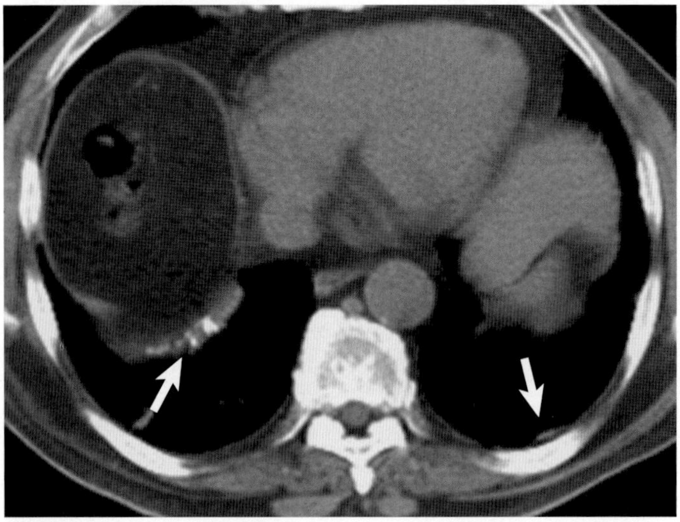

Fig. 73.14 Asbestos-related pleural plaques. CT image of the lower thorax shows the right diaphragmatic and left posterior pleural plaques *(arrows)*.

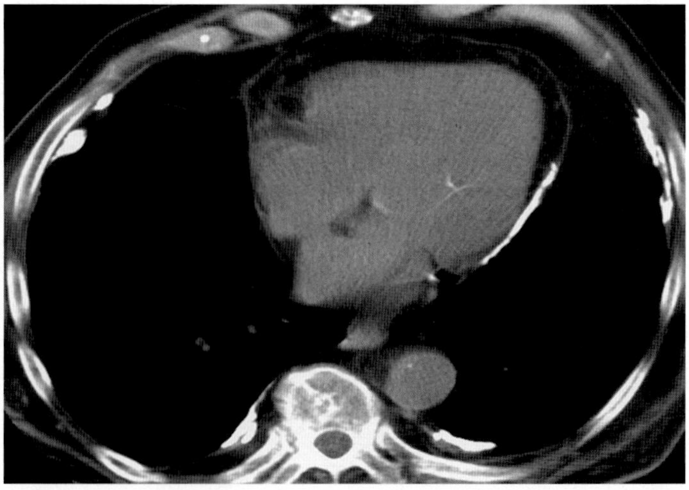

Fig. 73.15 Asbestos-related pleural plaques. CT image shows a calcified pericardial or mediastinal pleural plaque. Costal pleural plaques are also present.

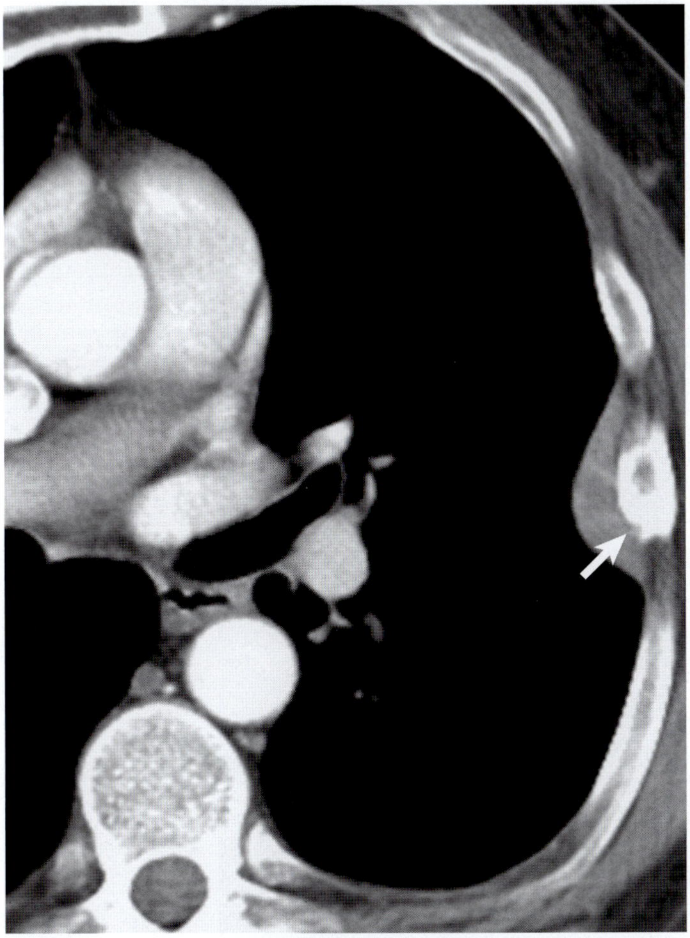

Fig. 73.16 Posttraumatic pleural plaque. CT image shows a single noncalcified pleural plaque adjacent to a healed rib fracture *(arrow)*. Biopsy finding was consistent with focal pleural fibrosis. The patient had sustained trauma 2 years previously.

POSITRON EMISSION TOMOGRAPHY–COMPUTED TOMOGRAPHY

Pleural plaques show no significant uptake of ^{18}F-fluorodeoxyglucose (FDG) on positron emission tomography (PET) imaging (Fig. 73.17).[58]

Differential Diagnosis

NORMAL ANATOMIC STRUCTURES

Because the combined thickness of the parietal and visceral pleura is approximately 0.2 mm, the pleura is not visible on the chest radiograph in the normal subject. With CT, a 1- to 2-mm-thick line of soft tissue attenuation is normally seen between the lung and chest wall between the inner edges of the ribs in the intercostal spaces. This line represents the combined thickness of the visceral pleura, normal pleural fluid, parietal pleura, endothoracic fascia, and innermost intercostal muscle.[53] The pleura and endothoracic fascia along the inner aspects of the ribs are too thin to be visible on the CT scan[53]; however, they may be identified as a thin, smooth line when there is increased extrapleural fat. The intercostal veins should not be confused with the pleura (Fig. 73.18).

The innermost intercostal muscle (intercostales intimi) passes between the internal surfaces of adjacent ribs and is relatively thin; two muscles may be mistaken for pleural thickening. Anteriorly, the transversus thoracis muscle is usually visible on CT as it extends to the end of a rib or its costal cartilage to the lower sternum or xiphoid.[53] This muscle is a 1- to 2-mm-thick line inside the most medial aspect of the ribs and is found at the level of the heart, external to the internal mammary vessels (Fig. 73.19). It is usually found bilaterally, which along with its characteristic location, helps distinguish it from pleural plaques. Posteriorly, the subcostal muscles are thin and variable and extend from the inner aspect of the angle of the lower ribs, crossing one or two ribs and intercostal spaces, to the inner aspect of a rib below.[53]

TALC PLEURODESIS

After pleurodesis with talc instillation in the pleural space, linear and/or nodular hyperattenuating talc deposits can be seen along the pleural surface (Fig. 73.20).[59] The hyperdensity related to talc tends to be amorphous and of lower attenuation than calcium. Unlike pleural plaques, talc incites a strong inflammatory reaction and is, therefore, associated with marked FDG uptake on PET (see also Chapter 68).

THORACOLITHIASIS AND PLEURAL FIBRIN BODY

Thoracolithiasis or thoracolith, defined as a mobile calcified intrapleural loose body, is rare. These can range from 5 to 15 mm and contain homogeneous diffuse calcification (Fig. 73.21). Some of the patients with thoracolithiasis have concomitant imaging findings of old granulomatous disease.[60] Pleural fibrin body, also known as "pleural mouse" or "pleural loose body,"[61–64] has been reported to consist of hypocellular hyalinized collagen and can be calcified or noncalcified. The terms "thoracolithiasis" and "pleural fibrin body" have been used interchangeably by some authors,[65] although thoracolithiasis is usually used to refer to lesions that are entirely calcified. Both may be single or multiple and are round, oval, or irregularly shaped. They tend to occur near the basilar thorax and change in position in serial imaging examinations (see Fig. 73.21) and when viewed en face on chest radiography can simulate a parenchymal nodule. These lesions usually do not cause symptoms and are found incidentally on imaging.[60,65–67]

KEY POINTS: PLEURAL PLAQUES

- Focal soft tissue thickening of the pleura
- Incomplete border sign, holly leaf sign
- Best seen in profile on chest radiograph; difficult to see en face when not calcified
- Typical location: posterolateral, diaphragmatic, and pericardial parietal pleura; spare apices and costophrenic sulci
- Typically bilateral if caused by asbestos exposure; unilateral if related to prior hemothorax or infection
- Plaque calcification in approximately 15%, which is likely underestimated

Diffuse Pleural Fibrosis

Etiology, Prevalence, and Epidemiology

Thickening of the pleura usually occurs after an episode of pleuritis and almost always as a result of fibrosis of the visceral

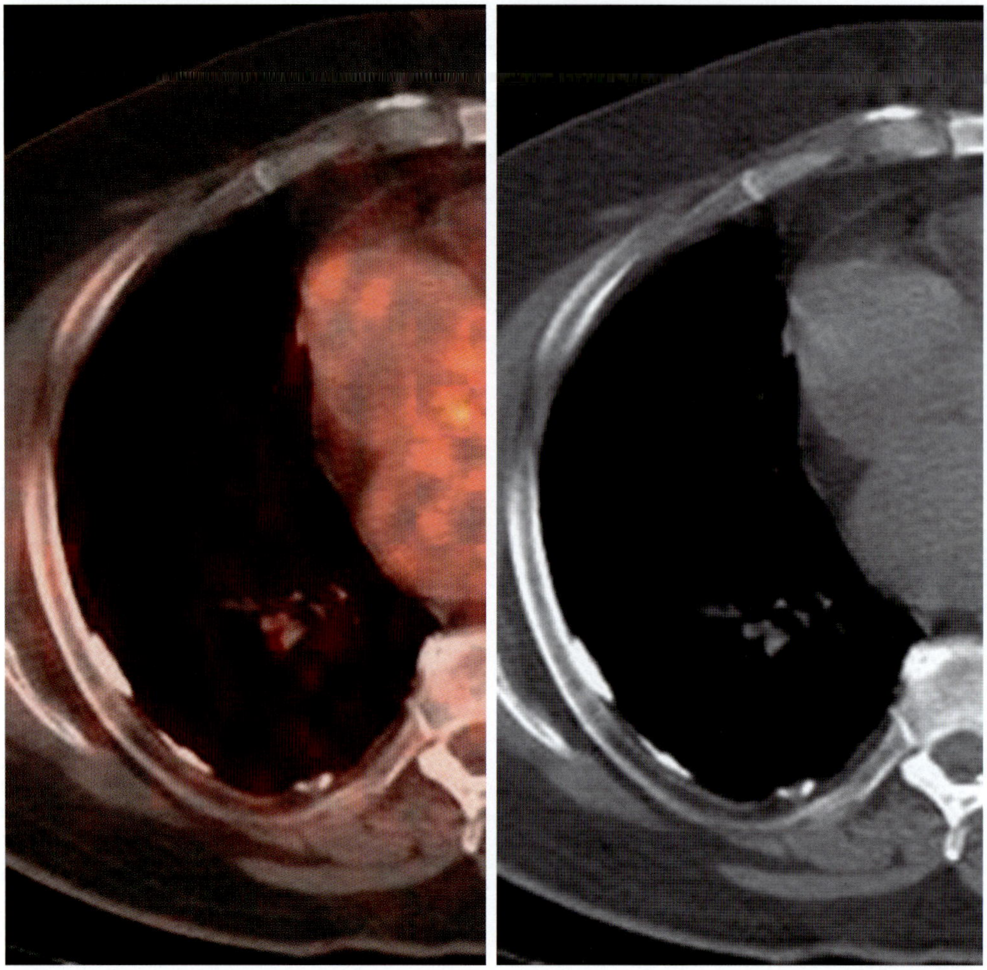

Fig. 73.17 Asbestos-related pleural disease. Composite image with fused fluorodeoxyglucose (FDG)–positron emission tomography–computed tomography scan *(left)* and axial CT scan *(right)* shows no significant FDG uptake by the right posterior pleural plaques.

TABLE 73.1 CAUSES OF DIFFUSE PLEURAL FIBROSIS

Causes	Unilateral	Bilateral	Incidence
Uremia	+	++	20%
Asbestos	++	+++	7%–13%[22]
Tuberculosis	++	+	Rare
Coronary artery bypass surgery	++ (left)	–	Unknown; higher with internal mammary artery grafts[109]
Hemothorax	++	+	1% (higher with hemopneumothorax or empyema[43])
Cryptogenic fibrosing pleuritis	–	+++	Rare, HLA-B44 positive[75]
Rheumatoid arthritis	++	+	38%–70%[70]
Systemic lupus erythematosus	++	+	30%[70]
Drugs	+	++	Unknown[76]

HLA, Human leukocyte antigen.

pleural surface with associated adhesions to the parietal pleura. This is different from the pleural plaque formation of asbestos exposure, which occurs almost exclusively along the parietal pleura.[10] Causes of diffuse pleural fibrosis include asbestos exposure,[22,68] systemic lupus erythematosus,[69] rheumatoid arthritis,[70] tuberculous pleurisy,[71] coronary artery bypass surgery,[72] hemothorax,[73] uremia,[74] cryptogenic fibrosing pleuritis (human leukocyte antigen [HLA]-B44 positive),[75] drugs,[76] and thoracic irradiation (Table 73.1).[77] More recently, visceral pleural thickening and fibrosis with pleural effusion have also been described in patients with immunoglobulin G4–related disease.[78,79]

Fibrothorax represents the most severe form of pleural fibrosis. Fibrothorax is dense fibrosis and fusion of the visceral and parietal pleura.[2] As a result, there is contracture of the involved hemithorax and reduced mobility of the lung and thoracic cage resulting from progressive fibrosis and fusion of the pleural membranes.

LUNG FUNCTION

Involvement of the visceral pleura through adherence or retractile fibrosis is responsible for the shrinking, folding, or incomplete inflation of the underlying lung parenchyma.[80] Patients with extensive pleural involvement can have significant restrictive impairment with no or only minimal interstitial lung disease. For any degree of pulmonary parenchymal disease, the lung function is more impaired when pleural thickening is present.[55] Patients with diffuse pleural thickening without asbestosis had significantly lower forced vital capacity and diffusing lung capacity for carbon monoxide (DLCO) than normal control subjects and those with confluent pleural plaques.[81] Multivariate analysis demonstrated that subjects with both diffuse pleural thickening and interstitial fibrosis have a significantly lower DLCO than those with interstitial fibrosis alone and those with diffuse pleural thickening alone.[82]

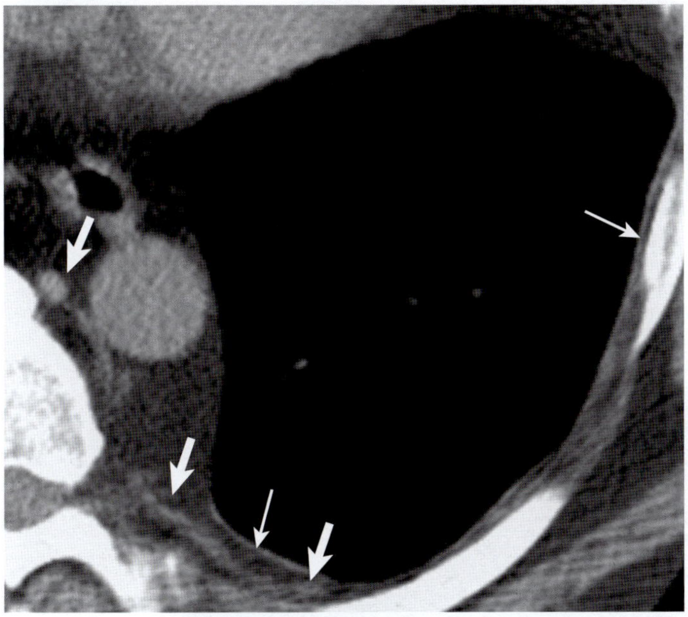

Fig. 73.18 Intercostal vein. CT scan through the left lower lobe demonstrates the thin line *(thin arrows)* along the inner aspect of the rib that represents the combined thickness of visceral pleura, normal pleural fluid, parietal pleura, endothoracic fascia, and innermost intercostal muscle. It should be less than 2 mm and is discontinuous on normal CT scans. The normal intercostal vein *(thick arrows)* coursing in the extrapleural fat is seen draining into the hemiazygos vein *(most medial thick arrow)*.

Pathophysiology

Diffuse pleural thickening results from thickening and fibrosis of the visceral pleura, with fusion to the parietal pleura, often over a wide area.[83] The development of pleural fibrosis follows severe pleural inflammation that is typically associated with an exudative pleural effusion.[84] A critical factor in pleural fibrosis is the formation of a fibrinous intrapleural matrix. This neomatrix results from a disorder in fibrin turnover, whereby fibrin is upregulated and fibrin dissolution is downregulated.[2] With asbestos exposure, many studies confirm that diffuse pleural thickening is preceded by a benign asbestos-related pleural effusion.[25,81,85,86]

Manifestations of the Disease

RADIOGRAPHY

On the chest radiograph diffuse pleural thickening is ill defined and irregular from all angles, whereas plaques are usually well defined.[87] Pleural thickening often extends over more than four rib interspaces.[87] The costophrenic angles are frequently partly or completely obliterated, particularly laterally.[81] The obliterated costophrenic sulcus is usually angulated rather than meniscus shaped, which distinguishes fibrosis from pleural effusion. Evidence of underlying parenchymal disease is usually seen in patients with previous tuberculosis or empyema (Fig. 73.22).

Two definitions have been used to characterize diffuse pleural thickening on posteroanterior chest radiographs: (1) pleural thickening associated with obliteration of the costophrenic angle and (2) pleural thickening at least 5 mm wide extending over more than one-quarter of the chest wall.[88] Agreement between readers was significantly better with use of the first definition.[88] The ILO has established a classification that allows epidemiologic comparison of radiographic pleural abnormalities by means of comparison with a standard set of radiographs.[49]

The latest 2011 edition of ILO guidelines states that diffuse pleural thickening extending up the lateral chest wall is recorded only in the presence of, and in continuity with, an obliterated costophrenic angle. A minimum width of about 3 mm is required for in-profile diffuse thickening to be considered present (Fig. 73.23).[89]

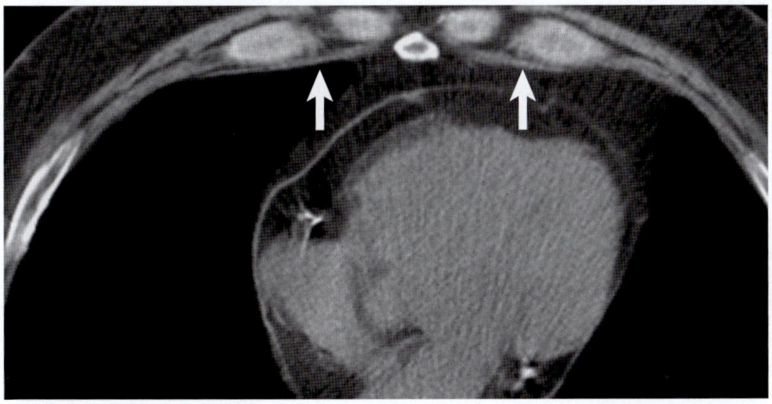

Fig. 73.19 Transversus thoracis muscle. CT image shows a 2-mm-thick line *(arrows)* inside the ribs, external to the internal mammary vessels, bilateral, at the level of the heart. This location is characteristic for the transversus thoracis muscle.

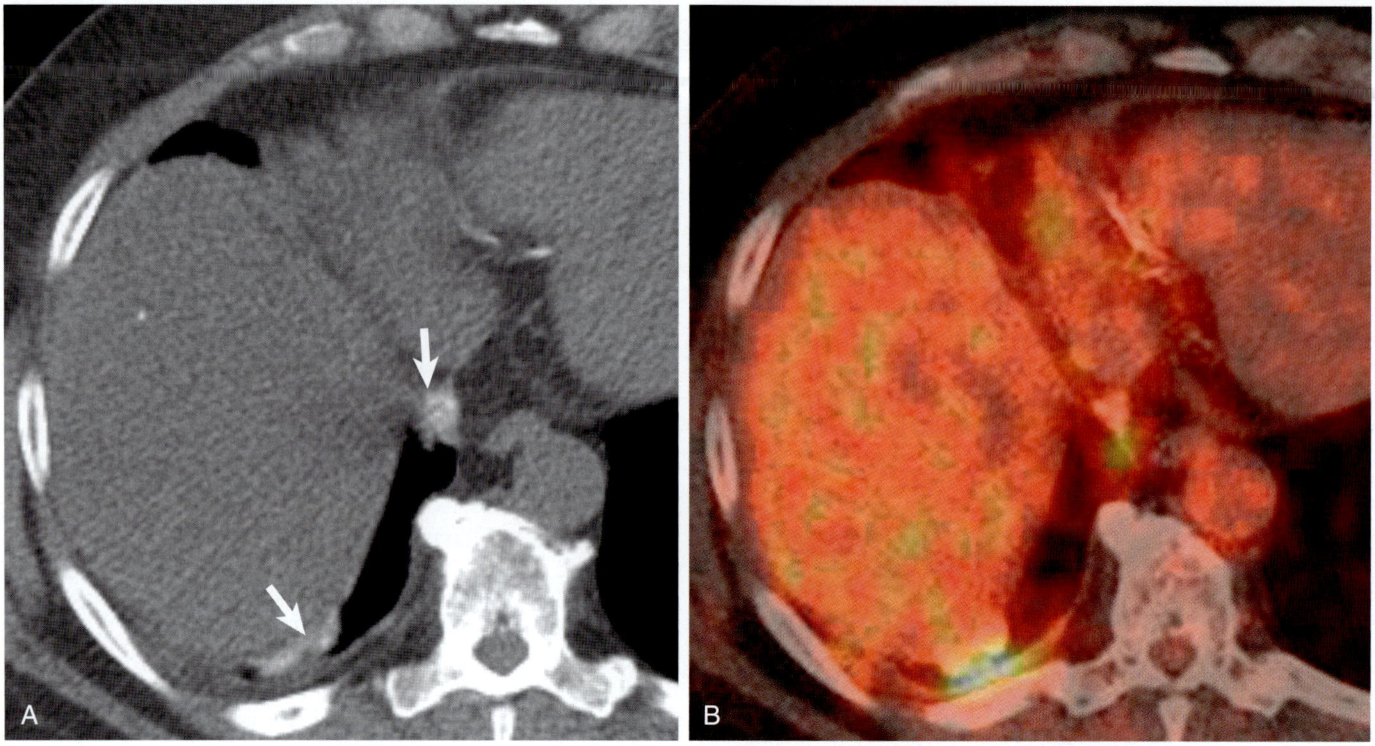

Fig. 73.20 Talc pleurodesis. (A) Noncontrast CT scan demonstrates hyperdense talc deposits *(arrows)* along the diaphragmatic and medial pleura. Talc deposits tend to be less dense than calcified pleural plaques. (B) Fused positron emission tomography–computed tomography image shows fluorodeoxyglucose avidity at the sites of talc deposits due to inflammatory reaction incited by talc.

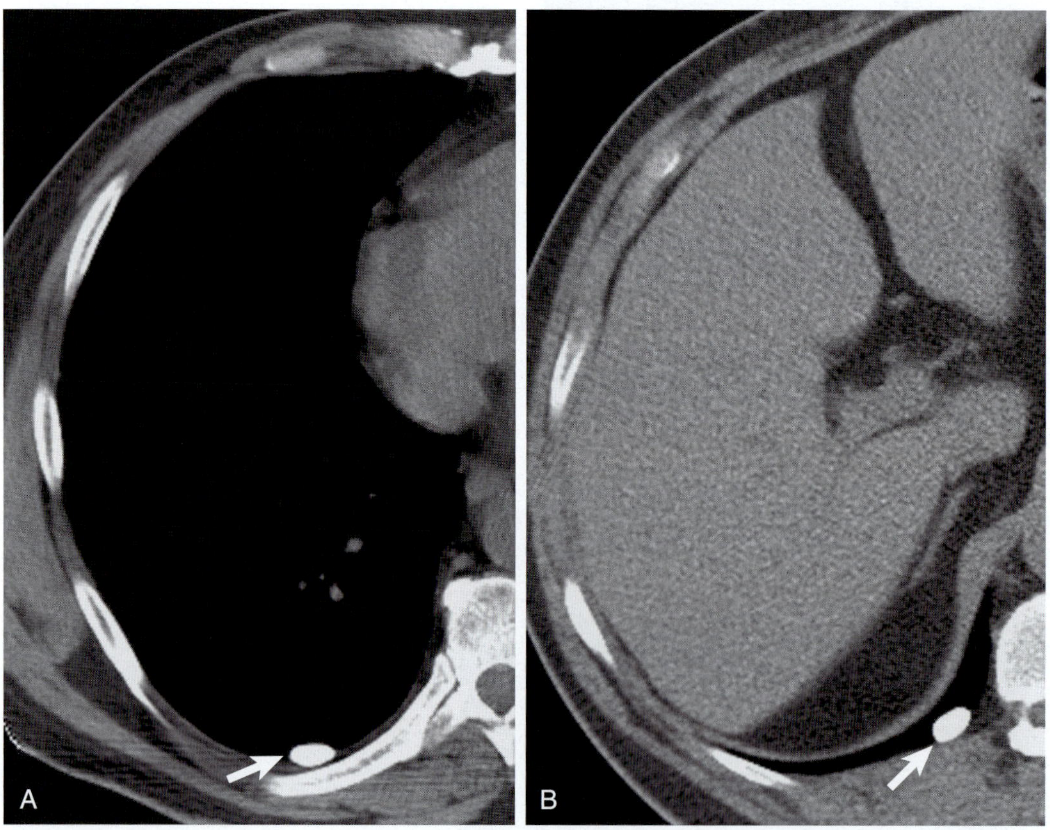

Fig. 73.21 Thoracolithiasis. (A) CT scan shows a solitary calcified lesion *(arrow)* that simulates a pleural plaque. (B) A follow-up CT scan shows that the solitary calcified lesion *(arrow)* has moved medially and inferiorly.

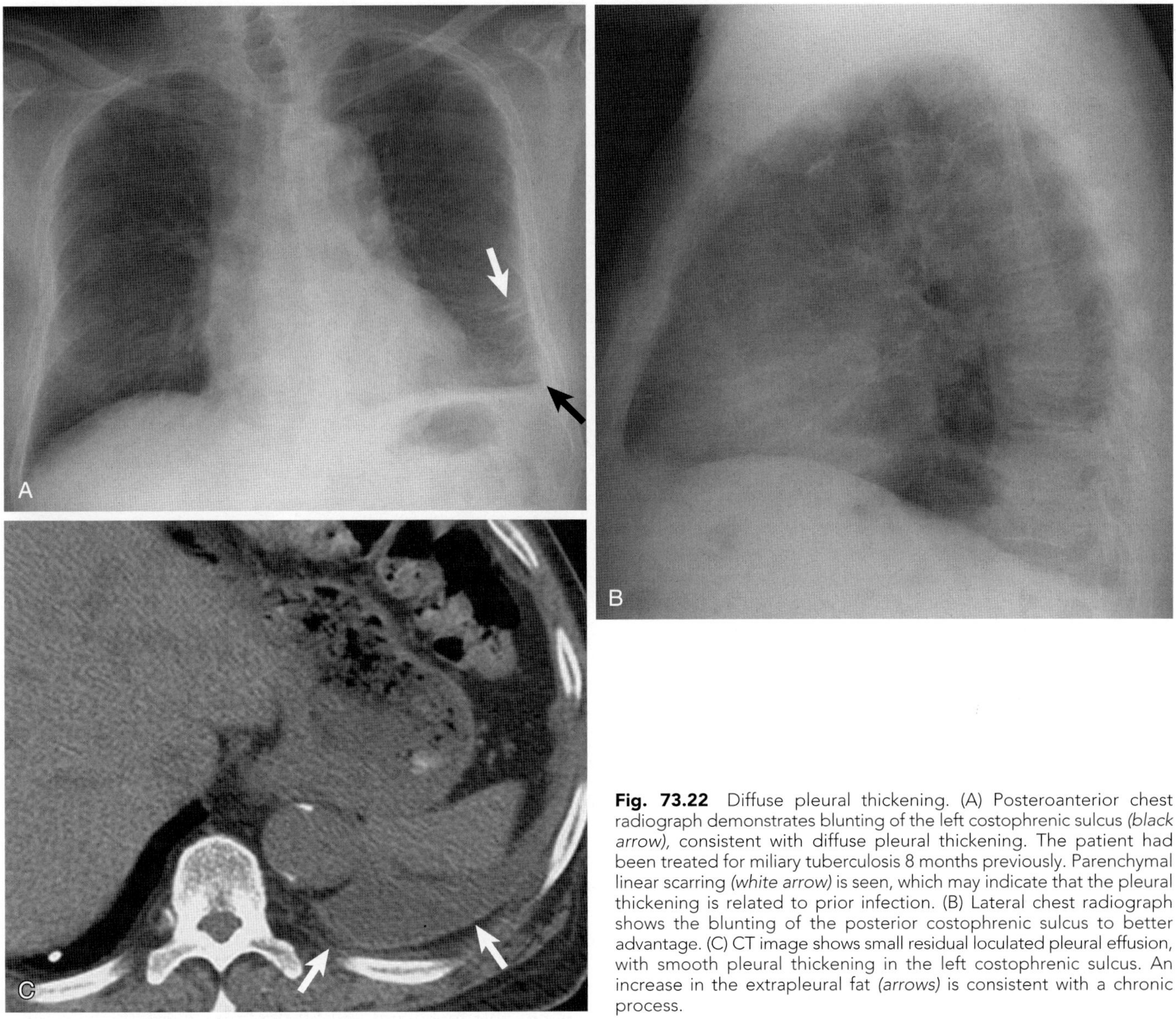

Fig. 73.22 Diffuse pleural thickening. (A) Posteroanterior chest radiograph demonstrates blunting of the left costophrenic sulcus *(black arrow)*, consistent with diffuse pleural thickening. The patient had been treated for miliary tuberculosis 8 months previously. Parenchymal linear scarring *(white arrow)* is seen, which may indicate that the pleural thickening is related to prior infection. (B) Lateral chest radiograph shows the blunting of the posterior costophrenic sulcus to better advantage. (C) CT image shows small residual loculated pleural effusion, with smooth pleural thickening in the left costophrenic sulcus. An increase in the extrapleural fat *(arrows)* is consistent with a chronic process.

In cases of fibrothorax the intercostal spaces narrow, the size of the ipsilateral hemithorax diminishes, and the mediastinum is displaced ipsilaterally (Fig. 73.24).[10] Fibrothorax is frequently associated with an accumulation of extrapleural fat.[35]

COMPUTED TOMOGRAPHY

Diffuse pleural thickening has been defined on CT as a continuous sheet of pleural thickening more than 5 cm wide, more than 8 cm in craniocaudal extent, and more than 3 mm thick.[90] Proliferation of the overlying extrapleural fat is commonly demonstrated, presumably drawn inward by pleural retraction (see Fig. 73.24).[35] Diffuse pleural thickening usually appears continuous, commonly involving the posterior and lateral surfaces of the lower hemithorax (Fig. 73.25).[35,91] Pleural thickening/fibrosis involves the mediastinal pleura very rarely, an important differentiating factor from malignant pleural thickening (Fig. 73.26).[34,45,92,93] Pure parietal pleural thickening is usually sharply defined on CT, whereas visceral pleural fibrosis is associated with fine fibrous strands extending into the underlying lung, giving a "blurred" or "fluffy" demarcation to the pleural process.[22]

Parenchymal bands and rounded atelectasis have been associated with diffuse visceral pleural fibrosis (Fig. 73.27) (see Chapter 61). When focal, visceral changes of pleural fibrosis appear on chest radiographs as small pleural-parenchymal fibrous strands known as crow's feet.[80] A CT study of asbestos-exposed workers revealed a strong association between visceral pleural thickening and parenchymal bands.[80]

MAGNETIC RESONANCE IMAGING

The morphologic features of pleural thickening are similar on MRI and CT. MRI and CT features most suggestive of a malignant cause are mediastinal pleural involvement, circumferential pleural thickening, nodularity, irregularity of pleural contour, and infiltration of the chest wall or diaphragm. Benign pleural thickening tends to be isointense or hypointense to intercostal muscles on T2-weighted and contrast-enhanced T1-weighted

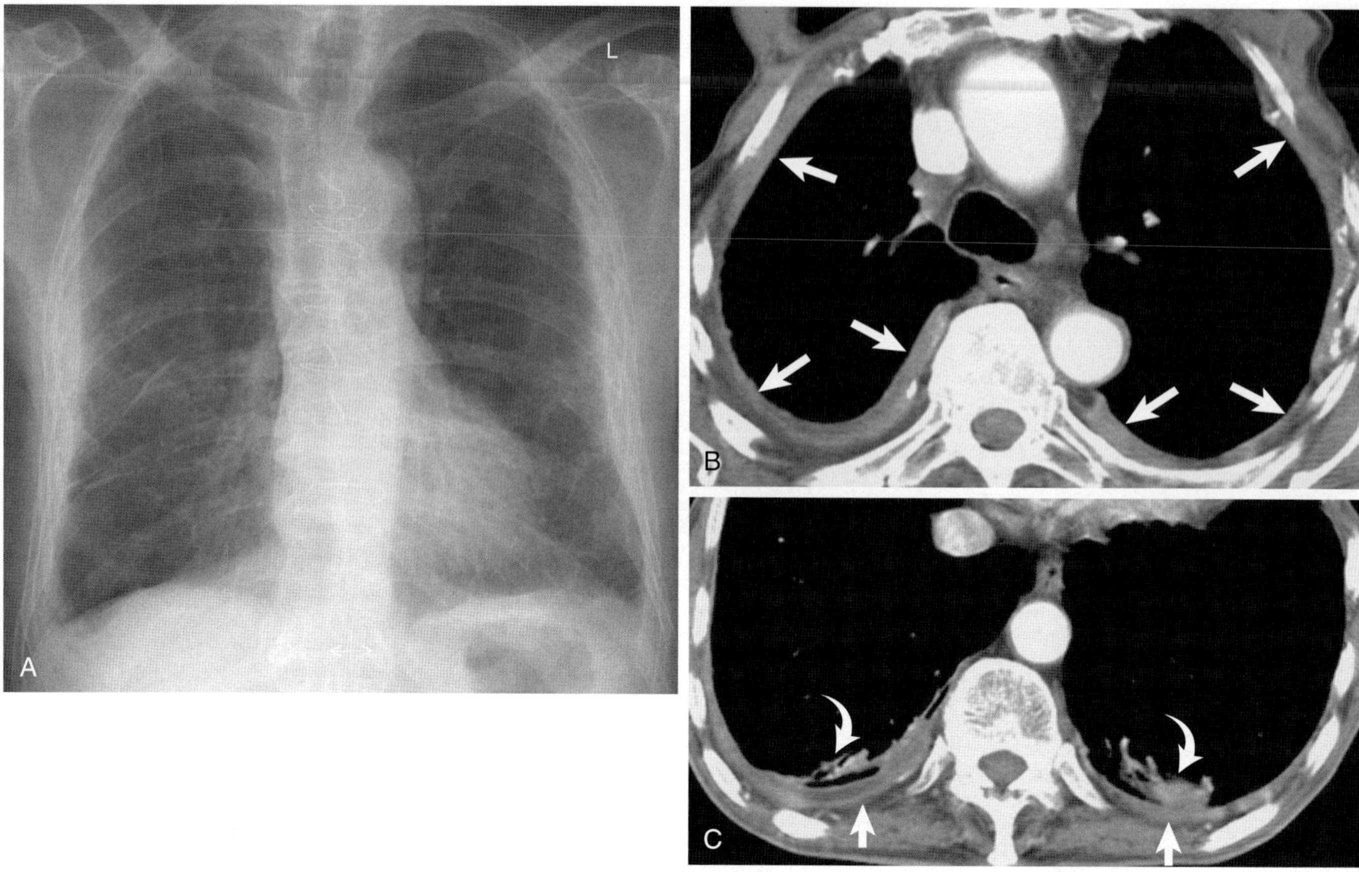

Fig. 73.23 Diffuse pleural thickening. (A) Posteroanterior chest radiograph in an asbestos-exposed man illustrates bilateral diffuse pleural thickening that is more than 50% of each hemithorax, is greater than 5-mm thick, and obliterates the costophrenic sulci. This meets the International Labour Organization criteria for bilateral diffuse pleural thickening. (B) Contrast-enhanced CT scan depicts extensive bilateral pleural thickening involving costal and paravertebral pleura *(arrows)* but sparing the mediastinal pleura. Focal pleural calcification is seen bilaterally. (C) CT lower in the hemithorax depicts bilateral rounded atelectasis *(curved arrows)* adjacent to pleural thickening *(straight arrows).*

images, whereas malignant pleural thickening tends to have hyperintense signal and more marked contrast enhancement.[94] The combination of morphologic features with signal intensity features on MRI usually allow correct identification of malignant pleural thickening (sensitivity of 100% and specificity of 93%).[94] Signal hypointensity with long repetition time (TR) sequences is a reliable predictive sign of benign pleural disease.[95]

POSITRON EMISSION TOMOGRAPHY–COMPUTED TOMOGRAPHY

A recent meta-analysis shows sensitivity of 95% and specificity of 82% of FDG-PET in the differential diagnosis between malignant and benign pleural lesions. Several studies have shown that most malignant pleural lesions exhibit significant, usually intense uptake of FDG (Fig. 73.28).[96–99] However, false-negative findings can occur with small malignant lesions or low-grade malignancies.

TRAPPED LUNG

Visceral pleural thickening and fibrosis may lead to lung entrapment, which results in restrictive physiology and associated dyspnea or even respiratory failure in severe cases. As the lung is not able to expand and fill the thoracic cavity, the resultant negative pressure of the pleural space leads to a transudative pleural effusion.[2] Trapped lung should be suspected after thoracentesis when there is an unexpected air lucency in the pleural space resulting from inability of the lung to fully expand.[100] The thickened visceral pleura can often be seen on postthoracentesis radiograph outlined by pleural and alveolar air.

IMAGING ALGORITHMS

Diffuse pleural thickening is usually first detected on the chest radiograph. Contrast-enhanced CT is the imaging modality of choice for further characterization of the extent and nature of pleural thickening and to distinguish benign from malignant causes. In those with benign-appearing diffuse pleural thickening, follow-up CT allows assessment of progression and development of malignancy.[101] FDG–PET-CT can be considered if malignancy is suspected. In the absence of FDG uptake, invasive procedures can be avoided, and follow-up CT would be preferred.[102] Confirmatory pleural biopsy is occasionally necessary despite negative PET-CT, particularly in the setting of concerning symptoms, such as chest wall pain or weight loss, to exclude malignancy.[103]

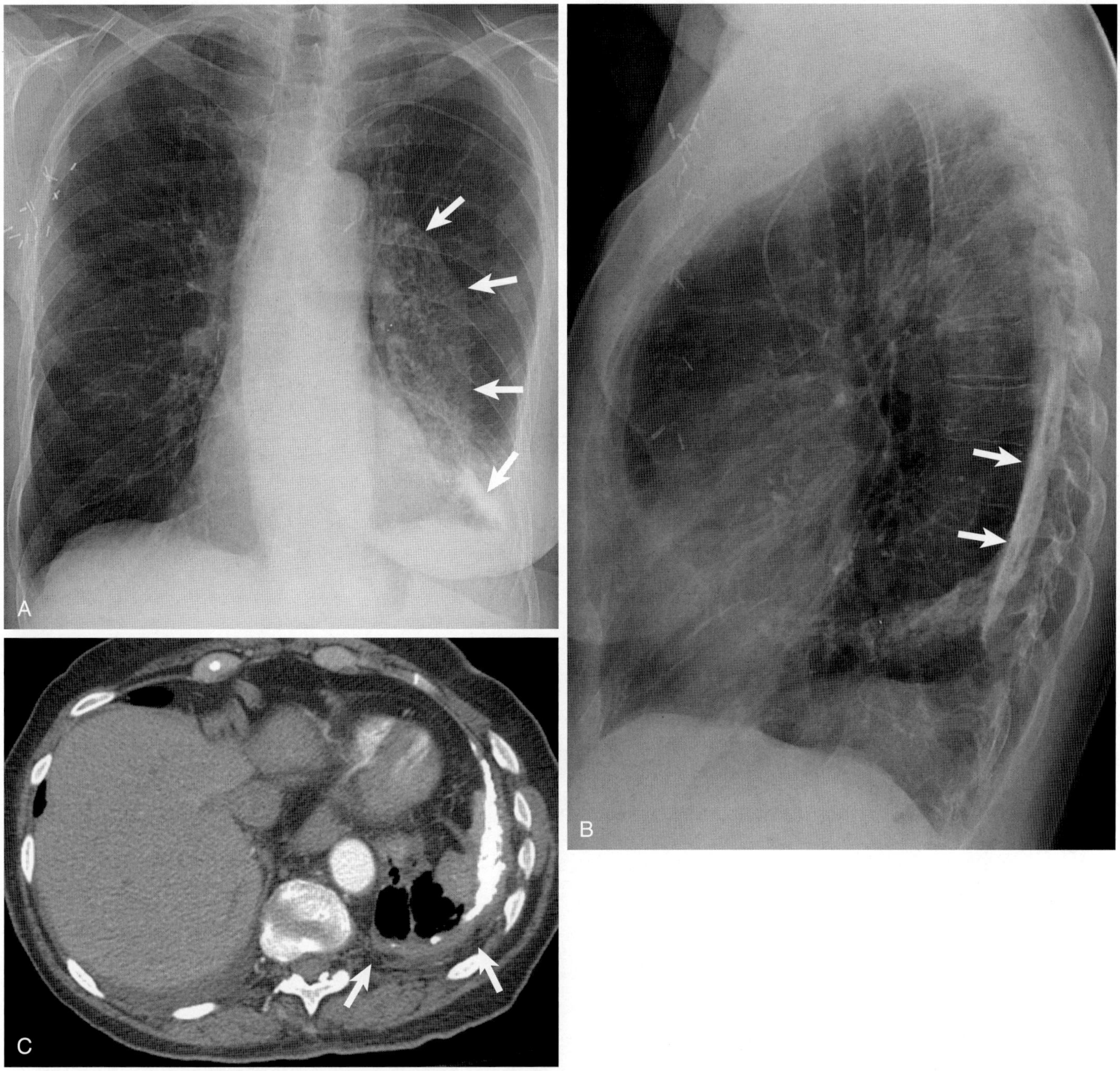

Fig. 73.24 Fibrothorax in patient with prior tuberculosis infection. (A) and (B) Posteroanterior and lateral chest radiographs show extensive left lower and posterior pleural calcification *(arrows)* associated with left lung volume loss. Note narrowed left intercostal spaces compared to the right. (C) Axial CT image shows left pleural thickening with dense calcification. Note extrapleural fat hypertrophy *(arrows),* presumably drawn inward by pleural retraction.

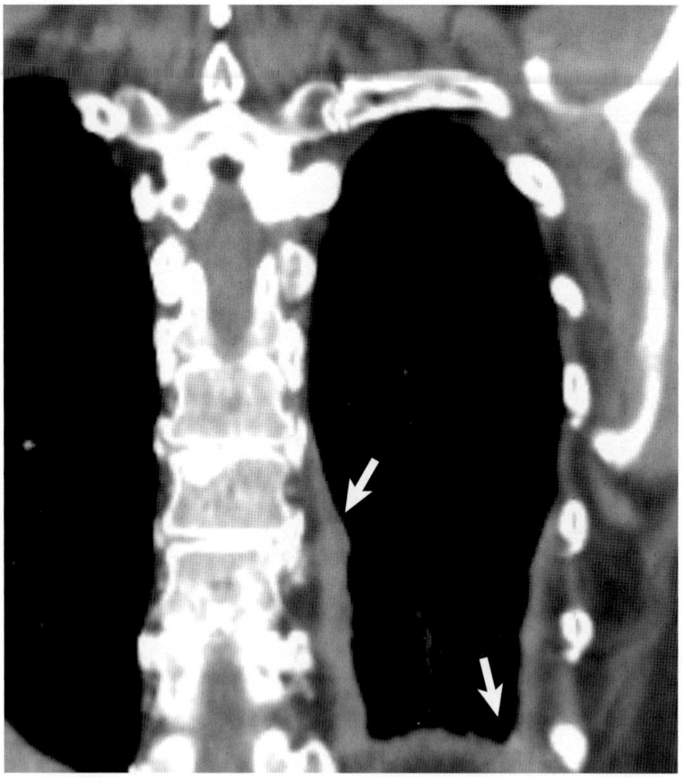

Fig. 73.25 Pleural thickening from prior hemothorax. Coronal reformatted CT image shows smooth pleural thickening *(arrows)* involving the mediastinal, diaphragmatic, and costal pleura.

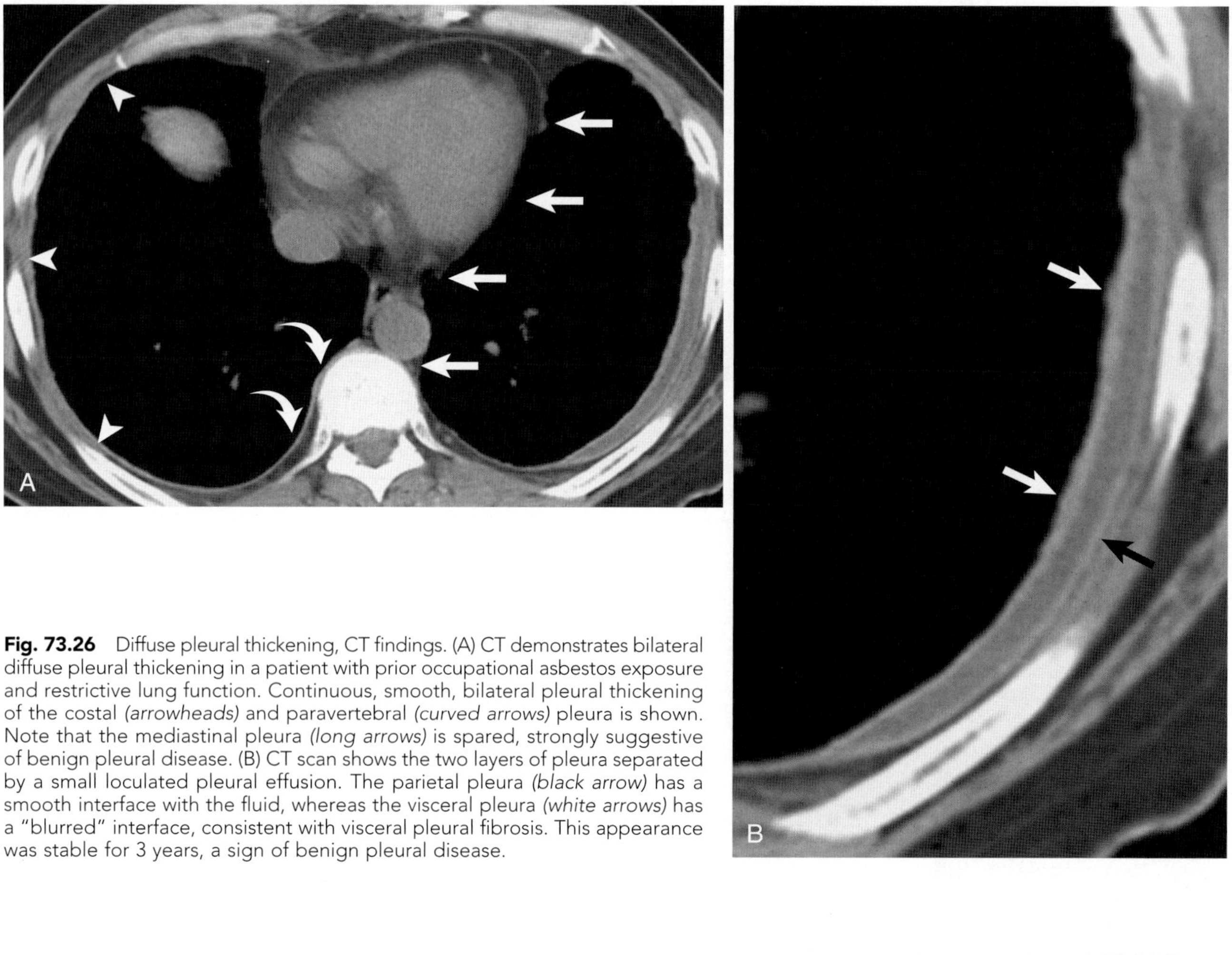

Fig. 73.26 Diffuse pleural thickening, CT findings. (A) CT demonstrates bilateral diffuse pleural thickening in a patient with prior occupational asbestos exposure and restrictive lung function. Continuous, smooth, bilateral pleural thickening of the costal *(arrowheads)* and paravertebral *(curved arrows)* pleura is shown. Note that the mediastinal pleura *(long arrows)* is spared, strongly suggestive of benign pleural disease. (B) CT scan shows the two layers of pleura separated by a small loculated pleural effusion. The parietal pleura *(black arrow)* has a smooth interface with the fluid, whereas the visceral pleura *(white arrows)* has a "blurred" interface, consistent with visceral pleural fibrosis. This appearance was stable for 3 years, a sign of benign pleural disease.

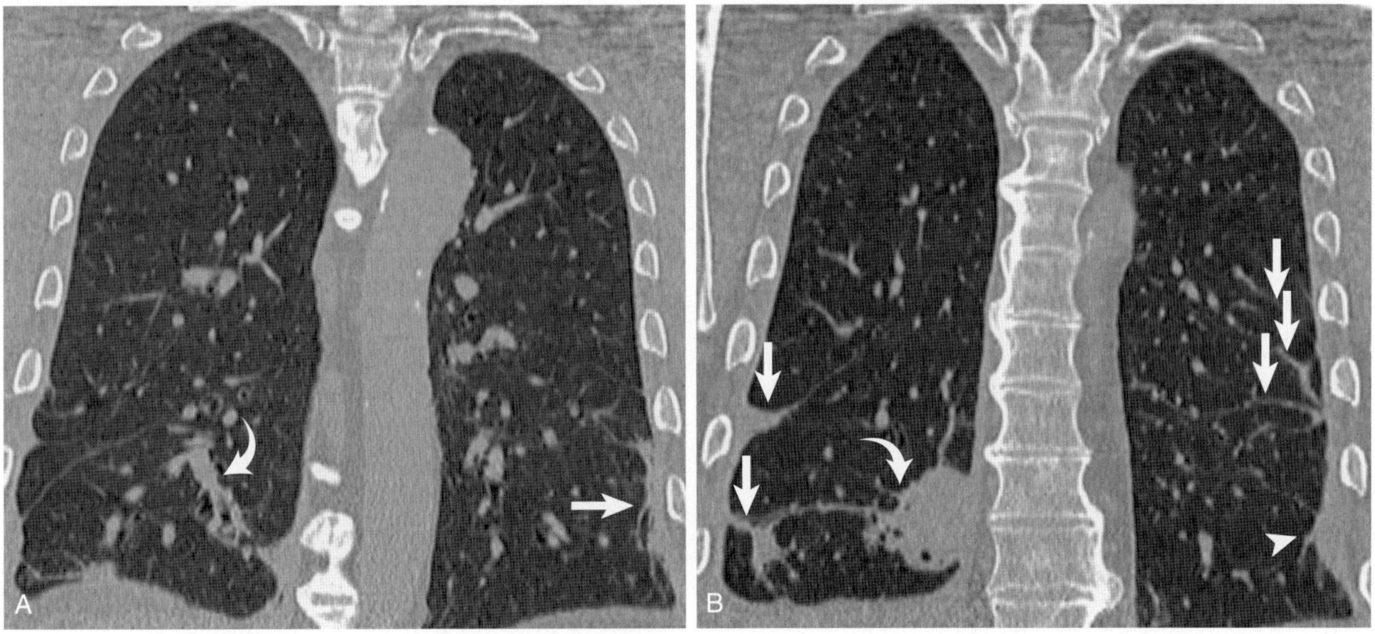

Fig. 73.27 Asbestos-related bilateral diffuse pleural thickening, parenchymal bands, and rounded atelectasis. (A) Coronal reformatted CT image demonstrates a curved band in the lower medial right lung *(curved arrow)* and subpleural atelectasis *(straight arrow)* in the left lower lobe. (B) Slightly more posterior reformatted CT image shows a rounded mass *(curved arrow)* abutting the pleura in the right lower lobe, consistent with rounded atelectasis. A smaller area of atelectasis *(arrowhead)* is seen in the left lower lobe. Also evident are parenchymal bands bilaterally *(straight arrows)*.

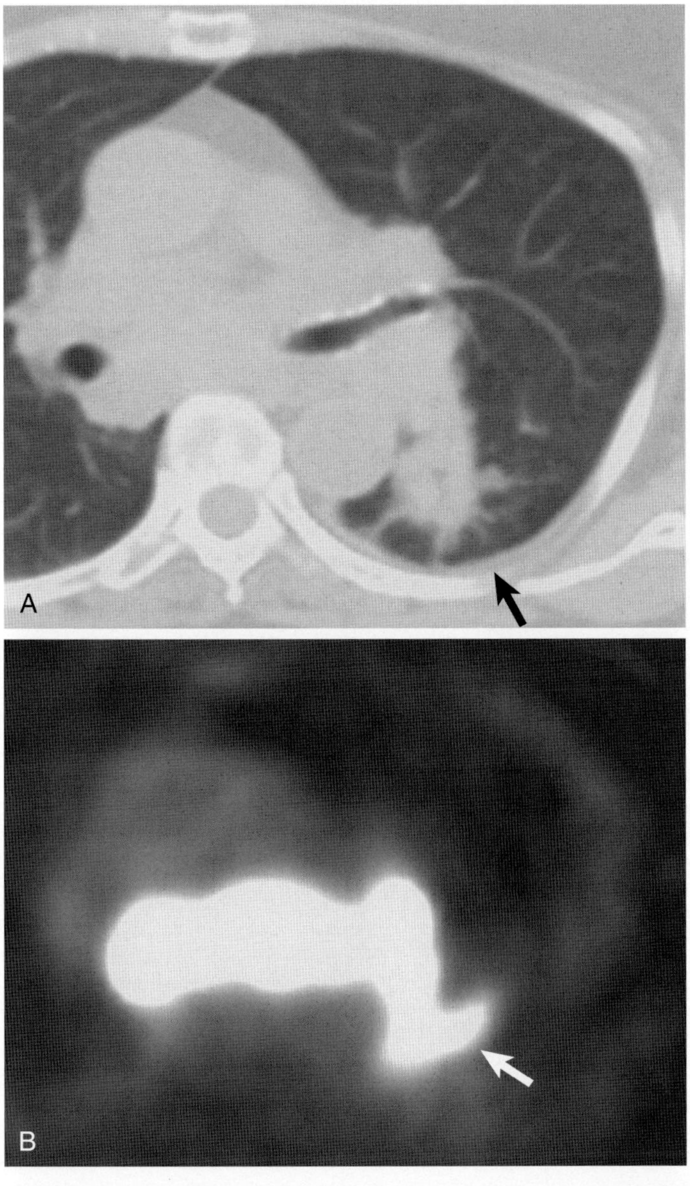

Fig. 73.28 Malignant pleural thickening best shown on fluorodeoxyglucose–positron emission tomography (FDG-PET). (A) Axial CT scan shows a left lower lobe spiculated mass with extensive left hilar and mediastinal lymph node metastases. Note subtle posterior left pleural thickening and/or effusion *(arrow)*. (B) FDG-PET scan shows extensive uptake of radiotracer in the left lung mass, mediastinal and hilar lymph nodes, and left posterior pleural thickening *(arrow)*. This is compatible with malignant pleural disease.

Synopsis of Treatment Options

SURGICAL

For patients with severe respiratory compromise of trapped lung, the only potentially effective treatment of fibrothorax or other forms of diffuse pleural thickening is decortication (removal of the fibrinous peel along the visceral pleura).[2] The timing of decortication is important because pleural thickening in some conditions does resolve. Therefore decortication is usually considered only in symptomatic patients, after the pleural thickening has been stable or progressive for a 6-month period.[2]

MEDICAL

Single case studies have described variable success with systemic and intrapleural corticosteroids for rheumatoid pleural fibrosis.[2] There was insufficient evidence to know whether steroids are effective in tuberculous pleural effusion.[104]

Differential Diagnosis

EXTRAPLEURAL FAT

On the chest radiograph the main differential diagnosis of diffuse pleural thickening is extrapleural fat, which typically occurs bilaterally and symmetrically, along the midlateral chest wall from the fourth to the eighth ribs (Fig. 73.29). There is often fat deposition along the pericardium and in the mediastinum. Extrapleural fat may also be differentiated on radiography as the "pseudo" pleural thickening gradually tapers, has indistinct edges, does not have adjacent parenchymal linear opacities, and usually does not extend into the costophrenic angles.

PLEURAL FLUID

Diffuse pleural thickening can be difficult to distinguish from pleural effusion, empyema, hemothorax, or chylothorax on radiography. Comparison with prior imaging can be helpful as

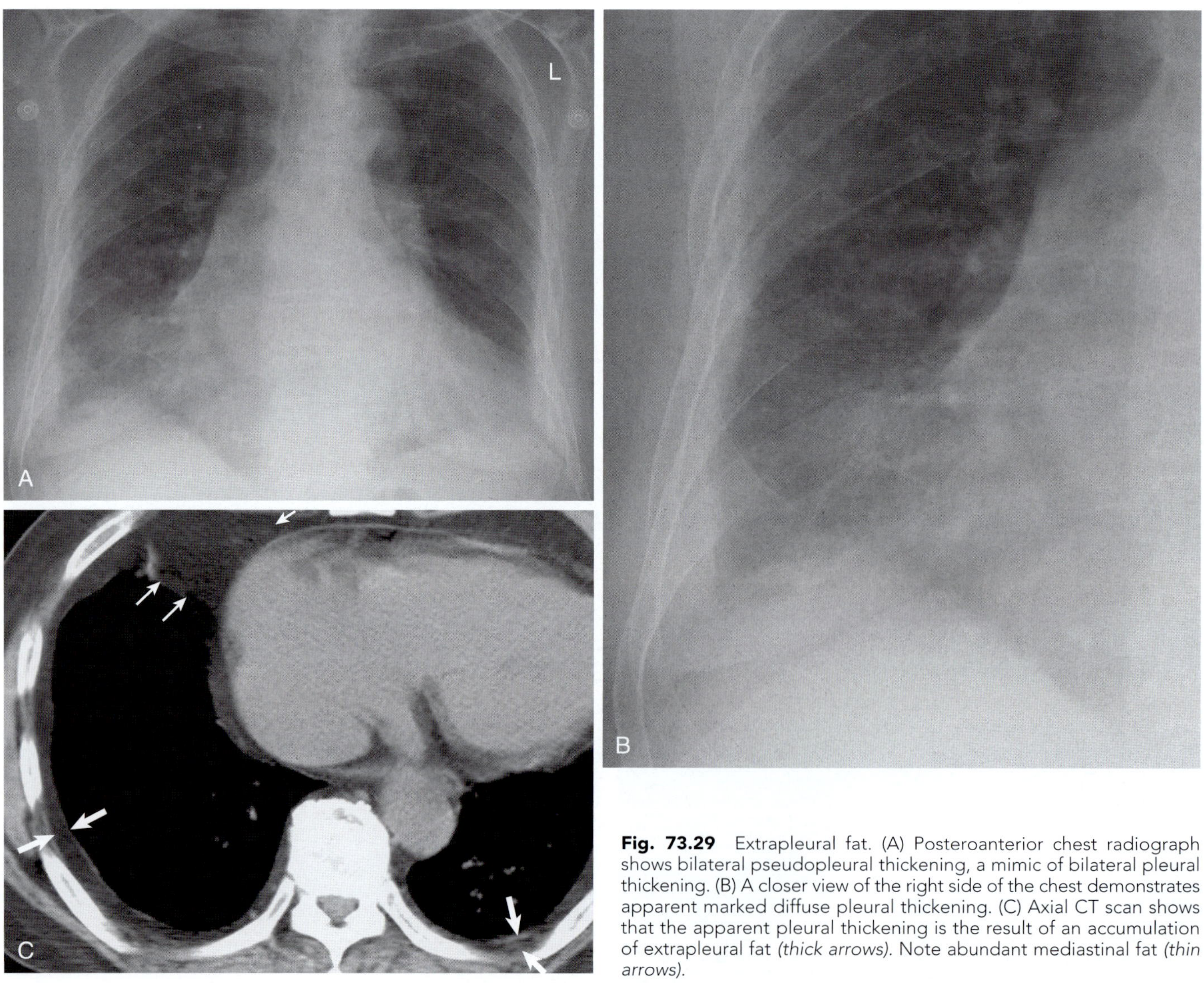

Fig. 73.29 Extrapleural fat. (A) Posteroanterior chest radiograph shows bilateral pseudopleural thickening, a mimic of bilateral pleural thickening. (B) A closer view of the right side of the chest demonstrates apparent marked diffuse pleural thickening. (C) Axial CT scan shows that the apparent pleural thickening is the result of an accumulation of extrapleural fat *(thick arrows)*. Note abundant mediastinal fat *(thin arrows)*.

TABLE 73.2 DISTINGUISHING FEATURES BETWEEN DIFFUSE PLEURAL THICKENING AND PLEURAL PLAQUES

	Diffuse Pleural Thickening	Pleural Plaques
Location	Visceral pleura	Parietal pleura
Involvement of costophrenic angle	Often	No
Borders	Ill-defined, irregular	Well-defined, discrete
Involvement of interlobar fissures	Typical	Rare
Loss of lung function	Typical	No

diffuse pleural thickening is a chronic process, whereas pleural fluid often develops or increases more acutely. CT allows differentiation of soft tissue attenuation of pleural fibrosis from various causes of pleural fluid accumulation.

PLEURAL PLAQUES

Plaques typically spare the costophrenic sulci and apices. Diffuse pleural thickening is ill defined and irregular, whereas plaques have well-defined borders. Pleural thickening tends to have tapering edges, whereas plaques often have raised margins. Plaques rarely extend over more than four rib interspaces (Table 73.2).[27,87]

ERDHEIM-CHESTER DISEASE

Erdheim-Chester disease is a non–Langerhans-cell histiocytosis caused by infiltration of various organs by foamy lipid-laden histiocytes (see Chapter 38). Most patients with Erdheim-Chester disease have symmetric long bone sclerosis. The disease is associated with symmetric, circumferential pleural thickening or effusion,[105,106] whereas diffuse pleural fibrosis is usually unilateral and spares the mediastinal pleura. Other findings of Erdheim-Chester disease include pericardial thickening, perirenal soft tissue thickening, and smooth pulmonary interlobular septal thickening.[107]

DIFFUSE PULMONARY LYMPHANGIOMATOSIS

A rare disorder with proliferation and dilatation of lymphatic channels in the pleura, interlobular septa, and mediastinum, diffuse pulmonary lymphangiomatosis can cause diffuse pleural thickening. Unlike diffuse pleural fibrosis, this entity affects young patients and is usually associated with thickening of interlobular septa and peribronchovascular interstitium and increased attenuation of mediastinal fat.[106,108]

MALIGNANT PLEURAL DISEASE

Mesothelioma and metastatic pleural disease may simulate benign diffuse pleural thickening. The study reported by Leung and colleagues[92] demonstrated that nodular, circumferential, and mediastinal pleural thickening were associated with a higher likelihood of malignant pleural disease; so in the presence of one or more of these characteristics, there should be a high level of suspicion for malignant pleural disease. FDG–PET-CT is useful in distinguishing benign from malignant pleural thickening as previously discussed.

KEY POINTS: DIFFUSE PLEURAL FIBROSIS

- Blunting of costophrenic sulci
- Continuous pleural thickening >5 cm wide, 8 cm in height, 3 mm thick
- Frequent accumulation of extrapleural fat
- Typically located along posterolateral hemithorax
- Often bilateral with asbestos exposure
- If unilateral, more likely from infection, hemothorax, connective tissue disease
- Uncommonly calcifies
- Often associated with parenchymal bands and rounded atelectasis

SUGGESTED READINGS

Downer NJ, Ali NJ, Au-Yong IT. Investigating pleural thickening. *Br Med J*. 2013;346:e8376.

Huggins JT, Sahn SA. Causes and management of pleural fibrosis. *Respirology*. 2004;9:441–447.

Kim JS, Lynch DA. Imaging of nonmalignant occupational lung disease. *J Thorac Imaging*. 2002;17:238–260.

Myers R. Asbestos-related pleural disease. *Curr Opin Pulm Med*. 2012;18(4):377–381.

Qureshi NR, Gleeson FV. Imaging of pleural disease. *Clin Chest Med*. 2006;27:193–213.

Walker CM, Takasugi JE, Chung JH, Reddy GP, Done SL, Pipavath SN, Schmidt RA, Godwin JD 2nd. Tumorlike conditions of the pleura. *Radiographics*. 2012;32(4):971–985.

The full reference list for this chapter is available at ExpertConsult.com.

74 Pleural Neoplasms

BRETT W. CARTER | PATRICIA M. DE GROOT | JEAN M. SEELY

The pleura may be affected by primary neoplasms or become involved by secondary spread of intrathoracic or extrathoracic tumors. Primary pleural tumors account for approximately 10% of all pleural neoplasms, the most common of which include malignant pleural mesothelioma (MPM) and solitary fibrous tumor. Other primary neoplasms include lymphoma, lipomatous tumors such as lipoma and liposarcoma, synovial sarcoma, and vascular sarcomas such as epithelioid hemangioendothelioma. Secondary neoplasms account for approximately 90% of pleural tumors and include metastatic disease and lymphoma.[1] In this chapter we discuss the etiology, clinical presentation, and imaging of these neoplasms, with specific attention given to their appearance on computed tomography (CT), magnetic resonance imaging (MRI), and fluorodeoxyglucose (FDG)–positron emission tomography (PET)-CT.

Malignant Pleural Mesothelioma

ETIOLOGY, PREVALENCE, AND EPIDEMIOLOGY

Malignant mesothelioma (MPM) is an uncommon, but increasingly recognized, neoplasm derived from mesothelial cells of the pleura, pericardium, peritoneum, or tunica vaginalis of the testis[2]; rare cases apparently derived from mediastinal mesothelial cysts have been reported.[3] Mesothelioma is the most common primary malignant neoplasm of the pleura, and it has importance not only because of its poor prognosis but also because of its impact on litigation and worker's compensation related to occupational asbestos exposure.[4]

In North America and Europe mesothelioma is estimated to account for 20 deaths per million men per year.[5] In Europe the cancer incidence is expected to peak between 2010 and 2030, despite regulatory restrictions adopted during the 1980s and 1990s, and there are 2000 to 3000 new cases per year reported in the United States.[6,7] Epidemiologic data suggest that the incidence of mesothelioma has already peaked in the United States.[8] In Israel the incidence increased sevenfold from 1.17 per million per year from 1978 to 1980 to 8.5 per million per year from 1993 to 1996.[9] Mesothelioma incidence rates have increased progressively in New Zealand since the 1960s and reached 25 per million for men in 1995.[10] In Japan analyses predict that there will be about 100,000 deaths caused by pleural mesothelioma in the next 40 years.[11] Despite the ban on asbestos use in Western countries, asbestos is still being used in many developing countries.[12] Mesothelioma occurs in both men and women, but overall the incidence is much higher in men. In Denmark, for example, the incidence rate of mesothelioma was 1.33 per 100,000 person-years from 1983 to 1987 among men and 0.51 from 1973 to 1977 among women.[13] The sex predominance is largely related to the increased likelihood of occupational asbestos exposure in men. The industries with the highest risks of mesothelioma are construction and ship repair, asbestos industry, and manufacture of metal construction materials; the occupations at highest risk are plumbers, pipe fitters, and sheet-metal workers. The mean age at diagnosis is 63 years.[4,14] It is estimated that only 2% to 5% of tumors appear in childhood or adolescence.[15]

ASBESTOS

There is strong evidence that more than 80% of mesotheliomas are related to the carcinogenic effect of asbestos. However, only approximately 10% of those with asbestos exposure develop mesothelioma.[16] Even minimal exposure to asbestos may result in mesothelioma. Exposure history may be difficult to obtain but can be confirmed by detection of asbestos fibers in the lung.[17] For example, exposure may occur by living in the household of an asbestos worker and coming into contact with fibers brought home on his or her body or clothing.[18] Most exposure to asbestos is by occupation, with the exception of environmental exposure in areas of Greece, Turkey, and New Caledonia, where tremolite exists naturally in the soil in substantial quantities and is used by villagers to whitewash their homes.[19,20] There is a latency period of 35 to 40 years from time of exposure to development of mesothelioma. Of interest, in the environmental exposure to asbestos in Turkey, a longer latency period of 55 years has been observed.[19] A few cases have been reported after shorter latency periods, but this may be related to earlier unobserved exposures to asbestos.[21]

The principal forms of asbestos include chrysotile, crocidolite, amosite, tremolite, actinolite, and anthophyllite. All but chrysotile (serpentine form) are classified as amphiboles, which tend to have a thin, needle-like appearance. Asbestos is classified as a known human carcinogen by US state, federal, and international agencies, as well as by the World Health Organization.[22] The most carcinogenic fiber is crocidolite, also known as blue asbestos, but the other amphiboles are also associated with mesothelioma. The amphiboles are more likely to be associated with mesothelioma than is chrysotile, or white asbestos, which has a two to four times less potent risk of mesothelioma[22]; however, the risk for development of lung cancer is equipotent for all types of asbestos.[23,24] Chrysotile accounts for more than 99% of the world production of asbestos and commonly is contaminated with tremolite and other asbestos fibers.[22]

Asbestos was used in many household and building products in the past, as it is a fibrous silicate that is strong and flexible and does not burn. It was used in insulation, cement, textiles, and ceiling and floor tiles.[25] It is one of the most pervasive environmental hazards in the world, present in more than 3000 manufactured products. The first reported association of mesothelioma with asbestos was published in 1960 by Wagner and colleagues.[26] In 1989 the Environmental Protection Agency announced an asbestos ban and phaseout, but in 1990 the ban was overturned by a US Circuit Court of Appeals. Unfortunately, although the industrialized countries show a steady decrease in asbestos use, the poorer developing countries show an increase.[25] Because of this indiscriminate dispersal of asbestos in the human environment in past years, it is common to find hundreds of thousands to millions of fibers in human lungs. In general, those with heavy exposures have greater asbestos lung burdens. For example, lung tissue taken from patients with mesothelioma often contains more than a million fibers per gram of tissue.[27–29]

OTHER RISK FACTORS

Other fibrous materials, such as a fibrous zeolite and erionite, are strongly associated with mesothelioma, most notably in central Turkey.[20,30] There is also increased risk of mesothelioma with prior irradiation,[31] with chronic inflammation such as tuberculosis,[32] and in association with the simian virus SV40.[33] This virus was inadvertently transmitted to humans in contaminated poliovirus vaccines in the late 1950s and early 1960s. It is estimated that perhaps 10% to 20% of mesotheliomas may be accounted for by the SV40 virus.[34] It is found in 80% of patients with mesothelioma.[33] Hamster studies indicate that mineral fibers and SV40 are cocarcinogens, which may explain why lower amounts of asbestos are sufficient to cause mesothelioma in individuals infected with SV40.[35] There is also a familial occurrence of mesotheliomas in both asbestos- and erionite-exposed individuals, with mortality rates from mesothelioma as high as 50% in some villages.[36] Whereas cigarette smoking and asbestos are clearly synergistic in the etiology of lung cancer, there is no evidence of a similar role for tobacco in the etiology of mesothelioma.

CLINICAL PRESENTATION

The onset of MPM is often insidious, and the most common first symptoms are dyspnea and chest pain. Chest pain is often vague and may be referred to the shoulder but typically is nonpleuritic. A substantial number of patients, up to one-third in one series, may present with unilateral pleural effusion.[37] Patients may be asymptomatic, with the presence of the pleural effusion noted incidentally on physical examination or chest radiography. The effusion may be recurrent and present for more than 3 years before the onset of symptoms.[38] An unusual presentation is spontaneous pneumothorax, first described in association with MPM in 1956.[39] In a recent series as many as 10% of MPM cases (9 of 92) presented with a spontaneous pneumothorax.[40] As the disease progresses, patients may develop dry cough, fever, fatigue, and weight loss. Physical examination reveals finger clubbing; retraction and dullness on percussion of the chest are common. The patient may adapt to functioning with only one lung and remain fairly free of symptoms for months or even years, but eventually the tumor usually results in severe pain by invading the chest wall, intercostal nerves, mediastinum, spine, or abdomen. Late manifestations include ascites and chest wall deformity.[41] Median survival time from symptom onset is approximately 1 year, depending on initial stage and various prognostic factors.[41,42] Local invasion of the chest wall and surrounding structures can cause increasing pain that is difficult to palliate, as well as functional abnormalities, including dysphagia, superior vena cava syndrome, Horner syndrome, vocal cord paralysis, and diaphragmatic paralysis.[43] Death is rarely a result of metastatic disease; it is usually caused by infection or respiratory failure along with constitutional symptoms associated with progressive malignant disease.

PATHOLOGY

The mesothelial cell is pluripotent because of its origin from the mesoderm, which is formed from both ectodermal and endodermal layers. Various irritants can cause metaplastic changes of the epithelial type, even squamous metaplasia and connective tissue types.[44] There are three separate histologic subtypes of MPM: the epithelial (epithelioid), sarcomatous (sarcomatoid), and mixed (biphasic) type.[45] The epithelioid type is most common, accounting for approximately 50% to 60% of cases; the sarcomatoid, 35%; and the biphasic form, 15%. On cytologic examination the cells of most epithelioid MPMs are relatively monotonous. On occasion, cells have a foamy, clear, or signet-ring appearance.[46] Sarcomatoid forms resemble sarcomas, most commonly malignant fibrous histiocytoma, although forms resembling osteosarcoma and chondrosarcoma have been reported. Biphasic MPMs can show any combination of the patterns seen in either form.

At the time of surgery and on gross pathologic examination, the parietal pleura is involved to a greater degree than the visceral pleura, as the disease occurs initially on the parietal surface of the pleural mesothelium. The right hemithorax is involved more often than the left. Tumors may be focal or coalesce into sheet-like pleural masses. In the largest postmortem case series of patients with MPM, extrathoracic metastatic disease was present in 55% of cases.[47]

DIAGNOSIS

The histopathologic diagnosis of MPM can be difficult and may require the opinion of an expert pathologist. Common diagnostic dilemmas for the pathologist include differentiation between adenocarcinoma and tubulopapillary MPM, between reactive mesothelial hyperplasia and early MPM, and between desmoplastic MPM and benign pleuritis or pleural plaque. Use of immunohistochemistry stains by an experienced pathologist who has access to sufficient fresh and formalin-fixed tissue will optimize results. In difficult cases electron microscopy remains the gold standard. Epithelioid MPMs possess large numbers of desmosomes and long, slender, branching microvilli, whereas adenocarcinomas have fewer desmosomes and short, stubby, unbranched microvilli.[48] The special stains reported to be most useful include periodic acid–Schiff with diastase, hyaluronic acid, mucicarmine, carcinogenic embryonic antigen, Leu-M1,[49,50] and more recently calretinin and cytokeratin 5/6.[51]

The diagnosis of MPM can be established by means of thoracentesis with cytology, closed pleural biopsy, and open pleural biopsy by video-assisted thoracic surgery. However, the result of cytology is positive in only 30% to 35% of cases.[52] This diagnostic yield may be improved with the help of immunohistochemistry and electron microscopy.[51] Closed pleural needle biopsy also has a low yield, largely because the biopsy is done in a blinded fashion and may easily miss the tumor. It increases the yield of cytology by only 7% to 26%.[53,54] Video-assisted thoracic surgery or thoracoscopy has become the favored diagnostic procedure for suspected MPM; it has sensitivity of 91% to 98% but is a costly and invasive technique.[55,56] The procedure requires 24- to 36-hour admission to the hospital and has a low rate of major complications.[55,56] An important aspect of MPM is its propensity to spread along tracks of chest tubes, thoracoscopy trocars, and surgical incisions.[57] These implantation metastases are extremely painful and difficult to treat. Seeding along the track after video-assisted thoracoscopic surgery may occur in up to 50% of patients, whereas the highest reported incidence after image-guided biopsy is only 22%.[58] Image-guided needle biopsy has therefore been evaluated as a viable alternative to surgical diagnosis, with a high diagnostic accuracy.[59,60] It is essential that enough tissue be obtained to permit a reliable diagnosis; fine-needle aspiration biopsy technique is inadequate, but core-needle biopsy is diagnostic in up to 86% of cases.[61] Image-guided biopsy can be performed with ultrasonography, fluoroscopy, or CT; the operator must adequately visualize the tumor and obtain an optimal amount of tissue. In the presence of an effusion, larger samples with use of 16- to 20-gauge cutting needles may be obtained, as the risk of pneumothorax is low. Immunostaining allows a pathologic diagnosis of MPM to be made from a relatively small tissue sample, such as that provided by image-guided core needle biopsy.[62]

IMAGING

General Imaging Features

In general, the most common imaging manifestations of MPM include pleural effusion, pleural thickening with or without nodules/masses, ipsilateral volume loss, intrathoracic and extrathoracic lymphadenopathy, and metastatic disease. Findings related to asbestos-related pleural disease may also be seen. Although individual imaging findings may be nonspecific for MPM, the presence of one or more of these features should raise suspicion for MPM, especially in the appropriate clinical scenario.[63]

Radiography

Because of its widespread use and availability, the first modality to depict imaging abnormalities of MPM is often chest radiography. The appearance of MPM on chest radiography ranges from normal in early disease to complete opacification of a hemithorax. A unilateral pleural effusion is one of the most common manifestations and is present in 30% to 80% of patients (Fig. 74.1). Diffuse pleural thickening and pleural nodules/masses are seen in 60% and 45% to 60% of cases, respectively (Fig. 74.2).[64] Extension of tumor along the interlobar fissures may be identified. Encasement of the lung may produce volume loss, resulting in elevation of the ipsilateral hemidiaphragm, ipsilateral mediastinal shift, and narrowing of the intercostal spaces. Osseous or cartilaginous differentiation may produce regions of ossification or calcification in the tumor. An indistinct or "shaggy" cardiac silhouette or ill-defined diaphragmatic contours may be seen in the setting of asbestos-related pleural disease.

Intrathoracic lymphadenopathy may manifest as abnormal thickening of lines and stripes, and the normal mediastinal contours may be absent. Extrathoracic lymphadenopathy and intrathoracic and extrathoracic metastatic disease are better assessed with cross-sectional imaging.

Computed Tomography

CT allows differentiation between benign and malignant pleural disease in most cases. Leung and colleagues[65] studied 74 consecutive patients with diffuse pleural disease. Features that were helpful in distinguishing malignant from benign pleural disease were circumferential pleural thickening, nodular pleural thickening, parietal pleural thickening of more than 1 cm, and mediastinal pleural involvement, with specificities of 100%, 94%, 94%, and 88% and sensitivities of 41%, 51%, 36%, and 56%, respectively.

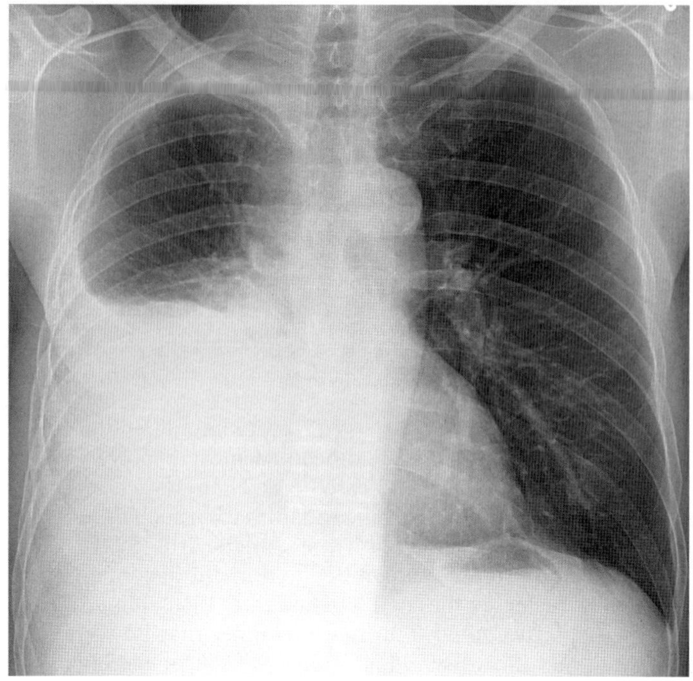

Fig. 74.1 Malignant pleural mesothelioma (MPM): radiographic features. Frontal chest radiograph demonstrates a large right pleural effusion. A unilateral pleural effusion is one of the most common manifestations of MPM and is present in 30%–80% of patients on chest radiography.

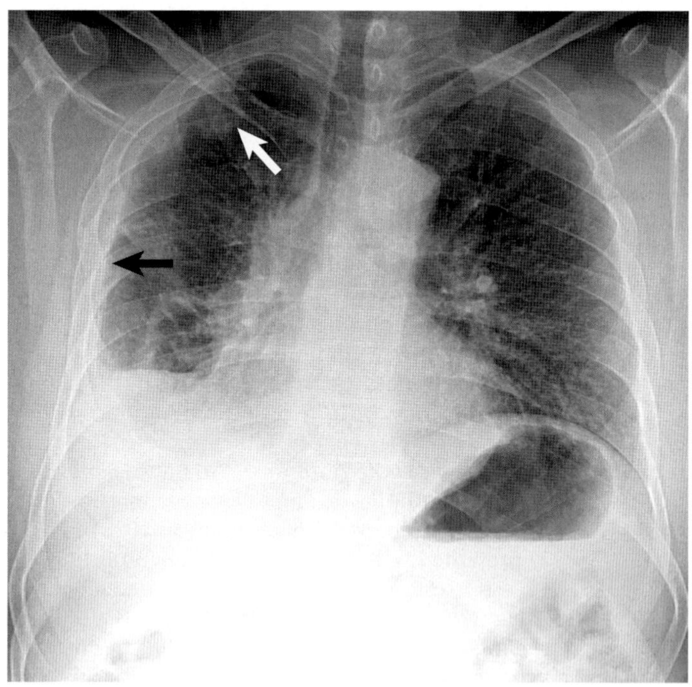

Fig. 74.2 Malignant pleural mesothelioma: radiographic features. Frontal chest radiograph demonstrates pleural thickening *(black arrow)* and focal pleural nodules *(white arrow)* in the right hemithorax.

Of 39 malignant cases, 28 were identified correctly by the presence of one or more of these criteria (sensitivity, 72%; specificity, 83%). Metintas and colleagues[66] reviewed the CT findings of 215 patients, 99 with MPM, 39 with metastatic pleural disease, and 77 with benign pleural disease. Sensitivities for circumferential thickening and mediastinal pleural involvement were 70% and 85%, respectively; pleural thickness of more than 1 cm was 47% sensitive and 64% specific.[66] Mediastinal pleural involvement had a lower specificity of 67%, probably explained by the large number of patients with tuberculous pleural infection (42% of benign pleural disease), which may also involve the mediastinal pleura.

CT is the imaging modality of choice to evaluate MPM as it reliably demonstrates the extent of tumor, lymphadenopathy, and intrathoracic and extrathoracic spread and is often sufficient for disease staging and treatment planning. With the administration of intravenous contrast material, malignant or inflammatory pleural disease enhances strongly, enabling differentiation between thickened pleura and effusions as well as atelectasis. Unenhanced CT also allows differentiation of thickened pleura from fluid, whereby the attenuation of the pleura is increased relative to that of the fluid. This may be accentuated by changing the window setting to a narrower window width, such as the liver window. With modern CT scanners, the use of narrow collimation (1 mm or less) allows high-quality multiplanar reconstructions and can be helpful in visualizing involvement of the interlobar fissures or extension below the diaphragm. A unilateral pleural effusion is seen in up to 74% of patients (Fig. 74.3). Pleural thickening can be nodular or lobular in configuration and is identified in 92% of cases (Fig. 74.4).[67] Pleural thickening that is nodular, circumferential, and greater than 1 cm in thickness is highly suggestive of malignant pleural disease, including MPM.[65] In cases of osseous or cartilaginous differentiation, ossification or calcification may be seen in regions of pleural abnormality, and the extent may be scattered or diffuse.[68] MPM with osseous or cartilaginous differentiation appears as large or punctate foci of mineralization within the tumor. Calcified pleural plaques are seen in 10% to 52% of cases and should not be mistaken for MPM with osseous or cartilaginous differentiation.[65,69,70] Calcification associated with pleural plaques is linear and can be identified on thickened plaques. There may be other features of asbestos exposure, such as rounded atelectasis and asbestosis in the lungs.

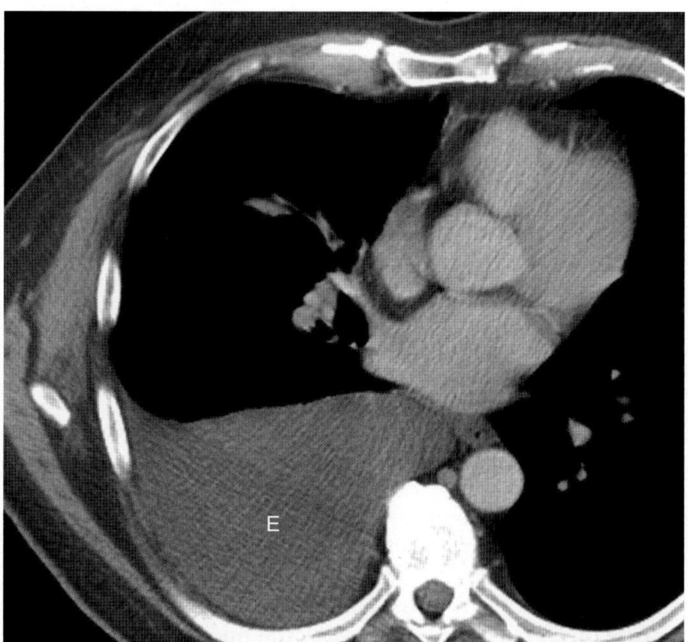

Fig. 74.3 Malignant pleural mesothelioma (MPM) manifesting as pleural effusion. Contrast-enhanced axial CT demonstrates a right pleural effusion (E). A unilateral pleural effusion is seen on CT in up to 74% of patients with MPM.

MPM may invade the mediastinum and result in the loss of fat and tissue planes between mediastinal structures. Invasion should also be suspected when MPM encases greater than 50% of the circumference of the trachea, esophagus, or other mediastinal structures (Fig. 74.5).[71] Involvement of the pericardium, which may be nontransmural or transmural, may produce pericardial effusion, pericardial thickening, pericardial nodules/masses, and/or infiltrating soft tissue (Fig. 74.6). Differentiating between nontransmural and transmural involvement may be difficult, although identification of epicardial fat suggests nontransmural involvement. A tumor that extends to the internal surface of the pericardium or involves the myocardium is consistent with transmural disease. Chest wall involvement is commonly seen at the site of previous intervention, including biopsy, drain, and surgical sites.[61] MPM that invades the chest wall may manifest as loss of normal extrapleural fat planes, invasion of intercostal muscles, rib displacement, or osseous destruction (Fig. 74.7). The accuracy of CT for transdiaphragmatic extension remains poor; however, the presence of a distinct fat plane between the inferior surface of the diaphragm and the adjacent abdominal organs is the most reliable indication that MPM is limited to the chest (Fig. 74.8). MPM with multifocal or diffuse invasion of the chest wall, invasion of the mediastinal structures, transmural pericardial disease, involvement of the contralateral pleura, transdiaphragmatic extension, or metastatic disease is typically considered unresectable.[71]

CT remains one of the primary methods for identifying lymph node metastases. Mediastinal lymph nodes, such as paratracheal, hilar, subcarinal, paraesophageal, and paraaortic lymph nodes, that measure 10 mm or larger in short-axis dimension are usually considered abnormal. Internal mammary, retrocrural, and extrapleural lymph nodes have no specific size criteria, and identification of these lymph nodes is often considered abnormal. In MPM different patterns of intrathoracic lymphadenopathy may be encountered, depending on the presence, location, and extent of pleural and diaphragmatic involvement.[72] The anterior pleura is drained by the internal mammary and peridiaphragmatic lymph nodes, the posterior pleura is drained by extrapleural lymph nodes, the anterior and lateral diaphragm is drained by the internal mammary and anterior peridiaphragmatic nodes, and the posterior diaphragm is drained by the paraaortic and posterior mediastinal nodes. The anterior and lateral chest wall lymphatics drain to the anterior or pectoral nodes, and the posterior chest wall lymphatics drain to the axillary nodes (Fig. 74.9).[73]

Intrathoracic and extrathoracic metastatic disease may be demonstrated on CT. Pulmonary metastases appear as nodules or masses, and lymphangitic carcinomatosis manifests as thickening and nodularity of the interlobular septa.

Magnetic Resonance Imaging

A number of studies have assessed the role of MRI in distinguishing malignant from benign pleural disease. By use of the CT

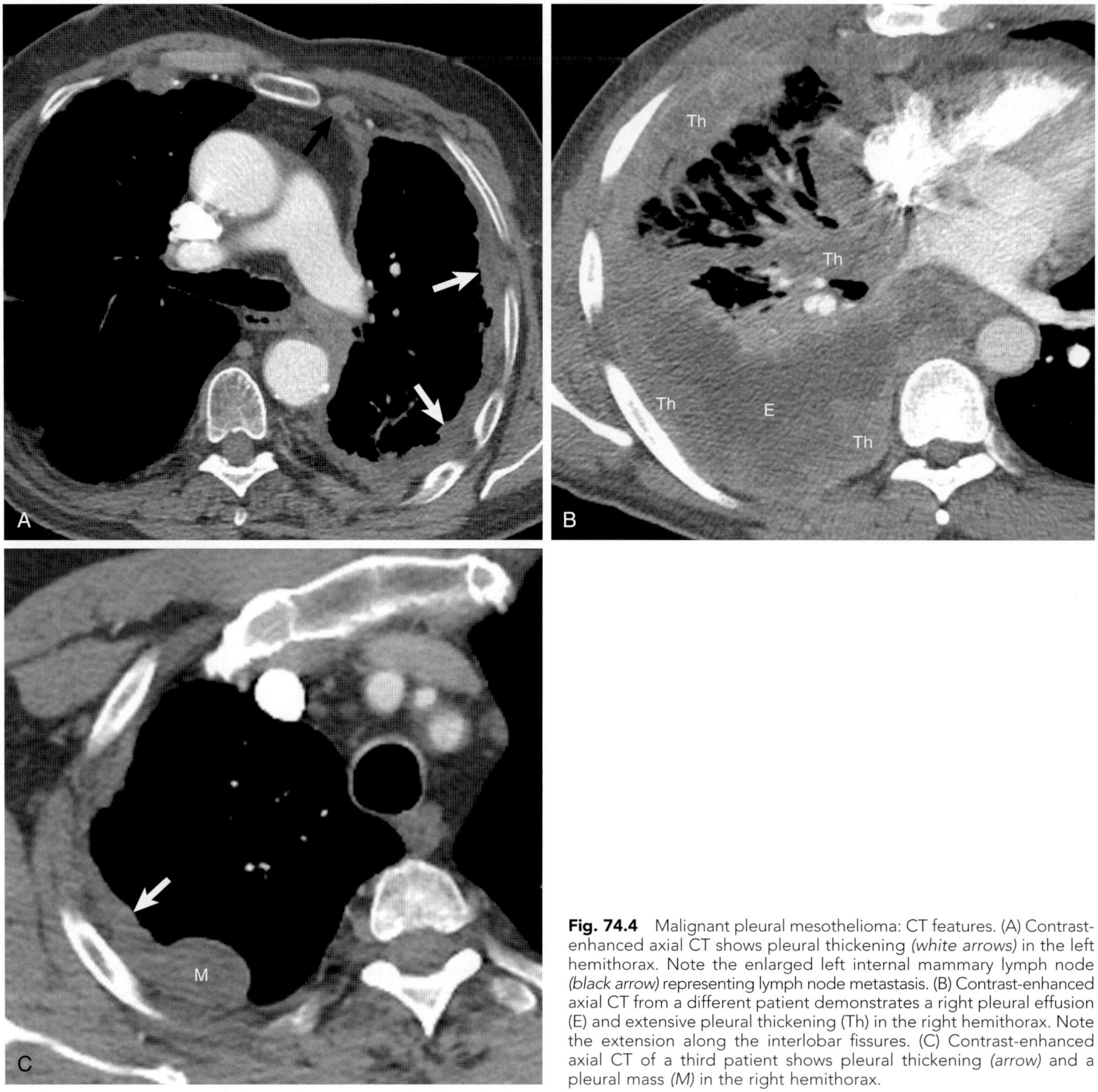

Fig. 74.4 Malignant pleural mesothelioma: CT features. (A) Contrast-enhanced axial CT shows pleural thickening *(white arrows)* in the left hemithorax. Note the enlarged left internal mammary lymph node *(black arrow)* representing lymph node metastasis. (B) Contrast-enhanced axial CT from a different patient demonstrates a right pleural effusion (E) and extensive pleural thickening (Th) in the right hemithorax. Note the extension along the interlobar fissures. (C) Contrast-enhanced axial CT of a third patient shows pleural thickening *(arrow)* and a pleural mass *(M)* in the right hemithorax.

criteria for malignant pleural thickening described previously, as well as signal intensity characteristics, sensitivities and specificities of MRI were equivalent to those of CT.[74,75] High–signal intensity on proton density/T2-weighted MRI in comparison with intercostal muscles provides a valuable additional feature to differentiate benign from malignant pleural disease (100% sensitivity, 87% specificity; negative predictive value, 100%).[74]

A recent study evaluated the ability of texture and shape features on CT and MRI to differentiate benign and malignant pleural lesions and assessed if radiomic models could improve the confidence and accuracy of radiologists with different subspecialty backgrounds.[76] This group found that quantitative textural and shape analysis may help distinguish malignant from benign lesions and concluded that a radiomics-based approach may increase diagnostic confidence of abdominal radiologists and potentially improve radiologists' accuracy in the assessment of pleural lesions characterized by MRI.[76]

MRI is not routinely used to evaluate patients with MPM but may provide more precise staging information in certain scenarios. Pleural effusions related to MPM are typically hyperintense on T2-weighted images. Pleural thickening is isointense to mildly hyperintense relative to muscle on T1-weighted images and moderately hyperintense relative to muscle on T2-weighted and proton density–weighted images (Fig. 74.10). After the administration of intravenous gadolinium-based contrast material, enhancement is typical (see Fig. 74.10). MRI is more sensitive

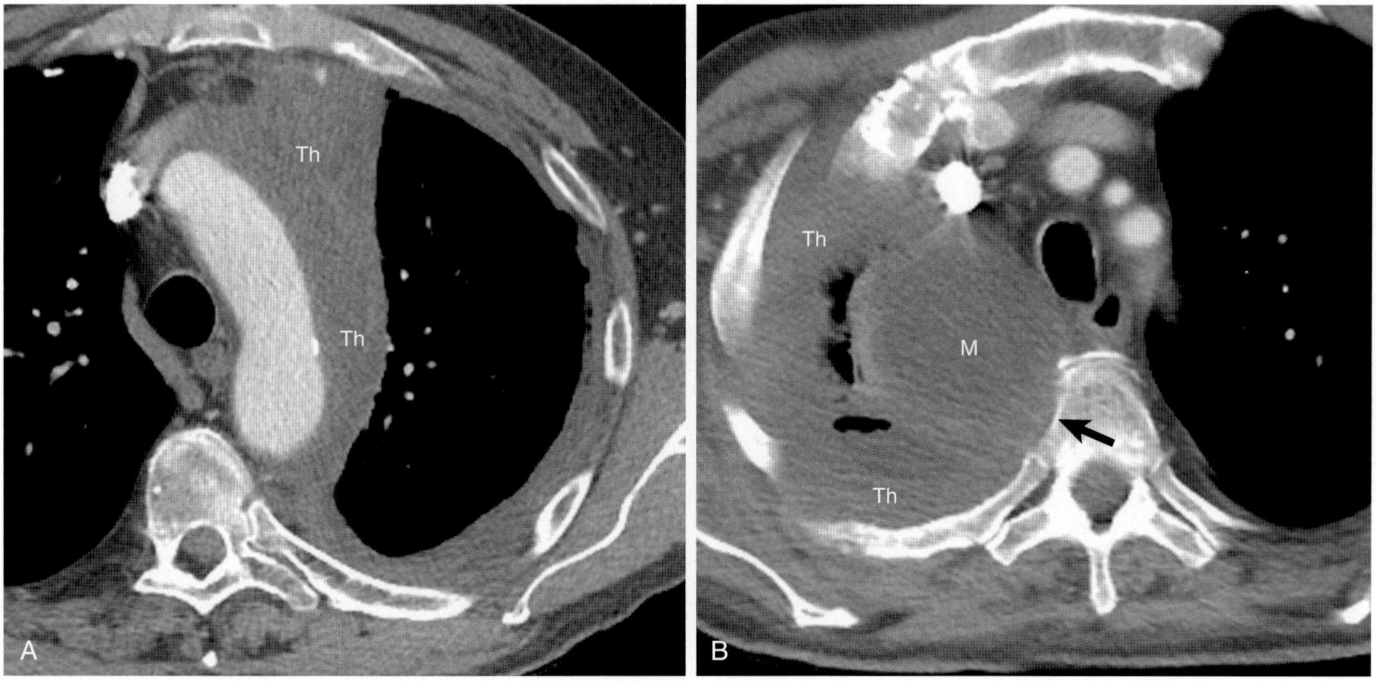

Fig. 74.5 Malignant pleural mesothelioma (MPM) with mediastinal invasion. (A) Contrast-enhanced axial CT demonstrates extensive pleural thickening (Th) in the left hemithorax that invades the mediastinum and the aortic arch. (B) Contrast-enhanced axial CT of a different patient shows pleural thickening (Th) in the right hemithorax and a focal mass (M) that invades the adjacent thoracic spine *(arrow)*. MPM may invade the mediastinum and result in the loss of fat and tissue planes between mediastinal structures. Invasion should also be suspected when the mass encases >50% of the circumference of the trachea, esophagus, or other mediastinal structures.

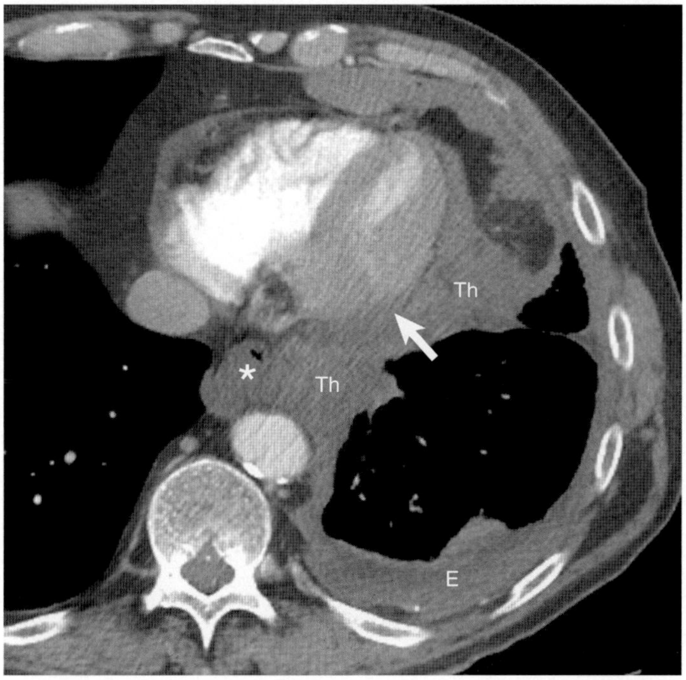

Fig. 74.6 Malignant pleural mesothelioma with pericardial involvement. Contrast-enhanced axial CT demonstrates a left pleural effusion (E) and pleural thickening (Th) that invades the esophagus *(asterisk)* and pericardium *(arrow)*. Involvement of the pericardium, which may be nontransmural or transmural, may produce pericardial effusion, pericardial thickening, pericardial nodules/masses, and/or infiltrating soft tissue.

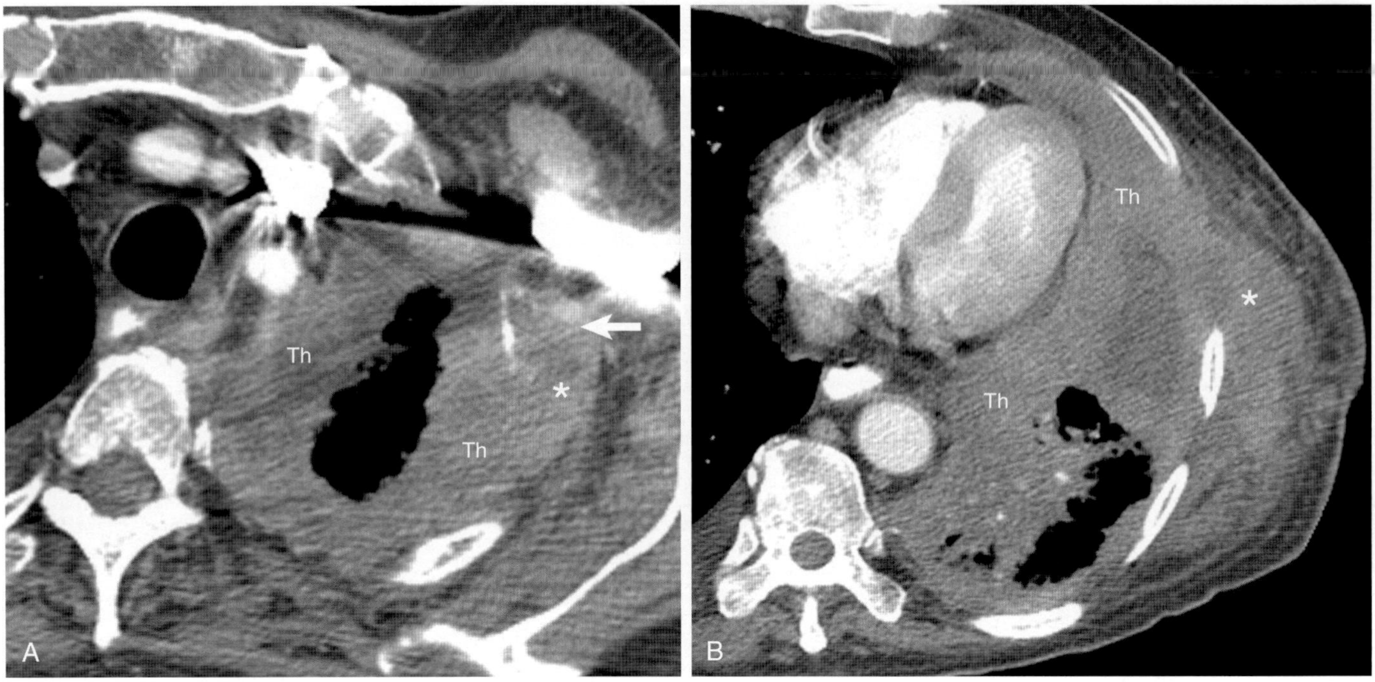

Fig. 74.7 Chest wall invasion of malignant pleural mesothelioma (MPM). (A) Contrast-enhanced axial CT shows extensive pleural thickening (Th) in the left hemithorax that invades an adjacent rib *(arrow)* and the chest wall *(asterisk)*. (B) Contrast-enhanced axial CT from a different patient demonstrates pleural thickening (Th) in the left hemithorax and a large region of chest wall invasion *(asterisk)*. On CT, MPM that invades the chest wall may manifest as loss of normal extrapleural fat planes, invasion of intercostal muscles, rib displacement, or osseous destruction.

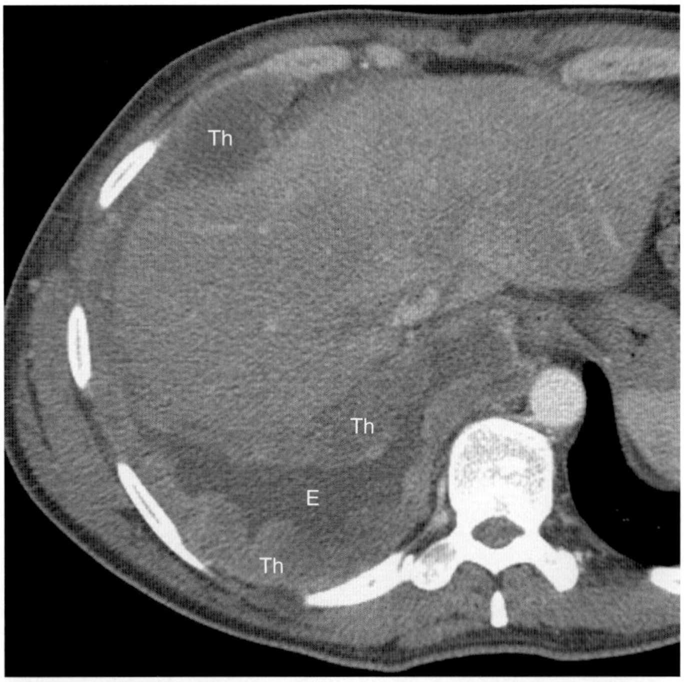

Fig. 74.8 Transdiaphragmatic extension of malignant pleural mesothelioma (MPM). Contrast-enhanced axial CT demonstrates a pleural effusion (E) and extensive pleural thickening (Th) in the right hemithorax. Note the loss of the normal fat plane between the inferior surface of the diaphragm and the liver, suggestive of transdiaphragmatic extension. The accuracy of CT for transdiaphragmatic extension remains poor; however, the presence of a distinct fat plane between the inferior surface of the diaphragm and the adjacent abdominal organs is the most reliable indication that MPM is limited to the chest.

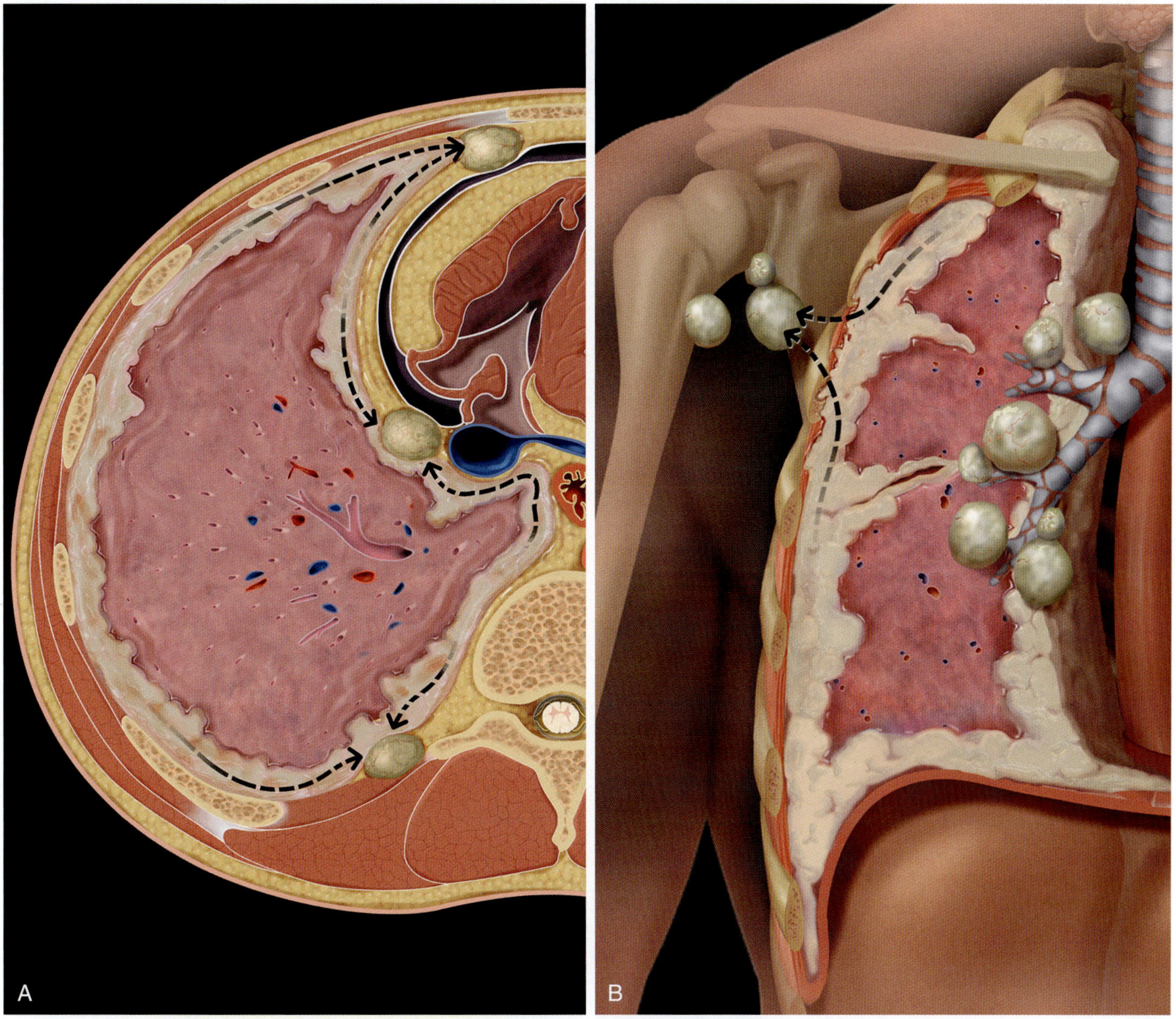

Fig. 74.9 Patterns of lymph node spread in malignant pleural mesothelioma (MPM). (A) Graphic shows drainage pattern of MPM involving the lower thoracic pleura and hemidiaphragm (not shown). The anterior pleura/diaphragm drain to anterior and middle peridiaphragmatic lymph nodes. The posterior pleura drains to posterior intercostal lymph nodes. (B) Graphic shows MPM with circumferential pleural thickening, chest wall invasion, and the corresponding lymphatic drainage. Chest wall invasion, in this case, results in lymphatic drainage to ipsilateral axillary lymph nodes, consistent with metastatic disease (stage M1). *(From Walker CW. Pathways of lymph node spread for mesothelioma. In: Rosado-de-Christenson ML, Carter BW, eds.* Specialty Imaging: Thoracic Neoplasms. *1st ed. Philadelphia: Elsevier Amirsys; 2015.)*

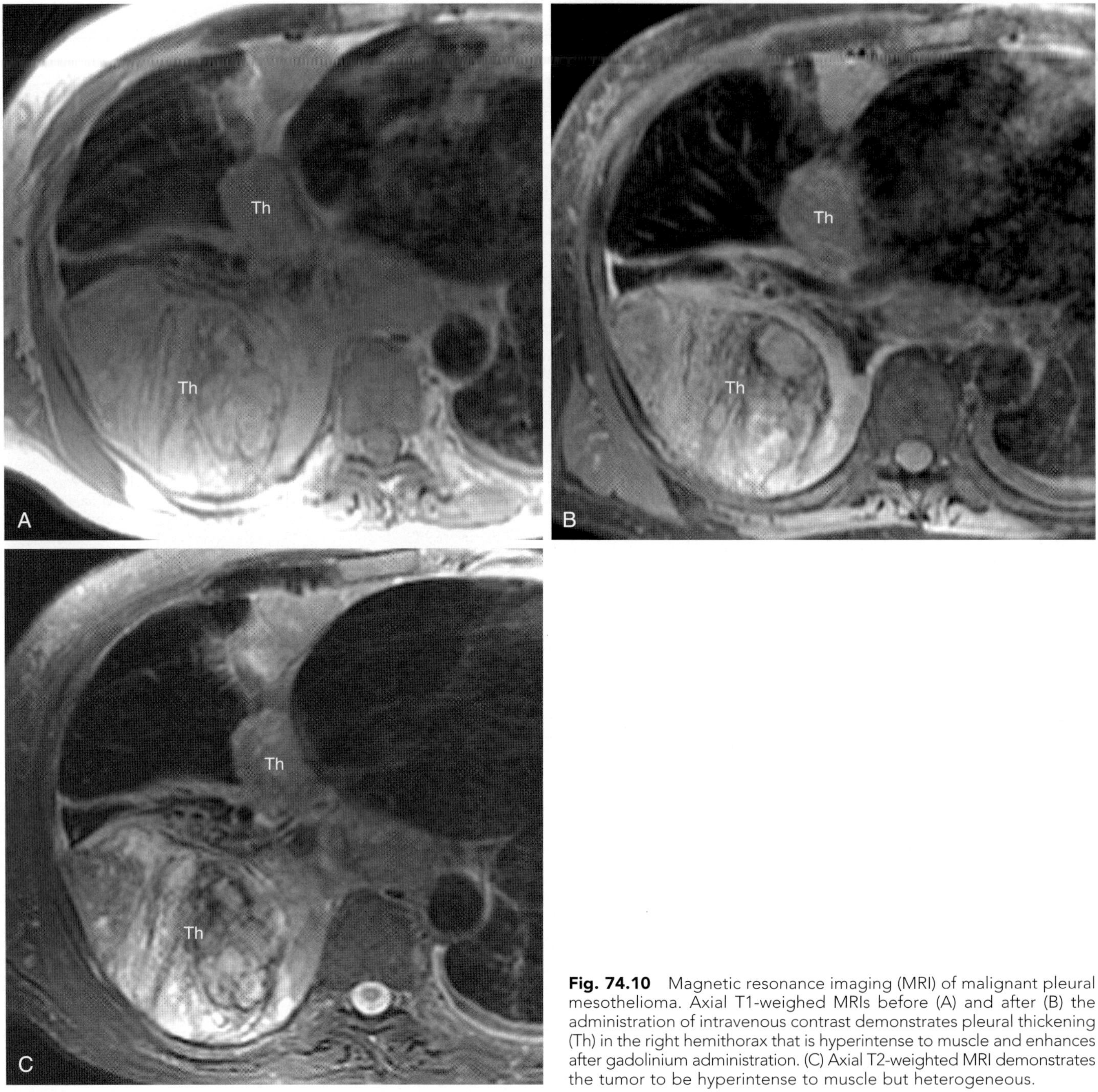

Fig. 74.10 Magnetic resonance imaging (MRI) of malignant pleural mesothelioma. Axial T1-weighed MRIs before (A) and after (B) the administration of intravenous contrast demonstrates pleural thickening (Th) in the right hemithorax that is hyperintense to muscle and enhances after gadolinium administration. (C) Axial T2-weighted MRI demonstrates the tumor to be hyperintense to muscle but heterogeneous.

than CT and other imaging modalities in detecting invasion of the chest wall, mediastinum, and diaphragm (Fig. 74.11).[77] Loss of the normal fat planes, extension into mediastinal fat, and tumoral encasement of more than 50% of the circumference of a mediastinal structure are some of the MRI features that suggest tumor invasion.

More recently, it has been shown that diffusion-weighted imaging (DWI) and dynamic contrast-enhanced MRI can further help characterize the histologic cell types of MPM, with the epithelial subtype showing higher apparent diffusion coefficient (ADC) value than the sarcomatoid subtype.[78] It has been proposed that an ADC value of 1.31×10^{-3} mm^2/s can be used as a cutoff to differentiate the two histologic cell types. Giesel and colleagues[79] were able to correlate perfusion parameters in mesothelioma with angiogenesis in these tumors.

Fluorodeoxyglucose–Positron Emission Tomography–Computed Tomography

FDG–PET-CT is an important adjunctive examination that is often used for the diagnosis and staging of MPM, as it combines valuable metabolic information and anatomic detail. FDG uptake in MPM and other causes of malignant pleural disease is significantly higher than in benign pleural diseases, and greater FDG uptake has been associated with a shorter survival time (Fig. 74.12).[80] The extent of FDG uptake is associated with median time to tumor progression and survival. Although PET-CT is

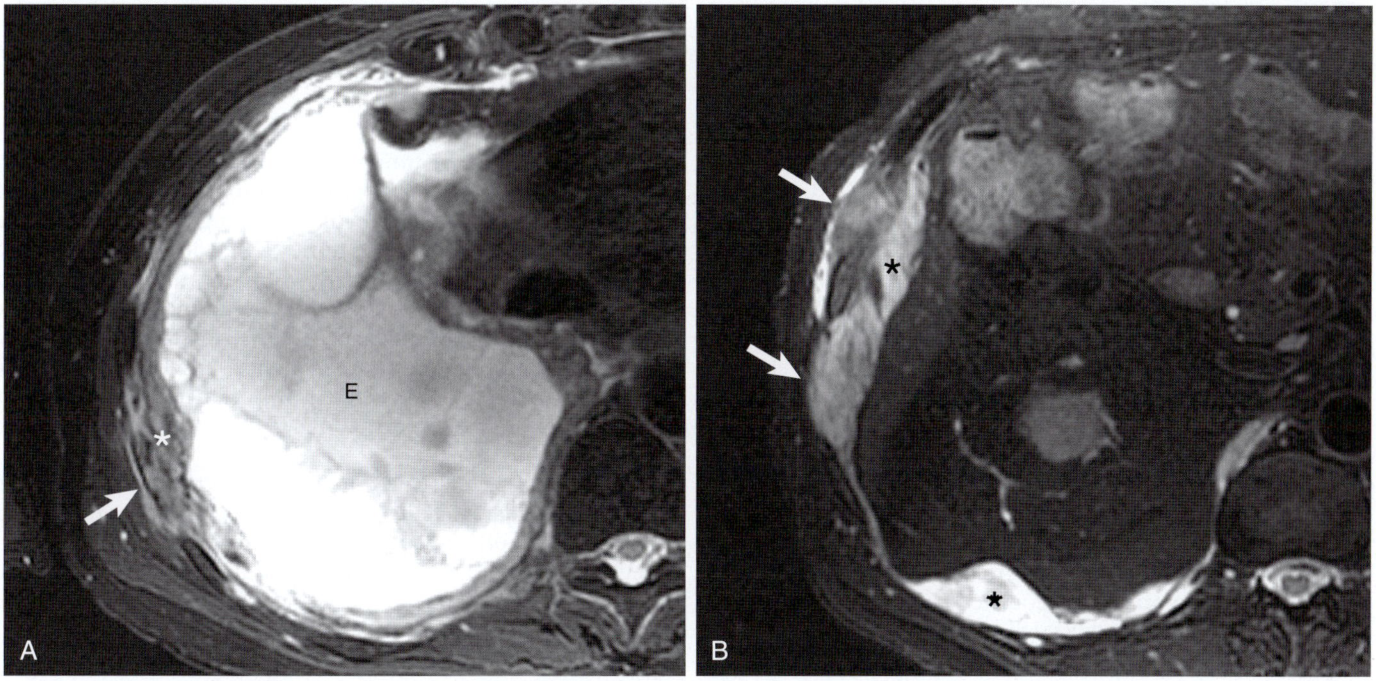

Fig. 74.11 Chest wall invasion of malignant pleural mesothelioma (MPM) on magnetic resonance imaging (MRI). (A) Axial T2-weighted MRI shows focal invasion of the right chest wall *(arrow)* by tumor *(asterisk)* with associated large pleural effusion (E). (B) Axial T2-weighed MRI from a different patient demonstrates multifocal invasion *(arrows)* of the right chest wall and a small right pleural effusion *(asterisk)*. MPM with multifocal or diffuse invasion of the chest wall is typically considered unresectable.

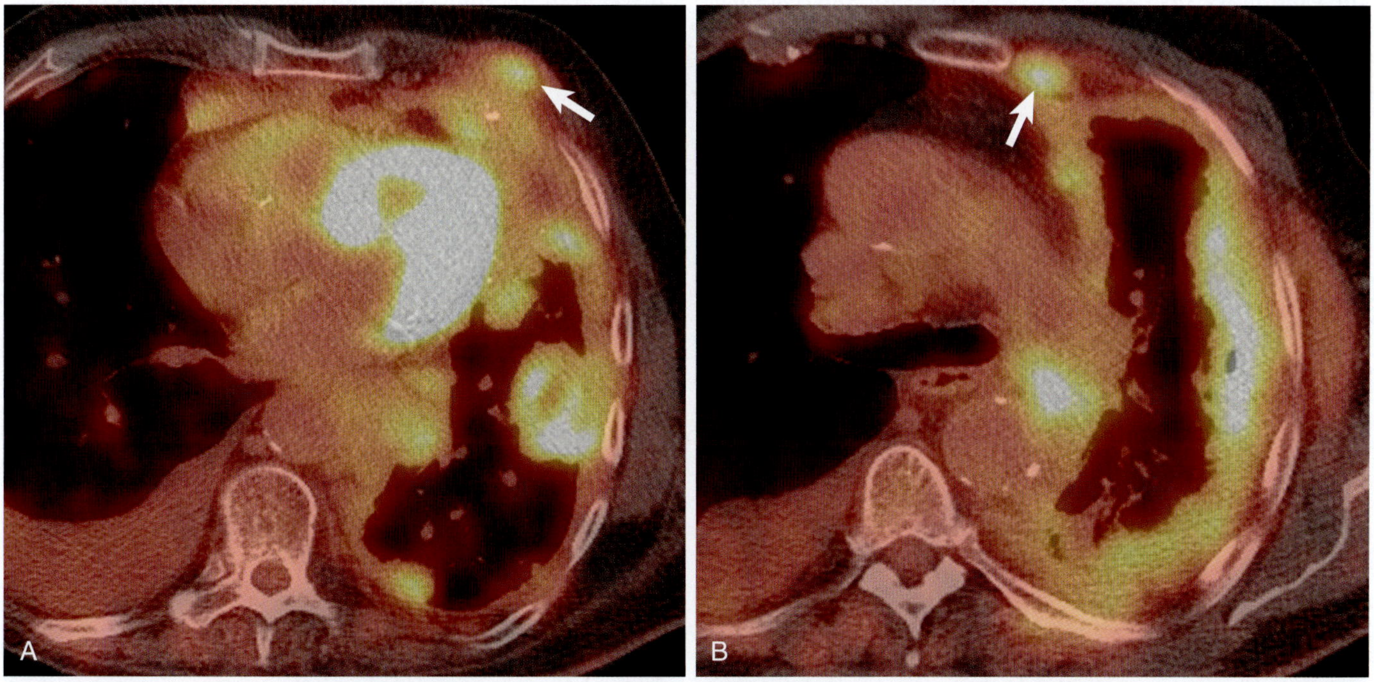

Fig. 74.12 Positron emission tomography (PET)-CT of malignant pleural mesothelioma. Fused axial fluorodeoxyglucose (FDG)–PET-CT images demonstrate extensive FDG-avid pleural thickening, nodules, and masses in the left hemithorax with focal invasion of the chest wall (*arrow*, A) and an FDG-avid left internal mammary lymph node (*arrow*, B) compatible with lymph node metastasis.

suboptimal compared with CT and MRI in delineating the extent of local tumor, it may depict invasion of the mediastinum and chest wall. PET-CT is better than CT and MRI for demonstrating intrathoracic and extrathoracic lymphadenopathy (see Fig. 74.12) and most cases of metastatic disease. In addition, PET-CT is more accurate than CT, MRI, and PET alone for the staging of MPM.[81]

PET-CT can be used to plan image-guided and surgical biopsies as the locations of greatest FDG uptake and/or those that are most accessible can be identified and targeted for tissue sampling. Another role for PET is in helping to predict prognosis.[82,83] Higher FDG uptake is associated with significantly shorter survival time.[82,83] Another study showed good correlation between FDG uptake and surgical stage.[84] This information may be useful clinically in determining the most appropriate treatment. PET-CT is also beneficial for evaluating treatment response (Figs. 74.13 and 74.14) and detecting recurrent disease (Fig. 74.15).

Ultrasonography

Ultrasonography can be useful in identifying disease of the pleura. The pleural effusion acts as an acoustic window and can enable detection of intrapleural nodules. Ultrasonography-guided biopsy of pleural thickening (reported accuracy of 80% for diagnosis of MPM) and drainage of effusions are well-established, safe techniques.[60]

STAGING

The eighth edition of the tumor-node-metastasis (TNM) staging system for MPM is effective as of January 1, 2018, by the American Joint Committee on Cancer (AJCC)/Union for International Cancer Control (UICC). Recommendations for the eighth edition are the result of an international collaboration and analysis of databases under the auspices of the International Association for the Study of Lung Cancer (IASLC) (Tables 74.1 to 74.4).[85–88]

T Classification

The extent of primary tumor spread, which includes tumor size, invasion, and location, is of primary importance in determining prognosis.[89] The T component of staging for MPM is based entirely upon the location of tumor tissue and anatomic site of invasion. In contrast to the staging of other malignancies, measurements are not used. However, unidimensional measurements of pleural thickness suggest that quantitative measures of disease burden may have prognostic value, and further work is planned to assess whether this limited preliminary data may add important information to the staging system in the future.[86,88]

Regarding specific T descriptors, T1 describes tumor affecting the ipsilateral parietal plus/minus visceral plus/minus mediastinal plus/minus diaphragmatic pleura. T2 lesions involve all ipsilateral pleural surfaces and at least one additional feature, such as invasion of the diaphragm or extension into the lung parenchyma. T3 disease includes all ipsilateral pleural surfaces and at least one additional feature, such as involvement of the endothoracic fascia, invasion of the mediastinal fat, a solitary, resectable focus of chest wall invasion, or involvement of the pericardium without transmural invasion. Finally, T4 tumors involve all pleural surfaces and at least one additional feature, such as multifocal chest wall invasion, with or without rib destruction; direct transdiaphragmatic extension into the peritoneum; direct extension to the contralateral pleura; direct invasion of mediastinal organs; direct invasion of the spine; and transmural involvement of the pericardium, with or without pericardial effusion.

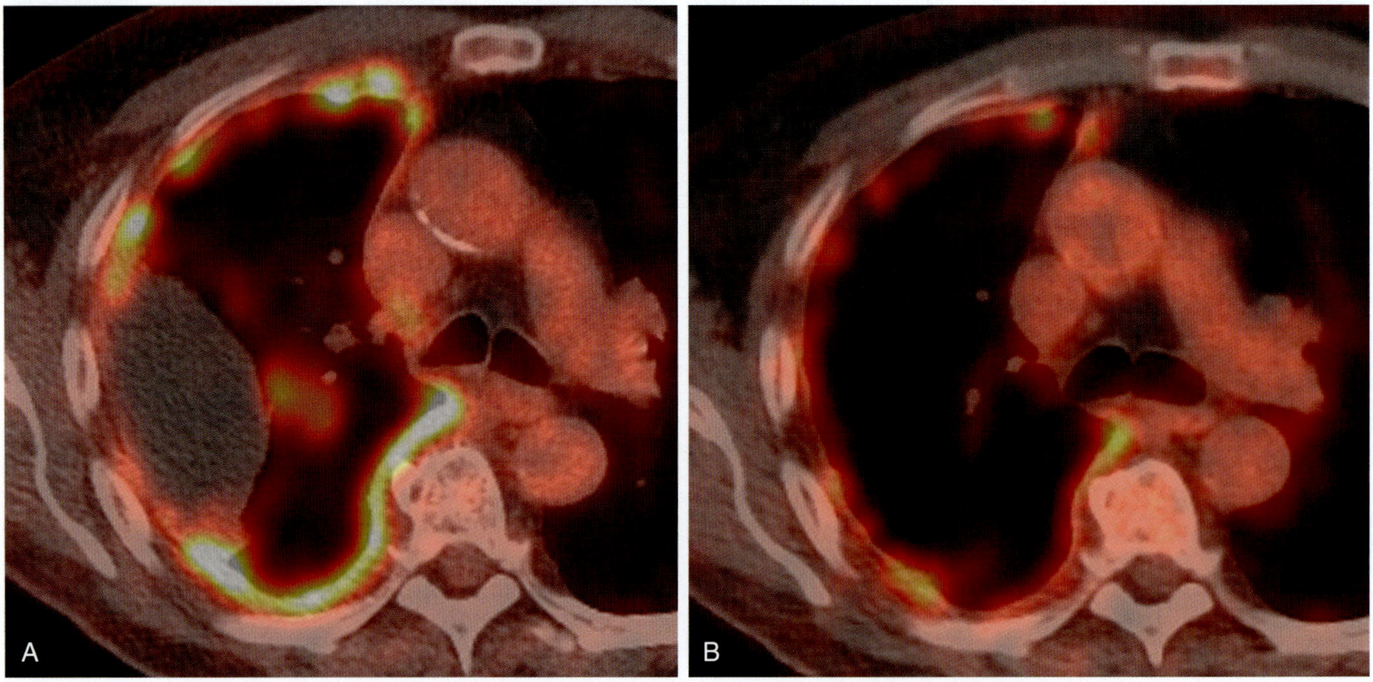

Fig. 74.13 Positron emission tomography (PET)-CT for treatment response evaluation of malignant pleural mesothelioma. Fused axial fluorodeoxyglucose (FDG)–PET-CT images at baseline (A) and after one cycle of chemotherapy (B) demonstrate FDG-avid pleural thickening in the right hemithorax that improves after treatment.

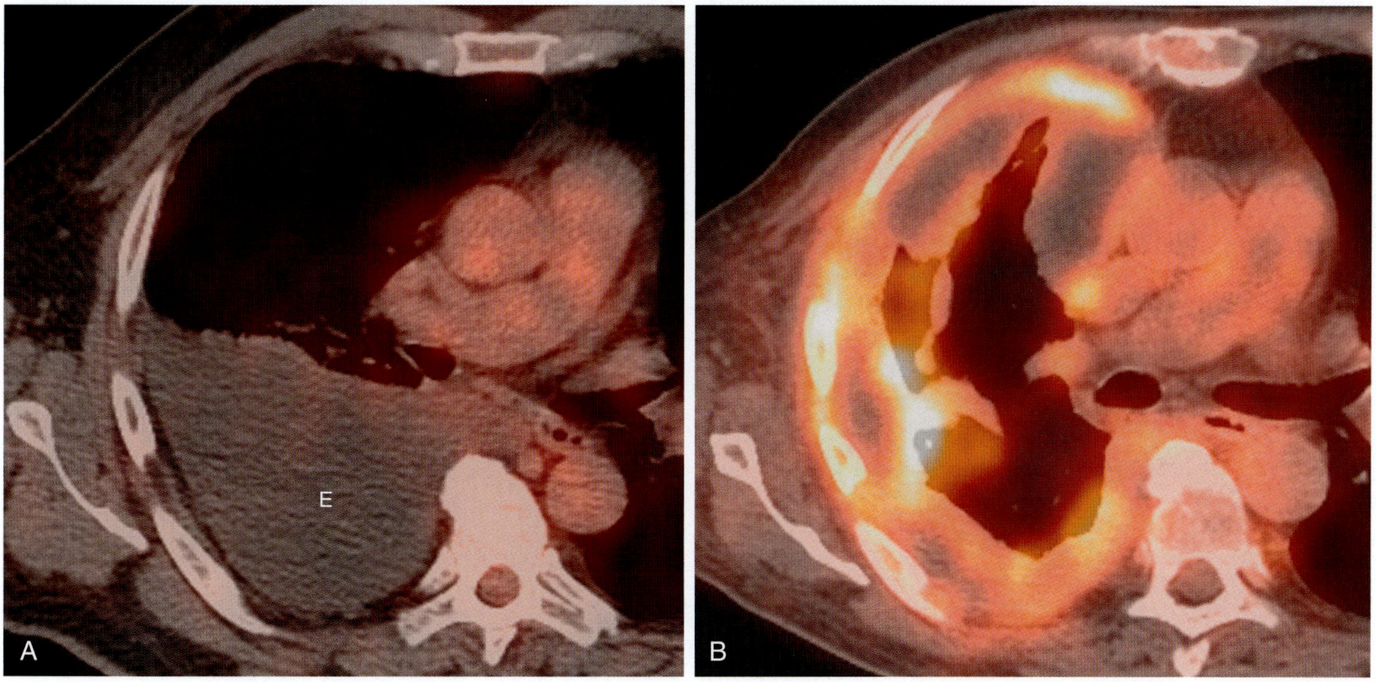

Fig. 74.14 Positron emission tomography (PET)-CT for treatment response evaluation of malignant pleural mesothelioma. Fused axial fluorodeoxyglucose (FDG)–PET-CT images at baseline (A) and at 6-month follow-up demonstrate a right pleural effusion (E in A) and progression to extensive FDG-avid pleural thickening in the right hemithorax (B).

TABLE 74.1 T CLASSIFICATION OF MALIGNANT PLEURAL MESOTHELIOMA

T Classification	Definition
TX	Primary tumor cannot be assessed
T0	No evidence of primary tumor
T1	Tumor limited to the ipsilateral parietal ± visceral ± mediastinal ± diaphragmatic pleura
T2	Tumor involving each of the ipsilateral pleural surfaces (parietal, mediastinal, diaphragmatic, and visceral pleura) with at least one of the following features: (1) involvement of diaphragmatic muscle or (2) extension of tumor from visceral pleura into the underlying lung parenchyma
T3	Describes locally advanced but potentially resectable tumor involving all of the ipsilateral pleural surfaces (parietal, mediastinal, diaphragmatic, and visceral pleura) with at least one of the following features: (1) involvement of the endothoracic fascia; (2) extension into the mediastinal fat; (3) solitary, completely resectable focus of tumor extending into the soft tissues of the chest wall; (4) nontransmural involvement of the pericardium
T4	Describes locally advanced technically unresectable tumor involving all of the ipsilateral pleural surfaces (parietal, mediastinal, diaphragmatic, and visceral pleura) with at least one of the following features: (1) diffuse extension or multifocal masses of tumor in the chest wall, with or without associated rib destruction; (2) direct transdiaphragmatic extension of tumor to the peritoneum; (3) direct extension of tumor to the contralateral pleura; (4) direct extension of tumor to mediastinal organs; (5) direct extension of tumor into the spine; (6) tumor extending through to the internal surface of the pericardium with or without a pericardial effusion; or (7) tumor involving the myocardium

Adapted from Nowak AK, Chansky K, Rice DC, et al. The IASLC Mesothelioma Staging Project: proposals for revisions of the T descriptors in the forthcoming eighth edition of the TNM classification for pleural mesothelioma. *J Thorac Oncol.* 2016;11:2089–2099.

N Classification

The N component of the MPM staging system was originally based on the N staging for lung cancer; however, it should be noted that lymphatic drainage of the pleura is distinct from that of the lung.[63] The eighth edition is the first evidence-based system for staging of lymph nodes in MPM. Lymph node metastases occur in 35% to 50% of MPM patients who undergo surgical resection; an autopsy series found lymph node involvement in 76%. Lymph node metastases can decrease long-term survival by up to 50%.[87]

N1 disease includes metastases involving ipsilateral bronchopulmonary, hilar, mediastinal, internal mammary, peridiaphragmatic/pericardial, and intercostal lymph nodes. N2 comprises metastases involving contralateral bronchopulmonary, hilar, and mediastinal lymph nodes, as well as metastases involving any supraclavicular lymph node. Metastatic disease to the axillary lymph nodes is considered M1 disease and is not included in the N descriptor. The staging of lymph nodes is difficult, given the limited accuracy of the size criteria used on CT, and metastases may be present in lymph nodes measuring less than 1 cm. Mediastinoscopy has been

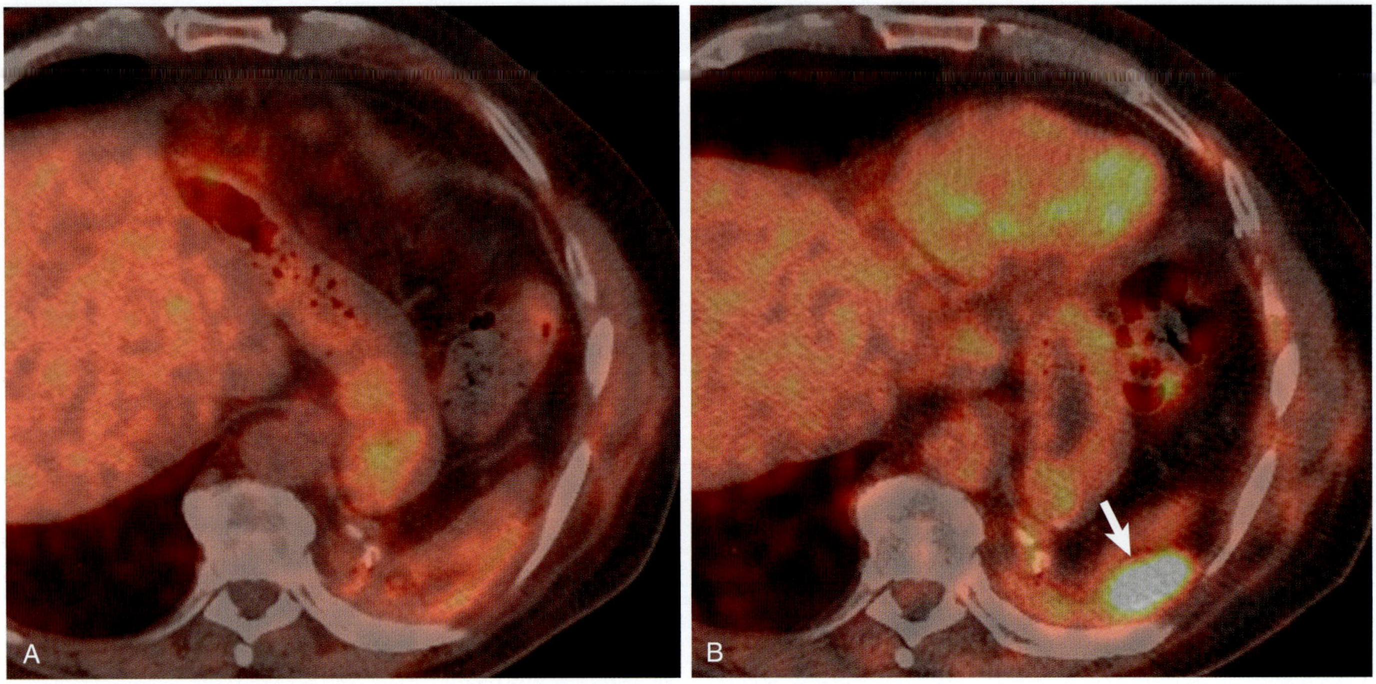

Fig. 74.15 Recurrent malignant pleural mesothelioma on positron emission tomography (PET)-CT. Fused axial fluorodeoxyglucose (FDG)–PET-CT images after initial therapy with surgery and radiation (A) and at 12-month follow-up demonstrate development of FDG-avid recurrence (*arrow*, B) at the site of therapy.

TABLE 74.2 N CLASSIFICATION OF MALIGNANT PLEURAL MESOTHELIOMA

Regional Lymph Nodes (N)	Definition
NX	Regional lymph nodes cannot be assessed
N0	No regional lymph node metastases
N1	Metastases in the ipsilateral bronchopulmonary, hilar, or mediastinal lymph nodes (including the internal mammary, peridiaphragmatic, mediastinal fat pad, or intercostal lymph nodes)
N2	Metastases in the contralateral bronchopulmonary, hilar, or mediastinal lymph nodes or ipsilateral or contralateral supraclavicular lymph nodes

Adapted from Rice D, Chansky K, Nowak A, et al. The IASLC Mesothelioma Staging Project: proposals for revisions of the N descriptors in the forthcoming eighth edition of the TNM classification for pleural mesothelioma. *J Thorac Oncol.* 2016;11:2100–2111.

TABLE 74.3 M CLASSIFICATION OF MALIGNANT PLEURAL MESOTHELIOMA

Metastasis (M)	Definition
M0	No distant metastasis
M1	Distant metastasis present

Adapted from Rusch VW, Chansky K, Kindler HL, et al. The IASLC Mesothelioma Staging Project: proposals for the M descriptors and for revision of the TNM stage groupings in the forthcoming (eighth) edition of the TNM classification for mesothelioma. *J Thorac Oncol.* 2016;11:2112–2119.

TABLE 74.4 STAGE GROUPINGS OF MALIGNANT PLEURAL MESOTHELIOMA

	N0	N1	N2
T1	IA	II	IIIB
T2	IB	II	IIIB
T3	IB	IIIA	IIIB
T4	IIIB	IIIB	IIIB
M1	IV	IV	IV

M, Metastasis; *N*, node; *T*, tumor.
Adapted from Rusch VW, Chansky K, Kindler HL, et al. The IASLC Mesothelioma Staging Project: proposals for the M descriptors and for revision of the TNM stage groupings in the forthcoming (eighth) edition of the TNM classification for mesothelioma. *J Thorac Oncol.* 2016;11:2112–2119.

shown to be more accurate than CT in the staging of MPM, with a sensitivity of 80% (vs. 60% for CT), a specificity of 100% (vs. 71% for CT), and an accuracy of 93% (vs. 67% for CT), although some lymph node groups are not accessible with this method.[90] Cervical mediastinoscopy allows evaluation of the 2R (upper right paratracheal), 2L (upper left paratracheal), 4R (lower right paratracheal), 4L (lower left paratracheal), and 7 (subcarinal) stations.[91] Extended mediastinoscopy permits evaluation of the 5 (subaortic) and 6 (paraaortic) stations.[92]

M Classification

The M component of the staging system is binary—distant metastases are present (M1) or absent (M0). Metastatic disease is a late manifestation of disease, and some of the most common sites of metastatic spread include the contralateral pleura, contralateral lung, peritoneum/abdomen, extrathoracic lymph nodes (apart from supraclavicular lymph nodes), bone, liver, and brain. Initial results of the IASLC Mesothelioma Staging Project suggest that the number of metastatic lesions may have an effect on prognosis, and further research on this topic may inform future editions of the TNM classification.[88]

PROGNOSIS

The prognosis overall is extremely poor. Most patients die within the first year of the onset of symptoms, and "long-term survival" is rare. In two series of 167 patients[93] and 114 patients,[35] only 7 (2.5%) lived for more than 5 years. Two-year and 5-year survival rates are reported as 23% and 0%, respectively, in another study of 80 patients.[94] As for most other cancers, prognosis is related to the extent of local or distant tumor spread.[95] Prognosis is better in tumors with an epithelioid subtype than with sarcomatoid histology and appears to be independent of stage.[96,97] Many factors are also reported to be prognostic in MPM, including histologic features, age, gender, and performance status, as well as chest pain, dyspnea, platelet count greater than 400,000/µL, weight loss, serum lactate dehydrogenase level greater than 500 U/L, low hemoglobin level, high white blood cell count, and increasing age older than 75 years all carry a worse prognosis.[41]

TREATMENT

Different treatment strategies may be used for MPM, depending on tumor factors, such as histology and stage at diagnosis, and patient factors, such as age and performance status. Single-modality therapy (i.e., surgery, chemotherapy, or radiation therapy alone) has demonstrated limited survival benefit. Therefore current treatment regimens focus on multimodality therapy, which has shown greater survival benefit.[43]

Chemotherapy

Most patients with MPM are diagnosed at advanced stages of disease. Thus chemotherapy is the mainstay of therapy, and a regimen of platinum-based cisplatin and the antifolate pemetrexed is considered first-line therapy for unresectable disease. This combination results in longer median survival and longer time to disease progression than treatment with cisplatin alone.[98] Other treatment regimens include gemcitabine and vinorelbine, alone or in combination with cisplatin. Neoadjuvant cisplatin may be used with pemetrexed or gemcitabine before extrapleural pneumonectomy and adjuvant radiation therapy.[99]

Surgery

Surgical treatments are typically used early on (stages I and II) and include pleurectomy and decortication and extrapleural pneumonectomy. Pleurectomy and decortication involve removal of the parietal and visceral pleura from the lung surface, mediastinum, pericardium, diaphragm, and chest wall. Extrapleural pneumonectomy is characterized by en bloc resection of the lung, parietal and visceral pleura, ipsilateral hemidiaphragm, and ipsilateral pericardium. A recent study showed no statistically significant differences in survival for either procedure at any stage of disease. However, multivariate analysis demonstrated significant survival benefit for pleurectomy and decortication versus extrapleural pneumonectomy. Pleurectomy and decortication are associated with a higher postsurgical recurrence rate than extrapleural pneumonectomy, although metastatic disease is less common.[100]

Radiation Therapy

Radiation therapy is typically used for palliative purposes in MPM.[101] One study showed decreased tumor seeding of procedural tracts with use of radiation therapy; however, prophylactic radiation therapy for this purpose is not currently recommended.[57] Adding intensity-modulated radiation therapy to extrapleural pneumonectomy may result in a decrease in local-regional recurrence.[102] Radiation treatment plans include all preoperative pleural surfaces, the ipsilateral mediastinal lymph nodes, the retrocrural space, and the deep margin of the surgical incision.

KEY POINTS: MALIGNANT PLEURAL MESOTHELIOMA

- Asbestos exposure is the main risk factor for malignant pleural mesothelioma (MPM). MPM incidence is decreasing in developed countries where asbestos is banned.
- Patients with MPM can present with chest pain, dyspnea, or asymptomatic pleural effusion.
- Typical imaging findings of MPM include nodular pleural thickening with or without pleural effusion.
- CT is the imaging modality of choice for evaluation of MPM, particularly in determining the extent of the primary tumor. Positron emission tomography–CT is useful for evaluation of nodal and distant metastatic disease. Magnetic resonance imaging is performed in selected cases for evaluation of mediastinal, chest wall, or diaphragmatic invasion.
- There should be a high level of suspicion for mesothelioma with history of asbestos exposure even in the absence of pleural plaques.
- Histologic diagnosis requires core-needle biopsy.
- Early-stage MPM can be treated surgically with pleurectomy and decortication or extrapleural pneumonectomy. Chemotherapy is used for advanced-stage disease, and radiation therapy is used for palliation or as adjuvant treatment postsurgery.
- Overall prognosis for MPM remains poor.

Solitary Fibrous Tumor of the Pleura

PREVALENCE AND EPIDEMIOLOGY

Solitary fibrous tumor is a relatively uncommon neoplasm, accounting for 5% to 10% of primary tumors of the pleura. The prevalence is approximately 2.8 cases per 100,000 population.[103] It is a mesenchymal tumor that has been increasingly recognized in the past few years. The tumor has been given a variety of names, the most common of which include solitary or localized fibrous tumor of the pleura. Others such as local, fibrous, or benign mesothelioma; subpleural, submesothelial, subserosal, or pleural fibroma; and fibrosarcoma are no longer used.[104] The etiology is unknown in most cases; occasional tumors have been reported after chest wall irradiation.[105] There is no known association with cigarette smoking. A case has been reported in association with asbestos exposure.[106]

CLINICAL PRESENTATION

Fibrous tumors occur equally in men and women. They have been described in all age groups from 5 to 87 years, but the peak incidence is in the sixth and seventh decades of life.[107–109] About 54% of patients are symptomatic; the most frequent symptoms are dyspnea, cough, and chest pain, present in 40% of patients.[108,110,111] Most small tumors are asymptomatic, discovered incidentally on radiographs obtained for other reasons. The tumors have traditionally been considered to have a high incidence of clubbing of the fingers and hypertrophic osteoarthropathy; in 1981, on the basis of a review of 360 cases reported, Briselli and colleagues[107] concluded that it was present in 35% of patients. However, it was noted that earlier reported cases were more likely to be symptomatic. More recent studies suggest that the incidence of finger clubbing and hypertrophic osteoarthropathy is only 4%.[108] Symptomatic hypoglycemia is present in 4% to 5% of cases and is more common with malignant tumors.[107,108] Some fibrous tumors have been associated with the presence of an insulin-like growth factor (IGF-II) in the tumor[112] and in the serum.[113] Once the tumor is removed, symptoms of osteoarthropathy and hypoglycemia resolve.[113] Hemoptysis and obstructive pneumonitis may rarely be observed, the results of airway obstruction.[114]

PATHOLOGY

Fibrous tumors most commonly occur in the pleura but have also been described in the pericardium, mediastinum, lung, peritoneum, chest wall, orbits, and other sites.[115–117] About 12% of solitary fibrous tumors of the pleura are malignant and eventually lead to death through local recurrence or metastatic disease.[107] Approximately 65% to 80% of solitary fibrous tumors of the pleura originate in the visceral pleura and 20% to 35% in the parietal pleura.[108] The tumors are usually well circumscribed. They range in size from 1 to 36 cm, with a mean of 6 cm.[107] Approximately 50% have a pedicle attached to the pleura, 1 cm in length, that contains hypertrophic arteries and veins.[108] The pedicle is associated with a lower risk of malignancy.[110,118]

The tumors appear as low-grade neoplasms of variable cellularity. A variety of architectural patterns have been described, the two most common being the “patternless pattern” (62%), with a random intermingling of tumor cells and collagen and the hemangiopericytoma-like pattern (25%), characterized by hypercellular zones that contain a network of open anastomosing or staghorn-shaped vessels.[106] Other less common patterns have an angiofibroma-like, fibrosarcoma-like, or neural pattern.[108]

Because of the highly variable light microscopic appearances of solitary fibrous tumor of the pleura, the histologic differential diagnosis is broad and includes primary and metastatic spindle cell carcinoma, spindle cell melanoma, sarcomatoid MPM, and a wide spectrum of primary and metastatic soft tissue neoplasms.[106] Immunohistochemical studies are helpful in excluding these other tumors. The criteria used to diagnose malignancy were described by England and colleagues[108] and include the following: bundles of high cellularity with crowding and overlapping of nuclei; high mitotic activity of more than four mitoses per 10 high-power fields; pleomorphism, based on nuclear size, irregularity, and nuclear prominence; presence of necrotic or hemorrhagic zones; and stromal or vascular invasion.[108,110] Enough tissue must be provided to ensure adequate diagnosis; definitive diagnosis may only be obtained at complete surgical resection.[106]

IMAGING

Radiography

Solitary fibrous tumor manifests as a peripheral solitary, smoothly marginated, homogeneous, rounded nodule or mass (Fig. 74.16). The tumor may be located within a fissure, where it may simulate a parenchymal mass.[108] They often have an incomplete border sign, the well-defined portion abutting the lung and the poorly defined margin abutting the chest wall.[119] Tapering margins form

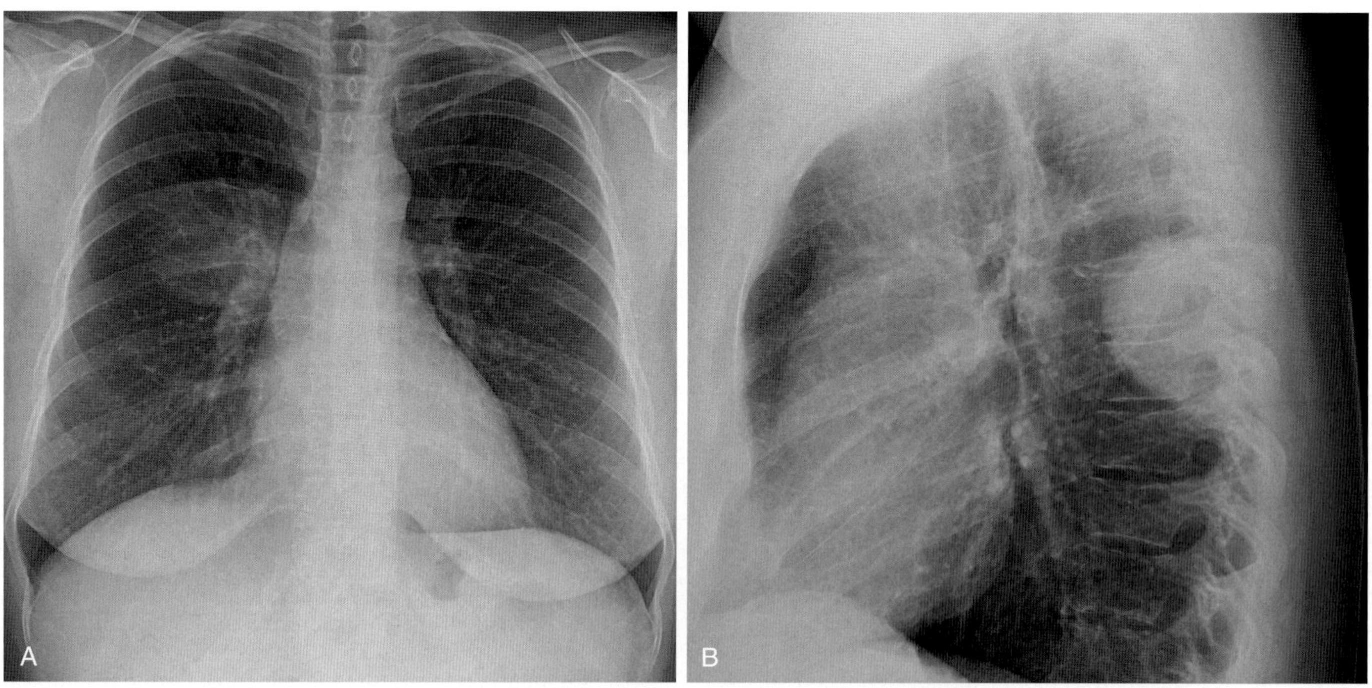

Fig. 74.16 Solitary fibrous tumor of the pleura: radiographic features. Frontal chest radiograph (A) demonstrates a lobular opacity projecting over the right hilum with well-defined inferior and left margins but ill-defined superior and right margins. Lateral chest radiograph (B) shows the opacity in the posterior right hemithorax with ill-defined posterior margin. These findings represent the "incomplete border sign," suggesting that the lesion is extrapulmonary.

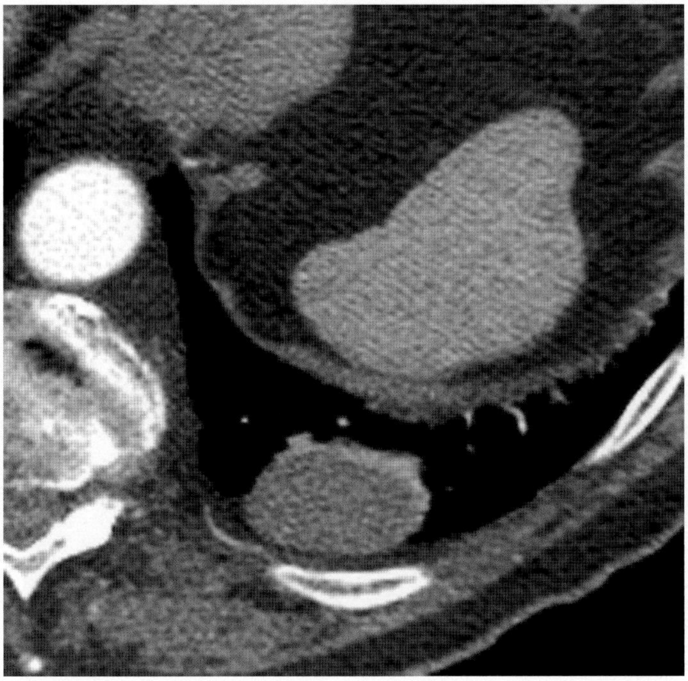

Fig. 74.17 Solitary fibrous tumor of the pleura: CT features. Contrast-enhanced axial CT shows a well-defined, homogeneous mass in the inferior left hemithorax with adjacent compressive atelectasis.

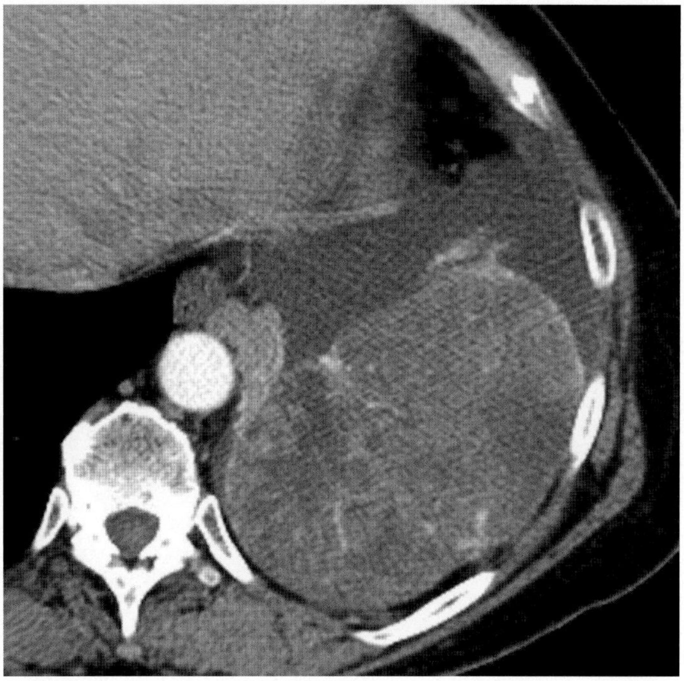

Fig. 74.18 Solitary fibrous tumor of the pleura: CT features. Contrast-enhanced axial CT demonstrates a large, heterogeneous mass in the inferior left hemithorax. Note the internal vascularity and regions of low attenuation indicative of necrosis. A small left pleural effusion is also present. On CT specific tumor characteristics suggesting malignancy are based primarily on size.

obtuse angles with the chest wall or mediastinum, such that en face radiography results in an ill-defined margin. Fibrous tumors of the pleura more typically occur in the middle or lower chest.[106] When they are in contiguity with the diaphragm, they may simulate diaphragmatic eventration or a Bochdalek hernia. Pedunculated tumors may be mobile, changing in position with respiration or posture.[120] Pleural effusions are reported in 6% to 17% of cases; if it is large enough, the effusion may obscure the mass.[106,108]

Computed Tomography

On CT a small solitary fibrous tumor of the pleura typically appears as a single well-defined, noninvasive, lobular soft tissue mass that abuts a pleural surface; it may form obtuse angles against the adjacent pleura or be located within a fissure.[106,121] The size of these tumors ranges from 1 to 36 cm.[106,108] When small, tumors are of homogeneous soft tissue density (Fig. 74.17). As tumors enlarge, they appear more heterogeneous; areas of necrosis, hemorrhage, and cystic changes are typically identified within the lesions (Figs. 74.18 and 74.19). Calcification occurs in 7% to 25% of cases, typically in larger tumors.[106,108,122] It is usually reported in association with necrosis.[123] Very rarely, a pedicle will be visualized on CT.[106] Mass effect on the adjacent lung or mediastinum is commonly seen.[106,108,121] Associated pleural effusions are seen in 25% to 37% of cases on CT.[106,108]

Solitary fibrous tumors of the pleura demonstrate intermediate to high attenuation on unenhanced CT scans.[106] This appearance has been attributed to the high density of collagen and abundant capillary network within the lesions. Contrast enhancement tends to be intense and homogeneous as a result of the rich vascularization of the tumor.[124] However, CT may show nonenhancing areas that correspond to necrosis, myxoid degeneration, or hemorrhage within the tumor.[124,125] This may have a geographic appearance or be focal or linear. In a series of 82 solitary fibrous tumors of the pleura from the Armed Forces Institute of Pathology, only benign lesions exhibited homogeneous attenuation, which was more commonly seen on unenhanced scans.[106] This has been indirectly related to size, as small lesions exhibit necrosis less frequently. In this series there was no difference in lesion size when benign and malignant tumors were compared; however, all malignant lesions demonstrated low-attenuation areas on both enhanced and nonenhanced CT scans. These areas correlated with the presence of hemorrhage, necrosis, or cystic change.[106] More recently, a comparison of the CT findings in benign and malignant solitary fibrous tumors of the pleura revealed that large size, lobulated margins, the presence of calcification, and ipsilateral pleural effusion were predictive but not diagnostic of malignancy.[126]

Magnetic Resonance Imaging

MRI may better characterize fibrous tumors of the pleura.[106,127,128] With large tumors, it can help differentiate the tumor from adjacent mediastinal and vital vascular structures. It may distinguish tumor from pleural effusion. MRI characteristics conform to the expected findings of fibrous tissue, predominantly of low– to intermediate–signal intensity on T1- and T2-weighted images.[1,127,129] However, high heterogeneous–signal intensity on T2-weighted sequences is frequently observed, which is thought to relate to necrosis and cystic or myxoid degeneration, with prominent vascular structures and areas of high cellularity (see Fig. 74.19).[106,130] A particularly common finding on T2-weighted images is the presence of septa of low–signal intensity (see Fig. 74.19).[106,129] Intense heterogeneous enhancement after intravenous injection of gadolinium is typical. There is no way to differentiate benign from malignant pleural tumors on MRI

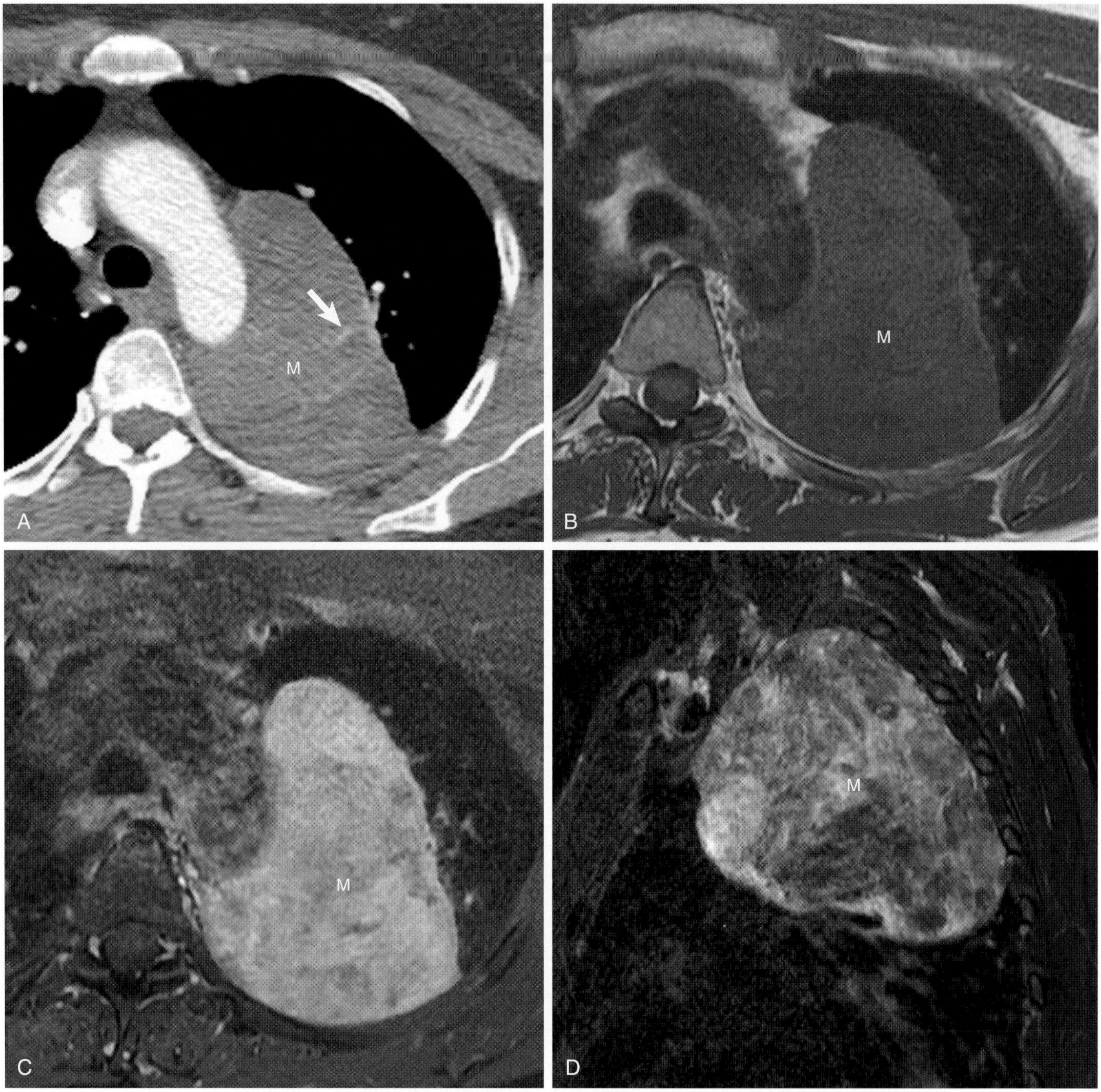

Fig. 74.19 Malignant solitary fibrous tumor of the pleura. (A) Contrast-enhanced axial CT demonstrates a large mass (M) in the left hemithorax with internal vascularity *(arrow)* that invades the adjacent mediastinum. Axial (B) and (C) and sagittal (D) MRIs demonstrate a soft tissue mass (M) in the left hemithorax that is isointense to muscle on T1-weighted imaging (B), enhances after the administration of intravenous contrast (C), and is heterogeneous on T2-weighted imaging (D).

unless there is local invasion of the chest wall or diaphragm, a feature that is rarely seen.[111] Sagittal and coronal images permit tumor localization within the chest and assessment of the diaphragm.[106]

Ultrasonography

Ultrasonography may help identify lesions in the lower hemithorax by demonstrating that the tumor is located just above the diaphragm.[106,128] Few reports of the sonographic features of fibrous tumors of the pleura are available, but one case was hypoechoic,[128] and another peritoneal fibrous tumor had cystic areas within a well-circumscribed solid mass.[131]

Fluorodeoxyglucose–Positron Emission Tomography–Computed Tomography

A few studies have evaluated the role of FDG–PET-CT in characterizing solitary fibrous tumors of the pleura.[132,133] In both of these studies, benign solitary fibrous tumors demonstrated

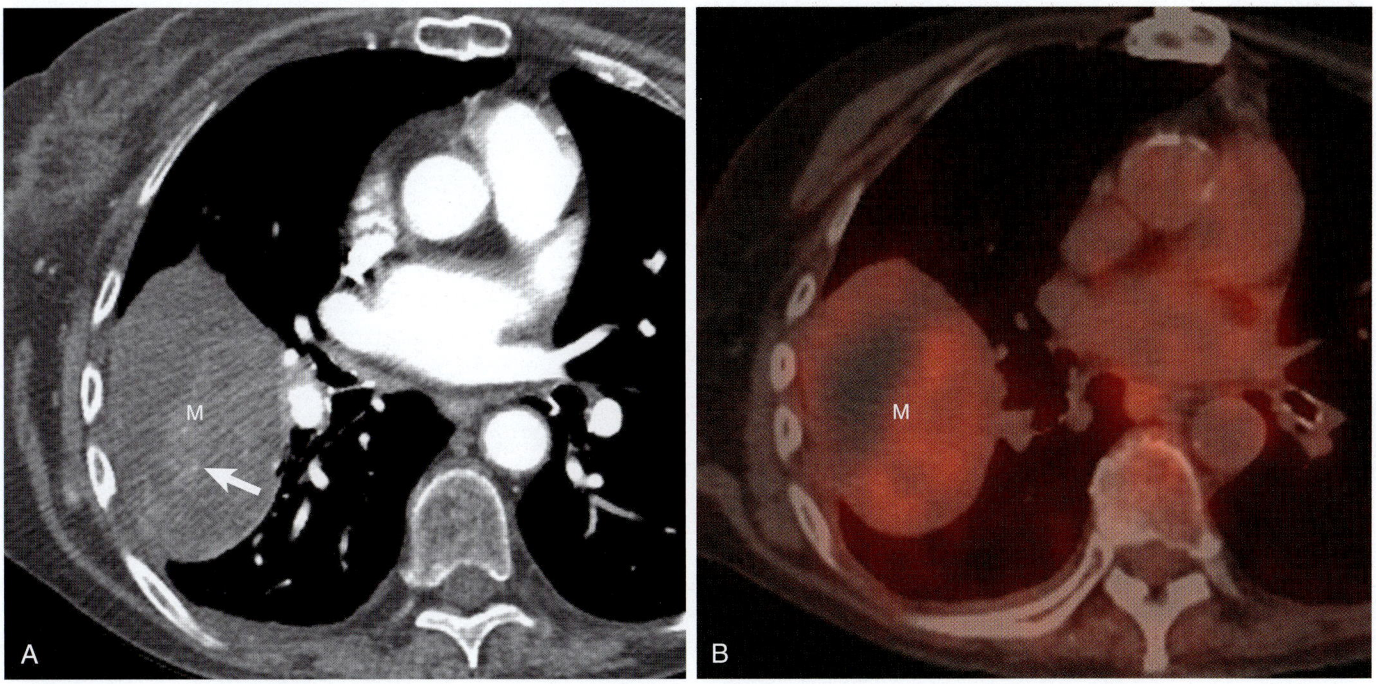

Fig. 74.20 Solitary fibrous tumor of the pleura: positron emission tomography (PET)-CT features. (A) Contrast-enhanced axial CT shows a heterogeneous mass (M) with internal vascularity *(arrow)* in the right hemithorax. (B) Fluorodeoxyglucose (FDG)–PET-CT demonstrates low-grade FDG uptake in the mass. On PET-CT benign solitary fibrous tumors tend to demonstrate low-grade FDG uptake, and malignant lesions usually show greater FDG uptake compared with benign lesions.

low-grade FDG uptake, and malignant solitary fibrous tumors demonstrated somewhat greater FDG uptake based on standardized uptake values; however, the overall role of PET-CT in evaluating these lesions is considered limited (Fig. 74.20).

TREATMENT

The treatment of all fibrous tumors of the pleura is complete en bloc surgical excision.[110] Aggressive surgery is recommended because of the possibility of recurrent or malignant disease. A distance of 1 to 2 cm from the tumor is usually recommended in healthy tissue.[110] Pedunculated and smaller tumors may be completely resected with video-assisted thoracoscopic surgery.[134] However, large tumors usually require a thoracotomy.[106] These may occasionally require a lobectomy or a pneumonectomy for complete resection to be achieved.[135] Long-term imaging follow-up is recommended in all cases to exclude tumor recurrence or metastatic disease as recurrence can occur more than 15 years postresection.[114,136] However, there are no established guidelines for the frequency and duration of imaging follow-up. Recurrent disease typically affects the ipsilateral pleura and manifests as nodule(s) and/or mass(es). If recurrent disease is identified, it must be resected; at present, there is no clear role for adjuvant therapy, although it may be useful for recurrent malignant fibrous tumors.[110] Metastatic disease to the bone, lung, and liver can occur.[136]

KEY POINTS: SOLITARY FIBROUS TUMOR

- Solitary fibrous tumor of the pleura is an uncommon mesenchymal tumor. A small percentage of affected patients have finger clubbing (hypertrophic osteoarthropathy) or hypoglycemia
- Solitary fibrous tumor typically appears as a pleural soft tissue mass that can change in position.
- On magnetic resonance imaging solitary fibrous tumors have low– to intermediate–signal intensity of T1- and T2-weighted images.
- Complete surgical resection is the treatment of choice.

Miscellaneous Mesenchymal Neoplasms

A variety of soft tissue neoplasms may develop in the pleura and tend to arise in the submesothelial mesenchymal cells. The most common is benign lipoma arising from the submesothelial layer of the parietal pleura and can extend into the subpleural, pleural, or extrapleural space. CT allows a confident diagnosis by demonstrating uniform fat density (−50 to −120 Hounsfield units) within a lesion (Fig. 74.21), and MRI can also demonstrate intensity similar to that of subcutaneous fat. Liposarcomas may be differentiated from lipomas by a heterogeneous mixture of fat and soft tissue attenuation (Fig. 74.22). Pleural liposarcomas are rare; only 12 cases were reported in the literature by 2000.[137] Other sarcomas can arise in the pleura and include rhabdomyosarcoma, angiosarcoma, epithelioid hemangioendothelioma, chondrosarcoma, and pleuropulmonary synovial sarcoma (Fig. 74.23).[138]

Pleural Metastases

Eighty percent of all malignant pleural effusions are caused by metastatic tumor from lung, breast, ovary, or stomach or by a lymphoproliferative disorder.[139] The most common finding in patients with pleural metastases is pleural effusion. Lung cancer accounts for approximately 40% of cases, breast cancer for 20%,

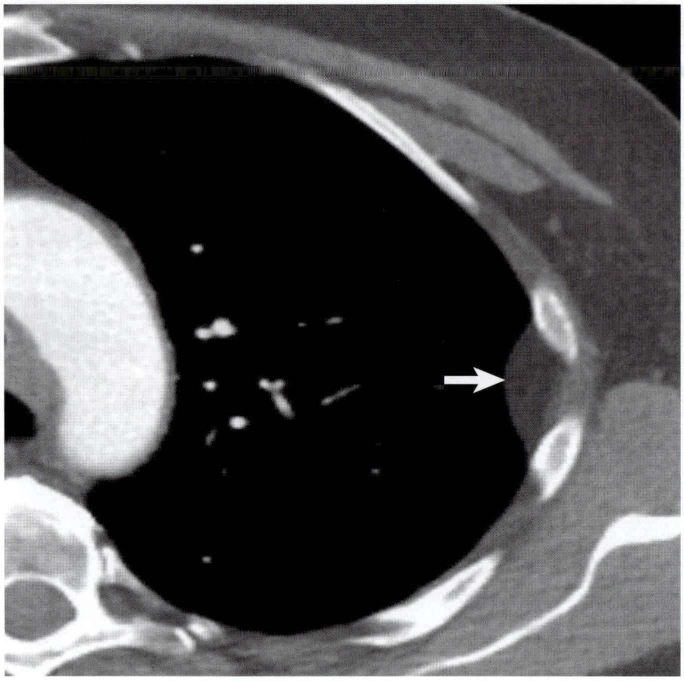

Fig. 74.21 Lipoma. Contrast-enhanced axial CT demonstrates a fat-containing lesion *(arrow)* in the left hemithorax compatible with a benign lipoma.

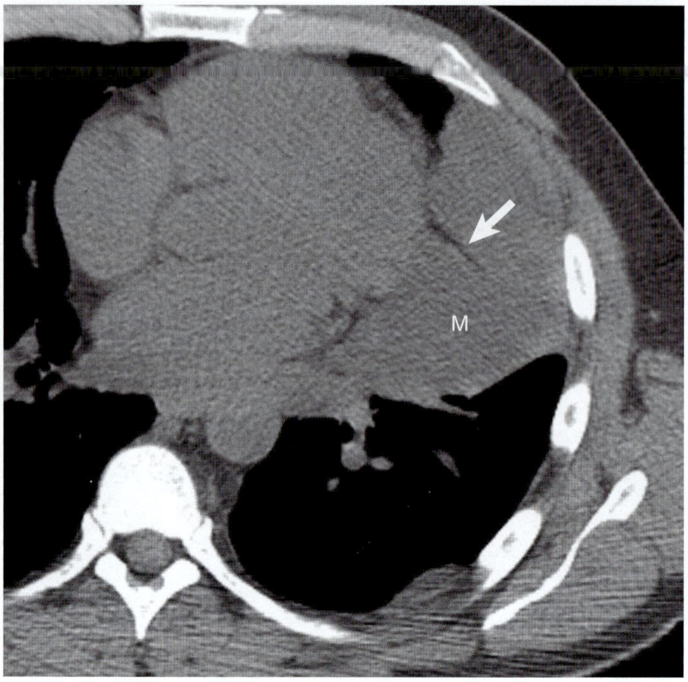

Fig. 74.22 Liposarcoma. Contrast-enhanced axial CT demonstrates a large soft tissue mass (M) containing a small amount of fat *(arrow)* in the left hemithorax. CT-guided biopsy revealed pleural liposarcoma.

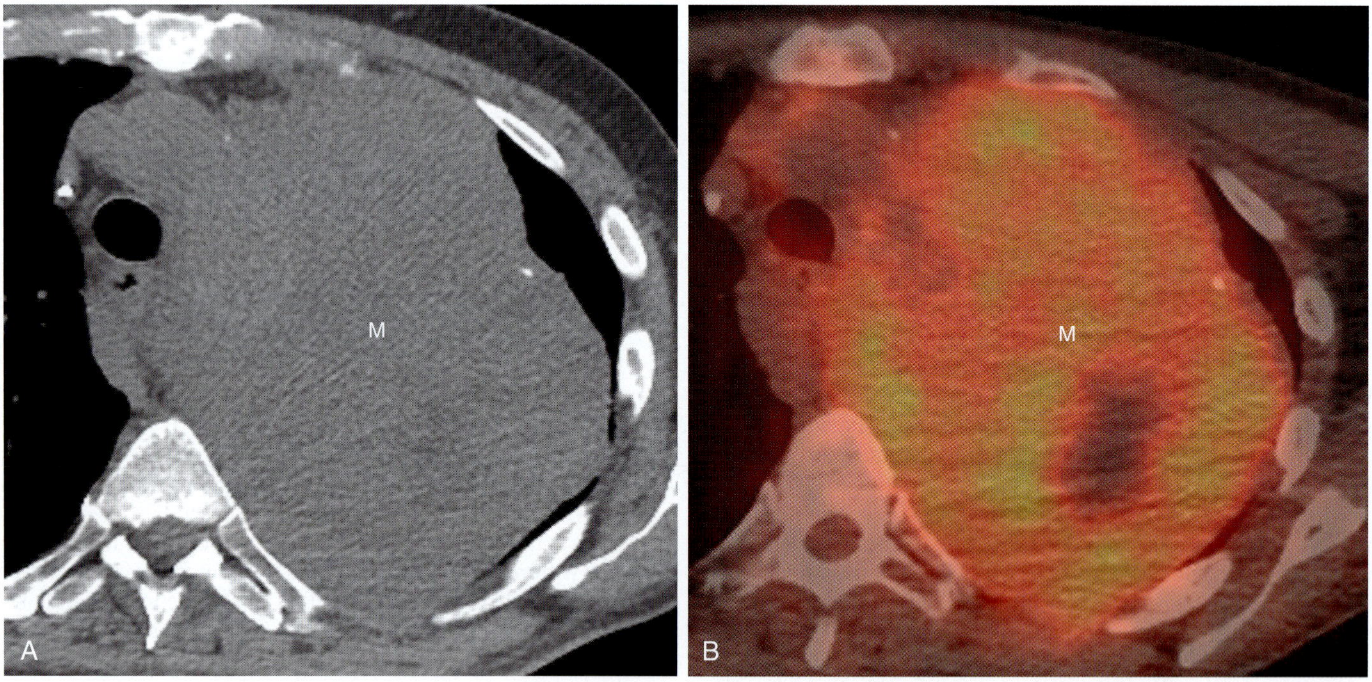

Fig. 74.23 Pleural sarcoma. Noncontrast axial CT (A) and fused axial fluorodeoxyglucose (FDG)– positron emission tomography (PET)-CT (B) show a large soft tissue mass (M) in the left hemithorax that is FDG-avid and compatible with malignancy. CT-guided biopsy revealed pleuropulmonary sarcoma.

lymphoma for 10%, and ovarian and gastric carcinoma for 5%.[140] The mechanism is most often contiguous spread and invasion of tumor into the pulmonary vasculature and lymphatics.[141] Invasive thymoma can also involve the pleura in a contiguous manner or with drop metastases. It can be impossible to differentiate pleural metastases from mesothelioma radiologically.

Adenocarcinoma of the lung is the most common cell type to involve the pleura because of its peripheral nature and its propensity to invade the vasculature.[1] Most pleural metastases involve the visceral pleura through pulmonary artery invasion and embolization.[1] Invasion of the pleura modifies staging of lung cancer. It behooves the radiologist and thoracic surgeon to prospectively identify malignant pleural disease to avoid unnecessary thoracotomy. PET-CT has been shown to be helpful for reliable differentiation of benign from malignant pleural effusion in patients with lung cancer.[141]

The most common findings on chest radiography include pleural nodules and/or masses and circumferential nodular pleural thickening (Fig. 74.24). Pleural effusions are present in approximately 50% of cases. Findings on chest CT include pleural nodules and/or masses and pleural thickening that is typically greater than 1 cm in thickness (see Fig. 74.24). High-density calcification may be present, resulting from bone-forming neoplasms, such as osteosarcoma or chondrosarcoma (Fig. 74.25). Metastatic disease may spread along the mediastinal pleura and along the interlobar fissures. FDG–PET-CT typically shows FDG uptake within pleural thickening, nodules, and masses (Fig. 74.26). The overall sensitivity and specificity of ^{18}F-FDG–PET-CT for the detection of pleural metastases is 96.8% and 88.5%, respectively. Pleural metastases are usually hyperintense to the intercostal muscles on T2-weighted MRI sequences and demonstrate enhancement after the administration of gadolinium. It can be impossible to differentiate pleural metastasis from MPM radiologically, but helpful features to suggest the diagnosis include the following[142–144]:

1. Metastatic pleural disease is far more common than MPM (9:1).
2. Asbestos pleural plaques are helpful as they suggest MPM but are not definitive for this diagnosis because asbestos exposure also increases the risk of lung carcinoma.
3. The presence of systemic metastases is more suggestive of metastatic pleural disease; mesothelioma has a low incidence of distant metastases (<15%).
4. Shrinkage of the hemithorax is more common in MPM (50%) than in metastatic adenocarcinoma.
5. Metastatic adenocarcinoma more commonly involves the visceral pleura.
6. Chest wall invasion is more likely with MPM (25%), particularly if more than one site is identified.

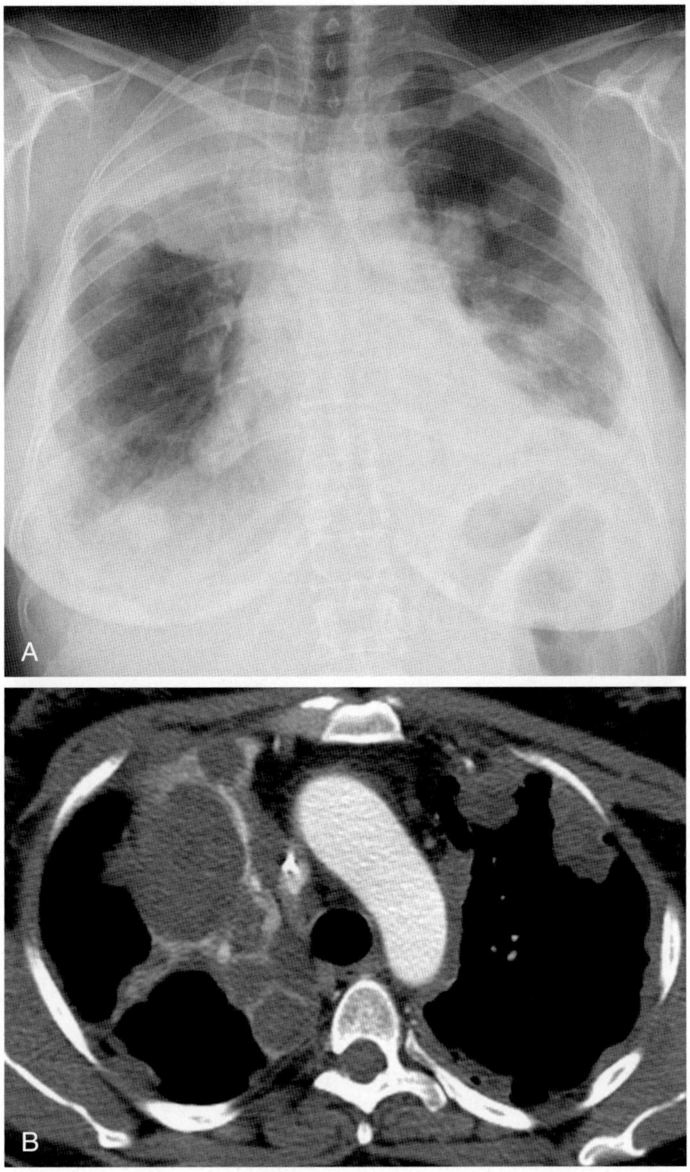

Fig. 74.24 Pleural metastases. Frontal chest radiograph (A) and contrast-enhanced axial CT (B) demonstrate extensive pleural thickening and masses bilaterally consistent with metastatic disease. Pleural metastases most commonly result from lung cancer (40%), gastrointestinal and genitourinary malignancies (30%), breast cancer (20%), and lymphoma (10%).

KEY POINTS: METASTATIC PLEURAL DISEASE

- Pleural metastases from lung, breast, ovarian, and gastric cancer account for the majority of malignant pleural disease. Invasive thymoma can also cause pleural metastases.
- Differentiation of pleural metastases from malignant pleural mesothelioma by imaging is difficult.

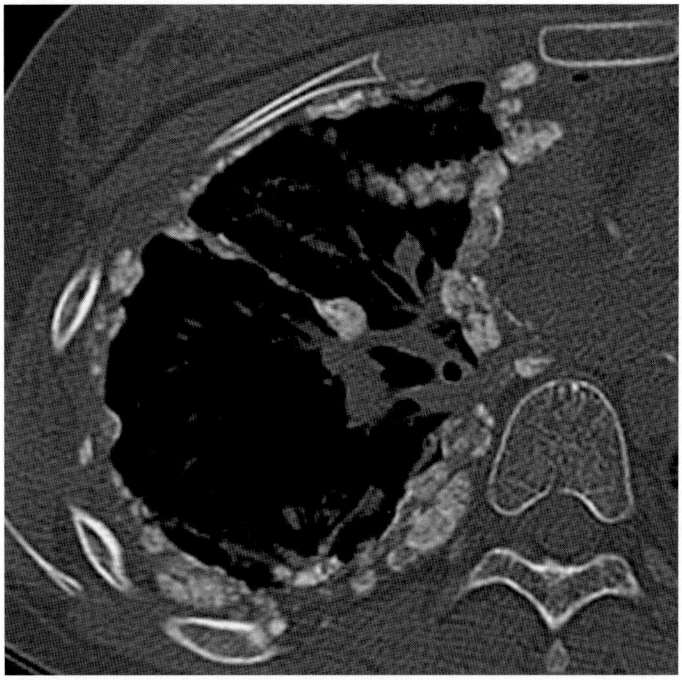

Fig. 74.25 Pleural metastases with calcification. Contrast-enhanced axial CT shows innumerable calcified pleural nodules in the right hemithorax consistent with metastases. Calcification or ossification may be present in metastases related to osteosarcoma, chondrosarcoma, and mucinous tumors of the gastrointestinal or genitourinary tract.

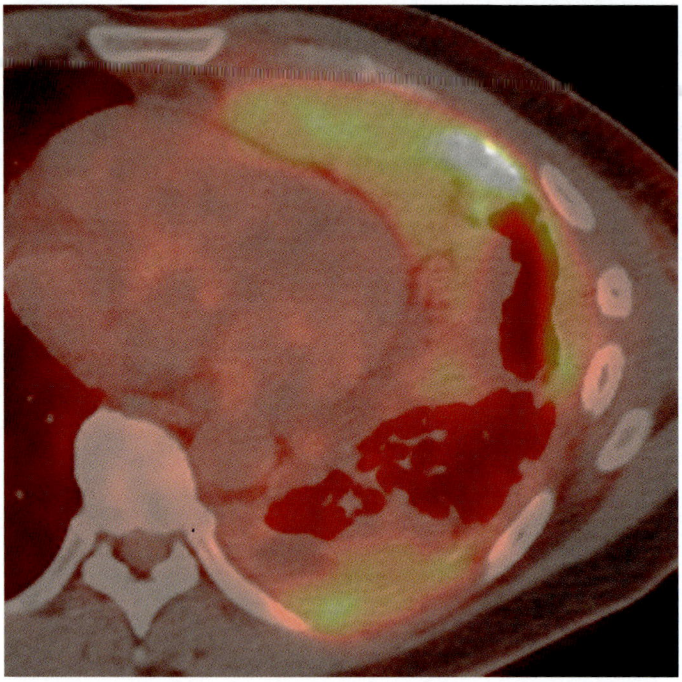

Fig. 74.26 Positron emission tomography (PET)-CT of pleural metastases. Fused axial PET-CT demonstrates extensive pleural thickening in the left hemithorax with increased fluorodeoxyglucose (FDG) uptake in the most mass-like regions of disease. FDG–PET-CT can reliably distinguish between malignant and benign pleural disease and has high sensitivity and specificity for detecting metastatic disease.

Lymphoma

Pleural lymphoma usually occurs as part of disseminated disease.[145] The prevalence of pleural disease in lymphoma is reported to be around 26% to 31%,[1,146–148] and it occurs in both Hodgkin (11.4% to 30%) and non-Hodgkin lymphoma (3.7% to 33%).[1] Typically, this is seen in conjunction with mediastinal lymphadenopathy (70%),[146] but it may occur as an extension of pulmonary lymphoma.[148]

Primary pleural lymphoma represents about 7% of primary lymphoma cases, and patients with human immunodeficiency virus (HIV) infection or long-standing diseases of the pleura, such as chronic tuberculous pyothorax, are typically affected.[149,150] Most primary pleural lymphomas are B-cell lymphomas, and the proposed mechanism for the development of the disease is chronic stimulation of B cells by long-standing pleural disease.[151] Primary effusion lymphoma (PEL) is a rare form of lymphoma found in HIV-infected males, patients who have undergone solid-organ transplantation, and other immunocompromised individuals. PEL is associated with human herpesvirus 8 and Epstein-Barr virus infection.[152] Pyothorax-associated lymphoma (PAL) may develop in patients with chronic pyothorax or long-standing pleural inflammation resulting from prior artificial pneumothorax used to treat tuberculosis.[145] As chemotherapeutic agents for the treatment of *Mycobacterium tuberculosis* became widely available, the artificial pneumothorax was generally abandoned in the 1950s, and PAL is rapidly becoming a rare disease.

PATHOLOGY

Lymphoma has a propensity to involve the subpleural lymphatics.[147] It may occur in both non-Hodgkin and Hodgkin lymphoma. This was first demonstrated in an autopsy series of 50 patients with Hodgkin disease of the lung.[148] The lymphomatous deposits arise from the lymphatic channels and lymphoid aggregates in the subpleural connective tissue below the visceral pleura. True visceral pleural invasion is uncommon.[147]

On histologic examination pyothorax-associated lymphoma shows a diffuse proliferation of large cells of B-cell type (diffuse large B-cell lymphoma).[153] Autopsies carried out in 23 cases revealed the disease to have been localized to the thorax in 11 patients. These findings indicated that malignant B-cell lymphoma arose as a monoclonal growth from a pool of proliferating polyclonal B lymphocytes in tissues affected by the chronic tuberculous pyothorax.[154]

CLINICAL PRESENTATION

The most common symptoms of pleural involvement in lymphoma are chest pain and fever. In 40% of patients with pyothorax-associated lymphoma, the presenting complaint is chest wall swelling.[155] Chest pain is a helpful sign to suggest the development of a tumor in a patient with chronic pyothorax; pain is not a common feature of pyothorax.[123] When tumor invades the spinal cord, patients may present with paralysis of the lower limbs.[123]

IMAGING

Radiography

The main radiologic finding is unilateral or bilateral pleural effusion, with or without pleural thickening.[146] Effusions are reported in 80% to 100% of patients with Hodgkin lymphoma.[156,157] In non-Hodgkin lymphoma, 20% to 70% of patients are reported to have associated lymphadenopathy.[158] In 50% of patients the effusions are bilateral.[146] On occasion, secondary pleural lymphoma appears either as a solitary nodule or as diffuse tumor infiltration.[147] Just as mediastinal Hodgkin nodes can calcify after treatment, so may subpleural deposits of lymphoma.[147] When effusions associated with lymphoma are present, radiography usually demonstrates coexisting mediastinal disease, reported in 80% to 100% of patients with Hodgkin disease[156,157] and 20% to 70% of patients with non-Hodgkin lymphoma.[146]

Computed Tomography

The most typical finding is pleural effusion, which is bilateral in 50% of patients.[146] Tumor involvement of parietal pleura and extrapleural space is also common, seen in approximately 4%, and pleural thickening is seen in approximately 25%.[146] Pleural thickening may appear focal or diffuse, nodular, or smooth (Fig. 74.27). It typically involves the parietal pleura.[146] Most patients have posterior mediastinal lymphadenopathy. This is related to the lymphatic drainage pattern of the parietal pleura and chest wall. Lymphatics of the pleura, extrapleural space, and paraspinal region communicate with the posterior mediastinal (paravertebral, paraaortic, and paraesophageal) lymph nodes, which then drain into the thoracic duct and cisterna chyli.[4] This explains why lymphomatous pleural effusions may be chyliform.[4]

PEL manifests as an effusion that affects one body cavity in the absence of a solid tumor mass.[145] The pleural space is most commonly involved, followed by the pericardial and peritoneal spaces. The CT appearance of pyothorax-associated lymphoma is that of an inhomogeneous soft tissue mass. This type of lymphoma usually manifests with a pleural mass of more than

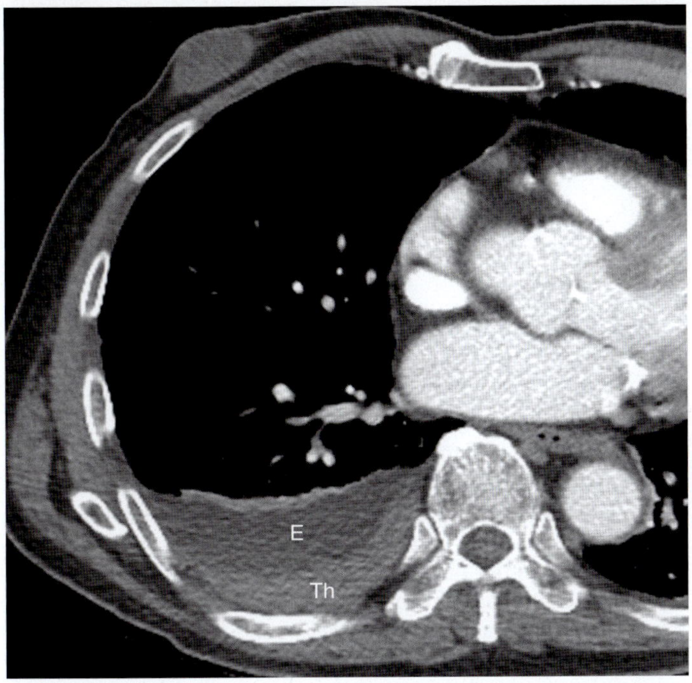

Fig. 74.27 Pleural involvement by lymphoma. Contrast-enhanced axial CT demonstrates a right pleural effusion (E) and pleural thickening (Th). A sebaceous cyst is incidentally noted in the anterior chest wall. With involvement of the pleura by lymphoma, effusion is the most common finding, and thickening may appear focal or diffuse, nodular, or smooth.

10 cm in size in more than 50% of cases but tends to be localized to the thoracic cavity at the time of diagnosis.[123] Rib destruction may be present. Contrast enhancement may be helpful to distinguish lymphoma from empyema, as chronic empyema does not enhance.[154] There is usually no lymphadenopathy, and evidence of chronic empyema is present.

TREATMENT

Secondary involvement of the pleura is treated with chemotherapy and radiation therapy, as dictated by the primary disease. With pyothorax-associated lymphoma, the prognosis is poor and related to age and performance status.[159] Complete surgical excision is required, and patients may be treated with radiation therapy and chemotherapy, but overall average survival after symptom onset is about 5 months.[160]

KEY POINTS: LYMPHOMA OF THE PLEURAL SPACE

- Lymphomatous involvement of the pleura can occur with both Hodgkin and non-Hodgkin lymphoma.
- Primary effusion lymphoma is rare and occurs in immunocompromised individuals. It presents with body cavity effusions without soft tissue masses.
- Pyothorax-associated lymphoma occurs in patients with chronic pyothorax or long-standing pleural inflammation resulting from prior artificial pneumothorax used to treat tuberculosis. It typically manifests as a pleural soft tissue mass.

SUGGESTED READINGS

Armato SG 3rd, Blyth KG, Keating JJ, Katz S, Tsim S, Coolen J, Gudmundsson E, Opitz I, Nowak AK. Imaging in pleural mesothelioma: a review of the 13th International Conference of the International Mesothelioma Interest Group. *Lung Cancer*. 2016;101:48–58.

Bibby AC, Tsim S, Kanellakis N, Ball H, Talbot DC, Blyth KG, Maskell NA, Psallidas I. Malignant pleural mesothelioma: an update on investigation, diagnosis and treatment. *Eur Respir Rev*. 2016;25(142):472–486.

Galateau-Salle F, Churg A, Roggli V, Travis WD, World Health Organization Committee for Tumors of the Pleura. The 2015 World Health Organization Classification of Tumors of the Pleura: advances since the 2004 classification. *J Thorac Oncol*. 2016;11(2):142–154.

Kruse M, Sherry SJ, Paidpally V, Mercier G, Subramaniam RM. FDG PET/CT in the management of primary pleural tumors and pleural metastases. *AJR Am J Roentgenol*. 2013;201(2):W215–W226.

Mordenti P, Di Cicilia R, Delfanti R, Capelli P, Paties C, Cavanna L. Solitary fibrous tumors of the pleura: a case report and review of the literature. *Tumori*. 2013;99(4):e177–e183.

The full reference list for this chapter is available at ExpertConsult.com.

75 Pneumomediastinum

TOMÁS FRANQUET

Etiology, Prevalence, and Epidemiology

Pneumomediastinum, also known as *mediastinal emphysema*, refers to the presence of free air or other gas in the mediastinal space. Pathologically, the major sources of entry of air to the mediastinum are (1) through the skin and chest wall, as commonly seen in penetrating trauma; (2) from the neck; (3) from a tear or defect in the esophagus or the trachea, allowing air to enter the mediastinum directly; (4) from ruptured alveoli; and (5) from the abdominal cavity.[1–3]

Most cases of pneumomediastinum are related to alveolar rupture and can be clinically divided into two categories: (1) "spontaneous" pneumomediastinum and (2) "barotrauma," or pneumomediastinum occurring during positive-pressure ventilation or associated with other externally applied distending pressures.[4–6]

The term *pneumomediastinum* usually refers to the presence of abnormal air within the mediastinum without associated infection. However, gas can form in the mediastinum during acute bacterial mediastinitis caused by gas-producing microorganisms or resulting from communication with the esophagus (e.g., Boerhaave syndrome), respiratory tract (e.g., necrotizing pneumonia), or head-neck soft tissue infection (e.g., cervical adenitis).[3,7] Moreover, acute mediastinitis may also occur with cardiovascular or other thoracic surgical procedures.[8–10]

Primary pneumomediastinum, also known as spontaneous pneumomediastinum, is generally described as a benign condition, manifesting in young adults exposed to a sudden pressure change within the intrathoracic cavity.[11] It may occur after involuntary alterations in the breathing pattern, such as asthma, violent coughing or vomiting, and athletic competition.[2,12–14] Other conditions associated with spontaneous pneumomediastinum include seizures, croup,[15] marijuana or crack cocaine smoking,[16,17] nitrous oxide inhalation,[18] pneumonia, diabetic ketoacidosis,[19] diffuse interstitial pulmonary fibrosis,[20–22] and parturition.[23] The majority of patients with spontaneous pneumomediastinum have predisposing factors that cause a sudden rise in alveolar pressure leading to alveolar rupture.[24]

Idiopathic spontaneous pneumomediastinum (Hamman syndrome or Macklin syndrome) is a rare self-limited condition described in young adult men without a history of a potential predisposing cause and normal lung parenchyma at computed tomography (CT).[25,26] The physical examination usually reveals subcutaneous air in the suprasternal notch and the Hamman sign, which is a crunching or clicking noise synchronous with the heartbeat and is best heard in the left lateral decubitus position.

Mechanical ventilation with positive end-expiratory pressure has long been recognized as a traumatic source of pneumomediastinum in intensive care unit patients.[5] In some cases extraalveolar air originating from disrupted alveoli may appear below the diaphragm as either pneumoperitoneum or pneumoretroperitoneum. In addition, gas from the anterior mediastinum can dissect through the diaphragm into the anterior abdominal extraperitoneal space resembling intraperitoneal air.[27] Loculated thoracic air collections can develop in mechanically ventilated neonates with acute lung injury or acute respiratory distress syndrome.[28,29] Barotrauma-associated posterior tension pneumomediastinum is a rare cause of cardiac tamponade in a ventilated neonate.[30] Moreover, on the chest radiograph, the cardiac shadow may be obscured because of flattening of the heart from tension pneumomediastinum ("vanishing heart").[31]

Secondary pneumomediastinum has been identified as a result of a specific injury or pathologic condition, such as blunt or penetrating trauma, recent interventions in the esophageal or tracheobronchial tree, rupture of a hollow viscus, tissue dissection originating from a spontaneous pneumothorax, or pulmonary or mediastinal infection caused by gas-forming organisms.[11,32,33]

The causes of pneumomediastinum are shown in Table 75.1. The reported clinical settings associated with alveolar rupture are shown in Table 75.2.

Clinical Presentation

Often misdiagnosed because of its vague manifestations, spontaneous pneumomediastinum must be part of the differential diagnosis of a patient presenting with chest pain or discomfort. Chest pain occurs in 80% to 90% of patients with spontaneous pneumomediastinum and represents the second most common cause of admission of young, healthy individuals experiencing sudden chest pain or shortness of breath.[34] The clinical presentation depends on the amount of air in the mediastinum and on the presence or absence of associated infection. Chest pain is characteristically retrosternal and aggravated by breathing and position changes[2]; dyspnea is present in about 50% of the cases.[25] On occasion, patients are asymptomatic.[14] Pneumomediastinum occurring in a patient on mechanical ventilation is potentially disastrous because of its frequent association with tension pneumothorax. In this clinical setting the diagnosis may be suggested by a history of sudden deterioration marked by hypotension and increased pulmonary pressures.

Tension pneumomediastinum is a rare, potentially fatal complication caused by large amounts of air in the mediastinum and a substantial increase in intramediastinal pressure that can

TABLE 75.1 CAUSES OF PNEUMOMEDIASTINUM
HEAD AND NECK
Perforation of nasopharynx, esophagus, and trachea (iatrogenic or traumatic)
Facial fractures (zygomaticomaxillary)
Facial surgery
Dental procedures
Neck surgery (thyroid, tonsils, tracheostomy)
MEDIASTINUM
Perforation of trachea, bronchi, or esophagus (achalasia, Boerhaave syndrome)
Mediastinal surgery, mediastinoscopy, sternal bone marrow aspiration
Lung transplantation
ABDOMEN
Intraperitoneal or retroperitoneal perforation of bowel (perforated diverticulitis, perforated retroperitoneal hernia, perforated duodenal ulcer, rectosigmoid surgery, trauma, rectal foreign bodies)
Postcolonoscopy or postpolypectomy
PULMONARY
Associated With Abnormal Lung Parenchyma
Atelectasis
Pneumonia (measles, influenza, smallpox, varicella, pneumocystis)
Tuberculosis
Lung abscess
Acute respiratory distress syndrome
Silicosis
Emphysema
Idiopathic pulmonary fibrosis
Associated With Airway Anomalies
Asthma
Foreign body
Laryngeal disease
Acute obstructive laryngitis
Congenital stenosis
ELEVATED INTRAALVEOLAR PRESSURE ASSOCIATED WITH CLINICAL ABNORMALITIES
Ventilation assistance
Anesthesia
Blunt chest trauma
Heimlich maneuver
Caisson disease
Seizure
Diabetic ketoacidosis
Marijuana, crack cocaine, or heroin use
Anorexia nervosa
ELEVATING INTRAALVEOLAR PRESSURE WITHOUT CLINICAL ABNORMALITY
Coughing
Vomiting
Straining, as in children or defecation
Parturition
Idiopathic

Modified from Rohlfing BM, Webb WR, Schlobohm RM. Ventilator-related extra-alveolar air in adults. *Radiology*. 1976;121:25–31.

lead to hemodynamic compromise.[35] Although uncommon, tension pneumomediastinum may result in acute diastolic dysfunction,[36] cardiac tamponade,[37] impaired venous return to the heart, and airway distortion that impedes air flow. Percutaneous CT-guided insertion of a mediastinal drainage catheter is a useful procedure to perform before the development of cardiac tamponade.[38]

TABLE 75.2 CLINICAL SETTINGS ASSOCIATED WITH ALVEOLAR RUPTURE
SPONTANEOUS
Deliberate Alteration in Breathing Pattern
Marijuana smoking and cocaine inhalation
Pulmonary function testing
Mountain climbing
Wind instrument playing
Yelling, shouting, and singing
Straining and Other Involuntary Alterations in Breathing Pattern
Childbirth
Vomiting
Seizures; status epilepticus
Violent coughing; sneezing; hiccupping
Heavy lifting; athletic competition
Straining at stool
Associated Lung Diseases
"Idiopathic" (Hamman Syndrome)
CAUSED BY EXTERNAL PRESSURE CHANGES (BAROTRAUMA)
Decompression: Gas Expansion
Scuba diving
Air travel
Positive Intrathoracic Pressure of External Origin
Asthma
Foreign body
Laryngeal disease
Acute obstructive laryngitis
Congenital stenosis
Elevated Intraalveolar Pressure Associated With Clinical Abnormalities
Mechanical ventilation
Continuous positive airway pressure
Manual ventilation during resuscitation, anesthesia, or transport
Equipment malfunction or misconnection in anesthesia or oxygen therapy
Heimlich maneuver
Deceleration injury

Modified from Rohlfing BM, Webb WR, Schlobohm RM. Ventilator-related extra-alveolar air in adults. *Radiology*. 1976;121:25–31.

Pathologic Findings and Pathophysiology

The pathophysiology of pneumomediastinum depends on the different clinical scenarios in which it is seen. Anatomically, the mediastinum communicates with several structures, including the submandibular space,[39] the retropharyngeal space, and the vascular sheaths in the neck.[40] There is a tissue plane that extends anteriorly from the mediastinum to the retroperitoneal space through the sternocostal attachment of the diaphragm.[41] This space is continuous with the flanks and extends to the pelvis.[42] The mediastinum also communicates directly with the retroperitoneum by way of the periaortic and periesophageal fascial planes.

In the presence of a pressure gradient between an alveolus and the interstitium, air ruptures from the alveolus into the perivascular and peribronchial fascial sheath.[1,43] The Macklin effect relates to a three-step pathophysiologic process: blunt traumatic alveolar rupture, air dissection along bronchovascular sheaths, and spreading of this pulmonary interstitial air into the mediastinum.[44,45] Because the mean pressure in the mediastinum is always somewhat negative with respect to the pressure in the pulmonary parenchyma, air tends to move centrally, perhaps facilitated by the pumping action of breathing.[44,45] On occasion, air will dissect peripherally, resulting in subpleural air cysts.[46,47] Pulmonary interstitial emphysema is typically a transient phenomenon; it rarely persists, and CT is helpful in making this diagnosis.[48–50]

Spontaneous pneumomediastinum commonly occurs in healthy young men in whom an increased intraalveolar pressure (e.g., Valsalva maneuver, cough, emesis) leads to the rupture of marginal pulmonary alveoli. On occasion, asymptomatic spontaneous epidural emphysema has been incidentally described in asthmatic patients.[51]

Blunt thoracic trauma is usually associated with simultaneous injuries to adjacent structures, such as great vessels, the esophagus, and osseous structures.[52] Tracheobronchial injuries occur in less than 1% of blunt chest trauma patients.[53] Pneumomediastinum in trauma patients may occur from alveolar rupture or fracture of a central airway. Isolated tracheobronchial injury is unusual because of the proximity of other major structures, such as great vessels, but has been reported in young individuals in whom the blood vessels are more compliant. Sudden deceleration injury resulting from a motor vehicle accident or fall from great heights may result in a tear or a total disruption of either the right or left main bronchus. Because of the relative fixation at the carina, the majority of airway injuries are within 3 cm of the carina.[46,47,53,54] Pneumomediastinum may also be a consequence of airway or bronchial laceration during bronchoscopy,[55–58] tracheotomy, endotracheal intubation, and overinflation of the endotracheal tube cuff.[59–61]

Pneumomediastinum may occur with esophageal perforation during upper gastrointestinal endoscopy,[62,63] after the ingestion of a caustic substance such as paraquat, or from spontaneous esophageal rupture as occurs in Boerhaave syndrome.[64] Pneumomediastinum has also been described after treating esophageal varices with endoscopic intravascular sclerotherapy.[65]

A continuum of fascial planes connects cervical soft tissues with the mediastinum and retroperitoneum, permitting aberrant air arising in any one of these areas to spread elsewhere.[41] Air dissecting downward into the mediastinum may be secondary to different head-neck infections. The most common causes include retropharyngeal or dental abscess, cervical adenitis, salivary gland infection, tonsillitis, and osteomyelitis of the facial bones. Surgical procedures involving the upper respiratory tract may produce air in the neck through breaches either in the oropharyngeal mucosa or in the trachea.[66]

Mediastinal air can also arise from below the diaphragm. Air may dissect into the mediastinum from the retroperitoneal space after perforation of a hollow viscus, ulcerative colitis, sigmoid diverticulitis, pneumatosis cystoides intestinalis, "rectal barotrauma," and procedures such as sigmoidoscopy, colonoscopy, and barium enema.[41,67–69]

Imaging Findings

RADIOGRAPHIC FINDINGS

Chest radiography has a low sensitivity to detect pneumomediastinum. The typical radiographic appearance is that of linear interstitial air collections.[70] Dissection of air along tissue planes may be more obvious on the lateral projection, showing an increase in the depth and lucency of the retrosternal space.[71] It is also recognized by streaks of gray-black density separating portions of mediastinal pleura from mediastinal contents or focal bubble-like or larger collections of gas outlining the mediastinal structures (Fig. 75.1).[70,72] Abnormal mediastinal air appears as vertical streaks of radiolucency just within the lateral borders of the mediastinal shadow. The parietal pleura is peeled off from the mediastinal structures and is seen as a line, parallel to and separated from the heart and mediastinum by a band of translucent air[73]; this line is best seen on the left side but may be easily overlooked (Figs. 75.2 and 75.3). In addition, the borders of the heart, aorta, and thymus appear more sharply outlined. Streak-like areas of radiolucency produced by mediastinal air are sometimes more clearly appreciated on the lateral view.

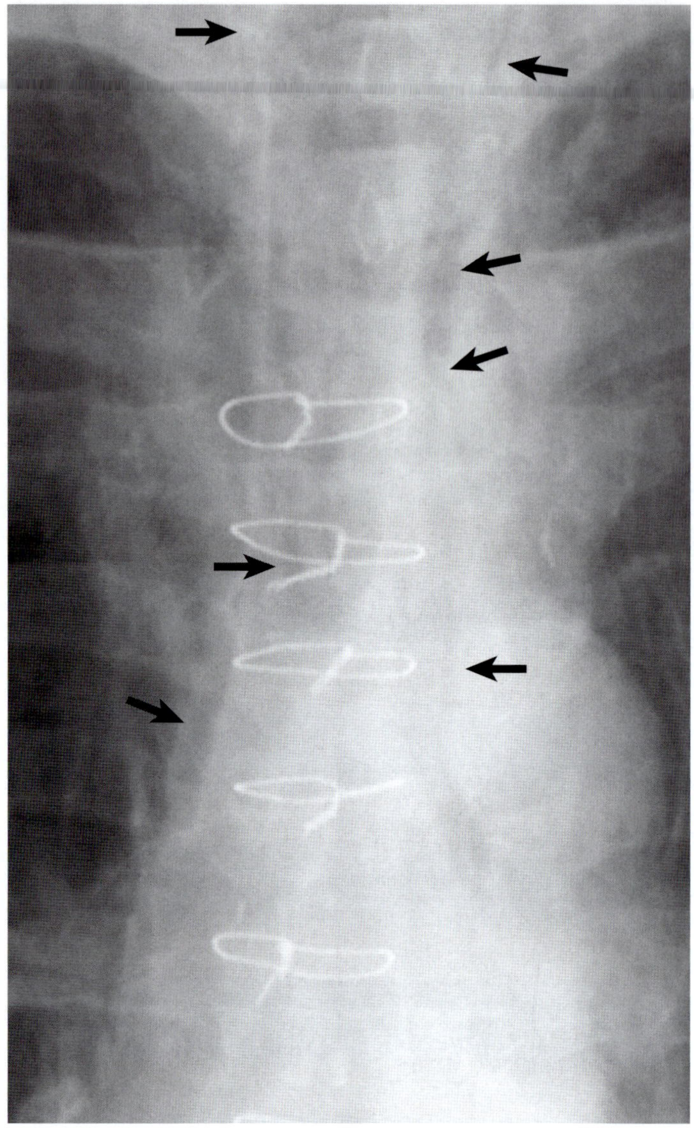

Fig. 75.1 Postsurgical pneumomediastinum. Close-up view from a posteroanterior chest radiograph shows multiple streaks of air outlining the mediastinal structures *(arrows)*.

Sometimes, air in the peribronchial sheaths can be detected radiographically, most commonly in premature infants with surfactant deficiency. Unlike air bronchograms, pulmonary interstitial emphysema does not branch and is usually subtle

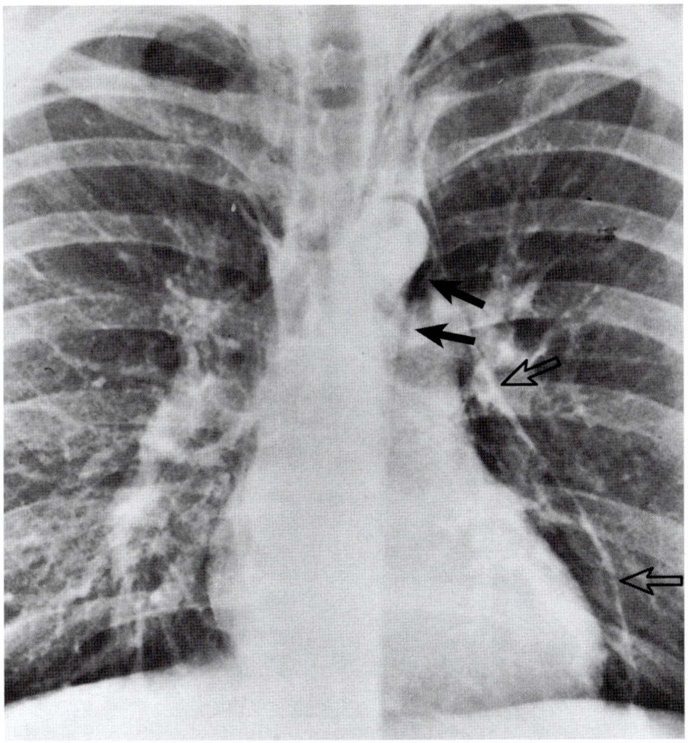

Fig. 75.2 Spontaneous pneumomediastinum in a young man with an abrupt onset of severe retrosternal chest pain. Posteroanterior chest radiograph shows a long linear opacity roughly paralleling the left heart border *(open arrows)*, representing the laterally displaced mediastinal pleura. Considerable gas is present around the aortic arch and proximal descending thoracic aorta *(solid arrows)*. *(From Müller NL, Fraser RS, Colman NC, et al.* Radiologic Diagnosis of Diseases of the Chest. *Philadelphia: Saunders; 2001.)*

and disorganized.[74] In neonates a loculated mediastinal air collection appears as a rounded hyperlucent cystic lesion adjacent or overlying the mediastinum (Fig. 75.4).

Alveolar rupture from the high airway pressures used in the treatment of acute respiratory distress syndrome (ARDS) may cause interstitial dissection of gas peripherally and the formation of "subpleural air cysts."[75,76] These thin-walled, rounded air collections are occasionally detected radiographically, and their recognition is an early manifestation of pulmonary barotrauma.[75,76] Although these findings are difficult to identify on radiographs, they can be easily seen on CT scans (Figs. 75.5 and 75.6).[77]

Various chest radiographic features of pneumomediastinum have been described.[28,31,73,78–82] These include the following: (1) *continuous diaphragm sign:* mediastinal air is visible along the diaphragm and below the heart, permitting identification of the central portion of the diaphragm in continuity with the lateral portions, a finding that gives the appearance of a continuous diaphragm (Fig. 75.7); (2) longitudinal line shadow parallel to the heart border (see Figs. 75.2 and 75.3); (3) *Naclerio V sign:* mediastinal air extends between the parietal pleura and the medial portion of the left hemidiaphragm, outlining the descending aorta and having a configuration that resembles a V; (4) *ring-around-the-artery sign:* a circular gas shadow surrounds the right pulmonary artery as visualized on the lateral projection (Fig. 75.8); (5) *thymic spinnaker-sail sign:* mediastinal air displaces one lobe of the thymus, creating a crescentic shape (Fig. 75.9); and (6) *vanished heart:* disappearance of the heart shadow secondary to a large pneumomediastinum that compresses and displaces the heart anteriorly.

Pneumomediastinum often decompresses superiorly into the neck and chest wall soft tissues. Air may also dissect inferiorly into the mesentery and gut wall, producing pneumatosis cystoides

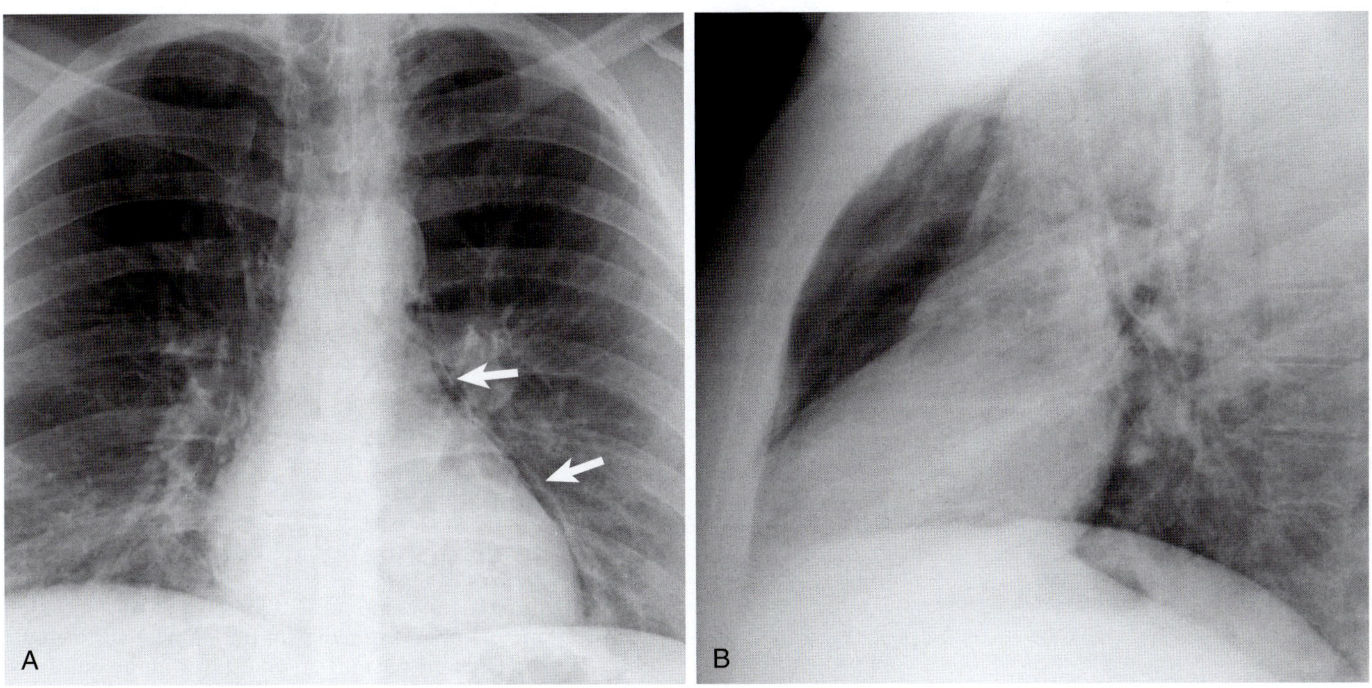

Fig. 75.3 Pneumomediastinum after balloon dilation for esophageal stricture. (A) Posteroanterior chest radiograph shows linear foci of air along the left heart border *(arrows)* and outlining the descending thoracic aorta. (B) Lateral chest radiograph shows mediastinal air outlining the retrosternal vascular structures and fat.

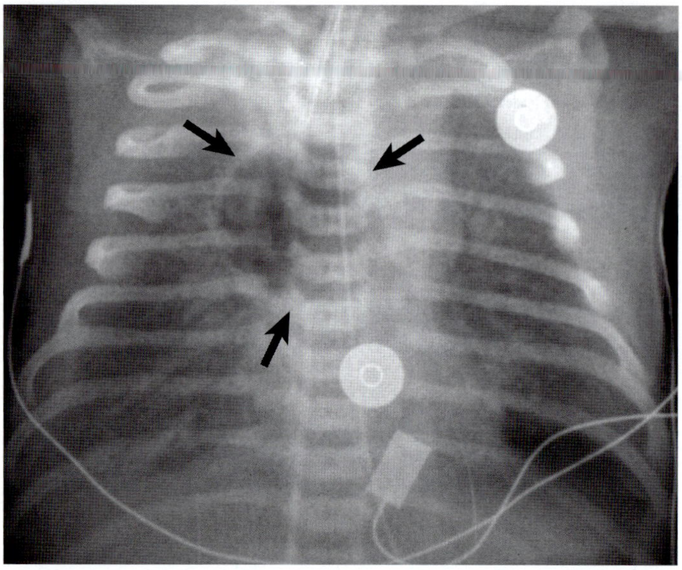

Fig. 75.4 Loculated pneumomediastinum in an infant with respiratory distress. Frontal chest radiograph obtained 5 days after birth shows a rounded air collection *(arrows)* overlying the mediastinum. This air collection was not present on a previous chest radiograph done 2 days prior (not shown).

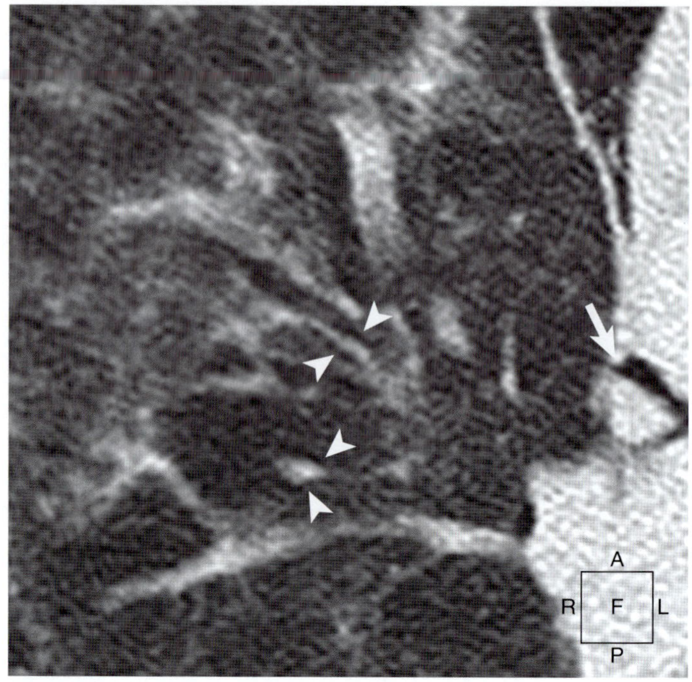

Fig. 75.6 Pulmonary interstitial emphysema. Close-up view from a CT scan shows interstitial emphysema surrounding the bronchovascular structures *(arrowheads)*. Air surrounding mediastinal vessels is also seen *(arrow)*.

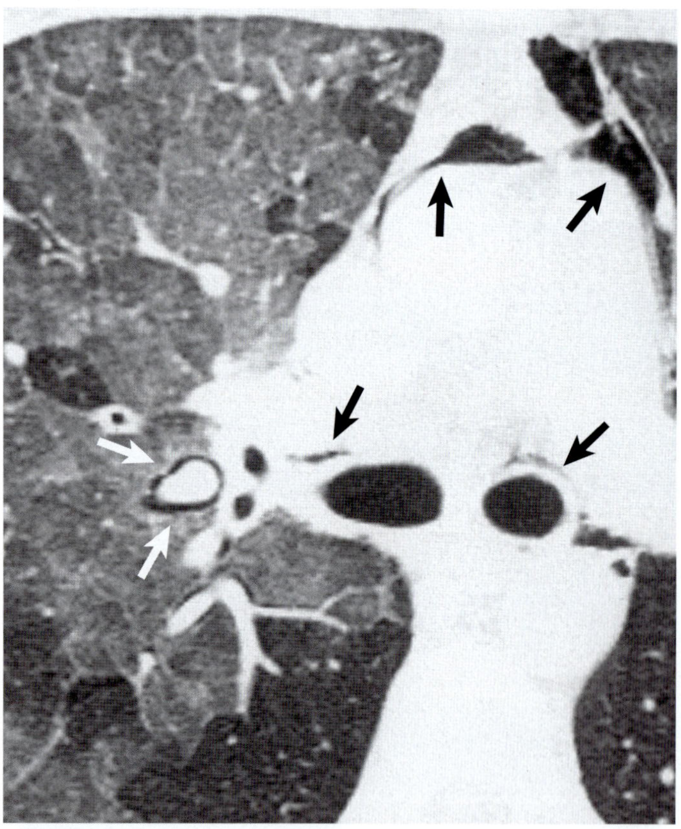

Fig. 75.5 Pulmonary interstitial emphysema and pneumomediastinum in a young man with acquired immune deficiency syndrome and *Pneumocystis* pneumonia. Close-up view from a CT scan shows mediastinal air in the anterior mediastinum and surrounding the main bronchi *(black arrows)*. Air is also seen surrounding the intrapulmonary vessels *(white arrows)*. Pulmonary interstitial emphysema leads directly to pneumomediastinum (Macklin effect).

intestinalis and may even break through the peritoneum or mesocolon to produce free intraabdominal air, simulating a perforated viscus. On occasion, pneumomediastinum will dissect into the pleural or pericardial space, resulting in pneumothorax and pneumopericardium, respectively.

KEY POINTS: RADIOGRAPHIC FINDINGS OF PNEUMOMEDIASTINUM

- Increase in the depth and lucency of the retrosternal space
- Streaks of gray-black density separating portions of mediastinal pleura from mediastinal contents
- Focal bubble-like or larger collections of gas outlining the mediastinal structures
- Rounded hyperlucent paramediastinal lesions (loculated pneumomediastinum)
- Longitudinal line shadow parallel to the heart border
- Continuous diaphragm sign
- Naclerio V sign
- Ring-around-the-artery sign
- Thymic spinnaker-sail sign
- Vanished heart

COMPUTED TOMOGRAPHY

Underlying lung diseases are present in 25% to 44% of patients with spontaneous pneumomediastinum.[11,83] The abnormal air collections can be easily recognized on CT. Air in the pulmonary interstitium, which leads to pneumomediastinum, may be associated with severe underlying lung disease, such as ARDS (Fig. 75.10), chronic graft-versus-host disease after stem cell transplant, or idiopathic pulmonary fibrosis (Fig. 75.11).[20,84,85]

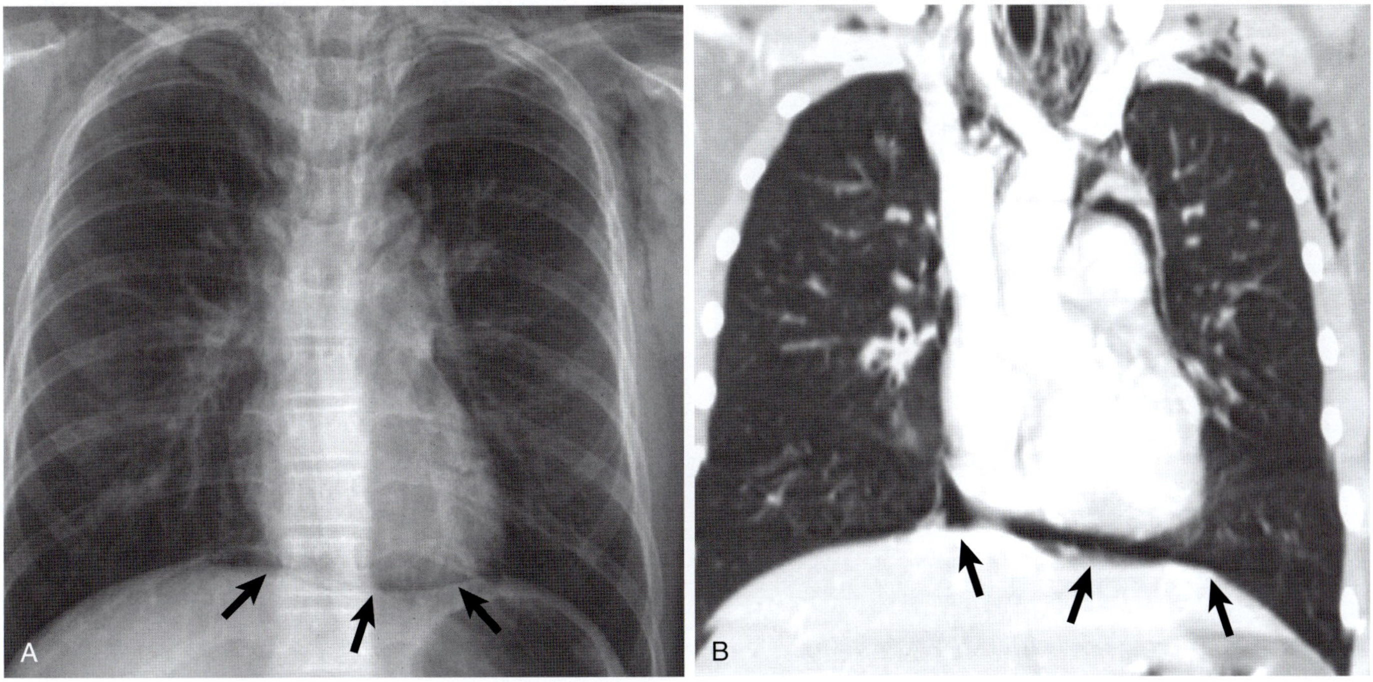

Fig. 75.7 Pneumomediastinum with continuous diaphragm sign after blunt chest trauma. Posteroanterior chest radiograph (A) and coronal CT scan (B) show pneumomediastinum outlining the central portion of the diaphragm *(arrows)*, a finding known as the continuous diaphragm sign.

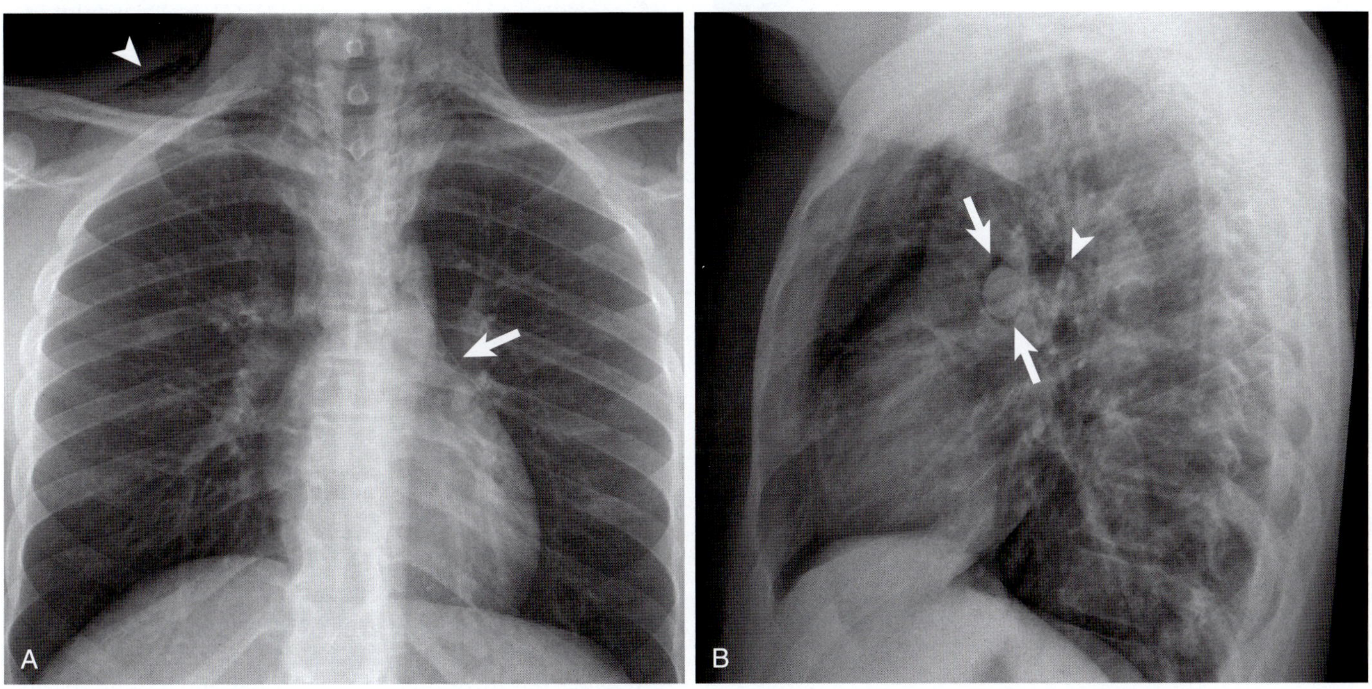

Fig. 75.8 Pneumomediastinum with "ring-around-the-artery" sign. (A) Posteroanterior chest radiograph shows subtle pneumomediastinum *(arrow)* adjacent to the left heart border and subcutaneous air in the right neck *(arrowhead)*. (B) Lateral chest radiograph shows air *(arrows)* surrounding the right pulmonary artery and, to a lesser extent, the left pulmonary artery *(arrowhead)*. There is also air in the retrosternal mediastinum.

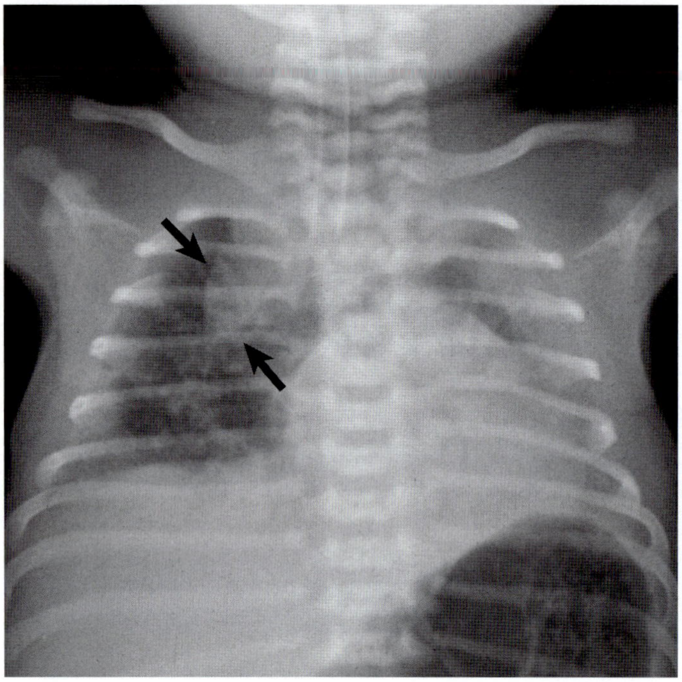

Fig. 75.9 Pneumomediastinum with spinnaker-sail sign. Anteroposterior chest radiograph shows a crescentic sail-like shadow *(arrows)* extending out over the right lung, representing the uplifted and displaced right lobe of the thymus.

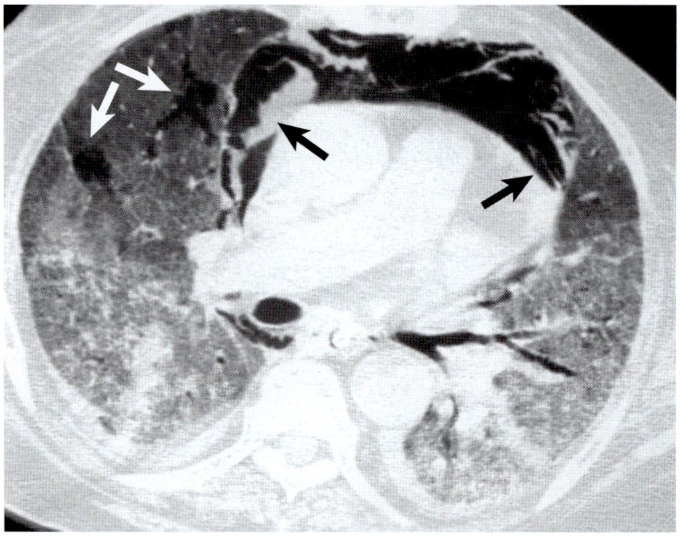

Fig. 75.10 Pneumomediastinum in acute respiratory distress syndrome from trauma. High-resolution CT scan shows diffuse bilateral areas of ground-glass opacity with a superimposed linear pattern ("crazy paving"). Irregular hyperlucent areas, representing pulmonary lacerations, are seen in the right upper lobe *(white arrows)*. Extensive pneumomediastinum *(black arrows)* and small bilateral pleural effusions are also visible.

CT is the gold standard in the evaluation of patients with clinical suspicion of spontaneous barotrauma and normal or nonspecific radiographic findings and in the assessment of suspected complications of ARDS or blunt chest trauma. In traumatic patients small lacerations of the pulmonary parenchyma may lead to pneumomediastinum (Fig. 75.12). Tension pneumomediastinum is rare, leading to cardiac compression by mediastinal air (Fig. 75.13). Percutaneous CT-guided insertion of a mediastinal drainage catheter is a useful therapeutic adjunct after confirmation of tension pneumomediastinum.[38]

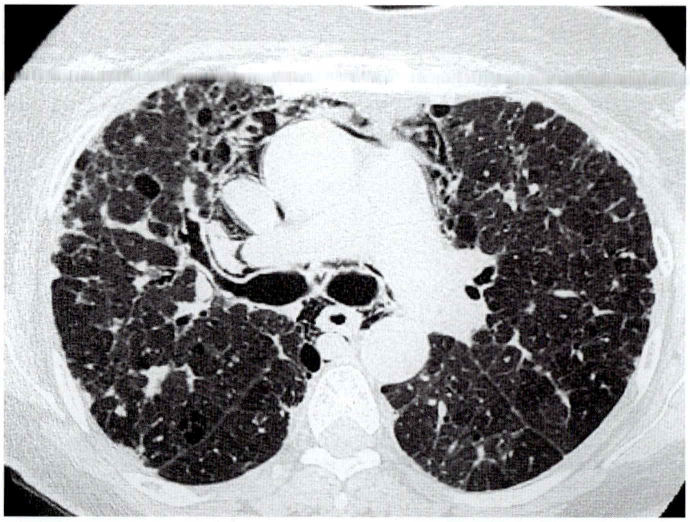

Fig. 75.11 Pneumomediastinum in pulmonary fibrosis. High-resolution CT scan obtained at the level of the carina shows findings of pulmonary fibrosis. Extensive mediastinal air is visible surrounding the large airways, vasculature, and esophagus.

After endoscopic procedures, such as sclerotherapy of esophageal varices or balloon dilation of a stenosis, CT is indicated in those patients with normal radiographs and clinical suspicion of esophageal perforation (Fig. 75.14). CT is also helpful in the early diagnosis of postsurgical cardiovascular infections.

DIFFERENTIAL DIAGNOSIS

A thin line of apparent radiolucency is frequently seen along the heart borders and aorta in healthy individuals resulting from the "Mach band" phenomenon. The Mach band might be misinterpreted as pneumomediastinum.[86]

In some cases displacement of the thymus is so great that its lateral border reaches the chest wall. This appearance may be confused with consolidation or collapse of the upper lobe. Air surrounding the thymus gland is a pathognomonic sign of pneumomediastinum. Pneumomediastinum may be overlooked in the setting of extensive subcutaneous air. Air in a distended esophagus may occasionally mimic pneumomediastinum.

On chest radiographs, depending on the anatomic extent of the air, it may be difficult to distinguish pneumomediastinum from pneumothorax or pneumopericardium.[72] In the lateral decubitus position pneumomediastinum will not shift rapidly, as opposed to a pneumothorax or pneumopericardium, which will rapidly shift to a nondependent location (unless loculated). Pneumopericardium typically extends from the diaphragm to just below the aortic arch but will not extend around the aortic arch or into the superior mediastinum.[72] In adults pneumopericardium is very rare in the absence of penetrating trauma or iatrogenic intervention.

Finally, it is important to differentiate the continuous diaphragm sign with pneumomediastinum from the cupola sign with free intraperitoneal air. The cupola sign generally has a curved interface, whereas the continuous diaphragm sign is generally straight.

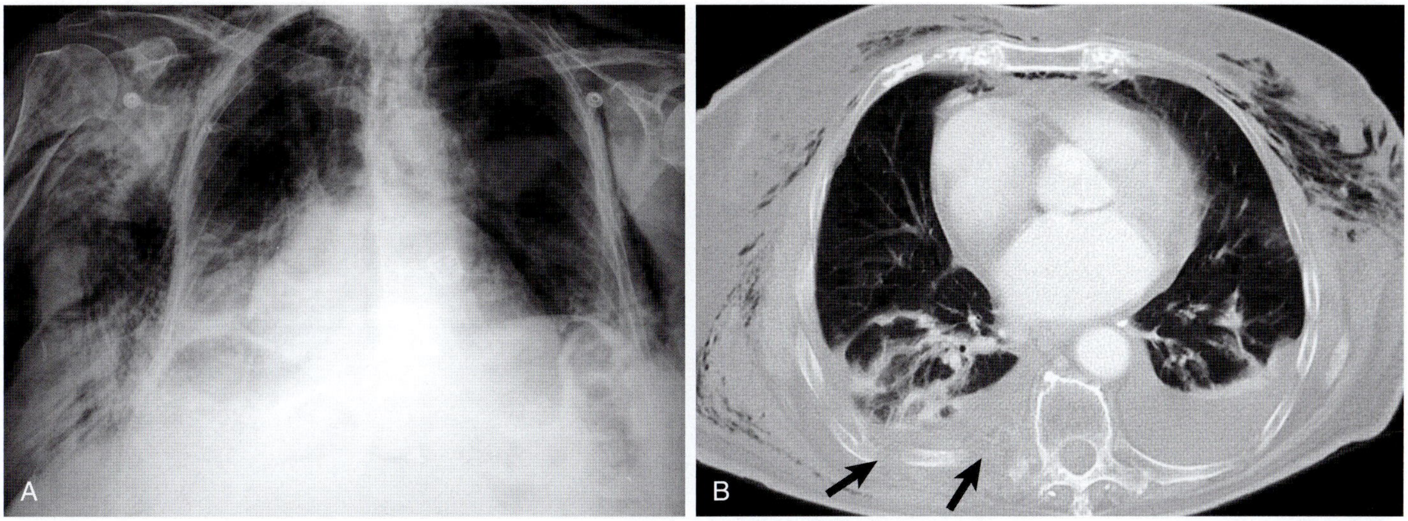

Fig. 75.12 Posttraumatic pneumomediastinum after blunt chest trauma. (A) Frontal chest radiograph shows diffuse soft tissue air. (B) Corresponding CT scan shows mediastinal air, subcutaneous air, and bilateral hemothoraces. Rib fractures are also visible *(arrows)*.

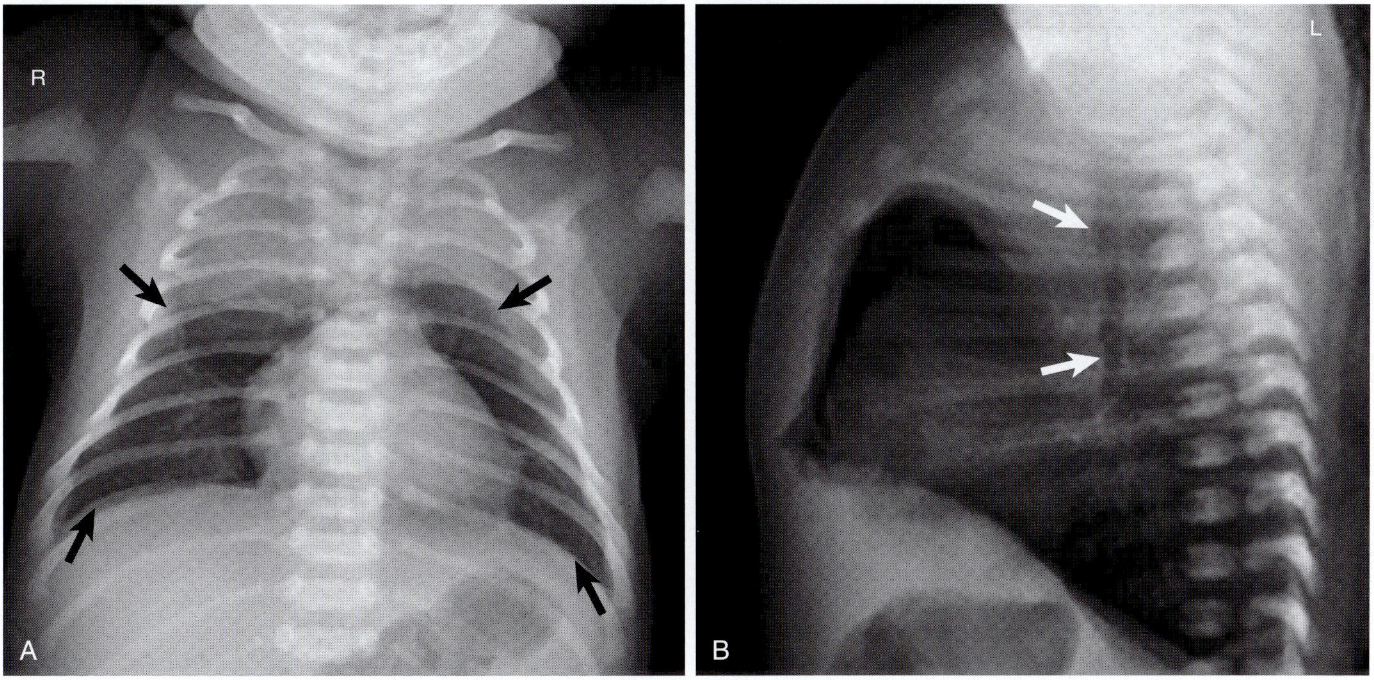

Fig. 75.13 Massive tension pneumomediastinum. (A) Frontal chest radiograph shows a large air collection *(arrows)* overlying the mediastinal cardiovascular structures. (B) On the lateral radiograph both lungs and the trachea *(arrows)* are pushed posteriorly.

IMAGING ALGORITHM

In patients in whom the chest radiograph is diagnostic of pneumomediastinum and the clinical history does not indicate a perforated intrathoracic viscus or another severe underlying condition, no further investigations are required. If there is suspicion of pneumomediastinum and the radiographic findings are not diagnostic, a CT scan of the chest is recommended.

Patients with suspected esophageal perforation require further evaluation with water-soluble or barium esophagram or CT with ingested oral contrast and, commonly, esophagoscopy.

SYNOPSIS OF TREATMENT OPTIONS

Pneumomediastinum usually resolves spontaneously. Acute interventions, such as needle decompression, CT-guided catheter drainage of loculated mediastinal air collections, and ventilatory assistance, are seldom needed. It is important, however, to identify the underlying condition, leading to pneumomediastinum because in many cases the cause of the pneumomediastinum may require acute intervention and treatment. The main conditions that need to be excluded are trauma, gas-forming organisms, and perforated esophagus. Boerhaave syndrome must be

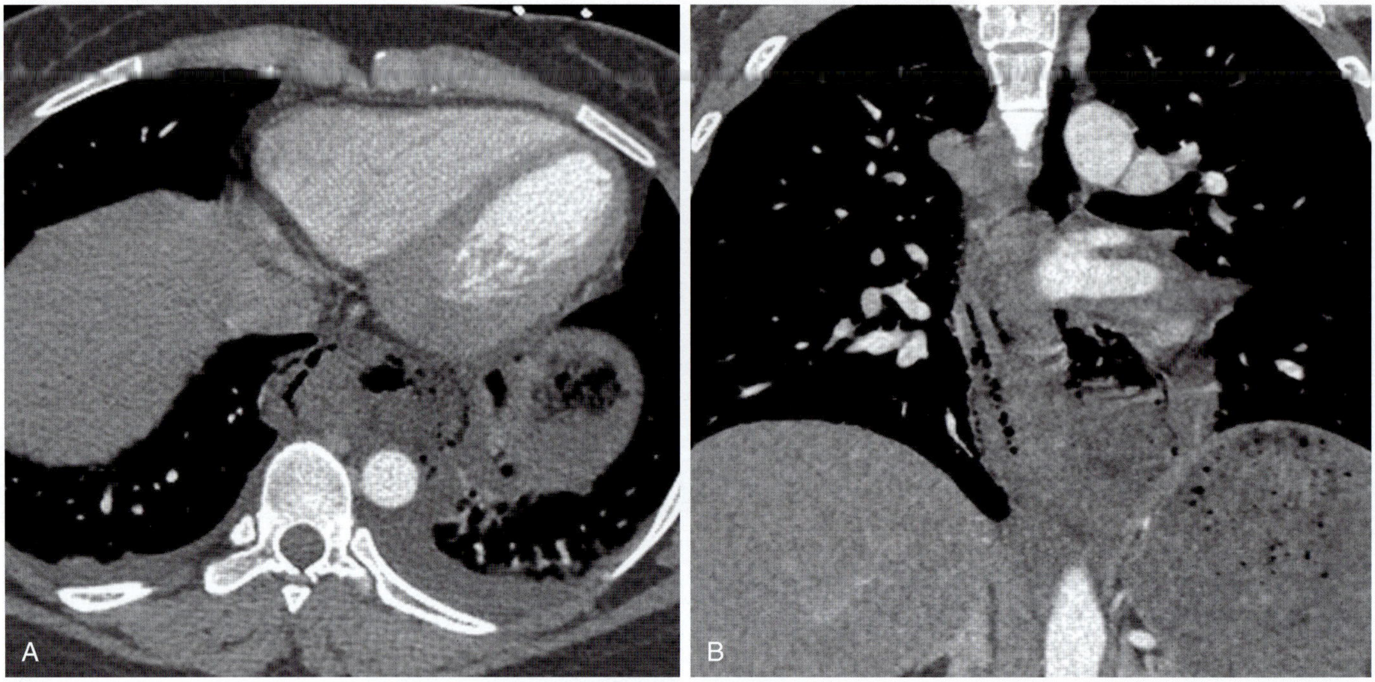

Fig. 75.14 Localized periesophageal hematoma and pneumomediastinum after traumatic esophageal rupture. Axial (A) and coronal (B) CT scans show a retrocardiac mediastinal mass comprised of an irregular solid component (hematoma and gastric contents) and streaky linear and small air-bubble collections (pneumomediastinum). Esophageal tear was confirmed at fluoroscopy (not shown).

KEY POINTS

- Air or gas may reach the mediastinum from ruptured alveoli, mediastinal airways, the esophagus or neck, and occasionally the abdominal cavity.
- The most common cause of pneumomediastinum is rupture of alveoli; gas passes into the perivascular or peribronchial interstitium and tracks through the interstitial tissue to the hilum and mediastinum.
- Common causes of pneumomediastinum include asthma, violent coughing or vomiting, marijuana or crack cocaine smoking, mechanical ventilation, and trauma.
- Patients may be asymptomatic or may present with variable degrees of chest discomfort.
- On occasion, large amounts of air in the mediastinum may result in tension pneumomediastinum with associated acute diastolic dysfunction, cardiac tamponade, and impaired venous return to the heart.
- The radiographic manifestations of pneumomediastinum consist of radiolucent streaks or focal bubble-like or larger collections of gas outlining the mediastinal structures.
- Pneumomediastinum displaces the mediastinal pleura laterally (most commonly the left), creating a longitudinal line shadow parallel to the heart border.
- Signs associated with pneumomediastinum include continuous diaphragm sign, Naclerio V sign, ring-around-the-artery sign, and thymic spinnaker-sail sign.
- Radiographic distinction between pneumomediastinum and pneumopericardium is as follows:
  - Pneumopericardium does not extend above the aortic arch or into the superior mediastinum.
  - Air within the pericardium moves freely on decubitus views.

considered in any patient with a history of vomiting, followed by chest pain and pneumomediastinum.

SUGGESTED READING

Caceres M, Ali SZ, Braud R, Weiman D, Garrett HE Jr. Spontaneous pneumomediastinum: a comparative study and review of the literature. *Ann Thorac Surg*. 2008;86(3):962–966.

Zylak CM, Standen JR, Barnes GR, Zylak CJ. Pneumomediastinum revisited. *Radiographics*. 2000;20(4):1043–1057. Erratum in *Radiographics* 2001;21(6):1616.

The full reference list for this chapter is available at ExpertConsult.com.

76 Mediastinitis

TOMÁS FRANQUET

Mediastinitis refers to a focal or diffuse inflammation of the tissues located in the mediastinum. The mediastinum lies between the right and left pleural cavities and extends from the thoracic inlet to the diaphragm. Mediastinitis can be classified into acute and chronic forms. Acute mediastinitis is usually a catastrophic disorder manifesting with a sudden and dramatic onset and a high mortality rate when the diagnosis is delayed.[1] The chronic forms of mediastinitis (fibrosing mediastinitis) comprise a spectrum of disease ranging from active granulomatous inflammation to "burned-out" mediastinal fibrosis.[2]

There are infectious and noninfectious causes of mediastinitis.[1,3] Mediastinal infection occurs through direct contamination and hematogenous or lymphatic spread or extension from the head, neck, lung, pleura, chest wall, or peritoneum.[4,5] The clinical presentation is variable, depending on the chronicity of the underlying process.[6] Acute mediastinitis is usually caused by bacteria, and chronic mediastinitis is most often related to tuberculous or fungal infections.[3,7–9]

Acute Mediastinitis

ETIOLOGY, PREVALENCE, AND EPIDEMIOLOGY

Acute mediastinitis may be classified, on the basis of its cause, as being postoperative, secondary to esophageal perforation, a result of the spread of osteomyelitis from adjacent bone, a direct extension of head and neck infection, or a result of hematogenous spread of infection.[3,10] Acute mediastinitis is a potentially life-threatening condition that necessitates aggressive surgical intervention, drainage of the mediastinum, and aggressive therapy with broad-spectrum parenterally administered antibiotics. The mortality ranges from 10% to 20%[11,12] to 40% to 50%[12,13] and increases drastically with delay in diagnosis and treatment.

The most common cause (90%) of acute mediastinitis is iatrogenic esophageal perforation during diagnostic or therapeutic endoscopic procedures (Box 76.1).[14–18] Esophageal perforation is an uncommon and life-threatening event that occurs more frequently in association with the use of endoscopic instruments and surgical thoracic procedures. This complication has been reported in about 1 per 1000 patients who undergo endoscopic examinations. The mortality associated with acute mediastinitis from esophageal disruption is 5% to 30%, even with appropriate treatment.[19] Perforation has been described after rigid esophagoscopy, dilatation of a stricture, pneumatic dilatation for achalasia, after variceal sclerosis, and esophageal tube placement (nasogastric and Sengstaken-Blakemore).[20] In one review of 114 cases of esophageal rupture, the cause was iatrogenic in 55%.[21] Esophageal perforation may also occur in association with a necrotic esophageal carcinoma, radiation esophagitis, and ulceration of a hiatal hernia.[11,22–24] Outcome after esophageal perforation is dependent on the cause and location of the injury, the presence of underlying esophageal disease, and the interval between injury and initiation of treatment.[20] Late complications of acute mediastinitis resulting from esophageal perforation include esophagocutaneous, esophagopleural, and esophagobronchial fistulas.[25]

Infectious mediastinitis also may occur after major airways perforation secondary to trauma or instrumentation.[26] Other causes of acute mediastinitis include odontogenic infections,[27] perforation of the superior vena cava (SVC) by a central venous catheter,[28] and the leakage of parenteral nutrition from a migrated central venous catheter.[29]

Postoperative acute mediastinitis occurs in 0.5% to 5% of patients who underwent median sternotomy for cardiothoracic surgery.[18,30–33] Nearly 700,000 median sternotomies are performed each year in the United States, leading to approximately 8300 deep sternal wound infections.[34] The risk of infection is increased in obesity, insulin-dependent diabetes, internal mammary artery grafting (especially bilaterally), and reoperation.[35] Commonly isolated organisms are *Staphylococcus epidermidis* and *Staphylococcus aureus*, various gram-negative organisms, fungi, and atypical mycobacteria.[36]

Boerhaave syndrome refers to spontaneous esophageal perforation associated with forceful vomiting after a sudden rise in intraesophageal pressure.[37] It represents a diagnostic challenge and remains a major consideration in patients with otherwise unexplained mediastinitis. Patients with significant pleural and mediastinal contamination are at high risk for sepsis and systemic inflammatory response syndrome.[38]

Descending necrotizing mediastinitis refers to a primary complication of oropharyngeal infections that can spread to the mediastinum through the anatomic fascial planes and cervical spaces (prevertebral, retrovisceral, pretracheal, or retropharyngeal).[39–41]

Pancreatitis can extend from the retroperitoneum into the mediastinum, resulting in mediastinitis.[42,43] On occasion, osteomyelitis of the spine and ribs may lead to mediastinitis.[42–44] In 2001 hemorrhagic mediastinitis was found in 5 of 11 patients with inhalational anthrax related to a bioterrorism attack in the United States.[45]

CLINICAL PRESENTATION

The characteristic clinical findings of acute mediastinitis consist of a sudden and dramatic onset with chills, high fever, tachycardia, tachypnea, and prostration. Retrosternal pain, worsened by breathing or coughing, is common; radiation to the neck and ear may occur. The Hamman sign, a crunching sound heard over the anterior chest wall, synchronous with cardiac systole, may be secondary to pneumomediastinum associated with acute mediastinitis. Accurate diagnosis depends on an appropriate degree of clinical suspicion. Although a history of a potential predisposing event or disease process can be elicited in most patients, cases

BOX 76.1 ETIOLOGY OF ACUTE MEDIASTINITIS

Perforation or rupture of esophagus
- Iatrogenic: diagnostic or therapeutic endoscopic procedures, sclerotherapy of esophageal varices, surgery
- Spontaneous: Boerhaave syndrome, labor, asthmatic attack
- Direct penetrating or blunt trauma
- Impacted foreign body
- Erosion: caustic ingestion, esophageal carcinoma, necrotizing infection, radiation esophagitis

Perforation or rupture of airways
- Direct penetrating or blunt trauma
- Iatrogenic: intubation, bronchoscopy
- Foreign body
- Broncholithiasis
- Erosion: bronchogenic carcinoma

Perforation of vessels
- Iatrogenic: indwelling central venous catheters

Direct extension
- Adjacent tissues: oropharyngeal infections, periodontal tissues, paraspinous abscess, retroperitoneal and subphrenic infection
- Anterior chest wall: drug abuse, closed-chest cardiopulmonary resuscitation
- Retroperitoneum: pancreatitis

Infection
- Tuberculosis

Postsurgical
- Cardiothoracic surgery, esophageal surgery

Primary
- Inhalational anthrax: hemorrhagic mediastinitis

without these associations may occur. In such circumstances the diagnosis may be delayed because symptoms may mimic those of myocardial infarction, aortic dissection, and pulmonary thromboembolism. In one review of 54 patients with esophageal perforations related to endoscopy, the diagnosis of perforation was made within 2 hours in 94.4% of cases.[46] Descending necrotizing mediastinitis has been linked with significant morbidity and mortality, and early recognition is important for a good prognosis for this potentially fatal condition.[47]

A distinctive clinical picture results from acute mediastinitis secondary to a spontaneous rupture of the esophagus as a result of a violent vomiting episode (Boerhaave syndrome). This condition affects approximately 1 in 6000 patients. Rupture is typically posterior, near the left hemidiaphragmatic crus.[48,49] Clinically, esophageal perforation must be suspected on the basis of the history in association with vomiting, chest pain, fever, and subcutaneous air. In spontaneous esophageal perforation (Boerhaave syndrome), hematemesis also is common.[37]

During October and November 2001, public health authorities investigated 11 patients with inhalational anthrax related to a bioterrorism attack in the United States.[45] Clinically, patients presented with a biphasic illness characterized by an initial insidious flu-like illness lasting 2 to 4 days and characterized by fever, malaise, myalgias, and nonproductive cough. This was followed by a fulminant acute mediastinitis with respiratory distress and chest pain. Serosanguineous pleural effusions and hemorrhagic mediastinitis were found in 5 patients who died. Immunohistochemical assays demonstrated abundant intracellular and extracellular bacilli, bacillary fragments, and granular antigen staining in mediastinal lymph nodes, surrounding soft tissues, and pleura.[45]

PATHOLOGIC FINDINGS AND PATHOPHYSIOLOGY

Acute mediastinitis is usually infectious in etiology and sometimes progresses to abscess formation. The organisms detected in acute mediastinitis vary with the underlying cause. Mixed infections containing aerobic and anaerobic organisms are commonly associated with acute mediastinitis resulting from esophageal perforation and spread from oropharyngeal sources.[50] Anaerobic bacteria are common in infections from esophageal perforation and oropharyngeal sources. *Candida* mediastinitis is an uncommon complication of a cardiothoracic surgery but is associated with a high mortality rate.[51]

IMAGING FINDINGS

Radiography

In acute mediastinitis chest radiography may show widening and poor definition of the margins of the superior mediastinum with or without pneumomediastinum (Fig. 76.1). Subcutaneous air may also be seen in the soft tissues of the neck.

Most cases of acute mediastinitis result from esophageal perforation.[20] Radiologically, detection of esophageal perforation relies on the presence of indirect signs, including pneumomediastinum, left-sided pneumothorax, and pleural effusion. Pneumomediastinum typically manifests as delineation of the pleura as a white line adjacent to the mediastinum, linear streaks of radiolucency in the mediastinum and cervical soft tissues, focal retrosternal air collections, linear extrapleural air collection outlining the diaphragm ("continuous diaphragm" sign), and a focal, sharply marginated area of radiolucency in a paraspinal location on the left side immediately above the diaphragm (V sign of Naclerio) (Fig. 76.2).[49] Although contrast-enhanced esophagram has been the standard technique for diagnosis of esophageal perforation, 10% of patients can have a false-negative result.[49,52] Extravasation of oral contrast material into the mediastinum or into the pleural cavity is an unequivocal sign of perforation (Figs. 76.3 and 76.4). Direct extension of sternal infection after surgery is another common cause of acute mediastinitis. Radiographic findings of sternal dehiscence include displacement, rotation, and fracture of the sternal wires on serial chest radiographs.[10]

Computed Tomography

Computed tomography (CT) is the imaging modality of choice in the evaluation of patients with suspected acute mediastinitis and mediastinal abscess (see Fig. 76.1).[53,54] Common CT findings secondary to esophageal perforation include esophageal thickening, extraluminal gas, pleural effusion, single or multiple abscesses, and extraluminal contrast medium (Figs. 76.5 to 76.7).[49,54] Pleural effusion tends to be right-sided in patients with iatrogenic, midesophageal perforation and left-sided in patients with spontaneous, distal esophageal perforation.[49] CT esophagography with ingested water-soluble contrast agent is more sensitive than fluoroscopic esophagram in the detection of esophageal perforation.[55,56]

In descending necrotizing mediastinitis, CT shows solitary or multiple fluid collections, which may be contiguous with other collections in the cervical region, increased attenuation and diffuse obliteration of normal mediastinal fat planes related to fasciitis, cellulitis, or myositis. CT also may depict associated abnormalities, such as pleural and pericardial effusions, vein thrombosis, and lymphadenopathy.[57]

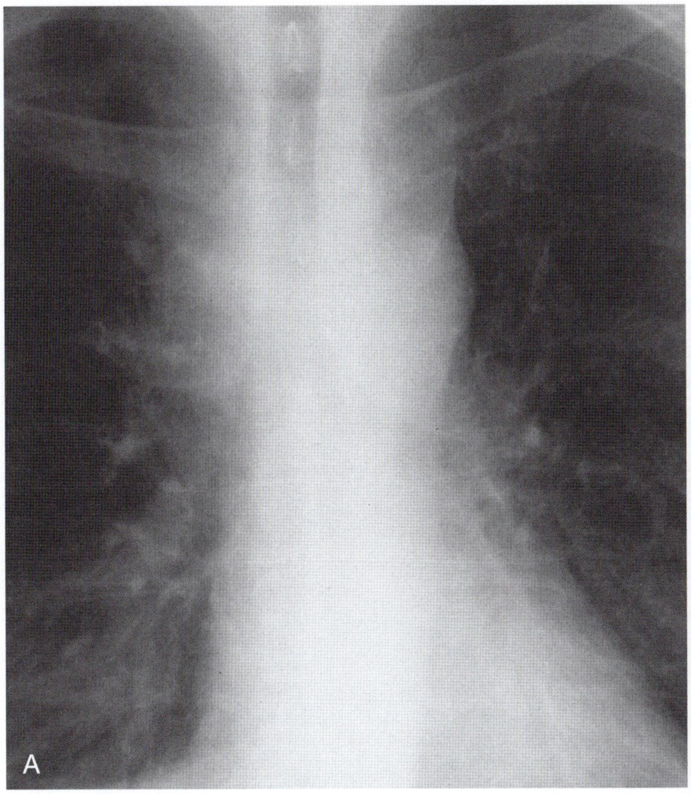

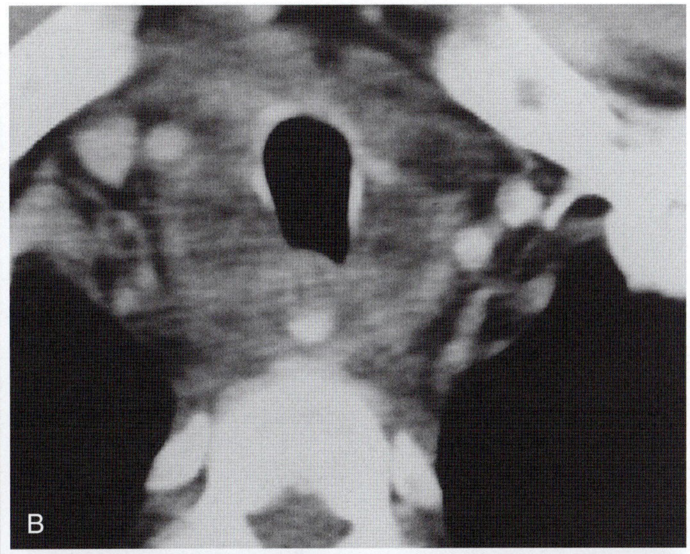

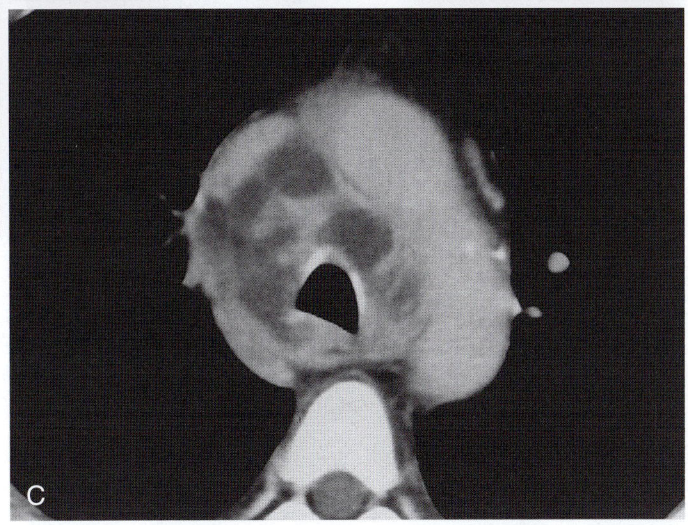

Fig. 76.1 Acute mediastinitis secondary to retropharyngeal abscess in a middle-aged man who presented with acute dysphagia and high fever. (A) Close-up view from posteroanterior chest radiograph shows smooth widening of the upper mediastinum. (B) Contrast-enhanced CT at the level of the thoracic inlet shows inhomogeneous areas of attenuation surrounding the trachea. (C) CT at the level of the aortic arch shows localized areas of low attenuation consistent with abscess formation anterior and lateral to the trachea. *(From Müller NL, Fraser RS, Colman NC, et al.* Radiologic Diagnosis of Diseases of the Chest. *Philadelphia: Saunders; 2001.)*

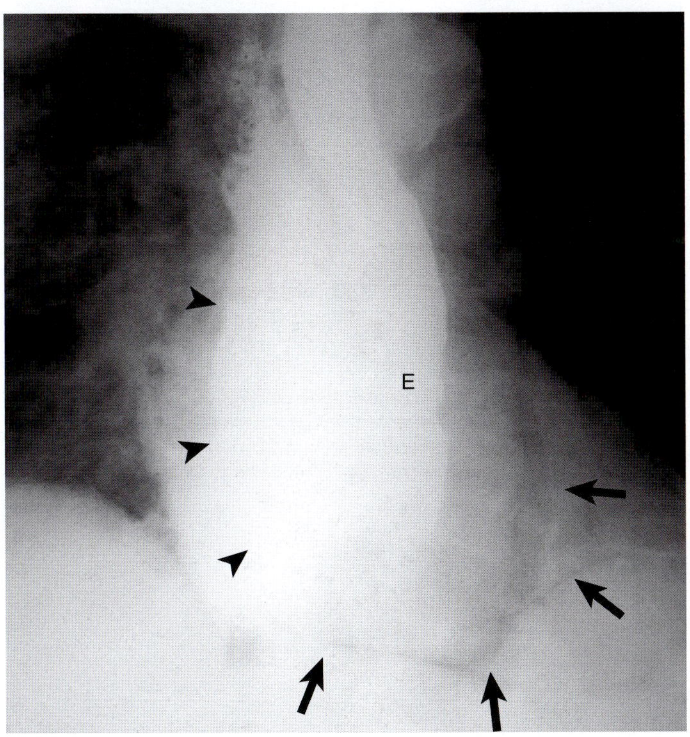

Fig. 76.2 Traumatic esophageal rupture with pneumomediastinum. Esophagram shows esophageal rupture with a right-sided paraesophageal collection of contrast *(arrowheads)*. Linear streaks of mediastinal air and extrapleural air *(arrows)* outline the diaphragm ("continuous diaphragm" sign). *E,* Esophagus. *(From Giménez A, Franquet T, Erasmus JJ, et al. Thoracic complications of esophageal disorders.* Radiographics. *2002;22: S247–S258.)*

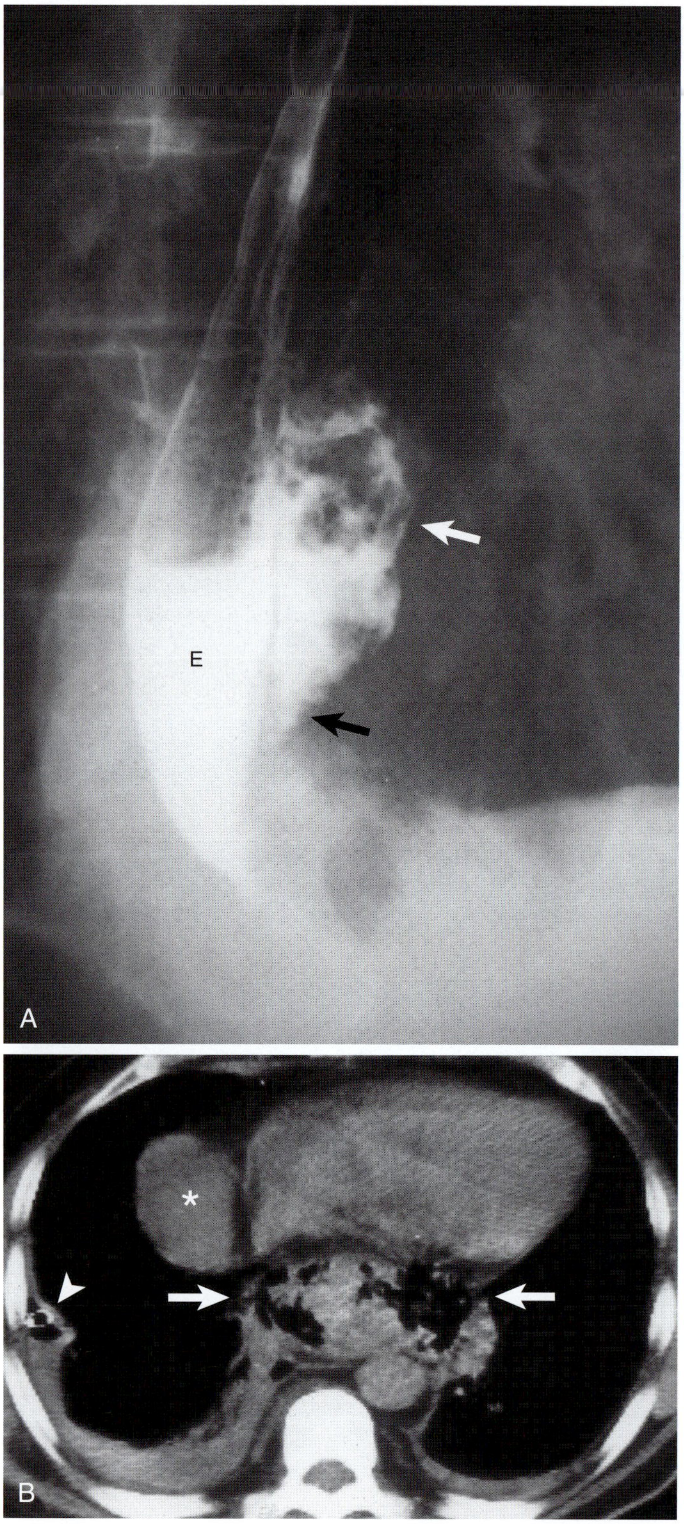

Fig. 76.3 Spontaneous perforation of the esophagus (Boerhaave syndrome) with mediastinal abscess in a man with burning substernal pain. (A) Esophagram shows a massive leak of barium into the left lower mediastinum *(arrows)*. *E*, Esophagus. (B) CT shows a periesophageal mediastinal abscess *(arrows)* with bilateral pleural effusions. Note right-sided chest tube *(arrowhead)* and a right paracardiac collection *(asterisk)*. *(From Giménez A, Franquet T, Erasmus JJ, et al. Thoracic complications of esophageal disorders.* Radiographics. *2002;22:S247–S258.)*

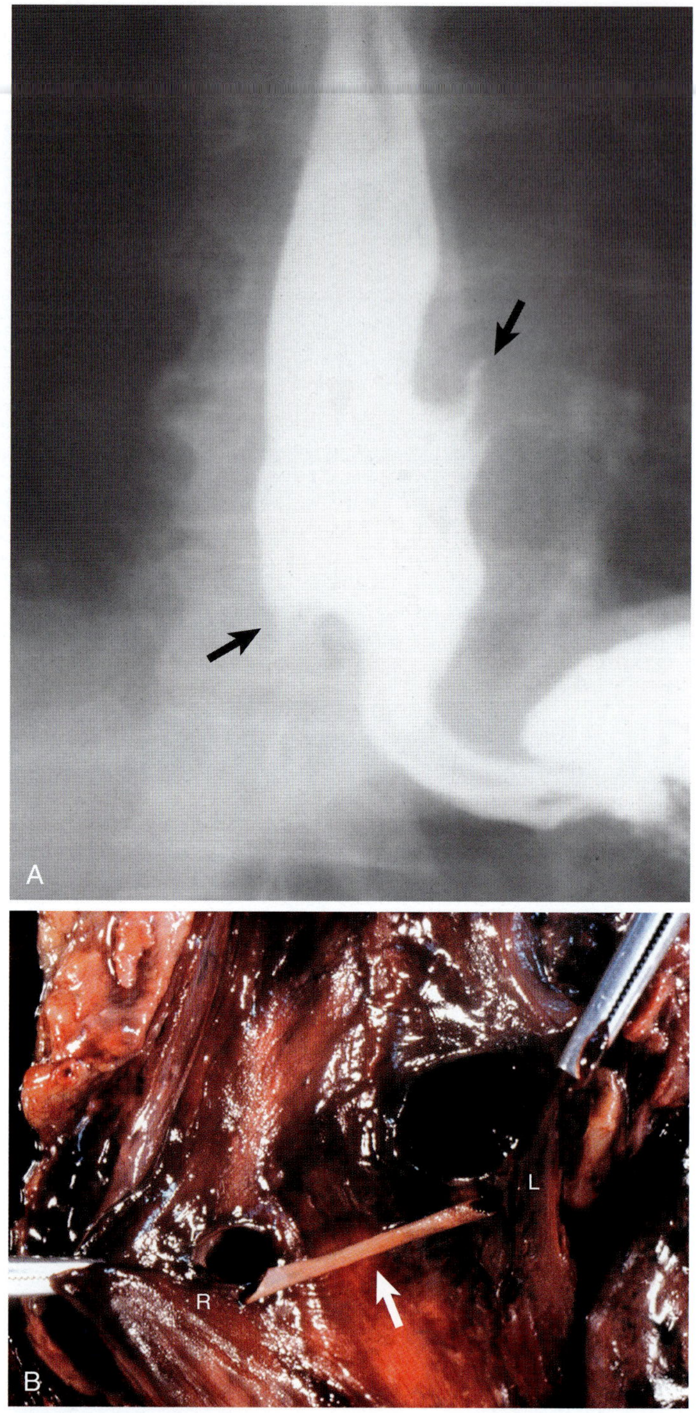

Fig. 76.4 Multifocal esophageal perforation resulting from chicken bone impaction in a woman with sensation of a foreign body, dysphagia, odynophagia, and drooling. (A) Barium esophagram reveals a double esophageal tear *(arrows)*. (B) Photograph of an autopsy specimen shows chicken bone *(arrow)* and esophageal perforations. *L*, Left perforation; *R*, right perforation. *(From Giménez A, Franquet T, Erasmus JJ, et al. Thoracic complications of esophageal disorders.* Radiographics. *2002;22: S247–S258.)*

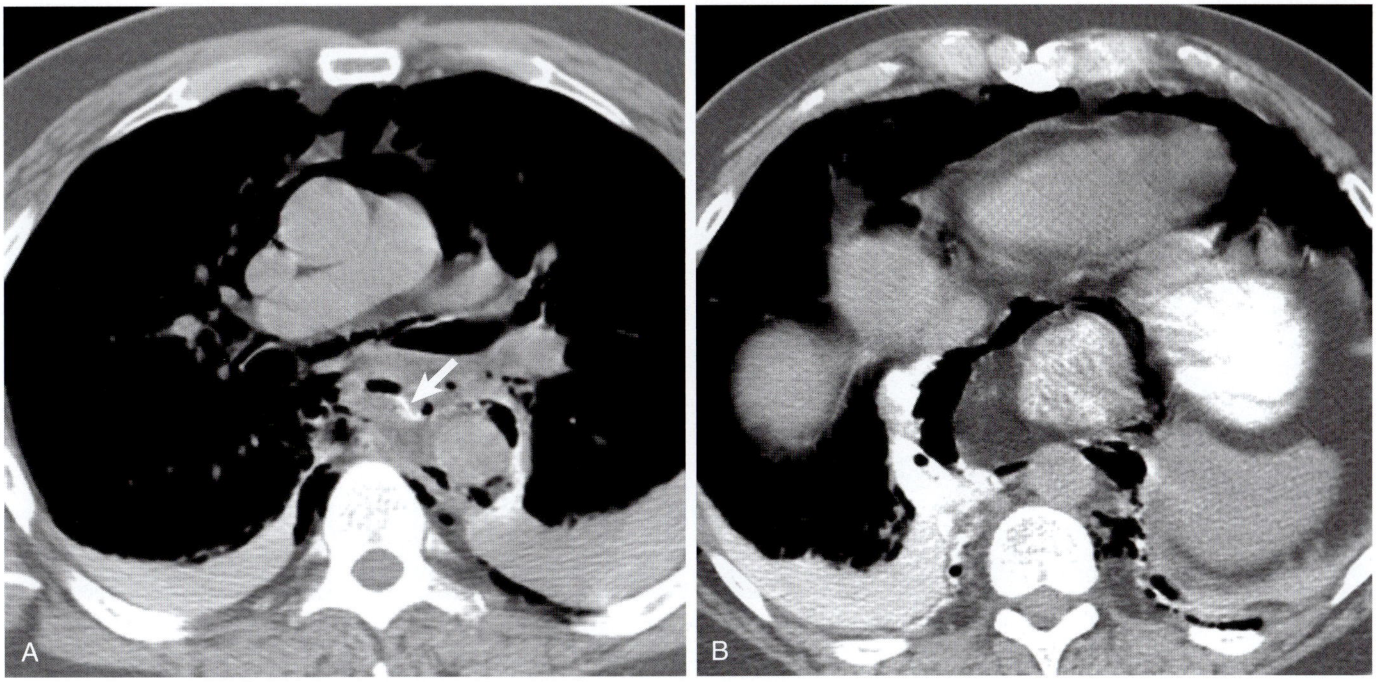

Fig. 76.5 Acute mediastinitis secondary to esophageal perforation. Axial CTs at the level of the right pulmonary artery (A) and lung bases (B) show extensive pneumomediastinum and contrast extravasation *(arrow)* from the posterior wall of the midesophagus. Note contrast within both pleural spaces and the mediastinum.

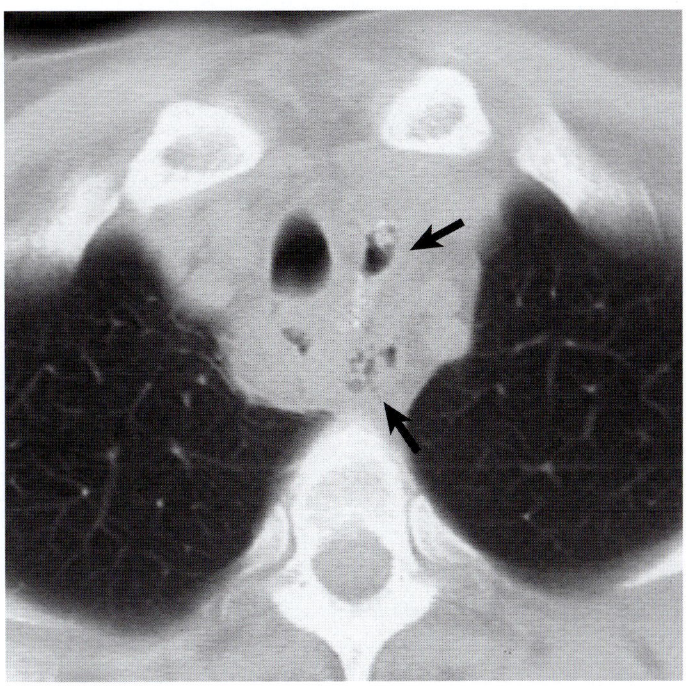

Fig. 76.6 Acute mediastinitis secondary to esophageal perforation. CT shows multiple bubbles of air *(arrows)* in the superior mediastinum.

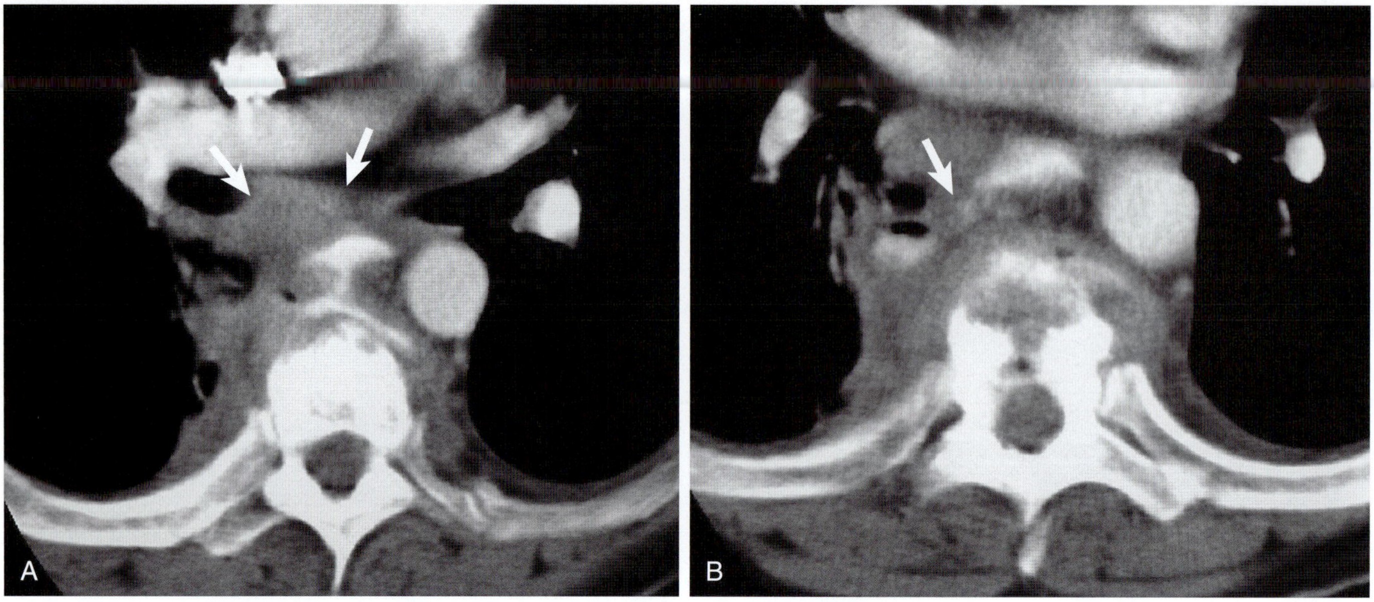

Fig. 76.7 Hodgkin disease (nodular sclerosis) in a man with esophagopulmonary and esophagomediastinal fistulas. (A) Contrast-enhanced CT shows mediastinal lymphadenopathy *(arrows)* with esophageal involvement and esophagomediastinal fistula. (B) Contrast-enhanced CT shows an esophagopulmonary fistula *(arrow)*. Extensive vertebral body involvement is also shown. *(From Giménez A, Franquet T, Erasmus JJ, et al. Thoracic complications of esophageal disorders.* Radiographics. *2002;22:S247–S258.)*

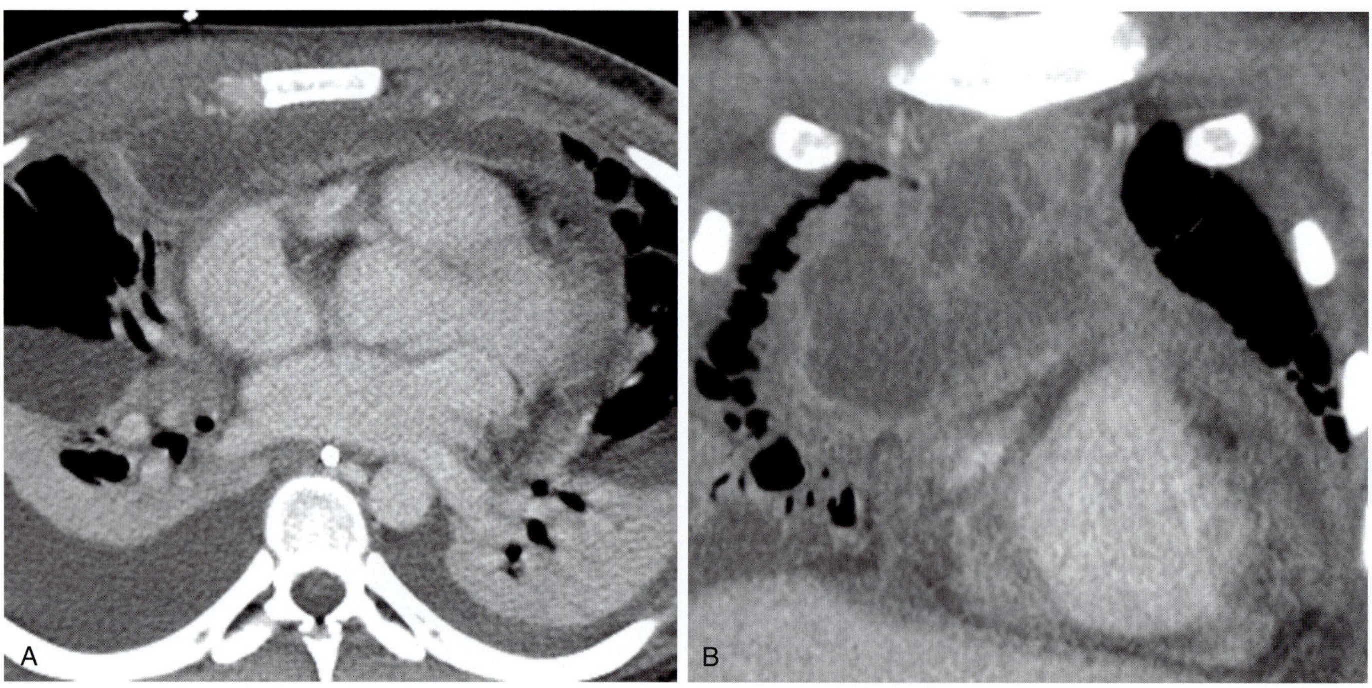

Fig. 76.8 Mediastinitis. Axial (A) and coronal (B) contrast-enhanced CT shows a rim-enhancing, multiloculated fluid collection in the anterior mediastinum (prevascular mediastinum) compatible with mediastinitis and abscess formation. Note bilateral pleural effusions with associated relaxation atelectasis.

CT is a valuable tool in diagnosing complications after sternotomy because it accurately depicts the extent and depth of the wound infections (Fig. 76.8).[58,59] Fluid and air collections, hematomas, pleural effusion, and increased attenuation of mediastinal fat are common findings in the immediate postoperative period (Fig. 76.9).[58,60,61] Distinguishing these normal postoperative findings from superimposed infection can be difficult or impossible on CT performed within the first few days after surgery. Timing of the CT examination is important in determining the clinical value of the imaging findings, such as cortical destruction of the sternum

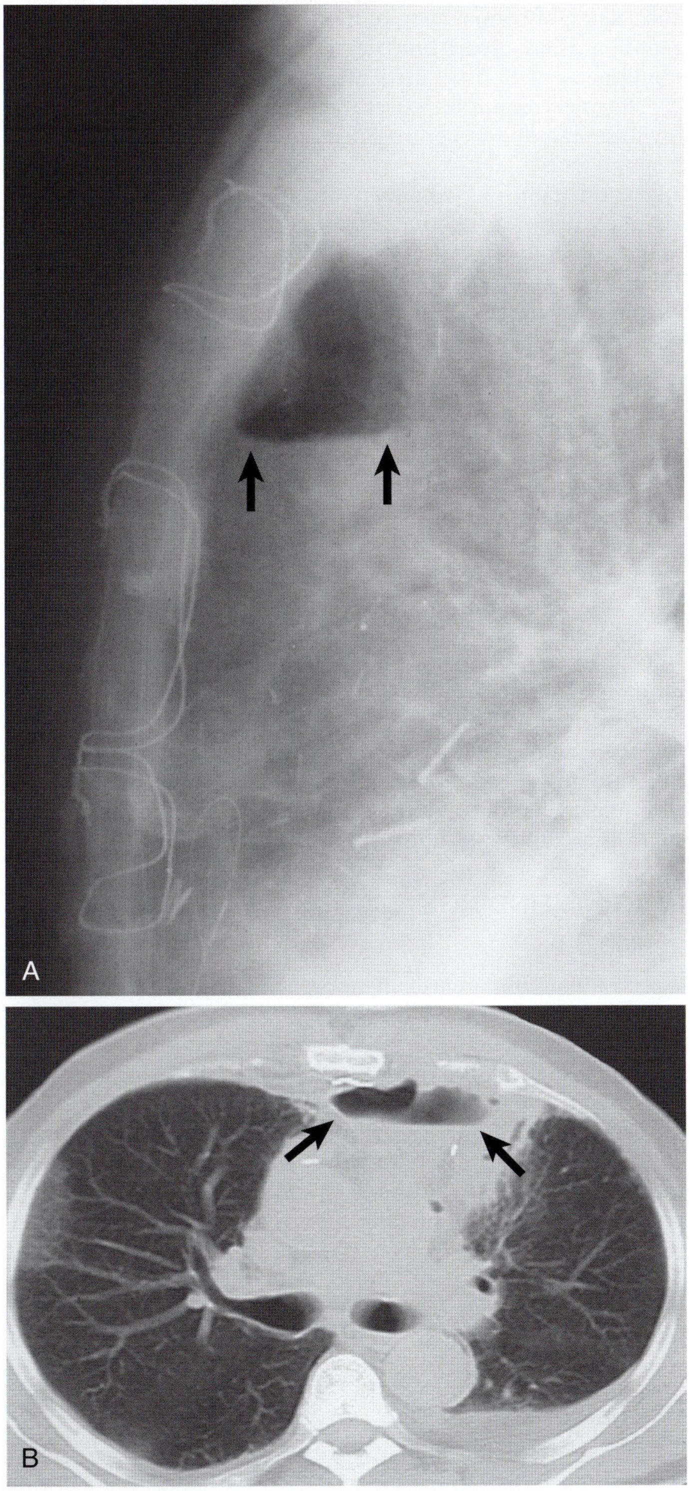

Fig. 76.9 Poststernotomy mediastinitis after bypass surgery. (A) Lateral chest radiograph shows a retrosternal air-fluid level *(arrows)*. (B) Noncontrast CT shows extensive air and fluid in the mediastinum *(arrows)*. A left pleural effusion is also visible.

and the adjacent sternoclavicular joint, widening of the joint space, irregular sternal contours, peristernal soft tissue swelling, and gas or fluid collections.[10] In one series of 50 patients with clinically suspected mediastinitis, these CT findings were nonspecific for mediastinitis until postoperative day 14; however, such findings were highly indicative of mediastinitis after the first 2 weeks.[18]

CT is also a valuable technique in the management of mediastinal abscesses and fluid collections.[62,63] Percutaneous catheter aspiration and drainage of mediastinal fluid collections, under CT guidance, can be useful as a diagnostic and therapeutic approach.[64]

Imaging Algorithm

In most patients with acute mediastinitis, a confident diagnosis can be made based on clinical and imaging findings. Acute mediastinitis is encountered clinically in two main settings: the rupture or perforation of the esophagus as a complication of instrumentation and the extension of infections from neighboring tissues in the neck. In these circumstances the chest radiograph may show widening of the mediastinum and air within the mediastinum and in the soft tissues of the neck. Esophagram with a water-soluble contrast agent, such as diatrizoate meglumine (Gastrografin), is safe and effective for evaluating the esophagus to rule out esophageal perforations.[65] Esophagram can also be performed safely with barium.[66] A typical esophagram protocol would include both water-soluble contrast to rule out frank rupture and then dilute barium to increase the sensitivity for a small esophageal leak.

Cross-sectional imaging techniques generally are required for diagnosis and evaluation of the site and extent of mediastinal involvement. The main utility of CT is in the evaluation of patients with clinical suspicion of acute mediastinitis and normal or nonspecific radiographic findings. In complications of median sternotomy and closed blunt chest trauma, CT is of great value in determining whether the infection is limited to the presternal tissues, the anterior mediastinum, or both.[60,67] CT and magnetic resonance imaging (MRI) also may guide the choice of the optimal therapeutic approach.[3]

DIFFERENTIAL DIAGNOSIS

The main role of imaging in the diagnosis of acute mediastinitis is in confirming the presence of mediastinal abnormalities consistent with the clinical diagnosis. The radiographic finding of a widened mediastinum in the clinical setting of fever and pleuritic chest pain strongly suggests acute mediastinitis.

Fibrosing Mediastinitis

ETIOLOGY, PREVALENCE, AND EPIDEMIOLOGY

Fibrosing mediastinitis, also known as sclerosing mediastinitis and mediastinal fibrosis, is a rare entity characterized by excessive fibrotic reaction usually caused by granulomatous infection, most commonly histoplasmosis and tuberculosis. It also may be idiopathic or secondary to the exposure to methysergide (Box 76.2).[68] Less common causes are silicosis, sarcoidosis, autoimmune disorders, immunoglobulin G4 (IgG4)-related disease, and familial multifocal fibrosclerosis.[69]

The most common abnormality on the chest radiograph is mediastinal widening, which is usually most marked in the right paratracheal region. The compression of the vessels and bronchi is usually smooth. Pulmonary venous and arterial obstruction may cause localized edema, cor pulmonale, and death.

PATHOLOGIC FINDINGS AND PATHOPHYSIOLOGY

Fibrosing mediastinitis is a rare benign disorder caused by extensive fibrous tissue throughout the visceral or middle

BOX 76.2 ETIOLOGY OF FIBROSING MEDIASTINITIS

Infection
- *Histoplasma capsulatum* (mainly in the United States)
- Tuberculosis
- Actinomycosis
- *Blastomyces dermatitidis*
- Zygomycosis
- *Aspergillus* species
- *Treponema pallidum*
- *Wuchereria bancrofti*
- *Rhodococcus equi*

Sarcoidosis
Silicosis
Behçet syndrome
Drugs: methysergide
Malignancy
Radiation therapy
Trauma
Iatrogenic: pacemakers, central venous catheter
Connective tissue disease: systemic lupus erythematosus, rheumatoid disease
IgG4-related disease
Keloids

mediastinum causing compression, encasement, or invasion of the large bronchi, SVC, pulmonary veins, or esophagus.[70] The histologic appearance varies, depending on the underlying cause. Most cases of fibrosing mediastinitis are associated with *Histoplasma capsulatum* infection (especially in North America) or tuberculosis; histologic findings consist of necrotizing granulomatous inflammation.[71]

Sometimes the pathogenesis is unclear and associated with fibroinflammatory and autoimmune disorders involving other structures.[72] In one review of 15 consecutive surgical biopsies of histoplasmosis or granulomatous-disease–associated fibrosing mediastinitis, one-third of cases with the same clinical and radiologic features demonstrated histopathologic features of IgG4-related disease.[73] Whether these changes occur as the host immune response against *Histoplasma* or represent a manifestation of IgG4-related disease remains to be determined.[73] In those cases in which an infectious organism is not identified, the granulomatous component is minimal or absent, and the abnormal tissue is composed predominantly of mature fibrous tissue containing a mononuclear inflammatory cell infiltrate.

The genesis of granulomatous mediastinitis and mediastinal fibrosis in patients who have infection is not completely understood. It has been hypothesized that infection begins as a primary focus in the lung that drains to mediastinal lymph nodes and leads to mediastinal lymphadenitis. Spillage of necrotic material from affected lymph nodes is followed by mediastinal infection and secondary fibrosis.[74] Fibrosing mediastinitis also has been suggested to result from a hypersensitivity reaction to antigenic material released from involved lymph nodes.[75–77]

The term *idiopathic fibroinflammatory lesion of the mediastinum* has been proposed to describe cases in which cultures and special stains for organisms are negative.[78]

CLINICAL PRESENTATION

Clinical manifestations are variable and depend on the degree of invasion or compression of mediastinal structures. Affected patients are typically young and present with signs and symptoms of obstruction or compression of the SVC, major pulmonary vessels, central airways, mediastinal nerves, or esophagus. In some cases more than one of these mediastinal structures is compressed.

The most common clinical manifestations resulting from involvement of the central airways are dyspnea, cough, and hemoptysis.[76,78,79] Esophageal involvement may result in dysphagia and chest pain. Entrapment or compression of the recurrent laryngeal nerve can produce hoarseness, and involvement of one or both phrenic nerves may cause diaphragmatic paralysis. Horner syndrome can be produced from impingement on autonomic ganglions or nerves.[2,80] Chylothorax and chylopericardium may result from involvement of the thoracic duct.[81]

Although malignancy is the most common cause of SVC syndrome, the most common etiologies of benign obstruction of SVC are fibrosing mediastinitis and iatrogenic causes, especially with the increasing use of intravascular devices.[81–83] Because obstruction develops gradually, collateral veins tend to divert much of the venous flow, and symptoms include face or neck swelling, upper extremity swelling, dyspnea, cough, and dilated chest vein collaterals. Dyspnea at rest, cough, and chest pain are less common than in patients with SVC syndrome from malignancy.[83]

Obstruction of one or both central pulmonary arteries may result in pulmonary hypertension, cor pulmonale, and refractory right-sided heart failure.[84,85] Stenosis of proximal pulmonary veins can manifest with a clinical picture similar to severe valvular mitral stenosis ("pseudomitral stenosis" syndrome).[86] Percutaneous stenting has been used as a treatment for pulmonary artery stenosis secondary to fibrosing mediastinitis.[87]

IMAGING FINDINGS

Radiography

Chest radiographs are usually nonspecific and frequently underestimate the extent of mediastinal disease. Granulomatous mediastinitis, generally secondary to histoplasmosis or tuberculosis, typically results in a localized calcified mass, usually in the right paratracheal region (Fig. 76.10). Noninfectious fibrosing mediastinitis results in a nonspecific widening of the mediastinum, with distortion and obliteration of normally recognizable mediastinal interfaces or lines.[88] In some cases of focal or diffuse disease the mediastinal silhouette is normal, and the radiographic manifestations result from narrowing of the trachea or major bronchi, obstruction of pulmonary veins or arteries, or narrowing of the esophagus (Fig. 76.11). Involvement of the SVC frequently results in a prominent aortic nipple as a result of a dilated left superior intercostal vein.

Computed Tomography

CT allows excellent evaluation of the extent of mediastinal soft tissue infiltration and calcification and can identify the degree of narrowing of the tracheobronchial tree. Two distinctly different CT patterns of fibrosing mediastinitis may be seen: a localized form that frequently contains foci of calcification and a diffuse form that does not contain calcifications (Fig. 76.12).[75] The focal form of fibrosing mediastinitis manifests on CT scans as a soft tissue mass that infiltrates the mediastinum, most commonly in the paratracheal regions, and causes narrowing or occlusion of adjacent vessels or airways (Fig. 76.13). Foci of calcification are evident on CT in 60% to 90% of cases. The diffuse form manifests on CT as a diffuse infiltrative mass of soft tissue attenuation that obliterates normal mediastinal fat planes and

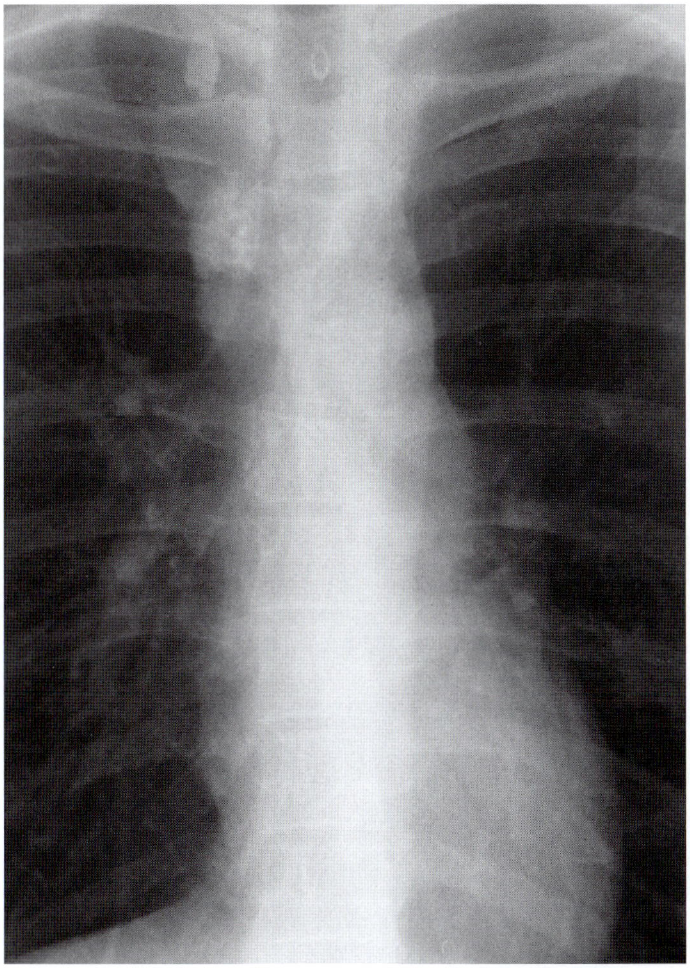

Fig. 76.10 Fibrosing mediastinitis related to histoplasmosis. Close-up posteroanterior chest radiograph shows enlarged and calcified right paratracheal lymph nodes. The patient presented with superior vena cava syndrome. *(Courtesy Dr. Robert Tarver, Indiana University Medical Center, Indianapolis, IN; from Müller NL, Fraser RS, Colman NC, et al.* Radiologic Diagnosis of Diseases of the Chest. *Philadelphia: Saunders; 2001.)*

encases or invades adjacent structures (Fig. 76.14).[88] The focal form of fibrosing mediastinitis is usually secondary to granulomatous infection, and the diffuse form is often secondary to other causes, such as drug reactions or autoimmune disease. CT allows assessment of the location and extent of the vascular and airway narrowing. Bronchial narrowing most commonly affects the right main bronchus, followed in decreasing frequency by the left main bronchus, bronchus intermedius, right upper lobe bronchus, left upper lobe bronchus, and right middle lobe bronchus. Bronchial obstruction frequently is associated with obstructive pneumonitis, atelectasis, or both. Contrast-enhanced CT with multiplanar reconstructions can help determine the severity of obstruction involving the pulmonary arteries, veins, and SVC as well as the presence of superimposed thrombosis.[89] Obstruction or narrowing of a pulmonary artery may result in localized areas of decreased opacification and vascularity, volume loss, or thrombosis. Findings of pulmonary venous hypertension, including interlobular septal thickening and airspace pulmonary edema, may occur (see Fig. 76.13).

Magnetic Resonance Imaging

MRI is similar to CT in the assessment of airway involvement and is superior to it in the assessment of vascular involvement.[90,91] The main disadvantage of MRI is that it does not allow confident assessment of the presence of calcification, a finding highly suggestive of previous histoplasmosis or tuberculosis as the cause of the fibrosing mediastinitis. MRI has a limited role in the diagnostic evaluation. MRI of fibrosing mediastinitis typically shows heterogeneous signal intensity on T1-weighted and T2-weighted images.[59]

^{18}F-Fluorodeoxyglucose–Positron Emission Tomography–Computed Tomography

^{18}F-Fluorodeoxyglucose–positron emission tomography–computed tomography (^{18}F-FDG–PET-CT) is not helpful in differentiating fibrosing mediastinitis from a neoplastic process as both are FDG avid. In proven fibrosing mediastinitis FDG uptake has been used to monitor the posttreatment disease response.[72,92]

Digital Subtraction Angiography

Digital subtraction angiography is used primarily in the treatment of SVC obstruction. SVC angioplasty with or without stent placement can provide rapid relief by restoring venous return.[93]

DIFFERENTIAL DIAGNOSIS

Chronic obstruction of pulmonary arteries can be due to a variety of disease processes, including chronic thromboembolic disease, fibrosing mediastinitis, and tumor. Pulmonary hilar fibrosis can mimic thromboembolic pulmonary hypertension, pulmonary

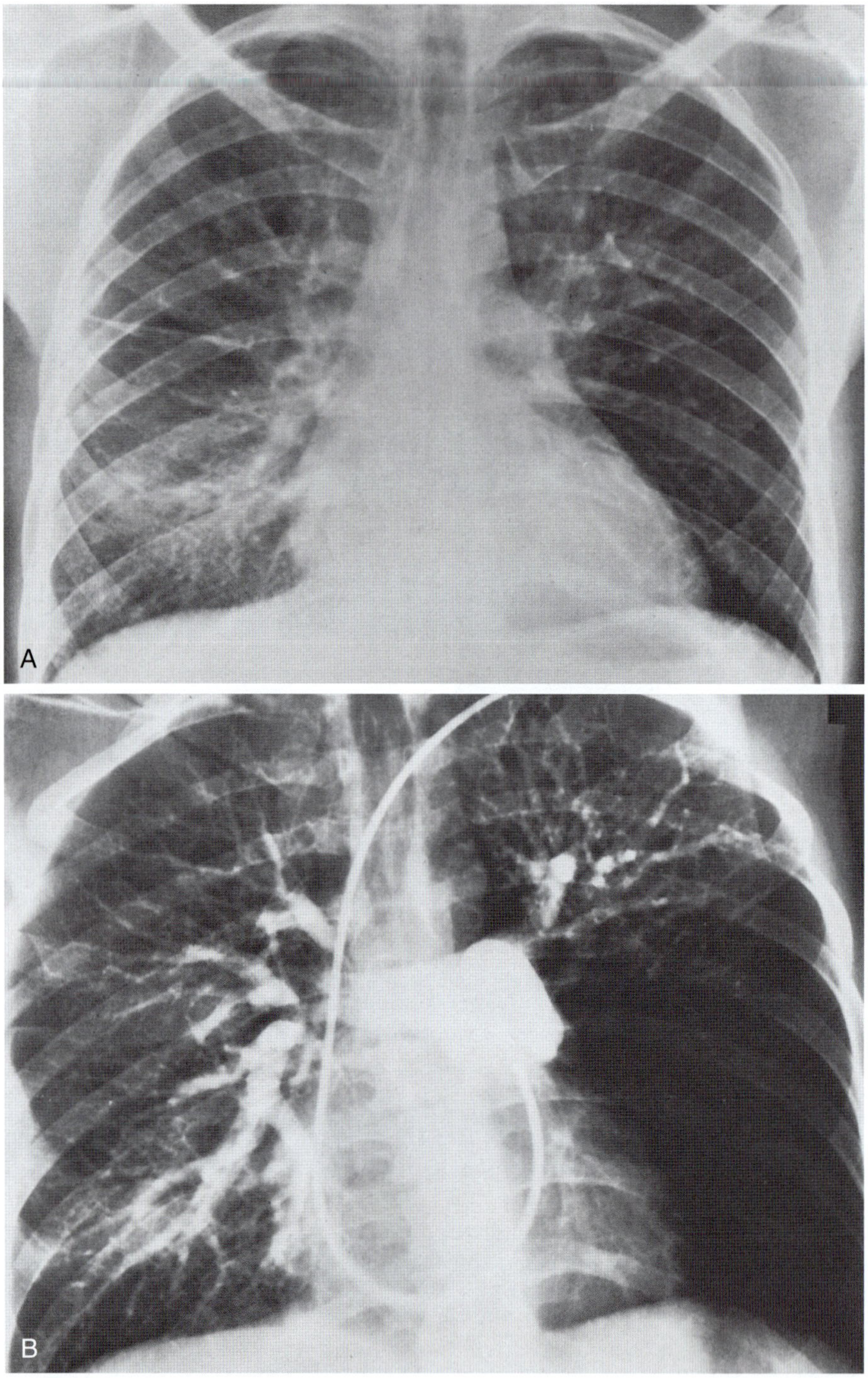

Fig. 76.11 Fibrosing mediastinitis with encasement of pulmonary arteries and veins. (A) Posteroanterior chest radiograph reveals interstitial edema throughout the right lung and left upper zone. Septal lines are present in the right costophrenic angle. A striking disparity in density of the lower half of the two lungs is observed, the left being radiolucent and oligemic. (B) Pulmonary arteriogram shows almost complete occlusion of the left interlobar artery with virtually no perfusion of the left lower lobe and lingula. Although there appears to be good opacification of the arteries of the right lung, the truncus anterior and interlobar arteries show concentric narrowing medial to the hilum. The venous phase of the angiogram is unavailable, but it is almost certain that the pulmonary veins were affected in the same manner, resulting in venous hypertension and the interstitial edema apparent on chest radiography. The cause of the fibrosis was *Histoplasma capsulatum* infection. *(Courtesy Dr. M.J. Palayew, Jewish General Hospital, Montreal, Quebec, Canada; from Müller NL, Fraser RS, Colman NC, et al.* Radiologic Diagnosis of Diseases of the Chest. *Philadelphia: Saunders; 2001.)*

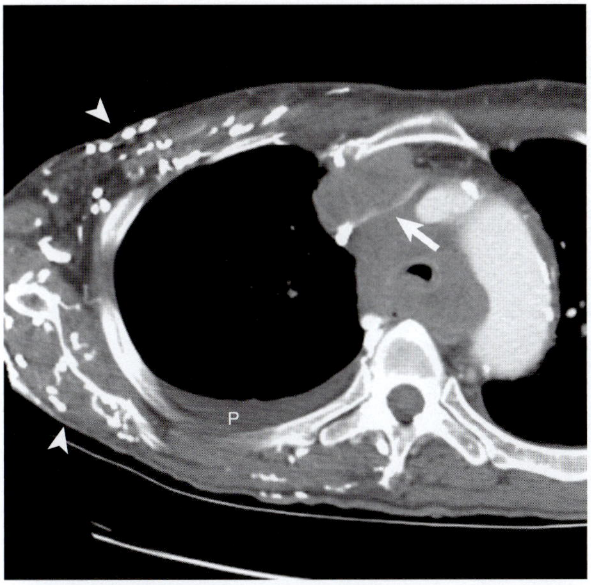

Fig. 76.12 Extensive fibrosing mediastinitis with encasement of brachiocephalic vein and stenosis of superior vena cava (SVC). Contrast-enhanced CT at the level of the aortic arch shows extensive mediastinal fibrosis with marked stenosis of the left brachiocephalic vein *(arrow)* and stenosis of the SVC. Note significant collateral circulation in the right subcutaneous tissues *(arrowheads)*. *P*, Pleural effusion.

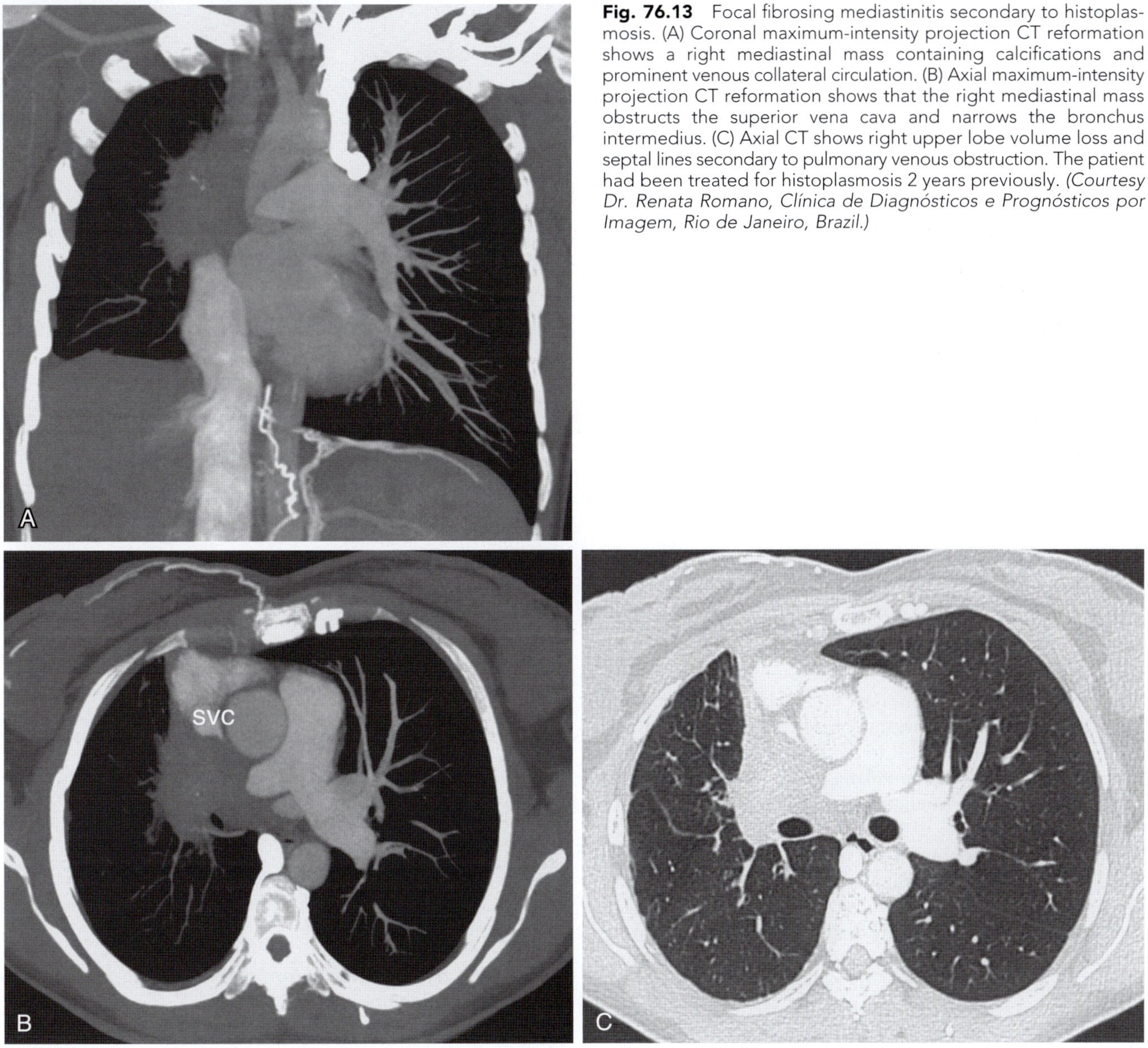

Fig. 76.13 Focal fibrosing mediastinitis secondary to histoplasmosis. (A) Coronal maximum-intensity projection CT reformation shows a right mediastinal mass containing calcifications and prominent venous collateral circulation. (B) Axial maximum-intensity projection CT reformation shows that the right mediastinal mass obstructs the superior vena cava and narrows the bronchus intermedius. (C) Axial CT shows right upper lobe volume loss and septal lines secondary to pulmonary venous obstruction. The patient had been treated for histoplasmosis 2 years previously. *(Courtesy Dr. Renata Romano, Clínica de Diagnósticos e Prognósticos por Imagem, Rio de Janeiro, Brazil.)*

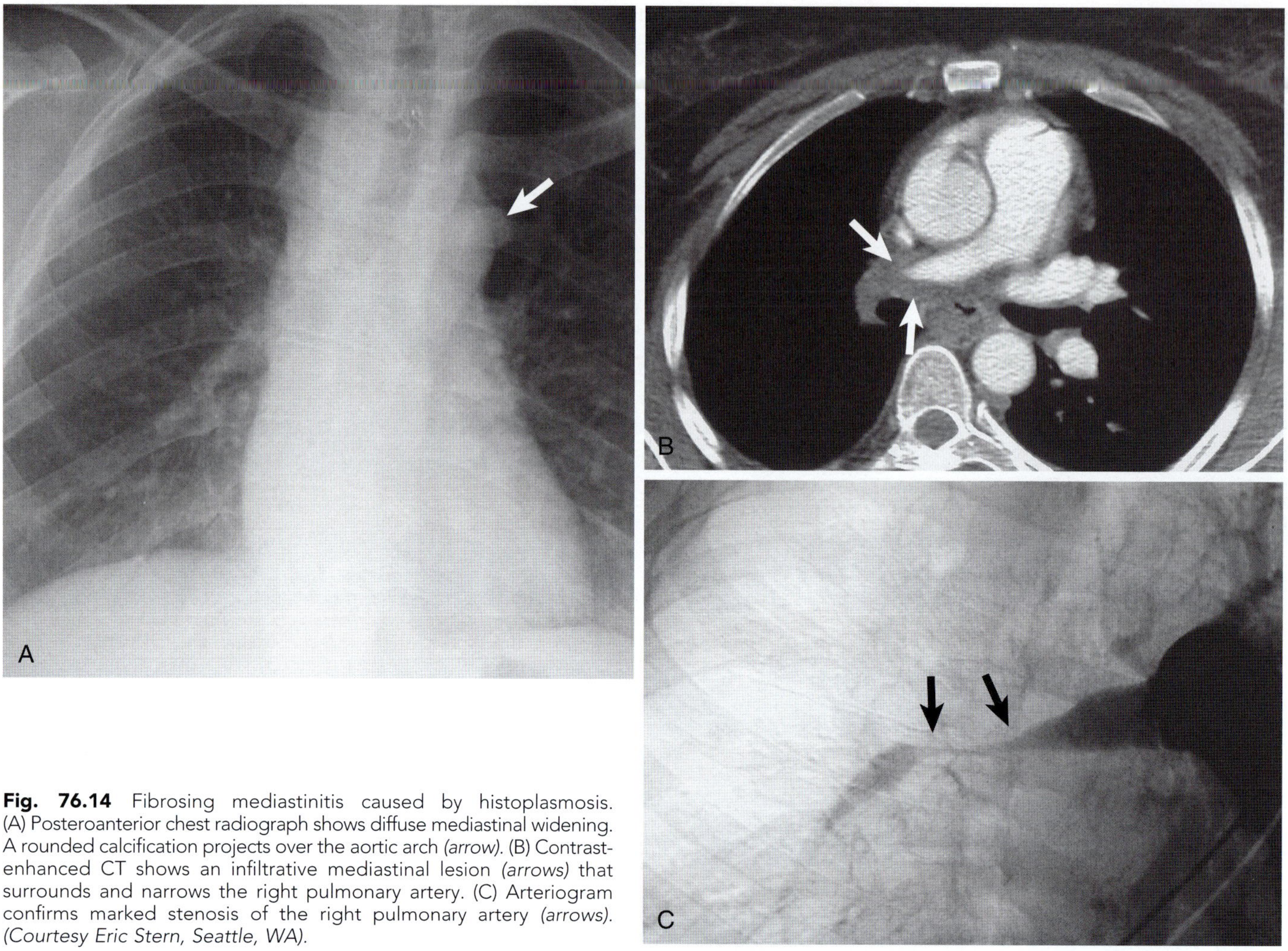

Fig. 76.14 Fibrosing mediastinitis caused by histoplasmosis. (A) Posteroanterior chest radiograph shows diffuse mediastinal widening. A rounded calcification projects over the aortic arch *(arrow)*. (B) Contrast-enhanced CT shows an infiltrative mediastinal lesion *(arrows)* that surrounds and narrows the right pulmonary artery. (C) Arteriogram confirms marked stenosis of the right pulmonary artery *(arrows)*. *(Courtesy Eric Stern, Seattle, WA)*.

KEY POINTS

- The most common cause of acute mediastinitis is esophageal perforation.
- The most common cause of chronic (fibrosing) mediastinitis is histoplasmosis infection.
- Common CT manifestations of acute mediastinitis include mediastinal fat stranding, obliteration of soft tissue planes, and focal areas of low attenuation surrounded by rim enhancement consistent with mediastinal abscess formation.
- In patients with clinical findings suggesting fibrosing mediastinitis, the presence of a localized partially calcified mediastinal soft tissue mass is virtually diagnostic of fibrosing mediastinitis secondary to previous histoplasmosis or tuberculosis infection.

venoocclusive disease, and pulmonary venous hypertension. Large vessel arteritis is another unusual cause of pulmonary artery obstruction and can be difficult to distinguish from the entities listed above.[94] The main differential diagnosis of SVC obstruction is lung cancer or another malignancy of the mediastinum such as lymphoma.

CT is performed almost routinely in the assessment of patients suspected to have fibrosing mediastinitis. In the appropriate clinical context the presence of a localized mediastinal soft tissue mass with calcification is virtually diagnostic of granulomatous fibrosing mediastinitis and obviates the need for tissue sampling. If the mass is not calcified, or if there is clinical or radiologic evidence of disease progression, biopsy may be required to exclude a neoplasm.

SUGGESTED READINGS

Akman C, Kantarci F, Cetinkaya S. Imaging in mediastinitis: a systematic review based on aetiology. *Clin Radiol.* 2004;59:573–585.
Exarhos DN, Malagari K, Tsatalou EG, et al. Acute mediastinitis: spectrum of computed tomography findings. *Eur Radiol.* 2005;15:1569–1574.
Giménez A, Franquet T, Erasmus JJ, et al. Thoracic complications of esophageal disorders. *Radiographics.* 2002;22:S247–S258.
McNeeley MF, Chung JH, Bhalla S, Godwin JD. Imaging of granulomatous fibrosing mediastinitis. *AJR Am J Roentgenol.* 2012;199(2):319–327.
Rossi SE, McAdams HP, Rosado-de-Christenson ML, et al. Fibrosing mediastinitis. *Radiographics.* 2001;21:737–757.

The full reference list for this chapter is available at ExpertConsult.com.

77 Mediastinal Masses*

BRETT W. CARTER

Mediastinal masses are relatively uncommon and include a wide variety of abnormalities of neoplastic, congenital, vascular, and lymphatic etiology that most radiologists encounter infrequently. Imaging plays a critical role in the identification and evaluation of mediastinal lesions, facilitating the formulation of focused differential diagnoses and guiding clinical management. In some cases mediastinal masses demonstrate imaging characteristics that can suggest a specific diagnosis; in other instances the imaging findings alone are inconclusive, and a combination of radiologic and clinical information is necessary to determine the next step in management.

Division of the mediastinum into specific compartments has traditionally served as a helpful tool for the identification and characterization of mediastinal masses and other abnormalities. Several different classification systems have been developed and used by anatomists, surgeons, and radiologists. The most commonly used scheme in clinical practice is the Shields classification system, whereas the traditional Fraser and Paré, Felson, Heitzman, Zylak, and Whitten models have been used to varying degrees in radiologic practice.[1–7] One model has been proposed in an attempt to bridge the gap between the various schemes.[8] Fundamental differences in the methods of mediastinal compartmentalization and terminology used in these systems have caused confusion and resulted in miscommunication among health care providers evaluating patients with mediastinal masses.

The existing models typically used in radiologic practice represent arbitrary divisions of the chest based primarily on the lateral chest radiograph that are nonanatomic. A classification scheme based on cross-sectional imaging techniques, principally computed tomography (CT) but also magnetic resonance imaging (MRI) and fluorodeoxyglucose (FDG)–positron emission tomography (PET)-CT, is necessary as these modalities are typically used to evaluate and diagnose mediastinal abnormalities, and a growing number of lesions are detected with CT studies performed for lung cancer screening, cardiac screening, and other purposes.[9,10] In 2014 the Japanese Association for Research on the Thymus (JART) developed a four-compartment model based on CT, which was derived from a retrospective study of 445 nonconsecutive pathology-proven mediastinal masses.[11] Based on discussions with experts in the field of mediastinal diseases, the International Thymic Malignancy Interest Group (ITMIG) has modified the JART model and introduced a new definition of mediastinal compartments to be used with cross-sectional imaging that has been accepted as a new standard.[12]

In this chapter the new ITMIG mediastinal compartment classification system based on cross-sectional imaging is presented along with detailed information regarding the wide variety of masses and other abnormalities that may be encountered in the mediastinum and their predominant manifestations on imaging studies.

*The editors and the publisher would like to thank Drs. Kiminori Fujimoto and Nestor L. Müller for contributing material on this topic to the prior edition of this work. It has served as the foundation for the current chapter.

International Thymic Malignancy Interest Group Definition of Mediastinal Compartments

The ITMIG classification includes specific prevascular (anterior), visceral (middle), and paravertebral (posterior) compartments (Table 77.1) and compartment boundaries, and the anatomic structures they contain can be readily identified on cross-sectional imaging (Fig. 77.1).

PREVASCULAR COMPARTMENT

The boundaries of the prevascular compartment include (1) superiorly: the thoracic inlet, (2) inferiorly: the diaphragm, (3) anteriorly: the posterior border/cortex of the sternum, (4) laterally: the parietal mediastinal pleura, and (5) posteriorly: the anterior aspect of the pericardium (see Table 77.1). This compartment contains the thymus, fat, lymph nodes, and the left brachiocephalic vein. Therefore the most common abnormalities encountered in the prevascular compartment include thymic lesions (cysts, hyperplasia, and thymic epithelial neoplasms, such as thymoma, thymic carcinoma, and thymic carcinoid), germ cell neoplasms, lymphoma, metastatic disease, and intrathoracic goiter.

VISCERAL COMPARTMENT

The boundaries of the visceral compartment include (1) superiorly: the thoracic inlet, (2) inferiorly: the diaphragm, (3) anteriorly: the posterior boundaries of the prevascular compartment, and (4) posteriorly: a vertical line connecting a point on the thoracic vertebral bodies 1 cm posterior to the anterior margin of the spine, referred to as the visceral–paravertebral compartment boundary line (see Table 77.1). This compartment includes vascular structures such as the heart, superior vena cava (SVC), thoracic aorta, intrapericardial pulmonary arteries, and the thoracic duct, and nonvascular structures, including the trachea, carina, esophagus, and lymph nodes. It should be noted that the ITMIG model includes all structures enclosed by the pericardium in the visceral compartment. The extrapericardial pulmonary arteries and veins are considered pulmonary structures and are not included in this compartment. Lymphadenopathy caused by lymphoma or metastatic disease, duplication cysts, esophageal lesions, and cardiovascular abnormalities are responsible for most abnormalities that arise from the visceral compartment.

PARAVERTEBRAL COMPARTMENT

The boundaries of the paravertebral compartment include (1) superiorly: the thoracic inlet, (2) inferiorly: the diaphragm,

TABLE 77.1 ITMIG CLASSIFICATION OF MEDIASTINAL COMPARTMENTS

Compartment	Boundaries	Major Contents
Prevascular	Superior: thoracic inlet Inferior: diaphragm Anterior: sternum Lateral: parietal mediastinal pleura Posterior: anterior aspect of the pericardium as it wraps around the heart in a curvilinear fashion	Thymus Fat Lymph nodes Left brachiocephalic vein
Visceral	Superior: thoracic inlet Inferior: diaphragm Anterior: posterior boundaries of the prevascular compartment Posterior: vertical line connecting a point on each thoracic vertebral body at 1 cm posterior to its anterior margin	Nonvascular: trachea, carina, esophagus, lymph nodes Vascular: heart, aorta, superior vena cava, intrapericardial pulmonary arteries, thoracic duct
Paravertebral	Superior: thoracic inlet Inferior: diaphragm Anterior: posterior boundaries of the visceral compartment Posterolateral: vertical line against the posterior margin of the chest wall at the lateral margin of the transverse process of the thoracic spine	Thoracic spine Paravertebral soft tissues

ITMIG, International Thymic Malignancy Interest Group.

(3) anteriorly: the posterior boundaries of the visceral compartment, and (4) posterolaterally: a vertical line along the posterior margin of the chest wall at the lateral aspect of the transverse processes (see Table 77.1). This compartment contains the thoracic spine and paravertebral soft tissues. Therefore neurogenic neoplasms that arise from the dorsal root ganglia/neurons adjacent to the intervertebral foramina comprise most lesions in the paravertebral compartment. Other abnormalities that may be encountered include infectious (diskitis/osteomyelitis) or traumatic (hematoma) lesions, as well as miscellaneous conditions, such as extramedullary hematopoiesis.

Imaging of Mediastinal Masses

GENERAL CONSIDERATIONS

Greater than half of all mediastinal masses arise from the anterior/prevascular compartment, whereas one-fourth each are identified in the middle/visceral and posterior/paravertebral mediastinal compartments.[10,13–21] In many instances localization and characterization of a mediastinal abnormality using CT are sufficient to make the diagnosis. In other cases correlation between imaging findings and clinical context, as well as additional imaging examinations, such as MRI and PET-CT, and histologic sampling through image-guided or surgical biopsy, is necessary to make a definitive diagnosis and guide further management.

RADIOGRAPHY

Chest radiography is the most commonly performed imaging examination and is often the first modality demonstrating findings suggestive of mediastinal pathology. Small lesions may not be visible or result in subtle abnormalities of mediastinal lines, stripes, and interfaces. For instance, a thymic epithelial neoplasm in the anterior mediastinum may only result in thickening of the anterior junction line. Therefore close evaluation of these landmarks is necessary on radiography. The lateral chest radiograph can be useful in identifying abnormalities that may not be visible on the posteroanterior radiograph, usually those that are only visible in the retrosternal space or overlying the upper thoracic spine. Large lesions can manifest in myriad ways, including more extensive irregularity of normal mediastinal contours or interfaces or one or multiple soft tissue masses.

Multiple radiographic signs have been described that can be useful in alerting the radiologist that a mediastinal mass may be present. One of these is the silhouette sign, which describes the loss of normal borders of intrathoracic structures and can assist the radiologist in identifying various mediastinal abnormalities. For instance, a mass in the right anterior mediastinum may obscure the right heart border, whereas a mass in the posterior mediastinal compartment may result in loss of the normal paraspinal line. The hilum overlay sign may help differentiate a mediastinal lesion from other abnormalities, such as cardiomegaly or enlarged pulmonary vessels.

Computed Tomography

CT is the imaging modality of choice for identifying, localizing, and characterizing mediastinal masses, and imaging features often enable the radiologist to formulate a focused differential diagnosis based on imaging alone. Tomiyama and colleagues[22] evaluated 127 mediastinal masses of various etiologies in the prevascular compartment and demonstrated that CT was equal or superior to MRI in correctly diagnosing most of the lesions, apart from thymic cysts.

Specific information regarding mediastinal masses that should be noted on CT and reported include (1) location, size, and configuration; (2) density, heterogeneity, and enhancement; (3) fat, cystic components, soft tissue, and calcification; and (4) connection with or invasion of adjacent structures. Some of these findings are more diagnostically relevant than others. For instance, the presence of fat in a prevascular mediastinal mass on CT is highly suggestive of a small number of lesions, such as mature teratoma, thymolipoma, and others, whereas calcifications are nonspecific and may be associated with benign or malignant lesions.

Magnetic Resonance Imaging

MRI is rarely the first imaging modality used to evaluate chest symptomatology or abnormalities identified on chest radiography but is the most effective modality for distinguishing cystic from solid lesions (e.g., thymic cysts from solid tumors), identifying

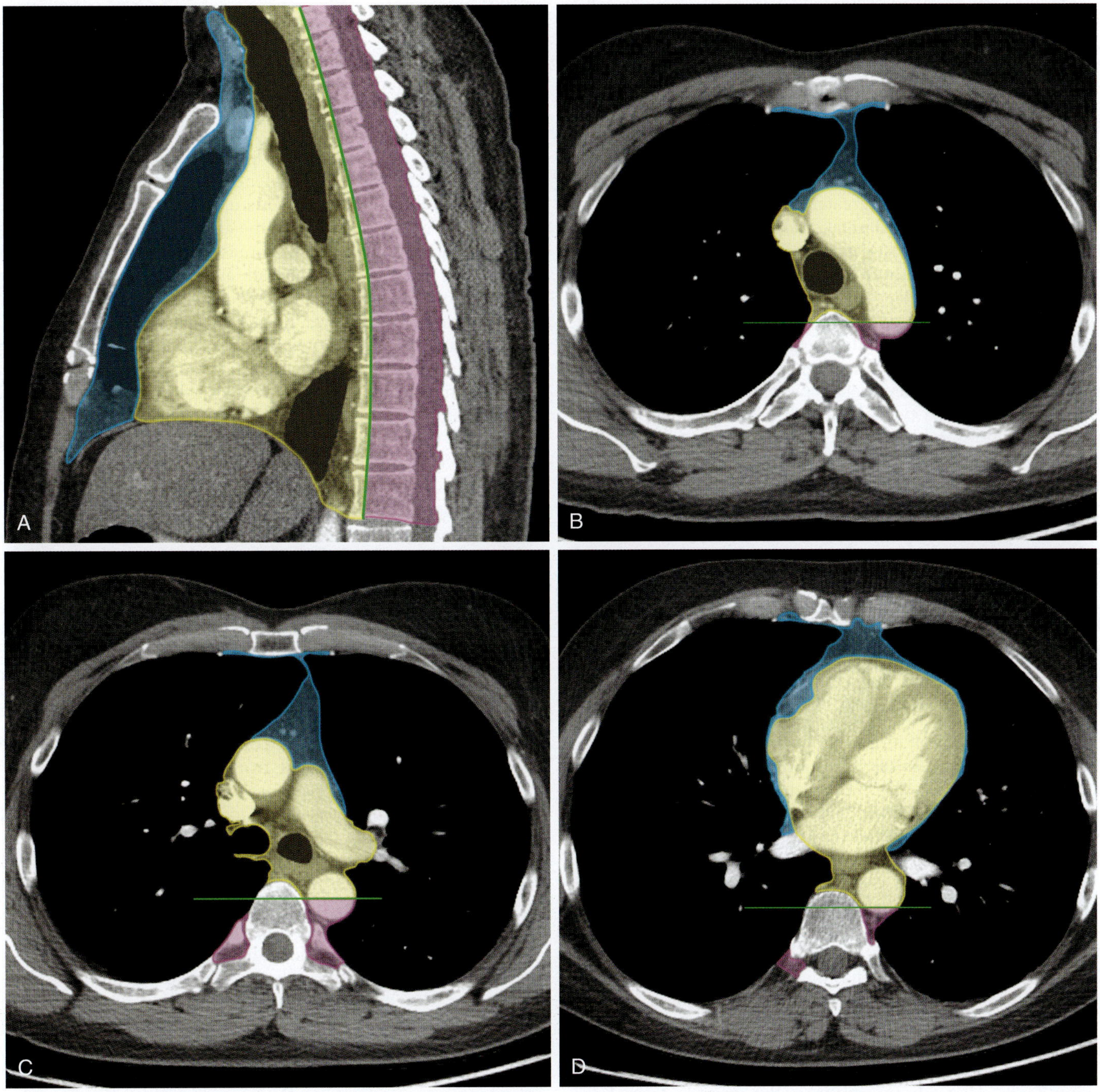

Fig. 77.1 International Thymic Malignancy Interest Group definition of mediastinal compartments. Sagittal reformatted CT (A) and axial CT images at the level of the aortic arch (B), at the level of the left pulmonary artery (C), and at the level of the left atrium (D) demonstrate the classification scheme. *Blue,* Prevascular compartment; *yellow,* visceral compartment; *purple,* paravertebral compartment; *green line,* visceral–paravertebral compartment boundary line.

cystic and/or necrotic components within solid masses, identifying septations and/or soft tissue within cystic lesions, and distinguishing thymic hyperplasia and normal thymus from solid neoplasms. Unenhanced MRI with specific fluid-sensitive sequences can be performed to evaluate mediastinal masses and identify vascular involvement when patients are unable to receive intravenous (IV) contrast for CT examinations because of severe allergy and/or impaired renal function. Finally, chemical shift MRI using in-phase and out-of-phase sequences is the technique of choice for diagnosing thymic hyperplasia and distinguishing it from thymoma and other thymic neoplasms, as the former is characterized by the loss of signal intensity on out-of-phase imaging resulting from the presence of microscopic fat interspersed between thymic tissue.[23–25]

Fluorodeoxyglucose–Positron Emission Tomography–Computed Tomography

The role of FDG–PET-CT in the evaluation of mediastinal masses is controversial, and several studies have been performed to investigate its efficacy in differentiating benign from malignant lesions and among specific types of malignant tumors. Kubota and colleagues[26] showed that malignant mediastinal neoplasms demonstrated significantly greater FDG uptake than benign lesions using a standardized uptake value (SUVmax) equivalent cutoff of 3.5. Others investigations have used higher SUVmax thresholds, and the authors have suggested that PET-CT is complementary to conventional imaging modalities such as CT but noted that histologic sampling is required to confirm PET-CT findings.[27] Luzzi and colleagues[28] reported significant overlap between the SUVmax of FDG-avid malignant neoplasms, including high-risk thymic epithelial neoplasms (World Health Organization [WHO] types B2 and B3), lymphoma, paraganglioma, and nonseminomatous germ cell tumors (NSGCTs). Thymic epithelial neoplasms tend to exhibit variable FDG uptake on PET-CT, with some lesions demonstrating little to no FDG uptake. Sung and colleagues[29] suggested that PET-CT could be used to distinguish low-risk thymomas (WHO types A, AB, and B1) from thymic carcinoma, and other investigators have reported that PET-CT could distinguish low-risk thymomas from high-risk thymomas (WHO types B2 and B3) and thymic carcinoma.[29,30] However, other studies have been less definitive, with PET-CT not demonstrating clear benefit in staging.

LOCALIZATION OF MEDIASTINAL MASSES

Although localization of mediastinal masses to specific compartments is critical, precise identification of the compartment of origin may be difficult in some instances. For instance, a large lesion may involve multiple compartments or extend from one compartment to another, making the delineation of the precise site of origin challenging. The ITMIG has defined and recommends the use of two specific tools that can help in lesion localization: (1) the "center method" and (2) the "structure displacement tool." The center method states that the center of a lesion, which is defined as its center point on the axial CT image on which the mass has the greatest diameter, localizes the mass to a specific compartment. This tool was used in the JART study and resulted in the accurate localization of all 445 mediastinal lesions. The structure displacement tool is particularly helpful when large mediastinal lesions displace organs from other mediastinal compartments. For example, a very large prevascular mediastinal mass may result in the posterior displacement of visceral compartment structures, such as the trachea or heart.

Imaging of the Prevascular Compartment

THYMIC EPITHELIAL NEOPLASMS

Thymic epithelial neoplasms are malignant tumors that affect 0.13 per 100,000 individuals in the United States and are the most common nonlymphomatous primary neoplasms of the prevascular/anterior mediastinum. The most common thymic epithelial neoplasms include thymoma, thymic carcinoma, and thymic neuroendocrine tumors.

Thymoma

Thymoma is the most common thymic epithelial neoplasm and primary malignancy of the prevascular mediastinum, with 1 to 5 cases per million individuals per year in the United States. The incidence is higher in Asians and African Americans compared with Hispanic and Caucasian populations, and men and women are affected equally.[31] The incidence of thymoma increases with advancing age such that patients older than 40 years are most commonly affected, although the incidence starts to decrease after the age of 60 years. Thymomas are typically slow-growing neoplasms but may demonstrate aggressive behavior, such as invasion of adjacent structures and involvement of the pleura and pericardium; however, distant metastases are rare.[32]

Symptomatic patients typically report clinical symptoms related to local effects of the primary tumor, including dysphagia, diaphragmatic paralysis, or SVC syndrome resulting from compression and invasion of adjacent structures. Approximately one-third of affected patients report chest pain, dyspnea, or cough.[33] Systemic symptoms and paraneoplastic syndromes resulting from the release of hormones, antibodies, and cytokines by the neoplasm may be reported. The most common paraneoplastic syndrome associated with thymoma is myasthenia gravis. Although 30% to 50% of patients with thymoma exhibit clinical signs and symptoms of myasthenia gravis, only 10% to 15% of patients with myasthenia gravis have thymoma.[34] Other associated paraneoplastic syndromes include hypogammaglobulinemia and pure red cell aplasia, which are present in 10% and 5% of cases, respectively.[35] Several autoimmune disorders have been described in association with thymoma, including systemic lupus erythematosus, polymyositis, and myocarditis.[36]

CT is the imaging modality of choice to evaluate thymoma and can help differentiate it from other prevascular masses. Thymoma typically manifests as a soft tissue mass with smooth or lobulated margins measuring 1 to 10 cm that characteristically arises from one lobe of the thymus (Fig. 77.2),[37] although involvement of the bilateral prevascular mediastinum has been described.[38] After the administration of IV contrast, thymoma typically demonstrates homogeneous enhancement, although heterogeneity is present in approximately one-third of patients resulting from necrosis, cystic change, and/or hemorrhage. Several patterns of calcification have been observed, including punctate, linear along the capsule, and within the lesion. Thymomas may invade adjacent vessels, resulting in direct signs, such as irregularity of the vessel lumen contour, enhancement or obliteration of vessels, and endoluminal soft tissue. Other findings on CT, such as extensive mediastinal lymphadenopathy, pleural effusions, and pulmonary metastases, are more characteristic of other thoracic malignancies, such as lung cancer, or other thymic epithelial neoplasms with more aggressive behavior (thymic carcinoma and thymic neuroendocrine tumors). Tomiyama and colleagues[39] demonstrated that the presence of lobulated or irregular contour, areas of low attenuation, and multifocal calcification are suggestive of invasive thymoma. Another study determined that tumor size greater than 7 cm, infiltration of surrounding fat, and lobulated tumor contours were useful in predicting higher-stage thymomas that often are best treated with neoadjuvant therapy. A standardized TNM (tumor, node, metastasis) staging system has recently been developed by the International Association for the Study of Lung Cancer (IASLC) and the ITMIG.[40]

On MRI thymomas typically demonstrate low to intermediate signal intensity on T1-weighted sequences and high signal

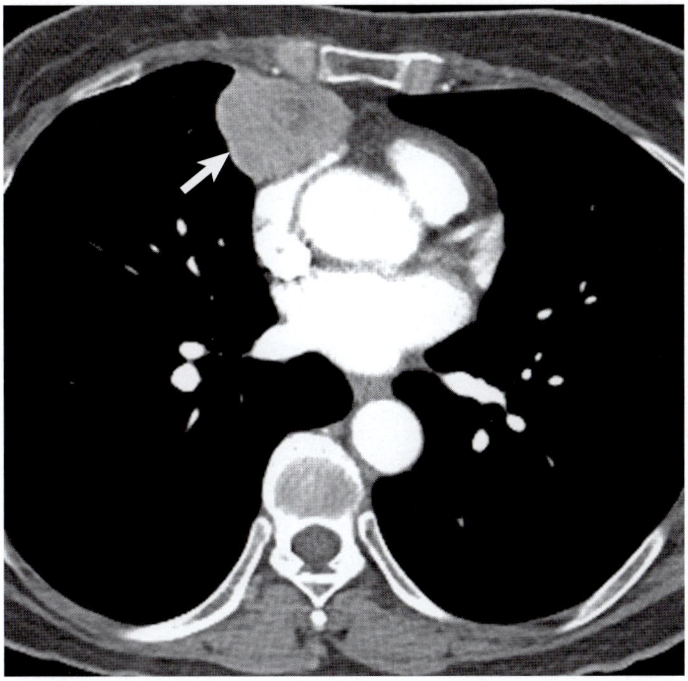

Fig. 77.2 Thymoma. Contrast-enhanced axial CT of a 62-year-old woman with chest pain and myasthenia gravis demonstrates a soft tissue mass *(arrow)* in the right prevascular mediastinum. Biopsy revealed thymoma. In the clinical setting of a paraneoplastic syndrome, such as myasthenia gravis, hypogammaglobulinemia or pure red cell aplasia, and a prevascular mediastinal mass, thymoma should be suspected.

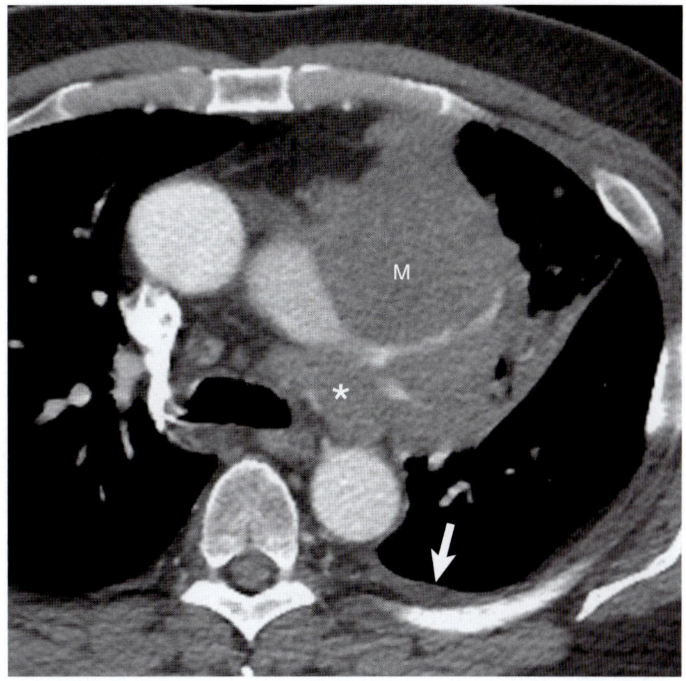

Fig. 77.3 Thymic carcinoma. Contrast-enhanced axial CT of a 53-year-old man with chest pain shows a large soft tissue mass (M) in the left prevascular mediastinum invading the left pulmonary artery and left upper lobe and extending into the visceral compartment *(asterisk)*. Biopsy revealed thymic carcinoma. Note the small left pleural effusion *(arrow)*. In contrast to thymoma, thymic carcinoma and thymic neuroendocrine neoplasms tend to demonstrate aggressive features, such as local invasion, intrathoracic lymphadenopathy, and distant metastases.

intensity on T2-weighted sequences.[41,42] Fat-suppression techniques may be beneficial in distinguishing thymoma from the adjacent mediastinal fat on T2-weighted sequences as the signal intensity of thymoma may approach that of fat. Cystic changes and necrosis result in low signal intensity on T1-weighted sequences and high signal intensity on T2-weighted sequences. Intratumoral findings, such as fibrous septations and nodules, are of low signal intensity, whereas hemorrhage demonstrates highly variable signal intensity depending upon age.

Thymic Carcinoma and Thymic Neuroendocrine Neoplasms

Thymic carcinoma is the second most common thymic epithelial neoplasm (after thymoma), representing 20% of such lesions.[43] The most common symptoms described at clinical presentation include those related to compression and invasion of adjacent structures. Neuroendocrine neoplasms of the thymus are the least common type of thymic epithelial neoplasm, most of which are carcinoid tumors.[43] Approximately 25% of these lesions develop in patients with multiple endocrine neoplasia syndrome type 1.[44] Most patients are symptomatic, with reported clinical symptoms at presentation including cough, dyspnea, and chest pain, SVC syndrome, and hoarseness.[45] Affected patients may report symptoms related to paraneoplastic syndromes, the most common of which is Cushing syndrome, characterized by ectopic production of adrenocorticotropic hormone; acromegaly and syndrome of inappropriate antidiuretic hormone are uncommon, and carcinoid syndrome is rare.[46,47] In contrast to thymoma, thymic carcinoma and thymic neuroendocrine neoplasms tend to demonstrate aggressive features, such as local invasion, intrathoracic lymphadenopathy, and distant metastases.[48]

On CT thymic carcinoma manifests as a soft tissue mass that tends to be more heterogeneous than thymoma because of regions of necrosis/cystic change, hemorrhage, and calcification (Fig. 77.3). Thymic neuroendocrine neoplasms may demonstrate invasion of mediastinal fat or vascular structures with a tendency to result in SVC syndrome, and heterogeneous enhancement or hyperenhancement may be present after the administration of IV contrast (Fig. 77.4). The presence of lymphadenopathy and distant metastases suggests an aggressive malignancy, such as thymic carcinoma or thymic neuroendocrine neoplasms; however, pleural metastases are less common than in thymoma.

On MRI thymic carcinoma and thymic neuroendocrine tumors typically appear hyperintense to muscle on both T1- and T2-weighted sequences.[49] Heterogeneous signal intensity secondary to cystic changes, necrosis, and hemorrhage may be present.[50] In contrast to thymic carcinoma, carcinoid tumors may demonstrate hyperenhancement after the administration of IV contrast.

FAT-CONTAINING MASSES

Fat-containing masses of the mediastinum demonstrate macroscopic or gross fat measuring between –40 and –120 Hounsfield units (HU) on CT. The most common prevascular masses that manifest with macroscopic intralesional fat include mature teratoma, thymolipoma, lipoma, and liposarcoma.

Mature Teratoma

Mature teratomas are benign neoplasms that usually contain fat, fluid, calcification, and soft tissue on CT, with intralesional

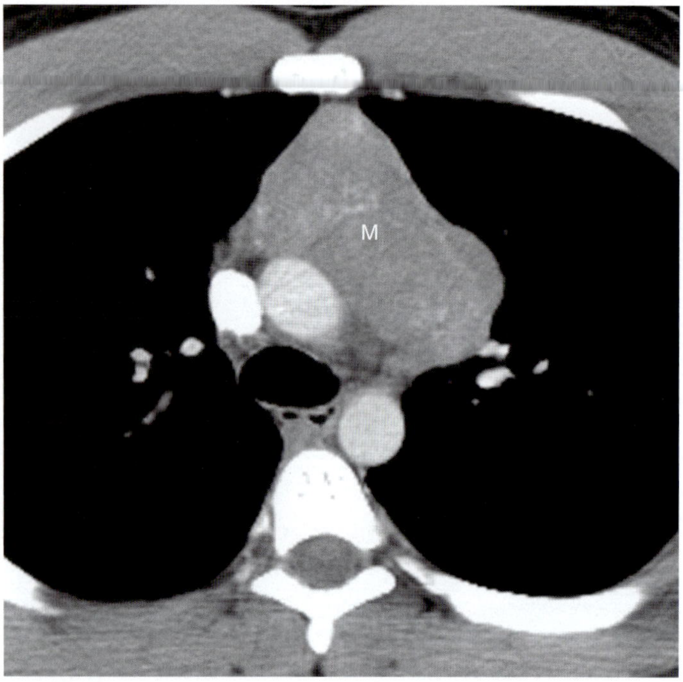

Fig. 77.4 Thymic carcinoid. Contrast-enhanced axial CT of a 39-year-old man demonstrates a heterogeneous soft tissue mass (M) in the prevascular mediastinum with internal regions of enhancement. Biopsy revealed thymic carcinoid. Thymic neuroendocrine neoplasms, such as carcinoid, may show heterogeneous enhancement or hyperenhancement after the administration of intravenous contrast.

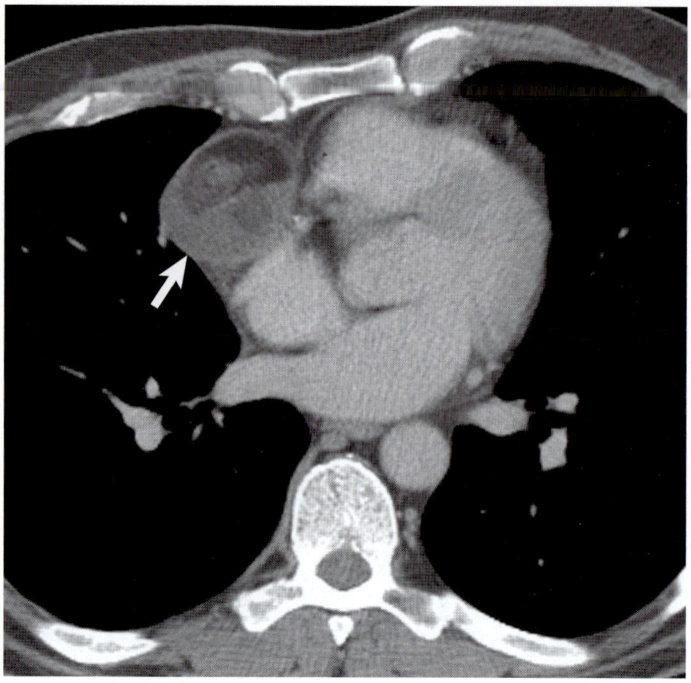

Fig. 77.5 Mature teratoma. Contrast-enhanced axial CT of a 57-year-old man shows a heterogeneous mass *(arrow)* in the right prevascular mediastinum with macroscopic fat, fluid, and a small amount of soft tissue. When a mass containing fat, fluid, calcification, and/or soft tissue is present in the prevascular mediastinum, the most likely diagnosis is mature teratoma.

fat present in 50% of cases[51,52] (Fig. 77.5). Fat-fluid levels are highly specific but are much less common.[53] Bone and tooth-like elements may rarely be identified. Mature teratoma accounts for 25% of prevascular masses in patients 10 to 19 years of age.[10] On MRI the prominent fat components are hyperintense on T1-weighted sequences and lose signal on T1-weighted fat-saturated sequences. Proteinaceous fluid and hemorrhage may demonstrate high signal intensity on T1-weighted sequences. Fluid or cystic components demonstrate low signal intensity on T1-weighted sequences and high signal intensity on T2-weighted sequences.

Thymolipoma

Thymolipoma is a benign encapsulated neoplasm composed of 50% to 85% fat and scattered regions of soft tissue and fibrous septa that is usually encountered in a cardiophrenic angle on CT[52] (Fig. 77.6). These lesions account for less than 5% of prevascular mediastinal masses in all age groups and tend to be very large at presentation, with an average reported size of 20 cm. On MRI the regions of fat are hyperintense on T1-weighted sequences and lose signal on T1-weighted fat-suppressed sequences. The soft tissue components demonstrate intermediate signal intensity of T1- and T2-weighted sequences. A direct connection with the thymus may be visible.

Lipoma and Liposarcoma

Lipomas account for 2% of all primary mediastinal neoplasms and are encapsulated lesions composed predominantly of fat with a small amount of soft tissue and blood vessels on CT. Although liposarcomas are also comprised predominantly of

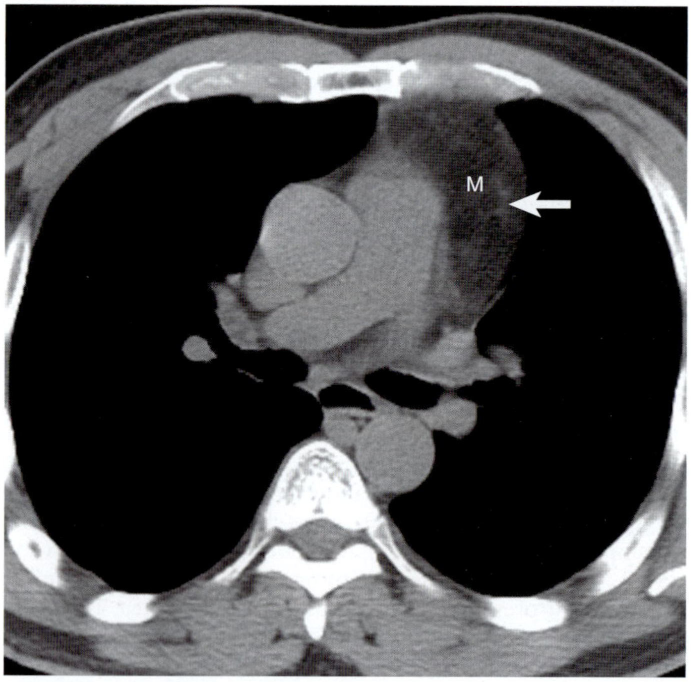

Fig. 77.6 Thymolipoma. Contrast-enhanced axial CT of a 48-year-old man demonstrates a predominantly fat-containing mass (M) in the left prevascular mediastinum with a small amount of soft tissue *(arrow)*. As this patient presented with chest pain, surgical resection was performed and revealed thymolipoma. Thymolipoma manifests as a mass primarily composed of fat with scattered regions of soft tissue and fibrous septa that is usually encountered in a cardiophrenic angle.

fat, these lesions may be distinguished from lipomas, thymolipomas, and other fat-containing lesions by a greater amount of soft tissue, local invasion, intrathoracic lymphadenopathy, and metastatic disease.[54] On MRI lipoma follows the signal intensity of subcutaneous fat on all sequences. The thin capsule and septations are hypointense on T1- and T2-weighted sequences. In contrast, liposarcoma appears as a more heterogeneous mass, the soft tissue components of which typically enhance after the administration of IV contrast.

THYMIC HYPERPLASIA

Normal thymic tissue is typically present in the prevascular mediastinal compartment in young individuals and decreases with advancing age. In most cases complete fatty replacement is achieved by 40 years of age; however, thymic hyperplasia may result in diffuse thymic enlargement or a focal soft tissue mass in the thymic bed. Two histologic types of thymic hyperplasia have been described: true and thymic lymphoid (or follicular) hyperplasia. True thymic hyperplasia is usually encountered in patients who have been treated with chemotherapy, radiation therapy, or corticosteroids or exposed to stresses such as burns or injuries. This form of thymic hyperplasia is also known as "rebound hyperplasia," defined as an increase in thymic volume of greater than 50% over baseline after a causative stressor, and affects approximately 10% to 25% of patients undergoing chemotherapy.[10,55] Follicular hyperplasia is characterized by an increased number of lymphoid follicles, which may or may not be associated with an increase in the size of the gland, usually associated with immunologic diseases, such as myasthenia gravis, hyperthyroidism, collagen vascular diseases, or human immunodeficiency virus (HIV) infection.[10]

True thymic hyperplasia manifests as diffuse symmetric enlargement of the thymus on CT, whereas follicular hyperplasia may result in a normal appearance of the thymus, thymic enlargement, or a focal soft tissue mass in the region of the thymus. Rarely, a heterogeneously hypodense prevascular mediastinal mass may be present on CT because of the deposition of fat between hyperplastic thymic tissue. Thymic hyperplasia may occasionally manifest as a focal soft tissue mass and mimic thymic epithelial neoplasms and other tumors, and chemical shift imaging can be performed to demonstrate the presence of microscopic or intravoxel fat (Fig. 77.7). Chemical shift imaging has been shown to distinguish thymic hyperplasia and normal thymus from other apparent soft tissue masses, as the former demonstrate loss of signal on out-of-phase sequences because of the suppression of microscopic fat interspersed between nonneoplastic thymic tissue, but the latter do not.[56,57] The chemical shift ratio (CSR) is a tool that can be used to calculate the signal loss and is defined as follows: CSR = (thymus SI OP/paraspinal muscle SI OP)/(thymus SI IP/paraspinal muscle SI IP), in which SI = signal intensity, IP = in-phase sequences, and OP = out-of-phase sequences. The signal loss with thymic hyperplasia and normal thymus results in CSRs of 0.5 to 0.6, whereas thymic epithelial tumors, lymphoma, and other lesions exhibit higher CSRs of 0.9 to 1.0.[56,57]

CYSTIC LESIONS

Cystic lesions of the mediastinum demonstrate water or fluid attenuation on CT, with HU values between 0 and 20. Prevascular masses that are purely cystic with no soft tissue components or internal septations can reliably be diagnosed as unilocular thymic cysts. When cystic lesions contain soft tissue components or internal septations, the differential diagnosis includes multilocular thymic cyst, cystic teratoma, lymphangioma, and cystic thymoma.

Thymic Cysts

Thymic cysts may be congenital and unilocular or acquired and unilocular or multilocular.[10] Acquired thymic cysts are typically due to inflammation; iatrogenic processes such as surgery, radiation therapy, or chemotherapy; or malignant neoplasms. A well-circumscribed homogeneous lesion in the prevascular mediastinum near the thymic bed that is round, oval, or saccular in appearance on CT likely represents a thymic cyst, although some may demonstrate internal high attenuation resulting from hemorrhagic or proteinaceous components. MRI should be performed to evaluate such lesions because of its ability to distinguish between cystic and solid lesions and identify solid internal components (Fig. 77.8). Thymic cysts typically manifest as well-circumscribed masses in the prevascular mediastinum with low signal intensity on T1-weighted sequences and high signal intensity on T2-weighted sequences. Regions of high signal intensity on T1-weighted sequences may be seen in cysts complicated by hemorrhage or infection. The cyst wall is typically visible as a low–signal intensity rim on T2-weighted images. The absence of internal septations and/or soft tissue components is suggestive of unilocular thymic cyst and allows differentiation from other lesions. Minimal enhancement along the peripheral aspect of the cyst may be visualized, although no enhancing internal components should be present. The management of thymic cysts is controversial and highly variable. Cystic lesions demonstrating soft tissue are often evaluated with biopsy and/or surgical resection. In our experience, purely cystic lesions can be reevaluated with follow-up MRI.

Mature Teratoma

Although mature teratomas often manifest as heterogeneous masses with varying degrees of fat, fluid, soft tissue, and calcification, a large percentage of these lesions manifest as predominantly or entirely unilocular or multilocular thin-walled cystic masses in the prevascular mediastinum. In contrast to simple cysts, cystic teratomas are typically associated with additional features, such as internal septations and soft tissue components that may enhance after the administration of IV contrast.

Other Cystic Lesions

A well-circumscribed unilocular mass of fluid attenuation with thin or imperceptible walls localized to a cardiophrenic angle can be confidently diagnosed as a pericardial cyst. These benign nonneoplastic lesions arise from aberrations in the formation of coelomic or somatic cavities and arise in the costophrenic angles, more commonly on the right than the left; however, pericardial cysts may be seen as high as the pericardial recesses at the level of the proximal aorta and pulmonary arteries.[58] Although pericardial cysts are connected to the pericardium, this is only identifiable at the time of surgery in a small number of cases. In the setting of a large multilocular cystic lesion with internal septa and/or soft-tissue components that extends into the neck, axilla, or chest wall, the diagnosis of lymphangioma should be considered (Fig. 77.9). Lymphangiomas are malformations of the lymphatic system characterized by cysts that may be macroscopic or microscopic that account for 0.7% to 4.5% of all mediastinal neoplasms in adults.[58] In the clinical setting

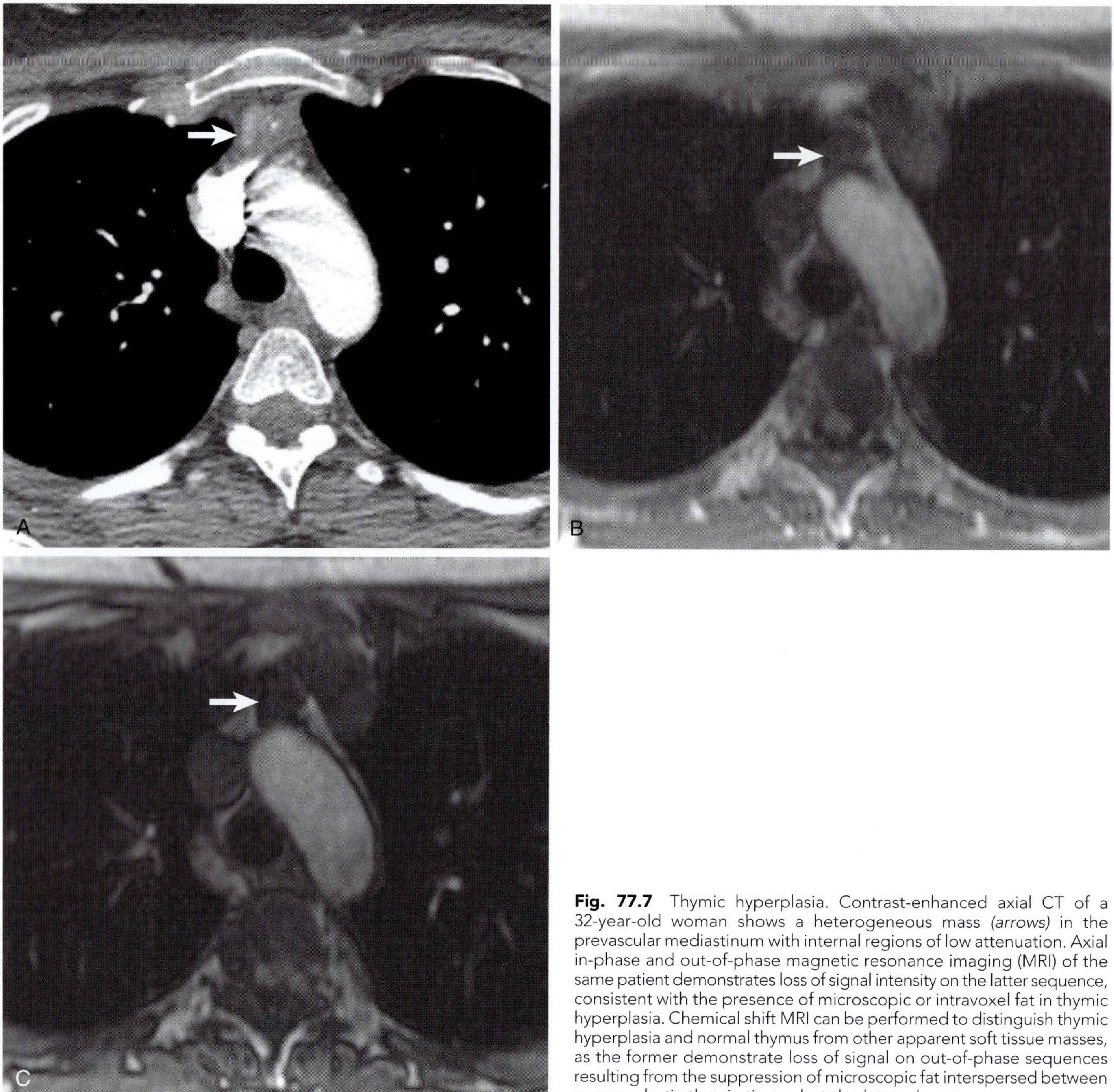

Fig. 77.7 Thymic hyperplasia. Contrast-enhanced axial CT of a 32-year-old woman shows a heterogeneous mass *(arrows)* in the prevascular mediastinum with internal regions of low attenuation. Axial in-phase and out-of-phase magnetic resonance imaging (MRI) of the same patient demonstrates loss of signal intensity on the latter sequence, consistent with the presence of microscopic or intravoxel fat in thymic hyperplasia. Chemical shift MRI can be performed to distinguish thymic hyperplasia and normal thymus from other apparent soft tissue masses, as the former demonstrate loss of signal on out-of-phase sequences resulting from the suppression of microscopic fat interspersed between nonneoplastic thymic tissue, but the latter do not.

of symptoms related to myasthenia gravis or other paraneoplastic syndromes and a cystic prevascular mass, cystic thymoma should be considered, especially when internal septations and/or soft tissue components are present (Figs. 77.10 and 77.11).

LYMPHOMA

Hodgkin and non-Hodgkin lymphoma may affect the mediastinum, either arising as a primary malignancy or a manifestation of systemic disease. Lymphomas that can manifest as a focal prevascular mediastinal mass include Hodgkin lymphoma and primary mediastinal non-Hodgkin lymphomas, including diffuse large B-cell lymphoma, gray zone lymphoma, and T-cell lymphoblastic lymphoma.

On CT lymphoma should be suspected when a mildly enhancing lobular soft tissue mass or group of enlarged lymph nodes is present in the prevascular mediastinum, especially in the setting of lymphadenopathy in the neck, axilla, or elsewhere in the body. Although differentiation between lymphoma and other soft tissue mediastinal masses may be challenging, the infiltrative nature of some types of lymphoma enables it to be distinguished from thymic epithelial neoplasms and germ cell tumors. In many cases lymphomas encase or encircle vascular structures but do not result in invasion. When such findings are present in young

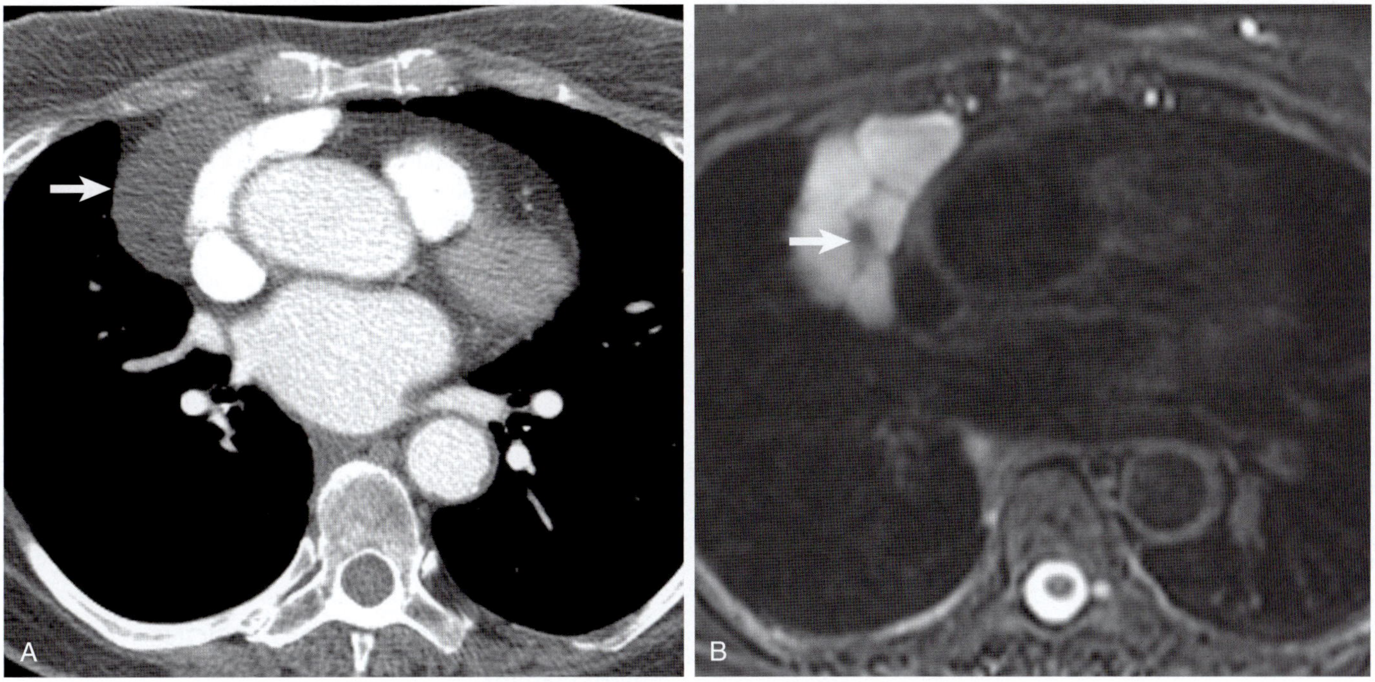

Fig. 77.8 Thymic cyst. (A) Contrast-enhanced axial CT demonstrates a homogeneous low-attenuation mass *(arrow)* in the right prevascular mediastinum. (B) Axial short time inversion recovery magnetic resonance imaging demonstrates a high–signal intensity lesion *(arrow)* with foci of low signal intensity representing multiple septations in this multilocular thymic cyst. Thymic cysts may be unilocular or multilocular, the former of which are usually congenital and the latter of which are associated with inflammation; iatrogenic processes, such as surgery, radiation therapy, or chemotherapy; or malignant neoplasms.

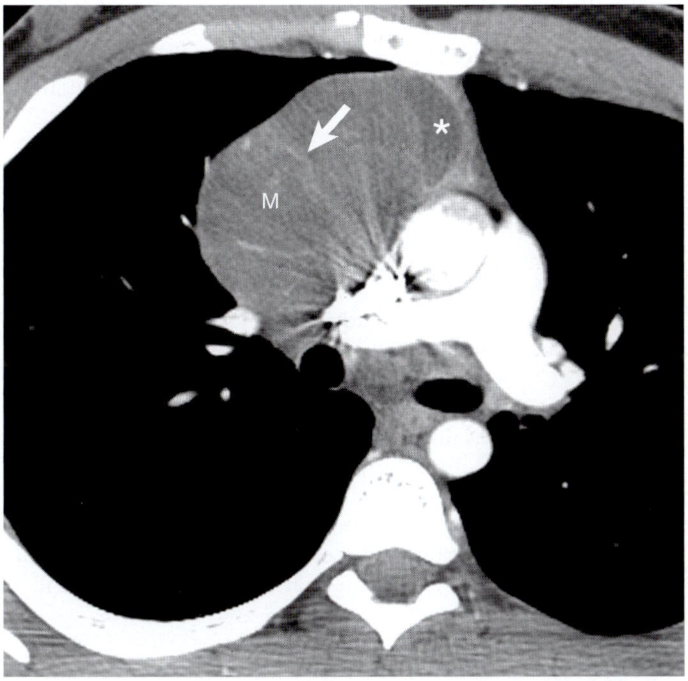

Fig. 77.9 Lymphangioma. Contrast-enhanced axial CT of a 19-year-old woman demonstrates a homogeneous low-attenuation mass (M) in the right prevascular mediastinum with regions of high and low attenuation (*) and linear foci of enhancement *(arrow)*. Lymphangiomas are characterized by cysts that may be macroscopic or microscopic and may be unilocular or multilocular.

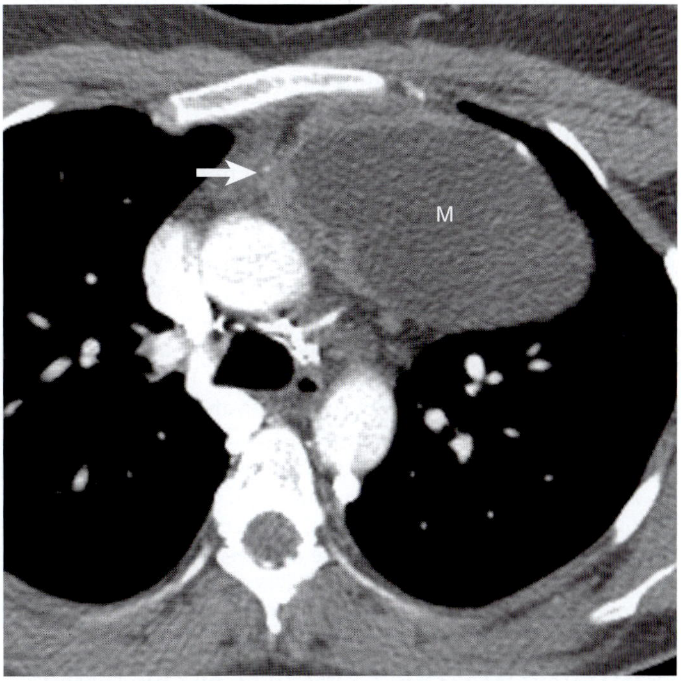

Fig. 77.10 Cystic thymoma. Contrast-enhanced axial CT of a 30-year-old woman with chest pain and myasthenia gravis demonstrates a predominantly low-attenuation cystic mass (M) in the left prevascular mediastinum, although peripheral soft tissue *(arrow)* is present. In the clinical setting of myasthenia gravis or other paraneoplastic syndrome and a cystic prevascular mass, cystic thymoma should be suspected.

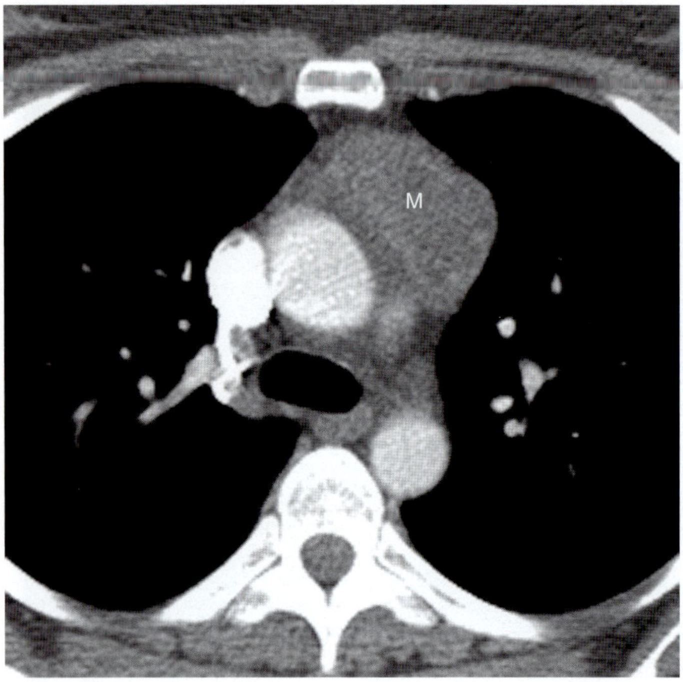

Fig. 77.11 Cystic thymoma. Contrast-enhanced axial CT of a 36-year-old woman shows a heterogeneous mass (M) in the left prevascular mediastinum that is predominantly soft tissue but also contains cystic components. Although cystic thymoma may manifest as a predominantly cystic lesion, some tumors may demonstrate significant soft tissue components.

patients who present with "B" symptoms, such as fever, weight loss, and night sweats, which occur in approximately 50% of cases, the diagnosis of mediastinal lymphoma should be strongly considered. Further evaluation is typically performed with core needle biopsy combined with aspiration for flow cytometry or surgical biopsy.

The MRI appearance of lymphoma depends on the type of lymphoma and treatment, although most untreated lymphomas demonstrate homogeneous hypointensity on T1- and T2-weighted sequences. After the administration of IV contrast, enhancement is usually homogeneous, although heterogeneity secondary to necrosis may be present.[59] During and after therapy, a decrease in water content and an increase in collagen or fibrotic content results in lower T2 signal intensity, and there is a decrease in enhancement on postcontrast sequences.[60–65] FDG–PET-CT has become the modality of choice for staging and restaging of types of lymphoma, as it is more accurate than CT in detecting involvement of lymph nodes, with sensitivity of 94% and specificity of 100% compared with 88% and 86%, respectively, for CT (Fig. 77.12). In addition, PET-CT effectively demonstrates intranodal and extranodal disease and end-organ involvement within the body, with sensitivity of 88% and specificity of 100% compared with 50% and 90%, respectively, for CT.[66]

NONTERATOMATOUS GERM CELL NEOPLASMS

The most common nonteratomatous germ cell neoplasms include seminomas and NSGCTs, which tend to manifest as large soft tissue masses in the prevascular mediastinal compartment on CT. Differentiation between these lesions and lymphoma can be difficult; however, in many cases clinical and serologic information can assist in securing the diagnosis. Most seminomas affect young men 10 to 39 years of age, and 10% of patients demonstrate slightly elevated serum levels of β–human chorionic gonadotropin (β-HCG).[67] Although elevated serum levels of lactate dehydrogenase levels are usually present, this is a nonspecific finding and has been associated with other lesions.[68,69] In contrast to seminomas, 90% of patients with NSGSTs present with markedly elevated serum levels of α-fetoprotein or β-HCG.[70,71]

On CT seminoma manifests as a large, lobular, homogeneous soft tissue mass in the prevascular mediastinum (Fig. 77.13). Pulmonary metastases are frequently identified, but pleural effusions are rare. NSGCTs tend to be more heterogeneous in appearance (Fig. 77.14). On MRI seminoma manifests as a homogeneous mass in the prevascular mediastinum with internal septations that enhance after the administration of IV contrast and are hypointense on T2-weighted imaging. As on CT, NSGCTs manifest as large heterogeneously enhancing masses. Internal foci of hemorrhage can appear as high–signal intensity regions on T1-weighted sequences.

THYROID AND PARATHYROID LESIONS

Thyroid Goiter

Thyroid goiters are often readily identified as heterogeneous prevascular mediastinal masses that are hyperdense (with HU values of 70 to 85 because of the presence of iodine), demonstrate intense and sustained enhancement after the administration of IV contrast, and exhibit a connection to the cervical thyroid gland (Fig. 77.15). Cystic changes manifesting as internal foci of low attenuation and calcifications may be identified. For instances in which a connection with the cervical thyroid gland cannot be identified, the other findings of goiter on CT should strongly suggest the diagnosis. When more aggressive features, such as loss of mediastinal tissue planes or associated cervical or mediastinal lymphadenopathy accompany a mediastinal goiter, then thyroid malignancy should be suspected and further work-up initiated.

Parathyroid Adenoma

Parathyroid adenoma should be considered when a soft tissue nodule is present in the prevascular mediastinum on CT in a patient with a clinical history of primary hyperparathyroidism, elevated serum calcium levels, and/or elevated serum parathyroid hormone, with or without prior surgical parathyroidectomy. Most parathyroid adenomas are juxtathyroid in location, although these lesions may occur in the mediastinum. High-resolution ultrasonography (US) with color Doppler, technetium-99m (^{99m}Tc) sestamibi, single-photon emission CT (SPECT), CT, and MRI can all be used to evaluate these lesions. Recent work has demonstrated that four-dimensional CT is more sensitive than US and scintigraphy for preoperative identification and localization of adenomas, with characteristic findings including intense contrast enhancement in the arterial phase, washout of contrast material in the delayed phase, and low attenuation on unenhanced CT.[72,73]

Imaging of the Visceral Compartment

FOREGUT DUPLICATION CYSTS

The most common cystic lesions in the visceral compartment include bronchogenic and esophageal duplication cysts. Bronchogenic cysts result from abnormal budding of the primitive

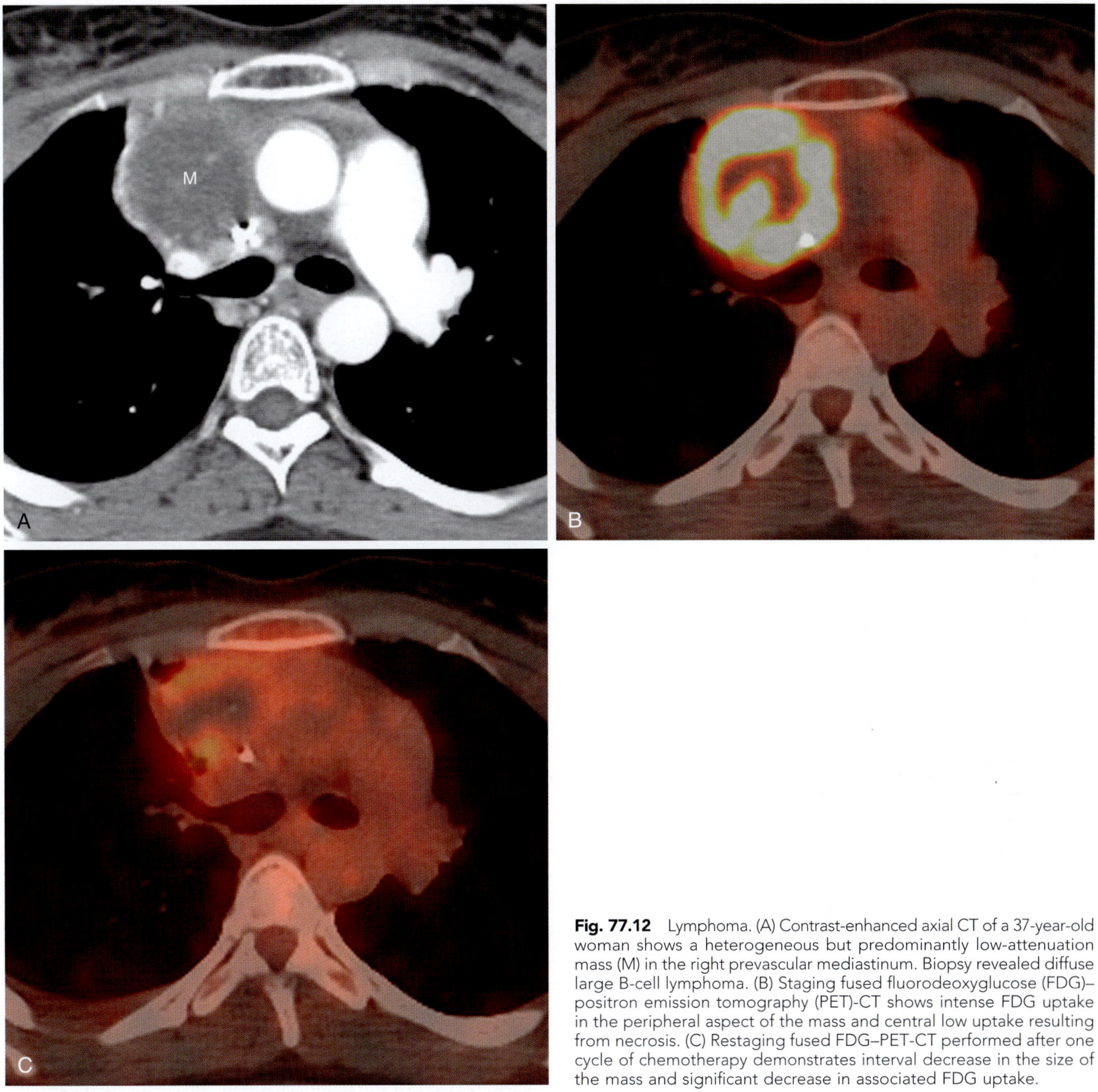

Fig. 77.12 Lymphoma. (A) Contrast-enhanced axial CT of a 37-year-old woman shows a heterogeneous but predominantly low-attenuation mass (M) in the right prevascular mediastinum. Biopsy revealed diffuse large B-cell lymphoma. (B) Staging fused fluorodeoxyglucose (FDG)–positron emission tomography (PET)-CT shows intense FDG uptake in the peripheral aspect of the mass and central low uptake resulting from necrosis. (C) Restaging fused FDG–PET-CT performed after one cycle of chemotherapy demonstrates interval decrease in the size of the mass and significant decrease in associated FDG uptake.

foregut during embryologic development and typically occur in the visceral compartment near the carina or, less commonly, the right paratracheal region.[58] Esophageal duplication cysts are uncommon developmental anomalies that are located adjacent to the esophagus or associated with the esophageal wall. Duplication cysts are usually recognized easily on CT as they manifest with fluid or water attenuation (Figs. 77.16 and 77.17). Hemorrhagic or proteinaceous components or cyst infection may result in an atypical appearance with heterogeneity on CT.[58] In this setting MRI can be performed to confirm the cystic nature of the lesion, which demonstrates high signal intensity on T2-weighted sequences regardless of the other contents, and identify hemorrhagic, proteinaceous, or mucoid content that is often variable in terms of signal intensity on T1-weighted sequences (Fig. 77.18). The walls of bronchogenic cysts have variable perceptibility and may enhance or demonstrate intrinsic calcifications. In contrast, the walls of esophageal duplication cysts tend to be thicker.

ESOPOHAGEAL CANCER AND OTHER MASSES

Esophageal malignancy must be considered when regions of esophageal wall thickening or a focal soft tissue mass are identified. Although any portion of the esophagus may be involved, the distal esophagus is typically affected because of the increasing incidence

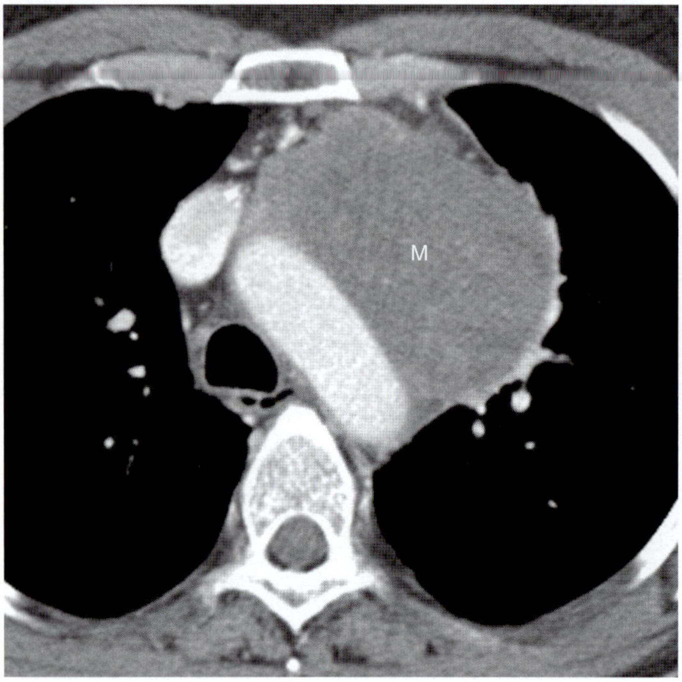

Fig. 77.13 Seminoma. Contrast-enhanced axial CT of a 28-year-old man with elevated serum levels of β–human chorionic gonadotropin demonstrates a homogeneous soft tissue mass (M) in the prevascular mediastinum. Biopsy revealed seminoma. Most seminomas affect young men 10–39 years of age and appear as homogeneous soft tissue masses on CT.

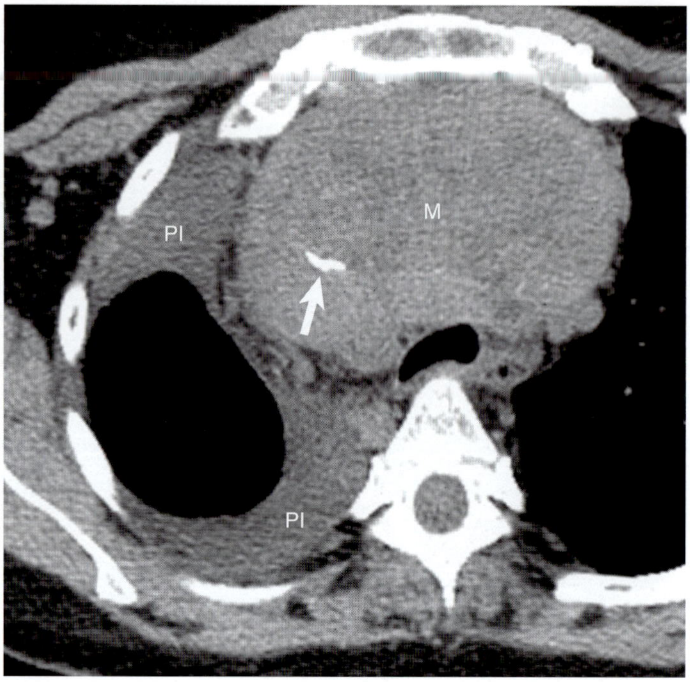

Fig. 77.15 Thyroid goiter. Unenhanced axial CT of a 61-year-old woman demonstrates a large mass (M) in the prevascular mediastinum that is intrinsically hyperdense and contains calcification *(arrow)* consistent with intrathoracic extension of a goiter. Note the right pleural effusion (Pl).

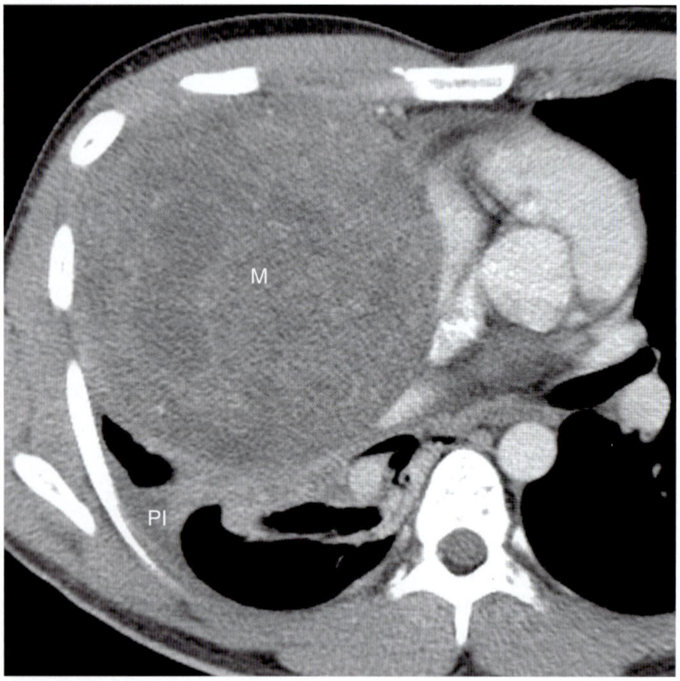

Fig. 77.14 Nonseminomatous germ cell tumor. Contrast-enhanced axial CT of a 33-year-old man shows a large heterogeneous mass (M) arising from the right prevascular mediastinum. Note the small right pleural effusion (Pl). In contrast to seminomas, nonseminomatous germ cell tumors tend to be larger and more heterogeneous in appearance.

of adenocarcinoma in the setting of gastroesophageal reflux disease. Unfortunately, CT may not allow differentiation between malignant and benign esophageal lesions, and further evaluation with upper endoscopy and endoscopic ultrasound with tissue biopsy is ultimately required for diagnosis. Nevertheless, some benign lesions, such as lipoma and fibrovascular polyp, may be differentiated from esophageal cancer, as the former manifests as an intraluminal mass with smooth margins, compared with the irregular margins and lobulated appearance of many esophageal cancers, and both of these benign lesions may demonstrate internal fat attenuation because of the presence of intralesional fat.

The role of MRI in the evaluation of esophageal cancer continues to expand. High-resolution T2-weighted sequences obtained with cardiorespiratory gating can be used to show the various layers of the esophageal wall and delineate the extent of invasion by esophageal cancers, thus enabling tumor staging. Leiomyomas, the most common benign neoplasms of the esophagus, are somewhat hyperintense on T2-weighted sequences and demonstrate homogeneous enhancement without necrosis on postcontrast imaging.[74]

ENHANCING LESIONS

When an enhancing mass is present in the visceral compartment, several entities should be considered, including paraganglioma, Castleman disease, and metastatic lymphadenopathy. Paraganglioma or extraadrenal pheochromocytoma is a highly vascular neoplasm that arises from chromaffin tissue located in the paraaortic ganglia and may secrete catecholamines, although most are nonfunctional. Clinical symptoms include hoarseness, dysphagia, shortness of

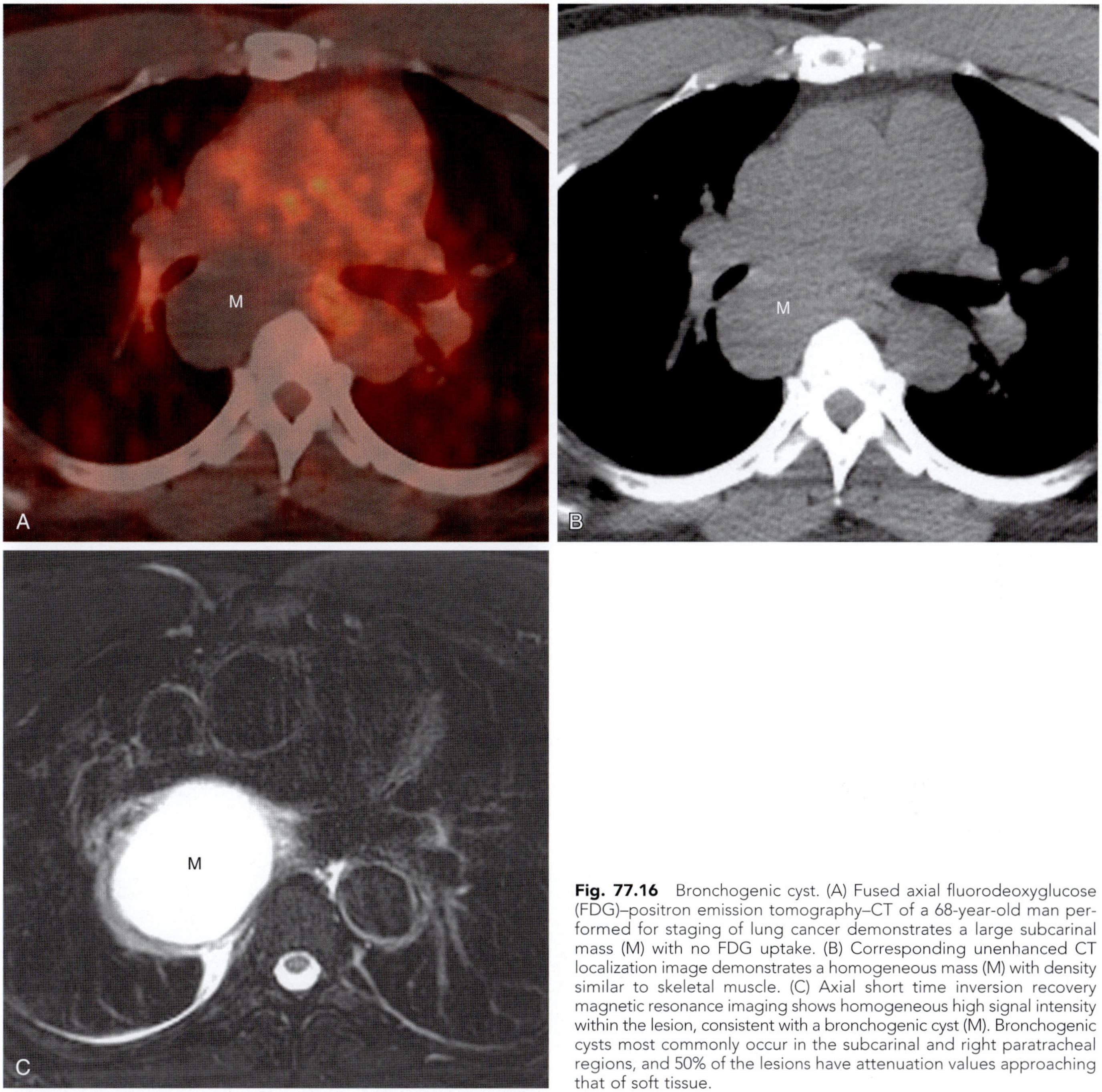

Fig. 77.16 Bronchogenic cyst. (A) Fused axial fluorodeoxyglucose (FDG)–positron emission tomography–CT of a 68-year-old man performed for staging of lung cancer demonstrates a large subcarinal mass (M) with no FDG uptake. (B) Corresponding unenhanced CT localization image demonstrates a homogeneous mass (M) with density similar to skeletal muscle. (C) Axial short time inversion recovery magnetic resonance imaging shows homogeneous high signal intensity within the lesion, consistent with a bronchogenic cyst (M). Bronchogenic cysts most commonly occur in the subcarinal and right paratracheal regions, and 50% of the lesions have attenuation values approaching that of soft tissue.

breath, and chest pain.[75,76] On CT paraganglioma manifests as an intensely and homogeneously enhancing mass, although regions of internal heterogeneity caused by necrosis can often be identified (Fig. 77.19). On MRI these neoplasms demonstrate intermediate signal intensity on T1-weighted sequences and high signal intensity on T2-weighted sequences.

Castleman disease is a form of nonclonal lymph node hyperplasia classified as hyaline vascular, plasma cell, or human herpesvirus 8 types and may be unicentric or multicentric.[77] The unicentric hyaline vascular type is the most common form and may appear as a focal enhancing mediastinal mass, an infiltrative mass with associated lymphadenopathy, or matted lymphadenopathy with intense enhancement after the administration of IV contrast (Fig. 77.20).[78]

Enhancing metastatic lymph nodes may complicate vascular primary malignancies, such as renal cell and thyroid neoplasms, melanoma, choriocarcinoma, and some sarcomas, and the diagnosis can be surmised when such clinical history is present. In the absence of such history, further evaluation with histologic sampling may be necessary; however, this should be done carefully, as biopsy of mediastinal vascular lesions may result in significant hemorrhage.

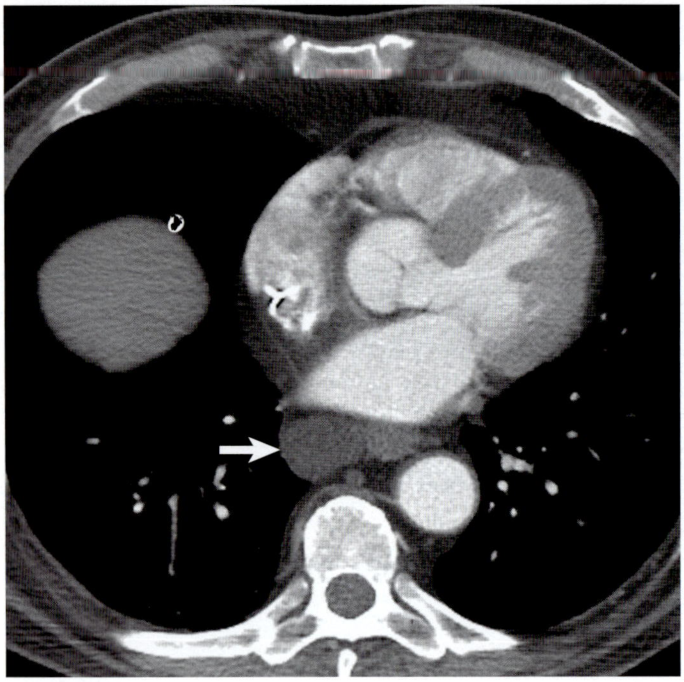

Fig. 77.17 Esophageal duplication cyst. Contrast-enhanced axial CT of a 32-year-old man demonstrates a well-circumscribed, homogeneous, and low-attenuation mass *(arrow)* in the visceral compartment adjacent to the distal esophagus. Esophageal duplication cysts appear as fluid or water-attenuation lesions adjacent to the esophagus or associated with the esophageal wall.

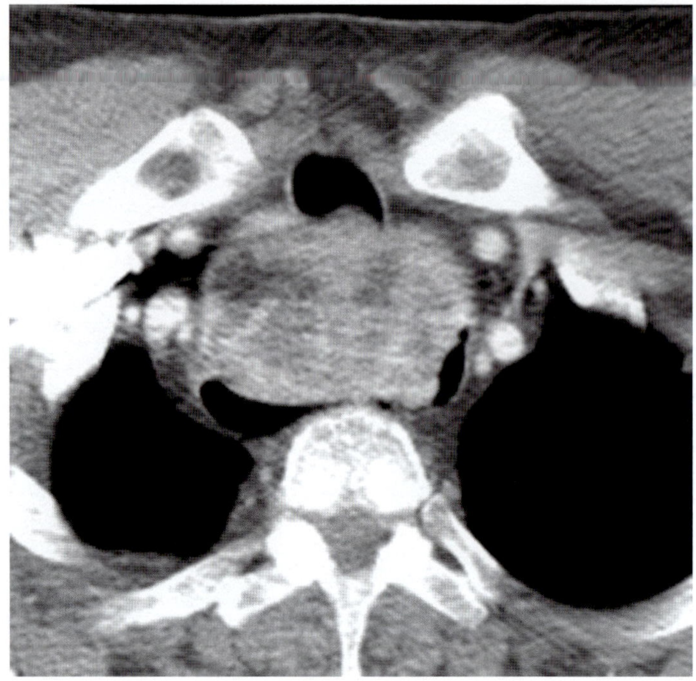

Fig. 77.19 Esophageal paraganglioma. Contrast-enhanced axial CT shows a hypervascular heterogeneously enhancing mass intimately associated with the esophagus, simulating the appearance of an intrathoracic thyroid gland.

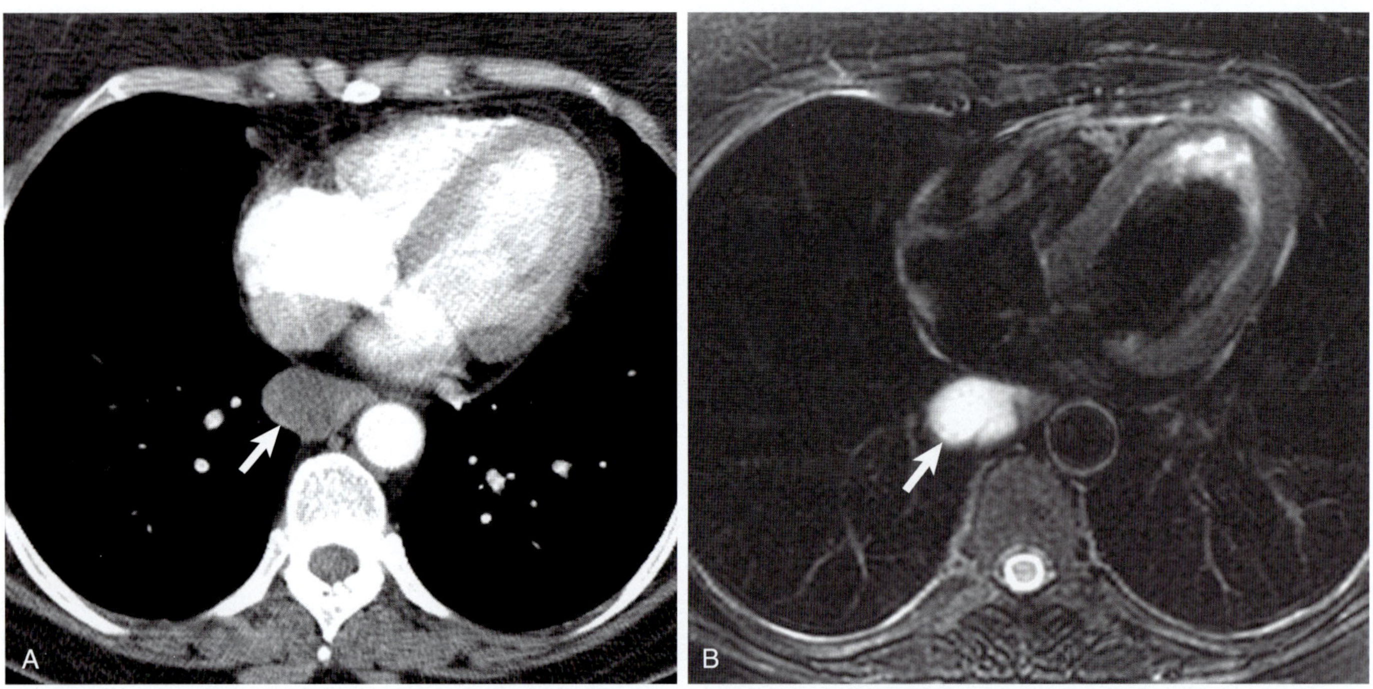

Fig. 77.18 Esophageal duplication cyst. (A) Contrast-enhanced axial CT of a 41-year-old woman demonstrates a heterogeneous mass *(arrow)* in the visceral compartment adjacent to the distal esophagus. Internal Hounsfield units were not consistent with a simple cyst, and magnetic resonance imaging (MRI) was performed for further evaluation. (B) Axial short T1 inversion recovery MRI demonstrates homogeneous high signal intensity in the lesion *(arrow)* consistent with an esophageal duplication cyst. Hemorrhagic or proteinaceous components or cyst infection may result in an atypical appearance with heterogeneity on CT, and MRI can be performed to confirm the cystic nature of the lesion.

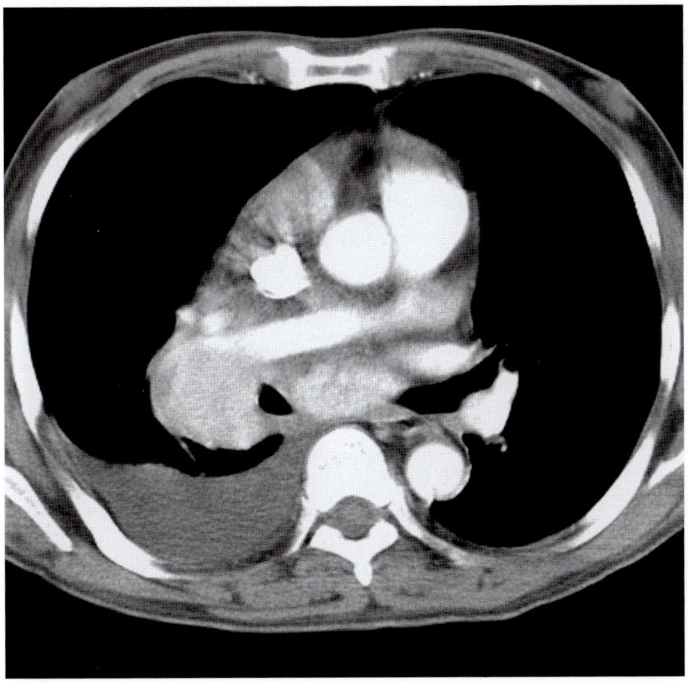

Fig. 77.20 Castleman disease. Contrast-enhanced axial CT shows enlarged, avidly enhancing subcarinal and right hilar lymph nodes. The major differential considerations would include Castleman disease and hypervascular metastases from malignancies such as renal cell carcinoma. *(Reproduced from Walker CM. Unilateral hilar mass. In: Stern EJ, Gurney JW, Walker CM, et al, eds.* ExpertDDX: Chest. *1st ed.. Philadelphia: Amirsys; 2011.)*

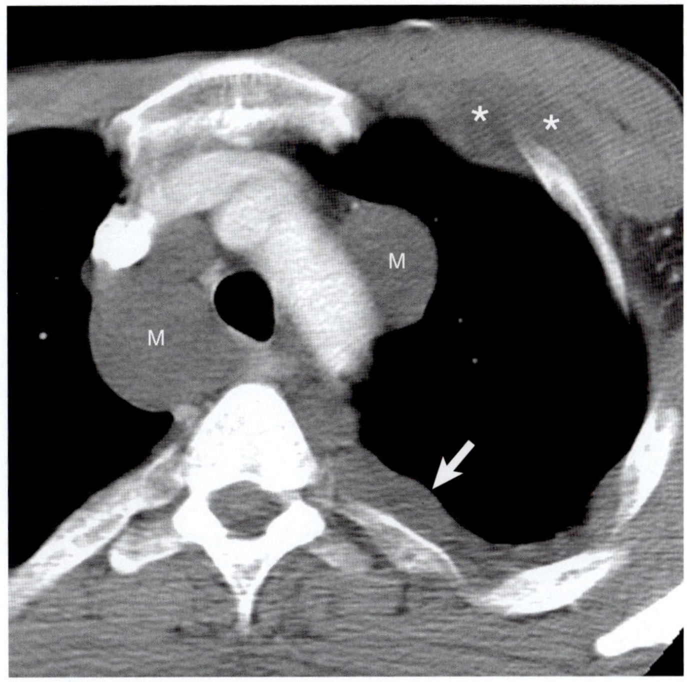

Fig. 77.21 Neurofibroma. Contrast-enhanced axial CT of a 33-year-old man with neurofibromatosis type 1 demonstrates multiple neurofibromas (M) arising from the prevascular and visceral mediastinal compartments, the left paravertebral compartment *(arrow)*, and left chest wall *(asterisks)*.

Imaging of the Paravertebral Compartment

NEUROGENIC NEOPLASMS

Neurogenic neoplasms, 70% to 80% of which are benign, are the most common cause of paravertebral compartment masses and account for 20% and 35% of all adult and pediatric mediastinal neoplasms, respectively.[79] Peripheral nerve sheath neoplasms typically arise from spinal or proximal intercostal nerves, less commonly from the vagus, recurrent laryngeal, or phrenic nerves, and account for 70% of mediastinal neurogenic tumors.[79] Peripheral nerve sheath neoplasms may demonstrate a dumbbell morphology and communication with the spinal canal on CT. Cystic changes or hemorrhage may result in internal regions of heterogeneity. Associated findings such as benign pressure erosion of adjacent ribs or vertebrae and enlargement of the neural foramina may be identified.[79] Numerous lesions may be present in patients with neurofibromatosis type 1 (NF-1) (Fig. 77.21).

MRI optimally demonstrates the extent of intraspinal/extradural extension and osseous changes. Schwannomas demonstrate variable signal intensity on T1-weighted imaging and intermediate to high signal intensity on T2-weighted sequences. After the administration of IV contrast, enhancement may be homogeneous or heterogeneous depending on regions of cellular and acellular components (Fig. 77.22). Neurofibromas show variable signal intensity on T1-weighted sequences, although central high signal may be present, and intermediate to high signal intensity on T2-weighted sequences, although low central signal may be present because of the presence of collagen.

Several imaging signs for peripheral nerve sheath tumors have been described, including the "fascicular sign" and "target sign."[80] The "fascicular sign" describes multiple hypointense, small, ring-like structures corresponding to fascicular bundles and is typically associated with schwannomas. The "target sign" is characterized by central low signal intensity and surrounding peripheral high signal intensity and is more commonly seen with neurofibromas than with schwannomas. Transformation of a benign peripheral nerve sheath neoplasm to a malignant peripheral nerve sheath tumor (MPNST) should be suspected when a previously stable neurofibroma suddenly increases in size, develops regions of heterogeneity, and/or invades adjacent tissues. There is a 10% lifetime risk of developing a malignant peripheral nerve sheath neoplasm for patients with NF-1. MPNSTs appear as variable signal intensity on T1-weighted sequences and intermediate to low signal on T2-weighting sequences, depending on the amount of collagen, although high–signal intensity cystic regions may be present. FDG–PET-CT is helpful for differentiating between benign and malignant peripheral nerve sheath tumors, with sensitivity of 95% and specificity of 72%.[81] Another study revealed sensitivity of 97% and specificity of 87% for detection of malignant peripheral nerve sheath tumors and suggested that lesions with SUVmax less than 2.5 should be considered benign, those with SUVmax greater than 3.5 should be considered malignant, and those with SUVmax of 2.5 to 3.5 should be followed with surveillance imaging.[82]

Additional neurogenic neoplasms that may originate in the paravertebral compartment include sympathetic ganglion neoplasms, such as ganglioneuromas, ganglioneuroblastomas, and neuroblastomas, and neuroendocrine neoplasms, such as paragangliomas. Ganglioneuroma manifests as a homogeneous

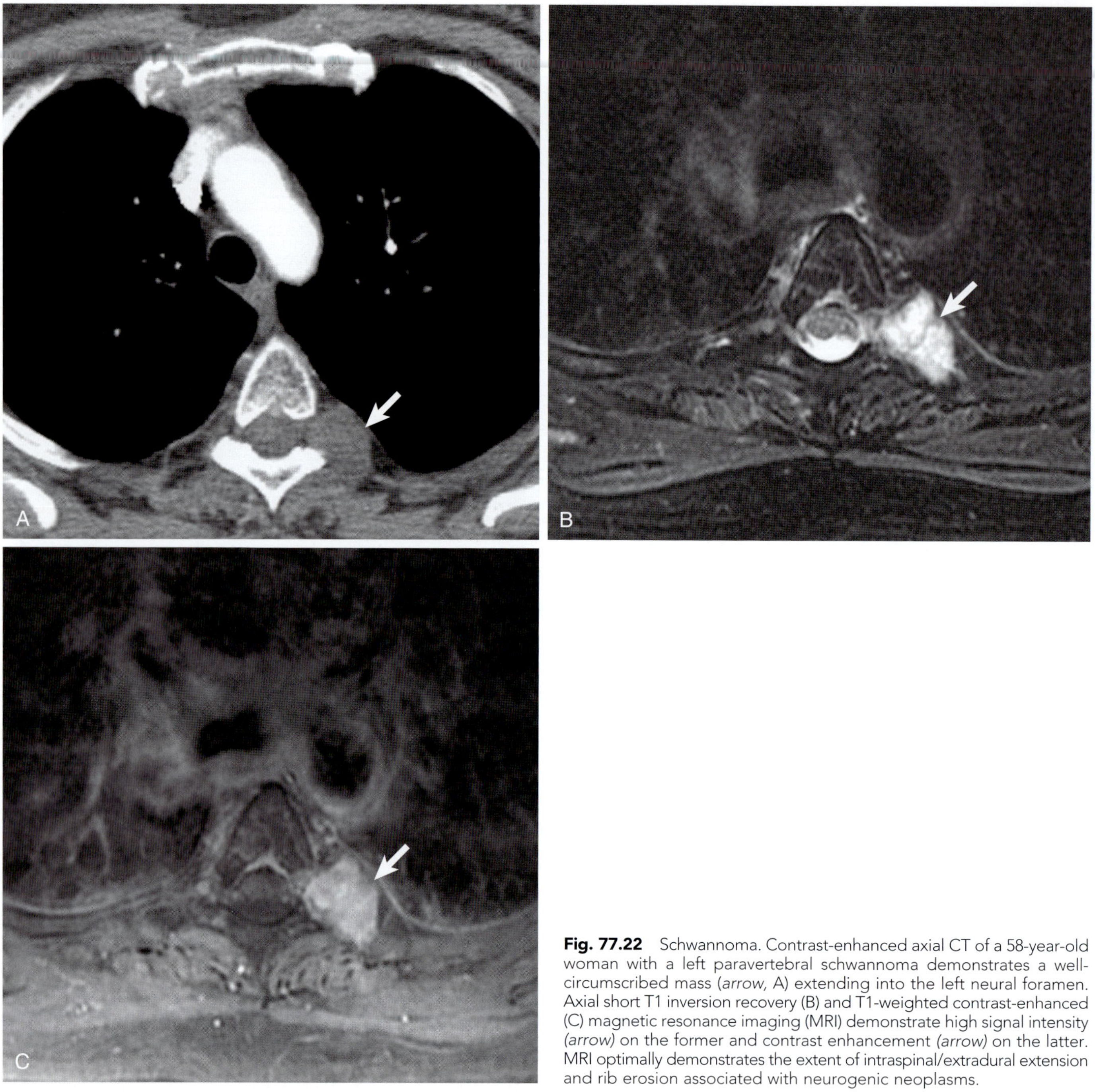

Fig. 77.22 Schwannoma. Contrast-enhanced axial CT of a 58-year-old woman with a left paravertebral schwannoma demonstrates a well-circumscribed mass (*arrow*, A) extending into the left neural foramen. Axial short T1 inversion recovery (B) and T1-weighted contrast-enhanced (C) magnetic resonance imaging (MRI) demonstrate high signal intensity (*arrow*) on the former and contrast enhancement (*arrow*) on the latter. MRI optimally demonstrates the extent of intraspinal/extradural extension and rib erosion associated with neurogenic neoplasms.

mass that is intermediate signal intensity on T1- and T2-weighted sequences and demonstrates homogeneous enhancement. Regions of high signal intensity on T2-weighted sequences correspond to mucinous matrix. Paragangliomas demonstrate high signal intensity on T1-weighted sequences with flow voids, hyperintensity relative to liver on T2-weighted imaging, and enhancement after the administration of IV contrast.

SPINAL INFECTIONS

Infections of the thoracic spine are typically due to bacterial organisms, and significant risk factors include diabetes, autoimmune diseases, malignancy, immunosuppression, and IV drug use.[83] Patients may present with symptoms such as back pain, fever, and malaise, and the diagnosis should be considered when ill-defined soft tissue, unorganized fluid, and/or a loculated collection is present in the paravertebral compartment. Early CT findings include fat infiltration and intervertebral disk hypoattenuation, whereas osseous erosion, disk space narrowing, and sequestrum formation may be present in later stages[83] (Fig. 77.23).

In the setting of immunodeficiency, such as HIV infection, tuberculous involvement of the spine should be considered. Approximately 60% of HIV-positive patients with tuberculosis have osseous involvement, and the spine is the most commonly

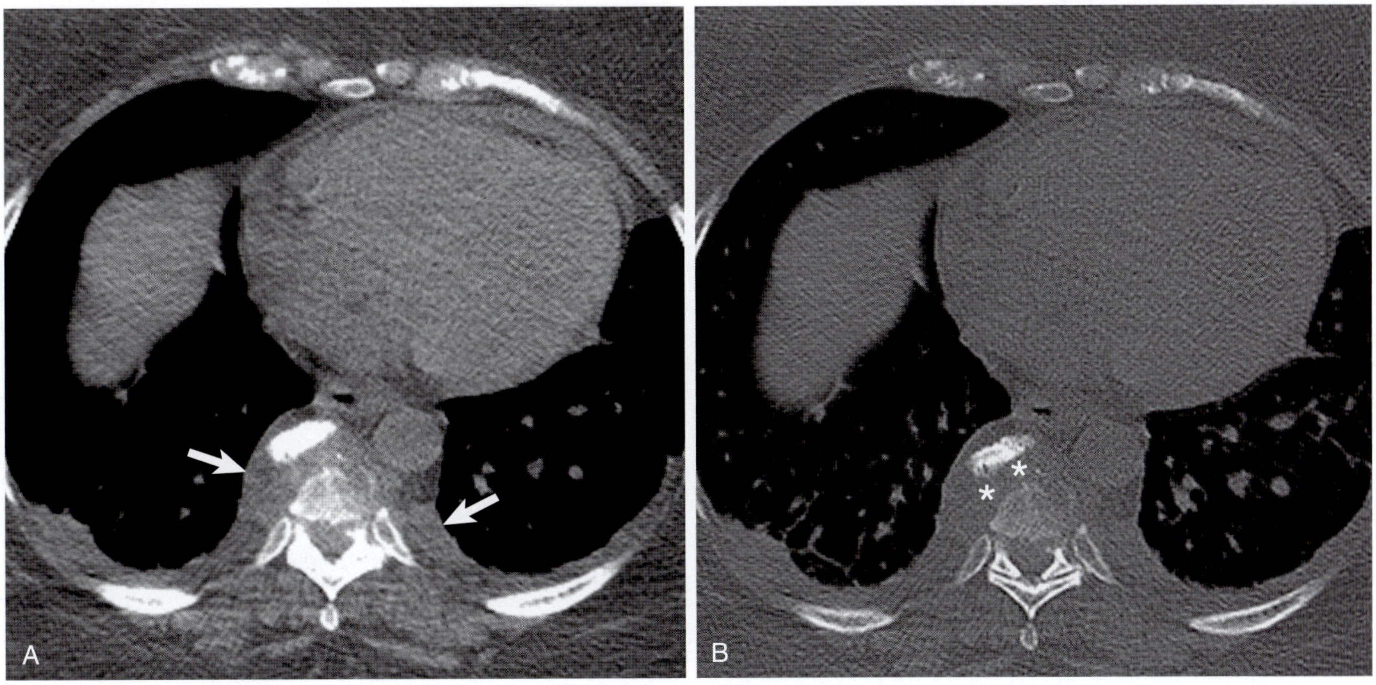

Fig. 77.23 Diskitis/osteomyelitis. Unenhanced axial CT of a 56-year-old woman in soft tissue (A) and bone (B) windows demonstrates ill-defined paravertebral soft tissue (*arrows*, A) and osseous destruction (*asterisks*, B) compatible with diskitis and osteomyelitis. Fat infiltration and intervertebral disk hypoattenuation may be present in the early stages of diskitis/osteomyelitis, whereas osseous erosion, disk space narrowing, and sequestrum formation may be present in later stages.

affected site. Tuberculosis associated with involvement of the posterior elements, the presence of a large prevertebral and paravertebral soft tissue component out of proportion to the degree of osseous destruction, and disk space narrowing enable differentiation of tuberculous from pyogenic infection. The presence of calcification without new bone formation or sclerosis strongly suggests the diagnosis of Pott disease.[84,85]

On MRI osteomyelitis may result in bone marrow edema with low signal intensity on T1-weighted sequences, high signal intensity on fluid-sensitive sequences, and diffuse enhancement of the involved bone. Abnormalities usually begin at the end plate and are best detected on T1-weighted sequences. Paraspinal edema and phlegmon result in high signal intensity in the paraspinal fat and musculature. After the administration of IV contrast, phlegmon demonstrates diffuse enhancement. Abscess formation may occur, which manifests as a focal hypointense (to muscle) region on T1-weighted sequences and high signal intensity on fluid-sensitive sequences. After the administration of IV contrast, peripheral enhancement is characteristic. Involvement of the posterior elements, the presence of a large prevertebral and paravertebral soft tissue component out of proportion to the degree of osseous destruction, and disk space narrowing enable differentiation of tuberculous from pyogenic infection.

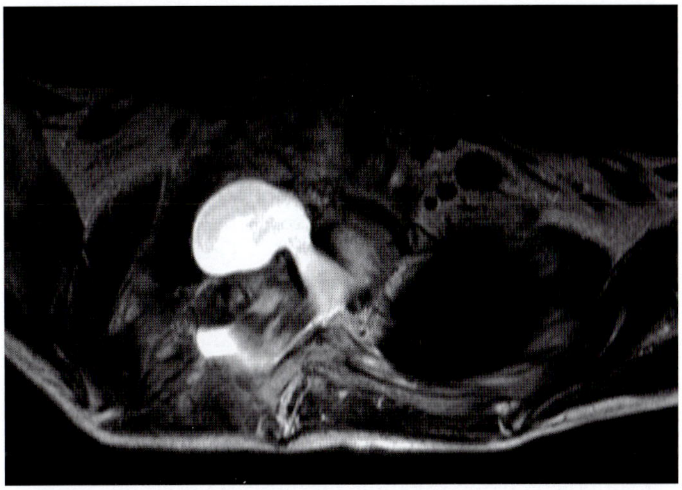

Fig. 77.24 Lateral intrathoracic meningocele of a patient with neurofibromatosis type 1. Axial T2-weighted magnetic resonance imaging shows a cystic lesion extending out of the spinal canal into the right paravertebral mediastinum. Note the associated thoracic scoliosis. *(Reproduced from Walker CM. Cystic mediastinal mass. In: Stern EJ, Gurney JW, Walker CM, et al, eds.* ExpertDDX: Chest. *1st ed. Philadelphia: Amirsys; 2011.)*

CYSTIC LESIONS

Intrathoracic Meningocele

An intrathoracic meningocele results from anomalous herniation of the leptomeninges through an intervertebral foramen or vertebral body defect and is typically associated with NF-1.[86] This abnormality typically occurs as a unilocular mass with fluid attenuation in the paravertebral mediastinum on CT. Associated findings include enlargement of intervertebral foramina and vertebral and/or rib anomalies or scoliosis. On MRI intrathoracic meningoceles are hypointense on T1-weighted sequences and hyperintense on T2-weighted sequences without evidence of enhancement after the administration of IV contrast (Fig. 77.24). Imaging can also be performed after intraspinal injection of contrast material, which demonstrates filling of the meningocele.[87]

Neurenteric Cyst

Neurenteric cysts are intraspinal cysts lined by enteric mucosa that most commonly affect the thoracic spine and associated with vertebral abnormalities, such as segmentation and fusion anomalies.[58] These lesions are well circumscribed and demonstrate fluid intensity on T1-weighted sequences and are isointense or hyperintense to cerebrospinal fluid depending on the content of protein and mucin. On T2-weighted sequences neurenteric cysts demonstrate fluid signal intensity and are hypointense or isointense to cerebrospinal fluid.

Other Cystic Lesions

Mediastinal abscess should be considered when a low-attenuation mass is present in the paravertebral compartment on CT in a patient after surgery or esophageal perforation or in the setting of infection in the adjacent thorax. Internal foci of air may be present, and connection with a coexisting subphrenic abscess or empyema may be identified.[88] In most situations the clinical context permits definitive diagnosis; however, in selected cases percutaneous needle aspiration may be necessary to differentiate between abscess and other postoperative fluid collections, such as seroma or hematoma.

Pancreatic pseudocyst should be considered when a cystic paravertebral mass is present that develops over a short period of time in the clinical setting of pancreatitis.[89] These lesions contain pancreatic secretions, blood, and necrotic material and spread through the esophageal or aortic hiatus and typically are located in the lower mediastinum. Pseudocysts typically manifest as thin-walled masses that may be low or high density depending on the internal contents.

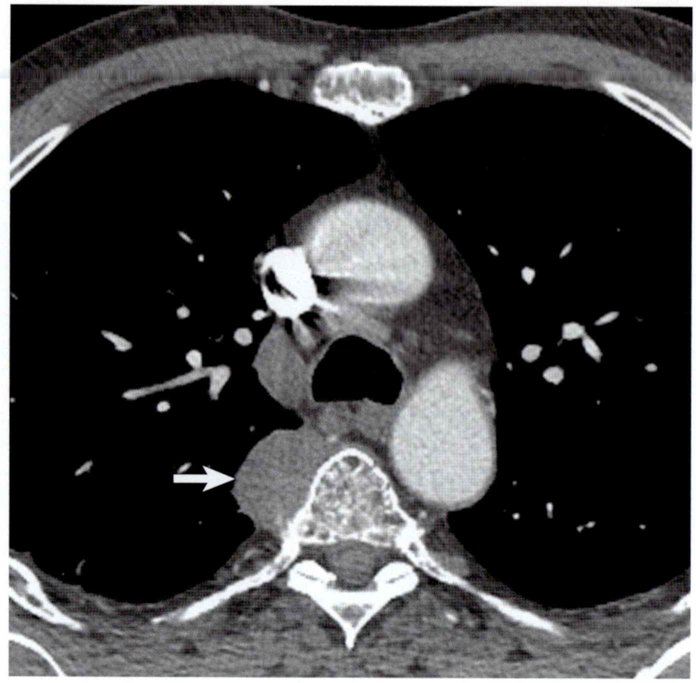

Fig. 77.25 Extramedullary hematopoiesis. Contrast-enhanced axial CT of a 34-year-old man with myelofibrosis demonstrates a homogeneous soft tissue mass *(arrow)* in the right paravertebral mediastinum. Extramedullary hematopoiesis typically affects individuals with hematologic disorders, resulting in bone marrow replacement (myelofibrosis or chronic myelogenous leukemia) or hemolytic anemia (thalassemia, sickle cell anemia, or hereditary spherocytosis).

EXTRAMEDULLARY HEMATOPOIESIS

Extramedullary hematopoiesis should be considered when a paravertebral mass is present adjacent to thoracic vertebrae and/or ribs on CT in a patient with hematologic disorder resulting in bone marrow replacement (myelofibrosis or chronic myelogenous leukemia) or hemolytic anemia (thalassemia, sickle cell anemia, or hereditary spherocytosis).[90] These lesions may be large or small and unilateral or bilateral and usually enhance after IV contrast administration secondary to high vascularity (Fig. 77.25). Heterogeneous attenuation and/or enhancement may be seen in the setting of iron deposition, and chronic lesions may demonstrate fat infiltration[91] (Fig. 77.26). Functional imaging with ^{99m}Tc sulfur colloid bone marrow scanning and SPECT-CT bone marrow scanning may noninvasively confirm functioning hematopoietic tissue when the diagnosis is uncertain.

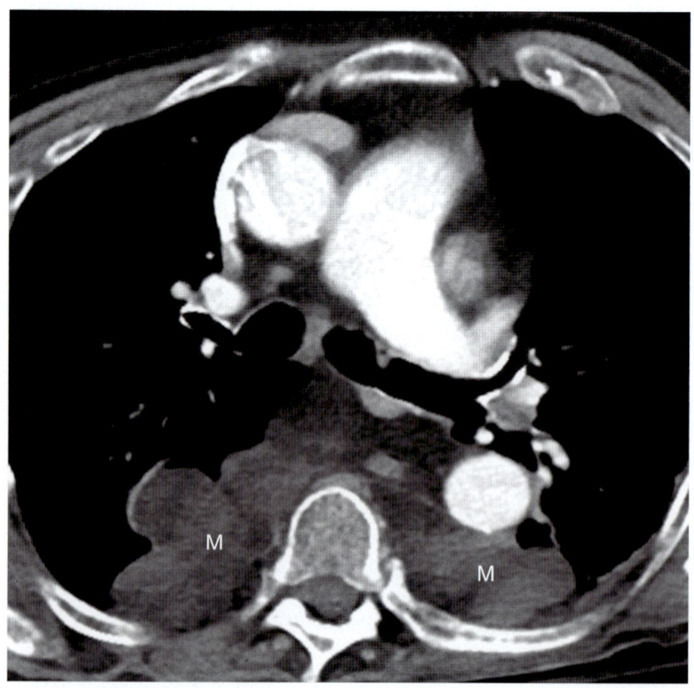

Fig. 77.26 Extramedullary hematopoiesis. Contrast-enhanced axial CT of a 62-year-old woman with extramedullary hematopoiesis demonstrates lobulated paravertebral masses (M) with intermixed fat and heterogeneously enhancing soft tissue. These lesions may demonstrate heterogeneous attenuation and/or enhancement in the setting of iron deposition and fat infiltration when chronic.

Conclusions

Mediastinal masses are relatively uncommon and include a wide variety of abnormalities that most radiologists encounter infrequently. Although chest radiography may be the first imaging modality to suggest the presence of mediastinal pathology, CT is considered the imaging modality of choice for evaluating most mediastinal masses and differentiating among the various lesions. In addition, the role of MRI continues to expand. Radiologists must be familiar with the strengths and limitations of each imaging modality in evaluating mediastinal masses and the new ITMIG classification of mediastinal compartments based on cross-sectional imaging, to accurately communicate with health care providers and guide appropriate management.

SUGGESTED READINGS

Carter BW, Benveniste M, Madan R, et al. ITMIG/IASLC staging system and lymph node map for thymic epithelial neoplasms. *Radiographics*. 2017;37(3):758–776.

Carter BW, Benveniste M, Madan R, et al. ITMIG classification of mediastinal compartments and multidisciplinary approach to mediastinal masses. *Radiographics*. 2017;37(3):758–776.

Carter BW, Tomiyama N, Bhora FY, et al. A modern definition of mediastinal compartments. *J Thorac Oncol*. 2014;9(9 suppl 2):S97–S101.

Tomiyama N, Müller NL, Ellis SJ, et al. Invasive and noninvasive thymoma: distinctive CT features. *J Comput Assist Tomogr*. 2001;25(3):388–393.

The full reference list for this chapter is available at ExpertConsult.com.

78 Diaphragm*

CHRISTOPHER M. WALKER | JONATHAN H. CHUNG | J. DAVID GODWIN

Abnormalities of Diaphragmatic Motion: Diaphragmatic Paralysis, Weakness, and Eventration

Etiology, Prevalence, and Epidemiology

The diaphragm is the primary muscle of ventilation, and dysfunction of the diaphragm is an underrecognized cause of dyspnea. Dysfunction of the diaphragm can be classified as paralysis, weakness, or eventration and is usually suggested by elevation of a hemidiaphragm on chest radiography.[1] Some of the more common causes of unilateral diaphragmatic paralysis are compression or invasion of the phrenic nerve by a neoplasm or iatrogenic injury during birth or open heart surgery.[2,3] Other common causes include trauma (natural or surgical) and cardioplegia for cardiac surgery ("phrenic frostbite").[2] Less common causes are herpes zoster, West Nile virus, cervical spondylosis, poliomyelitis, amyotrophic lateral sclerosis, and pneumonia.[1] However, in many cases the etiology is unknown.[2]

The most common cause of bilateral diaphragmatic paralysis is spinal cord injury. Bilateral diaphragmatic paralysis or weakness can also be caused by generalized neuromuscular syndromes, such as amyotrophic lateral sclerosis or myasthenia gravis.[2] Bilateral paralysis occurs occasionally after cardioplegia for cardiac surgery; this form is usually reversible with time.[2]

Eventration is a congenital anomaly consisting of failure of muscle development of part or all of one or both hemidiaphragms. On pathologic examination a totally eventrated hemidiaphragm consists of a thin membranous sheet attached peripherally to normal muscle at points of origin from the rib cage. Complete eventration almost exclusively affects the left hemidiaphragm. Partial eventration is much more common than the complete form. It affects men and women with equal frequency. It usually involves the anteromedial portion of the right hemidiaphragm and only rarely the left, but it can involve the central portion of either cupola.

Clinical Presentation

Unilateral diaphragmatic paralysis or weakness is usually asymptomatic and is found incidentally on chest radiographs obtained for a different reason.[2] Dyspnea with mild to moderate effort may develop in patients with underlying lung disease.[2] Patients with bilateral diaphragmatic paralysis or weakness usually have severe respiratory symptoms, mainly dyspnea and orthopnea, sometimes with a sense of suffocation when supine or when immersed in water.[2,4] Most patients eventually develop respiratory failure.[2] Bilateral hemidiaphragmatic weakness can also occur after prolonged mechanical ventilation and may signal that the patient cannot be weaned from the ventilator.[5]

Eventration is usually asymptomatic but may become symptomatic if the eventration is large or the patient is obese because obesity can raise intraabdominal pressure and further compromise diaphragmatic function.

Manifestations of Diaphragm Dysfunction

RADIOGRAPHY AND FLUOROSCOPY

The paralyzed or weak hemidiaphragm is elevated and has an accentuated domed shape on the posteroanterior radiograph. Elevation of the posterior aspect of the hemidiaphragm, best shown on the lateral radiograph (Fig. 78.1), is a helpful radiographic feature of a paralyzed or weak hemidiaphragm but is usually absent in a large eventration. The lung adjacent to a paralyzed hemidiaphragm often has subsegmental atelectasis resulting from elevation and reduced motion. If the paralysis is on the left, the stomach and splenic flexure of the colon relate to the inferior surface of the hemidiaphragm and usually contain more gas than normal.

Complete eventration of a hemidiaphragm is a rare, congenital abnormality that is almost always on the left. On the other hand, partial eventration is common; it may be acquired, and it usually affects patients older than 60 years, typically involving the anteromedial portion of the right hemidiaphragm.[6] For the rest of this chapter we will use *eventration* to mean *partial eventration*.

A small eventration usually has two distinct arcs on the lateral projection, with the higher arc representing the thinned portion (Fig. 78.2). A large eventration may be mistaken for a paralyzed or weak hemidiaphragm, but the pattern of elevation is different; in eventration the hemidiaphragm has a steeper arc and descends posteriorly to normal height, whereas a paralyzed or weak hemidiaphragm has a shallower arc and stays elevated posteriorly all the way to the chest wall. Subsegmental atelectasis near the elevated hemidiaphragm is often not as great as with paralysis because the hemidiaphragm usually maintains some degree of motion.

Eventration involving the anterior right hemidiaphragm can be distinguished from a Morgagni hernia by its contour on the lateral radiograph. With eventration, the entire contour of the hemidiaphragm is visible on lateral view, whereas with Morgagni

*The editors and the publisher would like to thank Drs. Nestor L. Müller and C. Isabela Silva Müller for contributing material on this topic to the prior edition of this work. It has served as the foundation for the current chapter.

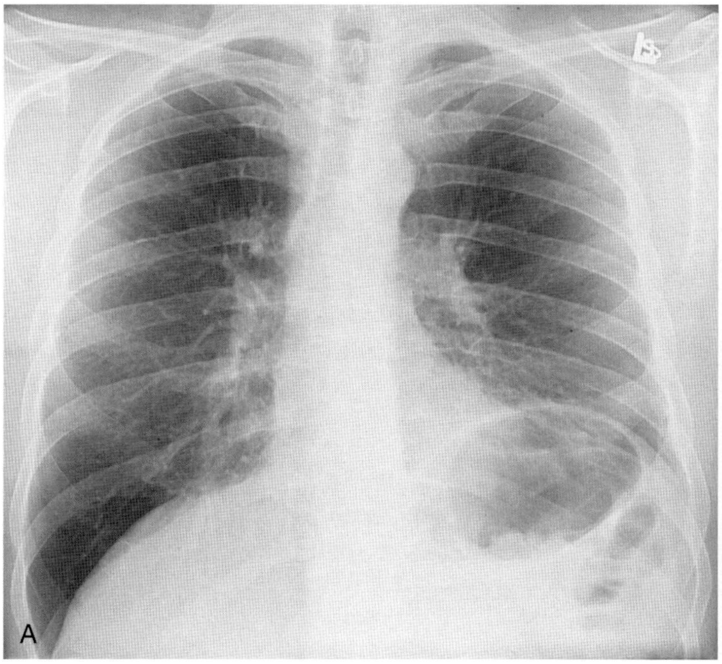

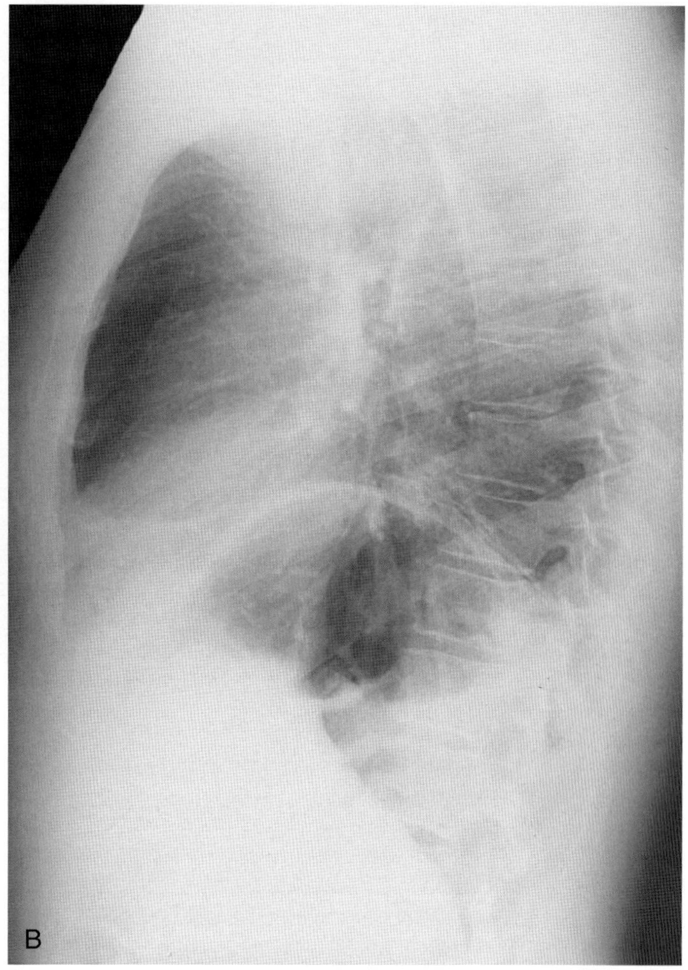

Fig. 78.1 Paralysis of left hemidiaphragm. Posteroanterior (A) and lateral (B) chest radiographs show marked elevation of the left hemidiaphragm with associated left basilar linear subsegmental atelectasis. The elevation extends all the way to the posterior chest wall on lateral view, unlike with large eventration. Fluoroscopy (not shown) demonstrated absent downward motion on deep inspiration and paradoxical upward motion of the left hemidiaphragm on sniffing.

hernia the contour is obscured by the hernia contents and surrounding mediastinal tissue.[3]

The usual imaging test to demonstrate hemidiaphragmatic paralysis, weakness, or eventration is fluoroscopy, but ultrasonography or dynamic magnetic resonance (MRI) can be used.

Although diaphragm fluoroscopy is often called the sniff test, sniffing is not the most important part, and sniffing by itself does not diagnose paralysis. The diagnosis of paralysis requires observing quiet and deep inspiration. Absence of downward motion on slow, deep inspiration is the critical finding that indicates paralysis. Sniffing is best viewed as a stress test that elicits relative weakness (not only paralysis) of a hemidiaphragm. In pitting one hemidiaphragm against the other, sniffing is analogous to arm wrestling, in which the arm of the stronger opponent pushes forward, forcing the weaker opponent's arm backward (i.e., paradoxically), even though the weaker arm is not paralyzed.

A thorough fluoroscopic examination includes watching the hemidiaphragms in both frontal and lateral projections with the patient upright and often also supine, particularly if the patient complains of dyspnea when lying down or is suspected to have bilateral paralysis. The lateral view is needed to show the excursion of the posterior portion of the diaphragm, which is usually more vigorous than the anterior portion. The lateral view also shows the anterior and upward movement of the chest wall on inspiration. The supine view is needed to reveal bilateral hemidiaphragmatic paralysis when the apparently normal diaphragm excursion on upright views is actually passive movement from use of the abdominal muscles. The supine view can also reveal weakness because the supine position provides a stress test of the diaphragm by making it work against the weight of the abdomen. Even decubitus positioning can be used if clinically relevant.

Performing the Fluoroscopic Sniff Test[a]

This technique includes upright frontal and lateral views followed by semisupine and fully supine frontal views.

1. Practice breathing maneuvers before fluoroscopy. Coach the patient in taking in a slow deep breath with the mouth open and then letting it out without forcing it or pursing the lips. Then coach the patient in sniffing. After exhalation of a slow deep breath, the patient should close the mouth and breathe in through the nose as hard, fast, and deeply as possible. Note that this maneuver should be a single long sniff, not a series of short sniffs.
2. With the patient upright, adjust collimation to show the entire chest. Observe a couple of quiet breaths.
3. Then observe a slow, deep breath. ("Take in a deep breath… now let it out.")
4. Observe a second deep breath and at the end of the expiration, tell the patient to close the mouth and sniff. "Take in a deep breath…now let it out.…now close your mouth and sniff!").
5. Repeat steps 3 and 4.

[a]Modified from reference 1.

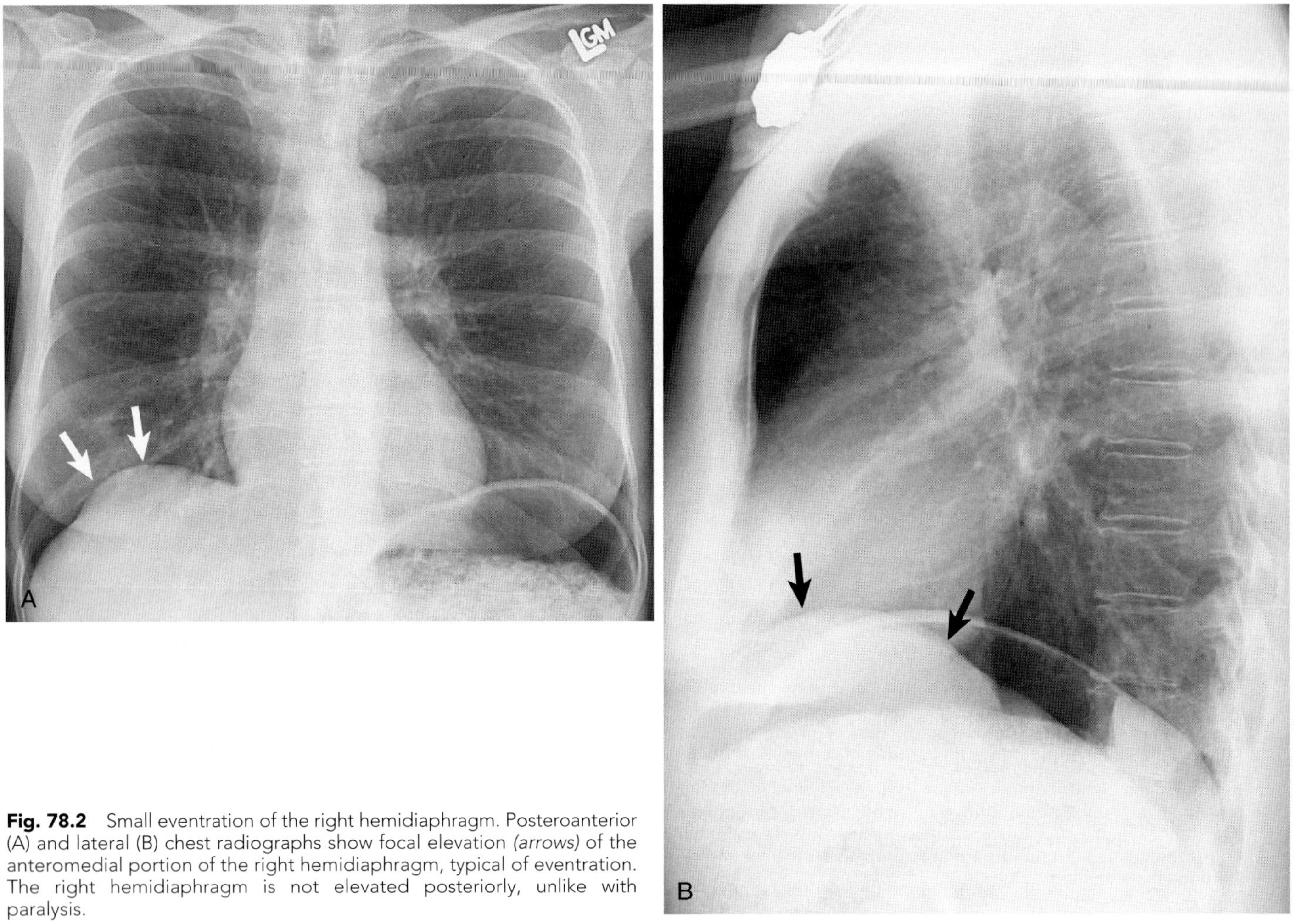

Fig. 78.2 Small eventration of the right hemidiaphragm. Posteroanterior (A) and lateral (B) chest radiographs show focal elevation *(arrows)* of the anteromedial portion of the right hemidiaphragm, typical of eventration. The right hemidiaphragm is not elevated posteriorly, unlike with paralysis.

6. Turn the patient into the lateral position, with arms out of the field of view. Observe two quiet breaths, and then observe two deep breaths with the second one followed by the sniff. Repeat.
7. Turn the patient back into the frontal position. Observe two deep breaths. Then observe two quiet breaths and note the resting positions of both hemidiaphragms at end expiration.
8. Tilt the fluoroscopic table to 45 degrees elevation. Observe two deep breaths, then two quiet breaths, and again note the resting positions of both hemidiaphragms at end expiration.
9. Tilt the fluoroscopic table to the supine position. Again observe two deep breaths, then two quiet breaths, and note the resting positions of both hemidiaphragms at end expiration.
10. The examination can be recorded on video loops sent to a picture archiving and communication system or with movies burned to a digital video disc.

Interpreting the Fluoroscopic Sniff Test[a]

1. Normal findings
   A. On quiet and deep inspiration both hemidiaphragms move downward as the anterior chest wall moves upward. Excursion is usually one rib interspace or more. On lateral view excursion is usually greater posteriorly, particularly on the right; it may be slightly asymmetric, and the right side may lag, particularly anteriorly.[7]
   B. On sniffing both hemidiaphragms move downward as the chest wall moves upward. (Chest wall motion may be attenuated compared to that on slow deep inspiration.) Excursion is again greater posteriorly. Some asymmetry is common, and the right hemidiaphragm may lag, particularly anteriorly. There may even be transient upward (paradoxical) motion, particularly of the right anterior hemidiaphragm.[7]
   C. When the patient is lowered to 45 degrees elevation and then to the supine position, excursion of both hemidiaphragms is usually less than with the patient upright. Also, there is often 1 to 2 cm upward displacement of the resting position of the hemidiaphragms.
2. Paralysis of one hemidiaphragm
   A. On deep breathing downward excursion is nearly or completely absent. There may be upward (paradoxical) motion on deep or even quiet breathing, and the mediastinum usually shifts away from the side of paralysis during inspiration.
   B. On sniffing there is usually upward (paradoxical) motion.
   C. On supine position there may be excess elevation of the resting position of the hemidiaphragm.
3. Paralysis of both hemidiaphragms
   A. Both hemidiaphragms are elevated, often with atelectasis in the lung bases.[7]
   B. Motion of the anterior chest wall in some cases may cause both hemidiaphragms to move upward on inspiration—that

[a]Modified from reference 1.

is, in the same (upward) direction as the chest wall rather than in the opposite (downward and orthograde) direction. It is important to recognize that the diaphragm is moving paradoxically when it moves in the same direction as the chest wall.

C. On upright views the excursion of both hemidiaphragms may appear to be normal if the patient is using abdominal muscles to passively move the diaphragm. (Tightening abdominal muscles on expiration pushes the diaphragm up, and relaxing them on inspiration allows the diaphragm to fall.) On supine and semisupine views this mechanism is defeated, and excursion of the hemidiaphragms is severely reduced.

D. On supine views there is excess elevation of the resting positions of both hemidiaphragms.

4. Weakness of one or both hemidiaphragms
   A. On deep inspiration downward excursion is less than one rib interspace. There may be upward (paradoxical) motion on deep or even quiet breathing. Hemidiaphragmatic weakness often becomes more obvious on rapid, deep inspiration, with the weak hemidiaphragm lagging behind the normal side.
   B. On sniffing there may be upward (paradoxical) motion.
   C. On supine views there may excess elevation of the resting position of the hemidiaphragm.
5. Eventration of a hemidiaphragm
   A. On deep breathing excursion of the eventrated segment is less than the rest of the hemidiaphragm. There may be transient upward motion of the segment on deep or even quiet breathing.
   B. On sniffing there may be upward (paradoxical) motion of the segment. A rocking motion may ensue on lateral view, with the anterior eventrated segment moving upward while the posterior portion moves downward.
   C. On supine position there may be excess elevation of the resting position of the eventrated segment.

Again, because upward (paradoxical) motion on sniffing could reflect weakness, eventration, or paralysis, the fluoroscopic diagnosis of hemidiaphragmatic paralysis is not based on sniffing but instead on the absence of downward motion on slow, deep inspiration.[1,8] Diaphragm fluoroscopy is positive in more than 90% of patients with unilateral phrenic nerve paralysis.[2,9] See Table 78.1 for a summary of fluoroscopic findings in the various conditions.

COMPUTED TOMOGRAPHY

An important role of computed tomography (CT) in the assessment of patients with diaphragmatic paralysis is to rule out tumor, lymphadenopathy, aneurysm, or other lesion that may be compromising the phrenic nerve (Fig. 78.3). The main role of CT in patients with eventration is in distinguishing the abnormality from a focal bulge along the diaphragm that might represent hernia or even tumor. In eventration the diaphragm, although thin, remains visible as a continuous layer over the elevated abdominal viscera and retroperitoneal or omental fat. There is often a sharp transition and undercutting at the edges of an eventration (Fig. 78.4).[1]

CT also is important in assessing the thickness of diaphragm muscle. The easiest place to observe muscle thickness is the crus of the hemidiaphragm. The left crus is normally slightly thinner than the right. The crus atrophies with paralysis but not with eventration (Fig. 78.5).[10] Thus the finding of an elevated hemidiaphragm with normal thickness of the crus likely reflects eventration rather than paralysis. If both hemidiaphragms are elevated, but the thicknesses of the crura are preserved, bilateral paralysis is unlikely, and some cause of abdominal distension, such as mass, ascites, or excess fat, is more likely.

MAGNETIC RESONANCE IMAGING

Normal and abnormal diaphragmatic motion and diaphragmatic paralysis can be assessed with dynamic MRI.[11] The advantage of MRI is avoiding ionizing radiation, as well as screening for central thoracic tumors that could be invading the phrenic nerve, but its disadvantages are high cost and lack of widespread availability.

ULTRASONOGRAPHY

Normal and abnormal diaphragmatic motion and diaphragmatic paralysis can be assessed with ultrasonography, which is often preferred for examination in children and young adults.[1,12,13] At ultrasonography the diaphragm appears as a thick echogenic line. M-mode ultrasound is used to measure diaphragmatic motion, and interpretation is similar to that used in fluoroscopy. A paralyzed hemidiaphragm will lack downward motion on inspiration and may have paradoxical motion on sniffing. In fact, the ability of ultrasonography to assess diaphragmatic

TABLE 78.1 FINDINGS ON DIAPHRAGMATIC FLUOROSCOPY

Condition	Deep Inspiration	Sniffing	Ancillary Findings
Normal	Downward motion > 1 rib interspace	Usually downward motion	Occasional transient upward motion of right anterior hemidiaphragm during strong sniffing
Unilateral weakness	Downward motion < 1 rib interspace	May be upward or downward	Weakness more evident on rapid deep inspiration with weak hemidiaphragm lagging behind normal side
Unilateral paralysis	Absent downward motion or upward motion	Usually upward motion	Adjacent basal atelectasis; ipsilateral crus thinning on CT
Bilateral paralysis	Absent downward motion or bilateral upward motion	Usually upward motion	Adjacent basal atelectasis; supine imaging necessary to show absent motion; bilateral crus thinning on CT
Eventration	Reduced downward motion of affected segment; occasional upward motion	Downward or upward motion of segment	Normal ipsilateral crus thickness on CT

CT, Computed tomography.

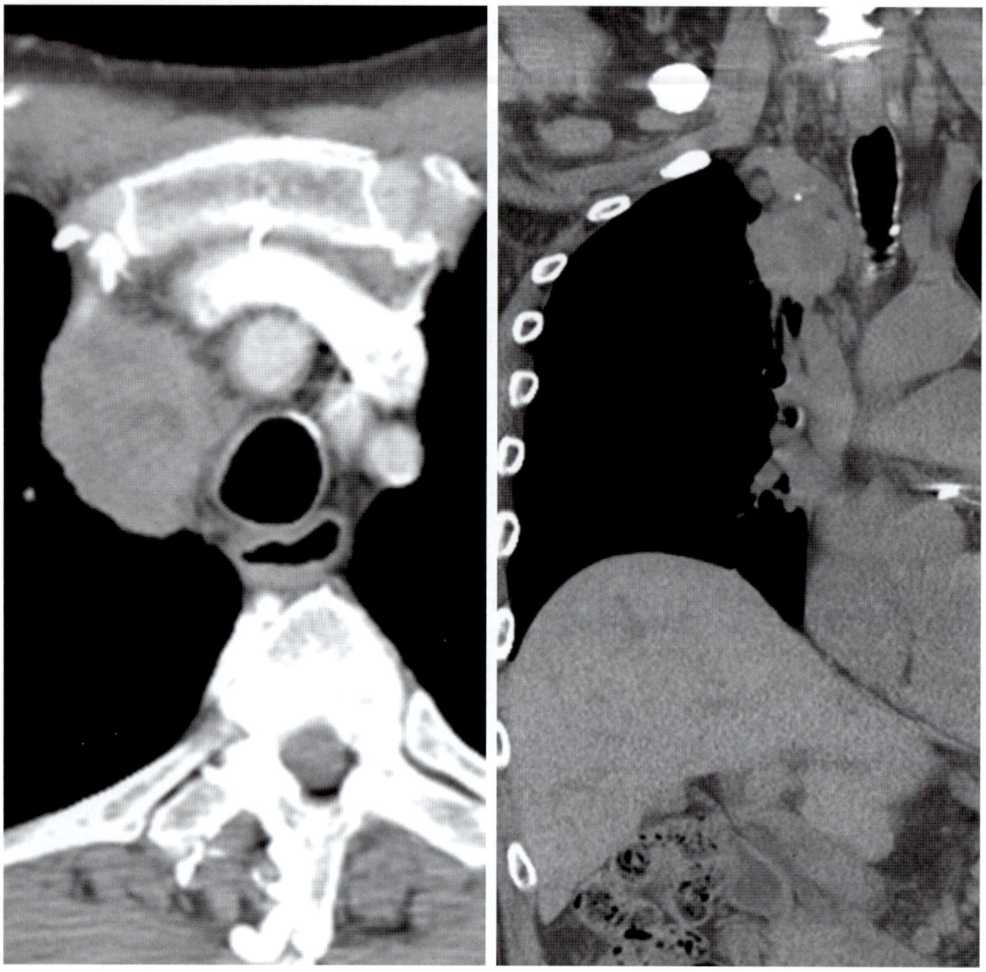

Fig. 78.3 Paralysis of right hemidiaphragm resulting from phrenic nerve injury by lung cancer. Axial and coronal CT images show a large right upper lobe mass that has invaded the adjacent mediastinum, injured the phrenic nerve, and paralyzed the right hemidiaphragm. *(Coronal image reproduced from Nason LK, Walker CM, McNeely MF, et al. Imaging of the diaphragm: anatomy and function. Radiographics. 2012;32:E51–E70.)*

thickness and changing thickness with respiration is a potential advantage over fluoroscopy.[12] Ultrasonography can be used in intubated patients to detect diaphragmatic thinning, which can influence weaning the patient from the ventilator.[5]

TREATMENT

Conservative management is indicated for asymptomatic patients with hemidiaphragmatic weakness or paralysis. Diaphragmatic plication is usually reserved for symptomatic patients with irreversible unilateral phrenic nerve dysfunction or large eventration. Prophylactic diaphragmatic plication may also be beneficial in patients with phrenic nerve involvement by lung cancer or if phrenic nerve injury is recognized during surgery on the heart, mediastinum, or lung.[14] Phrenic nerve stimulation may benefit patients with intact phrenic nerve function and absence of myopathy, such as those with high cervical spine injuries causing bilateral hemidiaphragmatic paralysis.[15]

Diaphragmatic Hernias

Etiology, Prevalence, and Epidemiology

Herniation of abdominal or retroperitoneal organs or tissues into the thorax may occur through congenitally weak areas of the diaphragm, through acquired weak areas, or through traumatic tears. The most frequent nontraumatic hernia is through the esophageal hiatus; hernias through the pleuroperitoneal hiatus (Bochdalek hernia) or the parasternal hiatus (Morgagni hernia) are less common.

The prevalence of esophageal hiatal hernia increases with age; the abnormality is found on CT in about 5% of patients younger than 40 years, 30% between 40 and 59 years, and 65% between 60 and 79 years.[16] Most hernias are asymptomatic and are discovered on radiographs or CT performed for unrelated complaints.

In infants herniation through a persistent embryonic pleuroperitoneal hiatus (i.e., congenital Bochdalek hernia) is both the most common and the most serious form of diaphragmatic hernia, with an incidence of about 1 in 2200 live births[17]; 75% to 90% are on the left.[18]

The size of the defect varies. When the defect is small, a sac lined by pleura contains retroperitoneal fat, part of the spleen or kidney, or only omentum. When the defect is large and the hemidiaphragm is almost or completely absent, a large amount of abdominal contents, including the stomach, can enter the left hemithorax, impairing development and leaving the lung hypoplastic.[19] Most large hernias have no peritoneal sac, so communication between the pleural and the peritoneal cavities is wide open. A large hernia is associated with high mortality; even after successful surgical correction, mortality is about 30% because of lung hypoplasia and pulmonary arterial hypertension.[18]

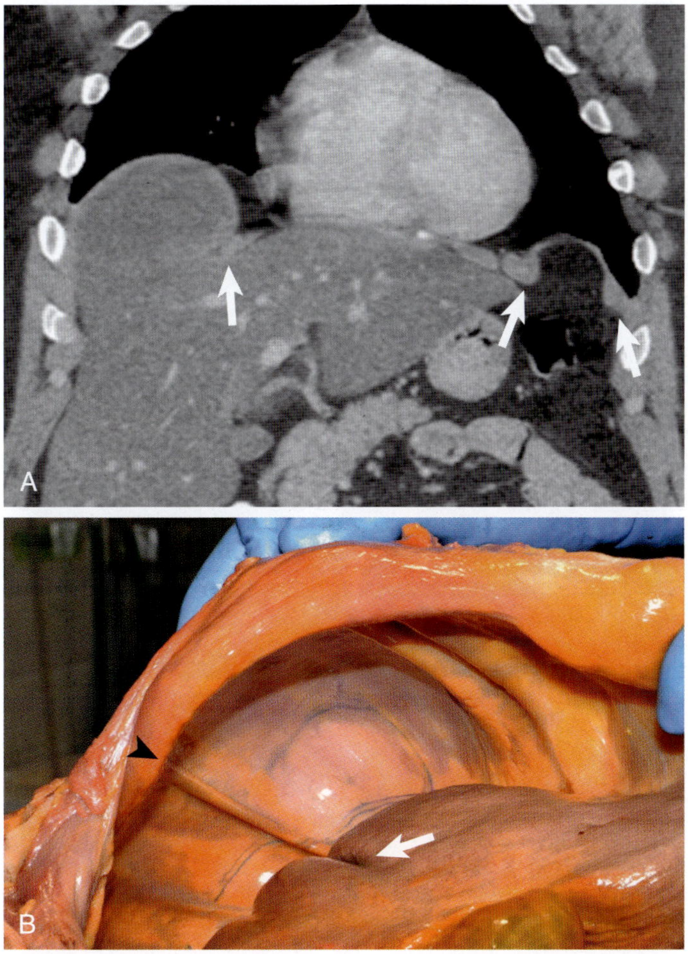

Fig. 78.4 Bilateral eventration. (A) Coronal CT shows focal elevation of both hemidiaphragms with undercut edges *(arrows)* resulting in a mushroom-like appearance. Although the mushroom-like appearance can also occur with diaphragmatic hernia, the diaphragm in eventration is continuous but thinned. (B) Specimen photograph from a different patient shows the medial *(arrowhead)* and lateral muscle bands of the right hemidiaphragm with a corresponding groove in the liver *(arrow)*. At CT (not shown) the medial muscle band formed the sharp edge of the eventration. *(Reproduced from Nason LK, Walker CM, McNeely MF, et al. Imaging of the diaphragm: anatomy and function.* Radiographics. *2012;32:E51–E70.)*

In adults small Bochdalek hernias are much more common than in infants; in fact, small ones are found on CT in 5% to 10% of adults,[16,20] but they are rarely symptomatic. As in children, most are on the left, presumably because the liver covers and protects the right pleuroperitoneal canal.[21] The incidence increases with age; rare in patients younger than 40 years, they affect about 5% of patients between 40 and 49 years, 15% between 50 and 69 years, and 35% of those older than 70 years.[16] This progression with age suggests that they are acquired, probably through enlargement of a persistent pleuroperitoneal canal.

Morgagni (parasternal) hernia is less common than Bochdalek hernia. Most are on the right, probably because the left foramen is covered by the heart. Although the underlying defect is developmental, hernias are more common in adults than in children and are often associated with abdominal obesity or other causes of increased intraabdominal pressure, such as severe effort or trauma.[22] In contrast to Bochdalek hernia, a peritoneal sac is usually present. The sac contains, in decreasing order, omentum, colon, stomach, liver, and small intestine.[23]

KEY POINTS: ABNORMALITIES OF DIAPHRAGMATIC MOTION

- The diagnosis of paralysis depends on an absence of downward excursion on slow deep inspiration, *not* on paradoxical motion on sniffing. If there is any downward movement during inspiration, the hemidiaphragm is not paralyzed but may be weak or eventrated.
- If bilateral paralysis is suspected, supine views are essential to prevent misinterpretation of passive motion of the diaphragm from use of abdominal muscles.
- Unilateral diaphragmatic paralysis
  - Common causes: invasion or injury of phrenic nerve by tumor, trauma, surgery
  - Radiologic findings: elevation of the hemidiaphragm extending all the way posteriorly on lateral view; basal atelectasis common; absence of downward excursion on deep breathing on fluoroscopy with or without upward (paradoxical) motion on sniffing; unilateral crus thinning on CT
- Unilateral diaphragmatic weakness
  - Radiologic findings: elevation of the hemidiaphragm extending posteriorly on lateral view; reduced or delayed downward motion on deep inspiration on fluoroscopy with or without paradoxical upward motion on sniffing
- Bilateral diaphragmatic paralysis
  - Common causes: spinal cord injury, generalized neuromuscular disorders
  - Radiologic findings: elevation of both hemidiaphragms; absent downward motion on deep inspiration on fluoroscopy (when supine); upward (paradoxical) motion on sniffing; basal atelectasis common; bilateral crus thinning on CT
- Eventration of diaphragm
  - Congenital failure of muscle development of part of one or both hemidiaphragms; often acquired disorder in adults
  - Usually unilateral in adults
  - Radiologic findings: eventration of the hemidiaphragm typically involving anteromedial portion of right hemidiaphragm; eventrated segment possibly showing upward (paradoxical) motion on sniffing; basal atelectasis usually mild; posterior aspect of hemidiaphragm usually descending to normal height and having normal excursion on deep inspiration; normal crus thickness on CT

Traumatic diaphragmatic hernia is diagnosed in 1% to 8% of hospital admissions for blunt trauma and in about 5% of those that subsequently undergo laparotomy or thoracotomy.[24,25] In a review of 1000 diaphragmatic injuries in 980 patients, 75% of diaphragmatic ruptures were caused by blunt trauma and 25% by penetrating injury.[24] The main mechanism of rupture by blunt trauma is believed to be a sudden increase in intrathoracic or intraabdominal pressure against a fixed diaphragm.[24,26] The majority of traumatic hernias are on the left, and most occur posterolaterally along the embryonic fusion lines.[24,26] Atypical locations result from penetrating trauma or from puncture by a fractured rib.[25]

Clinical Presentation

Most nontraumatic diaphragmatic hernias are asymptomatic. Hiatal hernia may cause heartburn or regurgitation, and chronic reflux may lead to scarring and narrowing of the lower esophagus and even to obstruction. Similarly, adult patients with Morgagni and Bochdalek hernias are usually asymptomatic, but some experience epigastric or lower sternal discomfort and sometimes cardiorespiratory or gastrointestinal symptoms.

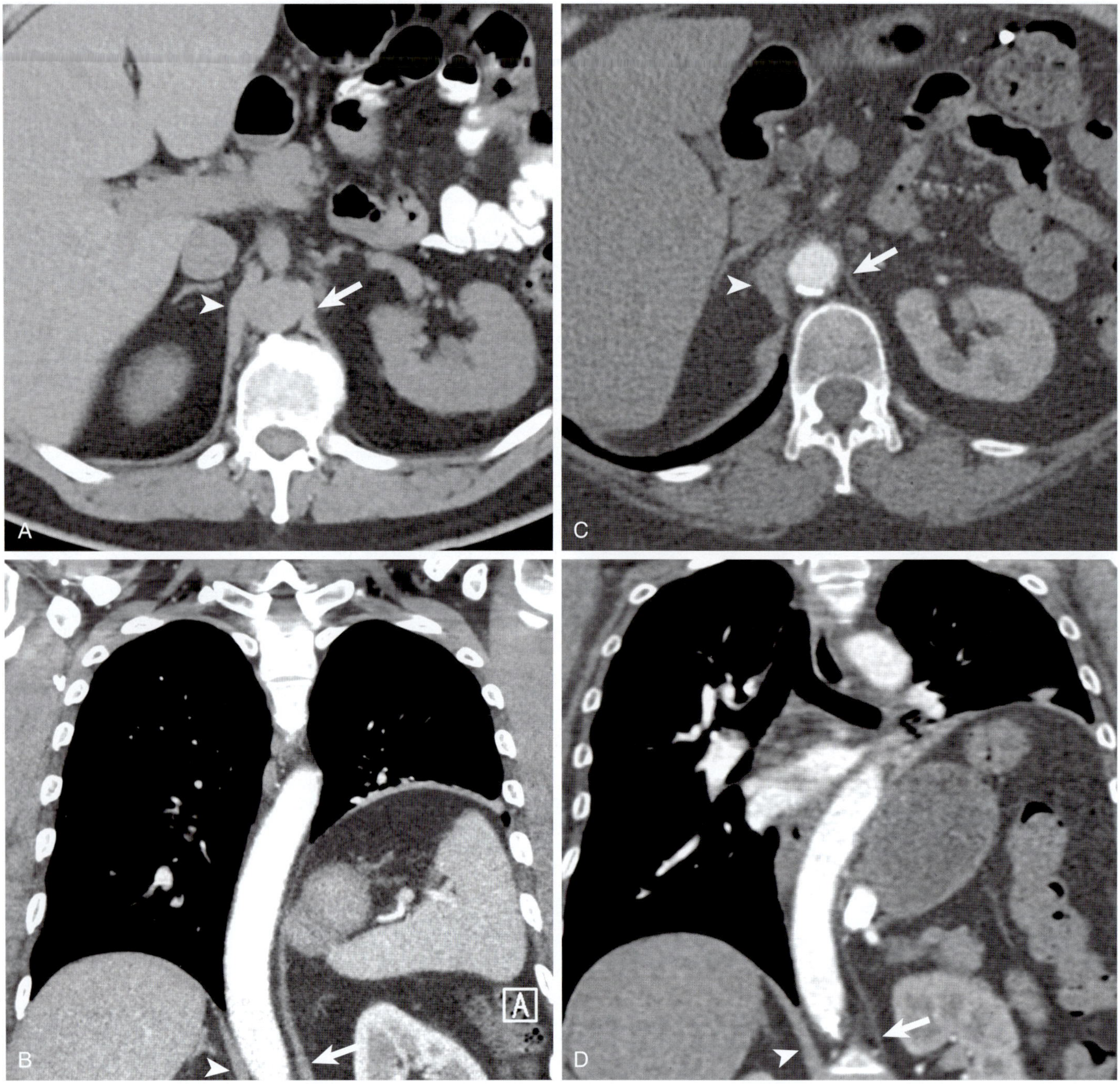

Fig. 78.5 Diaphragmatic crural thickness in eventration and paralysis. Axial CT (A) near level of celiac artery and coronal reformat (B) in a patient with elevation of the left hemidiaphragm by large eventration show normal thickness of the right crus *(arrowheads)* and left crus *(arrows)*. The left crus is often slightly thinner than the right. Axial (C) and coronal reformat CT (D) at similar levels in a patient with paralysis of the left hemidiaphragm show thinning of left crus *(arrows)* compared to the right crus *(arrowheads)*. The elevation of the left hemidiaphragm is similar to the case of eventration, but crus thinning helps in recognizing paralysis.

Signs and symptoms of traumatic diaphragmatic hernia can be immediate or delayed. Bleeding from the torn edge of the diaphragm is seldom of sufficient severity to cause hemodynamic compromise. Respiratory distress can be caused by mechanical displacement of lung, by pneumothorax, or by intrathoracic rupture of an abdominal viscus. Strangulation of herniated abdominal viscera can cause nausea and vomiting.

Manifestations of Diaphragmatic Hernia

RADIOGRAPHY

Hiatal hernia typically manifests on radiographs as a retrocardiac mass, usually with an air bubble or fluid level (Fig. 78.6). If most of the stomach has herniated, the stomach may undergo volvulus, creating a large mass with a double fluid level; incarceration and

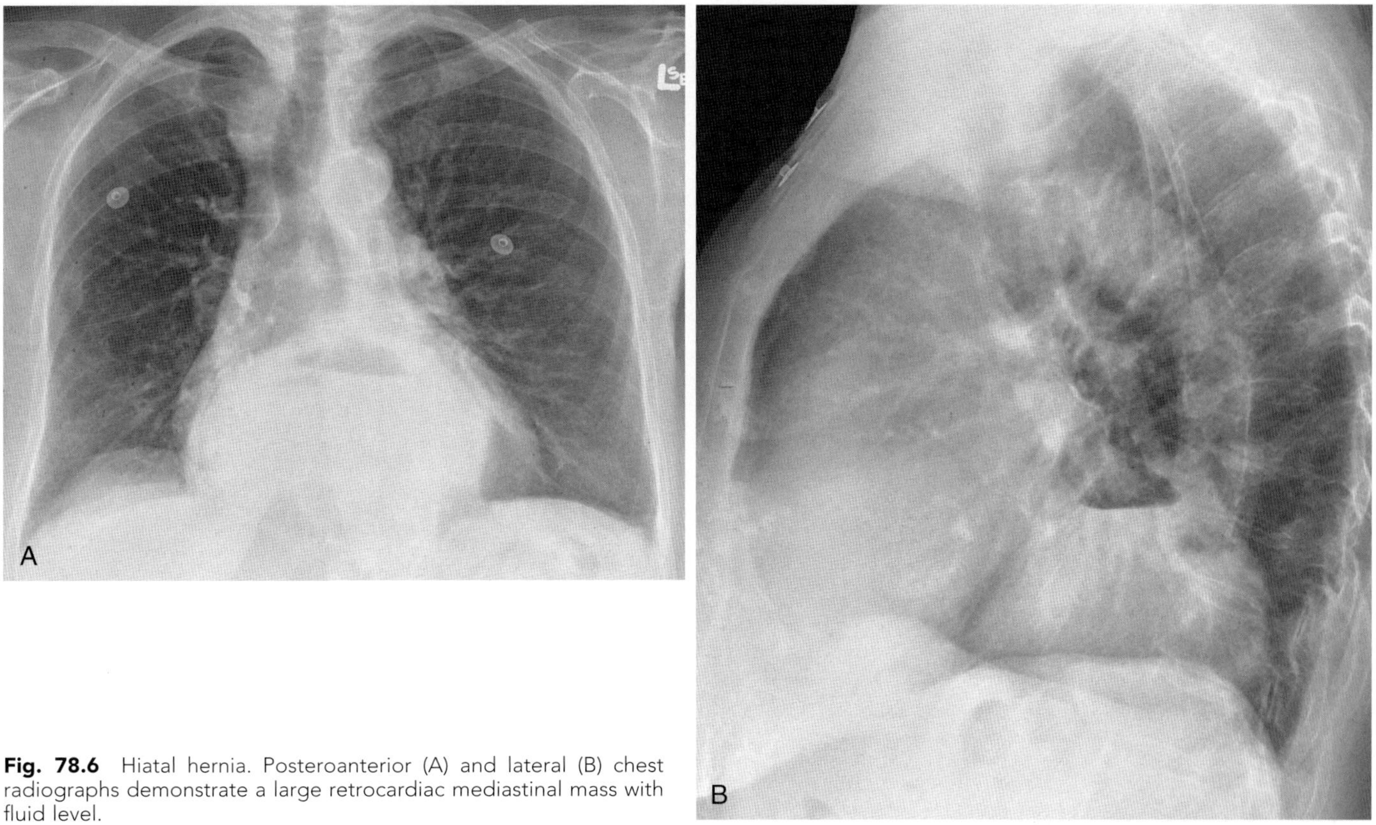

Fig. 78.6 Hiatal hernia. Posteroanterior (A) and lateral (B) chest radiographs demonstrate a large retrocardiac mediastinal mass with fluid level.

strangulation may occur but are uncommon. The stomach is the most common herniated viscus, but the transverse colon, omentum, and liver can also herniate.

Bochdalek hernia manifests as a focal bulge in the posterior hemidiaphragm or as a mass adjacent to the posteromedial aspect of either hemidiaphragm. Although the diagnosis can often be suspected on radiographs by the typical location, Bochdalek hernia can be mimicked by a mass in the lung, pleura, mediastinum, diaphragm, or paravertebral tissue.[27] The diagnosis is usually clear on CT.[27,28] Because its prevalence increases with age, a Bochdalek hernia can develop in a patient with previously normal radiographs (Fig. 78.7).

Morgagni hernia typically manifests as a smooth, well-defined opacity in the right anterior cardiophrenic angle. Most often, its density is homogeneous (Fig. 78.8), but it can be heterogeneous if it contains bowel (Fig. 78.9) or fat. Herniated fat is usually omentum, and the transverse colon is then situated high in the abdomen with an anterior and superior peak as it enters the hernia; this finding is virtually diagnostic of Morgagni hernia. In the rare case in which the hernia penetrates into the pericardial sac, loops of air-containing bowel may be visible anterior to the heart.[29]

Traumatic diaphragmatic hernia manifests as herniated stomach or bowel in the chest and cephalad extension of a gastric tube above the normal level of the diaphragm (Fig. 78.10).[24,30] A diagnostic radiographic finding is a focal constriction (collar sign) in the stomach or bowel loops caused by the edges of the diaphragmatic defect. Suggestive findings include irregularity or obscuration of the diaphragmatic contour, a persistent basal opacity (which can mimic atelectasis or a supradiaphragmatic mass), an elevated hemidiaphragm (>4 cm higher than the other side), and contralateral shift of the mediastinum in the absence of large pleural effusion or pneumothorax.[30,31] With rupture of the right hemidiaphragm, a portion of the liver may herniate and create a mushroom-shaped mass in the right hemithorax. In this case the diagnosis is suggested by the high position of the lower liver edge as indicated by the position of the hepatic flexure of the colon.

Chest radiography has relatively low sensitivity in diagnosing traumatic diaphragmatic hernia.[24,30] In one study of 50 patients with surgically proven rupture, chest radiographs were diagnostic in only 20 (46%) of 44 patients with rupture on the left and were considered suggestive in an additional 8 (18%).[30] Chest radiographs were strongly suggestive in only 1 (17%) of 6 patients with rupture on the right.[30] The sensitivity of radiographs is even lower for penetrating injury.[31] Repeat chest radiography may help reveal rupture that was initially obscured by lung or pleural abnormalities or by positive pressure ventilation.[25]

COMPUTED TOMOGRAPHY

CT with coronal and sagittal reformatted images is currently the most effective and useful imaging technique for assessing diaphragmatic hernia.[32]

In hiatal hernia the widening of the esophageal hiatus allows the stomach, omentum, and occasionally other organs to enter the chest (Fig. 78.11). The esophageal hiatus is just to the left of the midline and is marginated by the right and left diaphragmatic crura. It is elliptical, and its width (the distance between the medial crura) is normally 15 mm or less.

Hiatal hernias are classified as sliding (type I) or paraesophageal (types II–IV). Type I, or sliding hernia, is the most common, about 90% to 95% of all cases. It is characterized by herniation of the gastric cardia into the lower mediastinum along with the gastroesophageal junction, which maintains its position above

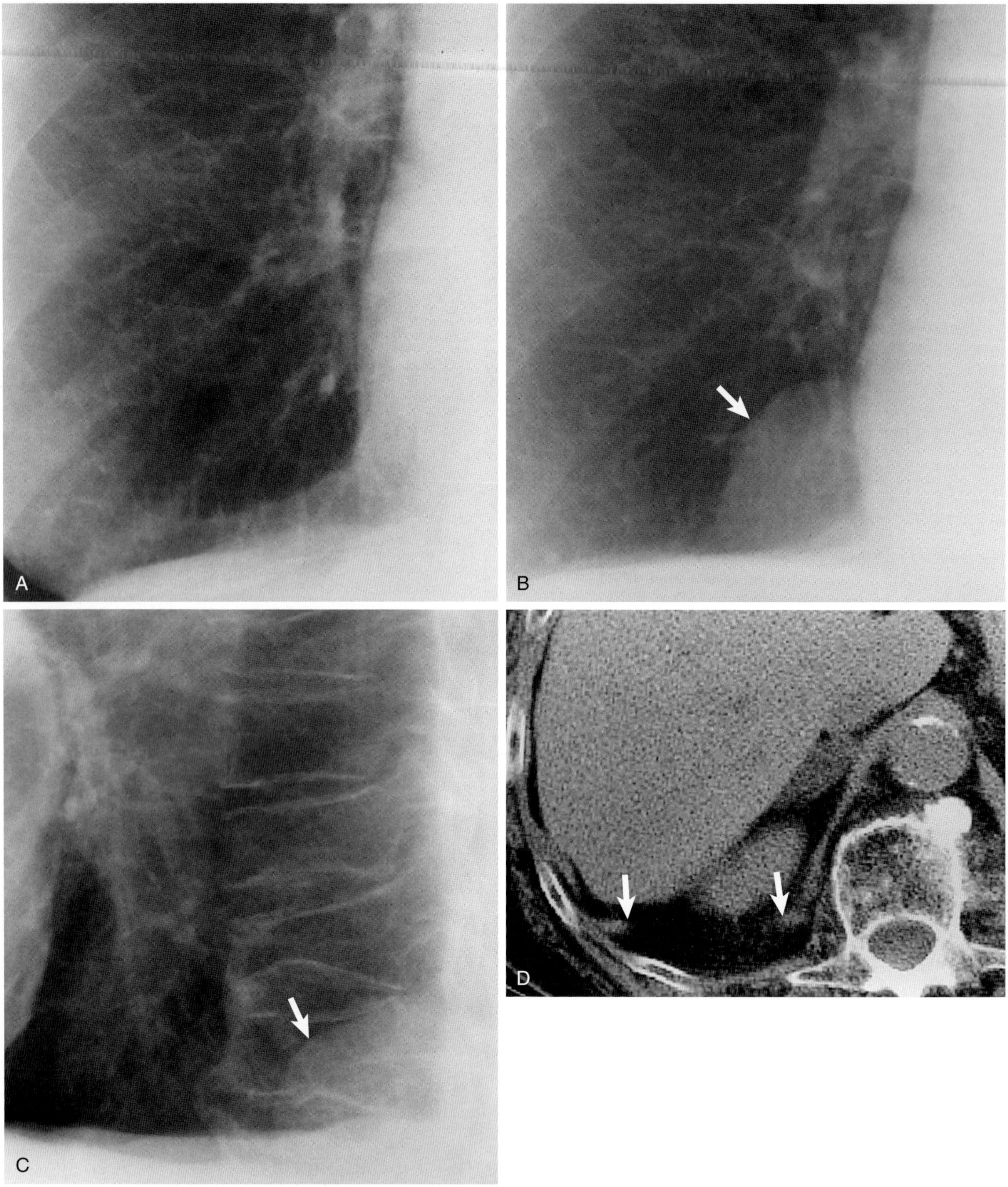

Fig. 78.7 Development of a Bochdalek hernia in an elderly woman. (A) Posteroanterior radiograph of the right medial lower chest is unremarkable. Five years later, posteroanterior (B) and lateral (C) radiographs show a large mass *(arrows)* adjacent to the posteromedial aspect of the right hemidiaphragm. (D) CT shows the focal defect *(arrows)* in the posterior aspect of the right hemidiaphragm with herniation of omental fat. The hernia caused no symptoms. *(From Müller NL, Fraser RS, Colman NC, Paré PD.* Radiologic Diagnosis of Diseases of the Chest. *Philadelphia: WB Saunders; 2001.)*

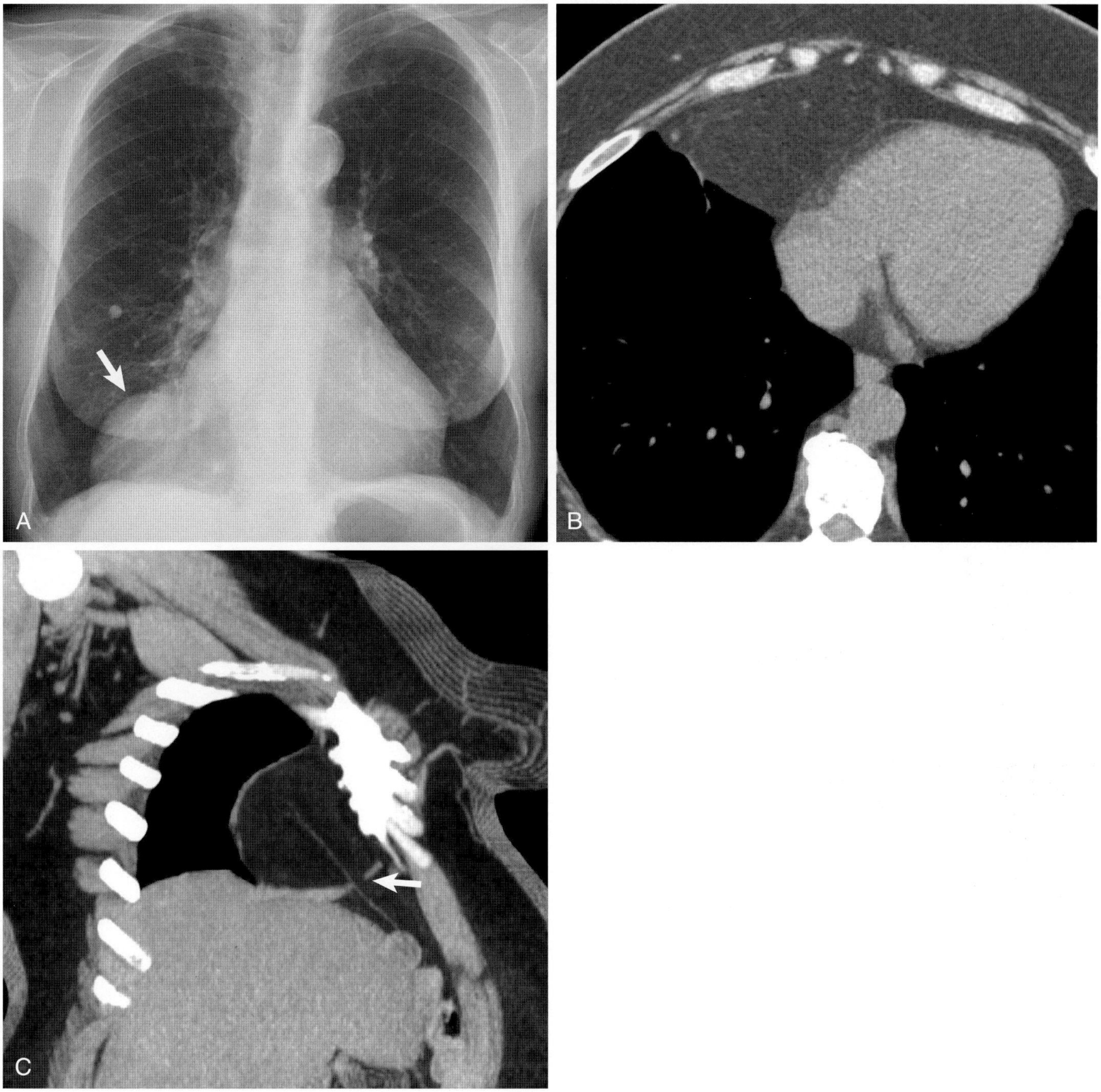

Fig. 78.8 Morgagni hernia containing omental fat. (A) Posteroanterior chest radiograph shows a mass *(arrow)* in the right cardiophrenic angle. Axial CT (B) and oblique maximum-intensity projection CT (C) show omental fat and vessels herniating through the right lower parasternal diaphragm *(arrow),* diagnostic of Morgagni hernia.

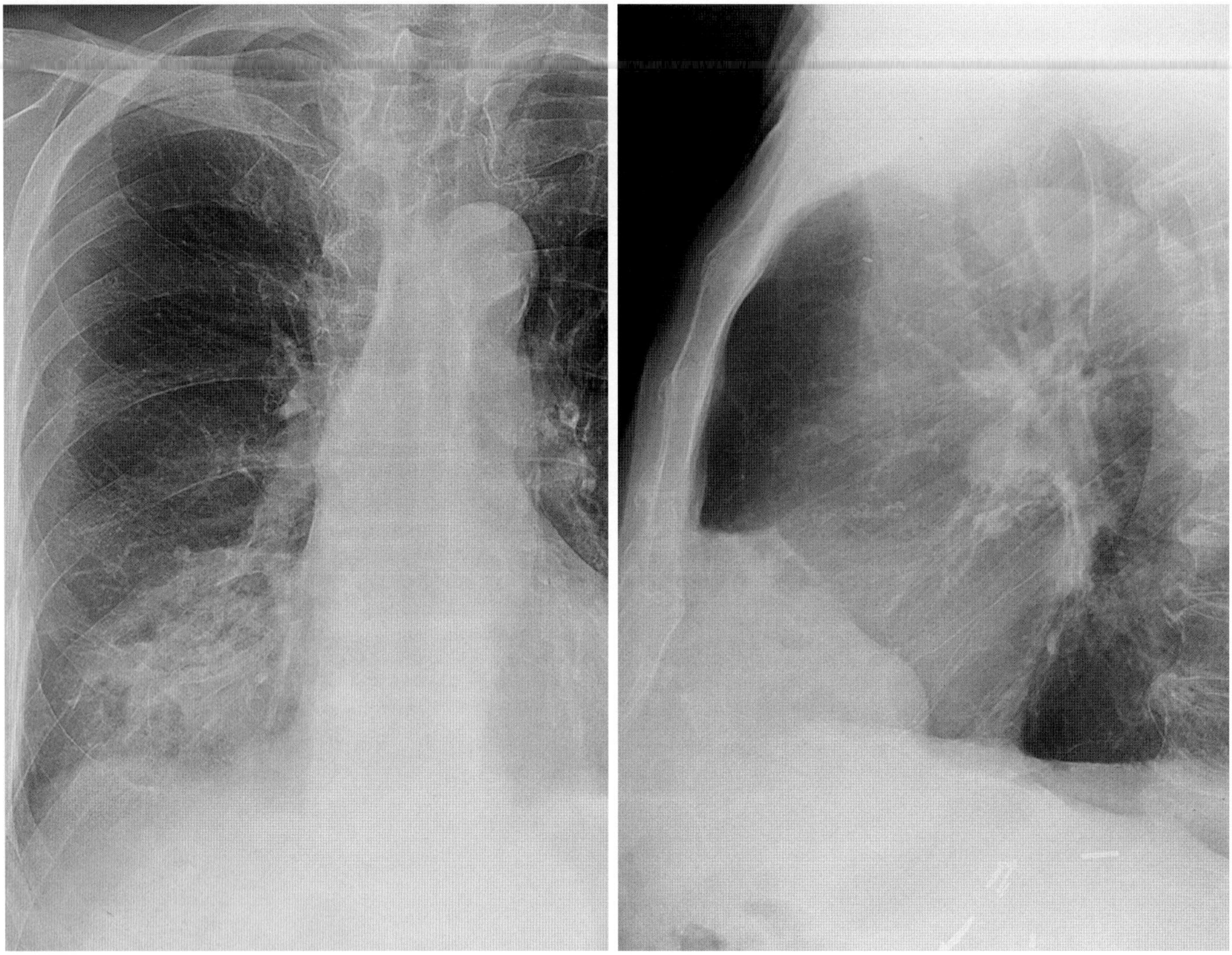

Fig. 78.9 Morgagni hernia containing transverse colon. Posteroanterior *(left)* and lateral *(right)* chest radiographs show a mass in the right cardiophrenic angle. Its inhomogeneity is caused by bubbles of colonic gas, as confirmed on CT (not shown).

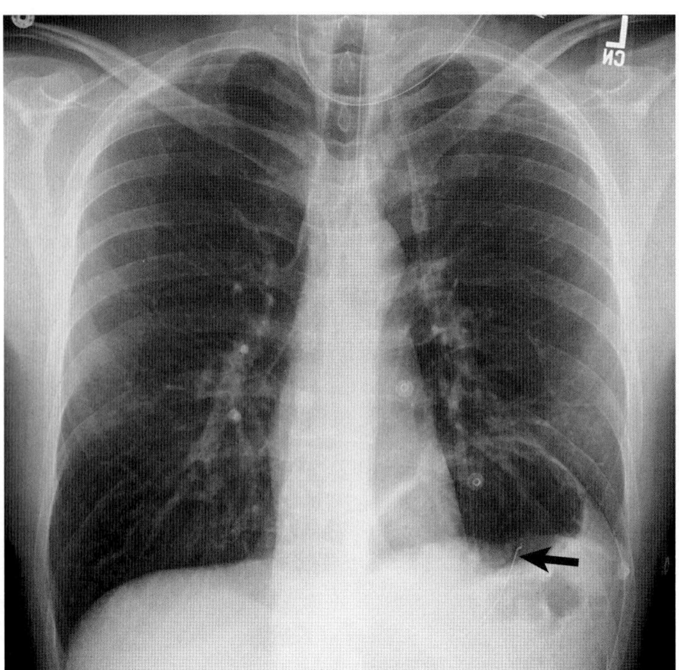

Fig. 78.10 Delayed presentation of traumatic diaphragmatic hernia. Frontal radiograph shows an intrathoracic stomach with cephalad extension of the gastric tube *(arrow)*.

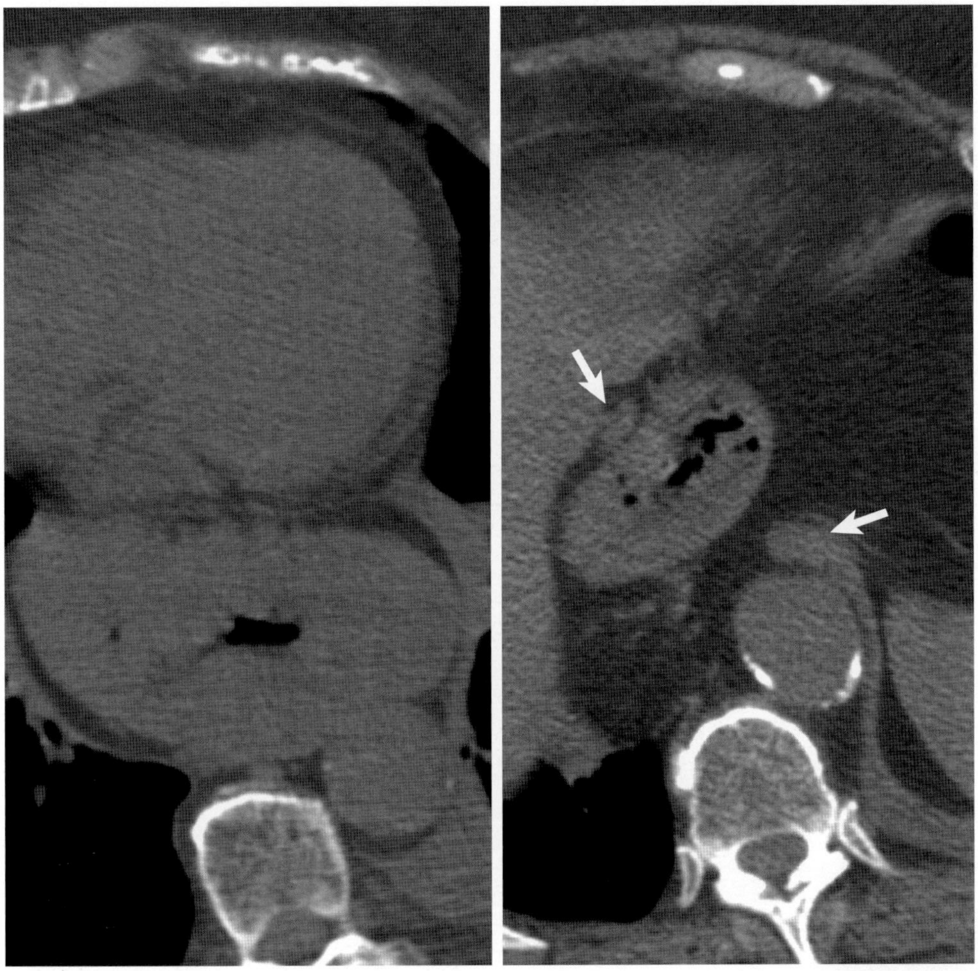

Fig. 78.11 Hiatal hernia. Axial CT images show herniation of stomach and omentum into the retrocardiac mediastinum. The left image shows the herniated stomach behind the heart. The right image, at the level of the esophageal hiatus, shows the stomach entering the widened space between the right and left hemidiaphragmatic crura *(arrows)*.

the stomach. Type II, or pure paraesophageal hernia, is rare and characterized by herniation of the gastric fundus into the lower mediastinum, with the gastroesophageal junction remaining in normal position below the esophageal hiatus. Type III, the second most common type, combines elements of paraesophageal and sliding hernias, with both the fundus and gastroesophageal junction herniated into the mediastinum; a type III hernia is distinguished from a type I hernia by having any part of the gastric fundus above the gastroesophageal junction. Type IV is characterized by herniation of an additional viscus (colon, omentum, or pancreas) into the mediastinum along with the stomach.

Bochdalek hernias in adults are found lateral to the crura (Fig. 78.12; see also Fig. 78.7). Most contain only perinephric fat, but when large, they can contain portions of the kidney and even stomach and small bowel.

Morgagni hernias are found anteromedially between the costal and sternal attachments of the diaphragm (Fig. 78.13; see also Fig. 78.8). Most are on the right and most contain only omental fat, but if large, they can contain portions of the liver, colon (see Fig. 78.13), or small intestine.

Characteristic findings of traumatic diaphragmatic hernia on CT include a sharp discontinuity of the diaphragm (Fig. 78.14); herniated abdominal viscera; obscuration of the hemidiaphragm (absent diaphragm sign); constriction of bowel or stomach at the site of herniation (collar sign); and contact between the stomach, bowel, spleen, or upper third of the liver with the posterior ribs

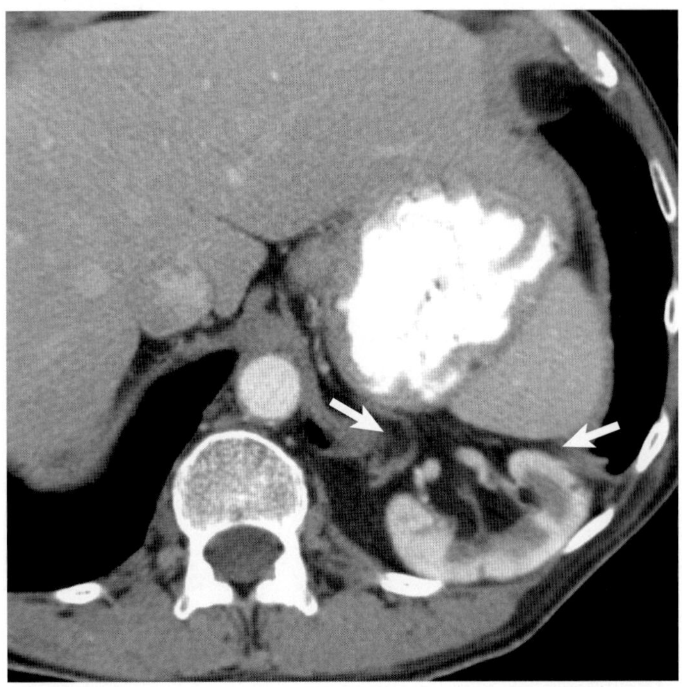

Fig. 78.12 Bochdalek hernia. Axial contrast-enhanced CT shows focal discontinuity of the left hemidiaphragm *(arrows)* and herniation of perinephric fat and part of the left kidney. Bochdalek hernias in adults are generally acquired, and their prevalence increases with age.

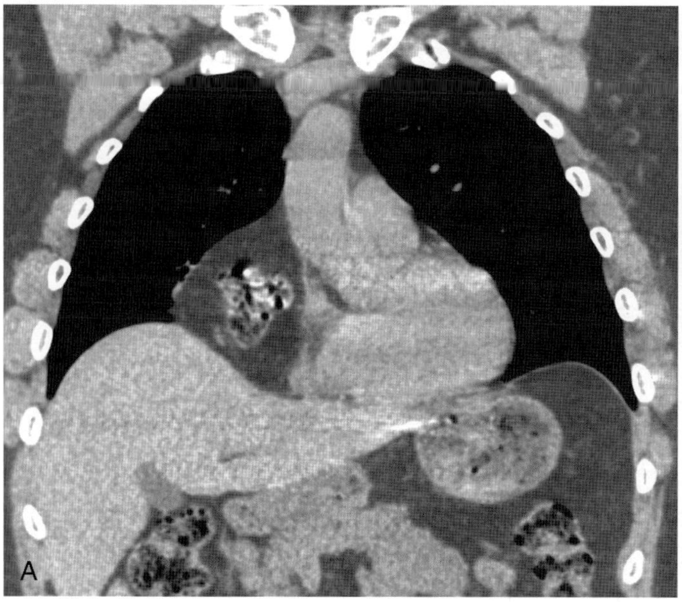

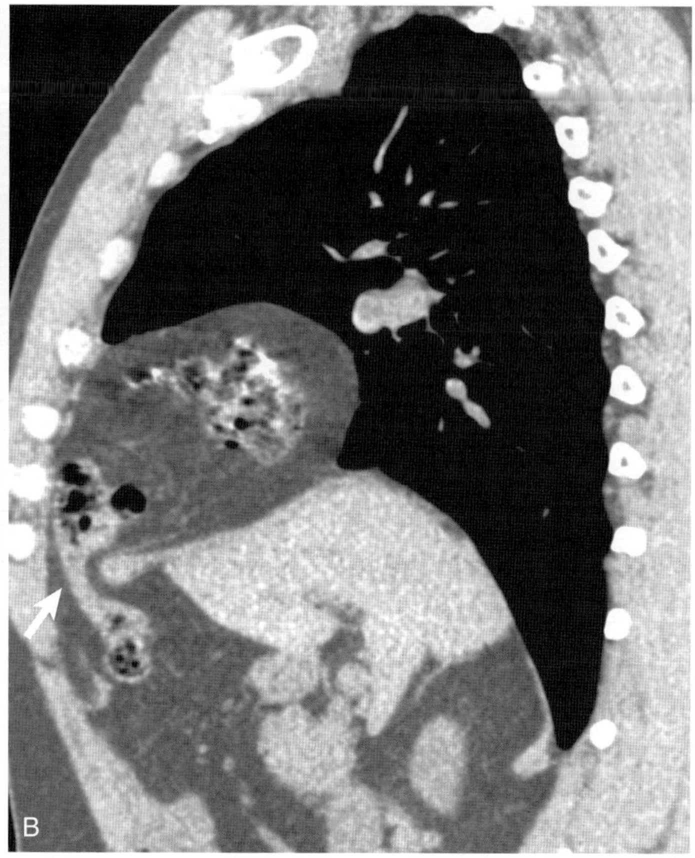

Fig. 78.13 Morgagni hernia: CT findings. (A) Coronal CT shows fat and colon adjacent to the right border of the heart. (B) Sagittal CT shows anterior herniation *(arrow)* of omentum and colon into the chest. Sagittal and coronal reformatted images are often better than axial images for showing the diaphragmatic defect and the continuity of vessels and intestine extending from the abdomen into the chest.

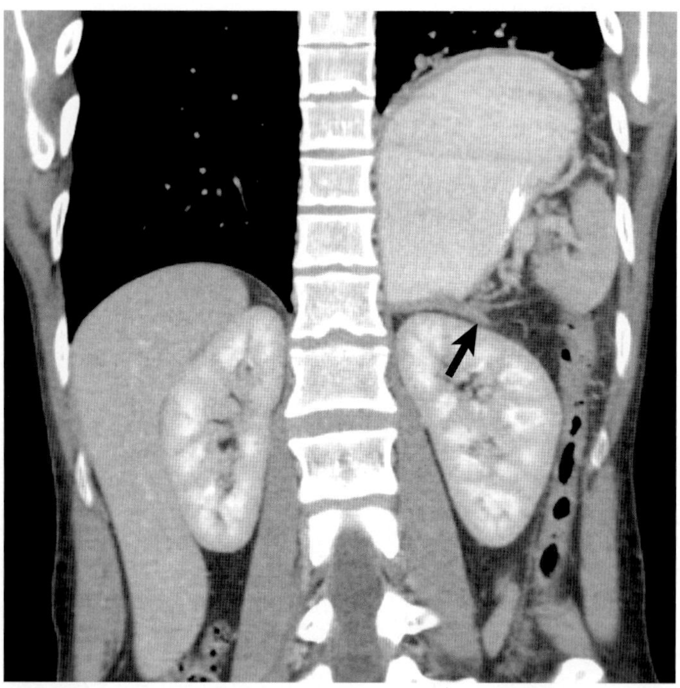

Fig. 78.14 Traumatic diaphragmatic hernia: CT findings. Contrast-enhanced coronal CT shows a focal tear of the left hemidiaphragm *(arrow)* with herniation of the stomach, omentum, spleen, and a portion of the splenic flexure of the colon.

(dependent viscera sign) (Fig. 78.15).[33–35] Focal discontinuity of the diaphragm is found on CT in 17% to 80% of cases of diaphragmatic rupture, but similar defects can occur in healthy persons, particularly the elderly, diminishing the specificity of this finding.[25,34,35] A more reliable sign is herniation of omental fat or abdominal viscera, which occurs in 50% to 60% of patients.[34,35] The collar sign, the waist-like narrowing of stomach, bowel, or liver by the edges of the diaphragmatic defect, occurs in 16% to 63% of patients, and it may be the sole abnormality on CT.[25,33–35]

The dependent viscera sign is one of the most sensitive CT signs of diaphragmatic rupture. It consists of contact of the stomach, bowel, or upper third of the liver with the posterior ribs. In a study of 28 patients with blunt trauma who had abdominal CT and subsequent laparotomy, 10 had diaphragmatic rupture[33]; the dependent viscera sign was found in 100% of the hemidiaphragmatic ruptures on the left and 83% of those on the right.[33]

In most cases the diagnosis of traumatic hernia can be made on cross-sectional CT images. In a one study of 42 confirmed diaphragmatic injuries, CT showed the injuries in 57%, with higher accuracy for injuries on the left than the right.[36] Multiplanar reformatted images in the sagittal and coronal planes are probably better than cross-sectional images in demonstrating small diaphragmatic tears and hernias (see Figs. 78.14 and 78.15).[37,38]

An unusual complication of thoracoabdominal trauma associated with diaphragmatic rupture is thoracic splenosis. Splenosis is the autotransplantation of viable splenic tissue, most often after splenic rupture. Thoracic splenosis usually results from combined diaphragmatic and splenic injury and may develop in up to 18% of such cases; it is usually detected years after

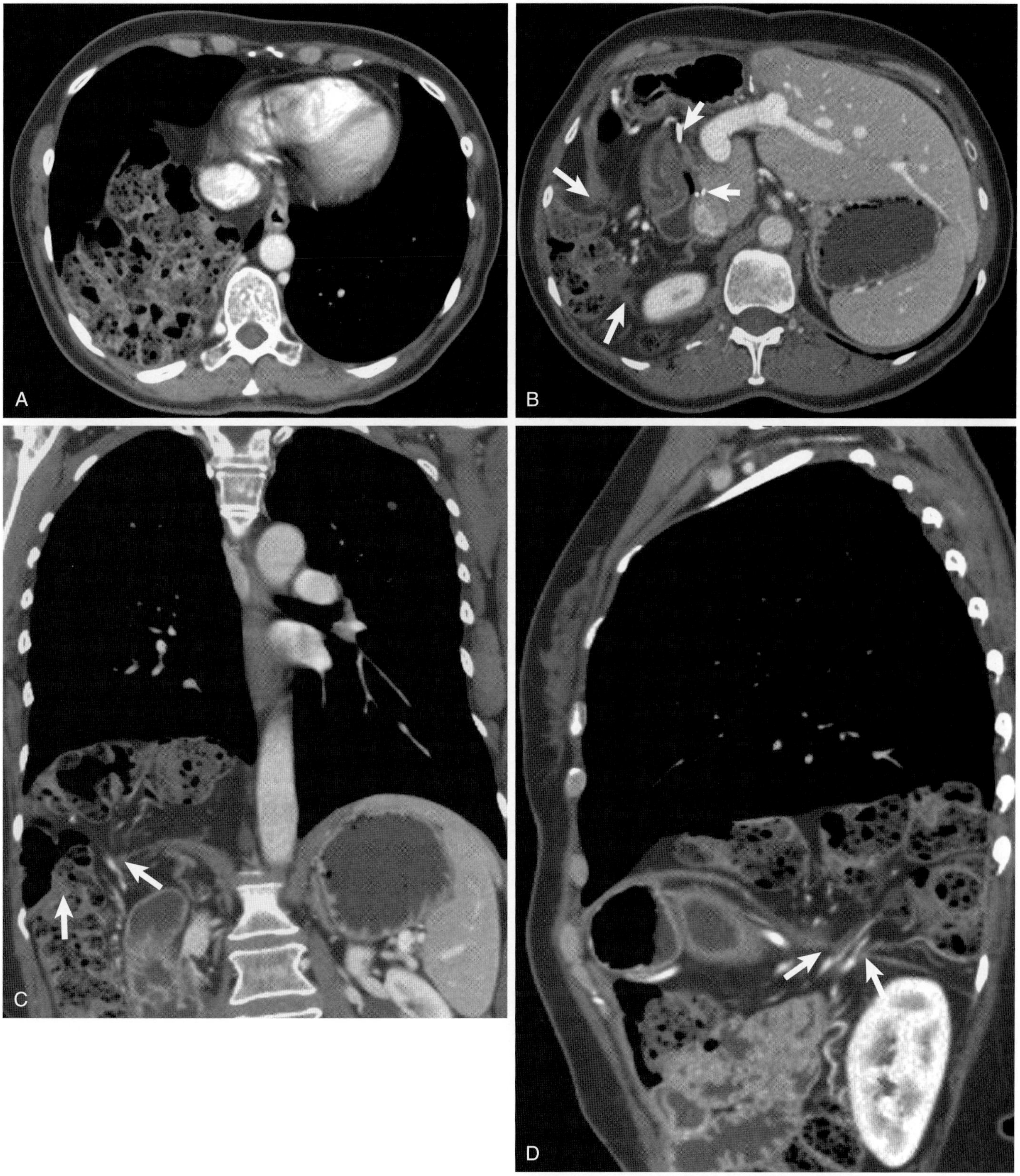

Fig. 78.15 Iatrogenic diaphragmatic hernia after partial hepatectomy for hepatoma. (A) Contrast-enhanced axial CT shows bowel loops and omentum in the right hemithorax. Note that the bowel loops contact the posterior ribs ("dependent viscera" sign). (B) Axial CT at the level of the liver shows surgical clips *(small arrows)*, discontinuity of the right hemidiaphragm *(large arrows)*, and intrathoracic herniation of omentum and bowel. Coronal (C) and sagittal (D) CT better show the discontinuity of the right hemidiaphragm *(arrows)* and the herniated viscera.

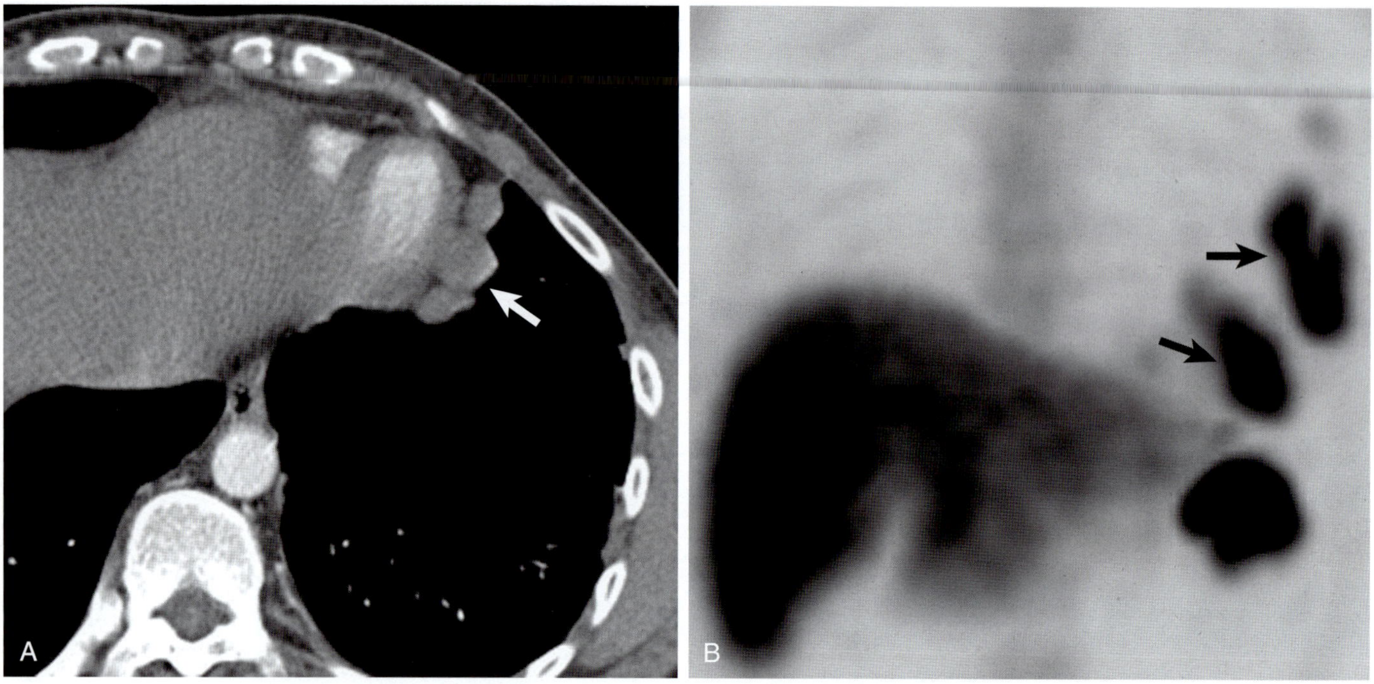

Fig. 78.16 Thoracic splenosis after remote gunshot injury. (A) Axial CT shows multiple nodules *(arrow)* in the anterior left lower pleural space. (B) Coronal radionuclide image obtained with heat-damaged red blood cells tagged with technetium-99m confirms that the pleural nodules *(arrows)* represent splenic tissue. The radiotracer accumulation below the left hemidiaphragm indicates abdominal splenosis, which often accompanies thoracic splenosis. *(Reproduced with permission from Walker CM, Takasugi JE, Chung JH, et al. Tumorlike conditions of the pleura.* Radiographics. *2012;32:971–985.)*

injury.[39,40] The splenic nodules may be solitary or multiple and are almost always located on left pleural surfaces and occasionally in subcutaneous tissues.[40] Radiographic and CT findings are nonspecific and include single or multiple pleural or paraspinal soft tissue nodules (Fig. 78.16).[41] The attenuation of the splenic implants is similar to that of the spleen. The diagnosis can be made with reticuloendothelial scintigraphic scans using indium-111–labeled platelets, technetium-99m (^{99m}Tc)-labeled sulfur colloid, ^{99m}Tc-labeled white blood cells, and ^{99m}Tc heat-damaged red blood cells.[42,43] ^{99m}Tc heat-damaged red blood cells are considered to be the most specific marker of splenic tissue. Another imaging technique is ferumoxide-enhanced MRI.[42] Ferumoxides are superparamagnetic iron oxides that are cleared by the reticuloendothelial system.[42]

MAGNETIC RESONANCE IMAGING

Diaphragmatic hernias can be diagnosed by MRI.[32] Although MRI is seldom used to assess hernia and is seldom used to assess acute chest injury, it can be used in stable patients or to clarify ambiguous findings on CT (Fig. 78.17).

KEY POINTS: DIAPHRAGMATIC HERNIAS

- Hiatal hernia
  - Prevalence increases with age; usually asymptomatic
  - Classified anatomically into types I–IV: type I (sliding) and type III (sliding + paraesophageal) are most common
- Bochdalek hernia
  - Congenital: herniation through pleuroperitoneal hiatus; incidence 1:2000 births; 75%–90% left-sided; associated with severe respiratory distress
  - Acquired: herniation through small diaphragmatic defect; found in 5%–10% of adults older than 40 years; prevalence increases with age; usually asymptomatic
- Morgagni hernia
  - Uncommon; associated with obesity, severe effort, or trauma
- Traumatic diaphragmatic hernia
  - Found in 1%–8% of patients with blunt chest trauma; most are on the left
  - Radiographic findings: irregularity of diaphragmatic contour; herniation of stomach or bowel; contralateral shift of mediastinum
  - CT findings: sharp discontinuity of the hemidiaphragm; herniation of omental fat or abdominal viscera; waist-like narrowing of herniated viscera (collar sign); contact between the stomach, bowel, spleen, or upper third of the liver and the posterior ribs (dependent viscera sign)

Neoplasms of the Diaphragm

Etiology, Prevalence, and Epidemiology

Primary neoplasms of the diaphragm are uncommon.[44,45] Most develop from the tendinous or anterior muscular portion. The most common benign tumor is lipoma; neural tumors, leiomyomas, hemangiomas, and other soft tissue tumors are rare.[46,47] Fat pads and herniated omental fat are common in the vicinity of the diaphragm; thus the diagnosis of lipoma requires demonstration of a true capsule.[48] Fibrosarcoma is the most common malignant tumor; other soft tissue sarcomas are rare.[48] Other nonneoplastic nodules or masses, such as lymphangioma and endometrioma (Fig. 78.18), are found occasionally.[44]

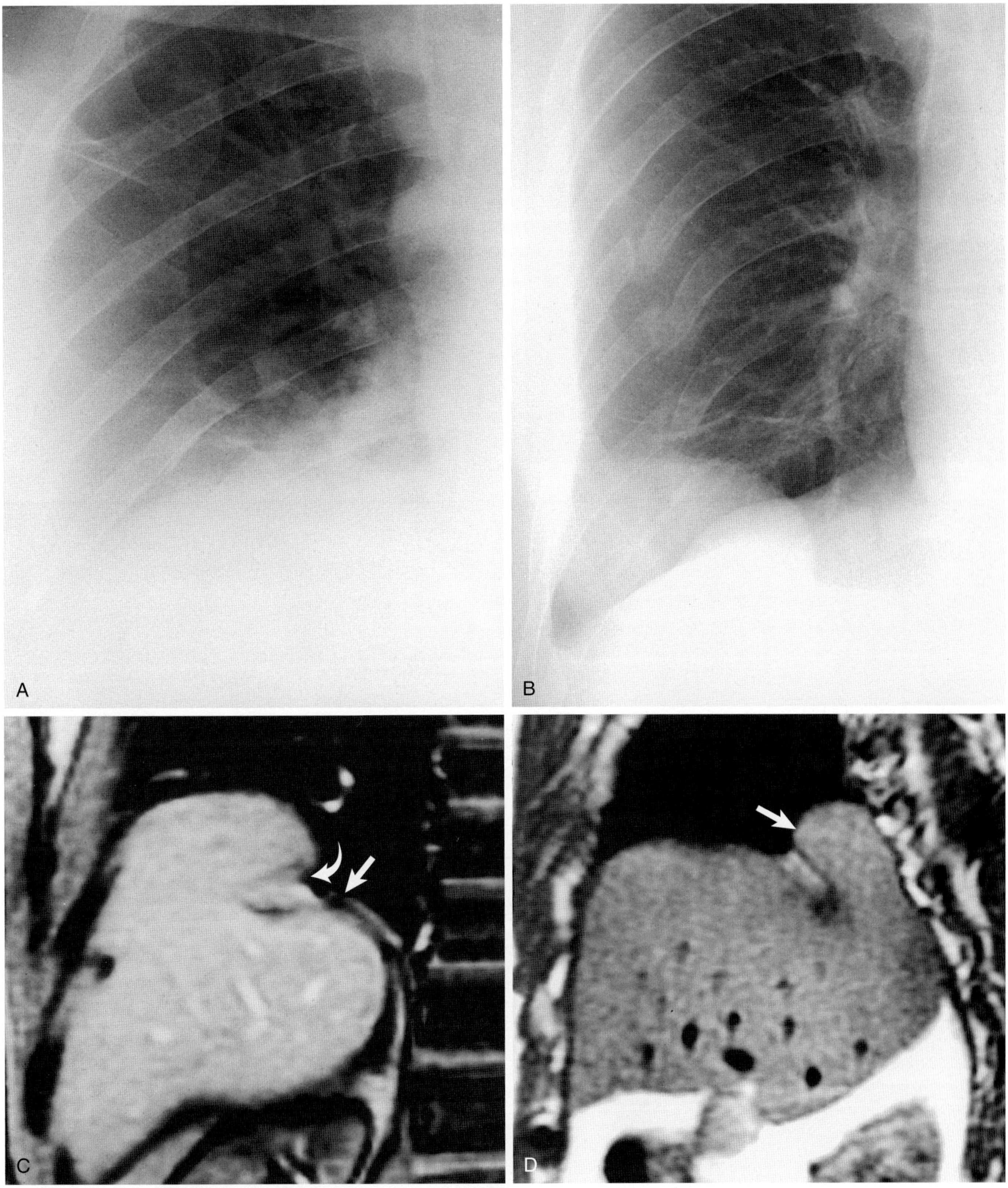

Fig. 78.17 Traumatic diaphragmatic hernia: magnetic resonance imaging (MRI) findings. (A) Anteroposterior radiograph after motor vehicle accident shows right rib fractures, pleural effusion, and apparent elevation of the right hemidiaphragm. The patient recovered and was discharged without further evaluation. Eleven months later and after 4 months of right upper quadrant pain, posteroanterior radiograph (B) shows interval development of a mushroom-like mass in the right lower hemithorax. Old rib fractures and blunting of the right hemidiaphragm are evident. (C) Coronal spin-echo T1-weighted MRI shows discontinuity of the right hemidiaphragm *(straight arrow)* and waist-like constriction of the liver *(curved arrow)* as it traverses the diaphragmatic tear. (D) Sagittal MRI shows the posterior location of the herniated liver *(arrow)*. *(From Müller NL, Fraser RS, Colman NC, Paré PD.* Radiologic Diagnosis of Diseases of the Chest. *Philadelphia: WB Saunders; 2001.)*

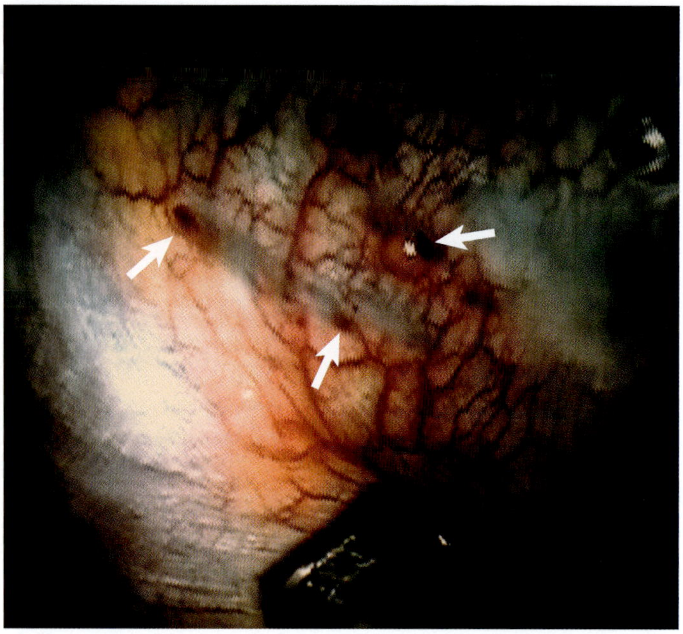

Fig. 78.18 Endometrial implants on the right hemidiaphragm causing recurrent catamenial pneumothorax. Image obtained at video-assisted thoracoscopic surgery shows round brown endometrial implants *(arrows)* on the right hemidiaphragm. *(Reproduced with permission from Walker CM, Takasugi JE, Chung JH, et al. Tumorlike conditions of the pleura.* Radiographics. *2012;32:971–985.)*

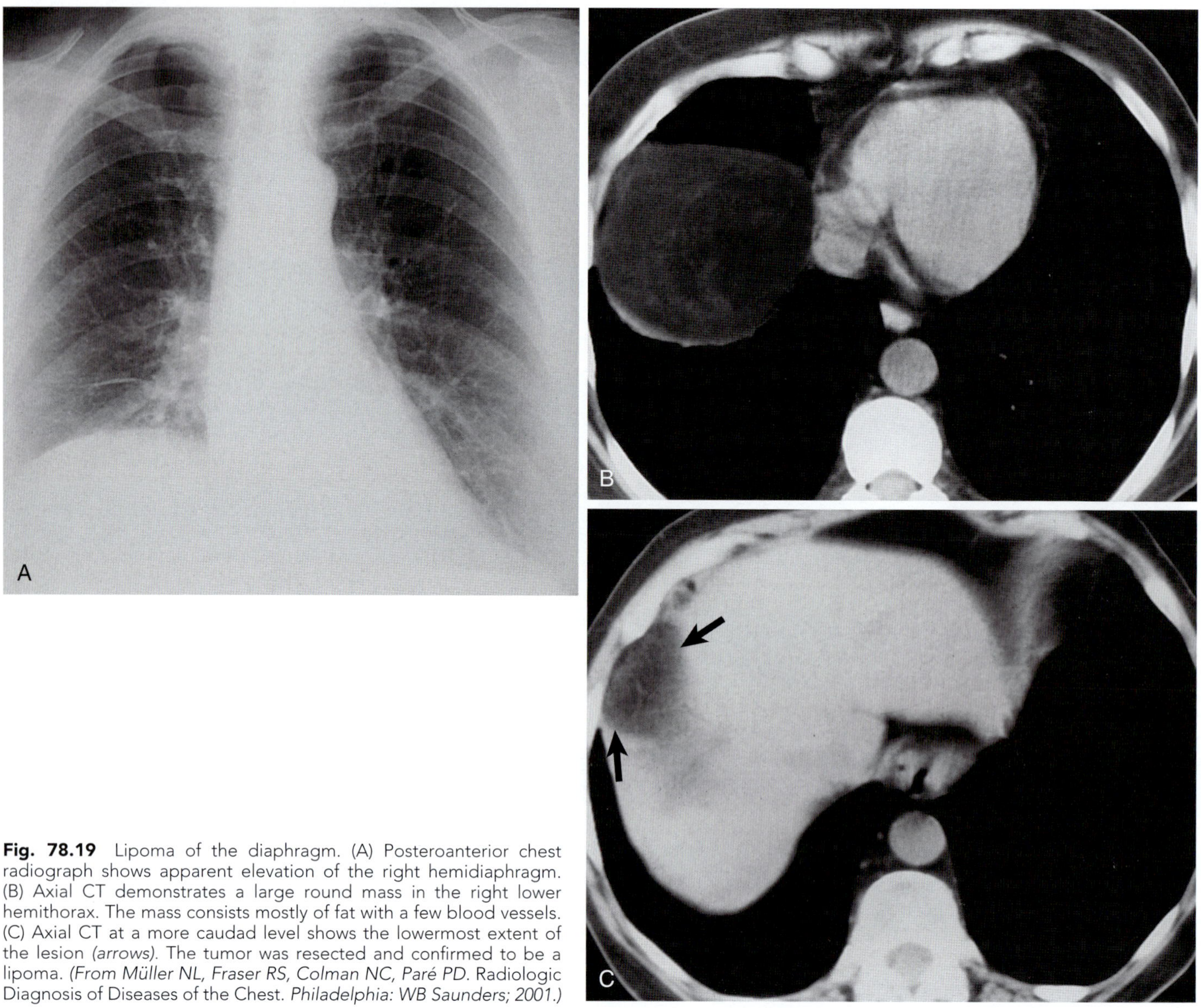

Fig. 78.19 Lipoma of the diaphragm. (A) Posteroanterior chest radiograph shows apparent elevation of the right hemidiaphragm. (B) Axial CT demonstrates a large round mass in the right lower hemithorax. The mass consists mostly of fat with a few blood vessels. (C) Axial CT at a more caudad level shows the lowermost extent of the lesion *(arrows)*. The tumor was resected and confirmed to be a lipoma. *(From Müller NL, Fraser RS, Colman NC, Paré PD.* Radiologic Diagnosis of Diseases of the Chest. *Philadelphia: WB Saunders; 2001.)*

Metastatic neoplasm of the diaphragm usually results from direct extension from the basal pleura in cases of lung cancer or mesothelioma. However, lymphoma or any neoplasm that metastasizes to the pleura or that involves the basal lung, the liver, or the subphrenic peritoneum can spread to the diaphragm.

Clinical Presentation

Benign neoplasms typically cause no symptoms unless they are large enough to cause shortness of breath or respiratory failure.[49] Patients with primary malignancies may experience epigastric or chest pain, cough, dyspnea, or gastrointestinal discomfort.[45]

Manifestations of Neoplasms

RADIOGRAPHY

Most diaphragmatic tumors manifest radiographically as smooth or lobulated soft tissue masses indenting or protruding into the inferior portion of the lung. If the tumor involves enough of the hemidiaphragm, it may simulate diaphragmatic elevation; associated pleural effusion is common.

COMPUTED TOMOGRAPHY

CT is the easiest way to show a diaphragmatic mass (Fig. 78.19).[48] When the tumor is large, it may not be clear whether it originates in the diaphragm, pleura, lung, or liver.[48] A diaphragmatic lipoma appears as a homogeneous mass with fat attenuation (≈100 Hounsfield units) on CT.[22] Other primary and metastatic diaphragmatic tumors manifest on CT as nonspecific masses with soft tissue attenuation.

SUGGESTED READINGS

Desir A, Ghaye B. CT of blunt diaphragmatic rupture. *Radiographics.* 2012;32(2):477–498.

McCool FD, Tzelepis GE. Dysfunction of the diaphragm. *N Engl J Med.* 2012;366(10):932–942.

Nason LK, Walker CM, McNeeley MF, Burivong W, Fligner CL, Godwin JD. Imaging of the diaphragm: anatomy and function. *Radiographics.* 2012;32(2):E51–E70.

Walker CM, Takasugi JE, Chung JH, Reddy GP, Done SL, Pipavath SN, Schmidt RA, Godwin JD 2nd. Tumorlike conditions of the pleura. *Radiographics.* 2012;32(4):971–985.

The full reference list for this chapter is available at ExpertConsult.com.

79 Chest Wall

TOMÁS FRANQUET | JAUME LLAUGER

The chest wall is a complex anatomic structure composed of muscles, bones, joints, and soft tissues that make up the area of the body between the neck and the abdomen. Pathologic processes that may involve the chest wall include congenital and developmental anomalies, trauma, inflammatory and infectious diseases, and soft tissue and bone tumors.[1] Because the clinical presentation of patients with chest wall disorders is diverse and nonspecific, imaging plays a key role in establishing the diagnosis. Diseases that affect the chest wall are difficult to evaluate with radiography.[2] The introduction of cross-sectional imaging techniques, including computed tomography (CT) and magnetic resonance imaging (MRI), has enabled precise localization of chest wall lesions and, in some cases, definitive diagnosis.[3–5] ^{18}F-fluorodeoxyglucose (FDG)–positron emission tomography (PET)-CT provides information regarding the metabolic status of chest wall masses but adds only limited additional diagnostic information.[2]

KEY POINTS: CHEST WALL

- It is formed by bones, joints, and soft tissues located between the neck and the abdomen.
- It is involved in developmental anomalies, trauma, inflammatory diseases, and neoplasms.
- Chest wall tumors may originate in the skeleton or soft tissues.

Normal Variants, Congenital Diseases, and Chest Wall Deformities

Congenital rib anomalies may be found on 1% to 2% of chest radiographs. Most of these anomalies are isolated findings that occur sporadically and lack clinical significance.[6] Representative examples include, among others, cervical rib, bifid or forked rib, fused ribs, hypoplastic rib, pseudoarthrosis of the first rib, and intrathoracic rib.

A cervical rib is a supernumerary rib that usually arises from the seventh cervical vertebra (Fig. 79.1).[7] It is present in about 0.5% of the general population and is bilateral and often asymmetric in 45% to 70% of cases. When unilateral, it is generally on the right. Most cervical ribs are detected incidentally, may articulate with the superior aspect of the first rib, and are asymptomatic. In less than 10% of patients, cervical ribs may result in thoracic outlet syndrome, which consists of symptoms resulting from pressure on nerves and vessels at the thoracic inlet, including paresthesias, pain, muscular atrophy, and claudication in the ipsilateral limb. Other anatomic causes of thoracic outlet syndrome include an abnormal scalene muscle, congenital fibromuscular bands, and an elongated transverse process of the seventh cervical vertebra.[8,9]

Rib notching usually affects the lower margin of one or more ribs. The most common and important cause is coarctation of the thoracic aorta. The notches result from rib erosion by dilated intercostal arteries taking part in collateral arterial flow. These arteries may become extremely tortuous and may extend to and erode the superior aspects of contiguous ribs. Rib notching secondary to coarctation of the aorta seldom is seen in patients before age 6 to 7 years and usually is not well developed until the early teens. Focal rib notching also may be due to an intercostal nerve tumor (Fig. 79.2).

KEY POINTS: THORACIC OUTLET SYNDROME

- Clinical signs: pain in the neck and shoulder area, paresthesias, and weakness in the arm
- Pathogenesis: compression of nerves (90%) and/or vessels at the superior thoracic aperture
- Causes: trauma, postural distortions, and congenital conditions (cervical rib, scalene triangle, congenital fibromuscular bands)
- Differential diagnosis: carpal tunnel syndrome, spinal disorders with nerve root compression, cord tumors, brachial plexopathy, and neuromuscular disorders
- Magnetic resonance angiography: useful, noninvasive, and safe method for evaluating the subclavian vessels if vascular compression is suspected

POLAND SYNDROME

Poland syndrome is a rare autosomal-recessive condition classically consisting of the combination of unilateral partial or complete absence of the pectoralis major muscle and an ipsilateral hypoplastic hand with simple syndactyly and short fingers. The incidence has been estimated at between 1 : 30,000 and 1 : 80,000 of live births. Bilateral involvement is rare. It is three times more common in boys than in girls and involves the right side in 75% of patients. Associated conditions include osseous dysostoses affecting the ipsilateral hand (brachymesophalangy with syndactyly, biphalangy, ectrodactyly), pectus excavatum, anomalies of the upper limb, and other anomalies of the anterior chest wall (absence of the pectoralis minor muscle, hypoplasia of latissimus dorsi and serratus anterior, hypoplasia or aplasia of nipple and breast, lung herniation, and hypoplasia of hemithorax and ribs). Increased incidences of leukemia, non-Hodgkin lymphoma, lung cancer, and breast cancer have been reported in these patients.

Chest radiography usually shows unilateral hyperlucency with absence of the normal axillary fold on the affected side. Rib deformities are found occasionally (Fig. 79.3). The diagnosis usually can be established on CT or MRI, both of which show absence or hypoplasia of pectoral girdle musculature (see Fig. 79.3).[10] With these techniques, absence of the sternocostal

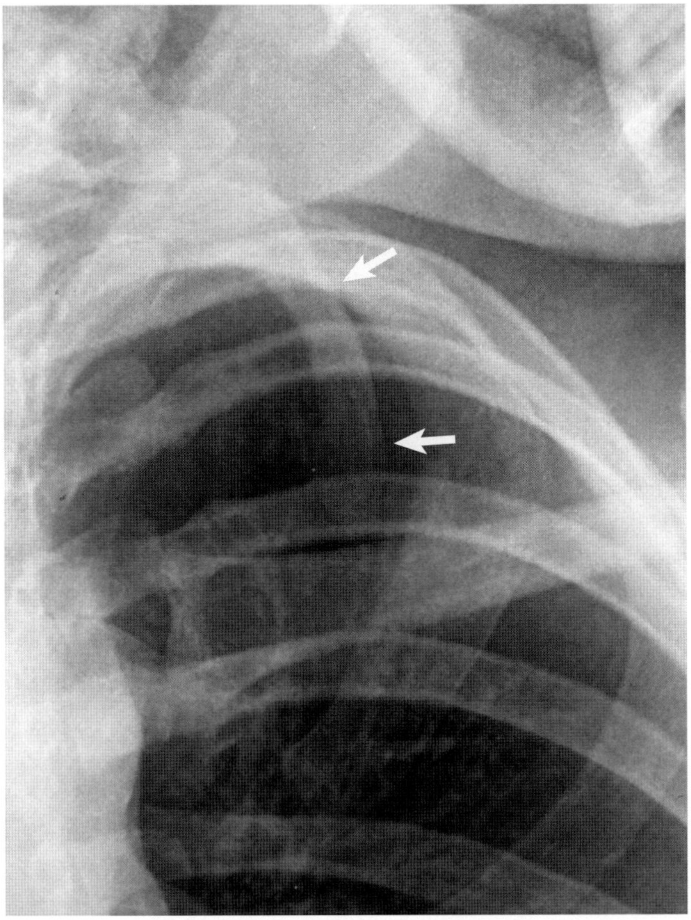

Fig. 79.1 Cervical rib. Close-up view from chest radiograph shows a supernumerary bone *(arrows)* arising from the left side of the seventh cervical vertebra.

head of the pectoralis major muscle is always noted, and associated chest wall defects are best depicted.[11]

Differential diagnosis of a diffuse hyperlucent hemithorax on chest radiograph includes radiographic artifact, patient rotation, extrapulmonary conditions (Poland syndrome, previous mastectomy, contralateral pleural effusion, and contralateral soft tissue thickening), pneumothorax, and pulmonary conditions (Swyer-James-MacLeod syndrome, overinflation, and unilateral diminished pulmonary blood flow owing to vascular abnormality or partial bronchial obstruction).

KEY POINTS: POLAND SYNDROME

Autosomal-recessive disorder characterized by:
- Unilateral partial or complete absence of pectoralis major muscle.
- Common association with other anomalies of chest wall or ipsilateral upper limb.
- Increased radiolucency of one hemithorax on posteroanterior chest radiography.
- Computed tomography and magnetic resonance imaging evaluation may help reconstructive surgical planning.

PECTUS EXCAVATUM

Pectus excavatum, also known as funnel chest, consists of depression of the anterior chest wall of variable severity that may be mild, moderate, or severe. It is the most common chest wall deformity, occurring in approximately 1 in 1000 live births with a strong male predominance (3–5 : 1). Approximately 90% of patients with developmental chest wall disorders have pectus excavatum.[12,13] A family history is known in about 35% to 45% of cases. Pectus excavatum is generally present at birth, or it arises shortly thereafter. It is often progressive, and the depth of sternal depression increases as the patient grows, especially during puberty. Pectus excavatum can be associated with other congenital abnormalities, including scoliosis (15%), osteogenesis imperfecta, Ehlers-Danlos syndrome, diaphragmatic abnormalities, and mitral valve prolapse (20%–60%). In 2% of patients it is associated with congenital cardiac anomalies. Approximately 2% of patients with this condition have Marfan syndrome; these patients typically have the most severe forms of pectus excavatum.

Patients with pectus excavatum are usually asymptomatic or present with chest or back pain, frequently exacerbated by exercise. Physical examination reveals sternal depression so that ribs protrude more anteriorly than the sternum.

On posteroanterior chest radiography, pectus excavatum causes obscuration of the right heart border. The heart is displaced to the left and rotated, and a spurious cardiomegaly may be noted. On lateral chest radiography a depression and deformity of the lower portion of the sternum may be noted (Fig. 79.4).[14] The severity of the defect can be best quantified with CT or MRI. A "pectus or Haller index" (transverse thoracic diameter/anteroposterior thoracic diameter) higher than 3.25 usually requires surgical correction.[15,16]

The differential diagnosis of obscuration of the right heart border on posteroanterior chest radiography includes right middle lobe atelectasis, right middle lobe pneumonia, large mediastinal fat pad, and Morgagni hernia. In all these conditions the lateral radiograph shows a normal sternum.

PECTUS CARINATUM

Pectus carinatum, also known as pigeon breast, is a protrusion deformity of the anterior chest wall consisting of anterior displacement of the sternum. It may involve the body of the sternum or, more rarely, the manubrium (chondromanubrial prominence). Pectus carinatum is less frequent than pectus excavatum (1 : 5) and accounts for 5% to 7% of all chest wall deformities. It occurs more frequently in men than women (4 : 1); a family history of chest wall deformities is present in about 25% of cases.

Patients with pectus carinatum are usually asymptomatic. Exertional dyspnea or cardiac arrhythmias may occur. The diagnosis is established on the basis of physical examination. Lateral chest radiography shows anterior prominence of the sternum.

KYPHOSCOLIOSIS

Kyphoscoliosis is an abnormal posterior (kyphosis) and lateral (scoliosis) curvature of the thoracic spine. Approximately 80% of cases are idiopathic. Congenital causes include, among others, type 1 neurofibromatosis, hemivertebra, Friedreich ataxia, muscular dystrophy, Morquio syndrome, and Marfan syndrome. The paralytic group includes spinal deformities secondary to poliomyelitis, muscular dystrophy, or cerebral palsy.

Severe forms of kyphoscoliosis cause decreased compliance of the lung and chest wall and result in restrictive lung disease with hypoventilation, hypoxic vasoconstriction, and eventually

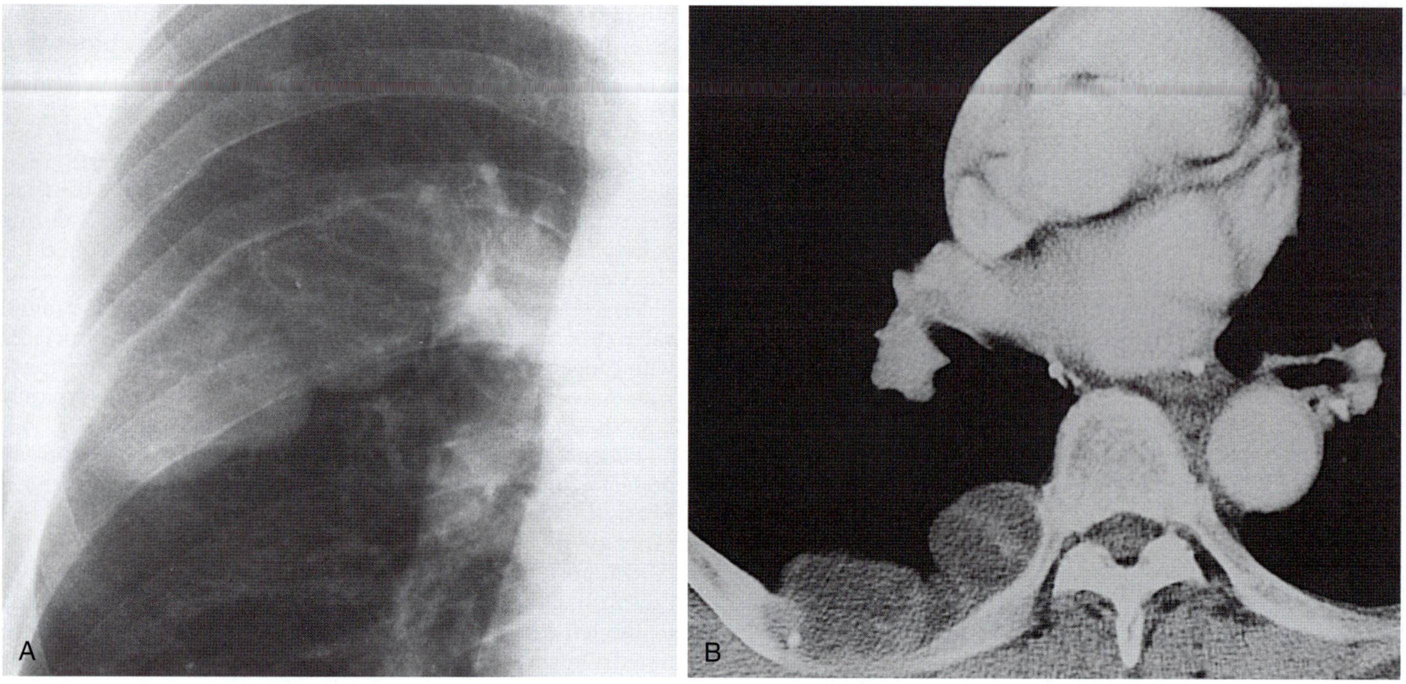

Fig. 79.2 Intercostal neurilemoma. (A) Close-up view of right chest from anteroposterior chest radiograph shows a soft tissue tumor adjacent to and parallel to the right seventh rib. Also note notching and sclerosis of the undersurface of the rib and widening of the interspace between the seventh and the eighth ribs. (B) Contrast-enhanced CT scan shows the tumor to have heterogeneous attenuation and to contain cystic areas. Note erosion of the posterior seventh rib. *(Case courtesy Dr. Eun-Young Kang, Department of Radiology, Korea University Guro Hospital, Seoul, South Korea; from Müller NL, Fraser RS, Colman NC, et al.* Radiologic Diagnosis of Diseases of the Chest. *Philadelphia: Saunders; 2001.)*

pulmonary hypertension, cor pulmonale, and respiratory failure. In cases of severe kyphoscoliosis the chest radiograph is difficult to evaluate because of rotation of the thorax and heart. The scoliotic curvature is usually convex to the right. About 60% of patients with type 1 neurofibromatosis have kyphoscoliosis, usually involving a short segment of the lower thoracic spine.

Blunt Chest Trauma

Blunt chest trauma most commonly results from high-energy mechanisms, such as motor vehicle accidents, motorcycle collisions, and falls.[17–19] Motor vehicle collisions are responsible for 80% of cases of blunt chest trauma and are associated with a wide range of injuries, many of which are life threatening (Fig. 79.5). Rib fracture is the most common thoracic injury, present in 10% of all blunt chest traumas and almost 40% of patients who sustain severe nonpenetrating trauma.[20] Posteroanterior chest radiography should be the initial, and often the only, imaging study in patients with suspected rib fracture after minor trauma.[20] In the workup of patients with high-mechanism blunt trauma, CT is more sensitive than radiography and may demonstrate traumatic injuries in patients with "normal" chest radiographs.[21,22] Blunt chest trauma is discussed in further detail in Chapter 67.

Inflammatory and Infectious Diseases

There are a wide variety of inflammatory and infectious diseases that can affect the chest wall. These lesions range from inflammatory conditions of uncertain etiology to acute or chronic infections involving bone, joints, or soft tissues. Infections include pyogenic, tuberculous, fungal, and some other unusual infections. The most common infections are those that follow median sternotomy. Infections and hematomas may affect the presternal (cellulitis, sinus tracts, abscess), sternal (osteomyelitis), or retrosternal (mediastinitis, abscess) compartments. Although radiography remains the first imaging method in suspected cases of chest wall infection, ultrasound, CT, and MRI are all useful and complementary; bone destruction is more accurately detected with CT, whereas soft tissue involvement is better visualized with ultrasound and MRI. Infections in the presternal or retrosternal compartments manifest as stranding, sinus tracts, soft tissue thickening with gas bubbles, or fluid collections with peripheral enhancement (abscess). Sternal osteomyelitis must be suspected when soft tissue anomalies are associated with bone destruction, dehiscence, or severe demineralization (Fig. 79.6).[23]

Primary chest wall soft tissue infections are rare and can occur either by direct inoculation (puncture) or by contiguous spread from other areas and occasionally by hematogenous spread of infection.[24] Soft tissue infections may be classified as necrotizing fasciitis, when they involve the subcutaneous fat and superficial fascia, and pyomyositis, if they involve the muscles alone.[25]

Necrotizing fasciitis is a rapidly spreading infection of the subcutaneous tissue characterized by spontaneous necrosis and gas formation. CT scans provide superior information about the true extent of disease and associated fluid collections, thus facilitating correct diagnosis and treatment (Fig. 79.7).[26]

Empyema necessitatis results from leakage of empyema through the parietal pleura with discharge of its contents into the

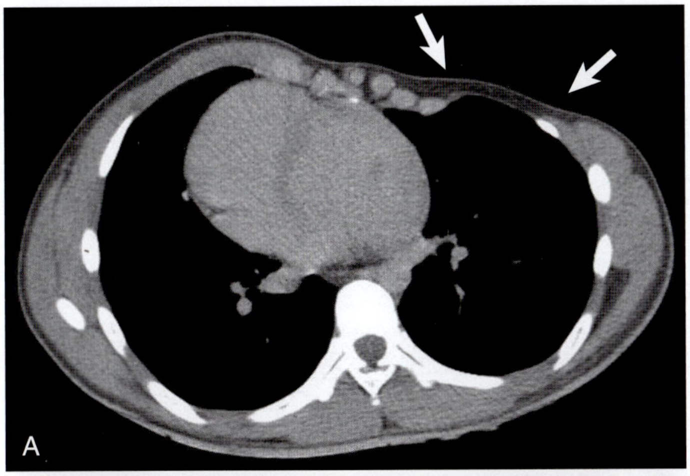

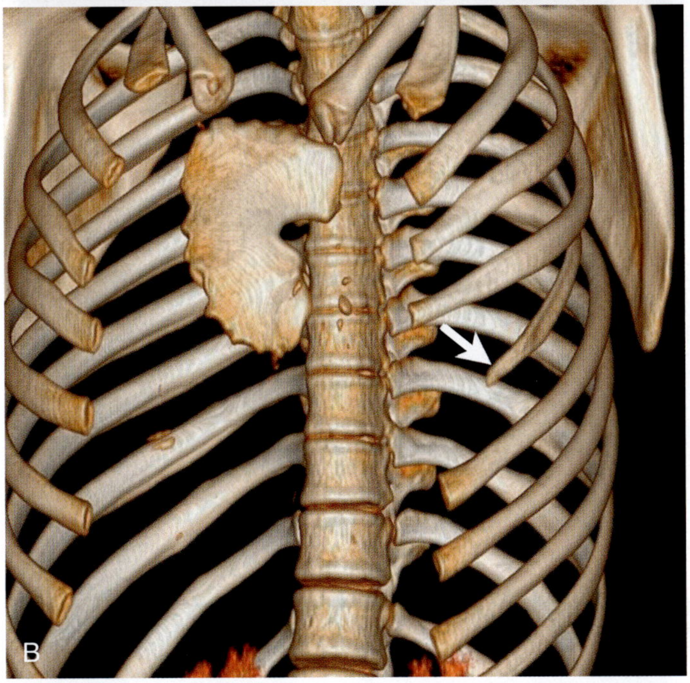

Fig. 79.3 Poland syndrome. (A) CT scan shows complete absence of the left pectoralis major muscle *(arrows)*. (B) Volume-rendering three-dimensional reconstruction shows hypoplastic rib *(arrow)* in the ipsilateral hemithorax.

subcutaneous tissues of the chest wall (Fig. 79.8). Although tuberculosis is the most commonly reported etiology, other pathogens, such as *Actinomyces* spp., *Staphylococcus aureus, Mycobacterium avium-intracellulare,* and *Aspergillus fumigatus,* have also been described.[27]

SAPHO SYNDROME

SAPHO syndrome (synovitis, acne, palmoplantar pustulosis, hyperostosis, and osteitis)[28] is a rare chronic autoimmune disease with hidradenitis suppurativa and severe acne that is sometimes associated with unusual noninfectious skeletal conditions.[29] SAPHO syndrome occurs with equal frequency in men and women and has been reported in patients of all ages but mainly affects young and middle-aged adults. The clinical manifestations of SAPHO syndrome vary. Osteoarticular lesions cause pain and soft tissue swelling and can occur without associated skin lesions.

The most common site of the lesions is the sternocostoclavicular region, involved in 70% to 90% of patients.[30] Imaging manifestations typically include hyperostosis and osteosclerosis with narrowing or ankylosis of the joint space (Fig. 79.9). Destructive changes, including osteolytic areas and erosions, may also be noted. Less frequently, involvement of spine, sacroiliac joint, or long tubular bones may be noted. Differential diagnosis includes osteomyelitis, spondylitis, osteosarcoma, Ewing sarcoma, Paget disease, metastasis, and avascular necrosis of bone.

KEY POINTS: SAPHO SYNDROME

Synovitis, acne, pustulosis, hyperostosis, and osteitis:

- Unknown etiology.
- Hyperostosis and osteosclerosis involving sternocostoclavicular region.
- Spine and appendicular skeleton may also be involved.
- Skin lesions may be absent, precede, or follow bone lesions.

PAGET DISEASE

Paget disease (PD), or osteitis deformans, is a chronic benign metabolic bone disease of unknown etiology that affects approximately 3% to 4% of the population older than 40 years. PD exhibits a predilection for the axial skeleton, but any bone may be affected.[31] It may affect a single bone (monostotic disease) or many bones (polyostotic forms). Monostotic PD disease is usually an incidental finding on radiographs obtained for unrelated purposes. The spine is the second most common site of involvement with PD (29%–57% of cases), after the pelvis (30%–75%).[32] Involvement of the ribs (1%–4%), scapula, or clavicle is uncommon. Sarcomatous degeneration of PD disease of the spine or the rib into osteosarcoma has been reported.[33]

Radiographs in PD disease are frequently sufficiently characteristic for diagnosis. It manifests as areas of enlargement of the bone with a thickened, coarsened trabecular pattern (Fig. 79.10).[34] Technetium-99m–labeled bisphosphonate tracer is more sensitive than radiography for the identification of PD lesions.[34] The differential diagnosis of a sclerotic rib includes chronic osteomyelitis, SAPHO syndrome, Paget disease, osteochondroma, fibrous dysplasia, and sclerotic metastases.

Chest Wall Tumors

Chest wall tumors are uncommon lesions that represent approximately 5% of all thoracic malignancies.[35,36] They may arise from any of the chest wall tissues—bone, cartilage, muscle, fat, fibrous connective tissue, nerves, and vessels (blood or lymphatic).[35,37] It is often difficult to make an accurate presurgical diagnosis and differentiate benign from malignant tumors. Although more than 20% of lesions are visible on chest radiography,[38] cross-sectional techniques, such as multidetector CT and MRI, are the imaging modalities of choice in the management of chest wall tumors.[5] A combination of clinical, radiologic, and histopathologic information is often necessary to establish the correct diagnosis.[5] In adults the most common benign chest wall tumors are lipoma and osteochondroma,[39] and the most common malignant chest wall tumor is undifferentiated pleomorphic sarcoma (formerly malignant fibrous histiocytoma). In children the most common primary chest wall malignancies are small round-cell tumors,

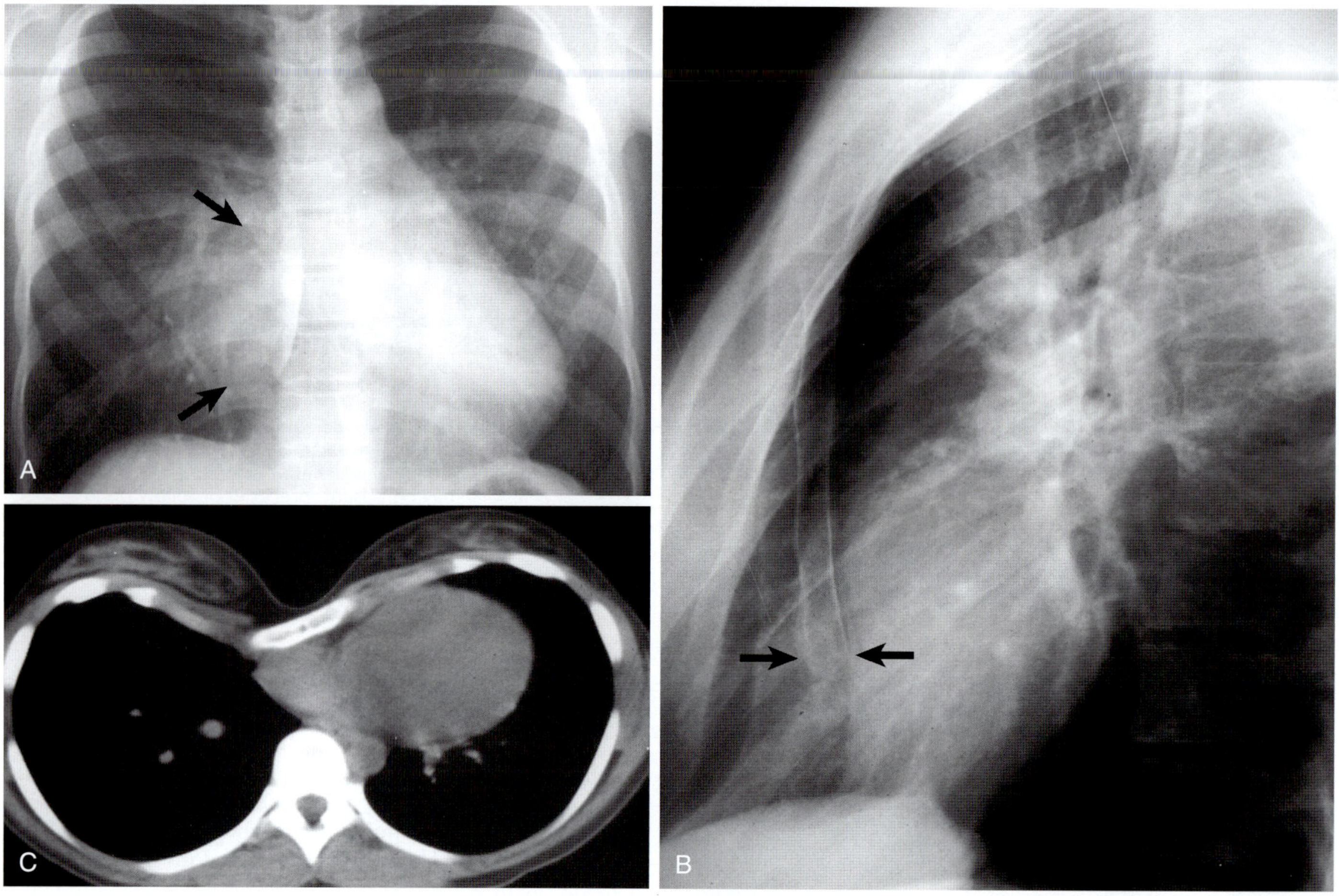

Fig. 79.4 Pectus excavatum. (A) Posteroanterior chest radiograph shows obscuration of the right heart border *(arrows)* and displacement of the heart to the left. (B) Lateral chest radiograph shows posterior displacement of the sternum *(arrows)*. (C) CT scan shows severe pectus excavatum with compression of the lungs and displacement of the heart to the left.

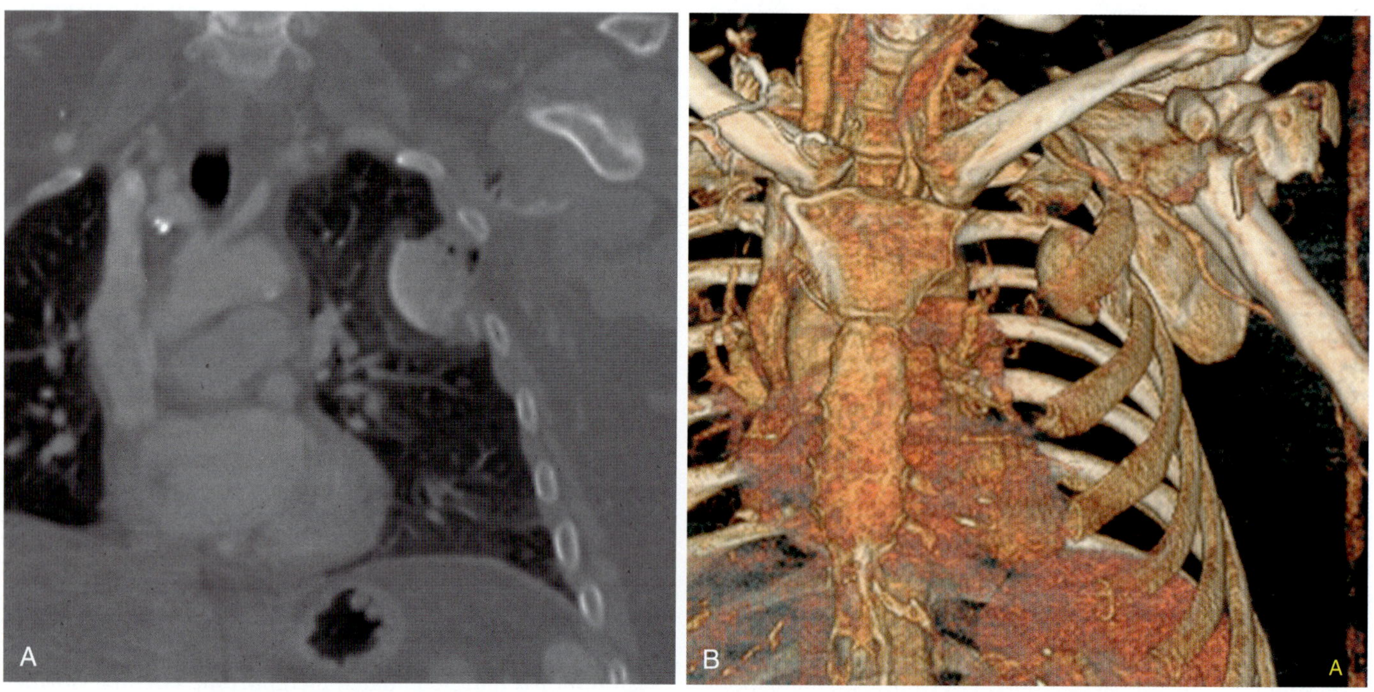

Fig. 79.5 Intrathoracic humeral head fracture and dislocation after chest wall trauma. Coronal chest CT scan (A) and three-dimensional reformatted image (B) show an intrathoracic dislocation of a portion of the fractured left humeral head.

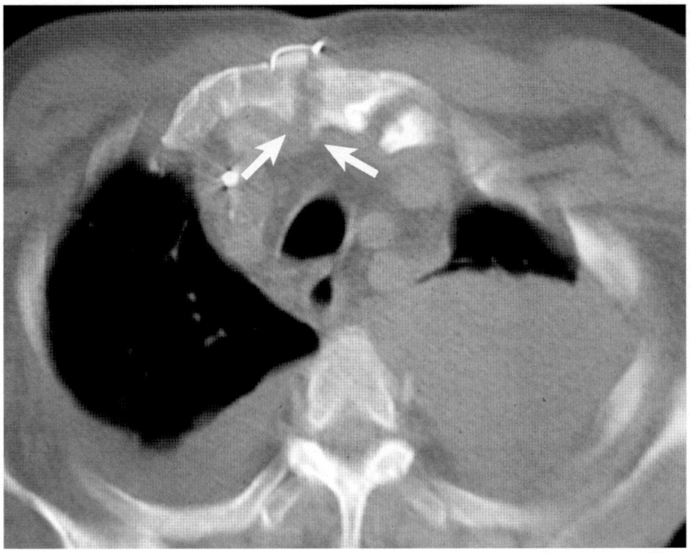

Fig. 79.6 Sternal dehiscence and infection from *Staphylococcus aureus* after coronary artery bypass graft surgery. CT image shows sternal dehiscence *(arrows)*. Bilateral pleural effusions are also noted.

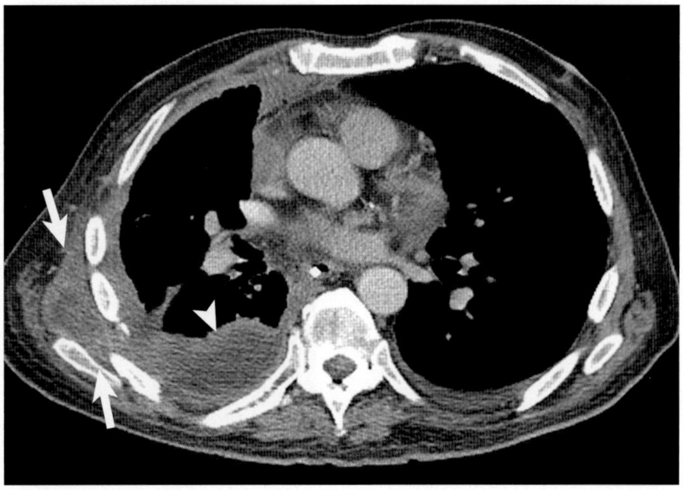

Fig. 79.8 Empyema necessitatis from tuberculosis. Contrast-enhanced CT scan shows a right pleural effusion *(arrowhead)* and a lentiform right chest wall lesion showing central low attenuation *(arrows)* consistent with focal tuberculous chest wall abscess.

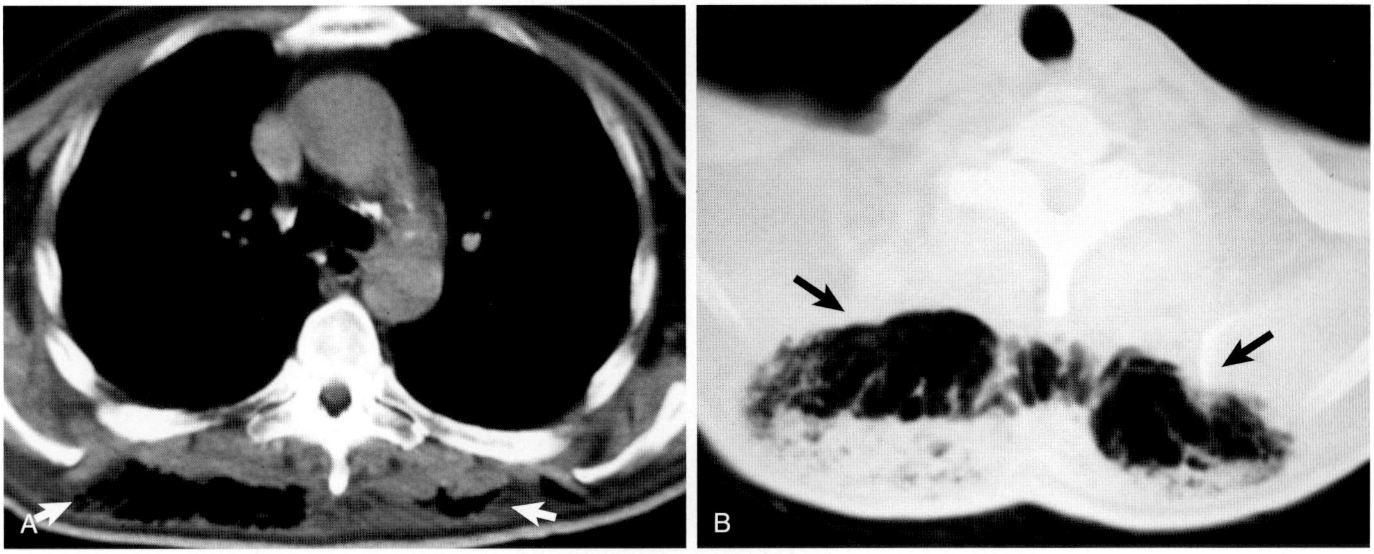

Fig. 79.7 Necrotizing fasciitis. (A) and (B) CT images show large gas collections *(arrows)* dissecting the fascial planes of the posterior chest wall.

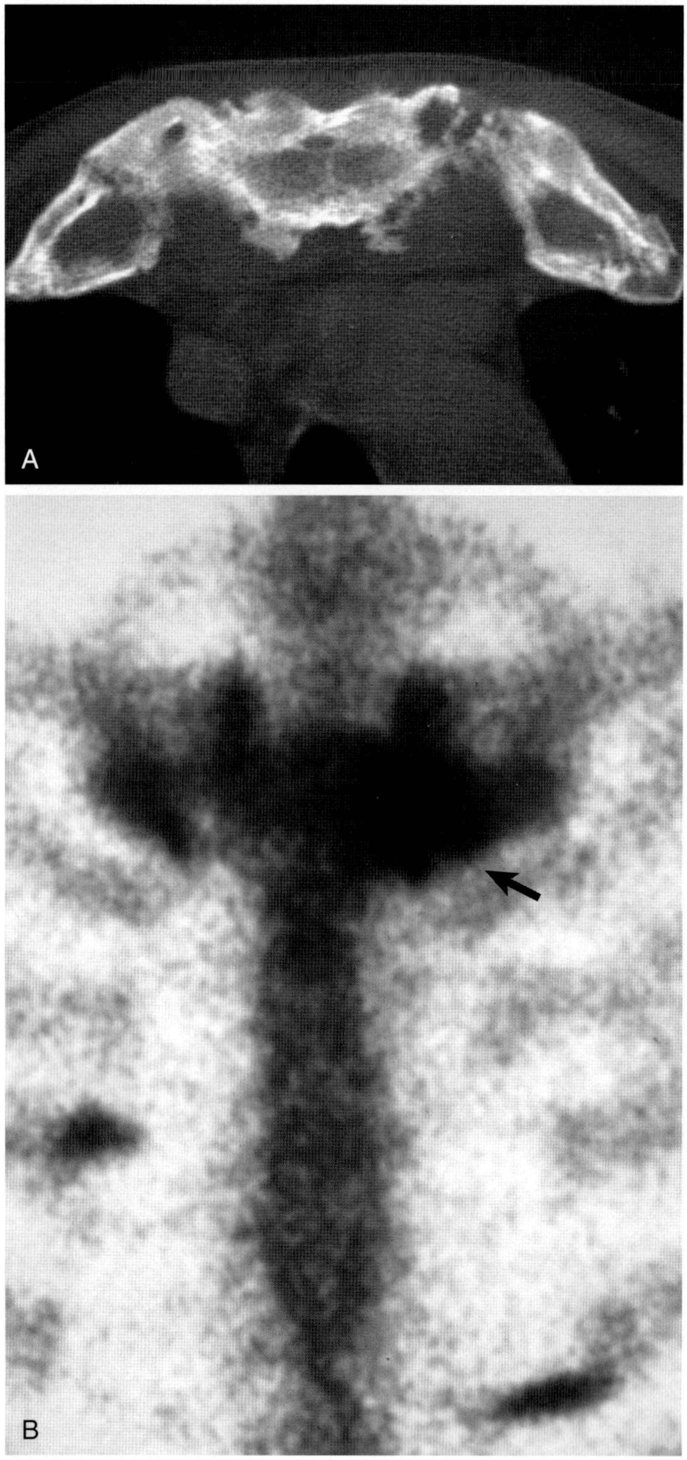

Fig. 79.9 SAPHO (synovitis, acne, palmoplantar pustulosis, hyperostosis, and osteitis) syndrome. (A) CT scan shows hyperostosis and osteosclerosis of the sternum and medial clavicles. (B) Technetium-99m bone scan shows marked tracer accumulation in the sternocostoclavicular region *(arrow)*.

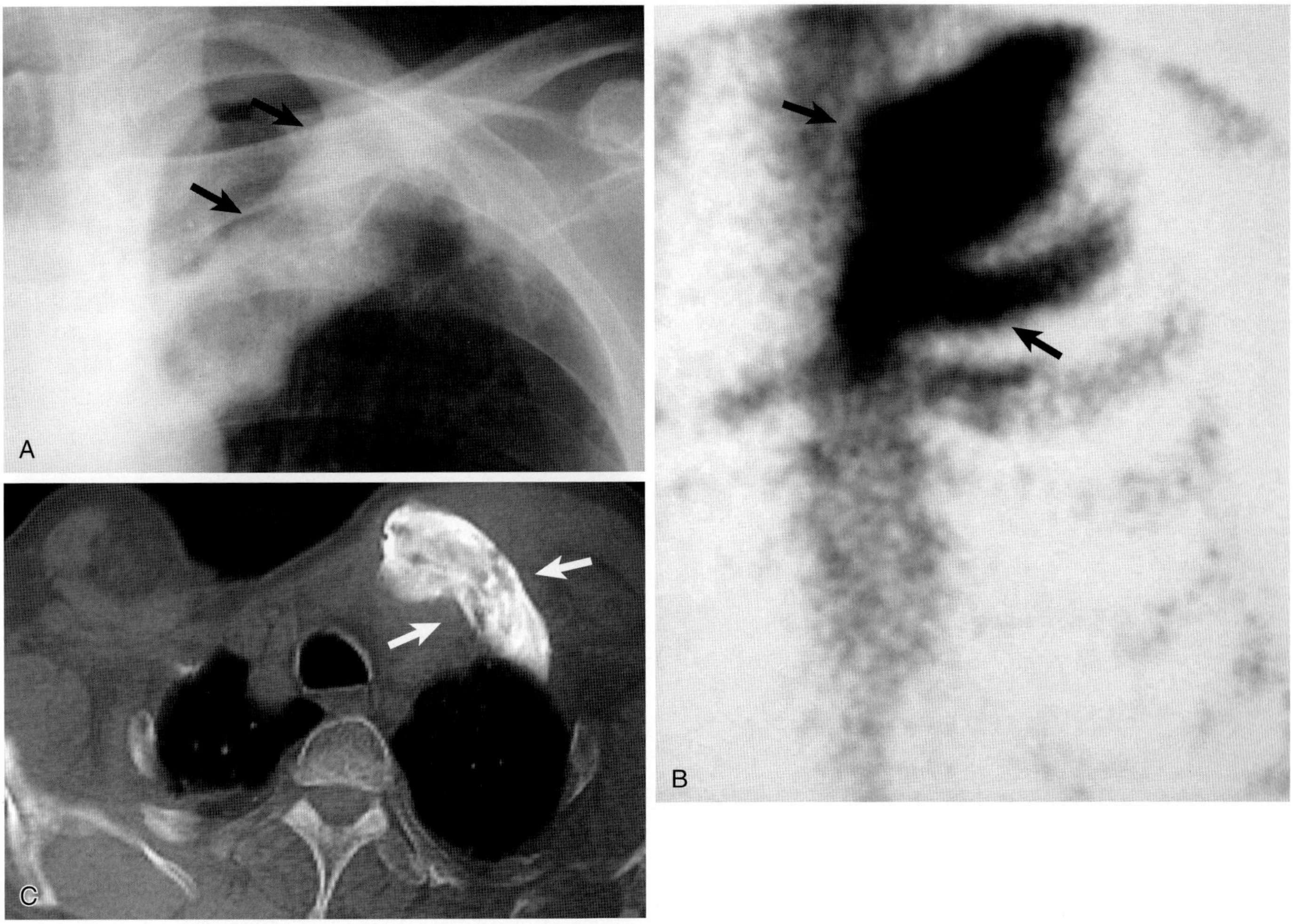

Fig. 79.10 Paget disease (PD) of the chest wall. (A) PD of the first rib. Close-up view from chest radiograph shows characteristic bone involvement, with enlargement of the rib, increased density, cortical thickening, and narrowing of the medullary cavity *(arrows)*. (B) PD of the left clavicle. Technetium-99m bone scan shows marked tracer accumulation in the left clavicle and adjacent rib *(arrows)*. (C) On corresponding CT scan obtained at the level of the upper thorax, the inner third of the clavicle is enlarged and shows trabecular coarsening and increased cortical thickness *(arrows)*.

including peripheral neuroectodermal tumors (PNETs) and rhabdomyosarcoma.[40]

BENIGN BONE TUMORS

Benign bone tumors of the chest wall are uncommon lesions less frequently encountered than malignant neoplasms.[39] They originate from blood vessels, nerves, bone, cartilage, or fat. Some of these tumors have characteristic radiographic features that allow a preoperative diagnosis. In other cases imaging plays a major role in tumor management, including staging, biopsy planning, and follow-up evaluation. Fibrous dysplasia and osteochondroma are the most common benign bone lesions of the chest wall. More unusual lesions include enchondroma, chondromyxoid fibroma, osteoid osteoma, aneurysmal bone cyst, and giant-cell tumor (Fig. 79.11).

Fibrous Dysplasia

Fibrous dysplasia is a nonhereditary skeletal anomaly in which the medullary bone is replaced by fibrous tissue during the period of skeletal growth. Fibrous dysplasia is the most common primary bone tumor of the chest wall, accounting for approximately 30% of all benign chest wall osseous lesions.[41] Virtually any bone in the body can be affected. There are two forms of the disease: monostotic (80% of cases) and polyostotic (20% of cases). Polyostotic involvement may be a part of McCune-Albright syndrome (fibrous dysplasia, patchy cutaneous pigmentation, and precocious puberty) or Mazabraud syndrome (fibrous dysplastic lesions in close proximity to soft tissue myxomas).[42]

Monostotic fibrous dysplasia occurs most frequently in the ribs (28%), femur (23%), tibia, or craniofacial bones (10%–25%). Pathologic fractures and bone deformities are common complications.

The usual radiologic appearance of fibrous dysplasia includes an osteolytic lesion in the medullary cavity of bone, with endosteal scalloping and possible bone expansion (Fig. 79.12). Periosteal reaction is typically absent. The lesion may be surrounded by a layer of thick sclerotic reactive bone (rind sign). Usually, the matrix of the lesion is smooth and relatively homogeneous; classically, this finding is described as a ground-glass appearance. Irregular

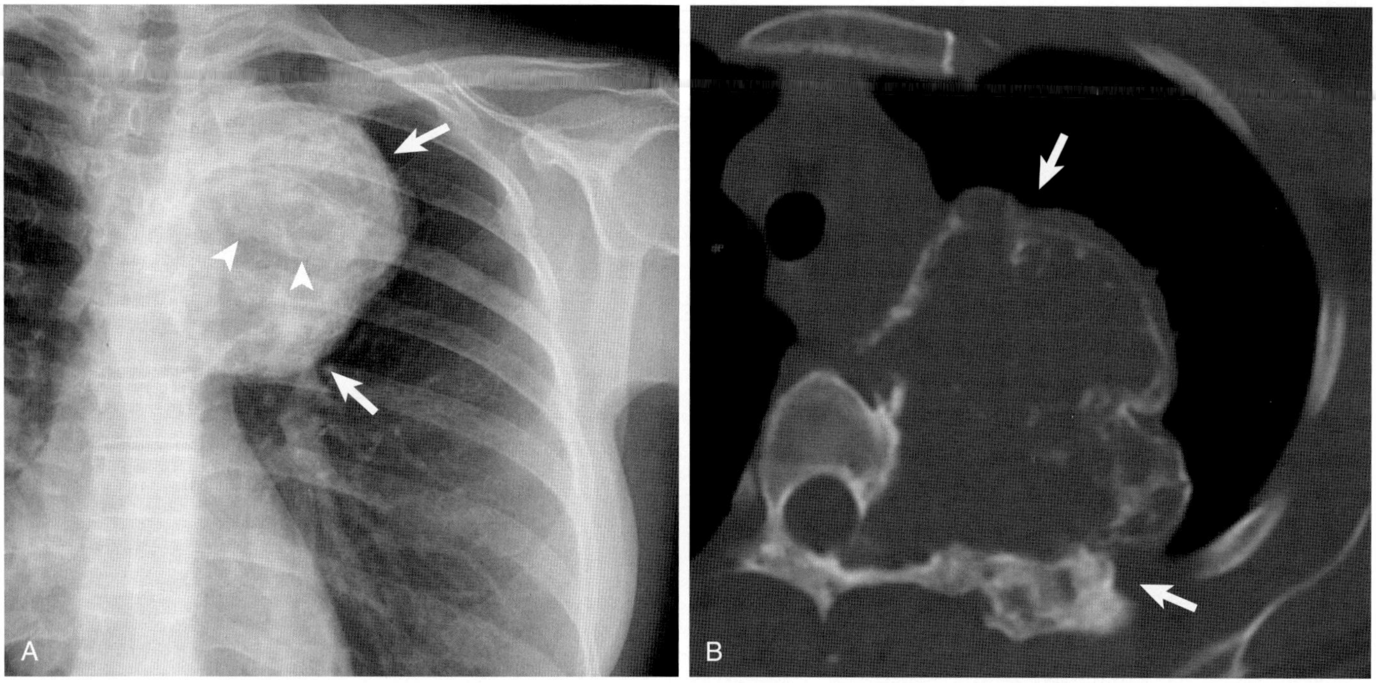

Fig. 79.11 Giant-cell tumor. (A) Close-up view from chest radiograph shows a large polylobulated hyperdense mass arising from the left costovertebral junction *(arrows)*. Note enlargement and increased density of the left posterior fifth rib *(arrowheads)*. (B) Unenhanced CT scan shows a large mass *(arrows)* extending into the paravertebral mediastinum that originates from a lytic lesion in the costovertebral junction.

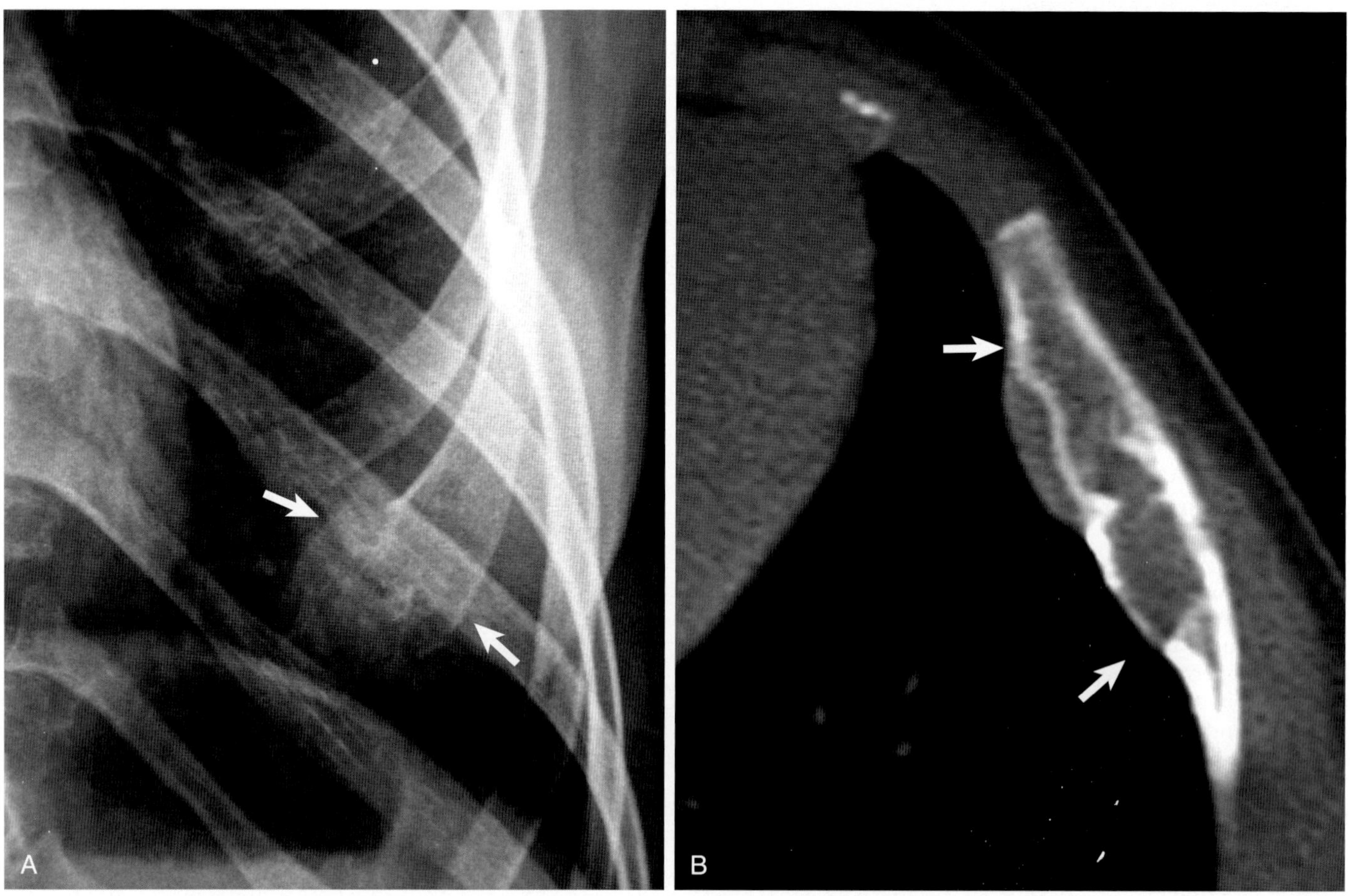

Fig. 79.12 Fibrous dysplasia. (A) Close-up view from chest radiograph shows an expansile, osteolytic lesion in the anterior aspect of the sixth rib *(arrows)*. (B) Corresponding CT scan shows a large lytic lesion in the rib. The lesion has caused cortical thinning and expansile remodeling of the rib *(arrows)*.

areas of sclerosis may be present with or without calcification. CT and MRI enable more accurate assessment of lesion morphology, location, and extent.

Osteochondroma

Cartilage-forming tumors are the most common primary bone tumors.[43] Osteochondroma is a cartilage-capped osseous growth that projects from the surface of the affected bone and accounts for 10% to 15% of all bone tumors.[43] Its central core of bone marrow is continuous with the marrow of the underlying bone and is surrounded by a cortex and periosteum that are continuous with those of the affected bone. Most osteochondromas are seen in the metaphyseal regions of the long bones. Patients are commonly in the second decade of life at diagnosis.

Osteochondroma is the second most common benign rib lesion after fibrous dysplasia. Solitary osteochondromas of the chest wall are uncommon lesions. In cases of multiple familial exostoses, nearly half of patients have a costal or scapular osteochondroma, however.[44] Osteochondromas appear on the chest radiograph as a deformity or expansion of the rib with calcification of the cartilaginous cap. CT is particularly useful in the assessment of osteochondromas in the spine, ribs, or shoulder (Fig. 79.13). Unusual complications secondary to osteochondromas of the ribs include spontaneous hemothorax,[45]

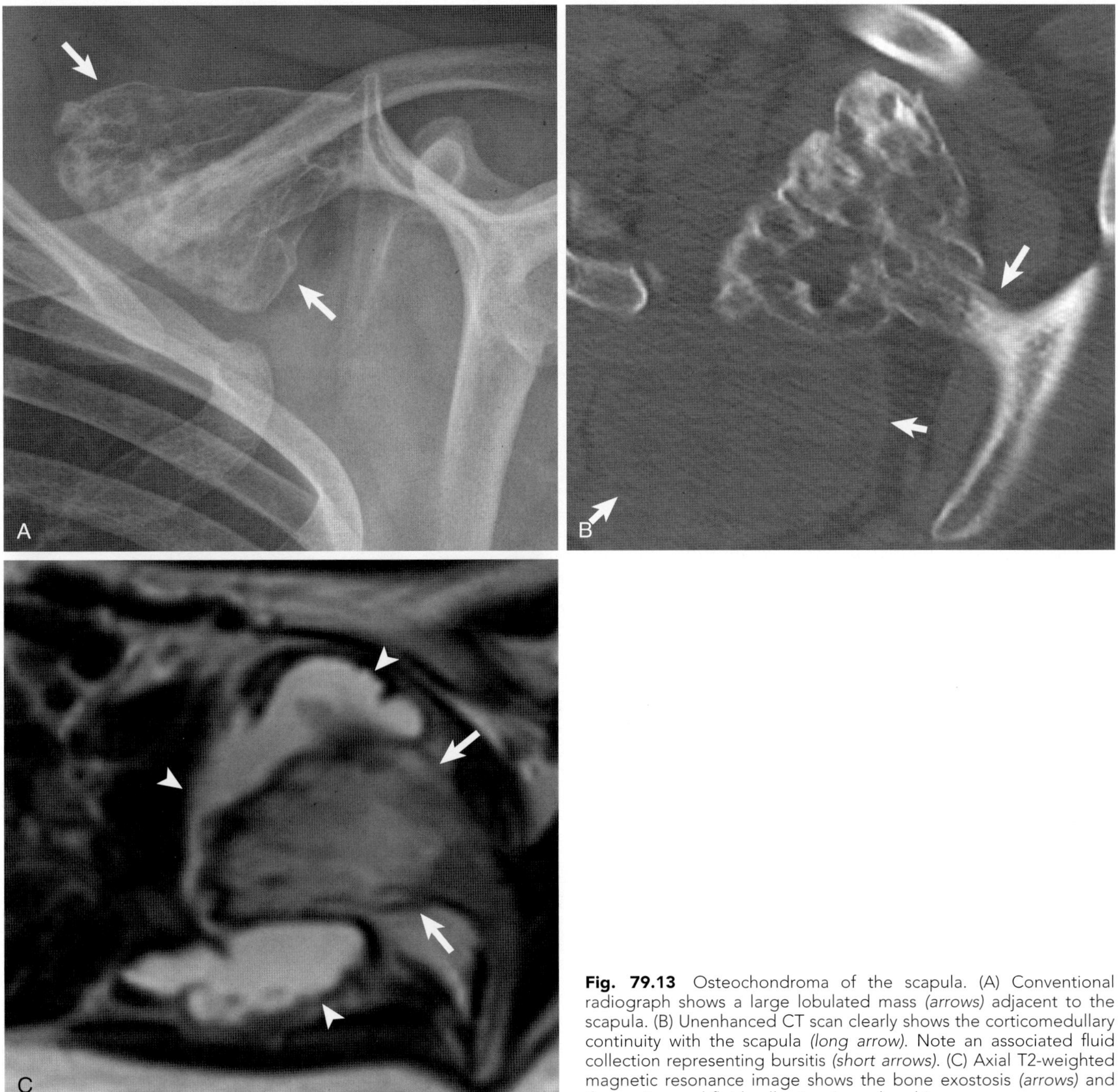

Fig. 79.13 Osteochondroma of the scapula. (A) Conventional radiograph shows a large lobulated mass *(arrows)* adjacent to the scapula. (B) Unenhanced CT scan clearly shows the corticomedullary continuity with the scapula *(long arrow)*. Note an associated fluid collection representing bursitis *(short arrows)*. (C) Axial T2-weighted magnetic resonance image shows the bone exostosis *(arrows)* and the peritumoral fluid collection *(arrowheads)*.

empyema,[46] extradural spinal cord compression, Horner syndrome, and malignant transformation.

Chondromyxoid Fibroma

Chondromyxoid fibroma (CMF) is a rare, slow-growing benign tumor of the bone that constitutes 0.5% to 1% of primary bone neoplasms.[47,48] It typically affects older children and young adults and is most often found in the metaphysis of long tubular bones, especially the tibia and femur near the knee joint.[47] Chest wall and rib CMFs are exceptionally rare. Radiographs in cases of chondromyxoid fibroma show a lytic lesion with well-defined margins.[49] The tumor usually has a sclerotic margin of bone and a lobulated contour (Fig. 79.14). The differential diagnosis includes chondrosarcoma and periosteal chondroma. Unlike other more common chondral lesions, matrix calcifications appear in only 2% to 13% of lesions. MRI typically reveals relatively homogeneous signal intensity on T1-weighted images, high signal intensity on T2-weighted images, and heterogeneous enhancement after administration of contrast. Chondromyxoid fibromas with areas of secondary aneurysmal bone cyst formation contain fluid-fluid levels and manifest as more heterogeneous lesions.

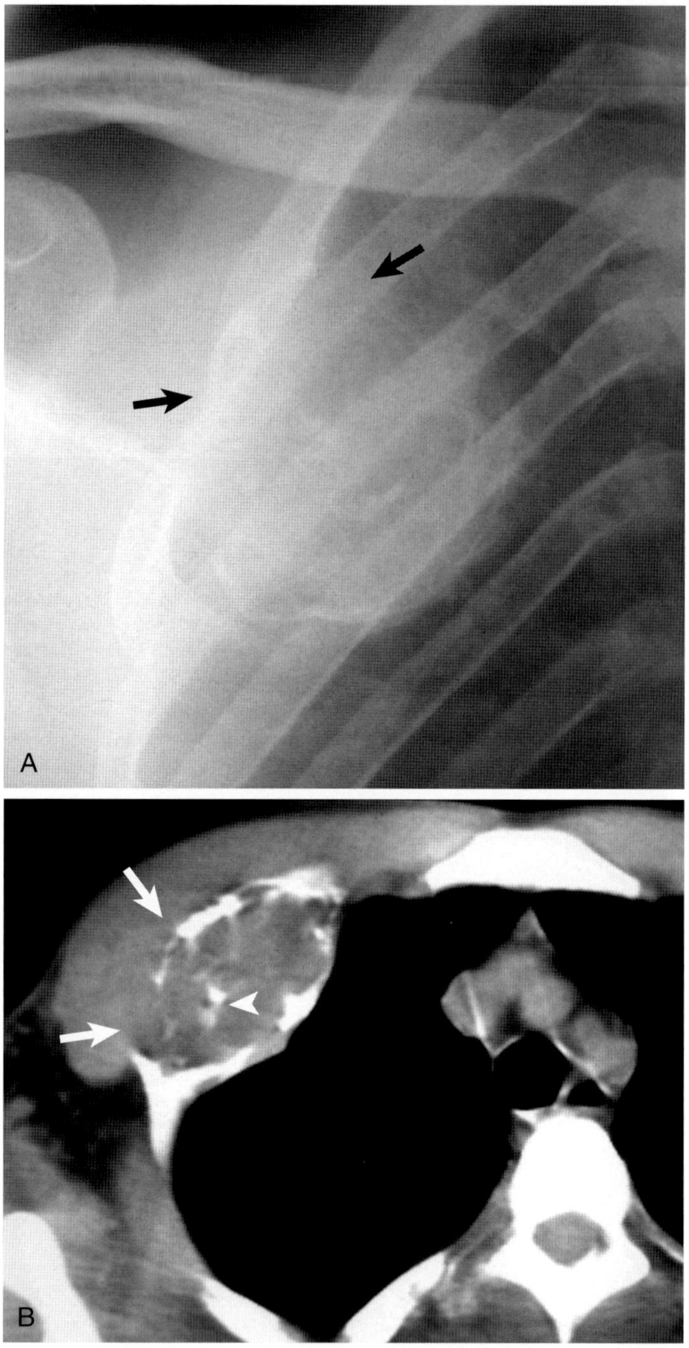

Fig. 79.14 Chondromyxoid fibroma of the rib. (A) Close-up view from chest radiograph shows an osteolytic expansile rib lesion *(arrows)*. (B) Unenhanced CT scan shows an expansile lytic mass in the anterior chest wall. Tumor causes bone expansion and cortical thinning *(arrows)* and contains coarse calcifications *(arrowhead)*.

KEY POINTS: BENIGN BONE TUMORS OF THE CHEST WALL

Uncommon lesions:

- The lesions usually are incidental findings on chest radiographs.
- Fibrous dysplasia commonly involves the ribs.
- Osteochondroma is the most common benign bone tumor of the chest wall.
- Chest wall osteochondromas are frequently found in multiple hereditary exostoses.

MALIGNANT BONE TUMORS

Chondrosarcoma is the most common primary malignant neoplasm of the ribs, followed by plasmacytoma and lymphoma.[50] Osteosarcoma and undifferentiated pleomorphic sarcoma (formerly malignant fibrous histiocytoma) are more rarely seen. Malignant chest wall tumors typically manifest clinically as large, painful, and rapidly growing masses.[51]

CHONDROSARCOMA

Chondrosarcoma is the most common primary osseous malignancy of the chest wall, representing 30% of all primary malignant osseous lesions and 33% of all primary rib neoplasms.[36,52] The vast majority of chondrosarcomas are classified as primary and arise in the medullary cavity of a previously normal bone. Secondary chondrosarcomas arise in benign chondral tumors, such as enchondroma or osteochondroma. Patients with primary chondrosarcoma are commonly in the fourth to sixth decades of age at diagnosis.

Unlike benign cartilaginous lesions, chondrosarcoma has a predilection for the trunk bones. The most common sites of the tumor are the long tubular bones (45%) and the axial skeleton (25% in the pelvis). The ribs (8%), scapula (5%), and sternum (2%) are less frequently involved. About 90% of thoracic chondrosarcomas arise from the anterior rib or costochondral junction, especially along the upper five ribs.[53]

Radiographs of costal or sternal chondrosarcomas typically reveal a large mineralized mass with a characteristic rings-and-arcs pattern of calcification. CT and MRI always demonstrate a destructive lesion, often with a large soft tissue component (Fig. 79.15). On MRI nonmineralized areas are isointense relative to skeletal muscle on T1-weighted images. On T2-weighted MRI cartilaginous lobules have high signal intensity and are surrounded by low–signal intensity septa (Fig. 79.16). Matrix mineralization manifests as areas of low signal intensity on all pulse sequences. After contrast administration, a characteristic pattern of peripheral and septal enhancement can be noted.[54]

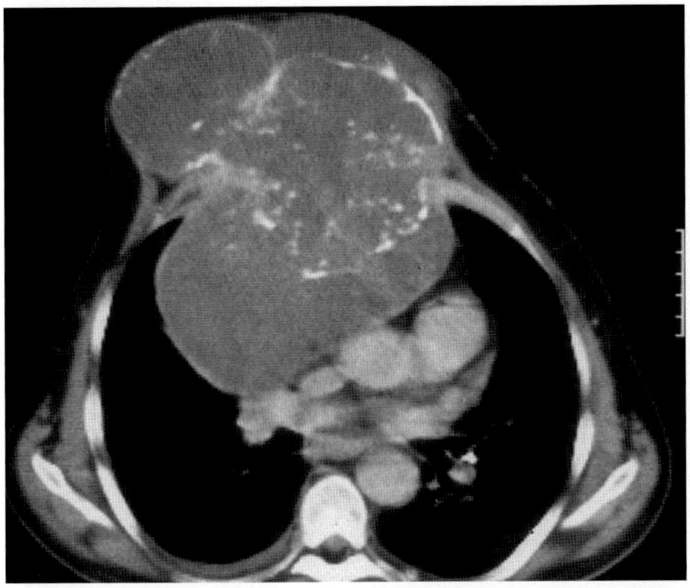

Fig. 79.15 Chondrosarcoma of the sternum. Contrast-enhanced CT scan shows a large, low-attenuation, and partially mineralized mass replacing the sternum and displacing mediastinal structures.

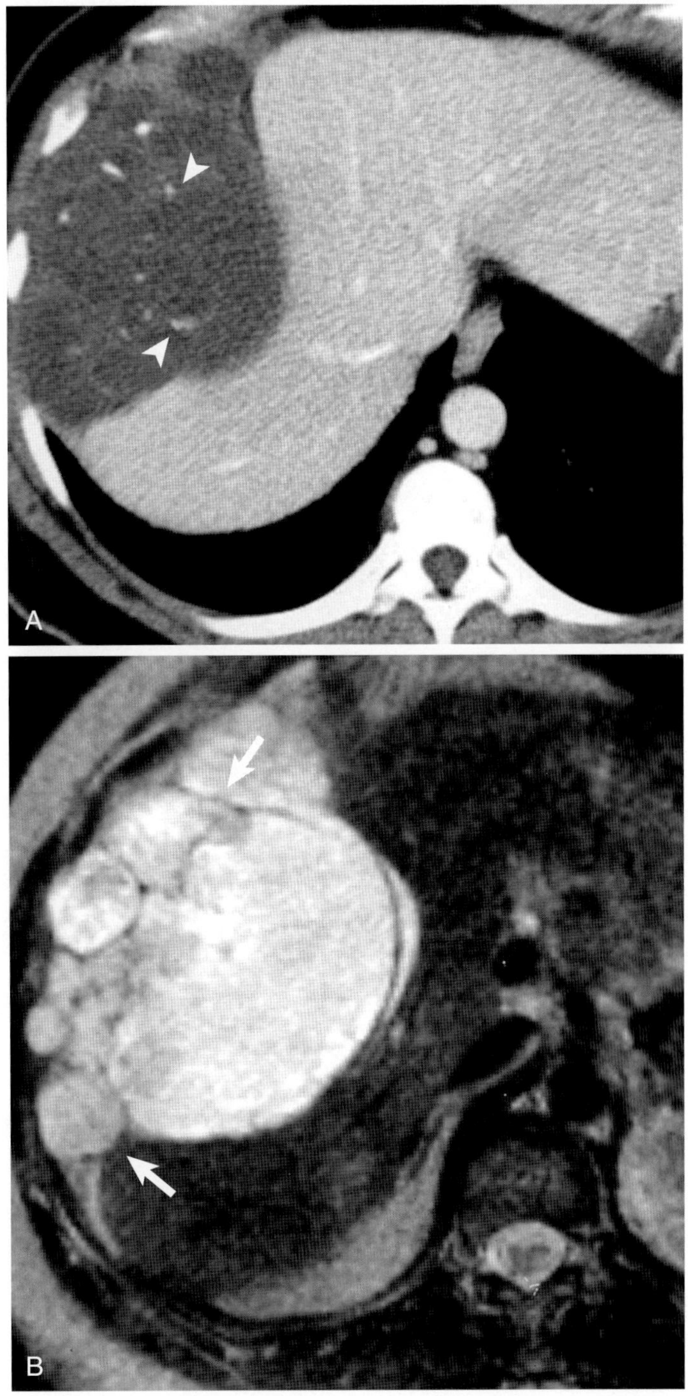

Fig. 79.16 Chondrosarcoma in a man with a painless, slowly growing chest wall mass. (A) Contrast-enhanced CT scan obtained at the level of the liver shows a heterogeneous and low-attenuation mass with chondroid mineralization *(arrowheads)* between the right hepatic lobe and chest wall. (B) T2-weighted magnetic resonance image shows high–signal intensity heterogeneous mass with lobulated appearance and low–signal intensity septa *(arrows)* between cartilaginous lobules.

In general, these tumors are not responsive to chemotherapy or radiotherapy, and a complete wide local surgical resection is the primary treatment modality.[55] The size and location of the tumor determine the extent of resection that should include any involved adjacent structures, including lung, pericardium, or vessels.[56]

KEY POINTS: CHONDROSARCOMA

Most common malignant primary tumor of the chest wall:

- The majority of chest wall lesions with chondroid mineralization are chondrosarcomas.
- Rib lesions usually arise from the costochondral junctions.
- There are large destructive tumors with a rings-and-arcs pattern of calcification.
- It is best evaluated with computed tomography or magnetic resonance imaging.

OSTEOSARCOMA

The term *osteosarcoma* defines a heterogeneous group of malignant bone tumors in which malignant mesenchymal cells produce osteoid or immature bone. Osteosarcoma is the most common primary sarcoma of bone and accounts for approximately 20% of all primary osseous sarcomas. Most patients with osteosarcoma are in the second and third decades of life, during the period of most active skeletal growth. Typical sites of involvement are the femur (42%), the tibia (19%), and the humerus (10%). Only 1% to 2% of primary osteosarcomas occur within the chest wall; the rib and the scapula are the most commonly involved chest wall sites.

Usually, osteosarcoma shows a mixed pattern of sclerosis and lucent areas within the medullary cavity. It shows an aggressive pathologic behavior, manifested as cortical disruption, aggressive periosteal reaction, and soft tissue mass. On occasion, osteosarcoma may be completely blastic or lytic. The radiographic appearance of osteosarcoma of the rib typically demonstrates an extrapleural mass with bone involvement. CT findings include a heterogeneous mass because of central ossification, necrosis, and hemorrhage.[57] Osteosarcoma should be suspected if CT reveals dense calcification within a mass that is centered in a rib (Fig. 79.17).[58] MRI features

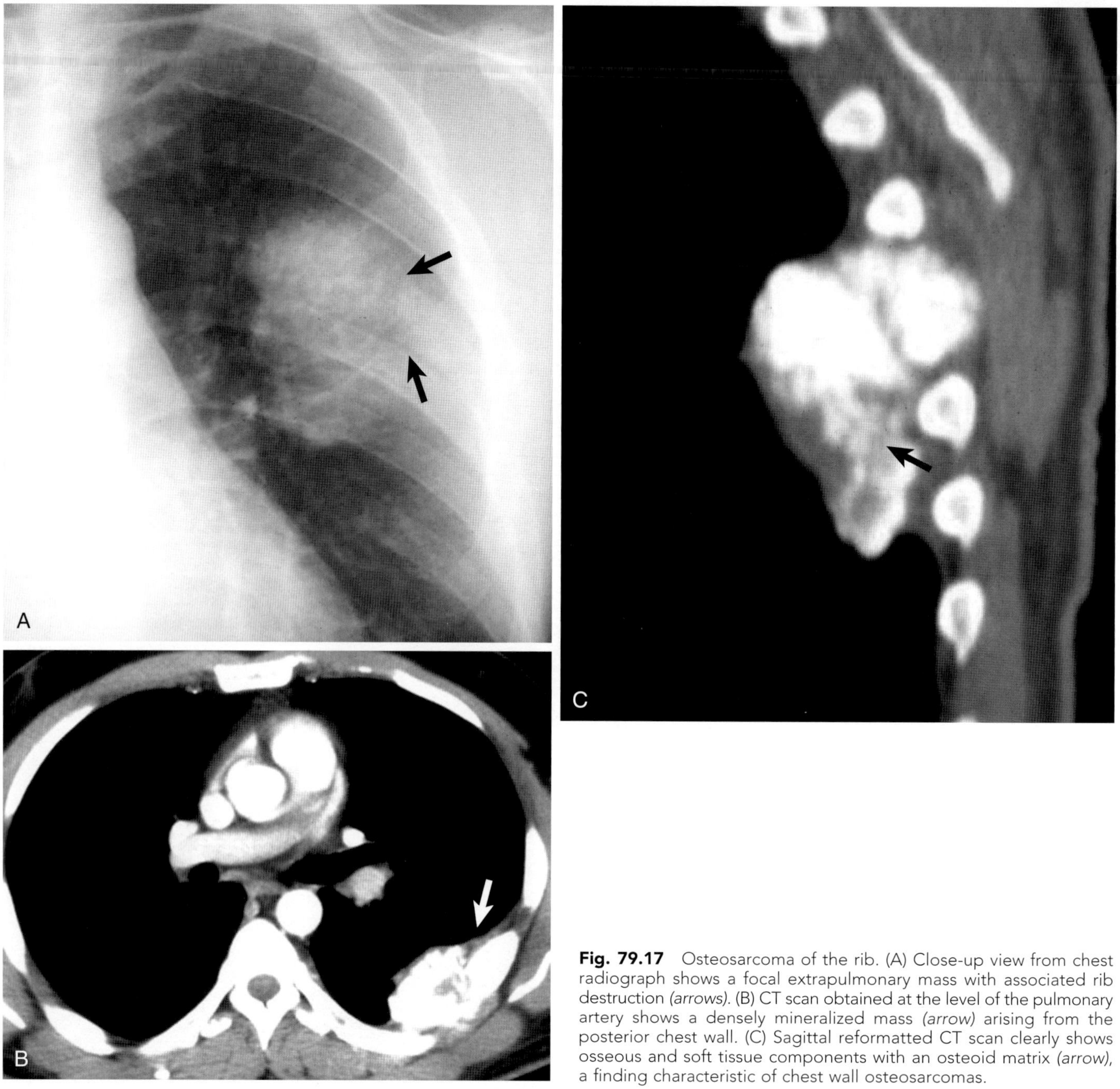

Fig. 79.17 Osteosarcoma of the rib. (A) Close-up view from chest radiograph shows a focal extrapulmonary mass with associated rib destruction *(arrows)*. (B) CT scan obtained at the level of the pulmonary artery shows a densely mineralized mass *(arrow)* arising from the posterior chest wall. (C) Sagittal reformatted CT scan clearly shows osseous and soft tissue components with an osteoid matrix *(arrow)*, a finding characteristic of chest wall osteosarcomas.

include a large soft tissue component with higher T1 signal and mixed to higher T2 signal than muscle[40]; matrix mineralization will be seen as signal void.[59]

PRIMITIVE NEUROECTODERMAL TUMORS

PNETs of the chest wall are rare, small, round-cell, rapidly progressive tumors with a poor prognosis. They usually occur in children and adolescents and share a similar histology, immunohistology, and cytogenetics with Ewing sarcoma. Boys are affected twice as frequently as girls. About 40% of these tumors involve flat bones, most commonly the pelvis, scapula, and ribs.[60] Tumors involving flat or short tubular bones usually contain areas of mixed sclerosis. Cortical destruction, periosteal reaction, and soft tissue masses are very common associated findings. On radiography there is usually an osteolytic lesion associated with a large soft tissue mass that is disproportionately large compared with the extent of bone involvement (Fig. 79.18). On CT most tumors show large lesions, often with a heterogeneous appearance, representing hemorrhage and necrosis or cystic degeneration.[61,62] On MRI the signal intensity is similar to or greater than muscle on T1-weighted MRI. There is more variability on T2-weighted MRI with heterogeneous high signal intensity (Fig. 79.19).[63,64] Differential diagnosis in children and adolescents should include neuroblastoma, rhabdomyosarcoma, and non-Hodgkin lymphoma.

KEY POINTS: PRIMITIVE NEUROECTODERMAL TUMORS

Most common malignant primary tumor of the chest wall in children:

- May occur in the rib, scapula, sternum, clavicle, or in an extraskeletal site
- Often originate in the paravertebral region
- Cause large soft tissue masses with intrathoracic and extrathoracic extension, including lung and pleural involvement
- Best evaluated with computed tomography or magnetic resonance imaging

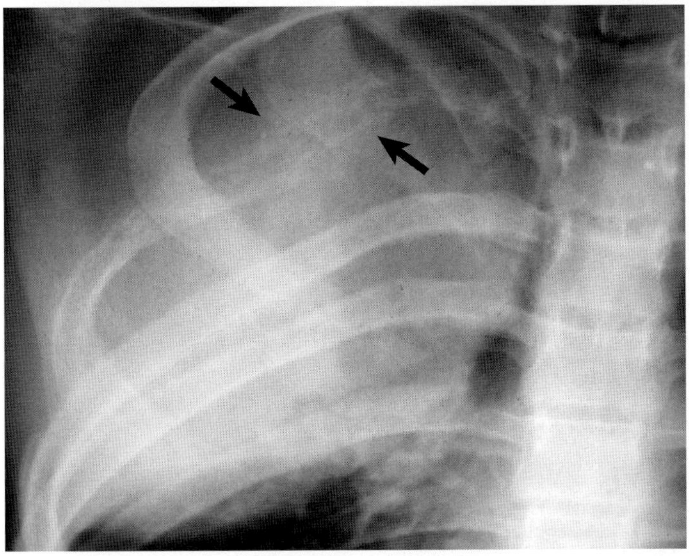

Fig. 79.18 Primitive neuroectodermal tumor of the rib in a 16-year-old boy. Close-up view from chest radiograph shows a large extrapulmonary mass with associated rib destruction *(arrows)*.

SOLITARY AND MULTIPLE MYELOMA

Solitary myeloma and multiple myeloma are plasma cell tumors characterized by a neoplastic proliferation of plasma cells, bone destruction, and presence of increased monoclonal immunoglobulin and light-chain proteins in the blood and urine. Solitary myeloma manifests radiologically as a multicystic expansile mass or purely osteolytic focus without expansion (Fig. 79.20). Multiple myeloma, the abnormal accumulation of plasma cells in bone marrow, is the most common primary osseous malignancy in the elderly population. The average age of involved patients is 60 to 70 years; the median age at diagnosis is 66 years. It is associated with multiple osteolytic lesions with discrete margins. The axial skeleton is the most common site of involvement. The most frequently affected sites are the vertebral column (66%), ribs (44%), skull (41%), pelvis (28%), femur (24%), clavicle (10%), and scapula (10%).[65]

Although it is well known that radiographs are limited for evaluating early disease, multiple myeloma typically manifests with osteolytic lesions appearing as punched-out holes without surrounding reactive sclerosis.[66] Whole-body low-dose CT has been demonstrated to be superior to conventional radiography for the detection of osteolytic lesions, and it is suggested to replace it in the workup of patients with multiple myeloma.[67–69] MRI and ^{18}F-FDG–PET-CT scan are also useful imaging techniques in assessing the extent of multiple myeloma at the time of initial diagnosis; FDG–PET-CT is also useful for evaluating therapy response.[70]

PRIMARY MUSCULOSKELETAL LYMPHOMA

Primary lymphoma of the musculoskeletal system is rare and may involve bone, subcutaneous tissue, and muscle.[71] Osseous lymphoma typically shows aggressive bone destruction, which

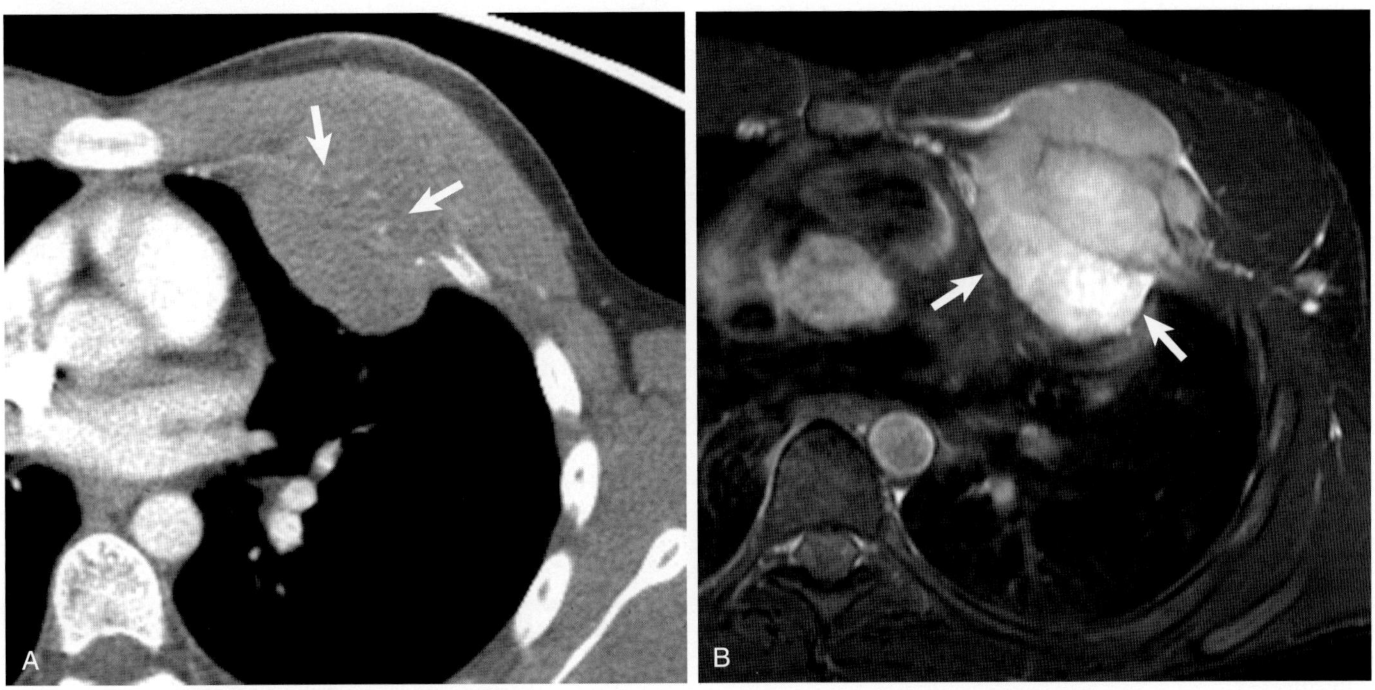

Fig. 79.19 Primitive neuroectodermal tumor of the rib. (A) Contrast-enhanced CT shows a large soft tissue mass arising from the left chest wall. Note osseous involvement manifesting with aggressive rib destruction *(arrows)*. (B) T1-weighted fat-suppressed magnetic resonance image after the administration of intravenous contrast shows diffuse homogeneous enhancement of the tumor *(arrows)*.

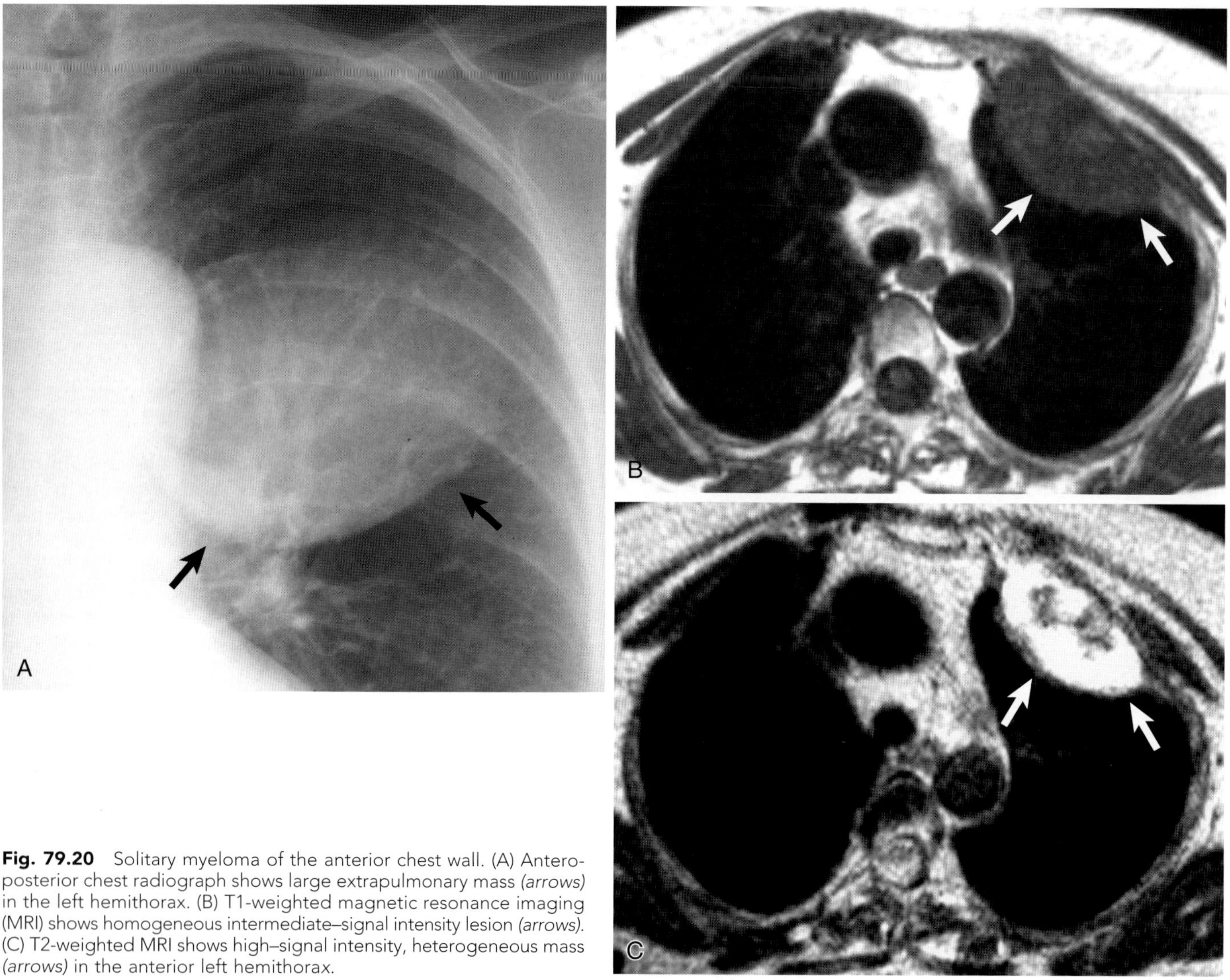

Fig. 79.20 Solitary myeloma of the anterior chest wall. (A) Anteroposterior chest radiograph shows large extrapulmonary mass *(arrows)* in the left hemithorax. (B) T1-weighted magnetic resonance imaging (MRI) shows homogeneous intermediate–signal intensity lesion *(arrows)*. (C) T2-weighted MRI shows high–signal intensity, heterogeneous mass *(arrows)* in the anterior left hemithorax.

can be associated with a soft tissue mass. Cortical destruction and connection between bone and adjacent soft tissues may be apparent (Fig. 79.21).[71] Primary malignant lymphomas of the chest wall account for less than 2% of soft tissue tumors.[72] The most typical sites of involvement are the femur (27%), pelvis (15%), and tibia/fibula (13%).[72,73]

BONE METASTASES

Metastases from carcinoma are by far the most common malignant tumors involving the skeleton. Carcinomas are much more likely to metastasize to bone than are sarcomas.[74] Cancers most likely to metastasize to bone include breast, lung, prostate, thyroid, and kidney. The axial skeleton is affected more commonly than the appendicular skeleton, partly because of the persistence of red bone marrow in the former, although the lesions may be found anywhere in the skeletal system. The ribs, pelvis, and spine are the most commonly involved bones, and distal bones are rarely affected.

Pain, pathologic fractures, and hypercalcemia are the most common clinical manifestations in patients with osseous metastases.

On radiographs bone metastases may be osteolytic, sclerotic, or mixed. Osteolytic metastases are encountered most frequently, especially in breast and lung carcinomas. Metastases from certain primary sites (renal cell or thyroid carcinomas) are almost always osteolytic, whereas those from other sites (prostate carcinoma) are predominantly sclerotic. The most common radiographic features are a lytic destructive process in the medullary cavity with ill-defined margins, erosion of the cortex, and frequent extension into the soft tissues (Fig. 79.22). Pathologic fractures are common.

On chest radiograph costal metastases frequently appear as well-defined extrapulmonary masses with destruction of the underlying rib. Whole-body MRI is more sensitive than skeletal scintigraphy for osseous metastasis detection.[75]

KEY POINTS: BONE METASTASES

- They are the most common malignant bone tumor.
- Breast, prostate, and lung are the most common primary malignancies.
- There are lytic, sclerotic, or mixed bone lesions.
- The axial skeleton is the most commonly affected.

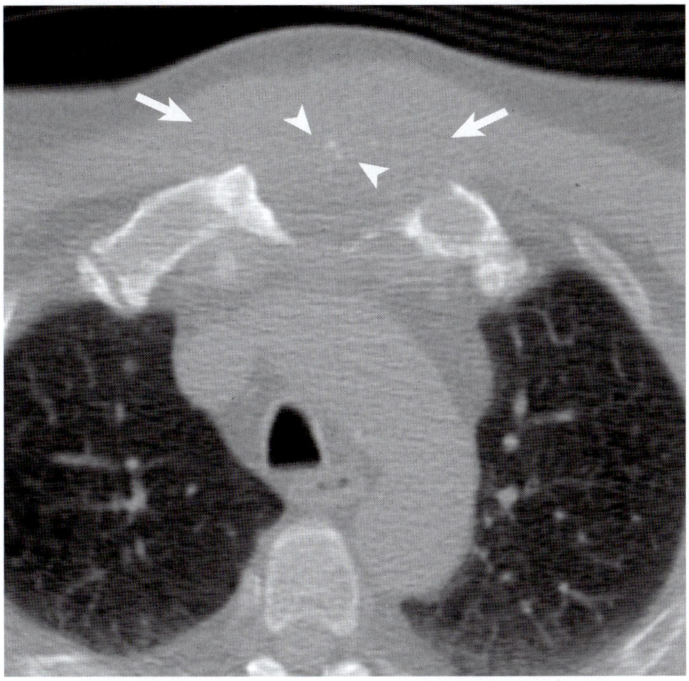

Fig. 79.21 Primary lymphoma of the sternum. Unenhanced CT scan shows an aggressive destructive lesion of the sternum with a large soft tissue mass *(arrows)*. Note a focal area of calcification *(arrowheads)* in the soft tissue component.

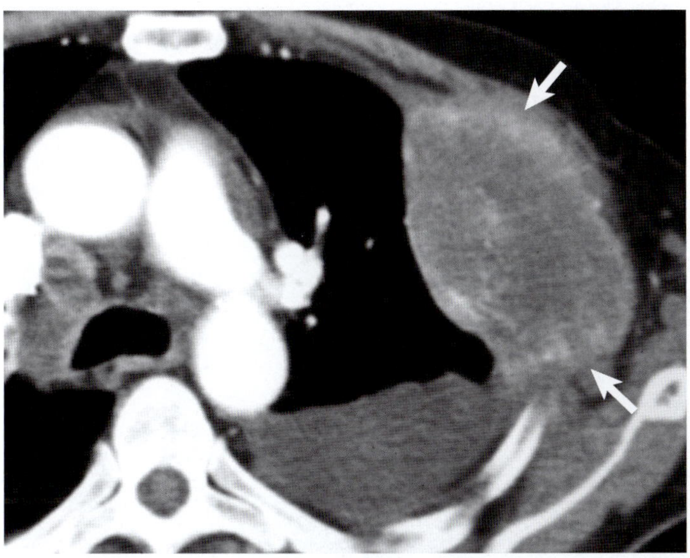

Fig. 79.22 Rib metastasis from colon carcinoma. Contrast-enhanced CT image shows an expansive large soft tissue lesion *(arrows)* causing rib destruction in the anterior left chest wall. The mass shows a peripheral rim of enhancement and central low attenuation consistent with necrosis.

Benign Soft Tissue Tumors

The soft tissues are composed of fat, skeletal muscle, fibrous tissue, peripheral nervous system, and the vessels that supply them. The vast majority of soft tissue tumors are benign and include the following main categories: lipomatous (lipoma and lipoma variants, hibernoma), fibrous histiocytoma, nodular fasciitis, hemangioma, desmoid-type fibromatosis, neurogenic tumors, and giant-cell tumors of the tendon sheath.[76,77]

Benign soft tissue tumors of the chest wall are relatively uncommon lesions that typically manifest as painless, slow-growing, palpable masses.[78] MRI, because of its multiplanar capability and superior contrast characterization, is the method of choice for evaluating soft tissue tumors. Frequently, these lesions may have imaging findings that are specific enough to establish the diagnosis.[78] Such features include, among others, isointensity relative to fat on all pulse sequences (lipoma), target-like appearance and evidence of neural origin (neurofibroma), and areas of very low signal intensity on all pulse sequences (desmoid-type fibromatosis). Benign soft tissue tumors with special predilection for involvement of the trunk include elastofibroma and fibromatoses.

The lipoma is the most common soft tissue tumor. Lipomas are composed of mature fat cells and are usually encapsulated. On MRI signal intensity of lipoma is similar to that of subcutaneous fat on all pulse sequences. Superficial or subcutaneous lipoma is the most common type. These tumors are usually small and may be indistinguishable from adjacent subcutaneous fat. In some cases, however, a thin surrounding fibrous capsule of low signal intensity may be observed. Intramuscular lipomas are typically larger in size and less well defined, with tumoral fat infiltrating the skeletal muscle fibers. In these cases MRI demonstrates the fatty nature of the mass and the poorly defined margins and, occasionally, thin fibrous septations of low signal intensity.

Hibernoma is a rare benign soft tissue tumor with no malignant potential that arises from rests of fetal brown fat. The lesion often occurs in adults with proximal extremity/truncal predilection. Grossly, it appears as a well-demarcated, mobile, encapsulated, soft, greasy to rubbery, brown to yellow lobulated mass.[79] Hibernoma can be difficult to differentiate from other lipomatous neoplasms. On radiographs it may manifest as a radiolucent mass with no osseous abnormalities or mineralization. Hibernoma can be suspected when a lipomatous mass demonstrates intermediate density on CT or intermediate high T1 and T2 signal intensities with incomplete fat suppression (Fig. 79.23).[80] Differentiation from dedifferentiated liposarcoma may be established when obvious nonadipocytic soft tissue masses and, occasionally, areas of mineralization or ossification are observed. However, because of its metabolic activity on FDG–PET-CT, its presence can lead to false-positive interpretations.[81]

Cavernous hemangioma is a benign vascular tumor composed of dilated spaces filled with blood and lined by endothelium. Most cavernous hemangiomas contain nonvascular elements, such as fat, smooth muscle, fibrous tissue, bone, hemosiderin, and thrombus. Calcified thrombus manifests as phleboliths, the most specific finding on radiographs. Reactive fat overgrowth within cavernous or arteriovenous hemangiomas may be a prominent feature both histologically and radiologically (Fig. 79.24). Cavernous hemangioma is usually a poorly marginated intramuscular mass. On T1-weighted images cavernous hemangioma manifests as a low– to intermediate–signal intensity mass. When present, fat manifests as linear or nodular areas of high signal intensity that predominate peripherally. On T2-weighted images most hemangiomas show a characteristic imaging appearance. Lesions are well marginated and show a lobulated morphology. Typically, slow-flowing spaces manifest as very-high-intensity areas of circular or serpiginous morphology separated by areas of decreased signal intensity corresponding to fibrous septations.

ELASTOFIBROMA DORSI

Elastofibroma dorsi is a slow growing, benign, soft tissue pseudotumor of unclear pathogenesis, typically located at the subscapular region of elderly women.[82] The etiology of this lesion remains unclear. Repeated trauma resulting from mechanical friction of the scapula against the ribs has been suggested to induce the process. Bilateral lesions are seen in up to 66% of patients.[83] It occurs in all age groups, but most patients are older adults. Clinically, patients usually present with a large well-circumscribed tumor in the subscapular area that most often does not adhere to the overlying skin.

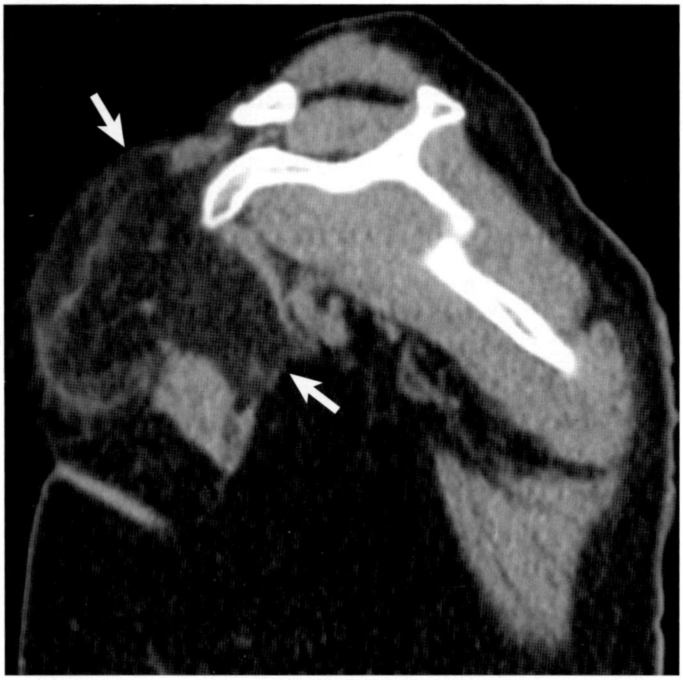

Fig. 79.23 Periscapular hibernoma. Unenhanced CT image shows a fatty mass *(arrows)* with slightly increased density compared with subcutaneous fat.

CT reveals a lenticular, unencapsulated, soft tissue mass with skeletal muscle attenuation interspersed with strands of fat attenuation. On MRI elastofibroma shows a lenticular or ovoid morphology and a typical striated appearance reflecting the presence of adipose tissue entrapped between bands of fibrous tissue (Fig. 79.25). Signal intensity of fat is similar to that of subcutaneous tissue on all pulse sequences; the fibrous component displays low signal intensity on T2-weighted sequences. On FDG–PET-CT scans most of the tumors have diffuse metabolic activity equal to or less than liver blood pool.[84]

KEY POINTS: ELASTOFIBROMA

Fibroblastic pseudotumor of unknown etiology:

- It is typically located between the chest wall and scapular tip.
- Bilateral lesions are seen in 10%–66% of cases.
- It is a common autopsy finding; most patients are asymptomatic.
- There is a characteristic layered appearance on magnetic resonance imaging.

MUSCULOSKELETAL FIBROMATOSES

Musculoskeletal fibromatoses represent a wide spectrum of fibroblastic and myofibroblastic neoplasms that are grouped together because of their similar pathologic appearances.[85] The musculoskeletal fibromatoses are classified as superficial and

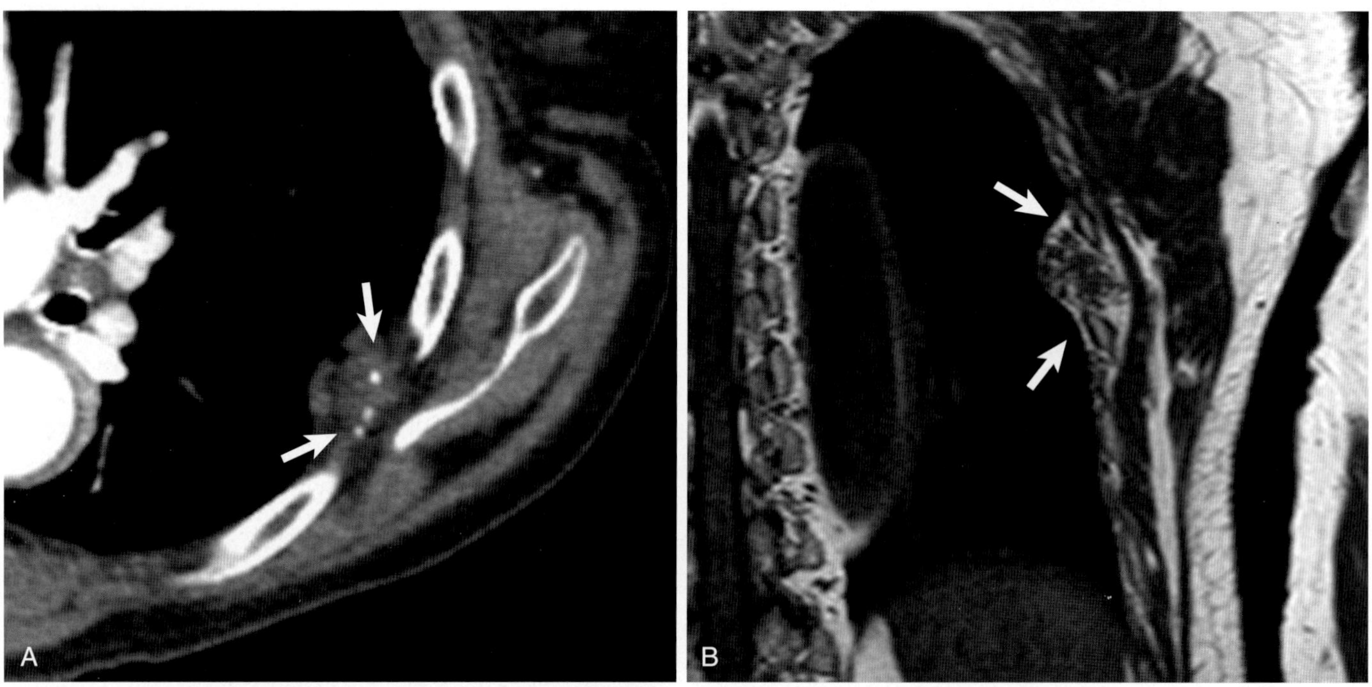

Fig. 79.24 Hemangioma. (A) Contrast-enhanced axial CT image shows an ill-defined intercostal heterogeneous mass *(arrows)* containing fat and punctate calcifications corresponding to phleboliths. (B) Coronal T1-weighted magnetic resonance image shows regions of internal high signal intensity because of the presence of fat *(arrows)*.

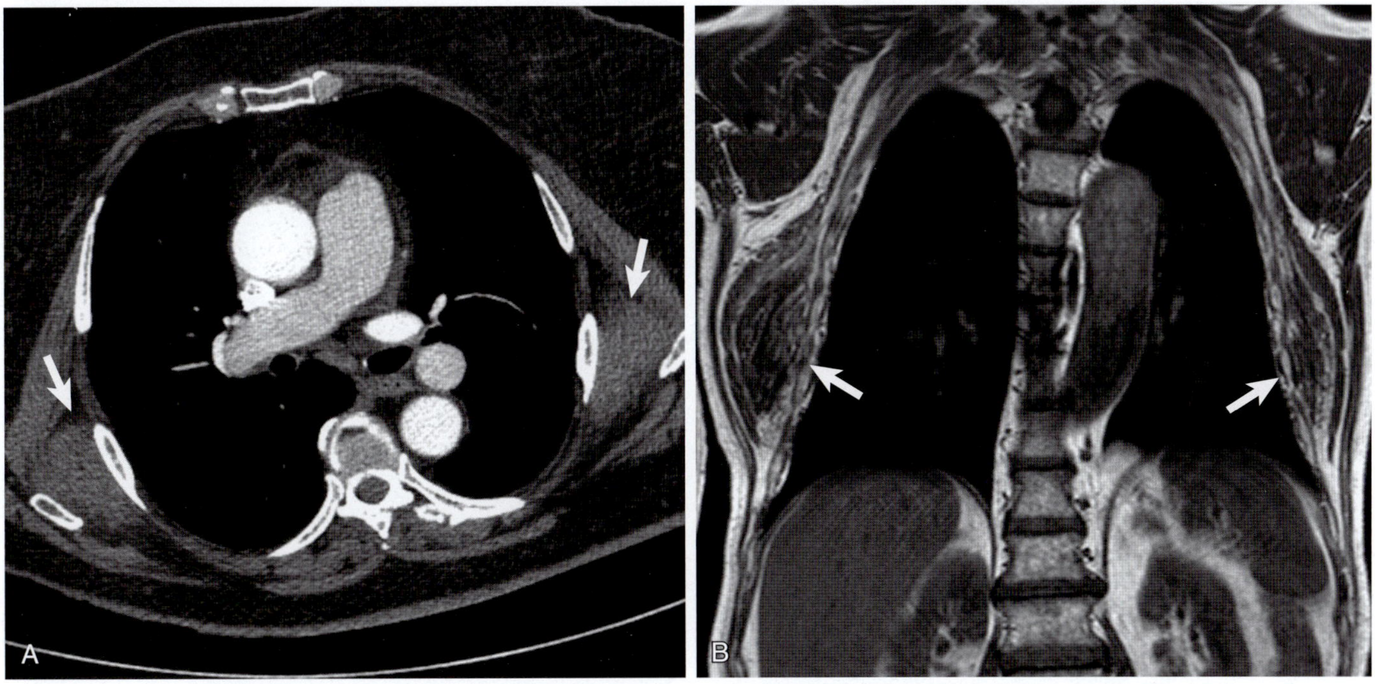

Fig. 79.25 Elastofibroma. (A) Contrast-enhanced CT image shows symmetric elastofibromas manifesting as bilateral homogeneous, lenticular, well-defined masses *(arrows)* in a characteristic subscapular location. (B) Coronal T1-weighted magnetic resonance image shows bilateral striated, ill-defined soft tissue masses *(arrows)* closely associated with the intercostal muscles.

deep. Superficial fibromatoses in adults (palmar and plantar) and children (calcifying aponeurotic fibroma, lipofibromatosis, and inclusion body fibromatosis) are often small slow-growing lesions. The deep fibromatoses in adults (desmoid type and abdominal wall) and children (fibromatosis colli, myofibroma, and myofibromatosis) are frequently large and more rapidly enlarging nonmetastasizing tumors.[85] The fibromatoses may be a component of the Gardner syndrome (familial adenomatous polyposis). Deep musculoskeletal fibromatoses involve the chest wall in 10% to 28% of cases. The shoulder area is the most commonly affected (Fig. 79.26). Women are more commonly affected than men. The majority of patients range from 10 to 40 years of age. They manifest as solitary or multicentric soft tissue masses with poorly defined margins. Local recurrence after surgery is very common. Bone involvement occurs in 6% to 30% of patients.[86] On MRI lesions are homogeneous low to intermediate signal intensity on T1W images (Fig. 79.27). On T2W images lesions are more heterogeneous and may show very low, intermediate, and very high signal intensity, according to the varying proportion of collagen and spindle cells.[87]

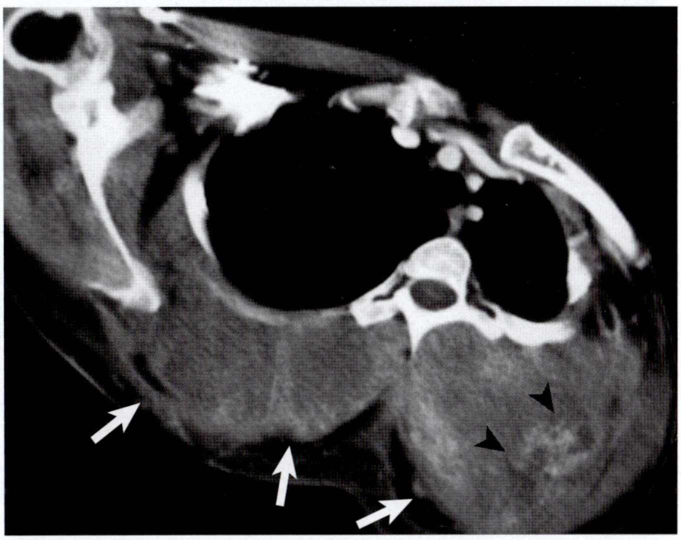

Fig. 79.26 Fibromatosis of the chest and abdomen in a 36-year-old woman with Gardner syndrome. Axial contrast-enhanced CT scan shows a large mass in the thoracic wall with marked enhancement *(arrowheads)*. Note extension into the right hemithorax *(arrows)*.

Soft Tissue Sarcomas

Soft tissue sarcomas, in contrast to benign soft tissue tumors, are uncommon lesions that account for approximately 1% of all malignant tumors. Soft tissue sarcomas of the chest wall are rare and typically manifest as painful and rapidly growing masses. Sarcomas belonging to this group are often high grade and include tumors such as undifferentiated high-grade pleomorphic sarcoma (UHPS, formerly known as malignant fibrous histiocytoma), leiomyosarcoma, liposarcoma, osteosarcoma, synovial sarcoma, rhabdomyosarcoma, fibrosarcoma, and malignant peripheral nerve sheath tumors.[88] These different types of sarcomas are frequently indistinguishable on imaging. The well-differentiated liposarcoma is the most common histologic variant of liposarcoma.[89] On MRI this tumor manifests as a predominantly fatty mass containing irregular septa and/or soft tissue areas that show decreased signal intensity on T1-weighted images and increased signal on T2-weighted images. Myxoid liposarcoma, as occurs with round-cell, pleomorphic, and dedifferentiated variants, usually does not contain significant amounts of fat. Most of these tumors are low- to intermediate-grade lesions and show

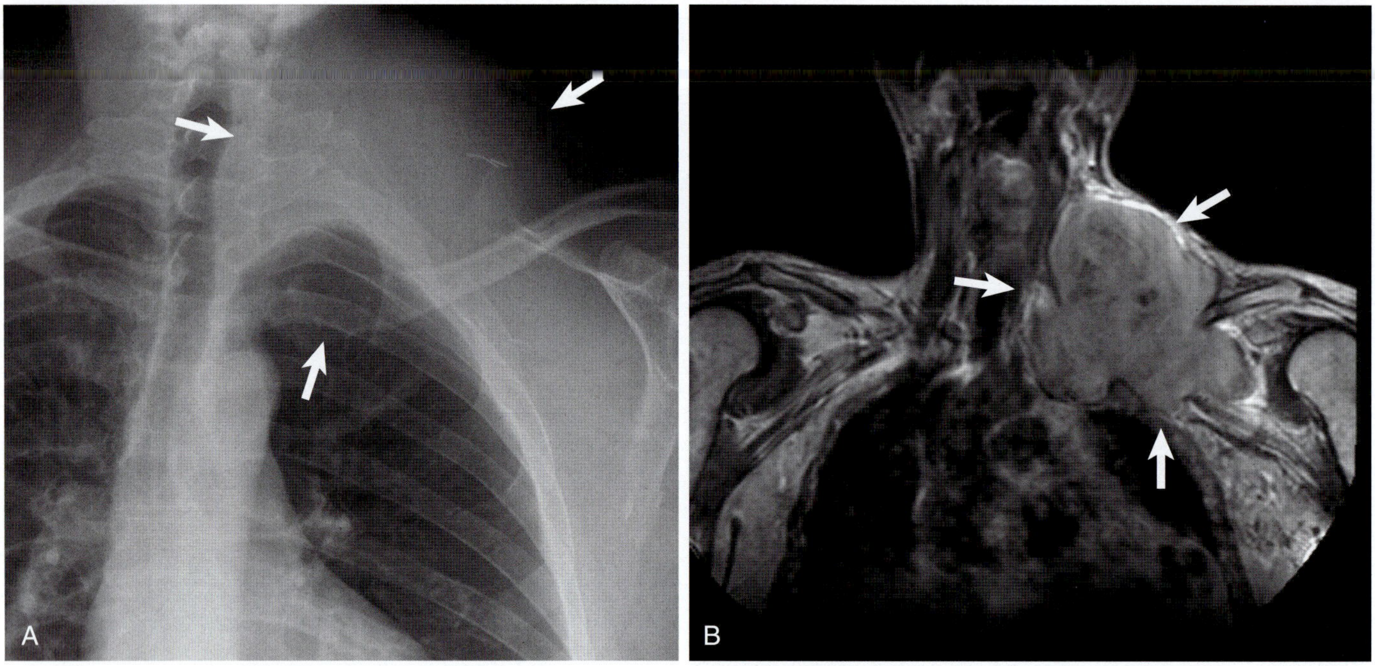

Fig. 79.27 Desmoid-type fibromatosis of the left cervicothoracic junction. (A) Posteroanterior radiograph shows a soft tissue mass *(arrows)* near the left cervicothoracic junction. (B) Coronal T1-weighted magnetic resonance image after contrast administration shows a large lobular-shaped mass *(arrows)* containing multiple low-signal areas corresponding to dense collagen fibrosis.

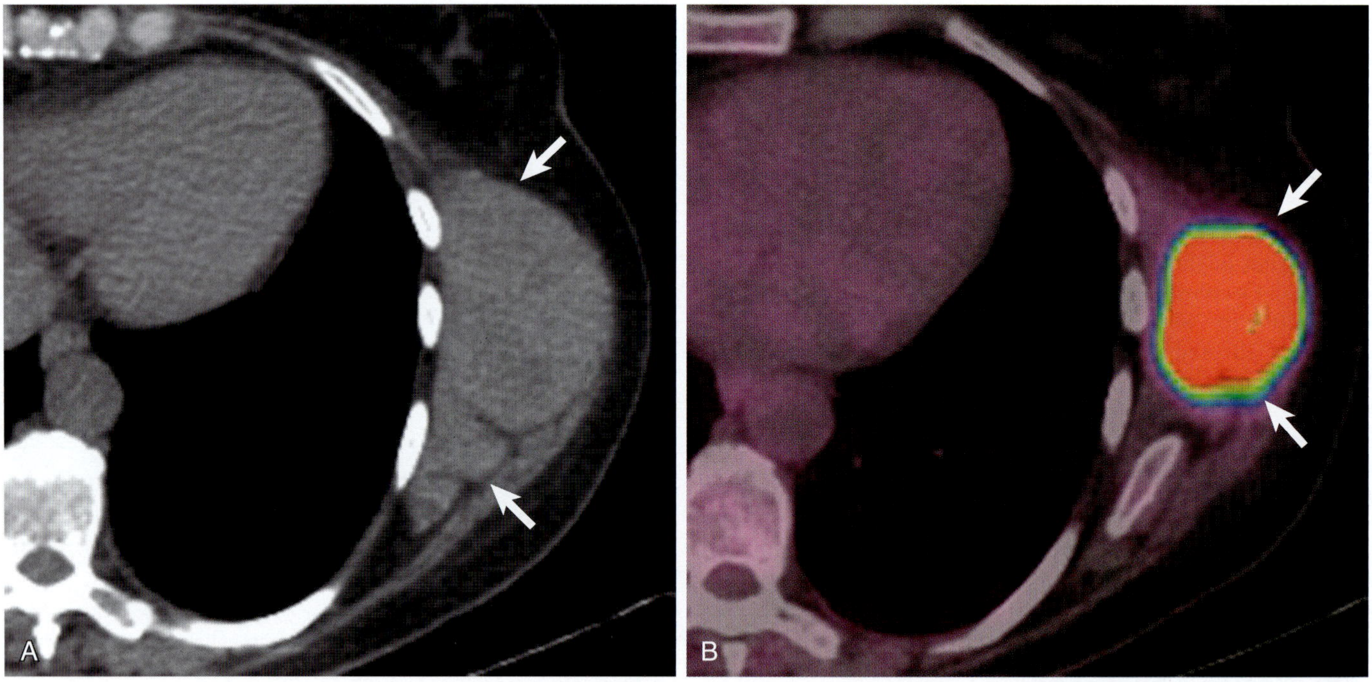

Fig. 79.28 Undifferentiated pleomorphic sarcoma. (A) Unenhanced CT shows a polylobular left axillary soft tissue mass *(arrows)*. (B) Axial fused fluorodeoxyglucose (FDG)–positron emission tomography–CT shows homogeneous marked FDG avidity *(arrows)*.

a heterogeneous and nonspecific imaging appearance. Myxoid liposarcoma, however, has a "cyst-like" appearance in approximately 25% of cases, in the form of a well-defined homogeneous mass, with high signal on T2-weighted images. UHPS is the most common soft tissue sarcoma of late adult life and accounts for 20% to 30% of all soft tissue sarcomas; the mean age at presentation is approximately 60 years, although patient ages range from 10 to 90 years. There is a male predominance in most series. Approximately 75% of soft tissue UHPS occur in the extremities; the thigh is the single most common location. Less commonly, they arise in the retroperitoneum (15% of all cases), head and neck (5%), or other unusual locations. Thoracic UHPS is uncommon and usually arises from the soft tissues of the chest wall (Figs. 79.28 and 79.29).

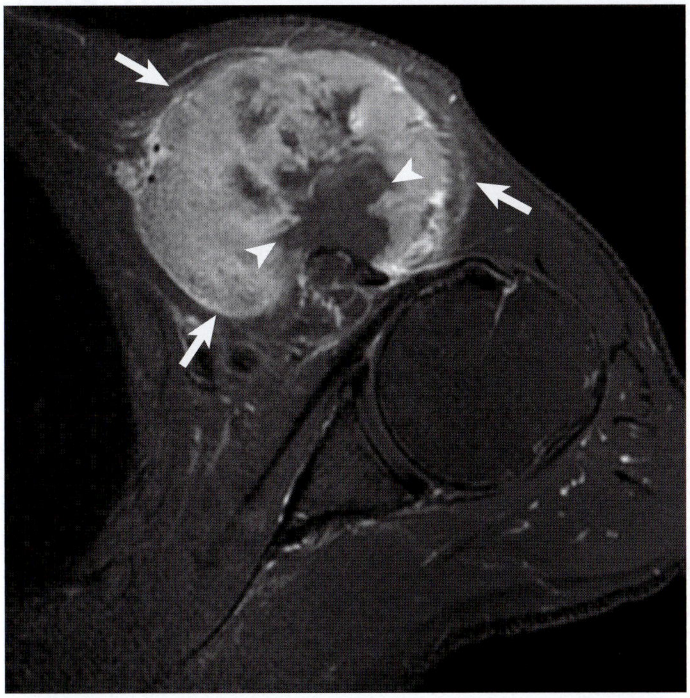

Fig. 79.29 Undifferentiated pleomorphic sarcoma. T1-weighted fat-suppressed magnetic resonance image after the administration of intravenous contrast shows a large well-defined tumor *(arrows)* containing multiple hypointense areas *(arrowheads)* representing necrosis.

Radiographs may reveal a nonspecific soft tissue mass. Calcification or ossification can be seen in 5% to 20% of cases. In contradistinction with other types of soft tissue sarcomas, cortical erosion or frank osseous invasion is frequently observed. Undifferentiated high-grade pleomorphic sarcoma typically shows areas of low, intermediate, and high signal intensity on T2-weighted images, reflecting the variable proportions of cells, myxoid tissue, calcification, fibrosis, necrosis, and hemorrhage. Hemorrhagic components may be very prominent and may be recognized as areas of high signal intensity on T1- and T2-weighted images or by the presence of fluid-fluid levels.

SUGGESTED READINGS

Carter BW, Benveniste MF, Betancourt SL, et al. Imaging evaluation of malignant chest wall neoplasms. *Radiographics.* 2016;36(5):1285–1306.

Jeung MY, Gangi A, Gasser B, et al. Imaging of chest wall disorders. *Radiographics.* 1999;19:617–637.

Nam SJ, Kim S, Lim BJ, et al. Imaging of primary chest wall tumors with radiologic-pathologic correlation. *Radiographics.* 2011;31(3):749–770.

The full reference list for this chapter is available at ExpertConsult.com.

Page numbers followed by *f* indicate figures; *t*, tables; *b*, boxes.

E

J

K

L

T